PRINCIPLES OF
SURGERY

PRINCIPLES OF SURGERY

EDITOR-IN-CHIEF

Seymour I. Schwartz, M.D.
Professor of Surgery
University of Rochester School of Medicine and Dentistry

ASSOCIATE EDITORS

G. Tom Shires, M.D.
Professor and Chairman
Department of Surgery
Cornell University Medical College

Frank C. Spencer, M.D.
Professor and Director
Department of Surgery
New York University School of Medicine

Edward H. Storer, M.D.
Professor of Surgery
Yale University School of Medicine

THIRD EDITION

McGRAW-HILL BOOK COMPANY
New York   St. Louis   San Francisco   Auckland   Bogotá   Düsseldorf
Johannesburg   London   Madrid   Mexico   Montreal   New Delhi
Panama   Paris   São Paulo   Singapore   Sydney   Tokyo   Toronto

NOTICE

Medicine is an ever-changing science. As new research and clinical experience broaden our knowledge, changes in treatment and drug therapy are required. The editors and the publisher of this work have made every effort to ensure that the drug dosage schedules herein are accurate and in accord with the standards accepted at the time of publication. Readers are advised, however, to check the product information sheet included in the package of each drug they plan to administer to be certain that changes have not been made in the recommended dose or in the contraindications for administration. This recommendation is of particular importance in regard to new or infrequently used drugs.

To students of surgery,
at all levels,
in their quest for knowledge

PRINCIPLES OF SURGERY

2 3 4 5 6 7 8 9 0   7 8 3 2 1 0 9

This book was set in Times Roman by York Graphic Services, Inc.
The editors were J. Dereck Jeffers, Stuart D. Boynton,
and Bob Leap; the designer was Barbara Ellwood;
the production supervisor was Robert C. Pedersen.
New drawings were done by J & R Services, Inc.
The cover was designed by Nicholas Krenitsky.

Library of Congress Cataloging in Publication Data

Main entry under title:

Principles of surgery.

    Bibliography: p.
    Includes index.
    1. Surgery. I. Schwartz, Seymour I.
[DNLM: 1. Surgery. W0100.3 P957]
RD31.P88 1979b   617   78-13763
ISBN 0-07-055735-7

LC CIP DATA (2 vol ed.)

RD31.P88 1979   617   78-6763
ISBN 0-07-055736-5

Contents

vi   CONTENTS

List of Contributors

James T. Adams, M.D.
Professor of Surgery, University of Rochester School of Medicine and Dentistry

R. Peter Altman, M.D.
Associate Professor of Surgery, George Washington University; Senior Attending Surgeon, Children's Hospital National Medical Center

Kathryn D. Anderson, M.D.
Assistant Professor of Surgery, George Washington University; Senior Attending Surgeon, Children's Hospital National Medical Center

Richard M. Bergland, M.D.
Associate Professor of Neurosurgery, Harvard; Chief, Division of Neurosurgery, Beth Israel Hospital

George H. Bornside, Ph.D.
Professor of Surgical Research and Microbiology, Louisiana State University School of Medicine

Thomas J. Brobyn, M.D.
Clinical Assistant Professor of Plastic Surgery, Thomas Jefferson University; Associate Chief of Plastic Surgery, Chesnut Hill Hospital

Lester R. Bryant, M.D.
Professor and Chairman, Department of Surgery, East Tennessee State University

Peter C. Canizaro, M.D.
Associate Professor of Surgery, Cornell University Medical College

C. James Carrico, M.D.
Professor of Surgery, University of Washington School of Medicine

Robert A. Chase, M.D.
Professor, Department of Surgery, Stanford University School of Medicine

Isidore Cohn, Jr., M.D.
Professor and Chairman, Department of Surgery, Louisiana State University School of Medicine

William F. Collins, Jr., M.D.
Professor and Chairman, Section of Neurological Surgery, Yale University School of Medicine

Robert E. Condon, M.D.
Professor of Surgery, The Medical College of Wisconsin

Lester M. Cramer, M.D.
Clinical Professor of Plastic Surgery, University of Colorado Medical Center; Chief of Plastic Surgery, Chesnut Hill Hospital

Joseph N. Cunningham, M.D.
Associate Professor, Department of Surgery, New York University School of Medicine

P. William Curreri, M.D.
Professor of Surgery and Director, Burn Center, The New York Hospital—Cornell Medical Center

Louis R. M. Del Guercio, M.D.
Professor and Chairman, Department of Surgery, New York Medical College

James A. DeWeese, M.D.
Professor of Surgery, University of Rochester School of Medicine and Dentistry

J. Herbert Dietz, Jr., M.D.
Associate Professor of Rehabilitation (Surgery), Cornell University Medical College; Chief, Rehabilitation Service (Surgery), Memorial Sloan-Kettering Cancer Center

Robert B. Duthie, M.D., M.B.
Nuffield Professor of Orthopedic Surgery, Nuffield Orthopedic Center, Oxford, England

F. Henry Ellis, Jr., M.D., Ph.D.
Chairman, Department of Thoracic and Cardiovascular Surgery, Lahey Clinic Foundation and New England Deaconess Hospital; Associate Clinical Professor of Surgery, Harvard Medical School

John E. Foker, M.D.
Assistant Professor of Surgery, University of Minnesota

John H. Foster, M.D.
Professor of Surgery, Vanderbilt University School of Medicine

Irwin N. Frank, M.D.
Professor of Surgery, Urology Division, University of Rochester School of Medicine and Dentistry

Donald S. Gann, M.D.
Professor of Surgery, The Johns Hopkins School of Medicine; Director of Emergency Medicine, Johns Hopkins Hospital

Adolph H. Giesecke, Jr., M.D.
Professor and Chairman, Department of Anesthesiology, The University of Texas Southwestern Medical School at Dallas

Stanley M. Goldberg, M.D.
Clinical Professor of Surgery, Director and Head, Division of Colon and Rectal Surgery, Department of Surgery, University of Minnesota Health Sciences Center

Nicholas M. Greene, M.D.
Professor, Department of Anesthesiology, Yale University School of Medicine

Timothy S. Harrison, M.D.
Professor of Surgery and Physiology, The Milton S. Hershey Medical Center, The Pennsylvania State University

Charles M. Haskell, M.D.
Associate Professor of Medicine and Surgery, Department of Medicine, UCLA School of Medicine, University of California at Los Angeles

Arthur L. Herbst, M.D.
Professor and Chairman, Department of Obstetrics and Gynecology, The University of Chicago

Franklin T. Hoaglund, M.D.
Professor and Chairman, Department of Orthopedic Surgery, University of Vermont College of Medicine

Anthony M. Imparato, M.D.
Professor of Clinical Surgery, New York University School of Medicine

E. R. Johnson, M.D.
Associate Professor of Physical Medicine and Rehabilitation, The University of Texas Southwestern Medical School at Dallas

Robert F. Jones, M.D.
Professor of Surgery, University of Washington School of Medicine

Ronald C. Jones, M.D.
Professor of Surgery, The University of Texas Southwestern Medical School at Dallas

Edwin L. Kaplan, M.D.
Professor of Surgery, Pritzker School of Medicine, University of Chicago

James F. Lee, M.D.
Professor of Anesthesiology, The University of Texas, Southwestern Medical School at Dallas

Richard R. Lower, M.D.
Professor and Chairman, Division of Thoracic and Cardiac Surgery, Medical College of Virginia

Robert N. McClelland, M.D.
Professor of Surgery, The University of Texas Southwestern Medical School at Dallas

Donald F. McDonald, M.D.
Professor, Division of Urology, University of Texas Medical Branch at Galveston

René B. Menguy, M.D.
Professor of Surgery, University of Rochester School of Medicine and Dentistry

Calvin Morgan, M.D.
Clinical Assistant Professor of Surgery, East Tennessee State University

Donald L. Morton, M.D.
Professor of Surgery and Chief, Divisions General Surgery and Oncology, UCLA School of Medicine, University of California at Los Angeles

John H. Morton, M.D.
Professor of Surgery, University of Rochester School of Medicine and Dentistry

John S. Najarian, M.D.
Professor and Chairman, Department of Surgery, University of Minnesota Health Sciences Center

Santhat Nivatvongs, M.D.
Assistant Professor, Division of Colon and Rectal Surgery, Department of Surgery, University of Minnesota Health Sciences Center

W. Spencer Payne, M.D.
Professor of Surgery, Mayo Medical School, Mayo Graduate School of Medicine, Consultant Section of Thoracic, Cardiovascular and General Surgery in the Mayo Clinic and Mayo Foundation

Erle E. Peacock, Jr., M.D.
Professor of Surgery, Plastic Surgery Section, Tulane University School of Medicine

Malcolm O. Perry, M.D.
Professor of Surgery and Chief, Division of Vascular Surgery, Cornell University Medical College

Judson G. Randolph, M.D.
Professor of Surgery, George Washington University; Surgeon-in-Chief, Children's Hospital, National Medical Center

Benjamin F. Rush, Jr., M.D.
Professor and Chairman, Department of Surgery, College of Medicine and Dentistry of New Jersey at Newark

Howard A. Rusk, M.D.
Professor of Rehabilitation Medicine, New York
University School of Medicine

Seymour I. Schwartz, M.D.
Professor of Surgery, University of Rochester School of
Medicine and Dentistry

G. Tom Shires, M.D.
Professor and Chairman, Department of Surgery,
Cornell University Medical College

William Silen, M.D.
Chief of Surgery, Beth Israel Hospital; Professor of
Surgery, Harvard Medical School

Richard L. Simmons, M.D.
Professor of Surgery and Microbiology, Department of
Surgery, University of Minnesota Health Sciences
Center

William H. Snyder, III, M.D.
Associate Professor of Surgery, The University of Texas
Southwestern Medical School at Dallas

Frank C. Sparks, M.D.
Professor and Chairman, Department of Surgery,
University of Connecticut Health Center, School of
Medicine

Dennis D. Spencer, M.D.
Assistant Professor, Section of Neurosurgery, Yale
University School of Medicine

Frank C. Spencer, M.D.
Professor and Director, Department of Surgery, New
York University School of Medicine

Edward H. Storer, M.D.
Professor of Surgery, Yale University School of
Medicine

Erwin R. Thal, M.D.
Associate Professor of Surgery, The University of Texas
Southwestern Medical School at Dallas

Donald R. Tredway, M.D., Ph.D.
Associate Professor and Chief, Section of Reproductive
Endocrinology, Department of Obstetrics and
Gynecology, The University of Chicago

Howard Ulfelder, M.D.
Joe V. Meigs Professor of Gynecology, Harvard Medical
School

Joan L. Venes, M.D.
Associate Professor, Section of Neurosurgery, Yale
University School of Medicine

Franklin C. Wagner, Jr., M.D.
Associate Professor, Section of Neurosurgery, Yale
University School of Medicine

Preface
to the Third Edition

The science of surgery continues to expand and change at a rate which makes only the title of a textbook immutable. The editors remain devoted to the concept of a *modern* source of information and therefore offer this third edition as evidence of their concern. The third edition of *Principles of Surgery* maintains its consistent format, while reflecting the changes which have evolved over the past five years.

There are 15 new authors and approximately 35 percent of the text has been altered. Chapters which were rewritten by new authors include: Endocrine and Metabolic Responses to Injury; Shock; Burns; Chest Wall, Pleura, Lung, and Mediastinum; Peritonitis and Intraabdominal Abscesses, Pituitary and Adrenal; Pediatric Surgery; and Urology. All other chapters have been extensively revised and updated. Each of the chapters in the "Basic Considerations" section have undergone major change—particularly those concerned with oncology and transplantation—reflecting the explosion of knowledge in these areas. The specific organ system chapters have been revised with an emphasis on newly introduced diagnostic techniques and current consensus of opinion regarding management. The References of each chapter have been brought up to date.

The editors wish to thank the readers for their past reception of our efforts, and offer the present work as a statement of our appreciation in the hopes that the third edition serves the same purpose as its two predecessors and is equally well received.

Seymour I. Schwartz

Acknowledgments

The editors appreciate the efforts of all the contributors whose expertise, lucid presentation, and promptness have eased our task. This statement is an expression of particular thanks to Ms. Wendy Husser, Administrative Assistant, who devoted her intellectual energies throughout the entire development of this edition. Finally, once again, the four editors would like to acknowledge the patience, cooperation, and sacrifice on the part of our families, permitting us uncompromised devotion to this project which has now extended over twelve years.

Seymour I. Schwartz

Preface to the First Edition

The raison d'etre for a new textbook in a discipline which has been served by standard works for many years was the Editorial Board's initial conviction that a distinct need for a modern approach in the dissemination of surgical knowledge existed. As incoming chapters were reviewed, both the need and satisfaction became increasingly apparent and, at the completion, we felt a sense of excitement at having the opportunity to contribute to the education of modern and future students concerned with the care of surgical patients.

The recent explosion of factual knowledge has emphasized the need for a presentation which would provide the student an opportunity to assimilate pertinent facts in a logical fashion. This would then permit correlation, synthesis of concepts, and eventual extrapolation to specific situations. The physiologic bases for diseases are therefore emphasized and the manifestations and diagnostic studies are considered as a reflection of pathophysiology. Therapy then becomes logical in this schema and the necessity to regurgitate facts is minimized. In appreciation of the impact which Harrison's *Principles of Internal Medicine* has had, the clinical manifestations of the disease processes are considered in detail for each area. Since the operative procedure represents the one element in the therapeutic armentarium unique to the surgeon, the indications, important technical considerations, and complications receive appropriate emphasis. While we appreciate that a textbook cannot hope to incorporate an atlas of surgical procedures, we have provided the student a single book which will satisfy the sequential demands in the care and considerations of surgical patients.

The ultimate goal of the Editorial Board has been to collate a book which is deserving of the adjective "modern." We have therefore selected as authors dynamic and active contributors to their particular fields. The *au courant* concept is hopefully apparent throughout the entire work and is exemplified by appropriate emphasis on diseases of modern surgical interest, such as trauma, transplantation, and the recently appreciated importance of rehabilitation. Cardiovascular surgery is presented in keeping with the exponential strides recently achieved.

There are two major subdivisions to the text. In the first twelve chapters, subjects that transcend several organ systems are presented. The second portion of the book represents a consideration of specific organ systems and surgical specialties.

Throughout the text, the authors have addressed themselves to a sophisticated audience, regarding the medical student as a graduate student, incorporating material generally sought after by the surgeon in training and presenting information appropriate for the continuing education of the practicing surgeon. The need for a text such as we have envisioned is great and the goal admittedly high. It is our hope that this effort fulfills the expressed demands.

Seymour I. Schwartz

Chapter 1

Endocrine and Metabolic Responses to Injury

by Donald S. Gann

Injury comes in so many variegated forms that it is no small wonder that response to injury may also be quite variable. There are, however, endocrine and metabolic changes that are common to many kinds of injury and that, when taken together, constitute one aspect of the body's response to trauma. These responses are sometimes greatly modified by anesthesia, by fluid and electrolyte replacement, by transfusion, and by other surgical and anesthetic iatrogens, so that identical injuries produced, on the one hand, by an automobile accident and, on the other, during a planned and controlled operation under general anesthesia may lead to courses which vary considerably either in magnitude or direction of response.

Furthermore, adaptation to certain kinds of injury may occur—e.g., to Noble-Collip drum shock or hemorrhagic shock in the rat, altitude hypoxia and poisons in man—thus increasing an already marked individual variation in response. As will be seen later, such adaptations may lead either to attenuated or to enhanced response to a subsequent insult.

In this initial chapter consideration will be given to some of the factors producing the changes consequent upon injury, to the mechanisms through which they are known or thought to act, and to the changes themselves. Some specific examples will be given to illustrate patient management problems related to trauma, together with their suggested solutions.

STIMULI INDUCING CHANGE

Once an injury has been incurred, a series of endocrine and metabolic events follow. Although it is clear that the neuroendocrine response to injury involves changes in the secretion of a large number of hormones, most of the studies of the details of this response have focused on changes in the secretion of ACTH and of cortisol. Accordingly, the mechanisms controlling secretion of these hormones are emphasized in this section. It seems likely that the neural mechanisms subserving control of other hormones involved in the neuroendocrine response are analogous to those subserving control of ACTH. Our own finding that every central nervous area receiving afferent signals from cardiovascular receptors signaling changes in blood volume is in turn involved in control of ACTH implies that the same areas must share in part in the

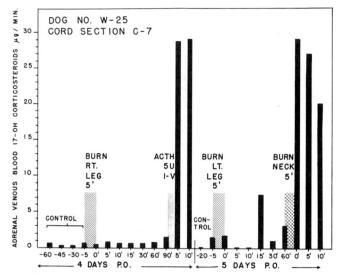

Fig. 1-1. Adrenocortical response to a burn following section of the cord at the level of C_7. A burn below the level of section produced no increase in the adrenocorticosteroid secretion over the control values. Five units of ACTH given intravenously produced an immediate marked rise in adrenocortical output. With the dog under Nembutal anesthesia a burn of the left hind leg leg produced no significant increase in adrenocorticosteroid output. In contrast, a burn of the neck above the level of cord section produced a marked and immediate increase in adrenocortical secretion. (*From D. M. Hume and R. H. Egdahl, Ann Surg, 150:697, 1959.*)

control of several hormones. Such a sharing provides a neural basis for a coordinated multihormonal response.

AFFERENT NERVE STIMULI FROM THE INJURED AREA. This is a major factor in the initiation of many of the endocrine changes that follow injury, particularly those related to increased ACTH and cortisol secretion. Abdominal laparotomy, burns, or severe trauma in dogs failed to

Fig. 1-2. Comparison of the adrenal venous blood 17-hydroxycorticosteroid (17-OHCS) response to a gastric operation in a patient with spinal cord transection at T_4 with that seen in a normal patient. The paraplegic patient fails to release endogenous ACTH in response to the operation but shows a marked rise in adrenal 17-OHCS secretion following ACTH. The normal patient shows a maximal secretion of 17-OHCS in response to the operation, and no further increase is seen with ACTH. (*From D. M. Hume et al., Surgery, 52:174, 1962.*)

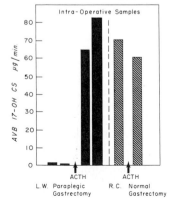

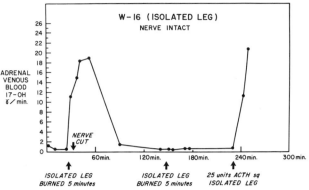

Fig. 1-3. Effect of limb denervation on ACTH secretion following trauma. The hind leg has been isolated so that it is attached to the body only by one artery, one vein, and one nerve. The burn of the isolated leg produces a marked and immediate response in adrenal venous blood corticosteroid secretion. During the height of the response the nerve was cut, and the secretion dropped rather promptly to control levels. A second burn of the same leg now produced no adrenocortical response. ACTH injected subcutaneously into the isolated leg produced a prompt and marked increase in adrenocorticosteroid secretion. (*From D. M. Hume and R. H. Egdahl, Ann Surg, 150:697, 1959.*)

produce an increased ACTH release if the traumatized area had been denervated so that afferent impulses from it failed to reach the brain. Trauma to the area which remained innervated continued to produce a normal response. This absence of increased ACTH release was also shown to be true for paraplegic or quadriplegic patients undergoing traumatic plastic or orthopedic procedures in the denervated area, or abdominal laparotomy for gastric resection (Figs. 1-1 and 1-2). Egdahl performed an ingenious experiment which confirmed these observations. In a series of dogs he divided the skin, muscle, and bone of one hind leg, thus isolating it from the body except for the femoral artery, vein, and nerve. Trauma to the innervated portion of the leg continued to evoke an increased secretion of ACTH and cortisol. The nerve was then divided, leaving the artery and vein intact. Following this, trauma no longer produced an increased secretion of ACTH (Fig. 1-3).

HEMORRHAGE AND HYPOVOLEMIA. The most prominent characteristic of trauma is a loss of circulating body fluids. Naturally, many severe injuries are accompanied by hemorrhage and thus direct loss of blood. In addition, as pointed out by Blalock, there is a sequestration of fluids in an injured region with formation of a so-called "third space." This sequestration leads to a loss of extracellular fluid available for exchange and thus to further hypovolemia. The cardiovascular system, acting through receptors in the atria and arteries (baroreceptors), exerts a tonic, inhibitory influence over the release of certain hormones which may be controlled either directly through the central nervous system or through peripheral sympathetic nerves. When blood volume decreases, the extent of cardiovascular inhibition of nervous function decreases. As the inhibition is released, there is direct central neural stimulation of the secretion of ACTH, vasopressin (ADH), and growth hormone (GH) from the anterior and posterior pituitary gland. Furthermore, with the release of inhibition, sympathetic neural activity increases and there is thus enhanced secretion of epinephrine and norepinephrine from the adrenal medulla, of renin from the kidney, and of glucagon from the pancreas. The same sympathetic stimulation or circulating catecholamines may inhibit release of insulin from the pancreas. The effect of hemorrhage on secretion of cortisol is shown in Fig. 1-4. This multihormonal response to hypovolemia is entirely analogous to the reflex changes in myocardial contractility, heart rate, and peripheral resistance which occur in response to the classic baroreceptor reflex in the presence of hypovolemia. In addition, changes in renal hemodynamics brought about by sympathetic stimulation may lead to changes in the renal handling of salt and water on a nonhormonal basis. These changes are further augmented by the secretion of aldosterone, stimulated by the renin angiotensin system, and by vasopressin. These changes are discussed below.

LOCAL WOUND FACTORS. As indicated above, afferent nerve impulses are required to convey signals from a wounded area to initiate direct release of hormones. Thus it might appear that local wound factors are unimportant in the metabolic response to injury. However, this does not appear to be the case, although local changes in a wounded area seem to evolve more slowly than do afferent signals conveyed over nerves. The blood sequestered in an injured area, together with decreased tissue perfusion brought about by local vascular injury and by edema, leads to local acidosis and results in the movement of potassium out of cells. In the presence of infection, bacterial toxins also accumulate in the wound area. Furthermore, the synthesis of kinins and prostaglandins may be accelerated in the presence of acidosis. With the return of adequate perfusion to the injured areas, these factors may be washed into the general circulation, where they may potentiate or initiate portions of the response to injury. Finally, there may be specific neuroendocrine responses to injury of critical areas such as the heart, great vessels, or brain.

SHOCK. When, as a consequence of severe hypovolemia, bacterial toxins, or myocardial infarction, or for any other reason, tissue perfusion drops to shock levels, profound metabolic disturbances occur. The decrease in tissue perfusion is made worse by direct damage to vital organs, particularly the brain, liver, heart, lungs, and kidneys. Until shock becomes profound, the chain of events set in motion by hypovolemia may appear first, followed then by changes due to organ failure and acidosis.

CHANGES IN BLOOD pH. Severe acidosis may be produced by some types of trauma including bacterial infection, prolonged shock, open heart surgical procedures with the pump-oxygenator, operations on diabetics who are out of control, temporary respiratory and cardiac arrest, and ingestion of acid, to name but a few. Acidosis itself interferes further with cellular function, and if compensatory mechanisms are blocked or if the change occurs too rapidly, death may supervene. Alkalosis also may occur with trauma, particularly in patients who are on gastric suction or those with cirrhosis, who are frequently alkalotic when they go to the operating room. The development of marked alkalosis is sometimes seen in patients who are

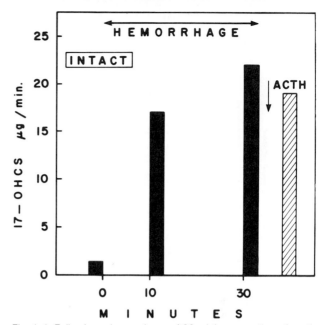

Fig. 1-4. Following a hemorrhage of 30 ml/kg, secretion of cortisol (measured as 17-OHCS) increases rapidly to rates equal to that elicited by a supramaximal dose of ACTH. Increased secretion of cortisol is sustained in the presence of this degree of hypovolemia.

hyperventilated or those overtreated with bicarbonate. In addition, pain may induce hyperventilation and thus lead to alkalosis. A marked change of pH in either direction from normal may be hazardous or even fatal to the patient. Respiratory alkalosis may convert rapidly and catastrophically to metabolic acidosis.

INFECTION. Bacterial endotoxin is capable of providing direct hypothalamic stimulation with attendant release of ACTH, epinephrine, norepinephrine, ADH, and GH (Fig. 1-5). In addition to this, of course, severe infection has profound influences on the cardiovascular system and can, if unchecked, lead to shock and ultimately to renal, hepatic, cardiac, and cerebral failure and to death.

ANESTHESIA AND OTHER DRUGS. Anesthesia has an effect upon the endocrine system, the cardiovascular system, the pulmonary and renal systems, the brain, and in fact the entire metabolism of the body. Depending upon the anesthetic agent employed, it may depress or abolish certain of the endocrine responses or else stimulate or augment them. It may produce a relative hypoxia or improve oxygenation. It may produce vasodilatation or vasoconstriction, stimulate the heart or depress it. Almost all anesthetic agents, however, depress hepatic function to a greater or lesser degree. No operative trauma ought to be thought of without a consideration of the particular anesthetic agent employed, as well as the depth and duration of anesthesia.

Morphine and Nembutal tend to depress hypothalamic stimulation of ACTH and GH release, but this depression can be overcome by operative trauma. They also depress respiration and gastrointestinal motility. Atropine produces tachycardia and decreases salivary gland activity. Antihy-

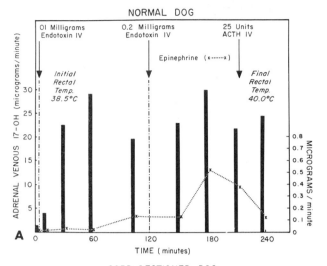

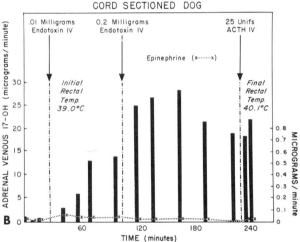

Fig. 1-5. Effects of endotoxin on 17-OHCS and epinephrine secretion. *A.* In the normal dog, a small dose of endotoxin produces a marked increase in the adrenal venous blood secretion of 17-OHCS, with almost no increase in the adrenal medullary output of epinephrine. A larger dose of endotoxin produces an increase both in 17-OHCS and epinephrine secretion in the adrenal venous blood. *B.* When the same experiment is repeated in the dog with section of the spinal cord, the endotoxin again produces a marked increase in the secretion of adrenal venous blood 17-OHCS, but now there is no increase at all in epinephrine secretion.

The experiments in *A* and *B* demonstrate that endotoxin acts at the level of the hypothalamus to stimulate the release of ACTH and also to stimulate the cells controlling the secretion of epinephrine via the spinal cord and sympathetic nerves. When the cord is cut, although the hypothalamic effect of endotoxin on ACTH release is retained, impulses can no longer pass down the cord and into the sympathetic nerves to bring about a release of epinephrine. (*From R. H. Egdahl, J Clin Invest, 38:1120, 1959.*)

pertensive drugs may lead to a marked hypotension with the induction of anesthesia, and many other commonly used drugs may have important effects in altering the response to injury.

CENTRAL NERVOUS SYSTEM INJURY. The endocrine and metabolic responses to injury may be greatly altered

if the central nervous system itself is injured. Thus the patient who is in a coma from a head injury may respond very differently to a severe injury elsewhere in the body than he would without an associated head injury. Head injury can produce diabetes insipidus, abnormal salt metabolism, inappropriate secretion of ADH, depressed pulmonary and cardiac action, or arrest, shock, and death. The patient whose spinal cord is transected may have tremendous vasodilatation of the vessels in the lower part of the body and cannot compensate for blood loss. In addition, as noted above, the patient will not respond to severe trauma below the level of cord section with an increased ACTH secretion.

EMOTIONAL TRAUMA. The emotional trauma of an injury may either inhibit or stimulate the endocrine response, although it usually does the latter. The effect of emotional trauma on endocrine secretion was originally demonstrated by Harris, who showed indirect evidence for an increased adrenocortical secretion in rabbits who were restrained. It was subsequently demonstrated by Ganong et al. that a tremendous rise in adrenal venous blood corticosteroid output accompanied restraint in nervous dogs (Fig. 1-6).

Everyone is familiar with the effect which emotional factors have on epinephrine release (sweating, tachycardia, dry mouth, pallor, intestinal motility, blood pressure, etc.). This factor may contribute to some of the differences between the effects of injury in the conscious state versus those of the same type of injury in the anesthetized patient.

ANOXIA. Anoxia caused, for example, by a pneumothorax due to a penetrating wound or a flail chest with rib fractures may produce profound change through tissue hypoxia. It is a strong stimulant to release of catecholamines and of ACTH.

IMMOBILIZATION. Immobilization leads to metabolic change by muscle wasting and mobilization of skeletal calcium and phosphorus. Bed rest reduces the secretion of renin, aldosterone, and to some extent epinephrine and norepinephrine. It promotes thrombosis in the deep veins of the pelvis and lower extremities.

STARVATION. Many types of severe trauma are accompanied by a negative nitrogen balance. This negative balance is augmented by starvation. Inadequate intake of vitamins and calories may produce considerable metabolic change, particularly if starvation is present over a long period of time.

HYPOGLYCEMIA. Hypoglycemia is a potent stimulus to the hypothalamic centers controlling the secretion of ACTH, GH, epinephrine, and norepinephrine. If it is persistent and profound, it will produce marked interference with central nervous system activity.

ENVIRONMENTAL TEMPERATURE CHANGES AND FEVER. If the trauma has a thermal component, profound general changes can be brought about by heat or cold alone. A hot or cold environment produces striking change in skin circulation with concomitant compensatory changes in other parts of the body. Heat and cold by themselves can each produce changes in the output of many hormones, including ACTH, cortisol, aldosterone, ADH, epinephrine, norepinephrine, thyroxine, and others. Respiration may be increased, fluid and electrolyte losses occur, and many other changes may ensue (Fig. 1-7). Fever increases catabolism, oxygen consumption, cardiac work, and water and salt loss. Ambient temperature alterations were shown by Redding and Mueller to have a profound effect on survival following tourniquet shock.

POISONS. Some injuries are accompanied by the addition of poisons, which may act locally or systemically. The bite of a poisonous snake is an example in which the local and general changes wrought by the injury itself are minor compared with those caused by the poison. Crush injury may be accompanied by the release of methemoglobin. Toxic bacterial products occur in injury associated with infections. Various other poisons, such as methyl alcohol, may have been ingested prior to the injury, giving rise to widespread metabolic changes.

WITHDRAWAL SYMPTOMS. The injured patient may be an alcoholic, and the early postoperative course may be complicated by the severe withdrawal symptoms of delirium tremens with its profound metabolic complications. The same may be said of narcotic withdrawal, or even withdrawal of commonly used drugs, such as insulin—for example, in patients who are unconscious and not known to be diabetics.

Fig. 1-7. Effects of hypothermia on ACTH and 17-OHCS secretion. *A.* The plasma ACTH levels and adrenal venous blood 17-OHCS output in a dog traumatized under ether anesthesia and then subjected to hypothermia. There is a marked depression of corticosteroid secretion during hypothermia with an increase again after rewarming. Blood ACTH, which is elevated before the induction of hypothermia, becomes too low to measure during hypothermia and is again easily detected after rewarming. *B.* Epinephrine, norepinephrine, and corticosteroid secretion in the adrenal venous blood of a dog traumatized under ether anesthesia before, during, and after induction of hypothermia. A marked decrease in epinephrine and norepinephrine output occurs during hypothermia, while a marked increase in the secretion of these substances is seen on rewarming. The output of 17-OHCS follows a similar pattern. (*From D. M. Hume and R. H. Egdahl, Ann NY Acad Sci, 80:435, 1959.*)

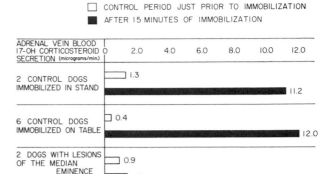

Fig. 1-6. Effect of forced immobilization on adrenal venous blood 17-OHCS secretion. This is shown in two groups of control dogs. Fifteen minutes after the introduction of the restraint there is an output of adrenal venous blood 17-OHCS secretion equivalent to that seen during major operative trauma as a consequence of the emotional stress of forced immobilization in untrained dogs. Lesions of the median eminence abolish this response, indicating that it is mediated by the hypothalamus. (*From W. F. Ganong et al., Fed Proc, 14:54, 1955.*)

ANAPHYLAXIS. Under some circumstances the overreactive response of the body to the injury can be much more devastating than the injury itself. A typical example of this is a bee sting in a patient who is hypersensitive to bee stings. Under these circumstances a bee sting may produce shock, coma, and death, the devastating chain of events occurring because of the body's pathologic hypersensitivity response to the antigen.

Thus it may be seen that there are many stimuli producing their effects through many different pathways in different kinds of trauma. Very frequently there are several stimuli to endocrine and metabolic change working simultaneously in the same patient.

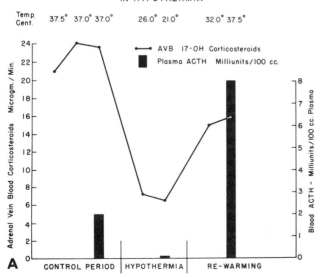

ADRENAL CORTICOSTEROID OUTPUT AND BLOOD ACTH LEVELS IN HYPOTHERMIA

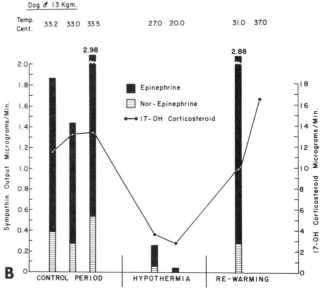

ADRENAL SYMPATHIN AND CORTICOSTEROID OUTPUT IN HYPOTHERMIA

CENTRAL NERVOUS SYSTEM AND ENDOCRINE CHANGES

As indicated above, the principal signals to initiate the endocrine response to injury are those of hypovolemia and of pain. The hormonal response is diffuse, including increased release of ACTH, cortisol, growth hormone, epinephrine, norepinephrine, glucagon, renin, and aldosterone. In each case the prompt initiation of hormonal release depends upon a reflex activated by afferent nerves. Although the reflex initiation of increased sympathetic activity may take place at the level of the medulla or spinal cord, it appears that even for these reflexes hypothalamic coordination is involved, as it is in the control of the release of the anterior pituitary hormones. The precise pathways from afferent nerve endings to the hypothalamus have been studied in detail only for ACTH and to some extent for vasopressin. However, where they are available, data for the control of other hormones seem analogous; and it is highly likely that the afferent pathways are shared to a considerable extent, providing a basis for coordinated neuroendocrine response to injury.

The central pathways have been best delineated for the neural control of ACTH in response to hypovolemia. The principal afferent receptors lie in the right atrium (Fig. 1-8) and in the carotid arteries. The afferent nerves converge on the lateral solitary nucleus and related structures in the dorsolateral medulla. From this point, they project without synapsing to the nuclei of the coeruleus complex in the dorsal pons, with medial projections to the tegmental and raphe nuclei. From this point, they project, apparently again without synapsing, to the hypothalamus in three principal pathways, two stimulatory and one inhibitory. A dorsal stimulatory pathway courses through the dorsal longitudinal fasciculus to end in the dorsal hypothalamus, including the paraventricular nucleus. A ventral stimulatory pathway courses through the ventral tegmental area of the midbrain to enter the medial forebrain bundle and terminate in the anteroventral hypothalamic nuclei, including the suprachiasmatic and ventromedial nuclei. The intermediate inhibitory pathway passes up the central tegmental tract to terminate in the posterior hypothalamic area. These stimulatory and inhibitory signals then converge on the medial basal hypothalamus to control release of corticotropin-releasing factor, the agent which controls pituitary release of ACTH, from the median eminence. These multiple pathways provide a basis for the observation of different degrees of steroid suppressibility in response to small and large hemorrhage, as discussed below.

In the case of pain transmission, neurophysiologic studies have not been coordinated with endocrine ones, but it is possible to piece together a likely pattern. In this case, afferent pain endings in the tissues synapse first in the substantia gelatinosa of the dorsal horn of the spinal cord. From here, fibers pass up the spinothalamic tract to terminate in the gigantocellular tegmental field of the medulla and pons. The degree of interaction at the pontine level with volume signals is unclear at present, but fibers appear to pass from the pontine level to the hypothalamus along the same pathways described above, with a major projection to the anteroventral hypothalamus through the medial forebrain bundle and a possible additional projection above the dorsal longitudinal fasciculus as well. There is no evidence at this time that the inhibitory pathway is involved in the control of ACTH release in response to pain.

Within the hypothalamus, specific nuclei control the release of releasing factors, which in turn govern the secretion of various anterior pituitary hormones or sympathetic activity, but there is clear overlap of function. For example, the posterior hypothalamic area is involved in the control of ACTH and of descending sympathetic activity. The paraventricular nucleus is involved in the control of vasopressin, of oxytocin, and of ACTH. The ventromedial nucleus is involved in the control of growth hormone and of ACTH. The supraoptic nucleus has been shown to be active in the control of vasopressin and oxytocin. The suprachiasmatic nucleus appears to control ACTH release and to contain corticotropin-releasing factor, but it has been shown to effect secretion of gonadotropins as well (Fig. 1-9). Hypothalamic control of the anterior pituitary is accomplished by secretion of neurohormones onto capillary loops in the median eminence (Fig. 1-10). Although this view focuses on the role of the hypothalamus in neuroendocrine control, it is clear that this region of the brain

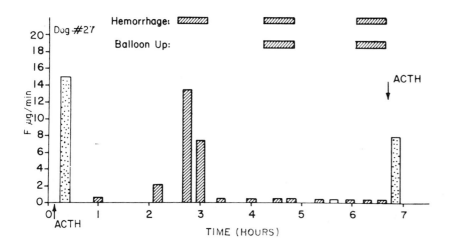

Fig. 1-8. Secretion of cortisol (F) after supramaximal doses of ACTH (stippled bars) and after sequential hemorrhages of 5 ml/kg in a dog with an inflatable balloon in the right atrium. Inflation of the balloon prevents the response to small hemorrhage, indicating mediation of this response by right atrial receptors. (*From G. L. Cryer and D. S. Gann, Am J Physiol, 227:325, 1974.*)

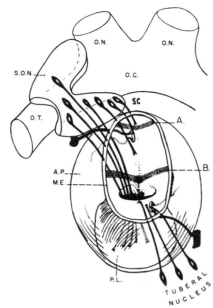

Fig. 1-9. Horizontal view through the median eminence. This indicates some of the relationships of the supraoptic nucleus (SON) and the tuberal nucleus to the hypophyseoportal blood vessels. The laterally placed axons of the supraoptic nucleus concerned with the production and release of ADH travel down into the posterior lobe (PL), as shown in the diagram. The more mediad placed cells of the suprachiasmatic nucleus (SC) terminate in the anterior portion of the median eminence on the hypophyseoportal capillaries. A lesion made at the point indicated by A will abolish the ACTH response to trauma without producing diabetes insipidus. A lesion made at the point indicated by B will produce diabetes insipidus without interfering with ACTH release. If a lesion is made at the level indicated by A but is somewhat larger, extending laterally, it will produce both diabetes insipidus and a failure of ACTH release in response to trauma. The cells of the tuberal nucleus which control gonadotropin release terminate in the posterior part of the median eminence on capillary loops of the posterior portion of the hypophyseoportal system. Their action is unaffected by lesions located either at A or B.

is important in the coordination of other autonomic functions as well in the control of other hormones which appear to be less affected by injury.

Modulation of Neuroendocrine Response

CORTISOL FEEDBACK

As indicated above, injury leads to the increased secretion of ACTH and of cortisol. Elevated plasma levels of cortisol lead in turn to inhibition of further release of ACTH. This effect is exerted primarily through action within the central nervous system, although there is almost certainly some direct effect on the pituitary gland as well. Thus one would expect to see diminished secretion of ACTH and cortisol after a second stimulus. Under appropriate circumstances this is the case (Fig. 1-11). This feedback effect takes approximately 90 minutes to work in most species studied. As indicated below, however, this feedback effect is not usually seen with respect to cortisol because of

potentiation. However, increased plasma levels of cortisol also lead to inhibition of release of vasopressin, growth hormone, and prolactin. Thus the feedback effect of cortisol may be general and may extend far beyond the control of ACTH release per se. The coordinated neuroendocrine response that is an important feature of host defense against injury may be disrupted by recent previous injury. This feature is especially important, since for most patients who have been traumatized, surgery may constitute a second injury, often taking place just at the time when cortisol feedback might be expected to have its principal effect on

Fig. 1-10. Sagittal section of the hypothalamus and pituitary of the dog. A. The brain has been injected with India ink to show the vascular supply. The open area above is the third ventricle, while the clear area with the capillary loops is the median eminence. A portion of the posterior lobe is shown to the right, and the anterior lobe is the dark area to the left and below. At the extreme left, superiorly, is the optic chiasm. Connections can be seen between the vessels of the posterior lobe of the pituitary and the capillary loops in the median eminence. The capillary loops transmitting the hormones controlling gonadotropin secretion to the anterior lobe are in the extreme upper right hand corner of the picture, while those controlling ACTH and TSH secretion are in the anterior portion of the median eminence. B. High-powered view of the median eminence superiorly and the anterior lobe below. The optic chiasm is to the right, but out of view. The capillary loops may be seen projecting up into the median eminence and then descending down into the anterior pituitary.

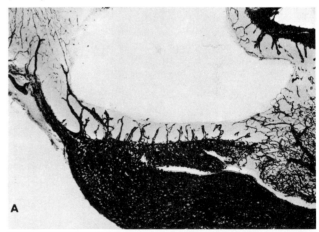

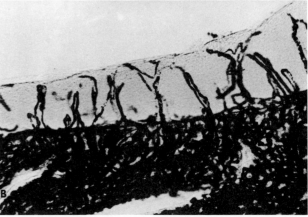

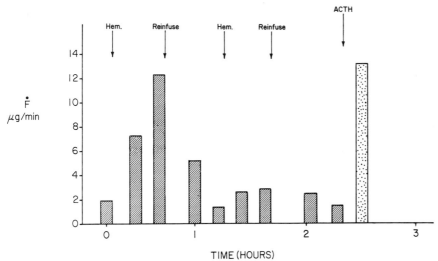

DOG #51

Sequential Hemorrhage; 10ml/kg/1.5min to Hypovolemia

the neuroendocrine response to the surgical intervention. Feedback inhibition of ACTH release can under appropriate circumstances be demonstrated for most stimuli, including pain, tissue trauma, and small hemorrhage. However, the response to some stimuli cannot be inhibited by even very high plasma levels of cortisol. The most common physiologic insult which cannot be suppressed by cortisol is large hemorrhage, although the response to intestinal traction also appears to be insuppressible by cortisol. In the presence of significant hypovolemia, ACTH release will

Fig. 1-11. Effects of two successive hemorrhages of 10 ml/kg, of reinfusion of shed blood, and of ACTH on secretion of cortisol. The response to the second hemorrhage 90 minutes after the first is attenuated, a reflection of cortisol feedback. Adrenal responsiveness to ACTH is maintained. (*From D. S. Gann et al., Am J Physiol, 232:R5, 1977.*)

Fig. 1-12. Effect of two successive rapid hemorrhages (10 ml/kg/45 seconds) on secretion of cortisol in a dog whose blood volume had been previously expanded by dextran so that hemorrhage would not lead to hypovolemia. The initial response, to rate of hemorrhage, is small and there is no significant cortisol feedback. The response to the second identical hemorrhage 90 minutes later is increased, an indication of physiologic facilitation. (*From D. S. Gann et al., Am J Physiol, 232:R5, 1977.*)

Dog #200

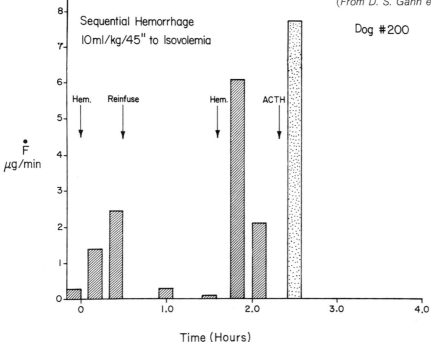

Sequential Hemorrhage
10ml/kg/45" to Isovolemia

persist until blood volume is restored. Thus hypovolemia seems to hold a preferential position among the various stimuli to ACTH release. The question of whether or not cortisol may suppress the release of hormones other than ACTH in the presence of hypovolemia has not been studied.

PHYSIOLOGIC FACILITATION

Under most circumstances, the adrenocortical response to a second stimulus appears unchanged from that to an initial stimulus. Because the feedback effect described above might be expected to inhibit this second response, the lack of inhibition has been ascribed to a physiologic facilitation. Under appropriate circumstances this facilitation can be demonstrated, provided that the initial stimulus is small enough to prevent high levels of cortisol (Fig. 1-12). The facilitation mechanism also appears to take 60 to 90 minutes and appears to be of sufficient magnitude to offset the feedback effect under most circumstances. The sites of action of facilitative mechanisms are not yet clear, but some data suggest that the adrenal cortex has an enhanced sensitivity to ACTH. There are also suggestions that this increased sensitivity is controlled by the central nervous system through a mechanism independent of ACTH release. Physiologic facilitation has also been observed in the adrenal medullary response to injury. In this case there is not only increased secretion of catecholamines but increased activity of several enzymes involved in catecholamine biosynthesis, including tyrosine hydroxylase. This effect appears to be mediated by increased corticosteroids as well as by increased nervous activity, since it is prevented by hypophysectomy. Cortisol, and possibly a history of increased sympathetic activity, appears to increase release of other hormones under sympathetic control, including glucagon and renin. Thus physiologic facilitation may lead to further imbalance among hormonal responses resulting from repeated injury. Again, the pattern of response to a second injury may be different from the response to the first.

Hormones with Generally Increased Secretion in Trauma

ACTH—CORTISOL

Most types of trauma are characterized by an increased secretion of ACTH and thus of cortisol. A more profound response is seen when the magnitude of the trauma is great, when infection, hemorrhage, and emotional trauma are present, and when stimulating anesthetic agents such as ether are used. The response may be diminished or abolished by cord section or by preexisting pituitary or adrenal disease (Figs. 1-13–1-16).

ADRENAL INSUFFICIENCY. The exogenous administration of corticosteroids partially inhibits ACTH, as described under Cortisol Feedback, and leads to decreased adrenal stimulation, atrophy, and finally very little production of corticosteroid. If the adrenal is sufficiently atrophic, even a large dose of ACTH will fail to arouse the adrenal cortex acutely to produce an increased output of

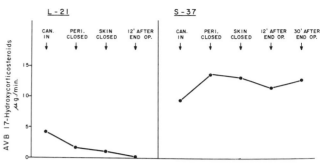

Fig. 1-13. Effects of anterior median eminence lesion on 17-OHCS secretion with operative trauma. Adrenal venous blood corticosteroid secretion in response to operative trauma. At the left are the values obtained in a dog with a lesion of the anterior median eminence. At the right are the values obtained in a normal control animal. A very minimal response was seen in the animal with the hypothalamic lesion, and the values declined during the course of the operation. In contrast, there was an excellent response in the normal animal which continued throughout the operative and immediate postoperative period. This illustrates the importance of the hypothalamus to the release of ACTH in response to trauma. (*From D. M. Hume, "Reticular Formation of the Brain," p. 231, Little, Brown and Company, Boston, 1958.*)

corticosteroids. Patients who have been on steroid administration for long periods of time, whose adrenal has become atrophic, and who are not given corticosteroids to support them during an operation have sometimes died because of the failure of cortisol release from an adrenal rendered temporarily inactive by atrophy. Patients should be questioned for a history of corticosteroid therapy. If acute adrenal insufficiency occurs, the most prominent features are fever and hypotension.

Fig. 1-14. Effect of anterior median eminence lesion on 17-OHCS and ACTH secretion during laparotomy: the adrenal venous blood 17-OHCS secretion and the blood ACTH level in response to operative trauma in normal dogs contrasted to dogs with lesions of the anterior median eminence. The solid bars represent mean values and the vertical lines the range of values. It may be seen that the animals with hypothalamic lesions show a markedly reduced pituitary and adrenal response to trauma. (*From D. M. Hume, "Reticular Formation of the Brain," p. 231, Little, Brown and Company, Boston, 1958.*)

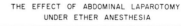
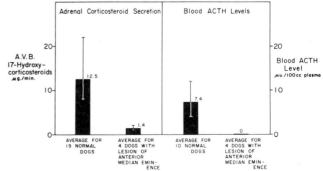

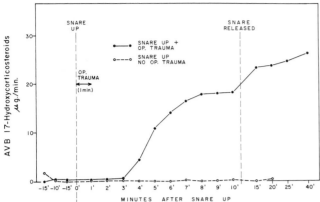

Fig. 1-15. Effect of nerve impulses from injured area on 17-OHCS secretion. This experiment was performed on an animal with a unilateral adrenalectomy and a cannula placed in the adrenal vein of the opposite side. The animal was put to sleep under Nembutal anesthesia, and after a series of base-line measurements a snare around the medial end of the adrenal view was pulled up so that all of the secretion of the only remaining adrenal drained to the outside over a period of 20 minutes. This had the effect of suddenly stopping all adrenal secretion into the blood of the animal, but this sudden hypoadrenalism did not produce a stimulus to ACTH release or increase in the secretion of 17-OHCS. After releasing the snare again, and following a suitable control period, the experiment was repeated exactly as before except that this time after the control period and the pulling up of the snare the animal was suddenly severely traumatized. Within 2 minutes there was a marked increase in adrenal venous blood 17-OHCS secretion. This indicates that the release of ACTH in response to trauma is not brought about as a consequence of a sudden diminution in blood levels of 17-OHCS but is instead stimulated by nervous impulses originating in the injured area.

Similarly, if a patient with unsuspected adrenal insufficiency is inadvertently operated upon without being supported with exogenous corticosteroids, death is likely to ensue. Thus cortisol is necessary for the normal response in trauma. Severe adrenal insufficiency (Addison's disease) is more fully discussed in the section on the adrenal (see Chap. 37). For purposes of the present discussion it is important to recognize that severe insufficiency may be seen in several forms. It may first be noted in the immediate newborn period, when it occurs as part of the adrenogenital syndrome. It is particularly hard to recognize in males, who, unlike females, do not show any physical stigmata of the syndrome. In females, the syndrome may be suspected because of enlargement of the clitoris. Adrenal insufficiency in the infant may be manifested by fever, weight loss, vomiting, hyponatremia, shock, and marked salt loss in the urine. These symptoms usually appear in the first week after birth but sometimes do not become manifest for 5 or 6 weeks. The disease is caused by an enzymatic defect in the adrenal cortex which leads to failure of hydroxylation at the C_{11}, C_{20}, or C_{21} positions. Addison's disease is particularly apt to occur when the defect is in C_{20} or C_{21} hydroxylation. A C_{20} block produces a general deficiency of corticosteroids. No survivals have ever been

reported. A C_{21} defect with Addison's disease can be successfully treated if recognized (Fig. 1-17).

If chronic adrenal insufficiency is present prior to the time of surgical treatment and is unrecognized, death is likely to occur within a matter of hours after operation has begun. Typically, chronic adrenal insufficiency is characterized by pigmentation, weakness, weight loss, hypotension, easy fatigability, nausea, vomiting, abdominal pain, hypoglycemia, hyponatremia, and hyperkalemia. Opera-

Fig. 1-16. Comparison of 17-OHCS increases following surgical procedures and ACTH injection. *A.* The response to cholecystectomy in an eighty-two-year-old patient. There is a marked increase in the level of plasma 17-OHCS during the operative procedure which rapidly returns to normal levels on the day after operation. The response to operative trauma is not quite as high as the response to an injection of ACTH. *B.* The plasma 17-OHCS response to a vagotomy and subtotal gastrectomy. There is a marked increase in the levels of 17-OHCS on the operative day, the values returning to normal the day after operation. The peak response was even greater than that seen with ACTH. This operation was of somewhat greater magnitude than the cholecystectomy shown in *A.*

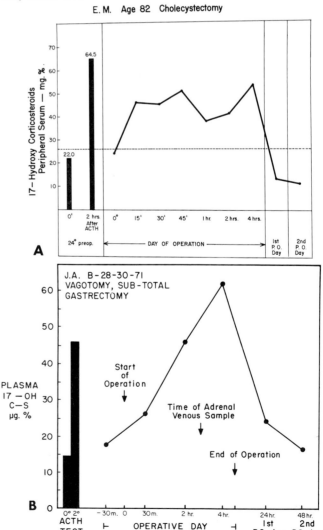

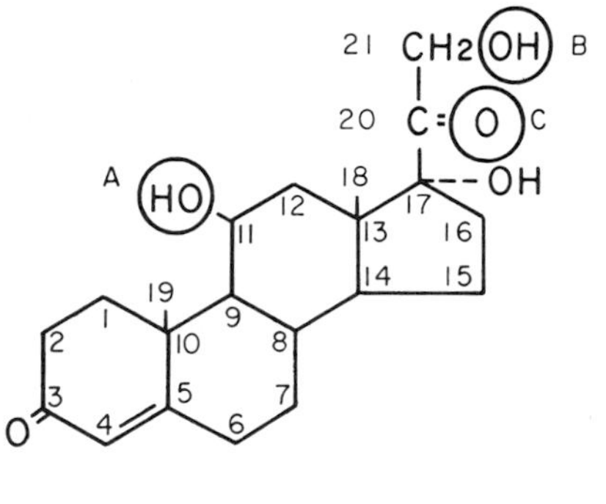

CORTISOL

Fig. 1-17. Steroid nucleus showing, in the circles, three of the defects which may be seen with congenital adrenal hyperplasia. A defect located at *A* produces hypertension, one located at *B* produces severe salt wasting and hypotension, and one located at *C* is usually fatal.

Table 1-1. DAILY SECRETION RATES OF HORMONES

Compound	Mean 24-hr secretion rate
Cortisol, mg	15–30
Corticosterone, mg	2–5
Aldosterone, μg	50–150
Dehydroepiandrosterone, mg	15–30
Androstenedione, mg	0–10
Hydroxyandrostenedione, mg	0–10
Progesterone, mg	0.4–0.8
Pregnenolone, mg	0.5–0.8
17-OH pregnenolone, mg	0.2–0.4
Estradiol, mg	Trace

SOURCE: From P. H. Forsham, The Adrenal Cortex, in R. H. Williams (ed.); "Textbook of Endocrinology," p. 287, W. B. Saunders Company, Philadelphia, 1968.

tive intervention will precipitate an acute Addisonian crisis leading to death if treatment is not promptly instituted.

A semiacute type of adrenal insufficiency occurs when the adrenal damage takes place at the time of, or shortly after, the operative event. This has occasionally been seen in patients who were given heparin and developed bilateral adrenal hemorrhages in the postoperative period, and of course it occurs automatically when the operation is a bilateral adrenalectomy. Here, however, exogenous corticosteroids are administered to compensate for the failure of endogenous secretion. If the condition is unrecognized, the patients tend to get along fairly well for 3 or 4 days, after which increasing difficulties develop which may lead

to severe hyponatremia, hypoglycemia, and death if untreated.

The hormones secreted by the adrenal cortex are shown in Fig. 1-18, and their relative secretion rates are shown in Table 1-1 and Fig. 1-19. The adrenal androgens and estrogens seem relatively unimportant in the response to trauma, but cortisol and aldosterone are of the utmost importance. A diagram showing the pathways for the control of secretion of cortisol may be seen in Fig. 1-20. The degradation of cortisol takes place by reduction (A-ring reduction) to tetrahydrocortisol and conjugation with glucuronic acid or sulfuric acid. When these steps have taken place, the cortisol becomes highly water-soluble and can be readily excreted in urine. Since the liver is responsible for

Fig. 1-18. Principal steroids secreted by the adrenal cortex.

GLUCOCORTICOIDS   MINERALOCORTICOIDS   ANDROGENS   ESTROGEN   PROGESTIN

CORTISOL   ALDOSTERONE   ANDROSTENEDIONE   ESTRADIOL   PROGESTERONE

CORTICOSTERONE   DEHYDROEPIANDROSTERONE   II-B HYDROXYANDRO-STENEDIONE   PREGNENOLONE

17α-HYDROXYPREGNENOLONE

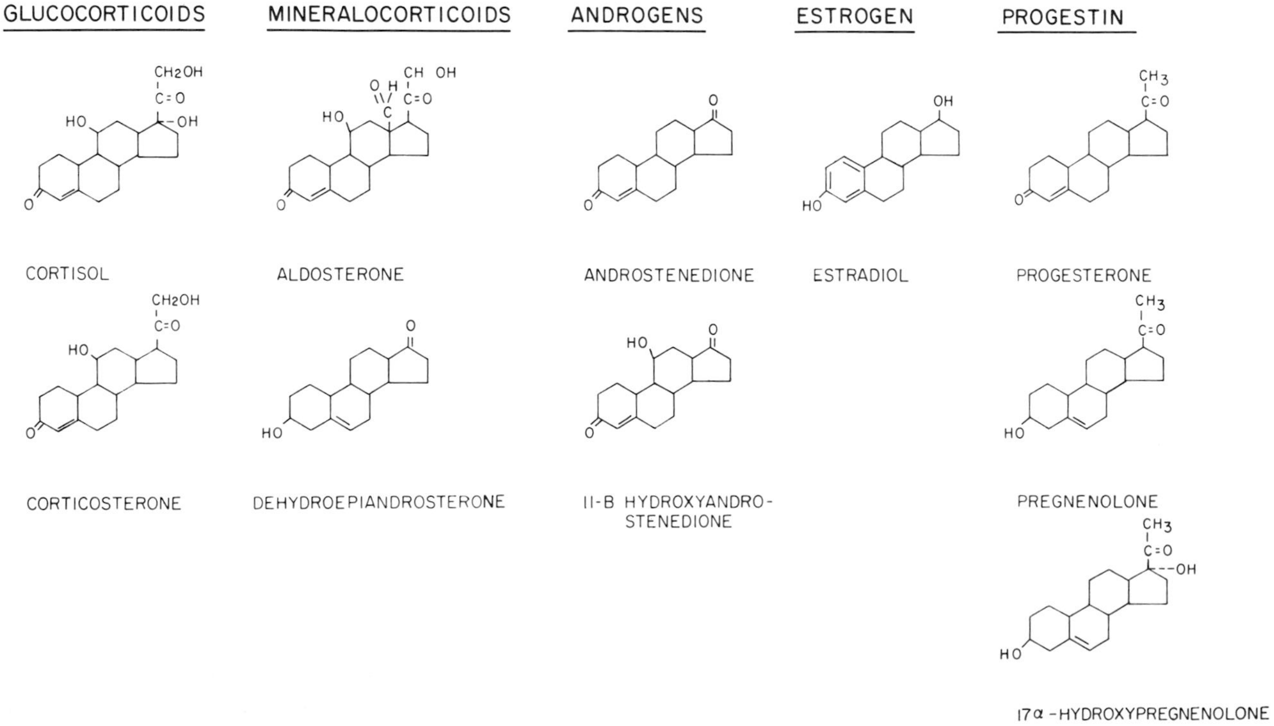

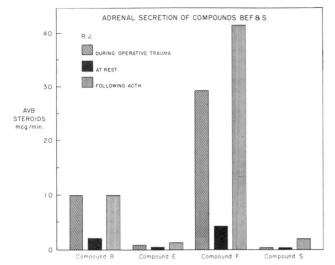

Fig. 1-19. Adrenal venous blood glucocorticoid secretion in man during operative trauma, at rest, and after an injection of ACTH. The principal glucocorticoid is cortisol (compound F), and the second is corticosterone (compound B). Only small amounts of cortisone (compound E and compound S) are secreted. (*From D. M. Hume et al., Surgery, 52:174, 1962.*)

reduction and conjugation of corticosteroids, severe liver disease may interfere with this step, and the level of blood conjugates may be very low. The kidney is responsible for excreting the greater part of the conjugated cortisol, so that the presence of kidney disease permits extremely high levels of the conjugates to build up in the bloodstream. The reduced and conjugated corticosteroid is no longer biologically effective.

Despite the obvious demonstration that an increased secretion of cortisol occurs in response to almost all types of trauma, that cortisol is necessary for the organism to withstand trauma successfully, and that patients with unrecognized adrenal insufficiency die following trauma whereas patients with bilateral adrenalectomy can tolerate trauma if given exogenous cortisol, adrenal insufficiency is rarely the cause of death after injury.

Fig. 1-20. Control of ACTH and cortisol. The cardiovascular system signals atrial and arterial receptors by means of pressures ($\overline{P}_{at}$ and $\overline{P}_a$), and atrial volume and rate of change of that volume (V, $\dot{V}$). Signals are first processed in the nuclei of the solitary tract (NTS) and then ascend to the hypothalamus for control of CRF. Both ACTH and cortisol (F) are distributed, bound, and metabolized (D, B, M), and the results of these processes establish the plasma concentrations. Cortisol feedback may inhibit release of ACTH at hypothalamic and pituitary sites. Cortisol acts with other hormones to increase blood volume. Other stimuli reach the hypothalamus as shown.

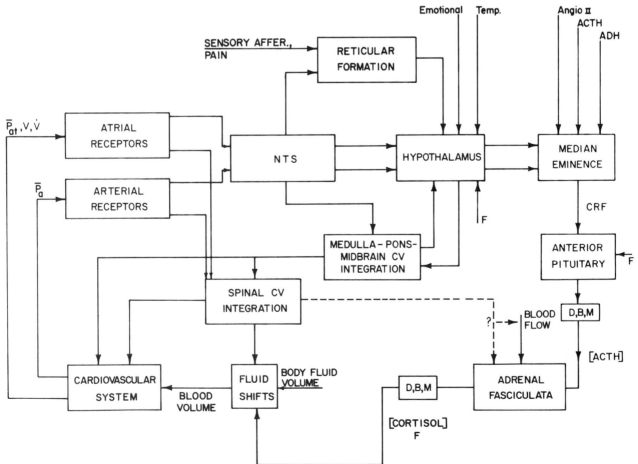

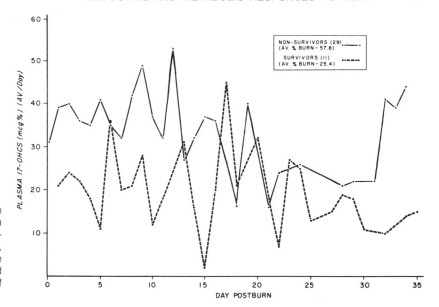

Fig. 1-21. Plasma 17-OHCS values in burn patients. It may be seen that the values in those patients who ultimately recovered gradually declined during the postburn period, whereas those patients who did not survive had higher values at first and later showed gradually increasing values up to the time of death.

It was demonstrated by Ingle that adrenalectomized animals traumatized while on a constant dose of corticosteroids showed some of the metabolic changes formerly ascribed to an *increased* secretion of these hormones, and this effect has been termed by him the "permissive" action of corticosteroids. Recent observations in our own laboratory indicate that restitution of blood volume required *increased* cortisol, so that the permissive action cannot be the sole explanation of the effect of cortisol in trauma. However, paraplegic patients, who fail to respond to operative trauma with an increased secretion of cortisol, generally tolerate the operative procedure well. These seeming paradoxes may be explained, at least in part, in the following ways:

In severe trauma, hepatic conjugation of corticosteroids into the inactive form may be reduced, so that larger amounts of unconjugated (active) corticosteroids are suddenly available even though the rate of infusion or secretion remains constant. The secretion of cortisol in the paraplegic remains low despite trauma because of the absence of afferent nerve impulses, but it can still increase if uncompensated hemorrhage or infection supervenes or if hypothalamic stimulation results from hypoglycemia or an excitatory anesthetic agent. Finally, an operative trauma is far better tolerated in patients whose body cells have not been deprived of the adrenal corticosteroids preoperatively than in those in whom preexisting deficiency is present. For this reason the patient who has adrenal insufficiency because of Addison's disease will tolerate the immediate operative event less well than a normal patient whose adrenals are removed without his being given cortisol or one whose adrenals are suppressed by prolonged corticosteroid administration which is stopped abruptly at operation. Nevertheless it should be emphasized that when in the past bilateral adrenalectomy was attempted in patients prior to the availability of cortisone, it was universally fatal, and hypophysectomy without corticosteroid support was likewise accompanied by an increased mortality.

However, in the absence of corticosteroid administration, hypophysectomy is tolerated far better than adrenalectomy.

Adrenal exhaustion, which was once thought to occur following prolonged trauma, probably never occurs. Most patients who die following injury, sepsis, burns, infection and other forms of severe prolonged trauma die with very high blood levels of corticosteroids (Fig. 1-21). In fact the very existence of continued high levels of plasma corticosteroids in the severely burned patient is usually a bad prognostic sign, suggesting that the trauma of burns is continuing and severe (Figs. 1-21 and 1-22). Nonetheless there is an occasional burned patient who shows evidences of adrenal insufficiency; there is an occasional patient in whom it develops in response to bilateral adrenal hemor-

Fig. 1-22. Relationship between plasma 17-OHCS and percentage of burn. It may be seen that the more severe the burn, the higher in general were the plasma 17-OHCS values.

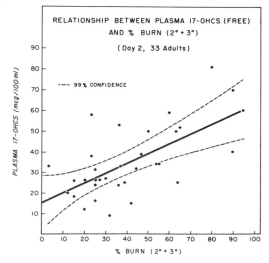

rhage due to anticoagulant therapy; and there is an occasional patient in whom prolonged corticosteroid administration or preexisting Addison's disease has been unrecognized at the time of operation. Since the operative event is so apt to be fatal under these circumstances and since excellent replacement therapy is now available, adrenal insufficiency becomes an important and preventable cause of postoperative demise, despite its rarity. The causes and manifestations of adrenal insufficiency are dealt with further in the chapter on the adrenal (Chap. 37).

The Waterhouse-Friderichsen syndrome, which consists of bilateral adrenal hemorrhage in patients, usually children, with meningococcal septicemia, was originally thought to produce death as a consequence of adrenal failure. When death occurs in this condition, however, it occurs very rapidly and is due to the meningococcal septicemia—the adrenal hemorrhage occurring as a terminal complication and an almost incidental finding. These patients die with elevated blood cortisol levels.

When the patient has been found to have adrenal insufficiency, replacement therapy is given. While orally or intravenously administered cortisol is effective almost at once, intramuscularly administered cortisol acetate is slowly absorbed and does not become maximally effective until 12 to 18 hours after administration. Initial therapy therefore always should be intravenous and should consist of 100 to 200 mg of cortisol as the 21-hemisuccinate or phosphate. These two conjugates are lysed quickly in blood.

RENIN

Most traumatic events lead to increased secretion of renin from the cells of the juxtaglomerular apparatus of the renal afferent arterioles. The secretion of renin is under the control of multiple factors. The principal factors that

lead to increased secretion of renin are increased sympathetic stimulation of the juxtaglomerular cells through a beta adrenergic mechanism, decreased renal arterial perfusion pressure, and decreased delivery of sodium chloride to the macula densa (a collection of modified distal tubular cells which have a constant proximity to the juxtaglomerular apparatus of the afferent arteriole) of the distal tubule. Following trauma, all three of these factors may stimulate increased secretion of renin as sympathetic nervous activity is increased, as arterial pressure falls, and as renal mechanisms for conservation of sodium and water in the proximal tubule come into effect. The principal factors leading to inhibition of renin release are angiotensin II, vasopressin, and potassium. Again, the plasma levels of all these factors are elevated after trauma, but in general the stimulatory factors outweigh the inhibitory ones. Renin released into the circulation acts as an enzyme to convert angiotensinogen (a hepatic α_2-globulin) to angiotensin I. The latter is converted by an enzyme to the active form angiotensin II, an octapeptide. The converting enzyme appears to have its major activity in the lung but is present in other tissues as well. Angiotensin II stimulates the adrenal cortex to secrete aldosterone. It is also the most potent hyperten-

Fig. 1-23. Signal flow in the control of secretion of aldosterone (+, stimulation; −, inhibition). *RF*, reticular formation; *C*, corticotropin-releasing factor; *NTS*, nucleus tractus solitarius; *VMC*, vasomotor center; *SNS*, sympathetic nervous system; *BV*, blood volume; *BP*, blood pressure; *MAP*, mean arterial pressure; *Na DELIV.*, sodium delivery; *MD*, macula densa; *JG*, juxtaglomerular apparatus; *TBW*, total body water; *DOC*, desoxycorticosterone; *B*, corticosterone; *18-OH-B*, 18-hydroxycorticosterone; *ECF*, extracellular fluid. (*From T. S. Harrison, D. S. Gann, A. J. Edis, and R. H. Egdahl, "Surgical Disorders of the Adrenal Gland," p. 13, Grune & Stratton, New York, 1975.*)

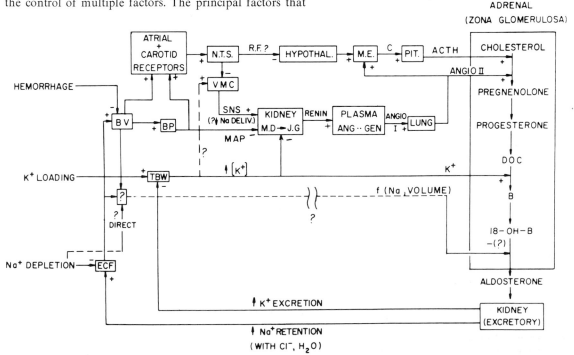

sive agent known. In addition, angiotensin acts to increase the secretion of vasopressin and of ACTH from the pituitary to constrict the veins, thus decreasing vascular compliance, and to limit excretion of sodium and water by decreasing glomerular filtration.

ALDOSTERONE

The increased secretion of aldosterone seen in response to injury results from increased stimulation of the zona glomerulosa of the adrenal cortex by three factors: angiotensin II, ACTH, and potassium. As indicated previously, the levels of all three of these factors are elevated in injury. The effect of angiotensin II is certainly more potent than that of ACTH in stimulating secretion of aldosterone in the chronic state, but both factors appear important in the acute response of the adrenal cortex to hypovolemia. The control of aldosterone synthesis and secretion is illustrated in Fig. 1-23. Aldosterone acts on the distal nephron to increase reabsorption of sodium, in part together with chloride and water and in part in exchange for potassium and hydrogen. The latter effect is critical for life, since it is the principal mechanism by which the kidney may excrete the potassium and acid which build up in severe trauma.

EPINEPHRINE AND NOREPINEPHRINE

Epinephrine and norepinephrine are both secreted in response to trauma, although the amounts of these substances secreted during operative trauma depend to a considerable extent on the anesthesia employed. Ether, for example, is a strong stimulus to epinephrine release, whereas Nembutal inhibits it almost entirely. The increased secretion of epinephrine and norepinephrine is quite short-lived and is usually limited to the day of trauma unless the injury is a very severe and continuing one. During operative trauma, with the anesthetic agents commonly employed, there is a greater total secretion of norepinephrine than of epinephrine. This is probably because the entire source of epinephrine is from the adrenal medulla, whereas norepinephrine is also secreted from the sympathetic nerve endings. There is a greater secretion of epinephrine in the adrenal venous blood than of norepinephrine, though this is not striking (Fig. 1-24).

Epinephrine and norepinephrine both increase cardiac output and elevate the blood pressure; epinephrine stimulates glycogenolysis and lipolysis and inhibits release of insulin. Increased secretion of the catecholamines is brought about by both changes in blood volume and by afferent sensory impulses. Cells in the posterior hypothalamus are stimulated and send impulses down through the parabrachial region of the pons to the lateral reticular nucleus of the medulla. From this point, impulses travel down the cord to the intermediolateral cell columns and out into the sympathetic efferents. Adrenal medullary secretory activity is brought about through the splanchnic sympathetics. Denervation of the adrenal stops the secretion of catecholamines in the adrenal venous blood. Some noxious stimuli, such as endotoxin, can act directly upon the hypothalamic sympathetic control centers to produce epinephrine and norepinephrine release (see Fig. 1-5). Hypoglycemia is also a stimulus to epinephrine and nor-

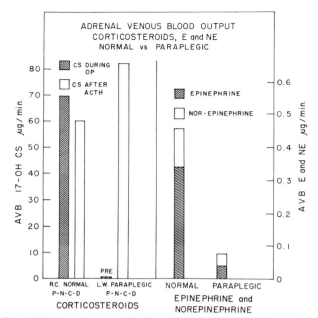

Fig. 1-24. Adrenal venous blood corticosteroids, epinephrine, and norepinephrine in normal versus paraplegic patients. It may be seen that the intraoperative production of 17-OHCS in the paraplegic patient was so low as to be nearly unmeasurable whereas after the injection of ACTH it rose promptly to a very high level. The secretion of epinephrine and norepinephrine too was greatly reduced in paraplegic patients.

epinephrine release. This apparently acts at a hypothalamic level. Although histamine in large doses is a potent stimulus to epinephrine release, it is doubtful whether the amounts of histamine released physiologically play any role in the increased secretion of catecholamines seen in response to trauma.

VASOPRESSIN (ANTIDIURETIC HORMONE, ADH)

Most trauma is accompanied by an increased secretion of ADH brought about by afferent neural stimuli impinging upon the hypothalamus. Stimulation of the supraoptic and paraventricular nuclei leads to a release of ADH from the posterior pituitary. Hypovolemia is also a potent stimulus to ADH release, acting through receptors and pathways similar to those controlling secretion of ACTH. Vasopressin acts on the distal tubule and collecting duct to increase water reabsorption and also has an important role in effecting splanchnic vasoconstriction. In the presence of increased vasopressin, administration of water without salt will lead to dilutional hyponatremia and, in the extreme, to water intoxication.

With head injury two additional peculiarities in ADH secretion sometimes occur. The first of these is called *inappropriate ADH secretion.* This is a term given to excessive secretion of ADH beyond that needed to promote homeostasis. The ADH secretion continues after the initial period of damage and produces a low urinary output with high osmolarity and a profound dilutional hyponatremia (see Chap. 42). The converse phenomenon of diabetes insipidus is sometimes seen with head injury, particularly basilar skull fractures. This may be either temporary or permanent and results from damage to the supraoptico-hypophyseal system. It may cause severe dehydration or even death in patients with head injury and coma who are given tube feedings. Since the patient is comatose, he cannot express thirst, and a continued excessive polyuria dehydrates him, leading to hypernatremia. This is compounded by the use of tube feedings high in sodium, small protein fractions, and glucose, which thus combines an excessive sodium load with an osmotic diuresis, further dehydrating the patient.

GROWTH HORMONE (GH)

The hypothalamic mechanisms controlling release of growth hormone involve both stimulation and inhibition. Pituitary release of growth hormone is stimulated by growth-hormone-releasing factor, coming principally from the ventromedial, arcuate, and perhaps dorsomedial nuclei. The growth-hormone-inhibiting hormone, somatostatin, comes principally from the preoptic area and from the amygdala. The release of growth hormone is promoted by hypoglycemia and also especially by blood loss and tissue injury. Meyer and Knobil found hemorrhage to be a potent stimulus to growth-hormone release in monkeys, and Carey et al. found war wounds to be strong stimuli to growth-hormone release in man. Carey et al. postulated that the elevated levels of plasma amino acid that were seen in injury were responsible for the increase in GH secretion. This seems unlikely, however, as plasma amino acid levels usually are not elevated in injury, and arginine concentration, which is the best stimulus to GH release, decreases. Growth hormone may act in trauma to increase glucose levels by opposing the action of insulin, by promoting gluconeogenesis, by promoting the synthesis of certain specific proteins, and by promoting lipolysis.

GLUCAGON

Glucagon is a diabetogenic hormone made by the alpha cells of the pancreatic islets. A glucagonlike substance is also made in the upper small intestine. Glucagon secretion is stimulated by hypoglycemia and by sympathetic stimulation acting directly on the alpha cell. There is increasing interest in the role of glucagon in the metabolism of injury. Some of its effects are listed in Tables 1-2 and 1-3.

Glucagon is a marked stimulus to lipolysis, increasing cyclic adenosine monophosphate (cyclic AMP) in fat, which in turn increases the activity of the lipolytic enzyme that hydrolyzes triglyceride to fatty acid and glycerol. The elevated free fatty acid levels stimulate gluconeogenesis, but glucagon has a direct effect on gluconeogenesis as well. Glucagon also promotes glycogenolysis through cyclic AMP activation of phosphorylase.

The main results of increased glucagon secretion in trauma are to produce increases in blood glucose through stimulation of glycogenolysis, gluconeogenesis, and lipolysis. Glucagon also promotes ketogenesis and ureagenesis and decreases lipoprotein release, but these effects are less striking than those relating to glucose and fat mobilization.

Glucagon also produces ionotropic cardiovascular effects when given to patients or animals in shock. These effects consist of an increase in cardiac output and stroke volume,

and a decrease in peripheral vascular resistance despite β-receptor blockade. To what degree these effects are part of the physiologic response to injury is unknown.

Hormones with Unaltered or Decreased Secretion in Trauma

TSH—THYROXIN

Because there is a hypermetabolic state in the immediate postoperative or posttraumatic period, it was originally thought that TSH secretion led to increased thyroid activity. More recent studies seem to indicate that this is not so. Although the presence of thyroid hormone is necessary for the normal functioning of organs in response to a traumatic stress, an increased secretion is apparently not necessary to meet this challenge, and release of thyroid hormones may actually decrease after trauma.

INSULIN

Insulin secretion is not usually increased in response to trauma. Epinephrine, which is, inhibits the release of insulin, and many factors are working to produce an elevation of the blood sugar level and to make carbohydrate available. The administration of glucose intravenously may call forth an insulin secretion, but there is a relatively diabetic glucose tolerance curve in the immediate posttraumatic period. The relative hypoinsulinism of trauma augments the hyperglycemia, gluconeogenesis, decreased amino acid

Table 1-2. REPORTED EFFECTS OF GLUCAGON ON ISOLATED LIVER

Process	Change	Involvement of cyclic AMP
Glycogenolysis	Increase	Yes
Phosphorylase	Increase	Yes
Gluconeogenesis	Increase	Yes
Glycogen synthesis	Decrease	Yes
Glycogen synthetase	Decrease	Yes
Ureogenesis	Increase	Yes
Protein synthesis	Decrease (?)	?
Protein breakdown	Increase (?)	?
Ketogenesis	Increase	Yes
Lipolysis	Increase	Yes
Amino acid uptake	Increase	Yes
Tyrosine aminotransferase	Increase	Yes
p-Pyruvate carboxykinase	Increase	Yes
Lysosome activation	Increase	?
K^+ release	Increase	Yes
Ca^{++} release	Increase	Yes
Mitochondrial pyruvate uptake	Increase	?
Krebs cycle	Increase	?
Transamination	Increase	?
Lipoprotein release	Decrease	Yes

SOURCE: J. H. Exton, M. Vi, S. B. Lewis, and C. R. Park, Mechanism of Glucagon Activation of Gluconeogenesis, in H. D. Soling and B. Willms (eds.), "Regulation of Gluconeogenesis," p. 160, Academic Press, Inc., New York, 1971.

Table 1-3. SOME METABOLIC EFFECTS OF HORMONES WITH GENERALLY INCREASED SECRETION IN TRAUMA

	Proteolysis (in muscle)	Gluconeogenesis (in liver & kidney)	Glycolysis		Glycogenolysis		Lipolysis (adipose tissue, liver, muscle)	Insulin antagonism	Insulin secretion	Sodium retention	Potassium loss	Water retention
			Muscle	Adipose tissue	Liver	Muscle						
ACTH-cortisol	+++	+++	0	0	......	0	++	++	++	++	++	0
Renin-aldosterone .	......	......	..	......	......	......	......	......	......	+++	+++	++
Epinephrine, norepinephrine .	+	++*	0	++	++++	++	++++*	+++	0	+	0	
ADH	......	......	..	......	......	......	......	......	......	......	......	++++
Growth hormone .	0	+	0	++	......	......	++*	+	+++			
Glucagon	++	+++*	0	......	++†	......	++*	++	+++			

* Only in the presence of the adrenal corticosteroids.
† By stimulating catecholamine secretion.

uptake, and lipolysis stimulated by epinephrine, ACTH, cortisol, GH, and glucagon.

FSH-LH AND SEX HORMONE SECRETION

No increased secretion of FSH or LH occurs in response to trauma, and there is some evidence to indicate that the secretion of these substances may even be inhibited somewhat during this period. Menstrual periods may be missed in the immediate postoperative period but may also occur on schedule or early. The emotional response to the trauma may to some extent influence cyclic activity. It is much more common to note amenorrhea in patients with chronic renal failure, however, than in the otherwise healthy woman who undergoes a severe trauma.

There are few data on the secretion of androgens of either testicular or adrenal origin in the posttraumatic period. No good data indicate whether or not adrenal androgens are increased following trauma. In the immediate posttrauma period there is only a very modest increase in urinary 17-ketosteroids.

Goals of Endocrine Changes

Survival after injury depends critically upon continued delivery of oxygen and nutrients to the brain and heart. The initial trend toward cardiovascular stabilization in the presence of hypovolemia is brought about by baroreflex increase in sympathetic nervous activity. The resulting increase in peripheral vasoconstriction may be augmented by the actions of angiotensin II, vasopressin, and circulating catecholamines. The increase in myocardial contractility may be augmented by circulating epinephrine and glucagon. Other hormonal changes also seem organized to promote the restitution of blood volume and thus cardiovascular stabilization. Increased secretion of cortisol, glucagon, and probably growth hormone appear to be required to bring about the prompt increase in extracellular osmolality that follows volume loss and that promotes the movement of fluids from the cells to the interstitium to

promote restitution of blood volume on protein, as discussed below. Many of the detrimental metabolic consequences of injury follow upon this immediate and homeostatic hormonally induced change in plasma osmolality. The renal effects of hormones increased after injury also tend to support the restitution of blood volume by limiting renal loss of salt and water. In the absence of such conservative mechanisms, homeostatic increases in blood volume would be negated by continuing renal loss. Thus the actions of the catecholamines in promoting salt and water reabsorption in the proximal tubule and of aldosterone and vasopressin in promoting reabsorption of salt and water in the distal nephron can again be viewed in terms of circulatory support. As indicated previously, the release of many of these hormones can be brought about by tissue injury per se. Such reflexly induced release of hormones may anticipate the hormonal response to loss of plasma volume. Most of these anticipatory responses can be inhibited by increased cortisol, whereas severe hypovolemia leads to a responsive ACTH release which is not cortisol-suppressible. Thus the general hormonal response to injury can be viewed in one sense as part of a cardiovascular reflex aimed at restitution of blood volume and ultimate stabilization of the cardiovascular system, as shown diagrammatically in Fig. 1-25. Some of these effects are brought about by the metabolic effects outlined in Table 1-3.

One may summarize the endocrine changes which occur in response to injury by saying that they seem to be directed toward water and salt conservation, blood pressure maintenance, gluconeogenesis, glycolysis, general mobilization of carbohydrate, lipolysis, the outpouring of hormones essential for cell life, and the providing of ready energy to the muscles, heart, and brain.

METABOLIC CHANGES

Following a severe injury there is marked tissue wasting and weight loss. This is partly due to semistarvation and partly to the extreme catabolism which occurs in the immediate postinjury period. The intensity and duration of the catabolic period depends upon the severity of the injury and on whether or not the injury is protracted by sepsis and other serious complications. The protein loss is far greater in healthy young men than in elderly patients, women, or children (Fig. 1-26), but it can be greatly decreased by the administration of amino acids and calories intravenously.

The metabolic changes which accompany trauma depend not only upon the intensity and duration of the injury but upon the presence or absence of shock, the degree of anoxia, the type of repair solutions administered to the patient, and the success or failure of the body in adapting itself to the injury. In order to understand the metabolic response to injury it becomes necessary to examine the energy sources available to the body, the effect of starvation and hyperalimentation, the changes produced by increased hormone secretion, and the adaptive mechanisms essential to recovery from profound injury.

Fig. 1-25. The neuroendocrine response to injury (pain, hemorrhage, and ECF loss) viewed as a homeostatic reflex organized for the control of blood volume and for cardiovascular stabilization. In response to volume loss the inhibition of the central nervous system (CNS) by the cardiovascular system (CVS) is released, leading to increased activity of the sympathetic nervous system (SNS) and to the endocrine changes described in the text. The autonomic and multihormonal reflexes are coordinated for the restitution of blood volume and for cardiovascular stability. (*From D. S. Gann, Ann NY Acad Sci, 297:591, 1977.*)

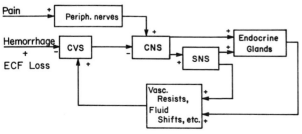

Energy Metabolism

Energy is stored in the body in the form of carbohydrate (glycogen), protein, and fat (triglycerides). Glycogen is stored in muscle and liver in combination with water and electrolytes, so that 1 Gm of glycogen yields only 1 or 2 kcal instead of the 4 kcal found in 1 Gm of dry carbohydrate. Protein is stored primarily in muscle, and, like carbohydrate, in combination with water. Therefore, muscles are only one-quarter to one-fifth protein. Furthermore, body protein is not designed primarily as a source of fuel, but performs other important functions in the form of enzymes, plasma protein, structural protein, cardiac and skeletal muscle, etc. Ingested protein beyond that needed to replenish body stores is metabolized, the nitrogen is excreted as urea, and the calories thus created are expended or, if unneeded, stored as fat.

Lipid is not stored in combination with water, and body fat therefore yields lipid contents as high as 90 percent of total weight. One gram of body fat thus provides nearly the full 9.4 kcal present in one gram of pure triglyceride.

Table 1-4 is modified from a concise and lucid review by Cahill on the metabolic effects of starvation in man. It may be seen that extracellular fluids and muscle and liver glycogen make very small contributions to the body energy pool when compared to muscle protein, and especially to fat—the major energy depot. During starvation man attempts to conserve protein by burning fat instead, and to preserve muscle and liver glycogen by accelerating gluconeogenesis. Cahill did not list plasma protein as a potential source of fuel, because in simple, short-term starvation the body is able to replenish plasma protein at a rate equal to its degradation. Plasma protein can probably be used as fuel, however, as demonstrated by the experiments of Allen et al., in which puppies were maintained and grew while receiving protein only in the form of intravenous plasma. With prolonged fasting in the face of trauma and marked catabolism, endogenous plasma proteins are burned, and the liver is incapable of synthesizing albumin at a rate equal to its loss, necessitating the

Table 1-4. FUEL COMPOSITION OF NORMAL
70-kg MAN

Fuel	Kilograms	Calories
Tissues:		
Fat (adipose triglyceride)	15.0	141,000
Protein (mainly muscle)	6.0	24,000
Glycogen (muscle)	0.150	600
Glycogen (liver)	0.075	300
Total	. . . . . .	165,900
Circulating fuels:		
Glucose (extracellular fluid) . . .	0.020	80
Free fatty acids (plasma)	0.0003	3
Triglycerides (plasma)	0.003	30
Plasma proteins	0.210	840
Total	. . . . . .	953

SOURCE: Adapted from G. F. Cahill, Jr., *N Eng J Med,* **282**:668, 1970.

replacement of plasma proteins from exogenous sources. Red blood cells probably are consumed as well. It is extremely important, therefore, to administer amino acids, albumin, plasma, or whole blood to surgical patients who are in a catabolic state and unable to eat, not only to replace plasma protein and blood lost externally or to the third space but also that which is burned as fuel.

With acute trauma, anoxia, and exercise muscle and liver glycogen are used as emergency fuels, and with severe or prolonged injury muscle protein is used as well, unless attempts are made to conserve it by the vigorous intravenous administration of protein or amino acids, and calories.

Starvation

An understanding of the metabolic changes seen following injury in man requires a consideration of the effects of starvation, which may accompany injury of a progressive or long-term nature. These are shown in Figs. 1-27 and 1-28. Glucose is derived from glycogenolysis of liver glycogen and from gluconeogenesis. The new glucose formed from gluconeogenesis derives in part from amino acids and in part from glycerol, which comes from the triglycerides of body fat. In the early fasting state, shown in Fig. 1-27 and in Table 1-5, a 70-kg man would be expected to make about 16 Gm of new glucose from glycerol and about 43 Gm from muscle protein for a total of 59 Gm a day. In addition to this he would obtain 85 Gm of glucose from glycogen breakdown and 36 Gm from recycled glucose, for a total of 180 Gm a day. Whereas the brain normally completely metabolizes glucose to carbon dioxide and water, other glycolytic tissues such as peripheral nerve, erythrocytes, leukocytes, bone marrow, renal medulla, and to a lesser extent normal muscle metabolize glucose mainly by converting it to lactate and pyruvate. These substances are released into the bloodstream and carried back to the liver and kidney, where they are remade into glucose, thus contributing to the total available glucose without creating any net gain of glucose. This process is known as the *Cori cycle;* its effect is to provide energy for the peripheral tissues by the anaerobic glycolysis of glucose, while the energy thus given up is regained in the liver by the reconversion of lactate into glucose utilizing energy derived from the oxidation of fat (Fig. 1-29). The entire process of gluconeogenesis requires energy, and this energy is sup-

Table 1-5. GLUCOSE AVAILABLE IN EARLY
STARVATION STATE IN A 70-kg MAN

Origin	Amount of glucose, Gm/24 hr
New glucose (gluconeogenesis):	
Fat (glycerol)	16
Protein	43
Stored or recycled glucose:	
Glycogen	85
Recycled glucose	36
Total	180

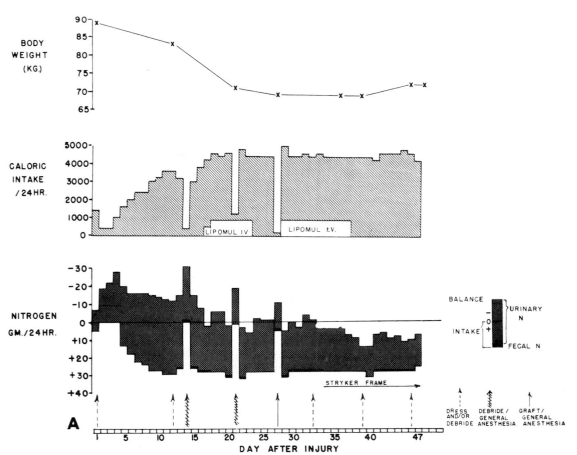

M.C.V. -26-06-68
WHITE, MALE, 28 YRS.
BURN 55% (40% 3°)
ADMISSION: 4/27/57

Fig. 1-26. A comparison of the nitrogen excretion in a burned woman and a burned man illustrating the far greater catabolism and nitrogen loss in the man. *A.* Twenty-eight-year-old white man with 55 percent burn. *B.* Thirty-one-year-old white woman with 55 percent burn.

plied by the oxidation of fatty acids. By means of the Cori cycle the amount of glucose that has to be supplied from protein breakdown is limited.

Whereas the brain and the other glycolytic tissues depend directly upon glucose for their energy, the rest of the organism derives its energy from fat, in the form of either fatty acids or ketone bodies created by the partial oxidation of fatty acids to acetoacetate or β-hydroxybutyrate. Although these tissues, especially muscle, readily utilize glucose in the presence of insulin in the nonfasting state or with vigorous exercise or anoxia, they abandon glucose metabolism during starvation, thus helping to conserve body protein.

The liver derives its energy from fatty acid oxidation in two stages: The partial oxidation of fatty acids to acetyl coenzyme A (acetyl CoA), and the terminal combustion of the acetate in the tricarboxylic acid cycle (Krebs cycle). About one-third of the total energy in fat is ordinarily derived from the first stage, but in starvation ketosis the first stage provides the major portion of the liver's energy, since the function of the tricarboxylic acid cycle is diminished and acetyl CoA is disposed of in the circulation as

acetoacetate and β-hydroxybutyrate. Ketogenesis generally, though not always, parallels the rate of gluconeogenesis.

In prolonged fasting rather profound changes in metabolism occur, as shown in Table 1-6 and in Fig. 1-28. It is apparent that liver and muscle glycogen cannot continue to supply glucose at all, since the total body store is only 225 Gm and this would be exhausted in a few days. Furthermore, body protein cannot continue to be converted to glucose at the rate of 75 Gm a day, since in about a month this would deplete the total body protein beyond the level which would permit survival. It thus becomes apparent that diminished utilization of glucose and sparing of body protein is essential for the survival of prolonged starvation.

If the brain is the one organ which needs glucose normally, it must either reduce its fuel consumption or substi-

NITROGEN METABOLISM FOLLOWING THERMAL INJURY

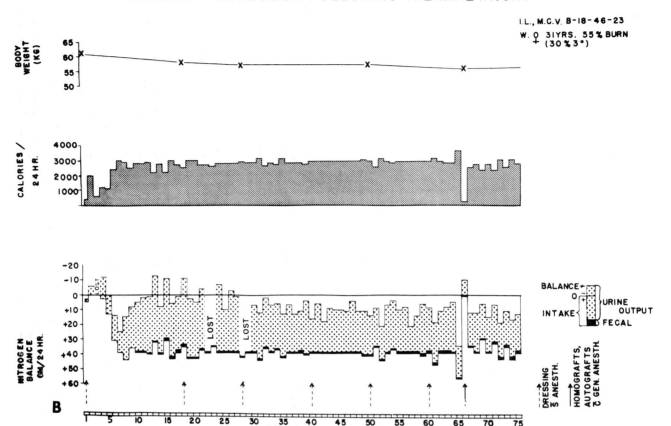

Fig. 1-26. Continued.

tute another fuel, or the body must make glucose directly from fatty acids, which it cannot do, since the enzymes required for this are not found in animals.

Owen and coworkers found that on prolonged fasting the ketone bodies, acetoacetate and β-hydroxybutyrate, replaced glucose as the predominant fuel for brain metabolism. This change of fuels by the brain did not produce any deficits in the function of the brain or change in the electroencephalogram. The amount of glucose completely utilized by the brain drops from 144 Gm to 30 Gm a day, 14 of the 44 Gm presented to the brain being recycled through the Cori cycle. The blood ketones are capable of being utilized by the brain in part because they, like glucose, are water-soluble and readily penetrate the blood-brain barrier.

The body not only manages to conserve protein, but also maintains almost normal levels of blood glucose, glycerol, amino acids, lactate, and pyruvate. The blood levels of free fatty acids and ketones are of course markedly increased.

One other striking change that occurs in prolonged fasting is a shift from the liver to the kidney of gluconeogenesis from protein sources. The liver continues to make glucose by recycling lactate and pyruvate, and it also continues gluconeogenesis from glycerol. Almost all of the gluconeogenesis from amino acids, however, takes place in the kidney, where there is a stoichiometric relation between ammoniogenesis and gluconeogenesis. The ammoniogenesis is required to maintain acid homoeostasis by titrating the ketone acids lost in the urine.

While there is only a slight change in concentration of total amino acids during starvation, there are striking changes in the values for individual amino acids. Glycine increases during starvation; valine, leucine, and isoleucine increase briefly and then decrease; arginine falls progressively; and lysine does not change at all. Alanine falls progressively, decreasing to less than one-third of the fed level. Alanine is the principal amino acid utilized by the liver for gluconeogenesis, and it is the decrease of alanine during fasting which limits gluconeogenesis in the liver.

Table 1-6. GLUCOSE AVAILABLE IN LATE STARVATION STATE IN A 70-kg MAN

Origin	Amount of glucose, Gm/24 hr
New glucose (gluconeogenesis):	
Fat (glycerol)	18
Protein	12
Stored or recycled glucose:	
Glycogen	0
Recycled glucose	50
Total	80

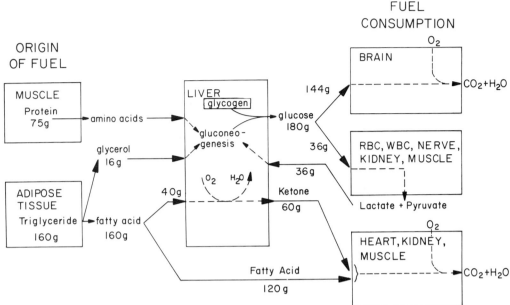

FASTING MAN
(24 hours, basal : –1800 calories)

Fig. 1-27. Scheme of fuel metabolism in a normal, fasted man. The two primary fuel sources are muscle protein and fat. The brain oxidizes glucose completely, the glycolyzers break down glucose by anaerobic metabolism into lactate and pyruvate, which are remade in the liver into glucose, and the rest of the body burns fatty acids and ketones. (*Adapted from G. F. Cahill, N Engl J Med, 282:668, 1970.*)

Alanine comes from muscle protein and also may be synthesized from pyruvate, as shown in Fig. 1-29.

ROLE OF THE HORMONES IN ALTERED METABOLISM OF STARVATION

The presence of cortisol is essential for a normal rate of gluconeogenesis, and this hormone participates in the hyperglycemia which occurs in the early posttraumatic period. The administration of large doses of cortisol analogues to fasting subjects did not result in an increased rate of nitrogen excretion, however.

GH likewise fails to increase daily nitrogen excretion in fasting subjects but elevates the level of insulin and blood glucose. Dwarfs having a congenital lack of growth hormones were found to be capable of mobilizing fatty acids and excreting nitrogen at rates similar to those observed in normal persons of the same size.

There is a marked rise in circulating glucagon in patients fasting for 2 or 3 days. Glucagon not only increases glycogenolysis in the liver but also increases gluconeogenesis, directly opposing insulin in this regard. Glucagon appears to have a role in regulating the level of circulating amino acids. The near absence of glucagon in totally pancreatectomized subjects may be the reason that such patients require less insulin to affect homeostasis than do most severely ill diabetics.

Insulin has at least two important effects on the regulation of fuel sources: it increases the rate of synthesis of triglycerides in adipose tissue, in which it opposes the catecholamines, ACTH, and glucagon; and it increases amino acid uptake by muscle and protein synthesis in which it appears to be opposed by glucagon and cortisol. Insulin, therefore, not only impedes fatty acid release but impedes amino acid release from muscle as well.

The hypothalamus controls all the hormones regulating glucose production, including glucagon and insulin. In addition, it contains an appetite-satiety center which is presumably responsive to the blood glucose level, and has been said by Conway et al. to regulate lipolysis in response to changes in glucose levels.

Gamble demonstrated many years ago that small amounts of administered glucose were capable of decreasing the excretion of nitrogen in the urine; this concept has recently been challenged by Blackburn et al. The classic concept is to maintain that the daily administration of 100 Gm of glucose given intravenously spares the proteolysis of about 50 Gm of protein. This effect presumably results from the increased secretion of insulin brought about by the elevated glucose level which in turn inhibits muscle proteolysis. The need for gluconeogenesis by the liver is no longer present, since the administered glucose takes care of the brain's need. Ketogenesis also ceases, and the rest of the body continues to utilize free fatty acids.

Clearly it is important to spare protein breakdown in the starved injured patient, since protein breakdown leads to muscle wasting, ineffective coughing, pneumonia, impaired wound repair, poor resistance to infection, and diminished synthesis of enzymes and plasma proteins. Blackburn et al. contend that they were unable to achieve nitrogen balance in fasting patients given an amino acid solution intravenously in combination with 100 Gm of glucose every 24 hours whereas they were able to achieve

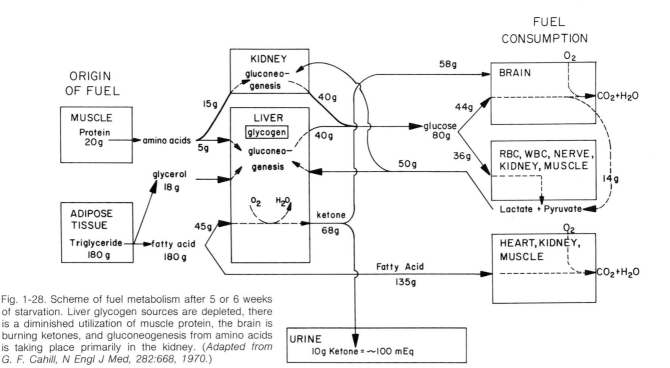

Fig. 1-28. Scheme of fuel metabolism after 5 or 6 weeks of starvation. Liver glycogen sources are depleted, there is a diminished utilization of muscle protein, the brain is burning ketones, and gluconeogenesis from amino acids is taking place primarily in the kidney. (*Adapted from G. F. Cahill, N Engl J Med, 282:668, 1970.*)

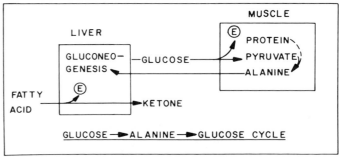

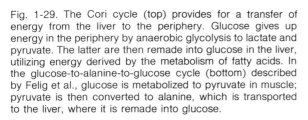

Fig. 1-29. The Cori cycle (top) provides for a transfer of energy from the liver to the periphery. Glucose gives up energy in the periphery by anaerobic glycolysis to lactate and pyruvate. The latter are then remade into glucose in the liver, utilizing energy derived by the metabolism of fatty acids. In the glucose-to-alanine-to-glucose cycle (bottom) described by Felig et al., glucose is metabolized to pyruvate in muscle; pyruvate is then converted to alanine, which is transported to the liver, where it is remade into glucose.

nitrogen balance in those patients given the same amount of amino acids without any added glucose. Their explanation is that the administration of glucose increases the output of insulin, which in turn exerts an antilipolytic effect which decreases the mobilization of fatty acids and makes it necessary to continue using muscle protein as a source of energy. By giving protein without glucose the insulin level remained low, and there was an increased mobilization of body fat with an associated ketosis, thus leading to a use of body fat as the energy source and sparing protein. Positive nitrogen balance could be achieved by administering 90 Gm of amino acid/day without any other caloric source. Although it may be true that small amounts of glucose, even in the presence of protein administration, may not lead to optimal utilization of body fat as an energy source, it is certainly true that the administration of hyperalimentation mixtures containing protein hydrolysates or amino acids in conjunction with an adequate caloric intake supplied by hypertonic glucose provides optimal protein sparing and improves wound healing and resistance to infection.

Metabolic Effects of Injury

The effects of trauma and sepsis on body metabolism are summarized in Table 1-7 and Fig. 1-30. In contrast to starvation, injury produces (1) hyperglycemia, unless the injury is overwhelming and fatal; (2) marked fatty acid mobilization and elevation of plasma free fatty acids; (3) a striking catabolism of muscle protein beyond that needed as a source for energy, in contrast to late starvation, where protein conservation is seen; (4) an increase in the synthesis of urea and the so-called "acute-phase reactants" (AP reactants) (Table 1-8); and (5) an increased extracellular osmolality.

Oxygen consumption is not increased in ordinary elective operations, but it is increased by as much as 25 percent after multiple fractures, and with severe sepsis may increase by 50 percent. Burns increase oxygen consumption by as much as 100 percent, partly because of sepsis and partly because of the break in the epidermis producing evaporative water loss which requires enormous expenditures of energy.

Carbohydrate Metabolism

The early elevation of blood glucose level after most types of injury is brought about primarily by the catecholamines and to a lesser extent by glucagon, cortisol, and growth hormone. There is an initial increase in hepatic glycogenolysis and an inhibition of insulin production. The elevated blood levels are also a consequence of enhancement of gluconeogenesis, brought about by cortisol and glucagon, and to a lesser extent by the catecholamines and GH. Cortisol also impedes the entry of glycolytic intermediates into the pentose shunt and into the tricarboxylic acid cycle, thus favoring increased release of glucose into blood. The increased plasma fatty acid concentrations also stimu-

Table 1-7. EFFECT OF TRAUMA ON CARBOHYDRATE, FAT, AND PROTEIN METABOLISM

Charge	Cause	Charge	Cause
Carbohydrate: Early hyperglycemia	Increased glycogenolysis produced principally by CA* and to lesser extent by glucagon. Increased gluconeogenesis produced by increased fatty acid level and by 17-OHCS and GH. Insulin inhibition produced by CA, glucagon, 17-OHCS and GH.	Triglycerides: no change	In trauma there is an increased ability to remove excess lipids from bloodstream, thus compensating for increased fat mobilization.
		Rise in β-hydroxybutyrate/acetoacetate ratio blood, liver, kidney, etc., in profound shock or sepsis	Hypoxia.
		Protein: Muscle:	
Hyperglycemia and glucose intolerance during convalescence	Moderate injury: insulin intolerance with decreased ability to oxidize glucose and block of conversion of pyruvate to two-carbon fragments. Severe injury: no change or an increase in rate oxidation glucose, but marked increase in glucose production.	Markedly increased catabolism Decreased protein synthesis	17-OHCS and glucagon promote catabolism muscle proteins to amino acids and inhibit protein synthesis. Starvation also leads to protein breakdown. Some breakdown due direct trauma, wound loss, etc. Protein catabolism above that needed for energy alone supplies carbohydrate intermediates, and is required to maintain level of circulating amino acids.
Hypoglycemia seen in profound shock or sepsis	Glycogen depletion. Utilization of glucose at rate faster than gluconeogenesis can provide it. Defect in gluconeogenesis.		Inhibition of increased insulin secretion. Insulin has an anabolic effect.

Table 1-7. Continued

Charge	Cause	Charge	Cause
Rise in lactate/pyruvate ratio in blood and tissue in profound shock or sepsis	Hypoxia, producing a block in conversion of pyruvate to acetyl CoA, rise in lactic acid level, and progressive tissue deficit of ATP.	Liver and kidney proteins: Increased turnover of protein, but no protein depletion	Increased protein synthesis involves largely "export" proteins like albumin and acute-phase (AP) reactants but probably involves intrinsic protein as well.
Fat: Fatty acid mobilization Elevated FFA plasma	CA and glucagon increase cyclic AMP in fat, thus increasing activity of lipolytic enzyme which hydrolyzes triglyceride to fatty acids and glycerol. GH and 17-OHCS have similar but much weaker effect. Insulin especially, and prostaglandins and metabolites (glucose, lactate, pyruvate, ketone bodies) to a lesser extent have opposite effect.		Whereas in starvation there may be a decrease in liver and kidney protein, in injury the 17-OHCS produces a preferential increase in catabolism of muscle protein, which leads to an increased synthesis of protein in liver and kidney—mainly through alanine release from muscle protein.
Elevation liver ketones	Moderate injury: FFA mobilization produces an increase in hepatic fatty acid oxidation to ketones. Glucagon stimulates this. Severe injury: Inhibition of liver citrate synthase due to ischemia, prevents acetyl CoA from entering tricarboxylic acid cycle, thus diverting it to synthesis of ketone bodies.	Plasma proteins: Increased catabolism Probably increased synthesis of albumin as well, but masked by catabolism γ-Globulin increased	Plasma proteins participate in protein catabolism seen in trauma. Liver increases synthesis of "export" proteins. γ-globulin increased by antibody production in response to sepsis.
Blood ketones unchanged or slightly elevated	Ketone metabolism unimpaired, some excess excreted urine.	Plasma amino acids: Decreased somewhat as gluconeogenesis uses up substrates; subsequently total kept fairly constant, although some glucogenic amino acids (such as alanine) tend to fail while lysine does not change at all and glycine rises	Exact mechanism unknown, though balance between insulin (which decreases amino acid release from muscle and decreases glucaneogenesis) and glucagon and 17-OHCS (which increase amino acid release from muscle and increase gluconeogenesis) plays an important regulatory role. If amino acids are infused at rates in excess of energy needs, the excess will be converted to fat and the nitrogen excreted in the urine, while the plasma level remains constant.
Lipoproteins: cholesterol falls	Cause unknown; related to albumin level; may be due to starvation, or to glucagon.		
		Urea: Urea synthesis greatly increased Urea excretion in urine greatly increased Plasma urea increased due to increased production; further increased if renal failure present	Increased deamination of alanine in liver to provide substrate for increased gluconeogenesis makes nitrogen available to the liver for synthesis into urea.
		AP reactants: Increased synthesis	Reason unknown.

*CA: catecholamines (epinephrine and norepinephrine).
17-OHCS: glucocorticoids (cortisol and corticosterone principally).
GH: growth hormone.
FFA: free fatty acids.

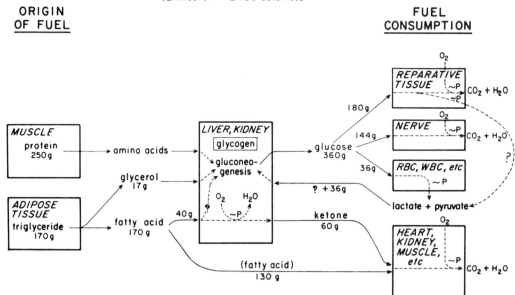

Fig. 1-30. Hypothetic scheme of rates of substrate flow in a traumatized individual excreting 40 Gm of nitrogen/day. Presumably reparative tissues are glucose utilizers, but the amount of glucose terminally combusted to carbon dioxide and that metabolized to lactate would depend both on the maturity of the tissue (presence of mitochondria) and on adequate perfusion and oxygenation. Fat still provides the bulk of the calories. (*From G. F. Cahill et al., in C. L. Fox, Jr., and G. G. Nahas [eds.]: "Body Fluid Replacement in the Surgical Patient," p. 286, Grune & Stratton, Inc., New York, 1970.*)

late gluconeogenesis, and the presence of available substrate, especially alanine, provides an additional stimulus to this reaction.

The presence of hyperglycemia provides a ready source of energy to the brain and thus may be important to early survival. Starvation reduces the ability of the body to tolerate shock. The administration of glucose prolongs survival after shock, as shown by Drucker and his colleagues in hypovolemic dogs and Berk and his associates in endotoxin shock. McNamara and his colleagues demonstrated that patients in hypovolemic shock who were resuscitated in the usual manner and at the same time received either 50% glucose, 25% mannitol, or 3% saline solution in equal total osmolar doses had a much greater increase in blood pressure and pulse pressure when they received glucose than with either of the other two agents. However, because of the different concentrations of the solutions, they may have induced different rates of leakage of protein into the interstitium. It appears quite possible that, as suggested by Järhult and by ourselves, the principal homeostatic significance of increased plasma glucose may be the resulting osmotic transfer of fluids, leading to restitution of blood volume.

While hemorrhagic shock has been found by some workers to be associated both with hyperglycemia and an

Table 1-8. ACUTE-PHASE (AP) REACTANTS

Haptoglobin
Fibrinogen
Ceruloplasmin
Seromucoid fraction
C-reactive protein
α_2-AP globulin
α_1-Acid glycoprotein
α_1-Antitrypsin

elevated insulin level, others have claimed that insulin levels are low. All agree, however, that there are elevated levels of anti-insulin hormones and that there is both a glucose intolerance and insulin resistance after injury.

During the recovery phase there continues to be a diabeticlike glucose tolerance curve which is more marked after severe injury. There is an insulin intolerance and a decrease in the ability to oxidize glucose. Drucker has demonstrated a partial block in the metabolic conversion of pyruvate to two-carbon fragments.

In profound shock or sepsis hypoglycemia may be present. This is due to depletion of glycogen stores and the utilization of glucose at a rate faster than gluconeogenesis can provide it. It is also due to a defect in gluconeogenesis. There may be a rise in the lactate/pyruvate ratio due to hypoxia, which produces a block in the conversion of pyruvate to acetyl CoA, a rise in the lactic acid level, and a progressive tissue deficit of adenosine triphosphate (ATP).

Fat Metabolism

Fat is the main energy source in trauma, as in starvation. The catecholamines, glucagon, ACTH, and GH increase cyclic AMP in fat, thus increasing the activity of the lipolytic enzyme which hydrolyzes triglyceride to fatty acid and glycerol. Lipolysis induced by these hormones requires the presence of cortisol.

The glycerol provides substrate for gluconeogenesis. The fatty acids are burned in the liver to supply energy for gluconeogenesis, and in the periphery to supply energy directly.

Liver ketone levels are elevated as a result of the increase in free fatty acids and the influence of glucagon. In very severe injury the level of ketones is further increased because of inhibition of liver citrate synthase, which prevents acetyl CoA from entering the tricarboxylic acid cycle, thus diverting it to the synthesis of ketone bodies.

In profound shock and sepsis there is a rise in the ratio of β-hydoxybutyrate to acetoacetate in blood, liver, kidney and other tissues as a consequence of hypoxia. As indicated above, the ketone bodies may provide an important source of energy to the brain. They may also contribute to the rise in extracellular osmolality.

Protein Metabolism

The daily intake of protein for a healthy young adult is usually about 80 to 120 Gm, or 13 to 20 Gm of nitrogen. Of this quantity of nitrogen about 2 to 3 Gm/day is lost in the stool and 11 to 17 Gm in the urine. Urinary nitrogen excretion increases greatly after injury, rising to as much as 30 to 50 Gm/day following severe trauma. This is nearly all in the form of urea nitrogen. In the patient with anuria or one whose kidneys have been removed preparatory to transplantation, operative trauma produces a very rapid rise in blood urea nitrogen (BUN) in comparison to that seen between dialyses in the nontraumatized state (Fig. 1-31).

The increase in nitrogen excretion begins shortly after injury, reaches a peak about the first week, and may continue for 3 to 7 weeks. In elective operative procedures the negative nitrogen balance is rapidly reversed, but in the burned patient the negative balance may be prolonged for a very considerable period of time. During this time the patient may lose 50 to 75 lb of weight. In the early postinjury period protein may be lost from the body surface if there is a large open or burned area, into the peritoneal cavity if there is peritonitis or ascites, into edema fluid if there is an extensive crush injury or burn, in tissue slough and necrotic muscle, and into areas where blood has been sequestered, or lost to the body economy.

The source of the great urinary protein loss is still not entirely certain. In studies of burned rats Levenson and his colleagues have demonstrated that the incorporation of labeled nitrogen in tissue protein was equal to, or greater than, that seen in the control animals, which means that they were synthesizing protein at the same time that they were losing large quantities of nitrogen in the urine. Therefore simple catabolism of body protein was not the only source for urinary nitrogen loss.

In a subsequent series of experiments it was found that the protein content of the liver and other active organs changed very little after burns whereas the muscle, which had a rather slow turnover rate, lost enough protein to

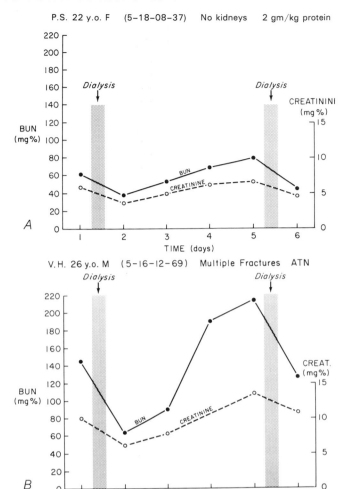

Fig. 1-31. Comparison of dialysis in patients with minimal and severe catabolism. *A.* Chronic dialysis in an anephric patient with very little catabolism, taking 2 Gm of protein/kg body weight daily. Note the slow rise in BUN and creatinine levels between dialyses despite high protein intakes. *B.* Dialysis in a patient with multiple fractures and acute tubular necrosis on no protein intake. Note the rapid rise in BUN and creatinine levels associated with marked catabolism. The patient recovered completely.

account for most of the urinary nitrogen loss. These experiments suggested that the integrity of the vital organs was maintained at the expense of skeletal muscle. Munro and Chalmers found that in rats fed on a protein-free diet until they were depleted negative nitrogen balance failed to develop after injury, and they hypothesized that the protein lost after injury was storage protein. If storage protein is largely muscle protein, this would account for the far greater protein loss seen in muscular young men than in women or debilitated elderly patients (see Fig. 1-26). It has also been noted by Browne and Schenker and by Howard et al. that if the patient has repeated injuries in close succession, the protein loss is less with each succeeding injury, perhaps because the storage protein has been wiped out by the previous trauma (Fig. 1-32). The striking muscle protein catabolism seen in trauma is far in excess of that

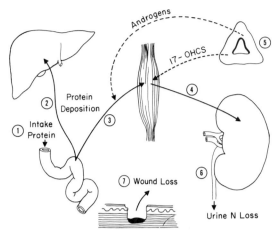

Fig. 1-32. Protein storage and catabolism. Protein may be preferentially deposited in the liver while it is being catabolized from muscle stores. Its catabolism is increased by glucocorticoids and decreased by insulin and adrenal androgens.

needed to supply energy. The magnitude of this response is related to the magnitude of the injury.

Protein contribution to the normal caloric requirement is in the range of 12 to 15 percent of the total, while Duke observed that this remained approximately 15 percent in most surgical conditions and did not rise much above 20 percent even with major increases in nitrogen excretion after extensive injury. Thus the major weight loss seen after surgery is not primarily the result of protein breakdown as a means of obtaining extra fuel. Although it has been claimed by Blackburn et al. that injury inhibits the mobilization and oxidation of fat from adipose tissue as a fuel source, Carlson and other investigators have shown that free fatty acids are readily mobilized in injury. They have even raised the question of whether excessive mobilization of fatty acids may sometimes occur.

The protein loss after injury does not result from impaired protein synthesis. Furthermore the protein loss occurs primarily from muscle, there being no decrease in the protein content of the liver and kidneys. Increased cortisol and glucagon and decreased insulin all limit the ability of muscle to take up amino acids. As catabolism of muscle continues, while anabolism is limited by these hormonal changes, there is a net release of amino acids from muscle cells. As mentioned earlier, alanine is the principal amino acid released from muscle, and this amino acid is the principal gluconeogenic precursor in the liver. Felig et al. have suggested that a cycle similar to the Cori cycle of glucose to lactate to glucose may be achieved through glucose to alanine to glucose. This cycle then provides a source for gluconeogenesis. Branched-chain amino acids are also lost from muscle, and their plasma concentration may increase for 2 hours to weeks after trauma. Increased concentrations of amino acids thus may contribute to the hyperosmolality of trauma.

There is some evidence that the increased nitrogen metabolism may be related to the need for carbohydrate intermediates via gluconeogenesis, rather than to the total energy needs of the body as indicated by its oxygen con-

sumption. This evidence as summarized by Kinney et al. is as follows: (1) the caloric contribution of protein to the fuel mixture of normal and injured man is rather small; (2) two-carbon fragments are readily available from adipose tissue and are utilized as the major energy source in most tissues after injury; (3) the body has a continuous requirement for carbohydrate intermediates for synthetic purposes, for which deamination of amino acids is the primary endogenous source; and (4) fatty acids cannot directly yield a net gain of carbohydrate intermediates, glucose, or glycogen.

Carbohydrate intermediates are used for the synthesis of nonessential amino acids, glycogen, glucose, and tricarboxylic acid cycle intermediates. As a by-product of the increased gluconeogenesis of trauma, there is an increased synthesis of urea, which is made from nitrogen stripped from alanine and other glucogenic amino acids as their carbon remains are used in the formation of glucose (Fig. 1-31).

The plasma proteins undergo increased catabolism, but there is an increased synthesis of albumin as well. γ-Globulin is likewise increased, presumably by antibody production against microorganisms. The total plasma amino acids decrease somewhat, but individual amino acids may increase or decrease depending on their utility as gluconeogenic substrates.

Acute-phase-reactant proteins (AP reactants) (Table 1-8) are those protein components of plasma whose concentration is significantly increased in the acute phase of trauma or inflammation. All these contain 5 to 20 percent carbohydrate in the molecule, and all are synthesized exclusively in the liver. An article by Koj summarizes our current knowledge of them.

Although most of the AP reactants are present normally and show an increased response to trauma, at least two of them, C-reactive protein in man and rabbit and α₂-AP globulin in the rat, do not appear to be present in healthy animals but appear only after injury. In some forms of trauma there may be an increase in the rate of synthesis of albumin as well as AP reactants, but because in severe trauma there is a marked increase in catabolism of albumin, the increased synthesis is not apparent. Increased synthesis of albumin is stimulated by cortisol and by growth hormone. However, this effect is not apparent for approximately 2 days, even after simple hemorrhage.

The AP-reactant glycoproteins appear at different time intervals after injury. C-reactive protein in man and α₂-AP globulin in rats respond most promptly, appearing in plasma soon after injury, while haptoglobin and fibrinogen appear 4 to 6 hours after, and seromucoid and ceruloplasmin reach maximal value several days after injury. The response of the various AP reactants to repeated injuries or to adrenalectomy or the administration of corticosteroids is very variable. Some of the AP reactants are inhibited and others are stimulated by adrenalectomy.

Presumably the AP reactants are of some benefit to the injured organism. Fibrinogen apparently improves clotting, and haptoglobins may help to prevent damage to the kidneys by binding hemoglobin released as a consequence of the injury. Other AP reactants may bind toxic products or inactivate lyzosomal enzymes whose release triggers production of toxins.

Restitution of Blood Volume

The restitution of blood volume in hypovolemia occurs in two major phases. The first phase is initiated by the fall in capillary pressure associated with hypotension and augmented by sympathetically mediated arteriolar vasoconstriction. In the presence of decreased capillary pressure, essentially protein-free fluid moves from the interstitium to the capillaries, leading to restitution of 20 to 50 percent of the lost volume. However, this fluid transfer leads to a fall in interstitial pressure and in capillary oncotic pressure, leading to the development of a pseudosteady state in which further restitution of blood volume is impossible. As shown first by Cope and Litwin, further restitution of blood volume depends upon restitution of plasma protein, primarily albumin. This second phase of blood volume restitution cannot depend upon the synthesis of new albumin, for, as indicated above, this does not occur for at least 2 days. Albumin loss from the circulation may be retarded in the presence of vasoconstriction, particularly of the splanchnic circulation, but this cannot account entirely for protein restitution. Thus the major source of albumin for blood volume restitution in the second phase must be the interstitium itself. The movement of protein from the interstitium to the circulation, either up the lymphatics or across the semipermeable capillary membranes, depends almost entirely upon interstitial pressure. Since the compliance of the interstitium is fixed, interstitial pressure can be increased only by the movement of fluid into the interstitium, primarily from cells. The movement of fluid between cells and interstitium is controlled exclusively by the osmotic gradient across the cell membrane. Because of this fact, the increased extracellular osmolality which occurs in the presence of injury and hypovolemia is critical for the second phase of blood volume restitution. As indicated above, the extracellular osmolality increases as a result of various metabolic effects of the hormones that are increased after injury. It depends critically upon increased concentrations of cortisol, but preliminary evidence has implicated glucagon, epinephrine, and growth hormone in this response as well. Both the extent and the duration of increased osmolality are functions of the extent of hypovolemia or injury, as shown by Boyd and Mansberger and by ourselves. The role of extracellular hyperosmolality and the ensuing second phase of restitution of blood volume appears critical in cardiovascular stabilization after injury. Its absence may account at least in part for the peculiar sensitivity to injury of patients with adrenal insufficiency. Of course, once hormonal changes have been initiated, the effects of the hormones will not cease merely because hormonal secretion is turned off by replacement of blood volume. Thus, once the metabolic effects of injury have begun, therapeutic or endogenous restitution of blood volume may lessen the severity of the metabolic consequences but cannot prevent them. In one sense, however, the protein loss, fat mobilization, and hypoglycemia and carbohydrate depletion of injury may be viewed as late

metabolic consequences of an initial attempt by the body to restore blood volume through this second phase of restitution. In this phase, the neuroendocrine response to injury induces a set of metabolic effects that serve to increase extracellular osmolality. Fluid then shifts from cells to interstitium, increasing interstitial pressure and thus leading directly to movement of fluid and protein into the vascular compartment.

Wound Healing

Wound healing is discussed in detail in Chap. 8. Many factors affect wound healing, chief among them being local factors of hematoma, dehiscence, infection, edema, blood supply, location, and extent. The administration of antibiotics can improve wound healing by decreasing sepsis, and the correction of clotting defects can promote healing by preventing hemorrhage in the wound. Various systemic metabolic factors are involved in wound healing.

Ascorbic acid is essential for collagen synthesis, and thus plays an important role in the healing of wounds. Cognizance is customarily taken of this by the intravenous administration of large doses of ascorbic acid after operation. It has been demonstrated by Levenson and his associates that injuries are accompanied by a decrease in plasma ascorbic acid concentration and by similar changes in thiamine and nicotinamide. This is associated with a decrease in urinary excretion of these substances. A decrease in the urinary excretion of riboflavin is also seen. It was found that the decrease in plasma ascorbic acid constituted a true physiologic scurvy and that this could be reversed by the administration of large doses of ascorbic acid, 500 to 2,000 mg daily. Sullivan and Eisenstein have noted ascorbic acid depletion during hemodialysis corrected by adding ascorbate to the dialysate concentrate.

There are considerable recent data on the effects of the fat-soluble vitamins on wound healing. Certain types of trauma are accompanied by a decrease in blood and hepatic concentrations of vitamin A. Chernov et al. reported that vitamin A depletion following thermal injury is associated with stress ulcers. Restoration of serum vitamin A levels markedly reduced the risk of ulceration. Hutcher et al. showed that vitamin A reduced the incidence of steroid-induced gastric ulcers. Collagen synthesis and wound healing are suppressed by corticosteroids, but collagen synthesis and tensile strength can be returned to normal by vitamin A administration, as shown by Hunt and his colleagues, and by Stein and Keiser. When steroids are used for immunosuppression, it was shown by Cohen and Cohen that vitamin A must be used with caution because it exerts an adjuvant-like effect and antagonizes steroid-induced immunosuppression.

It may be necessary to administer vitamin K in prolonged starvation, mild liver damage, biliary fistulas, or other circumstances in which intestinal absorption of this vitamin is chronically reduced. In the absence of preexisting vitamin K deficiency its acute depletion in trauma is not generally a problem. The same may be said for vitamin D, which is stored in the body for long periods of time.

Although the role of trace metals in wound repair and

metabolism awaits clearer definition, there is increasing evidence that zinc and copper are essential for normal healing. Hsu and Hsu have shown that zinc is necessary for both epithelialization and collagen synthesis. Cohen et al. have recently noted that zinc-depleted burned patients have decreased taste acuity and an associated anorexia, which is corrected by zinc repletion. While zinc depletion interferes with wound healing, this process cannot be speeded up by giving zinc to individuals with normal levels.

Abnormal wound healing in copper deficiency is detailed in Carnes' review. Copper is essential for lysyl oxidase, the enzyme that cross-links collagen. Drugs such as D-penicillamine which bind copper and block aldehyde cross-link sites will subsequently diminish collage cross linking and inhibit wound healing. They may be clinically useful in the treatment of diseases characterized by overabundant collagen deposition, such as cirrhosis, esophageal stricture, or keloids. D-Penicillamine has been clinically used by Harris and Sjoerdama for patients with scleroderma to inhibit skin collagen deposition.

Although various substances have been claimed to accelerate normal wound healing, there are no scientific data to show that cartilage extracts, vitamins, or metals accelerate healing in a normal healing wound.

The oxygen tension of the healing wound is said by Hunt and others to be directly related to the rate of healing. In the wound the oxygen reaches the area of injury by diffusion, and as the blood P_{O_2} is increased by breathing oxygen, the oxygen available in the wound is greater, and wound healing is accelerated. This is said to be because increases in wound P_{O_2} levels have three effects: (1) to increase the rate at which fibroblasts reproduce, (2) to increase the rate at which fibroblasts synthesize collagen, and (3) to increase the rate at which epithelial cells reproduce.

The studies of wound oxygen concentrations seem to give validity to the use of hyperbaric oxygen in the treatment of chronically unhealed wounds, supporting the claims that it improves wound healing.

Therapeutic Considerations

NUTRITIONAL SUPPLEMENTATION

The parenteral nutritional supplementation of the surgical patient has for many years included glucose solutions and blood and blood products, with abortive attempts to introduce amino acids intravenously to produce a positive nitrogen balance, and fat solutions to provide concentrated calories. In recent years, with the advent of parenteral "hyperalimentation" utilizing concentrated glucose and amino acid solutions introduced through an intraatrial catheter via the subclavian vein, there has been a plethora of papers devoted to the advantages and hazards of such therapy. Intravenous fat (Intralipid) was developed in Sweden and has received extensive experimental trial in this country. It seems to be a useful source of calories and of essential fatty acids.

Greenstein and his colleagues in 1960 produced a nutri-

tionally complete water-soluble liquid diet which when administered orally to rats maintained them for long periods without any detectable deficiencies. The diet contained 18 crystalline amino acids (9 essential and 9 nonessential), the water-soluble vitamins, the trace metals (Mg, Fe, Mn, Cu, Co, Zn) Na, K, Ca, ethyl linoleate, and sometimes vitamins A and D. Diets which did not include a linoleic acid source produced signs of essential fatty acid deficiency (scaling of skin, failure to grow well, occasionally cachexia).

Terry and his colleagues in 1948 first demonstrated that it was possible to maintain dogs for prolonged periods of time solely on oral glucose and parenteral plasma. The plasma proteins contributed to body tissue protein and did not produce a urinary nitrogen loss, but in fact decreased the urinary nitrogen loss seen in fasting. Total parenteral alimentation in dogs was described by Meng and Early in 1949. Allen et al. in 1956 used intravenously given plasma as the only protein source for littermate puppies and were able to obtain growth rates equivalent to those seen when the same amount of protein was given orally. Stemmer et al. republished these results 10 years later.

To Dudrick and his colleagues belongs the credit for pushing studies on parenteral hyperalimentation with amino acid and concentrated carbohydrate mixtures. In 1967–1968 these investigators demonstrated that it was possible to achieve normal growth in puppies supported entirely by intravenous feedings. The feedings consisted of amino acids, glucose, vitamins, Na, K, Ca, Cl, HPO_4, and trace metals with or without the addition of fat. They also reported 30 patients fed exclusively by vein for 10 to 200 days, using amino acids, 20% glucose, electrolytes, trace metals, and vitamins. Positive nitrogen balance was achieved, and the patients demonstrated better wound healing, weight gain, and increased strength and activity.

It seems clear that parenteral hyperalimentation is unnecessary for short-term surgical problems but is of great value for patients with long-term problems or for malnourished patients prior to surgery. It has also proved useful for putting the bowel at rest in severe diarrheal states such as ulcerative colitis and granulomatous colitis, and for maintaining patients with the short bowel syndrome.

The requirements for total parenteral alimentation solutions are given in Table 1-9. The amino acids may be supplied by any of the solutions shown in Table 1-10.

Table 1-9. REQUIREMENTS FOR PROLONGED INTRAVENOUS TOTAL ALIMENTATION

Essential amino acids
Possibly alanine and some other nonessential
    amino acids
Glucose
Na, K, Ca
Vitamins
Trace metals (Zn, Cu, Cr, Co,
    Mg, Mn, I, Fe)
Cl and HPO_4
Plasma or albumin
Linoleic acid

Table 1-10. AMINO ACID SOURCES FOR
INTRAVENOUS ALIMENTATION

Protein hydrolysates
Crystalline amino acid mixtures
Essential amino acids only
Plasma
Plasmanate
Albumin
Whole blood

Protein hydrolysates differ from mixtures of crystalline amino acids primarily by virtue of their contamination with trace elements and peptides, and (except for Aminosol) their content of phosphate (Table 1-11). The essential amino acids are listed in Table 1-12. The amino acid content of two of the commonly used commercial solutions are shown in Table 1-13, and a composition in which they are often administered is shown in Table 1-14.

Mixtures containing only the essential amino acids are used for patients with uremia or hepatic failure. In 1956 Rose and Dekker showed in rats that urea could be used for synthesis of nonessential amino acids when essential amino acids were supplied in the diet. This led to the clinical use by Giordano and by Giovannetti and Maggiore of similar diets for patients with uremia. The use of a parenteral essential amino acid–hypertonic glucose mixture has been described by Dudrick and his coworkers and others for surgical patients with renal failure and inability to eat. The blood urea nitrogen level falls, or remains stable after dialysis, and hyperphosphatemia, hypocalcemia, and acidosis are spontaneously reversed. Protein synthesis occurs, presumably from the metabolism of urea nitrogen. More recently, Walser and his associates have shown that administration of α-keto analogues of essential amino acids will lead to biosynthesis of those amino acids, in association with falls in plasma urea, ammonia, and glutamine concentrations. Infusion of the keto acids in starving subjects demonstrated a prolonged nitrogen-sparing effect. The possible usefulness of the keto acids after injury has not been evaluated at this time.

In liver failure the administration of protein hydrolysates is contraindicated because of their high ammonia content. Concentrated glucose solutions can be adminis-

Table 1-11. PHOSPHATE CONTENT OF AMINO
ACID SOLUTIONS

Amino acid solution	Percent	Phosphate, mEq/L
Protein hydrolysate:		
Amigen	5	30
CPH	5	14
Hyprotigen	5	25
Aminosol	5	0
Crystalline amino acid:		
Cutter	8	0
Freamine	8.5	0
Freamine-E	5.25	0

Table 1-12. ESSENTIAL AMINO ACIDS

Leucine	Threonine
Valine	Methionine
Lysine	Histidine
Isoleucine	Tryptophan
Phenylalanine	

tered using the techniques of hyperalimentation. Although mixtures containing only essential amino acids can sometimes be used, their effect on hepatic encephalopathy is unpredictable. It is preferable to use albumin, which is capable of directly entering into body protein tissues without deamination or increasing ammonia levels. Furthermore, the albumin exerts an oncotic force which helps to mobilize and excrete ascitic and edema fluid.

There are various well-known complications that occur with intravenous hyperalimentation. These can be divided into catheter problems—which include pneumothorax, sepsis, subclavian artery injury, or air or fat embolization—and metabolic problems. Chief among the metabolic problems is hyperglycemic, hyperosmolar dehydration usually secondary to too rapid administration, to too concentrated glucose solutions, to latent diabetes, or to administration during a state of glucose intolerance such as one sees soon after severe trauma or during continued sepsis. Reactive hypoglycemia also can be seen if the fluid is suddenly stopped, particularly if insulin has been used.

Table 1-13. AMINO ACID CONTENT OF TWO
COMMONLY USED PARENTERAL
AMINO ACID SOLUTIONS

Amigen (casein hydrolysate)

Essential	Nonessential
Leucine	Glutamic acid
Valine	Proline
Lysine	Serine
Isoleucine	Aspartic acid
Phenylalanine	Alanine
Threonine	Arginine
Methionine	Tyrosine
Histidine	Hydroxyproline
Tryptophan	Glycine
	Cystine

Freamine (synthetic amino acids)

Essential	Nonessential
Leucine	Alanine
Valine	Arginine
Lysine	Proline
Isoleucine	Serine
Phenylalanine	Cysteine
Threonine	Glycine
Methionine	
Histidine	
Tryptophan	

Table 1-14. COMPOSITION OF AMINO ACID–
SUGAR SOLUTIONS COMMONLY
ADMINISTERED

Amigen, 800 (5% Amigen; 12.5% fructose, 2.4% alcohol)

Protein, Gm	37.4
Nitrogen, Gm	5.54
Calories	800
Na, mEq	35
K, mEq	19
Ca, mEq	5
Mg, mEq	2
Cl, mEq	20
HPO₄, mEq	30

Freamine

Dextrose, Gm	250
Nitrogen, Gm	4.17
Calories	900
Na, mEq	23.6
K, mEq	40
Mg, mEq	5
Cl, mEq	35
Acetate, mEq	52
ZnSO₄, mEq	2.5

Five other metabolic complications are seen occasionally with long-term hyperalimentation. The first of these is an excessive plasma level of amino acids beyond that which the body can metabolize. This produces impairment of brain function, and stimulation of insulin secretion. The effect of excess aminoacidemia can be ameliorated in part by the concomitant administration of large amounts of carbohydrate.

The second complication is a metabolic hyperchloremic acidosis produced only by the synthetic amino acid mixtures. Heird and his colleagues ascribe this to the catabolism of positively charged amino acids. This problem is not seen with the hydrolysates because they have sufficient negatively charged amino acids and peptides to offset the hydrogen ion release by the cationic amino acids.

The third complication is hypophosphatemia, which occurs when fibrin hydrolysates or crystalline amino acids are used without added phosphate (Table 1-11). This can be corrected by adding Ca and P to the solutions.

The fourth complication is deficiency of essential fatty acids. Fatty acid deficiency was first described in animals by Burr and Burr in 1929. Pensler and his colleagues described the first clinical case in 1971. The essential defect

Table 1-15. ESSENTIAL FATTY ACID
DEFICIENCY

Fall in:
  Linoleic
  Arachidonic
  8,11,14-Eicosatetraenaic
Rise in:
  Palmitoleic
  Oleic
  5,8,11-Eicosatetraenoic

is a decrease in plasma linoleic, arachidonic, and linolenic acids, with an increase in oleic, palmitoleic, and 5,8,11-eicosatetraenoic acids. It is characterized clinically by scaly skin, itching, poor wound healing, weakness, lethargy, and thrombocytopenia. The thrombocytopenia appears to be due to a failure of separation of megakaryocyte buds.

Linoleic acid is the key essential acid, since arachidonic acid can be synthesized from it, and it has not been established whether linolenic acid is essential (Table 1-15). Although it has been recommended that patients on long-term hyperalimentation receive plasma on a weekly basis for its essential fatty acid content, it is doubtful whether this supplies enough linoleic acid to prevent the development of fatty acid deficiency. Intravenous fat in the form of Intralipid will correct the defect, but this substance is still available in this country only on an experimental basis.

The fifth complication is deficiency of trace elements. Although trace elements have often been added to pediatric hyperalimentation mixtures, they are not routinely added to mixtures for adults. The trace elements thought to be important are listed in Table 1-16. The administration of amino acid mixtures without trace elements led to the development of copper deficiency in one of our patients. This was characterized by dryness of the skin, weakness, and anemia, associated with a very low serum copper level. The symptoms were corrected by the intravenous administration of copper. As plasma and plasmanate contain trace elements, the periodic administration of plasma may prevent the development of deficiencies.

Alcohol, a component of some hyperalimentation solutions, probably should not be used. It potentiates ketosis, increases metabolic acidosis, uncouples oxidative phosphorylation (thus increasing oxygen consumption without energy production), depolarizes nerves, and may produce sedation and mild inebriation in children.

Fructose, also a component of some solutions, appears definitely inferior to glucose. It increases uric acid, lactic acid, amino acids, and bilirubin. The latter effect is apparently due to hepatic cell injury by fructose, which also increases the serum glutamic oxaloacetic transaminase (SGOT).

The elements are now available for the production of an ideal parenteral alimentation solution tailored to the individual patient. Long-term home hyperalimentation has

Table 1-16. TRACE METALS PRESENT IN
ENZYMES

Metal	*Enzymes*
Iron	Cytochromes, peroxidases
Copper	Tyrosinase, ascorbic oxidase
Zinc	Peptidase, carbonic anhydrase
Magnesium	Phosphatases, kinases
Maganese	Kinases, peptidases, arginase
Molybdenum	Xanthine oxidase, nitrate reductase
Cobalt	Vitamin B₁₂ coenzyme complexes
Potassium	Pyruvic kinase, β-methyl aspartase

SOURCE: Conn and Stumpf, "Outlines of Biochemistry," 3d ed., p. 233, John Wiley & Sons, Inc., New York, 1972.

been started, and a completely closed portable system has been devised. Provided the use of hyperalimentation solutions is not extended to patients who could do better without them and precautions are taken to avoid the complications, it will provide an exciting and important contribution to the care of the surgical patient.

COMPONENT THERAPY

Component therapy is a term for the intravenous administration of blood components, or substitutes for these components, instead of whole blood in order to create an intravenous mixture that offers some particular advantage over whole blood. To some extent this advantage may simply be that of greater availability, as for example reconstituted blood over fresh blood, but in some circumstances it may actually do a better job.

OXYGEN TRANSPORT. Traumatized patients may develop a shift of the oxygen dissociation curve to the left as a consequence primarily of alkalosis and lowered erythrocyte 2,3-diphosphoglycerate (2,3-DPG) levels. The reduced DPG level interferes with the ability of the red cell to give up its oxygen to the tissues. Old banked blood contains red cells with low 2,3-DPG content, and multiple transfusions of such blood tend to contribute to tissue anoxia. One may improve tissue oxygenation by correcting alkalosis or by providing erythrocytes high in 2,3-DPG content. Experiments have been made with free hemoglobin solutions and with chemical substitutes for hemoglobin.

Frozen erythrocytes are high in 2,3-DPG, in contrast to blood banked in the usual fashion, and have the advantage over fresh whole blood of not containing white cells (which are antigenic) and being far less likely to transmit hepatitis virus.

Free hemoglobin can also be used as an oxygen carrier. Although myoglobin produces renal damage, hemoglobin does not. Hemoglobin contaminated with red cell stroma produces a consumption coagulopathy, and pure hemoglobin produces anticoagulation as a result of reduced plasma factor VIII and factor V activity. Absorption with aluminum hydroxide was shown by Moss and his colleagues to remove the anticoagulant activity.

Fluorocarbons have been under investigation as an oxygen transport system, and there has been a recent symposium published on this subject. Clark and Galan first demonstrated that mice could be given liquid ventilation with an oxygenated fluorocarbon fluid at atmospheric pressure. Modell and his colleagues were able to ventilate dogs for 8 hours on liquid fluorocarbons with survival. Acidosis tends to develop because of poor CO_2 diffusion; however, mechanical hyperventilation produces pulmonary edema, and the chemicals themselves produce alveolitis, atelectasis, perivascular hemorrhage, and other lung changes.

Geyer and his coworkers have been able to replace almost all the erythrocytes in rats with emulsified perfluorochemicals and keep them alive on 50% oxygen for hours. It was found by Sloviter and his colleagues, however, that these substances produced a progressive anoxia and death in most laboratory animals, although frogs and mice could live several days with their erythrocytes re-

placed by circulating fluorocarbons. At least part of the damage caused by the perfluorochemicals is related to the fact that they produce pronounced platelet agglutination and microemboli, not prevented by heparin. Geyer has not confirmed these results and has shown that under some circumstances, increased numbers of platelets enter the circulation during perfusion.

While hemoglobin substitutes are an intriguing possibility, they do not yet seem to be serious contenders with red cells, or even free hemoglobin, for the honor of carrying the oxygen around the body. However, advances in this field are proceeding rapidly, and important progress is to be anticipated.

CLOTTING COMPONENTS. The clinically useful clotting components consist of fresh frozen plasma, cryoprecipitate, concentrates of factors II, VII, IX, X, antihemophilic globulin, platelet packs, and fibrinogen.

Fresh frozen plasma can be used to replenish the factors contributing to the prothrombin time and in bleeding patients in hepatic failure whose prothrombin times are low. It has the advantage over banked blood that it contains some labile factor V, which is characteristically low in liver failure and absent from banked blood, and the disadvantage that it contains no platelets. It is used in plasmapheresis for hepatic coma, where it is combined with the patient's own erythrocytes, and therefore it can be used for patients with rare blood types for whom the acquisition of multiple units of fresh whole blood might be difficult. Fresh frozen plasma is also useful for patients undergoing operations who develop bleeding tendencies secondary to deficiencies of clotting factors.

Cryoprecipitate contains factor VIII and some fibrinogen, while antihemophilic globulin contains only concentrated factor VIII. Both are used for hemophiliacs with factor VIII deficiency for whom replacement is desired.

Preparations containing factors II, VII, IX, and X (Konyne, Proplex) are used to treat Christmas disease.

Platelet packs are used to administer platelets to patients with hypersplenism, thrombocytopenic purpura, massive transfusions, and other deficiency states where thrombocytopenia can be demonstrated to be contributing to the bleeding disorder.

Fibrinogen is the specific therapy for patients with bleeding due to the presence of excessive amounts of fibrinolysin. It may be combined with steroids and EACA (ε-amino caproic acid).

PLASMA SUBSTITUTES. The risk of hepatitis from pooled plasma is so great that most hospitals have stopped using this preparation entirely. There is, of course, a significant risk from single blood or plasma transfusions, too, and for this reason transfusions or plasma infusions should never be given without a specific important indication. Apart from the administration of fresh frozen plasma discussed above, there is almost never a reason to administer plasma.

Ringer's lactate solution is, more or less, plasma without the plasma proteins, i.e., the immunoglobulins (IgG, IgA, IgM), albumin, fibrinogen, and the prothrombin-related clotting factors. The combination of Ringer's lactate solution (sometimes with modifications of the electrolyte content) and albumin makes a very satisfactory plasma substitute. Albumin itself is the therapy of choice in cirrhosis, not only because it replaces a specific loss, provides oncotic pull, and helps to promote diuresis, but also because its amino acids can enter muscle protein without deamination to create toxic nitrogen fragments. Furthermore hepatitis is not transmitted by albumin preparations.

Plasmanate is plasma with the clotting factors removed. It is made up as 5% protein in saline solution, and contains 88% albumin and 12% globulins. It is nearly free of hepatitis transmission.

The administration of fibrinogen to traumatized patients is seldom necessary, because there is an increased hepatic synthesis of fibrinogen in response to injury. It may be necessary, however, in patients with increased fibrinolysin.

ALIMENTATION MIXTURES. Special alimentation mixtures, discussed earlier in this chapter, offer a variety of combinations to fit the circumstances. Apart from hyperalimentation in severe, sustained, or septic trauma, the single most dramatic effect is that of essential amino acid mixtures in renal failure. This type of therapy makes possible the administration of amino acids which are not metabolized to release nitrogen but which are used in muscle synthesis—thus not contributing to urea formation—and in the presence of hypertonic glucose, even inducing the body to burn urea.

COMPONENT BLOOD. Frozen red cells are at present the best oxygen carrier available. Added to Ringer's lactate solution and albumin, they make a very acceptable blood substitute for patients not requiring clotting factors. Fresh frozen plasma is the best source of clotting factors but is the first component to introduce a risk of hepatitis. Platelet packs complete the clotting constituents, with the exception of fibrinogen which is needed only in the presence of excess fibrinolysins.

Apart from the leukocytes, which are specifically contraindicated in patients awaiting renal transplantation, and the ready availability of the constituents, there is no advantage attributable to component blood over fresh blood, which itself has the advantage of being cheaper and easier to prepare.

ACID-BASE BALANCE AND WATER AND ELECTROLYTE METABOLISM

Alkalosis

Attention has been directed to the development of alkalosis after trauma or operative insult. Some of the mechanisms involved have been summarized by Lyons and Moore, who find that alkalosis is observed more frequently than acidosis in patients with mild to moderate trauma who have not deteriorated to the point of severe renal circulatory or pulmonary decompensation. The criteria used by these writers to describe changes in acid-base balance are reproduced in Table 1-17, since they provide a handy guide for discussion of this subject. It was found that 64 percent of 105 patients operated upon developed

alkalosis on at least one determination in the postoperative period. Of the 67 patients in whom alkalosis developed, 29 demonstrated this change after open heart operations, 19 after ventilatory assistance, 8 had alkalosis from chronic pulmonary disease, 5 had so-called "residual posttraumatic alkalosis," and 6 had miscellaneous forms of alkalosis. It is of significance that the open heart surgical patients received 9 to 18 Gm of tris buffer routinely in the first few hours after bypass and were hyperventilated after operation. These pH changes were therefore not so much the consequence of trauma as of overenthusiastic use of the measures taken for the prevention of acidosis. Among the patients with ventilatory alkalosis only those with pulmonary disease had elevated buffer base values. Extreme hypocapnic alkalosis occasionally developed in patients with normal lungs.

Lyons and Moore point out that it is important to prevent severe alkalosis in the surgical patient because of its potential hazards and that by the same token it might be well to avoid creating it by the injudicious use of administered base or hyperventilation. Among the dangers listed by these writers was the production of tissue hypoxia through the effect of alkalosis on the oxygen-hemoglobin dissociation curve and on vasomotor tone. The rise in blood lactate level which accompanies respiratory alkalosis sets the stage for severe metabolic acidosis should hypocapnia suddenly yield to hypoventilation or hypoperfusion. Alkalosis tends to produce hypocalcemia and hypokalemia, and the latter may be extremely dangerous to the patient receiving digitalis or to patients who already have hypokalemia. Hypocapnic vasoconstriction tends to produce a reduced cerebral blood flow.

One of the mechanisms for the development of alkalosis is pulmonary arteriovenous shunting, which occurs in patients with cirrhosis or atelectasis. Patients with cirrhosis frequently have hypokalemia and a metabolic alkalosis to begin with, and this is further complicated by the respiratory alkalosis which develops as a consequence of the shunting. The shunting that occurs in atelectasis permits venous blood to traverse the pulmonary bed unoxygenated. The resultant hypoxia increases ventilation, thereby blowing off carbon dioxide and producing respiratory alkalosis.

Atelectasis can produce hyperventilation even in the absence of hypoxia by stimulation of the Hering-Breuer reflexes, whereas hypoxemia produces hyperventilation by stimulating the aortic and carotid body chemoreceptors. Furthermore a reduction in blood flow to the chemoreceptor bodies will stimulate hyperventilation, since these receptors extract oxygen from the blood rapidly and extensively. Thus respiration may be stimulated during hypotension and decreased cardiac output even though the arterial blood is adequately oxygenated. This, then, may be another mechanism for the production of respiratory alkalosis in surgical patients. Three of the patients described by Lyons and Moore had a metabolic alkalosis, one from overtreatment of diabetic acidosis and the others from gastrointestinal obstruction and vomiting.

Lactic acid accumulation occurs with hyperventilation and can be prevented by adding carbon dioxide to the

Table 1-17. COMPARISON OF SYSTEMS OF NOMENCLATURE USED TO DESCRIBE DISTURBANCES OF NEUTRALITY REGULATION*

Disturbance in conventional terms	pH (units)	$[H^+]$ (mEq/L)	P_{CO_2} (mm Hg)	Standard HCO_3^- (mM/L)	Actual HCO_3^- (mM/L)	CO_2 content (mM/L)	CO_2 combining power† (mM/L)	Buffer base (mM/L) Hemoglobin (Gm %)			Buffer base deviation (mM/L) Hemoglobin (Gm %)		
								10	15	20	10	15	20
Normal	7.40	39.8	40.0	23.9	23.9	25.1	25.1	45.7	48.0	50.1	0.0	0.0	0.0
Uncompensated respiratory alkalosis	7.53	29.5	25.0	23.9	20.2	20.9	22.9	45.0	48.0	50.9	− 0.7	0.0	+ 0.8
Uncompensated metabolic alkalosis	7.53	29.3	40.0	32.5	32.5	33.7	33.7	55.7	58.0	60.1	+10.0	+10.0	+10.0
Mixed respiratory and metabolic alkalosis	7.68	24.0	25.0	32.5	28.5	29.3	31.2	55.1	58.0	61.0	+ 9.4	+10.0	+10.9
Uncompensated respiratory acidosis	7.31	48.9	55.0	23.9	26.8	28.4	26.7	46.5	48.0	49.4	+ 0.8	0.0	− 0.7
Uncompensated metabolic acidosis	7.24	57.2	40.0	16.7	16.7	17.9	17.7	36.1	38.0	39.7	− 9.6	−10.0	−10.4
Mixed respiratory and metabolic acidosis	7.16	68.4	55.0	16.7	19.2	20.8	19.2	36.7	38.0	39.1	− 9.0	−10.0	−11.0
Mixed respiratory alkalosis and metabolic acidosis	7.40	39.8	25.0	18.4	15.0	15.7	17.5	37.7	41.5	43.1	− 8.0	− 7.5	− 7.0
Mixed respiratory acidosis and metabolic alkalosis	7.40	39.8	55.0	30.0	32.9	34.6	32.7	53.3	55.0	56.5	+ 7.6	+ 7.0	+ 6.4
Respiratory alkalosis with metabolic compensation	7.47	34.2	25.0	21.0	17.4	18.2	20.2	41.4	44.2	47.0	− 4.3	− 3.8	− 3.1
Metabolic alkalosis with respiratory compensation‡	7.47	34.2	50.0	32.5	34.8	36.3	35.0	56.2	58.0	59.7	+10.5	+10.0	+ 9.6
Respiratory acidosis with metabolic compensation	7.35	44.3	55.0	26.5	29.5	31.3	29.7	49.7	51.3	52.8	+ 4.0	+ 3.3	+ 2.7
Metabolic acidosis with respiratory compensation	7.35	44.3	25.0	16.7	13.5	14.2	16.0	35.4	38.0	40.4	−10.3	−10.0	− 9.7

* Actual bicarbonate obtained from Henderson-Hasselbalch equation with $pK^1 = 6.10$. Buffer base, buffer base deviation, standard bicarbonate, and CO_2 combining power obtained from Siggaard-Andersen blood acid-base curve and alignment nomograms. Equilibration temperature = 38°C, oxyhemoglobin saturation = 100 percent and hemoglobin = 15 Gm percent unless otherwise indicated.

† Expressed as total CO_2 of anaerobically collected separated plasma or serum.

‡ Some deny the clinical existence of this disturbance. Other studies indicate that respiratory compensation does occur but is weaker than the compensation accompanying metabolic acidosis.

SOURCE: J. H. Lyons, Jr., and F. D. Moore, *Surgery,* **60**:93, 1966.

inspired gas mixture. It is apparently dependent upon the reduction of carbon dioxide tension P_{CO_2} rather than the associated change in pH. Its exact mechanism is not known but may be related to the effect of hypocapnia on carbohydrate metabolism. If hyperventilation is suddenly stopped, the P_{CO_2} may rise more rapidly than the accumulated lactate can be cleared from the blood, leading to an acute metabolic acidosis. This is worsened by the accumulation of lactic acid of hypoxic origin.

The effects of alkalosis on ionized calcium and on potassium are important to myocardial irritability. It is claimed by Lyons and Moore that alkalosis generally promotes the renal excretion of sodium bicarbonate and an alkaline urine but that in the posttraumatic period this mechanism is blocked by adrenal cortical activity. This produces increased renal potassium loss and, acutely, aciduria. Administration of potassium and chloride permits the correction of the alkalosis. Chronic alkalosis cannot be corrected in the absence of exogenous potassium and chloride. These factors are of special importance in the management of the patient with pyloric obstruction.

Acidosis

Many articles have called attention to the development of acidosis in response to injury or operative trauma. Some of the patients alluded to above would have been acidotic had it not been for their vigorous treatment pushing them over into alkalosis.

BLOOD TRANSFUSION. Blood transfusion may produce either alkalosis or acidosis. Since citrated blood is intrinsically acid by virtue of the citric acid anticoagulant, it produces a metabolic acidosis upon rapid, massive infusion that persists until the fixed acid is metabolized. A standard acid citrate dextrose (ACD) solution also contains about 17 mEq of trisodium citrate per unit of blood, however. As the citrate is catabolized, sodium ions are released to the cation pool of the body and are balanced by newly formed bicarbonate. If renal bicarbonate excretion is inhibited, as it is following trauma, an "addition" metabolic alkalosis results. It takes about 135 mEq of sodium citrate, or the amount contained in 8 units of blood, to produce a discernible alkalosis. In the presence of hepatic impairment, whether brought about by preexisting disease, hypotension, hypoxia, or hypothermia, citrate metabolism is delayed, and transfusion acidosis then becomes more prominent. Transfusion alkalosis is postponed or never appears.

SHOCK. Severe shock, whether bacterial or hypovolemic, tends to produce acidosis. The mechanism for this is decreased tissue perfusion secondary to hypotension compounded by the release of catecholamines in response to hemorrhage, which further produces tissue anoxia by vasospasm. Arteriovenous shunting may increase further the hypoperfusion of tissues. Acidosis also increases coagulability of the blood and may produce capillary thrombosis. If the condition is allowed to persist, cellular death and terminal acidosis result. Hardaway and others have suggested that this condition can be reversed by the simultaneous administration of vasodilators to open up the arterioles together with blood or other fluid to maintain effective circulating blood volume. The increased blood flow to the organs improves tissue oxygenation and decreases the likelihood of capillary thrombosis. The acidosis can be further corrected by the administration of bicarbonate or other base.

Wilson et al. have used phenoxybenzamine, an α-adrenergic antagonist, in 19 patients with shock refractory to conventional treatment. The patients received doses varying between 0.2 and 2 mg/kg of body weight. This was administered over a 5-minute period in patients who were in pulmonary edema and over a 60-minute period in patients who were less severely ill. Large volumes of fluid were needed to maintain blood pressure, and attempts were made to correct acid-base changes when needed. The cardiac output increased in 8 of 9 patients studied, and urine output increased in 7 of 19. The use of vasodilators, or of vasoactive drugs of any kind, in patients with shock is waning in popularity, although phenoxybenzamine unquestionably improves renal cortical blood flow. This effect can be achieved equally well with dopamine, which also provides circulatory support. However, fluid and blood replacement, monitoring of venous pressure and blood gases, adequate ventilation, and treatment of sepsis remain the primary modalities for the treatment of shock.

The accumulation of lactic acid accounts in part for the progressive acidosis of shock, as shown by Broder and Weil. Likelihood of survival of patients in profound shock could be estimated by the levels of excess lactate in the blood. When it was less than 1 mM/liter, 82 percent survived; when it was 2 mM/liter, 60 percent survived; and when it was 2 to 4 mM/liter, only 26 percent survived. If the excess lactate was ever over 3 mM/liter, a fatal outcome could not be averted.

Boyd et al. have shown that nonlactate solutes may also accumulate in shock and that their accumulation indicates a poor prognosis. The presence of these substances, most of which have not been identified, may be demonstrated by measuring serum osmolality and then calculating by a formula using sodium, glucose, and blood urea nitrogen levels. The difference between the measured and calculated osmolality is called the *osmolal discriminant,* and it is only partly accounted for by lactic acid levels. If the osmo-

lality and the osmolal discriminant remain high after treatment, the prognosis is grave. The lactic acid concentration is also high in this group, of course.

MacLean and his coworkers reported studies on 56 patients in shock. These patients were divided into two groups according to whether the central venous pressure was above or below normal prior to treatment and were further subdivided into those patients who were alkalotic or normal and those who were frankly acidotic. The patients were treated with isoproterenol (2 μg/minute) combined with blood and saline solution, which produced an increase in cardiac output and blood pressure with a decline in central venous pressure and in arterial blood lactate.

If the patient was normovolemic before the onset of septic shock, the manifestations included hyperventilation, respiratory alkalosis, high cardiac index, elevated central venous pressure, low peripheral resistance, increased blood volume, hypotension, oliguria, warm, dry extremities, and arterial blood lactate accumulation. If this syndrome was recognized while the patient was still alkalotic, he responded to therapy designed to maintain the cardiac output at even higher levels. In contrast, if the patient was hypovolemic at the onset of sepsis, the clinical picture consisted of low central venous pressure, low cardiac output, high peripheral resistance, and cold, cyanotic extremities. These patients were also initially alkalotic and responded to treatment consisting of volume replacement and surgical procedures. If, however, they were not seen until they were acidotic, a low fixed output persisted and a high mortality rate ensued.

Acidosis is the result of shock, not the cause of it. Prevention or correction of acidosis seldom influences survival in hypovolemic shock. On the other hand, restoring fluid volume without correcting the acidosis does favorably influence the outcome. Severe acidosis (pH below 7.1) occurs in exhaustive exercise and in diabetic acidosis without producing shock, with good cardiac performance and ultimate recovery. The important thing is to remove the cause of the acidosis, not to treat the acidosis per se.

More patients with a normal or alkalotic pH survived than those with acidosis. In fact, of 18 patients with acidosis only 1 survived the shock episode, and none survived subsequently, whereas 33 of 48 who were normal or alkalotic survived the shock episode. It is postulated that in bacteremic shock hyperventilation occurs, leading to respiratory alkalosis. If the patient does not respond to treatment, a continued depression of tissue perfusion leads to the accumulation of large amounts of lactate with acidosis and death.

Bergentz and Brief showed that the development of refractory oligemic shock in dogs was accompanied by the production of acidosis and that the administration of a buffer prevented acidosis as well as the development of refractory shock. An identical volume of a concentrated sodium chloride solution also usually prevented the development of refractory shock without correcting the acidosis. It was felt that the improvement noted with hypertonic solutions was due to a redistribution of fluids from the intracellular to the extracellular space, thus perhaps preventing cellular swelling and promoting an expansion of the extracellular fluid volume. As noted above, expansion of the extracellular fluid volume leads to increased movement of albumin into the plasma and thus to sustained increased blood volume. Improved tissue perfusion might be expected to result.

CARDIAC ARREST. Chazan and his coworkers studied 22 patients during cardiac arrest and found that 10 had predominantly respiratory acidosis and 8 had metabolic acidosis. Most patients with a metabolic acidosis had had a myocardial infarction and had an arterial pH of 7.15 to 7.35. These patients appeared to be benefited by sodium bicarbonate with or without hyperventilation. In the 10 patients with respiratory acidosis, who were chiefly patients with pulmonary problems, the pH was 6.86 to 7.09 in 8. Hypercapnia was prevalent, alkalitherapy seemed less effective, and improved ventilation appeared to be the major therapeutic objective. Recent studies by Bishop and Weisfeldt suggest, in fact, that bicarbonate solutions may worsen the acidosis of cardiac arrest, and that they should not be used in this condition unless effective hyperventilation to remove CO_2 can be achieved. Acidosis tends to develop during cardiac arrest, because the cardiac index is markedly reduced during resuscitation by closed-chest massage; and this results in decreased tissue perfusion, hypoxia, anaerobic metabolism, and the production of lactic acid. In addition, many of the patients may be inadequately ventilated, causing a rise in P_{CO_2} and the development of respiratory acidosis. Only 2 patients in the group of 22 survived and left the hospital, although several others recovered temporarily, only to die later. In 4 patients, the acidosis could not be definitely classified as either metabolic or respiratory.

BURNS. Peaston demonstrated that although there is a paucity of information on acid-base disturbances in burn patients, acidosis is a frequent finding in these patients. He studied 14 consecutive unselected patients admitted to a regional burn unit and expressed the severity of acidosis in terms of the base deficit, after the method of Siggaard-Andersen et al., obtained by interpolation from the Siggaard-Andersen nomogram. Significant respiratory alkalosis was assumed when the arterial P_{CO_2} was below 30 mm Hg. Uncompensated acidosis was said to be present when the arterial pH fell below 7.35. It was found that 12 of the 14 patients had a base deficit at some stage after thermal injury and that in 7 of these the metabolic acidosis was maximal on admission and in 3 others within 24 hours of admission. The maximal degree of acidosis was found to correlate closely with the total extent of the body burn surface area. The severe degrees of base deficit observed were usually compensated by respiratory alkalosis. Acidosis was treated by the administration of sodium bicarbonate in doses as great as 400 mEq over 24 hours, or 2,750 mEq over a period of 11 days. The acidosis could not be attributed to the liberal use of normal saline solution, because in many patients it was maximal on admission before the patients had received any saline solution. It was felt that because of the unfavorable effect of acidosis on renal function the prompt correction of acidosis in the burn patient would help to prevent acute renal failure.

EFFECTS OF ACIDOSIS. Acidosis has profound effects on the cardiovascular system, producing a decreased myocardial contractility, a decreased response of the myocardium and peripheral vasculature to catecholamines, and a predisposition to cardiac arrhythmias. Acidosis predisposes to acute renal failure. Furthermore, it increases respiratory work.

Greenberg and Kittle have studied the effect of pH and P_{CO_2} changes on coronary blood flow and cardiac output, and find that both are increased by elevations of P_{CO_2} and that they are further increased by an elevation of pH. Thus both are increased in respiratory acidosis and metabolic alkalosis (particularly the latter), and both are reduced in metabolic acidosis and respiratory alkalosis.

Huckabee reported a series of 9 patients who had a syndrome of hyperpnea, tachypnea, and dyspnea with weakness and fatigue progressing to stupor and finally death. All these patients had acidosis characterized by a low serum bicarbonate level and a high value of unmeasured anion in the serum electrolyte pattern which turned out to be lactate. This group of patients had nothing else in common except for a very high level of lactic acidosis, which appeared to be due to widespread tissue hypoxia. This again illustrates the lethal nature of uncorrected acidosis.

A Problem in Acid-Base Balance. Figure 1-33 presents some of the findings from a very interesting patient who progressed from presumed metabolic acidosis to respiratory acidosis to respiratory alkalosis to metabolic alkalosis, all within a 24-hour period. This fourteen-year-old boy who had a large pheochromocytoma of the left adrenal was operated upon under general anesthesia, and the pheochromocytoma was removed. Within minutes after the last vein was tied off, the patient's blood pressure fell precipitously, and a severe bradycardia, hypotension, pulmonary edema, and cardiac arrest developed despite the administration of norepinephrine and all other attempts to support his blood pressure and cardiac action. It became necessary to open his chest in order to restore a cardiac beat, and there was a considerable period of hypotension and hypoxia, which almost certainly must have led to metabolic acidosis, although no measurements were made at this precise time.

When the operation was completed, the patient was removed to the recovery room, where because of continued poor ventilation and pulmonary edema he was placed on a respirator. He failed to regain consciousness, and it was then discovered that the respirator was defective. A blood pH taken at this time was 7.02, and the patient was found to have a profound respiratory acidosis. When the respirator was noted to be defective, the patient was placed on a manual bag and breathed vigorously. His respiration was further improved by placing him on a volume respirator, which lowered his P_{CO_2} from 72 to 26 and raised his pH to 7.54. A profound respiratory alkalosis then developed with a pH of 7.74, a P_{CO_2} of 33, and a potassium level of 2.3 mEq/L. At this point carpopedal spasm developed, and the respirator was stopped. Because of the alkalosis and because he had been receiving dexamethasone, large amounts of urinary potassium were lost. A spot check

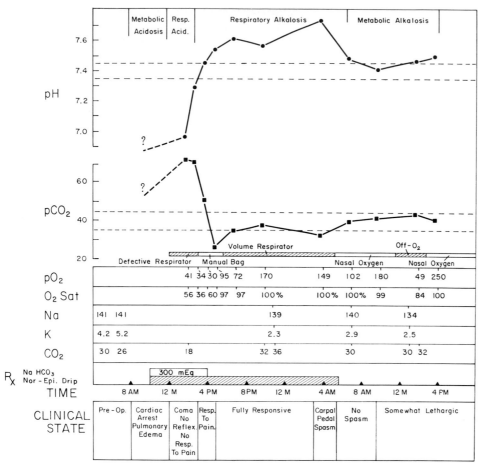

Fig. 1-33. Acid-base abnormalities in a patient with pheochromocytoma. The patient had a cardiac arrest on the operating table associated with peripheral vasoconstriction, overtransfusion with blood, tissue hypoxia, and pulmonary edema. It was necessary to open his chest to restore effective cardiac activity. During this time a severe metabolic acidosis was presumed to have developed, and the patient was given sodium bicarbonate intravenously. After getting his heart started again, the patient was maintained on intravenously administered norepinephrine and was returned to the recovery room and placed on a respirator. The respirator proved to be defective, producing a very severe hypoxia and a marked respiratory acidosis with a P_{CO_2} of 72. The patient's pH at this time was 7.02. When it was discovered that the respirator was defective, the patient was shifted to a manual bag, and this quickly brought the P_{CO_2} down, at which time the patient was placed on a volume respirator. This ventilated him so well that a rather marked respiratory alkalosis developed, with a pH of 7.74. Carpopedal spasm developed, and the respirator was discontinued. Subsequent to this a mild metabolic alkalosis developed, partly as a consequence of the administration of corticosteroids, and large amounts of potassium were lost in the urine, a rather significant hypokalemia developing. This was corrected by the administration of large amounts of potassium chloride intravenously, and the patient ultimately recovered completely.

showed 83 mEq/L of potassium in the urine, while the sodium concentration was 11 mEq/L. The marked potassium loss continued, and an acid urine developed. The pH, which had fallen to 7.42, rose to 7.51, with a P_{CO_2} of 250 (on oxygen), a P_{CO_2} of 41, a carbon dioxide level of 30, and a potassium level of 2.5 mEq/L in spite of the administration of large amounts of potassium intravenously. At this point an uncompensated metabolic alkalosis appeared to have developed. Still larger amounts of potassium were administered, and the dose of dexamethasone was reduced. He went on to make an uneventful recovery.

It is important to note that at times it may be necessary to administer very much larger doses of potassium than one is accustomed to give. Several cases of this type, all of them diabetics, were collected by Pullen et al., in which potassium was administered in doses of up to 860 mEq in 24 hours.

Water and Electrolyte Metabolism

Although it is axiomatic that the response to injury or operation depends upon the utilization and type of anesthetic agent, the preinjury state of the patient, the type of injury, and the particular fluid and electrolyte solutions used in the patient's treatment, nevertheless some generalizations can be made to serve as a frame of reference for the infinite variations produced by the factors just mentioned.

SODIUM METABOLISM

In the normal steady state, human beings excrete a quantity of sodium in the urine equal to the intake. In general, this quantity ranges between 60 and 100 mEq. Following injury, urinary sodium excretion falls to nearly zero, a direct consequence of the hormonal response to injury. If hypovolemia is severe and shock is present, there may also be a decrease in glomerular filtration in response to a fall in perfusion pressure. Filtration may also fall as a result of the action of angiotensin II, as described above. In the absence of any changes in glomerular filtration, however, nearly total sodium conservation is evident. Several mechanisms combine to produce this effect. Renal sympathetic nervous activity is enhanced in response to the injury itself, as well as in response to hypovolemia. In part, this sympathetic activity serves to maintain glomerular filtration in the presence of decreased total renal blood flow. However, as the fraction of blood which is filtered increases, the fraction that is contributed to peritubular blood flow in the renal cortex decreases. Since the glomerulus is nearly impermeable to protein, this change in filtration fraction results in an increase in protein concentration in the peritubular capillary perfusing the proximal tubule. The resulting rise in peritubular oncotic pressure results in

increased net transfer of water and accompanying sodium bicarbonate and sodium chloride from the proximal tubule back into the blood. This process may be further enhanced by a direct action of sympathetic nerves on sodium reabsorption and by decrease in a circulating natriuretic hormone. The net effect of these mechanisms is that a decreased proportion of filtered fluid is delivered to the loop of Henle. The reabsorption of sodium chloride in the loop of Henle is critical for the maintenance of medullary hyperosmolality, however, so that in the presence of enhanced proximal tubular reabsorption of sodium and sustained medullary blood flow, medullary osmolality falls. This fall in medullary hyperosmolality leads to a defect in urinary concentrating ability, so that more urine must be excreted to eliminate the same amount of solute. Gann and Wright have shown that in postoperative patients, expansion of the extracellular fluid can reverse the defect in sodium excretion and in concentrating ability, suggesting that hypovolemia, presumably as a result of sequestration of fluid in the third space, is the principal mechanism involved (Fig. 1-34). However, they also demonstrated that even if extracellular fluid volume is maintained, injury leads to the conservation mechanisms outlined.

Sodium that escapes reabsorption in the proximal tubule and in the loop of Henle is in general captured in the distal tubule and collecting duct under the influence of aldosterone. In the distal tubule, sodium is reabsorbed together with chloride and water to maintain osmotic equilibrium. In the collecting duct, however, sodium is reabsorbed in exchange for potassium and hydrogen, providing the principal mechanism for potassium excretion. If insufficient sodium is delivered to this site in the nephron, accumulated potassium and hydrogen cannot be excreted adequately and hyperkalemia and acidosis may ensue. Since

Fig. 1-34. Decreased extracellular fluid volume leads to sodium retention, reflected as decreased rate of sodium excretion ($U_{Na}V$). Since the increased reabsorption occurs in the proximal tubule, less sodium is delivered to the medulla and the urine cannot be concentrated maximally. Decreased urine osmolality (Uosm) and free water reabsorption ($T^c_{H_2O}$) follow despite administration of vasopressin. In this dog, the ECF was depleted 20 percent by intraperitoneal lavage with hypertonic glucose between two solute diureses. The latter allowed testing over a range of osmolar clearances (Cosm). (*From D. S. Gann and H. K. Wright, J Surg Res, 6:196, 1966.*)

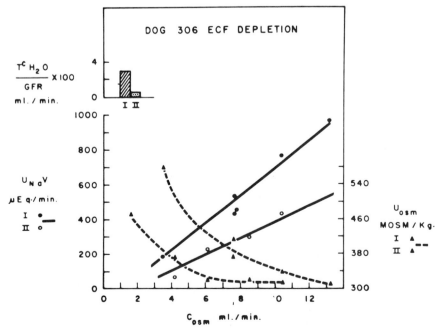

both potassium and acid accumulate in injury, maintained delivery of sodium to the most distal portions of the nephron and maintained urinary excretion are critical to the prevention of life-threatening hyperkalemia and acidosis.

WATER EXCRETION

One of the most constant responses to injury of all types is the release of vasopressin. This hormone produces oliguria unless specific steps are taken to overcome it. It was originally suggested that oliguria was a normal accompaniment of surgical trauma and that it did no particular harm. It is certainly reasonably well tolerated in most types of mild to moderate surgical trauma, but it is a potentially harmful condition in two ways: the first is that it predisposes to acute tubular necrosis in patients with severe trauma in whom hypovolemia and hypotension are apt to occur, and the second is that it sets the stage for the development of water intoxication if large amounts of nonsolute-containing fluids are given to the patient before, during, or immediately after the operative event.

The increased ADH activity persists for 3 to 5 days postoperatively, depending upon the severity of the trauma, and it is a very common event to see patients who have undergone rather severe operative trauma eliminate their water load with a very brisk diuresis, sometimes ranging up to 200 or 300 ml/hour on the third or fourth postoperative day.

Measurements of vasopressin levels in surgical patients were made by Moran et al.; they found that the night before the operation the blood level of ADH was 0.6 μU/ml of whole blood, while just prior to the induction of anesthesia the value had risen to 1.7 μU, apparently as a consequence of the standard practice of withholding fluids the night before the surgical procedure. The rise was greatest in those patients who had been placed on nasogastric suction. Adequate fluid replacement prior to the induction of anesthesia reduced these values to 0.7 μU/ml. The start of the operation was delayed for up to 40 minutes to note the effect of anesthesia per se on ADH levels. Anesthesia produced a slight increase in ADH levels, but this could be completely offset by the rapid administration of parenteral fluid, which led instead of falling ADH levels. The value for the anesthetic period was therefore 1.4 μU/ml, which was similar to that of the preinduction period.

The anesthetic agents used were halothane, Pentothal, methoxyflurane, and nitrous oxide. If the operation was performed under epidural anesthesia, no response to the abdominal incision was noted. In patients operated on under general anesthesia an increased output of ADH occurred within 5 minutes, and in all patients this increase occurred once traction was applied to the viscera innervated outside the area of effective block. A very minor response to skin incision alone took place, but a tenfold increase occurred when the incision was rapidly carried through all layers of the abdominal wall and traction was applied to the viscera.

The responses occurring during the intermediate portion of the operation were very variable. Sometimes the ADH level rose to a plateau which was maintained throughout the procedure, and at other times it simply rose and fell

according to visceral traction. Levels as high as 40 to 150 μU/ml occurred during visceral traction. The magnitude of response was related generally to the magnitude of the procedure. Levels of the sort observed are capable of producing a temporary complete cessation of urine flow. In two patients with high ADH values the creatinine clearance decreased 50 percent, whereas in a patient with a much smaller response there was no change in the creatinine clearance.

The postoperative period was characterized by two phases: the first phase began shortly after skin closure, lasted 6 to 12 hours, and was characterized by a plateau of moderately increased ADH output; this period was followed by a gradual decrease of ADH levels until normal levels were reached on the fourth or fifth postoperative day. In cases of lesser magnitude the return to normal levels occurred by the second postoperative day. The high levels of ADH could be correlated very well with a low urinary output, while the falloff in ADH levels corresponded with diuresis. While hydration was capable of suppressing the increased output of ADH preoperatively and during anesthesia alone, it was not capable of suppressing the elevated levels of ADH seen during operation and in the postoperative period.

The unopposed output of vasopressin leads to water retention, concentrated urine, and oliguria. If water is administered without salt to patients with high levels of ADH, hyponatremia will result. Maximum urine concentration often will not occur, however, because of limited medullary hyperosmolality, as discussed above. Wright and Gann showed that if the extracellular fluid volume was expanded in patients demonstrating postoperative antidiuresis, a dilute urine could be produced. These findings suggest strongly that volume expansion corrected the diuresis by inhibiting secretion of vasopressin and suggested, in addition, that hypovolemia dominates among the various stimuli to secretion of vasopressin as a result of injury or surgery.

Insensible Water Loss

Insensible water losses have been said by Hayes to be about the same after as before injury and of the order of 750 ml/m^2/day. This would be an insensible water loss of about 1,300 ml/day, which seems excessively high. Gump and Kinney report a loss of about 2 ml/m^2/hour, which comes to about 860 ml/day. Actually it is more frequently in the order of 500 ml/day. We have had an opportunity to carry a large number of patients through operative procedures in the complete absence of all renal tissue. Unless there are excessive losses into the wound or an exceptionally high fever, the patients are maintained in equilibrium on about 500 ml/day. Increased losses can occur in the presence of hyperventilation or fever, and huge losses occur from the skin wounds of burned patients and from the lungs of those with tracheostomies.

HYDRATION. It was shown by Hume and Egdahl that acute anuria after kidney transplantation in dogs could be prevented by sufficient hydration of the donor prior to and during operation in order to provide a brisk diuresis of the donor kidney before its removal. The same principle has been applied to renal homotransplantation in man. Barry and Malloy have stressed the value of preventing oliguria in the surgical patient by means of sustained hydration. These writers showed that at all concentrations of halothane anesthesia studied renal plasma flow, glomerular filtration rate, and urine flow were significantly depressed in fluid-restricted subjects. In contrast these measurements were normal in hydrated subjects, except when very high concentrations of halothane were used. The hydrated group was given a 0.3% saline solution. Sodium excretion in the hydrated and dehydrated groups were the same, but urine osmolality exceeded serum osmolality in all dehydrated subjects, whereas urine osmolality was considerably lower in the hydrated subjects.

During surgical procedures some sequestration of fluid occurs in the operative area (the so-called "third space"), and this produces a reduction in central circulatory volume which leads to a fall in renal blood flow. Renal blood flow can be restored to normal by the prompt administration of fluid, but if the deficit in central circulatory volume is allowed to persist beyond certain critical limits, the ability of renal circulation to respond promptly to restoration is lost. This reduction in central circulatory volume produces stimulation of the volume receptors, thus leading to the release of vasoconstrictor substances such as angiotensin II and catecholamines. This produces a further decrease in renal blood flow which may be resistant to change. Oliguria can be prevented by the routine administration of 1,000 to 1,500 ml of a balanced salt solution in the 2- to 3-hour period prior to the beginning of anesthesia or by the administration of mannitol during the operative event. Since solute diuresis leads to further loss of salt and water, mannitol should be given in 0.45% saline solution to prevent hyponatremia and hypovolemia, as suggested by Gann, Wright, and Newsome. It is very important that the diuresis be established before the introduction of anesthesia.

Postoperative Patterns

The two patterns that are perhaps most frequently seen in the postoperative patient are illustrated in Figs. 1-35 and 1-36. The first is that of a mild to moderate dilutional hyponatremia with hyperkalemia. This is primarily brought about by ADH secretion plus overhydration of the patient with non-salt-containing fluids. The potassium level may be elevated by the movement of potassium out of cells as a result of protein catabolism, by breakdown of red cells in a wound, or as a result of administration of old blood. This may pose a serious threat if renal function is impaired.

This response is made much worse if the trauma is severe and prolonged or if the patient has had a chronic wasting illness prior to operation. Other factors which make the response worse are starvation, which in itself can produce hyponatremia, preexisting renal impairment, which predisposes to a further elevation of potassium level and depression of sodium level, cardiac disease with edema, preexisting hyponatremia, a pronounced shift of sodium into the cell with severe trauma, and episodes of hypotension during the operation which may further im-

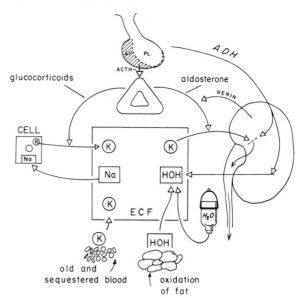

Fig. 1-35. Pattern of hyponatremia in the postoperative patient. Solute is diluted principally by excessive administration of water without salt. In addition, in severe trauma sodium will move into cells in exchange for potassium. The hyperkalemia may be further aggravated by acidosis, by the action of cortisol, and by the breakdown of blood and may be opposed by the action of aldosterone. The dilution may be aggravated by the oxidation of fat and sugar.

Fig. 1-36. Pattern of hypokalemic alkalosis in the postoperative patient. This is most commonly seen in patients who have been on gastric suction and who are alkalotic at the time of operation. The alkalosis produces an additional potassium loss in the urine. Hyperventilation increases the alkalosis and promotes further potassium loss. The administration of sodium bicarbonate, sometimes given in circumstances thought likely to produce acidosis, may further increase the alkalosis. These events then conspire to produce a severe hypokalemic alkalosis which, if renal function is good, may be made worse by the action of the corticosteroids in promoting potassium excretion.

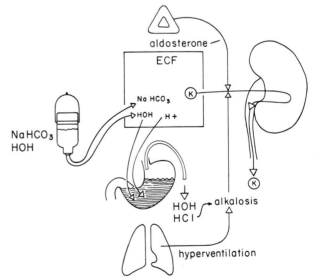

pair renal function. If a marked diuresis is induced by mannitol, this may produce considerable sodium diuresis and add to the hyponatremia if non-sodium-containing repair solutions are used. The cardiac patient needs sodium therapy postoperatively, even though he has an elevated total body sodium. Calcium can also be used but may potentiate digitalis effect if the potassium level remains high. These changes can be prevented or minimized by the use of sodium chloride-containing solutions in the preoperative, operative, and postoperative periods, and by the avoidance of potassium-containing solutions during periods of decreased renal perfusion or when such perfusion is uncertain, as during major surgery.

The second pattern is one of hypokalemic alkalosis. This is classically seen in the patient with an obstructing duodenal ulcer on gastric suction. The alkalosis created by the loss of hydrogen ion from the stomach produces marked urinary potassium loss. This condition is made worse by starvation; the intravenous administration of fluids without potassium; the administration of chlorothiazide diuretics; the administration of corticosteroids; the presence of diarrhea or a fistula; hyperventilation alkalosis; the preoperative existence of certain diseases, such as severe liver disease, where hypokalemia may frequently be present; the administration of sodium bicarbonate or tris buffer, particularly to open heart patients on extracorporeal circulation; or the presence of chronic pulmonary disease, where pulmonary arteriovenous shunts produce hypoxia and a secondary stimulus to hypocapnia. These changes can be prevented by avoidance of the factors listed above, which intensify the response, and by the administration of potassium-containing fluids as needed in the postoperative period. Chloride ion is a critical factor in the repair of hypokalemic alkalosis. In particular the restoration of acquired deficits prior to operation when possible helps to prevent development of these changes.

OXYGEN TRANSPORT

Certain organic phosphates in erythrocytes interact with deoxygenated hemoglobin, thereby altering the affinity of hemoglobin for oxygen. The most abundant of these phosphates in man is 2,3-DPG, the erythrocyte concentration of which has an inverse relationship to the affinity of hemoglobin for oxygen.

Blood stored in ACD at 4°C shows a progressive loss of 2,3-DPG, and after 15 days there is almost none at all. This shifts the oxyhemoglobin dissociation curve strikingly to the left. If such blood is infused into patients, it has a diminished ability to give up oxygen to the tissues.

There are other factors which lower erythrocyte 2,3-DPG levels and produce tissue anoxia. These include (1) acidosis, (2) alkalosis, (3) hypophosphatemia (especially seen with hyperalimentation with synthetic amino acids without added phosphate), (4) septic shock, and (5) trauma without hypotension.

Hemorrhagic shock in patients or baboons usually does not alter red cell 2,3-DPG levels, but resuscitation with old banked blood does. Less severe trauma is usually associated with respiratory alkalosis, and this may depress 2,3-DPG levels and reduce tissue oxygenation. Severe shock with acidosis or septic shock reduces 2,3-DPG and interferes with tissue oxygenation.

Hyperalimentation with essential amino acid solutions not containing added phosphate leads to severe hypophosphatemia, which in turn reduces erythrocyte 2,3-DPG and ATP levels and increases red cell avidity for oxygen, leading to tissue hypoxia.

Increases in erythrocyte 2,3-DPG occurs at high altitudes, with chronic anemia, and in congestive heart failure.

Changes in erythrocyte 2,3-DPG levels were not observed by Naylor and his colleagues in rhesus monkeys subjected either to endotoxin or hypovolemic shock.

In clinical settings, the use of old banked blood, marked alkalosis, septic shock, and hyperalimentation are the circumstances in which depressed erythrocyte 2,3-DPG levels are usually seen. All these except septic shock are easily reversed. The administration of fresh or frozen blood, correction of alkalosis, and addition of phosphate to hyperalimentation mixtures solve the other problems.

IMMUNOLOGIC PROTECTIVE MECHANISMS

After injury there is an acute fall in lymphocytes, an increase in polymorphonuclear leukocytes, and a transient suppression of the reticuloendothelial system (RES). Although some of these effects may be produced by cortisol, the decrease in immunologic competence occurs after injury in the absence of increased steroids, as shown by Munster and his colleagues.

Immediately after a severe trauma there is a surge of neuroendocrine activity designed to counteract the early effects of the injury, an event obviously of paramount importance to the survival of the organism. If the individual survives, this surge diminishes in favor of the mechanisms of orderly repair, and protein and fat repletion. If the injury is complicated by sepsis or repeated traumatic insult, there will be a continuous neuroendocrine stimulus, and cortisol levels will generally remain elevated right up to the point of death. The lymphocyte and eosinophil counts remain low, and cellular immunity continues to be suppressed.

Stetson showed that most of the effects of endotoxin could be produced by antigen-antibody complexes, and Pillemer and his colleagues showed that gram-negative bacterial endotoxins could activate complement. Weil and Spink noted a marked resemblance between endotoxin shock and anaphylactic shock. Schumer and his colleagues investigated the thesis that endotoxin shock was produced by antigen-antibody complexes and complement, which combined to produce an anaphylactic reaction, and found that corticosteroids exerted a protective effect by decreasing either complement or complement fixation. Schumer has recently demonstrated the efficacy of corticosteroid therapy in septic shock in man. While this may not be the sole explanation for the production of endotoxin shock or the beneficial effect of pharmacologic doses of corticosteroids, it seems likely that antigen-antibody complexes and complement play an important role in the production of this type of shock.

Polymorphonuclear leukocytes and platelets are increased in numbers by cortisol, so that although the lymphatic system is suppressed, the bone marrow is generally stimulated. The RES, like the lymphatic system, is suppressed early after severe injury, at which time there is an increased susceptibility to shock and infection. Later there is a recovery and even hyperactivity of the RES. These patterns of activity are frequently correlated with plasma cortisol, but the correlation may be accidental and is certainly not necessary.

The RES plays a role in resistance to certain types of shock which is quite apart from its antibacterial role. Stimulation of the RES by estrogen, choline, or zymosan increases phagocytic function and also increases the resistance to trauma. Adaptation to repeated trauma is accompanied by a marked hypertrophy and hyperfunction of the RES.

The RES aids in clearing away fibrin and other coagulation debris, and RES blockade leads to intravascular fibrin deposition and renal corticol necrosis. It also leads to increased susceptibility to shock.

In hemorrhagic shock the RES cell is said by Bell and his colleagues to undergo lysosomal disruption, a change which may lead to autolysis and RES failure.

Distant trauma increases the rate of wound or peritoneal infection in response to a bacterial inoculum. This is said by Hawley to be counteracted by dextran, which works by diminishing blood viscosity. The increased blood viscosity which normally accompanies trauma interferes with tissue perfusion and oxygenation, and thus increases susceptibility to infection.

Thus the obvious effects of trauma upon the immune system vary with the time after injury, the type of trauma, and the particular segment of the immune system which is studied. There are still many gaps in our knowledge of the response of the immune defense mechanisms to injury, and further work needs to be done to clarify this relationship.

ORGAN SYSTEM CHANGES

Cardiovascular Function

SURGERY. Many of the cardiovascular changes in severe trauma and shock have already been described. Clowes and Del Guercio followed the cardiac response in a series of patients before, during, and after operation. During operation the cardiac output fell an average of 33 percent from the preoperative level, mainly because of a decrease in stroke volume. This was accompanied by an elevation of central venous pressure. Immediately after the operation, following endotracheal extubation, the cardiac output rose on the average to 130 percent of the preoperative value and remained at somewhat elevated levels for the first postoperative week. This elevation of cardiac output after the end of the operation was characteristic of thoracic procedures but was not seen following abdominal laparotomy. Patients who died during the postoperative period

never achieved circulatory flows comparable to their preoperative levels.

BURNS. Berk and his colleagues studied eight severely burned patients and found a characteristic pattern consisting of a decrease in cardiac output with normal blood pressure and increased total peripheral resistance. The oxygen consumption was increased with a high arteriovenous oxygen difference, resulting from the low total cardiac flows. The central blood volume was increased, and central venous pressure showed no evidence of hypovolemia.

SHOCK. MacLean and Duff found that septic shock in dogs and man was accompanied by a fall in cardiac output, arterial pressure, and central venous pressure. In dogs, treatment with isoproterenol, blood, and hyperbaric oxygen restored cardiac output and decreased peripheral resistance but did not improve survival. In patients there was generally an increased peripheral resistance associated with hemorrhagic shock. Transfusion and isoproterenol restored venous pressure, cardiac output, and blood pressure to or toward normal and decreased peripheral resistance. Survival seems to have been favorably influenced by this treatment.

Wilson and coworkers evaluated the data in 31 patients in shock. Those in septic shock had a higher cardiac output and lower peripheral resistance than those in hypovolemic or cardiac shock, where the peripheral resistance was always high. No survival was noted in the septic shock group unless cardiac output was at least 2 liters/m^2/minute. It was stressed that although vasodilators, such as phenoxybenzamine, might be of value when peripheral resistance was increased, their use in patients with decreased peripheral resistance was of no definite benefit and might be deleterious.

Severe trauma is thus characterized by a decreased cardiac output and often an increased peripheral resistance. Tissue arteriovenous shunts may open up, partly as a consequence of epinephrine release, thus increasing venous oxygenation and further intensifying tissue anoxia. This increases acidosis and additionally reduces cardiac output.

The use of phenoxybenzamine in certain patients in septic shock to overcome some of the unfavorable cardiovascular changes has been championed by Hardaway and his associates. Before administering phenoxybenzamine the patients had been treated with volume replacement, antibiotics, correction of acid-base imbalances, corticosteroids, and vasopressors, with progressive deterioration on this regimen. It is emphasized that vasodilators should be used only when preceded by fluid volume replacement to the point of an elevated central venous or pulmonary artery pressure. At this time, when the cardiac index is low and peripheral resistance high, phenoxybenzamine may produce a dramatic increase in cardiac index, fall in peripheral resistance, and brisk diuresis (Fig. 1-37). Respiratory insufficiency, which is usually present, must be corrected and treatment instituted for sepsis and defects in coagulation. Apart from its peripheral effect of vasodilatation and improved tissue perfusion, phenoxybenzamine is believed to improve cardiac performance by direct inotropic action on the myocardium, vasodilating effect on

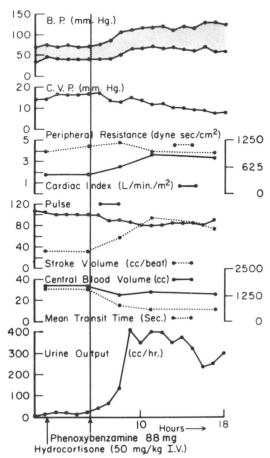

Fig. 1-37. Effect of phenoxybenzamine in septicemic shock. After raising the central venous pressure with colloids and after the failure of other modalities of treatment, phenoxybenzamine produced a rise of blood pressure, a fall in central venous pressure, a fall in peripheral resistance, an increase in cardiac index, a fall in pulse, an increase in stroke volume, and a marked increase in urinary output. (*From R. M. Hardaway et al., JAMA, 199:779, 1967.*)

to extract oxygen, and that the hyperdynamic state results as a compensatory mechanism.

After a period of time the hyperdynamic state gives way to deterioration of cardiac function and ultimately cardiac failure and death. During the period of deterioration of function Cann and his coworkers found that ouabain was the only agent they tested which was capable of improving myocardial function. Coalson and her colleagues, however, found that digoxin treatment provided functional protection for the heart and prevented the mitochondrial changes produced in the myocardium by endotoxin.

Interest has recently been renewed in the concept that there is a circulatory factor present in shock, particularly endotoxin shock, which is a specific myocardial depressant, and that this agent is responsible for the failure of the heart in septic shock. Attar et al. believe that plasma kallikreins are partly responsible for this effect. These are proteolytic enzymes activated by Hageman factor which release bradykinin from its precursor. The kallikreins were found to be increased in shock, and were assumed to release bradykinin, thus producing hypotension.

Solis and Downing, Lefer et al., Glenn and Lefer, and Wagensteen and his colleagues have written a series of papers reviving the concept that MDF is the primary agent producing myocardial depression in shock, particularly septic shock. MDF is a small peptide produced in the pancreas by the action of lysosomal proteases released during shock. They feel that the primary event in any type of shock is splanchnic hypoperfusion which then releases lysosomal hydrolases, primarily from the pancreas, giving rise to MDF, which in turn exerts strong negative inotropic effect on the heart.

Goodyer and his colleagues have shown that the canine myocardium, which usually extracts pyruvate from coronary blood, produces pyruvate in hemorrhagic shock, even when the ventricular function is still well preserved. The coronary sinus oxygen saturation falls below 20 percent at a time when the cardiac function is still quite good, and this may be responsible for the early abnormality in pyruvate metabolism, and the late impairment in contractile function. They feel that some factor present in the blood after 1 hour of shock may give rise to this change in oxygenation and in pyruvate metabolism and that their data generally support the concept of an MDF of some type. Low norepinephrine levels have been observed in the myocardium in shock by Hiott and Richardson, but the reduced myocardial effort could not be related to the levels of norepinephrine.

In the later stages of endotoxin shock there is universal agreement that cardiac failure supervenes. Hinshaw and his coworkers have noted a characteristic elevation of left ventricular end-diastolic pressure, decreased maximal change in the left ventricular pressure, and the need for a positive inotropic agent to drive the heart through an imposed after-load performance curve. Only slight improvement was noted with beta-adrenergic stimulatory agents.

Greenfield et al. and Hinshaw et al. have demonstrated normal myocardial performance in the early phases of

the coronary vessels and myocardial microvasculature, and relief of postcapillary pulmonary vasoconstriction with increased venous return to the left side of the heart. Most patients in septic shock, however, have peripheral vasodilatation, at least in the early and intermediate stages, and a hyperdynamic state. Therefore, the popularity of vasodilators has declined.

The cause of cardiac failure in shock, particularly in septic shock, is still being hotly debated. However, there is general agreement that septic shock induces initially a hyperdynamic state with a high cardiac output and a low peripheral resistance, unless the patient has previously had a reduced blood volume. Although those findings might be explained by arteriovenous shunting in the peripheral tissues or by defective oxygen transfer to the tissues as a consequence of the low erythrocyte 2,3-DPG levels known to be present in septic shock, Wright and his coworkers have developed evidence to suggest that there is instead a primary failure of the peripheral tissues in septic shock

endotoxin shock, and no adverse effects on cardiac work or metabolism during cross circulation with animals in the intermediate or late stages. These experiments did not, therefore, substantiate a primary role for MDF in endotoxin shock.

Levinson and Hume carried out exchange transfusions in animals and in four patients in refractory shock. In the animal experiments this procedure proved to be much more effective than administration of corticosteroids, isoproterenol, or Ringer's lactate solution. The four patients showed improvement in cardiac output, mean arterial pressure, urine output, and arterial pH—although all ultimately died. It was postulated that the exchange transfusions might have washed out substances interfering with cardiac function, including vasoactive polypeptides, histamine, serotonin, catecholamines, or MDF. The exchange also added erythrocytes containing normal amounts of 2,3-DPG to replace those with the depressed 2,3-DPG levels seen in septic shock, thus perhaps improving tissue oxygenation.

It is obvious that the question of the primacy of MDFs in septic shock has not yet been answered.

ANESTHESIA. Baez and Orkin studied the effect of various anesthetic agents on microcirculation and concluded that with cyclopropane anesthesia the compensatory mechanisms of vasomotion, epinephrine reactivity, and overall blood flow are well maintained whereas with ether these compensatory reactions, initially enhanced, are then depressed below normal. Halothane sustained compensatory vascular patterns until late in the course of observation. Methoxyflurane depressed compensatory mechanisms early. It was felt that these experiments confirmed the clinical observations of the utility of cyclopropane and halothane in shock.

Pulmonary Function

ANESTHESIA AND SURGERY. Hypoxia and hypercapnia following operation may be due to the continuing effects of anesthesia and muscle relaxants, together with the development of atelectasis. Significant decreases in pulmonary diffusion have been found following all types of operations, lasting as long as 5 days following operation. The ventilation perfusion defect or pulmonary arteriovenous shunting may involve 25 percent of the total pulmonary blood flow. This produces a considerable degree of hypoxia.

The work of breathing, which normally requires 1 to 2 percent of the cardiac output, may require as much as 30 to 50 percent of the total cardiac output after operation or trauma. Assisted respiration produces a decrease in oxygen consumption and cardiac output.

Anesthesia and surgical procedures alter respiration by depressing the pulmonary reflexes and the central nervous system response, thus depressing the patient's desire to breathe. This is true of both preoperative and postoperative medications, the general anesthetic agent, and of course the muscle relaxants. Patients may occasionally have very severe reactions to a muscle relaxant, so that they will not breathe on their own for several hours after the end of the operation. Respiratory excursion is also interfered with by spinal and epidural anesthesia and by disruption of the thorax, abdomen, or the respiratory tract itself. Secretions collect in the bronchial tree because of difficulty in coughing and moving, and this gives rise to atelectasis. Pulmonary arteriovenous shunts may be operative in atelectasis and in patients with cirrhosis, and profound acid-base changes may result as a consequence of hyperventilation or of prolonged cardiopulmonary bypass.

Peters and Hedgpeth have shown that an increase in airway resistance and pulmonary vascular resistance both cause increased respiratory work. They also lead to ventilation perfusion incoordination by changing the time constants for ventilation of the various areas of the lung. This causes more work. The increased respiratory work then leads to further acidosis in a vicious cycle, since acidosis leads to pulmonary vasoconstriction and further sensitizes the lung to vasoconstriction due to hypoxia. Metabolic acidosis superimposed on respiratory acidosis retards the increased cardiac output associated ordinarily with respiratory acidosis. Metabolic acidosis increases pulmonary vascular resistance, thus increasing respiratory work. Acidosis also leads to movement of potassium ion out of muscle cells, decreasing excitability and potentiating further the vicious cycle.

Prophylaxis. In an attempt to determine whether postoperative pulmonary complications can be prevented by the use of isoproterenol and intermittent positive pressure breathing (IPPB), Anderson and his colleagues studied 160 control patients and 42 patients receiving IPPB and isoproterenol. A very significant reduction in postoperative complications was encountered in the treated group. Roe has also urged the wider use of airway moisture, expectorants, tracheal aspiration, bronchoscopy, and tracheostomy as prophylaxis against pulmonary complications in postoperative patients. Should endotracheal intubation be required, effective prophylaxis against atelectasis and shunting is best achieved by constant positive pressure breathing (CPPB), together with maintained elevation of positive end-expiratory pressure (PEEP). The PEEP must be low enough to prevent decreased venous return.

High-Output Respiratory Failure. Burke and his coworkers have described the syndrome of high-output respiratory failure as that type of respiratory failure characterized by inability to produce adequate tissue oxygenation, and later carbon dioxide excretion, despite an initially increased gas exchange. In a study of 21 patients this type of failure frequently was associated with severe peritonitis or ileus. No deaths were directly attributable to the high-output failure. The syndrome of high-output respiratory failure may be suspected by persistent elevation of pulse and respiration with a normal blood pressure in an anxious exhausted patient. It is confirmed by a depressed arterial oxygen saturation. Previous lung disease, obesity, smoking, or severe debility predispose to it. Tracheostomy and assisted respiration may have to be used to treat it.

Nash and his coworkers have described a pulmonary lesion associated with oxygen therapy and artificial ventilation in 70 patients who died after prolonged artificial ventilation. These patients all showed characteristic pulmonary changes consisting of heavy, beefy, and edematous lungs. Microscopically these showed an early exudative phase characterized by congestion, alveolar edema, intra-alveolar hemorrhage, and a fibrin exudate, with formation of prominent hyaline membranes without any associated inflammatory component. A late proliferative phase was characterized by marked aveolar and interlobular septal edema, fibroblastic proliferation with early fibrosis, and prominent hyperplasia of the lining cells. These changes were not related to the duration of the ventilation but to high concentrations of inspired oxygen. It was felt that patients should receive inspired oxygen concentration sufficient to ensure normal or nearly normal arterial oxygen tension and that this should be reduced as soon as blood-gas measurements show that reduction can be accomplished safely.

SHOCK. Cook and Webb have studied the pulmonary changes in shock and found that there was a rise in transpulmonary vascular pressure and a great increase in pulmonary vascular resistance which persisted for several hours after the shock was corrected. There was congestive atelectasis, recruitment of pulmonary vascular segments, and alveolar capillary dilatation, suggesting venous constriction. Ventilation increased while compliance decreased, indicating a diminished gas exchange with increased ventilatory work. Veith and his coworkers found that shock and transfusion produced an initial active arteriolar vasoconstriction followed by secondary vasodilatation, congestion, hemorrhage, and edema. These changes may help to explain the frequent pulmonary complications accompanying hemorrhagic shock.

POSTTRAUMATIC PULMONARY INSUFFICIENCY. There has been a great deal of interest recently in the lung changes that occur in severe trauma not involving the thorax. The condition has often been called "shock lung," but as shock alone does not actually produce it, it is probably best called the *posttraumatic pulmonary insufficiency syndrome.* There are several different etiologic factors— some or all of them operative in each case. Among the factors most frequently incriminated in the syndrome are (1) oxygen therapy, (2) loss of pulmonary surfactant, (3) alveolar collapse, (4) platelet aggregate emboli induced by trauma, (5) platelet aggregates and other debris in infused blood, (6) viable immunologically competent leukocytes in fresh blood, (7) pump oxygenators, (8) fat emboli, (9) pulmonary arteriovenous shunting, (10) sepsis, endotoxin, (11) vomiting and aspiration, (12) fluid overload, and (13) vasoactive substances released into the pulmonary circulation.

Blaisdell and his colleagues have shown that microemboli of various types are probably a factor in most patients with the pulmonary insufficiency syndrome. Platelet microemboli tend to develop in vivo after hemorrhage and as a consequence of endotoxemia. They also develop in banked blood and increase as the storage period is extended, and in pump-oxygenator systems. They are caused by an increase in platelet adhesiveness. Micropore filters have been developed to remove the emboli from infused blood.

Nahas and his colleagues have claimed that viable leukocytes infused in fresh blood can mount a graft versus host reaction in the lung. This can be avoided by the use of frozen red cells. Fat emboli occur not only from bone marrow injury, but also from the reesterification of fatty acids mobilized by the catecholamines and glucagon.

Oxygen toxicity is capable of producing fatal pulmonary damage. When oxygen concentrations of 70 to 100% are used with respirators for prolonged periods of time (giving P_{O_2} values above 350 mm Hg), there is damage to the endothelial cells, with interstitial edema, hyaline membrane deposition, alveolar epithelial cell hypertrophy and desquamation, and alveolar hemorrhage. Arteriovenous shunting and hypoxemia result from this. These are similar to changes seen in the posttraumatic lung.

Sepsis is a major factor in the lung changes seen after trauma. The bacteria may be filtered out by the lung following their embolization from a distant site, they may enter directly through the airway, or they may affect the lungs by means of endotoxins. Endotoxin produces damage to pulmonary capillaries, thus initiating the changes of the pulmonary insufficiency syndrome.

Probably the most important cause of the lung changes of trauma is the loss of pulmonary surfactant with alveolar collapse, focal atelectases, decreased compliance, arteriovenous shunting, and interstitial edema.

Hypothalamic hypoxia is thought to contribute to the development of the syndrome by producing autonomically mediated pulmonary venular spasms leading to interstitial edema, intraalveolar hemorrhage, surfactant neutralization by plasma, hyaline membranes, and alveolar atelectasis.

The hypocapnia that normally develops as a consequence of the postinjury hyperventilation is thought by Trimble and associates to be an important etiologic agent in the production of pulmonary insufficiency. Hypocapnia is said to induce bronchoconstriction, and the alkalosis produced by blowing off carbon dioxide affects blood flow to the lung and unfavorably affects oxyhemoglobin dissociation. The addition of carbon dioxide to the inspired air is said to improve oxygenation and other parameters of pulmonary physiology.

Vomiting and aspirating stomach contents or blood and fluid overloading are contributing factors to the development of lung lesions after trauma.

The lysis of platelet aggregates and resulting reactions lead to release of serotonin, bradykinin, and prostaglandins (especially $F_{2\alpha}$) into the pulmonary circulation. Venular constriction and bronchoconstriction may result, leading in turn to interstitial movement of fluid and colloid, to a diffusion block for O_2, and thus to increased shunting.

The treatment and/or prevention of the pulmonary insufficiency syndrome consists of (1) the use of micropore filters for infused blood, (2) the avoidance of blood with viable leukocytes, (3) the treatment of sepsis, (4) the avoidance of aspiration or fluid overloading by administering corticosteroids if aspiration occurs and diuretics for fluid overloads, (5) the use of corticosteroids for massive fat embolization, (6) the use of oxygen mixtures of 45% or less, (7) the determination of serial blood gases, (8) the use of a volume respirator which "sighs" periodically, and especially (9) the application of continuous positive pressure to provide 6 cm water pressure at the end of expiration or, more appropriately, a level of PEEP that does not lead to a fall in arterial pressure. This helps to correct the alveolar collapse brought about by loss of surfactant.

The question of whether resuscitation with noncolloidal fluids is more damaging to the lung than if colloids had been used is still largely unresolved. While the functional differences between these two repair solutions is slight, there are more ultrastructural lung changes when noncolloids are used than when albumin is used.

The use of a membrane oxygenator and extracorporeal heart-lung machine for a severe case of pulmonary failure has been said by Hill and his colleagues to have resulted in survival. This may be an important therapeutic modality in the future.

The effects of the pulmonary insufficiency syndrome are to produce a progressive hypoxemia with arteriovenous shunting, acidosis, hypercapnia, interstitial edema, and sepsis, with stiff, beefy, heavy, wet lungs and, ultimately, death.

Hepatic Function

DRUGS AND ANESTHETIC AGENTS. Hepatic function may be depressed by many drugs and anesthetic agents administered to the patient prior to or during surgical procedures. If the liver is not diseased and the degree of trauma not too severe, these minor changes in function usually pass unnoticed and do not prove to be of any clinical significance. If the patient has cirrhosis or other liver damage, some of the commonly used drugs and virtually all the anesthetic agents may produce a depression of hepatic function which, because of inability of the damaged liver to detoxify them, leads to a profound generalized effect. Among these drugs are morphine, which may precipitate coma in patients with cirrhosis, and paraldehyde, which may produce a profound sleep or even death in such patients. This is also true of the barbiturates which are metabolized by the liver. Other drugs may interfere with bilirubin metabolism, such as the sulfonamides, which inhibit plasma binding; flavaspidic acid, which interferes with bilirubin transport through the cell; novobiocin, which interferes with glucuronide conjugation; cholecystographic media, which compete with the conjugated bilirubin for excretion into the biliary canaliculus; and methyltestosterone or chlorpromazine, which interfere with the excretion of the bilirubin into the canaliculus. In most instances these reactions are reversible. Direct hepatic toxicity sometimes results from the tetracyclines, particularly in malnutrition or pregnancy, ferrous sulfate, 6-mercaptopurine, methotrexate, and 5-fluoro-2-deoxyuridine. Cinchophen and iproniazid may cause a hepatitis-like reaction.

A great deal of debate has occurred over the effect of the anesthetic agent halothane as a hepatotoxin. Severe reactions and even death can occur occasionally with halothane anesthesia, although fortunately these reactions are rare. They usually depend upon a personal individual sensitivity and almost always occur only when anesthesia has been administered twice for separate operations. It is therefore probably not wise to repeat halothane anesthesia within 6 months. Some of the antituberculosis drugs may cause a hypersensitivity reaction; chief among this group is para-aminosalicylate. Chlorpropamide and tolbutamide can also cause this reaction.

If hepatic reserve is decreased, as it may be in severe cirrhosis, very minor trauma or brief anesthesia can precipitate hepatic failure, coma, and even death.

SHOCK. In severe trauma and shock there is an increased Bromsulphalein (BSP) retention, increased serum bilirubin, increased prothrombin time, decreased fibrinogen, increased SGOT, increased blood ammonia, and decreased urea formation. Glycogen stores are depleted, and lactate acid accumulates. Ketonemia follows and ultimately gives way to low blood ketone levels as hepatic function is further impaired. Blood amino acid nitrogen level rises. Impairment of enzyme systems occurs, and the liver content of high-energy stores such as ATP, ADP, thiamine pyrophosphate (TPP), and flavin adenine dinucleotide (FAD) as well as phosphocreatinine becomes depleted. CoA and succinate oxidase are reduced. There is a reduced capacity for aerobic metabolism.

Damage to the liver has been implicated as one of the causes of irreversibility in shock. It has been postulated that the inability of the liver to detoxify injurious agents released in shock is responsible for the trend toward irreversibility. Actually most of the experiments suggesting this possibility have been carried out in the dog, although differences in the splanchnic circulation and regular hepatic infection with microorganisms make this animal a poor model for the human system. The liver does seem to protect somewhat against intestinal ischemic shock. There is some depression of the RES of the liver in profound shock.

Holden and his coworkers carried out an electron microscopic study of the liver of the rat in shock. After 2 hours of shock there was a distortion of the endoplasmic reticulum, depletion of the glycogen granules, disorganization and swelling of the mitochondria, and in some cells an increase in the number and size of bodies thought to be lysosomes. Hypoxia produced by an atmosphere of 93% nitrous oxide and 7% oxygen for 1 hour failed to produce similar changes. It was suggested that the ultrastructural and biochemical changes observed in hypovolemic shock were not solely the result of cellular hypoxia but rather the result of the combined effects of cellular hypoxia, the neuroendocrine response to hypovolemia, and the altered physiochemical composition of extracellular fluid (ECF) resulting from diminished capillary perfusion.

A study of liver cell lysosomes in traumatic, ischemic, and endotoxin shock by Janoff showed that there was a disruption of lysosomes and the release of their contained enzymes in free active form in the liver of shocked animals. It was felt that the activation of lysosomal hydrolases within cells and their release into the circulation might play an important role in exacerbating tissue injury and accelerating the development of irreversible shock. In those animals rendered tolerant of shock or pretreated with cortisone there was a stabilization of lysosomes, and it was felt that this effect might constitute an important component of the resistance of such animals to shock. The exacerbating effect of reticuloendothelial blocking colloids on the lethality of shock procedures may be due in part to a direct action of these agents on lysosomes.

Blair and his colleagues have performed electron microscopic studies of the liver in shock and found that there was progressive hepatocellular damage during the first hour, characterized by reduction in glycogen, increased prominence of smooth endoplasmic reticulum, swelling of mitochondria, and a disarrangement of the rough endoplasmic reticulum. After 3 hours of shock there was a progressive increase in secondary lysosomes, and by $4\frac{1}{2}$ hours there was a marked prominence of secondary lysosomes which was related to the irreversible shock state. Clermont et al. demonstrated an increase in lysosomal enzyme acid phosphatase content of hepatic blood, lymph, and bile after the second hour of shock.

In addition to the changes in lysosomes, there is a decrease in cell transmembrane potential difference, a decrease in cyclic AMP, and a decrease in the energy-producing capabilities of mitochondria. The energy availability of the cell is dependent upon mitochondrial respiration, which in turn may be controlled by ATP-dependent membrane transport. Baue and his coworkers demonstrated that hepatic ATP-dependent membrane transport was progressively activated in shock, leading to increased sodium and decreased potassium in the mitochondria, with decreased mitochondrial respiration and energy depletion.

Patients with hepatic failure may have a buildup in the blood of substances profoundly toxic to cells throughout the body. Thus hepatic coma eventuates from the effect of these substances on the brain, oliguria appears as a consequence of their action on the kidney, and hypotension results from a depressed cardiac output as a consequence of a toxic effect on the myocardium. Further depression of hepatic function itself may also take place. These effects sometimes can be dramatically reversed by exchange transfusion, in which the toxic substances are washed out of the bloodstream as the patient's blood is replaced by large quantities of fresh donor blood. Fortunately, hepatic reserve in the normal patient is so great that liver failure is seldom a problem in severe trauma.

Gastrointestinal Function

The gastrointestinal changes in trauma range from the mild syndrome of ileus and temporary loss of appetite following intestinal operations, and mucosal changes in the intestinal tract brought about by shock, to stress ulcers of the stomach and duodenum.

SHOCK. Gurd has studied the metabolic and functional changes in the intestine in shock. He found that in dogs

with irreversible shock there was a profound depression of oxygen uptake by the intestine after retransfusion, despite a return of mesenteric blood flow to normal. This was in spite of the fact that oxygen consumption in the liver and limbs returned for a time to normal, as did the cardiac output. Studies with ^{32}P showed a depression of oxidative phosphorylation and nucleotide synthesis in the mucosa of the small intestine of these animals after retransfusion, while full recovery of these processes was noted in the liver. Hemorrhagic necrosis of the bowel was often seen in dogs and could be protected against by the injection of Trasylol, a trypsin inhibitor, into the lumen of the bowel. Hemorrhagic necrosis of this sort is seldom seen in man, where the amount of trypsin present in the intestinal chyme is far less than in dogs, but has been reported in cases of severe shock.

A higher metabolic activity was observed in bowel washed free of its fecal content, suggesting that contact with feces has a deleterious effect on cellular metabolism in ischemic anoxia. After curare was placed in the lumen, the bowel demonstrated an increased permeability in the metabolically depressed mucosa. If the pancreatic ducts were ligated 48 hours before the shock state was induced, hemorrhagic necrosis was prevented.

It could be demonstrated that the mucin coat over the villi was lost at the moment when signs of irreversibility appeared in hypovolemia. In time mucin production ceased. The first areas to lose the mucin coat were the tips of the villi. The loss of mucin permitted damage to the cells by trypsin and led to the development of hemorrhagic necrosis.

There is a striking species difference between the intestinal changes seen in shock in dogs and those in primates. In dogs endotoxin shock produces mesenteric vasoconstriction, intestinal ischemia, and epithelial necrosis, while in primates Barton and his colleagues found that endotoxemia was associated with a normal mesenteric blood flow, a fall in mesenteric vascular resistance, and no gross changes in the intestine. Hypovolemic shock in dogs characteristically produces intense mesenteric vasoconstriction, with diffuse necrosis of the epithelium. In primates mesenteric blood flow was decreased and vascular resistance was increased, but no lesions of the intestine were produced. Vyden and Corday, however, showed that in man gastrointestinal necrosis was sometimes seen in acute myocardial infarction, and that superior mesenteric artery blood flow fell under these circumstances. Drucker and his colleagues have reported a group of patients with hemorrhagic necrosis of the intestine and have suggested that the lesions were produced by anoxia brought about by decreased perfusion and vasospasm.

Intraluminal mucosal nutrients were shown to protect the mucosa of the ischemic bowel from necrosis. Chiu et al. achieved protection by using intraluminal glucose, and Bounous et al. by an elemental diet. This protection was thought to be afforded by direct utilization of the substrate by the mucosa.

In hypovolemic shock Cook and associates have shown that the intestine becomes a secretory rather than absorptive organ and that there can be huge fluid losses into the intestinal lumen.

In experiments on dogs in hemorrhagic shock the intestine has often been implicated as the cause of irreversibility due to the absorption of toxins from the ischemic intestine. This was first thought to be due to bacteria which escaped from the bowel lumen into the circulation as a consequence of ischemic destruction of the intestinal mucosal barrier. However, bacteremia is not found in standard irreversible shock, and Lillehei and coworkers have shown that pretreatment of the dogs with oral neomycin and other antibiotics to the point of sterilization of the stool cultures does not influence the result of hemorrhagic shock. The course prior to death and the hemorrhagic necrosis of the intestinal mucosa at autopsy do not differ in treated dogs from other dogs not receiving oral antibiotics.

Moreover, Zweifach and coworkers found no increased survival from shock in germ-free rats, and Carter and Einheber have shown that intestinal ischemia produced by occluding the superior mesenteric artery in germ-free rats was acutely lethal and there was no significant difference in survival times of germ-free, contaminated germ-free, and normal control rats. The mucosal destruction in dogs is considerably greater than in man, and this is apparently related in part to loss of protecting mucin and the presence of trypsin and other proteolytic enzymes.

Goodman and Osborn have discussed the problem of acute gastric ulceration and its diverse origins. In the neurogenic ulcer seen after head injury there is frequent perforation from esophagogastromalacia, whereas stress ulcers seen with shock rarely perforate. Corticosteroid ulcers are usually antral and respond to antacids, whereas stress ulcers are superficial linear fundic erosions unaffected by antacids and not associated with increased acid production. Postburn ulcers are located in the depths of rugal folds of the fundus as well as the duodenum, are round and deep, and may show bacterial colonies in the base.

Robert and coworkers and Menguy and Masters have shown that steroid ulcers are due to a loss of mucin protection of the epithelium, and Hutcher and his colleagues found that vitamin A prevented steroid ulcers by restoring mucin production. Stress ulcers show relatively little deficit in mucin, however, although Lev and his coworkers found some reduction. The main etiologic factor in stress ulcers is probably mucosal ischemia. Sepsis, in some unknown way, greatly increases the likelihood of the development of stress ulcers.

Intraluminal nutrients protect against stress ulceration, as shown by Voitk, and hyperalimentation does also; hypoglycemia and starvation increase the likelihood of ulceration.

Renal Function

As mentioned earlier in this section, renal function is generally depressed in operative trauma as a result of dehydration of the patient prior to operation, the cardiac depression produced by some anesthetic agents, the hypotension that may occur with blood loss, and the neuroendocrine effects on renal handling of salt and water. Renal function can usually be preserved at normal levels during operative trauma with proper hydration of the patient prior to operation, the avoidance of hypotension by the prompt replacement of blood loss, the monitoring of venous pressure, and the administration of mannitol to maintain an osmotic diuresis.

SHOCK. Severe shock may produce acute tubular necrosis or even cortical necrosis, with temporary or permanent renal failure. The treatment of this condition is considered in Chap. 40. It is now generally felt that the severely injured patient with acute tubular necrosis and severe oliguria or anuria should be treated with repetitive hemodialysis or peritoneal dialysis very early in the course of the renal insufficiency in order to ensure a smoother convalescence and to help prevent death from the complications of anuria. It is recognized that hyperkalemia is not the only indication for dialysis in renal shutdown, and the severely injured patient generally catabolizes tissue at such a rapid rate that early dialysis is mandatory to prevent demise. We have had occasion to dialyze patients within 48 hours of severe injury.

When cardiac output and aortic pressure are reduced experimentally by cardiogenic shock to 50 percent of normal, renal blood flow is 75 percent of normal, whereas similar conditions of cardiac function produced by hemorrhagic shock lead to renal blood flow that is 10 percent of normal. Gorfinkel and his colleagues conclude that this is a reflection of the intense renal vasoconstriction seen with hemorrhagic shock.

Severe oliguria and renal failure may occur in shock due to gram-negative septicemia. Under these circumstances renal function can often be restored by the administration of plasma until the venous pressure is at the upper limits of normal, of phenoxybenzamine to overcome peripheral vasoconstriction and improve renal plasma flow, and of mannitol to induce diuresis. More recently, dopamine has proved useful in producing vasodilation and maintained glomerular filtration; it may be used with furosemide to produce a natriuresis and diuresis. As with mannitol, this regimen requires care in replacing fluid volume to prevent secondary renal shutdown. In the traumatized patient who has become overly treated with fluids and who is edematous or in pulmonary edema, furosemide alone has been extremely valuable in promoting diuresis.

Staphylococcal toxin can produce shock and a profound depression of renal function consisting of reduction in total and effective renal plasma flow with congestion and secondary ischemia of the peripheral cortical zone. The free-water clearance falls, and the percentage of filtered sodium in the urine increases.

The depression of renal function in patients with severe shock differed in the survivors and nonsurvivors in a study by Strauch and coworkers in that the sodium and chloride clearances of the survivors reached levels of 1.2 to 1.4 ml/minute, whereas the values never exceeded 0.4 ml/minute in the nonsurvivors. There was a severe depression of glomerular filtration rate and urea clearance in all patients, but whereas this was transient in survivors, it was progressive in nonsurvivors.

Other aspects of renal function in trauma and shock have been considered in the preceding sections.

GENERAL CONSIDERATIONS

The foregoing discussion of the endocrine and metabolic response to injury has perhaps demonstrated that there are many gaps in our knowledge and that many areas of controversy still remain. The degree to which the body is able to compensate for injury is astonishing, although at times the compensating mechanisms may work to the patient's disadvantage.

Therapeutic trends which have perhaps excited the most interest among surgeons recently include the protection of renal function by hydration and osmotic diuresis; the monitoring of central venous pressure and left atrial pressure as an aid in the assessment of fluid replacement and cardiac action; the swing away from the use of vasoconstrictors in shock to the use of blood volume replacement, maintenance of normal venous pressure, and control of sepsis; the use of intravenously administered bicarbonate to correct situations in which acidosis is known to occur; the correction of clotting defects with specific coagulation agents and fresh blood; an appreciation of the lung problems associated with injury and their correction with proper respirators; the electronic monitoring of blood pressure and other vital parameters; the more exact determination of antibiotic sensitivity of microorganisms; the realization that complete intravenous therapy can be given to patients who are forced to undergo long periods of starvation by the administration of protein and calories; and the frequent measurement of blood gases and fluid and electrolyte flux to determine the pattern of the endocrine and metabolic response to injury. This chapter simply serves as an introduction to some of these subjects, most of which will be covered in more detail in other portions of the book.

References

Stimuli Inducing Change

Baertschi, A. J., Ward, D. G., and Gann, D. S.: Role of Atrial Receptors in the Control of ACTH, *Am J Physiol,* **231:**692, 1976.

Brown, R. S., Mohr, P. A., Carey, J. S., and Shoemaker, W. C.: Cardiovascular Changes after Cranial Cerebral Injury and Increased Intracranial Pressure, *Surg Gynecol Obstet,* **125:**1205, 1967.

Bursten, B., and Russ, J. J.: Preoperative Psychological State and Corticosteroid Levels of Surgical Patients, *Psychosom Med,* **27:**309, 1965.

Cryer, G. L., and Gann, D. S.: Right Atrial Receptors Mediate the Adrenocortical Response to Hemorrhage, *Am J Physiol,* **225:**1345, 1973.

Dallman, M. F., and Yates, F. E.: Anatomical and Functional Mapping of Central Neural Input and Feedback Pathways of the Adrenocortical System, *Mem Soc Endocrinol,* **17:**39, 1968.

Davis, J., Morrill, R., Fawcett, J., Upton, V., Bondy, P. K., and Spiro, H. M.: Apprehension and Elevated Serum Cortisol Levels, *J Psychosom Res,* **6:**83, 1962.

Gann, D. S.: Carotid Vascular Receptors and the Control of Adrenal Corticosteroid Secretion, *Am J Physiol,* **211:**193, 1966.

———— and Cryer, G. L.: Models of Adrenal Cortical Control, *Adv Biomed Eng,* **2:**1, 1972.

———— and Egdahl, R. H.: Responses of Adrenal Corticosteroid Secretion to Hypotension and Hypovolemia, *J Clin Invest,* **44:**1, 1965.

Ganong, W. F., Gold, N. I., and Hume, D. M.: The Effect of Hypothalamic Lesions on the Plasma 17-Hydroxycorticosteroid Response to Immobilization in the Dog, *Fed Proc,* **14:**54, 1955.

Gerich, J. E., Charles, M. A., and Grodsky, G. M.: Regulation of Pancreatic Insulin and Glucagon Secretion, *Annu Rev Physiol,* **38:**353, 1976.

Harris, G. W.: "Neural Control of the Pituitary Gland," Edward Arnold (Publishers) Ltd., London, 1955.

Hume, D. M.: The Method of Hypothalamic Regulation of Pituitary and Adrenal Secretion in Response to Trauma, in S. Curri and L. Martini (eds.), "Pathophysiologia Diencephalica," p. 217, Springer-Verlag OHG, Vienna, 1958.

Noble, R. L.: The Development of Resistance by Rats and Guinea-pigs to Amounts of Trauma Usually Fatal, *Am J Physiol,* **138:**346, 1943.

———— and Collip, J. B.: A Quantitative Method for the Production of Experimental Traumatic Shock without Hemorrhage in Unanaesthetized Animals, *Q J Exp Physiol,* **31:**187, 1942.

Redding, M., and Mueller, C. B.: Effect of Ambient Temperature upon Responses to Hypovolemic Insult in the Unanesthetized, Unrestrained Albino Rat. *Surgery,* **64:**110, 1968.

Central Nervous System and Endocrine Changes

Bowman, H. M., Cowan, D., Kovach, G., Jr., and Hook, J. B.: Renal Effects of Glucagon in Rhesus Monkeys during Hypovolemia, *Surg Gynecol Obstet,* **134:**937, 1972.

Carey, L. C., Cloutier, C. T., and Lowery, B. D.: Growth Hormone and Adrenal Cortical Response to Shock and Trauma in the Human, *Ann Surg,* **174:**451, 1971.

————, Lowery, B. D., and Cloutier, C. T.: Blood Sugar and Insulin Response of Humans in Shock, *Ann Surg,* **172:**342, 1970.

Cerchio, G. M., Moss, G. S., Popovich, P. A., Butler, E., and Siegel, D. C.: Serum Insulin and Growth Hormone Response to Hemorrhagic Shock, *Endocrinology,* **88:**138, 1971.

Cooper, C. E., and Nelson, D. H.: ACTH Levels in Plasma in Preoperative and Surgically Stressed Patients, *J Clin Invest,* **41:**1599, 1962.

Dallman, M. F., and Jones, M. T.: Corticosteroid Feedback Control of Stress-Induced ACTH Secretion, in A. Brodish and E. S. Redgate (eds.), "Brain-Pituitary-Adrenal Interrelationships," p. 176, Karger, Basel, 1973.

Egdahl, R. H.: Pituitary-Adrenal Response following Trauma to the Isolated Leg, *Surgery,* **46:**9, 1959.

Exton, J. H., Ui, M., Lewis, S. B., and Park, C. R.: Mechanism of

Glucagon Activation of Gluconeogenesis, in H. D. Soling and B. Willms (eds.), "Regulation of Gluconeogenesis," p. 160, Academic Press, Inc., New York, 1971.

Frohlich, J., and Wieland, O.: Dissociation of Gluconeogenic and Ketogenic Action of Glucagon in the Perfused Rat Liver, in H. D. Soling and B. Willms (eds.), "Regulation of Gluconeogenesis," p. 179, Academic Press, Inc., New York, 1971.

Gann, D. S.: Parameters of the Stimulus Initiating the Adrenocortical Response to Hemorrhage, *Ann NY Acad Sci,* **156:**740, 1969.

————: Endocrine Control of Plasma Protein and Volume, *Surg Clin North Am,* **56:**1135, 1976.

————, Baertschi, A. J., Ward, D. G., and Pirkle, J. C., Jr.: Homeostasis of Blood Volume through Hemodynamic Control of ACTH and Cortisol, Endocrinology—Proc V Int'l Congr Endocrinol, in V. H. T. James (ed.), *Excerpta Medica,* vol. 1, p. 245, Amsterdam, 1976.

———— and Cryer, G. L.: Feedback Control of ACTH Secretion by Cortisol, in "Brain-Pituitary-Adrenal Interrelationships," *op. cit.,* p. 197.

————, ————, and Pirkle, J. C., Jr.: Physiological Inhibition and Facilitation of Adrenocortical Response to Hemorrhage, *Am J Physiol,* **232:**R5, 1977.

————, Ward, D. G., Baertschi, A. J., Carlson, D. E., and Maran, J. W.: Neural Control of ACTH Release in Response to Hemorrhage, *Ann NY Acad Sci,* **297:**447, 1977.

Genuth, P., and Lebovitz, H. E.: Stimulation of Insulin Release by Corticotropin, *Endocrinology,* **76:**1093, 1965.

Grizzle, W. E., Dallman, M. F., Schramm, L. P., and Gann, D. S.: Inhibitory and Facilitatory Hypothalamic Areas Mediating ACTH Release in the Cat, *Endocrinology,* **95:**1430, 1974.

————, Johnson, R. N., Schramm, L. P., and Gann, D. S.: Hypothalamic Cells in an Area Mediating ACTH Release Respond to Right Atrial Stretch, *Am J Physiol,* **228:**1039, 1975.

Guillen, J., and Pappas, G.: Improved Cardiovascular Effects of Glucagon in Dogs with Endotoxin Shock, *Ann Surg,* **175:**535, 1972.

Halmagyi, D. F. J., Gillett, D. J., Lazarus, L., and Young, J. D.: Blood Glucose and Serum Insulin in Reversible Post Hemorrhagic Shock, *J Trauma,* **6:**623, 1966.

Henneman, D. H., and Henneman, P. H.: Effects of Human Growth Hormone on Levels of Blood and Urinary Carbohydrate and Fat Metabolites in Man, *J Clin Invest,* **39:**1239, 1960.

Herman, A. H., Mack, E., and Egdahl, R. H.: The Relationship of Adrenal Perfusion to Corticosteroid Secretion in Prolonged Hemorrhagic Shock, *Surg Gynecol Obstet,* **132:**795, 1971.

Hiebert, J. M., Soeldner, J. S., and Egdahl, R. H.: Altered Insulin and Glucose Metabolism Produced by Epinephrine during Hemorrhagic Shock in the Primate, *Surgery,* **74,** 1973.

Hume, D. M.: Hypothalamic Localization for the Control of Various Endocrine Secretions, in H. H. Jasper et al. (eds.), "International Symposium: Reticular Formation of the Brain," p. 231, Little, Brown and Company, Boston, 1958.

————, Bell, C. C., Jr., and Bartter, F.: Direct Measurement of Adrenal Secretion during Operative Trauma and Convalescence, *Surgery,* **52:**174, 1962.

———— and Egdahl, R. H.: Effect of Hypothermia and of Cold Exposure on Adrenal Cortical and Medullary Secretion, *Ann NY Acad Sci,* **80:**435, 1959.

———— and ————: The Importance of the Brain in the Endocrine Response to Injury, *Ann Surg,* **150:**697, 1959.

———— and Nelson, D. H.: Adrenal Cortical Function in Surgical Shock, *Surg Forum,* **5:**568, 1955.

————, ————, and Miller, D. W.: Blood and Urinary 17-Hydroxycorticosteroids in Patients with Severe Burns, *Ann Surg,* **143:**316, 1956.

Ingle, D. J.: Permissive Action of Hormones, *J Clin Endocrinol Metab,* **14:**1272, 1954.

Jones, M. T., Hillhowe, E., and Burden, J.: Secretion of Corticotropin-Releasing Hormone in Vitro, in L. Martini and W. F. Ganong (eds.), *Frontiers in Neuroendocrinology,* **4:**195, 1976.

Kaneto, A., Kajinuma, H. and Kosaka, K.: Effect of Splanchnic Nerve Stimulation on Glucagon and Insulin Output in the Dog, *Endocrinology,* **96:**143, 1975.

Krulich, L., and McCann, S. M.: Influence of Stress on the Growth Hormone (GH) Content of the Pituitary of the Rat, *Proc Soc Exp Biol Med,* **122:**612, 1966.

Kuetnansky, R., and Mikulaj, L.: Adrenal and Urinary Catecholamines in Rats during Adaptation to Repeated Immobilization Stress, *Endocrinology,* **87:**738, 1970.

————, Weise, V. K., and Kopin, I. J.: Effect of Dibutyryl Cyclic-AMP on Adrenal Catecholamine Synthesizing Enzymes in Repeatedly Immobilized Hypophysectomized Rats, *Endocrinology,* **89:**50, 1971.

Madden, J. J., Jr., Ludewig, R. M., and Wangensteen, S. L.: Failure of Glucagon in Experimental Hemorrhagic Shock, *Am J Surg,* **122:**502, 1971.

Martin, J. B.: Brain Regulation of Growth Hormone Secretion, in *Frontiers in Neuroendocrinology, op. cit.,* **5:**129, 1976.

Meyer, W., and Knobil, E.: Growth Hormone Secretion in the Unanesthetized Rhesus Monkey in Response to Noxious Stimuli, *Endocrinology,* **80:**163, 1967.

Moran, W. H., Jr., Miltenberger, F. W., Shuayb, W. A., and Zimmerman, B.: Relationship of Antidiuretic Hormone Secretion to Surgical Stress, *Surgery,* **56:**99, 1964.

Moss, G. S., Cerchio, G., Siegel, D. C., Reed, P. C., Cochin, A., and Fresquez, V.: Decline in Pancreatic Insulin Release during Hemorrhagic Shock in the Baboon, *Ann Surg,* **175:**210, 1972.

Newsome, H. H., Jr.: Pituitary-Adrenal Responsiveness in Surgical Patients on Acute and Chronic Corticosteroid Therapy, *Surgery,* **74,** 1973.

———— and Manalan, S. A.: Plasma Cortisol and Cortisone Concentrations following Postoperative Adrenal Steroid Replacement, *Surgery,* **73:**429, 1973.

Parmley, W. W., Gleck, G., and Sonnenblick, E. H.: Cardiovascular Effects of Glucagon in Man, *N Engl J Med,* **279:**12, 1968.

Price, H. L., Linde, H. W., Jones, R. E., Black, G. W., and Price, M. L.: Sympatho-adrenal Responses to General Anesthesia in Man and Their Relation to Hemodynamics, *Anesthesiology,* **20:**563, 1959.

Sachs, H., Share, L., Osindale, J., and Carpi, A.: Capacity of the Neurohypophysis to Release Vasopressin, *Endocrinology,* **81:**755, 1967.

Samols, E., Tyler, J., Megyesi, C., and Marks, V.: Immunochemical Glucagon in Human Pancreas, Gut, and Plasma, *Lancet,* **2:**727, 1966.

Unger, R. H., Ohneda, A., Valverde, I., Eisentraut, A. M., and Exton, J.: Characterization of the Responses of Circulating Glucagon-like Immunoreactivity to Intraduodenal and Intravenous Administration of Glucose, *J Clin Invest*, **47:**48, 1968.

VanderWall, D. A., Stowe, N. T., Spangenberg, R., and Hook, J. B.: Effect of Glucagon in Hemorrhagic Shock, *J Surg Oncol*, **2:**177, 1970.

Von Euler, U. S.: Adrenal Medullary Secretion and Its Neural Control, in L. Martini and W. F. Ganong (eds.), "Neuroendocrinology," vol. II, Academic Press, Inc., New York, 1967.

Ward, D. G., and Gann, D. S.: Inhibitory and Facilitatory Areas of the Rostral Pons Mediating ACTH Release in the Cat, *Endocrinology*, **99:**1220, 1976.

———, Grizzle, W. E., and Gann, D. S.: Inhibitory and Facilitatory Areas of the Dorsal Medulla Mediating ACTH Release in the Cat, *Endocrinology*, **99:**1213, 1976.

Webb, W. R., Degerli, I. U., Hardy, J. D., and Unal, M.: Cardiovascular Responses in Adrenal Insufficiency, *Surgery*, **58:**273, 1965.

Wilmore, D. W., Long, J. M., Mason, A. D., Shreen, R. W., and Pruitt, B. A.: Catecholamines: Mediator of the Hypermetabolic Responses to Thermal Injury, *Ann Surg*, **180:**653, 1974.

Metabolic Changes: General

Balegno, H. F., and Neuhaus, O. W.: Effect of Insulin on the Injury-stimulated Synthesis of Serum Albumin in the Rat, *Life Sci (II)*, **9:**1039, 1970.

Baue, A. E.: Metabolic Abnormalities of Shock, *Surg Clin North Am*, **56:**1059, 1976.

Bauer, W. E., Vigas, S. N. M., Haist, R. E., and Drucker, W. R.: Insulin Response during Hypovolemic Shock, *Surgery*, **66:**80, 1969.

Blackburn, G. L., Flatt, J. P., Clowes, G. H. A., O'Donnell, T. F., and Hensle, T. E.: Protein Sparing Therapy during Periods of Starvation with Sepsis or Trauma, *Ann Surg*, **177:**588, 1973.

Cahill, G. F., Jr.: Starvation in Man, *N Engl J Med*, **282:**668, 1970.

Carey, L. C., Cloutier, C. T., and Lowery, B. D.: Growth Hormone and Adrenal Cortical Response to Shock and Trauma in the Human, *Ann Surg*, **174:**451, 1971.

Clowes, G. H. A., Jr., O'Donnell, T. F., Blackburn, G. C., and Maki, T. N.: Energy Metabolism and Proteolysis in Traumatized and Septic Man, *Surg Clin North Am*, **56:**1169, 1976.

Conway, M. J., Goodner, C. J., and Werrbach, J. H.: Studies of Substrate Regulation in Fasting: II. Effect of Infusion of Glucose into the Carotid Artery upon Fasting Lipolysis in the Baboon, *J Clin Invest*, **48:**1349, 1969.

Cuthbertson, D., and Tilstone, W. D.: Metabolism during the Post-Injury Period, *Adv Clin Chem*, **12:**1, 1969.

Dale, G., Young, G., Latner, A. L., Goode, A., Tweedle, D., and Johnson, I. D. A.: The Effect of Surgical Operation on Venous Plasma Free Amino Acids, *Surgery*, **81:**295, 1977.

Drucker, W. R., Craig, J., Kingsbury, B., Hofmann, N., and Woodward, H.: Citrate Metabolism during Surgery, *Arch Surg*, **85:**557, 1962.

Duke, J. H., Jr., Jorgensen, S. B., Broell, J. R., Long, C. L., and Kinney, J. M.: Contribution of Protein to Caloric Expenditure following Injury, *Surgery*, **68:**168, 1970.

Exton, J. H., Lewis, S. B., and Park, C. R.: Mechanism of Glucagon Activation of Gluconeogenesis, in H. D. Soling and B. Willms (eds.), "Regulation of Gluconeogenesis," p. 160, Academic Press, Inc., New York, 1971.

Felig, P., Marliss, E., Owen, O. E., and Cahill, G. F., Jr.: Role of Substrate in the Regulation of Hepatic Gluconeogenesis in Fasting Man, *Adv Enzyme Regul*, **7:**41, 1969.

———, Owen, O. E., Wahren, J., and Cahill, G. F., Jr.: Amino Acid Metabolism during Prolonged Starvation, *J Clin Invest*, **48:**584, 1969.

Frohlich, J., and Wieland, O.: Dissociation of Gluconeogenic and Ketogenic Action of Glucagon in the Perfused Rat Liver, in H. D. Soling and B. Willms (eds.), "Regulation of Gluconeogenesis," p. 179, Academic Press, Inc., New York, 1971.

Gump, F. E., Long, C. L., Killian, P., and Kinney, J. M.: Studies of Glucose Intolerance in Septic Injured Patients, *J Trauma*, **14:**378, 1974.

Halmagyi, D. F. J., Neering, I. R., Lazarus, L., Young, J. D., and Pullin, J.: Plasma Glucagon in Experimental Posthemorrhagic Shock, *J Trauma*, **9:**320, 1969.

Hanson, R. W., Patel, M. S., Reshef, L., and Ballard, F. J.: The Role of Pyruvate Carboxylase and *P*-Enolpyruvate Carboxykinase in Rat Adipose Tissue, in H. D. Soling and B. Willms (eds.), "Regulation of Gluconeogenesis," p. 255, Academic Press, Inc., New York, 1971.

Heath, D. F., and Threlfall, C. J.: The Interaction of Glycolysis, Gluconeogenesis and the Tricarboxylic Acid Cycle in Rat Liver in Vivo, *Biochem J*, **110:**337, 1968.

Howard, J. M.: Studies of the Absorption and Metabolism of Glucose following Injury: The Systemic Response to Injury, *Ann Surg*, **141:**321, 1955.

Kinney, J. M., Long, C. L., and Duke, J. H.: Carbohydrate and Nitrogen Metabolism after Injury, in R. Porter and J. Knight (eds.), "Energy: Metabolism in Trauma," p. 123, J. & A. Churchill, London, 1970.

Koj, A.: Synthesis and Turnover of Acute-Phase Reactants, in R. Porter and J. Knight (eds.), "Energy: Metabolism in Trauma," p. 79, J. & A. Churchill, London, 1970.

Levenson, S. M., Pulaski, E. J., and Del Guercio, L. R. M.: Metabolic Changes Associated with Injury, in Zimmerman, L. M., and Levine, R. (eds.), "Physiologic Principles of Surgery," W. B. Saunders Company, Philadelphia, 1964.

McNamara, J. J., Molot, M. D., Dunn, R. A., and Stremple, J. F.: Effect of Hypertonic Glucose in Hypovolemic Shock in Man, *Ann Surg*, **176:**247, 1972.

Mallette, L. E., Exton, J. H., and Park, C. R.: Control of Gluconeogenesis from Amino Acids in the Perfused Rat Liver, *J Biol Chem*, **244:**5713, 1969.

Moss, G. S., Cerchio, G. M., Siegel, D. C., Popovich, P. A., and Butler, E.: Serum Insulin Response in Hemorrhagic Shock in Baboons, *Surgery*, **68:**34, 1970.

Owen, O. E., Morgan, A. P., Kemp, H. G., Sullivan, J. M., Herrera, M. G., and Cahill, G. F., Jr.: Brain Metabolism during Fasting, *J Clin Invest*, **46:**1589, 1967.

Schumer, W., and Sperling, R.: Shock and Its Effect on the Cell, *JAMA*, **205:**215, 1968.

Soling, H. D., Willms, B., and Kleineke, J.: Regulation of Gluconeogenesis in Rat and Guinea Pig Liver, in H. D. Soling and B. Willms (eds.), "Regulation of Gluconeogenesis," p. 210, Academic Press, Inc., New York, 1971.

Stoner, H. B., and Threlfall, C. J. (eds.): "The Biochemical Response to Injury," Charles C Thomas, Publisher, Springfield, Ill., 1960.

Threlfall, C. J., and Stoner, H. B.: Carbohydrate Metabolism in Ischemic Shock, *Q J Exp Physiol,* **39:**1, 1954.

Vaidyanath, N., Birkhahn, R., Border, J. R., McMenamy, R. H., Oswald, G., Trietleg, G., and Yuan, T. F.: The Turnover of Amino Acids in Sepsis and Starvation: Effects of Glucose Infusion, *J Trauma,* **16:**125, 1976.

Wilmore, D. W.: Hormonal Responses and Their Effect on Metabolism, *Surg Clin North Am,* **56:**999, 1976.

Energy Metabolism

Kinney, J. M.: Energy Significance of Weight Loss, in G. S. M. Cowan, Jr., and W. L. Scheetz (eds.), "Intravenous Hyper-alimentation" p. 84, Lea & Febiger, Philadelphia, 1972.

———, Long, C. L., and Duke, J. H.: Carbohydrate and Nitrogen Metabolism after Injury, in R. Porter and J. Knight (eds.), "Energy Metabolism in Trauma," p. 103, J. & A. Churchill, London, 1970.

———, ———, and ———: Energy Demands in the Surgical Patient, in C. L. Fox, Jr., and G. G. Nahos (eds.), "Body Fluid Replacement in Surgical Patient," Grune & Stratton, Inc., New York, 1970.

Mehlman, M. A., and Hanson, R. W., (eds.): "Energy Metabolism and the Regulation of Metabolic Processes in Mitochondria," Academic Press, Inc., New York, 1972.

Porter, R., and Knight, J. (eds.): "Energy Metabolism in Trauma," J. & A. Churchill, London, 1970.

Soling, H. D., and Willms, B. (eds.): "Regulation of Gluconeo-genesis," Academic Press, Inc., New York, 1971.

Wilmore, D. W.: Energy Requirements of Seriously Burned Patients and the Influence of Caloric Intake in Their Metabolic Rate, in G. S. M. Cowan, Jr., and W. L. Scheetz (eds.), "Intravenous Hyperalimentation," p. 96, Lea & Febiger, Philadelphia, 1972.

Starvation

Cahill, G. F., Jr.: Starvation in Man, *N Engl J Med,* **282:**668, 1970.

——— and Aoki, T. T.: The Starvation State and Requirements of the Deficit Economy, in G. S. M. Cowan, Jr. and W. L. Scheetz (eds.), "Intravenous Hyperalimentation," p. 21, Lea & Febiger, Philadelphia, 1972.

———, Felig, P., and Marliss, E. B.: Some Physiological Principles of Parenteral Nutrition, in C. L. Fox, Jr., and G. G. Nahas (eds.), "Body Fluid Replacement in the Surgical Patient," p. 286, Grune & Stratton, New York, 1970.

Owen, O. E., Felig, P., Morgan, A. P., Wahren, J., and Cahill, G. F., Jr.: Liver and Kidney Metabolism during Prolonged Starvation, *J Clin Invest,* **48:**574, 1969.

———, Morgan, A. P., Kemp, H. G., Sullivan, J. M., Herrera, M. G., and Cahill, G. F., Jr.: Brain Metabolism during Fasting, *J Clin Invest,* **46:**1589, 1967.

Sapir, D. G., Owen, O. E., Pozefsky, T., and Walser, M.: Nitrogen Sparing Induced by a Mixture of Essential Amino Acids Given Chiefly as Their Keto-Analogues During Prolonged Starvation in Obese Subjects, *J Clin Invest,* **54:**974, 1974.

Saudek, C. D., and Felig, P.: The Metabolic Events of Starvation, *Am J Med,* **60:**117, 1976.

Carbohydrate Metabolism

Berk, J. L., Hagen, J. F., Beyer, W. H., and Gerber, M. J.: Hypoglycemia of Shock, *Ann Surg,* **171:**400, 1970.

Drucker, W. R.: Carbohydrate Metabolism: The Traumatized versus Normal States, in G. S. M. Cowan and W. L. Scheetz (eds.), "Intravenous Hyperalimentation," p. 55, Lea & Febiger, Philadelphia, 1972.

———, Schlatter, J. E., and Drucker, R. P.: Metabolic Factors Associated with Endotoxin-induced Tolerance for Hemorrhagic Shock, *Surgery,* **64:**75, 1968.

Giddings, A. E.: The Control of Plasma Glucose in the Surgical Patient, *Br J Surg,* **6:**787, 1974.

Green, H. N., and Stoner, H. B.: Effects of Injury on Carbohydrate Metabolism and Energy Transformation, *Br Med J,* **10:**38, 1955.

Jordan, G. L., Jr., Fischer, E. P., and Lefrak, E. A.: Glucose Metabolism in Traumatic Shock in the Human, *Ann Surg,* **175:**685, 1972.

McCoy, S., and Drucker, W. R.: Carbohydrate Metabolism, in W. F. Ballinger, J. A. Collins, W. R. Drucker, S. J. Dadrich, and R. Zeppa (eds.), "Manual of Surgical Nutrition," p. 13, W. B. Saunders Company, Philadelphia, 1975.

Pappova, E., Urbaschek, B., Heitmann, L., Oroz, M., Steit, O. E., Lemeunier, A., and Lundsgaard-Hansen, P.: Energy-rich Phosphates and Glucose Metabolism in Early Endotoxin Shock, *J Surg Res,* **11:**506, 1971.

Rayfield, E. J., Carnow, R. T., George, D. T., and Beisel, W. R.: Impaired Carbohydrate Metabolism during a Mild Viral Illness, *N Eng J Med,* **289:**618, 1975.

Schumer, W.: Metabolic Considerations in the Preoperative Evaluation of the Surgical Patient, *Surg Gynecol Obstet,* **121:**611, 1965.

———: Localization of the Energy Pathway Block in Shock, *Surgery,* 1974.

Taylor, F. H. L., Levenson, S. M., and Adams, M. A.: Abnormal Carbohydrate Metabolism in Human Thermal Burns, *N Engl J Med,* **231:**437, 1944.

Fat Metabolism

Barton, R. N.: Ketone Body Metabolism after Trauma, in R. Porter and J. Knight (eds.), *Ciba Found Symp Energy Metab Trauma,* 1970, p. 173.

Carlson, L. A.: Mobilization and Utilization of Lipids after Trauma: Relation to Caloric Homeostasis, in R. Porter and J. Knight (eds), *Ciba Found Symp Energy Metab Trauma,* 1970, p. 155.

———: Fat Metabolism, in G. S. M. Cowan and W. L. Scheetz, (eds.), "Intravenous Hyperalimentation," p. 68, Lea & Febiger, Philadelphia, 1972.

Coran, A. G., Cryer, P. E., Horwitz, D. L., and Herman, C. M.: The Metabolism of Fat and Carbohydrate during Hemorrhagic Shock in the Unanesthetized Subhuman Primate: Changes in Serum Levels of Free Fatty Acids, Total Lipids, Insulin, and Glucose, *Surgery,* **71:**465, 1972.

Evarts, C. M.: The Fat Embolism Syndrome: A Review, *Surg Clin North Am,* **50:**493, 1970.

Farago, G., Levene, R. A., Lau, T. S., and Drucker, W. R.: Availability of Lipid for Energy Metabolism during Hypovolemia, *Surg Forum,* **22:**7, 1971.

Hansen, O. H.: Fat Embolism and Post-traumatic Diabetes Insipidus, *Acta Chir Scand,* **136**:161, 1970.

Lyman, R. L.: Endocrine Influences on the Metabolism of Polyunsaturated Fatty Acids, *Prog Chem,* **9**:193, 1968.

McGarry, J. D., Wright, P. H., and Foster, D. W.: Hormonal Control of Ketogenesis: Rapid Activation of Hepatic Ketogenic Capacity in Fed Rats by Anti-Insulin Serum and Glucagon, *J Clin Invest,* **55**:1202, 1975.

McKee, A., and Russell, J. A.: Effect of Acute Hypophysectomy and Growth Hormone on FFA Mobilization, Nitrogen Excretion and Cardiac Glycogen in Fasting Rats, *Endocrinology,* **83**:1162, 1968.

McNamara, J. J., Molot, M., Dunn, R., Burran, E. L., and Stremple, J. F.: Lipid Metabolism after Trauma: Role in the Pathogenesis of Fat Embolism, *J Thorac Cardiovasc Surg,* **63**:968, 1972.

Masoro, E. J.: The Effect of Physical Injury on Lipid Metabolism, in H. B. Stoner and C. J. Threlfall (eds.), "The Biochemical Response to Injury," p. 175, Charles C Thomas, Publisher, Springfield, Ill., 1960.

——————: Lipids and Lipid Metabolism, *Annu Rev Physiol,* **39**:301, 1977.

Moore, F. D., Haley, H. B., Bering, E. A., Jr., Brooks, L., and Edelman, I. S.: Further Observations on Total Body Water: II. Changes of Body Composition in Disease, *Surg Gynecol Obstet,* **95**:155, 1952.

Reichard, G. A., Owen, O. E., Huff, A. C., Paul, P., and Bortz, W. M.: Ketone-Body Production and Oxidation in Fasting Obese Humans, *J Clin Invest,* **53**:508, 1974.

Shafrir, E., and Steinberg, D.: The Essential Role of the Adrenal Cortex in the Response of Plasma Free Fatty Acids, Cholesterol, and Phospholipids to Epinephrine Injection, *J Clin Invest,* **39**:310, 1960.

Spergel, G., Bleicher, S. J., and Ertel, N. H.: Carbohydrate and Fat Metabolism in Patients with Pheochromocytoma, *N Engl J Med,* **278**:803, 1968.

Symbas, P. N., Abbott, O. A., and Ende, N.: Surgical Stress and Its Effects on Serum Cholesterol, *Surgery,* **61**:221, 1967.

Wadström, L. B.: Effect of Glucose Infusion on Plasma Lipids in Newly Operated Patients, *Acta Chir Scand,* **116**:395, 1958.

Wilmore, D. W.: Fat Metabolism, in W. F. Ballinger, J. A. Collins, W. R. Drucker, S. J. Dadrich, and R. Zeppa (eds.), "Manual of Surgical Nutrition," p. 33, W. B. Saunders Company, Philadelphia, 1975.

Protein Metabolism

Browne, J. S. L., and Schenker, V.: "Conferences on Metabolic Aspects of Convalescence Including Bone and Wound Healing: Transactions of Third Meeting," p. 162, Josiah Macy, Jr. Foundation Publications, New York, 1943.

Buse, M. G., and Reid, S. S.: Leacine: A Possible Regulator of Protein Turnover in Muscle, *J Clin Invest,* **56**:1250, 1975.

Cannon, P. R., Wissler, R. W., Woolride, R. L., and Benditt, E. P.: Relationship of Protein Deficiency to Surgical Infection, *Ann Surg,* **120**:514, 1944.

Clarke, H. C. M., Freeman, T., and Pryse-Phillips, W.: Serum Protein Changes after Injury, *Clin Sci,* **40**:337, 1971.

Costa, G., Ullrich, L., Kantor, F., and Holland, J. F.: Production of Elemental Nitrogen by Certain Mammals including Man, *Nature (Lond),* **218**:546, 1968.

Cuthbertson, D. P.: Further Observations on Disturbance of Metabolism Caused by Injury, with Particular Reference to Dietary Requirements of Fracture Cases, *Br J Surg,* **23**:505, 1936.

Davies, J. W. L., Bull, J. P., and Ricketts, C. R.: Catabolic Response to Injury, *Lancet,* **2**:320, 1971.

Flear, C. T. G., and Clarke, R.: The Influence of Blood Loss and Blood Transfusion upon Changes in the Metabolism of Water, Electrolytes and Nitrogen Following Civilian Trauma, *Clin Sci,* **14**:575, 1955.

Fleck, A.: Protein Metabolism after Injury, *Proc Nutr Soc,* **30**:152, 1971.

Fulks, R. M., Li, J. B., and Goldberg, A. L.: Effects of Insulin, Glucose and Amino Acids on Protein Turnover in Rat Diaphragm, *J Biol Chem,* **250**:290, 1975.

Hinton, P., Allison, S. P., Littlejohn, S., and Lloyd, J.: Insulin and Glucose to Reduce Catabolic Response to Injury in Burned Patients, *Lancet,* **1**:767, 1971.

Howard, J. E., Bingham, R. S., Jr., and Mason, R. E.: Studies on Convalescence: IV. Nitrogen and Mineral Balances during Starvation and Graduated Feeding in Healthy Young Males at Bed Rest, *Trans Assoc Am Physicians,* **59**:242, 1946.

Kekomaki, M., and Louhimo, I.: Observations on Plasma Amino Acid Concentrations during Haemorrhagic Shock in the Rabbit, *Ann Chir Gynaecol Fenn,* **60**:214, 1971.

Kukral, J. C., Riveron, E., Tiffany, J. C., Vaitys, S., and Barrett, B.: Plasma Protein Metabolism in Patients with Acute Surgical Peritonitis, *Am J Surg,* **113**:173, 1967.

Levenson, S. M., Howard, J. M., and Rosen, I. T.: Studies of the Plasma Amino Acids and Amino Conjugates in Patients with Severe Battle Wounds, *Surg Gynecol Obstet,* **101**:35, 1955.

—————— and Watkin, D. M.: Protein Requirements in Injury and Certain Acute and Chronic Diseases, *Fed Proc,* **18**:1155, 1959.

Munro, H. N., and Allison, J. B. (eds.): "Mammalian Protein Metabolism," Academic Press, Inc., New York, 1964.

—————— and Chalmers, M. I.: Fracture Metabolism at Different Levels of Protein Intake, *Br J Exp Pathol,* **26**:396, 1945.

Sherwin, R. S., Hendler, R. G., and Felig, P.: Effect of Ketone Infusions on Amino Acid and Nitrogen Metabolism in Man, *J Clin Invest,* **55**:1382, 1975.

Restitution of Blood Volume

Boyd, D. R., and Mansberger, A. R.: Serum Water and Osmolal Changes in Hemorrhagic Shock: An Experimental and Clinical Study, *Am Surg,* **34**:744, 1968.

Cope, O., and Litwin, S. B.: Contributions of the Lymphatic System to the Replenishment of the Plasma Volume Following a Hemorrhage, *Ann Surg,* **156**:655, 1962.

Deaux, E., and Kakolewski, J. W.: Emotionally Induced Increases in Effective Osmotic Pressure and Subsequent Thirst, *Science,* **169**:1226, 1970.

Gann, D. S.: Endocrine Control of Plasma Protein and Volume, *Surg Clin North Am,* **56**:1135, 1976.

—————— and Pirkle, J. C., Jr.: Role of Cortisol in the Restitution of Blood Volume after Hemorrhage, *Am J Surg,* **130**:565, 1975.

Pirkle, J. C., Jr., and Gann, D. S.: Restitution of Blood Volume After Hemorrhage: Mathematical Description, *Am J Physiol,* **228**:821, 1975.

—————— and ——————: Restitution of Blood Volume after Hemorrhage: Role of the Adrenal Cortex, *Am J Physiol*, **230**:1683, 1976.

——— and ———: Pituitary and Adrenal Glands Are Required for Full Restitution of Blood Volume after Hemorrhage, *Fed Proc*, **35**:637, 1976.

Skillman, J. J., Amwad, H. K., and Moore, F. D.: Plasma Protein Kinetics of the Early Transcapillary Refill after Hemorrhage, *Surg Gynecol Obstet*, **125**:983, 1967.

Stewart, J. D., and Rourke, M. G.: Intracellular Fluid Loss in Hemorrhage, *J Clin Invest*, **15**:697, 1936.

Zollinger, R. M., Jr.: Plasma Volume and Protein Restoration after Hemorrhage: Role of the Left Thoracic Duct versus Transcapillary Refilling, *J Surg Res*, **12**:151, 1972.

Wound Healing

Azar, M. M., and Good, R. A.: The Inhibitory Effect of Vitamin A on Complement Levels and Tolerance Production, *J Immunol*, **106**:241, 1971.

Calloway, D. H., Grossman, M. I., Bowman, J., and Calhoun, W. K.: Effect of Previous Level of Protein Feeding on Wound Healing and on Metabolic Response to Injury, *Surgery*, **37**:935, 1955.

Carnes, W. H.: Role of Copper in Connective Tissue Metabolism, *Fed Proc*, **30**:995, 1971.

Chernov, M. S., Hale, H. W., and Wood, M.: Prevention of Stress Ulcers, *Am J Surg*, **122**:674, 1971.

Cohen, B., and Cohen, I. K.: "Vitamin A: Adjuvant and Steroid Antagonist in the Immune Response," Plastic Surgery Research Council, St. Louis, May, 1973.

Cohen, I. K., Schechter, P. J., and Henkin, R. I.: Hypogeusia, Anorexia, and Altered Zinc Metabolism following Thermal Burn, *JAMA*, **223**:914, 1973.

Harris, E. D., and Sjoerdsma, A.: Effect of Penicillamine on Human Collagen and Its Possible Application in Treatment of Scleroderma, *Lancet*, **2**:996, 1966.

Hsu, T. H. S., and Hsu, J. M.: Zinc Deficiency and Epithelial Wound Repair: An Autoradiographic Study of 3H-Thymidine Incorporation, *Proc Soc Exp Biol Med*, **140**:157, 1972.

Hunt, T. K., Ehrlich, H. P., Garcia, J. A., and Dunphy, J. E.: Effect of Vitamin A on Reversing the Inhibitory Effect of Cortisone on Healing of Open Wounds in Animals and Man, *Ann Surg*, **170**:633, 1969.

———, Niinikoski, J., and Zederfeldt, B.: Role of Oxygen in Repair Processes, *Acta Chir Scand*, **138**:109, 1972.

Hutcher, N., Silverberg, S. G., and Lee, H. M.: The Effect of Vitamin A on the Formation of Steroid Induced Gastric Ulcers, *Surg Forum*, **22**:322, 1971.

Levenson, S. M., Green, R. W., Taylor, F. H. L., Robinson, P., Page, R. C., Johnson, R. E., and Lund, C. C.: Ascorbic Acid, Riboflavin, Thiamine, and Nicotinic Acid in Relation to Severe Injury, Hemorrhage and Infection in the Human, *Ann Surg*, **124**:840, 1946.

———, Pirani, C. L., Braasch, J. W., and Waterman, D. F.: The Effect of Thermal Burns on Wound Healing, *Surg Gynecol Obstet*, **99**:74, 1954.

———, Upjohn, H. L., Preston, J. A., and Steer, A.: Effect of Thermal Burns on Wound Healing, *Ann Surg*, **146**:357, 1957.

Niinikoski, J., Henghan, C., and Hunt, T. K.: Oxygen Tensions in Human Wounds, *J Surg Res*, **12**:77, 1972.

Quarantillo, E. P., Jr.: Effect of Supplemental Zinc on Wound Healing in Rats, *Am J Surg*, **121**:661, 1971.

Siegel, R. C., Pinnell, S. R., and Martin, G.: Cross-linking of Collagen and Elastin: Properties of Lysyl Oxidase, *Biochemistry*, **9**:4486, 1970.

Stein, H. D., and Keiser, H. R.: Collagen Metabolism in Granulating Wounds, *J Surg Res*, **11**:277, 1971.

Stephens, F. P., Hunt, T. K., Jawetz, E., Sonne, M., and Duphy, J. E.: Effect of Cortisone and Vitamin A on Wound Infection, *Am J Surg*, **121**:569, 1971.

Sullivan, J. F., and Eisenstein, A. B.: Ascorbic Acid Depletion during Hemodialysis. *JAMA*, **220**:1697, 1972.

Williamson, M. B., McCarthy, T. H., and Fromm, H. J.: Relation of Protein Nutrition to the Healing of Experimental Wounds, *Proc Soc Exp Biol Med*, **77**:302, 1951.

Udupa, K. N., Woessner, J. F., and Dunphy, J. E.: The Effect of Methionine on the Production of Mucopolysaccharides and Collagen in Healing Wounds of Protein-depleted Animals, *Surg Gynecol Obstet*, **102**:639, 1956.

Nutritional Supplementation

Abbott, W. E., Krieger, H., and Levey, S.: Postoperative Metabolic Changes in Relation to Nutritional Regimen, *Lancet*, **1**:704, 1958.

Abel, R. M., Beck, C. H., Jr., Abbott, W. M., Ryan, J. A., Jr., Barnett, G. O., and Fischer, J. E.: Improved Survival from Acute Renal Failure after Treatment with Intravenous Essential L-Amino Acids and Glucose, *N Engl J Med*, **288**:695, 1973.

Allen, J. G., Stemmer, E. A., and Head, L. R.: Similar Growth Rates of Littermate Puppies Maintained on Oral Protein with Those on the Same Quantity of Protein as Daily Intravenous Plasma for 99 Days as Only Protein Source, *Ann Surg*, **144**:349, 1956.

Blackburn, G. L., and Bistrian, B. R.: Nutritional Care of the Injured and/or Septic Patient, *Surg Clin North Am*, **56**:1195, 1976.

Brennan, M. F., Goldman, M. H., O'Connell, R. C., Kundsin, R. B., and Moore, F. D.: Prolonged Parenteral Alimentation: Candida Growth and the Prevention of Candidemia by Amphotericin Installation, *Ann Surg*, **176**:265, 1972.

Burr, A. O. and Burr, M. M.: A New Deficiency Disease Produced by the Rigid Exclusion of Fat from the Diet, *J Biol Chem*, **82**:345, 1929.

Cahill, G. F., Jr., and Aoki, T. T.: The Starvation State and Requirements of the Deficit Economy, in G. S. M. Cowan, Jr., and W. L. Scheetz (eds.), "Intravenous Hyperalimentation," p. 20, Lea & Febiger, Philadelphia, 1972.

———, Felig, P., and Marliss, E. B.: Some Physiological Principles of Parenteral Nutrition, in C. L. Fox, Jr. and G. G. Nahas (eds.), "Body Fluid Replacement in the Surgical Patient," p. 286, Grune & Stratton, Inc., New York, 1970.

Caldwell, M. D., Jonnsson, H. T., and Othersen, H. B., Jr.: Essential Fatty Acid Deficiency in an Infant Receiving Prolonged Parenteral Alimentation, *J Pediatr*, **81**:894, 1972.

Collins, F. D., Sinclair, A. J., and Royle, J. P.: Plasma Lipids in Human Linoleic Acid Deficiency, *Nutr Metabol*, **13**:150, 1971.

Cowan, G. S. M., Jr., and Scheetz, W. L. (eds.): "Intravenous Hyperalimentation," Lea & Febiger, Philadelphia, 1972.

Deitrick, J. E., Whedun, G. D., and Shorr, E.: Effects of Immobilization upon Various Metabolic and Physiologic Functions of Normal Men, *Am J Med,* **4:**3, 1948.

Dudrick, S. J., Wilmore, D. W., Vars, H. M., and Rhoads, J. E.: Long Term Total Parenteral Nutrition with Growth, Development and Positive Nitrogen Balance, *Surgery,* **64:**134, 1968.

———, MacFadyen, B. V., VanBuren, C. T., Ruberg, R. L., and Maynard, A. T.: Parenteral Hyperalimentation: Metabolic Problems and Solutions, *Ann Surg,* **176:**259, 1972.

———, Steiger, E., and Long, J. M.: Renal Failure in Surgical Patients: Treatment with Intravenous Essential Amino Acids and Hypertonic Glucose, *Surgery,* **68:**180, 1970.

———, ———, ———, Ruberg, R. L., Allen, T. R., Vars, H. M., and Rhoads, J. E.: General principles and techniques of intravenous hyperalimentation, in G. S. M. Cowan, Jr., and W. L. Scheetz (eds.), "Intravenous Hyperalimentation," p. 2, Lea & Febiger, Philadelphia, 1972.

Feller, I.: The Use of Plasma and Albumin in the Burned Patient, in C. L. Fox, Jr., and G. G. Nahas (eds.), "Body Fluid Replacement in the Surgical Patient," p. 153. Grune & Stratton, Inc., New York, 1970.

Fox, C. L., Jr., and Nahas, G. G. (eds.): "Body Fluid Replacement in the Surgical Patient," Grune & Stratton, Inc., New York, 1970.

Gann, D. S., and Robinson, H. B.: Salt, Water, and Vitamins, in W. F. Ballinger et al. (eds.), "Manual of Surgical Nutrition," p. 73, W. B. Saunders Company, Philadelphia, 1975.

Giordano, C.: Use of Exogenous and Endogenous Urea for Protein Synthesis in Normal and Uremic Subjects, *J Lab Clin Med,* **62:**321, 1963.

Giovannetti, S., and Maggiore, Q.: A Low Nitrogen Diet with Protein of High Biological Value for Severe Chronic Uremia, *Lancet,* **1:**1000, 1964.

Greenstein, J. P., Otey, M. C., Birnbaum, S. M., and Winitz, M.: Quantitative Nutritional Studies with Water-Soluble, Chemically Defined Diets: X. Formulation of a Nutritionally Complete Liquid Diet, *J Natl Cancer Inst,* **24:**211, 1960.

Hamilton, R. F., Davis, W. T., Stephenson, D. V., and McGee, D. F.: Effects of Parenteral Hyperalimentation on Upper Gastrointestinal Tract Secretions, *Arch Surg,* **102:**348, 1971.

Heird, W. C., Dell, R. B., Driscoll, J. M., Jr., Grebin, B., and Winters, R. W.: Metabolic Acidosis Resulting from Intravenous Alimentation Mixtures Containing Synthetic Amino Acids, *N Engl J Med,* **287:**943, 1972.

Holden, W. D., Krieger, H., Levey, S., and Abbott, W. E.: The Effect of Nutrition on Nitrogen Metabolism in the Surgical Patient, *Ann Surg,* **146:**563, 1957.

Holman, R. T.: Essential Fatty Acid Deficiency, *Prog Chem Toxicol,* **9:**279, 1968.

Host, W. H., Serlin, O., and Rush, B. F., Jr.: Hyperalimentation in Cirrhotic Patients, *Am J Surg,* **123:**57, 1972.

Jacobson, S., and Wretling, A.: The Use of Fat Emulsions for Complete Intravenous Nutrition, in C. L. Fox, Jr., and G. G. Nahas (eds.), "Body Fluid Replacement in the Surgical Patient," p. 334, Grune & Stratton, Inc., New York, 1970.

Kekomaki, M., Louhimo, I., Rahiala, E. L., and Suutarinen, T.: Comparison of Fructose and Glucose Solutions in the Treatment of Hypovolemic Shock in Rabbits, *Acta Chir Scand,* **138:**239, 1972.

Kinney, J. M., Long, C. L., and Duke, J. H., Jr.: Energy Demands in the Surgical Patient, in C. L. Fox and G. G. Nahas (eds.),

"Body Fluid Replacement in the Surgical Patient," p. 296, Grune & Stratton, Inc., New York, 1970.

Long, J. M., Dudrick, S. J., Steiger, E., Ruberg, R. L., and Allen, T. R.: Use of Intravenous Hyperalimentation in Patients with Renal or Liver Failure, in G. S. M. Cowan, Jr., and W. L. Scheetz (eds.), "Intravenous Hyperalimentation," p. 147, Lea & Febiger, Philadelphia, 1972.

Meng, H. C., and Early, F.: Study of Complete Parenteral Alimentation on Dogs, *J Lab Clin Med,* **34:**1121, 1949.

Munro, H. N.: Adaptation of Mammalian Protein Metabolism to Hyperalimentation, in G. S. M. Cowan, Jr., and W. L. Scheetz (eds.), "Intravenous Hyperalimentation," p. 34, Lea & Febiger, Philadelphia, 1972.

Ravdin, I. S., McNamee, H. G., Kamholz, J. H., and Rhoads, J. E.: Effect of Hypoproteinemia on Susceptibility to Shock Resulting from Hemorrhage, *Arch Surg,* **48:**491, 1944.

Rose, W. C., and Dekker, E. E.: Urea as a Source of Nitrogen for the Biosynthesis of Amino Acids, *J Biol Chem,* **223:**107, 1956.

Schumer, W.: High Calorie Solutions in Traumatized Patients, in C. L. Fox, Jr. and G. G. Nahas (eds.), "Body Fluid Replacement in the Surgical Patient, p. 326, Grune & Stratton, Inc., New York, 1970.

Scribbner, B. H., Cole, J. J., Christopher, P. H., Vizzo, J. E., Atkins, R. C., and Blagg, C. R.: Long Term Total Parenteral Nutrition: The Concept of an Artificial Gut, *JAMA,* **212:**457, 1970.

Stemmer, E. A., Allen, J. G., and Connolly, J. E.: Nutritional Value of Blood Plasma Protein: Growth in Puppies on Intravenous Diets of Plasma, Red Cells and Amino Acid, *Am Surg,* **32:**665, 1966.

———, ———, and ———: Value of Blood Plasma in Restoring Plasma Proteins in the Depleted Surgical Patient, *Am J Surg,* **112:**251, 1966.

Terry, R., Sandrock, W. E., Nye, R. E., and Whipple, G. H.: Parenteral Plasma Protein Maintains Nitrogen Equilibrium over Long Periods, *J Exp Med,* **87:**547, 1948.

Walser, M., Sapir, D. G., and Maddrey, W. C.: The Use of Alpha-Keto Analogues of Essential Amino Acids, in J. Fischer (ed.), "Total Parenteral Nutrition," Little, Brown and Company, Boston, 1976.

Whedon, G. D., Deitrick, J. E., and Shorr, E.: Modification of the Effects of Immobilization upon Metabolic Physiologic Functions of Normal Men by the Use of an Oscillating Bed, *Am J Med,* **6:**684, 1949.

Wilkinson, A. W.: Restriction of Fluid Intake after Partial Gastrectomy, *Lancet,* **2:**428, 1956.

Wilmore, D. W., Curreri, W., Spitzer, K. W., Spitzer, M. E., and Pruitt, B. A.: Supra-normal Dietary Intake in Thermally Injured Hypermetabolic Patients, *Surg Gynecol Obstet,* **132:**881, 1971.

Yuile, C. L., O'Dea, A. E., Lucas, F. V., and Whipple, G. H.: Plasma Protein Labeled with Lysine-E-D$_{14}$: Its Oral Feeding and Relating Protein Metabolism in the Dog, *J Exp Med,* **96:**247, 1952.

Component Therapy

Clark, I. C., Jr.: Symposium on Inert Organic Liquids for Biological Oxygen Transport, *Atlantic City, New Jersey, April 13, 1969, Fed Proc,* **29:**1698, 1970.

——— and Gollan, F.: Survival of Mammals Breathing Organic Liquids Equilibrated with Oxygen at Atmospheric Pressure, *Science,* **152:**1755, 1966.

Geyer, R. P.: Whole Animal Perfusion with Fluorocarbon Dispersions, *Fed Proc,* **29:**1758, 1970.

———: The Design of Artificial Blood Substitutes, in E. J. Ariens (ed.), "Drug Design," Academic Press, New York, 1976.

———, Monroe, R. G., and Taylor, K.: Survival of Rats Totally Perfused with a Fluorocarbon-Detergent Preparation, in J. Folkman, W. G. Hardison, L. E. Rudolf, and F. J. Veith (eds.), "Organ Perfusion and Preservation," p. 85, Appleton-Century-Crofts, New York, 1968.

Modell, J. H., Newby, E. J., and Ruiz, B. C.: Long Term Survival of Dogs after Breathing Oxygenated Fluorocarbon Liquid, *Fed Proc,* **29:**1731, 1970.

Moss, G. S.: Massive Transfusion of Frozen Processed Red Cells in Combat Casualties: Report of Three Cases, *Surgery,* **66:**1008, 1969.

———, Cochin, A., and DeWoskin, R.: "Pure" Hemoglobin Solution: Coagulability Changes Produced In Vitro, *Surgery,* **74,** 1973.

Patel, M. M., Patel, M. K., Szanto, P,, Alrenga, D. P., and Long, D. M.: Ventilation with Synthetic Fluids, *Surg Clin North Am,* **51:**25, 1971.

Sloviter, H. A.: Erythrocyte Substitutes, *Med Clin North Am,* **54:** 787, 1970.

———, Petkovic, M., Ogoshi, S., and Yamada, H.: Dispersed Fluorochemicals as Substitutes for Erythrocytes in Intact Animals, *J Appl Physiol,* **27:**666, 1969.

———, Yamada, H., and Ogoshi, S.: Some Effects of Intravenously Administered Dispersed Fluorochemicals in Animals, *Fed Proc,* **29:**1755, 1970.

Acid-Base Balance, Salt, and Water

Astrup, P., Jorgensen, K., Siggaard-Andersen, O., and Engel, K.: The Acid-Base Metabolism: A New Approach, *Lancet,* **1:**1035, 1960.

Barry, K. G., and Malloy, J. P.: Oliguric Renal Failure: Evaluation and Therapy by Intravenous Infusion of Mannitol, *JAMA,* **179:**510, 1962.

Bergentz, S.-E., and Brief, D. K.: The Effect of pH and Osmolality on the Production of Canine Hemorrhagic Shock, *Surgery,* **58:**412, 1965.

Bishop, R. L., and Weisfeldt, M. L.: Sodium Bicarbonate Administration during Cardiac Arrest, *JAMA,* **235:**506, 1976.

Blackburn, G. L., and Schloerb, P. R.: Intracellular Acid-Base Regulation in Hypoxia, *Arch Surg,* **93:**573, 1966.

Bleich, H. L., Tanner, R. L., and Schwartz, W. B.: The Induction of Metabolic Alkalosis by Correction of Potassium Deficiency, *J Clin Invest,* **45:**573, 1966.

Bradley, M. N.: Profound Shock Associated with Acidosis: Occurrence and Treatment, *Am Surg,* **30:**589, 1964.

Broder, G., and Weil, M. H.: Excess Lactate: Index of Reversibility of Shock in Human Patients, *Science,* **143:**1457, 1964.

Broido, P. W., Butcher, H. R., Jr., and Moyer, C. A.: A Bioassay of Treatment of Hemorrhagic Shock: II. The Expansion of Volume Distribution of Extracellular Ions during Hemorrhagic Hypotension and Its Possible Relationship to Change in Physical-Chemical Properties of Extravascular-Extracellular Tissue, *Arch Surg,* **93:**556, 1966.

Chazan, J. A., Stenson, R., and Kurland, G. S.: Acidosis of Cardiac Arrest, *N Engl J Med,* **278:**360, 1968.

Collins, J. A.: Effect of Massive Blood Transfusions on Acid-Base Status of Combat Casualties in Vietnam, in C. L. Fox, Jr., and G. G. Nahas (eds.), "Body Fluid Replacement in the Surgical Patient," p. 72, Grune & Stratton, Inc., New York, 1970.

———, Simmons, R. L., James, P. M., Bredenberg, C. E., Anderson, R. W., and Heisterkamp, C. A.: Acid-Base Status of Seriously Wounded Combat Casualties: II. Resuscitation with Stored Blood, *Ann Surg,* **173:**6, 1971.

Crandall, W. B., and Stueck, G. H., Jr.: Acid-Base Balance in Surgical Patients: I. A Survey of 62 Selected Cases, *Ann Surg,* **149:**342, 1959.

Cunningham, J. N., Shires, G. T., and Wagner, Y.: Changes in Intracellular Sodium and Potassium Content of Red Blood Cells in Trauma and Shock, *Am J Surg,* **122:**650, 1971.

DeWardener, H. E.: The Control of Sodium Excretion, in J. Orloff and R. W. Berliner (eds.), "Handbook of Physiology," sec. 8, Renal Physiology, p. 721, American Physiological Society, Washington, 1973.

Dillion, J., Lynch, L. J., Jr., Myers, R., Butcher, H. R., Jr., and Moyer, C. A.: Bioassay of Treatment of Hemorrhagic Shock, *Arch Surg,* **93:**537, 1966.

Dudley, H. F., Boling, E. A., LeQuesne, L. P., and Moore, F. D.: Studies on Antidiuresis in Surgery: Effects of Anesthesia, Surgery and Posterior Pituitary Antidiuretic Hormone on Water Metabolism in Man, *Ann Surg,* **140:**354, 1954.

Earley, L. E., and Schrier, R. W.: Intrarenal Control of Sodium Excretion by Hemodynamic and Physical Factors, in J. Orloff and R. W. Berliner (eds.), "Handbook of Physiology," sec. 8, Renal Physiology, p. 677, American Physiological Society, Washington, 1973.

Eichenholz, A., Mulhausen, R. O., Anderson, W. E., and MacDonald, F. M.: Primary Hypocapnia: A Cause of Metabolic Acidosis, *J Appl Physiol,* **17:**283, 1962.

Flemma, R. J., and Young, W. G., Jr.: The Metabolic Effects of Mechanical Ventilation and Respiratory Alkalosis in Postoperative Patients, *Surgery,* **56:**36, 1964.

Gann, D. S., and Wright, H. K.: Augmentation of Sodium Excretion in Postoperative Patients by Expansion of the Extracellular Fluid Volume, *Surg Gynecol Obstet,* **118:**1024, 1964.

——— and ———: Effects of Trauma on Sodium Metabolism and Urinary Concentrating Ability, *J Surg Res,* **6:**93, 1965.

——— and ———: Increased Renal Sodium Reabsorption After Depletion of the Extracellular or Nitrovascular Fluid Volumes, *J Surg Res,* **6:**196, 1966.

———, ———, and Newsome, H. H.: Prevention of Sodium Depletion during Osmotic Diuresis, *Surg Gynecol Obstet,* **119:**265, 1964.

Gill, J. R., Jr.: The Role of the Sympathetic Nervous System in the Regulation of Sodium Excretion by the Kidney, in W. F. Ganong and L. Martini (eds.), "Frontiers in Neuroendocrinology," p. 289, Oxford University Press, New York, 1969.

Greenberg, A. G., and Kittle, C. F.: The Effects of Acute Changes in Acid-Base Status on Coronary Blood Flow, *Surgery,* **64:** 315, 1968.

Gruber, U. F., Smith, L. L., and Moore, F. D.: The Effect of Acute Addition Metabolic Alkalosis on the Cardiovascular Response of the Dog to Hemorrhage, *J Surg Res,* **3:**21, 1963.

Gump, F. E., and Kinney, J. M.: Measurement of Water Balance: A Guide to Surgical Care, *Surgery,* **64:**154, 1968.

Hardaway, R. M., James, P. M., Jr., Anderson, R. W., Bredenberg, C. E., and West, R. L.: Intensive Study and Treatment of Shock in Man, *JAMA,* **199:**779, 1967.

Heaton, F. W., Clark, C. G., and Coligher, J. C.: Magnesium Deficiency Complicating Intestinal Surgery, *Br J Surg,* **54:**41, 1967.

Hoye, R. C., Ketcham, A. S., and Berlin, N. I.: Total Red Cell and Plasma Volume Alterations Occurring with Extensive Surgery in Humans, *Surg Gynecol Obstet,* **123:**27, 1966.

Huckabee, W. E.: Abnormal Resting Blood Lactate: I. The Significance of Hyperlactalemia in Hospitalized Patients, *Am J Med.,* **30:**833, 1961.

Kassirer, J. P., Berkman, P. M., Lawrenz, D. R., and Schwartz, W. B.: The Critical Role of Chloride in the Correction of Hypokalemic Alkalosis in Man, *Am J Med,* **38:**172, 1965.

Litwin, M. S., Smith, L. L., and Moore, F. D.: Metabolic Alkalosis following Massive Transfusion, *Surgery,* **45:**805, 1959.

Lyons, J. H., Jr., and Moore, F. D.: Posttraumatic Alkalosis: Incidence and Pathophysiology of Alkalosis in Surgery, *Surgery,* **60:**93, 1966.

MacLean, L. D., Mulligan, W. G., McLean, A. P. H., and Duff, J. H.: Patterns of Septic Shock in Man: A Detailed Study of 56 Patients, *Ann Surg,* **166:**543, 1967.

Peaston, M. J. T.: Metabolic Acidosis in Burns, *Br Med J,* **1:**809, 1968.

Pullen, H., Doig, A., and Lambie, A. T.: Intensive Intravenous Potassium Replacement Therapy, *Lancet,* **2:**809, 1967.

Rector, F. C., Jr., Bloomer, H. A., and Seldin, D. W.: Effect of Potassium Deficiency on the Reabsorption of Bicarbonate in the Proximal Tubule of the Rat Kidney, *J Clin Invest,* **43:**1976, 1964.

Robbins, H. S., and Dufrene, J. H.: Hyperkalemia in Anesthesia, *Pa Med,* **75:**77, 1972.

Schlobohm, R. M., and Holaday, D. A.: Prevention and Correction of Acidosis, in C. L. Fox, Jr., and G. G. Nahas (eds.), "Body Fluid Replacement in the Surgical Patient," p. 246, Grune & Stratton, Inc., New York, 1970.

Siggaard-Andersen, O.: The Acid-Base Status of Blood, *Scand J Clin Lab Invest,* **15**(*Suppl* 70):1, 1963.

Wacker, W. E. C., and Parisi, A. F.: Magnesium Metabolism, *N Engl J Med,* **278:**712, 1968.

Wright, H. K., and Gann, D. S.: Correction of the Force Water Defect in Postoperative Patients by Extracellular Fluid Volume Expansion, *Ann Surg,* **158:**70, 1963.

——— and ———: A Defect in Urinary Concentrating Ability during Postoperative Antidiuresis, *Surg Gynecol Obstet,* **121:**47, 1965.

Oxygen Transport

Benesch, R., and Benesch, R.: Intracellular Organic Phosphates as Regulators of Oxygen Release by Haemoglobin, *Nature,* (*Lond*), **221:**618, 1969.

Naylor, B. A., Welch, M. H., Shafer, A. W., and Cuenter, C. A.: Blood Affinity for Oxygen in Hemorrhagic and Endotoxic Shock, *J Appl Physiol,* **32:**829, 1972.

Plzak, L. F.: Hyperalimentation and the Oxy-hemoglobin Dissociation Curve, in G. S. M. Cowan, Jr., and W. L. Scheetz, (eds.) "Intravenous Hyperalimentation," p. 196, Lea & Febiger, Philadelphia, 1972.

Proctor, H. J., Lentz, R. R., and Johnson, G., Jr.: Alterations in Baboon Erythrocyte 2,3-Diphosphoglycerate Concentration Associated with Hemorrhagic Shock and Resuscitation, *Ann Surg,* **174:**923, 1971.

Shoemaker, W. C., Boyd, D. R., Kim, S. I., Brown, R. S., Dreiling, D. A., and Kark, A. E.: Sequential Oxygen Transport and Acid-Base Changes after Trauma to the Unanesthetized Patient, *Surg Gynecol Obstet,* **132:**1033, 1971.

Sugerman, H., Miller, L. D., Oski, F. A., Diaco, J., Delivoria-Papadopoulos, M., and Davidson, D.: Decreased 2,3-Diphosphoglycerate (DPG) and Reduced Oxygen (O_2) Consumption in Septic Shock, *Clin Res,* **18:**418, 1970.

Travis, S. F., Sugerman, H. J., Ruberg, R. L., Dudrick, S. J., Delivoria-Papadopoulos, M. D., Miller, L. D., and Oski, F. A.: Alterations of Red Cell Poikilitic Intermediates and Oxygen Transport as a Consequence of Hypophosphatemia in Patients Receiving Intravenous Hyperalimentation, *N Engl J Med,* **285:**763, 1971.

Immunologic Protective Mechanisms

Bell, M. L., Herman, A. H., Egdahl, R. H., Smith, E. E., and Rutenburg, A. M.: Role of Lysosomal Disruption in the Development of Refractory Shock, *Surg Forum,* **21:**10, 1970.

Greyson, N. D., Rhodes, B. A., Buchanan, J. W., and Wagner, H. N., Jr.: Local Increases in Reticuloendothelial Function during Healing, *J Reticuloendothel Soc,* **11:**293, 1972.

Hawley, P. R.: The Role of Trauma in the Development of Peritonitis and the Protection Afforded by Intravenous Dextran Solutions, *Br J Surg,* **58:**305, 1971.

Liedberg, C. F.: Antibacterial Resistance in Burns: II. The Effect on Unspecific Humoral Defense Mechanisms, Phagocytosis and the Development of Bacteremia, *Acta Chir Scand,* **121:**351, 1961.

Munster, A. M., Eurenius, K., Mortensen, R. F., and Mason, A. D.: Ability of Splenic Lymphocytes from Injured Rats to Induce a Graft-versus-Host Reaction, *Transplantation,* **14:**106, 1972.

———, ———, Katz, R. M., Canales, L., Foley, F. D., and Mortensen, R. F.: Cell-mediated Immunity after Thermal Injury, *Ann Surg,* **177:**139, 1973.

Palmerio, C., and Fine, J.: The Nature of Resistance to Shock, *Arch Surg,* **98:**679, 1969.

Pillemer, L., Schoenberg, M. D., Blum, L., and Wurz, L.: Properdin System and Immunity: II. Interaction of the Properdin System with Polysaccharides, *Science,* **122:**545, 1955.

Schildt, B. E.: Function of the RES after Thermal and Mechanical Trauma in Mice, *Acta Chir Scand,* **136:**359, 1970.

——— and Low, H.: Relationship between Trauma, Plasma Corticosterone and Reticuloendothelial Function in Anaesthetized Mice, *Acta Endocrinol* (*Kbh*), **67:**141, 1971.

Schumer, W.: Steroids in the Treatment of Clinical Septic Shock, *Ann Surg,* **184:**333, 1976.

———, Erve, P. R., and Obernolte, R. P.: Mechanisms of Steroid Protection in Septic Shock, *Surgery,* **72:**119, 1972.

Stetson, C. A., Jr.: Studies on the Mechanism of the Shwartzman Phenomenon: Similarities between Reactions to Endotoxins and Certain Reactions of Bacterial Allergy, *J Exp Med,* **101:**421, 1955.

Weil, M. H. and Spink, W. W.: A Comparison of Shock Due to Endotoxin with Anaphylactic Shock, *J Lab Clin Med,* **50:**501, 1957.

Zweifach, B. W.: Relation of the RES to Natural and Acquired Resistance to Shock, in S. G. Hershey (ed.), "Shock," Little, Brown and Company, Boston, 1964.

——, Benacerraf, B., and Thomas, L.: The Relationship Between the Vascular Manifestations of Shock Produced by Endotoxin, Trauma, and Hemorrhage, *J Exp Med,* **106:**403, 1957.

Organ System Changes: General

Bock, K. D. (ed.): "Shock: Pathogenesis and Therapy: An Internation Symposium, Stockholm, 27th-30th June, 1961," Ciba Symposium, Springer-Verlag OHG, Berlin, 1962.

Hardaway, R. M.: The Problem of Acute Severe Trauma and Shock, *Surg Gynecol Obstet,* **133:**799, 1971.

Hershey, S. G. (ed.): "Shock," Little, Brown and Company, Boston, 1964.

Jacobson, E. D.: A Physiologic Approach to Shock, *N Engl J Med,* **278:**834, 1968.

Landy, M., and Braun, W. (eds.): Bacterial Endotoxins, *Proc Symp Inst Microbiol Rutgers State Univ,* New Brunswick, N.J., 1964.

Mills, L. C., and Moyer, J. H. (eds.): "Shock and Hypotension: Pathogenesis and Treatment: The 12th Hahnemann Symposium," Grune & Stratton, Inc., New York, 1965.

Cardiovascular Function

Anderson, R. W., James, P. M., Bredenberg, C. E., and Hardaway, R. M.: Phenoxybenzamine in Septic Shock, *Ann Surg,* **165:**341, 1967.

Attar, S., McLaughlin, J., Hanashiro, P., and Cowley, R. A.: The Kallikreins in Human Shock and Trauma, *Surg Forum,* **22:**11, 1971.

Baez, S., and Orkin, L. R.: Microcirculatory Effects of Anesthesia in Shock, in S. G. Hershey (ed.), "Shock," p. 207, Little, Brown and Company, Boston, 1964.

Berk, J. L., Hagen, J. F., Beyer, W. H., and Niazmand, R.: Effect of Epinephrine on Arteriovenous Shunts in Pathogenesis of Shock, *Surg Gynecol Obstet,* **124:**347, 1967.

Cann, M. S., Stevenson, T., Fiallos, E. E., and Thal, A. P.: Effect of Digitalis on Myocardial Contractility in Sepsis, *Surg Forum,* **22:**1, 1971.

Clowes, G. H. A., Jr., and Del Guercio, L. R. M.: Circulatory Response to Trauma of Surgical Operations, *Metabolism,* **9:**67, 1960.

Coalson, J. J., Woodruff, H. K., Greenfield, L. J., Guemter, C. A., and Hinshaw, L. B.: Effects of Digoxin on Myocardial Ultrastructure in Endotoxin Shock, *Surg Gynecol Obstet,* **135:**908, 1972.

Cohn, J. N.: Central Venous Pressure as Guide to Volume Expansion, *Ann Intern Med,* **66:**1283, 1967.

Duff, J. H., Malave, G., Peretz, D. I., Scott, H. M., and MacLean, L. D.: Hemodynamics of Septic Shock in Man and in the Dog, *Ann Surg,* **162:**161, 1965.

Glenn, T. M., Herlihy, B. L., Ferguson, W. W., and Lefer, A. M.: Protective Effect of Pancreatic Duct Ligation in Splanchnic Ischemia Shock, *Am J Physiol,* **222:**1278, 1972.

—— and Lefer, A. M.: Protective Effect of Thoracic Lymph Diversion in Hemorrhagic Shock, *Am J Physiol,* **219:**1305, 1970.

—— and ——: Significance of Splanchnic Proteases in the Production of a Toxic Factor in Hemorrhagic Shock, *Circ Res,* **29:**338, 1971.

Goodyer, A. V. N., Hammond, G. L., Gross, C. C., and Kabimba, J.: Myocardial Production of Pyruvate in Hemorrhagic Shock, *J Surg Res,* **11:**501, 1971.

Greenfield, L. J., McCurdy, J. R., Hinshaw, L. B., and Elkins, R. C.: Preservation of Myocardial Function during Cross-Circulation in Terminal Endotoxin Shock, *Surgery,* **72:**111, 1972.

Hardaway, R. M., James, P. M., Jr., Anderson, R. W., Bredenberg, C. E., and West, R. L.: Intensive Study and Treatment of Shock in Man, *JAMA,* **199:**779, 1967.

Hermreck, A. S., and Thal, A. P.: Mechanisms for the High Circulatory Requirements in Sepsis and Septic Shock, *Ann Surg,* **170:**677, 1969.

Hinshaw, L. B., Greenfield, L. J., Archer, L. T., and Guenter, C. A.: Effects of Endotoxin on Myocardial Hemodynamics, Performance, and Metabolism during Beta Adrenergic Blockade, *Proc Soc Exp Biol Med,* **137:**1217, 1971.

——, ——, Owen, S. E., Black, M. R., and Guenter, C. A.: Precipitation of Cardiac Failure in Endotoxin Shock, *Surg Gynecol Obstet,* **135:**39, 1972.

Hiott, D. W., and Richardson, J. A.: Cardiac Norepinephrine Levels and Contractile Force Responses with Hemorrhagic Shock, Acidosis and Sympathetic Stimulation, *Res Comm Chem Pathol Pharmacol,* **2:**429, 1971.

Huberty, J. R., Schwarz, R. H., and Emich, J. P., Jr.: Central Venous Pressure Monitoring, *Obstet Gynecol,* **30:**842, 1967.

Lefer, A. M., Cowgill, R., Marshall, F. F., Hall, L. M., and Brank, E. D.: Characterization of a Myocardial Depressant Factor Present in Hemorrhagic Shock, *Am J Physiol,* **213:**492, 1967.

Levinson, S. A., and Hume, D. M.: Effect of Exchange Transfusion with Fresh Whole Blood on Refractory Septic Shock, *Am Surg,* **38:**49, 1972.

Longerbeam, J. K., Vannix, R., Wagner, W., and Joergenson, E.: Central Venous Pressure Monitoring: Useful Guide to Fluid Therapy during Shock and Other Forms of Cardiovascular Stress, *Am J Surg,* **110:**220, 1965.

MacLean, L. D., and Duff, J. H.: Use of Central Venous Pressure as Guide to Volume Replacement in Shock, *Dis Chest,* **48:**199, 1965.

Martin, A. M., Jr., Hackel, D. B., Entman, M. L., Capp, M. P., and Spach, M. S.: Mechanisms in the Development of Myocardial Lesions in Hemorrhagic Shock, *Ann NY Acad Sci,* **156:**79, 1969.

Mundth, E. D., Wright, J. E. C., Wanibuchi, Y., and Austen, W. G.: Effect of Varying After-load and Epinephrine Levels on the Ischemic Survival Time of the Dog Heart, *Surg Forum,* **22:**133, 1971.

Osborn, J. J., Rasson, J. C. A., Beaumont, J. O., Hill, J. D., Kerth, W. J., Popper, R. W., and Gerbode, F.: Respiratory Causes of Sudden Unexplained Arrhythmia in Post-Thoracotomy Patients, *Surgery,* **69:**24, 1971.

Rush, B. F., Jr., Rosenberg, J. C., and Spencer, F. C.: Effect of Dibenzyline Treatment on Cardiac Dynamics and Oxidative Metabolism in Hemorrhagic Shock, *Ann Surg,* **162:**1013, 1965.

Schumer, W.: Microcirculatory and Metabolic Effects of Dibenzyline in Oligemic Shock, *Surg Gynecol Obstet,* **123:**787, 1966.

Shires, G. T., Carrico, C. J., and Canizaro, P. C.: "Shock," W. B. Saunders Company, Philadelphia, 1973.

Solis, R. T., and Downing, S. E.: Effects of *E. Coli* Endotoxemia on Ventricular Performance, *Am J Physiol,* **211:**307, 1966.

Thal, A. P., Brown, E. B., Jr., Hermreck, A. S., and Bell, H. H.: "Shock: A Physiologic Basis for Treatment," Year Book Medical Publishers, Inc., Chicago, 1971.

Wangensteen, S. L., Geissinger, W. T., Lovett, W. L., Glenn, T. M., and Lefer, A. W.: Relationship between Splanchnic Blood Flow and a Myocardial Depressant Factor in Endotoxin Shock, *Surgery,* **69:**410, 1971.

Weil, M. H., Schubin, H., and Rusoff, L.: Fluid Repletion in Circulatory Shock: Central Venous Pressure and Other Practical Guides, *JAMA,* **192:**688, 1965.

Weinstein, L., and Klainer, A. S.: Septic Shock: Pathogenesis and Treatment: IV. Management of Emergencies, *N Engl J Med,* **274:**950, 1966.

Wilson, R. F., Jablonski, D. V., and Thal, A. P.: Usage of Dibenzyline in Clinical Shock, *Surgery,* **56:**172, 1964.

———, Thal, A. P., Kindling, P. H., Grifka, T., and Ackerman, E.: Hemodynamic Measurements in Septic Shock, *Arch Surg,* **91:**121, 1965.

Wright, C. J., Duff, J. H., McLean, A. P. H., and MacLean, L. D.: Regional Capillary Blood Flow and Oxygen Uptake in Severe Sepsis, *Surg Gynecol Obstet,* **132:**637, 1971.

Pulmonary Function

Anderson, W. H., Dossett, B. E., Jr., and Hamilton, G. L.: Prevention of Postoperative Pulmonary Complications: Use of Isoproterenol and Intermittent Positive Pressure Breathing on Inspiration, *JAMA,* **186:**763, 1963.

Ashbaugh, D. G., and Petty, T. L.: The Use of Corticosteroids in the Treatment of Respiratory Failure Associated with Massive Fat Embolism, *Surg Gynecol Obstet,* **123:**493, 1966.

———, ———, Bigelow, D. B., and Harris, T. M.: Continuous Positive-Pressure Breathing (CPPB) in Adult Respiratory Distress Syndrome, *J Thorac Cardiovasc Surg,* **57:**31, 1969.

———, Svitek, V., and Ambrose, P.: The Incidence and Effects of Particulate Aggregation and Microembolism in Pump-Oxygenator Systems, *J Thorac Cardiovasc Surg,* **55:**691, 1968.

Ayres, S. M., Mueller, H., Giannelli, S., Jr., Fleming, P., and Grace, W. J.: The Lung in Shock: Alveolar-Capillary Gas Exchange in the Shock Syndrome, *Am J Cardiol,* **26:**588, 1970.

Barber, R. E., Lee, J., and Hamilton, W. K.: Oxygen Toxicity in Man: Study in Patients with Irreversible Brain Damage, *N Engl J Med,* **283:**1498, 1970.

Barnes, R. W., and Merendino, K. A.: Post-traumatic Pulmonary Insufficiency Syndrome, *Surg Clin North Am,* **52:**625, 1972.

Bendixen, H. H., Hedley-Whyte, J., and Laver, M. B.: Impaired Oxygenation in Surgical Patients during General Anesthesia with Controlled Ventilation, *N Engl J Med,* **269:**991, 1963.

Bergofsky, E. H.: The Adult Acute Respiratory Insufficiency Syndrome following Nonthoracic Trauma: The Lung in Shock, *Am J Cardiol,* **26:**619, 1970.

Blaisdell, F. W., Lim, R. C., Jr., and Stallone, R. J.: The Mechanism of Pulmonary Damage following Traumatic Shock, *Surg Gynecol Obstet,* **130:**1, 1970.

——— and Lewis, F. R., Jr.: "Respiratory Distress Syndrome of Shock and Trauma," W. B. Saunders Company, Philadelphia, 1977.

Burke, J. F., Pontoppidan, H., and Welch, C. E.: High Output Respiratory Failure: An Important Cause of Death Ascribed to Peritonitis or Ileus, *Ann Surg,* **158:**581, 1963.

Calabresi, P., and Abelmann, W. H.: Porto-caval and Portopulmonary Anastomoses in Laennec's Cirrhosis and in Heart Failure, *J Clin Invest,* **36:**1257, 1957.

Carlson, L. A.: Lipid Mobilization in Trauma: Friend or Foe?, in A. P. Morgan (ed.), "Proceedings of Conference on Energy Metabolism and Body Fuel Utilization," p. 50, Harvard University Press, Cambridge, Mass., 1966.

Comroe, J. H., Jr., Forster, R. E., II, Du-Bois, A. B., Briscoe, W. A., and Carlsen, E.: "The Lung," Year Book Medical Publishers, Inc., Chicago, 1962.

Cook, W. A., and Webb, W. R.: Pulmonary Changes in Hemorrhagic Shock, *Surgery,* **64:**85, 1968.

Dowd, J., and Jenkins, L. C.: The Lung in Shock: A Review, *Can Anaesth Soc J,* **19:**309, 1972.

Eltringham, W. K., Schroder, R., Jenny, M., Matloff, J. M., and Zollinger, R. M., Jr.: Pulmonary Arteriovenous Admixture in Cardiac Surgical Patients, *Circulation,* **37, 38** (*Suppl* 2):207, 1968.

Geiger, J. P., and Gleichinsky, L.: Acute Pulmonary Insufficiency: Treatment in Vietnam Casualties, *Arch Surg,* **102:**400, 1971.

Hamilton, W. K.: Alterations in Pulmonary Functions, *JAMA,* **202:**116, 1967.

Hechtman, H. B., Weisel, R. D., and Berger, R. L.: Independence of Pulmonary Shunting and Pulmonary Edema, *Surgery,* **74,** 1973.

Hill, J. D., O'Brien, T. G., Murray, J. J., Dontigny, L., Bramson, M. L., Osborn, J. J., and Gerbode, F.: Prolonged Extracorporeal Oxygenation for Acute Post-traumatic Respiratory Failure (Shock-Lung Syndrome), *N Engl J Med,* **286:**629, 1972.

Hillen, G. P., Gaisford, W. D., and Jensen, C. G.: Pulmonary Changes in Treated and Untreated Hemorrhagic Shock, *Am J Surg,* **122:**639, 1971.

Hirsch, E. F., Fletcher, R., and Lucas, S.: Hemodynamic and Respiratory Changes Associated with Sepsis following Combat Trauma, *Ann Surg,* **174:**211, 1971.

Kumar, A., Falke, K. J., Gettin, B., Aldredge, C. F., Laver, M. B., Lowenstein, E., and Pontoppidan, H.: Continuous Positive-Pressure Ventilation in Acute Respiratory Failure: Effects on Hemodynamics and Lung Function, *N Engl J Med,* **283:**1430, 1970.

Lahdensuu, M.: Studies on Phospholipid Metabolism in the Lung and Alveolar Surfactant in Experimental Traumatic and Haemorrhagic Shock, *Ann Chir Gynaecol Fenn,* **60:**245, 1971.

Lawson, D. W., Defalco, A. J., Phelps, J. A., Bradley, B. E., and McClenathan, J. E.: Corticosteroids as Treatment for Aspiration of Gastric Contents: An Experimental Study, *Surgery,* **59:**845, 1966.

Levitsky, S., Annable, C. A., Park, B. S., Davis, A. L., and Thomas, P. A.: Depletion of Alveolar Surface Active Material by Transbronchial Plasma Irrigation of the Lung, *Ann Surg,* **173:**107, 1971.

McNamara, J. J., Melot, M. D., and Stremple, F. J.: Screen Filtration Pressure in Combat Casualties, *Ann Surg,* **172:**334, 1970.

Magilligan, D. J., Jr., Oleksyn, T. W., and Schwartz, S. I.: Pulmonary Intravascular and Extravascular Volumes in Hemorrhagic Shock and Fluid Replacement, *Surgery,* **72:**780, 1972.

Meagher, D. M., Piermattei, D. L., and Swan, H.: Platelet Aggregation during Progressive Hemorrhagic Shock in Pigs, *J Thorac Cardiovasc Surg,* **62:**823, 1971.

Moore, F. D., Lyons, J. H., Jr., Pierce, E. C., Morgan, A. P., Jr., Drinker, P. A., MacArthur, J. D., and Dammin, G. J.: "Post-traumatic Pulmonary Insufficiency," W. B. Saunders Company, Philadelphia, 1969.

Moseley, R. V., and Doty, D. B.: Physiologic Changes Due to Aspiration Pneumonitis, *Ann Surg,* **171:**73, 1970.

Moss, G., Staunton, C., and Stein, A. A.: Cerebral Hypoxia as the Primary Event in the Pathogenesis of the "Shock Lung Syndrome," *Surg Forum,* **22:**211, 1971.

Nahas, R. A., Melrose, D. G., Sykes, M. K., and Robinson, B.: Post-perfusion Lung Syndrome: Effect of Homologous Blood, *Lancet,* **2:**254, 1965.

———, ———, ———, and ———: Post-perfusion Lung Syndrome: Role of Circulatory Exclusion, *Lancet,* **2:**251, 1965.

Nash, G., Blennerhassett, J. B., and Pontoppidan, H.: Pulmonary Lesions Associated with Oxygen Therapy and Artificial Ventilation, *N Engl J Med,* **276:**368, 1967.

Pelter, L. F.: Fat Embolism: A Pulmonary Disease, *Surgery,* **62:** 756, 1967.

Peters, R. M., and Hedgpeth, E. McG., Jr.: Acid-Base Balance and Respiratory Work, *J Thorac Cardiovasc Surg,* **52:**649, 1966.

———, Hilberman, M., Hogan, J. S., and Crawford, D. A.: Objective Indications for Respiration Therapy in Post-Trauma and Postoperative Patients, *Am J Surg,* **124:**262, 1972.

Powers, S. R., Jr., Mannal, R., Neclerio, M., English, M., Marr, C., Leather, R., Ueda, H., Williams, G., Custead, W., and Dutton, R.: Physiologic Consequences of Positive End-Expiratory Pressure (PEEP) Ventilation, *Ann Surg,* **178:**265, 1973.

Ratliff, N. B., Wilson, J. W., Mikat, E., Hackel, D. B., and Graham, T. C.: The Lung in Hemorrhagic Shock: IV. The Role of Neutrophilic Polymorphonuclear Leukocytes, *Am J Pathol,* **65:**325, 1971.

Robb, H. J., Margulis, R. R., and Jabs, C. M.: Role of Pulmonary Microembolism in the Hemodynamics of Endotoxin Shock, *Surg Gynecol Obstet,* **135:**777, 1972.

Robin, E. D.: Abnormalities of Acid-Base Regulation in Chronic Pulmonary Disease, with Special Reference to Hypercapnia and Extracellular Alkalosis, *N Engl J Med,* **268:**917, 1963.

Roe, B. B.: Prevention and Treatment of Respiratory Complications in Surgery, *N Engl J Med,* **163:**547, 1960.

Siegel, D. C., Cochin, A., and Moss, G. S. The Ventilatory Response to Hemorrhagic Shock and Resuscitation, *Surgery,* **72:**451, 1972.

———, Moss, G. S., Cochin, A., and DasGupta, T. K.: Pulmonary Changes following Treatment for Hemorrhagic Shock: Saline versus Colloid Infusion, *Surg Forum,* **21:**17, 1970.

Suter, P. M., Fairley, H. B., and Isenberg, M. D.: Optimum End-Expiratory Airway Pressure in Patients with Acute Pulmonary Failure, *N Eng J Med,* **292:**284, 1975.

Trimble, C., Smith, D. E., Rosenthal, M. H., and Fosburg, R. G.: Pathophysiologic Role of Hypocarbia in Post-Traumatic Pulmonary Insufficiency, *Am J Surg,* **122:**633, 1971.

Veith, F. J., Hagstrom, J. W. C., Panossian, A., Nehlsen, S. L.,

and Wilson, J. W.: Pulmonary Microcirculatory Response to Shock, Transfusion, and Pump-Oxygenator Procedures: A Unified Mechanism Underlying Pulmonary Damage, *Surgery,* **64:**95, 1968.

Hepatic Function

Ballinger, W. F., Vollenweider, H., and Montgomery, E. H.: The Response of the Canine Liver to Anaerobic Metabolism Induced by Hemorrhagic Shock, *Surg Gynecol Obstet,* **112:**19, 1961.

Baue, A. E., Wurth, M. A., and Sayeed, M. M.: The Dynamics of Altered ATP-dependent and ATP-yielding Cell Processes in Shock, *Surgery,* **72:**94, 1972.

Blair, O. M., Stenger, R. J., Hopkins, R. W., and Simeone, F. A.: Hepatocellular Ultrastructure in Dogs with Hypovolemic Shock, *Lab Invest,* **18:**172, 1968.

Bloom, W. L.: Changes in Blood Ketones during Hemorrhagic Shock in Rats, *Metabolism,* **10:**171, 1961.

——— and Ward, J. A.: Changes in Carbohydrate Metabolism during Blood Loss, Shock, and Anoxia, *Metabolism,* **10:**379, 1961.

Buxton, R. W., Haines, B. W., and Michaelis, M.: Effects of Hemorrhagic Shock upon Succinic Oxidation in Dog, Liver and Brain Slices, *Bull School Med Univ Maryland,* **46:**3, 1961.

Clermont, H. G., Williams, J. S., and Adams, J. T.: Liver Acid Phosphatase as a Measure of Hepatocyte Resistance to Hemorrhagic Shock, *Surgery,* **71:**868, 1972.

DePalma, R. G., Holden, W. D., and Robinson, A. V.: Fluid Therapy in Experimental Hemorrhagic Shock: Ultrastructural Effects in Liver and Muscle, *Ann Surg,* **175:**539, 1972.

Holden, W. D., DePalma, R. G., Drucker, W. R., and McKalen, A.: Ultrastructural Changes in Hemorrhagic Shock: Electron Microscopic Study of Liver, Kidney, and Striated Muscle, *Ann Surg,* **162:**517, 1965.

Janoff, A.: Alterations in Lysosomes (Intracellular Enzymes) during Shock: Effects of Preconditioning (Tolerance) and Protective Drugs, in S. G. Hershey (ed.), "Shock," p. 93, Little, Brown and Company, Boston, 1964.

Kekomaki, M., and Louhimo, I.: Blood Ammonium Concentration during Hemorrhagic Shock in the Rabbit, *Acta Chir Scand,* **137:**745, 1971.

Lavine, L., Harano, Y., and DePalma, R. G.: ATPase Activity and Palmitate Oxidation of Hepatic Mitochondria in Energy Production in Endotoxemia, *Surg Forum,* **22:**5, 1971.

Murray, J. F., Dawson, A. M., and Sherlock, S.: Circulatory Changes in Chronic Liver Disease, *Am J Med,* **24:**358, 1958.

Rutenburg, A. M., Bell, M. L., Butcher, R. W., Polgar, P., Dorn, B. D., and Egdahl, R. H.: Adenosine 3′,5′-Monophosphate Levels in Hemorrhagic Shock, *Ann Surg,* **174:**461, 1971.

Selkurt, E. E.: Role of Liver and Toxic Factors in Shock, in S. G. Hershey (ed.), "Shock," p. 34, Little, Brown and Company, Boston, 1964.

Sherlock, S.: Disease of the Digestive System. Drugs and the Liver, *Br Med J,* **1:**227, 1968.

Shoemaker, W. C., and Fitch, L. B.: Hepatic Lesions of Hemorrhagic Shock, *Arch Surg,* **85:**492, 1962.

Smart, C. J., and Rowlands, S. D.: Oxygen Consumption and Hepatic Metabolism in Experimental Posthemorrhagic Shock, *Trauma,* **12:**327, 1972.

Wurth, M. A., Sayeed, M. M., and Baue, A. E.: (Na+ + K+)-ATPase Activity in the Liver with Hemorrhagic Shock, *Proc Soc Exp Biol Med,* **139:**1238, 1972.

Gastrointestinal Function

Abe, H., Carballo, J., Appert, H. E., and Howard, J. M.: The Release and Fate of the Intestinal Lysosomal Enzymes after Acute Ischemic Injury of the Intestine, *Surg Gynecol Obstet,* **135:**581, 1972.

Bacalzo, L. V., Jr., Parkins, F. M., Miller, L. D., and Parkins, W. M.: Effects of Prolonged Hypovolemic Shock on Jejunal Fluid and Sodium Transport, *Surg Gynecol Obstet,* **134:**399, 1972.

Barton, R. W., Reynolds, D. G., and Swan, K. G.: Mesenteric Circulatory Responses to Hemorrhagic Shock in the Baboon, *Ann Surg,* **175:**204, 1972.

Bounous, G.: Metabolic Changes in Intestinal Mucosa during Hemorrhagic Shock, *Can J Surg,* **8:**332, 1965.

———, McArdle, A. H., Hodges, D. M., Hampson, L. G., and Gurd, F. N.: Biosynthesis of Intestinal Mucin in Shock: Relationship to Tryptic Hemorrhagic Enteritis and Permeability to Curare, *Ann Surg,* **164:**13, 1966.

———, Sutherland, N. G., McArdle, A. H., and Gurd, F. N.: The Prophylactic Use of an "Elemental" Diet in Experimental Hemorrhagic Shock and Intestinal Ischemia, *Ann Surg,* **166:**312, 1967.

Carter, D., and Einheber, A.: Intestinal Ischemic Shock in Germfree Animals, *Surg Gynecol Obstet,* **122:**66, 1966.

Chiu, C. J., Scott, H. J., and Gurd, F. N.: Volume Deficit Versus Toxic Absorption: A Study of Canine Shock after Mesenteric Arterial Occlusion, *Ann Surg,* **175:**479, 1972.

Clermont, H. G., and Williams, J. S.: Lymph Lysosomal Enzyme Acid Phosphatase in Hemorrhagic Shock, *Ann Surg,* **176:**90, 1972.

Cook, B. H., Wilson, E. R., Jr., and Taylor, A. E.: Intestinal Fluid Loss in Hemorrhagic Shock, *Am J Physiol,* **221:**1494, 1971.

DenBesten, L., and Hamza, K. N.: Effect of Bile Salts on Ionic Permeability of Canine Gastric Mucosa during Experimental Shock, *Gastroenterology,* **62:**417, 1972.

Drucker, W. R., Davis, J. H., Holden, W. D., and Reagan, J. R.: Hemorrhagic Necrosis of the Intestine, *Arch Surg,* **89:**42, 1964.

Fine, J.: Intestinal Circulation in Shock, *Gastroenterology,* **52:**454, 1967.

Fischer, R. P., and Stremple, J. F.: Stress Ulcers in Post-traumatic Renal Insufficiency in Patients from Vietnam, *Surg Gynecol Obstet,* **134:**790, 1972.

Goodier, T. E. W., Horwich, L., and Galloway, R. W.: Morphological Observations on Gastric Ulcers Treated with Carbonoxolone Sodium. *Gut,* **8:**544, 1967.

Goodman, A. A., and Osborne, M. P.: An Experimental Model and Clinical Definition of Stress Ulceration, *Surg Gynecol Obstet,* **134:**563, 1972.

Gurd, F. N.: Metabolic and Functional Changes in Intestine in Shock, *Am J Surg,* **110:**333, 1965.

——— and McClelland, R. N.: Trauma Workshop Report: The Gastrointestinal Tract in Trauma, *J Trauma,* **11:**1089, 1970.

Howerton, E. E., and Kolmen, S. N.: The Intestinal Tract as a Portal of Entry of Pseudomonas in Burned Rats, *J Trauma,* **12:**335, 1972.

Hutcher, N., Silverberg, S. G., and Lee, H. M.: The Effect of

Vitamin A on the Formation of Steroid Induced Gastric Ulcers, *Surg Forum,* **22:**322, 1971.

Lev, R., Molot, M. D., McNamara, J., and Stremple, J. F.: "Stress" Ulcers following War Wounds in Vietnam: A Morphologic and Histochemical Study, *Lab Invest,* **25:**491, 1971.

Lillehei, R. C., Longerbeam, J. K., Bloch, J. H., and Manax, W. G.: The Nature of Experimental Irreversible Shock with Its Clinical Application, in S. G. Hershey (ed.), "Shock," p. 139, Little, Brown and Company, Boston, 1964.

Menguy, R., and Masters, Y. F.: Effect of Cortisone on Mucoprotein Secretion by Gastric Antrum of Dogs: Pathogenesis of Steroid Ulcer, *Surgery,* **54:**19, 1963.

——— and ———: Influence of Parathyroid Extract on Gastric Mucosal Content of Mucus, *Gastroenterology,* **48:**342, 1965.

Ritchie, W. P., and Fischer, R. P.: Studies on the Pathogenesis of "Stress Ulcer": Electrical Potential Difference and Ionic Fluxes across Canine Gastric Mucosa during Hemorrhagic Shock, *J Surg Res,* **12:**173, 1972.

———, Roth, R. R., and Fischer, R. P.: Studies on the Pathogenesis of "Stress Ulcer": Effect of Hemorrhage, Transfusion, and Vagotomy in the Restrained Rat, *Surgery,* **71:**445, 1972.

Robert, A., Bayer, R. B., and Nezamis, J. E.: Gastric Mucus Content during Development of Ulcers in Fasting Rats, *Gastroenterology,* **45:**740, 1963.

——— and Nezamis, J. E.: Effect of Prednisolone on Gastric Mucus Content and on Ulcer Formation, *Proc Soc Exp Biol Med,* **114:**545, 1943.

Shirazi, S. S., DenBesten, L., and Hamza, K. N.: Absorption of Bile Salts from the Gastric Mucosa during Hemorrhagic Shock, *Proc Soc Exp Biol Med,* **140:**924, 1972.

Swan, K. G., Barton, R. W., and Reynolds, D. G.: Mesenteric Hemodynamics during Endotoxemia in the Baboon, *Gastroenterology,* **61:**872, 1971.

——— and Reynolds, D. G.: Blood Flow to the Liver and Spleen during Endotoxin Shock in the Baboon, *Surgery,* **72:**388, 1972.

Voitk, A. J., Chiu, C. J., and Gurd, F. N.: Prevention of Porcine Stress Ulcer following Hemorrhagic Shock with Elemental Diet, *Arch Surg,* **105:**473, 1972.

Vyden, J. K., and Corday, E.: The Effect of Cardiogenic Shock on the Superior Mesenteric Circulation, *Geriatrics,* **26:**85, 1971.

Wilmore, D. W., Dudrick, S. J., Dailey, J. M., and Vars, H. M.: The Role of Nutrition in the Adaptation of the Small Intestine after Massive Resection, *Surg Gynecol Obstet,* **132:**673, 1971.

Zweifach, W. B., Gordon, H. A., Wagner, M., and Reyniers, J. A.: Irreversible Shock in Germ-free Rats, *J Exp Med,* **107:**437 1958.

Renal Function

Barry, K. G., Mazze, R. I., and Schwartz, F. D.: Prevention of Surgical Oliguria and Renal-Hemodynamic Suppression by Sustained Hydration, *N Engl J Med,* **270:**1371, 1964.

Baxter, C., and Powers, S. R., Trauma Workshop Report: Kidney Response to Trauma, *J Trauma,* **10:**1072, 1970.

Blagg, C. R., and Parsons, F. M.: Earlier Dialysis and Anabolic Steroids in Acute Renal Failure, *Am Heart J,* **61:**287, 1961.

Boba, A., and Landmesser, C. M.: Renal Complications after Anesthesia and Operation, *Anesthesiology,* **22:**781, 1961.

Gorfinkel, H. J., Szidon, J. P., Hirsch, L. J., and Fishman, A. P.:

Renal Performance in Experimental Cardiogenic Shock, *Am J Physiol,* **222:**1260, 1972.

Habif, D. V., Paper, E. M., Fitzpatrick, H. F., Lowrance, P., Smythe, C. McC., and Bradley, S. E.: Renal and Hepatic Blood Flow, Glomerular Filtration Rate, and Urinary Output of Electrolytes during Cyclopropane, Ether, and Thiopental Anesthesia, Operation, and Immediate Postoperative Period, *Surgery,* **30:**241, 1951.

Hatcher, C. R., Jr., Gagnon, J. A., and Clark, R. W.: Effects of Hydration on Epinephrine-induced Renal Shut Down in Dogs, *Surg Forum,* **9:**106, 1958.

Jones, L. W., and Weil, M. H.: Water, Creatinine and Sodium Excretion following Circulatory Shock with Renal Failure, *Am J Med,* **51:**314, 1971.

Knuth, O. E., Wagenknecht, L. V., and Madsen, P. O.: The Effect of Various Treatments on Renal Function during Endotoxin Shock, *Invest Urol,* **9:**304, 1972.

Logan, A., Jose, P., Eisner, G., Lilienfield, L., and Slotkoff, L.: Intracortical Distribution of Renal Blood Flow in Hemorrhagic Shock in Dogs, *Circ Res,* **29:**257, 1971.

Mazze, R. I., Schwartz, F. D., Slocum, H. C., and Barry, K. G.: Renal Function during Anesthesia and Surgery. I. Effects of Halothane Anesthesia, *Anesthesiology,* **24:**279, 1963.

Merrill, J. P.: "The Treatment of Renal Failure," Grune & Stratton, Inc., New York, 1965.

Moyer, C. A.: Acute Temporary Changes in Renal Function Associated with Major Surgical Procedures, *Surgery,* **27:**198, 1950.

Mueller, C. G.: Mechanism and Use of Mannitol Diuresis in Major Surgery and in Trauma, *South Med J,* **59:**408, 1966.

Nagy, Z., Bencsath, P., Tornyai, K., and Vaslaki, L.: Arterio-venous Anastomoses in the Kidney: IX. Intrarenal Circulation During Tourniquet Shock, *Acta Physiol Acad Sci Hung,* **40:**121, 1971.

————, Meszaros, A., and Vaslaki, L.: Arterio-venous Anastomoses in the Kidney: X. Effect of Phenoxybenzamine on Intrarenal Circulation of Dogs in Tourniquet Shock, *Acta Physiol Acad Sci Hung,* **40:**129, 1971.

Parry, W. L., Schaefer, J. A., and Mueller, C. B.: Experimental Studies of Acute Renal Failure. I. Protective Effect of Mannitol, *J Urol,* **89:**1, 1963.

Selkurt, E. E.: Atropine Influence on Altered Hemodynamics of the Primate Kidney in Hemorrhagic Shock, *Proc Soc Exp Biol Med,* **138:**497, 1971.

————: Influence of Aortic Constriction on the Positive Free-Water Clearance of Primate Hemorrhagic Shock, *Proc Soc Exp Biol Med,* **140:**221, 1972.

Skinner, D. G., and Hayes, M. A.: Effect of Staphylococcic Toxin on Renal Function: Irreversible Shock, *Ann Surg,* **162:**161, 1965.

Strauch, M., McLaughlin, J. S., Mansberger, A., Young, J., Mendonca, P., Gray, K., and Cowley, R. A.: Effects of Septic Shock on Renal Function in Humans, *Ann Surg,* **165:**536, 1967.

Stremple, J. F., Ellison, E. H., and Carey, L. C.: Osmolar Diuresis: Success and/or Failure: A Collective Review, *Surgery,* **60:**924, 1966.

Tobian, L.: Renin-Angiotensin Mechanisms in Shock, in L. C. Mills and J. H. Moyer (eds.), "Shock and Hypotension: Pathogenesis and Treatment, The 12th Hahnemann Symposium," Grune & Stratton, Inc., New York, 1965.

Uldall, P. R., and Kerr, D. N. S., Post-traumatic Acute Renal Failure, *Br J Anaesth,* **44:**283, 1972.

Chapter 2

Fluid, Electrolyte, and Nutritional Management of the Surgical Patient

by G. Tom Shires and Peter C. Canizaro

Anatomy of Body Fluids

Total Body Water
Intracellular Fluid
Extracellular Fluid
Osmotic Pressure

Classification of Body Fluid Changes

Volume Changes
Concentration Changes
Mixed Volume and Concentration Abnormalities
Composition Changes
    Acid-Base Balance
    Potassium Abnormalities
    Calcium Abnormalities
    Magnesium Abnormalities

Normal Exchange of Fluid and Electrolytes

Water Exchange
Salt Gain and Losses

Fluid and Electrolyte Therapy

Parenteral Solutions
Preoperative Fluid Therapy
    Correction of Volume Changes
    Correction of Concentration Changes
    Composition and Miscellaneous Considerations
Intraoperative Management of Fluids
Postoperative Management of Fluids
    Immediate Postoperative Period
    Later Postoperative Period
    Special Considerations in the Postoperative Patient

Nutrition in the Surgical Patient

Body Fuel Reserves
Starvation
Surgery, Trauma, Sepsis
Base-Line Requirements
Indications and Methods for Nutritional Support

One of the most critical aspects of patient care is management of the body composition of fluid and electrolytes. Most diseases, many injuries, and even operative trauma impose a great impact on the physiology of fluid and electrolytes within the body. These changes often exceed those brought about by acute lack of alimentation. There-fore, a thorough understanding of the metabolism of salt, water, and electrolytes and of certain metabolic responses is essential to the care of surgical patients.

An attempt will be made here to define the anatomy of body fluids and the physiologic principles governing function of fluids and electrolytes. In addition to these normal functions, a classification of derangements will be developed so that rational therapy may be described.

ANATOMY OF BODY FLUIDS

A prerequisite to the understanding of fluid and electrolyte management is knowledge of the extent and composition of the various body fluid compartments. Early attempts to define these compartments were relatively accurate, but a more precise definition has been obtained by many investigators through the use of isotope tracer techniques. The wide range of normal values is a function of body size, weight, and sex, but these compartments are relatively constant in size in the individual patient in the normal steady state. The figures used in this section, therefore, are approximate and presented as a percentage of body weight.

Total Body Water

Water constitutes between 50 and 70 percent of total body weight. Using deuterium oxide or tritiated water for measurement of total body water (TBW), the average normal value for young adult males is 60 percent of body weight and 50 percent for young adult females. A normal variation of ± 15 percent applies to both groups. The actual figure for each healthy individual is remarkably constant and is a function of several variables, including lean body mass and age. Since fat contains little water, the lean individual has a greater proportion of water to total body weight than the obese person. Thus, an extremely obese individual may have 25 to 30 percent less body water than a lean individual of the same weight. The lower percentage of total body water in females correlates well with a relatively large amount of subcutaneous adipose tissue and small muscle mass. Moore et al. have shown that total body water, as a percentage of total body weight, decreases steadily and significantly with age to a low of 52 and 47 percent in males and females respectively.

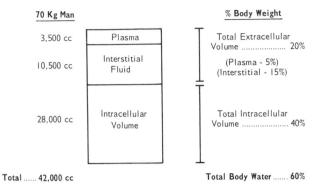

Fig. 2-1. Functional compartments of body fluids.

Conversely, the highest proportion of total body water to body weight is found in newborn infants, with a maximum of 75 to 80 percent. During the first several months following birth there is a gradual "physiologic" loss of body water as the infant adjusts to his environment. At one year of age, the total body water averages approximately 65 percent of the body weight and remains relatively constant throughout the remainder of infancy and childhood.

The water of the body is divided into three functional compartments (Fig. 2-1). The fluid within the body's diverse cell population, intracellular water, represents between 30 and 40 percent of the body weight. The extracellular water represents 20 percent of the body weight and is divided between the intravascular fluid, or plasma

(5 percent of body weight), and the interstitial, or extravascular, extracellular fluid (15 percent of body weight).

Intracellular Fluid

Measurement of intracellular fluid is determined indirectly by subtraction of the measured extracellular fluid from the measured total body water. The intracellular water is between 30 and 40 percent of the body weight, with the largest proportion in the skeletal muscle mass. Because of the smaller muscle mass in the female, the percentage of intracellular water is lower than in the male.

The chemical composition of the intracellular fluid is shown in Fig. 2-2, with potassium and magnesium the principal cations, and phosphates and proteins the principal anions. This is an approximation, since so few data concerning the intracellular fluid are available.

Extracellular Fluid

The total extracellular fluid volume represents approximately 20 percent of the body weight. The extracellular fluid compartment has two major subdivisions. The plasma volume comprises approximately 5 percent of the body weight in the normal adult. The interstitial, or extravascular, extracellular fluid volume, obtained by subtracting the plasma volume from the measured total extracellular fluid volume, comprises approximately 15 percent of the body weight.

The interstitial fluid is further complicated by having,

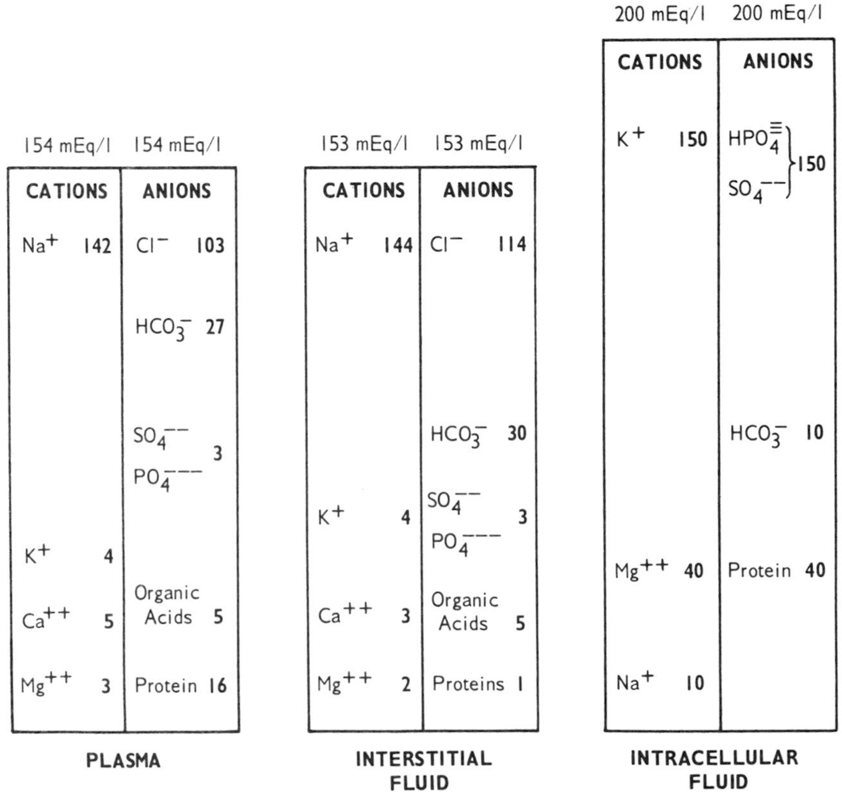

	PLASMA 154 mEq/l		INTERSTITIAL FLUID 153 mEq/l		INTRACELLULAR FLUID 200 mEq/l	
	CATIONS	ANIONS	CATIONS	ANIONS	CATIONS	ANIONS
	Na^+ 142	Cl^- 103	Na^+ 144	Cl^- 114	K^+ 150	$HPO_4^{\equiv}$ } 150
		HCO_3^- 27				SO_4^{--}
				HCO_3^- 30		
		SO_4^{--} 3				HCO_3^- 10
		PO_4^{---}	K^+ 4	SO_4^{--} 3		
				PO_4^{---}	Mg^{++} 40	Protein 40
	K^+ 4		Ca^{++} 3	Organic Acids 5		
	Ca^{++} 5	Organic Acids 5			Na^+ 10	
	Mg^{++} 3	Protein 16	Mg^{++} 2	Proteins 1		

Fig. 2-2. Chemical composition of body fluid compartments.

normally, a rapidly equilibrating, or functional, component, as well as several slower-equilibrating, or relatively nonfunctioning, components. The nonfunctioning components include connective tissue water as well as water that has been termed *transcellular,* which includes cerebrospinal and joint fluids. This nonfunctional component normally represents only 10 percent of the interstitial fluid volume (1 to 2 percent of body weight) and is not to be confused with the *relatively* nonfunctional extracellular fluid, often called a "third space," found in burns and soft tissue injuries.

The normal constituents of the extracellular fluid are shown in Fig. 2-2, with sodium the principal cation, and chloride and bicarbonate the principal anions. There are minor differences in ionic composition between the plasma and interstitial fluid occasioned by the difference in protein concentration. Because of the higher protein content (organic anions) of the plasma, the total concentration of cations is higher and the concentration of inorganic anions somewhat lower than in the interstitial fluid, as explained by the Gibbs-Donnan equilibrium equation.* For practical consideration, however, they may be considered equal. The total concentration of intracellular ions exceeds that of the extracellular compartment and would seem to violate the concept of osmolar equilibrium between the two compartments. This apparent discrepancy is due to the fact that the concentration of ions is expressed in milliequivalents (mEq) without regard to osmotic activity. In addition, some of the intracellular cations probably exist in undissociated form.

Osmotic Pressure

Relevant to a discussion of the complicated interactions between the various body fluid compartments is the definition of commonly used terms: The physiologic and chemical activity of electrolytes depend on (1) the *number of particles* present per unit volume [moles or millimoles (mM) per liter], (2) the *number of electric charges* per unit volume (equivalents or milliequivalents per liter), and (3) the *number of osmotically active particles,* or ions per unit volume [osmoles or milliosmoles (mO) per liter]. The use of the terms *grams* or *milligrams per 100 milliliters* expresses the weight of the electrolytes per unit volume but does not allow a physiologic comparison of the solutes in a solution.

A mole of a substance is the molecular weight of that substance in grams, and a millimole is that figure expressed in milligrams. For example, a mole of sodium chloride is 58 grams (Na—23, Cl—35), and a millimole is 58 milligrams. This expression, however, gives no direct information as to the number of osmotically active ions in solution or the electric charges that they carry.

The electrolytes of the body fluids then may be expressed in terms of chemical combining activity, or "equivalents." An equivalent of an ion is its atomic weight

expressed in grams divided by the valence, whereas a milliequivalent of an ion is that figure expressed in milligrams. In the case of univalent ions, a milliequivalent is the same as a millimole. However, in the case of divalent ions, such as calcium or magnesium, one millimole equals two milliequivalents. The importance of this expression is that a milliequivalent of any substance will combine chemically with a milliequivalent of any other substance; in any given solution, the number of milliequivalents of cations present is balanced by precisely the same number of milliequivalents of anions.

When the osmotic pressure of a solution is considered, it is more descriptive to employ the terms osmole and milliosmole. These terms refer to the actual number of osmotically active particles present in solution, but are not dependent on the chemical combining capacities of the substances. Thus, a millimole of sodium chloride, which dissociates nearly completely into sodium and chloride, contributes two milliosmoles, and one millimole of sodium sulfate (Na_2SO_4), which dissociates into three particles, contributes three milliosmoles. One millimole of an un-ionized substance such as glucose is equal to one milliosmole of the substance.

The differences in ionic composition between intracellular and extracellular fluid are maintained by the cell wall, which functions as a semipermeable membrane. The total number of osmotically active particles is 290 to 310 mO in each compartment. Although the total osmotic pressure of a fluid is the sum of the partial pressures contributed by each of the solutes in that fluid, the *effective* osmotic pressure is dependent on those substances which fail to pass through the pores of the semipermeable membrane. The dissolved proteins in the plasma, therefore, are primarily responsible for effective osmotic pressure between the plasma and the interstitial fluid compartments. This is frequently referred to as the *colloid osmotic pressure.* The effective osmotic pressure between the extracellular and intracellular fluid compartments would be contributed to by any substance that does not traverse the cell membranes freely. Thus sodium, which is the principal cation of the extracellular fluid, contributes a major portion of the osmotic pressure, but substances that fail to penetrate the cell membrane freely, such as glucose, also increase the effective osmotic pressure.

Since the cell membranes are completely permeable to water, the effective osmotic pressures in the two compartments are considered to be equal. Any condition that alters the effective osmotic pressure in either compartment will result in redistribution of water between the compartments. Thus, an increase in effective osmotic pressure in the extracellular fluid, which would occur most frequently as a result of increased sodium concentration, would cause a net transfer of water from the intracellular to the extracellular fluid compartment. This transfer of water would continue until the effective osmotic pressures in the two compartments were equal. Conversely, a decrease in the sodium concentration in the extracellular fluid will cause a transfer of water from the extracellular to the intracellular fluid compartment. However, depletion of the extracellular fluid volume without a change in the

---

*The product of the concentrations of any pair of diffusible cations and anions on one side of a semipermeable membrane will equal the product of the same pair of ions on the other side.

concentration of ions will not result in transfer of free water from the intracellular space.

Thus, the intracellular fluid shares in losses that involve a change in concentration or composition of the extracellular fluid but shares slowly in changes involving loss of isotonic volume alone. For practical consideration, most losses and gains of body fluid are directly from the extracellular compartment.

CLASSIFICATION OF BODY FLUID CHANGES

The disorders in fluid balance may be classified in three general categories: disturbances of (1) volume, (2) concentration, and (3) composition. Of primary importance is the concept that although these disturbances are interrelated, each is a separate entity.

If an isotonic salt solution is added to or lost from the body fluids, only the *volume* of the extracellular fluid is changed. The acute loss of an isotonic extracellular solution, such as intestinal juice, is followed by a significant decrease in the extracellular fluid volume and little, if any, change in the intracellular fluid volume. Fluid will not be transferred from the intracellular space to refill the depleted extracellular space as long as the osmolarity remains the same in the two compartments.

If water alone is added to or lost from the extracellular fluid, the *concentration* of osmotically active particles will change. Sodium ions account for 90 percent of the osmotically active particles in the extracellular fluid and generally reflect the tonicity of body fluid compartments. If the extracellular fluid is depleted of sodium, water will pass into the intracellular space until osmolarity is again equal in the two compartments.

The concentration of most other ions within the extracellular fluid compartment can be altered without significant change in the total number of osmotically active particles, thus producing only a *compositional* change. For instance, a rise of the serum potassium concentration from 4 to 8 mEq/L would have a significant effect on the myocardium, but it would not significantly change the effective osmotic pressure of the extracellular fluid compartment. Normally functioning kidneys minimize these changes considerably, particularly if the addition or loss of solute or water is gradual.

An internal loss of extracellular fluid into a nonfunctional space, such as the sequestration of isotonic fluid in a burn, peritonitis, ascites, or muscle trauma, is termed a *distributional* change. This transfer or functional loss of extracellular fluid internally may be extracellular (e.g., as in peritonitis) or intracellular (e.g., as in hemorrhagic shock). In any event, all distributional shifts or losses result in a contraction of the *functional* extracellular fluid space.

Volume Changes

Volume deficit or excess generally must be diagnosed by clinical examination of the patient. There are no readily available laboratory tests of benefit in the acute phase except measurement of the plasma volume. Changes secondary to long-standing derangements in volume, however, may be discernible by laboratory tests. For example, the blood urea nitrogen (BUN) level slowly rises with a long-standing extracellular fluid deficit of sufficient magnitude to reduce glomerular filtration. The concentration of serum sodium is *not* related to the volume status of extracellular fluid; a severe volume deficit may exist with a normal, low, or high serum sodium level.

VOLUME DEFICIT. Extracellular fluid volume deficit is by far the most common fluid disorder in the surgical patient. The loss of fluid is not water alone, but water and electrolytes in approximately the same proportion as that in which they exist in normal extracellular fluid. The most common disorders leading to an extracellular fluid volume deficit include losses of gastrointestinal fluids due to vomiting, nasogastric suction, diarrhea, and fistular drainage. Other common causes include sequestration of fluid in soft tissue injuries and infections, intraabdominal and retroperitoneal inflammatory processes, peritonitis, intestinal obstruction, and burns. The signs and symptoms of this state are easily recognized and are listed in Table 2-1. The central nervous system and cardiovascular signs occur early with acute rapid losses, whereas tissue signs may be absent until the deficit has existed for at least 24 hours. The central nervous system signs are similar to barbiturate intoxication and may be missed by the casual observer if the volume deficit is mild. The cardiovascular signs are secondary to a decrease in plasma volume and may be associated with varying degrees of hypotension in the patient with a severe extracellular fluid volume deficit. Skin turgor may be difficult to assess in the elderly patient or in the patient with recent weight loss and is not diagnostic in the absence of other confirmatory signs. The body temperature tends to vary with the environmental temperature. In a cool room, the patient may be slightly hypothermic and the febrile response to illness may be suppressed. This occurs frequently and can be very misleading during clinical evaluation of the septic patient. After partial correction of the volume deficit, the temperature will generally rise to the appropriate level.

VOLUME EXCESS. Extracellular fluid volume excess is generally iatrogenic or secondary to renal insufficiency. Both the plasma and interstitial fluid volumes are increased. In the healthy young adult, the signs are generally those of circulatory overload, manifested primarily in the pulmonary circulation, and of excessive fluid in other tissue (Table 2-1). In the elderly patient, congestive heart failure with pulmonary edema may develop rather quickly with a moderate volume excess.

Concentration Changes

Since the sodium ion is primarily responsible for the osmolarity of the extracellular fluid space, determination of the serum concentration of sodium generally indicates the tonicity of body fluids. Hyponatremia and hypernatremia can be diagnosed on clinical grounds (Table 2-2), but discernible signs and symptoms are not generally present until the changes are severe. Changes in concentration

Table 2-1. EXTRACELLULAR FLUID VOLUME

Type of sign	Deficit		Excess	
	Moderate	Severe	Moderate	Severe
Central nervous system	Sleepiness Apathy Slow responses Anorexia Cessation of usual activity	Decreased tendon reflexes. Anesthesia distal extremities Stupor Coma	None	None
Gastrointestinal	Progressive decrease in food consumption	Nausea, vomiting Refusal to eat Silent ileus and distension	At surgery: Edema of stomach, colon, lesser and greater omenta and small bowel mesentary	
Cardiovascular	Orthostatic hypotension Tachycardia Collapsed veins Collapsing pulse	Cutaneous lividity Hypotension Distant heart sounds Cold extremities Absent peripheral pulses	Elevated venous pressure Distension of peripheral veins Increased cardiac output Loud heart sounds Functional murmurs Bounding pulse High pulse pressure Increased pulmonary 2d sound Gallop	Pulmonary edema
Tissue	Soft, small tongue with longitudial wrinkling Decreased skin turgor	Atonic muscles Sunken eyes	Subcutaneous pitting edema Basilar râles	Anasarca Moist râles Vomiting Diarrhea
Metabolic	Mild decrease temperature, 97–99°R	Marked decrease temperature, 95–98°R	None	None

should be noted early by appropriate laboratory tests and corrected promptly. Clinical signs of hyponatremia or hypernatremia tend to occur early and with greater severity if the rate of change in extracellular sodium concentration is very rapid.

HYPONATREMIA. Acute symptomatic hyponatremia (sodium less than 130 mEq/L) clinically is characterized by central nervous system signs of increased intracranial pressure and tissue signs of excessive intracellular water. There are no cardiovascular signs per se. The hypertension is probably induced by the rise in intracranial pressure, since the blood pressure generally returns to normal with the administration of hypertonic solutions of sodium salts. Of importance with severe hyponatremia is the relatively rapid development of oliguric renal failure, which may not be reversible if therapy is delayed.

Many hyponatremic states are asymptomatic until the serum sodium level falls below 120 mEq/L. One important exception is the patient with increased cerebrospinal fluid pressure, as following closed head injury, in whom mild hyponatremia may be extremely deleterious, even fatal, because of the progressive increase in intracellular water as the extracellular fluid osmolarity falls.

HYPERNATREMIA. Central nervous system and tissue signs, listed in Table 2-2, characterize acute symptomatic

hypernatremia. This is the only state in which dry, sticky mucous membranes are characteristic. This sign does not occur with pure extracellular fluid volume deficit alone, and may be misleading in the patient who breathes through his mouth. Body temperature is generally elevated and may approach a lethal level, as in the patient with heatstroke.

While volume changes occur frequently without a change in serum sodium, the reverse is not true. The disease states that cause a significant acute alteration in the serum sodium frequently produce a concomitant change in the extracellular fluid volume.

Mixed Volume and Concentration Abnormalities

Mixed volume and concentration abnormalities may develop as a consequence of the disease state or occasionally may result from inappropriate parenteral fluid therapy. Moyer noted that the clinical picture associated with a combination of fluid abnormalities will tend to be an algebraic composite of the signs and symptoms of each state. Like signs produced by both abnormalities will be additive, and opposing signs will tend to nullify one another. For example, the tendency for the body temperature

Table 2-2. ACUTE CHANGES IN OSMOLAR CONCENTRATION

Type of signs	Hyponatremia (water intoxication)		Hypernatremia (water deficit)	
	Moderate:	Severe:	Moderate:	Severe:
Central nervous system	Muscle twitching Hyperactive tendon reflexes Increased intra-cranial pressure (compensated phase)	Convulsions Loss of reflexes Increased intra-cranial pressure (decompensated phase)	Restlessness Weakness	Delirium Maniacal be-havior
Cardiovascular	Changes in blood pressure and pulse secondary to increased intracranial pressure		Tachycardia Hypotension (if severe)	
Tissue	Salivation, lacrimation, watery diarrhea "Fingerprinting" of skin (sign of intracellular volume excess)		Decrease saliva and tears Dry and sticky mucous membranes Red, swollen tongue Skin flushed	
Renal	Oliguria progressing to anuria		Oliguria	
Metabolic	None		Fever	

to fall with an extracellular volume deficit may be counteracted by the tendency for it to rise with severe hypernatremia.

One of the more common mixed abnormalities is an extracellular fluid deficit and hyponatremia. This state is readily produced in the patient who continues to drink water while losing large volumes of gastrointestinal fluids. It may also occur in the postoperative period when gastrointestinal losses are replaced with only 5% dextrose in water or a hypotonic sodium solution. An extracellular volume deficit accompanied by hypernatremia may be produced by the loss of a large amount of hypotonic salt solution, such as sweat, in the absence of fluid intake.

The prolonged administration of excessive quantities of sodium salts with restricted water intake may result in an extracellular volume excess and hypernatremia. This may also occur when pure water losses (such as insensible loss of water from the skin and lungs) are replaced with sodium-containing solutions only. Similarly, the excessive administration of water or hypotonic salt solutions to the patient with oliguric renal failure may rapidly produce an extracellular volume excess and hyponatremia.

Normally functioning kidneys may minimize these changes to some extent and compensate for many of the errors associated with parenteral fluid administration. In contrast, the patient in anuric or oliguric renal failure is particularly prone to develop these mixed volume and osmolar concentration abnormalities. Fluid and electrolyte management in these patients, therefore, must be precise. Unfortunately, the fact that a patient with normal kidneys who develops a significant volume deficit may be in a state of "functional" renal failure is often not appreciated. As the volume deficit progresses, the glomerular filtration rate falls precipitously, and the kidneys' unique functions for maintaining fluid homeostasis are lost. These changes may occur with only a mild volume deficit in the elderly patient with borderline renal function. In these elderly patients, the blood urea nitrogen level may rise higher than 100 mg/100 ml in response to the fluid deficit with a concomitant rise in the serum creatinine level. Fortunately, these changes are usually reversible with early and adequate correction of the extracellular fluid volume deficit.

Composition Changes

Compositional abnormalities of importance include changes in acid-base balance and concentration changes of potassium, calcium, and magnesium.

ACID-BASE BALANCE

The pH (the negative logarithm of the hydrogen ion concentration) of the body fluids is normally maintained within narrow limits in spite of the rather large load of acid produced endogenously as a by-product of body metabolism. The acids are neutralized efficiently by several buffer systems and subsequently excreted by the lungs and kidneys.

The important buffers include proteins and phosphates, which play a primary role in maintaining intracellular pH, and the bicarbonate–carbonic acid system, which operates principally in the extracellular fluid space. The proteins and hemoglobin have only minor influence in the extracellular fluid space, but the latter is of prime significance as a buffer in the red cell.

A buffer system consists of a weak acid or base and the salt of that acid or base. The buffering effect is the result of the formation of an amount of weak acid or base equivalent to the amount of strong acid or base added to the system. The resultant change in pH is considerably less than if the substance were added to water alone. Thus, inorganic acids (e.g., hydrochloric, sulfuric, phosphoric) and organic acids (e.g., lactic, pyruvic, keto acids) combine with base bicarbonate producing the sodium salt of the acid and carbonic acid:

$$HCL + NaHCO_3 \longrightarrow NaCl + H_2CO_3$$

The carbonic acid formed is then excreted via the lungs as CO_2. The inorganic acid anions are excreted by the kidneys with hydrogen or as ammonium salts. The organic acid anions generally are metabolized as the underlying disorder is corrected, although some renal excretion may occur with high levels.

The functions of the buffer systems are expressed in the Henderson-Hasselbalch equation, which defines the pH in terms of the ratio of the salt and acid. The pH of the extracellular fluid is defined primarily by the ratio of the amount of base bicarbonate (majority as sodium bicarbonate) to the amount of carbonic acid (related to the CO_2 content of alveolar air) present in the blood:

$$pH = pK + \log \frac{BHCO_3}{H_2CO_3} = \frac{27 \text{ mEq/L}}{1.33 \text{ mEq/L}} = \frac{20}{1} = 7.4$$

pK represents the dissociation constant of carbonic acid in the presence of base bicarbonate and by measurement is 6.1. At a body pH of 7.4, the ratio must be 20:1, as depicted. From a chemical standpoint, this is an inefficient buffer system, but the unusual property of CO_2 to behave as an acid or change to a neutral gas subsequently excreted by the lungs makes it quite efficient biologically.

As long as the 20:1 ratio is maintained, regardless of the absolute values, the pH will remain at 7.4. When an acid is added to the system, the concentration of bicarbonate (the numerator in the Henderson-Hasselbalch equation) will decrease. Ventilation will immediately increase to eliminate larger quantities of CO_2 with a subsequent decrease in the carbonic acid (the denominator in the Henderson-Hasselbalch equation) until the 20:1 ratio is reestablished. Slower, more complete compensation is effected by the kidneys with increased excretion of acid salts and retention of bicarbonate. The reverse will occur if an alkali is added to the system. Respiratory acidosis and alkalosis are produced by disturbances of ventilation, with an increase or decrease in the denominator and a resultant change of the 20:1 ratio. Compensation is primarily renal, with a retention of bicarbonate and increased excretion of acid salts in respiratory acidosis and the reverse process in respiratory alkalosis.

The four types of acid-base disturbances are listed in Table 2-3. Use of the CO_2 combining power (approximates the plasma bicarbonate) or CO_2 content (includes bicarbonate, carbonic acid, and dissolved CO_2) and knowledge of the patient's disease may allow an accurate diagnosis in the uncomplicated case. However, use of the CO_2 content or CO_2 combining power alone is generally inadequate as an index of acid-base balance. Both these tests principally reflect the level of plasma bicarbonate, since

Table 2-3. ACIDOSIS-ALKALOSIS

Type of acid-base disorder	Defect	Common causes	$\frac{BHCO_3}{H_2CO_3} = \frac{20}{1}$	Compensation
Respiratory acidosis	Retention of CO_2 (Decreased alveolar ventilation)	Depression of respiratory center—morphine, CNS injury Pulmonary disease—emphysema, pneumonia	↑ Denominator Ratio less than 20:1	Renal Retention of bicarbonate, excretion of acid salts, increased ammonia formation Chloride shift into red cells
Respiratory alkalosis	Excessive loss of CO_2 (Increased alveolar ventilation)	Hyperventilation: Emotional, severe pain, assisted ventilation, encephalitis	↓ Denominator Ratio greater than 20:1	Renal Excretion of bicarbonate, retention of acid salts, decreased ammonia formation
Metabolic acidosis	Retention of fixed acids or Loss of base bicarbonate	Diabetes, azotemia, lactic acid accumulation, starvation Diarrhea, small bowel fistulae	↓ Numerator Ratio less than 20:1	Pulmonary (rapid) Increase rate and depth of breathing Renal (slow) As in respiratory acidosis
Metabolic alkalosis	Loss of fixed acids Gain of base bicarbonate Potassium depletion	Vomiting or gastric suction with pyloric obstruction Excessive intake of bicarbonate Diuretics	↑ Numerator Ratio greater than 20:1	Pulmonary (rapid) Decrease rate and depth of breathing Renal (slow) As in respiratory alkalosis

dissolved CO_2 and carbonic acid contribute no more than a few millimoles under most circumstances. In the acute phase, therefore, respiratory acidosis or alkalosis may exist without any change in the CO_2 content; determinations of the pH and P_{CO_2} from a freshly drawn arterial blood sample are necessary for diagnosis. Thus, measurements of pH, bicarbonate concentration, and P_{CO_2} are required for a more complete understanding of the acid-base status in most patients (Table 2-4).

Unfortunately, more complex acid-base disturbances are frequently encountered. Combinations of respiratory and metabolic changes occur and may represent compensation for the initial acid-base disturbance or may indicate two or more coexisting primary disorders (e.g., a *primary* respiratory acidosis complicated by a *primary* metabolic acidosis or alkalosis).

Usually primary acid-base disturbances are compensated to some extent. A primary metabolic disturbance is initially compensated by changes in pulmonary ventilation, while respiratory disturbances are compensated by renal mechanisms. For example, the initial compensation for an acute metabolic acidosis is an increase in the rate and depth of breathing to lower the arterial P_{CO_2}. As pointed out by Astrup et al., the actual state of the acid-base disorder may be characterized by the degree of compensation—*not compensated* (early or compensatory mechanisms not functioning), *partially compensated* (pH has not returned to a normal value), *compensated*, or *overcompensated*.

As previously noted, a knowledge of the pH, bicarbonate concentration, and P_{CO_2} will allow an accurate diagnosis of most acid-base disturbances. However, the clinical interpretation of these measurements is associated with some inherent problems. Although the arterial P_{CO_2} is considered an accurate index of primary respiratory disturbances, changes in the level may represent compensation for a primary metabolic alteration. Thus, a depressed P_{CO_2} (below 40 mm Hg) is characteristic of respiratory alkalosis

but also represents the normal compensatory response to a metabolic acidosis. Similarly, the level of plasma bicarbonate cannot be regarded exclusively as an index of metabolic disturbances. An elevated plasma bicarbonate level may indicate a primary metabolic alkalosis or a compensatory response to chronic respiratory acidosis.

In an effort to separate the respiratory and metabolic components of acid-base disorders, two other approaches have been introduced: in 1948 Singer and Hastings introduced the concept of *whole blood buffer base,* and later Astrup and his colleagues proposed the use of the *standard bicarbonate* and *base excess* values. The approach advocated by Astrup has been the more popular of the two, although both are attempts to quantify the metabolic, or nonrespiratory, component in an acid-base disturbance and separate it from the respiratory component.

The standard bicarbonate is defined as the concentration of bicarbonate in plasma, when whole blood with fully oxygenated hemoglobin has been equilibrated with CO_2 at a P_{CO_2} of 40 mm Hg at a temperature of 38°C. This value may be rapidly and accurately determined using the Astrup technique by measuring pH values at two known levels of P_{CO_2} and reading the standard bicarbonate directly from a nomogram. The normal mean value for standard bicarbonate is 24.5 mEq/L of plasma. As a measure of bicarbonate concentration in plasma, the standard bicarbonate is probably superior to both the CO_2 content and CO_2 combining power values, since the latter two determinations vary with the actual P_{CO_2} and oxygen saturation. Unfortunately, the standard bicarbonate, unlike the whole blood buffer base, does not indicate the total amount of surplus acid or base present, since the bicarbonate–carbonic acid system does not account for the entire buffering capacity of the blood. This information can be obtained by expressing the base content of the blood as *base excess* or *base deficit*. Base excess (or deficit) directly expresses the amount, in milliequivalents, of fixed base (or

Table 2-4. RESPIRATORY AND METABOLIC COMPONENTS
OF ACID-BASE DISORDERS

Type of acid-base disorder	Acute (uncompensated)			Chronic (partially compensated)		
	pH	P_{CO_2} (respiratory component)	Plasma HCO_3^-* (metabolic component)	pH	P_{CO_2} (respiratory component)	Plasma HCO_3^-* (metabolic component)
Respiratory acidosis...	↓↓	↑↑	N	↓	↑↑	↑
Respiratory alkalosis ..	↑↑	↓↓	N	↑	↓↓	↓
Metabolic acidosis...	↓↓	N	↓↓	↓	↓	↓
Metabolic alkalosis ..	↑↑	N	↑↑	↑	↑?	↑

*Measured as standard bicarbonate, whole blood buffer base, CO_2 content or CO_2 combining power. The *base excess value* is positive when the standard bicarbonate is above normal and negative when the standard bicarbonate is below normal.

fixed acid) added to each liter of blood. This value is obtained by multiplying the deviation of standard bicarbonate from the normal mean by a factor of 1.2. This factor corrects for the buffering capacity of the red cells and will vary slightly with changes in hemoglobin concentration. To avoid calculations, the base excess may be read directly from a nomogram. When the term *base excess* is used exclusively, the *positive* values represent the excess of base, and the *negative* values reflect the deficit of base (or excess of acid).*

In an excellent review of the Singer-Hastings and the Astrup systems, Schwartz and Relman state that neither system offers any advantage over the classic approach for the diagnosis of acid-base disorders. They question the validity of using an in vitro CO_2 titration curve as a measure of in vivo acid-base changes. Additionally, they note that the use of either of the two systems may be misleading in the analysis of chronic disorders. For example, a low pH with an elevated P_{CO_2}, a normal standard bicarbonate value, and a base excess value of zero are compatible with a diagnosis of primary uncompensated respiratory acidosis. After several hours or days, compensatory renal mechanisms would cause elevation of standard bicarbonate level above normal, resulting in a positive base excess value. This partially compensated respiratory acidosis, then, may be erroneously interpreted as a respiratory acidosis *plus* a metabolic alkalosis as indicated by a significant base excess.

Despite these shortcomings, either approach may be useful when properly interpreted as a single laboratory test. Other systems have been recommended, some with ingeniously devised nomograms, but all are subject to misinterpretation. Unfortunately, there are no shortcuts. Regardless of the methods used, the proper analysis of complex acid-base disorders requires a thorough knowledge of the clinical situation, good judgment, and a sound understanding of acid-base physiology.

RESPIRATORY ACIDOSIS. This condition is associated with retention of CO_2 secondary to decreased alveolar ventilation. The more common causes are listed in Table 2-3. Initially, the arterial P_{CO_2} is elevated (usually above 50 mm Hg), and the plasma bicarbonate concentration (measured as CO_2 combining power, CO_2 content, or standard bicarbonate) is normal. In the chronic form, the P_{CO_2} remains elevated, and the bicarbonate concentration rises as compensation occurs.

This problem may be particularly serious in the patient with chronic pulmonary disease in whom preexisting respiratory acidosis may be accentuated in the postoperative period. A number of conditions resulting in inadequate ventilation—airway obstruction, atelectasis, pneumonia, pleural effusion, hypoventilation due to the pain of upper abdominal incisions, or abdominal distension limiting diaphragmatic excursion—may exist singly or in combination to produce respiratory acidosis. Although restlessness, hy-

*The deficit or excess of base in the extracellular compartment can be estimated in milliequivalents by multiplying the negative or positive value for base excess, in milliequivalents per liter of blood, by 0.3 times the body weight in kilograms [Mellemgaard and Astrup].

pertension, and tachycardia in the immediate postoperative period may be due to pain, similar signs indicate inadequate ventilation with hypercapnia. The use of narcotics in this situation will compound the problem by further depressing respiration.

Management involves prompt correction of the pulmonary defect, when feasible, and measures to ensure adequate ventilation. Endotracheal intubation and mechanical ventilation are occasionally necessary to achieve this objective. Strict attention to tracheobronchial hygiene during the postoperative period is an important preventive measure in all patients, particularly those with chronic pulmonary disease. Encouraging deep breathing and coughing, using humidified air to prevent inspissation of secretions, and avoiding oversedation are all indicated.

RESPIRATORY ALKALOSIS. Respiratory alkalosis is a more common problem in the surgical patient than previously recognized. Hyperventilation due to apprehension, pain, hypoxia, central nervous system injury, and assisted ventilation are all common causes. Any of these conditions may cause a rapid depression of the arterial P_{CO_2} and elevation of the pH. The plasma bicarbonate concentration is normal in the acute phase, but falls with compensation if the condition persists.

Mild respiratory alkalosis secondary to hyperventilation during the operative procedure frequently occurs. This is of little consequence in the majority of patients and generally requires no therapy. One important exception is the patient with impaired cerebral blood flow from obstructive arterial disease (or during performance of carotid endarterectomy), in whom modest hypocapnia with cerebral vasoconstriction may cause irreparable damage.

The majority of patients who require ventilatory support in the postoperative period will develop varying degrees of respiratory alkalosis. This may be inadvertent, due to improper use of the mechanical respirator, or it may occur during attempts to raise the P_{O_2} in an hypoxic patient. Proper management of the patient on a mechanical ventilator requires frequent measurements of blood gases and appropriate corrections of the ventilatory pattern when indicated. The arterial P_{CO_2} should not be allowed to fall below 30 mm Hg, as serious complications may occur, particularly in the presence of a complicating hypokalemia or metabolic alkalosis. Generally, the P_{CO_2} can be maintained at an acceptable level by proper adjustments of the ventilatory rate and volume. Increasing the pulmonary dead space is of doubtful benefit, while adding 5 percent CO_2 to the inspired air is potentially dangerous and poorly tolerated by most patients.

The dangers of a severe respiratory alkalosis are those related to potassium depletion and include the development of ventricular arrhythmias and fibrillation, particularly in patients who are digitalized or have preexisting hypokalemia. Other complications include a shift of the oxygen dissociation curve to the left, which limits the ability of hemoglobin to unload oxygen at the tissue level except at low intracellular P_{O_2}, and the development of tetany and convulsions if the level of ionized calcium is significantly depressed. The development of hypokalemia may be quite sudden and is related to entry of potassium ions into the cells in exchange for hydrogen and an excessive urinary potassium loss in exchange for sodium. Severe and persistent respiratory alkalosis is often difficult to correct and may be associated with a poor prognosis because of the underlying cause of hyperventilation. Treatment is primarily directed toward preventing the condition by the proper use of mechanical respirators and correcting any preexisting potassium deficits.

METABOLIC ACIDOSIS. Metabolic acidosis results from the retention or gain of fixed acids (diabetic acidosis, lactic acidosis, azotemia) or the loss of base bicarbonate (diarrhea, small bowel fistula, renal insufficiency with inability to resorb bicarbonate). The excess of hydrogen ion results in lower pH and plasma bicarbonate concentration. The initial compensation is pulmonary, with an increase of the rate and depth of breathing and depression of the arterial P_{CO_2}.

Renal damage may interfere with the important role of the kidneys in the regulation of acid-base balance. The kidneys serve a vital function in this regard through the excretion of nitrogenous waste products and acid metabolites and the resorption of bicarbonates. If renal damage occurs and these functions are lost, metabolic acidosis develops rapidly and may be difficult to control.

With normal kidneys, metabolic acidosis may develop when the capacity of the kidneys for handling chlorides is exceeded. This is particularly common in patients who have excessive losses of alkaline gastrointestinal fluids (biliary, pancreatic, small bowel secretions) and are maintained on parenteral fluids for an extended period of time. Continued replacement of these losses with fluids having an inappropriate chloride/bicarbonate ratio, such as isotonic sodium chloride solution, will not correct the pH change; the use of a balanced salt solution, such as lactated Ringer's, is indicated.

One of the most common causes of severe metabolic acidosis in surgical patients is acute circulatory failure with accumulation of lactic acid. This is a reflection of tissue hypoxia due to inadequate perfusion, although it is only one of the manifestations of cellular dysfunction. Acute hemorrhagic shock may result in a rapid and profound drop in the pH, and attempts to raise the blood pressure with vasopressors will simply compound the problem. Similarly, attempts to correct the acidosis by the infusion of large quantities of sodium bicarbonate without restoration of flow are futile. Following restoration of adequate tissue perfusion by proper volume replacement, the lactic acid is quickly metabolized and the pH returned to normal. The use of lactated Ringer's solution to replace the extracellular fluid deficit incurred with hemorrhagic shock concomitant with administration of whole blood does not accentuate the lactic acidosis. Instead, there is a rapid decrease in the lactate level and return of pH toward normal, as opposed to the results when whole blood alone is used.

The indiscriminate use of sodium bicarbonate during the resuscitation of patients in hypovolemic shock is discouraged for several reasons. A mild metabolic alkalosis is a common finding following resuscitation, in part due to the alkalinizing effects of blood transfusions and the administration of lactated Ringer's solution. After infusion (and partial restoration of hepatic blood flow), the citrate contained in the transfused blood and the lactate in lactated Ringer's solution are metabolized and bicarbonate is formed. The organic acidosis (lactic acid) that developed during the shock episode is rapidly cleared once adequate tissue perfusion is restored. Lactic acid production ceases, the hydrogen ion load is buffered and excreted via the lungs as CO_2, and the organic anion, lactate, is metabolized by the liver. If excessive quantities of sodium bicarbonate are administered simultaneously, severe metabolic alkalosis can result. An alkaline pH may be highly undesirable in this situation, particularly in patients with hypoxia or low fixed cardiac outputs, because it shifts the oxygen dissociation curve to the left. Other factors that tend to shift the oxygen dissociation curve to the left in this situation include the depressed level of erythrocyte 2,3-diphosphoglycerate in the transfused blood and the development of hypothermia. If the curve shifts far enough to the left, significant interference with oxygen unloading at the cellular level may occur.

The treatment of metabolic acidosis, therefore, should be directed toward correction of the underlying disorder when possible. Bicarbonate therapy properly may be reserved for the treatment of severe metabolic acidosis, particularly following cardiac arrest, when partial correction of the pH may be essential to restore myocardial function. However, recent studies indicate that the acidosis accompanying cardiac arrest is well compensated for a significant period of time if the patient is well ventilated and not previously acidotic. In addition, the administration of bicarbonate in the usual recommended doses may induce an acute and severe hypernatremia and hyperosmolarity. Thus bicarbonate should be used judiciously during cardiac arrest. Mattar et al. recommended that the initial dose of bicarbonate not exceed 50 ml of 7.5% solution (45 mEq $NaHCO_3$ containing 90 mO) and that the decision for additional doses be based on measurements of pH and P_{CO_2} when possible.

Similarly, pH correction of more protracted states of metabolic acidosis may be indicated but should be accomplished slowly. Frequent measurements of serum electrolytes and blood pH are the best guides to therapy, since a satisfactory formula to estimate the amount of alkali needed has not been devised.

METABOLIC ALKALOSIS. Metabolic alkalosis results from the loss of fixed acids or the gain of base bicarbonate and is aggravated by any preexisting potassium depletion. Both the pH and plasma bicarbonate concentration are elevated. Compensation for metabolic alkalosis is primarily by renal mechanisms, since respiratory compensation is generally small and cannot be detected in most patients. Rarely, hypercapnia may represent a compensatory response to metabolic alkalosis in patients without chronic pulmonary disease. When this is suspected, rapid reduction in P_{CO_2} by mechanical ventilation should be avoided. Rather, the P_{CO_2} will fall as the metabolic alkalosis is corrected.

The majority of patients with metabolic alkalosis have some degree of hypokalemia. Depletion of cellular potassium results in entry of hydrogen and sodium ions into the cells with resultant lowering of intracellular pH and an extracellular alkalosis. Metabolic alkalosis, in turn, results in excessive urinary potassium loss in exchange for sodium, which further accentuates the alkalosis. The dangers of metabolic alkalosis are the same as discussed with respiratory alkalosis.

An interesting and not infrequent problem in the surgical patient is hypochloremic, hypokalemic metabolic alkalosis resulting from persistent vomiting or gastric suction in the patient with pyloric obstruction. Unlike vomiting with an open pylorus (involving a loss of gastric, pancreatic, biliary, and intestinal secretions), this entity results in loss of fluid with high chloride and hydrogen ion concentration in relation to sodium. The loss of chloride causes accelerated loss of sodium and bicarbonate in the urine and partial compensation of the alkalosis. In addition, the alkalosis itself causes increased renal excretion of potassium. As the volume deficit progresses, potassium and hydrogen ions are excreted into the urine in increasing quantities in an attempt to conserve sodium, resulting in an uncompensated alkalosis and hypokalemia. The initially alkaline urine becomes acid after a period of time due to the hydrogen ion excretion ("paradoxic aciduria"). Proper management includes replacement of the extracellular fluid volume deficit with isotonic sodium chloride solution in addition to replacement of potassium. A severe potassium depletion is invariably present but may be overlooked due to concentration of the serum potassium by a severe volume deficit. However, volume repletion should be started and a good urine output obtained before potassium is administered.

Rarely, severe hypokalemic metabolic alkalosis in a patient with pyloric outlet obstruction may be refractory to standard therapy. This occurs most often in patients who also have severe hypochloremia and several liters of nasogastric drainage daily. In the past, the infusion of ammonium chloride or arginine hydrochloride was the usual method for increasing the level of nonvolatile acids. However, infusion of the first may produce ammonia toxicity, and the latter solution is no longer available commercially. Recently, the use of $0.1N$ to $0.2N$ hydrochloric acid has been shown to be safe and effective therapy for correction of severe, resistant metabolic alkalosis. The technique for infusion of hydrochloric acid, as described by Abouna et al., involves the preparation of an isotonic solution by the addition of 150 ml of $1N$ hydrochloric acid (300 mEq of hydrogen and chloride) to 1 liter of sterile water. The hydrochloric acid can be added to a liter of isotonic saline or 5% dextrose solution if desired. The infusion should be administered over a 6- to 24-hour period, with measurements of pH, P_{CO_2}, and serum electrolytes every 4 to 6 hours. Generally, 1 or 2 liters of solution over a period of 24 hours is sufficient, although one should not hesitate to infuse additional hydrochloric acid when the need is based on appropriate clinical and laboratory evidence. Temporary control of the alkalosis with this method is usually successful, but underlying cause should be controlled as soon as possible.

The initial dose of hydrochloric acid solution can be roughly calculated from the estimated chloride or hydrogen ion deficit. The chloride deficit is calculated from the plasma chloride concentration and the chloride space (approximately 20 percent of body weight). The hydrogen ion deficit can be calculated from the plasma base excess and the hydrogen ion space (approximately 60 percent of total body weight). As an example, for a 70-kg patient with a metabolic alkalosis and a plasma chloride of 80 mEq/L the initial dose of hydrochloric acid is calculated as follows:

$$
\begin{aligned}
\text{Chloride deficit} &= (20\% \text{ of body weight}) \\
&\quad \times (\text{normal plasma chloride} \\
&\quad - \text{observed plasma chloride}) \\
&= (0.2 \times 70\,\text{kg}) \\
&\quad \times (103\,\text{mEq/L} - 80\,\text{mEq/L}) \\
&= 322\,\text{mEq}
\end{aligned}
$$

This amount of chloride (as hydrochloric acid) would be contained in approximately 2 liters of the solution described above. It is emphasized that while calculations of this type are helpful, close monitoring of pH and serum electrolytes is essential.

POTASSIUM ABNORMALITIES

The normal dietary intake of potassium is approximately 50 to 100 mEq daily, and in the absence of hypokalemia, the majority of this is excreted in the urine. Ninety-eight percent of the potassium in the body is located within the intracellular compartment at a concentration of approximately 150 mEq/L, and it is the major cation of intracellular water. Although the total extracellular potassium in a 70-kg male would approximate only 63 mEq (4.5 mEq/L $\times$ 14L), this small amount is critical to cardiac and neuromuscular function. In addition, the turnover rate in the extracellular fluid compartment may be extremely rapid.

The intracellular and extracellular distribution of potassium is influenced by many factors. Significant quantities of intracellular potassium are released into the extracellular space in response to severe injury or surgical stress, acidosis, and the catabolic state. A significant rise in serum potassium may occur in these states in the presence of oliguric or anuric renal failure, but dangerous hyperkalemia (greater than 6 mEq/L) is rarely encountered if renal function is normal. After severe trauma, however, normal or excessive urinary volumes may not reflect the ability of the kidney to clear solutes or to excrete potassium. (See the section High-Output Renal Failure.)

HYPERKALEMIA. The signs of a significant hyperkalemia are limited to the cardiovascular and gastrointestinal systems. The gastrointestinal symptoms include nausea, vomiting, intermittent intestinal colic, and diarrhea. The cardiovascular signs are apparent on the electrocardiogram initially, with high peaked T waves, widened QRS complex, and depressed ST segments. Disappearance of T waves, heart block, and diastolic cardiac arrest may develop with increasing levels of potassium.

Treatment of hyperkalemia consists of immediate measures to reduce the serum potassium level, withholding of exogenously administered potassium, and correction of the

Table 2-5. COMPOSITION OF GASTROINTESTINAL SECRETIONS

Type of secretion	Volume (ml/24 hr)	Na (mEq/L)	K (mEq/L)	Cl (mEq/L)	HCO₃ (mEq/L)
Salivary	1,500 (500–2,000)	10 (2–10)	26 (20–30)	10 (8–18)	30
Stomach	1,500 (100–4,000)	60 (9–116)	10 (0–32)	130 (8–154)	
Duodenum	(100–2,000)	140	5	80	
Ileum	3,000 (100–9,000)	140 (80–150)	5 (2–8)	104 (43–137)	30
Colon	. . . .	60	30	40	
Pancreas	. . . . (100–800)	140 (113–185)	5 (3–7)	75 (54–95)	115
Bile	. . . . (50–800)	145 (131–164)	5 (3–12)	100 (89–180)	35

underlying cause if possible. Temporary suppression of the myocardial effects of a sudden rapid rise of potassium level can be accomplished by the intravenous administration of a solution containing 80 mEq of sodium lactate, 100 ml of calcium gluconate, and 100 ml of 50% dextrose in water. The administration of dextrose stimulates the synthesis of glycogen, resulting in an uptake of potassium. Insulin may also be given, but it should be limited to 1 unit per 5 Gm or more of glucose, since rebound hypoglycemia may be fatal. The sodium lactate raises the pH and shifts potassium intracellularly, and the calcium gluconate tends to counteract the myocardial effects of hyperkalemia. Administration of this solution over a 2-hour period allows time to prepare for definitive removal of the excess potassium by hemodialysis or peritoneal dialysis. A slow rise of potassium level (less than 1 mEq/L/day) can be controlled by the use of cation-exchange resins, preferably in the sodium cycle,* administered by rectum in doses of 24 Gm every 12 hours. To prevent rapid absorption of water from the colon, 200 ml of 10% dextrose in water is used as the vehicle.

HYPOKALEMIA. The more common problem in the surgical patient is hypokalemia, which may occur as a result of (1) excessive renal excretion, (2) movement of potassium into cells, (3) prolonged administration of potassium-free parenteral fluids with continued obligatory renal loss of potassium (20 mEq/day or more), (4) parenteral hyperalimentation with inadequate potassium replacement, and (5) loss in gastrointestinal secretions.

Potassium plays an important role in the regulation of acid-base balance. Increased renal excretion occurs with both respiratory and metabolic alkalosis. Potassium is in competition with hydrogen ion for renal tubular excretion in exchange for sodium ion. Thus, in alkalosis, the increased potassium ion excretion in exchange for sodium ion permits hydrogen ion conservation. Hypokalemia itself may produce a metabolic alkalosis, since an increase in excretion of hydrogen ions occurs when the concentration

of potassium in the tubular cell is low. In addition, movement of hydrogen ions into the cells as a consequence of potassium loss is partly responsible for the alkalosis. In metabolic acidosis the reverse process occurs, and the excess hydrogen ion exchanges for sodium with retention of greater amounts of potassium.

Renal tubular excretion of potassium ion is increased when large quantities of sodium are available for excretion. The more sodium ion available for resorption, the more potassium is exchanged for it in the lumen. Potassium requirements for prolonged or massive isotonic fluid volume replacement are increased, probably on this basis. The same mechanism may also explain the increased potassium ion excretion with steroid administration.

The renal excretion of potassium may be small when compared to the amount of potassium that may be lost in gastrointestinal secretions. The amount per liter in various types of gastrointestinal fluids is shown in Table 2-5. Although the average potassium concentration of some of these fluids is relatively low, significant hypokalemia will result if potassium-free fluids are used for replacement.

Hypokalemia also may be a serious problem in the patient maintained on intravenous hyperalimentation. Large quantities of supplemental potassium generally are necessary to restore depleted intracellular stores and to meet the requirements for tissue synthesis during the anabolic phase. (See the section Nutrition.)

In summary, most of the factors that tend to influence potassium metabolism result in excess excretion, and a tendency toward hypokalemia occurs frequently in the surgical patient except when shock or acidosis interferes with the normal renal handling of potassium.

The signs of potassium deficit are related to failure of normal contractility of skeletal, smooth, and cardiac muscle and include weakness that may progress to flaccid paralysis, diminished to absent tendon reflexes, and paralytic ileus. Sensitivity to digitalis with cardiac arrhythmias and electrocardiographic signs of low voltage, flattening of T waves, and depression of ST segments are characteristic. However, signs of potassium deficit may be masked

*Kayexalate.

by those of a severe extracellular fluid volume deficit. Repletion of the volume deficit may further aggravate the situation by lowering the serum potassium level secondary to dilution.

The treatment of hypokalemia involves, first, prevention of this state. In the replacement of gastrointestinal fluids, it is safe to replace the upper limits of loss, since an excess is readily handled by the patient with normal renal function. Potassium is available in 20-mEq and 40-mEq ampules for addition to intravenous fluids. No more than 40 mEq should be added to a liter of intravenous fluid, and the rate of administration should not exceed 40 mEq/hour unless the electrocardiogram is being monitored. In the absence of specific indications, potassium should not be given to the oliguric patient or during the first 24 hours following severe surgical stress or trauma.

CALCIUM ABNORMALITIES

The majority of the 1,000 to 1,200 Gm of body calcium in the average-sized adult is found in the bone in the form of phosphate and carbonate. Normal daily intake of calcium is between 1 and 3 Gm. Most of this is excreted via the gastrointestinal tract, and 200 mg or less is excreted in the urine daily. The normal serum level is between 9 and 11 mg/100 ml (depending on the individual laboratory's normal range), and approximately half of this is not ionized and is bound to plasma protein. An additional nonionized fraction (5 percent) is bound to other substances in the plasma and interstitial fluid, whereas the remaining 45 percent is the ionized portion that is responsible for neuromuscular stability. Determination of the plasma protein level, therefore, is essential for proper analysis of the serum calcium level. The ratio of ionized to nonionized calcium is also related to the pH; acidosis causes an increase in the ionized fraction, whereas alkalosis causes a decrease.

Disturbances of calcium metabolism generally are not a problem in the uncomplicated postoperative patient, with the exception of skeletal loss during prolonged immobilization. Routine administration of calcium to the surgical patient, therefore, is not needed in the absence of specific indications.

HYPOCALCEMIA. The symptoms of hypocalcemia (serum level less than 8 mg/100 ml) are numbness and tingling of the circumoral region and the tips of the fingers and toes. The signs are of neuromuscular origin and include hyperactive tendon reflexes, positive Chvostek's sign, muscle and abdominal cramps, tetany with carpopedal spasm, convulsions (with severe deficit), and prolongation of the Q-T interval on the electrocardiogram.

The common causes include acute pancreatitis, massive soft tissue infections (necrotizing fasciitis), acute and chronic renal failure, pancreatic and small intestinal fistulas, and hypoparathyroidism. Transient hypocalcemia is a frequent occurrence in the hyperparathyroid patient following removal of a parathyroid adenoma, owing to atrophy of the remaining glands. Asymptomatic hypocalcemia may occur with hypoproteinemia (normal ionized fraction), whereas symptoms may appear with a normal serum calcium level in a patient with severe alkalosis. The latter is due to a decrease in the physiologically active or ionized fraction of total serum calcium. Calcium levels also may fall with a severe depletion of magnesium.

Treatment is directed toward correction of the underlying cause with concomitant repletion of the deficit. Acute symptoms may be relieved by the intravenous administration of calcium gluconate or calcium chloride. Calcium lactate may be given orally, with or without supplemental vitamin D, in the patient requiring prolonged replacement. The routine administration of calcium during massive transfusions of blood remains controversial and reflects a paucity of studies where calcium *ion* levels are measured. In the majority of studies, calcium ion concentrations have been estimated from measured *total* serum calcium levels. Presently, available data indicate that the majority of patients receiving blood transfusions do not require calcium supplementation. The binding of ionized calcium by citrate is generally compensated for by the mobilization of calcium from body stores. For patients receiving blood as rapidly as 500 ml every 5 to 10 minutes, however, calcium administration is recommended. An appropriate dose, from the data of Moore, is 0.2 Gm of calcium chloride (2 ml of 10% calcium chloride solution), administered intravenously in a separate line, for every 500 ml of blood transfused. To avoid dangerous levels of hypercalcemia, this dose of calcium is recommended only while blood is being transfused at the rate noted above. Additionally, the total dose of calcium generally should not exceed 3 Gm unless there is objective evidence of hypocalcemia. Larger doses are rarely indicated, since there is some mobilization of calcium and citrate breakdown with release of calcium ion even with shock and inadequate peripheral perfusion. During massive transfusions, some attempt should be made to monitor the calcium level. A rough approximation of calcium ion concentration can be obtained by monitoring the Q-T interval on the ECG, although techniques for the rapid measurement of calcium ion concentration are now available.

HYPERCALCEMIA. The symptoms of hypercalcemia are rather vague and of gastrointestinal, renal, musculoskeletal, and central nervous system origin. The early manifestations of hypercalcemia include easy fatigue, lassitude, weakness of varying degree, anorexia, nausea, vomiting, and weight loss. With higher serum calcium levels, lassitude gives way to somnambulism, stupor, and finally coma. Other symptoms include severe headaches, pains in the back and extremities, thirst, polydypsia, and polyuria. The critical level for serum calcium is between 16 and 20 mg/100 ml, and unless treatment is instituted promptly, the symptoms may rapidly progress to death. The two major causes of hypercalcemia are hyperparathyroidism and cancer with bony metastasis. The latter is most frequently seen in the patient with metastatic breast cancer who is receiving estrogen therapy.

The treatment of acute hypercalcemia crisis is an emergency. Measures to lower the serum calcium level are instituted immediately while preparations are being made for more definitive treatment. Of particular importance is the rapid repletion of the associated extracellular fluid volume deficit, which will immediately lower the calcium level by dilution. Other measures which have been used and may be of temporary benefit include the use of a chelating agent (EDTA), steroids, sodium sulfate solution, and hemodialysis. Recently, intravenous mithromycin has been shown to reduce the serum calcium level in normocalcemic and hypercalcemic patients. The definitive treatment of acute hypercalcemic crisis in patients with hyperparathyroidism is immediate surgery.

Treatment of hypercalcemia in the patient with metastatic cancer is primarily that of prevention. The serum calcium level is checked frequently; if it is elevated, the patient is placed on a low-calcium diet, and measures to ensure adequate hydration are instituted.

MAGNESIUM ABNORMALITIES

The infrequent occurrence of magnesium deficiency and the previous lack of a rapid, precise technique for measurement of magnesium ion concentration accounts for the late appreciation of this entity. The total body content of magnesium in the average adult is approximately 2,000 mEq, about half of which is incorporated in bone and only slowly exchangeable. The distribution of magnesium is similar to that of potassium, the major portion being intracellular. Plasma magnesium concentration normally ranges between 1.5 and 2.5 mEq/L. The normal dietary intake of magnesium is approximately 20 mEq (240 mg) daily. The larger part is excreted in the feces, and the remainder in the urine. The kidneys show a remarkable ability to conserve magnesium; on a magnesium-free diet, renal excretion of this ion may be less than 1 mEq/day.

MAGNESIUM DEFICIENCY. Magnesium deficiency is known to occur with starvation, malabsorption syndromes, protracted losses of gastrointestinal fluid, and prolonged parenteral fluid therapy with magnesium-free solutions, and during parenteral hyperalimentation when inadequate quantities of magnesium have been added to the solutions. Other causes include acute pancreatitis, diabetic acidosis during treatment, primary aldosteronism, chronic alcoholism, and burns (late stage).

The magnesium ion is essential for proper function of most enzyme systems, and depletion is characterized by neuromuscular and central nervous system hyperactivity. The signs and symptoms are quite similar to those of calcium deficiency, including hyperactive tendon reflexes, muscle tremors, and tetany with a positive Chvostek sign. Progression to delirium and convulsions may occur with a severe deficit. A concomitant calcium deficiency occasionally is noted, particularly in those with clinical signs of tetany.

The diagnosis of magnesium deficiency depends on an awareness of the syndrome and clinical recognition of the symptoms. Laboratory confirmation is available but not reliable, as the syndrome may exist in the presence of a normal serum magnesium level. The possibility of magnesium deficiency should always be considered in the surgical patient who exhibits disturbed neuromuscular or cerebral activity in the postoperative period. This is particularly important in patients who have had protracted dysfunction of the gastrointestinal tract with long-term maintenance on parenteral fluids and in patients on parenteral hyperalimentation. Routine magnesium is always indicated in the management of these patients.

Treatment of magnesium deficiency is by the parenteral administration of magnesium sulfate or magnesium chloride solution. If renal function is normal, as much as 2 mEq of magnesium/kg of body weight can be administered in a day in the face of severe depletion. Magnesium sulfate (50% solution contains approximately 4 mEq of magnesium ion per milliliter) may be given intravenously or intramuscularly. The intravenous route is preferable for the initial treatment of a severe symptomatic deficit. The solution is prepared by the addition of 80 mEq of magnesium sulfate (20 ml of 50% solution) to a liter of intravenous fluid and is administered over a 4-hour period. If the patient is not symptomatic, the infusion should be given over a longer period of time. The possibility of acute magnesium toxicity should be kept in mind when giving this ion intravenously. When large doses are given, the heart rate, blood pressure, respiration, and ECG should be monitored closely for signs of magnesium toxicity, which could lead to cardiac arrest. It is advisable to have calcium chloride or calcium gluconate available to counteract any adverse effects of a rapidly rising plasma magnesium level.

Partial or complete relief of symptoms may follow this infusion as a result of increased concentration of magnesium ion in the extracellular fluid compartment, although continued replacement over a 1- to 3-week period is necessary to replenish the intracellular compartment. For this purpose and for the asymptomatic patient who is likely to have significant magnesium depletion, 10 to 20 mEq of 50% magnesium sulfate solution is given daily by the intramuscular route or in infusion fluids. When magnesium sulfate is used, it should be given in divided doses or at multiple sites, since the intramuscular injection of this salt is painful. Following complete repletion of intracellular magnesium and in the absence of abnormal loss, balance may be maintained by the administration of as little as 4 mEq of magnesium ion daily. The amount of magnesium supplementation required for patients on parenteral hyperalimentation varies but approximates 12 to 24 mEq daily for the average patient.

Magnesium ion should not be given to the oliguric patient or in the presence of severe volume deficit unless actual magnesium depletion is demonstrated. If given to a patient with renal insufficiency, considerably smaller doses are used, and the patient is carefully observed for signs or symptoms of toxicity.

MAGNESIUM EXCESS. Symptomatic hypermagnesemia, although rare, is most commonly seen with severe renal insufficiency. Retention and accumulation of magnesium may occur in any patient with impaired glomerular or renal tubular function, and the presence of acidosis may rapidly compound the situation. Serum magnesium levels tend to parallel changes in potassium concentration in these cases. Therefore, magnesium levels should be carefully monitored in cases of acute and chronic renal failure and in selected patients with borderline renal function. Randall et al. have shown that in patients on ordinary dietary intakes of magnesium, increased serum concentrations of the ion do not occur until the glomerular filtration rate falls below 30 ml/minute. As noted by Henzel et al., however, magnesium-containing antacids and laxatives (milk of magnesia, epsom salts, Gelusil, Maalox) are commonly administered in quantities sufficient to produce toxic serum levels of magnesium where impaired renal function is present. Other conditions which may be associated with symptomatic hypermagnesemia include early-stage burns, massive trauma or surgical stress, severe extracellular volume deficit, and severe acidosis.

The early signs and symptoms include lethargy and weakness with progressive loss of deep tendon reflexes. Interference with cardiac conduction occurs with increasing levels of magnesium and changes in the electrocardiogram (increased P-R interval, widened QRS complex, and elevated T waves) resemble those seen with hyperkalemia. Somnolence leading to coma and muscular paralysis occur in the later stages, and death is usually caused by respiratory or cardiac arrest.

Treatment consists of immediate measures to lower the serum magnesium level by correcting any acidosis, replenishing any preexisting extracellular volume deficit, and withholding exogenously administered magnesium. Acute symptoms may be temporarily controlled by the slow intravenous administration of 5 to 10 mEq of calcium chloride or calcium gluconate. If elevated levels or symptoms persist, peritoneal dialysis or hemodialysis is indicated.

NORMAL EXCHANGE OF FLUID AND ELECTROLYTES

Knowledge of the basic principles governing both the internal and external exchanges of water and salt is mandatory for care of the patient undergoing major operative surgery. The stable internal fluid environment, which is maintained by the kidneys, brain, lungs, skin, and gastrointestinal tract, may be compromised by severe surgical stress or direct damage to any of these organs.

Water Exchange

The normal individual consumes an average of 2,000 to 2,500 ml water/day; approximately 1,500 ml water is taken by mouth, and the rest is extracted from solid food, either from the contents of the food or as the product of oxidation (Table 2-6). The daily water losses include 250 ml in stools, 800 to 1,500 ml as urine, and approximately 600 to 900 ml as insensible loss. A patient deprived of all external access to water must still excrete a minimum of 500 to 800 ml urine/day in order to excrete the products of catabolism, in addition to the mandatory insensible loss through the skin and lungs.

Insensible loss of water occurs through the skin (75 percent) and the lungs (25 percent) and is increased by hypermetabolism, hyperventilation, and fever. The insensible water loss through the skin is not from evaporation of water from sweat glands but from water vapor formed

Table 2-6. WATER EXCHANGE (60–80 kg man)

Routes	Average daily volume, ml	Minimal, ml	Maximal, ml
H$_2$O gain:			
Sensible:			
Oral fluids.......	800–1,500	0	1,500/hr
Solid foods	500–700	0	1,500
Insensible:			
Water of oxidation ..	250	125	800
Water of solution. . .	0	0	500
H$_2$O loss:			
Sensible:			
Urine	800–1,500	300	1,400/hr (diabetes insipidus)
Intestinal	0–250	0	2,500/hr
Sweat	0	0	4,000/hr
Insensible:			
Lungs and skin	600–900	600–900	1,500

within the body and lost through the skin. With excessive heat production (or excessive environmental heat), the capacity for insensible loss through the skin is exceeded, and sweating occurs. These losses may, but seldom do, exceed 250 ml/day/degree of fever. An unhumidified tracheostomy with hyperventilation increases the loss through the lungs and results in a total insensible loss up to 1.5 liters/day.

A frequently overlooked source of gain is the water of solution, which is the water that holds carbohydrates and proteins in solution in the cell. Normally, gain of water from this source is zero, but after 4 to 5 days without food intake, the postoperative patient may begin to gain significant quantities of water (maximum 500 ml daily) from excessive cellular catabolism. The amount depends on the degree of trauma and the complications occurring postoperatively.

Salt Gain and Losses

In the normal individual, the salt intake per day varies between 50 and 90 mEq (3 to 5 Gm) as sodium chloride (Table 2-7). Balance is maintained primarily by the normal kidneys that excrete the excess salt. Under conditions of reduced intake or extrarenal losses, the normal kidney can reduce sodium excretion to less than 1 mEq/day within 24 hours after restriction. In the patient with salt-wasting kidneys, however, the loss may exceed 200 mEq/L of urine. Sweat represents a hypotonic loss of fluids with an average sodium concentration of 15 mEq/L in the acclimatized patient. In the unacclimatized individual, the sodium concentration in sweat may be 60 mEq/L or more. Insensible fluid lost from the skin and lungs, by definition, is pure water. For practical considerations then, normal losses may be relatively free of salt in the healthy individual with normal renal function.

The volume and composition of various types of gastrointestinal secretions are shown in Table 2-5. Gastrointesti-

Table 2-7. SODIUM (SALT) EXCHANGE
(60–80 kg man)

Sodium exchange	Average	Minimal	Maximal
Sodium gain:			
Diet	50–90 mEq/day	0	75–100 mEq/hr (oral)
Sodium loss:			
Skin (sweat) . .	10–60 mEq/day*	0	300 mEq/hr
Urine	10–80 mEq/day	<1 mEq/day†	110–200 mEq/L‡
Intestines . . .	0–20 mEq/day	0	300 mEq/hr

*Depending on the degree of acclimatization of the individual.
†With normal renal function.
‡With renal salt wasting.

nal losses are usually isotonic or slightly hypotonic, although there is considerable variation in the composition. These should be replaced by an essentially isotonic salt solution. It is also important to reiterate that distributional or sequestration losses of extracellular fluid at any point in the operative or postoperative course also represent isotonic losses of salt and water.

FLUID AND ELECTROLYTE THERAPY

Parenteral Solutions

The composition of various parenteral fluids available for administration is shown in Table 2-8. There is sufficient variety to satisfy the majority of fluid requirements in the surgical patient. The proper choice of parenteral fluid in a given situation will correct the abnormalities but impose minimal demands on the kidneys.

A good available isotonic salt solution for replacing

Table 2-8. COMPOSITION OF PARENTERAL FLUIDS
Electrolyte content (mEq/L)

Solutions	Cations					Anions		
	Na	K	Ca	Mg	NH₄	Cl	HCO₃⁻	HPO₄⁻
Extracellular fluid	142	4	5	3	.3	103	27	3
Lactated Ringer's	130	4	2.7			109	28*	
0.9% sodium chloride (saline)	154					154		
M/6 sodium lactate	167						167*	
M (molar) sodium lactate	1,000						1,000*	
3% sodium chloride	513					513		
5% sodium chloride	855					855		
0.9% ammonium chloride					168	168		

*Present in solution as lactate which is converted to bicarbonate.

gastrointestinal losses and repairing preexisting volume deficits, in the absence of gross abnormalities of concentration and composition, is lactated Ringer's solution. This solution is "physiologic" and contains 130 mEq sodium balanced by 109 mEq chloride and 28 mEq lactate. This fluid has minimal effects on normal body fluid composition and pH even when infused in large quantities. The chief disadvantage of lactated Ringer's solution is the slight hyposmolarity with respect to sodium. Each liter of lactated Ringer's solution furnishes approximately 100 to 150 ml free water. This rarely presents a clinical problem if it is considered in calculating water replacement. The remainder of the solutions listed in Table 2-8 are used to correct specific defects. Choice of a particular fluid depends on the volume status of the patient and the type of concentration or compositional abnormality present.

Isotonic sodium chloride contains 154 mEq sodium and 154 mEq chloride/L. The high concentration of chloride above the normal serum concentration of 103 mEq/L imposes on the kidneys an appreciable load of excess chloride which cannot be rapidly excreted. Thus, a dilutional acidosis may develop.* This solution is ideal, however, for the initial correction of an extracellular fluid volume deficit in the presence of hyponatremia, hypochloremia, and metabolic alkalosis. In a similar situation with moderate metabolic acidosis, M/6 sodium lactate (167 mEq/L each of sodium and lactate) may be given. Another solution for this purpose can be made by adding one ampule of sodium bicarbonate (40 ml solution containing 40 mEq each of sodium and bicarbonate) to 1,000 ml lactated Ringer's solution.

Molar sodium lactate solution or 3 or 5% sodium chloride may be used to correct symptomatic hyponatremic states. The choice of anion (lactate or chloride) is determined by the accompanying acid-base derangement. The need for ammonium chloride solutions in the treatment of an uncompensated metabolic alkalosis is extremely rare. Indications for their use include very shallow or slow breathing with cyanosis or severe tetany. Following the correction of concentration or compositional abnormalities using specific repair solutions, a balanced salt solution is used to replenish the remaining volume deficit.

Preoperative Fluid Therapy

Preoperative evaluation and correction of existing fluid disorders is an integral part of surgical care. An orderly approach to these problems requires an understanding of the common fluid disturbances associated with surgical illness and adherence to a few simple guidelines. There are no shortcuts; close observation of the patient and frequent reevaluation of the clinical situation is the most rewarding approach.

The analysis of a fluid disorder may be facilitated by categorizing the abnormalities into *volume, concentration,*

*Infusion of a large volume of isotonic sodium chloride solution may induce or aggravate a preexisting acidosis by reducing the amount of base bicarbonate in the body relative to the carbonic acid content.

and *compositional* changes. Although some disease states produce characteristic changes in fluid balance, much confusion may be avoided by regarding each disturbance as a separate entity. For example, volume changes cannot be accurately predicted from a knowledge of the level of serum sodium, since an extracellular fluid volume deficit or excess may exist with a normal, low, or high sodium concentration. Similarly, any of the four primary acid-base disturbances may be associated with any combination of volume and concentration abnormalities.

CORRECTION OF VOLUME CHANGES

Changes in the volume of extracellular fluid are the most frequent and important abnormalities encountered in the surgical patient. Depletion of the extracellular fluid compartment without changes in concentration or composition is a common problem. The diagnosis of volume changes is made almost entirely on clinical grounds. The signs that will be present in an individual patient depend not only on the relative or absolute quantity of extracellular fluid which has been lost but also on the rapidity with which it is lost and the presence or absence of signs of associated disease.

Volume deficits in the surgical patient may result from external loss of fluids or from an internal redistribution of extracellular fluid into a nonfunctional compartment. Generally, it involves a combination of the two, but the internal redistribution is frequently overlooked.

The phenomenon of internal redistribution or translocation of extracellular fluid is peculiar to many surgical diseases; in the individual patient, the loss may be quite large. Although the concept of a "third space" is not new, it is generally considered only in relation to patients with massive ascites, burns, or crush injuries. Of more importance, however, is the "third space" loss into the peritoneum, the bowel wall, and other tissues with inflammatory lesions of the intraabdominal organs. The magnitude of these losses may not be fully appreciated without realization of the fact that the peritoneum alone has approximately 1 m² of surface area. A slight increase in thickness from sequestration of fluid, which would not be appreciated on casual observation, may result in a functional loss of several liters of fluid. Swelling of the bowel wall and mesentery and secretion of fluid into the lumen of the bowel will cause even larger losses. Similar deficits may occur with massive infection of the subcutaneous tissues (necrotizing fasciitis) or with severe crush injury.

These "parasitic" losses remain a part of the extracellular fluid space and may be measured as a slowly equilibrating volume. The term *nonfunctional* is used because the fluid is no longer able to participate in the normal functions of the extracellular fluid compartment and may just as well have been lost externally. Any transfer of intracellular fluid to the extracellular compartment for replenishment of the loss is insignificant in the acute phase. The patient with ascites may have an enormous total extracellular fluid volume although the functional component is severely depleted. The same is true of extensive inflammatory or obstructive lesions of the gastrointestinal tract, although the loss is not as obvious. These losses will

evoke the signs and symptoms of an extracellular fluid volume deficit with or without the concomitant external loss of fluids.

Exact quantification of these deficits is impossible and, at the present time, probably unnecessary. The defect can be estimated on the basis of the severity of the clinical signs. A mild deficit represents a loss of approximately 4 percent of body weight, a moderate loss is 6 to 8 percent of body weight, and a severe deficit is approximately 10 percent of body weight. It is important to reemphasize the fact that cardiovascular signs predominate when there is acute rapid loss of fluid from the extracellular fluid compartment with few or no tissue signs. In addition to the estimated deficit, fluids lost during the period of treatment must be replaced.

Fluid replacement should be started and changed according to the response of the patient noted on frequent clinical observation. Reliance on a formula or single clinical sign to determine adequacy of resuscitation is fraught with danger. Rather, reversal of the signs of the volume deficit, combined with stabilization of the blood pressure and pulse, and an hourly urine volume of 30 to 50 ml are used as general guidelines. An adequate hourly urine output, although usually a reliable index of volume replacement, may be totally misleading. The excessive administration of glucose (over 50 Gm in a 2- to 3-hour period) may result in osmotic diuresis, while an osmotic agent such as mannitol tends to produce urine at the expense of the vascular volume. Patients with chronic renal disease or incipient acute renal damage from shock and injury also may have inappropriately high urinary volumes. In addition, the rapid administration of salt solutions may transiently expand the intravascular volume, increase the glomerular filtration rate, and result in an immediate outpouring of urine, although the total extracellular fluid space remains quite depleted.

The choice of the proper fluid for replacement depends on the existence of concomitant concentration or compositional abnormalities. With pure extracellular fluid volume loss or when only minimal concentration or compositional abnormalities are present, the use of a balanced salt solution, such as lactated Ringer's, is desirable.

CORRECTION OF CONCENTRATION CHANGES

If severe *symptomatic* hyponatremia or hypernatremia complicates the volume loss, prompt correction of the concentration abnormality to the extent that symptoms are relieved is necessary. Volume replenishment then should be accomplished with slower correction of the remaining concentration abnormality. For immediate correction of severe hyponatremia, 5% sodium chloride solution or molar sodium lactate solution is used, depending on the patient's acid-base status. In any case, the sodium deficit can be estimated by multiplying the decrease in serum sodium concentration below normal (in milliequivalents per liter) *times* the liters of total body water. Total body water averages 60 percent of the body weight in young adult males and 50 percent in young adult females. Initially, up to one-half of the calculated amount of sodium may be administered slowly, followed by clinical and chemical reevaluation of the patient before any additional infusion of sodium salts.

> Example: A twenty-four-year-old female with symptomatic hyponatremia, weight = 60 kg, serum sodium = 120 mEq/L:
>
> Total body water = 60 kg × 0.50 = 30 liters
> Sodium deficit = (140 − 120 mEq/L) × 30 liters
>   = 600 mEq
>
> Half of this amount (300 mEq) could be given by slowly infusing approximately 350 ml 5% sodium chloride solution.

Note that this estimate is based on total body water, since the effective osmotic pressure in the extracellular compartment cannot be increased without increasing this function proportionately in the intracellular compartment. Although absolute reliance on any formula is undesirable, proper use of this estimate will allow a safe quantitative approximation of the sodium deficit. Generally, only a portion of the total deficit is replaced initially to relieve acute symptoms. Further correction is facilitated when renal function is restored by correction of the volume deficit. If the total calculated deficit were given rapidly, severe hypervolemia might occur particularly in patients with limited cardiac reserve. In practice, the infusion of small, successive increments of hypertonic saline solution with frequent evaluation of the clinical response and serum sodium concentration is recommended.

In the treatment of moderate hyponatremia with an associated volume deficit, volume replacement can be started immediately with concomitant correction of the serum sodium deficit. Isotonic sodium chloride solution (normal saline) is used initially in the presence of metabolic alkalosis, whereas $M/6$ sodium lactate is used to correct an associated acidosis. Only a few liters of these solutions may be necessary to correct the serum sodium concentration; the remainder of the volume deficit may be repaired with lactated Ringer's solution.

Treatment of hyponatremia associated with volume excess is by restriction of water. In the presence of severe symptomatic hyponatremia, a small amount of hypertonic salt solution may be infused cautiously to alleviate symptoms. As this will cause additional volume expansion, it is contraindicated in patients with limited cardiac reserve; peritoneal dialysis or hemodialysis is preferred in this situation.

For the correction of severe, symptomatic hypernatremia with an associated volume deficit, 5% dextrose in water may be infused slowly until symptoms are relieved. If the extracellular osmolarity is reduced too rapidly, however, convulsions and coma may result. For this reason, correction of hypernatremia concomitant with repletion of the volume deficit by half-strength sodium chloride or half-strength lactated Ringer's solution is safer in most cases. In the absence of a significant volume deficit, water should be administered cautiously since dangerous hypervolemia may result; constant observation and frequent determinations of the serum sodium concentration are indicated. The problem is somewhat simplified once a sufficient quantity of fluid has been given to permit renal excretion of the solute load.

RATE OF FLUID ADMINISTRATION. This varies considerably, depending on the severity and type of fluid disturbance, the presence of continuing losses, and the cardiac status. In general, the most severe volume deficits may be safely replaced initially with isotonic solutions at a rate of 2,000 ml/hour, reducing the rate as the fluid status improves. Constant observation by a physician is mandatory when the administration exceeds 1,000 ml/hour. At these rates, a significant portion may be lost as urinary output owing to a transient overexpansion of the plasma volume.

In elderly patients, associated cardiovascular disorders do not preclude correction of existing volume deficits, but they do require slower, more careful correction with constant monitoring of all functions including the central venous pressure. Hypertonic salt solutions should be given under close supervision, and the rate of administration generally should not exceed 100 to 150 ml/hour.

COMPOSITION AND MISCELLANEOUS CONSIDERATIONS

Correction of existing potassium deficits should be started *after* an adequate urine output is obtained, particularly in the patient with metabolic alkalosis since this may be secondary to or aggravated by potassium depletion. Potassium chloride is available in 20-mEq and 40-mEq ampules for addition to intravenous fluids. A maximum of 40 mEq of potassium chloride per hour may be safely administered to the adult of average size who is not severely depleted of extracellular fluid volume, in frank hypovolemic shock, or in established oliguric or high-output renal failure. The concentration of potassium chloride should not exceed 40 mEq/L of intravenous fluids, with rare exception, such as the treatment of digitalis intoxication during which the electrocardiogram must be constantly monitored. Calcium and magnesium rarely are needed during preoperative resuscitation, but should be given if any doubt exists, particularly to patients with massive subcutaneous infections, those with acute pancreatitis, and those who have been chronically starved.

Fluid abnormalities also must be suspected in the patient for whom an elective procedure is planned. Chronic illnesses frequently are associated with extracellular fluid volume deficits, and concentration and compositional changes are not uncommon. Correction of anemia and recognition of the fact that a contracted blood volume may exist in the chronically debilitated patient is of obvious importance. The choice of whole blood versus packed cells for correction of anemia depends on the volume status. If there is any question, 1 unit of packed cells may be given and the hemoglobin and hematocrit determined subsequently. The hemoglobin generally increases approximately 1.5 following the infusion of 250 ml of packed cells into the adult of average size. The increase will be significantly greater than 1.5 Gm/100 ml in the patient with a contracted intravascular volume, indicating the probable need for whole blood transfusions. If available, measurement of the blood volume is obviously more accurate.

Of additional importance is the prevention of volume depletion during the preoperative period. Prolonged periods of fluid restriction in preparation for various diagnostic procedures, and the use of cathartics and enemas for preparation of the bowel may cause a significant acute loss of extracellular fluid. Prompt recognition and treatment of these losses is necessary to prevent complications during the operative period.

Intraoperative Management of Fluids

If preoperative replacement of extracellular fluid volume has been incomplete, hypotension may develop promptly with the induction of anesthesia. This can be quite insidious, as the ability of the awake patient to compensate for mild volume deficit is revealed only when the compensatory mechanisms are abolished with anesthesia. This problem is prevented by maintaining base-line requirements and replacing abnormal losses of fluids and electrolytes by intravenous infusions in the preoperative period.

Blood lost during the operative procedure should be replaced steadily. It is usually unnecessary to replace blood loss of less than 500 ml, but after the loss has exceeded this, replacement should begin. The warnings against the use of a single transfusion during operation have been somewhat confusing. There may be a very definite need for a single-unit transfusion in the patient who loses between 500 and 1,000 ml of blood during operation.

In addition to blood losses during operation, there appear to be extracellular fluid losses during major operative procedures. Some of these, including edema from extensive dissection, collections within the lumen and wall of the small bowel, and accumulations of fluid in the peritoneal cavity, are clinically discernible and well recognized. They generally are felt to represent distributional shifts, in that the functional volume of extracellular fluid is reduced but not externally lost from the body. These functional losses are often referred to as "a parasitic loss of extracellular fluid," "a third space edema," or "a sequestration" of extracellular fluid. Another source of extracellular fluid loss during major operative trauma is the wound itself. This is a relatively smaller loss and very difficult to quantify except in extensive and major operative procedures.

At the beginning of this century, surgeons became aware that many changes occurred in urinary output, blood volume, and fluid and electrolyte composition during and after surgery. Assessment of these changes, however, awaited the development of analytic techniques and their application to patient studies. In the following 25 years, saline solutions in varying combinations were given to patients undergoing operation, often in excessive amounts. Work in the late 1930s and early 1940s by Moyer and by many others indicated that during and after operative procedures, saline and water solutions should be withheld entirely, because most of the fluid administered was retained.

The possibility existed that the operative and postoperative retention of salt and water administered in relatively small amounts might simply be physiologic retention to replace a deficit of salt and water incurred by the operative procedure. Subsequent studies have revealed that functional extracellular fluid decreases with major abdominal operations, largely as sequestered loss into the operative site. This extracellular fluid volume deficit can be replaced during the operative procedure. These data have led to the conclusion that the need for an extracellular "mimic" in the form of balanced salt solution now can be clinically estimated. Intraoperative correction of the volume deficit with salt solution markedly reduces "postoperative salt intolerance," but is not intended to substitute for blood replacement. Rather, it is felt to be a physiologic supplement, or adjunct, to replace sequestered losses.

Thus, the pendulum has swung from indiscriminate use of salt solutions in the first quarter of this century to almost total withholding of fluid and electrolytes from surgical patients in the second quarter of the century; indications at present are that proper management lies somewhere between these two extremes. Some guidelines are necessary for the intraoperative administration of saline solutions as a "mimic" for the sequestered extracellular fluid. Since this varies from an almost imperceptible minimum to a high of approximately 3 liters during an uncomplicated procedure, quantification is extremely difficult with the presently available means of measuring functional extracellular fluid. Consequently, no accurate formula for intraoperative fluid administration can yet be derived. Some arbitrary but clinically useful guidelines are the following: (1) Blood should be replaced as lost, irrespective of any additional fluid and electrolyte therapy. (2) The replacement of extracellular fluid should begin during the operative procedure. Recent data reveal that if the operative replacement of extracellular fluid is delayed until the adrenal compensatory mechanisms have started to react to the operative trauma in the immediate postoperative period, dangerous overloads may be produced. (3) Balanced salt solution needed during operation is approximately $\frac{1}{2}$ to 1 liter/hour, but only to a maximum of 2 to 3 liters during a 4-hour major abdominal procedure, unless there are other measurable losses.

Using a similar fluid regimen, Thompson and associates reported experiences in a series of 670 patients undergoing major aortoiliac reconstructive procedures. In this group of patients, the average amount of Ringer's lactate solution administered was 3555 ml, giving an average intraoperative replacement of salt solution of 677 ml per hour of operative procedure. In the last 6 years of this study there were only two deaths in 298 operations, an operative mortality of 0.67 percent. Among the entire 670 patients, only two patients died of renal failure, an incidence of 0.3 percent. No patient died of pulmonary insufficiency. This extremely low incidence of renal failure, even in the presence of extensive operative trauma, is similar to the authors' data for major abdominal operative procedures.

Postoperative Management of Fluids

IMMEDIATE POSTOPERATIVE PERIOD

Orders for postoperative fluids are not written until the patient is in the recovery room and the fluid status has been assessed. Evaluation at this point should include a review of preoperative fluid status, the amount of fluid loss and gain during operation, and clinical examination of the patient with assessment of the vital signs and urinary output. Initial fluid orders are written to correct any *existing* deficit, followed by maintenance fluids for the remainder of the day. For the patient with complications who has received or lost large amounts of fluid, it is frequently difficult to estimate the fluid requirements for the ensuing 24 hours. In this situation, intravenous fluids are ordered 1 liter at a time and the patient checked frequently until the situation is clarified. Proper replacement of fluids during this relatively short period will facilitate subsequent fluid management.

Immediately after operation, extracellular fluid volume depletion may occur as a result of continued losses of fluid at the site of injury or operative trauma—for example, into the wall or lumen of the small intestine. Several liters of extracellular fluid may be slowly deposited in such areas within a few hours or more during the first day or so from the time of the injury. Unrecognized deficits of extracellular fluid volume during the early postoperative period are manifest primarily as circulatory instability. The signs of volume deficiency in other organ systems may be delayed for several hours with this type of fluid loss. Postoperative hypotension and tachycardia require prompt investigation, followed by appropriate therapy. The generally accepted adequate blood pressure of 90/60 and a pulse of less than 120 in postoperative patients may not be sufficient to prevent renal ischemia unless, in addition to lack of signs of shock, urine flow is adequate. Evaluation of the level of consciousness, pupillary size, airway patency, breathing patterns, pulse rate and volume, skin warmth, color, body temperature, and a 30- to 50-ml hourly urine output, combined with critical review of the operative procedure and the operative fluid management, usually is rewarding. Since operative trauma frequently involves loss or transfer of significant quantities of whole blood, plasma, or extracellular fluid which can be only grossly estimated, circulatory instability is most commonly caused by underestimated initial losses or insidious, concealed continued losses. Operative blood loss is usually estimated by the operating surgeon to be 15 to 40 percent less than the isotopically measured blood loss from that patient. In addition, several liters of extravascular, extracellular fluid can be sequestered in areas of injury and manifested only by oliguria and mild depression of the blood pressure with a rapid pulse. For a patient with circulatory instability, further volume replacement of an additional 1,000 ml isotonic salt solution, while determining whether continuing losses or other causes are present, often resolves the problem. Contributing causes must be vigorously pursued with all diagnostic aids before excessive volumes of fluid have been administered.

It is unnecessary and probably unwise to administer potassium during the first 24 hours postoperatively, unless a definite potassium deficit exists. This is particularly important for the patient subjected to prolonged operative trauma involving one or more episodes of hypotension and for the posttraumatic patient with hemorrhagic hypotension. Oliguric renal failure or the more insidious high-output renal failure may develop, and the administration of even a small quantity of potassium may be quite detrimental.

LATER POSTOPERATIVE PERIOD

The problem of volume management during the postoperative convalescent phase is one of accurate measurement and replacement of all losses. In the otherwise healthy individual, this involves the replacement of measured sensible losses, which are generally of gastrointestinal origin, and the estimation and replacement of insensible losses.

The insensible loss is usually relatively constant and will average 600 to 900 ml daily. This may be increased by hypermetabolism, hyperventilation, and fever to a maximum of approximately 1,500 ml daily. The estimated insensible loss is replaced with 5% dextrose in water. This loss may be partially offset by an insensible gain of water from excessive tissue catabolism in the complicated postoperative patient, particularly if associated with oliguric renal failure.

Approximately 1 liter of fluid should be given to replace that volume of urine required to excrete the catabolic end products of metabolism (800 to 1,000 ml/day). In the individual with normal renal function, this may be given as 5% dextrose in water, since the kidneys are able to conserve sodium with excretion of less than 1 mEq daily. It is probably unnecessary to stress the kidneys to this degree, however, and a small amount of salt solution may be given in addition to water to cover urinary loss. In the elderly patient with salt-losing kidneys or in patients with head injuries, an insidious hyponatremia may develop if urinary losses are replaced with water. Urinary sodium in these circumstances may exceed 100 mEq/L and result in a daily loss of significant amounts of sodium. Measurement of urinary sodium will facilitate accurate replacement.

Urine volume is not replaced on a milliliter-for-milliliter basis. A urinary output of 2,000 to 3,000 ml on a given day may simply represent diuresis of fluids given during surgery or may represent excessive fluid administration. If these large losses are completely replaced, the urine output will progressively increase, and this may logically progress to a unique situation resembling diabetes insipidus with urinary outputs in excess of 10 liters daily.

Sensible losses, by definition, can be measured or, as in the case of sweating, the amount can be estimated. Gastrointestinal losses are usually isotonic or slightly hypotonic, and they are replaced with an essentially isotonic salt solution. When the estimated loss is slightly above or below isotonicity, appropriate corrections can be made in the daily water administration, while isotonic salt solutions are used to replace these losses volume for volume. Sweating is not usually a problem except with the febrile patient in whom losses may, but seldom do, exceed 250 ml/day/degree of fever. Excessive sweating may, in addition, represent a considerable loss of sodium in the unacclimatized individual.

Determination of serum electrolyte levels is generally unnecessary in the patient with an uncomplicated postoperative course maintained on parenteral fluids for 2 to 3 days. A more prolonged period of parenteral replacement or one complicated by excessive fluid losses requires frequent determinations of the serum sodium, potassium, and chloride levels, and carbon dioxide combining power. Adjustments then can be made with intravenous fluids of appropriate composition. For example, gastrointestinal losses should be replaced with isotonic sodium chloride solution in a patient with hyponatremia, hypochloremia, and mild metabolic alkalosis, and this should be continued until these abnormalities are corrected. In the hyponatremic patient with obvious overload, the amount of water given is restricted. In the presence of hyponatremia and mild metabolic acidosis, $M/6$ sodium lactate or lactated Ringer's solution with added sodium bicarbonate may be used. In this way, severe concentration and compositional changes can be avoided while an adequate extracellular fluid volume is maintained by appropriate maintenance fluids.

Maintenance fluids are administered at a steady rate over an 18- to 24-hour period as the losses are incurred. If given over a shorter period of time, renal excretion of the excess salt and water may occur while the normal losses continue over the full 24-hour period. For the same reason, fluids of different composition are alternated, and additives to intravenous fluids (e.g., potassium chloride and antibiotics) are evenly distributed in the total volume of fluid given.

In summary, daily fluid orders should begin with an assessment of the patient's volume status and a check for possible concentration or compositional disorders as reflected by proper laboratory determinations. All measured and insensible losses are replaced with fluids of appropriate composition, allowing for any preexisting deficit or excess. The amount of potassium replacement is 40 mEq daily for renal excretion of potassium in addition to approximately 20 mEq/L for replacement of gastrointestinal losses. Inadequate replacement may prolong the usual postoperative ileus and contribute to the insidious development of a resistant metabolic alkalosis. Calcium and magnesium are replaced when needed, as previously discussed.

SPECIAL CONSIDERATIONS IN THE POSTOPERATIVE PATIENT

VOLUME EXCESSES. The administration of isotonic salt solutions in excess of volume losses (external or internal) may result in overexpansion of the extracellular fluid space. The otherwise normal person in a postoperative state tolerates an acute overexpansion extremely well. Excesses administered over a period of several days, however, will soon exceed the kidneys' ability to excrete sodium; since water losses continue, hypernatremia will ensue. Therefore, it is important to determine as accurately as possible from intake and output records and serum sodium concentrations the actual needs of the patient managed over several postoperative days. Attention to the signs and symptoms of overload usually prevents this fluid abnormality. It arises most frequently with attempts to meet excessive volume losses that are not measurable, such as those occurring from incompletely controlled fistula drainage.

The earliest sign is a weight gain (when measurable) during the catabolic period, when the patient should be losing $\frac{1}{4}$ to $\frac{1}{2}$ lb/day. Heavy eyelids, hoarseness, or dyspnea on exertion may rapidly appear. Circulatory and pulmonary signs of overload appear late and represent a rather massive overload. Peripheral edema may be a sign, but it does not necessarily indicate volume excess. In the absence of additional evidence for volume overload, other causes for peripheral edema should be considered. Of particular importance is the fact that overexpansion of the *total* extracellular fluid may coexist with *depletion* of the functional extracellular fluid compartment. Central venous pressure measurements may be helpful during volume replacement but may be misleading, as a rapid rise may indicate an excessive rate of fluid administration or primary pump failure but it does not accurately establish volume status.

HYPONATREMIA. Significant postoperative alterations in serum sodium concentration are not frequently observed if the fluid resuscitation during operation has included adequate volumes of isotonic salt solutions. The kidneys retain the ability to excrete moderate excesses of salt water administered in the early postoperative period if functional extracellular fluid has been adequately replaced during the operative or immediate postoperative period. Previous studies of sodium balance have revealed that patients do excrete sodium after the functional deficit incurred by the shift of extracellular fluid has been replaced. Wright and Gann have demonstrated normal capacity to excrete water postoperatively when isotonic salt solutions are administered prior to a challenge with a water load. Thus, the commonly described hyponatremia associated with surgical procedures and traumatic injury is prevented by the replacement of extracellular fluid deficits. The daily maintenance of normal osmolarity is simplified by the replacement of observable losses of known sodium content.

Hyponatremia may easily occur when water is given to replace losses of sodium-containing fluids or when water administration consistently exceeds water losses. The latter may occur with oliguria or in association with decreased water loss through the skin and lungs, intracellular shifts of sodium, or the cellular release of excessive amounts of endogenous water. Severe or refractory hyponatremia, however, is difficult to produce if renal function remains normal.

Replacement of Sodium Losses with Water. A common error is replacement of gastrointestinal and other salt losses with only water or a hypotonic solution. Patients with head injury or with preexisting renal disease (loss of concentrating ability) may elaborate urine with a high salt concentration (50 to 200 mEq/L).

Progressive hyponatremia in the patient with head injury, despite adequate salt administration, is believed to be due to excessive secretion of antidiuretic hormone with consequent water retention. The loss of renal concentrating ability due to impairment of renal tubular function ("salt-wasting kidneys") is a common problem in elderly patients. This source of sodium loss is frequently not anticipated, since the blood urea nitrogen and creatinine levels usually fall within normal limits. Continued replacement of these urinary losses with water only eventually may result in symptomatic hyponatremia. The urine sodium concentration should be determined if the diagnosis is in doubt; with hyponatremia and normal renal function, the urine should be virtually free of sodium.

Decreased Urinary Volume. Oliguria, from whatever cause (prerenal or renal), reduces the daily water requirements if not corrected. Cellular catabolism and the metabolic acidosis produced by the retention of nitrogenous waste products increases the cellular release of water. Therefore, the gain of endogenous water decreases the total water requirement beyond that expected when the urinary volume is low.

Decreased Insensible Loss. Cutaneous vasoconstriction from any cause decreases both insensible and evaporative water loss by this route. This condition most commonly accompanies generalized hypothermia.

Endogenous Water Release. The patient maintained on intravenous fluids without adequate caloric intake will, between the fifth and tenth days, gain significant quantities of water (maximum, 500 ml daily) from excessive cellular catabolism, thus decreasing the quantity of exogenous water required per day.

Intracellular Shifts. Systemic bacterial sepsis is often accompanied by a precipitous drop in serum sodium concentration. This sudden change is poorly understood, but usually accompanies loss of extracellular fluid as either interstitial or intracellular sequestrations. This can be treated by withholding free water, restoring extracellular fluid volume, and initiating treatment of the sepsis.

Many hyponatremic states are asymptomatic until the serum sodium level falls below 120 mEq/L. This moderate asymptomatic hyponatremia, however, signifies inappropriate therapy or indicates the basic underlying condition. Symptomatic hyponatremia, or water intoxication, is difficult to produce if renal function is normal. Convulsions and apnea from uncorrected water excesses occur most often in children and elderly adults. Within the limits imposed by the circulatory apparatus, these deficits should be corrected by the administration of hypertonic salt solution to a serum sodium level above 130 mEq/L. Mild or moderate degrees of hyponatremia may be simply corrected by temporary restriction of water intake.

In the presence of hyperglycemia, determination of the glucose concentration is necessary to evaluate the significance of a depressed serum sodium level. Since glucose does not enter cells by passive diffusion, it exerts an osmotic force in the extracellular compartment. This contribution to osmotic pressure is normally small, but with an elevated glucose concentration, the increased osmotic pressure causes the transfer of cellular water into the extracellular compartment, resulting in a dilutional hypo-

natremia. Hyponatremia therefore may be observed when the total effective osmotic pressure in the extracellular compartment is normal or even above normal. In terms of tonicity, each 100 mg/100 ml rise in the blood glucose *above normal* is roughly equivalent to a 3 mEq/L rise in the serum sodium concentration. Consider a patient with a serum sodium concentration of 125 mEq/L and a blood glucose level of 500 mg/100 ml. The glucose level is approximately 400 mg/100 ml above normal, which is equivalent to a 12 mEq/L rise in the serum sodium level. Thus, $125 + 12 = 137$ mEq/L; the tonicity is normal despite the marked reduction in sodium concentration. In this instance, therapy is directed toward lowering the blood glucose level. The sodium concentration will return toward normal as the excess water leaves the extracellular compartment. In practice, a true sodium deficit may be secondary to the underlying disorder and must be corrected.

HYPERNATREMIA. Hypernatremia (serum sodium concentration above 150 mEq/L), although uncommon, is a dangerous abnormality. In contradistinction to decreased serum sodium concentration, hypernatremia is easily produced when renal function is normal. The extracellular fluid hyperosmolarity results in a shift of intracellular water from within the cell to the extracellular fluid compartment; in this situation, a high serum sodium level may indicate a significant deficit of total body water. In surgical patients hypernatremia arises most often from excessive or unexpected water losses, although it may result from use of salt-containing solutions to replace water losses. The following classification of water losses may be helpful in preventing and treating this abnormality.

Excessive Extrarenal Water Losses. With increased metabolism from any cause, but particularly associated with fever, the water loss through evaporation of sweat may reach several liters daily. Patients with tracheostomy in dry environments can (with excessive minute volume air exchange) lose as much as 1 to 1.5 liters of water/day by this route. Increased water evaporation from a granulating surface is of significant magnitude in the thermally injured patient, and losses may be as great as 3 to 5 liters/day.

Increased Renal Water Losses. Extremely large volumes of solute-poor urine may result from hypoxic damage to the distal tubules and collecting ducts or loss of antidiuretic hormone stimulation from damage to the central nervous system. In both instances, facultative water resorption is impaired. The former occurs in high-output renal failure; in our experience, this is the most common type of renal failure following severe injury or operative trauma. The latter occurs with extensive head injuries accompanied by temporary diabetes insipidus.

Solute Loading. High protein intake may produce an increased osmotic load of urea, which necessitates the excretion of large volumes of water. Hypernatremia, azotemia, and extracellular fluid volume deficits follow. In general, these can be prevented by an intake of 7 ml of water/Gm of dietary protein.

Excessive glucose administration results in the need for a large volume of water for excretion. Osmotic diuretics such as mannitol and urea also result in the obligatory excretion of a large volume of water as well as increasing urinary sodium losses. In addition, isotonic salt solutions, if used to replace pure water losses, rapidly produce hypernatremia.

HIGH-OUTPUT RENAL FAILURE. Acute renal insufficiency following trauma or surgical stress is a highly lethal complication. The diagnosis is classically based on persistent oliguria and chemical evidence of uremia after stabilization of the circulation. The clinical course is characterized by oliguria lasting from several days to several weeks, followed by a progressive rise in daily urine volume until both the excretory and concentrating functions of the kidney are gradually restored.

Uremia, occurring without a period of oliguria and accompanied by a daily urine volume greater than 1,000 to 1,500 ml/day, is a more frequent but less well recognized entity. Clinical experience and laboratory experiments suggest that high-output renal failure represents the renal response to a less severe or modified episode of renal injury than that required to produce classic oliguric renal failure. Its importance lies in the fact that it is a milder form of renal insufficiency and that realization of its presence, by serial measurement of blood urea nitrogen and serum electrolytes, permits intelligent chemical and fluid volume management with a much greater latitude because of the daily urine volume excretion. Normal extracellular fluid volume and normal serum sodium concentration, therefore, are quite easily maintained when accurate daily outputs of each are obtained and replaced accordingly. The sodium-containing fluids may be administered as lactate to control the mild metabolic acidosis that occurs. Severe acidosis may develop if isotonic losses from the gastrointestinal tract or renal excretion of sodium are replaced with sodium chloride.

The chief dangers of high-output renal failure are failure to recognize its existence because of normal output, and the intravenous administration of potassium salts. Good urinary output and gastrointestinal involvement requiring suction usually indicate the need for daily potassium replacement. With this type of renal failure, however, potassium intoxication may be produced. As little as 20 mEq of potassium chloride given intravenously may rapidly produce myocardial potassium intoxication requiring resin or hemodialysis treatment.

The typical course of high-output renal failure begins without a period of oliguria. The daily urine volumes are normal or greater than normal, often reaching levels of 3 to 5 liters/day while blood urea nitrogen is increasing. An attempt to decrease urine output by water restriction rapidly results in hypernatremia without a change in urine volume. On the average, urea nitrogen continues to increase for 8 to 12 days before a downward trend occurs. The blood/urine urea ratio is about 1:10 until a decrease occurs in the blood urea concentration.

Functionally, the lesion is characterized by a glomerular filtration rate of less than 20 percent of normal and complete resistance to vasopressin for 1 to 3 weeks after the blood urea nitrogen has declined. During the next 6 to 8 weeks, the glomerular filtration rate gradually rises, and the response to vasopressin becomes normal. The early recognition of high-output renal failure by serial blood determinations of blood urea nitrogen is important. Failure to recognize its presence may result in death from hyperkalemia, hypernatremia, or acidosis. As alluded to previously, it is unwise to administer potassium during the first 24 postoperative hours unless a definite potassium deficit exists. This is particularly important in the patient subjected to prolonged operative trauma involving one or more episodes of hypotension and in the patient with posttraumatic hemorrhagic hypotension.

NUTRITION IN THE SURGICAL PATIENT

The majority of patients undergoing elective surgical operations withstand the brief period of catabolism and starvation without noticeable difficulty. However, maintaining an adequate nutritional regimen may be of critical importance in managing seriously ill surgical patients with preexisting weight loss and depleted energy reserves. Between these two extremes are patients for whom nutritional support is not essential for life but may serve to shorten the postoperative recovery phase and minimize the number of complications. Not infrequently a patient may become ill or even die from complications secondary to starvation rather than the underlying disorder. Therefore, it is essential that the surgeon have a sound grasp of the fundamental metabolic changes associated with surgery, trauma, and sepsis and an awareness of the methods available to reverse or ameliorate these events.

Body Fuel Reserves

The body must mobilize appropriate nutrients from fuel reserves in order to withstand the necessary periods of partial or complete starvation and to meet the additional requirements imposed by surgery, trauma, or sepsis. The extent and availability of these reserves may be of critical importance for successful recovery from an illness. Available information concerning body fuel composition and the rate of fuel consumption in man has recently been reviewed by Cahill and is summarized below.

Carbohydrates, proteins, and fats are the three sources of fuel in man. Their relative contributions both by weight and caloric potential are illustrated in Fig. 2-3. Carbohydrate stores, primarily in the form of liver and muscle glycogen, are relatively small and could supply basal caloric requirements for less than 1 day. However, this relatively small quantity is absolutely essential in the emergency situation for the production of high-energy phosphates during anaerobic metabolism. Although glucose yields approximately 4 kcal/Gm, its storage as glycogen requires the addition of 1 or 2 Gm of intracellular water and electrolytes. Therefore it yields only 1 or 2 kcal/Gm of wet weight.

Protein represents a considerably larger source of fuel, but, as emphasized by Cahill, every molecule of protein in the body has a specific purpose, such as an enzyme, a structural component, or a contractile protein in muscle. Thus, any protein loss represents loss of an essential function. Additionally, the amount of total body protein is

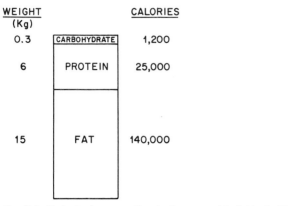

Fig. 2-3. Body fuel composition in the normal individual. (*From G. F. Cahill, Jr., Bull Am Coll Surg, 55:12, 1970.*)

relatively fixed in the normal healthy individual, and any additional protein is metabolized, the excess calories being stored as fat. Protein, like glycogen, represents an inefficient energy source relative to its wet weight, since it exists in an aqueous environment.

In contrast to glycogen and protein, fat is stored in a relatively anhydrous state. By weight, then, it is a relatively rich source of energy, supplying approximately 9 kcal/Gm. Most of the fat in the body serves as a readily available energy source; the few areas where fat serves a specific function (e.g., mechanical fat pads) are the last to be mobilized during starvation.

In summary, protein and fat are the only major sources of fuel. Total protein mass is relatively fixed in amount, and caloric excess or deficiency is met by an increase or decrease in the body's fat mass. Fat depots serve as sources of energy, protein stores represent *potential* sources of energy but only through the loss of some important function, and the small stores of carbohydrates are generally protected except for emergency use during anaerobic glycolysis.

Starvation

During the first several days of complete starvation, caloric needs are supplied by body fat and proteins; the small glycogen reserve is largely spared. Previous studies have shown an obligatory loss of approximately 10 to 15 grams of nitrogen daily in the urine during this period, indicating the utilization of approximately 60 to 90 grams of protein (each gram of nitrogen represents approximately 6.25 grams of muscle protein). The majority of this protein, which is largely derived from skeletal muscle, is converted to glucose in the liver by the process of gluconeogenesis; most of this endogenously produced glucose is used by the brain. The remainder is used by certain tissues such as red blood cells and leukocytes which convert the glucose to lactate and pyruvate. These are returned to the liver and resynthesized into glucose (the Cori cycle). This obligatory nitrogen loss, then, reflects the use of amino acids derived from muscle protein for gluconeogenesis to supply glucose to the brain. No patient, however, should be allowed to

starve completely. The administration of at least 100 Gm of glucose will obviate most of this gluconeogenesis and reduce the nitrogen loss by at least one-half—the well-known "protein-sparing effect" described by Gamble. Available evidence from Cahill indicates that this protein-sparing effect is regulated by insulin, which is released when exogenous glucose is infused for use by the brain. The slightly elevated insulin level reduces amino acid release from the muscle, amino acid extraction by the liver, and gluconeogenesis. In the diabetic with an absolute or relative lack of insulin, the infusion of glucose does not inhibit gluconeogenesis, and muscle breakdown to amino acids continues unabated. The liver derives its energy by oxidizing fatty acids to ketones, and the remainder of the body utilizes both fatty acids and ketones to meet caloric requirements. Generally a small quantity of the ketones is excreted into the urine.

If complete starvation continues for more than a few days, the obligatory nitrogen loss progressively decreases, as the brain begins to use fat as its fuel source. Unlike other body tissues, however, the brain cannot utilize free fatty acids, since they do not cross the blood-brain barrier. Instead, use of keto acids which are produced by the liver and readily cross the blood-brain barrier gradually displaces the use of glucose by the brain. After prolonged starvation, the net effect of this adaptation to ketone utilization is a protein-sparing effect with reduction of urinary nitrogen excretion to approximately 4 Gm/day. This 4 Gm of nitrogen represents approximately 25 Gm of protein, or about 100 Gm of lean wet muscle. Thus, the normal individual with an average supply of fat and muscle may survive total starvation for several months. Insulin again may be the signal for the reduction in muscle catabolism and gluconeogenesis (coincident with the increased use of keto acids by the brain), according to Cahill. However, changes in the blood level of alanine, which is quantitatively one of the more important amino acids, may also play a role. A fall in the blood level of this amino acid appears to decrease gluconeogenesis and glucose production by the liver.

Surgery, Trauma, Sepsis

The sequence of metabolic and endocrine events occasioned by surgery, trauma, or sepsis may be divided into several phases. As pointed out by Moore (1960), the magnitude of the changes and the duration of each phase vary considerably and are directly related to the severity of the injury.

CATABOLIC PHASE. This phase has also been termed the *adrenergic-corticoid phase* since it corresponds to the period during which changes induced by adrenergic and adrenal corticoid hormones are most striking. Immediately following surgery or trauma, there is a sudden increase in metabolic demands and urinary excretion of nitrogen beyond the levels associated with simple starvation. The patient generally cannot eat, cannot lower his metabolic rate, and cannot effectively alter the source of endogenous fuels to spare protein utilization. This is in distinct contrast to events in the normal individual subjected to prolonged starvation, where most body tissues use fat as their main source of fuel, thereby sparing protein. Trauma apparently results in a continued and excessive mobilization of protein; unfortunately, the administration of moderate amounts of glucose to these individuals produces little or no change in the rate of protein catabolism, although Blackburn has suggested that the administration of glucose-free crystalline amino acid solutions results in a decrease in urinary nitrogen excretion. During the hypermetabolic, reparative phase following injury, increased flow of glucose from the liver to the periphery has been documented by Wilmore and Dudrick. Simultaneously, increased Cori cycle activity is stimulated and three-carbon intermediates are converted back to glucose in the liver by pyruvate carboxylase and phosphoenolpyruvate carboxylase. Increased synthesis of these two enzymes occurs in the presence of elevated levels of glucagon, glucocorticoids, and catecholamines and low concentrations of insulin—the hormonal environment present during the catabolic phase of injury.

The extent of the negative nitrogen balance in these patients varies considerably and is largely related to the magnitude of the injury. In Fig. 2-4 daily net nitrogen losses during simple starvation with and without the administration of glucose are compared to losses sustained with moderate to severe surgical illness.

EARLY ANABOLIC PHASE. After several days or weeks, depending on the severity of injury, the body turns from a catabolic to an anabolic phase. This turning point, also known as the *corticoid-withdrawal phase*, is characterized by a sharp decline in nitrogen excretion and restoration of a positive potassium balance. Generally, this transition period lasts no more than a day or two.

The prolonged anabolic phase may last from a few weeks to a few months and generally coincides with the resumption of oral intake. Nitrogen balance is positive, indicating synthesis of proteins, and there is a rapid and progressive gain in weight and muscular strength. The patient is usually active, has an excellent appetite, and generally is discharged from the hospital at this point. Positive nitrogen balance reaches a maximum of approximately 4 Gm/day, which represents the synthesis of approximately 25 Gm of protein and the gain of over 100 Gm of lean body mass/day. The total amount of nitrogen gain will ultimately equal the amount lost during the catabolic phase, although the rate of gain will be much slower than the rate of initial loss.

LATE ANABOLIC PHASE. The final period of convalescence or the late anabolic phase may last from several weeks to several months after a severe injury. This phase is associated with the gradual gain of fatty tissue as the previously positive nitrogen balance declines toward normal. Weight gain is much slower during this phase because of the higher caloric content of fat and can be realized only if intake is in excess of caloric expenditure. In most individuals, the phase ends with a gradual return to the previously normal body weight. The patient who is partially immobilized during this period of time, however, may exhibit a marked gain in weight due to decreased energy expenditure.

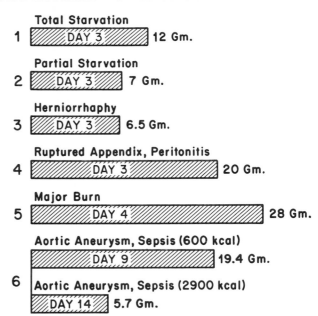

Fig. 2-4. The extent of negative nitrogen balance in adult patients during starvation alone and during various surgical illnesses associated with partial starvation. Note the difference in negative nitrogen balance in case 6 with low and high calorie parenteral supplementation. (*Cases 1 to 4 from W. D. Holden et al., Ann Surg, 146:563, 1957. Case 5 from J. M. Kinney, "Proceedings of a Conference on Energy Metabolism and Body Fuel Utilization," Harvard University Press, Cambridge, 1966. Case 6 from L. J. Lawson, Br J Surg, 52:795, 1965.*)

Base-Line Requirements

The normal caloric and protein requirements for individuals leading a sedentary life approximate 1 Gm of protein and 35 kcal/kg of body weight, or approximately 1400 kcal/m² of body surface area per day. These requirements, which have been recommended by the Food and Nutritional Board of the National Research Council, vary with age, sex, and the degree of daily activity.

These base-line requirements are totally inadequate for patients who have undergone surgery or who have suffered severe trauma or sepsis. The exact caloric and nitrogen requirements necessary to maintain an individual in balance after severe injury are unknown. However, guidelines for nutritional supplementation based on previous experimental data and clinical experience have been recommended. Moore has suggested that intakes in the region of 0.2 Gm of nitrogen/kg and 50 kcal/kg/day are necessary to maintain constant weight after moderate injury. Studies by Kinney suggest that a moderately positive caloric balance (1000 to 2000 kcal/day above resting expenditure) with a calorie-to-nitrogen ratio of approximately 150:200 may be appropriate for acutely ill surgical patients. Similarly, Dudrick et al. have noted that the average depleted or complicated major surgical patient requires between 2500 and 4000 kcal/day with approximately 12 to 24 Gm of nitrogen. These approximations are useful, although the quantity and composition of the nutrients must be tailored to meet individual needs.

The requirements for vitamins and essential trace minerals usually can be easily met in the average patient with an uncomplicated postoperative course, and vitamins usually are not given in the absence of preoperative deficiencies. The exception is vitamin C, essential for wound healing, which can be given orally or by subcutaneous or intravenous routes. The intravenous administration of vitamin C is associated with a large urinary loss, but since it is relatively nontoxic, large amounts (300 to 500 mg daily) can be given. Patients maintained on elemental diets or parenteral hyperalimentation require complete vitamin and mineral supplementation. Several commercial preparations are available for intravenous or intramuscular use, although most do not contain vitamin K and some do not contain vitamin B_{12} or folic acid. Supplemental essential trace minerals and essential fatty acids must also be administered to patients receiving all their nutrition via the parenteral route with hypertonic dextrose and crystalline amino acids.

Indications and Methods for Nutritional Support

The selection of patients who require partial or complete nutritional support has become increasingly important. The ability to provide complete nutritional support in the starving patient and to counteract the nitrogen losses in catabolic states with elemental diets or parenteral hyperalimentation represents a substantial contribution. However, it should be emphasized that the majority of surgical patients do not require special nutritional regimens. The reasonably well-nourished and otherwise healthy individual who undergoes an uncomplicated major surgical procedure has sufficient body fuel reserves to withstand the catabolic insult and partial starvation for at least 1 week. Adequate quantities of parenteral fluids with appropriate electrolyte composition and a minimum of 100 Gm of glucose daily to minimize protein catabolism will be all that is necessary in most patients. Assuming that the patient has a relatively uncomplicated postoperative course and resumes normal oral intake at the end of this period, elemental diets or parenteral hyperalimentation are unnecessary and probably inadvisable because of the associated risks. During the early anabolic phase, the patient must be provided with an adequate caloric intake of proper composition to meet the energy needs of the body and allow protein synthesis. A high calorie-to-nitrogen ratio (optimal ratio approximately 150 kcal/Gm nitrogen) and an adequate supply of vitamins and minerals are necessary for maximum anabolism during this period.

In contrast to this group, there is a small but significant number of surgical patients for whom an adequate nutritional regimen may be of critical importance for a successful outcome. This category includes preoperative patients who are chronically debilitated from their diseases or malnutrition and patients who have suffered trauma, sepsis, or surgical complications and cannot maintain an adequate caloric intake for any number of reasons.

The methods for partial or complete nutritional supple-

mentation in the surgical patient fall into three general categories: Nasopharyngeal, gastrostomy, and jejunostomy tube feedings are appropriate routes for alimentation in patients who have a relatively normal gastrointestinal tract but cannot or will not eat. Elemental diets may be administered by similar routes when bulk and fat-free nutrients requiring minimal digestion are indicated. Finally, parenteral hyperalimentation may be used for supplementation in the patient with limited oral intake or, more commonly, for complete nutritional management in the absence of oral intake.

NASOPHARYNGEAL TUBE FEEDING

Nasopharyngeal feedings, preferably through small, soft silastic tubes, should be used only in alert patients who are unable or unwilling to eat normally for various reasons; it is contraindicated in most other cases. The foremost contraindication for nasopharyngeal tube feeding is unconsciousness or lack of protective laryngeal reflexes, which may result in fatal pulmonary complications due to tracheal aspiration of regurgitated gastric content. Even with a tracheostomy, it is inadvisable to feed mentally obtunded patients via nasopharyngeal tubes, since such feedings often can be recovered from tracheostomy suction, indicating continued aspiration of gastric content even around a snugly fitting tracheostomy tube. An inflated tracheostomy tube cuff might prevent this, but the required constant inflation is inadvisable since it may cause pressure necrosis of the trachea. Furthermore, the prolonged use of a nasopharyngeal tube may cause severe discomfort, nasopharyngeal and laryngeal pressure necrosis, and esophagitis with stricture.

Pharyngeal tube feedings are often indicated for patients with oropharyngeal tumor; irritation may be prevented by inserting the tube into the pyriform sinus, as recommended by Graham and Royster. This technique also allows concealment of the feeding tube under the patient's clothing.

The nasopharyngeal tube may allow feeding beyond dysfunctional gastric stomas and high gastrointestinal fistulas. In such cases, it may be possible to maintain nutrition without a jejunostomy tube until stomal dysfunction relents or the fistula heals. This may be done by passing a Cantor tube or, preferably, a small polyethylene feeding tube weighted with a rubber finger cot filled with 1 ml of mercury distal to the faulty stoma or fistula, as recommended by Bachrach and Tecimer. The polyethylene feeding tube is prepared by passing a #1 silk thread through the tube with a wire. The mercury-filled finger cot is tied to the silk thread distad and the thread fixed to the tube proximally. The tube is then inserted through the nose into the stomach, and the patient is positioned so that the mercury weight tends to lead the small tube well into the jejunum. When the tube reaches the proper position (as noted on x-ray after the injection of a small amount of water-soluble opaque medium), the silk string is released proximally, and peristalsis carries the mercury-weighted finger cot and thread distad until they are passed per rectum. Feedings are started after a few hours when the string has cleared the tube. This small, flexible plastic tube and mercury weight may be more readily introduced into the intestine than the bulkier, more rigid, long intestinal tubes and is more conducive to patient comfort.

Whenever dietary preparations are administered into the gastrointestinal tract via tubes, it is advisable to employ bedside infusion pumps to ensure a constant rate of delivery over each 24-hour period. The utilization of such pumps decreases the incidence of gastrointestinal side effects induced by too rapid delivery of hyperosmolar solutions, while at the same time allowing safer administration of larger daily volumes of nutrients, since gastric distension is minimized.

GASTROSTOMY TUBE FEEDING

The administration of blended food through a gastrostomy tube is a good method for feeding patients with a variety of chronic gastrointestinal lesions arising at or above the cardioesophageal junction. However, gastrostomy tube feedings are contraindicated for mentally obtunded patients with inadequate laryngeal reflexes. This feeding method should be used only in alert patients or in patients with total obstruction of the distal esophagus.

Generally, gastrostomies of the Stamm (serosa-lined, temporary) or modified Glassman (mucosa-lined, permanent) type are constructed. The feeding mixture may be ordinarily prepared food converted by a blender into a semiliquid. Hyperosmolarity of the feeding formula is not generally a problem as long as the pylorus is intact. The jejunostomy formula outlined below also may be used.

JEJUNOSTOMY TUBE FEEDING

Jejunostomy tube feedings are generally required for patients in whom nasopharyngeal or gastrostomy tube feedings are contraindicated, e.g., comatose patients or patients with high gastrointestinal fistulas or obstructions. The jejunostomy may be of the Roux en Y (permanent) or the Witzel (temporary) type. The latter is constructed by inserting a #18 French rubber catheter into the proximal jejunum approximately 12 in. distal to the ligament of Treitz. The wall of the jejunum is inverted over the tube for about 3 cm as it emerges from the bowel to create a serosa-lined tunnel which allows rapid sealing of the jejunal opening when the tube is removed. The tube may then be brought out through a stab wound in the left upper quadrant of the abdomen. The jejunum is sutured to the anterior abdominal wall at the point of tube entry to seal it from the peritoneal cavity.

If the jejunostomy tube is inadvertently removed, blind attempts at reinsertion are contraindicated. If discovered within a few hours, the tube may be reinserted under fluoroscopic control to be sure it is in the bowel before feedings are resumed. The patient is observed for signs of peritonitis for 12 to 18 hours after feedings are restarted. If there is any doubt about the position of the tube, it should be replaced surgically. Feedings are safely begun 12 to 18 hours after jejunostomy construction, even though peristalsis is not audible. A progressive regimen of feeding modified from that recommended by Zollinger is prefera-

Table 2-9. JEJUNOSTOMY FEEDING REGIMEN

1. 12–18 hours after jejunostomy—nothing.
2. First day—50 ml/hr × 20 of 5% dextrose/water.
3. Second day—100 ml/hr × 20 of 5% dextrose/water.
4. Third day—50 ml/hr × 20 of homogenized milk.
5. Fourth day—100 ml/2hr × 10 of homogenized milk.
6. Fifth day—180 ml/2hr × 10 of homogenized milk.
7. Sixth day—240 ml/2hr × 10 of homogenized milk.
8. Continue same regimen as on sixth day but add an additional half cup of powdered milk to each quart of homogenized milk daily until 1.5 cups per quart of homogenized milk is being used as feeding formula. Thereafter, give 240 ml of this mixture q. 2 h. × 10 daily. Feedings should begin at 6 A.M. and continue through 12 midnight. Additional water may be given between feedings when indicated.

ble (Table 2-9). The full-strength formula suitable for most patients is simply a mixture of 1.5 cups of powdered milk, 1 qt of homogenized milk, and 1 ml of Tween 40 (an emulsifying agent allowing better fat absorption). This mixture contains about 1 kcal/ml, and, when given in the final volume recommended in Table 2-9, provides about 2500 kcal, 140 Gm of protein, and adequate carbohydrates. The fat content represents less than 4 percent of the total. Polyvisol and Fer-in-sol, 0.6 ml each, are added once daily to the formula. Many of the more complex jejunostomy feedings are difficult to prepare, likely to spoil before use, too high in fat content, and excessively hyperosmolar, leading to a greater incidence of patient intolerance.

With proper care, about 85 percent of jejunostomy patients tolerate their feedings. Diarrhea is usually controlled if the concentration and volume of formula are temporarily reduced. Failing this, feeding is halted for a day, then resumed from the beginning of the feeding regimen, progressing somewhat more slowly than before. If mild diarrhea or cramping persists, a pulverized Lomotil tablet or 8 to 10 drops of tincture of belladonna may be given through the tube 30 minutes prior to formula infusion. At times it may be necessary to give 5 ml paregoric 15 to 30 minutes before the formula to control cramping and diarrhea, but this should be employed sparingly and for as short a period as possible. In many cases, symptoms are relieved if the rate and volume of infusion are reduced and cold formula avoided. Each feeding should be infused in about 20 minutes.

If the patient with a jejunostomy has a proximal bowel or biliary fistula draining more than 300 ml daily for prolonged periods, the fistular drainage may be collected by sump suction, cooled in an ice basin at bedside, and promptly refed in small increments throughout the day. To avoid jejunal overloading, the fistular fluid is refed between formula feedings. It is not advisable to refeed aspirated gastric juice, for this may cause jejunal irritation and profuse diarrhea. If the fistular drainage is profuse, it is usually not possible to refeed more than 2 liters/day, and fluid and electrolyte losses must be replaced by appropriate intravenous supplements. Additional water may be given with the feedings or administered between the feedings as indicated. Occasionally, an elemental diet, as discussed below, may be indicated when other jejunostomy formulas are not tolerated.

ELEMENTAL DIETS

Clinical experience with chemically formulated bulk-free elemental diets has been encouraging. These diets may be used for complete nutritional support or as dietary supplements for patients who are unable to eat or digest enough food to meet their energy requirements. They may be preferable to high-caloric parenteral feedings for patients who have at least part of the small bowel available for the absorption of simple sugars and amino acids. As outlined by Randall et al., elemental diets have been found useful for patients with depleted protein reserves secondary to gastrointestinal tract disease, such as ulcerative or granulomatous colitis and malabsorption syndrome, and for patients with only partial function of the gastrointestinal tract, such as the short bowel syndrome or gastric or small bowel fistulas with feeding distal to the fistula. The diets also have been used during preoperative bowel preparation and in place of ordinary jejunostomy feedings when the latter cannot be tolerated.

Elemental diets differ from conventional foods in that they are formulated synthetically out of known chemical nutrients, such as purified amino acids and simple carbohydrates. As commercially prepared, these diets also contain base-line electrolytes, water- and fat-soluble vitamins (except vitamin K), and trace minerals. They contain no bulk and therefore produce a minimum of residue. The compositions of three elemental diets which are currently

Table 2-10. ELEMENTAL DIETS*
Approximate composition per 1,800 ml†

	W-T low-residue Food	Vivonex-100	Vivonex-100 HN (high-nitrogen)
Kilocalories. . . .	1800	1800	1800
Carbohydrates Gm	408 (dextrin)	407 (glucose)	379
Protein, Gm . . .	39	37	75
Nitrogen, Gm . .	5.4	5.9	12
Fat, Gm	1.3	1.3	0.8
Sodium, mEq . .	100	104	60
Potassium, mEq	54	54	32
Chloride, mEq. .	151	128	94
Calcium, mEq . .	50	40	24
Magnesium mEq	33	13	17
Osmolality, mOsm/L	650	1175	844

*All diets contain standard fat and water-soluble vitamins for normal daily requirements (based on 2000 kcal) and essential trace minerals. Contain only minimal quantities of vitamin K, which should be supplemented to the full therapeutic level. Additional quantities of B vitamins and vitamin C should also be added.

†Six 80-Gm packets diluted with water to a total of 1,800 ml.
SOURCE: VIVONEX-100, Eaton Laboratories, Norwich, N.Y.; W-I Low Residue Food, Warren-Teed Pharmaceuticals, Inc., Columbus, Ohio.

available are shown in Table 2-10. The diets with lower protein content may be taken orally or by tube, while the diet with higher protein content is unpalatable and intended primarily for tube feeding. Unfortunately, patient acceptance of the flavored diets has been only fair, and they frequently must be given by tube.

The amount of elemental diet required to maintain weight and nitrogen balance varies with the individual patient. In severe catabolic states the standard diet often fails to achieve positive nitrogen balance. The following guidelines are based on those recommended by Randall. For oral feedings, the diets are made up in standard dilution (25% weight/volume) and provide 1 kcal/ml of solution. The solution is cooled and ingested in small amounts of 100 to 150 ml at a time. Approximately 2,000 ml or more may be taken in a day, providing approximately 2000 kcal and 40 Gm of protein. Depending on patient tolerance, the volume of diet may be increased as indicated.

Either the high- or low-protein diets may be used for intragastric or jejunostomy tube feedings initially. The diet is mixed at half the standard dilution (12.5% weight/volume or less) and administered continuously by pump or gravity drip at a rate of 40 to 50 ml/hour. Once the individual has adjusted to the diet, the concentration may be gradually increased to the standard dilution and the volume increased in small increments until the desired caloric and protein intake is achieved. The development of nausea, vomiting, or diarrhea is an indication to slow or stop the infusion for a short period of time. The feeding may then be restarted at a slower rate or at a lower concentration. Lomotil tablets, tincture of belladonna, or paregoric may be indicated to control diarrhea as discussed previously. Using the high-protein diet, as much as 3000 ml/day may be administered, providing approximately 3000 kcal and 20 Gm of nitrogen.

Careful attention to water and electrolyte balance is mandatory, particularly when large quantities of fluid are being lost through fistulas or other routes. Additional sodium and potassium may be added to the mixture (not to exceed a total of 100 mEq), although they should be given in intravenous fluids when larger quantities are needed. Water may be added to the mixture in the face of excessive pure water losses.

Complications include nausea, vomiting, and diarrhea which develop because of the high osmolarity of the diets. This generally can be controlled by decreasing the rate and/or concentration of the mixture. Hypertonic nonketotic coma may occur in the presence of excessive water losses or if the diets are administered at concentrations above those recommended. Hyperglycemia and glycosuria may occur in any severely ill patient, particularly latent diabetics, and insulin may be indicated. Aspiration is a constant threat with intragastric feedings; for this reason, this route should not be used in the absence of laryngeal reflexes or in mentally obtunded patients.

PARENTERAL ALIMENTATION

The parenteral route for nutritional supplementation when oral or tube feedings into the gastrointestinal tract are not feasible has been tried for several decades but until recently has fallen short of expectations. Parenteral infusion of 5% dextrose solutions is totally inadequate to meet caloric requirements within the limits of fluid tolerance, while the use of hypertonic solutions of dextrose, fructose, or invert sugar has been limited by a high incidence of thrombophlebitis. The use of plasma and blood for nutritional supplementation is mentioned only to be condemned; they are very expensive and inefficient sources of calories, and their administration is associated with an unnecessary number of complications. High-caloric solutions, such as ethyl alcohol (7 kcal/Gm) and fat (9 kcal/Gm) have found limited use.

Recently, Dudrick et al. have demonstrated the clinical practicality of providing complete nutritional needs for an extended period of time using high-caloric parenteral feedings. Parenteral hyperalimentation involves the continuous infusion of a hyperosmolar solution containing carbohydrates, proteins, and other necessary nutrients through an indwelling catheter inserted into the superior vena cava. In order to obtain the maximum benefit, the ratio of calories to nitrogen must be adequate (at least 100 to 150 kcal/Gm nitrogen) and the two materials must be infused simultaneously. When the sources of calories and nitrogen are given at different times, there is a significant decrease in nitrogen utilization. These nutrients can be given in quantities considerably greater than the basic caloric and nitrogen requirements, and this method has proved to be highly successful in achieving growth and development, positive nitrogen balance, and weight gain in a variety of clinical situations.

INDICATIONS FOR THE USE OF INTRAVENOUS HYPER-ALIMENTATION. The principal indications for parenteral hyperalimentation are found in seriously ill patients suffering from malnutrition, sepsis, or surgical or accidental trauma when use of the gastrointestinal tract for feedings is not possible. The safe and successful use of this regimen requires proper selection of patients with specific nutritional needs, experience with the technique, and an awareness of the associated complications. The number of reported complications has increased significantly since this technique has become more popular; it has been used in many instances either where it is not needed or where use of the gastrointestinal tract is more appropriate. For this reason, Dudrick et al. have recently outlined specific goals and indications for parenteral hyperalimentation, listed below:

1. Newborn infants with catastrophic gastrointestinal anomalies, such as tracheoesophageal fistula, gastroschisis, omphalocele, or massive intestinal atresia
2. Infants who fail to thrive nonspecifically or secondarily to gastrointestinal insufficiency associated with the short bowel syndrome, malabsorption, enzyme deficiency, meconium ileus, or idiopathic diarrhea
3. Adult patients with short-bowel syndrome secondary to massive small bowel resection or enteroenteric, enterocolic, enterovesical, or enterocutaneous fistulas
4. Patients with high alimentary tract obstructions without vascular compromise, secondary to achalasia, stricture, or neoplasia of the esophagus; gastric carcinoma; or pyloric obstruction
5. Surgical patients with prolonged paralytic ileus following major operations, multiple injuries, or blunt or open abdominal trauma, or patients with reflex ileus complicating various medical diseases
6. Patients with normal bowel length but with malabsorption secondary to sprue, hypoproteinemia, enzyme or pancreatic insufficiency, regional enteritis, or ulcerative colitis
7. Adult patients with functional gastrointestinal disorders such as esophageal dyskinesia following cerebral vascular accident, idiopathic diarrhea, psychogenic vomiting, anorexia nervosa, or hyperemesis gravidarum
8. Patients who cannot ingest food or who regurgitate and aspirate oral or tube feedings because of depressed or obtunded sensorium following severe metabolic derangements, neurologic disorders, intracranial surgery, or central nervous system trauma
9. Patients with excessive metabolic requirements secondary to severe trauma, such as extensive full-thickness burns, major fractures, or soft tissue injuries
10. Patients with granulomatous colitis, ulcerative colitis, and tuberculous enteritis, in which major portions of the absorptive mucosa are diseased
11. Paraplegics, quadriplegics, or debilitated patients with indolent decubitus ulcers in the pelvic areas, particularly when soilage and fecal contamination are a problem
12. Patients who will eventually require surgery but in whom prolonged progressive malnutrition has greatly increased the risk of operation
13. Patients in whom protein deficiency states are to be avoided, reduced, or corrected
14. Patients with potentially reversible acute renal failure, in whom marked catabolism results in the liberation of intracellular anions and cations, inducing hyperkalemia, hypermagnesemia, and hyperphosphatemia

Conditions *contraindicating* hyperalimentation include the following:

1. Lack of a specific goal for patient management, or where instead of extending a meaningful life, inevitable dying is prolonged.
2. Periods of cardiovascular instability or severe metabolic derangement requiring control or correction before attempting hypertonic intravenous feeding.
3. Feasible gastrointestinal tract feeding. In the vast majority of instances, this is the best route by which to provide nutrition.
4. Patients in good nutritional status, in whom only short-term parenteral nutrition support is required or anticipated.
5. Infants with less than 8 cm of small bowel, since virtually all have been unable to adapt sufficiently despite prolonged periods of parenteral nutrition. Intravenous hyperalimentation must be seriously questioned until bowel transplantation has been perfected for these neonates.
6. Patients who are irreversibly decerebrate or otherwise dehumanized.

INSERTION OF CENTRAL VENOUS INFUSION CATHETER. The successful use of intravenous hyperalimentation generally depends upon the proper placement and management of the central venous feeding catheter. A 16-gauge, 8- or 12-in. radiopaque catheter is introduced percutaneously through the subclavian or internal jugular vein and threaded into the superior vena cava. Although the technique for subclavian vein puncture advocated by Dudrick and others has been quite popular, the internal jugular approach as described by Jernigan et al. has been equally satisfactory (Figs. 2-5 and 2-6).

For insertion of the intravenous catheter through the subclavian vein, the patient is placed on his back in a 15° head-down position with a small pad placed between the

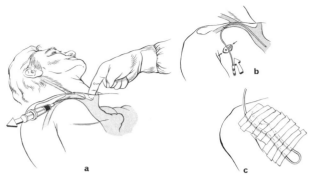

Fig. 2-5. Use of the subclavian vein for insertion of central venous catheter.

shoulder blades to allow the shoulders to drop posteriorly. This allows expansion of the subclavian vein and easier penetration. The skin is scrubbed with ether or acetone to defat the surface and then with an iodophor compound. Drapes are carefully placed, and *scrupulous* aseptic precautions are observed. Local anesthetic is infiltrated into the skin, subcutaneous tissue, and periosteum at the inferior border of the midpoint of the clavicle. A 2-in.-long, 14-gauge needle attached to a small syringe is inserted, beveled down through the wheal, and advanced toward the tip of the operator's finger, which is pressed well into the patient's suprasternal notch. The needle should hug the inferior clavicular surface and go over the first rib into the subclavian vein. With slight negative pressure applied to the syringe, entrance into the vein will be noted by the appearance of blood. The needle is advanced a few millimeters further to be sure that it is entirely within the lumen of the vein. The patient is asked to perform a Valsalva maneuver, or the thumb is held over the needle hub as the syringe is removed. A 16-gauge, 8- or 12-in. radiopaque catheter is then introduced through the needle and threaded into the superior vena cava. The needle is then withdrawn from the patient, and a small plastic splint is fitted over the junction of the catheter and needle to prevent catheter severance by the needle. The catheter is

Fig. 2-6. Use of internal jugular vein for insertion of central venous catheter.

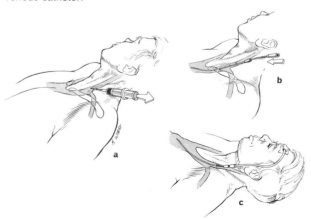

connected to a sterile intravenous administration tubing, and a slow infusion is begun while the catheter is sewn to the skin with a small synthetic suture. Antibiotic ointment is applied around the entrance of the catheter into the skin, and an occlusive dressing is applied over it including the junction of the intravenous tubing with the catheter. A chest film is immediately obtained to confirm the position of the radiopaque catheter in the vena cava and to check for a possible pneumothorax.

Every 2 or 3 days, the intravenous tubing is changed, the catheter site is scrubbed as for an operative procedure, and antibiotic ointment and a new occlusive dressing are applied. In general, withdrawal or administration of blood through the catheter or the use of the catheter for central venous pressure measurements should be avoided, since the risk of contamination and catheter occlusion are significantly increased.

The use of the internal jugular approach has also been quite satisfactory and is probably the preferred technique for the pediatric age group. It is probably unwise, unless absolutely necessary, to place catheters into the inferior vena cava from the lower extremities because of the greater likelihood of sepsis and thromboembolic phenomena. Additionally, cut-down catheter insertions into the cephalic or basilic veins have not proved satisfactory.

PREPARATION AND ADMINISTRATION OF SOLUTIONS. The basic solution contains between 20% and 25% dextrose and between 3% and 5% crystalline amino acids in water. The solutions are usually prepared in the pharmacy from commercially available kits containing the component solutions and transfer apparatus. Preparation in the pharmacy under laminar flow reduces the incidence of bacterial contamination of the solution. Proper preparation with suitable quality control is absolutely essential to avoid septic complications.

Since the formulation of commercially available hyperalimentation solutions varies considerably with regard to amino acid and electrolyte concentration, it is imperative that the physician become thoroughly familiar with the levels of the components within the solution utilized. Only in this manner may additives, in the form of additional electrolytes, be rationally planned to meet specific metabolic needs of the patient.

For the average adult patient without significant cardiac, renal, or hepatic disease, a typical hyperalimentation solution would contain components as outlined in Table 2-11. One should recognize that the recommended concentrations of electrolytes are only estimates and that actual requirements may vary considerably between individual patients, dependent on routes of fluid and electrolyte loss, renal function, metabolic rate, cardiac function, and the underlying disease state.

Intravenous vitamin preparations should be added to each bottle of solution as recommended in Table 2-11. In addition, phytonadione (vitamin K_1) 10 mg and folic acid 5 mg should be administered intramuscularly once a week, since these are unstable in the hyperalimentation solution. Cyanocobalamin (vitamin B_{12}) 1000 μg is given by intramuscular injection once a month. Intramuscular administration of iron may be required for patients with iron

Table 2-11. CONSTITUENTS OF SOLUTION FOR
TOTAL PARENTERAL NUTRITION
(PARENTERAL HYPERALIMENTATION)

(*Volume: 1050; osmolarity: 1900 mO; total caloric value:
1030 kcal; nitrogen content: 6.3 Gm*)

Protein equivalent (as crystalline aminoacid)	39 Gm
Dextrose	250 Gm
Calcium	4.7 mEq
Magnesium	8 mEq
Potassium	39 mEq
Sodium	49 mEq
Acetate	36 mEq
Chloride	35 mEq
Phosphate	29 mEq
Vitamin B complex*	2 ml
Ascorbic acid*	500 mg

*One day a week, these additives should be replaced by a
multiple vitamin preparation containing: Vitamin A, 10,000 units;
Ergocalciferol, 1,000 units; Vitamin E, 5 units; Thiamine HCl,
50 mg; Riboflavin, 10 mg; Pyridoxine HCl, 15 mg; Niacinamide,
100 mg; Dexpanthenal, 25 mg; Ascorbic acid, 500 mg.

deficiency anemia. After 30 to 40 days, essential fatty acid deficiency may become clinically apparent, manifested by a dry, scaly dermatitis and loss of hair. Chemical confirmation is obtained by noting an increase in the triene to tetraene ratio (>0.3) of total serum fatty acids. The syndrome may be prevented by weekly administration of a soybean fat emulsion. Essential trace minerals may be required after prolonged total parenteral nutrition and may be supplied by 1 or 2 units of plasma each week.

The infusion is started at 1 to 2 liters/day in the average adult and gradually increased to tolerance (3 to 4 liters/day). Rarely, additional intravenous fluids and electrolytes may be necessary with continued abnormal large losses of fluids. The patient should be carefully monitored for development of electrolyte, volume, acid-base, and septic complications. Vital signs and urinary output are regularly observed, and the patient should be weighed daily. Frequent adjustments of the volume and composition of the solutions are necessary during the course of therapy. Electrolytes are drawn daily until stable and every 2 or 3 days thereafter, and the hemogram and blood urea nitrogen are determined weekly.

The urine sugar level is checked every 6 hours and blood sugar concentration at least once daily during the first few days of the infusion and at frequent intervals thereafter. Relative glucose intolerance may occur following initiation of parenteral hyperalimentation, and blood sugar levels may rise as high as 400 mg/100 ml or more. Subsequently, blood sugar levels usually fall toward normal, urine sugar levels become negative to 2+, and insulin is not required in most cases. To avoid excessive glycosuria, the infusion is maintained at a rate which will allow urinary glucose level to exceed a 3+ reaction. However, if blood sugar levels remain elevated or urine sugar levels again become 3 or 4+, insulin (15 units) may be added to each liter of solution. The rise in blood glucose concentration observed after initiating a hyperalimentation program is generally temporary, as the normal pancreas increases its output of

insulin in response to the continuous carbohydrate infusion. In patients with diabetes mellitus, additional crystalline insulin may be required.

The administration of adequate amounts of potassium is essential to achieve positive nitrogen balance and replace depleted intracellular stores. In addition, a significant shift of potassium ion from the extracellular to the intracellular space may take place because of the large glucose infusion, with resultant hypokalemia, metabolic alkalosis, and poor glucose utilization. In some cases as much as 240 mEq of potassium ion daily may be required. Hypokalemia may cause glycosuria, which would be treated with potassium, not insulin. Thus, before giving insulin, the serum potassium level must be checked to avoid compounding the hypokalemia.

Often the blood urea nitrogen level rises, even in patients with normal renal function, but azotemia is not a contraindication to giving the solution if the elevation is moderate, does not continue to rise sharply, and does not rise over approximately 80 mg/100 ml. Wilmore and Dudrick, Abel, and Fischer have demonstrated the safety and efficacy of parenteral hyperalimentation in patients with renal failure and some forms of hepatic disease. For this purpose, special solutions of amino acids are required. Solutions for patients with acute renal failure contain 40 to 50% dextrose (to provide maximum caloric intake while restricting the volume of water infused) and only essential *l*-amino acids, which are efficiently utilized for protein synthesis. Solutions designed for patients with hepatic failure contain increased concentrations of branched-chain amino acids and decreased levels of the aromatic amino acids.

There is usually a delay of about a week before weight gain and positive nitrogen balance become apparent; the patient then may gain as much as $\frac{1}{2}$ to 1 lb daily. After several days, one frequently notes marked improvement in the patient's general appearance and healing of previously indolent wounds and intestinal fistulas. Dramatic recovery often ensues, whereas formerly death from inanition inexorably occurred.

FAT EMULSIONS. Recently a 10% fat emulsion, derived from soybean oil (Intralipid), has been marketed. The emulsion may be administered without many of the severe side effects previously observed after infusion of cottonseed oil emulsions two decades ago. The use of fat as an adjunctive nutrient prevents the development of essential fatty acid deficiency. In addition, the emulsion is not hypertonic and therefore may be delivered via a peripheral vein. A solution providing a source of nitrogen (5% crystalline amino acid) should be simultaneously infused. Fat emulsions may not be premixed with amino acid solutions, since the emulsion becomes unstable. Therefore the solutions are delivered via separate tubing joined together by a Y connector at the intravenous catheter. Patients with abnormal fat transport or metabolism, diabetes mellitus, liver disease, coagulopathy, or serious pulmonary disease should not receive fat emulsions, since inadequate clearance of fat from the bloodstream, additional hepatic or pulmonary dysfunction, or clinical hypocoagulability may be induced. Most investigators advise limitation of administered fat emulsion in adults to between 1.5 and 2.0 gm/kg body weight per day. Therefore caloric requirements of patients with major burns, severe trauma, and extensive surgical procedures cannot be met by the administration of fat emulsions alone. Furthermore, Long has recently demonstrated that infusion of fat is not as efficient in sparing protein as an isocaloric quantity of carbohydrate.

COMPLICATIONS. One of the more common and serious complications associated with long-term parenteral feeding is sepsis secondary to contamination of the solution, administration tubing, or the central venous catheter. This problem occurs more frequently in patients with systemic sepsis and in many cases is due to hematogenous seeding of the catheter with bacteria. More often, however, it is due to failure to observe strict aseptic precautions during preparation and administration of the solutions. One of the earliest signs of systemic sepsis may be the sudden development of glucose intolerance in a patient who previously has been maintained on parenteral hyperalimentation without difficulty. When this occurs or if fever develops without obvious cause, the solution and intravenous tubing are replaced. Other causes of fever should also be investigated; if fever persists, the infusion catheter should be removed and cultured. Antibiotics may be appropriate at this point in some cases. The catheter may be replaced in the opposite subclavian vein or into one of the internal jugular veins and the infusion restarted. In general, however, it is probably advisable to wait a short period of time before reinserting the catheter.

Other complications related to catheter placement include the development of pneumothorax, hemothorax, or hydrothorax; subclavian artery injury; cardiac arrhythmias if the catheter is placed into the atrium or the ventricle; air embolism or catheter embolism; and, rarely, cardiac perforation with tamponade. Thrombophlebitis or thrombosis of the superior vena cava has been an exceptionally rare complication. All these complications may be avoided by strict adherence to the techniques previously outlined.

Hyperosmolar nonketotic hyperglycemia may develop with normal rates of infusion in patients with impaired glucose tolerance or in any patient if the hypertonic solutions are administered too rapidly. This is a particularly common complication in latent diabetics and in patients following severe surgical stress or trauma. If blood and urine sugar concentrations are not monitored frequently, the blood sugar level may become markedly elevated with ensuing weakness, lethargy, and eventual coma. Treatment of the condition consists of volume replacement with correction of electrolyte abnormalities and the administration of insulin. This particularly serious complication can be avoided with careful attention to daily fluid balance and frequent determinations of urine and blood sugar levels and serum electrolyte content.

A number of volume, concentration, and compositional abnormalities may also develop, but these are largely avoided by careful attention to the details of patient management. This is particularly important for elderly patients and for patients with significant cardiovascular, renal, or hepatic disorders. Changes in the volume and composition of the administered solutions are often necessary to avoid complications. Additionally, the use of parenteral hyperalimentation in pediatric patients requires knowledge of the specific nutritional requirements of this age group and the special precautions that should be observed.

References

Fluid and Electrolyte Therapy

Abouna, G. M., Veazey, P. R., and Terry, D. B.: Intravenous Infusion of Hydrochloric Acid for Treatment of Severe Metabolic Alkalosis, *Surgery,* **75:**194, 1974.

Andersen, O. S., and Engel, K.: A New Acid-Base Nomogram: An Improved Method for the Calculation of the Relevent Blood Acid-Base Data, *Scand J Clin Lab Invest,* **12:**177, 1960.

Astrup, P., Jorgensen, K., Andersen, O. S., and Engel, K.: The Acid-Base Metabolism: A New Approach, *Lancet,* **1:**1035, 1960.

Bartlett, W. C.: Acute Hyperparathyroid Crisis, *Am J Surg,* **114:**796, 1967.

Baxter, C. R., Zedlitz, W. H., and Shires, G. T.: High-Output Acute Renal Failure Complicating Traumatic Injury, *J Trauma,* **4:**467, 1964.

Bishop, R. L., and Weisfeldt, M. L.: Sodium Bicarbonate Administration during Cardiac Arrest: Effect on Arterial pH, P_{CO_2} and Osmolality, *JAMA,* **235:**506, 1976.

Canizaro, P. C., Nelson, J., and Hennessy, J.: Alterations in Oxygen Transport, in G. T. Shires, C. J. Carrico, and P. C. Canizaro, "Shock," W. B. Saunders Company, Philadelphia, vol. XIII, 1973.

——, Prager, M. D., and Shires, G. T.: The Infusion of Ringer's Lactate Solution during Shock, *Am J Surg,* **122:**494, 1971.

Collins, J. A.: Problems Associated with the Massive Transfusion of Stored Blood, *Surgery,* **75:**274, 1974.

Cooper, N., Brazier, J. R., Hottenrott, C., Mulder, D. G., Maloney, J. V., and Buckberg, C. D.: Myocardial Depression Following Citrated Blood Transfusion, *Arch Surg,* **107:**756, 1973.

Elias, E. G., and Evans, J. T.: Hypercalcemic Crisis in Neoplastic Diseases: Management with Mithramycin, *Surgery,* **71:**631, 1972.

Harken, A. H., Gabel, R. A., Fencl, V., and Moore, F. D.: Hydrochloric Acid in the Correction of Metabolic Acidosis, *Arch Surg,* **110:**819, 1975.

Henzel, J. H., DeWeese, M. S., and Ridenhour, G.: Significance of Magnesium and Zinc Metabolism in the Surgical Patient. I. Magnesium, *Arch Surg,* **95:**974, 1967.

Jenkins, M. T., and Beck, G. P.: Differential Diagnosis of Hypotension Occurring during Anesthesia and Surgery, *Clin Anesthiol,* **3:**106, 1963.

Mattar, J. A., Weil, M. H., Shubin, H., and Stein, L.: Cardiac Arrest in the Critically Ill. II. Hyperosmolal States Following Cardiac Arrest, *Am J Med,* **56:**162, 1974.

McClelland, R. N., Shires, G. T., Baxter, C. R., Coln, C. D., and Carrico, C. J.: Balanced Salt Solution in the Treatment of Hemorrhagic Shock: Studies in Dogs, *JAMA,* **199:**830, 1967.

Mellemgaard, K., and Astrup, P.: The Quantitative Determination of Surplus Amounts of Acid or Base in the Human Body, *Scand J Clin Lab Invest,* **12:**187, 1960.

Mengoli, L. R.: Excerpts from the History of Postoperative Fluid Therapy, *Am J Surg,* **121:**311, 1971.

Moncrief, J. A., and Mason, A. D.: Water Vapor Loss in the Burned Patient, *Surg Forum,* **13:**38, 1962.

Moore, F. D., Olesen, K. H., McMurrey, J. D., Parker, H. V., Ball, M. R., and Boyden, C. M.: "Body Cell Mass and Its Supporting Environment: Body Composition in Health and Disease," W. B. Saunders Company, Philadelphia, 1963.

Moyer, C. A.: "Fluid Balance." Year Book Medical Publishers, Inc., Chicago, 1954.

Randall, R. E., Jr., Cohen, M. D., Spray, C. C., Jr., and Rossmeisl, E. C.: Hypermagnesemia in Renal Failure: Etiology and Toxic Manifestations, *Ann Intern Med,* **61:**73, 1964.

Schwarz, W. B., and Relman, A. S.: A Critique of the Parameters Used in the Evaluation of Acid-Base Disorders, *N Engl J Med,* **268:**1382, 1963.

Shavelle, H. S., and Parke, R.: Postoperative Alkalosis and Acute Renal Failure: Rationale for the Use of Hydrochloric Acid, *Surgery,* **78:**439, 1975.

Shires, G. T., Cunningham, J. N., Baker, C. R. F., Reeder, S. F., Illner, H., Wagner, I. Y., and Maher, J.: Alterations in Cellular Membrane Function During Hemorrhagic Shock in Primates, *Ann Surg,* **176:**288, 1972.

————, and Holman, V.: Dilutional Acidosis, *Ann Intern Med,* **28:**551, 1948.

————, and Jackson, D. E.: Postoperative Salt Tolerance, *Arch Surg,* **84:**703, 1962.

————, Williams, J., and Brown, F.: Acute Changes in Extracellular Fluids Associated with Major Surgical Procedures, *Ann Surg,* **154:**803, 1961.

Singer, R. B., and Hastings, A. B.: An Improved Clinical Method for the Estimation of Disturbances of the Acid-Base Balance of Human Blood, *Medicine,* **27:**223, 1948.

Thompson, J. E., Vollman, R. W., Austin, D. J., and Kartchner, M. M.: Prevention of Hypotensive and Renal Complications of Aortic Surgery Using Balanced Salt Solution, *Ann Surg,* **167:**767, 1968.

Tuller, M. A., and Mehdi, F.: Compensatory Hypoventilation and Hypercapnia in Primary Metabolic Alkalosis, *Am J Med,* **50:**281, 1971.

Wright, H. K., and Gann, D. S.: Correction of Defect in Free Water Excretion in Postoperative Patients by Extracellular Fluid Volume Expansion, *Ann Surg,* **158:**70, 1963.

Nutrition

Ballinger, W. F., Collins, J. A., Drucker, W. R., Dudrick, S. J., and Zeppa, R.: "Manual of Surgical Nutrition," W. B. Saunders Company, Philadelphia, 1975.

Boles, T., and Zollinger, R. M.: Critical Evaluation of Jejunostomy, *Arch Surg,* **65:**358, 1952.

Bury, K. D., Stephens, R. V., and Randall, H. T.: Use of a Chemically Defined, Liquid, Elemental Diet for Nutritional Management of Fistulas of the Alimentary Tract, *Am J Surg,* **121:**174, 1971.

Cahill, G. F., Jr.: Body Fuels and Their Metabolism, *Bull Am Coll Surg,* **55:**12, 1970.

Cuthbertson, D. P.: The Disturbance of Metabolism Produce by Bony and Non-bony Injury, with Notes on Certain Abnormal Conditions of Bone, *Biochem J,* **24:**1244, 1930.

Dudrick, S. J., Groff, D. B., and Wilmore, D. W.: Long-Term Venous Catheterization in Infants, *Surg Gynecol Obstet,* **129:**805, 1969.

————, Steiger, E., and Long, J. M.: Renal Failure in Surgical Patients: Treatment with Intravenous Essential Amino Acids and Hypertonic Glucose, *Surgery,* **68:**180, 1970.

————, ————, ————, Ruberg, R. L., Allen, T. R., Vars, H. M., and Rhoads, J. E.: General Principles and Techniques of Intravenous Hyperalimentation, in G. S. M. Cowan, Jr., and W. L. Scheetz (eds.), "Intravenous Hyperalimentation," Lea & Febiger, Philadelphia, 1972.

————, Wilmore, D. W., Vars, H. M., and Rhoads, J. E.: Long-Term Parenteral Nutrition with Growth, Development, and Positive Nitrogen Balance, *Surgery,* **64:**134, 1968.

Felig, P., Pozefsky, T., Marliss, E., and Cahill, G. F., Jr.: Alanine: Key Role in Gluconeogenesis, *Science,* **167:**1003, 1970.

Fischer, J. E.: "Total Parenteral Nutrition," Little, Brown and Company, Boston, 1976.

Graham, W. P., and Royster, H. P.: Simplified Cervical Esophagostomy for Long-Term Extraoral Feeding, *Surg Gynecol Obstet,* **125:**127, 1967.

Gump, F. E., Kinney, J. M., and Price, J. B., Jr.: Energy Metabolism in Surgical Patients: Oxygen Consumption and Blood Flow, *J Surg Res,* **10:**613, 1970.

Jernigan, W. R., Gardner, W. C., Mahr, M. M., and Milburn, J. L.: Use of the Internal Jugular Vein for Placement of Central Venous Catheter, *Surg Gynecol Obstet,* **130:**520, 1970.

Kinney, J. M.: A Consideration of Energy Exchange in Human Trauma, *Bull NY Acad Med,* **36:**617, 1960.

Long, J. M., Wilmore, D. W., Mason, A. D., Jr., and Pruitt, B. A., Jr.: Effect of Carbohydrate and Fat Intake on Nitrogen Excretion during Total Intravenous Feeding, *Ann Surg,* **185:**417, 1977.

McDougal, W. S., Wilmore, D. W., and Pruitt, B. A., Jr.: Glucose-Dependent Hepatic Membrane Transport in Nonbacteremic and Bacteremic Thermally Injured Patients, *J Surg Res,* **22:**697, 1977.

McMinn, R. M. H.: "Tissue Repair," Academic Press, Inc., New York, 1969.

Moore, F. D.: "Metabolic Care of the Surgical Patient," W. B. Saunders Company, Philadelphia, 1960.

White, P. L., and Nagy, M. E.: "Total Parenteral Nutrition," Publishing Sciences Group, Inc., Acton, Mass., 1974.

Wilmore, D. W., and Dudrick, S. J.: Treatment of Acute Renal Failure with Intravenous Essential L-amino Acids, *Arch Surg,* **99:**669, 1969.

Winters, R. W., and Hasselmeyer, E. G.: "Intravenous Nutrition in the High Risk Infant," John Wiley & Sons, New York, 1975.

Chapter 3

Hemostasis, Surgical Bleeding, and Transfusion

by Seymour I. Schwartz

Few events in clinical medicine are so ominous as the failure of hemostasis. For the surgeon, few failures in normal physiology are potentially so catastrophic. Disruption in normal hemostasis often can be anticipated, just as the physiologic failure usually can be identified and corrected. In this chapter the reader will become acquainted with the events of normal hemostasis. Advances in understanding in this area have come largely from the laboratory, not the clinic. As a consequence of this and because of the complex nature of some of the events involved, disproportionate emphasis often is placed upon the laboratory in attempting to solve what, primarily, are clinical problems. We shall try to provide a background whereby the problems encountered can be solved by careful evaluation of the patient and judicious use of the laboratory. A desired by-product will be the evolution of logical therapeutic programs. These may include methods for local control of bleeding, replacement for the loss of circulating blood volume, and selective transfusion of physiologic products necessary to provide normal hemostasis.

BIOLOGY OF NORMAL HEMOSTASIS

Cessation of blood flow from an injured vessel, the cumulative phenomenon we call hemostasis, occurs as a result of many events. Blood coagulation frequently is equated with hemostasis. Coagulation is not, however, always the central or most important factor. Clinical testimony to this heresy is supplied by the patient with congenital afibrinogenemia. This illness, characterized in the laboratory by incoagulability of the blood, may present clinically as a relatively minor hemostatic problem. This paradox is explained by the important role of the platelets, which, in this setting, are able to function in a near-normal manner because of the trace amount of fibrinogen present on their surface.

The accomplishment of hemostasis depends, to a variable degree, on the clinical condition of the patient, the nature of insult to the blood vessel, the type of vessel or vessels injured, the anatomic site of injury, the coagulation mechanism, and fibrinolytic activity. A lateral incision in a small artery may remain open because of physical forces and can be associated with extensive and continued bleeding. By contrast, a complete transection of a similar-sized vessel, as Hunter demonstrated centuries ago, contracts to the extent that the bleeding may cease spontaneously. Illustrative of the importance of anatomic site of injury is the fact that bleeding from a small venule ruptured by trauma in the thigh of a healthy athlete may be negligible because of the support of surrounding muscle. Bleeding from a similar vessel due to trauma of the nasal mucosa may be extensive in the same individual. An elderly person with atrophy of the subcutaneous connective tissue or a patient who has received corticosteroid therapy for a long time may sustain a large ecchymosis from minor trauma to the dorsum of the hand, while a younger person might note no change secondary to comparable trauma at the same site. Normal hemostasis, then, results from the interplay of multiple factors. A gross defect in one function or a lesser defect involving multiple functions usually

Fig. 3-1. Schematic representation of hemostasis.

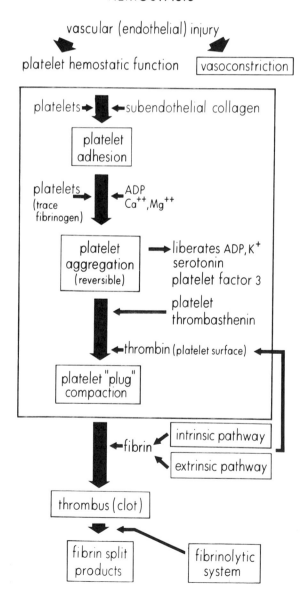

proves necessary to effect significant bleeding. Description of the events of normal hemostasis will permit consideration of the points at which failure may occur and also provides an opportunity to correlate laboratory tests with their physiologic counterparts.

VASCULAR RESPONSE. The initial vascular response to injury, even at the capillary level, is that of vasoconstriction. Experimental observation has demonstrated that adherence of endothelial cell to endothelial cell, with obliteration of microdefects, may, in itself, be sufficient to effect hemostasis. Whether vasoconstriction of these small vessels is neurogenically or humorally mediated remains unsettled. Human platelets normally carry vasoactive amines, some of which are liberated at the site of injury. The initial vasoconstriction described, however, occurs prior to platelet adherence at the site of injury. Animal experiments demonstrate that when platelets have been depleted of serotonin in vivo and vascular injury has been produced, vasoconstriction still occurs.

Patients with a mild bleeding disorder have been described in whom the only laboratory abnormality is a prolonged bleeding time. Capillary microscopy in certain of these patients reveals that the capillary loops do not constrict following injury. A capillary structural defect has been postulated, and support for this concept is provided by the observation that, even in the absence of trauma, the capillary loops are dilated and tortuous.

PLATELET FUNCTION. In less than 15 seconds following vascular injury, platelets (Fig. 3-1) adhere to the injured margins of the vessels. For many years it was believed that the platelets adhered directly to the injured endothelial cells. More recently, phase microscopy and electron microscopic observations have revealed that this early platelet adherence is to subendothelial collagen fibrils. The mechanism of attraction between collagen fibrils and platelets has not been defined, nor has the physiologic significance clearly been established. Two types of observations suggest that the platelet-collagen interaction is important. Quick demonstrated that the bleeding time, fastidiously performed, may be lengthened in patients taking aspirin. Platelet-rich plasma derived from patients taking aspirin demonstrates an impairment of the platelet-collagen reaction in vitro. The second observation, related to the first, is that of Vigliano and Horowitz. These writers described a patient with multiple myeloma and hemorrhagic tendency in whom the principal laboratory abnormality was impairment of the collagen-platelet interaction.

Within seconds of the collagen-platelet response, platelets begin to adhere to one another at the site of injury. The initial aggregation is loose. The loose aggregates may be fragmented and dispersed by the pressure of blood issuing from tiny arterioles. This platelet aggregation is thought to occur as a result of a platelet-ADP (adenosinediphosphate) interaction. Gaarder et al. initially demonstrated that ADP, added in minute amounts, results in rapid platelet aggregate formation in whole blood or platelet-rich plasma. Trace amounts of calcium or magnesium are necessary for this reaction. Interestingly, and probably significantly, heparin does not interfere with this reaction. The maintenance of normal hemostasis in the heparinized patient may well be explained by the platelets' ability to aggregate loosely at sites of minimal trauma, even when the blood is relatively incoagulable.

A relatively rare clinical entity, thrombasthenia of the Glanzmann type, may represent a naturally occurring failure of hemostasis at this level. Platelets from such patients fail to aggregate in the presence of ADP. This is not their only abnormality of platelet function, for blood clots from these patients also display poor retraction. The platelets lack fibrinogen, and it is possible that all these abnormalities are related.

Following the formation of the loose platelet aggregate the mass of platelets begins to compact. When observed microscopically, the platelets lose their individual identity and begin to fuse with one another. The platelet granules concentrate toward the center of the platelet, and fibrin strands now can be identified scattered throughout the platelet mass. These changes are described as viscous metamorphosis and have a biochemical counterpart. During compaction the platelets, normally rich in adenosinetriphosphate (ATP), suffer a drop in content of this energy-rich compound and liberate ADP. Potassium and serotonin, normally present in platelets, also are liberated at this time. Platelet factor 3 (phospholipid) is made available for the clotting process, but a small amount probably becomes available earlier. Platelet factor 3 is a normal component within the platelet membrane as well as in certain of the platelet granules.

The events initiating these morphologic and biochemical processes have not been established with certainty. Probably trace amounts of the enzyme thrombin are formed at the surface of the platelet. All the necessary plasma factors are present in the immediate plasmatic environment of the platelet. All the observed platelet changes can be produced in vitro by the addition of trace amounts of thrombin. Indirect experimental data suggest that this also occurs in vivo.

The events culminating in the compaction of the loose platelet aggregate into a "platelet plug" seem to correspond to what we measure with the bleeding time. Failure of any of the early events described above can result in lengthening of the bleeding time.

Approximately 15 percent of human platelet protein is contractile. This material is called *thrombosthenin*. It is very similar to muscle actomyosin and is an ATPase. Compaction of the platelet plug is credited to the contractile protein, which participates in the biochemical events as well. The platelets' responses to thrombin end in destruction of the platelets as intact cells. The sequential changes in the platelets have been described as preaggregation, aggregation, thrombocytorrhexis, and thrombocytolysis.

The platelet is equipped to enhance its function in many ways. Laboratory studies have demonstrated that platelets are capable of liberating enough ADP during hydrolysis of the energy-rich ATP to supply their own stimulus for the ADP aggregation. Interestingly, ADP aggregation is facilitated by amines which also are liberated from the platelets early in their hemostatic function. The serotonin which is released may induce vascular constriction in the immediate area. While evidence for the importance of serotonin in normal hemostasis is lacking, its presence is provocative.

BLOOD COAGULATION. Until this point in the hemostatic process, the role of blood coagulation has been inferential and invoked only to explain the initiation of viscous metamorphosis by the platelets. Microscopic clotting, assumed to take place at the platelet surface, is thought to evolve through the effects of tissue thromboplastin on the plasma procoagulant substances at the platelet surface. Reliance on the concept of a *tissue* thromboplastin leading to microscopic clotting at the platelet surface, rather than an *intrinsic* thromboplastin, is explained by the normal platelet function and bleeding time with defects in intrinsic thromboplastin formation.

The complex series of reactions that ultimately leads to the transformation of the soluble protein fibrinogen to the insoluble fibrin clot constitutes the process of coagulation. Failure at any one of the stages may manifest itself as a potential bleeding disorder. The importance of blood coagulation has been appreciated since antiquity. Allowable exceptions to the covenant of circumcision demanded by the Old Testament are described in the Babylonian Talmud. While our understanding of blood clotting has become somewhat more precise since that time, a degree of faith remains requisite in the student of the hemostatic process. Nowhere is this better demonstrated than in the earliest step in the coagulation process, activation of factor XII.

Factor XII (Hageman factor) deficiency results in lengthening of the whole blood clotting time. Despite this gross laboratory abnormality, the deficiency is not associated with significant hemostatic problems. A patient named Hageman, the first patient demonstrated to have this deficiency, underwent gastrectomy without bleeding complication. Interestingly, the same patient succumbed to complications of thromboembolic disease many years later.

The concept of the blood coagulation mechanism representing a "waterfall," or "cascade," phenomenon was developed simultaneously and independently by Davie and Ratnoff and by Macfarlane (Fig. 3-2). These writers view the activation of factor XII as the initiation of the coagulation sequence. In vitro studies demonstrate that activation of factor XII is accomplished by virtually any nonendothelial surface. The activated factor XII, which differs from the inactive form in certain physicochemical features, has enzymatic properties. The substrate for activated factor XII is believed to be factor XI (plasma thromboplastin antecedent, PTA). Factor XI seemingly can be changed to its activated form without depending upon activated factor XII. This could explain the absence of hemostatic problems in patients with factor XII deficiency.

Deficiency of factor XI clinically is associated with a mild bleeding disorder known as *Rosenthal's syndrome*. This is inherited as an incompletely recessive autosomal trait. Factor XI behaves as an enzyme when activated either by factor XII or by some unexplained process. Factor IX (Christmas factor, plasma thromboplastin component, PTC) serves as the substrate for activated factor XI. This step requires the presence of ionized calcium. Deficiency of factor IX is characterized clinically by the disorder known as *Christmas disease, PTC deficiency,* or *hemophilia B.* This sex-linked recessive trait will be discussed later in the chapter.

Activated factor IX is believed to have enzymatic activity interacting with its specific substrate factor VIII (antihemophilic factor, AHF). The effect of factor IX upon factor VIII requires the presence of phospholipid (platelet factor 3) as well as ionized calcium. Although the phospholipid normally is contributed by the platelets, it is clear from in vitro studies that other tissues may serve as a source. Under pathologic circumstances, such as massive intravascular hemolysis, it is possible that the phospholipid can be derived from the red blood cell membrane. Inherited deficiency of factor VIII clinically is represented by classical hemophilia, or hemophilia A.

The events in blood coagulation described until this point are relatively time-consuming. The steps leading to the activation of factor VIII probably consume 90 percent of the time that is required for blood to clot grossly. Accordingly, defects within this portion of the clotting sequence are characterized by prolonged whole blood clotting time when severe or by abnormalities in other test systems which relate to this slower phase of blood coagulation.

Activated factor VIII is believed to use factor X (Stuart-Prower factor) as its substrate. Factor X deficiency is a rare but potentially serious disorder which may manifest laboratory abnormalities characteristic of both the earlier and later phases of blood coagulation. Thus, severe deficiency of factor X may result in a prolonged whole blood clotting time and impaired prothrombin consumption. Such a deficiency also invariably will prolong the one-stage *prothrombin time.* Activated factor X appears to act upon, or act with, factor V (proaccelerin). When this stage is completed, the activator *prothrombinase* has evolved. In the presence of ionized calcium, prothrombinase will split the prothrombin molecule (factor II) to form the smaller molecular species thrombin. Figure 3-2 schematically depicts the foregoing discussion. Examples of each of the clinical deficiencies will be discussed subsequently.

Normal hemostasis also requires the integrity of the extrinsic system of blood coagulation (Fig. 3-3). This pathway of blood coagulation takes origin with the interaction of tissue lipoprotein (tissue thromboplastin) and factor VII (proconvertin). Factor X then is activated, and the sequence continues as previously described for the intrinsic system. The formation of the platelet hemostatic plug, described earlier, is believed to be triggered by the effect of thrombin on the platelet surface. An explanation for this early appearance of a trace amount of thrombin, too soon to be explained by the more leisurely intrinsic pathway of blood coagulation, is the "shortcut" provided by tissue thromboplastin and factor VII as the extrinsic clotting system.

The in vitro equivalent of the extrinsic pathway is the one-stage prothrombin determination. In this test an extrinsic source of tissue lipoprotein and calcium is added

Fig. 3-2. "Waterfall" phenomenon: intrinsic pathway for the formation of thrombin. The inhibitors of various steps and the alterations induced by thrombin in antihemophilic factor and proaccelerin are omitted from the diagram. (*From C. R. M. Prentice and O. D. Ratnoff, Semin Hematol, 4:93, 1967.*)

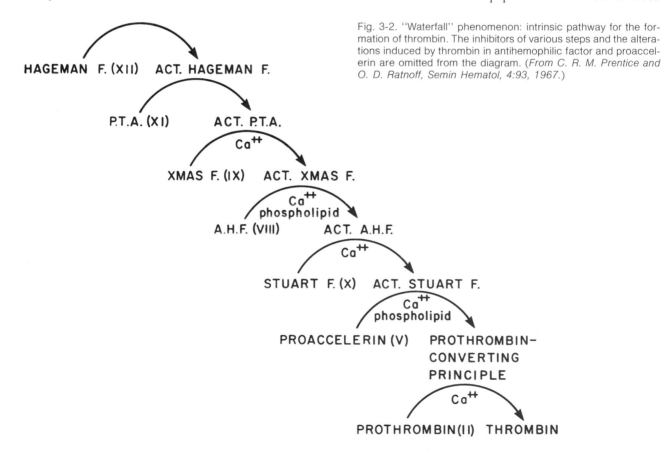

to plasma. Deficiencies in factor VII, factor X, factor V, or fibrinogen will lengthen the clotting time in this test. Since delays in clotting in this test are measured in seconds, it is clear that defects in this portion of the process will not noticeably lengthen the whole blood clotting time. The range of normal for the whole blood clotting time is appreciable, and even a substantial lengthening of the prothrombin time would be obscured within the variability of the whole blood clotting time.

The role of thrombin in the hemostatic mechanism has been the focus of much study. Thrombin probably serves as an initiator of the biochemical and functional platelet changes early in normal hemostasis. It has the ability to enhance strikingly the activation of certain of the blood clotting factors, e.g., factor V, factor VIII, and factor XIII (fibrin-stabilizing factor). The key position occupied by thrombin is emphasized further by our clinical approach to anticoagulation. On one hand the coumarin drugs are used to impair synthesis of those precursors that will lead to thrombin generation, while on the other hand the efficacy of heparin is its ability to impair or interfere with the effect of thrombin on fibrinogen.

The chemistry of the thrombin-fibrinogen reaction now is well characterized. Thrombin enzymatically cleaves two pairs of peptide chains from the fibrinogen molecule. The action of thrombin on fibrinogen ends at that point. Thereafter, the soluble fibrinogen monomers, which are the fibrinogen molecules minus the two pairs of peptide chains, unite by hydrogen bonding. This is a loose chemical bond that is easily separated. The weak formation is converted to a stable one through the enzymatic activity of factor XIII, fibrin-stabilizing factor. This enzyme probably works by facilitating conversion of sulfhydryl groups to disulfide bonds.

Inherited and acquired hemostatic abnormalities have been identified for these steps. Impaired organization of the fibrin monomers occurs in dysglobulinemic states, and the faulty clot structure has been blamed for the bleeding tendency. Congenital and acquired deficiencies of factor XIII have been described. Of interest to the surgeon is the repeated observation of impaired wound healing in patients with factor XIII deficiency. In vitro studies have suggested that fibroblasts grown on a medium lacking factor XIII show faulty organization, and it is possible that the biologic importance of factor XIII lies outside the immediate realm of hemostasis.

CLOT DISSOLUTION. Fibrinolysis (Fig. 3-4) is the mechanism by which dissolution of blood clots occurs. Although fibrinolysis is not necessarily part of the hemostatic mechanism, excessive fibrinolysis may cause failure of hemostasis. The process of clot dissolution is as complex as the clotting system itself but is not yet as thoroughly understood. The enzyme plasmin, which is derived from a precursor plasma protein (plasminogen), is essential to the mechanism of fibrinolysis. Under the influence of kinases, which may be blood activators, tissue activators, streptokinase, or urokinase, the precursor plasma protein (plasminogen) is converted into an enzyme with proteolytic activity (plasmin). There is some question as to whether the kinases act directly on plasminogen or transform a

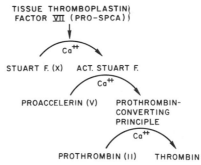

Fig. 3-3. Extrinsic pathway for the formation of thrombin. Inhibitors of the various steps and alterations induced by thrombin in proaccelerin are omitted from the diagram. (*From C. R. M. Prentice and O. D. Ratnoff, Semin Hematol, 4:93, 1967.*)

proactivator in the human plasma into an activator, which in turn converts plasminogen into plasmin. While fibrin is its preferred substrate, plasmin also can digest fibrinogen, factor V, and factor VIII. The fibrinolytic system can be activated in many ways, including by activated factor XII. It is likely that fibrinolysis progresses at the same time that the blood-clotting process itself is being activated. The initiation of fibrinolysis may arise from tissue sources, vascular endothelium representing a particularly likely possibility. Ischemia is a potent stimulator of the activation of the fibrinolytic system.

What Sherry has viewed as "physiologic proteolysis" results from the natural affinity of plasminogen for fibrin. The latter adsorbs the former during clot formation. The plasminogen then is in position to attack only the fibrin to which it is adsorbed, a locally controlled form of fibrinolysis resulting. On the other hand, pathologic proteolysis may occur when plasminogen free in the plasma is activated. The activated plasminogen may then attack other coagulant proteins as well.

The failure of hemostasis related to excessive activation or ineffective inactivation of the fibrinolytic system is due to several factors. The smaller fragments of fibrin liberated by proteolysis may interfere with normal platelet aggrega-

Fig. 3-4. Fibrinolytic system.

FIBRINOLYTIC SYSTEM

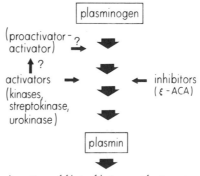

tion. The larger fibrin fragments are incorporated into the clot in lieu of normal fibrin monomers and create an unstable clot. When proteolysis is excessive, other plasma clotting factors also serve as substrates for protein digestion. Human blood normally has a high content of antiplasmin, which inhibits plasminogen activation, and platelets are also believed to possess an antifibrinolytic property.

TESTS OF HEMOSTASIS AND BLOOD COAGULATION

BLEEDING TIME. This is the time required for bleeding to cease after a standard skin incision has been made. The bleeding time probably corresponds to that time required for compaction of the platelet plug in the hemostatic process described above.

With the Duke technique, a clean 2- or 3-mm incision is made with a #11 Bard-Parker blade in the most dependent portion of the earlobe. A piece of filter paper is held below the wound, but not touching it, to catch each drop of blood as it forms and falls. The paper is held so that each drop strikes the margin of the filter paper serially. In this way, a permanent record of the bleeding time can be obtained and, if desired, entered in the patient's chart. The wound itself should not be disturbed, since this may prolong the bleeding time. When blood flow ceases, the time lapse following incision is recorded as the bleeding time. The upper limits of normal vary but probably should not exceed $3\frac{1}{2}$ minutes. The Ivy technique requires the placement of a blood pressure cuff above the elbow with inflation to 40 mm Hg pressure. A standard 5-mm incision is made to a depth of 2 mm on the volar surface of the forearm, taking care to avoid any obvious venules in the skin. Pressure within the cuff is maintained while a piece of filter paper is employed to touch the drops of blood carefully as they form. Once again, the wound must not be disturbed. With this method, a normal upper limit of 5 minutes is accepted. If the above tests are equivocal, an incision made through a template slit method of Mielke et al. will provide a more accurate result.

In our experience, abnormalities of bleeding time usually are fairly clear-cut. The bleeding time usually is normal in patients with a platelet count greater than 75,000/mm³. Patients with a qualitative platelet abnormality (thrombocytopathia or thrombasthenia), patients with defective capillaries as described earlier in this chapter, or patients with von Willebrand's disease all may have prolonged bleeding time. Aspirin ingested within 1 week will affect the results. Bleeding times as prolonged as 24 minutes have been related to aspirin alone.

RUMPEL-LEEDE (TOURNIQUET) TEST. This test, to our view, has little clinical application today. It is designed to estimate capillary fragility. A blood pressure cuff is applied to the upper arm and inflated to a pressure midway between diastolic and systolic pressure. The pressure is maintained at that level for a maximum of 5 minutes—less if many petechiae appear on the forearm before that time. Semiquantification of capillary fragility is obtained by counting the number of petechiae seen within a predeter-mined area, which should be at some distance from the blood pressure cuff. The antecubital space is not used, for some normal individuals will show petechiae in this area. No more than 2 to 4 petechiae should be seen in a circle of 2.5 cm diameter.

The test need not be performed on patients known to have a low platelet count or prolonged bleeding time. The demonstration of capillary fragility will not contribute to the diagnosis in such circumstances. Rather, it results in some discomfort to the patient, and the petechiae merely serve as a frightening reminder that something is grossly abnormal. The test characteristically is abnormal when thrombocytopenia is present, but this may be determined readily by inspection of the blood smear or a direct platelet count. It also may be abnormal in the group of patients with prolonged bleeding time as well as in elderly patients with poor tissue turgor. Severe vitamin C deficiency also may result in a positive tourniquet test.

PLATELET ESTIMATION AND COUNT. Thrombocytopenia is the most common abnormality of hemostasis encountered in the surgical patient. Microscopic examination of a properly stained blood smear can provide much information about such patients. When an area where the red blood cells display their customary central pallor and where few of the red blood cells overlap one another is examined, 15 to 20 platelets per oil immersion field should be noted. If the blood is not anticoagulated before the smear is prepared, as many as half of these may be in clumps of three or four platelets. A well-stained blood smear that fails to display more than three or four platelets in at least every other oil immersion field can be considered significantly thrombocytopenic. In this situation, the patient's platelet count generally is less than 75,000/mm³. Blood smears which must be searched because platelets appear in only every four or five oil immersion fields usually represent platelet counts of fewer than 40,000/mm³. If cover slip smears have been prepared, the cover slips always should be mounted as matched pairs. Platelets occasionally stick to one of the cover slips, and examination of both will obviate a false impression of thrombocytopenia. Lightly stained blood smears may appear thrombocytopenic in that the platelets are not prominent enough to attract the examiner's attention.

Inspection of the blood smear has the other obvious advantage of permitting the examiner to identify additional pathologic features which may have meaning in the care of the patient. The presence of nucleated red blood cells or abnormal white cells can provide information important to the diagnosis. The presence of giant platelets or large fragments of megakaryocyte cytoplasm also will alert the examiner to possible pathologic platelet function.

Direct enumeration of blood platelets can be accomplished quite accurately. The most reliable microscopic method is that described by Brecher and Cronkite, employing the phase contrast microscope. With this method, normal values ranging from 160,000 to 350,000/mm³ are obtained. Electronic particle counters recently have been adapted for platelet counting. The degree of precision matches that obtained by phase contrast microscopy. *Spontaneous* bleeding only rarely can be related to thrombocytopenia with platelet counts greater than 50,000/mm³. Platelet counts of 60,000 to 70,000/mm³ usually are sufficient to provide adequate hemostasis following trauma or surgical procedures if other hemostatic factors are normal.

CLOT RETRACTION. Normal platelet function is responsible for retraction of the clot, but this gross phenomenon has no clear function in hemostasis. The macroscopic event, however, may well have its microscopic equivalent in the compaction of the platelet plug.

Semiquantification of this platelet function can be obtained. If an applicator stick, string, or partially straightened paper clip is suspended in 5 ml of freshly drawn blood and the blood permitted to clot undisturbed about this object, the clot can be removed 1 hour following coagulation and the serum that has been expressed from the clot measured. Clot retraction then can be expressed as a percentage of the serum related to the original volume of blood. With blood of normal hematocrit, the usual range is 40 percent or slightly higher. Normally, clot retraction in a test tube is complete within 3 or 4 hours at room temperature. A rough relationship exists between the platelet count and clot retraction. Significant thrombocytopenia can exist in the presence of normal clot retraction, since the clot will retract well if the platelet count is slightly less than 100,000/mm³.

OTHER TESTS OF PLATELET FUNCTION. The ability of the platelets to liberate platelet factor 3 (phospholipid), essential in tiny amounts at several stages of the blood-clotting process (Fig. 3-2), also can be measured. Impairment of platelet factor 3 release has been reported in conditions described as *thrombocytopathia*. This defect can represent a primary disease entity, but similar impairment has been described as a secondary phenomenon in uremia and liver disease. Whether the impairment plays a functional role, for example, in the bleeding associated with uremia, remains uncertain. The inability of the platelet to make platelet factor 3 available for the clotting process may be a part of a more fundamental surface membrane abnormality.

The role of ADP in platelet aggregation during hemostasis has been mentioned earlier. The ability of platelets to aggregate in plasma upon the addition of ADP serves as another test of platelet function. Failure of platelets to aggregate following the addition of ADP is seen in patients with the Glanzmann type of thrombasthenia and also, artifactually, when anticoagulants, such as EDTA, which tightly bind divalent cations, are used.

The ability of platelets to adhere to a standardized glass bead column also has been used as a measure of platelet function. This test, refined by Salzman, is reported to be grossly abnormal in patients with von Willebrand's disease. The test requires meticulous preparation of the glass bead column and, while of great interest, does not yet enjoy total acceptance.

WHOLE BLOOD COAGULATION TIME. This test is of historical interest as a diagnostic aid but is quite insensitive as a detector of coagulation defects. The most commonly employed method is a modification of the Lee-White method, in which venous blood is removed by clean venipuncture and 1-ml volumes are delivered into each of three tubes. The first tube is tilted every 30 seconds until no flow of blood is observed. A similar procedure is carried out sequentially on the second and third tubes. The clotting time is taken as the elapsed time from the drawing of blood until coagulation is observed in the third tube.

The coagulation time of blood so studied is influenced by many factors. Several of these relate to the amount of surface activation occurring during the procedure. The smaller the amount of blood relative to the size of the tube, the greater the surface contact and activation. If the tube is tilted more frequently than every 30 seconds, surface activation also is increased. If the venipuncture has not been made cleanly, even minute amounts of tissue juice (tissue thromboplastin) may accelerate the clotting time. To obviate the latter a two-syringe technique may be used. Following successful venipuncture, 1 or 2 ml of blood is drawn into the first syringe, which is carefully disconnected while the needle is held in place and the second syringe attached. Blood is then drawn into the second syringe and provides the sample for the determination. When 1 ml of blood is added, with care to avoid bubbling, to 3 to 10 mm inner diameter clean glass test tubes, the normal range for clotting in the third tube is between 9 and 14 minutes. For practical purposes, only severe deficiencies of factors VIII, IX, XI, XII, and rarely X will be detected by this method. The sensitivity of the test can be increased by employing silicone-coated syringes and clotting tubes or by using plastic syringes and plastic (Lusteroid) tubes. When the latter are employed, the normal clotting time is up to 40 minutes. The test performed with untreated glassware finds its principal use in the control of patients receiving anticoagulation treatment with heparin.

ONE-STAGE PROTHROMBIN TIME (QUICK TEST). This test measures the speed of the events described earlier as the extrinsic pathway of blood coagulation. A tissue source of procoagulant, ideally derived from acetone-dehydrated rabbit brain, as described by Quick, is added with calcium to an aliquot of citrated plasma and the clotting time determined. The laboratory should establish a normal dilution curve and normal values daily. The 100 percent value using the method of Quick should be 15 seconds. Using other sources of tissue thromboplastin, the 100 percent value may be as low as 11 seconds. The prothrombin time will be prolonged in the presence of even minute amounts of heparin. The presence of heparin, by its antithrombin action, will artificially prolong the clotting time of the mixture so that it appears that the prothrombin complex is low. Accordingly, an accurate prothrombin determination cannot be carried out in a patient receiving anticoagulation treatment with heparin until the heparin has disappeared from the plasma. This should be at least 5 hours following the last intravenous dose.

The use of tissue procoagulants in the test eliminates the roles of factors VIII, IX, XI, XII, and platelets. Properly done, the test will detect deficiencies of factors II, V, VII, X, and fibrinogen. The one-stage prothrombin time is the preferred method of controlling anticoagulation with the coumarin and indandione drugs.

PARTIAL THROMBOPLASTIN TIME (PTT). The partial thromboplastin time technically is a variant of the one-stage prothrombin time but provides broader information. The tissue source of procoagulant, commercially available, is extracted and refined so that the in vitro clotting system now is sensitive to factors VIII, IX, XI, XII, as well as the factors normally detected by the one-stage prothrombin time. The range of normal with this test varies with the product used. Each laboratory should establish a normal dilution curve daily, and the patient's plasma must be compared with a normal control.

The partial thromboplastin time, when used in conjunction with the one-stage prothrombin time, can help to place a clotting defect in the first or second stage of the clotting process. If the partial thromboplastin time is prolonged and the one-stage prothrombin time is normal, factors VIII, IX, XI, or XII may be deficient. If the partial thromboplastin time is normal and the one-stage prothrombin time is prolonged, a single or multiple deficiency of factors II, V, VII, or X or of fibrinogen may be present. The partial thromboplastin time also is abnormal in the presence of circulating anticoagulants or during heparin administration. The sensitivity of the test is such that only extremely mild cases of factor VIII or IX deficiency may be missed. In one study of over 600 patients with clotting abnormalities, only two mild abnormalities failed to be detected with this test.

THROMBIN TIME. The test is of value in detecting qualitative abnormalities in fibrinogen, in the detection of circulating anticoagulants and inhibitors of fibrin polymerization. The clotting time of the patient's plasma is measured following the addition of a standard amount of thrombin to a fixed volume of plasma. Controls of normal plasma must be run in parallel. Failure of the clot to form, in the absence of circulating inhibitors such as heparin, is consistent with severe diminution of fibrinogen, usually well below 100 mg/100 ml.

THROMBOPLASTIN GENERATION TEST (TGT). The development of this test permitted a distinction of deficiencies in the hemophilia family of diseases without requiring use of plasma from patients with known abnormalities. The thromboplastin generation test, or modification of it, has been used with success in performing assays of specific clotting factors of the first stage. In most laboratories in this country, the test has been replaced by the partial thromboplastin time test, or variations of it. The thromboplastin generation test has facilitated understanding of current concepts in blood coagulation and continues to be used with success in Great Britain, where it was developed. Preparation of the reagents can be time-consuming, and the test must be done with great precision in order to be reproducible.

TESTS OF FIBRINOLYSIS. The most gross and earliest determination of fibrinolysis was that of observing the whole blood clot for dissolution. Normally, this may not occur for 48 hours or more. When fibrinolysis is a significant factor in hemostatic failure, dissolution of the whole blood clot is observed in 2 hours or less. The test has the disadvantage of being time-consuming in a circumstance where time may be of the essence. In addition, a false impression of increased fibrinolytic activity may be gained from clots formed in patients with high hematocrits

or in thrombocytopenia, where red cells may fall away from the clot. The euglobulin clot lysis time and dilute whole blood or plasma clot lysis time are more sensitive indices and permit more rapid evaluation of fibrinolysis.

OTHER TESTS OF HEMOSTASIS. Specific assays of all the known clotting factors now can be performed. The most popular of these assays are based upon modification of the partial thromboplastin time. The accuracy of these tests varies somewhat, but, on the average, the more accurate values are obtained when the factors are significantly reduced. Imprecision usually is found at the higher, clinically less important levels. These tests prove to be of significant clinical value but require an experienced laboratory staff.

Relatively simple tests permit identification of circulating anticoagulants. The simplest of these are based on the retardation of clotting of normal recalcified plasma by varying mixtures of the test plasma. The sensitivity of such tests usually can be increased by incubating the test plasma with the normal plasma for 30 minutes at body temperature prior to recalcification.

The *thrombotest*, devised by Owren, employs a refined tissue procoagulant which seems a little less sensitive than that used for the partial thromboplastin time but slightly more sensitive than that used for the standard one-stage prothrombin time. It has been credited with being more sensitive to factor X deficiency than the one-stage prothrombin time. While its developers have used it extensively, most laboratories will find the Quick one-stage prothrombin time test suitable.

The *thromboelastogram* is a graphic representation of clotting obtained by employing a special instrument, the thromboelastograph. The record obtained provides information about the clotting time, the speed of fibrin polymerization, and the strength and tendency toward dissolution of the clot. The instrument has provided information of research value but has not, in our experience, greatly aided the studies of clinical problems.

EVALUATION OF THE SURGICAL PATIENT AS A HEMOSTATIC RISK

General Considerations

Every patient viewed as a candidate for surgical treatment should be evaluated in terms of the risk of bleeding. The realities of time and economics dictate how exhaustive the approach to a given patient will be. For the patient requiring surgical intervention on an elective basis several points can be emphasized. The nondirective, open-ended patient interview has proved of value in many diagnostic settings. Direct questioning, however, is required to elicit most hints of a bleeding tendency.

The history should determine if circumcision was accompanied by unusual bleeding, since such bleeding is a frequent occurrence in patients who have inherited hemostatic problems. Hemophilic infants have been circumcised, however, without bleeding when the circumcision was performed immediately following delivery. Sufficient factor VIII may be supplied by transplacental transfer. The dental history can be of great significance. Many patients with inherited bleeding disorders may have bleeding with eruption of the teeth or bleeding after extraction. In the case of the hemophiliac, bleeding may begin hours after extraction and continue to be a problem for several days. The patient with a bleeding disorder, either acquired or inherited, who does not bleed after tonsillectomy sufficiently to require reexploration or transfusion is rare. It also is unusual for the patient with a hemorrhagic diathesis to have hematemesis, epistaxis, or hemoptysis without some other hemorrhagic manifestation. The gastrointestinal tract has been regarded as an area of poor resistance in patients with hemostatic difficulties, but isolated gastrointestinal bleeding, *in the absence of bleeding or bruising tendency elsewhere,* usually is not associated with generalized hemostatic failure. More often, it may be related to local disease or associated with lesions such as hereditary hemorrhagic telangiectasia. Excessive menstrual flow, rather than intermenstrual bleeding, is a common complaint in patients with generalized hemostatic problems. It is not infrequent for such a patient, usually with thrombocytopenia, to be subjected to uterine curettage. Such an oversight can result in catastrophic complications. A detailed history of drug ingestion is essential, and it is wise to specify products by name. The patient may not regard aspirin, tranquilizers, and other pharmacologic agents which can affect the hemostatic process as drugs.

Special emphasis must be made of the family history. It is not enough to question the health of siblings and parents. Appreciation of simple genetic principles, such as the sex-linked recessive mode of transmission of some of the more serious clotting disorders, requires that we inquire into the health of grandparents, occasionally great grandparents, and certainly uncles and cousins. Patterns for the genetic transmission of hemorrhagic disorders are presented later in this chapter.

Certain findings on the physical examination should alert the examiner to the possibility of a hemostatic problem. The entire body should be inspected for ecchymoses or petechiae. These lesions are likely to appear at pressure points, where snug foundation garments are worn, or under belts or garters. Purpuric lesions are characteristically spontaneous in origin, often multiple, and frequently bilateral. The lesions of senile purpura are most common on forearms and hands, where tissue support is loose, while lesions of Henoch-Schönlein purpura generally are distributed over the buttocks, backs of the legs, elbows, and ankles. Spider angiomas are suggestive of liver disease. While not related, they may be associated with reduction in the prothrombin complex. Lesions characteristic of hereditary hemorrhagic telangiectasia are often found on the lips, under the fingernails, or around the anus. Examination of these areas is indicated in patients with gastrointestinal bleeding. When inspecting the skin, the site of a recent venipuncture should be evaluated for petechiae, ecchymoses, or hematoma.

Widespread lymph node enlargement, the presence of an enlarged liver or spleen, may suggest the possibility of reticuloendothelial disease. Jaundice, hepatomegaly, ascites, distended abdominal veins, and splenomegaly may be stigmata of liver disease. Again, these may be associated with a significant reduction in the level of the prothrombin complex.

Evaluation of the Unsuspected Bleeder

The surest method of identifying an unsuspected bleeder is to obtain a complete history and perform a thorough physical examination. The ideal laboratory test to detect these patients has yet to be described. The single most productive laboratory procedure, unquestionably, is the examination of the peripheral blood smear. Since thrombocytopenia is the most common abnormality resulting in failure of hemostasis and is so easily identified by simple inspection of a well-stained blood smear, the importance of this examination cannot be overemphasized. Other important information derived from examination of the blood smear has already been described.

Measurement of the bleeding time is an imperfect screening test. When abnormal, one must heed its warning. When normal, as it frequently is in a variety of serious hemostatic disorders, little confidence should be derived. Regrettably, this test historically has been coupled with the whole blood clotting time as a screening battery for the detection of hemostatic defects. The limitations of the whole blood clotting time as a diagnostic screening test also have been noted earlier. Fully one-third of patients affected by blood-clotting disorders that theoretically might be identified by this test will be missed. Observation of the clot retraction is another time-honored test which is not recommended for reliable screening. Platelet counts as low as 60,000 to 70,000/mm^3 can result in respectable clot retraction. Significant thrombocytopenia may go undetected if one relies too heavily on this test. Its one virtue is its simplicity.

Simple tests with reliability are available. The partial thromboplastin time, performed with care and with normal controls, is of sufficient sensitivity that abnormalities likely to result in life-endangering bleeding at operation are unlikely to be missed. The partial thromboplastin time will detect not only those abnormalities that would be identified by the whole blood clotting time but also those abnormalities characterized by defects in the prothrombin complex. The Quick one-stage prothrombin time also is a simple and accurate test which will identify abnormalities of factors V, VII, and X and prothrombin (factor II). When used in conjunction with the partial thromboplastin time, it can separate an abnormality into problems of the first stage (hemophilia group) and those of the second stage (prothrombin complex). For screening related to problems of fibrinolysis, as in patients with metastatic prostatic carcinoma or pancreatic disease, the dilute whole blood or plasma clot lysis tests are applicable.

Evaluation of the Suspected Potential Bleeder

The patient who is suspected of having hemostatic dysfunction requires a more comprehensive evaluation. This includes a particularly detailed history, a thorough physical examination, and more complete study in the laboratory. Accordingly, time must be set aside to permit these efforts. These can usually be done on an outpatient basis, or if the patient is already hospitalized and scheduled for operation, scheduling of the case should permit time for the necessary evaluations. If suspicion of an abnormality is based on family history, every effort should be made to study other members of the family. If suspicion is based on previous bleeding following surgical treatment, every effort should be made to obtain the old hospital records, since they may provide important information. When the question of bleeding related to drug administration has been raised, identification of the drug through prescription files in pharmacies and obtaining the medications for inspection may be helpful.

If the history of drug exposure or the physical findings of petechiae or mucous membrane bleeding suggest the possibility of thrombocytopenia, in addition to the examination of the blood smear, direct platelet counting should be performed. Bleeding times should be determined using the template technique. Drug-related immunologic forms of thrombocytopenia can be evaluated with the clot retraction inhibition test. This takes advantage of the fact that antibody may remain in the patient's serum for 4 to 6 months. An aliquot of the patient's serum together with an aliquot of a saturated solution of the suspected drug are clotted together with an aliquot of the patient's blood. If the platelets are immunologically damaged in the presence of the drug, the clot retraction is inhibited. The use of appropriate normal controls is imperative. More detailed observations, such as the platelets' ability to aggregate in their native plasma following the addition of ADP, and measurements of platelet factor 3 release also can be performed.

If a blood coagulation defect is suspected, a combination of tests can help place the defect (Table 3-1). If the partial thromboplastin time is abnormal and the one-stage prothrombin time is normal, the defect is almost certainly in the first stage of clotting. One then has the option of

performing mixing and matching studies or, more desirably, specific clotting factor assays. The former require samples of plasma from patients with proved abnormalities. One then tests the patient in question by determining if a small amount of the patient's plasma will correct the abnormality of the known deficient sample in vitro. Such tests can give reliable qualitative results in terms of establishing a specific diagnosis. Assays for individual blood-clotting factors can be performed by many laboratories. In addition to the specificity of the test, quantitative values are obtained, permitting estimation of the severity of the disease process. The specific assays are of particular value in controlling the transfusion program of affected patients undergoing surgical treatment.

Evaluation of the Patient Who Begins to Bleed during or after Surgical Procedures

The patient who bleeds excessively during or shortly following surgical procedures is an emergency problem. The approach to this difficult situation must be prompt and well organized. Generally, bleeding at the time of operation ultimately is identified as being due to, singly or in combination, (1) ineffective local hemostasis, (2) complications of blood transfusion, (3) a previously present but unsuspected hemostatic defect, (4) sepsis, (5) induced fibrinolysis or defibrination.

Bleeding from one site only, such as the surgical wound, usually is not due to a generalized hemostatic defect. The patient who manifests bleeding at the primary incisional site, for example, but not at the site of a stab wound where drains have been placed or the patient who is bleeding from a thoracotomy wound but not at all from his tracheostomy site is more likely to have a local problem than a generalized defect. One exception to this generalization should be noted: Occasionally following prostatic surgical treatment excessive bleeding from the prostatic bed is noted. The plasminogen activator present in prostatic tissue is activated by the urokinase normally present in the

Table 3-1. DIAGNOSIS OF INHERITED DISORDERS OF COAGULATION

Deficient factor	Bleeding time	One-stage prothrombin time	Partial thromboplastin time	Thrombin time	Fibrinogen time	Platelet adhesiveness
I (fibrinogen)	Long or normal	Long	Long	Long	Low	Normal
II	Normal	Long	Long	Normal	Normal	Normal
V	Normal	Long	Long	Normal	Normal	Normal
VII	Normal	Long	Normal	Normal	Normal	Normal
VIII	Normal	Normal	Long	Normal	Normal	Normal
IX	Normal	Normal	Long	Normal	Normal	Normal
X	Normal	Long	Long	Normal	Normal	Normal
XI	Normal	Normal	Long	Normal	Normal	Normal
XII	Normal	Normal	Long	Normal	Normal	Normal
XIII	Normal	Normal	Normal	Normal	Normal	Normal
Von Willebrand's disease	Long	Normal	Long	Normal	Normal	Low

SOURCE: E. W. Salzman, Hemorrhagic disorders, in J. M. Kinney, R. H. Egdahl, and G. D. Zuidema (eds.), "Manual of Preoperative and Postoperative Care," p. 157, W. B. Saunders Company, Philadelphia, 1971.

urine as it washes over the raw prostatic bed. Increased fibrinolysis occurs locally on the raw surface of the wound, and bleeding is aggravated. This is a failure of local hemostasis based, not on any mechanical problem, but rather on the increased activation of the local fibrinolytic process. A 24- to 48-hour period of interruption of this plasminogen activation by the administration of ε-aminocaproic acid (ε-ACA) usually suffices to still the blood loss.

Although one may be reasonably certain on clinical grounds that surgical bleeding is related to local problems, laboratory investigation must be confirmatory. Prompt examination of the blood smear to determine the number of platelets and an actual platelet count if the smear is not clear-cut should be done. A partial thromboplastin time, one-stage prothrombin time, and thrombin clotting time all can be determined within minutes. Correct interpretation of the results should confirm the clinical impression or identify the exceptional problem.

Complications of blood transfusion are an occasional cause of hemostatic failure. Massive blood transfusion with banked blood is a well-documented cause of thrombocytopenia. Most patients who receive 10 units or more of banked blood within a period of 24 hours will be measurably thrombocytopenic, but usually not sufficiently so to result in hemostatic failure. Patients who receive 14 units or more of banked blood in a period of 24 hours or less invariably will be significantly thrombocytopenic and may have frank bleeding as a result. *The patient in whom signs of hemostatic failure develop during or following operation when large quantities of banked blood have been used should be assumed to be thrombocytopenic until demonstrated otherwise.* Treatment consists of supplying fresh platelets in the form of platelet concentrates or, if volume is also required, as fresh platelet-rich plasma. Following transfusion of 10 units of banked blood, prophylactic administration of fresh platelet packs is appropriate.

Another cause of hemostatic failure involving transfusion is that of the hemolytic transfusion reaction. This complication, usually so readily detected in the conscious patient, can be difficult to recognize in the anesthetized patient. The characteristic chilly sensation, muscle ache, backache, headache, and ultimate hemoglobinuria will not be evident. The first hint to the experienced surgeon that the patient is undergoing hemolytic transfusion reaction may be progressive failure of hemostasis. Tissues in the operative field which have previously been dry begin to ooze.

The pathogenesis of this bleeding is not perfectly established, but several probable causes have been suggested. The release of ADP from the hemolyzed red cells may be sufficient to cause platelet aggregation, and the platelet clumps then are swept out of the circulation. Red blood cells also are a rich source of the procoagulant platelet factor 3 (phospholipid) necessary at several stages of blood coagulation. Release of these substances during hemolytic transfusion reaction may result in progression of the clotting mechanism and intravascular defibrination. In addition, the fibrinolytic mechanism may be triggered by the intravascular clotting. Both defibrination and fibrinolysis have been documented clinically and experimentally following hemolytic transfusion reaction. Their incidence is low but must be considered when the clinical events are consistent. The bleeding problem associated with hemolytic transfusion reaction should be considered due to thrombocytopenia until other laboratory measures suggest defibrination or fibrinolysis.

Transfusion purpura, which has been described in detail by Shulman and associates, is an uncommon but interesting cause of thrombocytopenia and associated bleeding following transfusion. In this circumstance, the donor platelets are of the uncommon Pl^{A1} group. These platelets sensitize the recipient, who makes antibody to the foreign platelet antigen. The foreign platelet antigen does not completely disappear from the recipient circulation but seems to attach to the recipient's own platelets. The antibody, which attains a sufficient titer within 6 or 7 days following the sensitizing transfusion, then destroys the recipient's own platelets. The resultant thrombocytopenia and bleeding may continue for several weeks. This uncommon cause of thrombocytopenia should be considered if bleeding follows transfusion by 5 or 6 days. Platelet transfusions are of little help in the management of this syndrome, since the new donor platelets usually are subject to the binding of antigen and damage from the antibody. Corticosteroids may be of some help in reducing the bleeding tendency. Posttransfusion purpura is self-limited, and the passage of several weeks inevitably leads to subsidence of the problem.

The patient with a hemostatic defect which manifests itself first during surgical treatment is likely to have other evidence of bleeding, such as ecchymoses at the sites of injection or venipunctures, and bloody drainage from nasogastric tubes or bladder catheters.

A hemostatic defect may be imposed iatrogenically during surgical treatment employing extracorporeal bypass. Many etiologic factors may be involved, but the most commonly implicated is the introduction of heparin into the circulation. Bleeding after discontinuation of extracorporeal bypass may be due to inadequate neutralization of heparin with protamine sulfate. Since both protamine sulfate and Polybrene are themselves anticoagulants when large doses are used, it is possible that bleeding was caused by these drugs. This is a rare occurrence. Rapid tests can be performed in vitro by adding small amounts of protamine sulfate to see if the clotting time is shortened. Other abnormalities attributed to extracorporeal circulation are defibrination and fibrinolysis. Fibrinolytic activity is often increased. These changes usually are related to the duration of pumping. We are impressed by the *lack* of clinical bleeding in the patients with laboratory evidence of fibrinolysis. Thrombocytopenia, hypofibrinogenemia, and reduction in factors V and VIII have been demonstrated. The thrombocytopenia usually is not severe, and the platelet count generally remains above 50,000/mm³. Evaluation of the patient with intraoperative or postoperative bleeding suspected of being due to hemostatic defect follows the same course previously outlined for preoperative evaluation of these patients.

At times, an operation performed in a patient with sepsis is attended by continued bleeding. Severe hemorrhagic disorders due to thrombocytopenia have occurred consequent to gram-negative sepsis. The pathogenesis of endotoxin-induced thrombocytopenia has been studied in detail, and it is suggested that a labile factor, possibly factor V, is necessary for this interaction. Defibrination and hemostatic failure also may occur with meningococcemia, *Clostridium welchii* sepsis and staphylococcal sepsis. Hemolysis appears to be one mechanism in sepsis leading to defibrination.

The appearance of pathologic fibrinolysis during surgical treatment is an uncommon but potentially serious event. It can occur subsequent to shock, following intravascular defibrination, and in association with operation on tissues rich in activators of the fibrinolytic mechanism. These include pancreas, prostate, and lung. Defibrination also can occur as a consequence of hemolytic transfusion reaction and sepsis.

The thrombin time can be of value in detecting abnormalities in fibrinogen. When fibrinolysis is a significant factor, dissolution of the whole blood clot is observed in 2 hours or less, but the euglobulin clot lysis and dilute whole blood clot lysis are more sensitive indices and permit more rapid evaluation.

CLINICAL HEMOSTATIC DEFECTS

Inheritance

The importance of a detailed family history in the evaluation of the patient with a possible hemostatic defect has been emphasized. The sensible use of this information requires an understanding of genetic principles and knowledge of the specific genetic features of the hemostatic disorders.

The modes of inheritance of hemostatic disorders, with few rare exceptions, are three in type: (1) autosomal dominant, (2) autosomal recessive, and (3) sex-linked recessive. The 46 chromosomes of man consist of 22 autosomal pairs, plus a pair of sex chromosomes, the X and Y. Since one chromosome of each of the 22 autosomal pairs normally is derived from each parent, any gene inherited as a part of an autosomal chromosome normally will occur with equal frequency among males and females. Each child of a parent carrying an autosomal dominant gene has one chance in two of inheriting that trait. The most common hemostatic disorder transmitted by the autosomal dominant mode is von Willebrand's disease. Hereditary hemorrhagic telangiectasia and factor XI deficiency also appear to be transmitted in this fashion.

A normal individual should transmit no disease to his progeny. Occasionally, in a pedigree with an autosomal dominant gene, an *apparently* normal person may transmit disease to his or her child. The parent clearly carried the gene, which clinically expressed no defect. Explanation of this phenomenon is not at hand. The gene activity in the parent is referred to as "incompletely penetrant."

In inherited hemostatic disorders, the difference in clinical expression between dominant and recessive genes is a graded one rather than an "all-or-none" phenomenon. The heterozygous individual with an autosomal recessive trait may have a measurable deficiency of the factor governed by that gene, but no clinical disease. In order to demonstrate clinical expression of disease, the individual must be homozygous. This appears to be the case, for example, in factor X deficiency. The homozygote with clinical disease, as described by Hougie, has less than 5% of factor X activity, while heterozygotes have levels ranging from 21 to 50%. Since the presumed heterozygotes within the same pedigree vary in factor X activity, it is convenient to suggest that the gene shows variable expression. Other hemostatic disorders probably inherited in this mode are factor V, factor VII, and factor I deficiencies. This mode of transmission could be regarded as incompletely dominant inheritance, rather than incompletely recessive, depending upon one's view. Since these traits are not very common, it is difficult to resolve this problem.

Sex-linked recessive inheritance governs true hemophilia (factor VIII deficiency) and factor IX deficiency (Christmas disease). The genes for these diseases are recessive in expression and are carried on the female (X) chromosome. When paired with the normal X chromosome (the female carrier state), clinical disease is not present. When the affected X chromosome is paired with the normal male (Y) chromosome, clinical disease is expressed.

Theoretically, with the "graded" expression, the female carrier should be detectable in the laboratory. In fact, since the range of factor VIII activity normally is so broad, most female carriers *appear* to fall in the low-normal range. Estimates vary, but possibly as many as 50 percent of female carriers can be identified. Although the sex-linked recessive mode of inheritance has been confirmed repeatedly in true hemophilia, it seems likely that an *autosomal* gene also may influence factor VIII activity. This probability is emphasized by the autosomal dominant mode of inheritance of von Willebrand's disease, characterized by low factor VIII activity, and also by the patterns of variation in factor VIII activity among individuals within the same normal family and among different normal families.

Despite the lack of complete understanding of genetic determinants in hemostatic disorders, detailed consideration of the family history facilitates accurate diagnosis.

Factor VIII Deficiency (Classical Hemophilia)

Classical hemophilia (hemophilia A) is a disease of males. The failure to synthesize normal factor VIII activity is inherited as a sex-linked recessive trait. Incidence of the disease is approximately 1:25,000 population, and the clinical manifestations can be extremely variable.

CLINICAL MANIFESTATIONS. Characteristically, the severity of clinical manifestations is related to the degree of deficiency of factor VIII. Spontaneous bleeding and severe complications are the rule when virtually no factor VIII can be detected in the plasma. When plasma factor VIII concentrations are in the range of 25%, the patient may have no spontaneous bleeding yet may bleed severely with trauma or surgical treatment. Typically, members of the same pedigree with true hemophilia will have approximately the same degree of clinical manifestations.

While the severely affected patient may bleed during early infancy, significant bleeding typically is noted first when the child is a toddler. At that time, in addition to the classic bleeding into joints, bleeding may occur at other sites. Epistaxis and hematuria may be noted. Bleeding which is life-threatening may follow injury to the tongue or frenulum. We have seen tracheal compression following tonsillar infection and retropharyngeal bleeding. Vascular and neural compromise may occur in relation to pressure secondary to bleeding into a soft tissue closed space. Equinus contracture deformity may be seen in severely hemophilic patients secondary to bleeding into the calf. Volkmann's contracture of the forearm and flexion contractures of the knees and elbows are also disabling sequelae of deep soft tissue bleeding.

Hemarthrosis is the most characteristic orthopedic problem. Bleeding into the joint may cause few symptoms until distension of the joint capsule occurs. Muscle spasm and pain around the joint arise from involvement of periarticular structures. A large hemarthrosis generally is manifested by a tender, swollen, warm, and painful joint. These signs may mimic infection. The same orthopedic problems are noted in association with severe factor IX deficiency (Christmas disease).

Retroperitoneal bleeding may follow lifting of a heavy object or strenuous exercise. Signs of posterior peritoneal irritation and spasm of the iliopsoas suggest the diagnosis. Hypovolemic shock may occur, since the amount of blood loss that can take place in this setting is enormous. The potential space in the retroperitoneal area readily accommodates several liters of blood in the adult. An intramural hematoma within the intestine also can pose problems of differential diagnosis. The clinical manifestations of nausea and vomiting, crampy abdominal pain, and signs of peritoneal irritation mimic those of appendicitis. Fever and leukocytosis may be noted. Roentgenograms of the abdomen may fail to reveal an abnormality or may display a modest amount of ileus. Upper gastrointestinal examination may demonstrate a uniform thickening of mucosal folds which has been described as a "picket fence" or "stack of coins" appearance (Fig. 3-5). Intramural hematomas of the intestine occur with other hemostatic disorders and, therefore, should be considered when any patient with a hemostatic problem presents with findings suggesting an acute intraabdominal process.

TREATMENT. This requires an appreciation of the transfusion therapy necessary to correct factor VIII deficiency as well as the application of specific surgical principles.

Replacement Therapy. The plasma concentration of factor VIII necessary for maintenance of hemostatic integrity is normally quite small. Patients with as little as 2 to 3% of factor VIII activity usually do not bleed spontaneously. Once serious bleeding begins, however, a much higher level of factor VIII activity, probably approaching 30%, is necessary to achieve hemostasis.

Following transfusion, the plasma level of factor VIII

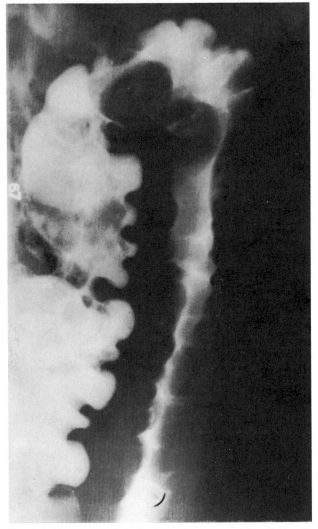

Fig. 3-5. Upper gastrointestinal roentgenogram of patient with "acquired hemophilia." Note thickening of mucosal folds indicative of an intramural hematoma. The spontaneous bleeding in this patient was ascribed to powerful circulating anticoagulant to factor VIII.

in vivo depends upon the potency of the administered preparation and the survival of the infused factor VIII. Many formulas have been developed as a guide to replacement. These should not be used in a cookbook fashion. We view laboratory control of the level of factor VIII as extremely important. This is particularly pertinent since the amount of factor VIII in individual aliquots of frozen plasma and cryoprecipitate varies considerably.

Following administration of a given dose of factor VIII, approximately one-half of the initial posttransfusion activity disappears from the plasma in 4 hours. This early disappearance is thought to be due, in large part, to diffusion from the intravascular space. The period of equilibration extends for as long as 8 hours, at which time only about one-quarter of the initial level remains in the circulating blood. From that time on, the slope of disap-

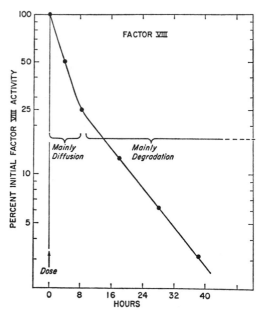

Fig. 3-6. Schematic representation of in vivo decay of a single dose of factor VIII. (*From N. R. Shulman, Mod Treat, 5:61, 1968.*)

in different lesions. Remembering the loss from the circulation, one-half the initial dose would need to be supplied every 12 hours. The use of fresh plasma in such a circumstance would require a volume that is excessive. Factor VIII concentrates now available circumvent this problem. Cryoprecipitate concentrates of factor VIII can be regarded as containing 9.6 units/ml. The amount of material to be given can be computed from the formula

$$\frac{\text{Patient's weight (kg)} \times \text{desired rise of factor VIII (\% average normal)}}{\text{Total units of factor VIII in dose}} = R$$

where R is a factor which is fairly constant for any given type of material and represents the rise of factor VIII obtained in the patient's plasma for every unit of transfused factor VIII per kg of the patient's body weight. Half that amount is subsequently administered every 12 hours to maintain a safe level. A promising factor VIII concentrate prepared as a glycine precipitate also is available. Concentrations as high as 70 or 80 units/ml are obtainable, simplifying the management of the hemophilic patient. Regardless of the preparation employed, continued laboratory assessment of circulating factor VIII level is an important element in the control of these patients.

Following major surgical treatment of the hemophiliac, transfusion replacement of factor VIII should be continued for at least 10 days. Wounds should be well healed and all drains removed prior to the termination of therapy. If sutures remain, transfusion should be reinstituted prior to their removal.

The virus of homologous serum hepatitis is transmitted by the various concentrates of plasma. Whether the new glycine precipitates are free of this virus remains to be demonstrated. Other complications of replacement therapy include the appearance of inhibitors of factor VIII, which may arise in the hemophiliacs who have had transfusion.

pearance is less steep (Fig. 3-6). Twenty-four hours after a given dose, no more than 7 to 8% of administered factor VIII activity remains within the circulation.

One unit of factor VIII activity is considered that amount present in 1 ml of normal plasma. Actually, fresh frozen plasma contains 0.60 units/ml. Theoretically, in a patient with 0% activity, to achieve an initial post-transfusion level of 60% of normal, using fresh plasma, a volume of plasma equal to 60% of the patient's estimated plasma volume would have to be administered. Table 3-2 shows approximate levels of factor VIII required for hemostasis

Table 3-2. APPROXIMATE LEVELS OF FACTOR VIII REQUIRED FOR HAEMOSTASIS IN DIFFERENT LESIONS

Lesion	Level of factor VIII desired in patient's blood immediately after transfusion (% average normal)	Dose of factor VIII (units/kg body weight)[a]
Minor spontaneous haemarthrosis and muscle haematomas	15–20 (0–5)	10–15
Severe haemarthrosis and muscle haematomas, haematomas in dangerous situations	20–40 (5–10)	15–20
Major surgery	80–100 (or less if transfusion given 8-hourly or 6-hourly)	40–50

Figures in parentheses are the approximate levels to which factor VIII will have fallen 24 hours after dose.

[a] 1 unit of factor VIII is the amount present in 1 ml of fresh average normal citrated plasma.

SOURCE: Clinics in Haematology, vol. 5, no. 1, February 1976. C. R. Rizza "Coagulation Factor Therapy," p. 113–133.

These inhibitors have been characterized as antibodies of the γ G variety. They tend to diminish in several weeks if further transfusion is not employed. Laboratory search for these factors should be carried out in every hemophilic patient who is considered a candidate for elective surgical treatment, as their presence enormously complicates transfusion management.

Adjunctive Management. Treatment of soft tissue bleeding is directed at the prevention of airway obstruction and vascular and neural damage. These are accomplished best by the administration of sufficient factor VIII. Bed rest and cold packs can be of some assistance. In general, results of fasciotomy to relieve pressure have varied from disappointing to disastrous. The occasional development of large cysts has resulted in sufficient deformity and disability to require amputation.

The primary treatment of hemophilic hemarthrosis is directed at maintaining full range of motion and minimal destruction of the cartilage. Aspiration of blood from the hemophilic joint is not uniformly endorsed, and when regarded as necessary, it should be considered a major surgical event. Elevation of factor VIII level by transfusion is necessary. The procedure should be carried out in the operating room under strict sterile precautions. In most instances, aspiration is not required, and the combination of factor VIII replacement and local cold packing proves sufficient. Physiotherapy plays a critical role and should consist of *active* exercises, since the patient is unlikely to move the extremity to a point where bleeding will recur. Passive exercises often result in recurrence of bleeding. The reader is referred to the review by Curtiss for details of orthopedic management.

The management of intramural intestinal hematoma and retroperitoneal bleeding is predicated on appropriate transfusion therapy and avoidance of surgical treatment. It is to be emphasized that even when a relatively minor procedure, such as tracheostomy, is performed, the plasma level of factor VIII should be raised above 25 to 30%. Since dental hygiene usually is poor in hemophilic patients, dental and oral surgical treatment frequently are necessary. The same principles of transfusion therapy pertain, and the procedures should be delegated to well-trained personnel working where optimal care can be provided.

Recently, the question of transplantation of the spleen as therapy for hemophilia has been raised. Norman and associates have suggested that the spleen may be a site of factor VIII synthesis and/or storage. Also, it has been reported that the spleen is receptive to circulating factor VIII–trophic substance in the plasma of human hemophiliacs. In hemophilic dogs receiving heterotrophic splenic transplants, factor VIII levels were increased thirtyfold, to levels more than that required to prevent spontaneous bleeding. In an independent study, Webster and associates reported dissimilar results and an absence of significant effect on factor VIII. They warned against clinical applicability of this procedure. This concern has been reinforced by one subsequent clinical case of splenic transplantation in a human being, with continued postoperative bleeding and splenic infarction necessitating removal of the transplanted spleen.

Von Willebrand's Disease (Pseudohemophilia)

Von Willebrand's disease occurs as commonly as true hemophilia. The increasing recognition is related to more reliable factor VIII assays. This hereditary disorder of hemostasis is transmitted as an autosomally dominant trait and, accordingly, appears in consecutive generations with males and females equally affected. The disease is characterized by a diminution of the level of factor VIII activity. The reduction of factor VIII activity usually is not as great as that seen in classical hemophilia. Also unlike classical hemophilia, where factor VIII activity remains constant, in the patient with von Willebrand's disease variation in the level of circulating factor VIII activity may be noted. Characteristically, these patients also have a prolonged bleeding time, but this is less constant than the factor VIII reduction. A given patient may have an abnormal bleeding time on one occasion and a normal bleeding time on another. Abnormalities of platelet adhesiveness in vitro, using Salzman's method, also have been described. Von Willebrand's disease can be distinguished from classical hemophilia by two findings: the level of factor VIII antigen is disproportionately lower than that of factor VIII, and ristocetin fails to cause platelet aggregation.

CLINICAL MANIFESTATIONS. The manifestations of bleeding usually are mild and often overlooked until trauma or the stress of surgical treatment makes them apparent. A careful clinical history is, therefore, of great importance in these patients. Spontaneous manifestations often are limited to bleeding into the skin or mild mucous membrane bleeding. Epistaxis and menorrhagia have been relatively common in our personal experience. Serious bleeding following dental extractions and tonsillectomy also are not uncommon. Fatal bleeding from the gastrointestinal tract has been described.

TREATMENT. The typical patient with von Willebrand's disease will produce factor VIII activity in response to transfusion of modest amounts of fresh frozen plasma, cryoprecipitate, or other factor VIII concentrates. This is unlike the classical hemophiliac in whom factor VIII concentration rises only in proportion to the amount of that substance actually transfused. In von Willebrand's disease, some 4 to 6 hours following transfusion an increase in circulating factor VIII activity to the range of five to eight times that which could be ascribed to transfusion alone is noted. This apparent synthesis continues for approximately 24 hours. Exceptions to this characteristic response recently have been described.

When a patient with von Willebrand's disease is scheduled to undergo surgical treatment, plasma transfusion should be instituted at least 48 hours prior to the operative procedure. In this manner, it can be determined whether the patient will respond to infusion with appearance of factor VIII activity. If factor VIII activity is not generated, a more ambitious program of transfusion is necessary to sustain the patient through the operative and postoperative period. In most patients, infusion of 10 ml of plasma/kg of body weight/24 hours will ensure hemostatically effective levels of factor VIII. Duration of treatment should be the same as that described for the patient with classical hemophilia.

Factor IX Deficiency (Christmas Disease)

Factor IX deficiency clinically is indistinguishable from factor VIII deficiency. These two entities were considered a single disease until 1952, when their unique deficiencies were documented. The incidence of factor IX deficiency is approximately 1:100,000 population.

TREATMENT. Factor IX, although not in the prothrombin complex, is dependent upon vitamin K for its synthesis in the liver. It is present in banked blood, plasma, and serum. Initially, the rate of disappearance of factor IX from the circulation is more rapid than that of factor VIII, but subsequently factor IX has a slower disappearance rate (Fig. 3-7). Half of the factor IX which is present 5 or 6 hours following transfusion remains after 24 hours. An infusion of plasma containing factor IX raises the recipient's factor IX level less than would be predicted. The extravascular space into which factor IX distributes itself may be larger than the distribution space for factor VIII. The longer survival of factor IX helps compensate for its more rapid initial disappearance following transfusion. Accordingly, a dose of 15 ml of plasma/kg of body weight administered over a 1- or 2-hour period 6 hours or more prior to operation usually serves to raise the plasma level to a suitable point. Half that volume then is administered every 12 hours as long as clinical indications require. An alternative method of treatment is that of administering 60 ml of plasma/kg over a 10- to 20-hour period 24 hours prior to anticipated surgical treatment and repeating doses of 7 ml/kg every 12 hours.

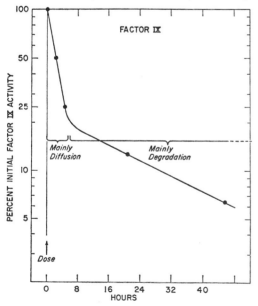

Fig. 3-7. Schematic representation of in vivo decay of a single dose of factor IX. (*From N. R. Shulman, Mod Treat, 5:61, 1968.*)

It should be emphasized that the patient with a mild factor IX deficiency, like the patient with a mild factor VIII deficiency, can bleed massively with surgical treatment and requires planned replacement therapy. There are now several preparations of factor IX concentrate available for replacement therapy.

Factor XI (PTA) Deficiency (Rosenthal's Syndrome)

This uncommon and relatively mild disorder is inherited in an autosomally dominant fashion. Without careful laboratory testing, the affected males and females may be confused with von Willebrand's disease patients. A majority of patients are of Jewish ancestry.

Epistaxis is a common spontaneous clinical manifestation. The disease usually is recognized as a result of bleeding during and after operation. The bleeding usually is minor. Some patients have undergone major procedures without significant hemorrhage.

TREATMENT. Factor XI actually may gain in potency during storage, so that plasma is a suitable therapeutic medium. This factor disappears slowly from the circulation, and its biologic half-life may be as long as 48 hours. An initial dose of 10 ml of plasma/kg of body weight can be given 6 or 8 hours prior to anticipated surgical treatment, followed by a maintenance dose of 5 ml/kg administered every 24 hours. Therapy usually can be discontinued several days earlier than with patients with more serious hemostatic disorders.

Factor V (Proaccelerin) Deficiency (Parahemophilia)

This extremely rare deficiency usually is associated with mild bleeding, but serious bleeding may be encountered. The disease is transmitted as an autosomal recessive trait and is found in males and females alike. Only patients who presumably inherit the gene from both parents seem to be bleeders.

Factor V is synthesized in the liver but differs from prothrombin and factors VII, IX, and X in that factor V synthesis is not dependent upon vitamin K or inhibited by the administration of the coumarin drugs. Patients with severe parenchymal liver disease may be deficient in factor V.

TREATMENT. Excessive bleeding may occur at the time of operation, usually in patients who have levels of less than 1% of normal factor V concentration. No more than 25% of normal activity is necessary for hemostasis during operative procedures. This level can be achieved by administering 15 ml of fresh or freshly frozen plasma per kg of body weight 12 hours prior to operation. The administration of 7 to 10 ml/kg every 24 hours will suffice to maintain hemostasis until healing has occurred. Once again, it is wise to administer the factor at the time of suture removal. Factor V, also known as labile factor, loses its activity during storage. Only fresh plasma or plasma freshly frozen is applicable as therapy.

Factor VII (Proconvertin) Deficiency

Factor VII (stable factor) deficiency is an uncommon but not rare disease. Mild clinical manifestations are the rule. The deficiency is inherited as an autosomal gene of "intermediate penetrance." The homozygous state results in significant deficiency and may be associated with serious bleeding. In these patients, spontaneous epistaxis, genitourinary and gastrointestinal bleeding, and even hemarthroses, may be seen. The heterozygotes have minimal, if any, clinical manifestations.

Factor VII, like factors II, IX, and X, requires vitamin K for synthesis. The synthesis is blocked by coumarin administration. Coumarin inhibition of synthesis is reversed by vitamin K administration. The administration of vitamin K to patients *congenitally* deficient in these activities will *not* result in synthesis and increased plasma levels.

As is also true for factor V–deficient patients and in patients with deficiencies of factors II and X, the one-stage prothrombin time is prolonged in patients with factor VII deficiency. Since factor VII is active only in the "extrinsic" blood-clotting system, deficient patients have a normal prothrombin consumption test. In contrast, patients with factor X deficiency have abnormal prothrombin consumption, significant prothrombin remaining in the serum 1 hour after coagulation. Another laboratory distinction between factor VII and factor X deficiency can be made by the use of the Stypven time test. Factor X is necessary for the effect of this viper venom in blood coagulation, while factor VII is not. Accordingly, the factor VII–deficient patient has a normal Stypven time.

TREATMENT. The biologic half-life of factor VII probably is the briefest of any of the blood-clotting factors. The initial half-life, thought to be due to equilibration between the intravascular and extravascular compartments, probably is no more than 30 minutes. The remainder of the disappearance time presumably represents catabolism and is estimated at between 5 and 6 hours. Despite this relatively rapid disappearance, the transfusion management of patients with factor VII deficiency is not a great problem. Factor VII levels of less than 4 to 5% of normal are necessary before significant bleeding occurs. Even at these low levels of plasma activity, replacement transfusion is not always necessary for surgical procedures. Although the one-stage prothrombin time recognizes deficiency of factor VII, this test is not an effective guide to the treatment of factor VII–deficient patients. The test is markedly abnormal at factor VII levels at which the deficient patient may not bleed. Transfusion of banked plasma, 10 ml/kg of body weight, on the day of the operation, followed by half that amount daily for the next 5 or 6 days, provides adequate factor VII for hemostasis during major surgical treatment.

Factor X (Stuart-Prower) Deficiency

This relatively rare deficiency is inherited as an autosomal recessive trait and has been described in amyloido-sis. Clinically, affected patients are homozygotes, while the heterozygotes are clinically well and only minimally affected. The latter may demonstrate mild abnormalities with the one-stage prothrombin test and the thromboplastin generation test.

TREATMENT. Little experience has been acquired in the surgical management of patients with factor X deficiency. Plasma levels of 15% of normal have proved sufficient to prevent significant bleeding following dental extractions. Plasma transfusion experiments in patients with factor X deficiency have demonstrated an 8- to 10-hour first-phase disappearance time of half the administered activity, followed by a disappearance time estimated at 40 hours. Applying these data, plasma levels of 15% or greater could be achieved by infusing 15 to 20 ml of normal plasma per kg of body weight initially, followed by half that amount per 24 hours for 5 days. It is always prudent to give an additional infusion at the time of removal of the operative sutures.

Inherited Hypoprothrombinemia (Factor II Deficiency)

This deficiency, inherited as an autosomal recessive trait, is perhaps the most rare of the inherited disorders of hemostasis. The prothrombin levels reported in affected patients have averaged about 10% of normal. Although the level of prothrombin activity required for hemostasis following surgical treatment is not precisely established, it seems likely that a level of 15% of normal is effective.

TREATMENT. The disappearance time of prothrombin from the intravascular compartment approximates that of factor X. An initial equilibration time of 9 hours has been estimated, followed by a much slower disappearance of activity with another half-life of up to 3 days. Stored plasma contains factor II. Surgical treatment without faulty hemostasis should be possible in affected patients if an initial plasma infusion of 15 ml/kg of body weight is administered 12 to 24 hours prior to the scheduled operation. This can be followed by an infusion of half this amount once daily until healing has occurred.

When the transfusion programs outlined above for deficiency of the prothrombin group of factors (factors II, V, VII, and X) are employed, the one-stage prothrombin time does not return to normal. Rather, a one-stage prothrombin time slightly less than twice the control value is achieved. This is sufficient to result in normal hemostasis. Of the four "prothrombin" factors, only factor V must be provided as fresh or freshly frozen plasma. Stored plasma is equally effective as therapy for factors II, VII, and X.

Inherited Fibrinogen Abnormalities

For nearly 50 years following the first description of a patient with congenital afibrinogenemia, this rare abnormality was considered the only inherited defect involving fibrinogen. More recently, families with qualitatively abnormal fibrinogen have been identified. These latter patients have varied in their clinical manifestations as well as in laboratory features.

Congenital afibrinogenemia is ascribed to an autosomal recessive mode of inheritance. The parents of patients with this entity usually have normal concentrations of fibrinogen. The affected individuals presumably are homozygous for the trait. Plasma fibrinogen levels of less that 5 mg/100 ml are usual, and, occasionally, immunochemical methods have been necessary to identify even trace amounts of fibrinogen in the plasma of these patients. The deficiency, however, usually is less of a clinical problem than classical hemophilia. Severely affected infants have bled following sectioning of the umbilical cord. More often the clinical manifestations include bleeding following lacerations, purpura, epistaxis, and bleeding following loss of deciduous teeth. The characteristic laboratory defect is the failure of the blood to clot in vitro, even following the addition of thrombin.

Less profound inherited deficiencies of fibrinogen have been observed. The bleeding usually is more modest, and therefore the treatment requires proportionately smaller amounts of fibrinogen concentrate or plasma. Patients with "dysfibrinogenemia" are uncommon. The characteristic abnormality is the retarded rate of clotting upon the addition of thrombin ("thrombin time"). Interestingly, thrombotic disease as well as bleeding disorders have been described in this heterogeneous group of patients. Although surgical experience with this type of patient has been negligible, the administration of normal fibrinogen should serve to diminish the hemorrhagic aspect of the problem.

TREATMENT. Approximately one-half of the transfused fibrinogen given to a deficient patient disappears from the intravascular compartment within the first 24 hours after administration. Following this, the biologic half-life is 3 days or more. The disappearance of fibrinogen is no more rapid in deficient patients than when fibrinogen is transfused into normal subjects, thus suggesting that accelerated fibrinogen catabolism is not a pathogenic mechanism. Although the hemostatically optimal level of fibrinogen is not known, a level of close to 100 mg/100 ml usually permits normal hemostasis. The patient's fibrinogen level should be raised above this prior to major surgical treatment. The volume of normal plasma necessary to accomplish this could sometimes exceed 50 ml/kg of body weight initially. Fibrinogen replacement has been made substantially easier by increasing the use of concentrates. A dose of 1 Gm of fibrinogen/10 kg/day has proved adequate. Approximately one-fifth of this then is administered daily following the initial loading dose. A substantial risk of homologous serum hepatitis is incurred when fibrinogen fractions are used. These concentrates are prepared from pooled plasma. The hepatitis risk can be reduced by using the cryoprecipitate preparation described for the treatment of hemophilia. Approximately one-half of the fibrinogen in the initial plasma is available in the precipitate. A 60-kg patient requires the precipitate obtained from approximately 25 units of plasma as a loading dose.

Acquired Hypofibrinogenemia

DEFIBRINATION SYNDROME

The largest proportion of patients with fibrinogen-related problems of surgical concern are in this group. The fibrinogen deficiency rarely is an isolated defect, as thrombocytopenia and factors II, V, and VIII deficiencies of variable severity usually accompany this state.

The majority of patients with acquired hypofibrinogenemia suffer from intravascular coagulation, more properly known as *defibrination syndrome* or *consumptive coagulopathy,* and it is to this group of patients that the term *disseminated intravascular coagulation* (DIC) has been applied. The syndrome, now recognized with increasing frequency, is caused by the introduction of thromboplastic materials into the circulation. Because this material is found in most tissues, many disease processes may activate the coagulation system. The hemorrhagic disasters of the perinatal period, e.g., retained dead fetus, premature separation of the placenta, and amniotic fluid embolus, primarily are due to this pathophysiologic mechanism. The hemorrhagic state following hemolytic transfusion reaction is also related to this process. Defibrination has been observed as a complication of extracorporeal circulation, disseminated carcinoma, lymphomas, thrombotic thrombocytopenia, rickettsial infection, snakebite, and shock. Release of thromboplastic material has long been a recognized complication of gram-negative sepsis and has been attributed to the effects of circulating endotoxin on platelets. More recently, it has been recognized that septicemia due to gram-positive organisms may also be associated with DIC.

The differentiation between DIC with secondary protective fibrinolysis from primary fibrinolytic states can be extremely difficult, as the thrombin time, which many consider to be the most useful single test in establishing the presence of significant DIC or fibrinolysis, is prolonged in both cases. The salient differentiating features are that DIC is more common and is associated with an increased amount of cold insoluble fibrinogen (cryofibrinogen) and, most important, thrombocytopenia.

TREATMENT. The most important facets of treatment are relieving the patient's primary medical or surgical problem and maintaining adequate capillary flow. The use of intravenous fluids to maintain volume and, at times, vasodilators to open the arterioles is indicated. If blood flow deficiency is related to inability of a damaged heart to pump, the use of drugs such as digitalis or Isuprel may be indicated. Viscosity may be affected by an increased hematocrit, and, therefore, a plasma expander may be beneficial.

In the past heparin has been regarded as the treatment of choice, since it provides the most direct interference with the coagulation process. However, there has been little evidence of success associated with this form of therapy. Administration of fibrinogen should be limited, since it may result in further intravascular coagulation, and the use of ε-aminocaproic acid to inhibit secondary fibrinolysis is contraindicated, since uncontrolled disseminated intravascular coagulation may result.

FIBRINOLYSIS

The acquired hypofibrinogenemic state in the surgical patient also can be due to pathologic fibrinolysis. This may occur in patients with metastatic prostatic carcinoma, shock, sepsis, hypoxia, neoplasia, cirrhosis, and portal hypertension.

The pathogenesis of this bleeding disorder is complex. Secondary to shock or hypoxia, a release of excessive plasminogen activator into the circulation occurs. This is thought to be endogenous kinases which can be released from vascular endothelium and other tissues. Pharmacologic activation of plasminogen also occurs with pyrogens, epinephrine, nicotinic acid, and acetylcholine. Electric shock and pneumoencephalopathy have also been reported to cause activation. Patients with cirrhosis and portal hypertension have a diminished ability to clear normal amounts of plasminogen activator from the blood.

In addition to the reduction in levels of plasma fibrinogen, diminution of factors V and VIII also occurs, since they also serve as substrates for the enzyme plasmin. Thrombocytopenia is not an accompaniment of the purely fibrinolytic state. Polymerization of fibrin monomers, a step in normal fibrin formation, is interfered with by the proteolytic residue of fibrinogen and fibrin. The fibrin and fibrinogen breakdown products usually disappear from the circulation in a matter of hours. The biologic half-life of the interfering products has been estimated at approximately 9 hours.

Streptokinase and urokinase have been used to induce therapeutic fibrinolysis, but enthusiasm for these drugs as treatment for venous thrombosis, pulmonary embolism, and clotted hemothorax is not widespread. As there is a limited endogenous supply of activator available, it is soon exhausted by the injections, and later injections fail to achieve the desired effect. Also, treatment with these drugs is frequently accompanied by chills and fever. Excessive bleeding has been noted in almost half the patients treated, and anemia has appeared beyond that anticipated by the amount of bleeding. At present, results of urokinase therapy for deep venous thrombosis should be regarded as encouraging but not conclusive.

TREATMENT. The successful treatment of the underlying disorder usually is followed by rapid spontaneous recovery, since the severity of fibrinolytic bleeding is dependent upon the concentration of breakdown products in the circulation. ϵ-Aminocaproic acid, a synthetic amino acid, interferes with fibrinolysis by inhibiting plasminogen activation. The drug may be administered intravenously or orally. An initial dose of 5 Gm for the average-sized adult is followed by another 5 Gm every 4 to 6 hours until the hemorrhagic state subsides. Treatment rarely is required for more than 2 or 3 days. Just as the administration of ϵ-aminocaproic acid to a patient with consumptive coagulopathy is potentially dangerous, the administration of heparin to the patient who has a primary pathologic fibrinolysis is fraught with danger. Thus, fine clinical judgment and reliable laboratories are needed to avoid therapeutic complications. Restraint in definitive treatment of both fibrinolysis and consumptive coagulopathy is recommended, while measures designed to reverse the shock and stabilize the patient are emphasized.

Thrombocytopenia

Thrombocytopenia, as stated earlier, is the most common abnormality of hemostasis resulting in bleeding in the surgical patient. A wide variety of diseases can lead to reduction in platelet count and purpuric bleeding. Thrombocytopenia may be primary and idiopathic (idiopathic thrombocytopenic purpura, or ITP) or secondary and symptomatic (lupus erythematosus, drug reaction, or portal hypertension). The lack of platelets may be associated with megakaryocytes in the bone marrow (ITP, congestive splenomegaly) or with absence of megakaryocytes (leukemia, following cytotoxic therapy).

Microscopic examination of a properly stained blood smear should suggest the diagnosis. The presence and extent of thrombocytopenia can be defined precisely by a quantitative platelet count. In general, 60,000 to 70,000 platelets per cubic millimeter are adequate for normal hemostasis, but often a poor correlation between bleeding and the platelet count is noted. The bleeding time may be prolonged with marked thrombocytopenia or, less commonly, with qualitative platelet abnormality. Clot retraction usually is abnormal when the platelet count is below 70,000. Thrombocytopenia obviously can exist in the presence of normal clot retraction. In patients with thrombocytopenia, the clotting time and one-stage prothrombin time are normal.

The numerous etiologic bases of thrombocytopenia create a therapeutic challenge for the surgeon. The problems can be reduced to manageable proportions by attempting to define the pathophysiology of the thrombocytopenic state. The patient whose bone marrow is replaced by leukemia, metastatic tumor, or fibrous tissue and is therefore not producing platelets will not benefit from splenectomy. If an immune mechanism is responsible for the thrombocytopenia, it is important to determine if this is related to an extrinsic stimulus, drug, or infection. If drug-related, the thrombocytopenia will correct itself within days to weeks of discontinuation of the medication. If thrombocytopenia is secondary to bacteremia, the repair usually occurs in a day or two. If thrombocytopenia is related to viral infection, the return of platelets may not take place for 3 weeks or longer. Occasionally, severe thrombocytopenia and bleeding are secondary to vitamin B_{12} or folic acid deficiency and are associated with a megaloblastic bone marrow. This may occur 2 or 3 years following total gastrectomy or in association with severe intestinal malabsorption. In either case, supplying the appropriate nutrient will correct the thrombocytopenia within 2 or 3 days. Thrombocytopenia has recently been reported in association with acute alcoholism in the noncirrhotic patient. The marrow megakaryocytes are normal, and the platelet count returns to normal 5 to 7 days after the alcohol intake ceases.

If the thrombocytopenia is associated with splenomegaly

and megakaryocytes remain in the marrow, removal of the spleen offers a good chance for relief of thrombocytopenia.

TREATMENT. Treatment must be based upon consideration of the patient at hand. Management of the thrombocytopenic patient takes one of four forms, separately or in combination. These include (1) careful observation alone, (2) steroid therapy, (3) splenectomy, and (4) transfusion therapy.

Careful observation, a form of management, is neglected too often in our anxiety to do something for the patient. This approach is applicable in the patient with chronic thrombocytopenia (75,000 to 85,000 platelets per cubic millimeter) and no bleeding symptoms or signs. The patient with drug-induced, immune-related thrombocytopenia or postinfectious thrombocytopenia also requires only careful observation if there is no significant bleeding.

Corticosteroid therapy is appropriate for the patient with thrombocytopenia who is having significant bleeding but is known to have a self-limited process. Although neither firm experimental data nor properly controlled clinical observations are available, a strong impression exists that corticosteroid administration to the thrombocytopenic patient reduces the bleeding tendency. This seems to be true even if there is no increase in the number of platelets in the peripheral blood. Corticosteroid administration to the patient with ITP can result in a partial or complete, temporary or permanent, remission. The incidence of success varies with the clinic. The most enthusiastic clinics do not report much more than 65 percent remission, either temporary or complete. Our experience suggests a figure of 50 percent or less, with fewer than 25 percent complete and permanent. The role of steroids in chronic ITP is to facilitate the management of acute bleeding episodes and to permit the scheduling of operations on a semielective basis.

Treatment of acute ITP is discussed in Chap. 33. Our approach is as follows: The patient is given 40 mg of prednisone daily in divided doses. If no return of platelets is noted after 4 weeks, the dose of prednisone is doubled. If no return of platelets occurs in 4 weeks with the higher dose, the patient then is considered a candidate for splenectomy. Should the platelets return during the course of prednisone treatment, the dose is decreased in a stepwise fashion over a 4- to 6-week period. If relapse occurs, the patient is considered a candidate for splenectomy rather than retreatment with steroids.

In certain patients, splenectomy may be considered because of relative contraindications to continued steroid therapy, e.g., an active peptic ulcer, serious psychologic changes, and diabetes in which difficulty of control is related to the steroid therapy.

Emergency splenectomy for ITP usually is limited to the patient who presents with central nervous system bleeding. If this is the case, the patient is given 200 mg of intravenous hydrocortisone immediately, and an intravenous infusion of 100 mg of hydrocortisone in 5% dextrose and water is administered over each 6-hour period. Platelet-rich plasma or platelet concentrates are administered preoperatively and during operation. Blood transfusions should consist of fresh whole blood. The platelet preparations and hydro-cortisone are continued postoperatively until the platelets return. Remission occurs in 65 to 70 percent of patients, usually within 3 to 4 days. Occasionally, return of platelets occurs more slowly, over 10 to 14 days.

To rapidly increase the platelet count in surgical patients with thrombocytopenia, particularly that which is associated with massive bleeding and replacement with banked blood, platelet packs are advised. Special platelet transfusion sets are used to reduce loss of platelets due to adherence. For the average patient an administration of 1×10^{11} platelets/m^2 of body surface area will increase circulating platelets by 12×10^9/l. Fever, infection, hepatosplenomegaly, and the presence of antiplatelet alloantibodies will decrease the effectiveness of platelet transfusion.

Recently it has been shown that normal survival of platelets can be obtained with platelets prepared and stored with agitation at room temperature for 72 hours. It has also been demonstrated that these stored concentrates are capable of producing satisfactory posttransfusion elevations in thrombocytopenic patients. Aster et al. have shown that the hemostatic effectiveness of platelets stored at 4°C for 24 hours is equivalent to that of fresh platelets and superior to that of platelets stored at room temperature.

In patients refractory to standard platelet transfusions, the use of HL-A–compatible platelets coupled with special processors has proved effective. Platelet aggregometry has been applied to screening for potential donors. When these refined techniques are not available, in most instances members of the family will provide suitable donors for otherwise refractory patients.

Myeloproliferative Diseases

POLYCYTHEMIA VERA

Surgical treatment of the patient with polycythemia vera is complicated by distinctly increased morbidity and mortality. This is particularly true for the untreated patient but also applies, to some extent, to the patient who has been treated successfully. Spontaneous thrombosis is a complication of polycythemia vera and can be explained, in part, by increased blood viscosity, increased platelet count, and increased tendency toward stasis. Paradoxically, a significant tendency to spontaneous hemorrhage also is noted in these patients. Approximately one-third of patients with polycythemia vera have some form of hemorrhagic complaint at the time of initial diagnosis. The tendency to bleed usually is a function of an excessively high platelet count. Patients with spontaneous bleeding characteristically have a platelet count of 1.5 million per cubic millimeter or greater. The bleeding time may be prolonged. Evidence has been offered that the platelets in these patients may be qualitatively defective. Despite intensive study, the seeming paradox of hemorrhagic tendency accompanied by thrombocytosis is poorly understood.

The polycythemic patient with marked thrombocytosis is a major surgical risk. Operation should be considered only for the most grave surgical emergency. If possible, operation should be deferred until medical management has returned the blood volume, hematocrit, and hemostatic process to normal.

TREATMENT. Thrombocytosis can be reduced by the careful administration of alkylating agents such as busulfan or chlorambucil. These measures are time-consuming. Surgical procedure should be delayed weeks to months following institution of treatment. Ideally, the hematocrit should be kept below 48 percent and the platelet count less than 400,000 per cubic millimeter. The blood volume also can be reduced more rapidly by phlebotomy. Prior to operation, a thorough laboratory investigation of hemostatic function should be conducted. Any gross defect, such as deficiency of vitamin K–dependent factors or low plasma fibrinogen values, should be investigated and corrected when possible. When surgical treatment is judged imperative in these patients, the erythremic state should be reduced by phlebotomy. Operation, at all times, must be performed fastidiously. Postoperative fibrinolysis also has been known to occur, further complicating the postoperative course.

In one series reported from a clinic with considerable experience, 46 percent of polycythemic patients undergoing major procedures had complications at the time of operation or during the postoperative course, and a 16 percent mortality was associated with the surgical procedures. Significantly, 80 percent of the deaths were encountered in patients on whom operations were performed while the disease was not under control. In operations on patients in whom hematocrit and platelet count had been reduced prior to operation the mortality and incidence of complications decreased. Hemorrhage is the most common complication occurring during or following operation and accounts for greater than two-thirds of the deaths. Thrombosis, either venous or arterial, is the next most frequent complication. Infection also is surprisingly common, occurring in approximately 20 percent of patients.

MYELOID METAPLASIA

Myeloid metaplasia frequently represents part of the natural history of polycythemia vera. Approximately 50 percent of patients with myeloid metaplasia are post-polycythemic, while in the remainder the condition apparently occurs as a separate, possibly related, disease entity. Myeloid metaplasia is characterized by many of the features of polycythemia vera. Splenomegaly usually is more prominent and may be massive. Laboratory features include leukocytosis, which may be severe, or, at times, severe leukopenia. Young myeloid forms may be present. Platelets may be strikingly increased in number, but thrombocytopenia also may be present. The latter is usually characteristic of the patient who has myelofibrosis rather than a hyperplastic bone marrow. Examination of the peripheral blood smear may reveal large, bizarre platelets, fragments of megakaryocyte nuclei, occasional nucleated red cells, and bizarre variations in red cell shape. Evidence suggesting qualitative platelet abnormalities has been described. This is considered as a factor in bleeding in some myeloid metaplasia patients. Abnormalities of platelet factor 3 release have been demonstrated, as have abnormalities in platelet aggregation with ADP.

The morbidity rate following surgical treatment in patients with myeloid metaplasia has been reported as high as 68 percent in a small series. The mortality rate in the same experience was greater than 42 percent. Relatively innocuous surgical procedures have been accompanied by nearly uncontrollable bleeding. Spontaneous bleeding from esophageal varices in patients with myeloid metaplasia and massive splenomegaly also has been reported. Preparation for an operation is similar to that described for polycythemia vera.

Other Diseases Associated with Increased Risk of Bleeding

A number of illnesses not primarily characterized by hemostatic failure may be associated with increased risk of bleeding. These diseases frequently involve organs of formation or synthesis of products essential to hemostasis. Diseases such as leukemia, lymphoma, or multiple myeloma may lead to thrombocytopenia because of the replacement of the megakaryocytes in the bone marrow. Illnesses resulting in severe impairment of hepatic function may limit synthesis of plasma factors essential to normal coagulation. The patient with advanced cirrhosis may be lacking in factors of the prothrombin complex (II, V, VII, X), as well as factor XIII.

Illnesses increasing the removal of products essential to hemostasis also occur. Representative of this problem is the patient with splenomegaly in whom sequestration and removal of platelets proceeds at an abnormally rapid rate. Accelerated removal of plasma factors necessary for coagulation has been mentioned in the discussion of the consumptive coagulopathies. The reciprocal of the latter problem has been identified in the case of the patients with cirrhosis and portal hypertension who fail to clear the activators of fibrinolysis from the circulation. This results in a longer biologic survival of these activators and attendant increased fibrinolytic activity.

Some illnesses are characterized by the production of substances which interfere with the normal hemostatic mechanism. These diseases are associated with the production of abnormal proteins which may coat the platelets, as in macroglobulinemia, or bind with certain of the normal blood-clotting factors, as in multiple myeloma or in states associated with the production of cryoglobulin.

Certain diseases may be associated with multiple hemostatic defects. These may include qualitative and quantitative platelet problems, vascular abnormalities, and impaired metabolism and excretion of administered anticoagulant. Any combination of these problems may be noted in patients with renal failure and uremia. The most common problem in this group of patients is thrombocytopenia concurrent with qualitative platelet defects which parallel the degree of azotemia. The hemostatic problems of patients with severe liver disease may be multiple. Major hemorrhagic episodes in these patients usually are accompanied by significant thrombocytopenia, but this is rarely the sole cause. Deficiencies of the coagulation factors normally synthesized in the liver may be present, and increased fibrinolysis also may be evident.

Iatrogenic disorders may result from the administration of drugs which directly or indirectly influence the hemostatic process. Agents which may damage or inhibit the bone marrow include alkylating agents used in malignant disease, antibiotics, such as chloramphenicol, or antibiotics which occasionally result in immunologic removal of platelets, e.g., penicillin, ristocetin, streptomycin. In the idiosyncratic patient, a wide variety of agents may precipitate immune responses leading to platelet removal, e.g., quinidine, quinine, chlorothiazides. Vasculitis and purpura may follow the use of sulfonamides. Salicylates and phenylbutazone may interfere with the platelet-collagen reaction early in the hemostatic process.

TREATMENT. The management of the patient with liver disease is discussed in Chap. 30. Transfusion with freshly drawn whole blood or freshly prepared platelet-rich plasma may be necessary. When thrombocytopenia is significant, the administration of corticosteroids may diminish the bleeding tendency, even though the platelet count is not raised. Bleeding encountered in patients with bone marrow replacement or bone marrow destruction is thrombocytopenic in origin. The use of whole fresh blood, fresh platelet-rich plasma, or fresh platelet concentrates is indicated for control of acute bleeding episodes. Corticosteroids also have been helpful in this situation. Patients with dysproteinemia and attendant bleeding are particularly difficult to manage. Generally, surgical treatment should be deferred until the basic disease is ameliorated and the production of abnormal protein is diminished. In some instances, diminution of the hemorrhagic potential has been accomplished by intensive plasmapheresis with reduction in the level of the abnormal circulating protein.

Anticoagulation and Bleeding

Spontaneous bleeding may be a complication of anticoagulant therapy with either heparin or the coumarin and indandione derivatives. An exaggerated response to oral anticoagulants may occur if dietary vitamin K is inadequate. The anticoagulant effect of coumarin is consistently reduced in patients receiving barbiturates, and increased coumarin requirements have also been documented in patients receiving contraceptives, other estrogen-containing compounds, corticosteroids, and ACTH. Therefore, reduced anticoagulant dosage should be anticipated following discontinuance of any of these drugs. Medications known to increase the effect of oral anticoagulants include phenylbutazone, the cholesterol-lowering agent clofibrate, anabolic steroids (norethandrolone), D-thyroxine, glucagon, quinidine, and a variety of antibiotics.

The history is all-important in recognizing these patients. Questioning should be specific. The patient should be asked if he is presently taking drugs to "thin out" his blood or prevent clotting. Unexplained bleeding in medical and paramedical personnel occasionally is due to surreptitious anticoagulation. The onset of hematuria or melena in the patient receiving anticoagulants should be investigated, since it has been shown that anticoagulants may unmask underlying tumors. Patients with bleeding secondary to anticoagulation may present with only epistaxis, gastro-

intestinal hemorrhage, or hematuria. Physical examination, however, almost always reveals other signs of bleeding such as ecchymoses, petechiae, or hematoma. Bleeding secondary to anticoagulation is not an uncommon cause of rectus sheath hematoma, simulating appendicitis, and intramural intestinal or retroperitoneal hematoma.

Surgical intervention may prove necessary in patients receiving anticoagulant therapy. The typical example is the patient with rheumatic heart disease receiving long-term anticoagulation because of repeated arterial emboli, who then is seen subsequent to a critical embolic episode. Increasing experience suggests that surgical treatment can be undertaken without discontinuing the anticoagulant program. The risk of thrombotic complications reportedly is increased when anticoagulant therapy is discontinued suddenly. If so, this may not be related to what has been called the "rebound phenomena" but may represent an event in a patient who has an underlying thrombotic tendency. When the clotting time is less than 25 minutes in the heparinized patient or when the prothrombin time is greater that 20% of normal in a patient on coumarin, reversal of anticoagulant therapy may not be necessary. Meticulous surgical technique is mandatory, and the patients must be observed closely.

Certain surgical procedures should not be performed in the face of anticoagulation. In sites where even minor bleeding can cause great morbidity, e.g., the central nervous system and the eye, anticoagulants should be discontinued and, if necessary, reversed. Because of the added problem of local fibrinolysis, prostatic surgical treatment should not be carried out in a patient on anticoagulants. Procedures requiring blind needle introduction should be avoided. Deaths have been reported following sympathetic block for peripheral vascular disease in patients receiving anticoagulation. Splenoportography has a markedly increased morbidity in patients in whom prothrombin times are less than 30% and who are thrombocytopenic.

Emergency operation occasionally is necessary in patients who have been heparinized as treatment for deep venous thrombosis. Reversal of heparinization may be desirable. The patient with repeated episodes of pulmonary embolization while fully heparinized is an example. Reversal of heparinization also can be a problem in cardiac surgical procedures employing extracorporeal circulation. The anticoagulant effect of heparin can be rapidly counteracted with protamine sulfate when the heparin has been given intravenously. Protamine sulfate also is administered intravenously. Theoretically, 1.28 mg should neutralize 1 mg of heparin. In fact, 1 milligram of protamine may be given for each milligram of heparin, provided the intravenous heparin was not given more than 2 hours previously. Protamine sulfate in large doses also has an anticoagulant activity. The formation of both extrinsic and intrinsic prothrombinase can be retarded, prolonging the one-stage prothrombin time test and the partial thromboplastin time test. Some patients exhibit the phenomenon of "heparin rebound" following apparently adequate heparin neutralization with protamine. Prolongation of the clotting time again recurs after adequate postoperative antagonism of the heparin. This can contribute to postoperative bleeding. In our experience, this is the major cause of "unexplained" postoperative bleeding following extracorporeal cardiac bypass surgical procedures. Activation of fibrinolysis and thrombocytopenia may also contribute to this problem.

Bleeding infrequently is related to hypoprothrombinemia if the prothrombin concentration is greater than 15%. We have successfully resected a ruptured aortic aneurysm and inserted a prosthetic graft in a patient with a prothrombin concentration at this level. Excessive bleeding was not encountered.

In the elective surgical patient receiving coumarin therapy adequately effecting anticoagulation, the drug can be discontinued several days prior to operation, and the prothrombin concentration then checked. A level greater than 50% is considered safe. If emergency surgical treatment is required, parenteral injection of vitamin K_1 can be used. Since the reversal effect may take 6 hours, transfusion of whole blood or, preferably, freshly frozen plasma may be required. Parenteral administration of vitamin K also is indicated in elective surgical treatment of patients with biliary obstruction, malabsorption, and hypoprothrombinemia. The drug should result in a normal prothrombin time. In contrast, if the hypoprothrombinemia is related to hepatocellular dysfunction, vitamin K therapy is ineffective and should not be prolonged over a week if no response is noted. Vitamin K is an oxidant, and one must be aware that patients with red cell enzyme deficiencies may sustain hemolysis following its administration.

LOCAL HEMOSTASIS

Surgical bleeding, even when alarmingly excessive, is usually caused by ineffective local hemostasis. The goal of local hemostasis is to prevent the flow of blood from incised or transected blood vessels. This may be accomplished by interrupting the flow of blood to the involved area or by direct closure of the blood vessel wall defect. The techniques may be classified as mechanical, thermal, or chemical.

Mechanical Procedures

The oldest mechanical device to effect closure of a bleeding point or to prevent blood from entering the area of disruption is digital pressure. When pressure is applied to an artery proximal to an area of bleeding, profuse bleeding is reduced, permitting more definitive action. The Pringle maneuver of occluding the hepatic artery in the hepatoduodenal ligament as a method of controlling bleeding from a transected cystic artery or from the surface of the liver is a classic example. Direct digital pressure over a bleeding site, such as a lateral rent in the inferior vena cava, is also effective. The finger has the advantage of being the least traumatic vascular hemostat. All clamps, including the so-called atraumatic vascular clamps, do result in damage to the intimal wall of the blood vessel. The obvious disadvantage of digital pressure is that it cannot be used permanently.

The hemostat also represents a temporary mechanical device to stem bleeding. In smaller and noncritical vessels, the trauma and adjacent tissue necrosis associated with the application of a hemostat are of little consequence. These minor disadvantages are outweighed by the mechanical advantage that the instrument offers to subsequent ligation. When bleeding occurs from a vessel which should be preserved, relatively atraumatic hemostats should be employed to limit the extent of intimal damage and subsequent thrombosis.

In general, a ligature replaces the hemostat as a permanent method of effecting hemostasis in a single vessel. When a vessel is transected, a simple ligature usually is sufficient. For large arteries with pulsation and longitudinal motion, transfixion suture to prevent slipping is indicated. When the bleeding site is from a lateral defect in the blood vessel wall, suture ligatures are required. The adventitia and media constitute the major holding forces within the walls of large vessels, and therefore multiple fine sutures are preferable to fewer larger sutures.

Historically, Aulus Cornelius Celsus devised the use of ligatures in 100 A.D. Because of the strong influence of Galen, who was inclined to cautery, this method did not gain popularity. Paré, in 1552, rediscovered the principle of ligature. In 1800, Physick used absorbable sutures of buckskin and parchment. In 1858, Simpson introduced the wire suture, and in 1881 Lister employed chromic catgut. Halsted, in the early 1900s, emphasized the importance of incorporating as little tissue as possible in the suture and indicated the advantages of silk. In 1911, Cushing reported on the use of silver clips to effect hemostasis in delicate vessels in critical areas. Recently, a wide variety of staples made of different metals, which are relatively inert in tissue, have been employed. The advantages of stapling are speed, accuracy, minimal tissue trauma, and the ability to effect hemostasis in otherwise inaccessible areas. Staples have not replaced the ligature, since they are less reliable and harder to apply to larger vessels.

All sutures represent foreign material, and the selection is based on the characteristics of the material and the state of the wound. Nonabsorbable sutures, such as silk, polyethylene, and wire, evoke less tissue reaction than absorbable materials, such as catgut. The latter are preferable, however, in the face of overt infection. The presence of nonabsorbable material in an infected wound can lead to extrusion or sinus tract formation. Wire is the least reactive of the nonabsorbable sutures but the most difficult to handle. Monofilament wire and coated sutures have an advantage over multifilament sutures in the presence of infection. The latter tend to fragment and permit sinus formation due to the interstices.

Diffuse bleeding from multiple transected vessels may be controlled by mechanical techniques which employ pressure directly over the bleeding area, pressure at a distance, or generalized pressure. These techniques are based on the premise that as pressure and flow are decreased in the area of vascular disruption, a clot will occur. Pressure at a distance was effected by application of tourniquets and other pressure devices at pressure points proximal to bleeding sites as a standard procedure by military surgeons in the seventeenth century. Now it is generally felt that direct pressure is preferable and is not attended by the danger of tissue necrosis associated with prolonged use of tourniquets. In our present aerospace age, gravitational suits have been employed to create generalized pressure and to decrease temporarily bleeding from rupture of major intraabdominal vessels.

Direct pressure applied by means of packs affords the best method of controlling diffuse bleeding from large areas. At times, hemostatic chemical materials, such as oxidized cellulose, are incorporated in the packing. Rarely is it necessary to leave a pack at the bleeding site and remove it at a second sitting. If this is done, several days should elapse before removal, and the possibility of recurrent bleeding should be anticipated. The question as to whether hot wet packs or cold wet packs should be applied has been investigated. Unless the heat is so great as to denature protein, it may actually increase bleeding, whereas cold packs promote hemostasis by inducing vascular spasm and increasing endothelial adhesiveness. Bleeding from cut bone may be controlled by packing beeswax in the area. This material effects pressure and is relatively nonirritative to the body.

Thermal Agents

Galen's favoring of cautery influenced medicine for 1,500 years, until the teachings of Paré were appreciated. The use of cautery was revitalized in 1928, when Cushing and Bovie applied this technique for effecting hemostasis of delicate vessels in recessed areas, such as the brain. Heat achieves hemostasis by denaturation of protein, which results in coagulation of large areas of tissue. With actual cautery, heat is transmitted from the instrument by conduction directly to the tissue, whereas with electrocautery, heating occurs by induction from an alternating-current source.

When electrocautery is employed, the amplitude setting should be high enough to produce prompt coagulation but not so high as to set up an arc between the tissue and the cautery tip. This avoids burns outside the operative field and prevents exit of current through electrocardiographic leads or other monitoring devices. A negative plate should be placed beneath the patient whenever cautery is employed to avoid severe skin burns. The advantage of cautery is that it saves time, whereas the disadvantage is that more tissue is necrosed than with precise ligature. Certain anesthetic agents cannot be used with electrocautery because of the hazard of explosion.

A direct current can also result in electrical hemostasis. Since the protein moieties and cellular elements of blood have a negative surface charge, they are attracted to the positive pole, where a thrombus is formed. Direct currents in the 20- to 100-ma range have been applied to control diffuse bleeding from large serous surfaces. High-power argon-laser treatment has been applied successfully to the control of bleeding from superficial erosions.

At the other end of the thermal spectrum, cooling has been applied to control bleeding, particularly from the mucosa of the esophagus and stomach. Generalized hypothermia is of little avail, since, in order to reduce the blood flow to visceral organs, the systemic temperature must be brought down to the level of $35°C$. At this point shivering and ventricular fibrillation may be encountered. Thrombocytopenia may also be a consequence of generalized cooling. Direct cooling is effective and acts by increasing the local intravascular hematocrit and decreasing blood flow by vasoconstriction. A variety of gastric balloons and cooling devices have been employed locally to cool the stomach and distal esophagus as treatment for bleeding esophagogastric varices and gastritis.

Extreme cooling, i.e., cryogenic surgery, has been applicable particularly in neurosurgery. Temperature ranges of -20 to $-180°C$ are used, and freezing occurs around the tip of the cannula within 5 seconds. At temperatures of $-20°C$ or below, the tissue, capillaries, small arterioles, and venules undergo cryogenic necrosis. This is caused by dehydration and denaturation of lipid molecules. The muscular walls of large arteries are an exception. Although the major arteries and blood may be frozen solid, the blood contained in these vessels does not clot. When thawing occurs, normal circulation is resumed.

Chemical Agents

Chemical agents vary in their hemostatic action. Some are vasoconstrictive, while others have coagulant properties. Still others are relatively inert but possess hygroscopic properties which increase their bulk and aid in plugging disrupted blood vessels.

Epinephrine, applied topically, induces vasoconstriction, but extensive application can result in considerable absorption and systemic effects. The drug generally is used on oozing sites in mucosal areas, during tonsillectomy, for example.

Historically, skeletal muscle was one of the first materials with locally hemostatic properties to be employed, its use having been introduced by Cushing in 1911. Shortly thereafter, hemostatic fibrin was manufactured. The properties required for local hemostatic materials include handling ease, rapid absorption, nonirritation, and hemostatic action independent of the general clotting mechanism. The most widely used of the commercially available materials are gelatin foam (Gelfoam), oxidized cellulose (Oxycel), and oxidized regenerated cellulose (Surgicel). All these materials act, in part, by transmitting pressure against the wound surface, and the interstices provide a scaffold on which the clot can organize.

Gelfoam is made from animal skin gelatin which has been denatured. In itself, Gelfoam has no intrinsic hemostatic action, but it can be used in combination with topical thrombin, for which it serves as an absorbable carrier. Its main hemostatic activity is related to the contact between blood and the large surface area of the sponge and to the pressure exerted by the weight of the sponge and absorbed blood. Prior to application of Gelfoam, the sponge should be moistened in saline or thrombin solution, and all the air should be removed from the interstices.

Oxycel and Surgicel are altered cellulose materials capable of reacting chemically with blood and producing a sticky mass which functions as an artificial clot. These substances are relatively inert and are removed by liquefaction in 1 week to 1 month. They should be dry when they are applied. Like Gelfoam, these materials are nontoxic and relatively nonirritating but are somewhat detrimental to wound healing and require phagocytosis to be removed. Surgicel has been shown to have an antibacterial effect.

Recently, adhesive chemicals have been developed to literally cement bleeding sites. One example is methyl-2-cyanoacrilate (Eastman 9-10), which is a rapidly polymerizing substance. These agents have little toxicity but do evoke a marked inflammatory response. Aneurysms have been reported subsequent to the application of cements to major blood vessels. Methyl-2-cyanoacrilate has been applied to the surface of the liver for hemostasis with reported success. Another local approach to the problem of bleeding from a large area is the application of tanned collagen sponge, which functions as a collagenous framework. This encourages the invasion and proliferation of fibroblasts while applying constant pressure against the wound to effect hemostatic action. Microcrystalline collagen has been shown to be more effective than other materials as a topical hemostatic agent.

TRANSFUSION

Background

In 1967, the tercentenarial anniversary of the transfusion of blood into human beings was celebrated. In June of 1667, Jean Baptiste Denis and a surgeon, Emmerez, transfused blood from a sheep into a fifteen-year-old boy who had been bled many times as treatment for fever. The patient apparently improved, and a successful experience was reported simultaneously in another patient. Because of two subsequent deaths associated with transfusion from animals to man, criminal charges were brought against Denis. In April of 1668, further transfusions in man were forbidden unless approved by the Faculty of Medicine in Paris. It was not until the nineteenth century that human blood was recognized as the only appropriate replacement. In 1900, Landsteiner and his associates introduced the concept of blood grouping and identified the major A, B and O groups. In 1939, the Rh group was recognized. Numerous other groups have been uncovered since that time. Development of sensitive cross-matching procedures took place in the 1940s, and with the impetus of World War II blood transfusion became a common procedure. The introduction of various preservative solutions, such as acid citrate dextrose (ACD) and citrate-phosphate-dextrose (CPD), contributed to the development of blood banking.

As the scope of surgery has expanded, the requirement for larger amounts of blood for transfusion has increased. Approximately 14 percent of all patients operated upon, exclusive of procedures performed in the outpatient department or emergency area, are transfused. Of 604 adults who received blood at a university medical center in association with surgical treatment, 125 required over 5,000 ml.

The record administration in this hospital in a patient who survived was 100 units within a 36-hour period. The logistics of the problem have resulted in modernization of transfusion practices, including the use of plasma expanders and component therapy. Preservation of blood and its constituents has been achieved by freezing. Cadaver blood has been used in large amounts in the U.S.S.R.

Characteristics of Blood and Replacement Therapy

BLOOD

Blood has been described as a vehicular organ which perfuses all other organs. It provides transportation of oxygen to satisfy the metabolic demands and removes the by-product carbon dioxide. Blood also transports chemical nutriments for, and waste products from, metabolic activity. Homeostatic governors, including hormones, coagulation factors, and antibodies, are carried to and from appropriate sites within the fluid portion of the blood. Red blood cells, with their oxygen-carrying capacity, white blood cells, which function in body defense processes, and platelets, which contribute to the hemostatic process, comprise the formed elements.

REPLACEMENT THERAPY

BANKED WHOLE BLOOD. Whole blood generally is collected in CPD solution and stored at 4°C. Such blood is considered suitable for administration any time up to 21 days of storage. Following this period, at least 70 percent of the transfused erythrocytes remain in the circulation 24 hours posttransfusion and are viable. Normal survival of red blood cells is 110 to 120 days. Sixty days after transfusion, approximately 52 percent of the cells will survive if the transfusion uses fresh blood. Fifty percent will survive if the transfusion is with CPD blood stored 14 days. In contrast, only 25 percent of erythrocytes survive at 60 days if the transfusion utilized blood stored for 28 days in CPD. The major loss occurs in the first 24 hours after transfusion, and subsequent to that time the survival slope for red cells from fresh blood and stored blood is identical.

Banked blood is a poor source of platelets, since they lose their ability to survive transfusion after 24 hours of storage. Among the clotting factors, factor II (prothrombin), factor VII, factor IX, and factor XI are stable in banked blood. Factor V is not stable in banked blood, while factor VIII also deteriorates during storage.

During the storage of whole blood, red cell metabolism and plasma protein degradation results in certain chemical changes in the plasma (Table 3-3). Lactic acid increases from 20 to 150 mg/100 ml, an amount which is insignificant in terms of transfusion at the end of 28 days. The pH decreases from 7 to 6.68 within 21 days. Little change in the sodium occurs, but the potassium concentration rises steadily to 32 mEq at the end of 21 days. This must be considered when transfusing patients with anuria, oliguria, or hyperkalemia. In these cases, fresh whole blood obviously is preferable. The ammonia concentration also rises steadily during storage from 50 to 680 μg at the end of

Table 3-3. CHARACTERISTICS OF PLASMA STORED IN
ACD SOLUTION AT $4 \pm 1°C$

Constituents	Unit value	Days stored				
		0	7	14	21	28
Dextrose	mg/100 ml	350	300	245	210	190
Lactic acid	mg/100 ml	20	70	120	140	150
Inorganic phosphate	mg/100 ml	1.8	4.5	6.6	9.0	9.5
pH*		7.0	6.85	6.77	6.68	6.65
Hemoglobin	mg/100 ml	0–10	25	50	100	150
Sodium	mEq/L	150	148	145	142	140
Potassium	mEq/L	3–4	12	24	32	40
Ammonia	μg/100 ml	50	260	470	680	

*Determined with glass electrode.
SOURCE: From M. M. Strumia, W. H. Crosby, J. G. Gibson II, T. J. Greenwalt, and J. R. Krevans, "General Principles of Blood Transfusion," J. B. Lippincott Company, Philadelphia, 1963.

21 days. This may be of significance for the patient with hepatic disease. The hemolysis which occurs during storage for 21 days is insignificant, since lysis of only about 1 percent of the red cells occurs and the free hemoglobin is rapidly cleared from the circulation following transfusion.

Typing and Cross Matching. In selecting blood for transfusion, serologic compatibility is established routinely for the recipients' and donors' A, B, O, and Rh groups. Cross matching between the donors' red cells and recipients' sera (the "major" cross match) is performed. The donor sera and recipient cells ("minor" cross match) also are checked. As a rule, Rh-negative recipients should be transfused only with Rh-negative blood. Since this group represents 15 percent of the donor population, the supply may be limited. If the recipient is an elderly male who has not been transfused previously, the transfusion of Rh-positive blood is reasonable if Rh-negative blood is unavailable. Anti-Rh antibodies form in several weeks of transfusion. If further transfusions are needed within a few days, more Rh-positive blood can be used. Rh-positive blood should not be transfused to Rh-negative females who are capable of childbearing. Administration of hyperimmune anti-Rh globulin to Rh-negative women shortly after Rh sensitization largely eliminates Rh disease in subsequent offspring. This promising observation may serve as a model to facilitate transfusions. At present, however, type-specific transfusions remain the basis for therapy. Any Rh-negative woman who has borne children may have been sensitized during pregnancy.

A variety of cell-serum interactions may be detected by careful cross matching. Incompatibility may be due to the fact that either the donor or recipient has been wrongly grouped. An interaction may be caused by a difference in a subgroup, e.g., a donor who is A_1 and a recipient who is A_2 with anti-A_1 in the serum. Interactions may also be due to other naturally occurring antibodies such as anti-P_1 or anti-Le.

In the patient who is receiving repeated transfusions,

serum drawn not more than 24 hours prior to cross matching should be utilized for matching with cells of the donor. The recipient cells used for the minor cross match also should be relatively fresh. Antigenic potency for certain blood groups is lost after several days of storage, and failure to detect minor incompatibility can result. Emergency blood transfusion can be performed with group O blood. If it is known that the prospective recipient is group AB, group A blood is preferable. The O donor blood should have low titers of anti-A and anti-B. Such emergency cases are extremely rare with the exception of battlefield casualties, and it should be possible to wait 45 minutes, during which time the patient's group can be determined and type-specific blood used. The use of plasma expanders in the meantime makes this particularly possible.

When the blood of multiple donors is to be transfused, such as in the case of extracorporeal circulatory procedures, the question arises as to whether all samples should be cross-matched with each other. In determining compatibility, screening is performed in the usual fashion. Major and minor cross matches are performed. Cold agglutinin titer of the recipient serum should be determined if hypothermia is to be employed. In patients with malignant lymphoma and leukemia cryoglobulins may be present, and the blood should be administered at room temperature. If these antibodies are present in high titer, hypothermia may be contraindicated.

In patients with thalassemia and, more particularly, with acquired hemolytic anemia, typing and cross matching may be difficult, and sufficient time should be allotted during the preoperative period to accumulate blood that may be required during the operation. Cross matching should always be carried out prior to the administration of dextran, since dextran interferes with the typing procedure.

FRESH WHOLE BLOOD. This refers to blood which is administered within 24 hours of its donation. In the patient who requires platelets, the blood must be transfused within

6 hours of donation. As noted earlier, such fresh blood also is a potential source of factors V and VIII.

PACKED RED CELLS AND FROZEN RED CELLS. Concentrated suspensions of red cells can be prepared by removing most of the supernatant plasma citrate from the blood following settling of the cells or centrifugation. A small amount of plasma citrate is left, so that the packed cell volume is approximately 70%.

The use of frozen red blood cells represents a recent addition to the transfusion armamentarium. The preparation is time-consuming and requires the addition of glycerol to assure uniform rate of intracellular crystal formation during freezing. At thawing, the cells are washed to remove the glycerol. An advantage of frozen red cells is that their use markedly reduces the risk of infusing hepatitis virus or antigens to which the patient has been previously sensitized. Either packed or frozen red cells are applicable in the treatment of anemia without hypovolemia. The use of packed red cells reduces the danger of circulatory overload. Reactions secondary to allergens in plasma to which the recipient is sensitive also can be minimized.

LEUKOCYTE AND PLATELET-POOR RED CELLS. These are prepared by aspirating the buffy coat and supernatant plasma, following slow centrifugation or settling. The red cells then are washed with sterile isotonic solution. The preparation is time-consuming and increases the possibility of bacterial contamination. This should be done only for patients with demonstrated hypersensitivity to either leukocytes or platelets (buffy coat reactions). Usually this syndrome is manifest by fever, chilly sensations, and urticaria in the absence of hemolysis.

PLATELET-RICH PLASMA AND PLATELET CONCENTRATES. The indications for platelet transfusion are as follows: thrombocytopenia due to massive blood loss and replacement with stored blood, thrombocytopenia due to inadequate platelet production, thrombocytopenia due to platelet destruction, and qualitative platelet disorders. The preparations should be used within 6 hours of blood donation. One unit of platelet-rich plasma has a volume of approximately 200 ml. The recovery of platelets in the recipient usually is no more than 60 percent of those present in the donor blood. The platelet concentrate consists of platelets prepared from a unit of platelet-rich plasma. These are resuspended in 30 ml of fluid and should be administered without a filter. The platelet concentrate has the advantage of obviating circulatory overload. Both preparations may harbor the hepatitis virus and account for allergic reactions similar to those due to whole blood. When treating thrombocytopenic bleeding or preparing thrombocytopenic patients for surgery, it is advisable to elevate the platelet levels to the range of 50,000 to 100,000/mm^3 in order to provide continued protection. The development of isoimmunity remains one of the most important factors limiting the usefulness of platelet transfusion. Isoantibodies are demonstrable in about 5 percent of patients after 1 to 10 transfusions, 20 percent after 10 to 20 transfusions, and 80 percent after more than 100 transfusions. The use of HL-A–compatible platelets addresses this problem.

POOLED PLASMA. Plasma prepared from pooled blood is associated with a high incidence of hepatitis. Some investigators suggest that this may be reduced by storage at 31.6°C for 6 months. Banked plasma has been used to treat certain coagulation defects. Frozen plasma prepared from freshly donated blood or fresh plasma is necessary to provide factors V and VIII. The other plasma clotting factors are present in banked preparations. The use of plasma for therapy in patients with hypovolemia rarely is indicated. Ringer's lactate or buffered saline solution, administered in amounts two to three times the estimated blood loss, is effective in an emergency and is associated with fewer complications. Dextran or a combination of Ringer's lactate solution and normal human serum albumin are preferred for rapid plasma expansion. Commercially available dextran preparations probably should not be administered in amounts exceeding 1 liter/day, since prolongation of bleeding time and hemorrhage can occur. Low-molecular-weight dextran, i.e., molecular weight of 30,000 to 40,000, has achieved recent popularity because it possesses a higher colloidal pressure than plasma and effects some reversal of erythrocyte agglutination.

CONCENTRATES. *Antihemophilic concentrates* are prepared from plasma and are available for the treatment of factor VIII deficiency. Some of these concentrates are twenty to thirty times as potent as an equal volume of fresh-frozen plasma. The simplest factor VIII concentrate, described initially by Pool and Shannon, is the plasma cryoprecipitate. Plasma is frozen rapidly by immersion of the plastic container in a dry ice–acetone mixture. The frozen plasma is thawed slowly (18 hours) at refrigerator temperature (4°C), and a sticky precipitate is found clinging to the bag. The thawed liquid plasma is expressed, and the precipitate, containing the bulk of the initial factor VIII activity, can be dissolved in 10 ml of sterile saline solution, pooled with other units if desired, and administered. *Desiccated human fibrinogen* is commercially available. The preparation is made from plasma pooled from many donors and carries a risk of transmitting the virus of hepatitis. *Albumin* also has been concentrated, so that 25 Gm may be administered and provide the osmotic equivalent of 500 ml of plasma. The advantage of albumin is that it is a hepatitis-free product. Salt-poor albumin is available for patients with sodium retention.

Indications for Replacement of Blood or Its Elements

VOLUME REPLACEMENT. The most common indication for blood transfusion in diseases of surgical interest is the replenishment of the circulating blood volume. It is difficult to evaluate the volume deficit accurately.

A variety of techniques employing dyes or isotopically tagged colloids have been introduced to determine the blood volume more precisely. Values for "normal blood volume" are variable, and the techniques are relatively inaccurate when there is a rapidly changing situation, such as hemorrhage. Chronically ill and elderly patients may have a diminution of blood volume. In patients with cardiac decompensation, the blood volume may be greater than normal. Many patients with chronically reduced blood volume are well accommodated to that volume. Blood volume, in itself, does not serve as an absolute indication for transfusion. Measurement of hemoglobin or hematocrit also is used to interpret blood loss. This is misleading in the face of acute blood loss, since the hematocrit may be normal in spite of a severely contracted blood volume. Ebert et al. showed that after a healthy adult male lost approximately 1,000 ml of blood rapidly, the venous hematocrit fell only 3 percent during the first hour, 5 percent at 24 hours, 6 percent at 48 hours, and 8 percent at 72 hours, thus indicating the time required for the body to restore blood volume.

A healthy person can lose 430 ml in 20 minutes with only minor effects on the circulation and little change in blood pressure or pulse, as evidenced by the normal blood donor. The normal person may lose 1 liter of blood rapidly without a fall in blood pressure as long as he remains supine. About 40% of blood volume, or 2 liters of blood, usually is lost before significant hypotension develops. Loss of blood may be evaluated in the operating room by estimating the amount of blood in the wound and on the drapes and by weighing sponges. The loss determined by weighing sponges is only about 70% of true loss.

IMPROVEMENT IN OXYGEN-CARRYING CAPACITY. This is primarily a function of the red cell. When anemia can be treated by specific therapy, transfusion should be withheld. Acute anemias, such as hemolytic anemia, are more disabling physiologically than chronic anemia, since most patients with chronic anemia have undergone an adjustment to the situation. In pregnancy, there is a moderate drop in hematocrit, and transfusions are not indicated to correct the physiologic anemia of pregnancy prior to surgical treatment. The correction of chronic anemia prior to surgical treatment, though often performed, is difficult to justify, and there is no indication that anemia predisposes to wound dehiscence. Peskin and associates have described a stroma-free hemoglobin solution which has the ability to carry and exchange oxygen and, in experimental animals, has demonstrated no toxicity. Blood volume may be replaced with dextran solution or Ringer's lactate solution with a reduction of the hemoglobin to levels below 10 Gm and little demonstrable change in the effects of a reduction in oxygen-carrying capacity or the capacity to remove metabolic gaseous by-products.

REPLACEMENT OF CLOTTING FACTORS. Transfusion of platelets and/or proteins contributing to coagulation may be indicated in specific patients either prior to or during operation. In the treatment of certain hemorrhagic conditions, it is to be appreciated that the clotting defects may be multiple and the injection of substitutes and extracts may be less effective than transfusion of fresh blood. Treatment with clotting factors requires an accurate diagnosis of the hemorrhagic disease with an appreciation of the changes which occur in the biologic properties of the factors during storage and the biologic effects and quantitative changes which occur after injection.

When transfusion with fibrinogen is deemed necessary, a plasma level greater than 100 mg/ml should be maintained. The hypofibrinogenemia encountered during surgical treatment is frequently related to excessive consumption. Adequate levels of fibrinogen frequently will return within hours without replacement therapy if the precipitating cause is corrected. Deficiency of factor V, per se, is relatively rare; although transfusion will increase the level, there is suggestion that the biologic half-life is short and may not exceed 12 hours.

Hypoprothrombinemia and deficiency of factor VII in patients on anticoagulant therapy can be reversed with injection of vitamin K_1. In patients who are deficient in prothrombin, such as those with cirrhosis, and who require surgical treatment, transfusion with banked blood may effect immediate benefit.

Transfusion therapy for patients with hemophilia subjected to trauma or surgical procedures requires sufficient quantities to raise and maintain the level of factor VIII in the plasma to above 30% of normal. Transfusion of small amounts of factor VIII is not justified. If a life-threatening situation exists, large amounts must be used. The factor IX–deficient patient subjected to surgery or trauma also requires levels of 20 to 30% for secure hemostasis. Such levels are difficult to attain with plasma infusions despite the stability of factor IX in stored plasma. Fortunately, factor IX concentrates now being tested offer considerable promise. The biologic half-life of factor IX is appreciably longer than that of factor VIII.

Usually, the hemostatic mechanism is not markedly altered with platelet counts greater than 50,000. If thrombocytopenia is more pronounced, however, the transfusion of fresh platelets may be indicated to prevent or treat active bleeding. The life span of freshly infused platelets is only about 10 days, and in some instances the recipient represents a hostile environment, and the survival is reduced to several hours.

SELECTIVE THERAPY

Johnson and Greenwalt have pointed out that less than 50 years ago we were concerned with making blood transfusions easier to administer while presently we are searching for arguments with which to discourage the administration of unnecessary transfusions and methods to place transfusion on a more logical basis. If the patient has severe anemia and hypovolemia, which are usually associated with massive hemorrhage, whole blood represents the treatment of choice, and ordinary banked blood generally can be used. An alternative to this approach is a combination of packed red cells plus a plasma volume expander. Operative blood losses of 1,000 to 1,500 ml may be replaced without untoward difficulty using Ringer's lactate or buffered saline solution. When anemia exists without hypovolemia, packed red cells represent the treatment of choice. This can be accomplished with the standard packed cells or with frozen cells, which, although presently expensive, provide a method of storage for many years, avoid the complication of hepatitis, and reduce the incidence of fever, chills, and allergic reactions. The use of packed red cells is particularly applicable in patients with severe anemia who have diminished cardiac reserve or hypervolemia.

Thrombocytopenic bleeding is treated with platelet con-

Table 3-4. REPLACEMENT OF CLOTTING FACTORS

Factors	Normal level	Life span in vivo ($\frac{1}{2}$ life)	Fate during coagulation	Level required for safe hemostasis	Stability in ACD bank blood (4°)	Ideal agent for replacing deficit
I (fibrinogen)	200–400 mg/ 100 ml	72 hr	Consumed	60–100 mg/ 100 ml	Very stable	Bank blood; concentrated fibrinogen
II (prothrombin)	20 mg/100 ml (100%)	72 hr	Consumed	15–20%	Stable	Bank blood; concentrated preparation
V (proaccelerin, accelerator globulin labile factor)	100%	36 hr	Consumed	5–20%	Labile (40% at 1 week)	Frozen fresh plasma; blood under 7 days
VII (proconvertin, serum prothrombin conversion accelerator [SPCA] stable factor)	100%	5 hr	Survives	5–30%	Stable	Bank blood; concentrated preparation
VIII (antihemophilic factor [AHF], antihemophilic globulin, [AHG]	100% (50–150)	6–12 hr	Consumed	30%	Labile (20–40% at 1 week)	Fresh frozen plasma; concentrated AHF; cryoprecipitate
IX (Christmas factor, plasma thromboplastin component [PTC], hemophilia B factor	100%	24 hr	Survives	20–30%	Stable	Fresh frozen plasma, bank blood, concentrated preparation
X (Stuart-Prower factor)	100%	40 hr	Survives	15–20%	Stable	Bank blood; concentrated preparation
XI (plasma thromboplastin antecedent [PTA])	100%	Probably 40–80 hr	Survives	10%	Probably stable	Bank blood
XII (Hageman factor)	100%	Unknown	Survives	Deficit produces no bleeding tendency	Stable	Replacement not required
XIII (fibrinase, fibrin-stabilizing factor [FSF])	100%	4–7 days	Survives	Probably less than 1%	Stable	Bank blood
Platelets	150,000–400,000/ mm³	8–11 days	Consumed	60,000–100,000/ mm³	Very labile (40% at 20 hr; 0 at 48 hr)	Fresh blood or plasma; fresh platelet concentrate (not frozen plasma)

SOURCE: E. W. Salzman, Hemorrhagic disorders, in J. M. Kinney, R. H. Egdahl, and G. D. Zuidema (eds.), "Manual of Preoperative and Postoperative Care," p. 157, W. B. Saunders Company, Philadelphia, 1971.

centrates or platelet-rich plasma (Table 3-4). Deficiencies of factors VII, IX, X, or XI unaccompanied by anemia can be treated with stored plasma or any plasma preparation. If patients with these defects are undergoing elective or emergency surgical treatment, stored blood may be preferable. Factor V deficiency requires fresh frozen plasma or fresh whole blood as therapy. Hemophilia without severe anemia should be treated with factor VIII concentrate or fresh frozen plasma as an alternative. If there is an accompanying severe anemia, the preferable treatment is packed red cells with either factor VIII concentrate or fresh frozen plasma, but fresh blood administered shortly after collection may be used. Congenital hypofibrinogenemia should be treated with whole blood or fibrinogen from small donor pools, while acute acquired hypofibrinogenemia requires, in addition to fibrinogen or whole blood, treatment of the underlying problem, i.e., heparin for defibrination and ϵ-aminocaproic acid for fibrinolysis.

SPECIFIC INDICATIONS

SINGLE-UNIT TRANSFUSION. There has been a general trend toward condemning all single-unit transfusion on surgical services. As has been previously mentioned, they are usually uncalled for. However, the Committee on Blood of the American Medical Association found it necessary to oppose this trend, pointing out that it is a poor practice to order 2 units of blood to escape criticism for using a single unit, and an appropriate volume of blood should be given whenever transfusion is required.

MASSIVE TRANSFUSION. The term *massive transfusion* implies a single transfusion greater than 2,500 ml or 5,000 ml transfused over a period of 24 hours. The approximate percentages of *original* blood volume remaining after varying degrees of hemorrhage and transfusion are shown in Table 3-5. A variety of problems may attend the use of massive transfusion. Dilutional thrombocytopenia, impaired platelet function, and deficiencies of factors V, VIII, and XI may occur. The acid load present in stored blood may have an additive effect in a patient with preexisting acidosis. Routine alkalinization is not advisable, since this could have an adverse effect on the oxyhemoglobin dissociation curve and presents an additional sodium load to a compromised patient. The increased potassium content of multiple units of stored blood does not provide clinical effects unless the patient is severely oliguric.

Table 3-5. PERCENTAGE OF ORIGINAL BLOOD VOLUME REMAINING
IN A PATIENT WITH A 5-LITRE BLOOD VOLUME TRANSFUSED WITH
500-ML UNITS

Situation*	Magnitude of hemorrhage and transfusion		
	1 Blood volume (10 units)	*2 Blood volumes* (20 units)	*3 Blood volumes* (30 units)
Best	37%	14%	5%
Usual	25–30%	10%	3–4%
Worst	18%	3%	0.4%

*The "best" situation requires simultaneous and equal replacement during hemorrhage; the "worst" situation means initial loss of one-half blood volume not replaced until the hemorrhage has stopped.

SOURCE: After Collins.

Citrate toxicity may be associated with massive transfusion, particularly in young children and patients with severe hypotension or liver disease. This is related to an excessive binding of ionized calcium and is usually corrected by spontaneous mobilization of calcium from bone. The availability of a calcium ion–sensing electrode should provide a base for intelligent calcium therapy and avoidance of iatrogenic hypercalcemia. The function of hemoglobin is altered by storage in that the concentration of 2,3-DPG (diphosphoglyceric acid) falls to a negligible level by the third week. This results in an increased affinity of the red blood cells for oxygen and a less efficient oxygen delivery system. The shift to CPD blood has a favorable consequence in that 2,3-DPG remains at normal levels for 1 week. Collins has shown that in itself reduction of 2,3-DPG may not have a significant effect but when combined with acute anemia may be an important factor.

When large transfusions are administered, a heat exchanger may be used to warm the blood, since hypothermia may cause a decrease in cardiac rate and output and a reduction in the blood pH. Warming the blood significantly decreases the frequency of intraoperative cardiac arrest.

The use of blood from many donors increases the possibility of hemolytic transfusion reaction due to incompatibility. This can be reduced by screening each potential donor in the pool and eliminating those who show possible incompatibility. Paradoxically, patients who survive a massive transfusion do not have a high probability of developing isoantibodies subsequently, and the risk is no greater than that from a single transfusion. The risk of homologous serum hepatitis increases progressively with each succeeding unit.

EXTRACORPOREAL CIRCULATION. Fresh, heparinized blood generally has been used for open heart operations and other applications of extracorporeal circulation in order to decrease the danger of citrate effect. Subsequent to the procedure, the excess heparin is usually neutralized with protamine. Johnson and Greenwalt indicate that their experience with over 2,000 replacement transfusions demonstrates that this can be performed adequately with ACD blood which is less than 5 days old and modified by the addition of heparin and calcium. Prior to its use, the ACD blood is heparinized with 20 to 25 mg/unit and treated with 500 to 600 mg of calcium chloride/unit. When treated ACD blood is compared with heparinized blood, the pH of the former is lower during the first few minutes of perfusion, and the platelet counts are significantly lower 10 minutes after perfusion. By the end of perfusion there is no difference in the two series. A variety of physiologic compatible fluids, such as Ringer's lactate solution, buffered saline solution, and dextran, may be applied to prime the pump during extracorporeal circulation and reduce the need for blood.

Methods of Administering Blood

ROUTINE ADMINISTRATION. The rate of transfusion depends upon the patient's status. Usually, 5 ml/minute is administered for 1 minute, following which 10 to 20 ml/min may be administered to complete routine transfusion. When marked oligemia is being treated, the first 500 ml may be given within 10 minutes, and the second 500 ml may be given equally rapidly in most cases. Cold blood may be used for this amount, but when larger amounts are administered, warm blood is desirable.

The gauge of the needle is a critical factor in the rate of flow. Flow also is determined by the height at which the bottle is suspended. In patients with peripheral circulatory failure, the veins may be constricted with resultant increased resistance to flow, necessitating raising of the bottle. Positive pressure may be applied by some form of rotary pump or fingers which compress the tubing of the transfusion set and drive the blood onward. If plastic bags have been used as containers for the blood, they may be surrounded with a blood pressure cuff and pressure applied. Air pumped into the transfusion bottle has been used extensively as a method of increasing pressure, but this technique is associated with a definite danger of air embolism.

When large transfusions are administered, it is important not to overload the circulation, and the use of central venous pressure monitoring is particularly pertinent. There is no practical advantage in the use of intraarterial transfusion as compared with the intravenous route in the treatment of oligemia. It has been shown that coronary flow and systemic arterial pressure respond as rapidly and to the same extent whether the blood is administered intravenously or intraarterially. The theoretical advantage of intraarterial infusion for patients in whom the blood cannot pass from the venous to the arterial side of the circulation because of cardiac arrest or ineffective ventricular contraction is offset by the delay in setting up an intraarterial transfusion.

OTHER METHODS. Blood may be instilled intraperitoneally or into the medullary cavity of the sternum and long bones. Intrasternal and intramedullary transfusion may be painful, and the rate of administration is limited. Approximately 90 percent of red cells injected intraperitoneally enter the circulation, but uptake is not complete for at least a week, and therefore the method is not suitable when immediate transfusion is required.

In 1934, Tiber reported 123 autotransfusions using intraperitoneal blood in patients with ruptured ectopic gestation. There was only one death. This technique has also been applied to patients with ruptured livers and spleens. Blood is suctioned gently from the peritoneal cavity and then reinfused after passing through a filter. A transient increase in free hemoglobin and thrombocytopenia results, but red blood cell survival is normal.

Complications

HEMOLYTIC REACTIONS. Hemolytic reactions due to incompatibility of A, B, O, and Rh groups or many other independent systems may result from errors in the laboratory of a clerical or technical nature or the administration of the wrong blood at the time of transfusion. Hemolytic reactions are characterized by intravascular destruction of red blood cells and consequent hemoglobinemia and hemoglobinuria. Circulating haptoglobin is capable of binding 100 mg of hemoglobin/100 ml of plasma, and the complex is cleared by the reticuloendothelial system. When the binding capacity is exceeded, free hemoglobin circulates, and the heme is released and combines with albumin to form methemalbumin. When free hemoglobin exceeds 25 mg/100 ml of plasma, some is excreted in the urine, but in most subjects hemoglobinuria occurs when the total plasma level exceeds 150 mg/100 ml. The renal lesions which may occur consist of tubular necrosis and precipitation of hemoglobin within the tubules.

Clinical Manifestations. There is an increased hazard in patients with a previous transfusion reaction. If the patient is awake, the most common symptoms are the sensation of heat and pain along the vein into which the blood is being transfused, flushing of the face, pain in the lumbar region, and constricting pain in the chest. The patient may experience chills, fever, and respiratory distress, hypotension, and tachycardia from amounts as small as 50 ml. In patients who are anesthetized and undergoing operation, the two signs which may call attention are abnormal bleeding and continued hypotension despite adequate replacement. Abnormal bleeding may be related to the fact that thromboplastic substances are released as the cells are

lysed. The mortality and morbidity resulting from hemolytic reactions is high if the patient receives a full unit of incompatible blood. Acute hemorrhagic diatheses occur in 8 to 30 percent of patients. There is a sudden fall in the platelet count, an increase in fibrinolytic activity, and consumption of coagulation factors, especially V and VIII, due to disseminated intravascular clotting.

Rudowski reported the following incidences of clinical manifestations in a large series with hemolytic posttransfusion reactions: oliguria, 58 percent; hemoglobinuria, 56 percent; arterial hypotension, 50 percent; jaundice, 40 percent; nausea and vomiting, 30 percent; flank pain, 25 percent; cyanosis and hypothermia, 22 percent; dyspnea, 20 percent; chills, 18 percent; diffuse bleeding, 16 percent; neurologic signs, 10 percent; and allergic reaction, 6 percent. The laboratory criteria are hemoglobinuria with a concentration of free hemoglobin over 5 mg/100 ml, a serum haptoglobin level below 50 mg/100 ml, and serologic criteria to show antigen incompatibility of the donor and recipient blood. The simplest clinical diagnostic test is insertion of a bladder catheter and evaluation of the color and volume of the excreted urine, since hemoglobinuria and oliguria are the most characteristic signs.

Treatment. If a transfusion reaction is suspected, the transfusion should be stopped immediately, and a sample of the recipient's blood should be drawn and sent along with the suspected unit to the blood bank for comparison with the pretransfusion samples. The residual blood from the transfusion should be cultured, and the serum bilirubin should be determined in the recipient. Each gram of hemoglobin is converted to about 40 mg of bilirubin. The hemolytic reaction is characterized by an increase in the indirect reacting fraction.

A Foley catheter should be inserted, and the hourly urine output recorded. Since renal toxicity is affected by the rate of urinary excretion and the pH and since alkalinizing the urine prevents precipitation of hemoglobin within the tubules, attempts are made to initiate diuresis and alkalinize the urine. This can be accomplished with 100 ml of 20% mannitol plus 45 mEq of bicarbonate. If marked oliguria or anuria occurs, the fluid intake and potassium intake are restricted, and the patient is treated as a case of renal shutdown. In some instances, dialysis is required. Following recovery from oliguria or anuria, diuresis is often copious and may be associated with significant losses of potassium and sodium which require replacement.

ALLERGIC REACTIONS. These are relatively frequent, occurring in about 1 percent of transfusions. Reactions are usually mild and are manifested by urticaria and fever. In rare instances, the reaction may be severe enough to cause anaphylactic shock. Allergic reactions are caused by transfusion of antibodies from hypersensitive donors or the transfusion of antigens to which the recipient is hypersensitive. Reactions may occur following the administration of whole blood, packed red cells, plasma, and antihemophilic factor. Treatment consists of antihistamines, epinephrine, and steroids, depending on the severity of the reaction.

BACTERIAL SEPSIS. Bacterial contamination of infused

blood is rare and may be acquired either from the contents of the container or the skin of the donor. Gram-negative organisms, which are capable of growth at 4°C, are the most common cause. Clinical manifestations include fever, chills, abdominal cramps, vomiting, and diarrhea. There may be hemorrhagic manifestations and increased bleeding if the patient is undergoing surgical treatment. In some instances, bacterial toxins can produce profound shock. If the diagnosis is suspected, the transfusion should be discontinued and the blood cultured. Emergency treatment includes adrenergic blocking agents, oxygen, antibiotics, and, in some cases, judicious transfusion.

EMBOLISM. Although air embolism has been reported as a complication of intravenous transfusion, healthy animals tolerate large amounts of air injected intravenously at a rapid rate. In experimental animals, the minimal lethal dose averages 7.5 ml/kg, and the mortality rate accompanying this amount of air injection can be halved by placing the animal on the left side at the time of injection. This displaces the air away from the outflow tract in the right ventricle. It has been suggested that the normal adult generally will tolerate an embolism of 200 ml of air. Smaller amounts, however, can cause alarming signs and may be fatal. The most common method of producing air embolism during transfusion is by injecting air under pressure into the container in order to increase rate of flow. Manifestations of venous air embolism include a rise in venous pressure and cyanosis, a "mill wheel" murmur heard over the precordium, hypotension, tachycardia, and syncope. Death usually is related to primary respiratory failure. Treatment consists of placing the patient on the left side in a head-down position with the feet up. Arterial air embolism is manifested by dizziness and fainting, loss of consciousness, and convulsions. Air may be visible in the retinal arteries, and bubbles of air may flow from transected vessels.

Plastic tubes used for transfusion also have embolized after they have broken off within the vein. Plastic tubes have passed into the right atrium and the pulmonary artery, resulting in death. Embolized catheters have been removed successfully.

THROMBOPHLEBITIS. Prolonged infusions into peripheral veins using either needles, cannulae, or plastic tubes are associated with superficial venous thrombosis. Intravenous infusions which last more than 8 hours are more likely to be followed by thrombophlebitis. There is an increased incidence in the lower limb as compared to upper limb infusions. Treatment consists of discontinuation of the infusion and local compressing. Embolism from superficial thrombophlebitis of this nature is extremely rare.

OVERTRANSFUSION AND PULMONARY EDEMA. Overloading the circulation is a complication which is avoidable. It may occur with rapid infusion of blood, plasma expanders, and other fluids, particularly in patients with heart disease. The central venous pressure should be monitored in these patients and whenever large amounts of fluid are administered in order to prevent this complication.

Circulatory overloading is manifested by a rise in the venous pressure, dyspnea, and cough. Râles generally can be heard at the bases of the lung. Treatment consists of stopping the infusion, placing the patient in a sitting position, and, occasionally, venous section for removal of blood.

Although acute pulmonary edema occurs more frequently following large transfusions, it has been reported in patients receiving small transfusions. A syndrome which can be confused with pulmonary edema consists of postoperative hypoxia seen in patients who have undergone cardiac surgical treatment and extracorporeal bypass procedures. A damaging factor apparently is carried by the perfusing blood, and immature plasma cells are found in the interalveolar tissue. The lesion represents an immune response to homologous blood. The incidence is reduced by employing the hemodilution technique of pump priming.

TRANSMISSION OF DISEASE. Malaria, Chagas' disease, brucellosis, and syphilis can be transmitted by blood transfusion. Positive serologic tests for syphilis may result 20 days after transfusion from donors with positive reactions.

Viral Hepatitis. Viral hepatitis is the most important disease transmitted by transfusion of blood components. Included in the general term are viral hepatitis A (formerly called infective hepatitis) and viral hepatitis B (formerly called serum hepatitis). The main clinical difference in the two types is in the incubation period, type A having an incubation of 15 to 50 days and type B 30 to 160 days. A serologic marker for either infection with or carriage of the virus of type B hepatitis is detectable. This serum antigen was formerly called Australian antigen but is now known as hepatitis B surface antigen (HB_sAg). A serum antigen specific for type A hepatitis has not been precisely defined.

In recipients who receive transfusions of an average of 2 units of blood, an incidence of hepatitis of approximately 0.5 percent has been reported. The clinical manifestations of hepatitis include lethargy and anorexia as part of anicteric disease, icterus, and chronic liver disease. HB_sAg persists in about 35 percent of patients who develop serum hepatitis of type B. The risk of hepatitis is definitely diminished by freezing the red cells in plasma. There is no risk from human serum albumin and other plasma protein fractions.

Krugman et al. have reported that immune serum globulin is effective in preventing type A hepatitis but inconsistent in regard to type B. Accidental self-inoculation with material which is definitely known to contain HB_sAg or the transfusion of blood which is HB_sAg-positive constitutes an indication for the immediate use of human specific immunoglobulin (HSI) anti-HB_sAg. The dosage is empirical, but the presently recommended dose is 0.5 IgG given by deep intramuscular injection. Another situation in which the HSI anti-HB_sAg may be of value is in chronic renal dialysis units.

References

General

Biggs, R. P., and Macfarlane, R. G.: "Human Blood Coagulation and Its Disorders," 3d ed., F. A. Davis Company, Philadelphia, 1962.

Hougie, C.: "Fundamentals of Blood Coagulation in Clinical Medicine," McGraw-Hill Book Company, New York, 1963.

Quick, A. J.: "Hemorrhagic Diseases and Thrombosis," Lea & Febiger, Philadelphia, 1966.

Ratnoff, O. D.: "Bleeding Syndromes," Charles C Thomas, Publisher, Springfield, Ill., 1960.

Ulin, A. W., and Gollub, S. S. (eds.): "Surgical Bleeding: Handbook for Medicine, Surgery, and Specialties," McGraw-Hill Book Company, New York, 1966.

Wintrobe, M. M.: "Clinical Hematology," Lea & Febiger, Philadelphia, 1967.

Biology of Normal Hemostasis

Astrup, T.: "Connective Tissue, Thrombosis, and Atherosclerosis," Academic Press, Inc., New York, 1959.

Davie, E. W., and Ratnoff, O. D.: Waterfall Sequence for Intrinsic Blood Clotting, *Science,* **145:**1310, 1964.

Gaarder, A., Jonsen, J., Laland, S., Hellem, A., and Owren, P. A.: Adenosine Diphosphate in Red Cells as a Factor in the Adhesiveness of Human Blood Platelets, *Nature (Lond),* **192:**531, 1961.

Macfarlane, R. G.: Enzyme Cascade in the Blood Clotting Mechanism and Its Function as a Biochemical Amplifier, *Nature (Lond),* **202:**498, 1964.

Quick, A. J.: Effect of Aspirin on the Bleeding Time, *Fed Proc,* **25:**498, 1966.

Rodman, N. F.: The Morphologic Basis of Platelet Function, in K. M. Brinkhous, R. W. Shermer, and F. K. Mostofi (eds.), "The Platelet," The Williams & Wilkins Company, Baltimore, 1971.

Sherry, S.: Present Concept of the Fibrinolytic System, *Ser Haemat,* **7:**70, 1965.

Vigliano, E. M., and Horowitz, H. I.: Bleeding Syndrome in a Patient with IGA Myeloma: Interaction of Protein and Connective Tissue, *Blood,* **29:**823, 1967.

Weiss, H. J.: Platelet Physiology and Abnormalities of Platelet Function, *N Engl J Med,* **293:**531, 1975.

——— Platelet Physiology and Abnormalities of Platelet Function, *N Engl J Med,* **293:**580, 1975.

Tests of Hemostasis and Blood Coagulation

Brecher, G., and Cronkite, E. P.: Morphology and Enumeration of Blood Platelets, *J Appl Physiol,* **3:**365, 1950.

Budtz-Olsen, A. E.: "Clot Retraction," Charles C Thomas, Publisher, Springfield, Ill., 1951.

Bull, B. S.: A Semiautomatic Micro Sample Dilutor, *Am J Clin Pathol,* **47:**549, 1967.

Cartwright, G. E.: "Diagnostic Laboratory Hematology," 4th ed., Grune & Stratton, Inc., New York, 1968.

DeNicola, P.: "Thromboelastography," Charles C Thomas, Publisher, Springfield, Ill., 1957.

Didisheim, P.: Screening Tests for Bleeding Disorders, *Am J Clin Path,* **47:**622, 1967.

Duke, W. W.: The Relation of Blood Platelets to Hemorrhagic Disease: Description of a Method for Determining the Bleeding Time and Coagulation Time, and Report of Three Cases of Hemorrhagic Disease Relieved by Transfusion, *JAMA,* **55:**1185, 1910.

Jim, R. T. S.: A Study of the Plasma Thrombin Time, *J Lab Clin Med,* **50:**45, 1957.

Lee, R. I., and White, P. D.: A Clinical Study of the Coagulation Time of Blood, *Am J Med Sci,* **145:**495, 1923.

Margolius, A., Jr., Jackson, D. P., and Ratnoff, O. D.: Circulating Anticoagulants: A Study of 40 Cases and a Review of the Literature, *Medicine (Baltimore),* **40:**145, 1961.

Mielke, C. H., Kaneshiro, M. M., Weiner, J. M., and Rapaport, S. I.: The Standardized Normal Ivy Bleeding Time and Its Prolongation by Aspirin. *Blood,* **34:**204, 1969.

Nye, S. W., Graham, J. B., and Brinkhous, K. M.: The Partial Thromboplastin Time as a Screening Test for the Detection of Latent Bleeders, *Am J Med Sci,* **243:**279, 1962.

Owren, P. A.: Thrombotest: A New Method for Controlling Anticoagulant Therapy, *Lancet,* **2:**754, 1959.

Quick, A. J.: Clinical Interpretation of the One-Stage Prothrombin Time, *Circulation,* **24:**1422, 1961.

Salzman, E. W.: Measurement of Platelet Adhesiveness: A Sample In Vitro Technique Demonstrating an Abnormality in von Willebrand's Disease, *J Lab Clin Med,* **62:**724, 1963.

Evaluation of the Surgical Patient as a Hemostatic Risk

Biggs, R., and Macfarlane, R. G.: "Human Blood Coagulation and Its Disorders," 3d ed., F. A. Davis Company, Philadelphia, 1962.

Hougie, C.: "Fundamentals of Blood Coagulation in Clinical Medicine," McGraw-Hill Book Company, New York, 1963.

Shulman, N. R., Aster, R. H., Leitner, A., and Hiller, M. C.: Immunoreactions Involving Platelets. V. Posttransfusion Purpura Due to Complement-fixing Antibody against Genetically Controlled Platelet Antigen: Proposed Mechanism for Thrombocytopenia and Its Relevance, in "Autoimmunity," The Year Book Medical Publishers, Inc., Chicago, 1962–1963.

Clinical Hemostatic Defects

Aster, R. H., Becker, G. A., Hamid, M., and Calvert, D. N.: Storage of Platelet Concentrates at 4°C; Use of Refrigerated Platelet Concentrates in the Treatment of Hemorrhage in Thrombocytopenic Patients, in M. G. Baldini and S. Ebbe (eds.), "Platelets: Production, Function, Transfusion, and Storage," Grune & Stratton, Inc., New York, 1974.

Baldini, M.: Idiopathic Thrombocytopenic Purpura, *N Engl J Med,* **274:**1245, 1966.

Biggs, R., and Macfarlane, R. G.: "Human Blood Coagulation and Its Disorders," 3d ed., F. A. Davis Company, Philadelphia, 1962.

Breckenridge, R. T., and Ratnoff, O. D.: Therapy of Hereditary Disorders of Blood Coagulation, *Mod Treat,* **5:**39, 1968.

Curtiss, P. H., Jr.: Orthopedic Management of Patients with Hereditary Disorders of Blood Coagulation, *Mod Treat,* **5:**84, 1968.

Griner, P. F.: Drug Effects on Oral Anticoagulants, in R. L. Weed (ed.), "Hematology for Internists," Little, Brown and Company, Boston, 1971.

Hardaway, R. M., III: Disseminated Intravascular Coagulation, *Thromb Diath Haemorrh [Suppl],* **56:**207, 1971.

Hoak, J. C., and Koepke, J. A.: Platelet transfusions, in "Clinics in Hematology," W. B. Saunders Company, Philadelphia, 1976.

Hougie, C.: "Fundamentals of Blood Coagulation in Clinical Medicine," McGraw-Hill Book Company, New York, 1963.

Hoyer, L. W.: Disseminated Intravascular Coagulation, in R. L.

Weed (ed.), "Hematology for Internists," Little, Brown and Company, Boston, 1971.

Klingensmith, W.: Surgical Implications of Hemorrhage during Anticoagulant Therapy, *Surg Gynecol Obstet,* **125:**1333, 1967.

Norman, J. C., Covelli, V. H. and Sise, H. S.: Experimental Transplantation of the Spleen for Classical Hemophilia: A Rationale and Long-Term Results, *Bibl Haematol,* **34:**187, 1970.

Prentice, C. R. M., and Ratnoff, O. D.: Genetic Disorders of Blood Coagulation, *Semin Hematol,* **4:**93, 1967.

Ratnoff, O. D.: Hereditary Disorders of Hemostasis, in J. B. Stanbury, J. B. Wyngaarden, and D. S. Fredrickson, "The Metabolic Basis of Inherited Disease," 2d ed., McGraw-Hill Book Company, New York, 1966.

————: An approach to the Diagnosis of Disorders of Hemostasis, *Mod Treat,* **5:**11, 1968.

Rizza, C. R.: Coagulation Factor Therapy, in "Clinics in Hematology," W. B. Saunders Company, Philadelphia, 1976.

Schwartz, S. I.: Myeloproliferative Disorders. *Ann Surg,* **182**(4):464, 1975.

Sherry, S.: Urokinase, *Ann Intern Med,* **69:**415, 1968.

Shulman, N. R.: Surgical Care of Patients with Hereditary Disorders of Blood Coagulation, *Mod Treat,* **5:**61, 1968.

Smith, W. W.: Bleeding Disorders in Surgical Patients, *Monogr Surg Sci,* **1:**3, 1964.

Stableforth, P., Hughes, J., Wilson, E., and Dormandy, K.: The von Willebrand Syndrome, *Br J Haematol,* **29:**605, 1975.

Wasserman, L. R., and Gilbert, H. S.: Polycythemia Vera and Myeloid Metaplasia, in A. W. Ulin and S. S. Gollub (eds.), "Surgical Bleeding: Handbook for Medicine, Surgery, and Specialties," McGraw-Hill Book Company, New York, 1966.

Webster, W. P., Zukoski, C. F., Hutchin, P., Reddick, R. L., Mandel, S. R., and Penick, G. D.: Plasma Factor VIII Synthesis and Control as Revealed by Canine Organ Transplantation, *Amer J Physiol,* **220:**1147, 1971.

Yankee, R. A.: HL-A Antigens and Platelet Therapy, in M. G. Baldini and S. Ebbe (eds.), "Platelets: Production, Function, Transfusion, and Storage," Grune & Stratton, Inc., New York, 1974.

Local Hemostasis

Abbott, W., and Austen, W. G.: The Effectiveness and Mechanism of Collagen-Induced Topical Hemostasis, *Surgery,* **78:**723, 1975.

Cushing, H.: The Control of Bleeding in Operations for Brain Tumor, *Ann Surg,* **54:**1, 1911.

Hait, M. R.: Microcrystalline Collagen: A New Hemostatic Agent, *Am J Surg,* **120:**330, 1970.

Halsted, W. S.: The Employment of Fine Silk in Preference to Catgut and the Advantages of Transfixing Tissues and Vessels in Controlling Hemorrhage, *JAMA,* **60:**1119, 1913.

Hinman, F., and Babcock, K. O.: Local Reaction to Oxidized Cellulose and Gelatin Hemostatic Agents in Experimentally Contaminated Renal Wounds, *Surgery,* **26:**633, 1949.

Jenkins, H. P., and Clarke, J. S.: Gelatin Sponge: A New Hemostatic Substance, *Arch Surg,* **51:**253, 1945.

Just-Viera, J. O., Puron-Del Aquila, R., and Yeager, G. H.: Control of Hemorrhage from the Liver without the Use of Sutures or Clamps: Preliminary Report, *Am Surg,* **28:**11, 1962.

Lindstrom, P. A.: Complications from the Use of Absorbable Sponges, *Arch Surg,* **73:**133, 1956.

Ravitch, M. M., Steichen, F. M., Fishbein, R. H., Knowles, P. W., and Weil, P.: Clinical Experiences with the Soviet Mechanical Bronchus Stapler (UKB-25), *J Thorac Cardiovasc Surg,* **47:**446, 1964.

Sawyer, P. N., and Wesolowski, S. A.: Electrical Hemostasis, in Conference on Bleeding in the Surgical Patient, *Ann NY Acad Sci,* **115:**455, 1964.

Schechter, D. S.: History of the Evolution of Methods of Hemostasis and the Study of Blood Coagulation, in A. W. Ulin and S. S. Gollub (eds.), "Surgical Bleeding: Handbook for Medicine, Surgery, and Specialties," McGraw-Hill Book Company, New York, 1966.

Schwartz, S. I., Muyshondt, E., and Penn, I.: Isotopic Evaluation of Bioelectric Factors Affecting Thrombogenesis, in Philip N. Sawyer (ed.), "Biophysical Mechanisms in Vascular Homeostasis and Intravascular Thrombosis," Appleton-Century Crofts, Inc., New York, 1965.

Silverstein, F. E., Auth, D. C., Rubin, C. E., and Protell, R. L.: High Power Argon Lazer Treatment Via Standard Endoscope. I. A Preliminary Study of Efficacy in Control of Experimental Erosive Bleeding, *Gastroenterology,* **71:**558, 1976.

Waltz, J. M., and Cooper, I. S.: Cryogenic Surgery, in A. W. Ulin and S. S. Gollub (eds.), "Surgical Bleeding: Handbook for Medicine, Surgery, and Specialties," McGraw-Hill Book Company, New York, 1966.

Wangensteen, S. L., Orahood, R. C., Voorhees, A. B., Smith, R. B., III, and Healey, W. V.: Intragastric Cooling in the Management of Hemorrhage from the Upper Gastrointestinal Tract, *Am J Surg,* **105:**401, 1963.

Willman, V. L., and Hanlon, C. R.: The Influence of Temperature on Surface Bleeding: Favorable Effects of Local Hypothermia, *Ann Surg,* **143:**660, 1956.

Transfusion

Aggeler, P. M.: Physiological Basis for Transfusion Therapy in Hemorrhagic Disorders: A Critical Review, *Transfusion,* **1:**71, 1961.

American Medical Association Committee on Blood: Single Unit Transfusions, *JAMA,* **189:**955, 1964.

Barry, K. G., and Crosby, W. H.: The Prevention and Treatment of Renal Failure following Transfusion Reactions, *Transfusion,* **3:**34, 1963.

Bennett, S. H., Geelhoed, G. W., Gralnick, H. R., and Hoye, R. C.: Effects of Autotransfusion on Blood Elements, *Am J Surg,* **125:**273, 1973.

Blakeley, W. R., Bennett, L. R., and Maloney, J. V., Jr.: An Evaluation of Preoperative Blood Volume Determination in the Debilitated Surgical Patient, *Surg Gynecol Obstet,* **115:**257, 1962.

Braude, A. I.: Transfusion Reactions from Contaminated Blood: Their Recognition and Treatment, *N Engl J Med,* **258:**1289, 1958.

Brzica, S. M., Pineda, A. A., and Taswell, H. F.: Autologous Blood Transfusion, *Mayo Clin Proc,* **51:**723, 1976.

Bunker, J. P., Stetson, J. B., Coe, R. C., Grillo, H. C., and Murphy, A. J.: Citric Acid Intoxication, *JAMA,* **157:**1361, 1955.

Caceres, E., and Whittembury, G.: Evaluation of Blood Losses during Surgical Operations: Comparison of the Gravimetric Method with the Blood Volume Determination, *Surgery,* **45:**681, 1959.

Carter, J. F. B.: Reduction in Thrombophlebitis by Limiting Duration of Intravenous Infusions, *Lancet,* **2:**20, 1951.

Case, R. B., Sarnoff, S. J., Waithe, P. E., and Sarnoff, L. C.: Intra-arterial and Intravenous Blood Infusions in Hemorrhagic Shock: Comparison of Effects on Coronary Blood Flow and Arterial Pressure, *JAMA,* **152:**208, 1953.

Chaplin, H., Jr., Brittingham, T. E., and Cassell, M.: Methods for Preparation of Suspensions of Buffy Coat–poor Red Blood Cells for Transfusion, including a Report of 50 Transfusions of Suspensions of Buffy Coat–poor Red Blood Cells Prepared by a Dextran Sedimentation Method, *Am J Clin Pathol,* **31:**373, 1959.

Collins, J. A.: Massive Blood Transfusions, in "Clinics in Hematology," W. B. Saunders Company, Philadelphia, 1976.

Durant, T. M., Oppenheimer, M. J., Lynch, P. R., Ascanio, G., and Webber, D.: Body Position in Relation to Venous Air Embolism: A Roentgenologic Study, *Am J Med Sci,* **277:**509, 1954.

Ebert, R. V., Stead, E. A., and Gibson, J. G.: Response of Normal Subjects to Acute Blood Loss, with Special Reference to the Mechanism of Restoration of Blood Volume, *Arch Intern Med,* **68:**578, 1941.

Gollub, S., and Bailey, C. P.: Management of Major Surgical Blood Loss without Transfusion, *JAMA,* **198:**1171, 1966.

Grady, G. F., Chalmers, T. C., and the Boston Inter-Hospital Liver Group: Risk of Post-transfusion Viral Hepatitis, *N Engl J Med,* **271:**337, 1964.

Grossman, E. B., Stewart, S. G., and Stokes, J. S., Jr.: Post-transfusion Hepatitis in Battle Casualties: A Study of Its Prophylaxis by Means of Human Immune Serum Globulin, *JAMA,* **129:**991, 1945.

Hoff, H. E., and Guillemin, R.: The Tercentenary of Transfusion in Man, *Cardiovasc Res Cent Bull,* **6:**47, 1967.

Holland, P. V., Rubinson, R. M., Morrow, A. G., and Schmidt, P. J.: Gamma Globulin in the Prophylaxis of Post-transfusion Hepatitis, *JAMA,* **196:**471, 1966.

Howland, W. S., Schweizer, O., and Boyan, O. P.: The Effect of Buffering on the Mortality of Massive Blood Replacement, *Surg Gynecol Obstet,* **121:**777, 1965.

Huggins, C. E: Frozen Blood: Principles of Practical Preservation, *Monogr Surg Sci,* **3:**133, 1966.

Ingram, G. I. C.: The Bleeding Complications of Blood Transfusion, *Transfusion,* **5:**1, 1965.

Johnson, S. A., and Greenwalt, T. J.: "Coagulation and Transfusion in Clinical Medicine," Little, Brown and Company, Boston, 1965.

Katz, R., Rodriguez, J., and Ward, R.: Posttransfusion Hepatitis: Effect of Modified Gamma-Globulin Added to Blood In Vitro, *N Engl J Med,* **285:**925, 1971.

Kliman, A.: Complications of Massive Blood Replacement, *NY State J Med,* **65:**239, 1965.

Krevans, J. R., and Jackson, D. P.: Hemorrhagic Disorder following Massive Whole Blood Tranfusions, *JAMA,* **159:**171, 1955.

Krugman, S., Giles, J. P., and Hammond, J.: Viral Hepatitis, Type B (MS-2 Strain): Prevention with Specific Hepatitis B Immune Serum Globulin, *JAMA,* **218:**1665, 1971.

Lalich, J. J., and Schwartz, S. I.: The Role of Aciduria in the Development of Hemoglobinuric Nephrosis in Dehydrated Rabbits, *J Exp Med,* **92:**11, 1950.

Langdell, R. D., Adelson, E., Furth, F. W., and Crosby, W. H.: Dextran and Prolonged Bleeding Time: Results of a Sixty-Gram, One-Liter Infusion Given to One Hundred and Sixty-three Normal Human Subjects, *JAMA,* **162:**346, 1958.

Lehane, D., Kwantes, C. M. S., Upward, M. G., and Thomson, D. R.: Homologous Serum Jaundice, *Br Med J,* **2:**572, 1949.

Luscher, E. F.: Biochemical Basis of Platelet Function, in K. M. Brinkhous, R. W. Shermer, and F. K. Mostofi (eds.), "The Platelet," The Williams & Wilkins Company, Baltimore, 1971.

MacCallum, F. O., McFarlan, A. M., Miles, J. A. R., Pollock, M. R., and Wilson, C.: Infective Hepatitis: Studies in E. Anglia during the Period 1943-7, *Med Res Counc Spec Rep Ser (Lond),* no. **273,** 1951.

Macon, W. L., and Pories, W. J.: The Effect of Iron Deficiency Anemia on Wound Healing, *Surgery,* **69:**792, 1971.

Maloney, J. V., Jr., Smythe, C. McC., Gilmore, J. P., and Handford, S. W.: Intra-arterial and Intravenous Transfusion, *Surg Gynecol Obstet,* **97:**529, 1953.

McNair, T. J., and Dudley, H. A. F.: The Local Complications of Intravenous Therapy, *Lancet,* **2:**365, 1959.

Med Lett Drugs Ther, vol. 9, no. 22, issue 230, Nov. 3, 1967.

Mollison, P. L.: "Blood Transfusion in Clinical Medicine," 4th ed., F. A. Davis Company, Philadelphia, 1967.

Morton, J. H.: Surgical Transfusion Practices, 1967, *Surgery,* **65:**407, 1969.

Moyer, C.: "Conference on Blood Groups and Blood Transfusion," Better Bellevue Association, New York, 1967.

Perrault, R., Jackson, J. R., Martin-Villar, J., and Smiley, R. K.: Experience with the Use of Frozen Blood, *Can Med Assoc J,* **96:**1504, 1967.

Peskin, G. W., O'Brien, K., and Rabiner, S. F.: Stroma-free Hemoglobin Solution: The "Ideal" Blood Substitute? *Surgery,* **66:**185, 1969.

Phillipps, E., and Fleischner, F. G.: Pulmonary Edema in the Course of a Blood Transfusion without Overloading the Circulation, *Dis Chest,* **50:**619, 1966.

Pruitt, B. A., Jr., Moncrief, J. A., and Mason, A. D., Jr.: Efficacy of Buffered Saline as the Sole Replacement Fluid following Acute Measured Hemorrhage in Man, *J Trauma,* **7:**767, 1967.

Reece, R. L., and Beckett, R. S.: Epidemiology of Single-Unit Transfusion: A One-Year Experience in a Community Hospital, *JAMA,* **195:**801, 1966.

Rigor, B., Bosomworth, P., and Rush, B. F., Jr.: Replacement of Operative Blood Loss of More than One Liter with Hartmann's Solution, *JAMA,* **203:**399, 1968.

Rudowski, W. J.: Complications Associated with Blood Transfusion, in M. Allgower, S.-E. Bergentz, R. Y. Calne, and U. F. Gruber (eds.), "Progress in Surgery," S. Karger, New York, 1971.

Schwartz, S. I., Adams, J. T., and Bauman, A. W.: Splenectomy for Hematologic Disorders, *Curr Probl Surg,* The Year Book Medical Publishers, Inc., Chicago, May, 1971.

Shields, C. E., Dennis, L. H., Eichelberger, J. W., and Conrad, M. E.: The Rapid Infusion of Large Quantities of ACD Adenine Solution into Humans, *Transfusion,* **7:**133, 1967.

Shires, T., Coln, D., Carrico, J., and Lightfoot, S.: Fluid Therapy in Hemorrhagic Shock, *Arch Surg,* **88:**688, 1964.

Strumia, M. M., Crosby, W. H., Gibson, J. G., II, Greenwalt, T. J., and Krevans, J. R.: "General Principles of Blood Transfusion," J. B. Lippincott Company, Philadelphia, 1963.

Tiber, L. J.: Ruptured Ectopic Pregnancy, *Calif Med,* **41:**16, 1934.

Tocantis, L. M., and O'Neill, J. F.: Infusion of Blood and Other Fluids into the General Circulation via the Bone Marrow: Technique and Results, *Surg Gynecol Obstet,* **73:**281, 1941.

Transfusion of Blood Components, *Med Lett Drugs Ther,* **9:**85, 1967.

Wallace, J.: Blood Transfusion and Transmissible Disease, in "Clinics in Hematology," W. B. Saunders Company, Philadelphia, 1976.

Wallace, J. M., and Henry, J. B.: Isoimmunization after Massive Transfusion for Open Heart Surgery, *Transfusion,* **5:**153, 1965.

Walter, C. W.: Blood Donors, Blood and Transfusion, in J. M. Kinney, R. H. Egdahl, and G. D. Zuidema (eds.), "Manual of Preoperative and Postoperative Care," W. B. Saunders Company, Philadelphia, 1971.

Waterman, D. F., Birkhill, F. R., Pirani, C. L., and Levenson, S. M.: The Healing of Wounds in the Presence of Anemia, *Surgery,* **31:**821, 1952.

Wilson, R. F., Bassett, J. S., and Walt, A. J.: Five Years Experience with Massive Blood Transfusions, *JAMA,* **194:**851, 1965.

Young, L. E.: Complications of Blood Transfusion, *Ann Intern Med,* **61:**136, 1964.

Chapter 4

Shock

by **G. Tom Shires, Peter C. Canizaro, and C. James Carrico**

CLINICAL MANIFESTATIONS OF SHOCK

Classification; Clinical and Physiologic Manifestations of Shock

DEFINITION AND WORKING CLASSIFICATION

The scope of modern medicine is increasing steadily. As understanding of physiologic and biochemical derange-ments is broadened, so is the horizon of possibilities for the relief of illness. As more seriously ill patients are pre-sented, the symptom complex of shock is more frequently encountered by the physician.

Although shock has been recognized for over 100 years, a clear definition and dissection of this complex and dev-astating state has emerged only slowly. Many attempts have been made over the years to define adequately the entity known as shock. In 1872 the elder Gross defined shock as a "manifestation of the rude unhinging of the machinery of life." Although the accuracy of this definition is unquestioned, it is obviously far from precise. In 1942 Wiggers, on the basis of an exhaustive examination of available evidence at that time, offered the definition: "Shock is a syndrome resulting from a depression of many functions, but in which reduction of the effective circulat-ing blood volume is of basic importance, and in which impairment of the circulation steadily progresses until it eventuates in a state of irreversible circulatory failure." Blalock offered the definition in 1940: "Shock is a periph-eral circulatory failure, resulting from a discrepancy in the size of the vascular bed and the volume of the intravascular fluid." A more modern definition has been devised by Simeone, who stated that shock may be defined as "a clinical condition characterized by signs and symptoms which arise when the cardiac output is insufficient to fill the arterial tree with blood under sufficient pressure to provide organs and tissues with adequate blood flow."

Shock of all forms appears to be invariably related to inadequate tissue perfusion. The low-flow state in vital organs seems to be the final common denominator in all forms of shock.

For purposes of a working clinical classification, the etiologic classification offered by Blalock in 1934 is still a useful and functional one. Blalock suggested four cate-gories:

1. Hematogenic (oligemic)
2. Neurogenic (caused primarily by nervous influences)
3. Vasogenic (initially decreased vascular resistance and increased vascular capacity)
4. Cardiogenic
   a. Failure of the heart as a pump
   b. Unclassified category (including diminished cardiac output from various causes)

It is now clear that shock invariably results from one or more of four separate but interrelated dysfunctions, in-volving (1) the pump (heart), (2) the fluid which is pumped (blood volume), (3) the arteriolar resistance vessels, and

(4) the capacity of the venous vessels. These dysfunctions may be correlated as follows with Blalock's etiologic classification:

1. Cardiogenic shock implies failure of the heart as a pump and may be brought about by primary myocardial dysfunction from myocardial infarction, serious cardiac arrhythmias, or a variety of causes resulting in myocardial depression; or by miscellaneous causes, including mechanical restriction of cardiac function or venous obstruction such as occurs in the mediastinum with tension pneumothorax, vena cava obstruction, or cardiac tamponade.

2. Reduction in blood volume may take the form of loss of whole blood, of plasma, or of extracellular fluid in the extravascular space or a combination of these three.

3. Changes in arterial resistance or venous capacity may be brought about by specific disorders. A decrease in resistance may result from spinal anesthesia or from neurogenic reflexes, as in acute pain, or may accompany the end stages of hypovolemic shock. Septic shock may produce changes in peripheral arterial resistance and in venous capacity, as well as peripheral arteriovenous shunting.

Therapy of shock will obviously revolve around the etiologic type or combination of types of shock present in a given patient who has undergone trauma.

CLINICAL MANIFESTATIONS

The signs and symptoms of hypovolemic shock, when they are well established, are classic and usually easy to recognize. Most of the signs of clinical shock are characteristic of low peripheral blood flow and are contributed to by the effects of excess adrenosympathetic activity. The signs and symptoms of human shock, according to the severity of the shock, were well described by Beecher et al., as summarized in Table 4-1.

On first inspection the patient in shock presents an anxious, tired expression, which early is that of restlessness and anxiety and later becomes a picture of apathy or exhaustion. Typically, the skin feels cool and is pale and mottled, and there is evidence of decreased capillary flow exhibited by easy blanching of the skin, particularly the nail beds.

There are varying discrepancies in the classic picture of shock. In neurogenic shock, particularly that in response to spinal anesthesia, the pulse rate is normal or, more often, decreased; the pulse pressure is wide, and the pulse feels strong rather than weak. The rapid pulse characteristic of early hemorrhagic or wound shock may be absent, even if the patient has lost blood rapidly. This is also true if the position is supine or prone, in which case a rapid pulse may not appear until the patient is moved or elevated to a sitting position. The varying clinical picture in septic shock is discussed subsequently.

In observing a large number of patients in hemorrhagic hypovolemic shock, one sees remarkably varied but typical responses of the sensorium to the shock episode. Most young, healthy patients who sustain wound or hemorrhagic shock, when seen early after the wounding, will appear to be restless and anxious and give the appearance of great fear. Shortly after being seen by a physician and started on treatment, this restlessness frequently gives way to great apathy and the patient appears sleepy. When aroused, he may complain of weakness or of a chilly sensation, although he does not actually have a chill. If blood loss is unchecked, the patient's apathy and sleepiness will rapidly progress into coma. In treating a large number of accident victims, it has been our experience that a patient who has bled into frank coma from which he cannot be aroused, resulting simply from blood loss alone (unassociated with other injuries such as brain damage), has usually sustained lethal blood loss. This sign usually indicates rapid massive hemorrhage for which compensations are inadequate to maintain sufficient cerebral blood flow to sustain consciousness.

Another characteristic of the wounded person, described

Table 4-1. GRADING OF SHOCK

Degree of shock	Blood pressure (approx.)	Skin				Thirst	Mental state
		Pulse quality	Temperature	Color	Circulation (response to pressure blanching)		
None	Normal	Normal	Normal	Normal	Normal	Normal	Clear and distressed
Slight	To 20% increase	Normal	Cool	Pale	Definite slowing	Normal	Clear and distressed
Moderate . . .	Decreased 20–40%	Definite decrease in volume	Cool	Pale	Definite slowing	Definite	Clear and some apathy unless stimulated
Severe	Decreased 40% to nonrecordable	Weak to imperceptible	Cold	Ashen to cyanotic (mottling)	Very sluggish	Severe	Apathethic to comatose, little distress except thirst

SOURCE: H. K. Beecher, F. A. Simeone, C. H. Burnett, S. L. Shapiro, E. R. Sullivan, and T. B. Mallory, The Internal State of the Severely Wounded Man on Entry to the Most Forward Hospital, *Surgery,* **22:**672, 1947.

by many investigators, is thirst. Thirst seems to be a characteristic of the injured person and is found in most emergency room patients brought in acutely ill from trauma with or without shock. The studies carried out to elucidate the nature of the thirst are many and varied. Most of these patients have intense adrenal medullary stimulation from trauma, not necessarily accompanied by shock. Consequently caution must be used in allowing water, since dangerous water intoxication may be induced by this intense stimulus to imbibe liquids in the face of altered renal function.

Another characteristic of the patient in hemorrhagic shock is the low peripheral venous pressure, manifested on inspection by empty peripheral veins. Indeed, the starting of a simple intravenous infusion in a patient in hemorrhagic shock can be quite difficult. Obviously there are exceptions, such as shock due to cardiac tamponade, in which there is restriction to inflow of blood to the right side of the heart. In this instance the peripheral veins, including the neck veins, are distended.

Nausea and vomiting from hypovolemic shock are common. It is true that other causes should be sought for, but shock alone may be first manifested in this manner.

Another classic finding in hemorrhagic hypovolemia is a fall in body "core" temperature. Whether this is due to a lowered metabolic rate or to lower perfusion in areas where body temperature is measured is debatable.

PHYSIOLOGIC CHANGES

BLOOD PRESSURE. Arterial blood pressure is normally maintained by the cardiac output and the peripheral vascular resistance. Thus, when the cardiac output is reduced because of loss of intravascular volume, the blood pressure may remain normal so long as the total peripheral vascular resistance can be increased to compensate for the reduction in cardiac output. The vascular resistance varies for different organs and in different parts of the same organ, depending on the local conditions that determine the state of vasoconstriction or vasodilatation at the time of the loss of intravascular volume. An example of the differential increase in peripheral resistance with reduction in cardiac output is seen in the change in distributional total blood flow to organs such as the heart and the brain, as opposed to that of most other organs which are not essential for immediate survival. In hemorrhagic shock the heart may receive 25 percent of the total cardiac output, as opposed to the normal 5 to 8 percent. The great increase in peripheral resistance in such organs as the skin and the kidney causes significant reduction in flow in these organs while providing a lifesaving diversion of the cardiac output to the brain and the heart. Consequently the blood pressure may not fall until the reduction in cardiac output or loss of blood volume is so great that the adaptive homeostatic mechanisms can no longer compensate for the reduced volume. As the deficit continues, however, there is a progressive hypotension.

PULSE RATE. Characteristically, reduction of the volume in the vascular tree is associated with tachycardia. A fall in pressure within the great vessels results in excitation of the adrenosympathetic division of the autonomic nervous system and, simultaneously, inhibition of the vagal-medullary center (Marey's reflex). Consequently, with hemorrhage or loss of circulating blood volume, the resulting fall in arterial blood pressure should cause an increase in heart rate.

This compensatory mechanism, however, is variable in its effectiveness. Obviously, the degree of loss of intravascular volume, the amount of reduction in venous return, and other variables such as ventricular function may markedly influence the ability of Marey's reflex to compensate for the reduction in blood volume. Work with slow hemorrhage in normal healthy volunteers by Shenkin et al. has shown that, as long as the supine position is maintained, as much as 1000 ml of blood may be lost without significant increase in pulse rate. Similarly, the pacemaker system of the heart within the sinoatrial node is obviously influenced by other stimuli, such as fear and anxiety, that may also accompany the trauma producing the loss of intravascular volume.

Consequently, during the course of observation and treatment of shock, changes in pulse rate are of value only when followed over an extended period. Change in pulse rate may indicate response to therapy once other external sources that may have changed cardiac rate are diminished or removed.

VASOCONSTRICTION. Increase in peripheral vascular resistance by production of peripheral vasoconstriction rapidly becomes maximal in an effort to compensate for the reduced cardiac output. Vascular resistance can be measured only indirectly in human beings and in animals. There is good evidence that early disproportionate reduction in vascular resistance in the heart occurs while there is still little change in vascular resistance in many organs. Subsequently, maximal vasoconstriction occurs in the skin, kidneys, liver, and finally, the brain. Concomitantly, there is generalized constriction of the veins in response to reduction in intravascular volume. Venoconstriction is a necessary homeostatic mechanism, since over half the total blood volume may be contained within the venous tree.

These vascular responses to hemorrhage are immediate and striking. Within seconds following the onset of hemorrhage there are unequivocal signs of sympathetic and adrenal activation. Serum catecholamine levels show prompt elevation, indicative of action of the adrenal medullary function. The adrenal cortical and pituitary hormones also show prompt increase in serum levels following shock. Many of the clinical signs associated with shock are simply signs of response of the sympathetic and adrenal medullary system to the insult sustained by the organism.

HEMODILUTION. All the responses to reduction of intravascular volume eventually result in decreased flow to tissues and initiation of compensatory mechanisms directed at correction of the low-flow state. One such compensation is movement of fluid into the circulation, resulting in hemodilution. This fluid, commonly known as extracellular fluid, has the composition of plasma but a lower protein content.

It is now clear, however, that the hematocrit reading, or hemoglobin concentration, in shock is simply an index of the balance between the amount of whole blood or plasma lost and the amount of extravascular extracellular fluid gained. For example, in hemorrhagic hypovolemia there is generally progressive hemodilution, which increases with the severity of the shock state. Obviously, in this circumstance there has been a greater movement of fluid from the extravascular to the intravascular space with progression of the shock. This is in contradistinction to shock associated with loss of intravascular volume due primarily to plasma loss. High-hematocrit shock may occur with massive losses of plasma and extravascular extracellular fluid, such as is associated with peritonitis, burns, large areas of soft tissue infection, and the crush syndrome.

The mechanism of hemodilution following hemorrhage is probably on the basis of the Starling hypothesis: that is, the reduction in hydrostatic pressure in the capillaries because of hypotension and arterial and arteriolar vasoconstriction results in a shift of the pressure gradient to favor the passage of fluid from the tissue extracellular space into the intravascular capillary bed.

It is worthy of note that the studies of Carey et al. do not demonstrate a significant reduction in serum protein content in patients following hemorrhagic shock and resuscitation.

BIOCHEMICAL CHANGES

The biochemically measurable changes that occur as a response to the stress invoked by shock fall into three fairly well-defined categories. These are (1) the changes invoked by the pituitary-adrenal response to stress, (2) the changes brought about by a net reduction in organ perfusion imposed by a low rate of blood flow, and (3) the changes brought about by failing function within specific organs.

PITUITARY-ADRENAL. The immediate effects seen from adrenosympathetic activity are those associated with high circulating epinephrine levels. Characteristically, these include eosinopenia and lymphocytopenia along with thrombocytopenia. This doubtless represents the laboratory reflection of increased circulating epinephrine that can be measured and has been found to be elevated as an early response to shock. These changes are nonspecific and are found early in a patient with shock or severe trauma. The phenomena usually disappear rapidly. Other evidences of the pituitary and hormonal response to shock are seen in the well-known stress reaction or metabolic responses so well described by Moore. These include a striking negative nitrogen balance and retention of sodium and water, as well as a notable increase in the excretion of potassium.

LOW-FLOW STATE. Those changes incident to the low rate of blood flow during shock are now becoming better understood. More evidence is accumulating to support the observation that, as a result of a decreased blood flow or low rate of perfusion, there is a reduction in oxygen delivered to the vital organs and, consequently, a mandatory change in metabolism from aerobic to anaerobic. In the switch from aerobic to anaerobic metabolism, energy made available by the oxidation of glucose is greatly reduced during shock. The most striking example of a shift in

metabolism is the production of lactic acid as the end product instead of the normal aerobic end product, carbon dioxide. This is reflected in a metabolic acidosis with a reduction in the carbon dioxide–combining power of the blood. The available buffer base is progressively decreased by combining with the increased lactic acid, and the respiratory compensation that occurs early in the course of hemorrhagic shock is frequently inadequate. Consequently the progressive decline in pH toward a striking acidosis is thereby hastened. Indeed, in several studies the ability of animals as well as human beings to recover from shock has been found to correlate rather closely with the degree of lactic acid production and the decrease in the alkali reserve and pH of the blood.

In some cases determination of blood pH may not accurately reflect changes in pH at the cellular level. After the induction of hemorrhagic shock in experimental animals, skeletal muscle surface pH changes precede those in blood, and minimal changes may be masked by the efficient blood buffer systems. Lactate and excess lactate levels correlate well with the clinical impression of the depth of shock, but the injuries producing the shock state have a much greater bearing on ultimate prognosis.

Drucker has pointed out that there is a consistent elevation of the blood sugar level in relation to the degree of blood loss and the severity of shock. This was earlier observed in battle casualties studied in World War II and has since been thoroughly confirmed by Simeone and others. It is Drucker's belief that this represents an increase in hepatic glycolysis in the change from aerobic or anaerobic metabolism, while Egdahl believes that there is decreased insulin secretion and decreased peripheral utilization of glucose.

Other evidences of failure of different parameters of cell metabolism have been presented by Thal, Schumer, Mela and Baue.

ORGAN FAILURE. The biochemical changes that appear incident to organ failure seem to be dependent in large part on the duration and severity of the shock. The changes in renal function induced by hypovolemia may vary from simple oliguria with a concentrated and acid urine to high-output renal failure with a urine of low specific gravity and high pH, or frank anuric renal failure. Similarly, the blood nonprotein nitrogen content depends on the degree of impairment in renal function. This may vary from slight or no retention of nitrogenous products to a steep and progressive rise that may require therapy.

Changes in ion concentration, including a rise of serum potassium, are dependent on many things, among them adrenal cortical response, the change in metabolism from aerobic to anaerobic with resultant release of potassium, and specific changes within tissues invoked by the shock. If renal function is maintained, the rise inevitably seen in serum potassium soon after the onset of shock is short-lived, in that the renal excretion of potassium is high during recovery from hemorrhagic shock. If renal function is impaired, the concentration of potassium and magnesium as well as creatine can rise to high levels in the serum.

PATHOPHYSIOLOGIC RESPONSES TO SHOCK

Experimental Studies of the Response of Extracellular Fluid

EARLY RESULTS

Hypovolemic shock is the most common form seen clinically and is also the form that has been studied most intensively both clinically and in the laboratory. Most of our own studies have been carried out using hypovolemic shock produced by external blood loss as the model. A method has been developed which allows the simultaneous measurement of total-body red cell mass with the use of ^{51}Cr-tagged red blood cells and total-body plasma volume with the use of ^{131}I-tagged and, later, ^{125}I-tagged human serum albumin. In addition, total-body extracellular fluid can be measured simultaneously with the use of ^{35}S-tagged sodium sulfate. The three isotopes are simultaneously injected intravenously, and with the use of appropriate energy-differentiating counting instruments, all three isotopes can be traced after equilibration. Volumes are then determined by the dilution principle, using multiple sampling.

In an early study the three volumes were measured; splenectomized dogs were then bled a sublethal, subshock amount of 10 percent of the measured blood volume. After hemorrhage the three volumes were again measured. The loss of the amount of red blood cells and plasma removed during the hemorrhage could be detected by the method described. It was shown that the decrease in extracellular fluid volume was only the amount lost as plasma removed during the hemorrhage.

By use of the same model, volumes were measured before and after hemorrhage of 25 percent of the measured blood volume. This hemorrhage was again sublethal but produced hypotension. In this group of animals also the loss of the amount of red blood cells and plasma removed could be detected. In addition, however, the functional extracellular fluid volume as measured by the ^{35}S-tagged sodium sulfate was found to have decreased by 18 to 26 percent of the original volume. Since there was no measurable external loss of ^{35}S sulfate, this reduction was presumed to be an internal redistribution of extracellular fluid. Subsequent studies of external bleeding of 35, 45, and even over 50 percent hemorrhage always produced the same reduction in functional extracellular fluid as long as the animal was in shock.

In subsequent studies, splenectomized dogs were subjected to "irreversible" hemorrhagic shock according to a modified method of Wiggers, which utilizes a reservoir. Return of shed blood in this severe preparation resulted in the return of blood pressure to near control levels, followed by a fall in blood pressure within 1 to 16 hours; death resulted in 80 percent of the dogs, i.e., a standard mortality rate.

In one group of animals the three volumes were measured and the dogs were then subjected to shock by the Wiggers method. The three volumes were remeasured by reinjection during the period of shock; then shed blood was returned. The decrease in blood volume was the amount which had been removed. Concurrently, the functional extracellular fluid exhibited a decided reduction. Immediately after the return of the shed blood, the red cell mass returned to essentially normal levels, as did the plasma volume; however, there remained a deficit of functional extracellular fluid. In dogs treated with shed blood plus plasma (10 ml/kg), the losses during shock were again similar. After therapy with plasma, plus return of shed blood, there was a return of blood volume to normal. There remained, however, a decrease in functional extracellular fluid volume.

Dogs treated with an extracellular "mimic," such as a balanced salt solution plus shed blood, had comparable losses during shock. As in the previous groups, the blood volume returned essentially to normal after treatment. But dogs treated with salt solution plus shed blood exhibited return of functional extracellular fluid volume to control levels.

In this study only 20 percent of those dogs treated with shed blood alone survived longer than 24 hours. When plasma was used in addition to whole blood as therapy, 30 percent of the dogs survived. Of the animals treated with lactated Ringer's solution plus shed blood, 70 percent survived (Fig. 4-1). The 80 percent mortality rate of a standard "irreversible" shock preparation was reduced to 30 percent by restoration of functional extracellular fluid volume in addition to return of shed blood.

All these early studies of the measurement of the functional extracellular fluid were based on volume distribution curves of sulfate measured for approximately 1 hour. At any point in the course of the curve there is a reduction in extracellular fluid in the untreated state of shock. Subsequent work has continued these volume distribution curves for many hours. In true untreated hemorrhagic shock there is a reduction in the total extracellular fluid, or final diluted volume of radiosulfate, when compared with preshock volumes (Fig. 4-2).

Even when a less severe shock preparation is used, there is still a reduction in early equilibrating extracellular fluid or early available extracellular fluid, whereas the total anatomic extracellular fluid may remain normal. Subsequent studies have shown that if shock is not of sufficient duration to produce reduction in both functional and total extracellular fluid, the reduction may be only in functional extracellular fluid. Furthermore, if therapy is instituted quickly and blood pressure is returned to normal, a long sulfate equilibration curve may fail to reveal the acute reduction which was corrected early.

Consequently, the current status of sulfate as a measure of the functional extracellular fluid must be interpreted as indicating that early sulfate volume measurement reveals functional or available extracellular fluid and that prolonged measurement of the volume distribution curves gives total extracellular fluid values. If therapy has been instituted or has been completed, then the reduction in

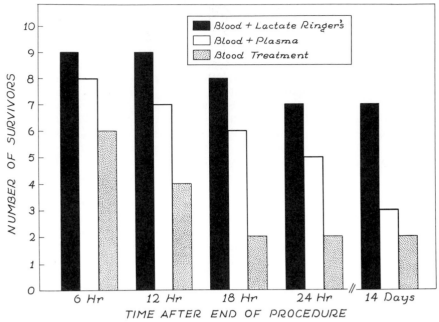

Fig. 4-1. Acute hemorrhagic shock: survival study.

total or even in the available extracellular fluid may not be measurable.

Unquestionably, some plasma, or transcapillary, refilling occurs in response to hemorrhage and to hemorrhagic shock. This response, however, is initially rather limited and, in severe hemorrhagic shock, is grossly inadequate to explain the reduction seen in interstitial fluid. Since there is no source for external loss, the question arose as to whether interstitial fluid might move into the cell mass in an isotonic fashion (Fig. 4-3).

CELLULAR STUDIES

Subsequently, studies of ion transport across the cell membrane were undertaken in order to determine the possibility of intracellular swelling in skeletal muscle in response to hemorrhagic shock. Using a Ling-Gerard ultramicroelectrode with glass tip diameter of less than 1μ (Fig. 4-4), intracellular transmembrane potential record-

Fig. 4-2. Radiosulfate equilibration curve: semilogarithmic plot, summary model.

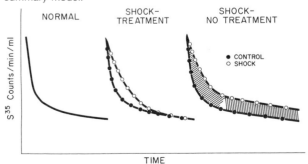

ings were made. The electrode was modified to record intracellular transmembrane potentials in vivo before, during, and after shock (Fig. 4-5).

Skeletal muscle measurements in acute hemorrhagic shock demonstrate a constant and sustained fall in the normally negative intracellular transmembrane potential. This may represent a reduction in efficiency of the sodium pump induced by tissue hypoxia; it is present only during shock-producing hypotension. Additional studies in splenectomized dogs showed that changes in variables such as pH, P_{CO_2}, and bicarbonate do not influence the transmembrane potential in shock. Even with progressive metabolic acidosis and its subsequent correction, the potential still follows the blood pressure and shock state.

Studies have been reported which utilized the ultramicroelectrode measurement of transmembrane potential combined with direct aspiration of skeletal muscle interstitial fluid by a modification of the technique of Hagberg. Using this technique, it was found that as blood pressure fell and transmembrane potential was reduced, plasma potassium rose slowly during the shock period (Fig. 4-6). However, the directly aspirated interstitial fluid potassium during the same period of time rose to a height of more than 15 mEq/L of interstitial fluid. This explained where potassium, moving out of skeletal muscle cells, was being sequestered as sodium chloride and water moved into muscle cells.

Additional studies have been performed in primates which show essentially the same phenomenon (Fig. 4-7). These studies also reveal that this cellular membrane transport is a reversible phenomenon, i.e., once the shock state is treated, transmembrane potential recovers. Concomitant muscle biopsies show clearly that muscle cells gain sodium, water, and chloride while losing potassium.

NORMAL

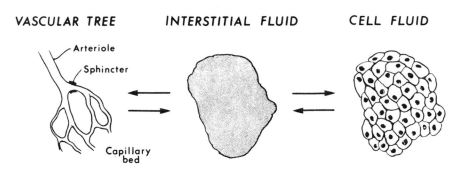

VASCULAR TREE   INTERSTITIAL FLUID   CELL FLUID

HEMORRHAGIC SHOCK

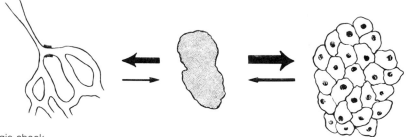

Fig. 4-3. Interstitial fluid response to hemorrhagic shock.

Fig. 4-4. Schematic of intracellular recording. (*From Ruch and Fulton,* eds., *Medical Physiology and Biophysics, 18th ed.,* W. B. Saunders Company, Philadelphia, 1960.)

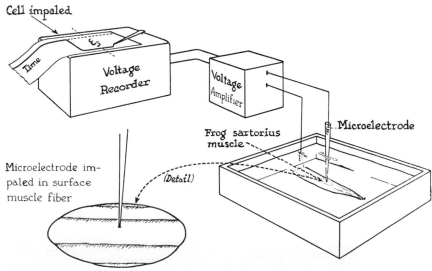

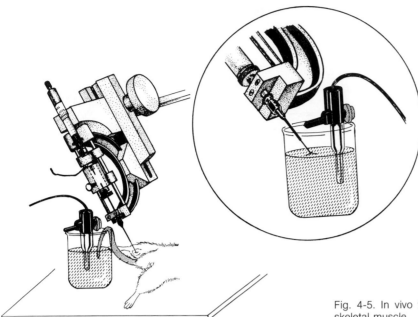

Fig. 4-5. In vivo transmembrane potential measurement in rat skeletal muscle.

Thus the data reveal an isotonic swelling of skeletal muscle cells in response to shock injury (Fig. 4-8).

Studies in human beings reveal the same response to shock injury. Interesting corroborative changes in action potentials of single cells in skeletal muscles have been revealed in primates (Fig. 4-9). One study shows a decrease in resting membrane potential, a decrease in amplitude of action potential, and prolongation of both repolarization and depolarization times. Resuscitation quickly reversed these changes, except for repolarization time, which remained prolonged for several days. This confirms in vitro the alterations in intracellular sodium and potassium con-

centrations which were measured by skeletal muscle biopsy and resting membrane potential measurements.

INTERPRETATION

Concisely stated, reduction in extracellular fluid in reversible hemorrhagic shock can consistently be shown (1) with extracellular fluid markers that enter cells slowly or not at all in the shock state when (2) reinjection of the extracellular fluid markers is utilized in the shock state, (3) extracellular fluid markers or tracers are allowed sufficient time for equilibration, (4) shock measurements are obtained while hemorrhagic shock is sustained, and (5) the shock preparation is sufficiently severe and is maintained until there is a change in cellular membrane transport.

The data obtained from prior experiments support the use of transmembrane potential measurements as an accurate indicator of cellular alterations resulting from the low-flow state of hemorrhagic shock. Severe hypotension is associated with depression of transmembrane potential difference (PD) which is sustained in the presence of a continued shock state.

Transmembrane PD is generally agreed to be the result of either an electrogenic sodium pump (with active outward extrusion of sodium from muscle cells by a redox system) or a coupled sodium-potassium exchange pump with diffusion of sodium and potassium down their respective chemical gradients. In the latter theory the relative permeabilities of the membrane to the two ions must be considered and the potential interpreted on the basis of the Hodgkin-Katz-Goldman equation in which pNa^+ (relative permeability to sodium) is 0.01. Since permeability to potassium is assumed to be much greater than permeability to sodium in the cell membrane, the PD is essentially a potassium diffusion potential.

The present data thus suggest that skeletal muscle cells

Fig. 4-6. Changes in membrane potential and interstitial K^+ in rats with hemorrhagic shock.

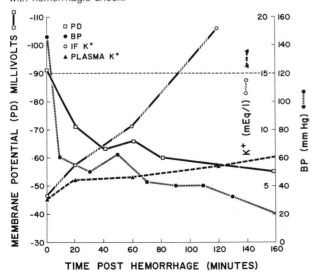

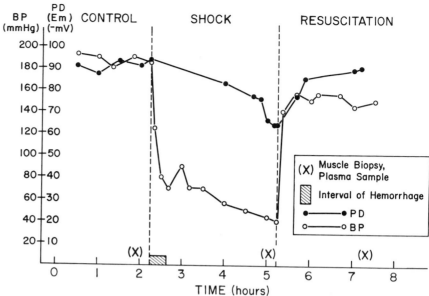

Fig. 4-7. Changes in membrane potential and blood pressure in primates during hemorrhagic shock and after resuscitation.

may be a principal site of fluid and electrolyte sequestration after severe, prolonged hemorrhagic shock. Adjunctive studies by Grossman suggest that similar changes in the intracellular mass of neurons in the brain also occur in response to hypovolemic shock. Furthermore, an increase in the cellular water content of both cellular and connective tissue components following hemorrhagic shock has been demonstrated by Slonim and Stahl, and Fulton has suggested that connective tissue may be the site of some sodium and water sequestration.

The exact mechanism for the production of electrolyte changes as well as for the notable diminution in extracellular water which occurs after hemorrhagic shock is not

Fig. 4-8. Changes in membrane potential, extracellular water, and intracellular Na+ in primates after resuscitation from hemorrhagic shock.

known. It appears that the changes may well represent a reduction in the efficiency of an active ionic pump mechanism or a selective increase in muscle cell membrane permeability to sodium, or both (Fig. 4-10).

With a reset membrane potential, extracellular fluid electrolyte concentrations are unchanged. Consequently, from the Nernst equation, intracellular Cl^- must rise from 3.5 to 10 mEq and intracellular Na^+ from 10 to 22 mEq. For transposition of these data to the previously cited measurements in hemorrhagic shock, a model is shown. This model shows a 10 percent isotonic swelling of muscle cells to explain the reduction in extracellular fluid measured in hemorrhagic shock. Studies are under way to determine the involvement of cell masses other than muscle during the course of hemorrhagic shock. One such study indicates that severe hemorrhagic shock of significant duration is associated with elevation of the internal sodium

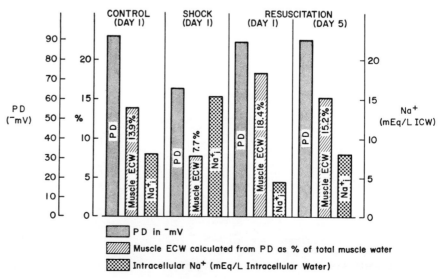

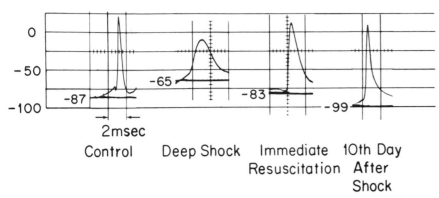

2msec

Control   Deep Shock   Immediate 10th Day
                           Resuscitation After
                                        Shock

Fig. 4-9. Action potentials in primates in hemorrhagic shock.

concentration of the red blood cells. The magnitude of these changes appears to be a function of both the severity and the duration of the shock process and seems to be well correlated with changes in clinical course when sequential sampling procedures are utilized.

There is a measurable reduction in extravascular extracellular fluid in response to sustained hemorrhagic shock. The cellular response to hypovolemic hypotension is characterized by a consistent change in active transport of ions. Evidence obtained directly from living cells indicates that sodium and water enter muscle cells, with resultant loss of cellular potassium to the extracellular fluid. The interstitial fluid holds the extruded potassium.

Replenishment of the depleted extracellular fluid counteracts these changes at the cellular level and is an important feature of therapy in patients with hypovolemic shock.

Renal Responses

The observation was made long ago that during severe shock, from any cause, renal function essentially stops in man. The kidneys, like the skin and the liver, share in the relative oligemia which is a rapid compensatory mechanism in shock to divert blood flow to those organs, such as the brain and the heart, most vital for maintaining life.

Consequently the relative oligemia suffered by the kidneys in response to shock is severe and immediate.

The development of oliguria and, indeed, even anuria is apparently a direct function of the severity and duration of the renal ischemia inevitably attendant on shock. In man, under normothermic conditions, normal kidneys will tolerate renal ischemia for periods varying from 15 minutes to a maximum of approximately 90 minutes. After this degree of ischemia, some functional and anatomic changes inevitably occur. With the use of hypothermia, the period of renal ischemia tolerated during hemorrhagic shock can be considerably prolonged.

SUBCLINICAL RENAL DAMAGE FOLLOWING INJURY AND SHOCK

In civilian and military practice, improved resuscitation with balanced electrolyte solution and blood and immediate corrective surgery have resulted in a great reduction in the incidence of primary oliguric renal failure. Recognition of nonoliguric renal failure as a less severe form of renal insufficiency suggested that graded renal damage might occur in association with systemic injury. Identification of patients with subclinical renal damage should be important in their postinjury care.

PATIENT STUDIES. A study was recently undertaken to determine the presence and degree of such renal damage during the early course of severely injured civilian patients. During the period of this study, 96,000 patients were treated in the emergency department, 988 of whom were admitted to the hospital for care of their injuries. Forty of the most severely injured were selected for continued care in a Trauma Research Unit after resuscitation and operative treatment of injuries. The criteria for inclusion in the study were hypotension following trauma and multiple long bone fractures.

All 40 patients showed generalized depression of renal function initially. Within 24 hours of admission, 30 demonstrated return of clearances to normal ranges. The patients were divided into groups according to blood urea nitrogen (BUN) values (Fig. 4-11). Group I, considered to show a characteristic renal response to trauma, was selected on the basis of BUN values continuously below 20 Gm/100 ml after the first hospital day. This group included 30 of the 40 patients. Eight patients with renal

Fig. 4-10. Theoretic transport mechanisms responsible for alterations in potential difference (*P.D.*) and fluid-electrolyte distribution in hemorrhagic shock.

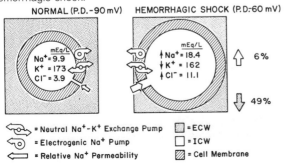

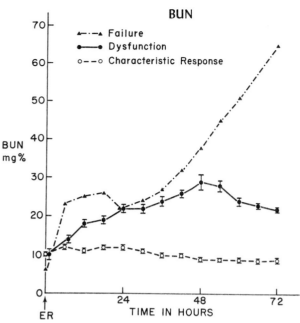

Fig. 4-11. Renal function after trauma: blood urea nitrogen values.

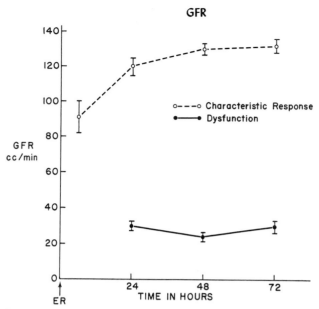

Fig. 4-12. Renal function after trauma: glomerular filtration rate.

dysfunction (Group II) showed persistent moderate elevation of BUN values above 20 mg/100 ml. Two patients showed frank renal failure with rapidly progressing azotemia. One of these patients had sustained a gunshot wound of the renal vein and vena cava and had had the renal pedicle on the involved side clamped for one hour. The other patient, with a gunshot wound of the aortic bifurcation, represented failure of resuscitation. These two patients with renal failure are not considered in the subsequent comparisons between patients with the characteristic renal response (Group I) and those with renal dysfunction (Group II). Three patients with direct renal injury requiring suture or partial nephrectomy were included in Group I.

As would be expected on the basis of the selection criteria for the groups, glomerular filtration rate (GFR) was quite different for the two groups (Fig. 4-12). Urea clearance (C_{urea}), another clearance primarily related to filtration, was depressed in both groups initially, with a rapid return to and above normal in the characteristic group and a slow return toward normal in the dysfunction group. Urine/plasma (U/P) urea ratio and osmolar clearances (C_{osm}) were different in the two groups only subsequent to 12 hours after admission (Fig. 4-13).

Tubular resorption of water (TcH_2O) was significantly different in the two groups only at 18 and 24 hours after admission. The trend in Group I was toward excretion of free water, while the trend in the dysfunction group was toward continued retention of free water. Cardiac output was not significantly different in the two groups.

Sodium clearances (C_{Na}) were similar in the two groups until after 12 hours following admission (Fig. 4-14). Subsequently C_{Na} fell in Group II. Postoperative sodium bal-

ance, represented as the difference between daily sodium intake and urinary sodium excretion, was different in the two groups. Group I showed positive sodium balance during day 1, balance during day 2, and negative balance during day 3. In Group II, the dysfunction group, increasing sodium retention occurred during each of the 3 days of the study.

There were no discernible differences between the two groups in age, type of injury, length of hypotensive episode, fluid administration, positive-pressure ventilation,

Fig. 4-13. Renal function after trauma: urine/plasma urea ratio.

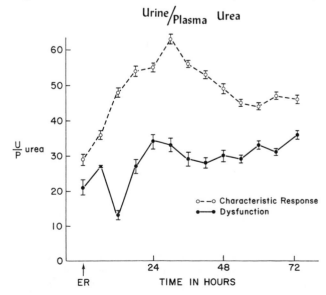

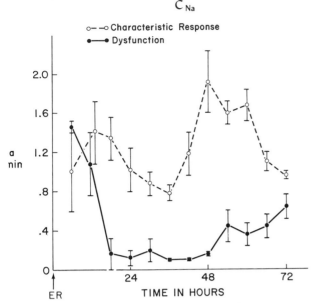

Fig. 4-14. Renal function after trauma: sodium clearance.

nephrotic antibiotics, minute urine volume, blood volume, or arterial P_{O_2} and pH.

Discussion

Classic renal clearance techniques have been used infrequently in surgical patients, partly because of errors inherent in the methods. All renal clearances are urine flow–sensitive. An increase in urine flow leads to a decrease in mean urine transit time. Consequently new filtrate washes out tubular and collecting system contents at a more rapid rate, yielding a factitiously high clearance. Conversely, a decrease in urine flow may lead to a factitiously low clearance. Errors in clearance measurements can be minimized by using constant mechanical infusion, long collection periods, and bladder washes. The long collection periods may obscure fluctuations during the period, but they provide accurate mean clearances.

In the normal human kidney, GFR may promptly increase 30 percent above basal level during diuresis. In the above-mentioned study, GFR was measured without fluid loading, yet six of the patients in Group I showed a GFR above 150 ml/minute, suggesting the presence of postinjury stimuli in the patients tending to increase GFR maximally. The patients with renal dysfunction (Group II) were presumably subject to similar stimuli but were unable to respond with any elevation in GFR because of renal damage or persistent nervous or humoral influences affecting GFR.

Endogenous creatinine clearance (C_{cr}) in both groups was always higher than GFR. Notable variation in C_{cr} in the injured patient was noted by Ladd, who concluded that endogenous C_{cr} was unsuitable for evaluation of GFR in battle casualties. Creatinine as determined by the Jaffe reaction overestimates the true creatinine in plasma, and since creatinine is secreted in human beings, the usual

agreement of endogenous C_{cr} with inulin or iothalamate ^{125}I clearance is coincidental. Twofold and threefold increases in endogenous C_{cr} occur in association with the changes in muscle metabolism following severe trauma. Apparently normal values for C_{cr} may lead to a false sense of security when, in fact, the GFR may be reduced by a factor of 2 or 3 in the severely injured patient.

Muscle metabolism is profoundly altered in the injured patient, resulting in increased loads of creatinine and creatine presented to the kidney. In the early postinjury period, many patients had metabolic changes similar to those found in patients placed on a high protein diet. Even with increases in urea nitrogen load from tissue injury, multiple transfusions, and gluconeogenesis, these patients did not undergo azotemia and creatinemia. Azotemia and creatinemia are not inevitable consequences of severe tissue injury, and other factors are operative in the injured patient who exhibits such changes.

Flear and Clarke demonstrated that transfused patients lost less nitrogen in the period following injury than similarly injured nontransfused patients. It is not surprising that catabolism and nitrogen excretion are inversely related to the adequacy of resuscitative therapy. The patients with the greatest catabolic responses had sustained a more severe injury than the patients who did not demonstrate such changes. Flear and Clarke also demonstrated that transfused patients had negative sodium balances after the first postoperative day. Patients with the most severely damaged kidneys demonstrate positive free water clearances, as do septic patients, so care must be taken in interpreting the finding of positive free water clearances. The earliest possible restoration of circulating volume with electrolyte solution and blood, combined with definitive treatment of injuries, should decrease the degree of secondary systemic injury.

Trueta first described arterialization of rabbit renal venous blood secondary to stimuli which led to renal failure when prolonged. From these and other observations he developed a concept of renal arteriovenous shunting as a main factor in the development of posttraumatic renal failure. Recent technical improvements in determining internal intrarenal blood flow support his earlier observations. Padula et al. evaluated the effect of equiosmolar loads of mannitol, glucose, urea, and sodium chloride on an isolated dog kidney preparation. The administration of each agent was followed initially by a decrease in renal resistance and an increase in directly measured renal blood flow. The administration of mannitol, glucose, or urea alone was followed by a decrease in renal O_2 utilization, while the administration of sodium chloride was followed by an increase in O_2 consumption. An interpretation differing from that of the author's would consider the saline-induced increase in O_2 utilization indicative of internal redistribution of renal blood flow to ischemic cortical areas.

Small transient increases of GFR were apparent after administration of the diuretic in some patients. In view of the demonstrated slow improvement in GFR which occurs after resuscitation and injury repair, it is difficult to ascribe increases in GFR during this early hospital period to furosemide. Further study of changes in GFR after administration of furosemide is indicated, however, in view of reports suggesting a beneficial effect of furosemide on renal function.

C_{urea}, C_{cr}, C_{osm}, and U/P urea, U/P creatinine, and U/P osmolarity ratios have each been proposed as good clinical determinants of renal damage. Objections to the use of creatinine determinations alone have been noted above. Otherwise there is little to recommend any one of these tests over the others, since all relate filtration to some aspect of tubular function. Recognition of the need to measure at least one of the foregoing in urine and plasma simultaneously is important. U/P ratios approaching unity and clearances below 10 ml/minute are diagnostic of some form of renal failure. Attempted diuresis with volume replacement and ethacrynic acid or furosemide is indicated early in the course of patients with apparent posttraumatic renal failure.

A spectrum of secondary renal injury exists after severe trauma, varying from oliguric renal failure to transient depression of glomerular filtration and tubular function. Tissue trauma and multiple transfusions do not lead to azotemia in the injured patient with normal renal function. Conversely, even minimal persistent elevations of BUN are uniformly associated with significant renal dysfunction and sodium and water retention.

The more severely injured patient can be readily identified in the early postoperative phase by serial evaluation of the renal metabolism of urea or sodium. Identification of such patients should lead to meticulous supportive care, since the general metabolic reserve of the more severely injured patients is diminished and further insults are poorly tolerated.

HIGH-OUTPUT RENAL FAILURE

Posttraumatic acute renal insufficiency is well recognized as a highly lethal complication. The diagnosis is classically based on persistent oliguria and chemical evidence of uremia after stabilization of the circulation. The clinical course is characterized by oliguria of several days' to several weeks' duration, followed by a progressive rise in daily urine volume until both the excretory and concentrating functions of the kidney are gradually restored.

It is less well recognized that renal insufficiency may occur without an observed period of oliguria. This variant of renal insufficiency has been reported infrequently after burns, head injury, and soft tissue trauma. The reported cases are characterized by increasing azotemia, while the daily urine volume remains normal or increased. Many of these patients have an apparently inappropriate increase in urine volume, and the term *high-output renal failure* may best describe this entity, despite a theoretical objection. Until recently, this type of renal failure has not been noted frequently after trauma, nor has the clinical course been described in sufficient detail for recognition or management.

PATIENT STUDIES. A report is here presented to describe the clinical course of acute renal failure without oliguria, to emphasize the problems encountered in management, and to suggest renal ischemia as the basic causative mechanism (Fig. 4-15).

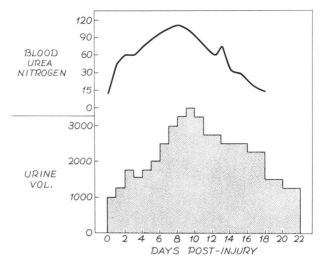

Fig. 4-15. High-output renal failure.

After severe abdominal trauma, the patients were in shock an average of 3.5 hours, the individual times varying from 1 to 6 hours. The average blood loss was 4.2 liters and average blood replacement 3.6 liters. The recorded blood loss was the amount measured at the time of operation. In most patients external bleeding was minimal. In addition to whole blood, they were given an average of 4 liters of Ringer's lactate solution per patient prior to and during the operative procedure.

After operation the diagnosis of renal failure was not immediately suspected, since urine volumes were above 30 ml/hour and few abnormalities were present in the initial values of blood urea nitrogen, potassium, sodium, carbon dioxide–combining power, and chlorides obtained on the first postoperative day.

In all cases not involving direct damage to the urinary tract, the urinalysis after operation showed specific gravities between 1.003 and 1.010, pH of 5.5 to 6.5, and urinary sediments containing at most a few red blood cells per high power field and an occasional cast. The urine:plasma ratio of urea nitrogen was found to be slightly less than 20:1.

The mean values of the daily urinary outputs for these patients can be seen in Fig. 4-16. On the day of operation the minimum urinary output was 730 ml. This represented the output for less than 12 hours in each case. There was a progressive increase in the mean urine volume for the first 6 to 8 days, reaching a height of 2350 ml and returning gradually to normal between the sixteenth and seventeenth days. The only low volumes were observed in an eight-year-old child with extensive blunt trauma requiring nephrectomy. The continued high output of 3 liters/day after the sixteenth day occurred in only one patient; the BUN in this patient did not return to normal for 37 days. The ranges denoted by the bars in Fig. 4-16 show the extremely high outputs in some patients compared to the relatively normal values in others during the period of azotemia. The highest urine volumes were found in patients with the highest BUN values.

Figure 4-17 shows a progressive rise of the mean BUN during the 6 to 8 days after injury and a gradual return to

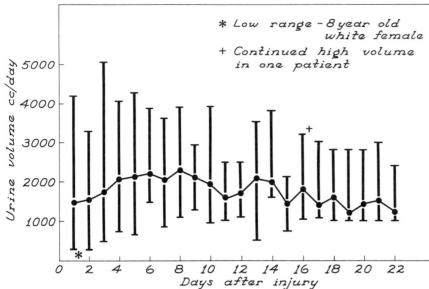

Fig. 4-16. High-output renal failure: urine volumes.

normal between the sixteenth and eighteenth days. The serum creatinine levels paralleled the azotemia, the highest value being 6.8 mg/100 ml. In all patients the increasing BUN level was paralleled by an increasing daily urinary volume. Similarly, the stepwise decline in blood urea was paralleled by a decreasing urinary volume.

In Fig. 4-18 the average values and ranges of the serum potassium levels are shown. In most instances the initial values after operation were slightly below normal. In some the serum potassium levels were above 6 mEq/L by the second or third postoperative day, while the remaining patients showed a slow but sustained rise. All the accelerated rises resulted from intravenous administration of potassium salts (not more than 60 mEq/day). When the serum potassium reached 6 mEq/L, treatment with cation exchange resins was instituted. This proved effective in preventing further rises in serum K. An increase of serum potassium from 5.5 to 9.2 mEq/L was caused by the intravenous administration of 60 mEq of KCl in a 12-hour

period. Extracorporeal hemodialysis was necessary to reduce the potassium intoxication that occurred. The bar graph represents the serum potassium levels resulting from the inability of the kidneys to excrete normal amounts of potassium and the administration of potassium salts, as well as the effective use of resins and the artificial kidney.

Moderately low values for the carbon dioxide–combining power were present for the first 4 or 5 days after injury and represent a mild to moderate metabolic acidosis. All isotonic losses were replaced with lactated Ringer's solution when acidosis persisted. In most patients the acidosis was well controlled by the administration of isotonic lactate solutions, which occasionally resulted in a mild metabolic alkalosis, although two patients had carbon dioxide–combining power values between 15 and 18 mEq/L despite lactate therapy and died on the tenth and twelfth postoperative days. After the eighth postoperative day carbon dioxide–combining powers were within a normal range without lactate administration. The serum chlorides did not show a reciprocal relationship to the carbon dioxide–combining powers.

Serum sodium determinations were made throughout the period of renal failure. The highest values of 150 to 154 mEq occurred during a trial of fluid restriction to determine whether the high urinary outputs were being induced by excessive administration of fluids. On these two occasions, hypernatremia was readily produced, indicating that the kidney was excreting a solute-poor urine.

Surviving patients were available for follow-up. Evaluation of renal function was carried out 1 to $1\frac{1}{2}$ years after injury. Determinations of blood urea nitrogen, creatinine, sodium, potassium, carbon dioxide, and chloride were normal. Intravenous pyelography was normal. The lowest urinary concentration obtained was 1.020, and excretion of phenolsulfonphthalein (PSP) exceeded 30 percent in 30 minutes in all patients studied. Within 3 months both tubular and glomerular functions had returned to normal.

Fig. 4-17. High-output renal failure: blood urea nitrogen values.

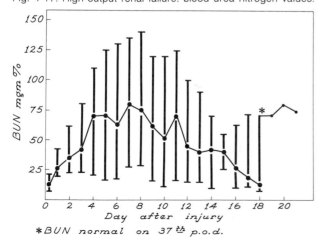

*BUN normal on 37th p.o.d.

Autopsy was performed on patients who died. Microscopic examination of the kidneys from these patients showed regenerating patchy tubular necrosis. The damage in each instance was principally to the distal nephron; less severe changes were seen in the proximal segments.

A typical course of high-output renal failure shows an increasing urea nitrogen which parallels the increasing urine volume, a mild metabolic acidosis, and an acute hyperkalemia produced by the administration of potassium salts. Recognition of the disease entity permits control of these abnormalities.

ANIMAL STUDIES. Animal experiments using dogs were carried out to determine the modifying effect of hypothermia on renal ischemia. After contralateral nephrectomy, the remaining renal pedicle was clamped for 2 hours in each day.

As seen in Fig. 4-19, Group A consists of normothermic controls. Group B dogs had regional renal hypothermia produced by irrigation of the peritoneal cavity with cold saline solution. Group C dogs had profound renal hypothermia to 25°C produced by circulating cold saline solution continuously around the kidney. This cooling technique has been previously described.

The results show progressive azotemia and death in untreated animals that are not cooled (Group A). There was only transient elevation of the BUN when the kidneys were cooled to 25°C (Group C). In Group B, regional hypothermia, the BUN rose to an average height of 60 mg/100 ml by the sixth to tenth day and gradually returned to normal between the twelfth and sixteenth days.

Utilizing this same model in six dogs with exteriorized ureters, minimum urine volumes of 400 ml/day were obtained without an observed period of oliguria. Usually the

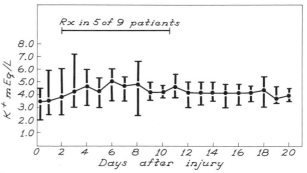

Fig. 4-18. High-output renal failure: serum potassium levels.

daily urine volume increased to between 600 and 900 ml/day before the BUN began to decline. Microscopic examination of these and six similarly treated animals, sacrificed between the fifth and tenth days, showed the tubular lesion to be confined principally to the distal tubules but with some proximal tubular involvement. These changes, both degenerative and regenerative, were scattered and irregular in distribution.

Consequently it can be seen that high-output renal failure in animals is an intermediate form of renal failure. With severe renal ischemia, unmodified oliguric renal failure inevitably resulted. When the kidney was protected with profound hypothermia, no significant renal failure resulted. On the other hand, with modest but practical protection to the kidney afforded by peritoneal sluicing with cold saline solution, moderate elevation of BUN associated with high urine volume was obtained. This protection resulted in recovery of the animal in each instance.

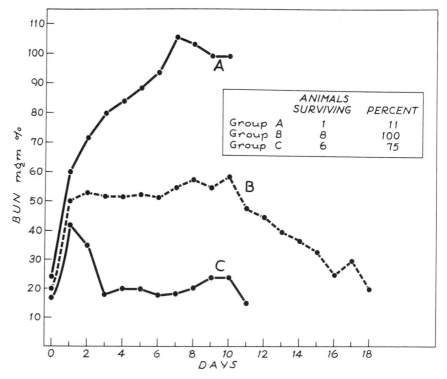

	ANIMALS SURVIVING	PERCENT
Group A	1	11
Group B	8	100
Group C	6	75

Fig. 4-19. Blood urea levels in dogs with renal ischemia, showing effect of hypothermia.

Discussion

Renal insufficiency without oliguria is important from the standpoint of recognition and clinical management of a variant of classic acute renal failure.

The clinical course of patients has been shown to be qualitatively the same as that occurring when oliguria is present. Quantitatively, however, these patients retain a limited ability to excrete acid products of metabolism, potassium, and urea. It is of primary importance that renal insufficiency of itself was not sufficient in terms of acidosis, uremia, potassium intoxication, or fluid volume control to cause death in this series.

The normal or high daily output of urine, although solute-poor, permits administration of fairly large quantities of water daily, in addition to replacement of isotonic salt losses such as those from gastrointestinal suction. The maintenance of normal extracellular fluid volume and normal serum sodium concentration is, therefore, easily accomplished when accurate daily outputs of each are obtained and losses are replaced accordingly. The quantity of fluids containing sodium may be administered as lactate to control the mild metabolic acidosis that occurs. The observations of Moore indicate that if the acidosis is not treated, it may become so severe as to become the outstanding abnormality in these cases.

The chief dangers of high-output renal failure are (1) failure to recognize the existence of renal failure because of normal output and (2) the administration of potassium salts intravenously. Good urinary output and gastrointestinal involvement requiring suction would usually indicate the need for daily replacement of potassium. When this type of renal failure exists, however, potassium intoxication may be produced. In the early patients studied, five of nine required therapy for hyperkalemia. One required emergency hemodialysis for control of excessively high serum potassium levels. It is important that the serum level be determined daily and prior to the administration of any potassium-containing solutions.

The factors involved in the production of acute renal failure following trauma are incompletely understood, but renal ischemia is of unquestioned importance. This concept implies that the ischemia produces damage to the nephrons, which results in failure of the kidneys to excrete urine. Diuresis is felt to represent the recovery phase. Allowing for the physiologic variation between individuals and between given degrees of renal ischemia, a spectrum of the length of the oliguric phase should occur. This has been well documented by Teschan and Mason. Presumably, a few cases of renal insufficiency without oliguria should occur. Although some theorize that renal failure without oliguria should be the most common type of renal failure observed, there is little documented support.

The frequency with which these cases occurred in relation to the small number of oliguric renal failures that were seen during the same period may represent differences in the therapy given during the ischemic episode. There are two outstanding differences in the therapy that we have routinely used. One is the administration of balanced salt solution along with whole blood in the resuscitation from hemorrhagic shock. It is well recognized that prolonged or severe extracellular fluid deficits are necessary for the production of renal failure in animals and may contribute to renal damage in man. The second difference in treatment is the use of renal hypothermia of a moderate degree to modify or prevent ischemic renal damage.

Clinical experience and laboratory experiments suggest that high-output renal failure represents the renal response to a less severe (or modified) episode of renal injury than that required to produce classic oliguric renal failure.

Pulmonary Responses

Acute respiratory failure following severe injury and critical illness has received increasing attention over the last decade. With advances in the management of hemorrhagic shock and support of circulatory and renal function in injured patients, it has become apparent that 1 to 2 percent of significantly injured patients develop acute respiratory failure in the postinjury period. Initially this lung injury was thought to be peculiar to the particular clinical situation. This is implied by such names as "shock lung" and "traumatic wet lung," which have been applied to acute respiratory insufficiency. It is now recognized that there are many similarities in the clinical presentation and the physiologic and pathologic findings of the pulmonary injury seen following a variety of insults. This has resulted in the concept that the lung has a limited number of ways of reacting to injury and that several different types of acute diffuse lung injury result in a similar pathophysiologic response. The common denominator of this response appears to be injury at the alveolar-capillary membrane, with resulting leakage of proteinaceous fluid from the intravascular space into the interstitium and subsequently into alveolar spaces. It has become acceptable to describe this entire spectrum of acute diffuse injury under the general term of *adult respiratory distress syndrome* (ARDS).

CLINICAL PRESENTATION. The syndrome of ARDS may occur under a variety of circumstances and result in a spectrum of clinical severity from mild dysfunction to progressive, eventually fatal, pulmonary failure. Fortunately, with proper management, the latter type is far less frequent than a milder type of abnormality.

For descriptive purposes the clinical picture can be divided into arbitrary stages. The first stage (injury, resuscitation, and alkalosis) immediately follows initial injury and is characterized by spontaneous hyperventilation with

Table 4-2. DIAGNOSTIC CRITERIA IN POST-INJURY PULMONARY INSUFFICIENCY

Major:
 Hypoxemia (unresponsive)
 Stiff lung (low compliance)
 Decreased resting volume (functional residual capacity)
 Diffuse interstitial pattern on x-ray
 Increased dead space ventilation

Minor:
 Increased cardiac output
 Hyperventilation
 Nonthoracic trauma

Table 4-3. BASIC TERMINOLOGY AND SYMBOLS

VO_2 . . . . Oxygen consumption
C.O. . . . . Cardiac output
VD/VT . . . . Physiologic dead space ventilation
                                        as a fraction of tidal volume
Qs/Qt . . . . Venous admixture as a fraction of
                                        total cardiac output
AaD . . . . Alveolar-arterial gradient
F_{IO_2} . . . . Fraction of inspired O_2
V/Q . . . . Ratio of ventilation to perfusion

hypocapnia, diminished pulmonary compliance, mixed metabolic and respiratory alkalosis, and a normal chest x-ray. After apparent stabilization of vital signs and adequate tissue perfusion, the patient enters Stage 2 (circulatory stability and beginning respiratory difficulty). This may persist for several hours to days. Persistent *hyperventilation,* progressive hypocapnia, increased cardiac output, progressive decrease in compliance, falling oxygenation, and increasing pulmonary shunt fraction all indicate that progressive pulmonary insufficiency will predominate in the subsequent clinical course. Recognition and therapeutic intervention at this point is believed to be extremely important. Stage 3 (progressive pulmonary insufficiency) and Stage 4 (terminal hypoxia with asystole) complete the syndrome.

The hallmarks of the clinical syndrome are

1. Hypoxemia which is relatively unresponsive to elevations of inspired oxygen concentration (indicating ventilation/perfusion imbalance and shunting).
2. Decreased pulmonary compliance (progressively increased airway pressure required to achieve adequate ventilation).
3. Chest x-ray changes, characteristically minimal in the early stages. With progression of the syndrome interstitial edema and diffuse infiltrates appear which may progress to widespread areas of consolidation.

Minor criteria for diagnosis include hyperventilation, increased cardiac output, and a history of nonthoracic trauma. The diagnostic criteria are summarized in Table 4-2.

MECHANISM. A review of a basic terminology is shown in Table 4-3.

The prominent derangements in pulmonary function associated with ARDS are (1) hypoxia which is unresponsive to increased inspired oxygen concentrations, (2) decreased pulmonary compliance (compliance defined as the amount of volume increase in the lungs obtained by a given change in pressure), which clinically appears as "stiff lungs," and (3) a fall in resting lung volume, specifically a fall in the functional residual capacity. The functional residual capacity, as shown in Fig. 4-20, is the amount of air remaining in the lungs after a normal expiration.

The possible causes of hypoxia (decreased arterial P_{O_2}) are shown in Table 4-4. All clinicians are familiar with

Table 4-4. CAUSES OF HYPOXEMIA

1. Hypoventilation
2. Diffusion defects
3. V/Q abnormalities
4. Shunting

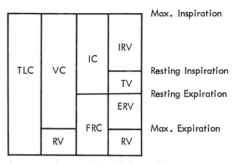

Fig. 4-20. Lung volumes and capacities: *TLC,* total lung capacity; *VC,* vital capacity; *IC,* inspiratory capacity; *FRC,* functional residual capacity; *RV,* residual volume; *ERV,* expiratory reserve volume; *TV,* tidal volume; *IRV,* inspiratory reserve volume.

hypoventilation as a cause of hypoxia, as seen in the recovery room, but it is unlikely that hypoventilation is responsible for the hypoxia in this syndrome. Hypoventilation significant enough to result in hypoxia is associated with a rise in the P_{CO_2}. These patients, however, have an abnormally low P_{CO_2}.

Although diffusion defects can theoretically result from interstitial edema and thickening, they should respond to the administration of 100 percent oxygen. This is not the case in the patients in question, so diffusion defects alone would appear to be unlikely causes of the clinical syndrome.

Ventilation/perfusion inequalities could explain the hypoxia seen in these patients, and shunting represents the ultimate ventilation/perfusion abnormality. This statement deserves further explanation. Normally, there is autoregulation of ventilation and perfusion within the lung so that a balance exists between ventilation and perfusion of alveolar groups. When a group of alveoli become nonventilated or have decreased ventilation, compensatory mechanisms bring about a reflex decrease in blood supply to these alveoli. This, in its extreme, results in no ventilation and no perfusion to these alveolar units; thus no abnormality in terms of dead space ventilation or shunting occurs. The effects of loss of this normal balance or loss of compensatory mechanisms are shown in Fig. 4-21. On the left, alternations in blood flow are demonstrated. It can be seen that progressive decrease in blood flow with continued ventilation affects primarily carbon dioxide elimination. This can be defined as high ventilation/perfusion ratio and is usually reflected by increases in dead space ventilation. Such changes do not result in hypoxia. On the right side of Fig. 4-21 is shown the effect of reduction in ventilation while perfusion is maintained. It can be seen that progressive lowering of ventilation can result in hypoxia until the ultimate reduction, i.e., nonventilation, occurs. In theory, as long as any ventilation of the alveolus occurs, the hypoxia should be responsive to oxygen. This, then, is generally referred to as a ventilation/perfusion abnormality characterized by a low V/Q ratio. When alveolar collapse or nonventilation occurs for any reason, the hypoxia secondary to this is no longer responsive to oxygen; this is defined as a shunt.

Causes of pulmonary shunting are shown in Fig. 4-22.

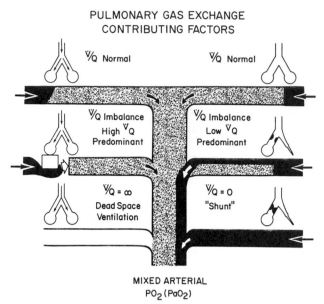

Fig. 4-21. Diagrammatic representation of ventilation/perfusion ratio (V/Q) abnormalities.

Shunting normally takes place, to the extent of about 3 percent of the cardiac output, through both intrapulmonary and extrapulmonary routes. Although pathologic shunts occur from extrapulmonary causes, intrapulmonary shunting appears to be the problem in posttraumatic pulmonary insufficiency. Basically, there is perfusion of alveoli which are collapsed or for other reasons cannot be ventilated. The alveoli, for example, may be filled with secretions, exudate, blood, edema, or protein.

Whatever the cause, the clinical picture appears to result from a distortion of the normal ventilation/perfusion balance. This concept is shown in Fig. 4-23. In some areas of the lung there appears to be perfusion with poor ventilation; in other areas there is ventilation of nonperfused alveoli. This combination of abnormalities will produce decreased resting lung volume (functional residual capacity, or FRC), shunting, and increased dead space ventilation.

The common denominator producing the abnormalities

Fig. 4-22. Mechanisms of arteriovenous admixture in pulmonary shunting.

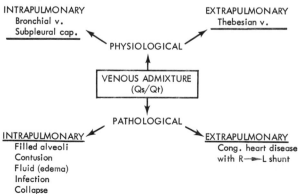

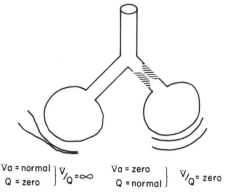

Fig. 4-23. Diagrammatic representation of mismatched ventilation and perfusion.

in ventilation and perfusion and other abnormalities seen in ARDS is thought to be injury to the alveolar-capillary membrane. This injury results in loss of integrity of the membrane, with increased permeability to albumin. The consequent leak of protein-rich fluid leads to *interstitial pulmonary edema* and decreased pulmonary compliance. With continued leakage, the alveolar units become fluid-filled and hypoxia (shunting) ensues. Thus the entire clinical picture of ventilation of poorly perfused segments (capillary injury), decreased compliance (interstitial edema), perfusion of poorly ventilated segments, and loss of lung volume (partially and completely fluid-filled alveoli) appears to result from capillary injury with a "capillary leak."

The majority of the causative factors listed in the next section cause such an alveolar-capillary injury.

ETIOLOGY. It appears likely that a variety of different injuries can produce a picture clinically indistinguishable from that described above. The most important of these are shown in Table 4-5.

Hemorrhagic Shock (Ischemic Pulmonary Injury). Pulmonary failure is commonly seen in severely injured patients, many of whom have been in shock. Initially, it was assumed that at least in part, the respiratory failure noted following injury was analogous to renal failure and was a result of ischemic injury to the lung. Support for this hypothesis came from early studies in animals and in human beings. Retrospective clinical reports implied a correlation between shock and pulmonary failure. Hemorrhage and congestion were noted in canine and human lungs after hemorrhagic shock and resuscitation. However, careful studies in dogs, primates, and other experimental animals, while demonstrating anatomic lesions of varying degree associated with hemorrhagic shock, do not demonstrate any measurable functional defect in the lung.

Table 4-5. POSSIBLE CAUSES OF ARDS
FOLLOWING INJURY

1. Ischemic pulmonary injury (?)	7. Fluid overload
2. Pulmonary infection	8. Oxygen toxicity
3. Systemic infection (sepsis)	9. Microatelectasis
4. Aspiration	10. Direct pulmonary injury
5. Fat embolism	11. Cerebral Injury
6. Microembolism	

Table 4-6. INCIDENCE OF PULMONARY
FAILURE AFTER INJURY

Group	Total no.	Significant pulmonary dysfunction	
		Number	Percent
All patients operated for trauma	978	21	2.1
Patients selected for study	49	21	43
Shock (all types)	28	11	39
No shock	21	10	48
Sepsis	10	8	80
No sepsis	39	13	33

Specifically, no significant or progressive hypoxia occurs. In fact, several studies have shown a decrease rather than an increase in pulmonary shunting in hemorrhagic shock. Adequate arterial oxygenation has been maintained during and up to several days following hypovolemic shock.

Only in extremely severe hemorrhagic shock preparations, lasting more than several hours, have preterminal decreases in arterial oxygen concentration been demonstrated. This is in contradistinction to sepsis and septic shock, in which hypoxia has been shown to occur regularly. Recent clinical studies have confirmed this finding. The highest incidence of pulmonary dysfunction is noted in those patients with sepsis, irrespective of the presence or absence of shock. The results of one prospective study are shown in Table 4-6. Thus, while hemorrhagic shock may compound other pulmonary injuries, it does not appear to be a primary cause of respiratory failure following trauma.

Pulmonary Infection. Pulmonary infection is eventually present in virtually all patients succumbing to respiratory insufficiency and usually becomes clinically apparent during the later stages of the syndrome. Although this can certainly compound the syndrome and produce further hypoxia and decreased compliance, it is probably a secondary event and not the initiating cause for the entire clinical picture. There is valid reason for concern about the role of ventilators and other respiratory equipment in the introduction of pulmonary infection. Without proper precautions, devices which are in line with the airway can be a source of bacteria. Pierce and his coworkers have shown that with appropriate measures this can be controlled so that the equipment used for respiratory assistance does not contribute to the incidence of bacterial pneumonia in patients.

Sepsis. Significant extrapulmonary infection with systemic sepsis appears to be a constant finding in a number of clinical studies of ARDS. In fact, acute respiratory failure may be the first manifestation of sepsis in a patient with burns, intracranial lesions, and pulmonary contusion. The syndrome of ARDS is rarely seen without severe sepsis. The concept that sepsis is an important causative agent is supported by a significant amount of laboratory evidence. A variety of septic insults, including injection of *Escherichia coli* endotoxin or live *E. coli* organisms and peritonitis-induced septicemia, produce significant derangements in pulmonary gas exchange.

The specific mechanism of septic lung damage is still speculative, but a number of factors appear to be operative:

1. Direct endothelial damage to the pulmonary capillaries with resultant loss of integrity and alveolar injury (see Mechanism)
2. Gross disturbances in the clotting mechanism as well as the release of a variety of vasoactive and bronchoconstrictive substances
3. Decrease in activity or amount of surfactant

Whatever the mechanism, available information supports the hypothesis that sepsis produces pronounced changes in vascular resistance, airway resistance, direct alveolar and vascular injury, interstitial and intraalveolar edema, hemorrhage, changes in surfactant, and progressive hypoxia. The association of sepsis and acute respiratory failure appears clear.

Aspiration. The syndrome produced by aspiration of gastric contents, blood, or mouth organisms with subsequent pneumonia can resemble the clinical picture described above. It would appear likely that in a small but significant number of patients, aspiration (recognized or unrecognized) occurs and may occasionally be the causative factor in posttraumatic pulmonary insufficiency.

Fat Embolism. A syndrome associated with multiple long bone fractures, which appears to be related to embolization of fat, can produce a clinical picture similar to that described above. Although mild x-ray differences may occur, these patients are difficult to distinguish from other patients with pulmonary insufficiency after injury. Fulminant fat embolism has been described in combat casualties. There is evidence that a more subtle form may occur in less severely injured patients, especially after significant soft tissue trauma and long-bone fractures. Again, the mechanism remains to be defined.

Microembolization. There is a growing body of evidence that microemboli of various sorts, with their attendant release of vasoactive substances, injury to pulmonary capillaries and adjacent alveoli, and hemodynamic effects can produce defects in pulmonary function. A number of theories are offered to explain the significance and source of such microscopic emboli.

One source of microemboli appears to be stored blood. Changes in screen filtration pressure due to particulate material in stored, banked blood have been reported. Several series have demonstrated a rough correlation between the number of transfusions and the incidence of pulmonary failure. The precise role of such filters remains to be established.

A second source of microemboli appears to be the formation of intravascular microaggregates. These have been demonstrated in the venous return following release of a cross-clamped aorta and following massive soft tissue injury. Recently they have been demonstrated in the venous effluent of limited nonhypotensive soft tissue injuries and in hypovolemic, nonhypotensive states. It now appears that arterial hypotension, hypovolemia, low-flow states, and trauma may all lead to the formation of microemboli. A third possible source of microembolism is disseminated intravascular coagulation.

In summary, many of these mechanisms appear to be operative in the trauma patient who develops pulmonary failure. However, the value of specific therapy in preventing or treating each entity has not been determined.

Fluid Overload. The role of fluid administration in the production of ARDS has created great controversy. It has been proposed that, in the severely injured patient, a point is reached at which maintenance of renal function and restoration of adequate tissue perfusion are gained at the cost of significant fluid overload to the detriment of pulmonary function.

Although there is little question regarding the deleterious effects of *massive* fluid overload, its role in the production of this syndrome remains questionable. Experimental animals massively transfused with balanced electrolyte solutions (amounts equivalent to 30 liters/hour in man) develop fulminant pulmonary edema. However, they respond briskly to assisted ventilation, and ventilatory therapy prevents hypoxia. Those that survive the insult clear the edema rapidly and do not develop the progressive pulmonary failure characteristic of the clinical syndrome. Similarly, clinical studies show no correlation between the amounts of fluids received and the development of pulmonary insufficiency.

While gross fluid overload is not desirable, excessive "drying out" of the lungs also may be dangerous. If excessive fluid restriction results in a fall of cardiac output, the degree of hypoxia resulting from any pulmonary damage will be compounded. At present the most reasonable course appears to be to maintain fluid balance as close to normal as possible.

An even more controversial subject is the administration of colloid versus electrolyte solutions in the production of the syndrome. If the pulmonary vasculature is normal, a fall in the serum oncotic pressure renders the lungs more susceptible to pulmonary edema. Some authors reason that if crystalloid solutions are used in resuscitation, a fall in oncotic pressure may occur and cause or compound a pulmonary abnormality. If this were the case, the administration of colloid might be potentially beneficial to these patients. Clinical reports on the use of colloid solutions in the therapy of this condition are scanty and the results difficult to evaluate. They do not conclusively demonstrate the clinical effectiveness of colloid or diuretic therapy in decreasing extravascular lung water and restoring normal serum oncotic pressure.

The available evidence implies that the pulmonary capillary membrane is abnormal in ARDS. Therefore colloids administered intravenously may gain access to the pulmonary interstitium and could potentially increase the interstitial oncotic pressure. This conceivably could compound the pulmonary problem in the healing phase.

Unfortunately, insufficient experimental data are available at present to resolve these conflicting hypotheses. A reliable experimental model of the syndrome is lacking. A large number of studies have evaluated pulmonary capillary permeability in hemorrhagic shock. Few changes in permeability or ultrastructural interstitial changes due to shock alone have been shown. This tends to support evidence that shock per se is not a primary factor in the etiology of this syndrome. Although large amounts of colloid have been shown to produce some changes in interstitial ultrastructure, no defect in oxygenation was produced. There is no significant difference in pulmonary function after resuscitation from hemorrhagic shock between crystalloid and colloid solution.

It is unlikely that the type of resuscitative fluid plays a primary role in the etiology of the syndrome. Hypervolemia produced by either type of fluid may produce pulmonary edema, but this responds quickly to standard treatment and should not be confused with the syndrome being described. Attempts at "drying out" the lung may be dangerous, because a decrease in cardiac output secondary to hypovolemia may compound any pulmonary functional defect present.

Oxygen Toxicity. Prolonged use of high oxygen concentrations can result in a clinical picture and pathologic findings identical to those seen in ARDS. Ventilation with high concentrations of oxygen is thought to poison cell enzyme systems and disrupt membrane integrity. It has also been shown to significantly reduce mucociliary clearance in the tracheobronchial tree. The critical level appears to be between 40% and 50% oxygen. There is also a time factor involved: the higher the oxygen tension, the less the time required to produce symptoms and evidence of damage. A conscientious attempt to keep inspired oxygen below these levels should prevent oxygen toxicity. It seems unlikely that oxygen toxicity is a major factor in the etiology of this syndrome, although it may compound the problem if oxygen is given in high concentrations for significant periods of time.

Microatelectasis. Microatelectasis can result from recumbency, sedation, operation, and anesthesia. Although not the primary factor responsible for the clinical picture, it may contribute to the hypoxia seen in these patients. Again, increased oxygen concentration increases the possibility of atelectasis.

Direct Pulmonary Injury. There is little doubt that direct pulmonary injury (pulmonary contusion) can produce the progressive syndrome previously outlined. Although many patients considered to have this syndrome are thought to have nonthoracic injury, unrecognized injury may well have occurred. A force applied to an animal's abdomen, comparable to that of a steering wheel blow received during a head-on collision, results in raising the diaphragm to the level of the second intercostal space posteriorly. Thus abdominal trauma may produce tremendous compressive pulmonary injury, which may not be immediately apparent.

Cerebral Injury. Massive head injury has been associated with acute pulmonary edema, and there is laboratory evidence of a cause-and-effect relationship. The progression of acute pulmonary edema to the clinical syndrome under discussion has not been established. A centrineurogenic basis for progressive pulmonary insufficiency has been proposed. There is some evidence that hypoxia in animals without direct head injury can produce the syndrome. The clinical significance of these observations has not been established.

TREATMENT. Therapeutic maneuvers could theoretically

Table 4-7. CONDITIONS INVOLVING GREATEST RISK FOR POSTINJURY RESPIRATORY FAILURE

1. Sepsis (systemic and pulmonary)
2. Massive soft tissue injury with or without long bone fractures
3. Direct pulmonary injury
4. Massive transfusion of whole blood
5. Aspiration of gastric contents

be directed at (1) manipulating pulmonary blood flow to increase the perfusion of well-ventilated units and decrease the perfusion of poorly ventilated units, (2) directly reducing the capillary leak by reversing the membrane injury, (3) indirectly reducing the interstitial edema, or (4) improving ventilation of poorly ventilated segments and preventing further alveolar filling or collapse. Often the one of these which is most practical and which is used clinically is the last. This involves using ventilatory support designed to support and increase alveolar volume.

The earlier in the course such therapy is applied, the more successful it is likely to be. Thus it is important to identify and closely monitor patients at high risk for developing ARDS after injury. Table 4-7 indicates patients in the high-risk category. Of these five groups, patients who have either systemic or pulmonary sepsis are most likely to develop acute respiratory failure. They should be admitted to an intensive care unit for repeated evaluation of pulmonary function.

Monitoring Pulmonary Functioning

Assessment of the adequacy of pulmonary function should begin immediately after injury in those patients at risk for developing ARDS. Endotracheal tubes inserted for airway control during surgery should not be removed prematurely. In many patients an additional 4 to 6 hours of intubation postoperatively will be sufficient to allow the physician to determine that ARDS is not a threat. Extubation should not be considered until adequate lung function

has been demonstrated (described below). If several days of intubation are contemplated, a nasotracheal tube may be substituted for the endotracheal tube in the operating room. This will allow for greater patient comfort and acceptance.

A prerequisite for optimal lung function is normal cardiovascular status. Hemodynamic monitoring, therefore, should be instituted routinely. This includes recording of heart rate, arterial pressure, electrocardiogram, central venous pressure, and pulmonary artery pressure if indicated. Serial body weight, intake and output balance, bacteriologic studies, coagulation profile, and chest x-rays are important data.

Monitoring of pulmonary function can be conveniently divided into three general areas: evaluation of oxygenation, ventilation, and lung-thorax mechanics. Table 4-8 details the most easily obtained tests and includes normal values. As a general principle, isolated determinations are not as valuable as serial measurements obtained at regular intervals. Hypoxemia is often detected in apparently normal patients who appear to be doing well clinically.

The partial pressure of oxygen in the arterial blood (Pa_{O_2}) is the hallmark of adequacy of oxygenation. This must be considered in the light of the inspired oxygen concentration $(F_{I_{O_2}})$. A simple means of establishing a measurable relationship between Pa_{O_2} and $F_{I_{O_2}}$ is their ratio $(Pa_{O_2}/F_{I_{O_2}})$. Ratios between 350 and 500 are considered adequate, while a value of less than 300 is definitely abnormal. This ratio provides the clinician with a gross estimate of the efficacy of oxygenation at the bedside during rapid changes in therapy. It appears to be most reliable when the $F_{I_{O_2}}$ is between 0.2 and 0.5.

The alveolar-arterial oxygen difference (AaD_{O_2}) may allow rapid differentiation of the cause of hypoxemia. Of the four causes of hypoxemia (hypoventilation, diffusion defects, ventilation/perfusion abnormalities, and pulmonary shunt), only the intrapulmonary shunt is theoretically

Table 4-8. ASSESSMENT OF PULMONARY FUNCTION

Function and measure	*Acceptable result*	*Indication for therapy*
Oxygenation:		
Partial pressure of oxygen, arterial blood (Pa_{O_2})	$Pa_{O_2} > 90$ mm on 40% $F_{I_{O_2}}$	< 90 mmHg on 40% $F_{I_{O_2}}$ or decreasing
Ratio of partial pressure of oxygen, arterial blood, to fraction of inspired oxygen (Pa_{O_2})	$Pa_{O_2}/F_{I_{O_2}} > 350$	< 300
Alveolar-arterial oxygen gradient	50–200 mmHg	> 200 mmHg or increasing
Ventilation:		
Partial pressure of carbon dioxide, arterial blood	35–40 mmHg	30 or decreasing
Minute volume	< 12 liters/min	Increasing
Mechanics:		
Rate	12–25/min	> 25 or increasing
Effective compliance	50 ml/cm H_2O	< 50 or decreasing

refractory to O_2 administration. In general, this relationship holds true. However, the AaD_{O_2} is affected by cardiac output, O_2 consumption, the position of the hemoglobin/O_2 dissociation curve, and the magnitude of the pulmonary shunt. If the three other variables are constant, the AaD_{O_2} is a good reflection of the amount of pulmonary shunting. Characteristically, the patient with ARDS will have hypoxemia resistant to oxygen administration and therefore an elevated shunt fraction.

The adequacy of ventilation is determined by the arterial partial pressure of carbon dioxide (Pa_{CO_2}). By definition, hypoventilation occurs when the Pa_{CO_2} is elevated. Postinjury pulmonary failure is usually associated with hypocapnia (hyperventilation). Therefore the patient with a decrease in both Pa_{CO_2} and Pa_{O_2} probably has ARDS. Tidal volume (VT)—the amount of air breathed during one respiratory cycle—is another indication of the adequacy of ventilation. This is readily measured with a modestly priced respirometer. VT multiplied by the respiratory rate is called the *minute ventilation*. This value is easily derived but by itself is only a rough guide to adequate ventilation. In many postinjury patients, high minute ventilations are recorded. It is not established whether this is a compensatory response or an indicator of a pathologic condition.

The effective compliance (C_{eff}) may be quite valuable as an assessment of the ease of distensibility of lung and thoracic cage. This derived value is obtained by dividing the VT by the peak airway pressure. C_{eff} indicates the "stiffness" of the lungs, i.e., how difficult they are to ventilate (low C_{eff} means increased stiffness). A decreased C_{eff} may indicate increased extravascular lung water, airway constriction, or increased chest wall resistance (impaired bellows activity). Low values are usually found in patients with ARDS.

An adequate assessment of pulmonary function can be achieved by serial measurement of arterial blood gases, tidal volume, minute ventilation, and effective compliance. Several other monitoring devices have been advocated. The work of breathing is almost always increased in ARDS. This value is a measure of the mechanical cost of achieving adequate ventilation. The major disadvantage of this test is that it requires an intraesophageal balloon to measure transthoracic pressure and the availability of an analog computer for usable results. Although highly desirable, the measurement of the work of breathing is difficult in the critically ill patient.

Although sophisticated and expensive equipment is available to continuously monitor arterial and venous blood gases and other pulmonary function tests, it has not been shown to significantly improve patient survival.

Ventilatory Support

Indications. There are no universal guidelines for the institution of ventilatory support. The indications outlined in Table 4-7 have been found reliable in treating a large number of patients. The most common indication for beginning ventilatory therapy is hypoxemia. Initial management should be to increase the F_{IO_2} both as a diagnostic test and to temporarily relieve hypoxemia if the Pa_{O_2} is less than 65 mmHg. For effective therapy, control of the airway must be achieved. The most rapid and reliable way to do this is the insertion of an endotracheal or nasotracheal tube. Mechanical ventilation may then be applied. Since a defect in the matching of ventilation to perfusion is present, therapy is directed at maintaining ventilation to marginally ventilated alveoli and the recruiting collapsed or partially occluded alveoli. This will directly increase the FRC of the lungs.

Technique. The volume ventilator is the device most often chosen for the treatment of ARDS. The initial tidal volume setting may be 10 to 15 ml/kg body weight at a rate of 12 to 14 breaths per minute, with an inspiration:expiration ratio of 1:2. The ventilator is adjusted so that the patient can "trigger" additional ventilator breaths. This can be described as assisted mechanical ventilation (AMV). An F_{IO_2} of 0.4 should be applied initially and blood gas determinations used to indicate the efficacy of this treatment. Humidification of the inspired air via a heated nebulizer is essential to avoid drying airway secretions.

Blood gases are checked within 10 to 20 minutes of beginning respiratory treatment to determine the patient's response. If hypoxemia persists on 40% oxygen, increasing the VT still further may be warranted in an effort to increase the FRC. The effect of this maneuver is best assessed by following serial compliance changes. If the C_{eff} is improving, benefit from increased VT may be expected. If C_{eff} decreases with an increase in VT, too much volume is being given to the patient. Lower tidal volume ventilation will then be required to minimize the risk of complications of ventilatory therapy. The compliance curve is shaped somewhat like the Starling curve of cardiac function, i.e., a plateau is reached, after which any increase in volume is achieved only at the expense of a marked increase in airway pressure.

Alternate methods of mechanical ventilatory support are available. One which is being used more frequently is intermittent mandatory ventilation (IMV). This is a technique of mechanical ventilation which allows the patient to breathe spontaneously and at the same time to receive periodic support from the ventilator.

Acceptable levels of Pa_{O_2} are between 65 and 80 torr. If this cannot be achieved with the treatment outlined above, there are two alternatives: manipulation of F_{IO_2} and support of lung volume.

The F_{IO_2} may be increased to higher levels. Since pulmonary shunting is caused by continued perfusion of nonventilated alveoli, simply increasing the concentration of oxygen will have no significant effect on the shunt. In addition, washout of nitrogen from poorly ventilated alveoli will make them more susceptible to collapse, thus converting low V/Q areas to areas of shunt resulting in more atelectasis. Although there is still controversy over the role of O_2 toxicity in the genesis of ARDS (see above), the literature clearly indicates that prolonged use of high O_2 concentrations can produce a clinical picture similar to ARDS. A concentration of more than 50% O_2 is required to produce deleterious effects in patients with normal lungs, depending on the amount of time alveolar hyperoxia is maintained. The higher the O_2 concentrations, the less the time required to produce damage. Therefore every effort should be made to limit the F_{IO_2} to less than 0.5.

Since acceptable manipulation of the F_{IO_2} is limited, the second alternative is to recruit collapsed or partially collapsed alveoli with some modification of ventilatory therapy. This can be done by applying continuous positive end-expiratory pressure (PEEP) to the airway. PEEP may be achieved by either inserting an airflow resistance during expiration or using a ventilator with an end-expiratory plateau of positive pressure. Providing positive pressure throughout the respiratory cycle prevents alveolar and small airway collapse and may recruit lung units which were previously collapsed. The beneficial effects of this modality are (1) increased FRC, compliance, and Pa_{O_2}; (2) increased V/Q ratio (when initially low); (3) decreased pulmonary shunting; and (4) decreased mortality from ARDS.

Technique of PEEP. The commonly used volume ventilators have the capability of instituting PEEP without modifying the equipment. Although there is some controversy about the absolute level required, incremental increases in pressure are advocated. The usual beginning level is 5 cm H_2O of PEEP. Cardiorespiratory function is monitored after 10 to 15 minutes to assess the effects. If no beneficial effect is noted, further increases in PEEP follow in increments of 3 to 5 cm H_2O pressure.

There may be variable response to PEEP. While some patients respond with an immediate increase in Pa_{O_2}, others may not show improvement for $\frac{1}{2}$ to 1 hour or longer. Therefore absence of immediate response should not be interpreted as an absolute failure of PEEP. Each patient has a different but demonstrable optimal PEEP level which correlates well with the highest compliance. Thus a practical bedside monitor of the effectiveness of PEEP may be compliance.

Complications of PEEP. It has been shown that cardiac output may be decreased secondary to an increase in intrathoracic pressure and decreased venous return. This is usually significant only when the intravascular volume is decreased. Therefore fluids should be given to assure a normal volume status before beginning PEEP therapy. Monitoring of the pulmonary wedge pressure is valuable in the assessment of volume prior to and during the administration of PEEP. Cardiac output may also be measured to assure normal values.

Excessive pressure applied to the terminal airways may overdistend and rupture normal alveoli, leading to pneumothorax. This complication of PEEP is uncommon below 20 cm H_2O pressure.

Close attention to the effective compliance can prevent excessive airway and alveolar pressure being applied during PEEP therapy. PEEP is most beneficial when FRC is low initially. In patients with a high FRC from preexisting lung disease (Chronic Obstructive Pulmonary Disease), any level of PEEP may be detrimental. This can be deter-

mined only by closely monitoring the patient's response to treatment, noting compliance especially.

Control of Pa_{CO_2}. Hyperventilation is a common problem in patients who are being artificially ventilated. Hypocarbia has been shown to be deleterious to the cerebral circulation (vasoconstriction) and the pulmonary circulation. Therefore ventilatory therapy should be set to maintain normal levels of Pa_{CO_2}. With high tidal volume ventilation, a compensatory decrease in respiratory rate is necessary to maintain a normal Pa_{CO_2}. Increasing the inspired concentration of CO_2 or adding dead space have both been advocated as methods of increasing the Pa_{CO_2} but are rarely effective in patients with ARDS. Effective control of the Pa_{CO_2} requires heavy sedation or muscle relaxation and control of the patient's respiration. Decrease of the Pa_{CO_2} below 30 is an indication for instituting respiratory control.

Adjunctive Therapy during Mechanical Ventilation. *Oxygen-carrying Capacity of Blood.* Although the Pa_{O_2} can be increased by higher levels of F_{IO_2}, it is the red blood cell that carries almost all the O_2 to the tissues. One unit of packed red cells carries more O_2 than plasma exposed to pure O_2 at hyperbaric pressure. The hemoglobin (Hb) concentration should therefore be maintained at 12 to 14 Gm/100 ml. Attention should also be given to the acid-base status of the patient. Both acidosis and alkalosis produce shifts of the Hb/O_2 dissociation curve, which can affect the ability of Hb to off-load O_2 at the tissue level (see Alterations in Oxygen Transport, below).

Fluid Management. As noted in the discussion of the etiology of ARDS, there is much debate concerning proper fluid management. It is our opinion that maintenance of normal fluid balance is important. This will obviate any deleterious effects of hypovolemia on the Pa_{O_2} and minimize any decrease in cardiac output which may occur with PEEP administration.

Diuretics. Diuretics have been suggested as a means for reducing the amount of pulmonary edema. There is no study which has randomly and prospectively shown that diuretics are as effective as or more effective than ventilatory therapy alone in ARDS. It is reasonable to give small doses of furosemide *when hemodynamic studies indicate that fluid overload has occurred* (elevated pulmonary artery wedge pressure). No attempt should be made to "dry out" the patient by long-term administration of diuretics.

Steroids. There is no conclusive proof that pharmacologic doses of steroids should be part of the specific therapy of the ARDS syndrome, although data indicate that steroids may be effective in treating pulmonary fat embolism, septic shock, and aspiration of gastric acid.

Heparin. If intravascular coagulation is shown to be a problem in the postinjury patient with ARDS, appropriate heparin therapy may be of benefit. Heparin is associated with significant side effects and should not be used indiscriminately in the patient who has recently sustained a traumatic injury.

Antibiotics. Prophylactic use of broad-spectrum antibiotics has no place in the primary therapy of ARDS. Indiscriminate use of these agents may allow the emergence of resistant strains of bacteria, which are very difficult to treat. Many patients will already have been given antibiotics because of certain types of injury. Specific antibiotics are used to treat pulmonary sepsis. Their choice is determined by serial cultures of the sputum.

Ancillary Pulmonary Care. Patients treated in the intensive care unit tend to be bound to the bed by numerous tubes, wires, and catheters. Change in position then becomes a difficult problem. It has been shown, however, that significant improvement in oxygenation results from frequent position changes. Maintenance of one position is likely to compound pulmonary abnormalities.

Routine pulmonary toilet, suctioning with sterile technique, and attempts to prevent pulmonary infection are important. These must all be done on a routine basis.

Weaning from Ventilatory Therapy. The criteria for discontinuing ventilatory therapy are the obverse of the indications for its institution, i.e., return of pulmonary function tests to normal. The primary requisites for weaning from ventilatory therapy are a stable cardiovascular system and the absence of cardiac arrhythmias. Monitoring must therefore continue during the process. The patient with chronic obstructive lung disease should meet these same criteria. Objective criteria for weaning are shown in Table 4-9. The recommended steps in weaning are as follows:

1. The F_{IO_2} is decreased to as close to room air as possible as rapidly as possible.
2. A stepwise decrease (3 to 5 cm H_2O at a time) in the level of PEEP is begun until intermittent positive pressure breathing (IPPB) is tolerated.
3. The tidal volume is decreased to normal values.
4. The patient is weaned from the mechanical ventilator.
5. The tracheostomy tube is removed.

Arterial blood gases should be analyzed at frequent intervals after each stage of the weaning process to assure that the patient does not become hypoxemic or hypercapnic. Several hours should elapse between steps so that the process is not carried out too rapidly.

A relatively new concept in weaning is the introduction of intermittent mandatory ventilation (IMV). IMV allows the patient to gradually resume the work of breathing, in contrast to conventional weaning, in which the entire burden is put on the patient for increasing periods of time. The rate of IMV may be varied from 30 respirations to 1 (at a preset tidal volume) per minute. We have been unable to demonstrate its superiority in our patients. Some patients require a great deal of time to be successfully

Table 4-9. MINIMAL CRITERIA FOR
WITHDRAWING VENTILATORY SUPPORT

1. Clinical stability
2. Inspiratory force < -15 torr
3. $Pa_{O_2} > 250$ torr ($F_{IO_2} = 1.0$) or equivalent oxygenation index
4. Dead space/tidal volume < 0.6
5. Vital capacity > 10 ml/kg

SOURCE: Adapted from T. W. Feeley and J. Hedley-Whyte, Weaning from Controlled Ventilation and Supplemental Oxygen, *N Engl J Med*, **292**:903, 1975.

weaned, particularly those with persistent sepsis and a severe catabolic state. Reeducation of the muscles of respiration may require repeated exercise by increasing the time off IPPB.

Once the patient is able to tolerate being off the ventilator, supplemental heated nebulized oxygen should be given by means of a T piece. If this is tolerable, the patient may be extubated or a fenestrated tracheostomy tube may be inserted. The supplemental O_2 may then be decreased over a period of several days to complete the weaning process.

Summary

The syndrome of acute pulmonary failure, as it occurs in the injured patient, has many possible causes. The definable causes are amenable to specific modes of therapy. The chief functional defect, hypoxemia unresponsive to increased F_{IO_2}, is treated with ventilatory therapy with or without PEEP on an empirical basis.

With early, aggressive ventilatory support, morbidity and mortality may be minimized. Adjunctive therapy may play a significant role when there are specific indications.

Alterations in Oxygen Transport

Cell hypoxia and eventually cell death may result from the complex changes induced by shock, regardless of the type, and restoration of delivery of oxygen to the tissues at an adequate concentration and pressure forms the basis for treatment. In the past, attention was directed primarily toward the factors affecting oxygen transport capability, including the concentration and partial pressure of oxygen in the inspired air, alveolar ventilation, ventilation/perfusion relationships, cardiac output, blood volume, and hemoglobin concentration. The demonstration that the level of organic phosphates in the red blood cell has a significant effect on the position of the oxygen/hemoglobin dissociation curve has served to focus attention on the processes responsible for release of oxygen at the tissue level. Because of the clinical implication of these findings, a knowledge of factors regulating both uptake and release of oxygen has assumed increasing importance in the care of critically ill patients.

OXYGEN TRANSPORT

The oxygen transport system consists of several component processes that function collectively to extract oxygen from inspired air and deliver it at a partial pressure sufficient to allow rapid diffusion from blood into the body cells. Each of the component processes has its own internal controls, and failure of any one may be compensated for by adjustments in the remainder of the system. The functions of the oxygen transport system are summarized in the following formula:

Oxygen consumption = arteriovenous oxygen difference
$$\times \frac{\text{cardiac output (liters/minute)}}{100}$$

The amount of oxygen in whole blood includes that bound to hemoglobin (1.38 ml O_2/Gm of hemoglobin) and a small amount dissolved in plasma (0.003 ml/mm of oxygen tension). The oxygen content of arterial (Ca_{O_2}) and venous blood CV_{O_2} are calculated by the formula

Oxygen content = (1.38 × Hb conc. × Hb sat.)
$$+ (0.003 \times P_{O_2})$$

Consider a person with a hemoglobin of 15 Gm/100 ml, an arterial oxygen tension of 100 mmHg, a venous oxygen tension of 40 mmHg, arterial and venous hemoglobin saturations of 97 and 75 percent respectively, and a cardiac output of 6 liters/minute. Substituting these values in the formulas above, arterial oxygen content is 20.4 vol%, venous oxygen content is 15.6 vol%, arteriovenous oxygen difference is 4.8 vol%, and oxygen consumption is 288 ml/minute.

Changes in any one of these factors are of variable significance regarding oxygen delivery. For instance, pulmonary gas exchange with 20% inspired oxygen concentration ($F_{I_{O_2}}$) normally produces an arterial oxygen tension (Pa_{O_2}) of approximately 100 mmHg, slightly less than average alveolar oxygen tension. Increasing the $F_{I_{O_2}}$ to 100% would raise Pa_{O_2} to approximately 650 mmHg. This would increase the amount of dissolved oxygen in the plasma from 0.3 to 2.0 vol% but would only increase the hemoglobin saturation from 97 to 100 percent. In contrast, even moderate changes in hemoglobin concentration or cardiac output have a strong influence on oxygen transport capability. A hemoglobin concentration of 10 Gm/100 ml (instead of 15) in the example above would reduce the oxygen-carrying capacity of the blood by one-third ($Ca_{O_2} = 13.7$ vol%). Coupled with a fall in cardiac output from 6 to 3 liters/minute, assuming that other variables remain unchanged, oxygen consumption theoretically would fall from 288 to 96 ml/minute. This is a not infrequent clinical occurrence, although oxygen consumption would be maintained at a higher level by adjustments in other parts of the system (e.g., increase of arteriovenous oxygen difference).

Therapy designed to improve tissue oxygenation, therefore, includes an evaluation of all factors affecting the oxygen transport system. Adjustment of inspired oxygen concentration and efforts to improve alveolar ventilation are of obvious importance; however, therapeutic attempts to maintain a normal hemoglobin concentration and cardiac output deserve special attention.

OXYGEN/HEMOGLOBIN DISSOCIATION CURVE

Another aspect of oxygen transport which deserves emphasis is the relationship between hemoglobin oxygen saturation and oxygen tension. The oxyhemoglobin dissociation curve describes hemoglobin affinity for oxygen, and its unusual sigmoid shape reflects the phenomenon of heme-heme interaction. Each of four heme groups in the hemoglobin molecule reacts with oxygen in a prescribed order, and uptake of an oxygen molecule by one heme group facilitates the oxygenation of the next heme group. The sigmoid configuration of this curve is particularly suitable for the uptake, transport, and subsequent release of oxygen. Since the upper portion of the dissociation

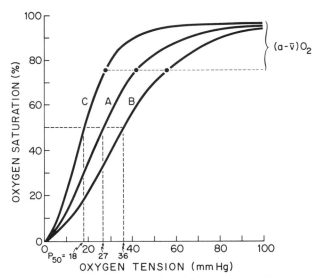

Fig. 4-24. Oxygen-hemoglobin dissociation curves in (A) normal, (B) rightward-shifted, and (C) leftward-shifted positions. The P_{50} value denotes the position of the curve along the horizontal axis and represents the oxygen tension (in mm Hg) necessary to saturate 50 percent of available hemoglobin with oxygen. Note that as the curve moves toward the left, the arteriovenous oxygen difference, (a-v̄) O_2, can be maintained only by decreasing venous oxygen tension. (*Adapted from S. D. Shappell and C. J. M. Lenfant, Anesthesiology, 37:127, 1972.*)

curve is relatively flat, oxygen loading by hemoglobin may remain relatively normal despite wide variations in the alveolar oxygen tension. As oxygenated blood traverses the peripheral capillary, however, P_{O_2} drops from approximately 100 to 40 mmHg, hemoglobin saturation falls from 97 to 75 percent, and the blood releases just over 22 percent of its oxygen load (Fig. 4-24). Since P_{O_2} values at the peripheral capillary level fall on the steep portion of the curve, significant changes in oxygen release are produced by only small alterations in oxygen tension.

The position of the oxyhemoglobin dissociation curve along the horizontal axis is characteristically termed the P_{50} value. This reflects the oxygen tension necessary to saturate 50 percent of the hemoglobin with oxygen; the normal value is approximately 27 mmHg.

The importance of positional changes of the curve is also related to its sigmoid shape. Within limits, rightward or leftward shifts have little effect on arterial oxygen saturation if Pa_{O_2} is above 80 mmHg. At the peripheral capillary level, however, even small shifts of the curve may be important. A rightward shift of the dissociation curve (P_{50} above 27 mmHg) indicates decreased hemoglobin affinity for oxygen, while a leftward shift (P_{50} below 27 mmHg) is associated with an increase of hemoglobin/oxygen affinity. Compared to the normally positioned curve, more oxygen is released at any given P_{O_2} with a rightward-shifted curve and less is released with a leftward-shifted curve. Therefore, if arterial and venous oxygen tensions remain constant, arteriovenous oxygen difference increases with a rightward shift of the curve and decreases with a leftward shift (Fig. 4-25).

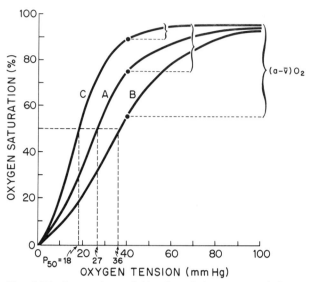

Fig. 4-25. Oxygen-hemoglobin dissociation curves similar to those in Fig. 4-24. Note that if arterial and venous oxygen tensions remain constant, arteriovenous oxygen difference decreases as the curve moves toward the left.

Changes in position of the oxygen/hemoglobin dissociation curve are significant in at least two respects. The transfer of oxygen from the blood to the sites of intracellular utilization is directly related to the oxygen pressure differential. Thus a rightward shift of the curve is theoretically advantageous, since an equivalent amount of oxygen is released at a higher P_{O_2} than with a leftward-positioned curve. (Note that in curve B of Fig. 4-24, half of the oxygen would be released at a P_{O_2} of 36 mmHg; in curve C, less than 10 percent of the oxygen would be released at the same P_{O_2}.) Secondly, the ability to maintain or enlarge the arteriovenous oxygen difference is dependent to some extent on the position of the curve. Normally, arterial hemoglobin saturation is near the upper limit and cannot be increased appreciably. Any enlargement of the arteriovenous oxygen difference necessitates reduction in venous hemoglobin saturation and venous oxygen tension Pv_{O_2}. As the curve moves to the left, maintenance of any given arteriovenous oxygen difference requires a progressive decrease in Pv_{O_2}. The fall in Pv_{O_2} is finally limited by the fact that a certain partial pressure is necessary for transfer of oxygen from the blood to the tissue cell. That level of oxygen pressure below which diffusion may be theoretically impaired and cellular function disturbed has been termed the "critical P_{O_2}."

Available data concerning the critical P_{O_2} are limited but suggest that it varies in individual organ systems and may depend on the level of activity of the tissues. Opitz and Snyder showed that oxygen uptake by the brain is impaired when venous oxygen tension falls below 20 to 25 mmHg, while Berne et al. indicated loss of myocardial function at oxygen tensions between 10 and 12 mmHg. With a leftward movement of the curve, therefore, maintaining or enlarging the arteriovenous oxygen difference is theoretically limited as the Pv_{O_2} approaches this critical level. Tissue oxygen delivery may be sustained in this instance by other mechanisms, principally by increasing cardiac output.

During hypovolemic shock, cardiac output is low and relatively fixed. Normally, enlargement of arteriovenous oxygen difference will partially compensate for the diminished blood flow; however, the response may be totally inadequate with a leftward shift of the dissociation curve. Continued survival and maintenance of essential organ function may be obtained only by shunting blood from tissues that tolerate a limited period of severe hypoxia (skin, skeletal muscle) to organs that require high oxygen flow rates (brain, heart).

FACTORS INFLUENCING THE POSITION OF THE OXYGEN/HEMOGLOBIN DISSOCIATION CURVE

Attempts to ensure a normal or rightward-positioned dissociation curve may be essential during treatment of patients with low-flow states. Factors affecting the position of the curve have been summarized by Shappel and Lenfant and are outlined in Table 4-10. The main in vivo influences include changes in pH, temperature, partial pressure of carbon dioxide, and level of red blood cell organic phosphates. Changes in hydrogen ion concentration and temperature have predictable and instantaneous effects on the position of the curve, while P_{CO_2} exerts its influence both by changing pH and by a pH-independent effect. The quantitative effects of these influences on the dissociation curve have been reviewed in several excellent publications.

The position of the dissociation curve is also influenced by interaction of hemoglobin with organic phosphates in the red blood cell. Both ATP and 2,3-diphosphoglycerate (DPG) bind to hemoglobin and lower the affinity of hemoglobin for oxygen, i.e., shift the dissociation curve to the right. In a quantitative sense, DPG is the more important of the two phosphates and exerts an additional influence in the intact red blood cell by lowering intracellular pH via Donnan equilibrium. Significant concentrations of DPG are found only in the red blood cell, and DPG is present in a concentration approximately equimolar with that of hemoglobin. DPG is a product of erythrocyte glycolysis, formed via a branch of the Embden-Myerhof pathway by conversion of 1,3-DPG to 2,3-DPG, catalyzed by diphosphoglycerate mutase.

Erythrocyte DPG undergoes considerable changes in response to several stimuli, with parallel changes in the position of the dissociation curve. Investigations have revealed that hypoxia increases erythrocyte DPG in conditions such as exercise, anemia, exposure to high altitude, cardiac failure, and various pulmonary diseases. The concomitant rightward shifts of the dissociation curve are thought to represent significant compensatory responses, allowing release of more oxygen at a higher P_{O_2}.

The regulation of DPG synthesis is complex and as yet not fully clarified. Although numerous factors influence the level of DPG (Table 4-10), the principal *mechanism* for increasing or decreasing its concentration appears to be related to the level of hydrogen ions in the red cell. DPG concentration increases as the red blood cell pH rises and decreases as the pH falls. These changes are due, in part, to

Table 4-10. FACTORS THAT ALTER HEMOGLOBIN/OXYGEN AFFINITY

Increase P_{50}	*Decrease P_{50}*

By direct effect:
  Increased [H⁺]
      temperature
      P_{CO_2}
      DPG, ATP
      Hb conc.
      Ionic strength
  Abnormal hemoglobin
  Aldosterone
	By direct effect:
	  Decreased [H⁺]
	      temperature
	      P_{CO_2}
	      DPG, ATP
	      Hb conc.
	      Ionic strength
	  Abnormal hemoglobin
	  Carboxyhemoglobin
	  Methemoglobin

By increasing DPG:
  Decreased [H⁺]
  Thyroid hormone
  Pyruvate kinase deficiency
  Increased inorganic phosphate
  Cortisol
  Cell age (young)
	By decreasing DPG:
	  Increased [H⁺]
	  Decreased thyroid hormone
	  Hexokinase deficiency
	  Decreased inorganic phosphate
	  Cell age (old)

SOURCE: Adapted from S. D. Shappell and C. J. M. Lenfant, Adaptive, Genetic and Iatrogenic Alterations of the Oxyhemoglobin Dissociation Curve, *Anesthesiology,* **37:**127, 1971.

the differential effects of pH on the activity of two red cell enzymes, DPG mutase and phosphatase. For instance, alkalosis stimulates DPG synthesis by increasing DPG-mutase activity and reducing the breakdown of DPG by DPG-phosphatase. The rise in red cell pH may be secondary to elevation of whole blood pH or, as in hypoxic states, a relative increase in the amount of deoxyhemoglobin. The pH also influences DPG binding to hemoglobin and may affect other enzymes in the glycolytic cycle. The net effect of pH changes on DPG concentration, therefore, probably represents a combination of these (and other unknown) influences. It should be noted that the pH-induced changes in DPG concentration tend to counteract the direct pH effects on the curve via the Bohr effect. Therefore the immediate rightward shift of the curve secondary to acute acidosis is eventually offset by a pH-induced reduction in DPG concentration.

DPG synthesis is also responsive to hormonal influences and the level of inorganic phosphate. The phosphate level is directly related to DPG concentration, and maintenance of a normal inorganic phosphate level during intravenous hyperalimentation is necessary to prevent a reduction in the level of erythrocyte 2,3-DPG. Thyroid hormone acts directly to increase DPG synthesis, a fact which probably explains the elevated levels of this compound in hyperthyroid patients. Cortisol and aldosterone both shift the dissociation curve to the right, thereby decreasing hemoglobin/oxygen affinity. The effects of cortisol are probably secondary to direct stimulation of DPG synthesis. Hemoglobin/oxygen affinity also increases as the erythrocyte ages, presumably owing to a decreasing DPG concentration.

BLOOD TRANSFUSIONS, ERYTHROCYTE DPG, AND OXYGEN DELIVERY

The acceptability for transfusion of blood which has been stored in ACD (acid citrate dextrose) solution for up to 3 weeks is based on survival of at least 70 percent of the cells in the recipient's circulation. During this 3-week period, however, there is a rapid decline in erythrocyte DPG and a progressive increase in hemoglobin/oxygen affinity. Following transfusion, several hours are required for the DPG levels to return to normal. These findings suggest that oxygen delivery may be impaired after the administration of large quantities of stored blood and have led to a re-evaluation of transfusion practices.

Several studies in both experimental animals and man have failed to show significant impairment of tissue oxygenation with markedly reduced levels of erythrocyte DPG and leftward shifts of the oxygen dissociation curve. Similar findings were noted in our study of 45 injured patients who received more than 5 units of whole blood stored in ACD solution during resuscitation and the subsequent operative procedure. Erythrocyte DPG levels were below normal in a majority of these patients and correlated well with the amount and storage time of the transfused blood. There were no consistent correlations, however, between DPG concentration and the measured parameters of oxygen delivery. This lack of correlation may be explained by two observations. First, the position of the dissociation curve cannot be reliably predicted from a knowledge of the DPG concentration alone. DPG represents only one of several factors that affect the curve, and the final P_{50} represents a composite of these influences. Normal or elevated P_{50} values noted in several patients with low DPG concentrations were probably due to other factors (e.g., pH and temperature) which tended to counteract the influence of DPG. A second observation is the lack of a consistent relationship between the P_{50} value and oxygen consumption. The majority of patients with leftward shifts of the dissociation curve had reasonably normal arteriovenous oxygen difference and oxygen consumption. Additionally, several of the patients with narrowed arteriovenous oxygen differences maintained oxygen delivery simply by increasing the cardiac output.

These findings do not imply that the position of the dissociation curve and the factors that influence it are unimportant. They do suggest that a person with reasonably intact cardiovascular and pulmonary systems is able to tolerate rather significant leftward shifts of the oxygen dissociation curve. The consequences may be quite different, however, in a patient with limited compensatory mechanisms and in some therapeutic regimens followed without understanding of their effects on the position of the curve. An example of this is shown in Fig. 4-26. Despite the sharp reduction in cardiac output following hemorrhage to a mean blood pressure of 50 mmHg, the control dog with a normal P_{50} value was able to maintain normal oxygen delivery by increasing the arteriovenous oxygen difference from 4.5 to 10.6 ml. In contrast the DPG-depleted dog was unable to expand the arteriovenous oxygen difference sufficiently (P_{50} value 15 mmHg). The problem was compounded by attempts to correct pH to normal by infusion of sodium bicarbonate solution. The dissociation curve moved further to the left (P_{50} value 8 mmHg), the hemoglobin concentration fell secondary to hemodilution, and oxygen consumption fell to near zero. Although extreme, the experimental conditions are not unlike those which may be found in the clinical setting.

In summary, available evidence suggests that changes in hemoglobin/oxygen affinity, as reflected by the position of the oxygen dissociation curve, may be important in several circumstances. The elevated DPG concentrations and rightward shifts of the dissociation curve observed in hypoxic states (pulmonary disease, cardiac failure, anemia, exposure to high altitude, and so on) probably represent compensatory responses that facilitate oxygen unloading in the tissue capillaries. Oxygenation can be maintained in these instances by other mechanisms (e.g., increasing cardiac output) but at greater expense to body economy.

Leftward shifts of the dissociation curve observed fol-

lowing transfusions of stored blood, acute alkalosis, hypothermia, and so forth are, at best, undesirable phenomena and may significantly impair oxygen unloading. Although leftward shifts are tolerated in many circumstances, maintenance of a normally positioned dissociation curve may be of singular importance in patients with hypoxia, anemia, or hypotension when compensatory responses are limited.

THERAPEUTIC IMPLICATIONS

Obtaining a sufficient quantity of fresh blood for resuscitation of the patient in hemorrhagic shock is difficult, and attempts are being made to find a suitable storage medium that will maintain the levels of organic phosphates in the red blood cells. At present, storage of blood in CPD (citrate phosphate dextrose) solution seems to be the most practical alternative. Survival of red blood cells is similar after transfusion of blood stored in either ACD or CPD solution. Compared to blood stored in ACD solution, however, blood stored in CPD media has a higher pH, and DPG and P_{50} are maintained at consistently higher levels. Conversion from ACD to CPD solution for blood storage is a simple matter for blood banks and has been accomplished in many areas. When large quantities of blood are administered, particularly in critically ill patients, some attention should be paid to the storage age of each unit of blood. If a significant portion of the blood administered has been stored for more than 7 to 10 days, every attempt should be made to obtain fresh blood for additional transfusion requirements. In our experience the institution of these simple changes, including conversion to CPD storage media, has been rewarding. The large reductions in DPG and P_{50} noted in the past are rarely seen today, even after massive transfusions.

Other factors that influence the position of the dissociation curve (Table 4-10) may also be important in the individual patient. For instance, the induction of respiratory alkalosis may produce an abrupt increase in hemoglobin/oxygen affinity. This is a common occurrence during operations and in patients requiring ventilatory assistance in the postoperative period; coupled with other factors that limit oxygen transport, the capacity to maintain tissue oxygenation may be sharply reduced. Similarly, the sudden correction of an acidosis, whether metabolic or respiratory, may have undesirable effects. In this regard the indiscriminate use of sodium bicarbonate during resuscitation of patients in hypovolemic shock is discouraged. The presence of a mild metabolic alkalosis is a common finding after resuscitation, owing in part to the alkalinizing effects of blood transfusions and the administration of lactated Ringer's solution. After infusion (and partial restoration of hepatic blood flow), the citrate and lactate contained in transfused blood and the lactate in lactated Ringer's solution are metabolized and bicarbonate is formed. If excessive quantities of sodium bicarbonate are administered simultaneously, a severe metabolic alkalosis may result. The alkaline pH may be highly undesirable, particularly in patients with hypoxia or low fixed cardiac output. Combined with other factors incident to blood replacement which increase hemoglobin/oxygen affinity (low DPG concentration and hypothermia), significant interference

Fig. 4-26. Effects of hemorrhagic shock and sodium bicarbonate infusion on oxygen consumption after exchange transfusion with fresh blood (dog A) and DPG-depleted blood (dog B). I, Control period; II, after exchange transfusion (DPG concentration 6.20 μM/ml RBC in dog B); III, after induction of hypotension; IV, continued hypotension and sodium bicarbonate infusion.

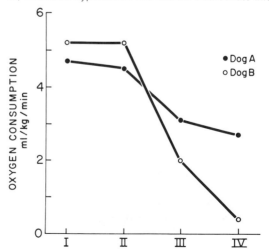

with oxygen unloading at the cellular level may occur.

The immediate and direct pH influences on the curve (via the Bohr effect) are eventually offset by reciprocal changes in DPG concentration. There is, however, a lag period of approximately 4 hours before any change in DPG concentration is noted, and the final level is not reached until 48 hours after induction of acidosis or alkalosis. The fact that the effects of sudden large changes in pH may persist for several hours should be considered during therapy. Correction of a metabolic acidosis, therefore, is properly directed toward correction of the underlying disorder. Bicarbonate therapy may be reserved for the treatment of severe metabolic acidosis, particularly following cardiac arrest, when *partial* correction of pH is essential to restore myocardial function. Similarly, pH correction in more protracted states of metabolic acidosis may be indicated but should be accomplished slowly.

Lowering body temperature also causes a leftward shift of the dissociation curve and an increase in hemoglobin/oxygen affinity, but any interference in oxygen delivery may be countered effectively by the hypothermia-induced reduction in metabolic requirements.

Rightward shifts of the curve are usually desirable and, unless extreme, rarely interfere with oxygen uptake in the lungs. Rightward shifts generally occur as a compensatory response to hypoxia, regardless of the cause. Nevertheless, in patients with severe arterial desaturation (exposure to high altitude, congestive failure, right-to-left cardiac shunts), any potential benefit from shifting the curve further to the right may be offset by interference with oxygen loading.

In a complex clinical setting, multiple factors that influence hemoglobin/oxygen affinity may be operative at any given time, and abrupt changes secondary to therapy or the disease process itself may occur. Evaluation of these multiple influences may be difficult, since few data concerning their cumulative effects are available. Nevertheless their *net* effect can be estimated by determining the position of the oxygen dissociation curve.

Techniques for constructing an oxygen dissociation curve are time-consuming and not readily available in most hospitals. For this reason we have developed a rapid, though less precise, method for estimating the position of the curve (the P_{50} value). Since the shape and slope of the curve do not change appreciably with changes in position, determination of a single point on the steep part of the slope should allow a rough estimate of the entire curve. To obviate the use of a tonometer, a single sample of venous blood is drawn anaerobically and the P_{O_2} and oxygen saturation are measured. (An arterial sample is unsuitable, since the values fall on the upper flat portion of the curve.) An estimated P_{50} value may then be obtained using the Severinghaus slide rule or a nomogram as depicted in Fig. 4-27. The nomogram represents a computer plot of a family of O_2 dissociation curves, using the correction factor for pH as suggested by Severinghaus. The point on the nomogram corresponding to the measured P_{O_2} and saturation values is found and traced to the line representing 50 percent oxygen saturation. This intersect represents the estimated P_{50}; the normal value is approximately

27 mmHg. A P_{50} above this level represents a rightward shift of the oxygen dissociation curve, while a lower value represents a leftward shift.

To test the validity of this technique, oxygen dissociation curves were constructed using a standard mixing technique on 50 occasions in 27 acutely ill patients. In each instance an estimated P_{50} was obtained from the nomogram using a single sample of venous blood drawn at the same time. Correlation between the two values was excellent (correlation coefficient .92).

Estimates of P_{50} have become routine in our care of critically ill patients. Combining this with measurements of both arterial and venous blood gases, a considerable amount of information may be obtained about the state of oxygenation and oxygen transport capability.

THERAPY OF SHOCK

Hypovolemic Shock

It is apparent from the previously described etiologic classification of shock that therapy will of necessity depend on detection of the causative mechanisms while providing support to the patient. Correction of the underlying causative factors can then be carried out. Consequently one sees again the usefulness of a practical clinical classification that includes (1) oligemic shock, (2) cardiogenic shock, and (3) shock caused by changes in peripheral resistance and

Fig. 4-27. Nomogram for estimation of P_{50} value (position of the oxygen-hemoglobin dissociation curve). The point on the nomogram corresponding to the measured P_{O_2} and saturation of a sample of venous blood is traced to the line representing 50 percent oxygen saturation. This intersect represents the estimated P_{50} (normal value approximately 27 mm Hg). In the example shown, the venous blood sample P_{O_2} is 39 mm Hg, the oxygen saturation 65 percent, and the P_{50} value 31 mm Hg (a rightward-positioned dissociation curve).

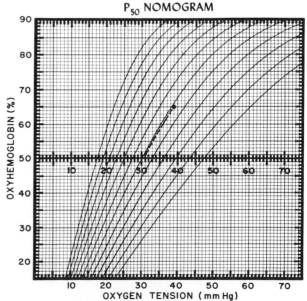

P_{50} NOMOGRAM

capacity vessels (neurogenic shock and septic shock). In a patient who has undergone trauma, more than one causative factor may be operating. Once the diagnosis of shock has been made and supportive therapy begun, a diligent search can be made for the causative factor or factors.

Treatment of shock, therefore, can best be thought of in relation to the type of shock that is present. As pointed out earlier, the pathogenesis of hypovolemic hypotension is varied. Recognition of deficits of total body water and electrolytes is usually subtle, and correction requires specific therapy with crystalloid solutions. Reductions in the extracellular fluid volume (plasma and interstitial fluids) primarily, as in burns, peritonitis, and some forms of crush injury, are more easily recognized. Specific therapy should be started with electrolyte solutions and rarely may require the use of plasma or some source of protein. External blood loss as seen in lacerations should be corrected immediately, as fluid therapy is begun, with first-aid measures, including pressure tamponade. Surgical procedures may then be carried out. Similarly, an external loss, such as bleeding from a duodenal ulcer, should be treated with the usual measures, including decompression of the stomach, while supportive therapy is begun.

The only other immediate concern in addition to control of the causative wounds is maintenance of an open airway. Pulmonary insufficiency rarely occurs from shock alone, but concomitant injuries may include crush injuries of the chest, pneumothorax, hemothorax, or specific obstruction of the airway from injuries to the head and neck. In these circumstances adequate respiratory exchange must be restored promptly.

VOLUME. The treatment of hemorrhagic shock continues to be the adequate replacement of whole blood, since this is the fluid that has been lost. Early use of properly cross-matched, type-specific whole blood is still the primary therapy when shock is due to whole blood loss. When available, type-specific or Rh-negative "universal donor" type O blood with low anti-A titer can be administered.

Extracellular Fluid Replacement

An effective therapeutic regimen for the treatment of hemorrhagic shock has now been used successfully in several thousand patients, taking into account the previously described changes in the peripheral circulation and interstitial fluid.

When patients are admitted to the emergency room in hemorrhagic shock, a large-gauge needle or catheter is inserted into an appropriate vein (preferably in the arm) and an infusion of lactated Ringer's solution is begun immediately. At the same time, blood is drawn for typing and cross matching. The lactated Ringer's solution is run at a rapid rate so that in a period of 45 minutes between 1,000 and 2,000 ml of lactated Ringer's solution is given intravenously. This approach has several advantages.

The procedure is a highly effective therapeutic trial to determine the preexisting amount of blood loss or the presence of continuing blood loss. It is often observed that blood pressure will return to normal, become stable, and remain so in patients with severe hypotension after infusion of 1 or 2 liters of a balanced salt solution. When such a

response is correlated with measurements of red blood cell mass, plasma volume, and extracellular fluid volume, the preexisting blood loss is shown to be relatively minimal. If blood loss has been minimal and hemorrhage is not continuing, hemorrhagic hypotension can be alleviated simply by the infusion of a balanced salt solution.

If blood loss has been severe or hemorrhage is continuing, the elevation of blood pressure and decrease in pulse rate that occur with rapid intravenous infusion of lactated Ringer's solution is usually transient. When this occurs, whole blood that has been accurately typed and cross-matched is available and can be given immediately. Consequently, the initial use of the balanced salt solution allows time for accurate typing and cross-matching.

In view of the disparate reduction in the extravascular, extracellular fluid as demonstrated in animals and man, it is felt that even though blood is needed, as it is in the majority of patients admitted in hemorrhagic hypovolemia, alleviation of the reduction in functional extracellular fluid is desirable.

Lactated Ringer's solution as initial therapy, both from the standpoint of a therapeutic trial and as a therapeutic adjunct, is a procedure that has been found to be effective. This is understandable, since lactated Ringer's solution is isotonic, essentially free from side reactions, and virtually harmless from the standpoint of aggravation of other fluid and electrolyte imbalances that may be present.

Further, it appears that the use of a balanced salt solution in this fashion significantly reduces the requirement of whole blood in the patient with hemorrhagic hypotension. This is true not only from the standpoint of proper hemoglobin and hemoconcentrations following therapy, but also from the standpoint of prevention of, or recovery from, renal failure.

A concern that Ringer's lactate solution may aggravate the existing lactate acidosis when used to treat patients in shock has been expressed by several investigators, but previous studies in both experimental animals and patients do not support this view. The use of blood plus Ringer's lactate solution to treat hemorrhagic shock in experimental animals results in a more rapid return to normal of lactate, excess lactate, and pH than does treatment with return of shed blood alone. Recently, serial determinations of lactate, excess lactate, pH, and base excess have been obtained in 52 patients in hemorrhagic shock. All patients received Ringer's lactate solution in addition to whole blood during the period of resuscitation. There was a significant reduction in lactate and excess lactate levels and a return of pH and base excess values toward normal during the period of shock while Ringer's lactate solution was being infused. After resuscitation, all these values rapidly returned to normal levels.

Blood Transfusions. Blood transfusions have been discussed above under Blood Transfusions, Erythrocyte DPG, and Oxygen Delivery.

Hemoconcentration. For many years the belief was held that hemorrhage and shock were separate entities, because hemorrhage was not accompanied by hemoconcentration and shock invariably was. As shown in Fig. 4-28 and as described previously under Pathophysiologic Responses to

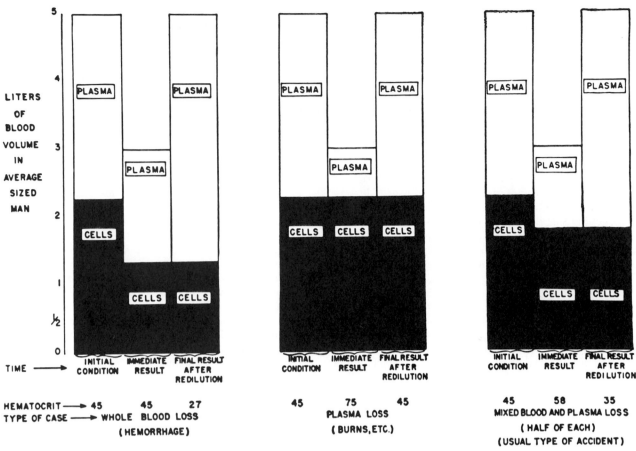

Fig. 4-28. Six possible results in shock cases, showing the fallacy of using hemoconcentration as the only guide to treatment. (*From H. N. Harkins, Surgery, 9:231, 1941.*)

Shock, the hemoconcentration is not a differentiating factor. The extent of concentration depends on the proportion of red blood cells and plasma lost in the hypovolemic episode, as well as on the compensatory adjustments that the interstitial fluid has been able to make to the intravascular volume reduction.

Blood Substitutes. In the absence of whole blood, many substances have been proposed as transient substitutes for the combination of red blood cells and plasma available in whole blood. The most popular and commonly used substitute has been human plasma. In some circumstances, e.g., battlefield conditions, plasma has been a highly serviceable substitute. Plasma carries with it the same risk of viral hepatitis that whole blood does. A unit of pooled plasma, however, carries a greater risk of harboring and transmitting the infective viral hepatitis than a unit of blood. As shown by Allen, storage of fresh plasma at room temperature for 6 to 8 months significantly reduces the attack rate and infectivity of the virus of infectious hepatitis. In any event, the administration of plasma carries with it some risk of hepatitis as well as the poorly understood antigen-antibody reactions that frequently occur from homologous plasma. Further, the volume of plasma required is such that for all practical purposes restoration of blood volume is not generally feasible with plasma alone. Plasma contains no hemoglobin and, therefore, no oxygen-carrying capacity beyond that of any non-erythrocyte-containing liquid. (Physically dissolved oxygen in plasma constitutes only 0.3 percent by volume.)

It should be pointed out that volume replacement with plasma is rapidly equilibrated into the total extracellular fluid. The albumin that remains in the vascular tree is easily degraded at a rapid rate. Moore estimates that plasma dispersal from the intravascular to the extravascular phase may proceed at a rate approaching 500 ml, or 2 units, per hour. Therefore plasma or albumin as a blood volume substitute is transient at best.

A number of other substances have been proposed for transfusion in hemorrhagic shock since early in World War I, when solutions of acacia were used. Several excellent review articles are available which summarize the problems with all these artificial solutions. Suffice it to say that at present the only acceptable one of the entire group continues to be dextran. This substance has been shown to be effective clinically in the absence of a severe need for hemoglobin and its oxygen-carrying capacity. Nevertheless, like all other plasma or blood substitutes, this substance still causes occasional severe antigen-antibody reactions and above all, regularly produces defects in the clotting mechanism. This has been shown in volunteers and patients when amounts of more than 1 liter of clinical dextran, with an average molecular weight of approximately 75,000, are used in man. The longest effect of dextran in maintaining an expanded plasma volume has been shown to be 24 to 48 hours. Low-molecular-weight dextran in the average range of 35,000 to 40,000 has recently received renewed interest because of data suggesting its ability to lower the viscosity of blood and possibly to prevent agglutination of erythrocytes during the low-flow state induced by hypovolemic shock. But work by Replogle indicates that the effect of low-molecular-weight dextran on blood viscosity is produced entirely by hemodilution or change in blood volume. When these parameters were controlled, no evidence of alterations in blood viscosity associated with infusions of low-molecular-weight dextran were observed. Although there are some theoretical advantages in using this plasma expander, investigative studies reveal serious clotting-mechanism defects with low-molecular-weight dextran, such as had been seen with the higher-molecular-weight dextrans.

POSITIONING. Positioning of the patient in shock has long been thought to be an adjunct in the treatment of hypovolemic shock. Most first-aid courses teach that the patient in shock should be placed in the head-down position. Although it is true that some forms of shock, particularly neurogenic shock, will respond to the head-down position, the effect of posture on the cerebral circulation in the face of true hypovolemia has not been defined. Frequently the patient with multiple trauma has sustained other injuries, within both the abdomen and the chest, so that the routine use of the Trendelenburg, or head-down, position may interfere with respiratory exchange far more than when the patient is left supine. The beneficial effect of the head-down position is probably the result of transient autotransfusion of pooled blood in the capacity or venous side of the peripheral circulation. This beneficial effect can be obtained easily by elevating both legs while maintaining the trunk and the remainder of the patient in the supine position. This is probably the preferable position, then, for the treatment of hypovolemic shock.

PULMONARY SUPPORT. In the past, most writings on the treatment of hypovolemic shock stated that breathing high oxygen concentrations is probably of little avail during a period of hypotension. These conclusions were based on the concept that the principal defect is in volume flow to tissues and decreased cardiac output. The oxygen saturation in the majority of patients with uncomplicated hypovolemic shock is generally normal, and the small increase in dissolved oxygen in the blood contributed by raising the P_{O_2} above this level is insignificant, particularly in the face of a markedly decreased cardiac output. This concept continues to be valid in terms of improvement of the shock state or tissue oxygenation itself. Nevertheless, in the small but significant group of patients in hypovolemic shock in whom the oxygen saturation is not normal, the *initial* use of increased oxygen concentrations may be extremely important, since the fall in cardiac output accompanying hemorrhagic shock has been shown to compound existing defects in oxygenation. This may occur in patients with preexisting defects, such as chronic obstructive lung dis-

ease, but more frequently problems in oxygenation arise directly from the patient's injury. Examples of this are a coexisting pneumothorax, pulmonary contusion, aspiration of gastric contents or blood, and larger obstructive problems. Thus, although oxygen is not routinely administered to patients in shock, if any doubt exists as to the possibility of one of these circumstances or as to the adequacy of oxygenation of arterial blood, the initial administration of oxygen until the injuries to the patient have been diligently assessed is certainly justified. If oxygen is to be administered to patients under these circumstances, it should be delivered through loose-fitting face masks designed for this purpose. If controlled airway is indicated for other reasons, an endotracheal tube is ideal. The use of nasal catheters, particularly those passed into the nasopharynx, is avoided because of potential complications of pharyngeal lacerations and gastric distension. Gastric rupture has been recorded secondary to such a catheter being inadvertently placed in the esophagus.

ANTIBIOTICS. Antibiotics were used in the treatment of hypovolemic shock for many years and were thought to exert a protective mechanism against the ravages of hypovolemia. Subsequent data fail to support this hypothesis. The use of antibiotics in patients who have open or potentially contaminated wounds, however, continues to be sound practice, when combined with good surgical debridement and care. Consequently the use of wide-spectrum antibiotics, as well as specific coverage against streptococci and staphylococci, is advisable as a preventive measure in the severely injured patient. Generally, penicillin is used in doses of 1 to 5 million units/24 hours, with parenteral administration of tetracycline in doses of 1 to 2 Gm for the first 24 hours. These are started immediately in patients who have sustained hypovolemic shock from trauma.

TREATMENT OF PAIN. Treatment of pain in the patient with hypovolemic shock is rarely a problem from the standpoint of shock itself. If, however, the causative injury produces severe pain, as in fracture, peritonitis, injury to the chest wall, and the like, control of pain becomes mandatory. Generally, when the patient is moved to the emergency facility where physicians and care are available, simple restorative measures, administration of intravenous fluids, passing of catheters, and so forth, will give reassurance. The need for analgesics is greatly reduced, since the need to allay fear and anxiety becomes markedly less. If, however, the patient continues to have severe pain, the observations made by Henry K. Beecher in World War II become extremely pertinent. Beecher pointed out that many battle casualties received morphine or other narcotic agents by subcutaneous administration early after wounding. Since these analgesics were not put into the circulation immediately, the pain continued and the patient ultimately received several doses that were not absorbed. Once effective therapy was begun for shock, the doses previously administered were absorbed and profound sedation resulted. As a result, the recommendation was made that small doses of narcotics be given *intravenously* for the management of pain in the patient with shock. This has been standard practice for 20 years and relieves pain without contributing significantly to the potentiation of the shock syndrome.

STEROIDS. Adrenocorticoid depletion was commonly regarded as a contributory factor in shock after it was learned that the presence of hypovolemic shock could in itself deplete the adrenal cortex of adrenocortical steroids. Subsequent studies, however, have shown that adrenocortical steroid production is stimulated maximally by the presence of hypovolemic shock. Steroid depletion with hypovolemic shock may possibly occur in the elderly patient or in patients who have specific adrenocortical diseases such as incipient Addison's disease, postadrenalectomy patients, or patients who have had adrenal suppression with exogenous adrenocortical steroids. In these specific instances the intravenous administration of hydrocortisone is desirable. In the general patient, with hypovolemic shock, however, administration of adrenocorticoids is probably not indicated.

DIGITALIS. Digitalis has been advocated in the treatment of hypovolemic shock. There is no doubt that in some patients, particularly elderly ones, the stress of hypovolemic shock will in itself induce or aggravate cardiac failure. In these patients, digitalis is found to be helpful. Over the years many have investigated the role of the heart as a cause of the irreversible form of hemorrhagic shock, but experimental data obtained in patients indicate that heart failure in response to hypovolemic shock is merely a terminal event. Further evidence of this is supplied by the fact that the central venous pressure does not rise except terminally in hypovolemic shock.

INTRAARTERIAL INFUSIONS. Intraarterial infusions were advocated for many years for the rapid replacement of intravascular volume in hypovolemic hypotension and shock. The weight of evidence at present, supplied by Hampson, Scott and Gurd, Harkins, and others, is that "the side of the circulation into which the blood is transfused is of no importance provided that the same rapid rate can be assured." Consequently the present-day usefulness of intraarterial transfusion resolves to a matter of convenience. If the operative procedure is in the area of a major artery, as in open-chest procedures, then a given quantity of blood may be delivered much faster via the intraarterial route. Otherwise no specific advantage seems to be offered by the arterial route of transfusion.

HYPOTHERMIA. Since the basic defect during shock is inadequate perfusion to tissues for maintenance of normal metabolism, a logical approach to supportive therapy would include some mechanism to lower the normal tissue metabolism. Hypothermia is available at present to lower metabolism. Experimental results in animals have demonstrated that induction of hypothermia prior to the onset of hemorrhagic shock will in fact protect against the lethality of the shock. Similarly, some experiments have shown that therapy of hemorrhagic shock with hypothermia has provided some beneficial effect. The available data for evaluation of hypothermia in human hypovolemic shock are meager. Since the induction of a hypothermic state is a serious undertaking, it is difficult to assess the effects on the severely injured patient. Some available data would indicate that under some circumstances, hypothermia may be desirable. These circumstances need to be further elucidated and are probably concerned with the later stages of prolonged hypovolemic or possibly septic shock.

RENAL HYPOTHERMIA. Local or regional cooling is of proved benefit in protecting the kidney from damage during ischemic periods. The methods of local cooling previously described have been developed in an attempt to reduce postoperative renal complications induced by the total ischemia necessary during renal artery repair, heminephrectomy, or stone removal, as well as aorticorenal surgery. Of far more common occurrence are the renal ischemia and resultant renal damage occasioned by hemorrhagic or hypovolemic shock. Since the kidney is rendered ischemic even in mild hypovolemic shock, rapid lowering of intrarenal temperature should afford protection during the prolonged periods of ischemia.

The effective methods of introducing local renal hypothermia previously described are limited for optimal use in emergency situations by requiring (1) the additional operative trauma of mobilization of the kidney; (2) cumbersome special equipment that is not readily available or is difficult to sterilize and maintain; and (3) careful attention to prevent interference with other operative procedures within the abdominal cavity.

The open peritoneal cavity affords a large surface area for heat exchange. Jaeger found that the introduction of a large volume of cold isotonic solution into the closed peritoneal cavity of dogs resulted in a rapid decrease in body temperature. If intraabdominal organs, particularly the kidneys, which are apparently the most sensitive to hypoxia, can be effectively cooled by the direct introduction of cold solution, then a simple, expedient, practical method of cooling is readily available in every operating room. This consists of filling the open abdominal cavity with isotonic salt solution that has been cooled in the operating-room refrigerator (Fig. 4-29).

Experiments in animals were undertaken (1) to compare the temperatures obtained and the protection afforded the ischemic kidney by this method with that of direct surface hypothermia, (2) to evaluate the depth of cooling obtained in the ischemic versus the intact kidney, and (3) to determine the depth of cooling obtained in the kidney during hemorrhagic shock. A summary of the results of these experiments follows.

1. Figure 4-19 shows the degree of protection afforded by surface cooling as opposed to formal hypothermic perfusion, as described earlier; surface cooling provided significant protection from renal ischemia (100 percent survival rate). Lower intrarenal temperatures could be obtained by circulating coolant; however, the survival rate was lowered, probably because of the necessary extensive mobilization of the kidney.

2. A subsequent experimental study was designed to evaluate the effect of intact blood supply on the degree of hypothermia obtained by peritoneal cooling. The results of this study are shown in Fig. 4-30, and a comparison between esophageal temperatures and renal temperatures

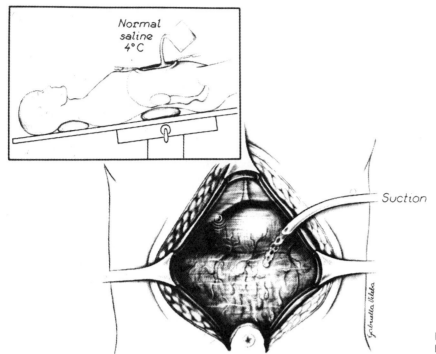

Fig. 4-29. Technique of regional abdominal hypothermia.

with and without intact renal blood supply is also seen. These results demonstrate that there is some decrease in total body temperature, especially with intact blood supply to the kidneys, but that the intrarenal temperature even with intact blood flow is decreased at more than twice the rate of the general body temperature. Without blood flow, the depth of renal hypothermia achieved is three times that of the esophageal temperature as long as cooling is continued. An equally important observation is that the ischemic

kidney rewarms only slowly as compared to the kidney with intact blood supply.

3. The results of the third study to determine the depth of cooling obtained during hemorrhagic shock are shown in Fig. 4-31. The depth of hypothermia obtained is seen to be approximately the same as that in the intact kidneys, without hemorrhagic hypotension. Similarly, there was a

Fig. 4-30. Degrees of peritoneal hypothermia obtained in dogs by introduction of intraperitoneal iced saline solution at 2 to 3°C (left renal pedicle occluded).

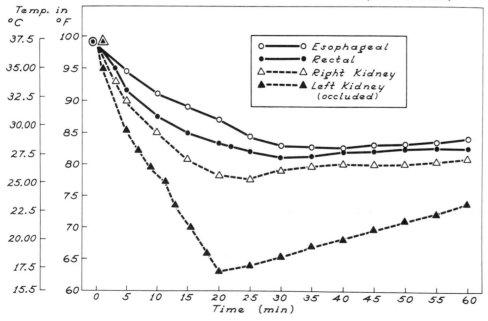

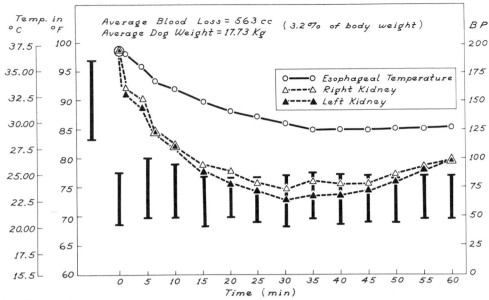

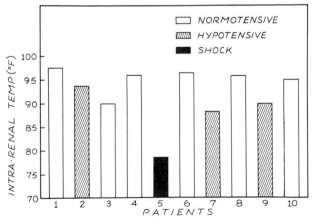

Fig. 4-31. Degrees of peritoneal hypothermia obtained in dogs by introduction of intraperitoneal iced saline solution at 2 to 3°C after blood loss shock (renal pedicle not occluded).

concomitant lowering of the total body temperature to approximately 88°F. But after the chilled solution had been removed from the abdominal cavity, the intrarenal temperatures in the hypotensive animals continued to decline, reaching 75°F in 30 minutes. Despite this, the total body temperatures did not reach significantly lower levels.

The studies indicate that intrarenal temperatures of approximately 25°C should furnish good protection with only transient mild suppression of renal function. Certainly 20°C offers complete protection to the ischemic kidney for periods extending to 6 hours. The effective cooling of the kidney with an intact blood supply versus the ischemic kidney emphasizes the importance of blood supply in determining the rate and depth of cooling.

Studies were then made in patients on the basis of the animal experiments. It was felt that this type of hypothermia could be used in patients with safety and could be expected to produce a sustained lowering of intrarenal temperatures during hypovolemic hypotension. Intrarenal hypothermia in patients was produced by filling the abdominal cavity with 2 liters of refrigerated (3°C) isotonic salt solution. The salt solution was allowed to remain in contact with the peritoneal cavity for approximately 1 to 2 minutes. The bulk of this was removed by suction, and this was repeated several times, employing a total of 4 to 6 liters of the cold solution during a 5-minute period. Intrarenal temperatures were measured by sterilized needle prior to the induction of hypothermia and at intervals during and after cooling.

Figure 4-32 shows the intrarenal temperatures of 10 patients taken 5 minutes after the beginning of peritoneal hypothermia. It can be seen that in those patients who were normotensive there was minimal lowering of the renal temperature. On the other hand, in patients with modest

hypotension, intrarenal temperatures were lowered to 88 to 90°F, and in the severely hypotensive patient the intrarenal temperature in 5 minutes had reached the level of 78°F.

Figure 4-33 depicts three patients in whom intrarenal temperatures were measured prior to induction of renal hypothermia and at 1-minute intervals thereafter. As would be expected from the studies just presented, the rate of fall of intrarenal temperature was directly proportional to the degree of hypotension present at the time of cooling.

Esophageal temperatures were monitored. In general, the fall in esophageal temperature was approximately half the fall in intrarenal temperatures in the first 10 minutes. The lowest temperature reached was 88°F in two patients. No untoward effects were noted other than a modest fall in blood pressure (less than 10 mmHg diastolic) in normotensive patients. There were no changes in cardiac rate or rhythm during this procedure.

The animal experiments show that an intrarenal tem-

Fig. 4-32. Intrarenal temperatures in 10 patients 5 minutes after beginning of peritoneal hypothermia.

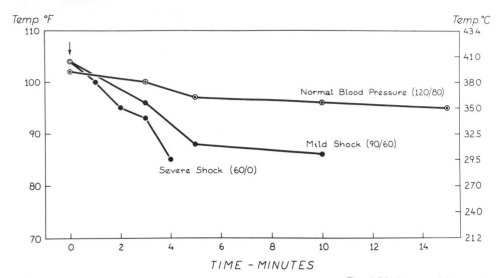

Fig. 4-33. Intrarenal temperatures of patients after induction of peritoneal hypothermia in relation to degree of hypotension.

perature of 28 to 30°C is easily attainable in the ischemic dog kidney by sluice-cooling of the peritoneal cavity. This moderate degree of hypothermia produced 100 percent survival, but with mild elevation of the BUN for a period of 12 to 15 days. All these animals excreted normal or increased amounts of urine.

The preliminary data suggest that cooling by means of peritoneal irrigation (1) produces sufficient lowering of intrarenal temperatures to afford protection to the kidney with decreased blood flow, (2) offers a rapid means of lowering total body temperature, and (3) should produce a decrease in intrarenal temperature in a kidney completely deprived of blood comparable to that obtained by other local techniques.

In the past the chief objection to peritoneal irrigation was the introduction of infection. Peritoneal dialysis for uremia has proved to be a safe procedure on a short-term basis, infection occurring only after prolonged use. In our experience the use of copious quantities of refrigerated salt solution in the operating room has been completely free from complications. Specifically, there have been no cases or peritonitis, abscess formation, wound disruption, or prolonged ileus in the patients studied.

VASOPRESSORS. In recent years the addition of substances that cause additional vasoconstriction in hypovolemic shock has been popular. These have been used largely because human blood pressure can usually be elevated somewhat by the addition of one of a series of pressor agents. Although it is true that blood pressure can be elevated, the objective in treating hypovolemic shock is to increase tissue perfusion. By the use of vasopressors, the blood pressure is raised by increasing peripheral vascular resistance and decreasing tissue perfusion. Therefore the injurious effects of shock may well be aggravated.

As experience has accumulated with the use of vasopressors, it is obvious that the alpha- and beta-stimulating functions of the vasopressors generally have a threefold action consisting of central inotropic and chronotropic effects and a peripheral vasoconstricting effect. In an evaluation of the comparative effects of a number of the cate-

cholamines, Waldhausen et al. demonstrated significant differences. Isoproterenol hydrochloride (Isuprel), levarterenol bitartrate (Levophed), epinephrine (Adrenalin), and phenylephrine hydrochloride (Neo-Synephrine) all produced a significant increase in contractility of the heart and an increase in heart rate. Isoproterenol had, in addition, a vasodilator effect on the peripheral vessels, while the other three amines were largely peripheral vasoconstrictors. Metaraminol (Aramine) produced a significant increase in myocardial contractility, further increasing the efficiency of the heart beat while the heart rate fell; this amine was also a moderate vasopressor. Of the drugs tested, phenylephrine showed the least efficient inotropic effect and was predominantly a peripheral vasopressor. Dopamine, a naturally occurring catecholamine biochemical precursor of norepinephrine, is similar to isoproterenol in exerting positive inotropic and chronotropic effects on the heart by stimulation of beta-adrenergic receptors. Because of its lower potential for causing tachyarrhythmias and its ability to enhance renal blood flow when infused at a dose below 30 μg/kg/minute, dopamine has virtually replaced isoproterenol as the agent of choice.

In 1923 Cannon condemned the use of vasopressors on this physiologic basis: "Damming the blood in the arterial portion of the circulation, when the organism is suffering primarily from a diminished quantity of blood flow, obviously does not improve the volume flow in the capillaries." In 1940 Blalock also condemned the use of vasopressors in treating shock. Recent studies have more clearly defined the hazards of using vasopressors in hypovolemic shock. Clowes and his associates demonstrated a sharp increase in the mortality of dogs rendered hypotensive by hemorrhage when norepinephrine was administered in sufficient doses to raise the blood pressure from 40 mmHg to 100 mmHg. Mortality in animals so treated was 64 percent compared with 33 percent in the untreated controls. Catchpole et al., using a drip of norepinephrine after 30 minutes of hypotension and again before reinfusion of shed blood, obtained no improvement in survival. Additionally, Hakstian, Hampson, and Gurd demonstrated no significant protection during hemorrhagic hypotension through the use of norepinephrine. On the other hand, studies by Lansing and Stevenson suggest that the use of norepinephrine for the maintenance of blood pressure and cardiac output *after* normovolemia has been restored may be advantageous. Simeone has similarly shown that the use of vasopressors after restoration of normal blood volume may be of some significant help if applied early. Probably the beneficial effects of these experimental studies can be related more properly to their inotropic effect on the heart than to their vasoconstrictor properties. This is especially true since these studies show benefit only after volume has been restored.

There is other available evidence that the administration of vasopressors during hypovolemia will reduce the already depleted plasma volume. Our own data tend to support this concept.

The use of vasopressors in hemorrhagic shock is rapidly disappearing. Suffice it to say that, as more and more data have become available, it is doubtful whether the use of vasopressors in the treatment of hypovolemic shock is ever warranted.

VASODILATORS. In 1948 Wiggers and his associates predicted that a significantly increased survival rate in animals treated with an adrenergic blocking agent and subjected to hemorrhagic shock would indicate the detrimental influence of protracted vasoconstriction in shock. Subsequently, in 1950, Remington and his associates reported an increased survival rate in dogs pretreated with Dibenamine before the induction of hemorrhagic shock. Zweifach, Baes, and Shorr similarly found that Diben-

amine protected rats against lethal-graded hemorrhage if the animals were pretreated, and Boba and Converse reported that ganglionic blocking agents increased the survival of experimentally shocked animals.

Webb et al. found that the administration of hydralazine during the hypovolemic hypotensive phase of experimental hemorrhagic shock was deleterious. In contrast, Hakstian, Hampson, and Gurd obtained 15 survivals out of 16 animals subjected to hemorrhagic shock and treated with hydralazine during the shock period. Collins, Jaffee, and Zahony reported survival in a study of 396 patients treated with chlorpromazine; 186 of these patients were treated after the onset of shock, and the survival rate was said to be twice that of the control group. Longerbeam, Lillehei, and Scott found that giving Dibenzyline (phenoxybenzamine) led to a remarkable improvement in the mortality rate of their animals. Thal recently reported encouraging results with Dibenzyline in the treatment of refractory normovolemic endotoxic shock (Fig. 4-34).

HEMODYNAMIC MEASUREMENTS. A patient in hemorrhagic or oligemic shock may rarely fail to respond to vigorous management as outlined above. Such a patient usually presents a complicated clinical picture. Frequently surgical procedures have been carried out for correction of the underlying causes of shock. Thus the problem is often compounded by massive fluid and blood administration, general anesthesia, and surgical trauma. At this point a comprehensive but rapid reevaluation of the patient must be carried out in order to institute effective therapy.

The basic defect underlying this "refractory shock" must be corrected. Possible causes are multiple: (1) continuing blood loss from the primary injury or disease or from another source, (2) inadequate replacement of fluids, (3) massive trauma and other derangements secondary to the trauma, especially cardiac tamponade and pneumothorax, (4) myocardial insufficiency either as a direct result

Fig. 4-34. Adrenergic mechanisms. (*From C. M. Lewis and M. H. Weil, JAMA, 208:1391, 1969. Copyright, 1969, American Medical Association.*)

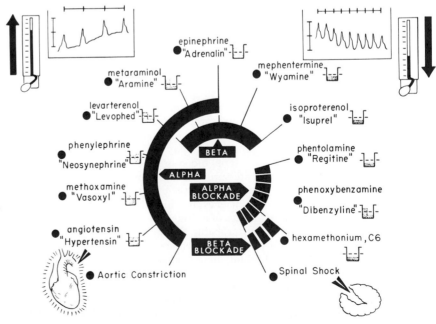

of inadequate perfusion for a prolonged period or secondary to anesthetic agents, and (5) even concomitant septic shock, as with intraperitoneal contamination from bowel perforation. The answers to this problem can best be obtained by careful clinical evaluation of the patient and evaluation of a few relatively simple hemodynamic parameters that may serve as a guide to satisfactory treatment (Chap. 13).

Cardiogenic Shock

In this form of shock the heart fails as a pump. Consequently primary therapy is directed toward the heart. Cardiac arrythmias, whatever their origin, should be treated promptly. Cardiac tamponade, if this is the cause, should be relieved by pericardiocentesis. When the origin of the pump failure is myocardial infarction or myocarditis, the primary therapy again is directed toward the myocardial damage. If the myocardial damage is sufficiently severe to produce reduction in blood pressure, and indeed in organ perfusion, to the point that organ functions begin to fail, drugs with positive inotropic action may be efficacious.

HEMODYNAMIC MEASUREMENTS

Hemodynamic measurements play an important role in the management of postoperative patients with this type of hypotension. As previously described, the classic findings are a central venous pressure that is elevated or rises briskly with fluid administration. This is accompanied by a cardiac output that is depressed and fails to respond to fluid administration. In evaluating postoperative hypotension, as after an extensive procedure in the elderly or especially after cardiac surgery, the measurement of hemodynamic parameters may be of great benefit in differentiating hypovolemic hypotension from hypotension due to depressed myocardial function.

When hemodynamic measurements suggestive of deficient pumping action are found, myocardial insufficiency is usually at fault. It should be stressed again, however, that this can be due to mechanical obstruction (e.g., cardiac tamponade or mediastinal compression in the injured patient or pulmonary embolism in the postoperative patient), and treatment directed at primary myocardial insufficiency can lead to unnecessary delay and catastrophic results. Although identification of abnormalities causing mechanical obstruction to venous return or myocardial function must rest largely on clinical grounds, hemodynamic measurements may be of some benefit in that one may find a slow increase in cardiac output and arterial blood pressure accompanying the rising venous pressure produced by rapid fluid administration. This is in contrast to the picture usually seen in pure myocardial insufficiency, in which the cardiac output frequently falls in the face of a rising venous pressure. The rise in cardiac output probably occurs because the rising venous pressure is partially effective in overcoming the obstruction and maintaining a nearer to normal cardiac filling.

It has been demonstrated that with myocardial injury and after cardiac surgery, differences in functional reserve of the two ventricles occur and the central venous pressure alone loses a great deal of its reliability. Thus in these patients the use of pulmonary artery pressure, pulmonary wedge pressure, and, when feasible, left atrial pressure have their greatest value. Left atrial pressure (or left ventricular end-diastolic pressure) is not necessarily the same as right atrial pressure (or central venous pressure, or right ventricular end-diastolic pressure) under these circumstances.

In patients with low cardiac output from low blood volume who also have certain forms of heart disease, left atrial pressure may be considerably higher than right atrial pressure. Examples of such conditions are mitral stenosis and insufficiency, aortic stenosis and insufficiency, severe hypertension, and coronary artery disease. In such patients, unless one is actually measuring left atrial pressure, rapid infusion should probably be stopped when right atrial or central venous pressure reaches 12 mmHg (150 mm saline solution). The relation between changes in atrial pressure and changes in stroke volume or cardiac output at relatively high atrial pressures is not known. In most patients, however, when atrial pressures are about 15 mmHg (230 mm saline solution), further increases do not seem to increase cardiac output. Thus when central venous or right atrial pressure is less than 6 mmHg (80 mm saline solution), augmentation of blood volume is indicated. As the infusion proceeds, if central venous pressure rises rapidly and there is little evidence of increase in cardiac output, the infusion should probably be discontinued as being ineffective.

ABNORMALITIES IN CONTRACTILITY

In the condition in which there is low cardiac output and high atrial pressures and in which tamponade and ventricular outflow obstruction have been ruled out, there is probably an acute reduction of myocardial contractility. Treatment must therefore be directed toward improving contractility.

The drugs to be considered are

1. *Digitalis.* If time permits, digitalis is given, and digoxin is recommended. The estimated digitalizing dose given intravenously to a child or adult is 0.9 mg/m^2 of body surface area (1.5 mg for average adult). Half or two-thirds of this may be given initially intravenously. An effect can be seen in 10 to 20 minutes, and the peak effect is reached in about 2 hours. After 1 to 3 hours, if no contraindication develops and further effect is desired, an additional one-sixth of the estimated digitalizing dose is given. This may be repeated after another 2 to 3 hours. In less acute situations the same drug may be given orally; the digitalizing dose is then 1 mg/m^2. The estimated daily maintenance dose is one-quarter of the estimated digitalizing dose, usually given in divided doses.

2. *Catecholamines.* Isoproterenol has a specific chronotropic effect on cardiac muscle and theoretically is the drug of choice when one needs a prompt and potent agent. It also has a peripheral vasodilating effect which may produce increased hypotension in a patient in shock. Because of a tendency to produce tachycardia and ventricular irritability, isoproterenol is particularly useful when the pulse rate is slow. It is administered by slow intravenous infu-

sion drop by drop of a solution of 0.5 mg of isoproterenol in 250 ml of 5% glucose in water (2 μg/ml). The rate of infusion is regulated to obtain the desired hemodynamic effect.

Norepinephrine or epinephrine may be used when undue hypertension results from isoproterenol. They increase systemic venous tone and therefore can increase both right and left atrial pressures strikingly; thus caution is indicated, since pulmonary edema can result. These drugs are given intravenously by drop-by-drop infusion of a solution containing 4 mg in 250 ml of 5% glucose in water. Prior to treating patients with low cardiac output and high atrial pressures with these drugs on the basis that the cause is poor myocardial contractility, one must rule out pericardial tamponade. If high intrapericardial pressure exists in patients with high atrial and ventricular end-diastolic pressure, transmural pressure is low, and the poor output is due to end-diastolic ventricular volume and fiber length. The treatment is relief of the pericardial tamponade, which is about the only acute cause of high atrial pressures and small end-diastolic ventricular volume. A clinical analysis and chest x-ray are helpful in establishing the diagnosis. The presence of a paradoxic pulse should suggest strongly the presence of tamponade, and needle aspiration or open pericardiotomy is indicated.

3. *Ganglionic Blocking Agents.* Some patients with low cardiac output and high atrial pressures have relatively high arterial blood pressure. Systemic arteriolar resistance is high (*afterload-load* resisting shortening of myocardial sarcomeres). In these circumstances systolic left ventricular pressure is relatively high, as is systolic ventricular wall stress. Theoretically, reducing arterial blood pressure and systolic ventricular wall stress increases cardiac output. This can be done with an agent such as Arfonad. One should measure cardiac output before and during administration of this drug, and only if a significant increase in cardiac output has accompanied the decrease in arterial blood pressure should the drug be continued. Because of present uncertainties with the use of this drug (such as the effect on coronary, cerebral, liver, and renal blood flow) in this situation, it should be given only under special circumstances.

ABNORMALITIES IN RATE

Rapid ventricular rates (over 150 to 180 beats/minute) are usually deleterious to cardiac output. Ventricular end-diastolic pressure is small because of the short period of ventricular filling with tachycardia, and ventricular extensibility is probably decreased because ventricular relaxation is not complete by the end of the extremely short diastolic period. Both tend to reduce stroke volume more than can be compensated for by the rapid heart rate, and cardiac output falls. If atrial fibrillation is the cardiac mechanism, digoxin is the drug of choice. Atrial flutter is more difficult to treat but likewise be treated with digoxin. If no progress has been achieved with the drug after two-thirds of the digitalizing dose has been given, electroversion should be considered. Atrial tachycardia and premature atrial contractions as causes of excessively rapid heart rates are still more difficult to treat. A continuous

intravenous infusion of a drug with pure peripheral vasoconstrictor properties may be helpful (Aramine, 500 mg in 500 ml of 5% glucose in water).

Premature ventricular contractions may on occasion cause fast ventricular rates. Their tendency to cause ventricular fibrillation is of even greater concern. Potassium chloride may be infused over a 10- to 20-minute period. If this is not effective or if the premature ventricular contractions are frequent, lidocaine (Xylocaine) should be given intravenously in a single injection of 50 mg. If further lidocaine is needed, a solution containing 2 mg/ml of lidocaine can be given continuously. If it is used excessively, central nervous system irritability and depression of myocardial contractility may result. If protection against premature ventricular contractions is needed later, Pronestyl (procainamide hydrochloride) can be given orally in doses of 250 to 500 mg every 3 hours.

Low output associated with ventricular rates of less than 60 to 70 beats/minute may occur in patients in whom cardiac performance is impaired. Because the myocardium is impaired, stroke volume cannot increase sufficiently to compensate for the slow rate. Regardless of whether the mechanism is sinus rhythm, atrial fibrillation with slow ventricular rate (too much digitalis or too little potassium), or complete atrioventricular dissociation, electrical pacing of the heart at a rate of 80 to 110 beats/minute is advantageous. If there is a sinus mechanism, atrial pacing is preferred. Otherwise, direct ventricular pacing is indicated.

MECHANICAL ASSISTANCE

Effective support for cardiogenic shock may eventually depend on mechanical assistance. Assistive devices are currently available in several centers. At present their use is restricted to patients who do not respond to more conventional therapy.

Neurogenic Shock

Neurogenic shock, or, by the older classification, "primary shock" is that form of shock which follows serious interference with the balance of vasodilator and vasoconstrictor influences to both arterioles and venules. This is the shock that is seen with clinical syncope, as with sudden exposure to unpleasant events such as the sight of blood, the hearing of bad tidings, or even the sudden onset of pain. Similarly, neurogenic shock is often observed with serious paralysis of vasomotor influences, as in high spinal anesthesia. The reflex interruption of nerve impulses also occurs with acute gastric dilatation.

The clinical picture of neurogenic shock is quite different from that classically seen in oligemic or hypovolemic shock. While the blood pressure may be extremely low, the pulse rate is usually slower than normal and is accompanied by dry, warm, and even flushed skin. Measurements made during neurogenic shock indicate a reduction in cardiac output, but this is accompanied by a decrease in resistance of arteriolar vessels as well as a decrease in the venous tone. Consequently there appears to be a normovolemic state with a greatly increased reservoir capacity in both arterioles and venules, thereby inducing a decreased venous return to the right side of the heart and subsequently a reduction in cardiac output.

If neurogenic shock is not corrected, a reduction of blood flow to the kidneys and damage to the brain result, and subsequently all the ravages of hypovolemic shock appear. Fortunately, treatment of neurogenic shock is usually obvious. Gastric dilatation can be rapidly treated with nasogastric suction. Shock in high spinal anesthesia can be treated effectively with a vasopressor such as ephedrine or phenylephrine (Neo-Synephrine), which will increase cardiac output as well as produce peripheral vasoconstriction. With the milder forms of neurogenic shock, such as fainting, simply removing the patient from the stimulus or relieving the pain will in itself be adequate therapy so that the vasoconstrictor nerves may regain the ability to maintain normal arteriolar and venous resistance.

There is rarely need for hemodynamic measurement in this usually benign and frequently self-limited form of hypotension. Correction of the underlying deficit usually results in prompt resumption of normal cardiovascular dynamics. The exception to this occurs when this form of shock results from injury, as with spinal cord transection from trauma. In this instance there may be significant loss of blood and extracellular fluid into the area of injury surrounding the cord and vertebral column. Considerable confusion can arise as to the relative need for fluid replacement, as opposed to the need for vasopressor drugs, under these circumstances. Similarly, if surgical intervention for any reason becomes necessary, hemodynamic measurements may be of great value in the management of these patients. In uncomplicated neurogenic shock, central venous pressure should be normal or slightly low, with a normal or elevated cardiac output. On the other hand, as hypovolemia ensues, central venous pressure decreases, as does cardiac output. Thus careful monitoring of central venous pressure may be of great aid. Fluid administration without vasopressors in this form of hypotension may produce a gradually rising arterial pressure and cardiac output without elevation of central venous pressure, by gradually "filling" the expanded vascular pool; therefore caution must be utilized during fluid administration.

In management of these patients balancing the two forms of therapy, slight volume overexpansion is much less deleterious than excessive vasopressor administration. The latter decreases organ perfusion in the presence of inadequate fluid replacement. Balance can best be obtained by maintaining a normal central venous pressure that rises slightly with rapid fluid administration (thus ensuring adequate volume) and using a vasopressor such as phenylephrine judiciously to support arterial pressure.

Septic Shock

During the past several years there has been a progressive increase in the incidence of shock secondary to sepsis, and the mortality rate remains in excess of 50 percent. This has occurred despite a better understanding of this entity, use of newer treatment regimens, and development of more potent antimicrobial agents. The most frequent causative organisms are gram-positive and gram-negative bacteria, although any agent capable of producing infection (including viruses, parasites, fungi, and rickettsiae) may initiate septic shock. Because of effective antibiotic control of most gram-positive infections, the majority of septic processes that result in shock are now caused by gram-negative bacteria. Among other causes, Altemeier and associates attribute this rising incidence of gram-negative sepsis to (1) the widespread use of antibiotics, with development of a reservoir of virulent and resistant organisms; (2) concentration in hospitals of large numbers of patients with established infections; (3) more extensive operations on elderly and poor-risk patients; (4) an increasing number of patients suffering from severe trauma; and (5) the use of steroids and immunosuppressive and anticancer agents.

GRAM-POSITIVE SEPSIS AND SHOCK

The shock state may be caused by gram-positive infections that produce massive fluid losses (necrotizing fasciitis) by dissemination of a potent exotoxin without evident bacteremia (*Clostridium perfringens, Clostridium tetani*) or, most often, by a fulminating infection from staphylococcus, streptococcus, or pneumococcus organisms. In the latter instance, shock is theoretically related to the release of exotoxins which many strains of staphylococcus and streptococcus (but not pneumococcus) are known to produce. The hemodynamic changes that occur are different from those seen in shock due to gram-negative organisms. Kwaan and Weil have noted hypotension of comparable severity in shock from both gram-positive and gram-negative infections, but their patients with gram-positive infections failed to show the other clinical manifestations of shock. Arterial resistance fell, but there was little or no reduction in cardiac output even with progressive hypotension. Urine flow was normal, sensorium clear, and perfusion of other organs was not grossly impaired, since neither acidosis nor a significant increase in serum lactic acid concentration appeared.

Treatment consists in the use of appropriate antibiotics, surgical drainage when indicated, and correction of any fluid volume deficit. A rapid and favorable response may be anticipated in many patients, and survival is substantially better than with gram-negative infections.

GRAM-NEGATIVE SEPSIS AND SHOCK

Gram-negative sepsis as a cause of shock is a more frequent and difficult problem. The highest incidence occurs during the seventh and eighth decades of life, and the response to treatment depends to a large extent on the age and previous health of the patient. There have been significant advances in the understanding of this entity, although much of the available information is still subject to controversy.

SOURCE. The most frequent source of gram-negative infections is the genitourinary system; almost half the patients have had an associated operation or instrumentation of the urinary tract. The second most frequent site of origin is the respiratory system, and many of the patients have an associated tracheostomy. Next in frequency is the alimentary system, with diseases such as peritonitis, intra-abdominal abscess, and biliary tract infections; and then diseases of the integumentary, including burns and soft tissue infections. Indwelling venous catheters for monitoring and hyperalimentation are an increasing source of contamination, particularly with prolonged use. The reproductive system continues to be a significant source of infection (principally from septic abortions and postpartum infections), although the incidence is variable, depending on the hospital population.

The severity of septic shock varies considerably and appears to be a time-dose phenomenon, depending on the type and site of infection. For instance, mild hypotension following instrumentation of the genitourinary tract may represent nothing more than a transient bacteremia which is self-limited or responds to minimal therapy. In contrast, the patient with necrotizing pneumonia or multiple intra-abdominal abscesses may have sepsis from an overwhelming number of organisms for a period of several days, and a much poorer prognosis. Similarly, the outlook is more favorable when the source of infection is accessible to surgical drainage, as in septic abortion, in which the infected products of conception can be removed readily. Variations in these factors must be considered when interpreting reported mortality rates and during the evaluation of new therapeutic regimens.

ASSOCIATED CONDITIONS. The presence of underlying disorders which limit cardiac, pulmonary, hepatic, or renal function increases the susceptibility to gram-negative infections and adversely affects the response to treatment. In Altemeier's reported series of 398 patients with gram-negative sepsis, almost half the patients had serious associated disease, including diabetes mellitus, malignant neoplasms, uremia, cirrhosis, burns, and malignant hematologic disorders. Of these conditions, cirrhosis of the liver appeared to have the most unfavorable prognosis. In addition, a small but significant number of patients were on corticosteroids or immunosuppressive agents, and corresponding mortality rates were 74 and 83 percent respectively.

BACTERIOLOGY. The common causative organisms are similar to those found in the human gastrointestinal tract and include (1) *E. coli;* (2) *Klebsiella aerobacter;* (3) *Proteus;* (4) *Pseudomonas;* and (5) *Bacteroides,* in order of decreasing frequency. Recently the *Klebsiella*-Enterobacteriaceae-*Serratia* groups have been isolated with increasing frequency, and many are resistant to more conventional antibiotics. It now appears that *Bacteroides* species may be the predominant organisms in the fecal flora. These anaerobic organisms are difficult to culture and may account for a far greater number of infections than was previously reported. The majority of infections are caused by a single gram-negative organism, although in 10 to 20 percent of cases more than one organism may be isolated. The isolates may be two or more gram-negative organisms or mixed cultures containing both gram-negative and gram-positive bacteria.

CLINICAL MANIFESTATIONS. Gram-negative infections are often recognized initially by the development of chills and elevated temperature above 101°F. The onset of shock may be abrupt and coincident with the signs and symptoms of sepsis or may occur several hours to days after recognition of an established infection. The complex hemody-

namic abnormalities that follow are incompletely understood but are probably initiated by endotoxins from the cell walls of gram-negative bacteria. Intravenous injection of this lipopolysaccharide-protein complex into experimental animals will produce a shock state, but the hemodynamic responses vary in different animal species. The use of experimental animal models has contributed to our understanding of this entity, but direct extrapolation of the findings to human septic shock is difficult. A single injection of endotoxin into dogs causes pooling of blood in the splanchnic circulation, decreased venous return to the heart, reduction in cardiac output, and an abrupt fall in blood pressure. This initial response is transient and apparently due to hepatic venous outflow obstruction. Shortly thereafter the blood pressure rises toward normal but then slowly declines over the next several hours until death of the animal. This pattern is different from that seen in the subhuman primate and in human beings. Injection of *E. coli* endotoxin into human volunteers has been shown to produce (1) no response; (2) chills, fever, and vasoconstriction; or (3) peripheral vasodilation and a rise in cardiac output. These observations emphasize our lack of understanding of the effects of gram-negative infections and septicemia on the human circulation and the need for the development of more realistic experimental animal models.

Clinically, the shock state may be characterized by a primary adrenergic response, as seen in hypovolemic shock, with hypotension, peripheral vasoconstriction, and cold, clammy extremities. Earlier in the course, however, there may be an absence of adrenergic effects, with warm, dry extremities and decreased peripheral resistance. These diverse responses, presumably to the same stimulus, have led to a considerable amount of confusion over the clinical manifestations of septic shock, although a report by MacLean and associates tends to shed some light on this subject. They have noted two distinct hemodynamic patterns, depending on the volume status of the patient, and believe that the natural history of septic shock is one of progression from respiratory alkalosis to metabolic acidosis. A syndrome of early septic shock occurs in patients who are *normovolemic* prior to onset of sepsis and exhibit a hyperdynamic circulatory pattern characterized by (1) hypotension, (2) high cardiac output, (3) normal or increased blood volume, (4) normal or high central venous pressure, (5) low peripheral resistance, (6) warm, dry extremities, (7) hyperventilation, and (8) respiratory alkalosis. A typical patient with this pattern is the young, previously healthy person with a septic abortion. The high cardiac output is often associated with a decrease in oxygen utilization per unit flow, i.e., a narrowed arteriovenous oxygen difference. These findings can be explained by any of several mechanisms, but the two most likely possibilities are arteriovenous shunting and a primary cellular defect in the utilization of oxygen due to a direct effect of sepsis. Data by Wright et al. suggest a primary cellular defect as the most likely cause. In either case the presence of oliguria, altered sensorium, and blood lactate accumulation reflects the need for a further increase in flow despite the high cardiac output. MacLean suggests that treatment include measures to increase the cardiac output even more, combined with appropriate antibiotic therapy and early surgical drainage. In his series all but 4 of 28 patients with this hemodynamic pattern survived the episode of shock. If control of the infection is delayed or unsuccessful, the patient may pass into an acidotic phase with evidence of cellular damage (narrowing arteriovenous oxygen difference, decreasing oxygen consumption) and become refractory to further therapy.

In contrast, if septic shock develops in a patient who is *hypovolemic*, a hypodynamic pattern emerges characterized by (1) hypotension, (2) low cardiac output, (3) high peripheral resistance, (4) low central venous pressure, and (5) cold, cyanotic extremities. This response is typically seen in a patient with strangulation obstruction of the small bowel and a moderate to severe extracellular fluid and plasma volume deficit. If seen early, these patients are also alkalotic and will respond favorably to treatment. In the absence of overt cardiac failure, prompt volume replacement will often increase cardiac output, and a more favorable hyperdynamic circulation may develop. If therapy to combat sepsis is delayed or unsuccessful, the patient will inevitably have cardiac and circulatory failure, with a low fixed cardiac output and a resistant metabolic acidosis. At this point the patient may not be salvageable.

Our own experience in the treatment of septic shock tends to confirm MacLean's findings, although the presence of a metabolic acidosis has not necessarily been an ominous finding. We have seen several patients with hypodynamic and hyperdynamic circulatory patterns and metabolic acidosis in the early phase who have responded satisfactorily to therapy. The clinical picture may also be influenced by the patient's ability to meet the increased circulatory requirements imposed by sepsis. The elderly patient with limited cardiac reserve may be unable to increase cardiac output and enter the hyperdynamic phase, even with prompt volume replacement and measures designed to increase cardiac efficiency. In this instance the typical adrenergic response may persist, and the patient may rapidly succumb to the disease process.

The laboratory tests of value for diagnosis will depend to a large extent on the specific disease causing sepsis. Generally, the white blood cell count is appropriately elevated, but in debilitated and hypovolemic patients, those on immunosuppressive agents, and those with overwhelming sepsis, the white blood cell count may be normal or low. However, there is usually a noticeable left shift in the white blood cell differential, with many immature cell types. Recent work by Rowe et al. indicates that a falling platelet count may be an early and sensitive indicator of gram-negative septicemia in pediatric patients. It has been suggested that endotoxin reacts with platelets, producing platelet aggregates which are subsequently trapped in the microcirculation. They suggest that patients at risk for sepsis have serial platelet counts; a fall in the platelet count below 150,000 suggests the presence of gram-negative septicemia, and measures to find and eradicate the source should be undertaken. Rarely, a sudden fall in the platelet count may be a manifestation of disseminated intravascular coagulation (DIC), a syndrome known to be initiated by several stimuli, including endotoxin.

Progressive pulmonary insufficiency is characteristically seen in many patients with septic shock. Mild hypoxia with compensatory hyperventilation and respiratory alkalosis are commonly seen early in the course of shock in the absence of clinical or x-ray evidence of pulmonary disease. The arterial desaturation has been attributed to a variety of causes, including the presence of physiologic arteriovenous shunts in the pulmonary circulation secondary to perfusion of atelectatic or nonaerated alveoli. Regardless of the cause, the picture is frequently that of rapid deterioration of pulmonary function, development of patchy infiltrates which become confluent, superimposed bacterial infection, severe hypoxemia, and death.

Finally, it is worth emphasizing that development of mild hyperventilation, respiratory alkalosis, and an altered sensorium may be the earliest signs of gram-negative infection. This triad may precede the usual signs and symptoms of sepsis by several hours to several days. The exact cause is not known, although the condition is thought to represent a primary response to bacteremia. Early recognition of these findings, followed by a prompt search for the source of infection, may allow proper diagnosis prior to the onset of shock.

TREATMENT. The only effective way to reduce mortality in septic shock is by prompt recognition and treatment of the associated infection prior to the onset of shock. Once shock occurs, the control of infection by early surgical debridement or drainage and use of appropriate antibiotics represents *definitive* therapy. Other recommended measures, including fluid replacement, steroid administration, and the use of vasoactive drugs, represent *adjunctive* forms of therapy and are useful to prepare the patient prior to surgical intervention or to support the patient until the infectious process is controlled. This point deserves special emphasis, since death of the patient is inevitable if the infection cannot be adequately controlled.

As soon as gram-negative sepsis and shock are apparent, a prompt and thorough search for the source of infection is made while instituting other supportive measures. Because of the multiple complicating factors that may accompany endotoxemia, the patient is preferably treated in an intensive care unit. Careful monitoring of direct arterial pressure, central venous pressure (preferably pulmonary artery and pulmonary wedge pressures measured via a Swan-Ganz catheter), urine output, and arterial and central venous blood gases may be essential for proper management.

If the infectious process is amenable to drainage, operation is performed as soon as possible after initial stabilization of the patient's condition. In some cases surgical debridement or drainage of the infection must be accomplished before the patient will respond; this may be performed under local or general anesthesia. For example, a patient with ascending cholangitis and shock secondary to sepsis may respond temporarily to supportive treatment. Improvement may be short-lived, however, unless prompt drainage of the biliary tract is instituted. The importance of surgical drainage is emphasized by the experience of

MacLean et al. in their treatment of 53 patients. Forty-eight percent of their patients with infections amenable to surgical drainage survived, while only 23 percent of those not amenable to surgical treatment survived.

Antibiotic Therapy. The use of specific antibiotics based on appropriate cultures and sensitivity tests is desirable when possible. The results may not be available for several days, but useful information may be gained from previous wound and blood cultures obtained during an earlier phase of the septic process and Gram stains of appropriate material. Antibiotics must often be chosen, however, on the basis of the suspected organisms and their previous sensitivity patterns. These patterns are sufficiently diverse to preclude selection of a single antibiotic agent which will be effective against all the potential pathogens.

At present an effective combination of antibiotics in our hospital population when gastrointestinal tract organisms are suspected includes cephalothin (6 to 8 Gm/day intravenously in four to six divided doses) or penicillin (10 to 20 million units daily) and gentamicin (5 mg/kg/day). These are average adult doses and should be reduced after initial control of the infection and modified in any patient with impaired renal function. This combination is effective against a majority of gram-negative organisms, with the notable exception of *Bacteroides* species. If presence of these organisms is suspected, an antibiotic of known effectiveness (e.g., clindamycin or Chloromycetin) should be added to the regimen.

When culture and sensitivity reports are available, more specific antibiotic coverage may be initiated if the infection is not under control. Altemeier and associates reported a mortality rate of 54 percent from sepsis in patients receiving inappropriate antibiotics and 28 percent when appropriate antibiotics were given.

Fluid Replacement. Prompt correction of preexisting fluid deficits is essential. A majority of patients will incur fluid losses from the disease processes that initiate sepsis and shock. "Third space losses," with massive sequestration of plasma and extracellular fluid, are characteristic of many surgical conditions, including peritonitis, burns, strangulation obstruction of the bowel, and extensive soft tissue infections.

The type of fluid used will vary, although most "third space losses" are properly replaced with a balanced salt solution such as Ringer's lactate. Any deficits in red blood cell mass should be corrected by the administration of packed cells or whole blood in order to maintain optimal oxygen-carrying capacity of the blood. Large quantities of replacement fluids are often needed in order to maintain an effective circulating volume. However, a fine balance exists between the need for volume replacement and the harmful effects that fluid overload may have on lungs already injured by the septic process. In this regard, attempts to increase pulmonary capillary osmotic pressure by the infusion of large volumes of plasma or albumin, in the absence of a specific need, may be deterimental. Because of the increase in pulmonary capillary permeability associated with severe sepsis, the use of large quantities of colloid solutions may result in an increase in extravascular pulmonary water. Careful replacement of "third space losses" with crystalloid solutions on the basis of patient response and continuous monitoring of the central venous or pulmonary artery and pulmonary wedge pressures are indicated.

Properly interpreted, the central venous pressure (CVP) will give a reliable estimate of the ability of the right side of the heart to pump the blood delivered to it. It is best used as an upper-limit guide; a rapid increase in central venous pressure, regardless of the initial level, may indicate that fluid is being administered too rapidly or that the heart is unable to handle additional volume. If central venous pressure is below 10 cm of water, fluids may be administered as rapidly as tolerated. If central venous pressure is above this level, fluids are still administered but at a slower rate of infusion. The central venous pressure may fall as blood pressure rises, owing to better perfusion of the coronary arteries and improved myocardial function. An abrupt rise in the central venous pressure or a fall in arterial pressure may indicate inability of the heart to respond, and the use of drugs that increase myocardial performance should be considered.

In many instances, measurement of the CVP alone during fluid resuscitation is not sufficient, since it gives no direct information regarding function of the left side of the heart. Insertion of a Swan-Ganz catheter (via a cutdown in an antecubital vein or by direct percutaneous insertion into the subclavian vein) for measurements of *both* pulmonary artery (PA) and pulmonary capillary wedge (PW) pressure, the latter a reflection of left ventricular end-diastolic pressure, is necessary. This is particularly true in patients on mechanical ventilation and positive end-expiratory pressure. Recently, Krausz et al. assessed the value of PWP monitoring during fluid resuscitation in patients in septic shock. In one group of patients the PW pressure prior to the administration of fluid was lower than the CVP, suggesting acute right ventricular failure due to increased pulmonary vascular resistance coexistent with relative hypovolemia. The intravenous administration of fluid in this group was accompanied by a significant rise in blood pressure and cardiac output without significant change in the pulse rate or the PA pressure. In a second group, the initial PW pressure was higher than the CVP, and signs of fluid overloading appeared after the administration of only a moderate amount of fluid without change in either blood pressure or cardiac output. Although not stated by the authors, the use of inotropic agents to improve myocardial performance may be indicated in the latter group of patients.

Many patients will respond favorably to fluid administration combined with prompt control of the infection with a rise in blood pressure, an increase in urine output, warming of the extremities, and clearing of the sensorium. In these instances no additional therapy may be indicated.

Steroids. The use of pharmacologic doses of corticosteroids in the treatment of septic shock is controversial but has become a common practice. There is no direct evidence that steroids are beneficial in these cases, although favorable responses, with improvement in cardiac, pulmonary, and renal functions and better survival rates, have been reported. Large doses of steroids are known to exert a modest inotropic effect on the heart and produce mild peripheral vasodilation. Although these salutary effects may be desirable, there are other, more potent drugs available with similar actions. Others have suggested that steroids protect the cell and its contents from the effects of endotoxin, for example, by stabilizing cellular and lysosomal membranes. In a recent prospective study of 172 consecutive patients in septic shock, Schumer noted a mortality rate of 10.4 percent in the steroid-treated patients, compared to a mortality rate of 38.4 percent in patients not receiving steroids. In a retrospective study of an additional 328 patients, the results were similar. Although impressive, evidence regarding the beneficial effects of steroids remains presumptive, because of many variables present in the clinical situation, including causes, associated conditions, and treatment.

Short-term, high-dose steroid therapy is associated with a minimal number of complications and is recommended in most cases that do not respond promptly to other measures. Steroids may be administered concomitant with volume replacement or reserved for use if the response to fluid administration is only temporary or produces a rapid rise in central venous pressure. Many dosage schedules have been recommended, and most stress the need for a large initial dose and cessation of therapy within 48 to 72 hours. Our current regimen is based on guidelines suggested by Lillehei. An initial dose of 15 to 30 mg/kg of body weight of methylprednisolone (or equivalent dose of dexamethasone) is given intravenously over a 5- to 10-minute period. The same dose may be repeated within 2 to 4 hours if the desired effects have not been achieved. If a beneficial response is obtained, additional injections are not given unless the effects are only short-lived. Used in this manner, there is rarely a need for more than two doses.

Vasoactive Drugs. Vasopressor drugs with prominent alpha-adrenergic effects are of limited value in treatment of this type of shock, since artificial attempts to maintain blood pressure without regard to flow are potentially harmful. Further, they are probably contraindicated in hypovolemic patients with increased peripheral resistance, in view of the known deleterious effects of prolonged vasoconstriction. Beneficial effects attributed to these agents are probably due to their inotropic effects on the heart, although better drugs are available for this purpose. Rarely, use of a vasoactive drug with mixed alpha- and beta-adrenergic effects (e.g., metaraminol) may be indicated in a patient with an elevated cardiac output and pronounced hypotension due to very low peripheral resistance. The increase in resistance (and slight increase in cardiac output) may produce a desired rise in blood pressure and improvement in flow.

Vasodilator drugs such as phenoxybenzamine have enjoyed some popularity, particularly when combined with additional fluid administration. Their use is based in part on improved survival of dogs when vasodilator drugs are given prior to the onset of endotoxic shock. These observations probably represent a specific canine response and cannot be directly extrapolated to human septic shock.

Vasodilator agents have also been used in conjunction with adrenergic agents (for their inotropic effects), but data on their usefulness are limited.

Since the heart is frequently unable to meet the increased circulatory demands of sepsis, the use of an inotropic agent such as isoproterenol or dopamine would seem ideal when volume replacement and other measures have failed to restore adequate circulation. Isoproterenol has potent inotropic and chronotropic effects on the heart and produces mild peripheral vasodilation. It is a relatively safe drug, but close observation of the patient is necessary, since severe tachycardia or cardiac arrhythmias may occur, particularly in digitalized patients. One or two milligrams of isoproterenol diluted in 500 ml of 5% dextrose in water may be administered by slow intravenous drip at a rate of 1 to 2 μg/minute, depending on the response. The infusion should be slowed or stopped completely if significant tachycardia or cardiac arrhythmias occur. In the absence of arrhythmias, a fall in blood pressure may result from the vasodilation induced by isoproterenol and indicates the need for additional volume replacement to maintain cardiac filling pressure. This combination may effectively restore blood flow even though systolic blood pressure remains less than 100 mmHg. The response is often temporary, but occasionally the infusion may be continued for 2 to 3 days without loss of effect or known deleterious effects. Dopamine, a naturally occurring catecholamine biochemical precursor of norepinephrine, is similar to isoproterenol in exerting positive inotropic and chronotropic effects on the heart by stimulation of beta-adrenergic receptors. Because of its lower potential for tachyarrhythmias and the ability to enhance renal blood flow when infused at a dose below 30 μg/kg/minute, dopamine has virtually replaced isoproterenol as the agent of choice.

In summary, a "polypharmacy" approach is discouraged, although proper selection and use of vasoactive drugs may offer needed support until infection can be controlled or eradicated. If eradication is not possible, response to any of these drugs is only temporary. Determination of cardiac output, combined with arterial, pulmonary artery, and pulmonary wedge pressure measurements can be of great benefit in establishing the nature of the hemodynamic alterations and evaluating responses to therapy.

Digitalis. Although Hinshaw et al. have shown that digitalis can prevent or reverse heart failure in septic animals, the clinical importance of this finding has yet to be established. We have not routinely administered digitalis to patients in septic shock in the absence of specific indications. Gram-negative sepsis and shock frequently occur in older patients with congestive failure or may precipitate cardiac failure in patients with limited cardiac reserve. In these instances digitalis can be administered cautiously in full doses, although toxicity may occur if the patient is hypokalemic or receiving isoproterenol.

Pulmonary Therapy. Many patients with sepsis and shock will develop significant pulmonary insufficiency and require maintenance of a controlled airway (via nasotracheal or endotracheal intubation) and assisted ventilation. (For a discussion of the adult respiratory distress syndrome as related to sepsis and the management of patients requiring ventilatory support, the reader is referred to the section Pulmonary Responses.)

Since inadequate tissue oxygenation is a consistent feature of shock, attention to all components of the oxygen transport system is essential (see the section Oxygen Transport). Efforts to maintain a normal or rightward-positioned oxygen/hemoglobin dissociation curve may be particularly important in view of reported reductions in red blood cell organic phosphates in late septic shock. The use of hyperbaric oxygen has also been suggested and would appear to be an ideal therapeutic approach. Limited experience with its use has been disappointing, however.

References

Clinical and Physiologic Manifestations of Shock

Baue, A. E., Wurth, M. A., and Sayeed, M. M.: The Dynamics of Altered ATP-dependent and ATP-yielding Cell Processes in Shock, *Surgery,* **72:**94, 1972.

Blalock, A.: Shock: Further Studies with Particular Reference to Effects of Hemorrhage, *Arch Surg,* **29:**837, 1937.

————: "Principles of Surgical Care, Shock and Other Problems," C. V. Mosby Company, St. Louis, 1940.

Canizaro, P. C., Prager, M. D., and Shires, G. T.: The Infusion of Ringer's Lactate Solution during Shock, *Am J Surg,* **122:**494, 1971.

Carey, L. C., Lowery, B. D., and Cloutier, C. T.: Treatment of Acidosis, *Curr Probl Surg,* January 1971, p. 37.

Cloutier, C. T., Lowery, B. D., and Carey, L. C.: The Effect of Hemodilutional Resuscitation on Serum Protein Levels in Humans in Hemorrhagic Shock, *J Trauma,* **9:**514, 1969.

Drucker, W. R., et al.: Metabolic Aspects of Hemorrhagic Shock: I. Changes in Intermediary Metabolism during Hemorrhage and Repletion of Blood, *Surg Forum,* **9:**49, 1959.

Gross, S. G.: "A System of Surgery: Pathological, Diagnostic, Therapeutic and Operative," Lea & Febiger, Philadelphia, 1872.

Hiebert, J. M., McCormick, J. M., and Egdahl, R. H.: Direct Measurement of Insulin Secretory Rate: Studies of Shocked Primates and Postoperative Patients, *Ann Surg,* **176:**296, 1972.

Lemieux, M. D., Smith, R. N., and Couch, N. P.: Surface pH and Redox Potential of Skeletal Muscle in Graded Hemorrhage, *Surgery,* **65:**457, 1969.

Mela, L. M., Miller, L. D., and Nicholas, G. G.: Influence of Cellular Acidosis and Altered Cation Concentrations on Shock-induced Mitochondrian Damage, *Surgery,* **72:**102, 1972.

Moore, F. D.: "Metabolic Care of the Surgical Patient," W. B. Saunders Company, Philadelphia, 1959.

Shenkin, H. S., et al.: On the Diagnosis of Hemorrhage in Man: A Study of Volunteers Bled Large Amounts, *Am J Med Sci,* **208:**421, 1944.

Shumer, W., Erve, P. R., and Obermolte, R. P.: Mechanisms of Steroid Protection in Septic Shock, *Surgery,* **72:**119, 1972.

Simeone, F. A.: Shock, in "Christopher's Textbook of Surgery," p. 58, W. B. Saunders Company, Philadelphia, 1964.

Thal, A. P., and Wilson, R. F.: Shock, *Curr Probl Surg,* September 1965.

Watts, D. T.: Arterial Blood Epinephrine Levels during Hemorrhagic Hypotension in Dogs, *Am J Physiol,* **184:**271, 1956.

Wiggers, C. J.: Present Status of Shock Problem, *Physiol Rev,* **22:**74, 1942.

Response of Extracellular Fluid

Baue, A. E., Wurth, M. A., and Sayeed, M. M.: The Dynamics of Altered ATP-dependent and ATP-yielding Cell Processes in Shock, *Surgery,* **72:**94, 1972.

Campion, D. S., et al.: The Effect of Hemorrhagic Shock on Transmembrane Potential, *Surgery,* **66:**1051, 1969.

Conway, E. J.: Nature and Significance of Concentration Relations of Potassium and Sodium Ions in Skeletal Muscle, *Physiol Rev,* **37:**84, 1957.

Cunningham, J. N., Jr., Shires, G. T., and Wagner, Y.: Cellular Transport Defects in Hemorrhagic Shock, *Surgery,* **70:**215, 1971.

————, ————, and ————: Changes in Intracellular Sodium and Potassium Content of Red Blood Cells in Trauma and Shock, *Am J Surg,* November 1971, p. 650.

Fulton, R. L.: Absorption of Sodium and Water by Collagen during Hemorrhagic Shock, *Am Surg,* **172:**861, 1970.

Goldman, D. E.: Potential, Impedance and Rectification in Membranes, *J Physiol,* **27:**37, 1943.

Grossman, R.: Intracellular Potentials of Motor Cortex Neurons in Cerebral Ischemia, *Electroencephalogr Clin Neurophysiol,* **24:**291, 1968.

Hagberg, S., Haljamas, H., and Rockert, H.: Shock Reactions in Skeletal Muscle: III. The Electrolyte Content of Tissue Fluid and Blood Plasma before and after Induced Hemorrhagic Shock. *Ann Surg,* **168:**243, 1968.

Hodgkin, A. L., and Katz, B.: The Effect of Sodium Ions on the Electrical Activity of the Giant Axon of the Squid, *J Physiol,* **108:**37, 1949.

Ling, G., and Gerard, R. W.: The Normal Membrane Potential of Frog Sartorius Fibers, *J Cell Sci,* **34:**383, 1949.

Mela, L. M., Miller, L. D., and Nicholas, G. G.: Influence of Cellular Acidosis and Altered Cation Concentrations on Shock-induced Mitochondrian Damage, *Surgery,* **72:**102, 1972.

Middleton, E. S., Mathews, R., and Shires, G. T.: Radiosulphate as a Measure of the Extracellular Fluid in Acute Hemorrhagic Shock, *Ann Surg,* **170:**174, 1969.

Shires, G. T., et al.: Alterations in Cellular Membrane Function during Hemorrhagic Shock in Primates, *Ann Surg,* **176:**288, 1972.

————, Brown, F. T., Canizaro, P. C., and Somerville, N.: Distributional Changes in Extracellular Fluid during Acute Hemorrhagic Shock, *Surg Forum,* **11:**115, 1960.

————, and Carrico, C. J.: Current Status of the Shock Problem, *Curr Probl Surg,* March 1966.

————, ————, and Canizaro, P. C.: "Shock," Chap. 4, Pulmonary Responses, W. B. Saunders Company, Philadelphia, 1973.

————, Coln, D., Carrico, C. J., and Lightfoot, S.: Fluid Therapy in Hemorrhagic Shock, *Arch Surg,* **88:**688, 1964.

Slonim, M., and Stahl, W. M.: Sodium and Water Content of Connective versus Cellular Tissue Following Hemorrhage, *Surg Forum,* **19:**53, 1968.

Van Leeuwen, A. M.: Net Cation Equivalency (Base Building Power) of the Plasma Proteins, *Acta Med Scand [Suppl],* **422:**3-206, 1964.

Welt, L. G., Sachs, J. R., and McManus, T. J.: An Ion Transport Defect in Erythrocytes from Uremic Patients, *Trans Assoc Am Physicians,* **77**:169, 1964.

Wilde, W. S.: The Chloride Equilibrium in Muscle, *Am J Physiol,* **143**:666, 1945.

Renal Responses

Baker, C. F., Baxter, C. R., and Shires, G. T.: The Evaluation of Renal Function Following Severe Trauma, *J Trauma.* (In press.)

Baxter, C. R., Crenshaw, C. A., Lehman, I., and Shires, T.: A Practical Method of Renal Hypothermia, *J Trauma,* **3**:349, 1963.

———, and Maynard, D. R.: Prevention and Recognition of Surgical Renal Complications, *Clin Anesth,* **3**:322, 1968.

———, Zedlitz, W. H., and Shires, G. T.: High Output Acute Renal Failure Complicating Traumatic Injury, *J Trauma,* **4**:567, 1964.

Brun, C., and Munck, O.: "Acute Renal Failure in The Kidney," Ed: F. K. Mostofi and D. E. Smith, International Academy of Pathology Monograph, Williams & Wilkins, Baltimore.

Defalco, A. J., Mundth, E. D., Brettschneider, L., Jacobson, Y. G., and McClenathan, J. E.: A Possible Explanation for Transplantation Anuria, *Surg Gynecol Obstet,* **120**:748, 1965.

Doberneck, R. C., Schwartz, F. D., and Barry, K. G.: A Comparison of the Prophylactic Value of 20 Per Cent Mannitol, 4 Per Cent Urea, and 5 Per Cent Dextrose on the Effects of Renal Ischemia, *J Urol,* **89**:300, 1963.

Finckh, E. S.: The Failure of Experimental Renal Tubulonecrosis to Produce Oliguria in the Rat, *Australas Ann Med,* **9**:283, 1960.

Flear, C. T. G., and Clarke, R.: The Influence of Blood Loss and Blood Transfusion upon Changes in the Metabolism of Water, Electrolytes and Nitrogen following Civilian Trauma, *Clinical Science,* **14**:575, 1955.

Fudenberg, H., and Allen, F. H., Jr.: Transfusion Reactions in Absence of Demonstrable Incompatibility, *N Engl J Med,* **256**:1180, 1957.

Graber, I. G., and Sevitt, S.: Renal Function in Burned Patients and Its Relationship to Morphological Changes, *J Clin Pathol,* **12**:25, 1959.

Ladd, M.: "Battle Casualties in Korea," vol. 4, p. 193, U.S. Army Medical Service Graduate School, Walter Reed Army Medical Center, 1956.

Meroney, W. H., and Rubini, M. E.: Kidney Function during Acute Tubular Necrosis: Clinical Studies and Theory, *Metabolism,* **8**:1, 1959.

Moore, F. D.: "Metabolic Care of the Surgical Patient," W. B. Saunders Company, Philadelphia, 1959.

Munck, O.: Renal Blood Flow and Oxygen Consumption in Acute Renal Failure Measured by Use of Radioactive ^{85}Krypton, in Proc. 1st Int. Cong. Nephrol. Geneve/Evian 1960, p. 230, 1961.

Oliver, J., MacDowell, M., and Tracy, A.: The Pathogenesis of Acute Renal Failure Associated with Traumatic and Toxic Injury: Renal Ischemia: Nephrotoxic Damage and the Ischemuric Episode, *J Clin Invest,* **30**:1307, 1951.

Padula, R. T., Camishion, R. C., Magee, J. H., Noble, P. H., and Cowan, G. S. M.: Evaluation of the Protective Effect of Osmotic Diuretics, *Adv Surg Res,* **1**:177, 1969.

Phillips, R. A., and Hamilton, P. B.: Effect of 20, 60 and 120

Minutes of Renal Ischemia on Glomerular and Tubular Function, *Am J Physiol,* **152**:523, 1948.

Powers, S. R.: Maintenance of Renal Function Following Massive Trauma, *Trauma,* **10**:554, 1970.

———: Renal Response to Systemic Trauma, *Am J Surg,* **119**:603, 1970.

Sevitt, S.: Distal Tubular Necrosis with Little or No Oliguria, *J Clin Pathol,* **9**:12, 1956.

Tanner, G. A., and Selkurt, E. E.: Kidney Function in the Squirrel Monkey before and after Hemorrhagic Hypotension. *Am J Physiol,* **219**:597, 1970.

Taylor, W. H.: Management of Acute Renal Failure Following Surgical Operation and Head Injury, *Lancet,* **2**:703, 1957.

Teschan, P. E., et al.: Post-traumatic Renal Insufficiency in Military Casualties: I. Clinical Characteristics, *Am J Med,* **18**:172, 1955.

———, and Mason, A. D.: Reproducible Experimental Acute Renal Failure in Rats, *Clin Res,* **6**:155, 1958.

Wright, H. K., and Gann, D. S.: Correction of Defect in Free Water Excretion in Postoperative Patients by Extracellular Fluid Volume Expansion, *Ann Surg,* **158**:70, 1963.

Pulmonary Responses

Ashbaugh, D. G., Bigelow, D. B., Petty, T. L., and Levine, B. E.: Acute Respiratory Distress in Adults, *Lancet,* **2**:319, 1967.

Bates, D. V., Macklem, P. T., and Christie, R. V.: The Normal Lung: Physiology and Methods of Study, in "Respiratory Function in Disease," Chap. 2, W. B. Saunders Company, Philadelphia, 1971.

Baue, A. E.: The Pushmi-Pullyu Syndrome, *Surgery,* **72**:655, 1972.

Berman, I. R., and Ducker, T. B.: Pulmonary, Somatic and Splanchnic Circulatory Responses to Increased Intracranial Pressure, *Ann Surg,* **169**:210, 1969.

Blaisdell, F. W., and Lewis, F. R.: Etiologic Factors in the Respiratory Distress Syndrome, in "Respiratory Distress Syndrome of Shock and Trauma," W. B. Saunders Company, Philadelphia, 1977.

———, Lim, R. C., Jr., and Stallone, R. J.: The Mechanism of Pulmonary Damage following Traumatic Shock, *Surg Gynecol Obstet,* **130**:15, 1970.

Boyd, D. R.: Monitoring Patients with Post-Traumatic Pulmonary Insufficiency, *Surg Clin North Am,* **52**:31, 1972.

Bredenberg, C. E., et al.: Respiratory Failure in Shock, *Ann Surg,* **169**:392, 1969.

Buckberg, G. D., and Dowell, A. R.: The Effects of Hemorrhagic Shock and Pulmonary Ischemia on Lung Compliance and Structure in Baboons, *Surg Gynecol Obstet,* **131**:1065, 1970.

———, Lipman, C. A., Hahn, J. A., Smith, M. J., and Hennessen, J. A.: Pulmonary Changes following Hemorrhagic Shock and Resuscitation in Baboons, *J Thorac Cardiovasc Surg,* **59**:450, 1970.

Burford, T. H., and Burbank, B.: Traumatic Wet Lung: Observations on Certain Physiologic Fundamentals of Thoracic Trauma, *J Thorac Surg,* **14**:415, 1945.

Burke, J. F., Pontoppidan, H., and Welch, C. E.: High Output Respiratory Failure: An Important Cause of Death Ascribed to Peritonitis or Ileus, *Ann Surg,* **158**:581, 1963.

Burnham, S. C., Martin, W. E., and Cheney, F. W., Jr.: The Effects of Various Tidal Volumes on Gas Exchange in Pulmonary Edema, *Anesthesiology,* **37**:27, 1972.

Cafferata, H. T., Aggeler, P. M., Robinson, A. J., and Blaisdell, F. W.: Intravascular Coagulation in the Surgical Patient, *Am J Surg,* **118:**281, 1969.

Camerson, J. L., Anderson, R. P., and Zuidema, G. D.: Aspiration and Pneumonia: A Clinical and Experimental Review, *J Surg Res,* **7:**44, 1967.

Carey, L. C., Lowery, B. D., and Cloutier, C. T.: "Hemorrhagic Shock," Current Problems in Surgery, Monograph, January 1971.

Churchill, E. D.: Pulmonary Atelectasis: With Especial Reference to Massive Collapse of Lung, *Arch Surg,* **11:**489, 1925.

Clauss, R. H., Scalabrini, B. Y., Ray, J. F., II, and Reed, C. E.: Effects of Changing Body Position upon Improved Ventilation-Perfusion Relationships, *Circulation,* **37–38** (Suppl II): 214, 1968.

Clowes, G. H. A., Jr., et al.: Observations on the Pathogenesis of the Pneumonitis Associated with Severe Infections in Other Parts of the Body, *Ann Surg,* **167:**630, 1968.

———, Farrington, G. H., Zuschneid, W., Cossette, G. R., and Saravis, C.: Circulating Factors in the Etiology of Pulmonary Insufficiency and Right Heart Failure Accompanying Severe Sepsis (Peritonitis), *Ann Surg,* **171:**663, 1970.

Coalson, J. J., Hinshaw, L. B., and Guenter, C. A.: The Pulmonary Ultrastructure in Septic Shock, *Exp Mol Pathol,* **12:**84, 1970.

Collins, J. A.: The Causes of Progressive Pulmonary Insufficiency in Surgical Patients, *J Surg Res,* **9:**685, 1969.

———, et al.: Inapparent Hypoxemia in Casualties with Wounded Limbs: Pulmonary Fat Embolism? *Ann Surg,* **167:**511, 1968.

Comroe, J. H., Jr., Forster, R. E., II, Dubois, A. B., Briscoe, W. A., and Carlsen, E. (eds.): The Pulmonary Circulation and Ventilation/Blood Flow Ratios, in "The Lung: Clinical Physiology and Pulmonary Function Tests." Chicago, Year Book Medical Publishers, 1962.

Ducker, T. B.: Increased Intracranial Pressure and Pulmonary Edema: Part I. Clinical Study of 11 Patients, *J Neurosurg,* **28:**112, 1968.

Eaton, R. M.: Pulmonary Edema: Experimental Observation on Dogs Following Acute Peripheral Blood Loss, *J Thorac Surg,* **16:**668, 1947.

Eiseman, B., and Ashbaugh, D. G. (eds.): Pulmonary Effects of Nonthoracic Trauma: Proceedings of a Conference Conducted by the Committee on Trauma, Division of Medical Sciences, National Academy of Sciences–National Research Council, *J Trauma,* vol. 8, 1968.

Elliot, T. R., and Dingley, L. A.: Massive Collapse of the Lungs following Abdominal Operation, *Lancet,* **1:**1305, 1914.

Falke, K. J., et al.: Ventilation with End-Expiratory Pressure in Acute Lung Disease, *J Clin Invest,* **51:**2315, 1972.

Feeley, T. W., and Hedley-Whyte, J.: Weaning from Controlled Ventilation and Supplemental Oxygen, *N Engl J Med,* **292:**903, 1975.

Fleming, W. H., and Bowen, J. C.: The Use of Diuretics in the Treatment of Early Wet Lung Syndrome, *Ann Surg,* **175:**505, 1972.

Fulton, R. L., and Jones, C. E.: The Cause of Post-traumatic Pulmonary Insufficiency in Man, *Surg Gynecol Obstet,* **140:**179, 1975.

Geiger, J. P., and Gielchinsky, I.: Acute Pulmonary Insufficiency, *Arch Surg,* **102:**400, 1971.

Gerst, P. H., Rattenborg, C., and Holday, D. A.: The Effects of Hemorrhage on Pulmonary Circulation and Respiratory Gas Exchange, *J Clin Invest,* **38:**524, 1959.

Gotoh, F., Meyer, J., and Takagi, Y.: Cerebral Effects of Hyperventilation in Man, *Arch Neurol,* **12:**419, 1965.

Greenfield, L. J.: Pulmonary Dysfunction in Shock, in L. B. Hinshaw and B. G. Cox (eds.): "The Fundamental Mechanisms of Shock: Advances in Experimental Medicine and Biology," vol 23, p. 47, Plenum Press, New York, 1972.

Guenter, C. A., Firoica, V., and Hinshaw, L. B.: Cardiorespiratory and Metabolic Responses to Live E. coli and Endotoxin in the Monkey, *J Appl Physiol,* **26:**780, 1969.

Gump, F. E., Mashima, Y., Ferenczy, A., and Kinney, J. M.: Pre- and Postmortem Studies of Lung Fluids and Electrolytes, *J Trauma,* **11:**474, 1971.

Halmagyi, D. F. J., Goodman, A. H., Little, M. J., Kennedy, M., and Varga, D.: Portal Blood Flow and Oxygen Usage in Dogs after Hemorrhage, *Ann Surg,* **172:**284, 1970.

Hedden, M., and Miller, G. J.: Mendelson's Syndrome and Its Sequelae, *Can Anaesth Soc J,* **19:**351, 1972.

Henry, J. N., McArdle, A. H., Scott, H. J., and Gurd, F. N.: A Study of the Acute and Chronic Respiratory Pathophysiology of Hemorrhagic Shock, *J Thorac Cardiovasc Surg,* **54:**666, 1967.

Herndon, J. H., Riseborough, E. J., and Fischer, J. E.: Fat Embolism: A Review of Current Concepts, *J Trauma,* **11:**673, 1971.

Hill, J. D., et al.: Acute Respiratory Insufficiency: Treatment with Prolonged Extracorporeal Oxygenation, *J Thorac Cardiovasc Surg,* **64:**551, 1972.

Hillen, G. P., Gaisford, W. D., and Jensen, C. G.: Pulmonary Changes in Treated and Untreated Hemorrhagic Shock: I. Early Functional and Ultrastructural Alterations after Moderate Shock, *Am J Surg,* **122:**639, 1971.

Hinshaw, L. B., Emerson, T. E., Jr., and Reins, D. A.: Cardiovascular Responses of the Primate in Endotoxin Shock, *Am J Physiol,* **210:**335, 1966.

Hirsch, E. F., Fletcher, R., and Lucas, S.: Hemodynamic and Respiratory Changes Associated with Sepsis Following Combat Trauma, *Ann Surg,* **174:**211, 1971.

Holcroft, J. W., Trunkey, D. D., and Lim, R. C.: Further Analysis of Lung Water in Baboons Resuscitated from Hemorrhagic Shock, *J Surg Res,* **20:**291, 1976.

Horovitz, J. H., and Carrico, C. J.: Lung Colloid Permeability in Hemorrhagic Shock, *Surg Forum,* **23:**6, 1972.

———, ———, Maher, J., and Shires, G. T.: Pulmonary Shunt Determination: A Comparison between Oxygen Inhalation (Berggren) and Xenon-133 Methods, *J Lab Clin Med,* **78:**785, 1971.

———, ———, and Shires, G. T.: The Pulmonary Response to Major Injury, *Arch Surg,* **105:**699, 1974.

Huller, T., and Bazini, Y.: Blast Injuries of the Chest and Abdomen, *Arch Surg,* **100:**24, 1970.

Jenkins, M. T., Jones, R. F., Wilson, B., and Moyer, C. A.: Congestive Atelectasis: A Complication of the Intravenous Infusion of Fluids, *Ann Surg,* **132:**327, 1950.

Kafer, E. R.: Pulmonary Oxygen Toxicity: A Review of the Evidence for Acute and Chronic Oxygen Toxicity in Man, *Br J Anaesthiol,* **43:**687, 1971.

Keller, C. A., Schramel, R. J., Hyman, A. L., and Creech, O., Jr.: The Cause of Acute Congestive Lesions of the Lung, *J Thorac Cardiovasc Surg,* **53:**743, 1967.

Kim, S. I., Desai, J. M., and Shoemaker, W. C.: Sequential Respiratory Changes in an Experimental Hemorrhagic Shock Preparation Designed to Simulate Clinical Shock, *Ann Surg,* **170:**166, 1969.

Kuman, A., et al.: Continuous Positive-Pressure Ventilation in Acute Respiratory Failure: Effects on Hemodynamics and Lung Function, *N Engl J Med,* **283:**1430, 1970.

Laennec, R. T. H.: "De l'auscultation médiate ou traité du diagnostic des maladies des poumons et du coeur, fondé principalement sur ce nouveau moyen d'exploration," Paris, 1819.

Lande, A. J., et al.: Prolonged Cardio-Pulmonary Support with a Practical Membrane Oxygenator, *Trans Am Soc Artif Intern Organs,* **16:**352, 1970.

Levine, M., Gilbert, R., and Auchingloss, J. H., Jr.: A Comparison of the Effects of Signs, Large Tidal Volumes, and Positive End Expiratory Pressure in Assisted Ventilation, *Scand J Respir Dis,* **53:**101, 1972.

Lim, R. C., Jr., Blaisdell, F. W., Choy, S. H., Goodman, J. R., and Hall, A. D.: Pulmonary Microvascular Changes Following Regional Shock: A Clinical and Experimental Study, *Bull Soc Int Chir,* **1:**22, 1968.

Markello, R., Winter, P., and Olszowka, A.: Assessment of Ventilation-Perfusion Inequalities by Arterial-Alveolar Nitrogen Differences in Intensive-Care Patients, *Anesthesiology,* **37:**4, 1972.

Martin, A. M., Jr., Soloway, H. B., and Simmons, R. L.: Pathologic Anatomy of the Lungs Following Shock and Trauma, *J Trauma,* **8:**687, 1968.

McLaughlin, J. S.: Physiologic Consideration of Hypoxemia in Shock and Trauma, *Ann Surg,* **173:**667, 1971.

McNamara, J. J., Molot, M. D., and Stremple, J. F.: Screen Filtration Pressure in Combat Casualties, *Ann Surg,* **172:**334, 1970.

Meyer, J. A.: Mechanical Support of Respiration, *Surg Clin North Am,* **54:**(5):115, 1974.

Michenfelder, J., Fowler, W., and Theye, R.: CO_2 Levels and Pulmonary Shunting in Anesthetized Man, *J Appl Physiol,* **21:**1471, 1966.

Mills, M.: The Clinical Syndrome, *J Trauma,* **8:**651, 1968.

Monaco, V., et al.: Pulmonary Venous Admixture in Injured Patients, *J Trauma,* **12:**15, 1972.

Moore, F. D., et al.: "Post-Traumatic Pulmonary Insufficiency," W. B. Saunders Company, Philadelphia, 1969.

Moseley, R. V., and Doty, D. B.: Changes in the Filtration Characteristics of Stored Blood, *Ann Surg,* **171:**329, 1970.

Moss, G., Staunton, C., and Stein, A. A.: Cerebral Etiology of the "Shock Lung Syndrome," *J Trauma,* **12:**885, 1972.

Motsay, G. J., Alho, A. V., Schultz, L. S., Dietzman, R. H., and Lillehei, R. C.: Pulmonary Capillary Permeability in the Post-traumatic Pulmonary Insufficiency Syndrome: Comparison of Isogravimetric Capillary Pressures, *Ann Surg,* **173:**244, 1971.

Naimark, A., Dugard, A., and Rangno, R. E.: Regional Pulmonary Blood Flow and Gas Exchange in Hemorrhagic Shock, *J Appl Physiol,* **25:**301, 1968.

Nash, G., Bowen, J. A., and Langlinais, P. C.: "Respirator Lung": A Misnomer, *Arch Pathol,* **21:**234, 1971.

Neeley, W. A., et al.: Postoperative Respiratory Insufficiency: Physiological Studies with Therapeutic Implications, *Ann Surg,* **171:**679, 1970.

Nichols, R. T., Pearce, H. J., and Greenfield, L. J.: Effects of Experimental Pulmonary Contusion on Respiratory Exchange and Lung Mechanics, *Arch Surg,* **96:**723, 1968.

Olcott, C., Barber, R. E., and Blaisdell, F. W.: Diagnosis and Treatment of Respiratory Failure after Civilian Trauma, *Am J Surg,* **122:**260, 1971.

Pierce, A. K., et al.: Long-term Evaluation of Decontamination of Inhalation Therapy Equipment and the Occurrence of Necrotizing Pneumonia. *N Engl J Med,* **282:**528, 1970.

Pinardi, G., Leal, E., and Sallas Coll, A.: Vascular Permeability to Red Blood Cells and Protein in Hemorrhagic Shock, *Acta Physiol Lat Am,* **17:**175, 1967.

Pontoppidan, H., Geffin, B., and Lowenstein, E.: Acute Respiratory Failure in the Adult, *N Engl J Med,* **287:**690, 1972.

———, Laver, M. B., and Geffin, B.: Acute Respiratory Failure in the Surgical Patient, *Adv Surg,* **4:**163, 1970.

Powers, S. R., Jr.: The Use of Positive and Expiratory Pressure (PEEP) for Respiratory Support, *Surg Clin North Am,* **54:**1125, 1974.

———, et al.: Studies of Pulmonary Insufficiency in Non-thoracic Trauma, *J Trauma,* **12:**1, 1972.

Proctor, H. J., Ballantine, T. V. N., and Broussard, N. D.: An Analysis of Pulmonary Function Following Non-thoracic Trauma, with Recommendations for Therapy, *Ann Surg,* **172:**180, 1970.

Robin, E. D., Carey, L. C., Grenvik, A., Glauser, F., and Gaudio, R.: Capillary Leak Syndrome with Pulmonary Edema, *Arch Intern Med,* **130:**66, 1972.

Rosen, A. J.: Shock Lung: Fact or Fancy? *Surg Clin North Am,* **55:**613, 1975.

Rounthwaite, H. L., Scott, H. J., and Gurd, F. N.: Changes in the Pulmonary Circulation during Hemorrhagic Shock and Resuscitation, *Surg Forum,* **3:**454, 1952.

Said, S. I., et al.: Pulmonary Gas Exchange during Induction of Pulmonary Edema in Anesthetized Dogs, *J Appl Physiol,* **19:**403, 1964.

Schloerb, P. R., Hunt, P. T., Plummer, J. A., and Cage, G. K.: Pulmonary Edema after Replacement of Blood Loss by Electrolyte Solutions, *Surg Gynecol Obstet,* **135:**893, 1972.

Schon, G. R., Delphin, E. S., Millan, P. R., and Labat, R.: Relationship of Blood Substitutes to Pulmonary Changes and Volemia, *Ann Surg,* **173:**504, 1971.

Sealy, W. C., Ogino, S., Lesage, A. M., and Young, W. G., Jr.: Functional and Structural Changes in the Lungs in Hemorrhagic Shock, *Surg Gynecol Obstet,* **122:**754, 1966.

Shires, G. T., Carrico, C. J., and Canizaro, P. C.: "Shock," Chap. 4, Pulmonary Responses, W. B. Saunders Company, Philadelphia, 1973.

Siegel, D. C., Cochin, A., and Moss, G. S.: The Ventilatory Response to Hemorrhagic Shock and Resuscitation, *Surgery,* **72:**451, 1972.

———, Moss, G. S., Cochin, A., and Das Gupta, T. K.: Pulmonary Changes following Treatment for Hemorrhagic Shock: Saline versus Colloid Infusion, *Surg Forum,* **21:**17, 1970.

Simeone, F. A.: Shock, in "Christopher's Textbook of Surgery," 8th ed., Ed: Loyal Davis, p. 58, W. B. Saunders Company, Philadelphia, 1964.

Simmons, R. L., Martin, A. M., Jr., Heisterkamp, C. A., III, and Ducker, T. B.: Respiratory Insufficiency in Combat Casualties: II. Pulmonary Edema following Head Injury, *Ann Surg,* **170:**39, 1969.

Skillman, J. J., Parikh, B. M., and Tanenbaum, B. J.: Pulmonary Arteriovenous Admixture Improvement with Albumin and Diuresis, *Am J Surg,* **119:**450, 1970.

Sladen, A., Laver, M. B., and Pontoppidan, H.: Pulmonary Complications and Water Retention in Prolonged Mechanical Ventilation, *N Engl J Med,* **279:**448, 1968.

Stallone, R. J., Herbst, H., Blaisdell, F. W., and Murray, J. F.: Pulmonary Changes following Ischemia of the Lower Extremities and Their Treatment, *Am Rev Respir Dis,* **100:**813, 1969.

Staub, N. C.: Pathogenesis of Pulmonary Edema, *Am Rev Respir Dis,* **109:**358, 1974.

Sterling, G. M.: The Mechanism of Bronchoconstriction Due to Hypocapnia in Man, *Clin Sci,* **34:**277, 1968.

Sugg, W. F., et al.: Congestive Atelectasis: An Experimental Study, *Ann Surg,* **168:**234, 1968.

Swank, R. L.: Alteration of Blood on Storage: Measurement of Adhesiveness of "Aging" Platelets and Leukocytes and Their Removal by Filtration, *N Engl J Med,* **265:**728, 1961.

Sykes, M. P., Adams, A. P., Finlay, W. E. I., Wightman, A. E., and Munroe, J. P.: The Cardiorespiratory Effects of Haemorrhage and Overtransfusion in Dogs, *Br J Anaesthiol,* **42:**573, 1970.

Terzi, R. G., and Peters, R. M.: The Effect of Large Fluid Loads on Lung Mechanics and Work, *Ann Thorac Surg,* **6:**16, 1968.

Trimble, C., Smith, D. E., Rosenthal, M. H., and Fosburg, R. G.: Pathophysiologic Role of Hypocarbia in Post-traumatic Pulmonary Insufficiency, *Am J Surg,* **122:**633, 1971.

Wahrenbrock, E. A., Carrico, C. J., Amundsen, D. A., Trummer, M. J., and Severinghaus, J. W.: Increased Atelectatic Pulmonary Shunt during Hemorrhagic Shock in Dogs, *J Appl Physiol,* **29:**615, 1970.

————, ————, Schroeder, C. F., and Trummer, M. J.: The Effect of Posture on Pulmonary Function and Survival of Anesthetized Dogs, *J Surg Res,* **10:**13, 1970.

Wangensteen, O. D., Wittmers, L. E., and Johnson, J. A.: Permeability of the Mammalian Blood-Gas Barrier and Its Components, *Am J Physiol,* **216:**719, 1969.

Willwerth, B. M., Crawford, F. A., Young, W. G., Jr., and Sealy, W. C.: The Role of Functional Demand in the Development of Pulmonary Lesions during Hemorrhagic Shock, *J Thorac Cardiovasc Surg,* **54:**658, 1967.

Wilson, J. W.: Treatment or Prevention of Pulmonary Cellular Damage with Pharmacologic Doses of Corticosteroid, *Surg Gynecol Obstet,* **134:**675, 1972.

Wilson, R. F., Kafi, A., Asuncion, Z., and Walt, A. J.: Clinical Respiratory Failure after Shock or Trauma, *Arch Surg,* **98:**539, 1969.

Wyche, M. Q., Marshall, B. E., Mehall, S. L., and Schuetze, M. M.: Lung Function, Pulmonary Extravascular Water Volume and Hemodynamics in Early Hemorrhagic Shock in Anesthetized Dogs, *Ann Surg,* **174:**296, 1971.

Alterations in Oxygen Transport

Bellingham, A. J., Detter, J. C., and Lenfant, C.: Regulatory Mechanisms of Hemoglobin Oxygen Affinity in Acidosis and Alkalosis, *J Clin Invest,* **50:**700, 1971.

Benesch, R., and Benesch, R. E.: The Effect of Organic Phosphates from the Human Erythrocyte on the Allosteric Properties of Hemoglobin, *Biochem Biophys Res Commun,* **26:**162, 1967.

Berne, R. M., Blackman, J. R., and Gardner, T. H.: Hypoxemia and Coronary Blood Flow, *J Clin Invest,* **36:**1101, 1957.

Beutler, E., Meul, A., and Wood, L. A.: Depletion and Regeneration of 2,3-Diphosphoglyceric Acid in Stored Red Blood Cells, *Transfusion,* **9:**109, 1969.

Bowen, J. C., and Fleming, W. H.: Increased Oxyhemoglobin Affinity after Transfusion of Stored Blood, *Ann Surg,* **180:**760, 1974.

Canizaro, P. C., Nelson, J. L., Hennessy, J. L., and Bright, P. B.: A Technique for Estimating the Position of the Oxygen-Hemoglobin Dissociation Curve, *Ann Surg,* **180:**364, 1974.

Chaunutin, A., and Curnish, R. R.: Effect of Organic and Inorganic Phosphates on the Oxygen Equilibrium of Human Erythrocytes, *Arch Biochem Biophys,* **121:**96, 1967.

Dawson, R. B., Edinger, M. C., and Ellis, T. J.: Hemoglobin Function in Stored Blood, *J Lab Clin Med,* **77:**46, 1971.

Dennis, R. C., Vito, L., Weisel, R. D., Valeri, C. R., Berger, R. L., and Hechtman, H. B.: Improved Myocardial Performance Following High 2-3 Diphosphoglycerate Red Cell Transfusions, *Surgery,* **77:**741, 1975.

Duhm, J., Deuticke, B., and Gerlach, E.: Complete Restoration of Oxygen Transport Function and 2,3-Diphosphoglycerate Concentration in Stored Blood, *Transfusion,* **11:**147, 1971.

Harker, A. H.: The Surgical Significance of the Oxyhemoglobin Dissociation Curve, *Surg Gynecol Obstet,* **144:**935, 1977.

Lenfant, C., et al.: Effects of Altitude on Oxygen Binding by Hemoglobin and on Organic Phosphate Levels, *J Clin Invest,* **47:**2652, 1968.

————, Ways, P., and Aucutt, C.: Effect of Chronic Hypoxic Hypoxia on the O_2-Hb Dissociation Curve and Respiratory Gas Transport in Man, *Respir Physiol,* **7:**7, 1969.

McConn, R., and Del Guercio, L. R. M.: Respiratory Function of Blood in the Acutely Ill Patient and the Effect of Steroids, *Ann Surg,* **174:**436, 1971.

Opitz, E., and Schneider, M.: Über die Sauerstoffversorgung des Gehirns und den Mechanismus von Mangelverhungerung, *Ergeb Physiol,* **46:**126, 1950.

Oski, F. A., et al.: The *in vitro* Restoration of Red Cell 2,3-Diphosphoglycerate Levels in Banked Blood, *Blood,* **37:**52, 1971.

Pollock, T. W., et al.: *In vivo* Effect of Inosine, Pyruvate, and Phosphate (IPP) on Oxygen-Hemoglobin Affinity, *Fed Proc,* **30:**546, 1971.

Rice, C. L., Herman, C. M., Kiesow, L. A., Homer, L. D., and John, D. A.: Benefits from Improved Oxygen Delivery of Blood in Shock Therapy, *Surg Res,* **19:**193, 1975.

Severinghaus, J. W.: Blood Gas Calculator, *J Appl Physiol,* **21:**1108, 1966.

Shappell, S. D., and Lenfant, C. J. M.: Adaptive, Genetic, and Iatrogenic Alterations of the Oxyhemoglobin-Dissociation Curve, *Anesthesiology,* **37:**127, 1972.

Valeri, C. R., and Hirsch, N. M.: Restoration *in vivo* of Erythrocyte Adenosine Triphosphate, 2,3-Diphosphoglycerate, Potassium Ion, and Sodium Ion Concentrations Following the Transfusion of Acid-Citrate-Dextrose-Stored Human Red Blood Cells, *J Lab Clin Med,* **73:**722, 1969.

Therapy of Shock

Alican, F., Dalton, M. L., Jr., and Hardy, J. D.: Experimental Endotoxin Shock, *Am J Surg,* **103:**702, 1962.

Altemeier, W. A., Todd, J. C., and Inge, W. W.: Gramnegative Septicemia: A Growing Threat, *Ann Surg,* **166:**530, 1967.

Baue, A. E.: The Treatment of Septic Shock: A Problem Intensified by Advancing Science, *Surgery,* **65:**850, 1969.

Blair, E., Ollodart, R., Esmond, W. G., Attar, S., and Crowley, R. A.: Effect of Hyperbaric Oxygenation (OHP) on Bacteremic Shock, *Circulation,* **29** (Suppl I):135, 1964.

Carey, J. S., et al.: Cardiovascular Function in Shock; Responses to Volume Loading and Isoproterenol Infusion, *Circulation,* **35:**327, 1967.

Clermont, G., Williams, J. S., and Adams, J. T.: Steroid Effect on the Release of the Lysosomal Enzyme Acid Phosphatase in Shock, *Ann Surg,* **179:**917, 1974.

Duff, J. H., Malave, G., Pertz, D. I., Scott, H. M., and MacLean, L. D.: The Hemodynamics of Septic Shock in Man and in the Dog, *Surgery,* **58:**174, 1965.

Grollman, A.: "Cardiac Output of Man in Health and Disease," Charles C Thomas, Springfield, Ill., 1932.

Hinshaw, L. B., Archer, L. T., Black, M. R., Greenfield, L. J., and Guenter, C. A.: Prevention and Reversal of Myocardial Failure in Endotoxin Shock, *Surg Gynecol Obstet,* **136:**1, 1973.

Iampietro, P. F., Henshaw, L. B., and Brake, C. M.: Effect of an Adrenergic Blocking Agent on Vascular Alterations Associated with Endotoxin Shock, *Am J Physiol,* **204:**611, 1963.

Krausz, M. M., Perel, A., Eimerl, D., and Cotev, S.: Cardiopulmonary Effects of Volume Loading in Patients in Septic Shock, *Ann Surg,* **185:**429, 1977.

Kwaan, H. M., and Weil, M. H.: Differences in the Mechanism of Shock Caused by Bacterial Infections, *Surg Gynecol Obstet,* **128:**37, 1969.

Loeb, H. S., Winslow, E. B. J., Rahimtoola, S. H., Rosen, K. M., and Gunnar, R. M.: Acute Hemodynamic Effects of Dopamine in Patients with Shock, *Circulation,* **44:**163, 1971.

MacLean, L. D., Mulligan, W. G., MacLean, A. P. H., and Duff, J. H.: Patterns of Septic Shock in Man: A Detailed Study of 56 Patients, *Ann Surg,* **166:**543, 1967.

Motsay, G. J., Dietzman, R. H., Ersek, R. A., and Lillehei, R. C.: Hemodynamic Alterations and Results of Treatment in Patients with Gram-negative Septic Shock, *Surgery,* **67:**577, 1970.

Ollodart, R. M., Hawthorne, I., and Attar, S.: Studies in Experimental Endotoxemia in Man, *Am J Surg,* **113:**599, 1967.

Rowe, M. I., Buckner, D. M., and Newmark, S.: The Early Diagnosis of Gram-negative Septicemia in the Pediatric Surgical Patient, *Ann Surg,* **182:**280, 1975.

Schuler, J. J., Erve, P. R., and Schumer, W.: Glucocorticoid Effect on Hepatic Carbohydrate Metabolism in the Endotoxin-Shocked Monkey, *Ann Surg,* **183:**345, 1976.

Schumer, W.: Steroids in the Treatment of Clinical Septic Shock, *Ann Surg,* **184:**333, 1976.

———, and Nyhus, L. M.: "Corticosteroids in the Treatment of Shock," University of Illinois Press, Urbana, 1970.

Shubin, H., and Weil, M. H.: Bacterial Shock: A Serious Complication in Urological Practice, *JAMA,* **185:**850, 1963.

Spath, J. A., Gorczynski, R. J., and Lefer, A. M.: Possible Mechanisms of the Beneficial Action of Glucocorticoids in Circulatory Shock, *Surg Gynecol Obstet,* **137:**597, 1973.

Spink, W. W.: The Ecology of Human Septic Shock, in S. G. Hershey, L. R. M. Del Guercio, and R. McConn (eds.), "Septic Shock in Man," Little, Brown and Company, Boston, 1971.

Swan, H. J. C., et al.: Catheterization of the Heart in Man with Use of a Flow-Directed Balloon-Tipped Catheter, *N Engl J Med,* **283:**447, 1970.

Waldhausen, J. A., Kilman, J. W., and Abel, F. L.: Effects of Catecholamines on the Heart: Myocardial Contractility, Cardiac Efficiency, and Total Peripheral Resistance, *Arch Surg,* **91:**86, 1965.

Weil, M. H., Shubin, H., and Rosoff, L.: Fluid Repletion in Circulatory Shock: Central Venous Pressure and Other Practical Guides, *JAMA,* **192:**668, 1965.

Wilson, J. N., Grow, J. B., Demong, C. V., Prevedel, A. E., and Owens, J. C.: Central Venous Pressure in Optimal Blood Volume Maintenance, *Arch Surg,* **85:**563, 1962.

Wilson, R. F., and Fisher, R. R.: The Hemodynamic Effects of Massive Steroids in Clinical Shock, *Surg Gynecol Obstet,* **127:**769, 1968.

———, Sukhnanden, R., and Thal, A. P.: Combined Use of Norepinephrine and Dibenzyline in Clinical Shock, *Surg Forum,* **15:**30, 1964.

Wright, C. J., Duff, J. H., MacLean, A. P. H., and MacLean, L. D.: Regional Capillary Blood Flow and Oxygen Uptake in Severe Sepsis, *Surg Gynecol Obstet,* **132:**637, 1971.

Chapter 5

Infections

by Isidore Cohn, Jr. and George H. Bornside

INTRODUCTION

Infection is a dynamic process involving invasion of the body by pathogenic microorganisms and reaction of the tissues to organisms and their toxins. Soon after birth, a variety of microorganisms colonize the external and internal surfaces of the human body. This indigenous microflora usually does no harm; it produces no detectable pathologic effects in tissues and may be beneficial. Indeed, current research indicates that the normal intestinal flora functions as a barrier providing natural resistance against enteric infections with pathogens such as *Salmonella* and *Shigella* species. Infection evolves into overt disease only when the equilibrium between host and parasite is upset. Of the thousands of species of microorganisms in nature, only a few hundred are known to be pathogenic for man.

Current thinking concerning clinical disease resulting from host and parasite interrelationships recognizes the role of the general health of the host, his previous contact with infectious microorganisms, his past clinical history, and various insults (toxic, traumatic, or therapeutic) of nonmicrobial origin. When the host's resistance is lowered, the indigenous microflora can become involved in infectious disease. This presents a dilemma to both the clinician and the microbiologist, as it must be decided which of the several microorganisms usually isolated from a clinical specimen are involved in the patient's disease. There are very few pathogenic species which cause disease at all times. Most organisms found in and on man often are harmless but are capable of causing disease in patients who are elderly, very young, or debilitated (Table 5-1).

Despite 80 years of aseptic surgery and more than 40 years of experience with antimicrobial agents, the surgeon finds that infections are as great a problem now as in the past. But the etiologic agents have changed. Streptococci and pneumococci are no longer the captains of death, because they can be controlled by antibiotics. Staphylococci con-

Table 5-1. SOME INDIGENOUS MICROORGANISMS AND SOME INFECTIONS WITH WHICH THEY MAY BE INVOLVED

Microorganism	Infection
Aerobic or facultative:	
Achromobacter spp.	Bloodstream, burns, meningitis, urethritis
Acinetobacter spp.	Bloodstream, burns, meningitis, urethritis, pneumonia
Alcaligenes fecalis	Bloodstream, conjunctivitis, meningitis, respiratory tract, urinary tract
Candida albicans and other yeasts	Bacterial endocarditis, pneumonitis, septicemia, thrush, vulvovaginitis, candidiosis
Corynebacterium spp.	Bacterial endocarditis, lung abscesses
Enterobacteriaceae (*Escherichia, Klebsiella, Enterobacter, Proteus,* etc.)	Abscesses, bloodstream, meningitis, peritonitis, pneumonia, wounds, urinary tract, endocarditis, pyelonephritis, cystitis
Hemophilus spp.	Bronchitis, conjunctivitis, meningitis, urinary tract
Moraxella spp.	Conjunctivitis
Nocardia spp.	Nocardiosis
Pseudomonas spp.	Bloodstream, burns, meningitis, urinary tract, wounds
Staphylococcus aureus	Abscesses, pneumonia, wounds, pseudomembranous enterocolitis
Staphylococcus epidermidis	Bacterial endocarditis, septicemia, thrombophlebitis
Streptococcus fecalis	Bacterial endocarditis, bloodstream, urinary tract, wounds, peritonitis, meningitis
Streptococcus viridans	Bacterial endocarditis
Anaerobic:	
Actinomyces spp.	Actinomycosis
Bacteroides spp.	Abscesses, bacterial endocarditis, peritonitis
Clostridium spp.	Cellulitis, myonecrosis
Fusobacterium spp.	Abscesses, myonecrosis, bacteremia
Lactobacillus spp.	Bacterial endocarditis
Peptostreptococcus spp.	Abscesses, myonecrosis
Veillonella spp.	Bacterial endocarditis

tinue to cause nosocomial (hospital-acquired) infections, and those gram-negative bacteria usually considered nonpathogens, opportunists, or secondary invaders have become a major problem. Nosocomial infection results from the transmission of pathogens to a previously uninfected patient from a source in the hospital environment (cross infection). Alternatively, the pathogens may come from the patient himself (autoinfection). He may be a carrier of the pathogen or become colonized with virulent hospital strains during hospitalization. Many nosocomial infections have a iatrogenic basis (i.e., result from treatment by the physician and his professional collaborators). Frequent or prolonged use of supportive procedures such as indwelling venous or urinary catheters, tracheostomies, and equipment for postoperative respiratory care are responsible for most iatrogenic infections. Nosocomial infection causes morbidity, mortality, expense to the patient, and increasing malpractice liability for the surgeon and hospital.

A surgical infection is an infection which requires surgical treatment and has developed before, or as a complication of, surgical treatment. Thus, a postoperative wound infection is also a specific nosocomial infection. Surgical infections may be analyzed in relation to procedures in clean or contaminated fields, the anatomic site or system involved, and the pathophysiologic activities of the causative microorganisms (Table 5-2). The microorganisms commonly encountered in surgical infections are the staphylococci, streptococci, clostridia, bacteroides, and the enteric bacteria. Most surgical incisions are contaminated but not infected with normal skin flora (bacteria such as coagulase-negative staphylococci and anaerobic diphtheroids). However, traumatic wounds are usually contaminated if not yet infected, and operations on infected or "contaminated" tissue usually result in infection. Postoperative infections present a double hazard: First, the infection itself may result in toxemia or produce extensive tissue damage and perhaps septicemia. Second, the local effects of infection delay healing of the wound and may cause hemorrhage or disruption of the wound. In either case, the patient's hospitalization is extended.

GENERAL PRINCIPLES

Pathogenic species of bacteria have the capacity to invade and produce disease. However, disease is a biologic accident and represents a complex interaction between the microorganism and the host which occurs only under special circumstances. Healthy people may harbor pathogenic bacteria and yet be clinically unaffected. They are referred to as carriers of the particular pathogen. The healthy carrier of pathogenic microorganisms is the principal reservoir of most diseases. Although species such as *Staphylococcus aureus* and *Escherichia coli* are examples of pathogens, individual strains may be too feeble to cause infection. Feeble or noninvasive strains may cause infection if the resistance of the host is extremely low or if tremendous numbers of bacteria are introduced. Some bacteria which are nonpathogenic under ordinary conditions are opportunistic and may be pathogenic when the host-parasite

Table 5-2. CLASSIFICATION OF
SURGICAL INFECTIONS

I. Relative to final outcome
  A. Self-limiting infections: The patient recovers completely without medical or surgical treatment, or despite it (e.g., a boil).
  B. Serious infections requiring treatment: The outcome depends largely on the nature of treatment, the time after outset that it is administered, and clinical judgment (e.g., septicemia, pneumonia, empyema, primary peritonitis).
  C. Fulminating infections: These prove to be fatal or permanently disabling (e.g., retroperitoneal cellulitis).
II. Relative to time of onset
  A. Anteoperative surgical infections: These include all infections in which the microorganisms have gained entrance to the body before any operative procedure.
    1. Time and portal of entry are known—accidents.
    2. Time and portal of entry are not known—disease (infection) is established before the surgeon treats the patient.
  B. Operative surgical infections: These include all in which microorganisms gain entrance to the body during an operative procedure or as an immediate result of it (i.e., surgery may be considered either directly or indirectly responsible for the development of infection).
    1. Preventable operative surgical infections—failure of the surgeon or operating-room personnel to adhere to the principles of sterile procedure and all accepted and accredited practices
    2. Nonpreventable operative surgical infections
      a. Pathogenic microorganisms already resident within body tissues (e.g., incision seeded with *Staphylococcus aureus* resident in ducts and glands of normal skin)
      b. Microorganisms from a deep focus of infection (e.g., peritoneal abscess, lung abscess, etc.)
      c. Microorganisms resident on the surface of normal mucous membranes (e.g., intestinal tract, respiratory tract, genitourinary tract)
      d. Microorganisms on dust particles and borne by air currents
  C. Postoperative surgical infections: These are complications of the operation or the postoperative management of the patient
    1. Surgical wound infection
    2. Respiratory tract infection
    3. Urinary tract infection

SOURCE: Modified from F. L. Meleney, "Treatise on Surgical Infections," Oxford University Press, New York, 1948.

equilibrium is upset, e.g., when normal flora is eliminated by antibiotics or when incision makes available a new area of the body. Antibiotic-resistant strains of *Staphylococcus aureus* of specific phage types, which cause nosocomial postoperative wound infections, may be endemic among carrier personnel of a particular hospital. The patient may become infected by direct contact with a carrier or may become infected with a hospital staphylococcus with which he has become colonized during hospitalization.

The term *virulence* refers to the tissue-invading powers of a specific strain of a pathogen and is used in two different ways: First, virulence describes quantitatively the smallest dose of a bacterial strain which will produce disease in a specified host. This assessment is usually conducted in experimental animals and may have no relation to human disease. Second, virulence describes an epi-

demiologic concept such as a given phage type of *Staphylococcus aureus* producing human disease more frequently than another. In this situation, virulence is based on ecologic advantage in the external environment but may not necessarily involve greater capacity to be virulent as measured by the critical dose of bacteria causing clinical infection.

A large infecting dose is favorable to the production of bacterial disease, because only a small number of bacteria may actually reach a favorable site in the host. A sudden change to a different environment or to a new site may injure most of the inoculum. Moreover, the defense mechanisms of the host often destroy a large proportion of the invading organisms before they can become established. The greater the number of bacteria introduced into the host, the greater the amount of preformed toxins that will be carried along. Preformed toxins may protect bacteria from destruction during the period when they are adapting to the new environment and are incapable of producing additional toxin. The resistance of the host is shown in his ability to keep bacteria out of the body initially and, failing in this, to localize and destroy them. A healthy, unbroken skin is the first line of resistance. Although mucous membranes are less resistant, even here minute breaks usually provide for bacterial entry. It is then that active defensive measures come into play. Primary defenses include the system of fixed phagocytic cells (i.e., the histiocytes of the reticuloendothelial system) and mobile phagocytes. These are aided by antibacterial substances in blood plasma, lymph, and interstitial fluid, by physical barriers to the spread of bacteria (i.e., ground substances, serous and fibrous membranes), and by local and systemic reactions such as hyperemia, fever, and leukocytosis. Secondary defenses are dependent upon the presence of specific antigenic stimuli (bacteria and bacterial products). The antibodies formed in response to these antigens inhibit or destroy bacteria, or neutralize their toxins. In the presence of sufficient antibodies, the primary defenses are greatly accelerated, bacteria are phagocytized and digested more quickly than before, and the ability of serum to neutralize bacterial toxins is increased many thousandfold. The presence of other disease may greatly reduce resistance to microbial infection. For example, diabetes predisposes to infection of the skin and the genitourinary tract. Influenza, measles, and other viral infections markedly predispose to secondary bacterial infections of the respiratory tract. Malignant disease, malnutrition, chronic alcoholism, or metabolic disease may interfere seriously with an individual's resistance to infectious disease.

Bacteria cause disease by invading tissues and producing toxins. Bacterial invasion leads to demonstrable damage of host cells and tissues in the vicinity of the invasion, whereas bacterial toxins are transported by the blood and lymph to cause cytotoxic effects at sites removed from the initial lesion. Species such as *Streptococcus pyogenes* are both invasive and toxigenic. *Staphylococcus aureus* produces local damage but has little tendency to spread, although the local inflammatory response may be severe as in the case of carbuncles. *Clostridium tetani* is almost solely toxigenic. Generally, invasiveness and toxigenicity are not completely separable, since invasion involves some degree of toxin production and toxigenicity requires some degree of bacterial multiplication. *Exotoxins* are specific, soluble, diffusible proteins produced by gram-positive bacteria as they multiply in a circumscribed area. Exotoxins lose their toxicity upon denaturation but retain much of their original antigenicity. Such modified exotoxins are called *toxoids*. Those prepared from *Clostridium tetani* are used to induce active immunity in man. The alpha toxin of *Clostridium perfringens* is a lecithinase which acts upon the membrane lipids of body cells and erythrocytes. *Endotoxins* are complex lipopolysaccharides of the bacterial cell wall produced by many gram-negative species. They are released only on partial or complete dissolution of the bacterial cell. Endotoxins are relatively heat-stable; many withstand temperatures of 60 to 100°C for 1 hour. They do not form toxoids. Their toxicity is associated with the phospholipid moiety of the molecule, whereas their antigenic determinants are associated with the polysaccharide moiety.

Diagnosis

The classic signs and symptoms of infection are redness, swelling, heat, and pain. Redness of the skin, due to intense hyperemia, is seen only in infections of the skin itself. Swelling accompanies infection unless the infection is confined to bone which cannot swell. Heat results from hyperemia and may be detected in the absence of redness. Pain is the most universal sign of infection. Along with pain goes tenderness, or pain to the touch, which is greatest over the area of maximal involvement. Loss of function is another sign of infection. It is brought about by reflex and by voluntary immobilization. The patient immobilizes the painful part in the most comfortable position he can find. For example, a finger with an infected tendon sheath is kept flexed. In peritonitis, the abdominal muscles are maintained in a state of tonic contraction to keep the inflamed peritoneum beneath from moving. Fever and tachycardia are additional, albeit nonspecific, signs of infection. Fever and chills indicate septicemia, while an elevated pulse rate is a sign of a toxic state.

Leukocytosis accompanies an acute bacterial infection more often than a viral infection. The more severe the infection, the greater is the leukocytosis. In most surgical infections, the total leukocyte count is only slightly or moderately elevated. However, a high leukocyte count ($35,000/mm^3$) occurs as a result of suppuration. The endotoxin released by gram-negative bacilli is thought to contribute to the production of high leukocyte counts. However, in the elderly, in the severely ill, and during therapy with antibiotic and immunosuppressive drugs, white cell counts may be normal or low. The leukopenia of overwhelming sepsis is probably due to exhaustion of the supply of leukocytes and to bone marrow depression. Although the total number of leukocytes is normal in some infections, there is a preponderance of immature granulocytes, which may be increased above 85 percent compared with the normal below 75 percent ("shift to the left"). A chronic infection may be evident only by fatigue, low-grade fever, and perhaps anemia. Moreover, massive pyogenic abscesses may occur without leukocytosis, fever, or tenderness.

Exudate from the area of infection should be examined for color, odor, and consistency. The microorganisms causing a surgical infection often may be seen microscopically on gram-stained smears. For each bacterial cell observed under the oil-immersion lens, there are approximately 10^5 similar organisms in each milliliter of exudate from which the smear was prepared. The staining and examination of slides are simple, rapid, inexpensive procedures which provide valuable and immediate information for the surgeon. Pus from deep-seated abscesses may be obtained by needle aspiration or at the time of definitive drainage. Exudate from surface infections may be examined directly. Specimens submitted to the bacteriologic laboratory should be collected before chemotherapy is begun and should be labeled adequately to identify the patient, the clinical diagnosis, and the nature and site of the specimen. The laboratory should be requested to do aerobic and anaerobic cultures and antibiotic-sensitivity tests. The surgeon must initiate treatment immediately upon clinical judgment, although the subsequent laboratory report will often enable him to make appropriate changes.

Biopsy is useful in establishing a diagnosis in granulomatous infections such as tuberculosis, syphilis, and mycoses. Additional sources of biopsy material are enlarged lymph nodes draining an area of infection or a sinus tract. Blood cultures are the single most definitive method of determining etiology in infectious disease and are often helpful in identifying the microorganisms causing surgical infection. Transient bacteremias accompany the early phase of many infections and may result from manipulation of infected or contaminated tissues (e.g., surgical incision of furuncles or abscesses, instrumentation of the genitourinary tract, and dental procedures). Bacteria usually enter the circulation via the lymphatic system. Consequently, when bacteria multiply at a site of local infection in tissues, the lymph drained from that area carries bacteria to the thoracic duct and eventually to the venous blood. However, a blood culture taken at the time of chill and fever may be negative for bacteria, as phagocytes promptly remove bacteria suddenly entering the bloodstream and chill and fever occur 30 to 90 minutes later. Thus, blood cultures should be taken at frequent intervals in a patient with febrile disease of unknown origin in an attempt to obtain blood before an expected chill and rise in temperature. A careful history and physical examination provide the basis for diagnosis and laboratory tests.

Surgical Therapy

It is necessary to distinguish between contamination and infection. Almost all wounds are contaminated with bacteria from the skin or from sources external to the patient. However, very few wounds become infected (i.e., exhibit disease manifested by inflammation, dehiscence, suppuration, and necrosis). The major clinical responses to wound infection are suppuration and invasion. Bacteria grow in the wound on substrates consisting of blood clots, lymph, leukocytes, and necrotic debris. Extension of the local inflammatory response to adjacent tissues is associated with a systemic reaction. The hazard of generalized infection is associated with all traumatic wounds. These and preoperative surgical infections are treated to overcome existing infection and to prevent postoperative infection. Local treatment consists of debridement of all necrotic or injured tissue, drainage of abscesses, removal of foreign bodies, and adjunctive therapy with antibiotics. Supportive measures governing the treatment of established surgical infections are bed rest, immobilization of the infected region, elevation to promote venous and lymphatic drainage, and relief of swelling and pain. Moist heat is applied to increase local blood supply, facilitate exudation, and hasten sloughing. The detailed management of wounds is discussed in Chap. 8 (Wound Healing and Wound Care).

Antibiotic Therapy

The adjunctive use of antibiotics in the treatment of infections is dependent upon an adequate blood supply and is most effective against acute infections such as cellulitis, septicemia, or peritonitis. Antibiotics have slight access to abscesses and penetrate by slow diffusion, if at all. In these situations, they should be used in conjunction with incision and drainage. Antibiotics are the primary treatment for acute spreading infections and should result in clinical improvement in 24 to 48 hours. Change to a more effective antibiotic may be based on the culture and sensitivity report.

Although clinical judgment frequently must be used to select an antibiotic and although the causative microorganism often is revealed on microscopic examination of a gram-stained smear of exudate or pus, the infecting microorganisms should be identified and antibiotic sensitivities determined by the laboratory. Accordingly, the specimen for culture (pus, exudate, blood, or urine) should be obtained before chemotherapy is begun. In severe infections, exudate can often be inoculated on a blood agar plate and antibiotic sensitivity discs positioned so that rapid, presumptive sensitivity information can be obtained after incubation overnight or for several hours. This crude procedure does not replace the official pure culture studies of all microorganisms isolated from the specimen.

Hyperbaric Therapy

Brummelkamp and associates in Amsterdam introduced the hyperbaric oxygen chamber for operative procedures. In 1963 they reported the first use of hyperbaric oxygen for gas-producing infections. Both the patient and medical personnel were placed in a room-sized chamber in which the air pressure was raised to three times that of the normal atmosphere (i.e., 2,280 mm Hg, or 3 atm absolute). For seven periods of $1\frac{1}{2}$ hours during 3 days, the patient inhaled 100% oxygen from a face mask. This increased the normal oxygen tension in plasma, lymph, and tissue fluids about fifteen to twenty times. Dramatic clinical improvement was described in most patients within the first day. Roding and colleagues advise that "operations be limited to opening the original wound and incising abscesses. Any further excision and removal of necrotic tissue can be done much later after clinical resolution. The advantage of postponement is that the operation can be performed in a dramatically improved patient who is no longer toxic." Large pressure chambers are available at only a few medical centers in the world and at special military and marine industrial facilities. In addition, much less expensive single-patient chambers are available and are also used to treat patients. Therapy with hyperbaric oxygen, antibiotics, and surgical debridement has been effective for clostridial myonecrosis. Hyperbaric oxygenation appears to reduce toxemia and diminish the amount of tissue requiring excision. However, gas-producing infection due to anaerobic streptococci, *Escherichia coli,* and *Klebsiella* species showed no improvement after exposure to high-pressure oxygen. The use of hyperbaric oxygen is advocated as an adjunct to the surgical treatment of clostridial infections. In cases of clostridial myonecrosis, all conventional means of treatment should be employed, including early surgical debridement and administration of antibiotics. The reliability of immediate surgical treatment and adjunctive antibiotic therapy remains unquestioned.

SOME COMMON SURGICAL INFECTIONS

Cellulitis is a nonsuppurative inflammation of the subcutaneous tissues extending along connective tissue planes and across intercellular spaces. There is widespread swelling, redness, and pain without definite localization. Central necrosis and suppuration may occur at a later stage. In severe infections, blebs and bullae form on the skin. Although a variety of aerobic and anaerobic bacteria produce cellulitis, the hemolytic streptococci are the classic etiologic agents. Treatment consists of antibiotic therapy and rest. Failure of the inflammatory swelling to subside after 48 to 72 hours of antibiotic therapy suggests that an abscess has developed, and that incision and drainage are needed.

Lymphangitis is an inflammation of lymphatic pathways which is usually visible as erythematous streaking of the skin. This is especially true in infections by hemolytic streptococci. Lymphangitis and the associated inflammatory swelling of lymph nodes (*lymphadenitis*) are a normal defense reaction against bacterial invasion and are frequently seen in the forearm of a patient with an infection of the hand or fingers. Most cases will respond to antibiotic therapy and rest.

Erysipelas is an acute spreading cellulitis and lymphangitis, usually caused by hemolytic streptococci which gain entrance through a break in the skin. There is a severe systemic as well as local reaction with abrupt onset, chills, fever, and prostration. The skin is red, swollen, and tender, and there is a distinct line of demarcation at the advancing margin of the infection. Erysipelas may develop on any cutaneous surface but commonly involves the face in a "butterfly lesion" over the nose and cheeks. Recurrent erysipelas in an extremity may lead to chronic lymphedema. Antibiotic therapy will usually halt the progress of the invasive infection, but the erythema disappears more slowly since it is a toxigenic consequence of bacterial invasion.

Infection in soft tissues is of paramount concern to the surgeon, and a variety of superficial infections will be discussed. An *abscess* is a localized collection of pus surrounded by an area of inflamed tissue in which hyperemia and infiltration of leukocytes is marked. A *furuncle*, or boil, is an abscess in a sweat gland or hair follicle. The inflammatory reaction is intense, leading to tissue necrosis and the formation of a central core. This is surrounded by a peripheral zone of cellulitis. An abscess beneath the corium of the skin is a *subepithelial abscess*. *Impetigo* is an acute contagious skin disease characterized by the formation of a series of intraepithelial abscesses. Gangrenous impetigo may occur as a complication in severe chronic debilitating diseases (e.g., chronic ulcerative colitis), and hemolytic streptococci and staphylococci can be cultured from the exudate. The lesions appear as multiple small pustules which extend and coalesce to form large areas of cutaneous gangrene and ulceration. Although management is similar to that of postoperative gangrene, favorable response is proportional to success in overcoming the primary disease.

A *carbuncle* is a multilocular suppurative extension of a furuncle into the subcutaneous tissues. The nape of the neck, dorsum of trunk, hands and digits, and hirsute portions of the chest and abdomen are apt to be involved. Individual compartments in a carbuncle are maintained through persistence of fascial attachments to the skin. As these numerous component locules rupture separately, individual fistulas appear. Most abscesses are caused by pyogenic cocci, usually *Staphylococcus aureus.* However, gram-negative bacilli and streptococci may be found coincidentally. Carbuncles may be more extensive than they appear and should be excised widely to prevent spread and to effect a cure. The wound contracts to a small scar, and a skin graft is not usually required.

The course of a furuncle is often self-limited and may require no specific therapy. However, furuncles can be serious and may become carbuncles. Large furuncles and abscesses should be incised and drained and the patient treated with antibiotics. Abscesses in the "dangerous" nasolabial area of the face bounded by the bridge of the nose and the angles of the mouth may become complicated by septic phlebitis with intracranial extension along the nasal veins to the cavernous sinus. The incidence of septic cavernous sinus thrombosis has declined since the introduction of antibiotics, and this lethal complication is now rare but unfortunately still occurs.

Bacteremia is defined as bacteria in the circulating blood with no indication of toxemia or other clinical manifestations. Bacteremia is usually transient and may last only a few moments, as the reticuloendothelial system localizes and destroys these organisms under favorable conditions. The normal individual probably experiences bacteremia, unknowingly, many times each year. This state follows dental procedures, major traumatic wounds, etc., and may be the means by which apparently isolated infections arise in internal organs, e.g., osteomyelitis, pyelonephritis (descending type), or subacute bacterial endocarditis.

Septicemia is a diffuse infection in which infectious bacteria and their toxins are present in the bloodstream. Septicemia may arise directly from the introduction of infecting organisms into the circulation but, as a rule, is secondary to a focus of infection within the body. The major routes by which bacteria reach the blood are (1) by direct extension and entrance into an open vessel, (2) by release of infected emboli following thrombosis of a blood vessel in an area of inflammation, (3) by discharge of infected lymph into the bloodstream following lymphangitis. Many specific diseases, e.g., typhoid fever and brucellosis, include a septicemic phase. In the absence of systemic disease, beta-hemolytic streptococci (*Streptococcus pyogenes*) are most frequently responsible. Septicemia caused by alpha-hemolytic streptococci (*Streptococcus viridans*) is usually a consequence of subacute bacterial endocarditis. The majority of bacteria that produce suppurative lesions may give rise to secondary septicemia. *Pyemia* is septicemia in which pyogenic microorganisms, most notably *Staphylococcus aureus,* and their toxins are carried in the bloodstream and sequentially initiate multiple focal abscesses in many parts of the body. Before the advent of chemotherapy, staphylococcic pyemia was almost always fatal; the mortality is still high. In *toxemia,* toxins are circulating in the blood, though the microorganism producing the toxin need not be. Toxemia is usually associated with infection by toxin-producing bacteria (e.g., the clostridia of gas gangrene and the diphtheria bacillus), but this is not always so. For example, botulinum toxin and staphylococcal enterotoxin may be ingested directly to cause a profound toxemia without true infection.

PRINCIPLES OF ANTIBIOTIC THERAPY

Basic Considerations

Chemotherapeutic agents act primarily upon the parasite and not upon the host. They include antibiotics and metabolic antagonists such as the sulfonamides. An antibiotic is a chemical compound derived from, or produced by, living organisms and capable, at low concentrations, of inhibiting the life processes of microorganisms. *Bacteriostatic* agents prevent the growth of bacteria but do not destroy them. The defense mechanisms of the body then eliminate the bacteria which are unable to multiply. If the defenses are insufficient or if the bacteriostatic drug is withdrawn prematurely, then the bacterial population will resurge, and the patient will suffer a relapse. *Bactericidal* agents actively kill bacteria and must be employed in patients whose defense mechanisms are impaired or altered by disease or immunosuppressive therapy. The distinction between bactericidal and bacteriostatic effects is sometimes relative to duration of therapy and dosage. Some drugs are bacteriostatic at low concentrations and bactericidal at high concentrations. With most bactericidal drugs, the rate of killing increases with concentration. Antibiotic agents exert their effects in a variety of ways (Table 5-3). They may inhibit the synthesis of the bacterial

Table 5-3. ANTIBIOTICS: MODES OF ACTION

Cellular site of inhibition	Bactericidal	Bacteriostatic
Cell wall synthesis . . .	Penicillins Cephalosporins Vancomycin Bacitracin	
Barrier function of cell membrane. . . .	Polymyxin B Colistin Amphotericin B	Nystatin
Protein synthesis in ribosome	Streptomycin Kanamycin Neomycin Gentamicin	Tetracyclines Chloramphenicol Erythromycin Lincomycin Clindamycin
DNA replication in chromosome	Griseofulvin	

cell wall and consequently interfere with the cell's osmotic defenses, or they may affect the barrier function of the cell membrane and cause loss of vital metabolites. An entirely different mode of action impairs the translation of genetic information and affects protein synthesis. Bacteriostatic drugs affect early stages of protein synthesis in the ribosome and result in an insufficiency, preventing growth and proliferation of bacteria without actually destroying them. However, bactericidal drugs cause the ribosome to miscode and consequently induce the manufacture of defective proteins or enzymes which poison the cell. Replication of deoxyribonucleic acid (DNA) in the chromosome at the level of the assembly of purine nucleotides may be affected by some antibiotics. Although their precise locus of action is not known, these drugs impede the replication of genetic information.

The addition of antibiotics to the armamentarium of the physician has revolutionized the practice of medicine, but has been a double-edged sword. It is pertinent to point out that the surgeon employs antibiotic drugs as adjunctive agents in the treatment of surgical infections, whereas the internist usually employs antibiotics as the primary treatment for medical infections. For the surgeon the aims of antibiotic therapy are much the same as those of surgical therapy, i.e., to control or eradicate bacterial infections acquired before or during hospitalization and to prevent infection from developing postoperatively. To obtain these goals, antibiotic agents are administered (1) systemically by either parenteral or oral routes, (2) preoperatively for preparation of the large intestine (intestinal antisepsis), or (3) locally by (*a*) topical irrigation, (*b*) topical application, (*c*) intraperitoneal, intrapleural, or intrathecal instillation or irrigation, and (*d*) intraluminal instillation into the large intestine. Antibacterial drugs may be administered preoperatively, peroperatively, and postoperatively to prevent infection (prophylaxis) or to treat already established infection.

The fundamental principles governing the use of antibiotics are (1) administration of an agent active against the infecting microorganism, (2) adequate contact between the drug and the infecting microbe, (3) absence of (or minimal) toxic side effects or complications, and (4) utilization of host defenses to augment antibacterial effects of the antibiotic. The specificity of the antibiotic for the infecting microorganism is based upon laboratory identification and antibiotic-sensitivity studies. Clinical judgment is called upon in serious, rapidly developing infections, such as gram-negative shock, to administer antibiotics known to be effective. However, cultures should be taken before antibiotic therapy is initiated, and the antibiotic changed, if necessary, when culture and antibiotic-sensitivity reports are available.

The antibiotic must come in contact with the infecting microorganism. In an acute, diffuse infection, blood flow into the area of infection will usually deliver adequate levels of systemic antibiotic. A spreading cellulitis with lymphangitis and lymphadenitis often responds within 24 hours to an appropriate antibiotic. However, since antibiotics cannot penetrate a thick-walled pyogenic abscess or an infected serous cavity, they should be used in conjunction with drainage of the abscess, debridement of necrotic tissue, and removal of any foreign bodies. These principles apply to every organ of the body. A spreading infection of the meninges responds to chemotherapy, but a brain abscess must be drained; a staphylococcal septicemia is treated by chemotherapy, but a pulp abscess of the fingertip must be drained.

The surgeon must be aware of toxic complications of antibiotics and should be prepared to treat them. Toxic effects range from minor skin rashes, drug fever, and gastrointestinal disturbances to renal tubular necrosis, loss of vision and hearing, irreversible blood dyscrasias, and anaphylactic shock. In addition, alterations in the normal flora of the body may occur in patients receiving prolonged antibiotic therapy. In most cases these changes produce no ill result, but in some the alterations of flora result in the rapid overgrowth of virulent, antibiotic-resistant bacteria which may have been present originally in small numbers (colonization). If the patient's general resistance to infection is depressed, a new infection may follow the antibiotic-induced alteration of flora (superinfection). The term *colonization* indicates an antibiotic-induced quantitative change in the resident microflora of the patient, a common consequence of antimicrobial therapy. There is no clinical evidence of secondary infection, and discontinuance of the antibiotic usually allows the normal flora to become reestablished. However, there is the risk that colonization will lead to superinfection, a clinical event which may be of great danger to the patient. The term *superinfection* usually refers to a new microbial disease induced by antibiotic therapy. Superinfection is most frequent with broad-spectrum antibiotics. Inhibition of the normal flora allows proliferation of species and strains of bacteria not inhibited by the antibiotic. Superinfection is often due to gram-negative bacilli and fungi which are more difficult to eradicate than are gram-positive streptococci and pneumococci. Superinfection may be fatal, usually occurs in elderly patients, and often follows therapy with aminoglycoside antibiotics (e.g., gentamicin and kanamycin) and other broad-spectrum drugs (either alone or in combination with penicillin). Clinical evidence of secondary infection (i.e., a rise in temperature, increased peripheral white blood cell count, and physical signs of a disease not present at the beginning of antibiotic therapy) indicates that colonization has progressed to superinfection. Serial superinfections with different antibiotic-resistant microbial species may occur in the same patient.

Secondary or opportunistic infections may also occur in patients with noninfectious diseases. For example, mycotic infections may develop in patients with lymphoma or leukemia. Deficiencies in host resistance as a result of disease (e.g., diabetes mellitus, hematopoietic disorders, renal failure, liver disease) or as a consequence of therapy with radiation, antimetabolites, or corticosteroids confer the potential for pathogenicity on many ordinary nonpathogenic microorganisms. Indwelling venous or urinary catheters also contribute to lowered host resistance. The term *suprainfection* designates a secondary infection unrelated to antibiotic therapy, and the term *antibiotic-induced suprainfection* describes secondary infections arising during treatment with antimicrobial agents.

Chemoprophylaxis

Prophylactic antibiotics are administered to an uninfected patient who is in jeopardy of acquiring a bacterial infection. There is controversy regarding prophylactic antibiotic therapy because prophylaxis has not been as valuable as therapeutic use. In surgical patients, prophylactic antibiotics are administered to treat contaminated wounds before infection occurs. However, the administration of antibiotic drugs cannot be substituted for sound surgical judgment and good surgical technique. Prophylactic antibiotic therapy has no place in clean operative procedures or in those carrying a minimal risk of sepsis, but it should be considered for traumatic injuries and severe burns and for operations in infected tissues or those associated with heavy contamination (e.g., operations involving the large intestine). An equally beneficial role for chemoprophylaxis is prior to operations on patients especially prone to infection because of malnutrition, impoverished blood supply, or preexisting infection remote from the operative site. The patient undergoing immunosuppressive therapy and/or requiring insertion of a permanent prosthetic device is particularly prone to infection.

Surgical wounds have been designated as "clean," "contaminated," or "dirty" depending upon the presence or absence of prior infection and contact with the interior of the respiratory, urinary, or gastrointestinal tracts. Traumatic wounds are generally grossly contaminated, whereas elective clean surgical procedures may be slightly contaminated during the operative procedure. Infection does not necessarily follow contamination, since host factors as well as microbial factors are involved. However, the greater the contamination, the greater the possibility of consequent infection. Accordingly, in surgery of traumatic wounds or in elective "contaminated" or "dirty" surgery, prophylaxis should be started before the operation so that adequate levels of antibiotic may be obtained in tissue and body fluids during the operative procedure. Bernard and Cole (1964) investigated the use of antibiotics administered intramuscularly 1 to 2 hours prior to surgery, intravenously during the operation, and postoperatively when the patient was in the recovery room. They found a reduced incidence of postoperative infection (5 percent) with prophylactic treatment compared with administration of a placebo (25 percent). However, a prophylactic antibiotic regimen may not be successful if the drug is not effective against all potential pathogens or if the agent does not come in contact with susceptible pathogens at the site of infection. The antibiotic should be administered parenterally and in sufficient dosage to achieve high circulating blood levels. For treatment of patients with severe trauma, antibiotic therapy should be started prior to operation, as manipulation of wounds causes transient bacteremia.

Intestinal Antisepsis

The protocol for preoperative preparation of the large intestine includes the specific prophylactic use of antibiotics. Bacterial infection following elective colonic surgery results from unavoidable seeding of the wound with contents of the colon. This is manifested by intraabdominal abscesses and anastomotic disruption with resultant peritonitis and fistula formation. The ideal antibiotic agent for preoperative preparation of the colon has rapid bactericidal activity against pathogens in the gastrointestinal tract, minimal absorption, and the absence of undesirable or toxic side effects. The protocol we employ involves a 3-day period of hospitalization during which the patient is placed on a low-residue diet (some surgeons prefer a clear diet), given a cathartic and daily enemas, and administered a suitable chemotherapeutic agent for 72 hours. Although mechanical cleansing alone diminishes the volume of feces and, consequently, the total number of fecal bacteria, the remaining feces contain the usual large numbers of bacteria (on the order of 10^{11} bacteria per gram), and the potential for postoperative infections remains a major hazard. Therefore, although there is no uniform agreement, we feel that antibiotic therapy along with mechanical cleansing is essential for effective preoperative preparation of the large intestine. The antibiotics most frequently employed are kanamycin (1 Gm every hour for 4 hours, and then every 6 hours for a total of 72 hours) and Sulfathalidine-neomycin in combination (every hour for 4 hours, and then every 4 hours for a total of 72 hours). Nichols et al. employ a combination of neomycin and erythromycin base in a three-day cleansing protocol which differs in administering the antibiotic on the third day only. One gram of each is given at 1:00, 2:00, and 11:00 P.M.; the operation is scheduled for 8:00 A.M. Intestinal antisepsis has been shown to reduce the incidence of postoperative complications related to bacteria but does not protect against errors of surgical skill or judgment.

Intraperitoneal Antibiotic Therapy

The most frequent indications for the intraperitoneal instillation of antibiotics are perforated and gangrenous appendicitis, perforated peptic ulcer, gangrenous intestinal obstruction, traumatic perforation of the gastrointestinal tract at any level, intraabdominal abscess, and excessive spillage associated with elective colonic, gastric, or small bowel surgery. Intraperitoneally administered antibiotics may be useful in pelvic inflammatory disease, acute pancreatitis, major intraabdominal vascular procedures, closure of evisceration, and repair of large abdominal incisional hernias. To be effective for routine intraperitoneal instillation, the antibiotic must provide adequate control of endogenous enteric bacteria that may be expected in the peritoneal cavity, with minimal accompanying pain and local or systemic reaction. Since intraperitoneal antibiotics are usually administered to anesthetized patients, the possible synergistic activity of the antibiotic and the anesthetic agent must be considered. This danger may be avoided if the catheter is placed in the peritoneal cavity after the operation, but before the incision is completely closed, and antibiotic instilled after the patient has recovered from anesthesia. Neomycin is safe for intraperitoneal administration only when the dosage is carefully controlled. Clinical success and safety have been achieved with kanamycin and also with cephalothin. Multiple postoperative instillations of kanamycin in patients with peritonitis reduce the incidence of wound infections and are more effective than a single instillation of the drug. The intraluminal administration of kanamycin into the colon to prevent perforation, slough, and leakage at the anastomosis has been recommended to support a colon anastomosis postoperatively.

ANTIMICROBIAL AGENTS

Antibiotics and chemotherapeutic agents which are currently useful in surgical practice are described briefly in this section. It is important to use an antibiotic agent for a sensitive microorganism and not to treat a particular disease. Precise antimicrobial therapy is based upon the laboratory culture and sensitivity report. Table 5-4 is a guide to the activities of antibiotics against microorganisms commonly involved in surgical infections. Table 5-5 summarizes the routes of administration and doses commonly employed. The selection of antibiotic and dosage for a specific infection depend upon clinical judgment, bacterial sensitivity tests, and awareness of the toxicity of the drug.

Table 5-4. ANTIBIOTICS USEFUL AGAINST MICROORGANISMS IN SURGICAL INFECTIONS

Microorganism	First choice	Alternate agents
Gram-positive cocci:		
Staphylococcus aureus		
Penicillinase-producing	Methicillin	Oxacillin, cloxacillin, cephalothin
Non-penicillinase-producing	Penicillin G	Erythromycin, cephalothin, kanamycin
Streptococcus pyogenes	Penicillin G	Erythromycin, cephalothin
Streptococcus pneumoniae	Penicillin G	Erythromycin, cephalothin
Streptococcus viridans	Penicillin G	Erythromycin, cephalothin
Streptococcus fecalis	Penicillin G + kanamycin	Ampicillin, kanamycin
Peptostreptococcus spp.	Penicillin G	Tetracycline
Gram-negative cocci:		
Neisseria gonorrhoeae	Penicillin G	Erythromycin, cephaloridine, kanamycin
Gram-positive rods:		
Clostridium spp.	Penicillin G	Tetracycline, erythromycin
Gram-negative rods:		
Acinetobacter calcoaceticus	Kanamycin	Gentamicin
Bacteroides fragilis	Clindamycin	Chloramphenicol, erythromycin
Bacteroides spp.	Penicillin G	Clindamycin, chloramphenicol, tetracycline
Escherichia coli	Kanamycin	Ampicillin, gentamicin, cephalothin
Fusobacterium spp.	Penicillin G	Clindamycin, chloramphenicol, tetracycline
Hemophilus influenzae	Ampicillin	Cephalothin, chloramphenicol
Klebsiella-Enterobacter-Serratia group	Gentamicin	Kanamycin, cephalothin, tetracycline
Proteus mirabilis	Ampicillin	Gentamicin, carbenicillin, cephalothin
Proteus spp. (indol-positive)	Kanamycin	Gentamicin, carbenicillin
Providencia spp.	Carbenicillin	Gentamicin, kanamycin
Pseudomonas aeruginosa	Gentamicin (± carbenicillin)	Carbenicillin, amikacin, tobramycin
Salmonella spp.	Ampicillin	Chloramphenicol, tetracycline
Actinomycetes:		
Actinomyces israelii	Penicillin G (± tetracycline)	Tetracycline, clindamycin, ampicillin
Nocardia spp.	Sulfadiazine (+ streptomycin)	Ampicillin
Fungi:		
Blastomyces dermatitidis	Amphotericin B	2-Hydroxystilbamidine
Candida albicans and other yeasts	Amphotericin B	5-Fluorocytosine, nystatin (oral or topical)
Coccidioides immitis	Amphotericin B	—
Cryptococcus neoformans	Amphotericin B	5-Fluorocytosine
Histoplasma capsulatum	Amphotericin B	—
Mucor spp; *Rhizopus* spp; *Aspergillus* spp.	Amphotericin B	—
Paracoccidioides brasiliensis	Amphotericin B	—
Sporotrichum schenckii	Potassium iodide	Amphotericin B

Table 5-5. ROUTES OF ADMINISTRATION AND DAILY DOSAGE OF
ANTIBIOTICS COMMONLY USED IN ADULT SURGICAL PATIENTS

Drug (trade name)	Oral	Dose (grams per day)	
		Intramuscular	Intravenous
Aminoglycosides:			
Amikacin (Amikin)	. . . . .	1–1.5	1–1.5
Gentamicin (Garamycin)	. . . . .	0.18–0.24	0.18–0.24
Kanamycin (Kantrex)	4–7*	0.5–1	0.5–1
Streptomycin	. . . . .	1–2	Not recommended
Tobramycin (Nebcin)	. . . . .	0.21–0.35	0.21–0.35
Cephalosporins:			
Cephalexin (Keflex)	1–4	. . . . .	. . . . .
Cephalothin (Keflin)		2–4	4–12
Cephaloridine (Loridine)		1–2	1–2
Chloramphenicol (Chloromycetin)	. . . . .	Not recommended	2–4
Clindamycin (Cleocin)	. . . . .	1.2–2.4	1.2–2.4
Erythromycin (Erythrocin)	1–2	0.2–0.6	1–4
Penicillin:			
Ampicillin (Amcill, Omnipen, Penbritin, Polycillin, Principen)	1–2	2–8	2–8
Carbenicillin (Geopen)	. . . . .	8–12	20–40
Cloxacillin (Tegopen)	4–6	. . . . .	. . . . .
Dicloxacillin (Dynapen, Pathocil, Veracillin)	2–3	. . . . .	. . . . .
Methicillin (Celbenin, Staphcillin)	. . . . .	4–6	4–24
Nafcillin (Nafcil, Unipen)	2–6	2–6	4–24
Oxacillin (Bactocill, Prostaphlin)	2–6	2–6	4–24
Penicillin G, potassium or sodium	0.5–2 million units/day	2–12 million units/day	4–20 million units/day
Tetracyclines:			
Doxycycline (Vibramycin)	0.1–0.2	. . . . .	. . . . .
Oxytetracycline (Terramycin)	1–2	0.2–0.8	1–2
Tetracycline (Achromycin, Panmycin, Sumycin, Tetracyn, Tetrex)	1–2	0.2–0.8	1–2

*Intestinal antisepsis only.

The white blood cell count is important in evaluating the response to antibiotic treatment and the appearance of adverse reactions in patients with infections. Individual drugs will be considered in terms of mechanism of antimicrobial action, absorption, distribution, metabolic fate, excretion, toxicity, and indications for use.

Antibiotics Active against Gram-positive Microorganisms

Penicillin G (benzyl penicillin) is active against almost all gram-positive pathogens. If necessary, very large doses can be given to combat infections by bacterial species which may be moderately resistant. Penicillin is bactericidal for susceptible bacteria; it blocks the synthesis of bacterial cell walls. Penicillin G is well absorbed but is not suitable for oral administration, because it is destroyed by gastric acidity. Therefore, it is injected intramuscularly or intravenously and becomes distributed throughout the body within a few minutes following injection. Excretion is mainly by the renal tubules. Hypersensitivity to penicillin is an important problem; it is usually manifested as urticaria, but almost any type of allergic response may develop. Anaphylactic reactions may occur in the highly sensitized patient within minutes after an injection and will require subcutaneous epinephrine. Penicillin G is recom-

mended (provided hypersensitivity does not exist) for severe infections produced by beta-hemolytic streptococci, enterococci, pneumococci, gonococci, meningococci, clostridia, actinomycetes, and treponemata.

Penicillin V (phenoxymethyl penicillin) is a natural penicillin obtained when phenoxyacetic acid is the precursor during fermentation. It is acid-stable and may be administered orally. Penicillin V is more active than penicillin G against resistant staphylococci because it is more slowly destroyed by penicillinase; it is slightly less active against streptococci. Penicillin V is not indicated for infections involving the respiratory tract or the urinary tract.

The natural penicillins have been superseded by several semisynthetic penicillins prepared by adding side chains to the 6-aminopenicillanic acid nucleus. The semisynthetic penicillins combine one or more of the following advantages: (1) they are acid-resistant and suitable for oral use; (2) they exert prolonged action in the body; (3) they are resistant to penicillinase produced by *Staphylococcus aureus* and some gram-negative bacilli; and (4) they are active against gram-negative bacteria.

Methicillin (Staphcillin) is sensitive to acid but resistant to staphylococcal penicillinase. It must be administered parenterally, and it is rapidly excreted by the renal tubules. Methicillin is inactivated by penicillinase 100 times more slowly than is penicillin G but has only one-tenth the potency of penicillin G. Methicillin is also the preferred parenteral semisynthetic penicillin against streptococci, pneumococci, and gram-negative bacteria.

Oxacillin, cloxacillin, and *dicloxacillin* are semisynthetic isoxazolyl penicillins combining resistance to penicillinase with resistance to acid. They can be administered orally and are effective against streptococcal infections complicated by the presence of penicillinase-producing staphylococci. *Nafcillin* is also resistant to penicillinase and to acid. It may be used either orally or parenterally, but relatively low blood levels are obtained due to inactivation in the liver.

These penicillinase-resistant penicillins are effective, specific agents for treatment of serious staphylococcal infections, such as pneumonia, septicemia, wound infection, and infections occurring as a consequence of malignant diseases or cardiac, hepatic, or renal disease. Although methicillin has the lowest activity against staphylococci, 60 percent of the dose is free in the blood. On the other hand, the acid-resistant penicillins have higher antibacterial activity, but only 5 percent is free. Accordingly, adequate doses of any one of these penicillins will achieve similar effects, and initial treatment of a severe staphylococcal infection should always be with one of these penicillins (unless the staphylococcus has been shown to be sensitive to penicillin G). Concomitant administration of probenecid, which partially blocks tubular excretion of penicillins, may be used to double blood levels.

Cephalothin is one of a group of exceedingly useful antibiotics known as the cephalosporins, which are structually similar to the penicillins and may be used as alternative agents for therapy in patients allergic to penicillin. However, they are often given in excessively high doses for prolonged periods. Their use is unwarranted in infections which can be readily treated with less expensive agents (e.g., penicillin for pneumococcal pneumonia) and in surgical prophylaxis. Cephalothin is effective against staphylococci, streptococci (except enterococci), and pneumococci. Most strains of *Escherichia coli, Proteus mirabilis,* and *Klebsiella* species are susceptible. *Enterobacter aerogenes, Pseudomonas aeruginosa, Hemophilus influenzae,* and group D streptococci (enterococci) are resistant. Cephalosporin antibiotics, like the penicillins, are bactericidal and inhibit the synthesis of bacterial cell walls. Cephalothin must be administered parenterally, as it is not absorbed orally. Excretion is by the renal tubules. Intramuscular injections may be painful, and frequent injections are required if adequate levels of antibiotic are to be maintained. Phlebitis occurs with intravenous use; rashes are sometimes produced. Cephalothin may be administered to patients who are allergic to penicillin without danger of cross reaction, but sensitization to cephalothin itself may occur. The antibiotic is active against penicillin-resistant staphylococci. However, antibiotic-induced suprainfection with gram-negative bacilli or fungi can occur if indiscriminately large doses are used for 1 to 3 weeks. Cephalothin has a broader spectrum than ampicillin and is useful in treating urinary tract infections caused by sensitive enterobacteria.

Cephaloridine is a derivative similar to cephalothin both in its properties and indications for use. It is more stable in the body and is cleared more slowly. Renal toxicity has been encountered following large doses. Although it is not effective orally, there is little or no pain when it is injected intramuscularly. Cephaloridine is not a substitute for cephalothin, since staphylococci are not uniformly susceptible. Antibiotic-induced suprainfections have occurred.

Cephalexin is a semisynthetic cephalosporin which is almost completely absorbed after oral administration. Food delays absorption. Cephalexin is excreted in urine by glomerular filtration and tubular secretion. High urinary concentrations are obtained. Some cephalexin is excreted in the bile of patients with normal gallbladders. Diarrhea, vomiting, cramps, and hypersensitivity reactions have been observed. Cephalexin has been used for urinary tract infections due to *Escherichia coli, Proteus mirabilis,* and *Klebsiella* species. It appears to be about as effective as ampicillin for these infections. However, use of any cephalosporin as the sole drug in treating gram-negative sepsis without in vitro evidence of susceptibility is not good practice.

Vancomycin is active against gram-positive organisms only, and it is of clinical importance against staphylococci and streptococci. Microorganisms sensitive to vancomycin do not acquire resistance. The antibiotic is bactericidal; it inhibits the incorporation of amino acids into the bacterial cell wall and suppresses the growth of protoplasts. Vancomycin is not absorbed from the alimentary tract and is administered intravenously; intramuscular injections cause pain and necrosis. The antibiotic becomes widely distributed, but little is found in bile or spinal fluid. Excretion is by glomerular filtration, but this is delayed in patients with impaired renal function. Because of serious ototoxicity and nephrotoxicity, vancomycin should not be used in patients with renal insufficiency or in patients who have significant hearing loss. Antibiotic-induced suprainfections with fungi and gram-negative bacteria may appear during treatment. Thrombophlebitis, fever, and rashes occur. Vancomycin is now regarded as a reserve drug which may be valuable for the treatment of serious staphylococcal or streptococcal disease in patients allergic or nonresponsive to other antibiotics (penicillin G, methicillin, cephalothin).

Erythromycin is active against pneumococci, beta-hemolytic streptococci, enterococci, many staphylococci, gonococci (although less effective as an alternative agent than tetracycline), and clostridia. Erythromycin is bacteriostatic but may be bactericidal in high concentrations, inhibiting bacterial protein synthesis. Erythromycin may be administered orally or intravenously. Most strains of *Bacteroides* can be inhibited by the high levels of erythromycin attained in serum after parenteral injection. The antibiotic is uniformly distributed throughout the body and is excreted in the urine and bile. However, the major portion of the drug is broken down in the body. Erythromycin base is generally well tolerated but may cause some gastrointestinal disturbance (nausea, vomiting, diarrhea, flatulence). Erythromycin estolate (the propionyl ester) can produce hepatic disease during prolonged administration. For this reason the plain erythromycin base is recommended. Erythromycin may be used as an alternative to penicillin for hemolytic streptococcal, staphylococcal, or pneumococcal infections in patients allergic to penicillin and for elimination of *Corynebacterium diphtheriae* from the pharynx of carriers. Bacterial resistance to erythromycin is common during long-term treatment.

Lincomycin resembles erythromycin in its antibacterial activity against staphylococci, hemolytic streptococci, and pneumococci. Bacteroides and anaerobic cocci are also sensitive. Enterobacteria and enterococci are resistant. Lincomycin is bacteriostatic; it inhibits protein synthesis. The antibiotic is absorbed from the gastrointestinal tract, but food delays absorption. The drug may also be administered intramuscularly and intravenously; it becomes widely distributed, and significant levels occur in tissues and fluids. Therapeutic levels of lincomycin are found in bone. Excretion is primarily biliary; urine levels are low. Diarrhea and pseudomembranous colitis have been reported as adverse reactions to this antibiotic. Lincomycin is recommended for the treatment of both acute and chronic osteomyelitis. Although the antibiotic is effective against severe staphylococcal and streptococcal infections, these diseases are readily treated with semisynthetic penicillins. Lincomycin resistance is easily induced, and the antibiotic has cross resistance with erythromycin.

Clindamycin is a synthetically modified lincomycin (7-chloro-7-deoxylincomycin-HCl hydrate) which is more thoroughly absorbed and produces higher blood levels. Diarrhea and pseudomembranous colitis have been reported as adverse reactions to this antibiotic. Clindamycin is also more active against staphylococci and pneumococci and equally active against other species susceptible to lincomycin. The lincosamines (*lincomycin* and *clindamycin*) are, however, no more effective than the penicillins or erythromycin for treatment of infections caused by gram-positive aerobes or *Clostridium* species. They are second-line agents for treatment of staphylococcal infections (except chronic osteomyelitis), since they appear to be as effective as the penicillinase-resistant penicillins and cephalosporins. In staphylococcal infections their use should be limited primarily to patients allergic to the preferred drugs. Use of vancomycin should also be considered in serious staphylococcal infections. The lincosamines can sometimes produce an illness with features indistinguishable from idiopathic ulcerative colitis. However, lincomycin and clindamycin are especially effective in the treatment of abdominal and pelvic infections due to *Bacteroides fragilis*.

Bacitracin is a polypeptide antibiotic active against gram-positive bacteria and pathogenic *Neisseria* species, but inactive against common gram-negative bacilli. It is bactericidal, and inhibits bacterial cell wall synthesis by binding to the cell membrane. Therefore, unlike penicillin, bacitracin is active against protoplasts. The antibiotic is not absorbed orally or by the skin. After intramuscular injection, which causes painful infiltrates at the site of injection, much of the antibiotic is bound by tissues so that systemic absorption is limited. Bacitracin does not cross the blood-brain barrier. It is excreted by the kidneys, and glomerular and tublar damage may occur. Bacitracin has no place in the systemic treatment of clinical infections, but it is useful for irrigating wounds, infected joints, or abscess cavities. It is used topically with neomycin and polymyxin in treating superficial infections of the skin, infected wounds, and suppurative conjunctivitis.

Antibiotics Active against Some Gram-positive or Some Gram-negative Microorganisms or Both

Ampicillin is a semisynthetic penicillin which is slightly less active than benzyl penicillin against most gram-positive bacteria, is slightly more active against enterococci, and is destroyed by penicillinase. It is not indicated for staphylococcal infections. Ampicillin is recommended for the treatment of gram-negative infections due to *Escherichia coli, Proteus mirabilis,* and *Salmonella* and *Shigella* species. It is bactericidal and well absorbed when administered orally. Excretion is mainly renal, although some biliary excretion occurs. The toxicity of ampicillin is similar to that of penicillin G, but macular rashes are more frequent.

Carbenicillin is a semisynthetic, bactericidal penicillin; it may be used parenterally or orally. It is active against *Pseudomonas aeruginosa,* all species of *Proteus,* and some other enterobacteria, but it is inferior to benzyl penicillin against gram-positive bacteria. Synergism with gentamicin has been demonstrated, and combination therapy has been recommended because *Pseudomonas aeruginosa* may become resistant during treatment with carbenicillin alone. Carbenicillin is one of the few drugs effective for the treatment of systemic *Pseudomonas* infections. Very large doses for prolonged periods are required. Probenecid elevates serum levels twofold to fourfold and is a useful adjunct to therapy.

Polymyxin B and *colistin* (polymyxin E) are basic polypeptide antibiotics having similar structure and antibacterial activity. Most species of gram-negative bacilli are sensitive to polymyxin. The exceptions are *Proteus* species, and *Neisseria* species. All species of gram-positive bacteria and fungi are resistant. Both these antibiotics are bactericidal and disrupt the cell membranes of susceptible bacteria. They are not absorbed from the alimentary tract but are well absorbed following intramuscular injection. The polymyxins are nephrotoxic in the presence of renal disease and may be associated with respiratory arrest. Polymyxin B was formerly recommended for pseudomonal meningitis and pseudomonal endocarditis and was also useful in treating infection by most strains of *Escherichia coli* and *Klebsiella-Enterobacter.* Colistin was formerly recommended for treatment of systemic pseudomonal infections and for the same infections as those responsive to polymyxin. The introduction of broad-spectrum penicillins, cephalosporins, and aminoglycosides has, however, lessened the importance of polymyxins. In particular, the availability of gentamicin and carbenicillin, either separately or in combination, for the treatment of pseudomonal infections has practically eliminated the need for polymyxins in clinical medicine.

Chloramphenicol is a broad-spectrum antibiotic; it is bacteriostatic and inhibits protein synthesis by interfering with messenger ribonucleic acid (mRNA). It is well absorbed orally and parenterally. Excretion is mainly renal;

about 90 percent can be detected in urine as an inactive conjugate with glucuronic acid; only about 10 percent appears as active antibiotic. Two different lethal toxic effects are known: First, a rare total aplasia of the bone marrow with aplastic anemia may occur during treatment or as long as 4 months afterward. Second, because of deficiency in detoxifying enzymes, premature infants may accumulate sufficient free chloramphenicol to cause an acute and usually fatal circulatory collapse (gray syndrome). Minor toxic effects include soreness of the mouth from overgrowth of *Candida albicans* resulting from depression of normal flora due to antibiotic in the saliva, and optic neuritis in children with cystic fibrosis of the pancreas receiving treatment with chloramphenicol for pulmonary infection. Chloramphenicol should not be used for trivial infections or as a prophylactic agent to prevent bacterial infection. It is effective for typhoid fever and other severe *Salmonella* infections, but since most *Salmonella* infections will respond to ampicillin, chloramphenicol should be used only if the patient does not respond to ampicillin or is allergic to it. Chloramphenicol is recommended for patients who cannot tolerate tetracyclines and for those who have rickettsial disease, psittacosis, or lymphopathia venereum. It can be a life-saving drug in the treatment of patients with meningitis when penicillin cannot be administered. Chloramphenicol is the drug of choice in *Bacteroides* sepsis, in treatment of typhoid fever, and in severe infections such as *Hemophilus influenzae* in patients allergic to penicillin. Prolonged usage and repeated exposure should be avoided. Leukocyte counts with a differential should be taken daily, and therapy should be discontinued if leukopenia occurs.

The aminoglycosides include streptomycin, neomycin, paromomycin, kanamycin, gentamicin, tobramycin, and amikacin. They possess a wide range of bactericidal activity against gram-negative and gram-positive bacteria and mycobacteria. Bacteria acquire resistance to aminoglycosides slowly. There is little absorption from the alimentary tract and fairly slow renal excretion in unchanged form after intramuscular injection. This affords therapeutic levels for 6 to 8 hours. Aminoglycosides exhibit a high degree of mutual cross resistance, a strong dose-related tendency to damage the auditory branch of the eighth nerve, and some possibility of damage to the kidney.

Streptomycin is bactericidal and particularly active against *Mycobacterium tuberculosis,* gram-negative bacilli, and some strains of *Staphylococcus aureus.* However, the introduction of other aminoglycosides has relegated streptomycin to a minor role in the treatment of infections by gram-negative and gram-positive bacteria. Bactericidal effects usually occur during the phase of multiplication. There is damage to the cell membrane and also interference with protein synthesis by disorganizing the proper attachments of mRNA to ribosomes. Streptomycin usually is administered intramuscularly for systemic treatment. It is completely absorbed following parenteral injection, but it is absorbed poorly from the intestinal tract. Streptomycin is rapidly excreted in the urine. Streptomycin combined with isoniazid and *p*-aminosalicylic acid is indicated for the treatment of tuberculosis. Streptomycin with sulfadiazine is used to treat nocardiosis.

Neomycin is bactericidal; it is active against gram-negative enteric bacteria, some strains of staphylococci, and mycobacteria, but has limited usefulness because of its toxicity. Its major use is in ointments and solutions for topical application although skin sensitivity may occur. Following oral therapy, neomycin-resistant staphylococci are often found in the stool, and enteritis or even pseudomembranous enterocolitis may result. Neomycin inhibits absorption of oral penicillin V and has caused malabsorption of fat (with or without diarrhea). There is considerable risk of ototoxicity and nephrotoxicity when neomycin is given parenterally. Neomycin is used in treating patients with cirrhosis who have elevated levels of ammonia, and it is used in combination with other agents, such as sulfathalidine, bacitracin, erythromycin, or polymyxin B, for intestinal antisepsis prior to abdominal surgery. *Paromomycin* is similar to neomycin and kanamycin but generally administered orally. The main difference between paromomycin and other aminoglycosides is its direct activity against *Entamoeba histolytica.*

Kanamycin is bactericidal. It is rapidly absorbed after intramuscular injection and acts like streptomycin with regard to blood levels, distribution, and excretion. It is necessary to limit the dose in accordance with renal function; the length of treatment should be limited to 7 to 10 days. Kanamycin is the drug of choice in the management of septicemias due to gram-negative bacilli and is recognized as a second-line drug for treatment of tuberculosis in patients whose infecting mycobacteria are resistant to primary antituberculous drugs. Kanamycin is not absorbed from the gastrointestinal tract and can be used for preoperative intestinal antisepsis. Ototoxicity may occur; it is related to duration of therapy, blood level, and dosage greater than 15 mg/kg body weight/day. However, in patients with meningitis or other serious infections, temporary increases above this level may be necessary. Kanamycin continues to be valuable for the treatment of infections due to *Escherichia coli, Proteus* species, and some strains of the *Klebsiella-Enterobacter-Serratia* group.

Gentamicin is another bactericidal aminoglycoside. It is administered by intramuscular injection but is not absorbed orally. It is well-distributed in most highly vascular organs, and excretion is mainly renal. Gentamicin may exhibit nephrotoxicity and ototoxicity (affecting both vestibular and auditory branches of the eighth nerve), particularly in patients with any impairment of renal function. It should not be administered with streptomycin, kanamycin, colistin, polymyxin B, or vancomycin, as additional toxicity may result. Gentamicin is useful in treating bacteremia and severe soft tissue infections due to *Escherichia coli, Serratia marcescens,* and many *Proteus* species (but not *Proteus vulgaris*), and it is most effective in treatment of infections due to *Pseudomonas aeruginosa.* However, it is not recommended as an initial therapy of severe infections of unknown cause, because many gram-negative bacteria are resistant.

Tobramycin is virtually identical with gentamicin. *Amikacin* is a semisynthetic aminoglycoside derived from kanamycin and possesses attributes of both kanamycin and gentamicin. Parenteral aminoglycosides are among the most valuable agents available for the treatment of life-threatening infections by enteric gram-negative bacteria. Because of the emergence of resistant strains of *Pseudomonas, Proteus rettgeri, Providencia,* and *Serratia,* hospitals should select a single aminoglycoside antibiotic for primary use and hold the others in reserve for use against infections caused by resistant bacteria. The tetracyclines are a family of closely related antibiotics. Those now widely used are *tetracycline, oxytetracycline,* and *doxycycline.* There is no good evidence that tetracycline has any advantage over oxytetracycline in the treatment of disease or in the production of fewer side effects in the adult. Doxycycline possesses the advantage, because of its slower excretion, of requiring only one dose daily. Members of this group are broad-spectrum and active against those gram-positive species which are also sensitive to penicillin, against many gram-negative species which are not sensitive to penicillin, against *Treponema pallidum* and other treponemata, and against *Mycobacterium tuberculosis.* They also inhibit the growth of actinomycetes, rickettsiae, mycoplasma, and agents of the psittacosis–lymphogranuloma venerum–trachoma group of *Chlamydia.* The tetracyclines are bacteriostatic. They interfere with protein synthesis by inhibiting amino acid transfer from RNA to microsomal protein. Resistance may be due to decreased permeability to the antibiotic. A microorganism resistant to one tetracycline is equally resistant to the others. Tetracyclines are usually administered orally; they become distributed throughout the body and appear to have affinity for fast-growing tissues, such as liver, tumors, and new bone. They are slowly filtered by the renal glomeruli and are excreted in the urine unchanged. Some biliary excretion occurs. Tetracyclines are deposited in teeth during early stages of calcification, causing a yellow to brownish discoloration which is undesirable cosmetically. Therefore, tetracycline treatment should be avoided in early childhood except for imperative reasons or unless a short course will suffice. Liver damage has resulted from excessive doses. Replacement of suppressed normal flora by tetracycline-resistant microorganisms (antibiotic-induced suprainfection) causes gastrointestinal disturbance such as nausea, vomiting, diarrhea, and flatulence. Suprainfection with *Candida albicans* may produce soreness of the mouth and even thrush, which may spread to the pharynx and bronchi, or diarrhea and pruritus ani. Suprainfection with *Proteus* and *Pseudomonas* species resistant to tetracycline commonly produces diarrhea. Suprainfection with *Staphylococcus aureus* may produce a fatal staphylococcal enterocolitis. Tetracycline is effective against 50 percent of strains of *Bacteroides.* Tetracycline with penicillin is recommended for actinomycosis and, with sulfadiazine, for nocardiosis. If penicillin cannot be used, tetracycline is recommended for treatment of gonorrhea and syphilis.

Antifungal Antibiotics

Nystatin is effective in the treatment of candidosis. It is fungistatic and damages the fungal cell membrane by binding to sterol sites in it. The antibiotic is not absorbed from the gastrointestinal tract, skin, or mucosal surfaces. It is used to treat gastrointestinal candidosis, which may result as a complication of therapy with broad-spectrum antibiotics. Such antibiotic-induced suprainfection often disappears with discontinuance of the antibacterial therapy which provoked it. Nystatin is available in topical powders, creams, and ointments which may be useful in treating cutaneous and mucocutaneous candidosis. Nystatin tablets may be sucked for candida stomatitis; vaginal tablets are available for treatment of vaginal candidosis. Nystatin is harmless by local application. There have been rare cases of diarrhea, nausea, and vomiting after administration of large oral doses.

Griseofulvin has its greatest activity against dermatophytes and is useful in treating superficial dermatomycoses of skin, hair, or nails due to species of *Microsporum, Epidermophyton,* and *Trichophyton.* Griseofulvin is fungicidal, impairs synthesis of nucleic acids and protein, and breaks down intracellular membranes of dermatophytes but not of fungi causing systemic mycoses. The antibiotic is administered orally, and it is incorporated into liver, fat, keratin, and skeletal muscle. The antibiotic is well tolerated even during long courses of treatment, and toxic effects (skin reactions, gastric discomfort, and neurologic reactions) are uncommon and rarely severe. Griseofulvin has value in the systemic treatment of chronic fungal infection of the nails and hair. Cultures are needed to determine that skin lesions are not due to *Candida* or bacteria, as these are not improved by griseofulvin and may be exacerbated by the antibiotic.

Amphotericin B is the only antifungal antibiotic effective in the treatment of systemic mycotic infections. It binds to sterols, specifically ergosterol, and interferes with the permeability of the fungal cell wall. Amphotericin B is the drug of choice for treatment of systemic candidosis, mucormycosis, disseminated active histoplasmosis, cryptococcosis, coccidioidomycosis, and pulmonary sporotrichosis. Amphotericin is not appreciably absorbed from the gastrointestinal tract or the skin; it is administered intravenously or intrathecally, or instilled directly into the site of infection. Initial toxic effects commonly include fever, chills, nausea, vomiting, and headache. Toxic effects brought on by continued usage may include anemia, thrombophlebitis at the site of injection, hypokalemia, rise of blood urea and serum creatinine levels, and permanent damage to the kidney.

5-Fluorocytosine is a halogenated pyrimidine inhibiting nucleic acid synthesis in fungi; it is not metabolized by mammalian cells. This compound is effective in systemic cryptococcosis and candidosis and has been used after failure of therapy with amphotericin.

Sulfonamides

Introduced in 1935, the sulfonamides initiated the modern antibacterial chemotherapeutic revolution in medicine. Their use antedates that of the antibiotics by several years, since penicillin did not become available until 1941. The sulfonamides are valuable agents in the management of some infections, particularly urinary tract infections due to *Escherichia coli,* and can be employed for the prophylaxis of recurrences of rheumatic fever. Although one of these compounds, mafenide acetate (Sulfamylon), has an important use in the topical therapy of severe burn wounds, the value of the sulfonamides in the treatment of surgical infections is severely limited by their inactivation by pus. The sulfonamides are bacteriostatic and active against both gram-positive and gram-negative bacteria. The drugs are strongly antagonized by *p*-aminobenzoic acid (PABA), an essential intermediate in the synthesis of folic acid by bacterial cells, and act as competitive inhibitors. Bacteria sensitive to the sulfonamides are unable to utilize preformed folic acid in the body and must synthesize it themselves. Folic acid acts as a coenzyme in the transfer of fragments containing one carbon atom, which are involved in the synthesis of amino acids (such as methionine and serine), purine, and thymine. These compounds also inhibit the activity of sulfonamides, but unlike PABA they are noncompetitive inhibitors, and their effect is not reversed by increasing the concentration of drugs. Accordingly, pus, which is rich in amino acids and purines made available by the breakdown of cellular protein and nucleic acids, inactivates the sulfonamides.

Some of the sulfonamides of use in surgical practice are sulfadiazine, which is the preparation of choice in treating nocardiosis; phthalylsulfathiazole (Sulfathalidine), which is poorly absorbed from the gastrointestinal tract and is used in combination with neomycin for preoperative preparation of the large intestine; sulfisoxazole (Gantrisin) and sulfamethoxazole (Gantanol), which are used for treating urinary tract infections; and mafenide (Sulfamylon), which is applied topically and used to treat burn wound infections. Mafenide is not inhibited by the products of tissue necrosis but causes pain. Of comparable value in the treatment of burns is the silver salt of sulfadiazine (Silvadene), which does not cause pain on application and is free of major toxicity.

Except for nonabsorbable sulfonamides, orally administered sulfonamides are rapidly absorbed in the stomach and duodenum and become distributed in all tissues and fluids. The sulfonamides are bound to either serum albumin or to tissue proteins, and they are detoxified in the liver. Both the drug and its less active metabolites are excreted by glomerular filtration. Sensitivity to one sulfonamide frequently confers sensitivity to others. Toxic reactions limiting sulfonamide therapy range from nausea, vomiting, and dermatitis to crystalluria, renal injury, hepatic damage, and hematologic disorders.

STREPTOCOCCAL INFECTIONS

Streptococci form the dominant aerobic flora of the mouth and pharyngeal areas of man. They are grampositive spherical or ovoid cells (rarely elongated into rods) arranged in pairs (short chains). Long chains are observed when the organism is cultured in fluid media. Although most species are aerobic or facultatively anaerobic, there are also species which are obligately anaerobic (e.g., *Peptostreptococcus putridus* and *Peptostreptococcus micros*) or microaerophilic. They may be divided into those which

produce a soluble hemolysin and those which do not. Aerobes producing a clear zone of hemolysis on blood agar (beta hemolysis) include most of the species associated with primary streptococcal infections in man and can be subdivided into 15 broad groups (Lancefield groups) which are identified by precipitin tests with group-specific antisera against specific carbohydrate haptens (C antigens) of the streptococci. Strains belonging to Lancefield group A (*Streptococcus pyogenes*) are responsible for over 90 percent of human streptococcal infections. These group A strains can be further subdivided for epidemiologic studies into Griffith types according to their surface protein antigens (M, T, and R) by capillary precipitin or slide agglutination tests.

Another group of streptococci produce an ill-defined zone of partial hemolysis having a green or brownish-green color (alpha hemolysis). These are strains of *Streptococcus viridans*. Streptococci which are without effect on blood agar (nonhemolytic) include the fecal enterococci (*Streptococcus fecalis*). Viridans and nonhemolytic streptococci are associated with chronic diseases or are nonpathogenic. *Streptococcus viridans* is part of the commensal flora of the mouth and throat and is dangerous in individuals with congenitally deformed or rheumatically damaged heart valves. It is the commonest cause of subacute bacterial endocarditis. *Streptococcus viridans* has been incriminated in apical tooth infections and is commonly found in carious teeth. Bacteremia frequently follows tooth extraction and even routine dental procedures. In otherwise healthy individuals the streptococci are rapidly removed from the circulation, but in those with heart lesions the organisms settle in or on the defective valves. Accordingly, patients with congenital or other valvular cardiac defects should be given penicillin prophylactically before and after any dental attention.

Nonhemolytic streptococci are always present in the colon and may be isolated from the terminal ileum and upper jejunum of 60 percent of surgical patients. These enterococci (*Streptococcus fecalis*) can cause suppurative lesions and urinary tract infections. In our hospital, enterococci are isolated from 12 percent of surgical wound infections and from 8 percent of urinary tract infections. Some strains of *Streptococcus fecalis* produce a true beta hemolysis; they belong to Lancefield group D.

Group A beta-hemolytic streptococci (*Streptococcus pyogenes*) are the principal causes of streptococcal pharyngitis, scarlet fever, and rheumatic fever. They also cause bacteremias following surgical procedures in patients with malignant disease. Groups B, C, D, F, and G are usually less virulent. Although group B streptococci are often isolated from patients with puerperal sepsis, with meningitis of the newborn, with diabetes mellitus, and/or with peripheral vascular insufficiency, they are also involved in pneumonias and infections of the male genitourinary tract. Since group C streptococci are part of the skin flora, they may be isolated from wounds and exudates more often than group B strains. The group G streptococci involved in infections usually originate in the genitourinary tract or skin, but they may also originate in the upper respiratory tract or gastrointestinal tract. We find streptococci in

4 percent of surgical wound infections and in 6 percent of nosocomial respiratory tract infections.

Streptococcus pyogenes is an invasive microorganism; it secretes two distinct hemolysins (streptolysins O and S) and several other products which aid in invasion. Streptolysin O is cardiotoxic and leukocidic and may be identical with leukocidin. Streptolysin S is a pure hemolysin responsible for beta hemolysis on blood agar plates. Hyaluronidase hydrolyzes hyaluronic acid and allows increased permeability of tissues. Streptokinase reduces fibrinolysis by activating the plasmin system. Streptodornase depolymerizes DNA. Erythrogenic toxin produces erythema when injected intradermally and is responsible for the punctate erythema of scarlet fever. The hyaluronidase and streptokinase produced by most strains of *Streptococcus pyogenes* are responsible for the spreading cellulitis (erysipelas) which is the typical streptococcal lesion. When abscess occurs, the pus is watery and often blood-stained due to the action of streptodornase and streptokinase, since the viscosity of pus is due to DNA and fibrin.

Erysipelas

Erysipelas is a spreading streptococcal cellulitis and lymphangitis with raised, sharply defined, irregular, reddish borders. The classic lesion of erysipelas is a "butterfly" erythema centered around the nose and extending onto both cheeks. Since erythrogenic toxin is produced in variable amounts by hemolytic streptococci, the development of cutaneous erythema is an inconstant manifestation of streptococcal infection. Minor skin abrasions and fissures predispose to these infections of the skin. The cutis is edematous and reddened, with a palpably raised border; the lesion is hot, tender, and painful. The systemic manifestations of erisipelas may be severe and suggest invasion via the lymphatics or bloodstream. Penicillin is usually effective against the invasive infection, but the erythema disappears more slowly.

Erysipeloid, a nonstreptococcal disease distinct from erysipelas, is a type of cutaneous cellulitis. Erysipeloid often is contracted after contamination of a cutaneous abrasion of the hand, particularly the fingers. The typical lesion is a violaceous nodule, often having a curved shape, which differs from that of erysipelas by its tendency to central clearing and the absence of suppuration. Human cases of erysipeloid may also occur as either a severe, generalized cutaneous disease or as septicemia with or without cutaneous involvement and often associated with endocarditis. Penicillin therapy is specific for most cases. Erysipeloid is due to infection by *Erysipelothrix rhusopathiae*, a gram-positive, nonsporulating, facultative anaerobe in the family Corynebacteriaceae. Erysipelothrix infection is considered an occupational disease of abattoir workers, fish handlers, and others exposed to meat, poultry, and fish products.

Necrotizing Fasciitis

This is a life-threatening infection which may occur in only one or two patients a year in large city-county hospitals. The most significant manifestation of the infection is extensive necrosis of the superficial fascia with resultant widespread undermining of surrounding tissue and extreme systemic toxicity. The bacteria involved in about 90 percent of cases have usually been beta-hemolytic streptococci, coagulase-positive staphylococci, or both. Gram-negative enteric pathogens alone have been associated with about 10 percent of cases of necrotizing fasciitis. The disease appears to be a clinical entity and not a specific bacterial infection. It has been described previously as hemolytic or acute streptococcal gangrene, gangrenous or necrotizing erysipelas, suppurative fasciitis, and hospital gangrene. Although necrotizing fasciitis may develop following surgical procedures such as appendectomy, the majority of cases have occurred outside the hospital following minor trauma such as abrasions, cuts, bruises, boils, and insect bites on the extremities, particularly in individuals with diabetes and peripheral vascular disease. The chief diagnostic criterion for necrotizing fasciitis is superficial and widespread fascial necrosis. Cellulitis as well as edema (mild to massive) are present in most patients. The involved skin is pale red without distinct borders and with blisters or bullae. Pale red areas progress to a distinct purple. The diagnosis is confirmed by observation of (1) serosanguinous exudate; (2) swollen, stringy, dull gray, necrotic fascia with extensive undermining; and (3) a gram-stained smear of the pus or fluid.

TREATMENT. This consists of multiple linear incisions over the affected area. In an open wound, the extent of undermining can be ascertained by passing a sterile hemostat along the plane just superficial to the deep fascia. In simple cellulitis or erysipelas, the hemostat cannot be passed. Before operation, the patient should be given a full dose of systemic antibiotic(s) effective against both hemolytic streptococci and penicillinase-producing staphylococci. Therapy is continued postoperatively until the infection is controlled. Repeated debridement may be necessary if the patient continues to be febrile. With the appearance of clean granulation tissue after 5 to 10 days, the wound may be closed by skin graft or suture. Rea and Wyrick (1970) report a 30 percent mortality.

Peptostreptococci (anaerobic streptococci) are also pathogenic. They are normal inhabitants of the mouth, intestine, and vagina. They are abundant in the presence of poor oral hygiene, and aspiration into the lungs and sinuses may lead to putrid lung abscess, empyema, and sinusitis. Brain abscesses often develop as complications of chronic or acute infections of the lungs, sinuses, or ears. *Peptostreptococcus putridus* has been isolated from cases of puerperal sepsis, brain abscess, and infected wounds. *Nonclostridial crepitant anaerobic cellulitis* is due to peptostreptococci, whereas *synergistic necrotizing cellulitis* with widespread involvement of deeper tissues is caused by the symbiotic activity of peptostreptococci, aerobic gram-negative rods, and frequently bacteroides.

Streptococcal Myonecrosis

Anaerobic streptococci also can cause gas gangrene. Facultative streptococci and *Staphylococcus aureus* may also be isolated. *Streptococcal myonecrosis* resembles subacute clostridial gas gangrene and was not described until World War II. After an incubation period of 3 to 4 days, there is swelling, edema, and purulent wound exudate. These signs are followed by pain which rapidly becomes severe. Gas is present, and the infected muscle changes from pale and soft to bright red, striped with purple, and finally purple and gangrenous. The seropurulent discharge has a sour odor. In this disease, muscle is involved, in contrast to necrotizing fasciitis, in which the fascia is affected. Treatment consists of incision and drainage, antibiotic therapy, and supportive measures.

Progressive Synergistic Gangrene

Frank L. Meleney (1889–1963) established the importance of microaerophilic and anaerobic streptococci in special wound infections known as progressive synergistic gangrene and chronic burrowing ulcer. *Meleney's progressive synergistic gangrene* characteristically develops in sutured, infected thoracic or abdominal incisions or around a colostomy, ileostomy, or simple abrasion. The initial lesion is a small, painful, superficial ulcer which gradually spreads. The central ulcerated area is surrounded by a rim of gangrenous skin, which is in turn encircled by a zone of purple erythema blending into a surrounding area of bright, painful erythema. There is seropurulent discharge. Cultures taken from the outer edematous part of the lesion yield microaerophilic or anaerobic nonhemolytic streptococci. Cultures taken from the central ulcerated area yield *Staphylococcus aureus* and sometimes gram-negative bacilli, such as *Proteus* species. However, clinical cases of progressive synergistic gangrene from which anaerobic or microaerophilic streptococci could not be isolated have been reported. Treatment involves wide excision and therapy with penicillin or chloramphenicol. Corticosteroids have been employed to aid healing. Ledingham and Tehrani find that the problem in acute dermal gangrene following surgery, such as necrotizing fasciitis and progressive synergistic gangrene, is no longer any apparent specificity of invading bacteria but rather a vicious cycle of infection, local ischemia, and diminished host defense mechanisms.

Meleney's Ulcer

Chronic burrowing or undermining ulcer, often designated as *Meleney's ulcer,* is caused by a nonhemolytic anaerobic or microaerophilic streptococcus. The lesion begins as a small, superficial ulcer following trauma or surgery and may also originate from an infected lymph node or subcutaneous abscess. The ulcer is only mildly painful, and systemic reaction is minimal. Slow, progressive enlargement of the lesion occurs over months or years. Infection of subcutaneous tissue is associated with ulceration of the overlying skin. Cutaneous gangrene is absent, and the edges of the undermined skin roll inward. The periphery of the lesion is erythematous, and the advancing edge of the lesion is characterized by pain and tenderness. Meleney's ulcer occurs most frequently after incision of a lymph node in the neck, axilla, or groin and after opera-

tions on the genital and intestinal tracts. As the lesion spreads, multiple ulcers and sinuses develop, producing epithelial strands and undermined bridges of skin. Treatment consists of debridement, drainage of sinuses, penicillin therapy, and split-thickness skin grafts over denuded areas as soon as the wound appears clean.

Peptostreptococci, either in pure culture or mixed with bacteroides, are frequently involved in appendiceal abscesses, peritonitis, abdominal wall sepsis, perirectal abscesses, and superficial abscesses related to infections of pilonidal and sebaceous cysts. Most abscesses are treated successfully by incision and drainage, and penicillin therapy. Peptostreptococcal infections, including septicemias, commonly occur in the female pelvic area following septic abortion and postpartum sepsis.

STAPHYLOCOCCAL INFECTIONS

Staphylococci form part of the permanent bacterial flora of the normal skin and nasopharynx and may cause a variety of infections, often characterized by suppuration, ranging from mild, localized pustules to lethal septicemias. Surgical and traumatic wounds are particularly susceptible to purulent infection. In stained preparations of pus, staphylococci appear as spherical cells occurring singly, in pairs, or in small clusters. They are gram-positive and nonmotile, and produce no spores. Staphylococci are aerobic or facultatively anaerobic and grow on ordinary unenriched bacteriologic media. They may produce pigmentation varying from white, orange, or yellow to golden. Blood agar is often hemolyzed (beta hemolysis). Two species are of medical importance: *Staphylococcus aureus* and *Staphylococcus epidermidis* (formerly called *Staphylococcus albus*). *Staphylococcus aureus* is usually associated with disease, and will be discussed subsequently. On the other hand, *Staphylococcus epidermidis* usually has not been considered a pathogen, but it has become recognized as an important cause of opportunistic infection following surgical procedures in which foreign materials and prostheses are placed in the patient. *Staphylococcus epidermidis* causes endocarditis following open heart surgery and occasionally produces septicemia.

The criteria identifying staphylococci are colonial appearance on blood agar, Gram-stain reaction, microscopic morphologic features, production of coagulase, and fermentation of mannitol. *Staphylococcus aureus* is coagulase-positive and produces acid from mannitol. *Staphylococcus epidermidis* produces neither coagulase nor acid from mannitol. Filtrates of cultures of *Staphylococcus aureus* contain hemolysins, dermonecrotic and lethal factors, leukocidins, and enzymes. Strains of *Staphylococcus aureus* may be classified into groups on the basis of their susceptibility to various bacteriophages. Although phage typing of isolates is of value in epidemiologic investigations, it is not employed by the diagnostic laboratory for routine identification of clinical isolates.

Staphylococci are readily phagocytized by polymorphonuclear leukocytes, which may then be killed by the bacteria, presumably by their leukocidins. Although leukocidins, hemolysins, and coagulase are antigenic, antibodies to these antigens provide little or no protection. Since the antigenic components of staphylococci responsible for virulence are unknown, it has not been possible to make effective vaccines.

Staphylococcal infections in man depend upon many factors, including the type and number of staphylococci, the route of introduction, and the toxic substances produced by the staphylococci. Of equal importance are the susceptibility of the host, his previous exposure to specific strains, his general health and nutritional state, and the amount of trauma he has sustained. Factors such as toxemia, allergic reactions, starvation, and diabetes influence the onset and course of staphylococcal infections. Foreign body reaction as a consequence of sutures is an important factor in staphylococcal infection.

The skin is the most common site of staphylococcal infections. Lesions range from furuncles (boils) and carbuncles to surgical wound infections. Hospital-acquired staphylococcal infection by antibiotic-resistant strains reached epidemic proportion during the 1950s. The development and use of semisynthetic penicillinase-resistant penicillins has controlled these infections. However, the antibiotic-resistant staphylococci are endemic in hospitals and pose a continual threat to the patient. A rapidly spreading cellulitis is sometimes seen with staphylococcal infections and should be treated vigorously with an appropriate antibiotic. Often there is pain, swelling, induration, patchy discoloration of the skin, and fever. Cellulitis may occur at the site of a venipuncture for intravenous cannulation. Staphylococcal abscesses characteristically begin in hair follicles or small sebaceous glands. An indurated area of cellulitis undergoes central necrosis and formation of an abscess having thick, odorless, and yellow or greenish pus. Staphylococci are a primary cause of acute wound sepsis and are involved in postoperative infections of "clean" incised wounds. The source of the infecting microorganisms is frequently exogenous. Virulent, antibiotic-resistant, hospital strains of *Staphylococcus aureus* may be carried in the nares and on the hands of physicians and hospital personnel, and these may be newly colonized on the skin of the patient. The air in the operating room may bear microorganisms from the nasopharynx, skin, hair, and clothing of the surgical staff and of the patient. Accordingly, it is essential to maintain strict, rigid rules for asepsis in the operating room. At our hospital, coagulase-positive staphylococci are isolated from 8 percent of postoperative surgical wound infections and account for 5 percent of nosocomial infections.

Infected incisions should be opened widely and allowed to drain. Therapy with antistaphylococcal antibiotics should be initiated. Fulminating septicemias may arise from severe wound infections. The patient is ill with high fever, leukocytosis, toxemia, and evidence of irritation of the central nervous system. The mortality rate in fulminating untreated infections may be as high as 90 percent. If the infection persists, metastatic abscesses form in lungs, heart, kidneys, gallbladder, appendix, liver, peritoneum, and bone. Meningitis and brain abscesses hasten death.

Endocarditis is a frequent complication of staphylococcal septicemia. Staphylococcal pneumonia is another nosocomial postoperative infection. It may be severe and is often associated with a tracheostomy. In fatal cases, the major finding at autopsy is marked pulmonary edema with little destruction of tissue.

Staphylococcal Enteritis

Enteritis with a drug-resistant staphylococcus following oral administration of a broad-spectrum antibiotic was first described by Kramer in 1948. Generally, this disease is benign with mild to moderate symptoms including nausea, vomiting, diarrhea, abdominal distension, fever, and weakness, but may be fulminating and lead to septicemia and death. Discontinuance of the oral antibiotic usually leads to disappearance of symptoms. The prognosis is good so long as the intestinal mucosa remains intact.

Staphylococcal enterocolitis (*pseudomembranous enterocolitis*) is an acute inflammatory disease of the small and large intestine characterized by foci of epithelial necrosis and erosion of the mucosa. There is profuse, continuous diarrhea which soon becomes watery, contains desquamated, membranous patches, and often is greenish. The disease is a complication in debilitated surgical patients following therapy with broad-spectrum antibiotics. The use of neomycin in debilitated patients for preoperative intestinal antisepsis and for treatment of hepatic coma has resulted in staphylococcal enterocolitis. The major etiologic factors are suppression of normal gastrointestinal flora by a broad-spectrum antibiotic and acquisition of an enterotoxic strain of *Staphylococcus aureus* possessing multiple antibiotic-resistance. Secondary factors are debilitation and an empty small bowel (as a result of preoperative starvation). Although stool cultures from some patients yield a pure culture of *Staphylococcus aureus*, pseudomembranous enterocolitis may exist without culturable *Staphylococcus aureus*. Conversely, *Staphylococcus aureus may exist in pure culture in the intestine of a patient with the symptoms of enteritis but in the absence of a pseudomembrane.*

TREATMENT. Treatment consists of discontinuing previous antibiotics and employing a specific antistaphylococcal drug such as methicillin, hydration with intravenously administered fluids, replacement of electrolytes, intramuscular administration of corticosteroids, and attempts to reestablish a normal flora. The fulminating form of enterocolitis may be refractory to all forms of therapy and result in death.

Peptococci and Disease?

Both obligately anaerobic staphylococci (peptococci) and facultatively anaerobic staphylococci grow in anaerobic cultures. However, the facultatives (e.g., *Staphylococcus aureus*) can be subcultured aerobically and separated from the peptococci which grow anaerobically only. In contrast to the role of pure cultures of staphylococci in disease, the peptococci may be found in wound infections, abscesses, and septicemias in association with bacteroides, clostridia, aerobic gram-negative bacilli, and aerobic cocci. These bacterial groups are major components of the normal flora of the skin and mucous membranes and can exert a role in mixed infections when these sites are disturbed. Peptococci (e.g., *Peptococcus magnus* and *Peptococcus asaccharolyticus*) account for approximately 20 percent of anaerobes found in clinical specimens from surgical patients (Holland et al.). Nevertheless, the peptococci have slight, if any, propensity to produce disease and seem unable to cause progressive infection in laboratory animals. This apparent nonpathogenicity is shared by many anaerobic species from normal flora found in anaerobic infections and has led to speculation that the unitarian theory of infection which has evolved from the monumental work of Koch and Ehrlich (one microbe, one disease, one drug) does not explain all infectious disease (Gorbach and Bartlett).

CLOSTRIDIAL INFECTIONS

The clostridia are large, gram-positive, rod-shaped microorganisms. They are ubiquitous. *Clostridium perfringens* is more widespread than any other pathogen. Its principal habitats are the soil and the intestinal tract of man and animals. The most characteristic feature of clostridia is the presence of an oval, central, or subterminal spore. In the case of *Clostridium tetani*, the spore is spherical and terminally located and produces a characteristic drumstick appearance. The clostridia are obligate anaerobes and can be cultured only on media having a low oxidation-reduction potential. This may be achieved by employing fresh media incubated in an anaerobic atmosphere in specially designed jars or with liquid media exposed to the atmosphere, but containing added reducing agents (such as sodium thioglycolate, powdered iron, or chopped meat).

The lesions produced by the pathogenic clostridia are due to their exotoxins. Gas gangrene is a necrosis of tissue along with putrefaction and is usually caused by clostridia derived from the intestine or soil. The infection is localized but its systemic effects are far-reaching. Gas gangrene is rarely a pure culture infection. It usually involves *Clostridium perfringens* along with other clostridial species, such as *Clostridium novyi, Clostridium septicum, Clostridium bifermentans (sordelli),* sometimes *Clostridium tetani* and *Clostridium botulinum,* and often nonpathogenic but proteolytic *Clostridium sporogenes* and *Clostridium histolyticum.* In addition, gram-positive cocci and gram-negative enterobacteria are often present.

Clostridium perfringens is, nevertheless, the most important organism. Five types, A through F, have been described. They are differentiated on the basis of production of lethal toxins. All types produce alpha toxin, a lethal, necrotizing, hemolytic exotoxin, which is also a lecithinase. *Clostridium perfringens* type A produces the greatest amount of alpha toxin. In addition, some strains of type A produce variable amounts of hemolysin (theta toxin), collagenase (kappa toxin), hyaluronidase (mu toxin), and deoxyribonuclease (nu toxin).

Clostridial Wound Infection

MacLennan in 1962 described three types of anaerobic wound infection: simple contamination, clostridial cellulitis, and clostridial myonecrosis.

SIMPLE CONTAMINATION

Simple contamination of a wound by clostridia is common. It causes no discomfort to the patient and is of little concern to the surgeon. When anaerobes are digesting dead tissue, there may be a thin seropurulent exudate. If the necrotic material is removed, there will be no subsequent invasion of underlying tissues. The relatively common occurrence of clostridia in accidental wounds in the absence of anaerobic infection is probably due to the ubiquitous presence of these anaerobes and their spores. The absence of subsequent anaerobic infections is most likely due to unsuitable conditions for further multiplication of the contaminant and for toxin production. MacLennan estimated that between 10 and 30 percent of all severe civilian wounds were infected with spore-forming anaerobic bacilli. A high oxidation-reduction potential (Eh) due to the surrounding healthy tissues prevents colonization of the tissues. In the absence of treatment, however, cellulitis or myonecrosis may develop from the simple contamination, and the three types of anaerobic wound infection may be considered as ascending grades of severity.

CLOSTRIDIAL CELLULITIS

This is a gassy, crepitant infection involving necrotic tissue (killed by ischemia or trauma, but not by bacterial activity). Intact, healthy muscle is not invaded. The cellulitis is characterized as a foul, seropurulent infection of the depths and crevices of a wound. There is often local extension along fascial planes, but involvement of healthy muscle and marked toxemia are absent. Although *Clostridium perfringens* may be present, the predominant organisms are proteolytic and nontoxigenic clostridia, such as *Clostridium sporogenes* and *Clostridium tertium.* Clostridial cellulitis generally has a gradual onset; the incubation period is from 3 to 5 days; systemic effects are usually mild; there is no toxemia; the skin is rarely discolored; and there is little or no edema. This distinguishes the infection from gas gangrene. The spread of the cellulitis in the tissue spaces often has been rapid and extensive, necessitating immediate radical surgical drainage.

CLOSTRIDIAL MYONECROSIS (GAS GANGRENE)

This infection is rapid-spreading. It may be crepitant, or noncrepitant and edematous, mixed, or toxemic. The lesion also has been described as a "myositis," which is not as precise a term as is *myonecrosis.* The infection occurs in association with severe wounds of large muscle masses that have become contaminated with pathogenic clostridia, especially *Clostridium perfringens.* Such wounds are most commonly caused by the high-velocity missiles of modern warfare and by accidental trauma. Sometimes clostridial myonecrosis follows clean elective surgical procedures.

Many patients with clostridial myonecrosis harbor a variety of anaerobic as well as aerobic bacteria. In fatal cases it is rare for only a single species to be present. Clostridial myonecrosis is most likely to develop in wounds in which there has been extensive laceration or devitalization of thick muscle masses, such as the buttock, thigh, and shoulder. Associated with such trauma is impaired arterial supply to the limb or muscle group and gross contamination of the wound by soil, clothing, and other foreign bodies. These conditions provide an ideal substrate for the development of clostridia. In anoxic muscle glycolysis continues, and the oxidation-reduction potential (Eh) of the muscle falls. With the accumulation of lactate, alkaline reservoirs become depleted, and the pH also falls. As a consequence of lowered Eh and pH, the proteinases present and the amino acids produced not only lower the pH further but provide substrate for the growth of clostridia. Once bacterial growth is established and toxins and other products of bacterial metabolism accumulate, the invasion of uninjured tissue is promoted, and the anaerobic infection is established. The infection is further aided by the fact that neither phagocytes nor antibodies can enter the necrotic lesion. Gas gangrene is considered to have begun when the infecting pathogenic anaerobes have produced sufficient toxins to overcome local defenses. Gas gangrene is relatively infrequent in clinical practice. The overall incidence is less than 2 percent, although from 4 to 40 percent of wounds may be contaminated with clostridia.

TREATMENT. Early and adequate surgery is the most effective means of treating gas gangrene. Because of the rapid spread of the infection, a 24-hour delay in treatment may be fatal. The diagnosis of gas gangrene is based on clinical evidence. Multiple longitudinal incisions for decompression and drainage and surgical debridement usually arrest the disease. If not or if early diagnosis was not made, then amputation is necessary. Antibiotic therapy with penicillin G and tetracycline has been most effective as an adjunct to operative treatment. Antitoxin is of no value therapeutically or prophylactically and should not be used. Adjunctive hyperbaric oxygenation has been used with success.

Infections of the Gastrointestinal Tract

Clostridia are usually present among the mixed flora in peritonitis, appendicitis, and strangulation intestinal obstruction. Quantitatively, the most numerous flora in peritoneal and loop fluids of dogs with experimental strangulation intestinal obstruction are clostridia, coliforms, bacteriodes, and streptococci, in that order. Although it appears reasonable to assume that *Clostridium perfringens* actively participates in the pathophysiology of severe cases of appendicitis and acute cases of strangulated intestinal obstruction, direct clinical evidence is lacking. Experimental studies demonstrate that clostridial exotoxins contribute to the lethal activity of filter-sterilized strangulation fluids. However, this finding does not preclude a role for combinations of varying proportions of viable bacteria, bacterial endotoxins, and clostridial exotoxins. In biliary tract infections due to clostridia, acute emphysematous cholecystitis (gas gangrene of the gallbladder) and postcholecystectomy septicemia, it is generally believed that clostridia are transported to the liver from the gastrointestinal tract via the portal circulation and then excreted with the bile into the biliary tract. In postoperative gas gangrene of the abdominal wall, a rare complication of abdominal surgery, intestinal clostridia contaminate the abdominal wound at the time of operation. It occurs less often after operations on the stomach and duodenum than after those involving the lower intestinal tract. These infections are usually due to *Clostridium perfringens* and are fatal; they require awareness and early treatment. Gas gangrene of the abdominal wall must be distinguished from Meleney's progressive synergistic gangrene of the abdominal wall following drainage of appendiceal abscesses. Synergistic gangrene is a chronic, superficial progressive gangrene characterized by a slow, relentless progression, severe local symptoms, and absence of severe systemic symptoms. It is due to anaerobic cocci mixed with *Staphylococcus aureus, Streptococcus pyogenes, Pseudomonas aeruginosa,* or *Proteus* species.

Urogenital Infections

Postoperative infections due to *Clostridium perfringens* have occurred following procedures such as nephrectomy, lithotomy, and prostatectomy. Almost all uterine clostridial infections are due to *Clostridium perfringens.* They generally occur following criminal abortion and are rare following normal childbirth. Introduction of the organisms into the uterus is favored by instrumentation and manipulation. In modern obstetrics, the use of prophylactic antibiotic therapy and the wide use of cesarean section probably account for the decreasing frequency of this already rare form of uterine infection. In contrast, in cases of criminal abortion both endogenous and exogenous sources of contamination occur as the result of unskilled manipulations and the use of unsterile and unclean instruments and abortifacients. Once the interior of the puerperal or postabortal uterus has been contaminated, fragments of blood clot and necrotic tissue provide conditions favorable for multiplication of clostridia. Early diagnosis depends upon clinical recognition of such signs as jaundice, hypotension, tachycardia, shock, hemoglobinuria, uterine or perianal tenderness, and offensive vaginal discharge. The simplest method for the rapid detection of *Clostridium perfringens* is the demonstration of gram-positive rods with rounded ends in direct smears from the cervical os or canal. The treatment of uterine gas gangrene involves immediate chemotherapy, hyperbaric oxygenation, treatment of shock, hysterectomy, and management of renal failure. Penicillin is the antibiotic of choice.

Tetanus

This disease is a toxemia resulting from the growth of contaminating *Clostridium tetani* at a traumatized site and consequent production of exotoxin. In contrast to the clostridia of gas gangrene, *Clostridium tetani* is noninvasive, and neurotoxin is responsible for the symptoms of tetanus.

The conditions necessary for the development of tetanus are the presence of the organisms or spores in the wound and favorable anaerobic conditions for bacterial growth and the elaboration of exotoxin. The presence of *Clostridium tetani* in soil and in the intestine of man and animals ensures that accidental wounds are exposed to the risk of contamination at the time of injury. However, as with other clostridial infections, the mere presence of *Clostridium tetani* or its spores in a wound is not followed by tetanus, and the organism may be isolated from wounds in individuals who never develop tetanus. A low oxygen tension is necessary if *Clostridium tetani* is to grow. Currently, tetanus commonly follows mild injuries because the routine protective measures employed in severe cases are frequently omitted. The type of lesions leading to the development of tetanus are penetrating wounds due to splinters, thorns, rusty nails, and even dirty abrasions. In about 50 percent of cases, it is presumed that the wound was slight and healed before evidence of intoxication developed. Such mild injuries may not induce significant local anoxia, but they may be accompanied by other infections which lower the oxidation-reduction potential of the tissues to a point at which the spores of *Clostridium tetani* can germinate. For example, chronic ulcers of the leg, measles rash, boils, paronychia, and dental extractions have been implicated as modes of entry. In the United States, tetanus has become a disease primarily of adults. The median age of patients with nonneonatal tetanus varies from fifty-five to fifty-seven years; the median age for those dying from tetanus is from fifty-five to sixty years.

Currently, tetanus is seen in urban centers of the United States as a complication of narcotic addiction; *urban tetanus* has a mortality of 90 percent. *Tetanus neonatorum* results from contamination of the cut surface of the umbilical cord and is an important cause of infant mortality in developing countries where primitive unhygienic obstetric practices prevail. There is often continuous crying for hours followed by cessation of sucking and crying, convulsions, and fever. Severe spasm of the respiratory muscles is a common cause of death. *Postabortal tetanus* and *puerperal tetanus* result from unsterile manipulation or instrumentation of the genital tract. *Postoperative tetanus* sometimes follows elective surgical procedures, and is usually due to some breakdown in sterile technique, but it may also be caused by contamination from the patient's intestinal tract.

CLINICAL MANIFESTATIONS. The average incubation period for tetanus is from 7 to 10 days after injury, but it may range between 3 and 30 days. The incubation period is followed by the *period of onset,* that is, the time interval between the first symptom (usually trismus) and the onset of spasms. In severe cases reflex spasms may begin 12 hours after onset, in moderately severe cases after 2 to 3 days, and in milder cases after 5 or more days. In general, the shorter the periods of incubation and onset, the worse the prognosis. Even with modern treatment, the mortality rate is rarely less than 30 percent.

Trismus is the most common early symptom. It often is combined with pain and stiffness in the neck, back, and abdomen. Occasionally dysphagia appears first. These symptoms increase according to the severity of the attack. Twenty-four hours after the onset, a patient with a moderately severe attack has a characteristically anxious expression (*risus sardonicus*) in which the eyebrows and the corners of the mouth are drawn up. The muscles of the neck and trunk are rigid to varying degrees, and the back is usually slightly arched. The patient is usually comfortable except for occasional pain in the neck or back, which tends to be made worse by movement. Manipulation of a limb or palpation of any part of the body tends to increase muscular rigidity and may bring on cramplike pain. Initially, reflex spasms are brought on by external stimuli, such as moving the patient or knocking the bed, but later they occur spontaneously at regular and increasingly shorter intervals until the height of the disease is reached. Spasms often begin with a sudden jerk. Every muscle in the body is thrown into intense tonic contraction, the jaws are tightly clenched, the head is retracted, the back is arched, the chest and abdomen are fixed, and the limbs are usually extended. A severe spasm may stop respiration. Spasms may last a few seconds or several minutes. When spasms occur frequently, they lead to rapid exhaustion and sometimes to death from asphyxiation. Without spasms, mortality is low; with severe spasms, few survive. Aspiration pneumonia is a common contributory cause of death.

Less common manifestations of the disease include local contracture of muscles in the neighborhood of the wound: *local tetanus.* This may precede the more generalized forms of involvement. *Cephalic tetanus* is a manifestation in which irritation or paralysis of cranial nerves appears early and dominates the picture. The facial nerve is affected most often, but ophthalmoplegia from involvement of the ocular nerves and spasm or paralysis of the tongue from involvement of the hypoglossal nerve may develop. Trismus and dysphagia may also be present. This condition, which is a type of local tetanus, follows wounds of the head and face, and the symptoms often appear first on the injured side.

Severe tetanus is terrible and often fatal, but those who recover do so completely. The patient who has survived tetanus is not immune and, unless immunized, is susceptible to a second attack. *Recurrent tetanus* in the same patient has been reported. Apparently a sublethal amount of tetanus toxin is not sufficient to provide an adequate antigenic stimulus for the production of active immunity.

The diagnosis of tetanus is a clinical one with bacteriologic confirmation sometimes possible. Frequently the presumed lesion has been so slight that it is not detectable at the time when clinical tetanus develops.

IMMUNIZATION. Prophylaxis with tetanus toxoid is the best means of preventing tetanus. For active immunization of individuals seven years old or over, the initial dose is 0.5 ml aluminum phosphate–adsorbed tetanus toxoid given intramuscularly, preferably in the left deltoid region, but it also may be given subcutaneously. This is repeated in 4 to 6 weeks, and a third injection is given in 6 to 12 months (or more). Only after this third injection is the basic series considered complete. For children six years old or under, diphtheria and tetanus toxoid combined with pertussis vaccine (DTP) is used. Delay in administering the second and third injections is not disadvantageous, and the series does not need to be restarted or repeated. Even after 25 years, a booster will rapidly recall complete active protection.

Following the initial dose of tetanus toxoid, nonimmunized individuals require approximately 30 days to acquire a safe antibody level (at least 0.01 I.U. of serum antitoxin per milliliter of blood). Patients are passively immunized in the interim by intramuscular administration of human hyperimmune globulin containing 250 units of tetanus antitoxin simultaneously with the toxoid. This protects for about 4 weeks. Passive immunization is not recommended for individuals who have received previous active immunization.

TREATMENT. Surgical care of wounds should be immediate. The most important features of surgical wound care are thorough cleansing and debridement. Foreign bodies and necrotic tissue can be massively contaminated with *Clostridium tetani* and establish wound conditions promoting growth and exotoxin production by *Clostridium tetani*. The wound should be left open until the patient has recovered from the convulsive stage of the disease. Antibiotic therapy with penicillin is effective against vegetative cells of *Clostridium tetani*. Oxytetracycline or chloramphenicol may be used if an allergy to penicillin exists. Antibiotics also are important as prophylaxis against respiratory infections, which are common in tetanus. Treatment of the patient with severe tetanus involves the use of muscle relaxants, sedation with Pentothal sodium, balance of fluid and electrolytes, control of respiratory secretions, and elimination of visceral stimuli such as distension of the urinary bladder and fecal impaction. A tracheostomy is performed if needed or when the period of onset is 1 day or less. Constant nursing care is required.

COMPLICATIONS. Tetanus is a particularly lethal disease, and death is generally due to respiratory arrest. Some complications of tetanus and its treatment are drug intoxication, especially from barbituates; bronchopneumonia or other pulmonary infection; compression fracture of vertebrae, especially the thoracic vertebrae; anemia; and exhaustion, which may be so severe as a result of repeated convulsions that the patient lapses into coma and expires. Before human tetanus immune globulin was available, the risk of anaphylaxis complicated the use of bovine or equine tetanus antitoxin.

PROPHYLAXIS. The Committee on Trauma of the American College of Surgeons recommends the following guidelines in management of the tetanus-prone wound:

I. General principles
   A. For each patient the attending physician must determine the adequate prophylaxis against tetanus.
   B. Meticulous surgical care, including removal of all devitalized tissue and foreign bodies, should be provided immediately for all wounds regardless of the active immunization status of the patient. Such care is an essential part of the prophylaxis against tetanus.
   C. Each patient with a wound should receive adsorbed tetanus toxoid intramuscularly at the time of injury, either as an initial immunizing dose or as a booster for previous immunization, unless he has received a booster or has com-

pleted his initial immunization series within the past 12 months. As the antigen concentration varies in different products, specific information on the volume of a single dose is provided on the label of the package.
   D. Need for passive immunization with homologous (human) tetanus immune globulin must be considered in relation to the characteristics of the wound, the conditions under which it was incurred, and the previous active immunization status of the patient.
   E. Every wounded patient should be given a written record of the immunization provided, and instructed to carry the record at all times and, if indicated, to complete active immunization. For precise tetanus prophylaxis, an accurate and immediately available history regarding previous active immunization against tetanus is required.
   F. Basic immunization with adsorbed toxoid requires three injections. A booster of adsorbed toxoid is indicated 10 years after the third injection or 10 years after an intervening wound booster.
II. Specific measures for patients with wounds
   A. For previously immunized individuals
      1. When the patient has been immunized within the past 10 years
         a. To the majority, give 0.5 ml of adsorbed tetanus toxoid as a booster unless it is certain that the patient has received a booster within the previous 12 months.
         b. To those with severe, neglected, and old (more than 24 hours) tetanus-prone wounds, give 0.5 ml of adsorbed toxoid unless it is certain that a booster was received within the previous 6 months.
      2. When the patient received active immunization more than 10 years previously and has not received a booster within the past 10 years
         a. To the majority, give 0.5 ml of adsorbed tetanus toxoid.
         b. To those with wounds which indicate an overwhelming possibility that tetanus might develop
           (1) Give 0.5 ml of adsorbed tetanus toxoid.
           (2) Give 250 units of tetanus immune globulin (human). Use different syringes, needles, and sites. For severe, neglected, or old wounds, 500 units of tetanus immune globulin (human) is advisable.
           (3) Consider administering oxytetracycline or penicillin prophylactically.
   B. For individuals not previously immunized
      1. With clean minor wounds in which tetanus is most likely, give 0.5 ml of adsorbed tetanus toxoid (initial immunizing dose).
      2. With all other wounds
         a. Give 0.5 ml of adsorbed tetanus toxoid (initial immunizing dose).
         b. Give 250 units of tetanus immune globulin (human). For severe, neglected, or old wounds, 500 units of tetanus immune globulin (human) is advisable.
         c. Consider administering oxytetracycline or penicillin prophylactically.

Medical students sometimes question on theoretical grounds the validity of administering toxoid and antitoxin (immune globulin) simultaneously to a previously unimmunized patient. The problem of interference during simultaneous active and passive immunization against tetanus has been studied quantitatively (Rubbo and Suri). There is some lowering of the antigenicity of toxoid, but the interference is not clinically significant if 250 units of tetanus immune globulin is injected. The antibody level in patients receiving immune globulin is protective for at least

4 weeks, and the second and third doses of toxoid produce an active antitoxin response. In addition, alum-adsorbed tetanus toxoid stimulates a quicker, higher, and more durable immunity than does plain toxoid because the aluminum in the preparation is an immunologic adjuvant. Use of the recommended adsorbed toxoid is, therefore, more reliable.

Wound Botulism

Botulism is an example of an intoxication resulting from the ingestion of exotoxin formed by *Clostridium botulinum* growing in improperly sterilized or inadequately preserved foods. Following gastrointestinal symptoms, botulism progresses to diplopia, blurred vision, and dysphagia and to a descending motor paralysis spreading to involve other cranial nerves and peripheral motor nerves. Although *C. botulinum* may be isolated from a wound as a simple contaminant, *wound botulism* occurs and is indicated by the presence of clinical signs of botulism. Thus wound botulism should be suspected in any patient with a wound who presents with clinical signs of descending paralysis and a negative food history. Therapy of the wound is routine; therapy of the botulism is supportive, with respiratory care and assisted ventilation if required. Equine trivalent antitoxin should be given after testing for sensitivity to equine serum.

INFECTIONS CAUSED BY GRAM-NEGATIVE BACILLI

The gram-negative bacilli of importance to surgery are for the most part indigenous to man and often found in the intestinal tract. They are non-spore-forming rods, and they may be aerobes, facultative anaerobes, or obligate anaerobes. The role of some gram-negative bacilli as primary pathogens has long been known, e.g., *Pseudomonas aeruginosa* and *Salmonella typhi*. Others have been recognized only rarely as primary pathogens in human beings, e.g., *Serratia marcescens* and *Enterobacter aerogenes* (formerly *Aerobacter aerogenes*). However, since the development of modern chemotherapy after World War II, the gram-negative bacilli have become increasingly important as causes of serious infection, particularly in hospitalized patients. Prior to the introduction of broad-spectrum antibiotics, the role of gram-negative bacilli as pathogens was usually overshadowed by the pneumococci, streptococci, and staphylococci. We now know that infection is most likely to occur when body defense mechanisms are either undeveloped or overtaxed, as in the case of infants and debilitated patients, and that therapeutic measures to combat one situation may provide an environment promoting the establishment of infection by almost any mixture of gram-negative bacilli. This situation prevails because of the great number of patients with impaired host defenses secondary to the use of multiple antibiotics, corticosteroids, immunosuppressive agents, antineoplastic drugs, and radiotherapy. Surgical procedures in which foreign bodies such as prosthetic valves or grafts are inserted appear to allow these less virulent species to become established and to produce infection. Indwelling venous and urethral catheters, endotracheal tubes and mechanical ventilators, peritoneal dialysis apparatus, and pump-oxygenators for extracorporeal circulation in cardiac surgery often serve as portals of entry for the gram-negative bacilli. The current taxonomic organization of gram-negative bacilli (aerobic, facultative, and anaerobic) is outlined in Table 5-6.

Aerobic and Facultative Bacteria

Pseudomonas aeruginosa is a strict aerobe; it is widely distributed and is frequently present in small numbers on healthy skin surfaces and in the normal intestinal flora of some individuals. *P. aeruginosa* is an opportunistic pathogen which can cause serious and lethal infections in debilitated or immunosuppressed patients, such as those with cancer, large burns, or cystic fibrosis, and is common in postoperative infections following the use of mechanical ventilators and indwelling urinary catheters. It is incriminated in primary infections such as meningitis resulting from lumbar puncture, traumatic injuries to the eye, and enteritis with associated bacteremia. Heroin addicts are subject to hematogenous pseudomonal osteomyelitis. Although *P. aeruginosa* is gram-negative and produces an endotoxin, its cell-wall lipopolysaccharides are not as toxic as those isolated from the enteric bacteria. It does, however, produce a variety of extracellular products that contribute to its pathogenicity, including hemolysins, proteases, an enterotoxin, and a heat-labile exotoxin. This exotoxin is more toxic than the other extracellular products or the endotoxin. *Pseudomonas* infections are treated with either gentamicin or carbenicillin, alone or in combination.

Escherichia coli is found in the intestinal tract of man and animals and is the predominant facultative commensal in the normal intestinal flora. Although more than 145

Table 5-6. TAXONOMY OF GRAM-NEGATIVE BACILLI

Family	Tribe	Genus
Pseudomonaceae. . . .	. . . .	*Pseudomonas*
Enterobacteriaceae. . .	Eschericheae	*Escherichia* (*E. coli,* including *Alkalescens-Dispar* group)
		Shigella
	Edwardsielliae	*Edwardsiella*
	Salmonelleae	*Salmonella*
		Arizona
		Citrobacter (including Bethesda-Ballerup group)
	Klebsielleae	*Klebsiella*
		Enterobacter (including *Hafnia*)
		Pectobacterium
		Serratia
	Proteae	*Proteus*
		Providencia
Bacteroidaceae	. . . .	*Bacteroides*
		Fusobacterium

different envelope capsular (K) antigens have been identified, the ability of a strain to be typed does not necessarily
denote pathogenicity or virulence. Nevertheless, certain
strains belonging to distinct antigenic types are *entero-
pathogenic,* others are *enterotoxigenic* by their capacity to
produce toxins, and others are *enteroinvasive* by their ability to penetrate mucosal cells. These strains produce diarrheal disease, especially in infants. Stool isolates may have
none, one, two, or all three of these pathogenic characteristics. *Escherichia coli* may produce meningitis, septicemia,
endocarditis, appendiceal abscess, peritonitis, septic
wounds, and pyogenic infections, chiefly urinary tract infections (pyelitis, cystitis, etc.) in pure culture or in association with fecal streptococci. *Escherichia coli* also has the
capacity to produce a potent endotoxin which enters the
circulation and induces shock. The antibiotic of choice in
the treatment of the patient seriously ill with *Escherichia
coli* sepsis is an aminoglycoside, such as kanamycin or
gentamicin.

The *Salmonella* species are a large group of enteric
pathogens transmitted via food and water. They cause
enteric fevers (particularly typhoid fever), gastroenteritis,
and septicemia. *Salmonella typhi* and *Salmonella enteritidis*
pass from the small intestine by way of the lymphatics to
the mesenteric glands. After multiplication there, they
invade the bloodstream via the thoracic duct. Complications which may result from this hematogenous dissemination include thrombophlebitis, lymphadenitis, pneumonia,
osteomyelitis, arthritis, endocarditis, and meningitis. Hemorrhage may occur from perforation of ulcers in lymphoid
tissue of the intestine. The specific surgical treatment for
perforation, i.e., simple closure or segmental resection, is
determined by the pathologic findings encountered at operation. Chloramphenicol has long been advocated in the
treatment of typhoid fever, but ampicillin is equally effective. Although postoperative wound infection due to *Salmonella typhi* is rare, recorded cases occur after gallbladder
surgery in patients who are unsuspected typhoid carriers.
Contaminated wound drainage and positive stools from
such patients are distinct hazards to other hospitalized
patients.

Before the introduction of modern chemotherapy,
gram-negative bacilli of the tribe Klebsielleae were rarely
noted as primary pathogens. However, along with other
gram-negative bacilli, they have assumed increasing importance as causes of serious hospital-acquired infections.
Klebsiella pneumoniae (Friedlander's bacillus) causes a
severe pneumonia having a propensity for debilitated (frequently alcoholic) patients. *Klebsiella* has also been implicated in endocarditis, septic thrombophlebitis, septicemia,
urinary tract infection, wound infection, crepitant cellulitis,
and myonecrosis. *Enterobacter aerogenes* (formerly *Aerobacter aerogenes*) is a commensal in the intestinal tract of
approximately 5 percent of healthy individuals. It has less
pathogenic potential than strains of *Klebsiella* but is commonly involved in hospital-acquired sepsis. *Serratia marcescens* is another species formerly considered to be nonpathogenic for man. Although it too has low virulence for
healthy individuals, it is now found primarily in hospitalized patients with some underlying disease. It may spread

like other "hospital bacteria," and infection may not always produce clinical symptoms. Classically, *Serratia marcescens* has been recognized by its ability to produce a
characteristic red pigment, and it has been thought to be an
obligate pigment producer. However, the majority of
strains of *Serratia marcescens* involved in hospital-acquired
infections are nonpigmented and often have been mistaken
for other enterobacteria. These nonchromogenic strains of
Serratia marcescens now can be identified by appropriate
biochemical tests. The *Klebsiella-Enterobacter-Serratia*
species are often isolated in mixed culture from sputum,
urine, blood, and wounds in which there are other potential pathogens such as streptococci, staphylococci, *Escherichia coli, Proteus* species, *Citrobacter* species, and *Pseudomonas aeruginosa.* Epidemiologic studies indicate that
the particular strains and types of the gram-negative species producing infection are nosocomial and acquired in
the intestinal tract of patients during hospitalization. They
are often highly drug-resistant, and the overall mortality
associated with bacteremia is approximately 50 percent.
The risk of bacteremia appears to be related to the underlying disease of the patient and the nature of his infection
(urinary tract, respiratory, wound infection, abscess, etc.).
Gentamicin is the antibiotic of choice in treatment of
infections caused by the *Klebsiella-Enterobacter-Serratia*
species. Kanamycin is a satisfactory alternate drug.

Gram-negative bacilli in the genera *Proteus* and *Providencia* also compete for prominence with the other aerobic
gram-negatives in infections. Rapid and abundant urease
production distinguishes *Proteus* from *Providencia.* These
organisms often occur in abscesses, in infected wounds,
and also in burns as one component of a mixed infection.
They are resistant to most antibiotics, and what was originally a mixed infection may be converted into a pure
proteus infection as a result of antibiotic therapy. Sepsis
due to indol-negative *Proteus* (*Proteus mirabilis*) is treated
with ampicillin, while that due to indol-positive species
(*Proteus vulgaris, P. morganii,* and *P. rettgeri*) is treated
with kanamycin or carbenicillin. *Providencia* species are
sensitive to carbenicillin. The genus *Acinetobacter* includes
gram-negative pleomorphic aerobes previously known by a
wide variety of names. *Acinetobacter calcoaceticus* var.
anitratus (formerly *Herellea vaginicola* and *Bacterium ani-
tratum*) and *Acinetobacter calcoaceticus* var. *lwoffi* (formerly *Mima polymorpha*) are opportunists capable of
causing therapy-potentiated infections in compromised
patients. Kanamycin or gentamicin constitute appropriate
therapy for these infections.

Anaerobic Bacteria

Obligately anaerobic bacteria, especially gram-negative
bacilli, are found as normal flora on skin and all mucous
membrane surfaces. They are by far the major component
of the normal flora. In the normal oral cavity, anaerobes
outnumber aerobes 10 to 1, and in the normal colon, 1000
to 1. When the mucous membrane barrier is disturbed by
disease, trauma, or surgical procedures, these bacteria can
invade adjacent tissue and may cause infection. In the
upper respiratory tract and lungs, the major anaerobic

pathogens are peptostreptococci, fusobacteria, and *Bacteroides melaninogenicus*. In intraabdominal infections, *Bacteroides fragilis* is the most frequent isolate; clostridia, peptostreptococci, and peptococci are also found. In infection of the female genital tract, the same anaerobes are also the principal pathogens. Although anaerobic infections often originate close to a mucosal surface, they may occur anywhere in the body as a result of direct or hematogenous spread. Clues to diagnosis include foul-smelling discharge, gas, necrotic tissue, abscess formation, and failure to obtain growth on aerobic culture despite the presence of organisms on Gram-stained direct smear. Anaerobes are associated with 90 percent of cases of intraabdominal abscess, 95 percent of appendiceal abscess, 90 percent of aspiration pneumonia, 95 percent of lung abscess, 85 percent of brain abscess, and 75 percent of upper tract female pelvic infections.

The bacteroides are obligately anaerobic, gram-negative, non-spore-forming bacilli. They are sometimes the only microorganisms found in clinical specimens but more often are found in association with other anaerobes and aerobes. Currently, human pathogens are assigned to the genus *Bacteroides* and the genus *Fusobacterium*. *Bacteroides* are rod-shaped cells with rounded ends and are sometimes coccobacillary; *Fusobacterium* may be bacilli with pointed ends or pleomorphic, filamentous forms with swellings and free, round bodies. Species causing infections in human beings are *Bacteroides fragilis, Bacteroides melaninogenicus, Fusobacterium fusiforme,* and *Fusobacterium necrophorus* (previously known as *Bacteroides fundiformis* and as *Sphaerophorus necrophorus*).

In circumstances such as chronic illness, malignant disease, surgical treatment, and cystoscopy, the bacteroides may invade the bloodstream to cause septicemia and penetrate tissue and organs to produce abscesses. The clinical spectrum of infections varies from superficial infections to deep abscesses with overwhelming bacteremia and shock. The gastrointestinal tract, especially the colon and appendix, appears to be the most frequent source of bacteroides infection. Gynecologic infections involve the vagina, uterus, and contiguous structures, and are related to malignancy of pelvic organs, septic abortions, and postpartum complications. Upper respiratory tract infections and those of the nasopharynx, mouth, and jaw (tonsillar and peritonsillar abscesses, chronic otitis media, and dentoalveolar abscesses) have become relatively uncommon since the widespread use of antibiotics (penicillin or tetracycline) for the treatment of undiagnosed pharyngitis. Brain abscesses are a well-known complication of these upper respiratory tract infections in which bacteroides are involved along with other microorganisms, such as anaerobic streptococci.

Bacteroides bacteremia is characterized by a spiking fever, jaundice, and leukocytosis. In the patient more than forty years old, it is associated with chronic debilitating disease, hypotension, and a high mortality. Bacteremias have followed primary infection in the gastrointestinal, pelvic, and pharyngeal areas, and may originate from thrombophlebitis in these sites of infection. An indication of *Bacteroides* infection is the presence of a foul-smelling exudate from wounds or abscesses which contain gram-

negative forms but produce no growth on aerobic culture. There appears to be a disposition toward *Bacteroides* infection in patients with underlying malignant disease. Often these patients have undergone elective intestinal surgery after preoperative intestinal antisepsis. This suggests that changes in the normal intestinal flora may predispose to *Bacteroides* infection. Therefore, the surgeon should be alert to the possibility of *Bacteroides* infection. A changing pattern of pyogenic abscesses of the liver has been characterized by an increased incidence of *Bacteroides* as the pathogen.

Treatment of anaerobic infections consists of surgical drainage of abscesses, excision of necrotic tissue, and appropriate antibiotic therapy. This should be based upon the results of sensitivity tests, since anaerobes can be divided into two groups on the basis of antibiotic susceptibility tests, i.e., *Bacteroides fragilis* and all other anaerobes. Penicillin G is the drug of choice for virtually all anaerobic infections except those caused by *Bacteroides fragilis*, which require chloramphenicol or clindamycin. However, the efficacy of penicillin in some infections in which *Bacteroides fragilis* is present in mixed culture is due to its effectiveness against the other members of the mixed flora.

PSEUDOMYCOTIC INFECTIONS

Among the actinomycetes, *Actinomyces israelii* and *Nocardia asteroides* are isolated most frequently as human pathogens, although other species of each genus may also be implicated in human infections. Actinomycetes are true bacteria but traditionally have been studied and grouped with the fungi because of their resemblance to mycotic agents and their involvement in diseases resembling mycoses. Infections caused by these false fungi (pseudomyces) may be called pseudomycoses to separate them from true fungal infections. They will therefore be considered separately from the true mycoses.

Actinomycosis

Actinomyces israelii is a strict anaerobe present in normal oral flora. Actinomycosis is therefore an endogenous infection. There are three clinical types of actinomycosis: cervicofacial (the most common type), thoracic, and abdominal. A dense fibroblastic reaction is produced, and connective and granulation tissue tend to form a wall around the abscess. Wherever lesions occur, abscesses expand into contiguous tissue and form burrowing, tortuous sinuses to the outside, where they discharge pus and necrotic material. This pus contains dense clusters of organisms and hyphae appearing as macroscopic, yellow-brown "sulfur granules," which facilitate diagnosis when examined microscopically and cultured. Actinomycosis can be cured with massive doses of penicillin G or ampicillin. Tetracycline, lincomycin, and clindamycin are alternative agents. Surgical drainage of abscesses and aggressive resection of damaged tissue are important adjuncts to long-term chemotherapy.

Nocardiosis

Nocardia, in contrast to actinomycetes, are aerobic inhabitants of soil and are not part of the normal flora of man. *Nocardia asteroides* and *Nocardia brasiliensis,* opportunistic pathogens for man, are less acid-fast than mycobacteria, and their filaments tend to branch. Nocardiosis tends to be progressive and fatal but is a rare disease. Pulmonary infection arises from inhalation of the organisms, while subcutaneous abscesses (mycetomas) result from contamination of skin wounds, usually of the hands and feet of laborers. Massive doses of sulfonamides, e.g., sulfadiazine 6 to 8 Gm/day orally for at least 4 to 6 months, is the preferred therapy; ampicillin is an alternate agent. Drainage of empyema and abscesses is an important surgical adjunct to chemotherapy.

MYCOTIC INFECTIONS

The relation of the surgeon to mycotic infection has changed in recent years. The need for surgical treatment has diminished because of more effective modern chemotherapy. However, the long-term use of cytotoxic agents, corticosteroids, and antibacterial drugs for patients with leukemia and neoplasms has increased the incidence of opportunistic mycotic infections. Among the pathogenic fungi to be discussed, *Blastomyces dermatitidis, Paracoccidioides brasiliensis, Histoplasma capsulatum, Cryptococcus neoformans,* and even *Coccidioides immitis* are frank pathogens but may be opportunistic to the extent that they cause progressive infections in debilitated patients more frequently than in healthy ones. Definite opportunistic infections are caused by species of *Mucor, Rhizopus, Aspergillus,* and *Candida.* Fungal infection threatens any compromised hosts, such as severely burned patients and those with implanted prosthetic devices and transplanted organs. Some of the symptoms of mycotic disease are chronic skin or mucous membrane lesions, low-grade fever, weight loss, chronic pulmonary or meningeal involvement, hepatosplenomegaly, and lymphadenopathy. Mycotic disease should be suspected unless another cause

is clearly established. A mycosis may coexist with a lymphomatous disease, e.g., the association of histoplasmosis and cryptococcosis with Hodgkin's disease. A presumptive clinical diagnosis of a mycosis must be confirmed in the laboratory. Serologic tests are useful in reaching a presumptive diagnosis. The morphologic features of the fungus in tissue and culture are significant in identification.

The majority of patients with fungal infections seen by the physician have serious illness and present with typical symptoms of infection. Symptoms of pulmonary involvement frequently are present. Hematogenous dissemination of the disease produces manifestations such as tender swollen joints, draining subcutaneous abscesses, ulcerative lesions of the oropharynx, and meningitis. Many patients with systemic mycoses, as well as those with dermatophytoses, have skin lesions which are painful, itching, weeping, crusting, malodorous, and disfiguring. Fungi of ever-increasing importance as agents of infection in surgical patients are grouped in Table 5-7 according to the type of disease they cause and will be discussed in the order shown.

Blastomycosis (North American Blastomycosis)

Blastomyces dermatitidis is a dimorphic fungus; it grows in tissues and in culture at 37°C as a spherical thick-walled, single-budding yeast and in culture at room temperature as a mold. Lateral, rounded conidia borne along hyphae are presumably the infectious spores. Demonstration of nonencapsulated, thick-walled, multinucleate yeast cells in pus, sputum, or tissue sections and their subsequent laboratory culture establish the diagnosis. Blastomycosis usually begins in the lungs as a subacute respiratory infection (pulmonary form) which gradually increases in severity over a period of weeks or months and sometimes resembles tuberculosis or carcinoma. Frequently, during the course of infection, patients develop skin lesions. These may be the only apparent signs of blastomycosis. Pulmonary blastomycosis spreads hematogenously to establish focal destructive lesions in other parts of the body. Spreading, ulcerated, crusted skin lesions in particular arise as metastases from the primary pulmonary lesions. Cure has been

Table 5-7. MYCOSES IMPORTANT IN SURGICAL INFECTIONS

Type of disease	Mycosis	Representative fungus	Dimorphism	Infected tissue	Laboratory culture
Systemic	Blastomycosis	*Blastomyces dermatitidis*	Yes	Yeast	Mycelia
	Paracoccidioidomycosis	*Paracoccidioides brasiliensis*	Yes	Yeast	Mycelia
	Histoplasmosis	*Histoplasma capsulatum*	Yes	Yeast	Mycelia
	Coccidioidomycosis	*Coccidioides immitis*	Yes	Spherules	Mycelia
	Cryptococcosis	*Cryptococcus neoformans*	No	Yeast	Yeast
Subcutaneous	Sporotrichosis	*Sporotrichum schenckii*	Yes	Yeast	Mycelia
Systemic, particularly opportunistic . .	Phycomycosis	*Mucor corymbifera*	No	Mycelia	Mycelia
		Rhizopus oryzae	No	Mycelia	Mycelia
	Aspergillosis	*Aspergillus fumigatus*	No	Mycelia	Mycelia
	Candidosis	*Candida albicans*	Yes	Yeast and hyphae	Yeast and hyphae

effected in many cutaneous cases by 2-hydroxystilbami-dine. However, amphotericin B is indicated in treating all forms of blastomycosis. If surgery is indicated for diagnosis to rule out bronchogenic carcinoma, amphotericin is used both pre- and postoperatively to minimize operative spread.

Paracoccidioidomycosis (South American Blastomycosis)

Paracoccidioides brasiliensis is dimorphic and grows in tissue as a multiple-budding yeast, in contrast to the single-budding yeast in blastomycosis. Paracoccidioidomycosis is characterized by primary pulmonary lesions with dissemination to visceral organs, by conspicuous ulcerative granulomas of the buccal and nasal mucosa, and by generalized lymphangitis. In blastomycosis, visceral organs are *not* involved. Treatment with amphotericin B is usually effective.

Histoplasmosis

Histoplasma capsulatum is dimorphic; it appears characteristically in infected tissues as many, small, oval yeast cells packed within macrophages and reticuloendothelial cells; at room temperature it forms slowly growing mycelial colonies. This pathogen is present in soil, especially that enriched by feces of birds and bats, and is endemic in the Mississippi and Ohio valleys and along the Appalachian mountains of the United States. Inhalation of conidia leads to pulmonary infection. The initial infection is mild and may be inapparent or may occur as a primary acute disease. Symptoms may include fever, cough, chest pain, dyspnea, and pleurisy with effusion. Localized pulmonary histoplasmosis resembles tuberculosis in its histopathology. In a few individuals the infection becomes progressive and widely disseminated and may simulate miliary tuberculosis. Disseminated histoplasmosis primarily involves the reticuloendothelial system in various tissues and organs and often coexists in individuals who have tuberculosis, leukemia, or Hodgkin's disease. Histoplasmosis is treated with high doses of intravenous amphotericin B. In chronic cavitary disease surgical resection should be performed, with amphotericin therapy given before and after surgery to reduce postoperative complications and avoid relapse.

Coccidioidomycosis

Coccidioides immitis is a somewhat different dimorphic fungus; it varies in structure between a hyphal form found in soil and a spherule or sporangium form found in infected tissues. The sporangia are thick-walled structures filled with globular endospores or sporangiospores. At maturity the sporangium bursts and releases hundreds of endospores, each of which can form a new sporangium in tissue. When sporangia are plated on Sabouraud agar, growth of the mycelial form occurs. Barrel-shaped arthrospores are formed in the mycelium. These arthrospores are highly infectious and become airborne easily. The mycelial

(saprophytic) form is readily converted into the sporangium (parasitic) form in man. *Coccidioides immitis* is endemic in the southwestern United States and adjacent Mexico, where it grows as a saprophyte in desert soils. Infection is established by inhalation of airborne arthrospores.

About 60 percent of infected individuals remain asymptomatic but become skin-sensitive to coccidioidin. The acute and most common form of coccidioidomycosis resembles influenza. When confined to the lungs, the disease is usually self-limited and heals with scarring. However, a chronic, progressive, granulomatous disease occurs in fewer than 1 percent of infected individuals. Years may elapse between primary infection and the more serious disseminated disease. Patients with disseminated coccidioidomycosis appear to have some defect in their immune response to the fungus. The symptoms are similar to those seen in advancing tuberculosis. Any organ or tissue of the body may be involved. However, the infection shows predilection for bone, skin, and subcutaneous tissue. This disease is not contagious, since it is spread only by saprophytic arthrospores. The majority of patients with primary infection recover without therapy or with only symptomatic care. Amphotericin B is used to treat disseminated coccidioidomycosis but is less effective than with blastomycosis, histoplasmosis, and cryptococcosis.

Cryptococcosis

Cryptococcus neoformans is *not dimorphic;* in both infected tissue and in culture it appears as encapsulated yeast cells. The yeast cells are thin-walled, but the large, clear polysaccharide capsules surrounding them are distinctive. *Cryptococcus neoformans* is found in dust and bird droppings. Inhalation of yeast cells is thought to initiate pulmonary infection, which may be inapparent or mild. There is little inflammatory response of invaded tissues. Cryptococcosis is a subacute or chronic mycotic infection most frequently involving tissues of the central nervous system but occasionally producing lesions in the lungs or skin. Cryptococcal meningitis is the most frequent form of disseminated disease and mimics tuberculous meningitis, brain abscess, or brain tumor. Pulmonary lesions are usually found at autopsy. Many patients with pulmonary or dermal cryptococcosis respond to therapy with 5-fluorocytosine. Surgical resection is indicated for both cavitary and nodular pulmonary disease. When diagnosis is established by surgery, therapy with amphotericin B is begun postoperatively to avoid meningitis and recurrence. Amphotericin B is the drug of choice for cryptococcosis of the central nervous system. Cryptococcosis is an opportunistic mycosis in debilitated patients, particularly those with Hodgkin's disease or leukemia.

Sporotrichosis

Sporotrichum schenckii is dimorphic. When found in tissues or exudate stained by the periodic acid–Schiff technique, this fungus appears as fusiform bodies or round budding cells, but these are rarely seen. When these materials are cultured on Sabouraud agar at room temperature, the mycelial form grows. Microscopically, hyphae are slender and septate, and conidia are individually attached by sterigmata to a common conidiophore. Hyphae are converted to the yeast form by injection into mice and by cultivation at 37°C on enriched media. Man becomes infected by accidental subcutaneous inoculation from thorns and splinters. Sporotrichosis is a chronic progressive infection of the skin and subcutaneous tissue which frequently begins as a primary lesion of the skin of the hand or forearm and secondarily involves lymphatic channels and lymph nodes draining the area, which become cord-like, resulting in a chain of ulcers. Generalized infection occurs in the compromised host by way of the blood, and any organ or tissue can be the site of lesions. Symptoms are then related to the region involved. Orally administered potassium iodide is specific in sporotrichosis and must be continued for several weeks after recovery seems complete. Intravenous amphotericin B is indicated for disseminated sporotrichosis. *Sporotrichum schenckii* has caused suprainfection in patients with underlying hematologic malignant disease who have been treated with antitumor agents and steroids.

Phycomycosis

Species of *Mucor* and *Rhizopus* are saprophytes common in nature and are *not dimorphic*. They can produce rapidly fatal disease when they invade the brain, lungs, or other organs of a compromised host. These fungi may also produce a superficial infection of the skin with occasional ulceration and granuloma or abscess formation. *Mucor* and *Rhizopus* are opportunistic and are held in check by normal serum factors which become diminished in individuals suffering from uncontrolled diabetes mellitus, blood dyscrasias, endocrine disturbances, malnutrition, and burns. Corticosteroid therapy and prolonged use of broad-spectrum antibiotics may also enhance susceptibility to phycomycosis. The local cutaneous lesions heal with proper hygiene and fungicides; extensive lesions may require debridement. Amphotericin B and correction of the underlying disease is the therapy for the acute form of phycomycosis. Amphotericin should be used to treat any patient not responding to other measures. Surgery should be considered for patients with pulmonary lesions not responsive to amphotericin.

Aspergillosis

Aspergillus has become an important pathogen in patients with impaired host defenses. These mycelial fungi are saprophytic and are not dimorphic but can cause local as well as disseminated disease. *Aspergillus fumigatus* is the most commonly reported species. Two forms of pulmonary aspergillosis are frequently seen: (1) pulmonary or bronchial aspergilloma (fungus ball), due to secondary invasion of a tuberculous or coccidioidal cavity, and (2) allergic bronchopulmonary aspergillosis. In the compromised host these may proceed to disseminated infection. Otomycosis is secondary to bacterial infection of the ear. The fungus grows on ear wax and macerated tissue. Systemic aspergillosis may complicate severe underlying diseases which are being treated with steroids, immunosuppressive drugs, or broad-spectrum antibiotics. Local superficial lesions often heal spontaneously with hygienic care. Localized abscesses and granulomas should be excised. Systemic infection requires treatment with amphotericin B. The prognosis in disseminated aspergillosis is poor; the patient often succumbs to the underlying disease.

Candidosis

Candida albicans is indigenous in man and is dimorphic; both yeast and mycelial forms are seen in infected tissue. *Candida albicans* affects mucous membranes and causes diseases ranging from thrush (oral candidosis) and vulvovaginal candidosis to systemic candidosis. The former are common medical problems, the latter an opportunistic infection of the compromised host. Patients with hemopoietic and lymphoreticular neoplasms, as well as those being treated with immunosuppressives, glucocorticoids, and broad-spectrum antibiotics, are particularly prone to systemic fungal infections. Patients with burns and those undergoing intravenous hyperalimentation are also prone to systemic candidosis. Candidal endocarditis, especially that due to *Candida parapsilosis,* is seen in drug addicts using intravenous heroin.

Thrush and other clinically distinctive candidal infections frequently result from antibacterial therapy, and discontinuance of the therapy will usually cause the antibiotic-induced suprainfection to disappear. Topical nystatin is effective in treating candidal infections of the skin, mouth, and vagina. Amphotericin B is the mainstay in treating systemic candidosis. Oral 5-fluorocytosine is considerably less toxic than amphotericin, but 50 percent of *Candida* strains are initially resistant.

SURGICAL ASEPSIS

Surgical asepsis, the prevention of the access of microorganisms to an operative wound, is achieved by methods designed to destroy bacteria or remove them from all objects coming in contact with the wound. Modern surgery is aseptic in the use of sterile instruments, sutures, and dressings and in the wearing of sterile caps, gowns, masks, and rubber gloves by the operating personnel. Although this is presently the extent of routine sterility in surgical asepsis, the technology of germ-free research is able to provide sterile flexible plastic isolation chambers in which neonates or antibiotic-decontaminated patients may be maintained in a sterile environment. Operations may be performed in "surgical" isolators cemented to the operative site of the patient. The surgeon makes his incision through the site of attachment of the isolator, and the operation may be conducted in the absence of all microorganisms. There is currently considerable interest in unidirectional (laminar) airflow systems as a less absolute means of limiting the number of bacteria to which a patient is exposed. These systems recirculate air through high-efficiency particulate air filters that assure unidirectional flow in either a downward or horizontal direction. However, the advantages or necessity of such systems in operating rooms are controversial, since there has not yet been substantial evidence to demonstrate their effectiveness in reducing postoperative infections. The Committee on Control of Operating Room Environment of the American College of Surgeons does not recommend laminar airflow for general use in operating rooms.

It is necessary to resort to the use of antiseptics to degerm the site of the operation on the patient's skin. The surgeon and operating-room personnel usually use soaps or detergents containing antiseptics for scrubbing their hands before donning gloves or else rinse in an antiseptic after the scrub. An *antiseptic* is a chemical agent which either kills pathogenic microorganisms or inhibits their growth so long as there is contact between agent and microbe. By custom as well as by federal law, the term "antiseptic" is reserved for agents applied to the body. The antiseptic may actually be a disinfectant used in dilute solutions to avoid damage to tissues. A *disinfectant* is a germicidal, chemical substance used on inanimate objects to kill pathogenic microorganisms but not necessarily all others. These germicidal agents are used to disinfect instruments and other equipment which cannot be exposed to heat. They are essential for good housekeeping practices in hospitals, where they are used to disinfect floors, fabrics, and excreta. The first step in any process of biologic decontamination is thorough mechanical cleansing with soap or detergent and water to remove all traces of blood, pus, proteins, and mucus before the antiseptic or disinfectant is employed.

Sterilization

Sterilization is the process of killing all microorganisms (bacteria, spores, viruses, mycotic agents, and parasites). It is the ultimate in disinfection. The practical criterion of sterility is the failure of microbial growth to appear on tests in suitable bacteriologic media. Sterilization can be achieved by either physical or chemical agents. *Steam under pressure* is the most reliable means of sterilizing surgical supplies because of its power of penetration, microbiologic efficiency, ease of control, and economy of operation. Application of steam under a pressure of 15 psi (pounds per square inch) for 15 to 45 minutes will destroy all forms of life. Free-flowing steam, like boiling water, has a temperature of 100°C, but the same steam under pressure of 15 psi exerts a temperature of 121°C. Steam gives up heat by condensing into water. Thus when a bundle containing surgical pads or sponges is sterilized, the steam contacts the outer layer. There a portion of it condenses into water and releases heat. The steam then penetrates to a second layer, where another portion condenses and gives up heat. The steam thus approaches the center of the package, layer after layer, until the whole package is sterilized. The time of exposure depends upon the size of the parcel and its wrappings. Sterilization by steam under pressure is carried out in an autoclave. A major caution to be recognized when operating an auto-

clave is that a mixture of air and steam has a lower temperature than does pure steam. Therefore, when air is present in the chamber, the killing power of the process is diminished in proportion to the amount of air present. Most autoclaves depend upon gravity displacement of air from the chamber and from within articles being sterilized. Thus, improperly packed and positioned articles in the autoclave may fail to become sterile even though all physical conditions of the run may be correct. A new development in autoclaves is the high-vacuum sterilizer. A vacuum pump is incorporated into the system, and a vacuum is pulled in the chamber at the beginning and end of the sterilizing cycle. There is a considerable shortening of the time needed for sterilization, as only 3 minutes are needed to achieve sterility rather than the 20 minutes on the regular systems. In addition, there appears to be less damage to rubber, fabrics, and sharp instruments because of reduced exposure to moisture. There is less danger of creating air pockets and less chance of the steam's failing to penetrate to the center of bundles. Materials emerge dry, and much greater tolerances in packing the chamber are afforded.

Dry-heat sterilization is commonly used for glassware, for items that are injured by moisture, and for materials that resist penetration by steam, such as talc, vaseline, fats, and oils. The process consists of baking the material to be sterilized in a hot-air oven. At a temperature of 121°C (250°F) it takes about 6 hours to sterilize glassware, but at 170°C (340°F) the time required is about 1 hour. *Gas sterilization* is practical with ethylene oxide, a gas employed as a sterilizing agent in specially designed chambers in which temperatures and humidity can be controlled and from which air can be evacuated. The killing action is slow, and an exposure period from 3 to 6 hours is needed. Sterilization employing ethylene oxide is used for delicate surgical instruments with optical lenses, for tubing and plastic parts of heart-lung machines and respirators, for prepacked commercial plastic products such as disposable syringes, and for blankets, pillows, and mattresses. Ethylene oxide is most reliable when applied to clean, dry surfaces that do not absorb the chemical. The gas dissolves in plastic, rubber, fabric, and leather, and chemical burns may occur when materials laden with ethylene oxide are applied to tissue. The dissolved chemical escapes from materials when they are exposed to air, and a minimum of 24 hours of aeration is necessary to ensure removal of the gas from sterilized articles. However, solid metal or glass items may be used immediately after sterilization. *Radiation sterilization* refers to ionizing radiation by cobalt 60 sources (γ-radiation) and by electron accelerators (high-energy electrons). It is currently used commercially to sterilize disposable hospital supplies, such as plastic hyperdermic syringes and sutures. Radiation sterilization of heat-sensitive pharmaceuticals has been recommended.

Chemical sterilization is currently achieved with a 2% aqueous solution of glutaraldehyde. This compound is an effective disinfectant for surgical, anesthetic, and dental equipment, rubber and plastic mouthpieces, catheters, and other heat-sensitive hospital equipment. Either a buffered alkaline solution (Cidex) or a potentiated acid solution

(Sonacide) of glutaraldehyde may be used. They are equally bactericidal, sporicidal, and virucidal. Isopropyl alcohol may also be used for the chemical sterilization of instruments if they are first cleansed of all blood, pus, and body fluids. Only in the absence of spores is alcohol an effective sterilizing agent.

Degerming of Skin

Antiseptics incorporated into soaps are used for preoperative preparation of the skin at the operative site and for surgical hand scrubs by operating personnel. The bacteriologic content of normal skin consists of a resident flora, composed of coagulase-negative *Staphylococcus epidermidis* and anaerobic diphtheroides (e.g., *Propionibacterium acnes*), which reside on the surface of the skin, in hair follicles, and in the ducts of sebaceous glands. These bacteria can be diminished temporarily, but they cannot be permanently eradicated. They are not usually responsible for surgical infections. Superimposed upon the resident flora is a transient flora consisting of bacteria picked up as a result of temporary colonizing of the skin. In the hospital, this transient flora often consists of pathogens resistant to antibiotics and is likely to be composed of pathogenic strains of *Staphylococcus aureus* and gram-negative enterobacteria. Therefore, pathogenic bacteria on the hands of operating personnel at the time of operation must be removed by scrubbing and destroyed by an antiseptic agent. The patient's skin must be degermed in the area of operation prior to the incision. The most efficient method is a vigorous scrub with liquid soaps containing either hexachlorophene or an iodophor.

Hexachlorophene is a bisphenol which disinfects the skin slowly. Commercial preparations containing 3% hexachlorophene, a detergent, and liquid soap are used for surgical scrubbing. Over a period of days, regular use of these surgical soaps brings about a progressive decrease in the number of bacteria on and in the skin. The hexachlorophene leaves an active film, which is renewed with each scrubbing. Consequently, its antibacterial activity persists so long as one continues to wash with soap containing hexachlorophene. A single washing with ordinary soap removes the antibacterial film. Hexachlorophene is effective against gram-positive pathogens such as *Staphylococcus aureus,* but it is without activity against gram-negative bacteria, such as the pseudomonas and the enterobacteria. This fact should be seriously considered by anyone using hexachlorophene, since gram-negative bacteria are currently responsible for the majority of nosocomial infections.

Iodophors are organic complexes of iodine and a synthetic detergent. About 1% iodine is available in the formula, whose germicidal action results from the liberation of free iodine when the compound is diluted with water. The detergent in the complex enhances the bactericidal activity of the iodine. Advantages of iodophors are that they destroy both gram-positive and gram-negative bacterial cells, but not spores; they do not stain skin and clothing; and they do not produce allergic reactions. Iodophors

have been incorporated into surgical scrub soaps for hands and for the operative site.

Other Surgical Antiseptics

No economical antiseptic or disinfectant is available to kill all microbial flora in a reasonable time at concentrations which will not irritate tissue or damage medical devices. However, there are several agents that have high reliability and low toxicity as surgical antiseptics. Among them are alcohol and iodine. The combination of inorganic iodine and alcohol, either as a tincture or as a mixture of 1% to 3% iodine with 70% ethyl or isopropyl alcohol, kills both gram-positive and gram-negative bacteria. Only a short contact time is needed, and the solution itself is not likely to be contaminated. Some patients, however, have adverse reactions to iodine, and most physicians hesitate to use this combination on mucous membranes or denuded skin. Aqueous iodophor solutions are available as an alternative. These also have a broad antimicrobic spectrum and are not likely to be contaminated, and they provoke adverse reaction less frequently than do inorganic tinctures of iodine. For patients sensitive to iodine, a thorough scrub with soap and water followed by a 2-minute scrub with 70% to 90% ethyl or isopropyl alcohol is effective surgical antisepsis. Isopropyl alcohol is slightly more effective than ethyl alcohol when used as a 70% solution and is less expensive and more readily obtained because it is not potable. As a group, alcohols exhibit many desirable features. They are bactericidal, have a cleansing action, and evaporate readily. They do not, however, kill spores, and the best one can hope to accomplish with alcohol is to reduce the number of viable bacteria and destroy pathogens which may be on the skin as transients.

Aqueous quaternary ammonium compounds such as benzalkonium chloride (Zephiran Chloride) are used diluted 1:750 for skin antisepsis for venipuncture and for disinfection of cystoscopes, bronchoscopes, and intravenous tubing. They are less expensive than many other products and are nontoxic and nonallergenic but *must* be used with caution. Although they are potent bactericides in vitro and are particularly active against gram-positive cocci, benzalkonium antiseptics have been implicated in nosocomial infections by resistant *Pseudomonas cepacia* and *Enterobacter* species which contaminate working solutions of these compounds. Accordingly, there are few applications for quaternary ammonium compounds in hospitals other than for environmental sanitation. Alternative surgical antiseptics such as iodine, iodophors, and alcohol have a broad antibacterial spectrum.

References

Introduction; General Principles; Surgical Infections

Alexander, J. W.: Emerging Concepts in the Control of Surgical Infections, *Surgery,* **75**:934, 1974.
American College of Surgeons, Committee on Control of Surgical

Infections: "Manual on Control of Surgical Infections," J. B. Lippincott Company, Philadelphia, 1976.

Brummelkamp, W. H., Boerema, I., and Hoogendyk, L.: Treatment of Clostridial Infections with Hyperbaric Oxygen Drenching: A Report of 26 Cases, *Lancet,* **1:**235, 1963.

Casaubon, J.-N., Dion, M. A., and Larbrisseau, A.: Septic Cavernous Sinus Thrombosis after Rhinoplasty, *Reconstr Surg,* **59:**119, 1977.

Dubos, R. J.: "Biochemical Determinants of Microbial Diseases," Harvard University Press, Cambridge, Mass., 1954.

Holland, J. A., Hill, G. B., Wolfe, W. G., Osterhout, S., Saltzman, H. A., and Brown, I. W.: Experimental and Clinical Experience with Hyperbaric Oxygen in the Treatment of Clostridial Myonecrosis, *Surgery,* **77:**75, 1975.

Meleney, F. L.: "Treatise on Surgical Infections," Oxford University Press, New York, 1948.

————: "Clinical Aspects and Treatment of Surgical Infections," W. B. Saunders Company, Philadelphia, 1949.

Noble, W. C., and Somerville, D. A.: "Microbiology of Human Skin," W. B. Saunders Company, Philadelphia, 1974.

Polk, H. C., Jr., and Stone, H. H. (eds.): "Hospital-acquired Infections in Surgery," University Park Press, Baltimore, 1977.

Pulaski, E. J.: Common Bacterial Infections: Pathophysiology and Clinical Management," W. B. Saunders Company, Philadelphia, 1964.

Roding, B., Groeneveld, P. H. A., and Boerema, I.: Ten Years of Experience in The Treatment of Gas Gangrene with Hyperbaric Oxygen, *Surg Gynecol Obstet,* **134:**579, 1972.

Rosebury, T.: "Microorganisms Indigenous to Man," McGraw-Hill Book Company, New York, 1962.

Slack, W. K., Hanson, G. C., and Chew, H. E. R.: Hyperbaric Oxygen in the Treatment of Gas Gangrene and Clostridial Infection: A Report of 40 Patients Treated in a Single-Person Hyperbaric Oxygen Chamber, *Br J Surg,* **56:**505, 1969.

Wangensteen, O. H., Wangensteen, S. D., and Klinger, C. F.: Surgical Cleanliness, Hospital Salubrity, and Surgical Statistics, Historically Considered, *Surgery,* **71:**477, 1972.

Basic Considerations of Antibiotic Therapy

Crofton, J.: Some Principles in the Chemotherapy of Bacterial Infections, *Br Med J,* **2:**137, 209, 1969.

Kabins, S.: Interactions among Antibiotics and Other Drugs, *JAMA,* **219:**206, 1972.

Kantor, H. S., and Shaw, W. V.: Microbial Suprainfection. Recognition and Management, *Med Clin North Am,* **55:**471, 1971.

Pratt, W. B.: "Fundamentals of Chemotherapy," Oxford University Press, New York, 1973.

Weinstein, L., and Musher, D. M.: Antibiotic-induced Suprainfection, *J Infect Dis,* **119:**662, 1969. (Editorial.)

Yale, C. E., and Peet, W. J.: Antibiotics in Colon Surgery, *Am J Surg,* **122:**787, 1971.

Chemoprophylaxis; Intestinal Antisepsis; Intraperitoneal Antibiotics

Bernard, H. R., and Cole, W. R.: The Prophylaxis of Surgical Infection: The Effect of Prophylactic Antimicrobial Drugs on the Incidence of Infection following Potentially Contaminated Operations, *Surgery,* **56:**151, 1964.

Bornside, G. H., and Cohn, I., Jr.: Stability of Normal Human Fecal Flora During a Chemically Defined, Low Residue Diet, *Ann Surg,* **181:**58, 1975.

Burke, J. F.: Use of Preventive Antibiotics in Clinical Surgery, *Am Surg,* **39:**6, 1973.

Cohn, I., Jr.: "Intestinal Antisepsis," Charles C Thomas, Publisher, Springfield, Ill., 1968.

————: Intestinal Antisepsis, *Surg Gynec Obstet,* **130:**1006, 1970.

————, Langford, D., and Rives, J. D.: Antibiotic Support of Colon Anastomoses, *Surg Gynecol Obstet,* **104:**1, 1957.

DiVincenti, F. C., and Cohn, I., Jr.: Prolonged Administration of Intraperitoneal Kanamycin in the Treatment of Peritonitis, *Amer Surg,* **37:**177, 1971.

MacLean, L. D.: Prophylactic Antibiotic Therapy in Surgery, *Can J Surg,* **18:**243, 1975.

Nelson, J. L., Kuzman, J. H., and Cohn, I., Jr.: Intraperitoneal Lavage and Kanamycin for the Contaminated Abdomen, *Surg Clin North Am,* **55:**1391, 1975.

Nichols, R. L., Broido, P., Condon, R. E., Gorbach, S. L., and Nyhus, L. M.: Effect of Preoperative Neomycin-Erythromycin Intestinal Preparation on the Incidence of Infectious Complications Following Colon Surgery, *Ann Surg,* **178:**453, 1973.

————, and Condon, R. E.: Preoperative Preparation of the Colon, *Surg Gynecol Obstet,* **132:**323, 1971.

Smith, E. B.: A Rationale for Intraperitoneally Administered Antibiotic Therapy, *Surg Gynecol Obstet,* **143:**561, 1976.

Antimicrobial Agents

Garrod, L. P., Lambert, H. P., O'Grady, F., and Waterford, P. M.: "Antibiotic and Chemotherapy," 4th ed., Churchill Livingstone, Edinburgh, 1973.

Kagan, B. M. (ed.): "Antimicrobial Therapy," 2d ed., W. B. Saunders Company, Philadelphia, 1974.

Kucers, A., and Bennett, N. McK.: "The Use of Antibiotics: A Comprehensive Review with Clinical Emphasis," 2d ed., J. B. Lippincott Company, Philadelphia, 1975.

Smith, H.: "Antibiotics in Clinical Practice," 3d ed., University Park Press, Baltimore, 1977.

Streptococcal Infections

Abrams, J. S.: Role of Steroids in the Management of Phagedenic Ulcer, *Surgery,* **66:**297, 1969.

Altemeier, W. A., and Culbertson, W. R.: Acute Non-clostridial Crepitant Cellulitis, *Surg Gynecol Obstet,* **87:**206, 1948.

Armstrong, D., Blevins, A., Louria, D. B., Henkel, J. S., Moody, M. D., and Sukany, M.: Groups B, C, and G Streptococcal Infections in a Cancer Hospital, *Ann NY Acad Sci,* **174:**511, 1970.

Brewer, G. E., and Meleney, F. L.: Progressive Gangrenous Infection of the Skin and Subcutaneous Tissues, following Operation for Acute Perforative Appendicitis: A Study in Symbiosis, *Ann Surg,* **84:**438, 1926.

Grieco, M. H., and Sheldon, C.: *Erysipelothrix rhusopathiae, Ann NY Acad Sci,* **174:**523, 1970.

Ledingham, I. McA., and Tehrani, M. A.: Diagnosis, Clinical Course and Treatment of Acute Dermal Gangrene, *Br J Surg,* **62:**364, 1975.

MacLennan, J. D.: Streptococcal Infection of Muscle, *Lancet,* **1:**582, 1943.

Meleney, F. L., Friedman, S. T., and Harvey, H. D.: The Treatment of Progressive Bacterial Synergistic Gangrene with Penicillin, *Surgery,* **18**:423, 1945.

———, and Johnson, B. A.: Further Laboratory and Clinical Experiences in the Treatment of Chronic, Undermining, Burrowing Ulcers with Zinc Peroxide, *Surgery,* **1**:169, 1937.

Rea, W. J., and Wyrick, W. J., Jr.: Necrotizing Fasciitis, *Ann Surg,* **172**:957, 1970.

Stone, H. H., and Martin, J. D., Jr.: Synergistic Necrotizing Cellulitis, *Ann Surg,* **175**:702, 1972.

Strasberg, S. M., and Silver, M. S.: Hemolytic Streptococcus Gangrene: An Uncommon but Frequently Fatal Infection in the Antibiotic Era, *Am J Surg,* **115**:763, 1968.

Staphylococcal Infections

Altemeier, W. A., Hummel, R. P., and Hill, E. O.: Staphylococcal Enterocolitis following Antibiotic Therapy, *Ann Surg,* **157**:847, 1963.

Andriole, V. T., and Lyons, R. W.: Coagulase-negative Staphylococcus, *Ann NY Acad Sci,* **174**:533, 1970.

Elek, S. D.: "Staphylococcus Pyogenes and Its Relation to Disease," Livingstone Ltd., London, 1959.

Gorbach, S. L., and Bartlett, J. G.: Anaerobic Infections: Old Myths and New Realities, *J Infect Dis,* **130**:307, 1974. (Editorial.)

Hardaway, R. M., III, and McKay, D. G.: Pseudomembranous Enterocolitis: Are Antibiotics Wholly Responsible? *Arch Surg,* **78**:446, 1959.

Holland, J. W., Hill, E. O., and Altemeier, W. A.: Numbers and Types of Anaerobic Bacteria Isolated from Clinical Specimens since 1960, *J Clin Microbiol,* **5**:20, 1977.

Kramer, I. R. H.: Fatal Staphylococcal Enteritis Developing during Streptomycin Therapy by Mouth, *Lancet,* **2**:646, 1948.

Wilson, T. S., and Stuart, R. D.: *Staphylococcus albus* in Wound Infection and in Septicemia, *Can Med Assoc J,* **93**:8, 1965.

Clostridial Infections

Altemeier, W. A., and Fullen, W. D.: Prevention and Treatment of Gas Gangrene, *JAMA,* **217**:806, 1971.

Altemeier, W. A., and Hummel, R. P.: Treatment of Tetanus, *Surgery,* **60**:495, 1966.

Athavale, V. B., Pai, P. N., Fernandez, A., Patnekar, P. N., and Acharya, V. S.: Tetanus Neonatorium; Tetanus in Children, *Prog Drug Res,* **19**:189, 209, 1975.

Brooks, G. F., Buchanan, T. M., and Bennett, J. V.: Tetanus Toxoid Immunization of Adults: A Continuing Need, *Ann Intern Med,* **73**:603, 1970.

Cherubin, C. E.: Clinical Severity of Tetanus in Narcotic Addicts in New York City, *Arch Intern Med,* **121**:156, 1968.

Clay, R. C., and Bolton, J. W.: Tetanus Arising from Gangrenous Unperforated Small Intestine, *JAMA,* **187**:856, 1964.

DeJongh, D. S.: Postoperative Synergistic Gangrene, *JAMA,* **200**:227, 1967.

Dickinson, K. M., and Edgar, W. M.: Anaerobic Cellulitis of the Abdominal Wall after Prostatectomy and Orchidectomy, *Lancet,* **1**:1139, 1963.

Faust, R. A., Vickers, O. R., and Cohn, I., Jr.: Tetanus: 2,449 Cases in 68 Years at Charity Hospital, *J Trauma,* **16**:704, 1976.

Grainger, R. W., MacKenzie, D. A., and McLachlin, A. D.: Progressive Bacterial Synergistic Gangrene: Chronic Undermining Ulcer of Meleney, *Can J Surg,* **10**:439, 1967.

Isenberg, A. N.: *Clostridium welchii* Infection, *Arch Surg,* **92**:727, 1966.

Lowbury, E. J. L., and Lilly, H. A.: Contamination of Operating-Theatre Air with *Cl. tetani, Br Med J,* **2**:1334, 1958.

MacLennan, J. D.: The Histotoxic Clostridial Infections of Man, *Bacteriol Rev,* **26**:177, 1962.

McNally, M. J., and Crile, G., Jr.: Diagnosis and Treatment of Gas Gangrene of the Abdominal Wall, *Surg Gynecol Obstet,* **118**:1046, 1964.

Meleney, F. L.: Bacterial Synergism in Disease Processes: With a Confirmation of the Synergistic Bacterial Etiology of a Certain Type of Progressive Gangrene of the Abdominal Wall, *Ann Surg,* **94**:961, 1931.

Oakley, C. L.: Gas Gangrene, *Br Med Bull,* **10**:52, 1954.

Rubbo, S. D., and Suri, J. C.: Combined Active-Passive Immunization against Tetanus with Human Immune Globulin, *Med J Aust,* **2**:109, 1965.

Treadway, C. R., and Prange, A. J., Jr.: Tetanus Mimicking Psychophysiologic Reaction: Occurrence after Dental Extraction, *JAMA,* **200**:891, 1967.

Vakil, B. J., Singhal, B. S., Pandya, S. S., and Irani, P. F.: Cephalic Tetanus, *Prog Drug Res,* **19**:443, 1975.

Willis, A. T.: "Clostridia of Wound Infection," Butterworth Scientific Publications, London, 1969.

Aerobic Infections

Artenstein, M. S., and Sanford, J. P. (eds.): Symposium on *Pseudomonas aeruginosa, J Infect Dis,* Vol. 130, Suppl, November 1974.

DiGioia, R. A., Kane, J. G., and Parker, R. H.: Crepitant Cellulitis and Myonecrosis Caused by Klebsiella, *JAMA,* **237**:2097, 1977.

Forkner, C. E., Jr.: "Pseudomonas Aeruginosa Infections," Grune & Stratton, Inc., New York, 1960.

Kaul, B. K.: Operative Management of Typhoid Perforation in Children, *Int Surg,* **60**:407, 1975.

Reisig, G., and Schaffner, W.: Postoperative Detection of *Salmonella typhi, Arch Surg,* **104**:349, 1972.

Steinhauer, B. W., Eickhoff, T. C., Kislak, J. W., and Finland, M.: The *Klebsiella-Enterobacter-Serratia* Division: Chemical and Epidemiologic Characteristics, *Ann Intern Med,* **65**:1180, 1966.

Thong, M. L.: Acinetobacter Anitratus Infections in Man, *Aust NZ J Med,* **5**:435, 1975.

Wilkowske, C. J., Washington, J. A., II, Martin, W. J., and Ritts, R. E., Jr.: *Serratia marcescens:* Biochemical Characteristics, Antibiotic Susceptibility Patterns, and Clinical Significance, *JAMA,* **214**:2157, 1970.

Anaerobic Infections

Altemeier, W. A., Schowengerdt, C. G., and Whiteley, D. H.: Abscesses of the Liver: Surgical Considerations, *Arch Surg,* **101**:258, 1970.

Anderson, C. B., Marr, J. J., and Ballinger, W. F.: Anaerobic Infections in Surgery: Clinical Review, *Surgery,* **79**:313, 1976.

Finegold, S. M.: "Anaerobic Bacteria in Human Disease," Academic Press, New York, 1977.

Gorbach, S. L., and Bartlett, J. G.: Anaerobic Infections, *N Engl J Med,* **290**:1177, 1237, 1289, 1974.

Gorbach, S. L., and Bartlett, J. G. (eds.): The Role of Clindamycin in Anaerobic Bacterial Infections, *J Infect Dis,* Vol. 135, Suppl, March 1977. (Symposium.)

Holland, J. W., Hill, E. O., and Altemeier, W. A.: Numbers and Types of Anaerobic Bacteria Isolated from Clinical Specimens since 1960, *J Clin Microbiol,* **5:**20, 1977.

Leigh, D. A.: Wound Infections Due to *Bacteroides fragilis* Following Intestinal Surgery, *Br J Surg,* **62:**375, 1975.

Meyer, R. D., and Finegold, S. M.: Anaerobic Infections: Diagnosis and Treatment, *South Med J,* **69:**1178, 1976.

Sinkovics, J. G., and Smith, J. P.: Septicemia with Bacteroides in Patients with Malignant Disease, *Cancer,* **25:**663, 1970.

Stone, H. H., Kolb, L. D., and Geheber, C. E.: Incidence and Significance of Intraperitoneal Anaerobic Bacteria, *Ann Surg,* **181:**705, 1975.

Swenson, R. M., Lorber, B., Michaelson, T. C., and Spaulding, E. H.: The Bacteriology of Intra-abdominal Infections, *Arch Surg,* **109:**398, 1974.

Mycotic Infections

Bennett, J. E.: Chemotherapy of Systemic Mycoses, *N Engl J Med,* **290:**30, 323, 1974.

Bernhardt, H. E., Orlando, J. C., Benfield, J. R., Hirose, F. M., and Foos, R. Y.: Disseminated Candidiasis in Surgical Patients, *Surg Gynecol Obstet,* **134:**819, 1972.

Emmons, C. W., Binford, C. H., Utz, J. P., and Kwon-Chung, K. J.: "Medical Mycology," 3d ed., Lea & Febiger, Philadelphia, 1977.

MacMillan, B. G., Law, E. J., and Holder, I. A.: Experience with *Candida* Infections in the Burn Patient, *Arch Surg,* **104:**509, 1972.

Moss, E., and McQuown, A. L.: "Atlas of Medical Mycology," 3d ed., The Williams & Wilkins Company, Baltimore, 1969.

Nash, G., Foley, F. D., Goodwin, M. N., Jr., Bruck, H. M., Greenwald, K. A., and Pruitt, B. A., Jr.: Fungal Burn Wound Infection, *JAMA,* **215:**1664, 1971.

Nelson, A. R.: The Surgical Treatment of Pulmonary Coccidioidomycosis, *Curr Probl Surg,* October 1974.

Schroter, G. P. J., Temple, D. R., Husberg, B. S., Weil, R., III, and Starzl, T. E.: Cryptococcosis after Renal Transplantation, *Surgery,* **79:**268, 1976.

Surgical Asepsis

Block, S. S. (ed.): "Disinfection, Sterilization, and Preservation," 2d ed., Lea & Febiger, Philadelphia, 1977.

Bornside, G. H., Crowder, V. H., Jr., and Cohn, I., Jr.: A Bacteriological Evaluation of Surgical Scrubbing with Disposable Iodophor-Soap Impregnated Polyurethane Scrub Sponges, *Surgery,* **64:**743, 1968.

Collins, F. M., and Montalbine, V.: Mycobactericidal Activity of Glutaraldehyde Solutions, *J Clin Microbiol,* **4:**408, 1976.

Crowder, V. H., Jr., Bornside, G. H., and Cohn, I., Jr.: Bacteriological Comparison of Hexachlorophene and Polyvinylpyrrolidine-Iodine Surgical Scrub Soaps, *Am. Surg,* **33:**906, 1967.

Frank, M. J., and Schaffner, W.: Contaminated Aqueous Benzalkonium Chloride: An Unnecessary Hospital Infection Hazard, *JAMA,* **236:**2418, 1976.

Kaslow, R. A., Mackel, D. C., and Mallison, G. F.: Nosocomial Pseudobacteremia: Positive Blood Cultures Due to Contaminated Benzalkonium Antiseptic, *JAMA,* **236:**2407, 1976.

Levenson, S. M., Trexler, P. C., Malm, O. J., LaConte, M. L., Horowitz, R. E., and Moncrief, W. H.: A Plastic Isolator for Operating in a Sterile Environment, *Am J Surg,* **104:**891, 1962.

Chapter 6

Trauma

by G. Tom Shires

GENERAL CONSIDERATIONS

(by G. Tom Shires and Ronald C. Jones)

The magnitude of the problem of trauma in the United States is probably not adequately appreciated. In this country trauma is the leading cause of death in the first three decades of life. It ranks overall as the fourth leading cause of death in the United States today; if arteriosclerosis is considered as a single entity, trauma is the third leading cause of death. Fifty million injuries occur annually in the United States, over ten million of them being disabling. Over 100,000 deaths occur each year from accidents. Automobile accidents alone kill more Americans each year than were lost during the entire Korean conflict. Unlike many serious disease entities in the United States, the incidence of and mortality from injuries are increasing each year.

Accident patients take up to 22 million hospital bed days a year in the United States—more than are needed to take care of the delivery of all the babies in a given year, more than are needed by all the heart patients, and four times more than are needed by all cancer patients. Even during wartime, deaths from accidents always exceed battle deaths. In World War II, United States battle deaths were 292,000; accidental civilian deaths during the same period in the United States alone were 450,000. And more military personnel die from accidents than from combat during a period of national involvement.

An attempt will be made in this chapter to cover certain principles related to injuries, as well as selected areas of bodily injury. The following discussions of certain specifics of the patient who has sustained trauma will, of necessity, omit several critical areas concerned with care of the traumatized patient. These related problems are being discussed elsewhere in the text and include related principles such as those of shock, cardiac arrest, transfusion problems, pulmonary ventilation, and surgical infections initiated by trauma. Other organ system injuries covered elsewhere include burns, injuries to central nervous system, thoracic trauma, and genitourinary trauma. Similarly, complications including renal failure and embolism are covered in detail in separate chapters.

Initial Resuscitation of the Severely Injured Patient

The patient with multiple injuries is best managed by one physician. When the responsibility is divided, evaluation of the patient's overall problems may be lacking, and complications may not be recognized for several hours.

PRIORITY BY INJURY

There are three categories of patients, according to immediacy of injury. The first group includes injuries which interfere with vital physiologic function and therefore immediately threaten life, such as obstruction of an airway or bleeding from a gunshot wound. The primary treatment is to establish an airway and control the bleeding. This type of patient may require surgical treatment for massive internal bleeding within 5 to 10 minutes following arrival in the emergency room. The operating room should be alerted when the patient is admitted to the emergency room, and no time is wasted in getting the patient into "operative" condition. Often the control of hemorrhage is dependent on a rapid thoracotomy or laparotomy to occlude injured major vessels.

A second group of patients are those with injuries which offer no immediate threat to life. These include patients who have received gunshot wounds, stab wounds, or blunt trauma to the chest and abdomen but whose vital signs are stable. The majority of injured patients are in this category. Although they will require surgical procedures within 1 to 2 hours, there is time for additional information to be obtained. Blood for typing and cross matching is drawn, and blood is made available if there is any possibility that the patient will require surgical intervention. If vital signs are stable, x-rays may be obtained to determine the course of the missile and the extent of possible associated injuries, such as fractures. Cystography and pyelography may be done to assess hematuria. Since patients with penetrating and blunt abdominal injuries may develop shock at any moment, a physician must be in constant attendance during all evaluations. Patients who suddenly go into shock are immediately taken to the operating room without additional diagnostic procedures.

The third group of patients are those whose injuries produce occult damage. This group is composed primarily of patients who have sustained blunt trauma to the abdomen which may or may not require surgical intervention and in whom the exact nature of the injury is not apparent. These patients usually have time for extensive laboratory studies, x-rays, and more complete physical examination.

Surgical intervention in this group may be delayed hours or days, as with delayed rupture of the spleen.

Patients who are severely injured should be admitted to the emergency room in a trauma area equipped for emergency resuscitation. This room should contain such items as intravenous fluids, overhead operating-room light, oxygen, cardiac monitor and defibrillator, and a portable carriage which is suitable for an operating-room table in an emergency situation. A cabinet should be in the room containing a tracheostomy tray, closed chest drainage tray, venous section tray, closed-chest drainage bottle, intravenous fluids with tubing and needles, and syringes for four-quadrant abdominal paracentesis and pericardiocentesis. The cabinet shelf should have clearly visible labels under each tray or set of instruments. These trays and instruments should be kept in this trauma room and not in central supply, as a waiting period of even 5 minutes may prove fatal.

ADEQUATE AIRWAY. The first and most important emergency measure in the management of the severely injured patient is to establish an effective airway. A cabinet should be available at the head of the emergency room carriage in which a laryngoscope and cuffed endotracheal tubes of various sizes are available. Endotracheal intubation is a most rapid method of obtaining an adequate airway. Once an airway is established, a means of positive-pressure breathing should be available, such as an Ambu bag or an intermittent positive-pressure breathing machine. A cuffed endotracheal tube is desirable, so that positive-pressure breathing may be accomplished if needed in the resuscitation or in the administration of anesthesia. Either wall suction or a portable suction machine must be available in the trauma room to remove pulmonary secretions, foreign bodies, and, frequently, blood from the upper respiratory tract. When an endotracheal tube cannot readily be inserted, a tracheostomy may be done.

SHOCK AND HEMORRHAGE. Shock is usually controlled while the patient's airway is being cleared by another person. Internal hemorrhage will require immediate surgical intervention. Hypovolemic shock is best prevented or controlled by starting intravenous infusions in at least two extremities, using 18-gauge needles or cutdown catheters of comparable size. At least one upper extremity should be chosen for the intravenous infusion in the presence of abdominal wounds. If the inferior vena cava or one of its major tributaries is partially severed, the intravenous fluid may pour from the lower extremity into the retroperitoneal space, depriving the heart of any infusion from the lower extremities. A balanced salt solution such as Ringer's lactate solution is usually started until blood is available. Blood for typing and cross matching is drawn at the time the intravenous fluid is started, and the balanced salt solution is given in addition to the blood. Shock resulting from a blood loss of 500 to 750 ml can usually be corrected by rapid administration of 2 liters of Ringer's lactate solution over a 15- to 20-minute period. Blood loss in excess of 750 ml usually requires the administration of whole blood in addition to balanced salt solution. Often, 2 liters of balanced salt solution will replace the volume and correct hypotension so that no blood is necessary, reducing the possibility of blood transfusion reaction. When a patient initially responds to 1 to 2 liters of balanced salt solution, as evidenced by a normal blood pressure and decrease in pulse rate, but subsequently becomes hypotensive, whole blood usually is indicated. However, by this time, type-specific blood usually is available and often cross-matched, which reduces the chances for a transfusion reaction. Should a patient not respond to the rapid administration of 2 liters of balanced salt solution, un-cross-matched, type O, Rh-negative blood is administered without hesitation. The administration of blood from plastic bags markedly decreases the possibility of an air embolus when blood is being pumped.

External bleeding is best controlled by direct finger pressure on the bleeding wound or vessel. Tourniquets are of little benefit in the control of major arterial bleeding and often injurious if they occlude collateral circulation. A frequent mistake is the placement of a tourniquet on an extremity tight enough to obstruct venous return but loose enough not to inhibit arterial flow; this only increases the blood loss and edema. The danger of tissue loss from tourniquet use is always present.

Superficial vessels may be ligated if they are readily seen; however, wounds are not probed in a blind attempt to place a hemostat on a vessel. As soon as bleeding is controlled, the wound is covered with a sterile dressing, and the patient is taken to the operating room, where the wound is more adequately visualized and proper instruments are available. The needless probing of wounds in the emergency room may lead to severe infection, which can be avoided by proper exploration including adequate irrigation and sterile surgical technique in the operating room.

NEUROLOGIC EVALUATION. After an adequate airway has been obtained and hemorrhage has been controlled, a gross neurologic evaluation of the patient is undertaken. Motor function in the four extremities should be verified. A progressing neurologic deficit following injury to the spinal cord may indicate an emergency laminectomy. Decompression of a hematoma may result in return of function. Thoracoabdominal injuries usually take precedence over orthopedic or neurologic injury.

CHEST INJURIES. Airway obstruction may be due to mucus, fragments of bone from facial fractures, dirt and debris, and, commonly, broken teeth or dentures. If the patient does not ventilate normally after an endotracheal tube is inserted or a tracheostomy has been performed, several injuries should be considered. These include pneumothorax, hemothorax, cardiac tamponade, flail chest, and a ruptured bronchus.

Pneumothorax. If a pneumothorax is questionable, an 18-gauge needle may be inserted into the chest in the anterior axillary line and aspiration done to reveal the presence of air. A chest x-ray is preferable, but often severe respiratory distress precludes time for x-ray confirmation. Tension pneumothorax with mediastinal shift is suggested by displacement of the trachea to the opposite side. Auscultation of the chest may reveal decreased breath sounds.

The patient with a pneumothorax is treated with closed-chest drainage. As there is little danger from the insertion of a chest tube in the absence of a pneumothorax, an anterior chest tube should be inserted if there is doubt.

Hemothorax. Diagnosis of hemothorax is similar to that of pneumothorax. If the patient on the emergency-room cart is in distress, a needle may be inserted in the eighth interspace in the posterior axillary line and aspiration done to reveal a hemothorax. This is best drained with both anterior and posterior chest tubes. The anterior chest tube is placed in the second interspace in the midclavicular line, and the posterior chest tube is placed in the eighth interspace in the posterior axillary line in the region between the midaxillary and posterior axillary line. Chest tubes are of large caliber and soft rubber so that adequate drainage may be maintained. Thoracotomy may be indicated, depending on the rate of bleeding or the presence of intrathoracic clots.

Cardiac Tamponade. During initial observation, an unsuspected cardiac tamponade may develop secondary to blunt or penetrating trauma. This is often not present on arrival in the emergency room but may develop after 1 to 2 hours of observation. The clinical signs pathognomonic for cardiac tamponade are increased venous pressure, decreased pulse pressure, particularly with a paradoxical pulse and with or without cyanosis, and subsequent development of hypotension and decreased heart sounds. Emergency treatment includes aspiration of the pericardial sac with an 18-gauge needle through the xyphocostal angle. As little as 20 ml of aspirated blood may make a remarkable difference in the patient's vital signs. Depending on the cause of cardiac tamponade, immediate thoracotomy may be required to repair the cardiac wound, or the patient may be observed until a second aspiration is necessary. Following the development of the second cardiac tamponade, almost all patients will require an emergency thoracotomy. When a patient arrives at the emergency room in shock without evidence of blood loss, this diagnosis should be suspected.

Flail Chest. Unless patients sustaining blunt trauma to the thorax and abdomen are fully disrobed in the emergency room, a flail chest may not be recognized. Patients sustaining flail chest are best treated immediately with tracheostomy and intermittent positive-pressure breathing (IPPB). This promptly expands the lungs and provides adequate ventilation, often preventing the development of atelectasis and pneumonia. Some type of stabilizing apparatus such as towel clips may be beneficial. However, towel clips alone may not be effective, since the patient may not ventilate as well without intermittent positive-pressure breathing. Sandbags are of little value and may lead to the development of pulmonary complications such as atelectasis.

Ruptured Bronchus. After rupture of a bronchus, respiratory distress, hemoptysis, cyanosis, and a massive air leak with both mediastinal and subcutaneous emphysema and/or tension pneumothorax may be observed. Often the diagnosis is not obvious. There is a close relationship between fractures of the first and second ribs and rupture of a bronchus. If extrapleural hematoma is noted, special views of the first ribs are indicated. A ruptured bronchus is treated initially with closed-chest drainage. If this does not effectively keep the lung expanded, open thoracotomy with repair of the bronchus is indicated.

Open Chest Wounds. The patient with a chest injury resulting in a sucking chest wound is best managed by immediately covering the open wound with whatever material is available, such as a large gauze bandage. This prevents further shifting of the mediastinum and allows ventilation of the opposite lung. Chest tubes are usually inserted prior to operation, and immediate surgical intervention is indicated.

Ruptured Thoracic Aorta. The diagnosis may be suspected from chest x-ray showing a widened mediastinum and confirmed by arteriography. Immediate operation usually is indicated.

PENETRATING WOUNDS OF THE ABDOMINAL WALL. All penetrating injuries to the abdominal wall are explored locally in the emergency room to determine if the peritoneal cavity is penetrated. Exploration is usually accomplished by extending the stab wound and determining its depth. In the event that the extent of penetration cannot be determined or if the stab wound violates the posterior rectus abdominis sheath, the abdominal cavity is explored. The use of radiopaque material to determine abdominal cavity penetration has been reported, but until the accuracy of this method is better confirmed, questionable penetrating injuries of the abdominal cavity should be explored. The mortality and morbidity from a negative abdominal exploration is negligible, but failure to discover such injuries as colon or liver injury for several hours may allow peritonitis and other complications to develop. All gunshot wounds of the abdomen should be explored whether penetration is evident or not. Shock waves from nonpenetrating gunshot wounds of the abdominal wall often easily transect bowel or lacerate the liver or spleen without entering the abdominal cavity.

THE UNCONSCIOUS PATIENT. Patients with closed head injuries who are unconscious must have an airway established immediately. Hypotension rarely' results from a closed head injury but is almost always caused by blood loss, usually in the thorax or abdomen. The cause of the blood loss is most rapidly determined by using an 18-gauge needle for immediate abdominal and chest taps, which may reveal nonclotting blood. The absence of blood does not rule out an intraabdominal or thoracic injury. Extreme care should be used in moving unconscious patients until injuries of the spine have been ruled out, as repositioning the head may result in transection of the spinal cord.

Immediate Nonoperative Surgical Care

HEMATURIA. A Foley catheter is routinely inserted, particularly following blunt trauma to the abdomen, to determine the presence of hematuria as well as to follow the urinary output during and immediately following the surgical procedure. Gross hematuria is evidence of urinary tract injury resulting from contusion, laceration, or rupture.

If the patient's vital signs are stable and hematuria is present, a combined cystogram and intravenous pyelogram should be done. A single 15-minute film is usually adequate to determine kidney function as well as indicate extravasation from the bladder, ureter, or kidneys. Failure to demonstrate extravasation does not rule out the possibility of a ruptured bladder or kidney. Should a nephrectomy be required during a laparotomy, functioning of the kidney on the opposite side should be proved. It is useless to attempt to visualize the kidneys by intravenous pyelogram when the patient is hypotensive. X-rays are delayed until the patient has been resuscitated and bleeding has been controlled in the operating room. If time is not available preoperatively for an intravenous pyelogram, a cassette may be placed under the patient prior to the start of surgical procedures and a pyelogram obtained intraoperatively.

FRACTURES. Fractures of the extremities are best managed immediately with splints, such as a Thomas splint for the lower extremities and an arm board for the upper extremities. Immobilization may prevent additional nerve and blood vessel injury and conversion of a closed fracture to an open one. The presence or absence of pulses in the fractured extremities should be noted on initial examination. Intravenous infusions should not be started in an injured extremity. Massive thoracoabdominal bleeding takes precedence over fractures, unless there is an accompanying arterial injury of such magnitude that there is danger of loss of limb. In such instances, it is often necessary to have two surgical teams working simultaneously.

Pelvic fractures usually are managed conservatively with a pelvic binder, traction, or only bed rest. Inability to insert a Foley catheter into the urethra following a pelvic fracture may indicate a fractured urethra.

ARTERIAL INJURIES. Any penetrating injury in the region of a major blood vessel or nerve requires surgical exploration. On initial examination, 18 percent of subsequently proved arterial injuries are noted to have a normal pulse distal to the arterial injury, and one-third of the patients have a palpable but diminshed distal pulse. Arteriography is time-consuming and often will not demonstrate extravasation if the vessel injury is covered by a clot. If the platysma muscle in the neck has been violated, the neck is explored, and carotid and/or subclavian vessels also are explored. Vessel exploration in the region of the neck should be done under endotracheal anesthesia and may require resection of a portion of the clavicle for adequate visualization. Early recognition of an arterial injury is the most important factor in preserving a viable extremity or functioning distal organ.

Diagnosis and Management of Unapparent Injury

Blunt trauma to the abdomen may produce severe intraperitoneal or retroperitoneal injury with minimal physical findings. Bowel sounds may not be lost for several hours, and evidence of retroperitoneal or intraabdominal injury may not become apparent for as long as 18 hours.

An abdominal paracentesis may be performed early in the observation period in patients with injuries from blunt trauma to the abdomen. A 95 percent diagnostic accuracy is associated with the positive abdominal tap, and even a tap which yields only a few drops of nonclotting blood is indication for abdominal exploration. A negative abdominal tap does not rule out intraabdominal injury; if injury is still suspected, peritoneal lavage is indicated. Strong suspicion of intraabdominal injury in the female with a negative abdominal tap calls for culdocentesis. Patients with signs of peritoneal irritation require exploratory laparotomy even in the absence of a positive abdominal tap.

ROENTGENOGRAMS. These are taken when a patient's vital signs remain stable but are omitted for patients in severe shock. X-rays of the chest and abdomen are routinely performed to rule out foreign bodies such as knife blades within the depths of the wound. Patients sustaining gunshot wounds should have x-rays when possible in an attempt to trace the course of the missile. Patients sustaining blunt trauma often require multiple x-rays to rule out obscure fractures of the vertebral spine and retroperitoneal injuries. X-rays of extremities will be of value in determining whether or not the missile struck bone, fractured bone, or passed near vital structures.

NASOGASTRIC INTUBATION. A Levin tube is routinely inserted in the severely injured patient. Passage of the tube may provoke vomiting and empty the stomach of large particles, preventing subsequent aspiration during anesthesia. Stomach injury from penetrating or blunt trauma may be diagnosed by finding bright red blood in the Levin tube drainage. Gastric intubation prevents gastric dilatation during tracheal intubation and aids in the prevention of postoperative distension of the small bowel.

PROPHYLACTIC ANTIBIOTICS. Antibiotics are administered preoperatively to all patients sustaining penetrating wounds of the abdomen, beginning as soon as possible after the injured patient arrives in the emergency room. They may be discontinued if exploratory laparotomy is negative. Considerable experimental evidence indicates that prophylactic antibiotics in trauma are of benefit if administered within the first 3 hours following injury. A recent review of a group of patients at Parkland Memorial Hospital, Dallas, Texas, who sustained penetrating abdominal injuries showed that there was a statistically significant decrease in the incidence of wound infection in those patients who received antibiotics preoperatively or intraoperatively as opposed to those who received antibiotics in the immediate postoperative period or therapeutically. Following injury, immunized patients are administered a tetanus toxoid booster. In unimmunized patients the wound is debrided, and 250 units of tetanus human immune globulin is administered. Patients who were previously immunized but are now taking steroids, immunosuppressive therapy, or chemotherapy or who have had extensive irradiation should receive human immune globulin, since they may not have normal antibody response. Contaminated wounds should be left open or converted to open wounds when feasible.

METABOLIC RESPONSE TO TRAUMA

(by Malcolm O. Perry)

Trauma acutely and extensively alters the delicate integration of endocrine and metabolic systems in man (see Chap. 1). The wide range of response correlates with the magnitude of injury and the metabolic adjustments of which the patient is capable. Moore has divided the metabolic response into four phases: (1) the initial injury reaction, lasting 2 to 4 days; (2) the turning point, requiring 1 to 2 days; (3) an anabolic period, characterized by protein synthesis and lasting 2 to 5 weeks; (4) a period of several months of final adjustment in which "fat gain" is preponderant. These metabolic responses can be conveniently grouped into two categories: endocrine and catabolic.

Endocrine Response

Following injury, there is increased urinary excretion of epinephrine, norepinephrine, and their metabolic products. Although the measurement of blood levels of catecholamines does not always correlate well with the clinical findings, sympathicoadrenal activity is present. During the early stages the patient frequently exhibits tachycardia, sweating, and vasoconstriction, and is pale and apprehensive. Although the clinical signs may disappear relatively rapidly, elevated urinary levels of catecholamines and their metabolic products may persist for 1 or 2 days. If no complications follow the initial traumatic episode, the primary effects of sympathicoadrenal action are noted only during the early stages of the injury and pass rather rapidly.

Many of the metabolic changes noted following injury are similar to those induced by the administration of excessive amounts of cortisone or hydrocortisone. Urinary excretion of conjugated steroids is increased in the posttraumatic period. The normal excretion of 10 to 20 mg of 17-hydroxycorticosteroids may be tripled during the first 3 to 4 days following an injury of moderate severity. If shock or liver injury has not occurred, peak blood levels of 17-hydroxycorticosteroids are obtained about 6 hours after trauma. This reaction appears to be nonspecific and more closely related to the severity of the injury than to the specific type of injury. There is a less exact correlation between the negative nitrogen balance and the increasing levels of corticosteroid production. It has been observed that even in adrenalectomized rats urinary nitrogen excretion increases after injury if the animals are maintained on constant amounts of adrenocortical extracts, suggesting that the metabolic changes which follow injury are not directly related to the absolute level of corticosteroid production. This observation accords with the concept of the corticosteroids exerting a "permissive" or "conditioning" action.

The exact relationship between injury and the function of other endocrine glands remains unclear. The increase in oxygen consumption and carbon dioxide production following injury suggests that the thyroid gland may play an essential role, but similar effects can be produced by a variety of influences in the absence of trauma. Various measurements of thyroid function fail to correlate well with energy changes in the traumatized patient. The increased calcium excretion following injury can be related quite well to immobilization, and parathyroid function need not be invoked to explain calcium loss. Somatotropin, or growth hormone, has a profound effect on body metabolism, particularly skeletal growth and the synthesis of protein. Normal growth and development seem to be directly related to its presence, but there is no evidence that this hormone is necessary for normal convalescence. At the present time, the exact reaction of these other endocrine glands to injury is unclear.

Catabolic Response

Catabolism is increased following injury. Dissolution of body protein is reflected by increased urinary nitrogen excretion; after extensive trauma or with infection, levels of 15 to 20 Gm/day may be reached. The increased rate of excretion may persist for 3 to 5 days in the uncomplicated case. This can be reduced by the administration of exogenous protein and other compounds which supply calories, thus decreasing the effect of starvation. The inability to prevent these nitrogen losses completely indicates a definite catabolic effect in excess of that produced by starvation.

If water gain and loss are kept at minimal rates, careful weight measurements will reveal a loss of body tissue. A urinary loss of approximately 10 Gm of nitrogen represents about 62 Gm of protein loss, or about 300 Gm of wet lean muscle. The protein in bone and connective tissue and in plasma less readily reflect these changes. There can be, in fact, large losses or gains in protein without detectable changes in the concentrations of plasma proteins.

As initial responses to injury dissipate, a relatively abrupt change toward normal occurs in urinary nitrogen excretion. With sufficient caloric intake, protein balance is restored. If subsequent complications do not occur, net protein gain is prominent, and recovery proceeds rapidly. This gain, however, is usually much slower than the initial loss. It will often require three to six times as long to repair the protein deficit as it took to create it. If protein and caloric intake are satisfactory, the level eventually obtained is quite close to that prior to the loss.

Metabolic Requirements

ENERGY. The normal person at rest may require 2000 kcal/day, but a febrile, severely injured patient may use 4000 kcal in a single day. Variable periods of starvation almost inevitably follow severe trauma, and weight loss in excess of water loss may reach as high as 100 Gm daily as the energy demands are met by the consumption of body tissue.

Initial energy needs are supplied by the body stores of carbohydrate, 300 to 500 Gm being present as liver and muscle glycogen. The supply is exhausted within 14 to 18 hours after severe trauma, and subsequent energy requirements must be supplied by body tissues. In the postinjury period, 200 to 500 Gm of fat may be oxidized daily to yield 1800 to 4500 kcal. This is greatly in excess of the 1000 to 1300 kcal liberated by the oxidation of 100 to 150 Gm of fat/day in starvation.

Although the major contribution to energy needs comes from the oxidation of fat, protein catabolism yields a significant number of calories. Normal daily intake of 70 Gm of protein results in the urinary excretion of some 10 Gm of nitrogen daily. Following extensive injury, urinary nitrogen may reach levels as high as 20 Gm/day, representing the liberation of more than 500 kcal.

The production of energy is dependent upon the oxidation of metabolites via the tricarboxylic cycle. The two carbon fragments, active acetate or coenzyme A (CoA), assume a pivotal position in this important process. Acetyl CoA combines with oxaloacetic acid to form citric acid, which is subsequently degraded stepwise to yield eight hydrogen atoms, two molecules of carbon dioxide, and oxaloacetic acid. The eight electrons liberated by specific dehydrogenases then are introduced into the electron transport charge for transfer to oxygen. By oxidative phosphorylation the energy of foodstuffs is thus converted to adenosinetriphosphate (ATP), which is the ultimate driving force for most of the energy reactions within the cells (Fig. 6-1).

Intravenously administered carbohydrate solutions may supply a significant portion of the caloric needs for these energy processes. These solutions also may exert a protein-sparing effect, thus reducing the dissolution of lean body tissue. Approximately 100 Gm of carbohydrate appears to be adequate to obtain maximal protein sparing. As the first phase of injury passes, parenteral feeding is replaced by oral intake, and anabolic processes approach normal although the need for increased caloric supply often continues. Moore indicates that approximately 1 Gm of nitrogen and 20 kcal/kg of body weight/day are necessary to ensure restoration of body tissues during early convalescence.

CARBOHYDRATES. Although present in relatively small amounts, the monosaccharide glucose occupies a very important position because of its ready availability for energy. The two carbon fragments are intermediates in fatty acid metabolism and energy production. Via transamination reactions, glucose eventually may be converted to amino acids and proteins. Thus, glucose is an important precursor to fat and protein, as well as a supplier of oxidative energy.

Approximately 55 percent of absorbed carbohydrate is rapidly introduced into the Krebs cycle and converted into energy, carbon dioxide, and water. A portion of the remaining carbohydrate is converted to fat or protein, and about 5 percent is stored as liver and muscle glycogen. The carbohydrate in muscle is not readily available for use except by the muscle, but liver glycogen can easily be broken down and used elsewhere in the body. This glycogen is rapidly depleted in periods of starvation and in less

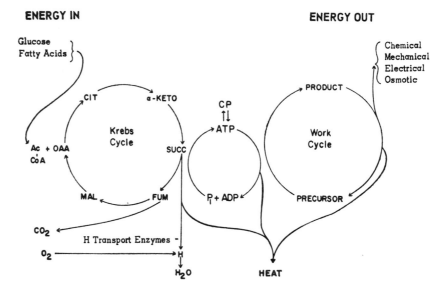

ENERGY IN   **ENERGY OUT**

Fig. 6-1. Schema of the mechanism of energy produced within the cell. OAA, oxalacetic acid; CIT, citric acid; α-KETO, α-ketoglutaric acid; SUCC, succinic acid; FUM, fumaric acid; MAL, malic acid; ADP, adenosinediphosphate; P_1, inorganic phosphate; ATP, adenosinetriphosphate; CP, creatine phosphate. (*From R. E. Olson, JAMA, 183:471, 1963.*)

than 5 hours may be exhausted if gluconeogenesis is interdicted. Without supplemental carbohydrate body tissues must be used to meet energy requirements.

FAT. Fat is rapidly oxidized to yield energy during starvation. From 75 to 100 Gm daily is mobilized under these conditions, but after extensive injury, as much as 500 Gm/day may be used. In addition to energy, free water is obtained. Although neutral fat contains little free water, the oxidation of 1 kg of fat liberates more than 1,000 ml of water.

VITAMINS. The suggested daily requirements of vitamins have been outlined by the National Research Council Committee on Nutrition. The exact vitamin requirements of the injured patient are not known, but it is probable that the vitamin C requirement is increased out of proportion to those of the other vitamins. There is a great individual variability in requirement for ascorbic acid in healthy adults, and it has been observed that blood level or buffy coat determinations for vitamin C do not necessarily reflect the magnitude of the deficit. It is widely held that the failure of wound healing and subsequent dehiscence is related more to the lack of vitamin C than to actual caloric starvation or protein depletion. It appears reasonable that the intake of vitamin C required to maintain normal body function in the posttraumatic patient is considerably higher than that customarily given for daily maintenance. If vitamin C is given intravenously in high levels, the renal threshold is soon exceeded, and a large portion of the administered dose is lost in the urine.

Most patients on parenteral therapy for short periods following surgical procedures for trauma will not require supplemental vitamins A and D. However, in addition to C, thiamine is certainly needed, as body stores of thiamine are rapidly depleted after the administration of large amounts of glucose. One of the important coenzymes in the tricarboxylic acid cycle necessary for oxidative decarboxylation of pyruvate to acetyl CoA is cocarboxylase, or thiamine pyrophosphate. The defect in oxidation of pyru-

vate therefore may be related to a preexisting thiamine deficiency in some patients.

Management

Most patients will reach the operating room in satisfactory nutritional status, but this desirable goal is not easily attained after extensive trauma. Preexisting nutritional and vitamin deficits may further complicate the severe metabolic response following trauma. Patients with hypoproteinemia may exhibit diminished tolerance to blood loss and reduced antibody production. There may be impaired wound healing and delayed union of fractures, and perhaps fatty infiltration of the liver in patients who are severely hypoproteinemic.

Although the normal patient at bed rest can be maintained easily on approximately 1 Gm of protein and 30 kcal/kg of body weight, after extensive trauma these requirements may be doubled or tripled. In the past it has been quite difficult to supply sufficient calories by the intravenous route.

Although protein may be supplied via administered blood plasma or albumin, these solutions are expensive, they require considerable metabolic work for their assimilation and caloric equilibrium for maximal use, and their caloric values are quite low. At one time there was widespread interest in the use of intravenous solutions containing protein hydrolysates and fat emulsions, which theoretically appeared to be more useful. However, this nutritional technique was not extensively employed because of doubtful effectiveness in preventing nitrogen losses and because of certain hazards attending their use. In 1968, Dudrick and associates reported that large quantities of protein hydrolysates and dextrose could be administered through a catheter inserted in the superior vena cava to consistently and safely achieve a positive nitrogen balance and weight gain. In over 300 patients, Dudrick and his colleagues induced weight gain and promoted healing of fistulas and wounds by this technique of *parenteral hyperalimentation.* Intravenous solutions containing adequate protein, essential amino acids, fat, carbohydrate, and vitamins to meet chronic nutritional requirements are now available. This important development in the pre- and postoperative care of patients is particularly useful when protein and caloric requirements are quite high and convalescence is prolonged.

Improvements in infusion technique are primarily responsible for the success of parenteral hyperalimentation, particularly the technique of catheterizing the subclavian vein to approach the superior vena cava for instillation of the concentrated solutions. As the subclavian vein is large, the catheter does not usually produce irritation of the vein wall and subsequent thrombosis, and the rapid blood flow prevents clotting and reduces bacterial growth. Placement of the catheter tip in the superior vena cava permits rapid dilution of the hypertonic solutions, thus decreasing the incidence of chemical phlebitis. Rigid sterile technique in placement and care of these catheters has allowed an acceptably low infection rate.

It is clear that with careful attention to strict asepsis and antisepsis in preparing and infusing these solutions (see Chap. 2) parenteral hyperalimentation may be considered a primary mode of both acute and long-term therapy, rather than a modified method of intravenous treatment, and can provide all essential nutrients without exceeding the daily fluid requirements. Initially, the solutions were prepared just prior to administration, but commercial products with a wide range of constituents now are available. Minor adjustments of essential amino acids, vitamins, and ion supplementation facilitate the preparation of individualized solutions.

ANESTHESIA

(by A. H. Giesecke, Jr., E. R. Johnson and James F. Lee)

Complicating Problems

Distinct problems differentiate the injured patient requiring emergency operation from the patient well prepared for elective operation (see Chap. 11). The major problems are possible airway difficulties, lack of comprehensive preoperative evaluation, multiple injuries, the full or nonemptied stomach, intoxication with alcohol or drugs, and shock.

AIRWAY OBSTRUCTION. Establishment and maintenance of the patient's airway may be the most important step in successful resuscitation. Some form of artificial airway is indicated for any patient with respiratory obstruction, inability to clear secretions, need for artificial ventilation, or unconsciousness. The type of airway must be individualized, but oropharyngeal or nasopharyngeal airways, orotracheal tubes, nasotracheal tubes, or tracheostomy should be considered.

Endotracheal intubation, if technically possible, is an effective method of rapidly clearing an airway obstruction to allow a more orderly, unhurried tracheostomy. Intubation should be performed under direct vision with a laryn-goscope so that loose fragments of bone, teeth, or tissue will not be carried into the trachea by the advancing tube. The tube may be left in place for 48 hours or longer, if necessary, to support ventilation or maintain the airway until the patient can satisfactorily perform these functions. Meticulous care is as important for the indwelling endotracheal tube as for the tracheostomy. Inspired gases should be completely humidified. Periodic saline solution instillation followed by suctioning with a sterile catheter and hyperinflation of the lungs every other hour are prerequisites for proper management. Chest physiotherapy consisting of postural drainage, percussion, and vibration are beneficial in preventing and treating atelectasis.

The period of induction of anesthesia is probably the most hazardous time in the anesthetic period. During this time, hypotension, hypoxia, arrhythmias, and vomiting are likely to occur. The patient should be preoxygenated, allowing time for placement of intravenous infusions, further appraisal of the patient's status, and protection against hypoxia during induction. If general anesthesia is selected for the emergency repair of trauma, tracheal intubation is necessary. After consideration of the preanesthetic condition, the patient may be intubated while awake or following rapid induction. Awake intubation may avoid many dangers which may occur on induction of anesthesia, is generally easily performed, and is far less distressing to the patient than most physicians anticipate. Use of topical anesthesia will facilitate awake intubation in the more alert patient with a full stomach or hypotension. Awake intubation is contraindicated in patients with penetrating eye injuries and in patients with elevated intracranial pressure.

Intubation under general anesthesia will require consideration of other factors such as restoration of circulating volume and identification of associated injuries. Rapid intravenous induction is accomplished, and a cuffed endotracheal tube is inserted. The lungs must not be manually ventilated until the endotracheal tube is in place and the cuff inflated, except when intubation has been unsuccessful and hypoxia must be prevented or treated.

Many recent developments have improved a trauma patient's chances of survival with respiratory obstruction. The use of the esophageal airway by the EMTs (Emergency Medical Technicians) and evacuation of the unconscious injured in the lateral or prone position have saved many lives. In the desperate asphyxial emergency from supraglottic obstruction, oxygenation can be established by insufflating oxygen at a high flow through a 15-gauge needle inserted into the larynx via the cricothyroid membrane. Catheter-guided endotracheal intubation and fiberoptic intubation have made intubation possible in cases in which it was previously felt to be impossible.

For desperate asphyxia with supraglottic obstruction, a rapid flow of oxygen can be administered via a 15-gauge needle inserted through the cricothyroid membrane into the tracheal lumen. This will provide sufficient oxygenation for establishing an adequate airway by tracheal intubation or tracheostomy.

LACK OF COMPREHENSIVE PREOPERATIVE EVALUATION. Morbidity and mortality of trauma are inversely related to the preinjury state of health, but no patient should be assumed to have been healthy before injury. Evidence of prior diseases, allergies, or chronic drug therapy should be sought from the patient or an available informant. The main categories of drugs which create hazardous interactions with anesthetics are hormones (corticosteroids, insulin), psychopharmacologics, antihypertensives (including diuretics), cardiac drugs (including digitalis), and anticoagulants.

MULTIPLE INJURIES. When injuries involve many areas, problems arise in establishing priorities for operative intervention. In patients with head injuries, associated injuries may compel initial consideration. However, one must be alert to change in the patient's neurologic status during the anesthesia. Usually the pupils are the best indicators, and reduced requirement for anesthesia may indicate progression of the neurologic deterioration. Conversely, if the head injury is the primary surgical target, the anesthesiologist should be alert for progression of associated trauma, such as tension pneumothorax, hemoperitoneum, and cardiac tamponade. As shock rarely is directly caused by head injuries, its occurrence in the presence of head injury should engender suspicion of other injury. Unusual diagnostic skill may be needed to assess associated injuries with effects that become apparent only after an operation is progressing in another area. For example, hemorrhage from a torn spleen or liver may be minimal at the beginning of operation to correct extremity trauma but will require careful consideration if hypotension occurs. The diagnosis may be masked and delayed by the empiric administration of vasopressors for hypotension of uncertain cause.

THE FULL OR NONEMPTIED STOMACH. The chief hazard of the unprepared stomach is vomiting and aspiration of the vomitus. Peristalsis may cease at the time of the accident because of shock, anxiety, or abdominal or central nervous system trauma. For this reason all traumatized patients should be managed as if the stomach were full regardless of the interval since the last oral intake. Where appropriate, regional anesthesia should be selected for these patients, although aspiration remains a hazard. Regional analgesia is technically contraindicated for agitated, intoxicated patients and for those with significant hypovolemia.

Awake intubation with or without topical anesthesia has been shown to be safe for the emergency patient with a full stomach. An alternative choice for a vigorous patient is rapid induction with an intravenous thiobarbiturate followed by a paralyzing dose of succinylcholine to facilitate tracheal intubation. The hazard of anesthetic overdosage exists if, following intubation, volatile inhalation agents are pumped into the lungs by controlled ventilation. The stomach should be previously decompressed with a nasogastric tube. Following administration of the thiobarbiturate, an assistant should exert continuous pressure on the cricoid cartilage to occlude the esophagus. This should not be released until the tube is securely in the trachea and the cuff inflated. The endotracheal tube should not be removed until the patient is conscious postoperatively and has protective laryngeal reflexes to prevent aspiration during extubation.

Two clinical pictures of aspiration have been described: First is the aspiration of undigested food resulting in respiratory obstruction and distress. Depending on the amount of material aspirated, patients may have acute respiratory distress with cyanosis and cardiac arrest or may exhibit a milder, chronic course leading to lobar pneumonitis and lung abscess. A second form, Mendelson's syndrome, is caused by aspiration of liquid acid gastric secretions. This is equally hazardous in terms of morbidity and mortality and is manifest by generalized bronchospasm, dyspnea, tachypnea, and cyanosis. In severe cases cardiac arrest may develop. Immediate therapy includes oxygen, endotracheal suctioning, methylprednisolone given intravenously, and broad-spectrum antibiotics. Bronchoscopy is indicated if particulate material is found in the vomitus or if signs of obstructive atelectasis develop. Tracheobronchial lavage with large volumes of saline solution is no longer recommended.

ALCOHOL AND DRUG INTOXICATION. Based largely on animal studies, the statement has been repeatedly made that the manifestations of shock are more severe in the drunk patient than in the sober patient. However, mild to moderate intoxication (blood alcohol less than 250 mg/100 ml) is reported to have no effect on the incidence of hypotension, morbidity, or mortality of surgical treatment for trauma. Higher levels of blood alcohol are expected to increase intraoperative anesthetic complications. Regional anesthesia is not technically feasible for the agitated and intoxicated patient; intravenous induction is preferred. The airway should be protected by rapid endotracheal intubation.

Patients intoxicated with cannabis, LSD, and/or amphetamines may exhibit altered responses to anesthetics. Intoxication with barbiturates and methyl alcohol may result in delayed emergence from anesthesia.

SHOCK. The severely hypovolemic patient, unresponsive to pain or verbal stimulus, should receive no anesthetic drugs which may depress the cardiovascular system. Such a patient needs endotracheal intubation, ventilation with oxygen, and restoration of circulating volume. Satisfactory operating conditions should be provided, with muscle relaxants and analgesic concentrations of nitrous oxide.

Other aspects of care for the severely hypotensive, hypovolemic patient include (1) simultaneous infusion of large quantities of blood and electrolyte solutions, warmed to avoid myocardial hypothermia and irreversible cardiac arrhythmias; (2) administration of calcium as an antagonist to hyperkalemia, to prevent citrate intoxication and to strengthen myocardial force; (3) administration of sodium bicarbonate to correct the acidosis produced by anaerobic metabolism and infusion of acidotic blood; and (4) administration of large doses of steroids, although their efficacy is not firmly established.

Simultaneous infusions of type-specific whole blood and balanced salt solutions are used for the resuscitation of patients in hypovolemic shock. Balanced salt solutions are infused to correct the deficit in functional extracellular fluid volume which has been demonstrated to occur in hypovolemic shock and severe tissue trauma. The following guidelines are followed in the rational and moderate approach to the treatment of hypovolemic shock: (1) balanced salt solutions are not a substitute for whole blood; (2) blood should be given whenever losses approach 10 percent of blood volume; (3) balanced salt solutions are intended to replace deficits in functional extracellular fluid; (4) balanced salt solutions should be given to hypotensive, emergency room patients while type-specific whole blood is being obtained; (5) during surgery, blood loss is replaced with blood plus balanced salt solution at a rate of 7 to 10 ml/kg/hour; (6) patients with cardiac or renal disease deserve special consideration and care in fluid therapy; (7) intravenous infusions should be warmed; (8) microfiltration may be employed in transfusions of whole blood or packed cells; (9) packed cells should be reconstituted with normal saline solution prior to infusion.

Assessment of the Patient's Status

Blood pressure, pulse, skin color, capillary filling time, and pupil size should be monitored during all anesthesia. In addition, the central venous pressure of the severely traumatized patient should be monitored to detect early failure of the myocardium and overload with colloid solutions. The hourly urine output should be monitored to determine the efficacy of fluid therapy. Output should be at least 50 ml/hour if the extracellular fluid volume is being sufficiently replaced with a balanced salt solution.

Premedication

The emphasis in anesthesia for trauma is on resuscitation. An obligation exists to relieve suffering of a patient whose physical condition will tolerate the effects of analgesic drugs. However, hypoxic agitation must be differentiated from suffering. Barbiturates should not be used if the patient is in pain, as in this circumstance they tend to produce the paradoxic response of excitement or depressed agitation rather than sedation. Narcotics are contraindicated for patients with closed head injuries, because they deepen the depression, produce miosis, and mask the progression of intracranial injuries. For its drying effects and vagal depressant characteristics, an anticholinergic drug should be used for nearly all patients.

Choice of Anesthetic

The choice of agent varies from oxygen alone for the patient in hypovolemic shock to the full range of anesthetic agents for the patient with intact homeostatic mechanisms. Those agents and techniques should be chosen which tend to facilitate successful resuscitation. The patient who is hypoxic preoperatively should be managed with an anesthetic which can be given with the highest concentration of oxygen. Nitrous oxide is acceptable for obtunded or inebriated patients. Spinal anesthesia is useful for patients with injuries of the lower extremities if the central nervous system is not involved, if the blood volume has been replaced, and if the patient is not otherwise unmanageable.

A guiding principle in the choice of anesthetic agents and techniques is that complete supression of sensation is not necessary and may be harmful if achieved by deep anesthesia. Extensive surgical procedures can be performed in analgesic planes of nitrous oxide, ether, cyclopropane, or halothane, or by combining light general and local anesthesia. Severely traumatized and unconscious patients will require oxygen only and perhaps a muscle relaxant.

Postoperative Management

Not all the effects of massive trauma may be apparent at the same time. Following definitive correction of damage in one area, the patient must be closely observed for evidences of injury in other areas. The usual principles of recovery-room care must be applied. These include oxygen by mask, at least until the patient is awake and oriented; periodic use of intermittent positive-pressure breathing; frequent turning from side to side; and monitoring of the blood pressure, pulse rate, adequacy of ventilation, urine output, fluid infusion, gastric suction, emergence from anesthesia, and evidences of continued or recurring blood loss.

Delayed emergence from anesthesia may be caused by many factors, including possible head injury from the initial trauma or brain damage from prolonged shock or hypoxia. Progression of nervous system lesions should be watched for even if head injury was not suspected prior to operation. If the patient remains motionless except for breathing, anesthetic overdosage may be the cause, but the differential diagnosis should include spinal cord injury, brain damage, persistent partial curarization, overdosage with curare antagonists, hypothermia, and alcohol or drug intoxication. Bizarre causes for failure to awaken include myasthenia gravis, hypothyroidism, hypoglycemia, sickle cell crisis, intermittent porphyria, and nonketotic hyperosmotic coma.

Hypoventilation is a difficult problem to assess clinically in the postoperative patient. It can be caused by one condition or by a combination of several perplexing conditions. The list of reasons for hypoventilation includes most of those considered in delayed emergence from anesthesia, i.e., anesthetic overdosage or idiosyncrasy, relaxant overdosage or idiosyncrasy, overdosage with narcotics given for postoperative pain, endocrinopathies including myasthenia gravis and hypothyroidism, fluid overload, shock, neomycin or streptomycin administered intraperitoneally, upper and/or lower airway obstruction, respiratory restriction by dressings or casts, pneumothorax or hemothorax, abdominal distension, and pain.

An informed suspicion is required for the early diagnosis of hypoventilation, since the classic syndrome appears late and may be masked. Signs include restlessness, stridor or retractions, air hunger, disorientation or stupor, diminution of respiration (volume and/or frequency), hypertension which progresses to hypotension, tachycardia changing to bradycardia, and pallor or cyanosis. Chest roentgenograms may show atelectasis, pneumonitis, pneumothorax, or hemothorax. Spirometer measurements will confirm diminished tidal ventilation. Arterial blood-gas analysis will show hypercapnia, acidosis, and arterial unsaturation.

The proper treatment for hypoventilation is directed primarily at respiratory assistance or control with a breathing apparatus. Other measures may be indicated for specific causes: atropine and neostigmine to reverse residual paresis from curare; levallorphan or naloxone to antagonize narcotics; and analeptics. All are useful but are secondary to good ventilatory support.

PRINCIPLES IN THE MANAGEMENT OF WOUNDS

(by Ronald C. Jones and G. Tom Shires)

Primary Wound Management

The most important single factor in the management of contaminated wounds is adequate debridement. This old surgical principle frequently has been forgotten since the advent of antibiotics. All tissue which is dead, has a poor blood supply, or is heavily contaminated should be removed if at all possible. This is particularly true of subcutaneous fat and muscle. Skin with impaired blood supply should be removed initially because of its tendency to suppurate and become infected. Granulation tissue formation and later grafting procedures are preferable. Following sharp debridement and hemostasis, the wound is irrigated with copious quantities of saline solution, depending on the area and degree of soft tissue injury and contamination. That the incidence of wound infection is inversely proportional to the amount of irrigation and debridement at the time of injury has been demonstrated by Singleton et al. and by Peterson and confirmed clinically many times.

LOCAL CARE OF WOUNDS

Glass or sharp instruments usually carry a minimal amount of foreign material into a wound and cause a minimal amount of tissue trauma. X-rays should be taken of any area in which the depth of the wound cannot clearly be seen. It is not uncommon for the deep portion of a stab wound to contain the tip of a knife blade or other foreign body. Stab wounds of soft tissues are explored in the emergency room with the gloved finger or under local anesthesia by extending the length of the laceration to determine the direction and extent of the wound and to rule out any major vessel, nerve, or organ injury. The wound is then irrigated with copious amounts of saline solution. If the solution is found not to penetrate the peritoneal cavity, a small, soft-rubber Penrose drain is inserted, and the wound is left open for drainage. The drain is removed in 24 hours. Gunshot wounds are debrided externally and left open for drainage. Suturing these wounds leaves a closed contaminated space, and the infection can easily spread to surrounding soft tissue structures. Deep lacerations involving the extremity with damage to major vessels and tendons and massive muscle injury are managed by controlling major vessel bleeding and immediately wrapping the wound in sterile dressings. An x-ray is taken, if indicated, but a severe laceration is not explored until the patient is in the operating room. This procedure prevents undue contamination of the wound in the emergency room before the patient is adequately prepared. Minor lacerations can be managed in the emergency room.

Muscles usually can be approximated and, depending on the type of wound, the skin and subcutaneous tissue may or may not be closed initially. These wounds are often left open and have delayed primary closure in 3 to 5 days. Damaged muscle due to gunshot wounds is debrided, hemostasis is obtained, and the wound is irrigated as outlined above. The wounds are packed open and closed with delayed closure. All patients with such wounds receive antibiotics and tetanus toxoid.

Antibacterial soaps or detergent materials are not used to irrigate wounds when muscle, tendon, or blood vessels are visible. Severe chemical irritation to these structures may occur, with resultant structure impairment and delayed wound healing.

Many factors, such as the number and virulence of organisms, blood supply of tissue, host resistance, shock, adequacy of surgical debridement, tissue tension, dead space, hemostasis, age, and associated diseases, are responsible for infection. Condie demonstrated in dogs that obliterating dead space reduced the occurrence of wound infection in the presence of contamination. Viable bacteria can be demonstrated in many surgical wounds at the time of closure; however, few incisions become infected. Therefore, the number of bacteria encountered in clean operations is not, in itself, sufficient to produce sepsis.

Cosmetic appearance is a secondary consideration; the primary aim is to avoid infection and cover vital structures. No attempt at plastic repair is made at the initial closure of a potentially contaminated wound. Jagged edges of skin with poor blood supply are trimmed, and any resulting unpleasant scar can be cared for at a later date when no infection is present. Most lacerations, regardless of location, will never need revision if they meet the criteria previously outlined for the primary closure.

PUNCTURE WOUNDS. The most frequent puncture injury is that caused by a rusty nail in the foot. Initial treatment consists of ellipsing a small area of skin and subcutaneous tissue around the puncture site. A simple method of excising a portion of skin uses cuticle nippers. The wound is then irrigated with copious amounts of saline solution and left open for drainage. The patient is started on antibiotics both to prevent secondary infection and to aid in the prevention of tetanus, since this wound is not completely open to the air.

Puncture wounds elsewhere in the body are debrided more conservatively if they involve only the skin and subcutaneous tissue. Human tetanus immune globulin is given (250 mg) to the unimmunized patient. Debridement with conversion to an open wound and the administration of antibiotics and tetanus toxoid, whether or not the patient has been previously immunized, is also performed.

POWER MOWER INJURIES. Injuries resulting from the use of power mowers have increased in recent years. These include injuries from flying objects thrown from the power mower and from the mower itself to the hands and feet, particularly the fingers and toes. Treatment has consisted of covering exposed bones with muscle and leaving the entire wound open. These injuries almost uniformly become infected if an attempt is made to close the wound primarily. Patients are treated with systemic antibiotics and tetanus prophylaxis, and the wounds are packed with fine-mesh gauze. Skin grafting and reconstructive procedures should be delayed.

Emergency Laparotomy

INCISIONS. A longitudinal midline incision is regularly used for exploratory laparotomy in patients with abdominal trauma and does not endanger the abdominal muscle blood supply or nerve supply, or damage aponeuroses. Skin towels are routinely sewn into place, if time permits, to prevent skin contamination and drying of subcutaneous tissues. Minimal ligatures are used on bleeders which are contained in small bits of tissue, as each extra ligature is a foreign body and enhances the chance of a wound infection. Tissues should be kept moistened and gently handled. Surgical technique governs the development of wound infection as significantly as any single factor.

SUTURE. Number 30 stainless steel wire is the suture material of choice for closing the uncomplicated midline abdominal incision, particularly in operations for traumatic lesions. This has been shown to cause the least reaction and is of sufficient strength. It has not been the cause of draining sinuses following postoperative wound infections. Suture placement is probably the most important factor in the prevention of wound dehiscence. There is no longer need to overlap fascia, since new tissue comes from surrounding tissue, and if fascia is freed to allow overlapping, this surrounding tissue is damaged. Sutures should not be placed at equal distances from the edge of the fascia, as they will fall in the same group of fibers; should one suture tear the fascia longitudinally, the tear may extend from suture to suture until dehiscence occurs. Sutures should be staggered or placed at varying intervals from the edge of the fascia. With such a closure, there should be no fear in having a patient cough vigorously for adequate postoperative pulmonary care. No problem has occurred with wire sutures protruding through the skin. An occasional patient with minimal subcutaneous tissue will complain of pain in the incision when the wire is

under a pressure point such as a belt. These sutures are easily removed under local anesthesia.

Simple interrupted suture is used to close the fascia and peritoneum in a single layer. This is felt to be superior to the figure-of-eight suture, because less tissue is gathered and the suture can be placed faster, thus reducing anesthesia time. Interrupted sutures are used instead of running sutures, because a break in the suture material will not loosen the entire incision. Regardless of the type of suture or method of placement, the fascia should be loosely approximated and not strangulated. Tightening fascial sutures may lead to necrosis with the suture subsequently cutting through the tissue. Retention sutures have not been regularly used. Routine antibiotic irrigation of the wound for the prevention of infection has not been necessary. Fragmentation of wire sutures has been described as a complication, but this must be quite rare; we have seen no patients with fragmentation with erosion into a viscus such as the small bowel.

Through-and-Through Closure. Several local and systemic factors noted at the time of the original operation may make through-and-through closure the procedure of choice (Fig. 6-2). This uses plastic bridges and #4 stainless steel wire swaged on a large cutting needle. The bridges prevent cutting of skin by the wire and allow for swelling which occurs in the first 24 to 48 hours postoperatively. These sutures usually do not require postoperative adjustment. Wounds massively contaminated from shotgun wadding and fecal material, in patients on steroids, or associated with massive infection and peritonitis are best handled with through-and-through closure. Often a single patient may have several indications for this type of closure such as chronic pulmonary disease, obesity, and/or chronic debilitating disease. Occasionally through-and-through closure is used at the end of a lengthy operation with a long incision to shorten anesthesia time if the patient is not tolerating the procedure well. This type of closure is routinely used in the patient requiring reoperation in the early postoperative period because of gastrointestinal bleeding or intestinal obstruction. The wires are left in place for 3 weeks. This measure has proved to be sure, safe, timesaving, and often lifesaving.

INFECTION. Infection and severe abdominal distension are frequently mentioned as causative factors in dehiscence. Routine use of the Levin tube may prevent the latter. A severe wound infection may be prevented in the markedly contaminated abdomen by leaving the skin and subcutaneous tissue open down to the fascia for delayed primary closure. This method is frequently used in long operations or with excessive contamination such as from feces. Staphylococcus remains the number one organism causing wound infections in trauma patients. Abdominal wounds freqently harbor coliform organisms if bowel injury has been sustained. These wounds are packed open with fine-mesh gauze, changed daily for debridement, and either closed at 5 days or allowed to granulate until closure. This procedure will usually result in an excellent scar. Reoperation in the same area of a previous wound infection, even months later, will frequently result in a second wound infection.

Fig. 6-2. Through-and-through wire closure. (*From G. T. Shires, "Care of the Trauma Patient," p. 37, McGraw-Hill Book Company, New York, 1966.*)

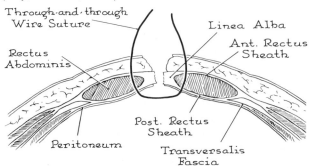

DRAINS. Subcutaneous drains will not substitute for good hemostasis. Failure to obtain hemostasis will give rise to a hematoma which is an excellent culture medium for an already contaminated wound. Drains from the abdominal cavity are usually brought out through a separate stab wound which will easily admit two fingers and by the most direct route, which occasionally may be through the midline incision. This is especially true for some liver and pancreatic injuries. Drainage of the free peritoneal cavity is not attempted unless drainage of a particular organ or a well-localized abscess is specifically indicated.

Antibiotics

Sepsis is related to the length of time which elapses between bacterial contamination of the traumatic wound or surgical incision and the start of treatment designed to prevent sepsis. The "golden period" for wound infection has been stated to be 6 hours, but the effectiveness of preventive antibiotics in surgical wounds has been shown to be no more than 3 hours. In fact, the shorter the time between contamination or surgical incision and the administration of antibiotics, the more effective are the antibiotics in preventing a bacterial infection.

Burke has demonstrated in animals injected with staphylococci that the steps which determine the size of a bacterial lesion take place very shortly after the bacteria reach the tissue. As the time interval between the injection of bacteria and the administration of an antibiotic increases, the antibiotic effect on the size of the lesion produced is decreased. Most of the antibiotic effect is over in 1 to 2 hours. As antibiotics injected more than 3 hours after staphylococci have been introduced have no effect on the size of the 24-hour lesion, it appears that there is little benefit from antibiotics administered 3 hours following the injection of staphylococci. This indicates that the antibiotic should be given early, so that it is in the tissue when the bacteria arrive. If given postoperatively, the antibiotic may reach the local dead tissue after the time period considered safe for traumatic injuries, and bacteria already may be beginning to multiply.

Viable bacteria can be demonstrated in many surgical wounds at the time of closure; however, only a minimal number later become infected. Therefore, the number of bacteria encountered in clean operations is not alone sufficient to produce sepsis. There is considerable evidence that other factors produce decreased host resistance.

Various regions of the body respond differently to wound contamination. Clinical experience has long shown an inverse relationship between the vascularity of an area and its susceptibility to infection. This probably is reflected in the low incidence of infection in head and neck operations, compared with the higher incidence with abdominal operations. Normal tissues have remarkable resistance to microorganisms, but devitalized tissues have limited resistance. Thus, the development of local wound infection depends greatly on the altered physiologic state of the wound. In addition, Ollodart and Mansberger have demonstrated in both animals and man that bacterial resistance is decreased following hypovolemic shock.

Surgical materials and technique are also important. Suture material enhances the virulence of staphylococci several-fold. Altemeier and Wulsin have shown that this occurs less with monofilament suture than with twisted or braided material. However, Condie and Ferguson have shown that dead space is more important in the production of wound infection than is increased amount of suture material.

Various regions of the body respond differently to wound contamination. Clinical experience has long shown an inverse relationship between the vascularity of an area and its susceptibility to infection. Normal tissues have remarkable resistance to microorganisms, but devitalized tissues have limited resistance. Thus, the development of local wound infection depends greatly on the altered physiologic state of the wound. Ollodart and Mansberger have demonstrated in both animals and human beings that bacterial resistance is decreased following hypovolemic shock. Routine antibiotic irrigation of the wound for the prevention of infection is not necessary if systemic antibiotics are being administered.

Approximately 80 percent of the organisms cultured from trauma patients with bacteremia are gram-negative. The mortality for polymicrobial bacteremia is almost twice that with single organisms. *Klebsiella pneumoniae, Bacteroides fragilis,* and *Pseudomonas aeruginosa* are the most frequent gram-negative organisms isolated. Enterococci remain the most common gram-positive organisms isolated from blood cultures on the trauma services, and are frequently associated with intraabdominal abscesses and wound infection. The treatment of choice for enterococcal infection is penicillin and an aminoglycoside such as gentamicin or tobramycin.

The systemic antibiotic treatment of choice for suppurative peritonitis in the absence of identification of organisms includes penicillin, Cleocin, and an aminoglycoside such as gentamicin or tobramycin. The combination of penicillin and an aminoglycoside is effective against the enterococci, and the aminoglycoside is effective against over 96 percent of gram-negative organisms. Clindamicin is effective against anaerobes, particularly *B. fragilis.* Two-drug combinations such as penicillin and an aminoglycoside or Cleocin and an aminoglycoside are also usually effective. If a single antibiotic is preferred, high-dose cephalothin, 12 Gm daily, is probably the drug of choice. Stone has demonstrated that cephalothin is as effective as clindamicin in the treatment of patients with peritonitis. The incidence of intraabdominal abscess formation appears to be common following the administration of penicillin and tetracycline since half the gram-negative organisms are resistant to tetracycline, and *Enterococcus* is a common pathogen. Penicillin and tetracycline appear to have little effect on the more resistant *E. coli* and *Klebsiella. Proteus mirabilis, Pseudomonas,* and *Providentia stuartii* are resistant to tetracycline, as are *B. fragilis* in most cases. After cultures are available, antibiotics can be stopped or changed, occasionally to a single antibiotic, although mixed gram-positive and gram-negative infections are common.

Following severe penetrating abdominal trauma, intraabdominal abscess formation is common, even with prophylactic antibiotic therapy. The organisms recovered from abscesses and peritonitis include *E. coli, Klebsiella,* and *B. fragilis.* Gram-positive organisms include enterococci, anaerobic streptococci, and *Clostridium.* Gorbach has demonstrated that *B. fragilis* is the most common anaerobe isolated following penetrating abdominal trauma, and these organisms were significantly altered by the administration of a combination of clindamycin and kanamycin. *B. fragilis* is the most significant anaerobic pathogen in infections below the diaphragm, and is the most common organism found in the colon, outnumbering gram-negative aerobes by a hundred times. Any abscess which fails to culture an organism is strongly suspected of containing anaerobes; this may be further supported by performing a Gram stain of the purulent material. Organisms present on Gram stain give some indication of which antibiotics are to be selected—i.e., antibiotics for gram-positive, gram-negative, or a mixed infection.

A sinogram through any drain tract or wound is the simplest and most direct method of detecting an intraabdominal collection. Unless the patient is producing large quantities of purulent material through a drain tract, routine cultures of the drain tract are of limited benefit. However, if large volumes of purulent material are produced, the organisms isolated in this instance frequently are those present in a deeper abscess. Occasionally a sump drain may be placed through this drain tract and the abscess aspirated without the necessity of a formal laparotomy; however, the majority of these cases require formal drainage. Prompt drainage and identification of the continued source of sepsis are most important.

INTRAPERITONEAL ANTIBIOTICS. Since the advent of sulfa drugs, the administration of antibiotics intraperitoneally has been advocated. Artz demonstrated in dogs that antibiotics administered intravenously 2 hours after a fecal suspension had been injected intraperitoneally gave the same degree of protection as did intraperitoneal administration, without its complications. Because of the degrees of respiratory depression following intraperitoneal administration of neomycin and kanamycin, the concentration should be no greater than $\frac{1}{2}\%$. Pittinger noted in 1959 the toxic responses that occur during anesthesia following administration of intraperitoneal antibiotics, and reported several instances of severe respiratory depression following intraperitoneal administration of neomycin. An effective antagonist of the respiratory and neuromuscular depressant actions of antibiotics is intravenous calcium gluconate and sodium bicarbonate. Intraperitoneal irrigations without systemic antibiotics reduce primary wound infection more than intraabdominal abscess formation. The question remains as to whether intraperitoneal antibiotics offer any value over systemic antibiotics.

Condon demonstrated, with the administration of 500 mg kanamycin intraperitoneally, that there was rapid absorption of the drug, producing serum levels comparable to those achieved with an intramuscular injection of kanamycin. Rambo has demonstrated the rapid absorption of cephalothin by intraperitoneal irrigation, resulting in a serum level comparable to that obtained by systemic administration and a high peritoneal fluid level following intravenous infusion of cephalothin. For single intraoperative instillation of cephalothin, 4 gm/liter may be used. Barnett has reported the effectiveness of cephalothin for established peritonitis; he believes it to be the drug of choice. The antibiotic used must be calculated into the total daily systemic dose unless rapidly removed.

Intraperitoneal antibiotic irrigation is not routine on a trauma service. Patients with significant intraperitoneal contamination are given systemic antibiotics, the abdomen is irrigated with saline solution, the fascia is closed, and the skin and subcutaneous tissue left open for delayed primary closure, usually within 3 to 4 days.

Singleton has shown that the incidence of infection in wounds already 4 hours old can be reduced by freshening with gauze sponges before irrigation, as opposed to irrigation without scrubbing the wound edges. Scrubbing the wound with a solution was significantly more effective than instillation of the solution intraperitoneally. Howes found that irrigation of a contaminated crushed wound in rabbits before 3 hours resulted in a significant reduction in infections, but that infection was not prevented after 3 hours unless the wound was freshened with debridement.

A review of 400 patients sustaining gunshot and stab wounds to the abdomen indicated that the incidence of infection in patients with abdominal injuries who received prophylactic antibiotics penicillin and tetracycline in the emergency room or intraoperatively was lower (4.5 percent) than in patients who did not receive antibiotics until the immediate postoperative period or therapeutically (9 percent). Patients receiving gunshot wounds are at a four times greater risk of infection than stab wound victims. If no significant injury is found at laparotomy, antibiotics are discontinued in the recovery room or postoperatively during the first 24 hours. With severe contamination, antibiotics are administered for 3 to 5 days.

If the patient develops an infection following topical or intraperitoneal irrigation with antibiotics, the organisms isolated are usually resistant to the antibiotic used. This has been almost uniformly true in those patients receiving prophylactic antibiotics following penetrating abdominal trauma.

BITES AND STINGS OF ANIMALS AND INSECTS

(by Ronald C. Jones and G. Tom Shires)

Rabies

INCIDENCE. In the United States an estimated 2 million human beings are bitten by animals yearly, and $\frac{1}{2}$ million are bitten by dogs. Any mammalian animal may carry rabies. In 1975 there were 2,674 laboratory-confirmed cases of rabies. The animals most frequently reported infected and the percentage of the cases they accounted for were skunks (46 percent), foxes (15 percent), bats (11 percent), cattle (9 percent), dogs (5 percent), cats (5 percent), and raccoons (4 percent). In 1971, 80 percent of the rabies in this country was in wildlife species. Wildlife rabies was also reported in coyotes, opossum, otter, bobcats, bear, squirrel, deer, mink, woodchucks, coatis, and a badger. Domestic rabies was reported in cattle, dogs, cats, horses, mules, sheep, goats, swine, and guinea pigs in 1971. The Communicable Disease Center estimates that this represents less than 10 percent of the cases that actually exist. In the past 5 years, there has been an average of two cases of human rabies per year. Table 6-1 shows the incidence and frequency of reported rabies in the United States in various animals and in human beings by states or territory in 1975. Many of the few cases of human rabies reported in the past 10 years have resulted from exposure abroad.

EPIDEMIOLOGY. Saliva from a rabid animal contains large numbers of the rabies virus and is inoculated through a bite, any laceration, or break in the skin. Animal experiments and at least two human infections indicate that animals and man can become infected by bats, without being bitten, by inhalation of rabies virus. Girard examined bats and demonstrated rabies virus in the brain, kidney, urine, salivary gland, adrenal gland, and liver using the fluorescent antibody test. Most cases of racoon rabies are reported from Florida and Georgia, the only part of the United States where a cycle of transmission in raccoons has been established.

The maintenance of wild and exotic animals such as skunks, raccoons, ocelots, and bobcats as household pets is discouraged since many of these animals are infected with rabies. If people insist on maintaining wild and exotic animals as household pets, these animals should be quarantined for a minimum of 90 days after capture and vaccinated at least 30 days prior to being released to an owner. Annual vaccination is recommended.

Dogs and cats bitten by a known rabid animal should be destroyed immediately. If the animal has been vaccinated within the previous 3 years, it should be revaccinated immediately and confined for 90 days.

DIAGNOSIS. Circumstances of the Bite. Circumstances surrounding the attack frequently furnish vital information as to whether or not vaccine is indicated. Most domestic animal bites are provoked attacks; if this history is obtained, rabies vaccine can usually be withheld if the animal appears healthy. Children are frequently bitten while attempting to separate fighting animals or while teasing or accidentally hurting the animal. Bites during attempts to feed or handle an apparently healthy animal should generally be regarded as provoked. Frequently the patient has attempted to handle a sick animal.

Although vaccination of the animal does not totally rule out the possibility of transmitting rabies, it is over 90 percent effective. A small number of dog rabies have apparently involved vaccine failure.

Bites from rodents, including squirrels, chipmunks, rats, and mice, seldom require specific rabies prophylaxis. Each case of possible exposure must be studied individually before a conclusion can be reached as to whether antirabies therapy is indicated. An unprovoked attack is more likely to indicate that the animal is rabid.

Extent and Location of Bite Wound. The likelihood that rabies will result from a bite varies with its extent and location. For convenience in approaching management,

two categories of exposure are widely accepted:

Severe: Multiple or deep puncture wounds, or any bites on the head, face, neck, hands, or fingers.
Mild: Scratches, lacerations, or single bites on areas of the body other than the head, face, neck, hands, or fingers. Open wounds, such as abrasions, suspected of being contaminated with saliva also belong in this category.

Laboratory Diagnosis. The fluorescent antibody test described by Goldwasser and his associates appears to be a more accurate test than the stain for Negri bodies. The intracerebral inoculation of mice combined with the microscopic examination of brain tissue for Negri bodies is still one of the most useful tests in the laboratory diagnosis of rabies and should be used whenever human beings have been bitten by suspect animals and the fluorescent antibody test is negative.

MANAGEMENT OF BITING ANIMALS. Most animal bites of human beings are caused by dogs and cats, and in most instances it is possible to observe the biting animal for the development of rabies. Domestic animals that bite a person should be captured and observed for symptoms of rabies for 10 days. If none develop, the animal may be assumed to be nonrabid. If the animal dies or is killed, the head should not be damaged but should be sent promptly to a public health laboratory for examination. The tissue requires refrigeration but not freezing, and transportation to the laboratory following death of the animal should be rapid. Clinical signs of rabies in wild animals cannot be interpreted reliably; therefore, any wild animal that bites or scratches a person should be killed at once (without unnecessary damage to the head) and the brain examined for evidence of rabies.

Information from the county health department regarding which animals, both domestic and wild, have been reported to be rabid within the past 10 years in the particular area may indicate a possible specific animal transmitting rabies.

EXPOSURE OF PERSONS PREVIOUSLY IMMUNIZED. For mild exposure of a person who has demonstrated an antibody response to antirabies vaccination received in the past, a single booster dose of vaccine is recommended. In the case of severe exposure, five daily doses of vaccine should be given followed by a booster dose 20 days later.

If it is not known whether an exposed person has had antibody, the complete postexposure antirabies treatment should be given. Because of variation in vaccine potency and individual response, immunization should not be considered complete until antibody is demonstrated in the serum. Farrar et al. have demonstrated that most persons receiving three or more injections of any rabies vaccine within 4 years will show antibody in the blood 30 days after a single booster injection of duck embryo vaccine (DEV), a killed virus.

PREEXPOSURE PROPHYLAXIS. The relatively low frequency of reactions to DEV has made it more practical to offer preexposure immunization to persons in high-risk groups, e.g., veterinarians, animal handlers, certain laboratory workers, and individuals, especially children, living in areas where rabies is a constant threat. Others whose vocations or avocations result in frequent contact with

Table 6-1. RABIES IN ANIMALS BY STATE AND BY TYPE OF ANIMAL, UNITED STATES, 1975

Area	Dog	Cattle	Other domestic	Fox	Skunk	Bat	Raccoon	Other wild	Total
United States	116	151	141	278	1,226	514	192	7	2,625
New England	2	7	2	36	5	26	..	..	78
Maine	2	7	2	36	4	1	..	..	52
New Hampshire	..	..	..	..	...	2	..	..	2
Vermont									
Massachusetts	..	..	..	..	1	11	..		12
Rhode Island	..	..	..	..		4	..		4
Connecticut	..	..	..	..	...	8	..	..	8
Middle Atlantic	2	5	2	21	25	64	1	..	120
New York	1	5	2	18	24	26	..	..	76
New Jersey	..	..	..	2	...	22	..	..	24
Pennsylvania	1	..	..	1	1	16	1	..	20
East North Central	20	8	12	5	87	41	2	..	175
Ohio	1	2	..	1	5	8	1	..	18
Indiana	1	..	1	1	1	6	..	..	10
Illinois	6	3	6	2	32	15	1	..	65
Michigan	..	..	3	..	2	5	..	..	10
Wisconsin	12	3	2	1	47	7	..	..	72
West North Central	27	66	52	3	402	24	4	1	579
Minnesota	10	12	7	..	143	10	1	..	183
Iowa	10	17	15	1	52	7	..	..	102
Missouri	4	2	4	1	24	6	1	..	42
North Dakota	1	16	11	..	74	..	1	..	103
South Dakota	..	12	11	1	60	..	..	1	85
Nebraska	..	2	1	..	...	1	..	..	4
Kansas	2	5	3	..	49	..	1	..	60
South Atlantic	7	6	8	113	6	54	175	1	370
Delaware	..	..	..	..	...	6	..	..	6
Maryland	..	..	..	..	...	15	..	..	15
District of Columbia									
Virginia	..	5	2	99	2	5	..	1	114
West Virginia	1	1	..	3	...	..	..	..	5
North Carolina	..	..	1	..	...	11	..	..	12
South Carolina	..	..	..	1	...	8	2	..	11
Georgia	4	..	3	10	3	7	143	..	170
Florida	2	..	2	..	1	2	30	..	37
East South Central	12	11	13	70	27	14	5	..	152
Kentucky	10	11	10	55	6	3	1	..	96
Tennessee	..	..	1	5	9	6	..	..	21
Alabama	2	..	2	10	12	4	4	..	34
Mississippi	..	..	..	..	...	1	..	..	1
West South Central	34	35	38	13	308	90	1	3	522
Arkansas	1	6	3	..	59	14	..	..	83
Louisiana	1	..	..	..	2	4	..	1	8
Oklahoma	8	15	8	..	70	4	..	..	105
Texas	24	14	27	13	177	68	1	2	326
Mountain	8	6	11	4	199	86	3	1	318
Montana	2	2	8	..	152	6	2	..	172
Idaho									
Wyoming	..	2	..	..	24	9	1	..	36
Colorado	..	..	..	1	5	26	..	..	32
New Mexico	5	2	3	1	13	18	..	..	42
Arizona	1	..	..	2	4	19	..	..	26
Utah	..	..	..	..	...	3	..	..	3
Nevada	..	..	..	..	1	5	..	1	7
Pacific	4	7	3	13	167	115	1	1	311
Washington	..	..	..	..	...	10	..	..	10
Oregon	..	..	..	..	...	6	..	..	6
California	4	7	3	7	167	99	1	1	289
Alaska	..	..	..	6	...	..	..	..	6
Hawaii	..	..	..	..	...	..	..	..	
Guam									
Puerto Rico	13	7	5	..	...	..	..	24	49
Virgin Islands									

SOURCE: Reported through the Rabies Surveillance Program, Center for Disease Control.

dogs, cats, foxes, skunks, or bats should also be considered for preexposure prophylaxis.

A significant number of citizens of the United States have been and, with increasing frequency, will continue to be exposed to rabies in other countries where rabies in dogs is a major problem. Because rabies in animals is widespread in large areas of Asia, Africa, and Latin America, the Foreign Quarantine Program of the United States Public Health Service has recently advised that preexposure immunization against rabies with DEV be suggested for Americans traveling in these areas.

Two 1-ml injections of DEV given subcutaneously in the deltoid area 1 month apart should be followed by a third dose 6 to 7 months after the second dose. This series of three injections can be expected to have produced neutralizing antibody in 80 to 90 percent of vaccinees by 1 month after the third dose. For more rapid immunization, three 1-ml injections of DEV should be given at weekly intervals with a fourth dose 3 months later. This schedule elicits an antibody response in about 80 percent of those vaccinated. All who receive the preexposure vaccination should have their serum tested for neutralizing antibody 3 to 4 weeks after the last injection. Tests for rabies antibody can be arranged with or through state health department laboratories. If no antibody is detected, booster doses should be given until a response is demonstrated. Persons with continuing exposure should receive 1-ml boosters every 2 to 3 years.

ACCIDENTAL INOCULATION WITH LIVE RABIES VIRUS VACCINE. Persons inadvertently inoculated with attenuated rabies vaccines for use in animals, such as the Flury strain vaccine, are not considered at risk, and antirabies prophylaxis is not indicated.

POSTEXPOSURE PROPHYLAXIS. Incubation Period. It is generally accepted that the incubation period for rabies in human beings ranges from 10 days to 1 year, most cases occurring within 4 months of the time of exposure. In cases of exposure of the head, neck, or upper extremities, the incubation period is potentially less than 30 days.

Immediate Local Care. Not all persons bitten by rabid animals contract the disease. Vigorous local treatment to remove possible rabies virus may be as important as specific antirabies therapy. Free bleeding from the wound is encouraged. Local care of an animal bite should consist of:

1. Thorough irrigation with copious amounts of saline solution.
2. Cleansing with a 20% soap solution.
3. Swabbing with a 1 or 2% solution of benzalkonium chloride (all soap should be removed before application of quaternary ammonium compounds, because soap neutralizes the activity of such compounds).
4. Debridement.
5. Administration of antibiotic when indicated to prevent bacterial infection.
6. Administration of tetanus toxoid.
7. Immediate suturing of the wound generally is not advised, since it may contribute to the development of rabies, but a severe laceration secondary to a dog bite may be sutured if exposure to rabies is unlikely.

Passive Immunization. RIG (rabies immune globulin) in combination with DEV is considered the best postexposure prophylaxis. RIG, 20 IU/kg body weight, is recommended

for most exposures classified as severe, for all bites by rabid animals or those suspected of having rabies, for unprovoked bites by wild carnivores and bats, and for nonbite exposure to animals suspected of being rabid. A portion of the RIG is used to infiltrate the wound, and the remainder administered intramuscularly. When indicated, RIG is used instead of equine serum and is used regardless of the interval between exposure and treatment. RIG is given only once, as early as possible following exposure. The use of human immune antirabies globulin is accompanied by 21 doses of vaccine over a 14-day period, with two doses given per day for the first 7 days (Table 6-2). If RIG is not available, the recommended dose of equine antibodies serum is 40 IU/kg body weight.

Active Immunization. *Primary Immunization.* At least 23 injections, including booster doses, of vaccine in the dose recommended by the manufacturer are administered. These are given subcutaneously in the abdomen, lower part of the back, or lateral aspect of the thighs; rotation of sites is recommended.

For severe exposure, 21 doses of vaccine are recommended. These 21 doses are administered as two doses per day for the first 7 days, followed by one dose per day for seven daily doses. This method is preferred to detect the slow responder. A shorter course of vaccine is not recommended, since passive immunity induced by serum may limit response to vaccine. The vaccine may be stopped if the animal is proved nonrabid.

Booster Doses. Two booster doses, one 10 days and the other 20 days after completion of the primary course, are administered. Two booster doses are particularly important if RIG or antirabies serum was used in the initial therapy. A serum antibody titer is drawn at the time of the second booster dose to detect the poor responder, and these poor responders are given additional boosters until an adequate titer is obtained. If two additional booster doses of vaccine do not result in demonstrable antibody, authorities at the state health department or Center for Disease Control should be consulted to determine if alternative procedures such as the use of experimental vaccine (human diploid rabies vaccine) should be used.

Factors that contribute to a poor antibody response include administration of steroid during postexposure prophylaxis and use of more than 55 IU/kg of equine antirabies serum.

Side Reaction to Vaccine and Antiserum. Rabies vaccine should not be given unless there is a definite indication for its use. Local reactions to DEV are frequent. These consist of erythema, pruritus, pain, and tenderness at the site of inoculation. Generalized reactions occasionally are observed, usually after five to eight doses.

Neurologic reactions following DEV are rare. Perhaps one death has been attributed to its use. Neurologic reactions to nerve tissue vaccine constitute the principal hazard to its use. They occur in three main types: peripheral neuritis, the spinal form, and the cerebral form with acute encephalitis. Dorsolumbar paralysis may be either flaccid or spastic. Peripheral neuritis may involve facial, oculomotor, glossopharyngeal, or vagal nerves.

Immediate reactions may occur in an individual sensi-

Table 6-2. POSTEXPOSURE ANTIRABIES TREATMENT GUIDE

The following recommendations are only a guide. They should be applied in conjunction with knowledge of the animal species involved, circumstances of the bite or other exposure, vaccination status of the animal, and presence of rabies in the region.

Species of animal	Condition of animal at time of attack	Treatment of exposed person
Skunk Fox Coyote Raccoon Bat	Regard as rabid	RIG + DEV*
Dog	Healthy	None†
	Unknown (escaped)	RIG + DEV
Cat	Rabid or suspected rabid	RIG + DEV*
Other	Consider individually—see Circumstances of the Bite	

*Discontinue vaccine if fluorescent antibody (FA) tests of animal killed at time of attack are negative.
†Begin RIG + DEV at first sign of rabies in biting dog or cat during holding period (10 days).
NOTE: RIG, rabies immune globulin, human; DEV, duck embryo vaccine.

tive to avian tissue. Epinephrine is helpful in anaphylactic reactions. Should a complication develop and if, in view of the severity of the exposure, the amount of immunization already obtained is considered adequate, the vaccine may be discontinued. If further immunization is indicated, steroids and antihistamines should be administered.

Antirabies serum is obtained from immunized horses and may be expected to produce side reactions in approximately 20 percent of persons. Serum sickness occurs in approximately 5 percent of persons.

Effectiveness of Vaccines in Human Beings. Over 30,000 people receive antirabies vaccine yearly. Comparative effectiveness of vaccines can be judged only by reported failures. During the years 1957 through 1968 when both nerve tissue vaccine and DEV were available, there were six rabies deaths among 125,000 individuals receiving the nerve tissue vaccine, or 1:20,800, and eight among the 225,000 treated with DEV, or 1:28,100. It is the opinion of the National Communicable Disease Center that the clinical effectiveness of the two vaccines has not been significantly different. Therefore, the lower frequency of central nervous system reactions with DEV makes it preferable to nerve tissue vaccine. Antibody tends to develop somewhat earlier following DEV than following nerve tissue vaccine, but the titers tend to be lower. Human beings may contract rabies even after 14 doses of DEV, particularly when the incubation period has been less than 30 days.

MANIFESTATIONS AND TREATMENT OF DISEASE. Rabid dogs are noted to have purposeless movements with snapping, drooling, and vocal cord paralysis. Death usually occurs in 2 to 5 days. Man dies essentially the same way. There are 2 to 4 days of prodromal symptoms before the patient reaches the excited stage. Paresthesia in the region of the bite is an important early symptom. Symptoms noted with the onset of clinical rabies include headaches, vertigo, stiff neck, malaise, lethargy, and severe pulmonary symptoms including wheezing, hyperventilation, and dyspnea. The patient may have spasm of the throat muscles with dysphagia. The outstanding clinical symptom of rabies is related to swallowing. Drooling, maniacal behavior, and convulsions ensue and are followed by coma, paralysis, and death.

Instead of sedation and symptomatic treatment only, it is now recognized that intensive respiratory supportive care may be beneficial, in view of a case of human rabies in which the patient survived. Strict attention was given to the management of airway, pulmonary care, cardiac arrhythmias, and seizures. This included tracheostomy, vigorous suctioning, Dilantin for seizures, close monitoring of blood gases, electrocardiograms, electroencephalograms, and a ventricular shunt. Nursing care is extremely important. Probably many organs are involved, including brain, heart, and lungs.

Snakebites

INCIDENCE. In North America all the poisonous snakes of medical importance are members of the family Crotalidae, or pit vipers, with exception of the coral snake. Coral snakes are scattered from Florida to southern Arizona, are biologically related to the Indian cobra, and produce a different envenomation syndrome than the crotalids. The pit vipers include the rattlesnake, cottonmouth moccasin, and copperhead.

Approximately 8,000 persons are bitten each year by poisonous snakes. Over 98 percent of snakebites occur on the extremities. Thirty-five percent of snakebites occur in children less than ten years of age, usually in an area around their homes. Since 1960, an average of 14 victims have died annually as a result of snakebites. Seventy percent of all such deaths occur in five states: Texas, Georgia, Florida, Alabama, and Southern California. Rattlesnakes are responsible for approximately 70 percent of all deaths due to snakebite. Death from the bite of a copperhead snake is extremely rare, probably not exceeding an incidence of 0.01 percent.

POISONOUS VERSUS NONPOISONOUS SNAKES. Pit vipers are named for the characteristic pit, a heat-sensitive organ, that is located between the eye and the nostril on each side of the head. As a rule, these snakes may be identified by their elliptical pupils, as opposed to the round pupil of harmless snakes. Nonpoisonous snakes do not have pits. However, the coral snake does have a round pupil and lacks the facial pit. Pit vipers have two well-developed fangs that protrude from the maxillae, whereas nonpoisonous snakes have rows of teeth without fangs. Pit vipers also may be identified by turning the snake's belly upward and noting the single row of subcaudal plates. Nonpoisonous snakes have a double row of subcaudal plates (Fig. 6-3). The coral snake is a brightly colored small snake with red, yellow, and black rings. This color combination occurs also in nonpoisonous snakes, but the alternating colors are different. Only the coral snake has a red ring next to a yellow ring; when red touches yellow, it is a coral snake. The nose of the coral snake is black.

The venoms of poisonous snakes consist of enzymatic, complex proteins which affect all soft tissues. Venoms have been shown to have neurotoxic, hemorrhagic, thrombogenic, hemolytic, cytotoxic, antifibrin, and anticoagulant effects. Phospholipase A is probably responsible for hemolysis. Most venoms contain hyaluronidase, which enhances the rapid spread of venom by way of the superficial lymphatics. There may be considerable variation in the venom effect. Either neurotoxic features such as muscle cramping, fasciculation, weakness, and respiratory paralysis or hemolytic characteristics may predominate depending on the snake and the patient.

CLINICAL MANIFESTATIONS OF POISONOUS SNAKE-BITES. Pain from the bite of a poisonous snake is excruciating and probably the symptom that most easily differentiates poisonous from nonpoisonous snakebites. Poisonous snakes characteristically produce one or two fang marks, whereas nonpoisonous snakes may produce rows of punctures. Swelling, tenderness, pain, and ecchymosis appear within minutes at the site of the venom injection. If no edema is present within 30 minutes following the injury, the pit viper probably did not inject any venom. Swelling may continue to increase for 24 hours. Hemorrhagic vesiculations and petechiae may appear in the first 24 hours, with thrombosis of superficial vessels and eventual sloughing of tissue.

Rattlesnake. Most rattlesnakes probably eject less than 50 percent of their venom during a single biting act. Following a rattlesnake bite ecchymosis, hemorrhagic vesiculations, swelling of the regional lymph nodes, weakness, fainting, and sweating commonly are reported. The venom produces deleterious changes in the blood cells, defects in blood coagulation, injuries to the intimal linings of vessels, damage to the heart muscles, alterations in respiration, and, to a lesser extent, changes in neuromuscular conduction. Pulmonary edema is common in severe poisoning, and hemorrhage into the lungs, kidneys, heart, and peritoneum may occur. Hematemesis, melena, changes in salivation, and muscle fasciculations may be seen. Urinalysis may reveal hematuria, glycosuria, and proteinuria. Red blood cells and platelets may decrease, and bleeding and clotting times are usually prolonged.

Coral Snakes. The coral snake contributes only 1.5 percent of all deaths from poisonous snakes. Bites by the coral snake occasionally provoke blurred vision, ptosis, drowsiness, increased salivation, and sweating. The patient may notice paresthesia about the mouth and throat, sometimes slurring of speech, and nausea and vomiting. Pain is not a constant complaint, nor is edema a constant finding. Thus coral snake venom causes more extensive changes in the nervous system, but death may occur from cardiovascular collapse.

CHARACTERISTICS OF SNAKES

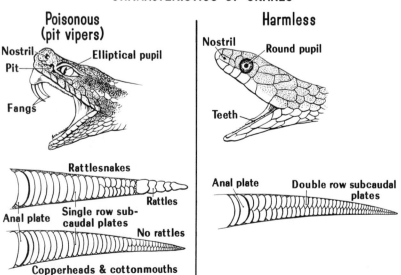

Fig. 6-3. Characteristics of poisonous and nonpoisonous snakes. (*From H. M. Parrish, Texas State J Med, 60:592, 1964.*)

LOCAL TREATMENT OF SNAKEBITES. The treatment of the bite of a poisonous snake varies considerably but is related to the length of time from the bite until treatment is instituted. The tourniquet, and incision and suction as well, are appropriate if employed within 1 hour from the time of the bite.

Immobilization. Patients are kept quiet, and the extremity is immobilized. Splinting the limb may inhibit the local diffusion of venom by stopping the movement of muscle bellies within their sheaths. Snyder and Knowles have shown in animals that exercise greatly enhances the absorption of venom, and as much as 30 percent may be absorbed within 30 minutes following vigorous exercise.

Tourniquet. The snake injects venom into the subcutaneous tissue, and this is absorbed by the lymphatics. As almost none of the venom is absorbed through the bloodstream, the tourniquet is applied loosely to obstruct only venous and lymphatic flow. The index finger should be easily inserted beneath the tourniquet after its application. The tourniquet is not released once applied and may be left in place during the 30 minutes that suction is being applied. Snyder and Knowles have injected ^{131}I-tagged venom into dogs and have demonstrated that if the tourniquet is applied promptly, less than 10 percent of the venom leaves the leg of the dog in 2 hours. The tourniquet may be removed as soon as an intravenous infusion is started and antivenin is ready for administration, if indicated.

Incision and Suction. Incision and suction should be accomplished as soon as possible after snakebite. Approximately 50 percent of subcutaneously injected venom can be removed when the suction is started within 3 minutes. Treatment in the first 5 minutes is important, since half the value of suction is lost after 15 minutes and almost all after 30 minutes. A 30-minute period of suction extracts about 90 percent of the venom which can be removed by this procedure. The incision should be $\frac{1}{4}$ in. long and $\frac{1}{8}$ to $\frac{1}{4}$ in. deep, longitudinal and not cruciate. When two fang marks are seen, the depth of the venom injection is generally considered to be one-third of the distance between the fang marks. A good rule of thumb has been to incise the skin and subcutaneous tissue the same distance between the fang marks to ensure adequate drainage. A superficial incision may be easily accomplished by raising the skin with a pinch between two fingers. This procedure rarely results in penetration of fascia or muscle. Incisions made proximal to the bite will usually recover venom insufficient to make the procedure worthwhile.

When a suction cup is not available after incisions have been made, mouth suction may be used if the mucosa of the mouth is intact. Snake venom is not absorbed through an intact oral mucosa but may be absorbed when there is any denuded area or minor laceration of the mucosa. The digestive juices neutralize poisonous snake venom if it is swallowed.

Russell has demonstrated that the serosanguinous fluid removed during suction contains substances which when injected into animals produced a fall in systemic blood pressure and changes in respiratory rates, and alterations in the electrocardiogram and electroencephalogram similar to those observed following injection of crude *Crotalus*

venom. If exudate removed during suction contains venom, its removal should increase the chances of survival.

Excision. Snyder and Knowles showed that wide excision of the entire area around the snakebite within 1 hour from the time of injection can remove most of the venom. Excision of the fang marks including skin and subcutaneous tissue should be considered in severe bites and in patients known to be allergic to horse serum who are seen within 1 hour following the bite.

Most fatalities from snakebites do not occur for 6 to 48 hours following the bite, giving time to institute these first-aid measures.

Cryotherapy. This form of therapy has been used but is not recommended, as it probably only increases the local area of necrosis. McCollough and Gennard analyzed cryotherapy in relation to amputation and noted that 75 percent of children requiring amputation following snakebite had received cryotherapy. In seven of nine snakebite cases requiring amputations in California, cryotherapy had been used. Cooling or refrigeration experimentally produces intense vasoconstriction and thus decreases the amount of antivenin getting into the area of the bite. Gill found that dogs developed edema and ecchymosis just as rapidly and extensively with cryotherapy as without it. There was no evidence to suggest inactivation of venom by tissue temperature of 15°C and below.

SYSTEMIC TREATMENT. The most important treatment for a snakebite is antivenin. Most snakebite fatalities in the United States during the past 20 years have involved either delay in obtaining treatment, no antivenin treatment, or inadequate dosage. Because antivenin contains horse serum, its administration requires prior skin testing.

Information concerning identification of a snake or proper antivenin frequently can be obtained from the nearest zoo herpetarium. A major problem with bites by exotic poisonous snakes is the choice and availability of suitable antiserum. Physicians confronted with this situation may obtain advice from the local poison control center or from the Antivenin Index Center of the American Association of Zoological Parks and Aquariums in Oklahoma City, Oklahoma (405-271-5454).

Because the rattlesnake, cottonmouth moccasin, and copperhead belong to the same biologic family, their bites can be treated by the same antivenin (antivenin Crotalidae polyvalent).

The coral snakebite is rare, and the antivenin is different from that for the pit vipers. A North American coral snake (*Micrurus fulvius*) antivenin has recently been developed and released. It effectively treats *Micrurus* coral snake bites but is not effective in treating bites of *Micruroides,* the genus native to Arizona and New Mexico. Coral snake antivenin can be obtained from many state public health departments. Also, a large supply has been stocked at the United States Public Health Service National Communicable Disease Center in Atlanta, Georgia.

The time of antivenin administration depends upon the snake involved. If the bite is from a snake with quick-acting venom, such as a king cobra or mamba, an initial dose of antivenin may be required as part of the first-aid treatment. However, for bites by most snakes, such as rattlesnakes and others with less virulent venom, antivenin should be withheld until a physician can determine if it is indicated. Approximately 30 percent of all poisonous snakebites in the United States result in no venenation.

The indication for antivenin is governed by the degree of venenation, as outlined by Wood et al. and modified by Parrish and by McCollough and Gennard:

Grade 0—no venenation: One or more fang marks; minimal pain; less than 1 in. of surrounding edema and erythema at 12 hours; no systemic involvement.
Grade I—minimal venenation: Fang marks; moderate to severe pain; 1 to 5 in. of surrounding edema and erythema in the first 12 hours after bite; systemic involvement usually not present.
Grade II—moderate venenation: Fang marks; severe pain; 6 to 12 in. of surrounding edema and erythema in the first 12 hours after bite; possible systemic involvement including nausea, vomiting giddiness, shock, or neurotoxic symptoms.
Grade III—severe venenation: Fang marks; severe pain; more than 12 in. of surrounding edema and erythema in first 12 hours after bite; grade II symptoms of systemic involvement usually present and may include generalized petechiae and ecchymoses.
Grade IV—very severe venenation: Systemic involvement is always present, and symptoms may include renal failure, blood-tinged secretions, coma, and death; local edema may extend beyond the involved extremity to the ipsilateral trunk.

Antivenin usually is not required for grades 0 or I venenation. Grade II may require three or four ampules, and grade III usually requires five ampules or more. If symptoms increase, several vials may be required during the first 2 hours. Because children are smaller, they receive relatively larger doses of venom, which places them in a higher-risk group. Thus, the smaller the patient, the relatively larger the required dose of antivenin. Proper dosage can be estimated by observing the clinical signs and symptoms. With frequent observations using this classification, the severity of the bite will be found to increase with time, and thus a change in grade is observed.

The injection of antivenin locally around the bite is not advised, as massive edema usually occurs in that area. Therefore, absorption from this area is poor, and additional antivenin fluid will further decrease perfusion and perhaps increase tissue anoxia.

Antivenin is given by intravenous drip in 250 ml of normal saline solution or 5% glucose solution. McCollough and Gennard have demonstrated in studies with radioisotopes that antivenin accumulates at the site of the bite more rapidly after *intravenous* than after *intramuscular* administration. The dose of intravenously administered antivenin can be more easily titrated with response to treatment. Antivenin is administered until severe local or systemic symptoms improve. When it is obvious that antivenin therapy will be instituted, the tourniquet should be left in place until antivenin is started intravenously.

Complications of Antivenin. If too much time has elapsed for excision to be effective and the patient is allergic to horse serum, a slow infusion of one vial of antivenin in 250 ml of 5% glucose solution may be given over a 90-minute period with constant monitoring of the blood pressure and electrocardiogram depending on the seriousness of the bite. If an immediate reaction occurs, the antivenin is stopped, and a vasopressor, epinephrine, and perhaps an antihistamine may be required, depending on the severity of the reaction.

The incidence of serum sickness is directly related to the volume of horse serum injected. Of patients receiving 100 to 200 ml of horse serum, 85 percent will have some degree of sensitivity in 8 to 12 days following injection. This complication will have to be dealt with at a later time since some patients may require from one to five vials of antiserum every 4 to 6 hours.

Steroids have been used but are of questionable benefit. Russell experimentally used doses of methylprednisone up to 100 mg/kg in mice and noted that steroids neither affected survival nor prevented tissue damage and inflammation. When used in association with the antivenin, there is a decreased incidence of serum sickness. According to Parrish, cortisone and ACTH do not affect the survival rate of animals poisoned with pit viper venom. Antibiotics are started immediately to prevent secondary infection, and tetanus toxoid is administered. Tracheal intubation and prolonged ventilation may be required for respiratory failure. Acute renal failure may require renal dialysis.

Intravenous fluids are frequently required to replace the decreased extracellular fluid volume resulting from edema formation. Fascial planes may become very tense, with obstruction of venous and later arterial flow, requiring fasciotomy.

Blood should be immediately drawn for typing and cross matching, since hemolysis may later make this difficult. Since hemolysis and injury to kidneys and liver may occur, it is important to follow alterations in clotting mechanism and renal and liver function as well as electrolyte status. Bleeding and clotting time, platelet count, prothrombin time, fibrinogen level, and partial thromboplastin times are included in the base-line studies. These patients may need blood, since anemia can develop from the hematologic effects. As afibrinogenemia has been reported, fibrinogen may be required. Vitamin K may also be required, according to Stahnke. The patient is started on antibiotics immediately to prevent secondary infection, and tetanus toxoid is administered on arrival at the emergency ward. Prolonged artificial ventilation may be required for respiratory failure.

Stinging Insects and Animals

HYMENOPTERA

The most important insects that produce serious and possibly fatal anaphylactic reactions are the arthropods of the order Hymenoptera. This group includes the honeybee, bumblebee, wasp, yellow and black hornet, and fire ant. The venom of these stinging insects is just as potent as that of snakes and causes more deaths in the United States yearly than are caused by snakebites. Davidson states that, drop for drop, the venom of the bee is just as potent as that of the rattlesnake. Parrish noted that, of 460 deaths between 1950 and 1959, 50 percent were due to Hymenoptera, 30 percent due to poisonous snakes, and 14 percent due to spiders. Scorpions accounted for eight deaths. No other poisonous creature killed more than five persons.

Insects of the Hymenoptera group, except the bee, retain their sting and are in a position to sting repeatedly, each time injecting some portion of the venom sac contents. The worker honeybee sinks its barbed sting into the skin, and it cannot be withdrawn. As the bee attempts to escape, it is disemboweled. The stinger with the bowel, muscles, and venom sac attached are left behind. The muscles controlling the venom sac, although separated from the bee, rhythmically contract for as long as 20 minutes, driving the sting deeper and deeper into the skin, and continuing to inject venom.

Bee venoms contain histamine, serotonin, acelytcholine, formic acid, phospholipase A, hyaluronidase, and other proteins. Once the proteins of these insects are injected, the patient may become sensitized and be a candidate for anaphylactic response with the next sting.

CLINICAL MANIFESTATIONS. Symptoms consist of one or more of the following: localized pain, swelling, generalized erythema, a feeling of intense heat throughout the body, headache, blurred vision, injected conjunctiva, swollen and tender joints, itching, apprehension, urticaria, petechial hemorrhages of skin and mucous membranes, dizziness, weakness, sweating, severe nausea, abdominal cramps, dyspnea, constriction of the chest, asthma, angioneurotic edema, vascular collapse, and possible death from anaphylaxis. Fatal cases may manifest glottal and laryngeal edema, pulmonary and cerebral edema, visceral congestion, meningeal hyperemia, and interventricular hemorrhage. Death apparently results from a combination of shock, respiratory failure, and central nervous system changes.

The acute, allergic phase of the simple reaction is thought to be due to protein allergens rather than to toxicity of venom. These allergens may be found in dust from the wings, bodies, venom, saliva, or feces of the insect. Most deaths from insect stings occur within 15 to 30 minutes following the bite or sting.

TREATMENT. Early application of a tourniquet may prevent rapid spread of the venom. Affected persons should be taught to remove the venom sacs if present, being careful not to squeeze the sac. It may be necessary for some patients to carry an emergency kit, which is commercially available, supplied with a tourniquet, sublingual isoproterenol in 10-mg tablets, epinephrine hydrochloride aerosol for inhalation to reduce bronchospasm and laryngeal edema, and tweezers to remove the sting and venom sac until a physician is available. The patient should be taught to give himself an epinephrine injection. Patients having severe reactions should first receive 0.3 to 0.5 ml of a 1:1,000 solution of epinephrine intravenously. Antihistamines also may be intravenously administered, and oxygen may be given. If wheezing continues, aminophylline may be given slowly intravenously. Occasionally the patient may require a tracheostomy.

DESENSITIZATION. The Insect Allergy Committee of the American Academy of Allergy noted that 50 percent of people who had a severe generalized reaction to stings had no previous history of a severe reaction. A sharp rise was noted in the proportion of serious reactions after the age of thirty, suggesting increasing sensitivity as the total number of stings increase. Patients with a history of severe local or systemic involvement following insect stings should be desensitized.

The efficacy of desensitization to insect stings has been demonstrated. Of persons desensitized and stung again, 88 percent experienced milder reactions than they had previously, and only 3 percent suffered more severe reactions. By comparison, 63 percent of those patients stung again but not desensitized suffered more severe reactions. It has been suspected that a refractory period of 10 to 14 days persists following an insect sting during which skin tests may be negative. Therefore, skin tests should be delayed several weeks after stinging and be performed with extreme caution. Cross reactions to the wasp, bee, and yellow jacket may occur.

Because the antigens eliciting hypersensitive reactions are present in the insect's body as well as its venom, whole insect extract should be used for skin testing before hyposensitization therapy is begun. The initial dilution should be weak, since shocklike reactions have been reported after intradermal testing with a 1:1 million dilution. Immunotherapy consists of weekly subcutaneous injections of whole body extract, containing equal parts of bee, hornet, wasp, and yellow jacket whole body extracts, administered for at least 3 years, perhaps indefinitely.

STINGRAYS

Approximately 750 persons each year are stung by stingrays. However, during the past 60 years, only two deaths in this country have been attributed to the venom of the stingray.

As the spine, which is curved and has serrated edges, enters the flesh, the sheath surrounding the spine ruptures, and venom is released. As the spine is withdrawn, fragments of the sheath may remain in the wound. The wound edges are often jagged and bleed freely. Pain is usually immediate and severe, increasing to maximum intensity in 1 to 2 hours and lasting for 12 to 48 hours.

TREATMENT. This consists of copious irrigation with water to wash out any toxin and fragments of the spine's integumentary sheath. Russell noted that the venom is inactivated when exposed to heat. Therefore, the area of the bite should be placed in water as hot as the patient can stand without injury for 30 minutes to 1 hour. After soaking, the wound may be further debrided and treated appropriately. Patients treated in this manner were shown to have rapid and uncomplicated healing of the wound. Patients not treated with heat had tissue necrosis with prolonged drainage and chronically infected wounds.

PORTUGUESE MAN-OF-WAR

This coelenterate is commonly found along our southern Atlantic coast. Its tentacles are covered with thousands of stinging cells, the nematocytes, capable of emitting microscopic organelles, the nematocysts, each of which consists of a small sphere containing a coiled hollow thread. When activated by touch, the thread is uncoiled with such force that it can penetrate skin and even rubber gloves. On contact, venom in the cyst is injected into the victim through the thread. This sting produces extreme pain and often signs of clinical shock; however, no deaths have been reported due to this sting alone.

Following a severe sting there may be almost immediate severe nausea, gastric cramping, and constriction and tightness of throat and chest with severe muscle spasm. There is intense burning pain with weakness and perhaps cyanosis with respiratory distress.

TREATMENT. The most important emergency treatment is to inactivate the nematocysts immediately, to prevent their continuous firing of toxins. This is accomplished by application to the involved area of a substance of high alcohol content, such as rubbing alcohol. This is followed by application of a drying agent, such as flour, baking soda, talc, or shaving cream. The tentacles may then be removed by shaving. Alkaline agents, such as baking soda, are then applied to the involved area in order to neutralize the toxins, which are acetic. Antihistamines may be helpful in controlling the inflammatory response after these emergency treatments. Demerol and Benadryl may dramatically relieve the pain and symptoms. Aerosol corticosteroid-analgesic balm is helpful.

Spider Bites

BLACK WIDOW SPIDER

The most common biting spider in the United States is the black widow (*Latrodectus mactans*) (Fig. 6-4). This spider is black and globular, with a red hourglass mark on the abdomen. The bite of this species in the 10-year period 1950–1959 accounted for 63 deaths. *Latrodectus* venom is primarily neurotoxic in action and appears to center on the spinal cord. Following a bite by the black widow spider, the patient usually experiences sudden pain, and in a few minutes a small wheal with an area of erythema appears. The most prominent physical finding is generalized muscle spasm. Even if bitten on an extremity, the spasm may involve the abdomen and chest. Although the abdomen is rigid, it is nontender. The severe symptoms last from 24 to 48 hours.

TREATMENT. Treatment has consisted of narcotics for the relief of pain and a muscle relaxant for relief of spasm. Either methocarbamol (Robaxin) or 10 ml of a 10% solution of calcium gluconate relieves symptoms. Methocarbamol can be administered intravenously, 10 ml over a 5-minute period, with a second ampule started in a saline solution drip. Specific treatment involves the use of antivenin. This is administered intramuscularly, after appropriate skin tests, since it contains horse serum.

NORTH AMERICAN LOXOSCELISM

The distinguishing mark of the *Loxosceles reclusa* is the darker violin-shaped band over the dorsal cephalothorax (Fig. 6-5). The spider is native to the South Central United States and is found both indoors and outdoors and under cliffs and overhanging rocks. The first recognized and documented case in the United States of a bite by *Loxosceles reclusa* was not published until 1957.

CLINICAL MANIFESTATIONS. The bite may go unnoticed because pain may not occur until 6 to 8 hours afterward.

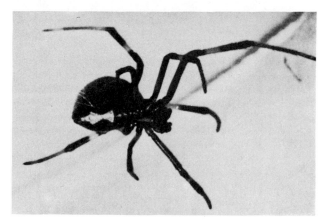

Fig. 6-4. Abdominal view of a female black widow spider showing the hourglass marking. (*From B. C. Paton, Surg Clin North Am, 43:537, 1963.*)

A generalized macular and erythematous rash may appear in 12 to 24 hours. Erythema develops, with bleb or blister formation surrounded by an irregular area of ischemia. A zone of hemorrhage with induration and a surrounding halo of erythema may develop peripherally. The central ischemia turns dark, an eschar forms by the seventh

Fig. 6-5. The distinguishing mark of the *Loxosceles reclusa* is the darker violin-shaped band over the dorsal cephalothorax. (*From C. J. Dillaha, G. T. Jansen, W. M. Honeycutt, and C. R. Hayden, JAMA, 188:33, 1964.*)

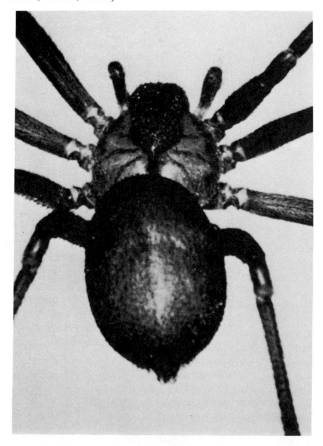

day, and by the fourteenth day the area sloughs, leaving an open ulcer. Approximately 3 weeks is required for the lesion to heal. Severe systemic manifestations may occur in 24 to 48 hours in small children, with fever, chills, malaise, weakness, nausea, vomiting, joint pain, and even petechial eruption. The two principal systemic effects, hemolysis and thrombocytopenia, have been responsible for two deaths. Hemoglobinemia, hemoglobinuria, leukocytosis, and proteinuria may also occur. *Loxosceles* venom is chiefly cytotoxic in action.

TREATMENT. Immediate excision with primary closure has been advocated as the treatment of choice. This usually is not possible since the patient rarely can be certain of what bit him or has failed to recognize the type of spider. Several writers immediately administered steroids. The dose has varied from 30 to 80 mg of methylprednisolone daily, tapered over a period of several days. This seems to be the preferred treatment. Excision of the necrotic area with skin grafting may be required at a later date.

PENETRATING WOUNDS OF THE NECK AND THORACIC INLET

(by Robert F. Jones, G. Tom Shires, and William H. Snyder III)

INCIDENCE. Although major wounds of the soft tissues of the neck are relatively uncommon in civilian surgical practice, the number of vital structures in the small volume of the neck makes it imperative that every penetrating neck wound be considered a serious surgical problem.

Prior to World War II, the treatment of penetrating wounds of the neck was largely nonsurgical unless major bleeding or deep injuries were obvious. Reported mortality rates were 18 percent of 188 cases in the Spanish-American War and 11 percent of 594 cases in World War I. During World War II the mortality rate fell to 7 percent, probably because of a variety of factors, including earlier tracheostomy, earlier and more frequent surgical exploration, antibiotics, and improvements in surgical and anesthetic techniques.

Since 1960, several civilian series have been reported with no further reduction in mortality rate, which seems to have leveled off at about 10 percent. In the three previous series, the total number of deaths was 57. Of these, 43 were a direct result of blood vessel injuries. The other 14 deaths were due principally to complications from wounds of the larynx, trachea, and esophagus. In the study of Shirkey et al. 6 of the 22 deaths occurred in the group in which exploration was delayed beyond 6 hours or omitted entirely. Fogelman and Stewart pointed out that the mortality rate for their cases which were promptly explored was 6 percent, whereas for those in which surgical intervention was omitted or postponed the mortality rate was 35 percent. Their overall mortality was 11 percent. Since the initial phase of the Fogelman and Stewart series, it has been the policy at Parkland Memorial Hospital to "treat the platysma like the peritoneum" and explore virtually all neck wounds that penetrate the platysma in the

operating room under general endotracheal anesthesia, regardless of preoperative opinion as to the extent and severity of the damage.

Recently, 274 penetrating wounds of the neck treated at Parkland Memorial Hospital have been reviewed. There were 11 deaths, for a mortality rate of 3.6 percent. Of the fatalities, four were due to complications from spinal cord injuries, three from massive hemorrhage, one from extensive aspiration of blood from a bleeding tracheal wound, one from blast injury to the brainstem, one from a cerebral embolus following repair of a common carotid artery injury, and one from blast injury to the trachea unrecognized at the original exploration and leading to laryngeal edema and obstruction in the absence of a tracheostomy.

Of the 274 cases, 103 explorations were negative, i.e., with no hematoma, no significant bleeding, and no damage to any named structure in the neck, although the tract of injury frequently was within millimeters of vital structures. Of these negative cases, there were no deaths and no complications except one superficial wound infection which cleared promptly with drainage. These patients usually were discharged within 72 hours to clinic follow-up if there were no associated injuries.

Table 6-3 summarizes the injuries found in 15 patients with clinically "negative" neck wounds, i.e., with no visible bleeding, no visible hematoma, no evidence of hemorrhagic shock. At some hospitals these wounds would not have been explored, and many probably would have healed uneventfully without surgical exploration. However, unexplored patients, apparently free of significant injury on examination in the emergency room, may bleed massively later when a blood clot is shaken loose, or a deep abscess may develop from a small perforation of the esophagus, or other complications may develop from unrecognized injuries. Even those less serious injuries associated only with damage to subcutaneous tissues and muscles will heal faster with less chance of infection if hemostasis, debridement, and adequate drainage are accomplished. It is a fundamental fact that bacteria thrive on extravasated blood and damaged tissue, and every penetrating wound is contaminated.

TREATMENT. The safest treatment for penetrating neck wounds appears to be prompt and thorough surgical exploration under local or general anesthesia.

Initial Treatment. On admission to the emergency room, all patients with neck injuries are immediately evaluated

Table 6-3. INJURIES IN 15 CLINICALLY "NEGATIVE"* NECK WOUNDS

Total series = 274 patients

Innominate vein	2
Subclavian vein	1
Internal jugular vein	5
Thyrocervical artery	3
Thoracic duct	2
Esophagus (blast injury)	2
Ascending pharyngeal artery	1

*No visible bleeding, no visible hematoma, no shock.

regarding their systemic condition, i.e., airway and adequacy of ventilation, blood pressure, pulse, mental state, and peripheral signs of shock such as sweating, cold skin, and collapsed veins. If there is external bleeding, some type of pressure is applied for temporary hemostasis. If there is upper airway obstruction, an endotracheal tube is passed immediately, or if there is sufficient time, a tracheostomy is performed. Meanwhile, one or two large-bore intravenous cannulas or needles are inserted in peripheral veins and Ringer's lactate solution is started while blood is drawn for typing and cross matching. If shock is present, the fluid is given rapidly, and if there is no evidence of significant blood loss, the intravenous infusions are kept going by slow drip. When indicated, whole blood is administered as soon as it is available. Usually the salt solution will temporarily reverse the shock state until cross-matched blood is available. If shock is severe and is not improved promptly by the Ringer's lactate solution, type O, Rh-negative low-titer unmatched blood is infused rapidly until the matched blood is available. Plasma has also been used, but there is little advantage over salt solutions; i.e., both are quite helpful temporarily, although neither is a substitute for whole blood.

If it is apparent that blood or air is free in a pleural cavity, closed-chest drainage is immediately instituted. If there is no clinical evidence or a pneumothorax or hemothorax and the missile or blade could have possibly reached the pleura, and if the patient's systemic condition is stable, an upright chest film is obtained with a physician in constant attendance. Special x-ray studies such as arteriograms have rarely been worthwhile.

If the depth of the injury is not apparent, the wound is very gently probed with a small hemostat only to the depth of the platysma muscle. If the platysma has been penetrated, the probing is discontinued. Nonbleeding neck wounds should not be deeply probed in an emergency room. The patient is then transferred to the operating room. No attempt is made to pass a nasogastric tube in the emergency room because of the danger of hemorrhage with coughing or gagging.

Anesthesia. Virtually all neck wounds are explored under general anesthesia, using an orotracheal airway with an inflatable cuff. The anesthetic agent varies considerably according to the specific problem, necessity for rapid induction, circulatory status, preexisting disease, etc. There are no specific contraindications in neck injuries per se to any of the commonly used anesthetic agents or relaxants.

The chest is again examined just prior to induction, since pneumothorax or hemothorax may develop slowly following a neck wound, appearing an hour or longer after an initially negative chest x-ray. Wounds at the root of the neck following a downward path may barely penetrate the pleura so that a pneumothorax is not apparent initially and may not be manifest until after the patient is intubated. This should be kept in mind as a cause for hypotension or hypoxia during anesthesia, especially if closed thoracotomy drainage has not been instituted.

Technique of Exploration. With adequate control of the ventilatory and cardiovascular systems, the surgeon can now safely and adequately explore the structures that are apparently or potentially injured. The incision is planned to allow full exposure of the tract of injury. Proximal and distal control of the major vessels must also be considered in the length and position of the incision. The sternocleidomastoid muscle and/or any other neck muscles are transected whenever necessary to provide adequate exposure. An oblique incision along the anterior border of the sternocleidomastoid muscle is often useful, or any transverse incision may be used if it gives adequate exposure. The tract of injury is followed to its depth, with systematic examination of each structure in or near the tract. It should also be pointed out that blast injury from gunshot wounds may not be immediately apparent in the tissues adjacent to the tract.

Specific Injuries

CERVICAL BLOOD VESSELS. If injuries to the major vessels are suspected, umbilical tapes are passed around the vessels proximal and distal to the point of suspected injury before local clots are removed if bleeding has previously occurred and stopped. This happens frequently with venous and occasionally with arterial injury. The vessels are then carefully inspected, all clots are removed, and repair is carried out.

When the injury involves the low anterior neck, it may be necessary to resect a portion of the clavicle or to split the sternum to obtain proximal control and prevent uncontrollable hemorrhage. The medial one-third or one-half of the clavicle is resected whenever necessary, disarticulating the sternoclavicular joint. There is no significant disability following this procedure, and if the periosteum is preserved, bony regeneration will usually occur. When this does not adequately expose the great vessels for repair or for proximal control, the entire clavicle is removed, or the sternum may be split with a Lebsche knife. The sternal incision may be carried off laterally into the second or third intercostal space to avoid opening the full mediastinum unnecessarily.

The internal carotid, common carotid, subclavian, and innominate arteries should be repaired if at all possible. An internal or external shunt may be utilized during carotid repair, as with carotid grafting or endarterectomy, or the vessel may be partially occluded with a curved vascular clamp to allow partial flow during repair. The vertebral artery is usually very difficult to repair in the bony canal but may be controlled by prolonged pressure, suture ligatures, and bone wax. The external carotid artery and/or its branches may be ligated except in patients with carotid arteriosclerosis with an occluded common or internal carotid vessel. In these cases, the external carotid may be a major source of collateral flow.

When the carotid arteries are to be handled or pressed upon in the region of the bifurcation, the adventitia of the carotid bulb is infiltrated with a local anesthetic to prevent hypotension from reflexes originating in pressor receptors of the carotid sinus. Atropine may be given at intervals during the procedure when hypotension results from such stimuli.

The internal jugular vein is repaired if feasible but may

be ligated unilaterally if necessary without adverse seque-lae. All other neck veins are routinely ligated if injured. Prompt pressure on an open vein and a slight head-down tilt to the table will prevent the occurrence of air embolism.

BLOOD VESSELS OF THORACIC INLET. Injuries to the major vascular structures in the base of the neck or thoracic inlet are a significant challenge in management. Rapid resuscitation, liberal surgical exploration, and a thorough knowledge of the operative approach are the necessary ingredients of success. The vascular structures involved are the common carotid, subclavian, and innominate arteries and their corresponding veins. A penetrating wound due to an act of violence is the usual cause. Indications for early surgical exploration are listed in Table 6-4. Diagnostic errors and subsequent inappropriately conservative management rarely occur with overt signs of major vascular injury. Unfortunately, a significant number of these injuries appear innocuous at the time of presentation, and a high index of suspicion is necessary. It is in this context that platysmal penetration and proximity of the wound to a major vascular structure must be regarded as absolute indications for surgical exploration. This concept is emphasized by data from a recent Parkland Memorial Hospital series, to be presented later. Arteriography to modify the principle of proximity and penetration exploration remains controversial. It may prove useful if always immediately available. However, valuable time should not be wasted obtaining studies if objective evidence of major vascular injury exists.

Immediate formal exploration in the operating room generally is recommended. Massive bleeding progressing to exsanguination can occur rapidly from a wound that initially appears innocent if increased intrathoracic pressure dislodges a tamponading clot. For this reason, every effort is made to avoid vomiting, coughing, or agitation. Smooth anesthetic induction is most important. Endotracheal intubation of patients with wounds in the base of the neck is most safely accomplished following infusion of muscle relaxants, thus minimizing the danger of "bucking the endotracheal tube" with a sudden increase in intravascular pressure.

As preoperative prediction of the specific vessels injured

Table 6-4. FINDINGS SUGGESTING MAJOR VASCULAR INJURY

Obvious or direct evidence of injury:
1. Circulatory instability
2. Excessive external bleeding
3. A large or progressing hematoma
4. Distal pulse deficit
5. Neurologic deficit involving nerves anatomically adjacent to major vascular structures
6. Massive or continued intrathoracic bleeding

Indirect evidence indicating exploration:
1. A wound above the clavicle or manubrium that penetrates the platysma muscle
2. Thoracic wounds whose trajectory traverses the superior mediastinum or thoracic inlet
3. Mediastinal widening demonstrated roentgenographically

often is inaccurate, a flexible operative approach is necessary. The entire neck, thorax, and proximal arms are included in the surgical field. The supine position with slight cervical extension provides the greatest flexibility for performing the primary incision and any necessary extensions. The major technical problem is to provide adequate exposure for establishing proximal and distal vascular control prior to dissecting the area of injury. Familiarity with several basic incisions and their extensions is necessary. These are demonstrated in Fig. 6-6. They include the oblique neck incision, the horizontal clavicular incision with resection of the medial portion of the clavicle, the median sternotomy, and the bilateral fourth intercostal space anterolateral thoracotomies.

The right oblique incision generally is adequate to expose the entire right common carotid artery. The horizontal clavicular incision with subperiostial resection of the medial half of the clavicle adequately exposes the right subclavian vessels. Extension to a median sternotomy generally is necessary to expose the innominate artery; the distal left common carotid artery is easily exposed through a left oblique neck incision. The proximal left common carotid and the distal left subclavian can be reached

Fig. 6-6. Incisions and extensions for base-of-the-neck vascular injuries.

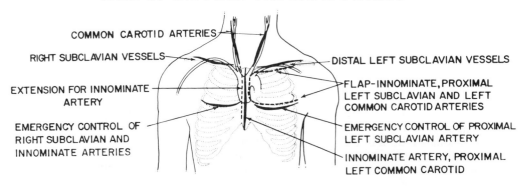

INCISIONS AND EXTENSIONS
FOR
BASE OF THE NECK VASCULAR INJURIES

through a horizontal clavicular incision; further exposure can be gained by extension to a median sternotomy. However, the proximal portion of the left subclavian artery is best approached through a left anterolateral thoracotomy. The entire left subclavian artery is adequately exposed through a combined left clavicular and left anterolateral thoracotomy incision. The construction of a musculoskeletal flap, or "trapdoor," has been used by some to expose the innominate and subclavian vessels. This is formed by combining horizontal clavicular, superior median sternotomy, and anterolateral thoracotomy incisions. As a general rule, the majority of these injuries are exposed through the oblique neck or horizontal clavicular incisions. Major extensions should be made without hesitation when these incisions provide inadequate exposure. The vascular repair seldom is difficult and most often can be accomplished by lateral arteriorrhaphy or end-to-end anastomosis. When graft interposition is required, autogenous material is preferred.

Important factors in the management of these injuries are emphasized by a recent series from Parkland Memorial Hospital. During a 10-year period, 99 patients with 122 injuries of the major vascular structures at the base of the neck were seen. Arterial injuries accounted for 40 percent, including 23 injuries to the subclavian artery, 21 to the common carotid, and 3 to the innominate artery. Of 74 venous injuries, there were 35 to the subclavian vein, 31 to the internal jugular, and 8 to the innominate vein. Signs and symptoms of significant vascular injury were equivocal in many patients and totally absent in 32 patients. These patients were explored on the basis of platysmal penetration and the proximity of the wound to a major vascular structure. The overall mortality was 5.1 percent, generally related to the magnitude of associated injuries or the extent of blood loss prior to operation. Eleven percent of the patients with arterial trauma died, compared with 1.3 percent of those with venous injuries. Postoperative complications were related to vascular injury or repair in only 20 percent of patients. Essentially all injuries of the common carotid arteries or internal jugular veins were exposed through oblique neck incisions. Extension into a median sternotomy or horizontal clavicular incision was required only with associated vertebral or subclavian vessel injuries or when the proximal left common carotid artery was involved. Horizontal clavicular incisions with resection of the medial portion of the clavicle adequately exposed injuries of the subclavian vessels in most instances. An anterolateral thoracotomy was necessary only for immediate control of bleeding or when the proximal portion of the left subclavian artery was involved. The majority of the innominate vein injuries could be managed through horizontal clavicular incisions. However, median sternotomy was necessary to adequately expose innominate artery injuries. Early and liberal surgical exploration with emphasis on adequate exposure has resulted in the low mortality and morbidity rates in this large series.

LARYNX AND TRACHEA. Whenever laryngeal or tracheal injury is apparent in the emergency room, tracheostomy is performed promptly, prior to transfer of the patient to the main operating suite. If the injury is not apparent until the time of exploration, a tracheostomy is done during exploration. When the patient is hoarse or the wound is near the thyroid or larynx, indirect laryngoscopy is performed preoperatively when feasible to determine the integrity of the recurrent laryngeal nerve. Laryngeal blast injury may result from a bullet tract near the larynx; in such a case, a tracheostomy is also performed.

Subcutaneous air may be present with such injuries and may increase rapidly under observation. However, air may spread subcutaneously from outside via the entrance wound in the absence of tracheal, pharyngeal, or esophageal penetration. Cervical extension of mediastinal air from an injured bronchus or lung may also occur.

Clean lacerations of the trachea or larynx are closed using a nonabsorbable suture, usually cotton or silk. If the defect cannot be closed primarily, a fascial flap may be used as a patch. Synthetic patch grafts such as Marlex have been successful. The tracheostomy is maintained until healing is complete and laryngeal or tracheal edema has subsided, usually 4 to 8 days.

PHARYNX AND ESOPHAGUS. If a small esophageal injury is suspected but cannot be demonstrated during exploration, an anesthetic mask may be applied to the nose and mouth and positive pressure exerted while the wound is filled with saline solution. Bubbles may disclose the point of injury. The pharynx and esophagus may be repaired primarily using chromic catgut suture, following debridement as necessary. It is vital to drain all such wounds, since infection and/or a salivary leak is not an infrequent complication. If there is massive loss of tissue, as with a close-range shotgun blast, it may be necessary to perform a cutaneous esophagostomy for feeding purposes and cutaneous pharyngostomy for salivary drainage. A secondary plastic reconstruction will be required after initial healing is complete. A small plastic nasogastric tube is used for feeding for 8 to 10 days following all esophageal injuries, unless for some reason a gastrostomy is deemed preferable.

NERVES. A preoperative neurologic examination is performed whenever possible to identify an injured nerve. The brachial plexus, the deep cervical plexus, the phrenic nerve, and the cranial nerves are systematically tested. The vagus and recurrent laryngeal nerves can be checked by examination of the vocal cords. A hypoglossal or spinal accessory nerve injury is particularly easy to miss unless a preoperative neurologic examination is performed. An associated head injury or alcoholic intoxication will frequently complicate the neurologic evaluation.

Whenever possible, all severed or lacerated nerves are debrided and repaired primarily, using interrupted fine silk sutures on the perineurium. If a motor nerve deficit is apparent, an expendable sensory nerve such as the great auricular nerve may be interposed as a nerve autograft to allow anastomosis without tension.

THYROID. After debridement of devitalized tissue, hemostasis may be secured by suture ligature. Adequate drainage is particularly important.

THORACIC DUCT. Wounds near the inferior segment of the left internal jugular vein may sever the thoracic duct at or below the point of entry; the location is quite variable. Repair of the duct is not feasible because of its friability, but simple ligation is adequate. Since the duct may divide just before entering the vein or there may be tributaries for the head and arm, multiple ligatures may be required for lymphostasis. The area should be thoroughly dried and inspected before closing, since a large collection of lymph may occur postoperatively from even a small leak. If lymph does accumulate, incision and drainage with the application of a bulky pressure dressing will usually allow closure of the lymph fistula within a few days. Occasionally, an injured right lymphatic duct is encountered on the opposite side in the same location and is treated in like manner.

SALIVARY GLANDS. A sialogram may be used preoperatively to establish the diagnosis, or it may be determined during exploration. Injuries to the gland may be handled by debridement, hemostasis, and simple drainage. In the absence of ductal obstruction, a salivary fistula will rarely occur following injury to the gland substance. When the major duct is injured, it may be repaired with fine silk over a ureteral catheter stent. The catheter should be removed after repair is effected. When repair is not feasible because of the patient's condition or for some other compelling reason, the duct may be ligated and the gland allowed to atrophy, or the duct may be reimplanted in the mucosa at a later time.

When the parotid gland is involved, the major facial nerve branches should be identified and repaired if injured. Primary repair has a better prognosis for nerve function than does delayed repair, unless there is gross bacterial contamination or massive loss of tissue.

If a salivary fistula does occur postoperatively and fails to close spontaneously, irradiation is usually effective in arresting salivary flow but is not used for this purpose in children or young adults.

CLOSURE. Almost all soft tissue neck wounds are drained for 24 to 48 hours using soft Penrose drains to prevent the accumulation of blood and serum. If the pharynx or esophagus is injured, drainage is continued for 4 to 8 days. All muscles are repaired. In the case of massive gunshot wounds, such as a close-range shotgun injury, the wound is left open initially and a delayed primary closure performed 3 to 4 days later, if possible.

ABDOMINAL TRAUMA

(*by Robert N. McClelland, Ronald C. Jones,*
Malcolm O. Perry, G. Tom Shires and Erwin R. Thal)

The incidence of abdominal trauma increases each year. About 5 million persons in the United States are injured yearly in automobile accidents, and many of these injuries are abdominal. Blunt abdominal trauma generally leads to higher mortality rates than penetrating wounds and presents greater problems in diagnosis. The spleen, liver, kidneys, and bowel are the most frequently injured abdominal viscera. In a review of several series of abdominal trauma by Griswold and Collier, the frequency of injury was determined (see Table 6-5).

Evaluation of Blunt Trauma

The greatest difficulty in the management of blunt abdominal trauma is in the diagnosis. This is largely due to masking of abdominal injury by associated injuries. The most frequently associated injuries are head trauma, chest trauma, and fractures. Often the patient is unconscious because of alcoholism, shock, or associated head injury. Another misleading factor in diagnosis, often not recognized, is that relatively trivial injuries may rupture abdominal viscera. The index of suspicion of abdominal trauma must be high, even in cases of supposedly minor abdominal trauma, if diagnostic errors are to be avoided.

CLINICAL MANIFESTATIONS. The evaluation of the patient with blunt abdominal trauma begins with a careful history and physical examination. The entire patient must be examined as well as the abdomen because of the high incidence of associated trauma. Fitzgerald et al. have reported extraabdominal injuries in 97 percent of patients with abdominal injuries who were dead on arrival at the hospital and in 70 percent of those admitted alive. When the diagnosis is doubtful, one must often depend on repeated physical examinations alone, done at frequent intervals by the same examiner to decide whether the patient requires laparotomy.

Abdominal pain and tenderness are the most frequent findings. Abdominal rigidity, or involuntary guarding, is the most helpful sign and even when present alone warrants exploratory laparotomy. Hinton, in 1929, recommended a period of watchful waiting before exploration because of fear of uncontrollable hemorrhage and infection, as well as the difficulty of performing the necessary surgical procedures under adverse conditions. There is no excuse for this course today, and a policy of watchful waiting frequently may be disastrous. Fitzgerald et al. reported no deaths of patients who had exploratory laparotomy without a finding of intraabdominal injury. However, three deaths in their series occurred from intraabdominal hemorrhage because abdominal injury was masked by associated head injuries. The absence of any mortality for negative abdominal exploration for suspected abdominal trauma has been reported from several trauma centers.

In patients with blunt abdominal trauma, determinations of alterations in blood pressure are often useful. In a series of patients with blunt trauma reviewed recently from this institution, approximately 65 percent had systolic

Table 6-5. FREQUENCY OF INJURY
IN ABDOMINAL TRAUMA

Viscera injured	Frequency, %
Spleen	26.2
Kidneys	24.2
Intestines	16.2
Liver	15.6
Abdominal wall	3.6
Retroperitoneal hematoma	2.7
Mesentery	2.5
Pancreas	1.4
Diaphragm	1.1

blood pressures below 80 mm Hg on admission to the emergency room. It was found that a valuable sign of continuing intraabdominal hemorrhage was transient elevation of the blood pressure to normal levels for a few minutes followed by return to hypotensive levels with rapid infusion of 500 to 1,000 ml of Ringer's lactate solution. Patients who are hypotensive from minimal blood loss or from neurogenic shock usually do not behave in this manner. The Ringer's lactate solution generally is infused over a period of 15 to 20 minutes while other measures, such as blood typing and cross matching, are being carried out. Postural hypotension, when the patient assumes the erect position, is another useful sign of continuing intraabdominal bleeding.

DIAGNOSTIC PROCEDURES. Berman et al. state that if the leukocyte count is greater than 15,000 following abdominal trauma, a ruptured solid viscus is likely, especially if other findings are compatible with that diagnosis. Knopp and Harkins and Williams and Zollinger, however, have not found the leukocyte count to be so helpful. Several studies of the hemoglobin and hematocrit done at intervals of 30 minutes to 1 hour in suspicious cases may be helpful, but they may be misleading if the findings are overinterpreted. Naffziger and McCorkle note that the serum amylase level is valuable in recognizing acute pancreatic trauma. Elevated amylase levels may also indicate injury to the upper small bowel and duodenum with leakage of amylase-containing fluid from the injured bowel into the peritoneal cavity, where the amylase is freely absorbed into the blood. Studies of urinary sediment are useful, since hematuria may indicate injury to the genitourinary tract. If the patient with abdominal injury cannot void, catheterization should be done to obtain urine for examination. Examination of vomitus or insertion of a nasogastric tube to obtain gastric contents to be checked for evidence of upper gastrointestinal tract bleeding is helpful.

Radiologic Findings. For patients who have sustained severe abdominal injury and in whom other clinical signs obviously point to such injury, roentgenography, for diagnosis, may dangerously delay surgical intervention. However, for about one-third of patients with stable vital signs and questionable diagnoses of intraabdominal injury, x-ray studies may be helpful. Roentgenography is of least aid in injury to solid viscera, notably the liver, spleen, and pancreas.

When a patient is suspected of having intraabdominal injuries, upright films of the chest should be made, in addition to supine films of the abdomen. Occasionally additional information may be obtained from lateral and left lateral decubitus films. In addition: (1) Skeletal parts are checked for fractures or dislocations. (2) Examination of the soft tissues may give information concerning alterations of size, shape, or position of many viscera. (3) Pneumoperitoneum may be diagnosed with the patient in the erect or lateral decubitus positions. (4) Indirect evidence of solid viscera rupture with secondary hemorrhage may be presumed by an increase in density in the region, by displacement of neighboring viscera, or by accumulation of fluid between the gas shadows of bowel loops. Also, if a gastric, duodenal, or upper jejunal rupture is possible, the frequency of pneumoperitoneum may be increased by injecting 750 to 1,000 ml of air into a nasogastric tube, after which the patient sits in a semierect position for 10 minutes before an upright chest film or left lateral decubitus film of the abdomen is made. Films should also be made prior to the air injection for purposes of comparison if the patient's condition permits.

Another study which may be useful is examination of the upper gastrointestinal tract by x-ray after ingestion of a water-soluble opaque medium, which may indicate injury of the stomach, duodenum, or upper small bowel. The use of barium mixtures for this is dangerous, since a severe peritoneal reaction is caused by barium if it leaks through a perforation in the gastrointestinal tract. This is especially true if there is fecal contamination in the peritoneal cavity from concomitant colon injury.

Intravenous or retrograde pyelograms should be done if feasible for patients with hematuria or other evidence of genitourinary injury, not only to establish the nature of the injury, but also to determine if both kidneys are functioning prior to surgical intervention in case an injured kidney must be removed. If necessary, intravenous pyelograms may be done during the surgical procedure to determine the presence of a functional kidney on one side before removing the other kidney.

Cystograms may also be useful for diagnosing bladder injury or perforation from blunt abdominal trauma, but normal cystograms do not rule out bladder injury.

Intravenous cholangiography has also been helpful at times in suspected trauma to the hepatobiliary system.

Levin Tubes. Levin tubes are inserted in all patients sustaining blunt abdominal trauma. The stomach contents are aspirated, and the aspirate is examined for the presence of blood. In addition, a Levin tube provides for decompression of the stomach, prevents gastric dilatation, and prevents aspiration with the induction of anesthesia.

Paracentesis. Needle abdominal paracentesis is a useful diagnostic aid only for those cases of abdominal trauma in which, after physical examination, the examiner continues to suspect intraabdominal hemorrhage. The abdominal tap has been particularly useful as a diagnostic adjunct for comatose patients with head injury in whom adequate physical examination of the abdomen is not possible. A recent review with this procedure shows a diagnostic accuracy of 95 percent with positive paracentesis. A negative tap is not definitive, particularly if other elements of the physical examination indicate other reasons for exploring the abdomen. In female patients with suspected intraabdominal hemorrhage, culdocentesis may be positive for blood when abdominal taps are negative.

The technique is well described by Drapanas and McDonald and illustrated in Fig. 6-7. The abdomen is surgically cleansed with pHisoHex or an iodophor compound. An 18-gauge short-bevel spinal needle is attached to a syringe and inserted through the abdominal wall after prior infiltration of the site of tap with a local anesthetic agent. Suction is applied to the syringe as the needle is slowly advanced into the abdomen at the sites illustrated. Return of a minimum of 0.1 ml of nonclotting blood constitutes a positive tap. Occasionally, an intraabdominal

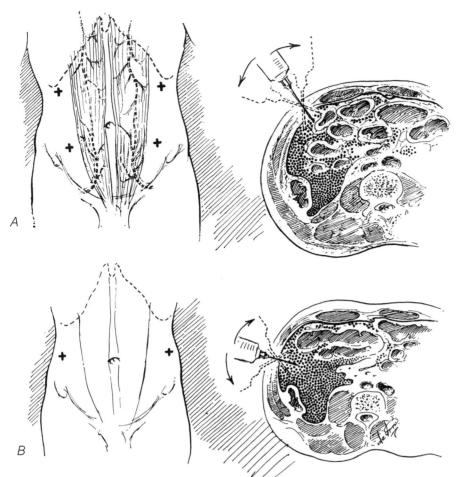

Fig. 6-7. *A.* Technique for four-quadrant peritoneal taps. Preferred location for aspiration of each quadrant is shown. Note that puncture through the rectus abdominis sheath is avoided. *B.* Technique for bilateral flank taps. Aspiration is performed in each flank midway between the costal margin and iliac spine. In our experience, bilateral flank taps are equally reliable as, and more easily performed than, four-quadrant taps in cases of abdominal trauma. (*From T. Drapanas and J. McDonald, Surgery, 50:742, 1961.*)

blood vessel may be entered, but this blood will clot and differentiate it from blood obtained from the free peritoneal cavity. Puncture of the rectus abdominis sheath anteriorly should be avoided to prevent a rectus abdominis sheath hematoma from injury to the epigastric vessels and to diminish the chance of the needle's penetrating the bowel, since gas-filled loops of bowel tend to float anteriorly in the abdomen containing fluid or blood. Actually, the danger of penetrating the intestine is slight; several studies have shown that penetration with an 18-gauge needle is harmless, as a hole in the bowel seals off quite rapidly with no leakage. Other technical considerations include the following:

1. Areas of abdominal scars or other points of possible bowel fixation to the abdominal wall should be avoided.
2. The direction of the needle inside the abdominal cavity should be changed only by withdrawing the point of the needle just superficially to the peritoneum, redirecting the needle, and reintroducing it into the peritoneal cavity.
3. Peritoneal taps should be avoided in the presence of markedly distended bowel, because abnormally elevated intraluminal pressure may cause continued leakage.

Paracentesis is simple and quick with relatively few complications. The major drawback is the high percentage of false-negative results.

Peritoneal Lavage. Because of the poor reliability of paracentesis, other procedures have been developed to detect intraabdominal injury. Canizaro et al. described in 1964 the use of intraperitoneal saline infusions in animals. Root et al. described in 1965 the technique of peritoneal lavage in human beings and subsequently reported a series of 304 patients with a 96 percent accuracy. A recent review of this procedure has proved peritoneal lavage to be a safe and reliable adjunctive procedure for evaluating patients with blunt abdominal trauma. The indications for this technique are closed head injuries, altered consciousness, spinal cord injuries, equivocal abdominal findings, and negative needle paracentesis. It is not recommended for patients with either gunshot or stab wounds to the abdomen, multiple abdominal procedures, dilated bowel, pregnancy, or positive needle paracentesis.

The technique used is similar to that described by Perry et al. A point is selected in the lower midline below the umbilicus approximately one-third of the distance between that and the pubic symphysis. After decompression of the urinary bladder, the skin is cleansed and prepared with an iodinated antiseptic solution. A wheal is raised with 1% lidocaine and the skin incised with a #11 scalpel. A standard peritoneal dialysis catheter (McGaw V-4900) is inserted, and the trocar is advanced carefully until it just penetrates the peritoneum (Fig. 6-8). Once the peritoneum is penetrated, the trocar is removed and the dialysis catheter advanced toward the pelvis. A syringe is then attached to the catheter and the peritoneal cavity aspirated.

Nonclotting blood often will be aspirated through the larger catheter even with a negative needle paracentesis. If no blood or fluid is aspirated, a liter of balanced saline solution (Ringer's lactate) is rapidly infused into the peritoneal cavity over 5 to 10 minutes, using 10 ml/kg for small adults and children. The patient is then turned from side to side in order to further mix the blood and fluid. If other injuries such as pelvic or long bone fractures are present, this step is eliminated.

The empty intravenous-fluid bottle is lowered and the fluid siphoned out of the peritoneal cavity. A sample is sent to the laboratory for quantitative analysis. In addition to obtaining red cell and white cell counts, it is important to determine the presence or absence of amylase, bile, or bacteria. Some have recommended colorimetric methods, but these do not appear to be as accurate as quantitative analysis of the fluid. The criteria for positive peritoneal lavage include the following determinations: gross blood in lavage fluid; greater than 100,000 RBC/mm^3; greater than 500 WBC/mm^3; elevated amylase level; bacteria or bile.

It must be emphasized that the lavage is very inaccurate in indicating retroperitoneal injuries. Unless the posterior peritoneum has been torn or considerable time has elapsed between the injury and lavage, most pancreatic injuries are not detected. The same is true for duodenal, urologic, and major vessel injuries which are retroperitoneal. Complications occur frequently enough that lavage is not recommended for every patient suspected of abdominal injury. However, a negative lavage may spare the patient exploratory laparotomy.

Arteriography. Selective arteriography is another available aid to the diagnosis of blunt abdominal trauma. This procedure, advocated by Freeark, employs percutaneous retrograde arteriography by the Seldinger method. Depending upon the skill of the technician, selective catheterization of celiac, mesenteric, or renal vessels may be performed. The arteriogram provides visualization of the arteries supplying the abdominal viscera and pelvis. A film taken several minutes after injection can be used as an excretory urogram.

The benefits of arteriography are directly related to the capabilities of the radiology department. Again, it must be emphasized that time should not be wasted on adjunctive procedures when surgical intervention is indicated.

Scintiscanning. Both liver and splenic scanning have been described in conjunction with blunt abdominal trauma. This technique primarily is limited to those patients whose diagnoses are uncertain and whose conditions remain stable. The radionuclide most frequently used is ^{99m}Tc sulfur colloid. Most series reporting results of this technique are small and emphasize the relative inaccuracy of the examination.

A filling defect representing a parenchymal hematoma frequently is seen with damage to the spleen or liver. In addition, displacement, increased size, and mottled ap-

pearance of the spleen may increase the suspicion of splenic trauma. Filling defects also may indicate cysts, abscesses, infarcts, or tumors secondary to trauma.

Other Procedures. Newer, noninvasive modalities, such as sonography and computerized tomography, may have a place in the diagnostic armamentarium, but their value is as yet unproved. Needleoscopy and laparoscopy provide a less than complete examination and cannot be recommended at this time for the multiply injured patient.

Penetrating Trauma

STAB WOUNDS

The diagnosis of penetrating injuries of the abdomen does not usually present the difficult problem often posed by blunt abdominal trauma. Three methods of managing stab wounds of the abdomen have evolved: (1) routine exploration of all abdominal stab wounds, (2) selective management, and (3) laparotomy following demonstration of peritoneal cavity penetration.

Abdominal stab wounds frequently were managed by routine exploration. Since the incidence of negative laparotomy results was as high as 60 percent in some series, a more conservative approach recommending selective management for those patients with abdominal stab wounds and no clinical evidence of intraabdominal injury has been advocated. The vital signs should be stable, with no evidence of upper or lower gastrointestinal bleeding, pneumoperitoneum, or signs and symptoms of peritoneal irritation if the patient is to be selectively managed. These patients are admitted to the hospital and reevaluated frequently, preferably by the same observer. If the patient's condition deteriorates or changes significantly, exploratory laparotomy is performed. Objections to selective management are that (1) minimal physical findings may be common in spite of significant visceral injury, (2) peritonitis may develop prior to laparotomy, and (3) the incidence of negative laparotomies may still run as high as 30 percent.

Instead of subjecting the patient to general anesthesia and exploratory laparotomy, it is often possible to deter-

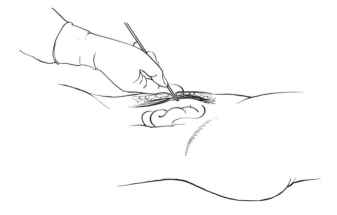

Fig. 6-8. Insertion of catheter for peritoneal lavage in the lower midline below the umbilicus.

mine by other means whether the wound has penetrated the peritoneal cavity. Cornell et al. have described the diagnostic injection of radiopaque contrast material. Following aseptic preparation of the wound site, a small catheter is inserted into the wound and held tightly by a purse-string suture. Fifty to one hundred milliliters of contrast media is injected, and anteroposterior, lateral, and oblique films of the abdomen are obtained. Contrast media seen within the peritoneal cavity is an indication for surgery. Objections to this technique are the following: (1) Some patients are hypersensitive to the radiopaque material. (2) Injection of this material may be quite painful, thereby masking further evaluation. (3) The incidence of false-positive and false-negative results may be as high as 15 to 25 percent in some series. (4) The technique is impractical for multiple stab wounds.

Local exploration may provide useful information. The abdominal wall is prepared with an antiseptic agent, and, with local anesthesia, the abdominal wound is opened sufficiently to visualize the complete course and depth of the wound. Often with adequate light, instruments, assistance, and exposure it is obvious that a wound thought to have penetrated the peritoneal cavity is actually superficial and not damaging to viscera. These patients are managed by simple drainage and outpatient follow-up if other injuries do not require hospitalization. Usually, local wound exploration involves more than simple instrument probing to determine penetration. This blind probing may be misleading since a tortuous wound tract may allow passage of the probe for only a short distance, creating a false impression of nonpenetration. In this case, the course of penetration must be directly visualized. If the end of the tract cannot be visualized or if the peritoneum is penetrated, the patient is taken to surgery. This technique is equally useful for stab wounds of the back, although the thickness of the paraspinous muscles may prevent visualization of the end of the wound tract and exploration in the operating room may be necessary. Frequently, innocuous small stab wounds of the back significantly damage such

retroperitoneal structures as the inferior vena cava, ureter, pancreas, or duodenum.

Many wounds which appear to penetrate only the thorax also penetrate the abdomen, injuring abdominal viscera as well as intrathoracic organs. Figure 6-9 indicates the diaphragmatic excursion on maximal expiration and maximal inspiration; it is apparent that certain penetrating wounds of the lower thoracic region often involve the diaphragm and adjacent abdominal viscera. Consequently, an exploratory laparotomy is performed when penetrating injuries involve the lower thoracic region.

Prior to abdominal exploration of these thoracic wounds, anterior and posterior chest tubes are inserted to drain air and blood from the thorax and to prevent pulmonary complications during the operative procedure from concurrent thoracic injuries. Although a pneumothorax or hemothorax may not be indicated by x-ray or physical examination, prophylactic insertion of an anterior chest tube will decrease the danger of a tension pheumothorax developing during induction of anesthesia and subsequent abdominal exploration.

GUNSHOT WOUNDS

Any bullet passing in proximity to the peritoneal cavity requires laparotomy, since visceral injury from "blast effect" may occur whether or not the cavity is entered. In a report by Edwards and Gaspard, 14 percent of 35 patients sustaining gunshot wounds to the abdomen without penetration of the peritoneal cavity sustained at least one visceral injury. It is not possible to predict the path of a missile by merely observing the entrance and exit wounds or by connecting a line between an entrance wound and the appearance of a bullet on the x-ray film. Missiles may bounce, tumble, ricochet, and embolize. If the patient's condition permits, anteroposterior and lateral films of the abdomen should be made to locate the missile and determine its probable trajectory. Selective management, the use of radiopaque material, or local exploration is not recommended.

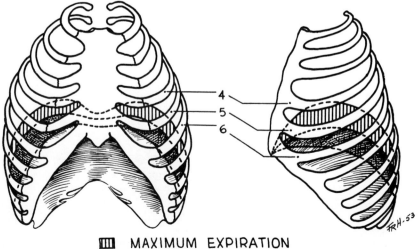

▦ MAXIMUM EXPIRATION
▨ MAXIMUM INSPIRATION

Fig. 6-9. Maximum diaphragmatic respiratory excursion. (*From L. M. Shefts, Surg Clin North Am, 38:1577, 1958.*)

Once the diagnosis of intraabdominal injury is established and resuscitation instituted, the abdomen is explored. A long midline incision is preferred for the following reasons: (1) It may be made much more rapidly than other incisions—a matter of vital importance when attempting rapid control of exsanguinating hemorrhage; (2) it gives wide access to all parts of the abdomen, which transverse incisions do not; (3) it may be readily extended into either side of the thorax in case of combined thoracoabdominal injury or when better abdominal exposure is required; and (4) it may be rapidly closed, which is of great importance in decreasing the anesthesia and operative time for gravely injured patients.

MANAGEMENT OF PATIENTS WITH EXSANGUINATING ABDOMINAL HEMORRHAGE. With improvement of prehospital care, more patients are arriving at the hospital in extremis. Frequently this condition is due to massive intraabdominal hemorrhage that is refractory to standard resuscitative measures. Ledgerwood and associates have recently advocated performing preliminary left thoracotomy and temporary thoracic aortic occlusion prior to opening the abdomen in patients with massive hemoperitoneum, tense abdominal distension, and persistent hypotension. The descending thoracic aorta is quickly and bluntly dissected circumferentially and occluded by a straight vascular clamp just above the diaphragm.

Once the abdomen is opened, the aortic clamp can be slowly released following stabilization of the patient, and proximal control gained at a lower level. A medium or large Richardson retractor may be used to obtain rapid temporary occlusion of the abdominal aorta just below the diaphragm. The lesser curvature of the stomach is pulled inferiorly and the flat surface of the retractor blade is compressed firmly against the abdominal aorta, thus occluding it against the vertebra just beneath the diaphragm.

With effective control of massive hemorrhage, resuscitation can be successfully completed, ensuring continuous perfusion to the heart and brain and minimizing the possibility of sudden cardiac arrest.

Stomach

Injuries to the stomach from blunt trauma are not frequent, perhaps because of the relative lack of fixation of the stomach and its protected position. However, penetrating injuries of the stomach from gunshot wounds occur frequently.

DIAGNOSIS. The diagnosis is generally suspected from the course of the penetrating object, and, at times, additional suspicion of gastric injury arises from the presence of bloody fluid aspirated from the Levin tube. Generally, wounds of the anterior stomach wall are easily seen at laparotomy. Because of the possibility of missing posterior stomach wall wounds, it is important in all cases of proved or possible gastric injury to open the lesser sac through the gastrocolic omentum. This allows the entire posterior aspect of the stomach to be searched for injury. The points of insertion of the greater and lesser omentum into the greater and lesser curvature of the stomach, respectively, should also be carefully inspected. If a hematoma is noted

at the mesenteric attachment, it should be evacuated and the stomach wall at that site carefully inspected for injury of that part of the wall located between the leaves of the greater or lesser omentum.

TREATMENT. Gastric wounds are repaired by first placing a continuous locked 2-0 chromic catgut suture through all the layers of the gastric wall; a purse-string suture does not give adequate hemostasis. This hemostatic stitch is very important to control extensive bleeding which may occur from the rich submucosal network of blood vessels in the stomach. Following the first layer closure, an outer inverting row of interrupted nonabsorbable mattress sutures of the Lembert or Halsted type is placed. The outer row of sutures provides adequate serosal approximation of the stomach wall, seals off readily, and prevents leaks. These sutures in the outer layer should not be through-and-through, as is the first row of sutures, but should extend through the seromuscular coat and the submucosal layer of the stomach. Wounds of the stomach are not drained, since they are unlikely to break down and leak, as duodenal wounds sometimes do. However, it is very important to suction the peritoneal cavity, with particular attention to the subhepatic and subphrenic spaces and the lesser sac, so that all food particles and gastric juice spilled into these areas are removed.

After operation for a gastric wound, Levin tube suction should be maintained for several days until active peristalsis has resumed and the danger of postoperative gastric dilatation has passed. The gastric aspirate should be observed for inordinate bleeding, which may occur if the hemostatic suture line is inadequate. If bleeding is brisk or persists, the patient should be immediately reexplored for control of the gastric bleeding point. After peristalsis resumes, gastric aspiration is discontinued, and the patient is started on clear liquids in the usual fashion and advanced to a normal diet over the next few days.

COMPLICATIONS. Complications which may develop following stomach wounds are hemorrhage from, or leakage of, the suture line and development of subhepatic, subphrenic, or lesser sac abscesses secondary to spilling of contaminated gastric contents. The development of such abscesses is suspected following gastric wounds in patients who fail to do well postoperatively and who persist with unexplainable fever for more than a few days. If contamination seems heavy, the skin should be left open until the wound appears clean.

Duodenum

Injuries to the duodenum and small bowel comprise about 24 percent of blunt and penetrating abdominal trauma. Lauritzen reported the mortality rate for retroperitoneal duodenal perforation as approximately 60 percent and related it to the difficulty in establishing an early diagnosis. A mortality of 55.9 percent has been reported for abdominal wounds with all types of duodenal injury. Burrus et al. have reported a series of 86 duodenal injuries with a total mortality of 26 percent.

Mortality rates for duodenal injuries have steadily decreased and are directly proportional to the number and severity of associated injuries as well as the time interval between injury and treatment. Lucas reported a mortality rate of 40 percent in those patients who were not operated upon in the first 24 hours after injury, as contrasted to a mortality rate of only 11 percent among the patients operated upon within less than 24 hours. The average overall mortality rate is about 20 percent. The mortality rate for simple stab wounds involving only the duodenum should be significantly less than five percent, while the mortality rate for severe blunt trauma or shotgun wounds to the duodenum ranges from about 35 percent to more than 50 percent, especially when such trauma is combined with serious pancreatic injuries.

DIAGNOSIS. The diagnosis of blunt trauma to the duodenum and small bowel is considerably more difficult than that of penetrating trauma to these organs. With duodenal or small bowel trauma, all the characteristic signs of trauma to abdominal viscera may be minimal or absent, particularly in the early period following injury for several reasons: (1) The injury of the duodenum following blunt trauma is frequently retroperitoneal, so that duodenal contents leak into the retroperitoneal area, rather than into the free peritoneal cavity. (2) Duodenal and small bowel fluid is generally sterile and does not lead to early signs of bacterial peritonitis, as occurs following colon injury. (3) The pH of the small bowel contents if frequently nearly neutral and, thus, produces only slight chemical irritation of the peritoneum. This is not true of injuries to the duodenum, in which duodenal fluid freely flows into the peritoneal cavity. The highly alkaline pH of this fluid causes immediate chemical irritation of the peritoneum and physical signs of such irritation.

One should be suspicious of injuries to the duodenum or upper small bowel in any patients who have received a blow to the upper abdomen or lower chest, such as from a steering wheel. Testicular pain should raise suspicion of a retroperitoneal duodenal rupture. Also, pain referred to the shoulders, chest, and back is associated with perforation of the duodenum and small intestine.

Several diagnostic aids may be helpful in determining rupture of the duodenum or small bowel. First, needle paracentesis of the abdomen, particularly in the right gutter region or in the upper quadrants, may be helpful if blood, bile, or abnormal amounts of small bowel content are aspirated. Roentgenograms are helpful and may be diagnostic, but the absence of free intraperitoneal air does not rule out bowel perforation. Retroperitoneal rupture of the duodenum is not often diagnosed by x-ray. The diagnosis may be based on finding a large accumulation of air about the right kidney. It is also important to inspect the psoas muscle margins on the plain film of the abdomen for the presence of air, indicating retroperitoneal rupture of a viscus. After x-ray films of the abdomen and upright chest films are made to search for free air collections, it is valuable to inject air through the Levin tube in order to produce or enlarge these air collections. Such a maneuver frequently increases the diagnostic accuracy of x-ray films for free air. An additional aid is to give the patient a water-soluble radiopaque dye orally and then to make abdominal x-ray films to detect any dye leak from the duodenum or small bowel. Such diagnostic procedures are unnecessary if other clinical signs indicate the need for exploratory laparotomy.

When laparotomy is done for suspected intraabdominal injury, duodenal lesions are often missed, especially retroperitoneal lesions of the third and fourth portions of the duodenum. This is due to superficial observation, inadequate exposure, and lack of persistence on the part of the surgeon. Hinton has reported that duodenal perforations have been missed initially in 33 to 50 percent of the various reported series of retroperitoneal duodenal injuries. To avoid overlooking duodenal trauma and contributing to the high mortality from duodenal wounds, it is important to inspect the entire duodenum during abdominal exploration for trauma. This is particularly true if a retroperitoneal hematoma is noted near the duodenum or if there is crepitation or bile-stained fluid along the lateral margins of the duodenum retroperitoneally. If these signs are noted or if the duodenum is contused, it should be widely mobilized by the Kocher maneuver, incising the peritoneum along its lateral margins, so that it is completely mobilized along with the head of the pancreas. Thus, small areas of perforation in the retroperitoneal aspect of the duodenum may be seen. Often retroperitoneal wounds of the duodenum which have been missed are not recognized until several days later, when bile-stained fluid drains from the abdominal wound of a patient who has continued to do poorly postoperatively. As Cohn et al. state, the following signs, in addition to those mentioned previously, indicate careful exploration of the duodenum and the retroduodenal area: elevation of the posterior peritoneum with a glassy edema; petechiae or fat necrosis over the ascending and transverse colon or mesocolon; retroperitoneal phlegmon; hematoma over the head of the pancreas extending into the base of the mesocolon; fat necrosis of the retroperitoneal tissues; and/or discoloration of retroperitoneal tissues—dark from hemorrhage, grayish from suppuration, or yellowish from bile.

TREATMENT. The local treatment of the duodenal perforation itself will depend more on the size of the perforation than any other single factor. Generally, an attempt is made to close the duodenal perforation if this can be done without decreasing the lumen of the duodenum. This closure is done with a continuous locking 3-0 chromic catgut suture through all layers of the duodenal wall, followed by an outer layer of nonabsorbable interrupted mattress sutures in the seromuscular layer of the duodenum. After this, the duodenum should be carefully palpated to exclude stenosis. If the perforation is so large that closure will cause a stricture of the duodenum, consideration should be given to (1) complete division of the duodenum and an end-to-end anastomosis or (2) division of the duodenum, closure of both ends, and gastroenterostomy.

Kobold and Thal have reported another method of handling large duodenal defects, which previously might have necessitated one of the above techniques of duodenal division. This consists of using a retrocolic loop of proxi-

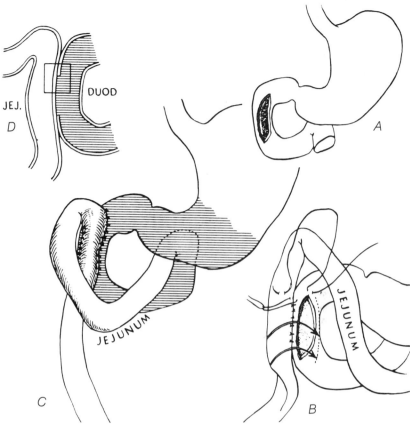

Fig. 6-10. *A.* Area of excision of duodenal wall. *B.* Technique of placement of intact jejunum over the wound to form a patch. *C.* The completed closure. *D.* Cross section of the completed closure showing the relationship of the intact jejunum to the duodenal perforation. The boxed area is the site from which tissue was subsequently removed for study. (*From E. E. Kobold and A. P. Thal, Surg Gynecol Obstet, 116:340, 1963.*)

mal jejunum with suture over the large defect in the duodenum, with an inner row of absorbable catgut sutures taken between the torn edge of the duodenum and the seromuscular layer of the jejunum and an outer layer of nonabsorbable mattress sutures taken between the seromuscular coats of the duodenum and the jejunum. Animal studies, as well as clinical usage, have demonstrated the feasibility of this "patching" technique in managing large duodenal defects (Fig. 6-10).

Large duodenal wounds and duodenal wounds which have dehisced also have been managed by anastomosing the open end of a defunctionalized Roux en Y loop of proximal jejunum over the duodenal defect.

The common bile duct should be identified with insertion of a T tube if the region of the ampulla is involved in a duodenal injury, since reimplantation of the common bile duct sometimes may be necessary. Approximately 75 to 80 percent of all duodenal injuries may be closed by debridement of the wound edges and simple suture. For the other 20 to 25 percent, however, one of the reparative procedures described above or recommended by Cleveland

and Waddell is used. Rarely, even a pancreatoduodenectomy may be necessary to manage large defects of the duodenum with extensive trauma to the duodenum and periampullary region (Fig. 6-11).

A recent report from the Lahey Clinic describes a technique for wide exposure of the third and fourth portions of the duodenum. This involves mobilizing the cecum, right colon, hepatic flexure of the colon, and mesenteries of these organs up to and including the ligament of Treitz, carrying the dissection of the mesocolon along the attachment at the root of the small bowel mesentery, as shown in Fig. 6-12.

It is also frequently important after duodenal injuries to establish adequate drainage. This is done by placing two or three Penrose drains near the injury, bringing them out of the abdomen by the most direct route possible. This reduced markedly the mortality from duodenal wounds in the several series in which drainage was evaluated. It is even more important to institute drainage if there appears to be associated pancreatic injury, as often occurs.

Fistulas. Fistula formation following duodenal injury occurs frequently because of poor blood supply, infection, excessive tension on suture lines, distal obstruction, etc., and leads to approximately a 50 percent mortality. The occurrence of a fistula may be related to the lack of a serosal surface in which to sew the retroperitoneal portion of the duodenum, so that an insecure closure is obtained.

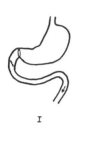
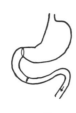
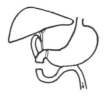
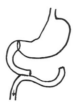
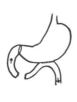

I   II   III   IV

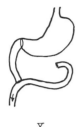
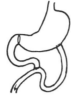

V   VI   VII

Fistulas may be prevented by prolonged decompression of the duodenum following closure of the wound. This is especially indicated in more severe injuries of the duodenum and is accomplished by several means:

1. A Levin tube may be threaded through the entire course of the duodenum with sufficient holes in the tube to allow simultaneous decompression of the duodenum and stomach. The tube may be brought through the anterior wall as a gastrostomy tube and placed on suction or may be inserted through the nasopharynx. A similar approach may be used via a retrograde jejunostomy (Witzel).

2. A #10 Foley catheter may be placed through a small stab wound in the duodenum, adjacent to the area of duodenal injury, to serve as a vent. The tube is maintained on gentle suction until active bowel sounds return. At this time, suction is discontinued, and the tube is attached to a glass Y tube fixed to a stand at the level of the duodenum. This arrangement does not allow siphonage of

Fig. 6-11. Diagrammatic representation of various operative procedures in a series of cases. I, Simple closure; II, end-to-end duodenoduodenostomy; III and IV, closure of both ends of duodenum and gastroenterostomy; V, closure of distal duodenum and duodenojejunostomy; VI, duodenojejunostomy and gastroduodenostomy; VII, resection of fourth part of duodenum and duodenojejunostomy. (*From H. C. Cleveland and W. R. Waddell, Surg Clin North Am, 43:413, 1963.*)

Fig. 6-12. A technique for the exposure of the third and fourth portions of the duodenum. *A and B.* Initial dissection for mobilization of the right side of the colon, small intestine, and mesentery. *C.* Exposure obtained of the third and fourth portions of the duodenum. (*From R. B. Cattell and J. W. Braasch, Surg Gynecol Obstet, 111:379, 1960.*)

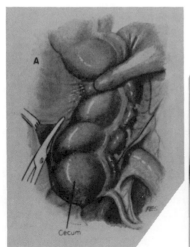
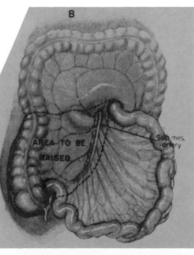
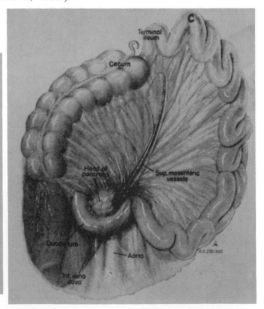

duodenal contents, as does gravity drainage, but does provide a decompressive vent if the pressure rises in the duodenum. After 9 or 10 days, at which time a fibrinous tract has formed about the small Foley catheter, the bag, which contains only 2 ml of water, is deflated. The Foley tube is again placed on gentle suction and is pulled just outside the duodenum, where it remains on suction for an additional 24 hours. At the end of the 24-hour period, the Foley catheter is removed if drainage is minimal. This small tube has been used for duodenal trauma at Parkland Memorial Hospital and also has been used to decompress the duodenum following gastric resection in which closure of the duodenal stump is insecure. In none of the approximately 75 cases in which the Foley tube was used following gastric resection and duodenal trauma has there been a significant complication, and no fistulas have occurred.

Postoperative Care. Postoperative care of these patients may be extremely difficult. Extracellular fluid volume deficits may be large, particularly if fistulas, retroperitoneal inflammation, or pancreatitis occur. It is very important to maintain the extracellular fluid volume with adequate infusions of balanced salt solution. In addition, these patients should be maintained on adequate doses of broad-spectrum intravenously administered antibiotics. Gastric and duodenal decompression should be continued for long periods of time in order to protect the suture lines. The average period of gastroduodenal decompression for duodenal wounds is about 5 to 7 days following exploration. If fistulas form, gastroduodenal decompression should be continued for longer periods, and a sump drain should be inserted into the drain site for continuous active suction of the fistular tract. This is instituted to prevent the collection of duodenal fluid with possible spread throughout the peritoneal cavity, to promote collapse and healing of the fistular tract, to prevent digestion of the skin by duodenal fluid draining onto the skin, and to aid calculation and replacement of fluid and electrolyte losses. Although several types of sump drains are now available commercially, recent experience with a simple sump drain made from two red rubber catheters has shown it to be more effective. A #18 French and a #14 French red rubber catheter are sewn together with nonabsorbable suture material at two or three points along the distal one-third of the catheters. Extra holes are cut in the sides of both tubes in their distal thirds. This sump drain is placed among several large Penrose drains through the abdominal drainage site. Postoperatively, suction is applied to the #18 catheter, and the smaller tube parallel to it serves as an effective air vent. This sump device was adapted from Waterman et al., although we have found it to be more effective when placed among several Penrose drains rather than through a single Penrose drain.

When a duodenal fistula develops, the patient should be placed on central intravenous hyperalimentation according to the principles of Dudrick and associates, which are discussed in Chap. 2. This regimen maintains excellent nutrition and may reduce the volume of gastrointestinal secretions.

With central intravenous hyperalimentation, it is now frequently unnecessary to perform feeding jejunostomies

to provide nutritional support for patients with duodenal fistulas. If for some reason central intravenous feeding is not possible or if copious fistular drainage persists, a jejunostomy may become necessary. Two tubes are inserted through separate Witzel (serosal-lined) tunnels in the proximal jejunum and brought out through separate sites in the left upper quadrant of the abdomen. One jejunostomy tube is inserted in a retrograde direction so that its tip lies within the duodenum just below the duodenal fistula, and the other tube is inserted in an antegrade direction into the upper jejunum. Suction is applied to the retrograde tube lying within the duodenum; this usually greatly reduces the volume of drainage and promotes closure. Standard jejunostomy feedings are given through the antegrade tube in the proximal jejunum. Also, the duodenal fluid is slowly refed through this tube as it is removed by suction from the sump drain in the fistula and from the retrograde jejunostomy tube. This feeding is ideally done with constant slow infusions through a Barron pump.

If, after 5 to 7 days of Levin tube or gastrostomy decompression of the duodenum, the patient is doing well, shows no evidence of duodenal leak, and has adequate bowel activity, he is given 1 oz of water orally every hour for approximately 12 hours, after the Levin tube is removed or the gastrostomy tube clamped. If water is tolerated, the diet is increased in the usual fashion. Also, after feeding has been instituted for 1 to 2 days and there has been little or no drainage, the Penrose drains are advanced and removed over 3 days unless further drainage ensues. In the face of continued drainage, the drains should be left for at least 2 or 3 weeks, or as long as any significant drainage continues. After about 3 weeks, if drainage persists, the Penrose drains may be removed; the only drainage tube which should remain is the previously described sump drain, which is removed when drainage has dropped to a minimum.

Occasionally, the duodenal fistula does not close despite adequate nonoperative treatment described above. In such cases, when a reasonable trial of conservative treatment has been made and the patient is in optimal condition for reoperation, the abdomen is opened and completely explored to rule out distal bowel obstruction which may be causing the fistula to persist. The fistula is exposed at its origin from the duodenum, and a Roux en Y defunctionalized limb of proximal jejunum is brought up to the fistula and anastomosed to it. This anastomosis may use either the end or the side (after closing the end of the jejunal limb) of the defunctionalized jejunum. This procedure permanently diverts the fistular drainage internally and has been very effective in treating persistent duodenal fistulas.

INTRAMURAL HEMATOMA

Another interesting but infrequently reported lesion of the duodenum secondary to trauma is intramural hematoma of the duodenum.

This lesion is generally caused by blunt abdominal trauma which causes rupture of intramural duodenal blood vessels with formation of a dark, sausage-shaped mass in the submucosal layer of the duodenal wall. This hematoma causes partial or complete duodenal obstruction, usually partial. The patient shows signs of a high small bowel obstruction, with nausea and vomiting associated with upper abdominal pain and tenderness, and sometimes a suggestion of a right upper quandrant mass. Flat films of the abdomen may show an ill-defined right upper quadrant mass and obliteration of the right psoas shadow. An upper gastrointestinal tract series is almost diagnostic, showing dilatation of the duodenal lumen with the appearance of a "coiled spring" in the second and third portions of the duodenum due to the crowding of the valvulae conniventes by the hematoma, according to Felson and Levin. The serum amylase level may be elevated. The lesion has occurred spontaneously in patients on anticoagulants.

Treatment generally consists of celiotomy, evacuation of the duodenal hematoma, and closure of the defect in the seromuscular coat of the duodenum with interrupted nonabsorbable sutures after control of any bleeding points. Fullen has recently recommended conservative treatment of this injury. Eleven patients treated with restriction of oral intake, nasogastric suction, and intravenous fluids and electrolytes all survived without complication. Nonoperative treatment is considered only after satisfactorily excluding the possibility of duodenal perforation or other associated injuries requiring celiotomy. The prognosis is excellent.

Small Bowel

Injuries to the small bowel are more frequent than injuries to the duodenum or colon. Counseller and McCormack, in a review of 1,313 cases of intestinal trauma, found that 80 percent of bowel injuries occur between the duodenojejunal junction and the terminal ileum, with approximately 10 percent each in the duodenum and large intestine. The usual mechanism of small bowel injury from blunt trauma is the crushing of the small bowel against the vertebral column. Rupture of the small bowel is also caused by shearing and tearing forces applied to the abdomen, and rarely by sudden elevation of the intraluminal pressure of the bowel with bursting from such sudden high pressure. Work by Williams and Sargent has shown that rupture due to sudden elevation of pressure is quite unusual.

In exploring the abdomen for injuries to the small bowel, it is important to inspect minutely the entire circumference of the small bowel and its attached mesentery from the ligament of Treitz to the ileocecal valve. The bowel may be completely transected in one or more places by blunt trauma with or without severe injury to the mesentery and its blood supply; at times, the mesentery may be torn from a segment of bowel, thus depriving the bowel of its blood supply. Penetrating trauma to the small bowel from a gunshot wound or stab wound is frequent, although, surprisingly, it has been noted at times that in patients with a stab wound of the abdomen the small bowel has been spared. This is probably because the great mobility of the small bowel allows it to slide away from the knife, a much less likely occurrence with gunshot wounds than with stab wounds.

TREATMENT. Small, single perforations of the small bowel may be closed safely with a single layer of interrupted nonabsorbable mattress sutures which include and invert the seromuscular and submucosal coats of the bowel. A hemostatic stitch, as required for stomach wounds, is not necessary for small bowel wounds, because the small bowel does not tend to continue bleeding from the submucosal plexus, as does the stomach. Individual bleeders, however, should be ligated with fine suture material. An advantage of a single-layer closure is its rapidity of performance, which is important in patients in precarious condition following multiple trauma.

Two small perforations of the bowel which are very close together may often be repaired by converting the wounds into one and closing the resulting defect as a single linear wound. This type of repair does not constrict the lumen of the bowel as much as two separate lines of suture placed close together and is more secure. Multiple perforations of the small bowel may occur following injury from shotgun pellets. Each one of these injuries should be carefully sought out and closed with interrupted rows of nonabsorbable mattress sutures.

Long linear lacerations of the lumen also should be closed with a single row of nonabsorbable sutures after ligating any persistent bleeders with small nonabsorbable suture. Longitudinal lacerations may be closed in a longitudinal direction or transversely according to the Heineke-Mikulicz principle.

Small bowel injuries produced by high-velocity missiles cause severe contusions of tissue surrounding the actual perforation. Because the contusion is a site of potential tissue necrosis and bowel leakage caused by thrombosis of vessels in the area of blast injury, it should be debrided. The debridement should extend into viable bowel where active bleeding is obtained.

If the wound is too large or is long and longitudinal, the bowel may not be adequately closed without loss of lumen, and the damaged segment should be resected. Also, if there are multiple wounds in a short segment of bowel, it is much safer and easier to resect the injured segment than to attempt to suture each of the closely spaced wounds, with resulting impairment of the bowel lumen and blood supply and subsequent obstruction and/or necrosis and leakage. Perforations or lacerations to the mesenteric border, unless they are quite small, are difficult to repair and frequently are associated with vascular impairment. They also should be managed by resection of the involved bowel if an adequate closure cannot be obtained without interference with blood supply. Bowel transections should be reanastomosed after debriding contused and damaged bowel on either side of the wound back to normal bowel with good blood supply. Careful attention should be given to leaving uninjured mesentery adjacent to the suture line of the reanastomosis. Extensive segments of bowel may be avulsed from the mesentery, so that the bowel loses its blood supply. All the necrotic or potentially necrotic bowel and injured mesentery must be resected and an end-to-end anastomosis made between uninjured bowel attached to uninjured mesentery.

Contusions of the small bowel should be assumed to

be larger than is apparent. Such injuries are dangerous, since they may lead to necrosis and perforation. Contusions up to 1 cm in diameter may be turned in with a row of fine, nonabsorbable mattress sutures. Larger contusions should be resected.

Postoperative care of patients with wounds of the small bowel includes maintenance on nasogastric suction and no oral intake until adequate bowel activity has returned. Also, these patients are usually maintained on antibiotics, most frequently penicillin and tetracycline, which are given preoperatively and postoperatively. Usually, the antibiotic is discontinued at about the time that the nasogastric tube is removed, unless there is some other indication to continue antibiotic treatment. Leakage from suture lines and intestinal obstruction are rarely seen if the wounds are properly managed. In the report of Giddings and McDaniel concerning wounds of the jejunum and ileum during World War II, leakage from suture lines occurred in only 1 percent and intestinal obstruction in 1.7 percent, in a series of 1,168 patients with small bowel injuries, most of whom had multiple visceral injury. Again, extracellular fluid volume deficits should be replaced in patients with small bowel injury, with adequate amounts of balanced salt solution given during the surgical procedure and in the postoperative period to maintain sufficient urine volume and prevent extracellular fluid volume deficit.

Colon Injuries

The morbidity and mortality from acute injuries to the colon and rectum have been significantly reduced by an aggressive surgical approach. This has been largely influenced by the experiences of military surgeons during World War II and the Korean conflict. In the American Civil War, wounds of the abdomen carried a mortality rate of approximately 90 percent; it was not until the Boer War that the mortality rate of 80 percent of cases treated conservatively was thought to be excessive and active intervention was viewed more favorably. During this time, the fatalities from wounds of the colon eventually dropped to less than 60 percent. In World War II, an impressive improvement in the mortality from wounds of the colon was noted. This was due to several factors including improved methods of triage and transportation, effective replacement of blood and fluid, and early surgical intervention combined with ancillary use of antibiotics.

The mortality rate for wounds of the colon of 37 percent in World War II was reduced to approximately 15 percent during the action in Korea. The majority of military surgeons treating acute injuries of the colon tended to exteriorize the wound as an artificial anus to prevent further soilage of the peritoneal cavity. This approach to these particular wounds was duly carried over into civilian practice and reflected in the subsequent reduction in mortality and morbidity. In the later phase of the Korean conflict, however, some modification of the aggressive technique was noted in that small, primary wounds treated early were handled by primary closure without exteriorization.

Acute wounds of the colon which occur in a civilian environment exhibit features that may modify the indications for exteriorization of the wound. The types of injury usually noted in a military situation resulted from either high-velocity missiles or fragmentation missiles in which there was massive destruction of tissue and usually gross soilage of the peritoneal cavity. In the civilian environment, the wounds more often are caused by low-velocity missiles and usually are unassociated with massive destruction of surrounding organs and tissue. The time from wounding to initial treatment in the civilian situation is generally somewhat less than that noted during military conflict. Similarly, associated injuries occurring in civilian accidents do not tend to be so numerous nor so massive as those in a military environment, and this has a definite influence on morbidity and mortality.

ETIOLOGY. Acute injuries of the colon and rectum may be divided into penetrating wounds and wounds resulting from blunt trauma. In the former group, accidental colon injuries may be the result of industrial accidents involving explosions resulting in impalement, penetrating injuries from flying objects, or blast injuries. These injuries may be either the direct result of explosives or the result of accidents involving sources of greatly compressed air. External acts of violence constitute an important source of injuries to the colon, and these are generally penetrating injuries caused by guns or knives or, on rarer occasions, blunt abdominal trauma. Wounds of the rectum, particularly, may be the result of instrumentation during the process of sigmoidoscopy or the administration of enemas. There may also be perforations of the colorectum by foreign bodies which pass through the alimentary canal into the colon. Inadvertent penetration of the colon or rectum may occur during difficult operations; this is especially true of operations in the pelvis for severe neoplastic or inflammatory disease. Falls resulting in impalement upon sharp objects may produce wounds of the rectum. Automobile accidents and other forms of blunt trauma may produce acute injuries to the colon and rectum.

DIAGNOSIS. A systematic diagnostic approach to problems of abdominal trauma is necessary, but specific examinations of the colon and rectum may be necessary to delineate an injury. This is particularly pertinent in those instances in which instrumentation is the cause of suspected perforation of the rectum or colon. Rectal examination and sigmoidoscopy should occupy a prominent place in the examination of these patients. Diagnostic abdominal x-ray studies should be employed to determine if there is a perforated colon with leakage of air into the free peritoneal cavity. Anteroposterior and lateral decubitus views are particularly helpful in these instances. Contrast studies of the colon should be employed rarely and cautiously in view of the high morbidity and mortality associated with leakage of barium and feces into the free peritoneal cavity. Aqueous opaque media, such as Gastrografin, are preferable when penetration of the colon is suspected.

TREATMENT. The general principles of management of patients with abdominal trauma apply to those patients who have acute injuries of the colon. It is important that the time from wounding to definitive operation be as short as possible, and aggressive replacement of fluid and blood losses should be undertaken at once. Preoperatively, penicillin and tetracycline should be started in all patients suspected of having penetrating injuries of the colorectum. Two million units of aqueous penicillin and 0.5 Gm of tetracycline are added to the intravenous solution.

These patients are explored through a midline incision in order to allow access to all parts of the abdominal cavity. A thorough and complete exploration of all abdominal viscera is made, for the morbidity and mortality vary directly with the number of associated injuries. Bleeding should be controlled as rapidly as possible and immediate efforts made to reduce peritoneal soilage from any penetrating wound of an abdominal viscus. The specific care of the wound of the colon should be approached by noting the anatomic differences between the intraperitoneal and extraperitoneal large intestine. Particular attention must be paid to the type of wound, its location, the amount of tissue destruction, the presence of associated injuries, and the time from wounding to definitive care.

Wounds of the intraperitoneal colon may be divided into two groups: First, small, primary wounds located on the antimesenteric border which are seen quite early, in which there is minimal tissue destruction, and minimal or no peritoneal soiling. These wounds, especially of the left colon and in the absence of associated injuries of other abdominal viscera, may often be adequately managed by a primary two-layer closure. The mucosa is approximated with a running lock suture of 3-0 chromic catgut, and the seromuscular layers are closed with interrupted #50 cotton sutures, the Lembert technique. Second, wounds of the right colon, containing liquid feces, are less amenable to this type of primary closure, for often gross and extensive peritoneal soiling follows the colon penetration. High-velocity missile wounds should rarely, if ever, be closed primarily, for tissue destruction is often excessive and may not be readily apparent. The injured area should be extensively debrided.

Acute injuries of the intraperitoneal colon resulting from high-velocity missiles which are associated with extensive destruction of tissues or which are large and ragged in nature and are located near or involve the mesenteric border should not be closed primarily. If located in the ascending, transverse, or descending colon, the wound may be exteriorized as a colostomy. Similarly, if the time from wounding to definitive care is relatively long, allowing seeding of the peritoneal cavity with a large number of bacteria, some type of colostomy should be performed either as a wound exteriorization or as a proximal diverting colostomy. Primary closure of the distal wounds is then permissible. Although a loop colostomy may be done for expediency, a completely diverting double-barrel colostomy is favored. It is preferable to open the loop colostomy immediately, usually with the cautery, and secure early, complete fecal diversion. This is performed in the operating room after all the wounds are closed and dressed. When there are associated massive injuries to other viscera, although the colon wound itself might fulfill the indications for primary closure, a colostomy is indicated. In some instances, there may be massive injury of the cecum or of the ileocecal area, in which case it will be necessary to resect the injured bowel and do an ileotransverse colostomy. This is preferable to an ileostomy and, with suitable antibiotic coverage and intraluminal antibiotics, is an adequate procedure.

Localized minor wounds of the right colon and cecum which do not produce extensive destruction of the large bowel and are not associated with massive soilage or serious injuries to other viscera may often be managed by primary closure and appendicostomy. In these instances, after debridement and careful closure of the laceration of the cecum, tube appendicostomy is performed to decompress this segment. Seromuscular sutures are placed about the base of the appendix and secured to the lateral parietal peritoneum in order to prevent intraperitoneal leakage about the area of tube insertion. By this technique, suitable decompression of the cecum and right colon may be obtained, and removal of the tube appendicostomy permits the vent to close spontaneously. This route may also be used for intraluminal installation of neomycin or kanamycin solutions, which may offer some protection from bacterial invasion of the suture line.

The extraperitoneal perforations of the rectum must be evaluated under the same principles employed for colon injuries within the peritoneal cavity. If clean lacerations with minimal spillage are seen early, primary bowel repair may be indicated if the wound is accessible. Presacral drains should then be inserted. Associated perineal wounds should be debrided and, if grossly contaminated, left open. If debridement is adequate and these wounds are clean, they may be closed with drainage. Any damage to the anal sphincter may be repaired at this time. When a perineal wound is present but not penetrating the colon, it should be debrided widely and if not grossly contaminated then may be closed with drainage. Where there is no perineal wound but there is significant tissue destruction about the extraperitoneal rectum, presacral drainage should be instituted.

For all injuries of the rectum, complete diversion of the fecal stream is mandatory and can be accomplished by constructing a proximal double-barrel colostomy. Even in those instances where the rectal wound has been closed and diverting colostomy performed, presacral drainage is necessary.

Drainage of the retrorectal area is extremely important. This can be established by making a curvilinear incision in the posterior perianal area, incising the anococcygeal ligament, and bluntly dissecting into the presacral space. Two Penrose drains will usually suffice, but with extensive injuries, it may be necessary to utilize sump drainage for a few days.

Lavenson and Cohen, on the basis of their experience in the Vietnam conflict, strongly recommend removal of all feces from the distal rectum. This is accomplished by irrigating copious amounts of saline solution through the defunctionalized segment until the return is clear. They report a significant decrease in mortality and complication rates when utilizing this technique. Military injuries are generally associated with higher-velocity missiles and cause more fecal contamination and blast injury to surrounding pelvic tissue. In civilian injuries, distal irrigation may not be as important, as evidenced by Trunkey and Shires, who report a lower morbidity and mortality rate in their series, in which distal irrigation was not employed but adequate drainage and diversion were used.

Serious perineal injuries are treated in a similar manner. Even in the absence of rectal injury, sepsis can be avoided by early fecal diversion. Failure to recognize this potential problem may lead to extensive soft tissue infections extending from the knee to the axilla, with potential involvement of the anterior and posterior abdominal wall.

Early closure of the colostomy is indicated in patients who have completely recovered and have no distal colon injury. It is desirable to close the simple colostomy in 2 or 3 weeks. Prior to closure, both limbs of the colon should be visualized radiographically to assure that no lesion persists. Mechanical and bacterial cleansing of the colon is effected preoperatively.

Adjunctive Measures. Aggressive replacement of fluid and blood loss should be undertaken immediately and general supportive measures instituted. Attention to possible injuries elsewhere is mandatory. The systemic antibiotics begun in the preoperative period are continued for 5 to 7 days postoperatively. The use of peritoneal and intraluminal instillation of antibiotics has been advocated by many. Certainly, removing all gross fecal material from the peritoneal cavity is indicated, but instillation of intraperitoneal antibiotics has been followed by some complications, notably respiratory depression. These have been most frequently seen in anesthetized patients who received intraperitoneal neomycin. Extensive lavage of the peritoneal cavity with saline solution may actually result in dissemination of fecal material and is not recommended. The use of an intraluminal catheter for postoperative instillation of antibiotics as advocated by Cohn may add further protection from late wound disruption. The antibiotics may be instilled through a small polyethylene catheter, which is inserted into the bowel proximal to the areas of injury. It is desirable to place the catheter through a taenia and secure it with a purse-string suture. The bowel is then sutured to the parietal peritoneum at the point of entrance of the catheter. A 1% solution of neomycin or 15 ml of sterile saline solution with 1 Gm of kanamycin may be instilled at 6-hour intervals for the first three or four postoperative days. The small polyethylene catheter may then be removed without difficulty. The use of antibiotics systemically and locally may reduce the incidence of septic complications, particularly septic shock.

Liver

Injury to the liver is suspected in all patients with penetrating or blunt trauma that involves the lower part of the chest and upper part of the abdomen. Among patients with penetrating abdominal trauma, the liver is second only to the small bowel as the structure most commonly injured; among those with blunt trauma, the liver is second only to the spleen as the most commonly injured organ. About 80 percent of liver injuries occur as a result of penetrating trauma from stab wounds or gunshot wounds; only 15 to 20 percent occur from blunt trauma. In the past decade, the incidence of stab wounds has diminished while the incidence of gunshot wounds, especially those caused by higher-velocity and larger-caliber missiles, and blunt trauma has increased. These changes in the types of liver injury, the more rapid transport of patients with hepatic trauma to treatment facilities, and better resuscitation methods have caused an increase in severity of liver injuries that are likely to confront the surgeon.

Early exploration, prompt replacement of blood and use of balanced electrolyte solution, use of antibiotics, proper choice of surgical treatment, and adequate drainage are all factors that have led to increased survival rates. The average overall mortality rate of patients with hepatic trauma is about 13 to 15 percent. However, this rate is directly related to the severity of the liver injury and the injury to other intraabdominal organs. The mortality rate of stab wounds to the liver without associated organ injury is only about 1 percent. When significant liver trauma is associated with injuries of more than five other intraabdominal organs, or when major hepatic resection is required to control bleeding, the mortality rate rises to about 45 to 50 percent.

TREATMENT. After initial resuscitation and diagnostic maneuvers, patients with suspected hepatic injuries are rapidly moved to the operating room. The entire abdomen and chest are "prepped" and draped, and a long upper midline incision is made. Sources of bleeding from the liver and the abdomen are quickly appraised, and temporary control of the bleeding is achieved by manual compression of packs placed over the bleeding sites and by temporary occlusion of appropriate major vessels. Digital compression of the hepatic artery and portal vein to occlude temporarily the blood flow to the liver (the Pringle maneuver) may control or slow hepatic hemorrhage in some patients, but more often it is necessary to combine the Pringle maneuver with compression packs placed over the liver injury to control hemorrhage effectively. There is general agreement that, in the normothermic liver, blood flow to the liver can be completely occluded for about 15 minutes without causing any hepatocellular damage. If it is necessary to occlude the hepatic blood supply for more than 15 minutes, the vascular occlusion can be briefly interrupted every 10 or 15 minutes to allow short periods of uninterrupted hepatic blood flow.

Definitive treatment may be accomplished by drainage alone, suture or hemostatic maneuvers and drainage, or variations of hepatic resection.

Drainage Alone. Hepatic hemorrhage will have ceased spontaneously by the time the abdomen is opened or stops soon after compression of the bleeding site in about 50 to 70 percent of patients with liver injuries. In such patients, the only treatment necessary is adequate drainage of the injury. Suturing of nonbleeding liver injuries is unnecessary. This is emphasized by Trunkey, Shires and McClelland, who reported no rebleeding among several hundred patients with liver injuries that stopped bleeding spontaneously or soon after temporary pack compression. Suturing of nonbleeding liver wounds may cause bleeding and needlessly traumatize hepatic tissue.

All liver injuries should be drained with large, 1-in. wide Penrose drains, and several drains should be used in patients with larger injuries. The drains are brought out posterolaterally, as dependently as possible, through an abdominal wall stab wound in order to achieve the best drainage by gravity. This greatly reduces the formation of infected collections of bile, blood, and tissue fluid in the subphrenic and subhepatic spaces. Also, dependent gravity drainage is more reliable than nondependent suction drainage. In most patients with liver injury it is unnecessary to resect the twelfth rib to achieve dependent drainage. Usually the drains can be brought through the stab wound at the tip of, or just below, the twelfth rib. However, in large patients with more extensive liver wounds, it may be preferable to resect the lateral half or two-thirds of the right twelfth rib, to achieve more effective drainage. An adequate opening, easily admitting two fingers, must be made in the abdominal wall to be certain that these injuries are effectively drained. The drains are left in place 5 to 10 days thereafter, being slowly removed over a 3-day period. Not until the end of this time is a firm, fibrinous tract formed about the drains which ensures adequate external drainage of any material that accumulates in the abdomen after the drain is removed.

Suture, Hemostatic Techniques, and Drainage. Bleeding persists despite temporary compression packing of the injury site in 30 to 50 percent of patients with liver injuries. Definitive hemostasis of persistently bleeding liver injuries usually can be achieved by liver sutures. Simple interrupted sutures are placed 2 cm from the wound margins, using 2-0 or 0 chromic suture swaged onto a 2-in. blunt-tipped "liver needle." This will allow gentle but firm approximation, thereby stopping most bleeding which originates from the outer 2 cm of the liver parenchyma immediately beneath the capsule of the liver. Larger wounds may require placement of figure-of-eight liver sutures to prevent cutting through the liver capsule. Passage of the liver suture through buttressing materials such as Surgicel, Gelfoam, or omentum is seldom needed if the sutures are placed 2 cm from the margin of the injury and tied gently. However, if a bolster is needed, it is preferable to use a vascularized pedicle of omentum instead of foreign material. Trunkey, Shires, and McClelland have abandoned the technique previously described using interlocking mattress sutures for hemostasis. These authors now recommend direct suture ligation of the bleeding vessel as an attempt to reduce the chance of strangulation and subsequent necrosis.

Recently, microcrystalline collagen powder (Avitene) has been reported to be successful in controlling bleeding from liver wounds. Unlike other material such as Gelfoam, Avitene can be left in liver wounds without inciting significant foreign body reaction. The use of other hemostatic agents as well as gauze packs to tamponade hemorrhage is not recommended.

The use of liver sutures to obtain hemostasis from both the entrance and exit sites of long gunshot tracts in the liver is controversial. However, Lucas and Ledgerwood state that this technique was successfully used in several of their patients who otherwise would have required extensive surgery. Placement of the liver sutures at both ends of the

bullet tract stops bleeding arising from the subcapsular area, which is the usual source. During their 5-year prospective review, Lucas and Ledgerwood found that only one patient developed an intrahepatic abscess following this technique, and no patients developed hemobilia after closure of both ends of a long gunshot tract. Continued bleeding which persists after closure of both ends of the tract is usually identified at the initial operation by blood oozing between the liver sutures or by an increase in the size of the liver within 10 minutes after placement of the sutures. If the persistently bleeding tract is short and close to an accessible surface of the liver, hemostasis can be achieved by limited wedge resection or by resectional debridement incorporating the tract as part of the debridement. Persistently active bleeding from deep bilobar tracts that do not lend themselves to resectional debridement is best controlled either by ligation of an appropriate branch of the hepatic artery or by tractotomy and ligation of the intraparenchymal bleeding vessels. However, tractotomy may cause further bleeding, and for this reason, ligation of one of the main hepatic artery branches is preferable, since it usually stops arterial bleeding from deep tracts and is likely to cause less morbidity than tractotomy.

Ligation of an appropriate major branch of the hepatic artery (i.e., the right or left branch) is a safe and effective means for controlling liver bleeding in patients with active arterial bleeding from wounds that do not permit suture ligature or wedge resection and in whom bleeding stops with temporary hepatic artery occlusion. Mays reported achieving liver hemostasis in 15 of 16 patients who underwent ligation of hepatic artery branches. Lucas and Ledgerwood did not find ligation of major branches of the hepatic artery as effective in arresting hemorrhage as Mays did, possibly because some of these patients were bleeding from major venous injuries. It is suggested that the right or left hepatic artery should not be ligated if a simple temporary compression pack or suturing of a bleeding liver injury controls the hemorrhage. However, if compression or suturing does not control bleeding and temporary occlusion of the hepatic artery branch supplying the injured area of the liver does stop hemorrhage, then the appropriate major hepatic artery branch should be ligated, especially if the alternative treatment is a hepatic resection.

Resection. Resectional debridement or limited wedge resection is recommended for control of bleeding from the ragged liver injuries that may be caused by shotgun wounds, high-velocity rifle wounds, and severe blunt injuries. Limited resectional debridement of shattered liver tissue usually achieves hemostasis from such injuries effectively and safely. The margins of resectional debridement should be 2 or 3 cm beyond the point of injury, and bleeding during debridement is controlled by digital parenchymal constriction and/or temporary occlusion of the inflow of blood to the liver at the porta hepatis. The liver parenchyma is separated bluntly by finger fracture, a suction tip, or a scalpel handle. Vessels and bile ducts are secured by individual suture ligation or by metal clips as they are encountered. It is not necessary to oppose the margins of resection with interrupted liver sutures if bleeding from the resected surface is controlled. This suture technique may be undesirable, since it may create a potentially infected closed space within the liver.

Anatomic hepatic lobectomy for control of bleeding, especially from the right lobe, is best reserved for patients in whom (1) hepatic suturing is unsuccessful; (2) resectional debridement of hepatotomy with intraparenchymal hemostasis is precluded by the anatomic location of the injury; (3) occlusion of the hepatic artery is ineffective in controlling hemorrhage. Although resectional debridement or sublobar hepatic resection may be required in about 4 or 5 percent of all patients with liver injuries, no more than 2 or 3 percent require anatomic, lobar resection to control hemorrhage. Most of the few patients with liver injuries who require major hepatic lobectomies to control bleeding have massive, shattering injuries of the liver, injuries of the retrohepatic vena cava, or injuries to the major hepatic vein (Fig. 6-13). If it becomes apparent that major lobar resection is necessary, the hepatic bleeding is temporarily controlled by manual compression packing and a Pringle maneuver while the midline abdominal incision is extended by performing a median sternotomy.

A median sternotomy is much more quickly and easily made and closed than a right thoracoabdominal incision, causes considerably less diaphragmatic injury, provides much easier access to the vena cava and hepatic veins, permits easier insertion of a retrohepatic vena caval shunt if this is required, and causes less postoperative pain and pulmonary morbidity than a right thoracoabdominal incision.

After wide exposure is obtained by the median sternotomy extension of the midline abdominal incision, Rumel tourniquets are placed about the vena cava superior and inferior to the liver. The superior tape is placed about the vena cava superior to the central tendon of the dia-

phragm after this portion of the vena cava is exposed by opening the pericardium. These tapes permit temporary occlusion of the vena cava for insertion of a retrohepatic intracaval shunt if vascular isolation of the liver is required during hepatic lobectomy because of major retrohepatic vena cava or major hepatic vein injury. The hepatic artery, portal vein, and bile ducts supplying the lobe to be resected are then suture-ligated and divided. After this, hepatic resection can be carried out by dividing Glisson's capsule with a cautery along the line appropriate for the lobe being removed. The lobe is removed by fracturing through the liver substance along the line of resection with the thumb and forefinger or with the tip of an abdominal suction tube from which the guard has been removed. The back of a scalpel handle may also be used to fracture through the liver parenchyma. As the blood vessels and bile ducts are encountered within the liver, they are isolated by passing a right-angle clamp around them and are then sharply divided. After the larger vessels and ducts are suture-ligated, the smaller ones are secured with tantalum (Weck) clips. No attempt is made to secure the hepatic veins at their junction with the retrohepatic vena cava before beginning the resection; instead, it is much easier and safer to isolate and suture-ligate or oversew the appropriate major hepatic veins as they are encountered posteriorly during the liver resection. The resection begins anteriorly and progresses posteriorly toward the right or left side of the vena cava, keeping to the right or left of the middle hepatic vein (depending upon whether a right or left lobectomy is being done). The middle hepatic vein demarcates the right from the left lobe of the liver and passes in a line from the middle of the gallbladder bed posteriorly to the midportion of the retrohepatic vena cava. The hepatic veins and other large vascular structures must be oversewn, since simple ligatures on these large structures often slip off and cause catastrophic bleeding.

Fig. 6-13. Typical liver injury requiring hepatic resection.

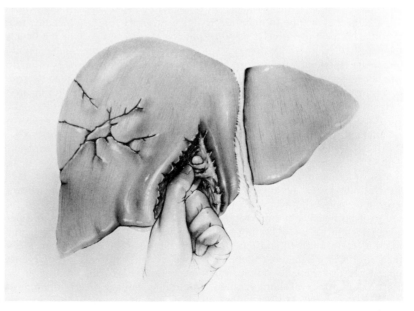

The recently described Lin liver clamp may be helpful in performing resections. There is considerable reduction in blood loss and operating time with the use of this clamp, but its availability should not cause a broadening of the indications for liver resection. The clamp can be used for resecting the liver only when the liver has been severely shattered and devitalized without injury to the retrohepatic vena cava or the major hepatic veins near the junction with the vena cava.

Although Merendino et al., Longmire and Marable, and Perry and LaFave suggest that T-tube drainage of the common bile duct should be carried out after hepatic resections, reports by Lucas and by Pinkerton et al., suggest that septic complications and bleeding from gastroduodenal stress ulcers are significantly increased by this practice. Although T-tube drainage may not lower pressures in the common bile duct and therefore probably does not prevent bile leakage from the liver and bile collections in the operative site, the T-tube does help identify the right and left hepatic ducts with certainty during liver resections, and thus aids in preventing operative injury to the remaining major bile duct. Also, the T-tube does provide a useful port through which such postoperative complications as hematobilia and biliary fistula formation can be recognized and the type of drainage observed. Cholangiography may also be done through the tube postoperatively, and this may be very useful in determining the cause of prolonged jaundice after hepatic resections. Lucas and Walt, in a well-controlled prospective study, support the position that effective biliary decompression is not achieved by the T-tube and that drainage of the common duct may, indeed, increase the incidence of complications in patients with hepatic trauma, especially those due to infection and bile duct obstruction (i.e., jaundice, cholangitis, and bile duct stricture). The increased likelihood of bleeding from gastroduodenal stress ulcers caused by T-tube drainage of the common bile duct after hepatic resection may be offset by frequently lavaging the stomach with antacid solution through the Levin tube to maintain a high gastric pH for several days postoperatively, as suggested by Curtis and associates.

Vascular Isolation. Vascular isolation may be required in a highly selected group of patients with liver injuries. This technique allows the surgeon to control bleeding from and to repair retrohepatic vena caval or major hepatic venous injuries. Vascular isolation of the liver is attained by using one of two techniques. The first technique was initially described and reported by Heaney in 1966; when this method of vascular isolation is used, occlusive vascular clamps are placed across the aorta just below the diaphragm, the porta hepatis, and the inferior vena cava above and below the liver. This technique may be associated with cardiac dysrhythmias and renal insufficiency. The second technique for obtaining vascular isolation of the liver was first described and reported by Shrock and associates in 1968. When this technique is used, retrohepatic vena caval and hepatic venous isolation is attained by inserting an intracaval shunt via the right atrial appendage of the heart; control of vascular inflow to the liver is obtained by placing a Rumel tourniquet or vascular clamp

on the porta hepatis. Defore and associates reported survival of 7 of 15 patients with major vena caval or hepatic vein injuries following vascular isolation and the introduction of intracaval shunts. The introduction of the intracaval shunt via the right atrial appendage is most expeditiously done via a median sternotomy. It is suggested that three equidistant "guy" sutures be placed in the right atrial wall somewhat outside the atrial purse-string suture before making the atrial opening in the center of the purse-string suture to insert the shunt. These "guy" sutures are then split apart and held up by assistants as the atrium is opened; this greatly facilitates the insertion of the shunt as the atrial wall is stabilized.

Another method for controlling hemorrhage from the retrohepatic vena cava or major hepatic veins has been described. If the major venous laceration is in such a position in the suprahepatic vena cava or the extrahepatic portion of the hepatic veins, a Foley catheter may be quickly inserted into the exposed laceration. The balloon of the Foley catheter is then inflated and pulled up against the wall of the vena cava or hepatic vein to occlude the laceration, arrest the hemorrhage, and thus permit repair of the venous laceration with relatively good exposure and little blood loss.

It is reemphasized that these methods should not be used except by a skillful and experienced surgeon in whose judgment exsanguination will occur unless vascular isolation is carried out.

SUBCAPSULAR HEMATOMA. The treatment of subcapsular hematomas is somewhat controversial. Left alone, these may (1) resolve spontaneously; (2) expand and burst with delayed intraperitoneal bleeding; (3) cause development of hepatic abscess; or (4) decompress into the biliary tree and cause hemobilia. The risk of inducing massive hemorrhage, at times uncontrollable, accompanies attempts at incision and evacuation.

Richie and Fonkalsrud reported on a series of patients treated nonoperatively. They emphasized that severe bleeding may result in some patients in whom hematomas of the liver are unroofed, and they further note that since some hematomas are centrally located within the liver, they often do not lend themselves to resection or control by hepatic artery ligation. These authors recommend performing an emergency liver scan on patients with probable blunt hepatic trauma who do not have evidence of persistent hemorrhage or shock and who do not have other indications for immediate celiotomy, such as positive needle paracentesis of the abdomen or positive peritoneal lavage. If the patient's condition remains stable, and a subcapsular hematoma is seen on liver scan, they recommend close observation of the patient in the hospital by means of frequent physical examinations, serial hematocrits, and performance of liver function studies. The status of the hematoma is appraised by serial liver scans to be certain it is resolving, not increasing in size.

Emergency hepatic arteriography for patients in stable condition with probable intrahepatic hematomas due to blunt trauma is probably preferable to emergency scanning. Arteriography more definitely delineates the size and location of a subcapsular or intrahepatic hematoma, indicates whether there is persistent intrahepatic or extrahepatic hemorrhage, and may show the source and severity of the bleeding.

Another notable advantage of hepatic arteriography, in some stable patients with intrahepatic hematomas, is that this technique may be used therapeutically as well as diagnostically. If a site of arterial hemorrhage is visualized arteriographically, the hemorrhage may be stopped non-operatively and atraumatically by embolizing several 2-mm^2 pieces of Gelfoam through the hepatic catheter. These emboli obstruct the bleeding site and thus prevent further bleeding.

Hemobilia. Hemobilia is caused by arterial hemorrhage into the biliary tract after liver trauma; it classically presents with a triad of findings consisting of upper or lower gastrointestinal hemorrhage, obstructive jaundice, and colicky abdominal pain. In the past the standard treatment for this condition has consisted of hepatic resection or hepatotomy with direct exposure and suture ligation of the bleeding artery. Such treatment is often associated with considerable blood loss and high operative mortality and morbidity rates. There are now several reports of successful management of traumatic hemobilia by ligation of the hepatic arteries supplying the involved lobe of the liver. Recent experience with hepatic artery ligation in the management of hepatic trauma and hepatic tumors has proved this to be a safe technique.

COMPLICATIONS. Major nonfatal complications occur in approximately 20 percent of patients with liver injuries. Since the thorax is involved in a large number of hepatic injuries, there is a high incidence of pulmonary complications. A large number of patients develop intraabdominal abscesses, and approximately 50 percent of these are associated with injuries to the colon.

Patients with major lobar resections may be expected to have some degree of postoperative bilirubin elevation, secondary probably to transient biliary obstruction by blood clots and temporary hepatic insufficiency (due to shock, loss of hepatic mass, operative trauma, and on occasion, perhaps secondary to postoperative sepsis). Such hyperbilirubinemia usually disappears in about 3 weeks, with no further surgical treatment for the relief of jaundice required. Liver function studies generally demonstrate hepatic impairment but usually return to normal after several weeks. Glucose metabolism is altered following resection, and in the early postoperative period it may be necessary to give the patient supplemental glucose solutions. Studies indicate that survival is possible with only 20 percent of the normal hepatic mass and that within 1 to 2 years most of the resected hepatic tissue is replaced as a result of hepatic regeneration.

Gallbladder

Although perforations of the gallbladder due to blunt trauma are very unusual, penetrating abdominal trauma frequently causes gallbladder injury. Penetrating or avulsion injuries of the gallbladder are best managed by cholecystectomy, but in unstable patients with other severe injuries when, in the surgeon's judgment, cholecystectomy is inadvisable, a tube cholecystostomy should be done, with placement of Penrose drains around the gallbladder in the subhepatic space. In general, simple suture of a gallbladder perforation is not recommended because of the probability of bile leakage. After about 4 weeks, if a patient who has had a tube cholecystostomy is doing well, a cholangiogram is performed through the cholecystostomy tube, and if this shows that the gallbladder and biliary ducts are normal, with free flow of contrast material into the duodenum, the cholecystostomy tube can be removed. Routine cholecystectomy after removal of the cholecystostomy tube in patients who have sustained gallbladder trauma is unnecessary, but it is probably advisable to perform an oral cholecystogram several months after injury to determine the status of the gallbladder.

Extrahepatic Biliary Tree

PENETRATING INJURIES

The diagnosis of penetrating injuries of the extrahepatic biliary tree generally presents no problem as compared with the diagnosis of blunt trauma of the biliary tree, which may be difficult unless intraabdominal hemorrhage occurs. When the hepatic artery and portal vein are involved, the mortality rate is inordinately high because of massive hemorrhage which may be virtually impossible to control before irreversible hypoxic damage occurs to the brain and myocardium. Probably most patients with injuries to the extrahepatic biliary tree and one of the major vessels in the hepatoduodenal ligament do not survive to come to surgical exploration. This is particularly true when the wounding agent is a large-caliber, high-velocity missile. In contrast, wounds of the gallbladder which are seen frequently following penetrating abdominal trauma have a low mortality rate and are not so frequently associated with injuries to the major vessels in the hepatoduodenal ligament.

On opening the abdomen, blood and bile seen issuing from the subhepatic region indicate possible injury to the biliary tree. At times, the amount of bile, blood, or contusion may be minimal, and the gallbladder, cystic duct, and hepatoduodenal structures must be carefully inspected to evaluate the significance of any subserosal hematoma or bile staining. If the patient has survived to be surgically explored, generally no massive bleeding from the subhepatic region will be noted initially. However, many times in obtaining exposure of the hepatoduodenal ligament structures, clots which have formed and caused tamponade of major bleeding sites may be dislodged, with recurrence of vigorous bleeding from the portal vein, hepatic artery, or their branches, which are so frequently injured when the bile ducts are injured.

Generally, the hemorrhage may be immediately arrested by placing the fingers in the foramen of Winslow and compressing the hepatoduodenal ligament. Following this, after removing the free blood and obtaining good exposure while maintaining finger tamponade as above, more definitive control of the hemorrhage may be obtained by placing vascular clamps or rubber-shod clamps across all structures in the hepatoduodenal ligament. One clamp should be placed as far distad as possible on the hepato-duodenal ligament, and this maneuver is aided by dividing the lateral serosal reflection of the duodenum and reflecting the duodenum and the head of the pancreas mediad. Another clamp is then placed on the hepatoduodenal ligament through the foramen of Winslow as near the liver hilus as possible.

After hemorrhage is controlled, the serosa of the hepato-duodenal ligament at the point of the hematoma formation is incised, and the disruption of the portal vein or hepatic artery is visualized by rapidly dissecting out these structures. When the defects in the major vessels are located, repair is done with 5-0 silk arterial sutures using the general principles and techniques of vascular surgery. The vascular repair should be done only after careful exposure of the defect but also with dispatch, since the safe occlusion period of hepatic vascular inflow is only 15 to 20 minutes unless the patient is under hypothermia.

After repair of any vascular injuries, the biliary tract is carefully dissected out along the course of the penetrating missile. Knife wounds of the bile ducts may be closed with interrupted 4-0 silk suture. The common duct should be decompressed with a T tube inserted through a separate incision in the ductal system a short distance above or below the injury, so that one arm of the T tube serves as a stent for the wounded portion of the bile duct. For injuries caused by bullets or other large penetrating objects which may produce destruction or avulsion of a segment of the biliary ductal system, the wound should be carefully debrided and all devitalized ductal tissue removed. This may require completing a partial transection of the bile ducts, so that an end-to-end anastomosis may be made between viable portions of the common duct. This anastomosis is again made with interrupted simple sutures of 4-0 silk, and the repair is stented with a rubber T tube placed through a separate incision in the duct, above or below the injury. Medial reflection of the duodenum relaxes tension and allows the ends of the divided ducts to come together more readily, particularly when duct tissue has been destroyed and the ducts are shortened.

If the loss of biliary ductal structure is extensive, end-to-end repair of the duct may not be possible, and a bypass procedure is necessary. Generally, the Roux en Y bypass is effective. This is done by bringing up a 30-cm Roux en Y limb of jejunum made by transecting the jejunum about 30 cm below the ligament of Treitz. The end of the defunctionalized limb of jejunum is closed with two layers of suture. Following this, the distal end of the common duct is doubly ligated with heavy nonabsorbable suture material, and the choledochojejunostomy is performed in the following manner: a small incision is made in the side of the defunctionalized limb of jejunum about 2 cm from the closed end, at a site where the free limb of jejunum comfortably opposes the divided proximal bile duct. The anastomosis is performed by placing a posterior row of 4-0 silk arterial sutures between the seromuscular coat of the jejunum and the common duct. Usually, it is possible to place only two or three silk sutures in the posterior layer of the anastomosis.

After this, the inner row of the anastomosis is made with 4-0 chromic gastrointestinal catgut sutures, placing the sutures so that the knots are tied within the lumen of the anastomosis. These catgut sutures are continued around from the posterior to the anterior row, and, again, it is usually possible with a small duct to place only about four of these catgut sutures. Following this, the anterior row of silk sutures is placed in the same manner as described above for the posterior row. It is best to perform this anastomosis over a T-tube stent to help prevent stenosis of the anastomosis and to reduce bile leakage from the anastomosis in the immediate postoperative period. The T tube should be placed in the bile duct, just above the anastomosis to the jejunum, so that one limb of the tube goes across the anastomosis. If the anastomosis is made so high in the hilus of the liver that it is impossible to place a T tube above it, then the T tube may be placed through a stab wound in the wall of the jejunal limb and one limb led through the anastomosis into the biliary ductal system. A purse-string suture should be placed in the jejunum about the T tube to secure it in position.

The abdomen should be closed with extensive drainage of the biliary-jejunal anastomosis. The T tube should be left in place for 3 or 4 weeks, following which cholangiography is performed to ensure adequate healing and patent anastomosis, and the T tube is removed. The drains are left in until all biliary drainage has ceased, or until a firm drainage tract has formed, which occurs about 3 weeks postoperatively.

If the gallbladder and cystic duct are intact, the bypass also may be done between the gallbladder and jejunum with ligation of the distal and proximal limbs of the damaged common duct. Also, it may be more expedient at times to use a simple loop of jejunum instead of a Roux en Y limb to perform the bypass procedure.

If the patient is in poor condition and cannot tolerate a prolonged procedure for definitive repair, then the defects of the biliary ductal structures may be repaired by simple bridging with a T tube fixed in place with a suture at either end of the ductal defect; secondary repair may be done later as soon as the patient can tolerate it. If possible, however, definitive repair should be done, since recurrent strictures are more likely to occur following the more difficult secondary repairs of the bile ducts.

Injuries to the gallbladder generally may be handled in one of two ways: (1) If the patient has other extensive injuries or is in poor condition from hemorrhagic shock and other complications, the most rapid means of dealing with the gallbladder injury is to suture the wound with a one-layer row of interrupted nonabsorbable mattress sutures and to decompress the gallbladder with a #28 to 30 French mushroom catheter, placed in the fundus of the gallbladder through a purse-string suture. The catheter is brought out through a separate stab wound in the right upper quadrant of the abdomen. This catheter remains for approximately 3 weeks, or until a good tract has formed around it in order to prevent bile leakage into the peritoneal cavity following removal of the tube. Before removing the tube, cholangiography should be done through it to demonstrate patent cystic and common ducts. (2) If the patient is in good condition, however, it is preferable to remove the gallbladder when it has been injured.

BLUNT TRAUMA

Blunt trauma to the biliary tree deserves separate discussion, not because the surgical management differs, but because of its relative rarity and difficulty of diagnosis. Barnes and Diamonon reported in 1963 that only 48 cases of traumatic rupture of the gallbladder due to blunt trauma to the abdomen had been reported up to that time. According to Rydell, complete division of the common duct by blunt trauma was reported in 25 cases up to 1970. The usual means of closed injury to the extrahepatic biliary tree is a shearing force applied to the common duct or impingement of the bile duct between the vertebral column and a crushing force applied to the abdominal wall.

When blunt trauma to the biliary tree is severe enough to result in a free flow of bile, the characteristic picture of bile peritonitis occurs. According to Sturmer and Wilt, the usual history reveals a crushing injury to the right upper quadrant, the epigastrium, or the lower part of the chest, which results in severe pain and is followed by shock. The shock usually is of relatively short duration, seldom more than a few hours. Generally during this period, the diagnosis of probable intraabdominal injury may be established by signs of peritoneal irritation, such as abdominal rigidity and guarding. Bile or nonclotting blood may be found on peritoneal tap or lavage. Shock is usually secondary to the marked outpouring of extracellular fluid into the peritoneal cavity due to the chemical irritation of the peritoneum by bile. The initial chemical peritonitis caused by bile may be followed shortly by a bacterial peritonitis. If biliary leakage is minimal, shock may be of relatively short duration or absent, and abdominal signs initially may be slight. This may be followed by the recovery and well-being of the patient, which lasts for periods up to 5 or 10 days. However, the onset of jaundice on about the third day is a fairly constant sign. The appearance of clay-colored stools and the presence of bile in the urine may be noticed from about the second to the fifth day after injury.

A considerable gradual increase in abdominal size occurs during the first 10 days that may be unattended by the usual signs of peritonitis. This condition is accompanied by progressive signs of extracellular fluid volume deficit and by evidence of infection, such as rising temperature and elevated white cell count. In the reported cases of complete transection of the common duct, the site of transection was uniformly in the retroduodenal area, thus again indicating the importance of extensive medial reflection of the duodenum to explore the retroperitoneal duodenum as well as the distal common duct and pancreas.

When blunt trauma to the extrahepatic biliary tract is diagnosed, the repair is generally the same as in the previous discussion of penetrating trauma. End-to-end repair of the ducts over a T tube should be done, if possible, or a bypass procedure between the ducts and the jejunum should be done by bringing up a Roux en Y limb or loop of jejunum to perform an anastomosis between the biliary tract and the jejunum as described in the discussion of penetrating trauma. The ducts should not be implanted in the duodenum, since anastomotic leaks occur more often with this than with the anastomosis to a defunctionalized limb of jejunum. Leak of a choledochoduodenal anastomosis produces not only a biliary fistula but a duodenal fistula as well, with all the grave consequences of such a fistula. If a biliary-jejunal anastomosis leaks, only a bile leak occurs, which is easier to manage generally and has a better prognosis than a biliary duodenal fistula.

The postoperative therapy of biliary tract injuries, in which bile peritonitis is an important complicating feature, should include adequate replacement of extracellular fluid volume deficits, which may require several liters of balanced salt solutions in 24 hours. These solutions should be given as soon as possible preoperatively and continued throughout the surgical procedure and postoperatively to avoid extracellular fluid volume deficit. Broad-spectrum antibiotics should be given prior to the surgical procedure and continued throughout the procedure and for several days after, until the chances of sepsis and infection have diminished.

Mortality from biliary tract injuries should be below 5 to 10 percent if they are discovered early and treated by adequate reconstruction, adequate drainage and decompression of the biliary tree, adequate coverage with antibiotics, and proper fluid replacement. Patients with more severe injuries probably do not survive to be diagnosed and treated.

Portal Vein

Approximately 90 percent of portal vein injuries occur because of penetrating trauma. They are frequently associated with other visceral injuries, most commonly to the inferior vena cava, liver, pancreas, and stomach. Mattox and associates recently reported a survival rate of 50 percent in their series of 22 patients.

Lateral venorrhaphy, if possible, is the preferred method of treatment. Mattox suggests performing a portacaval or mesocaval shunt as an alternate treatment of portal vein injury if suture repair is impossible and the patient's general condition is stable. Fish, on the other hand, reported that four of five patients who had portacaval shunts for portal vein reconstruction after trauma developed hepatic decompensation or encephalopathy, whereas these complications were not observed in patients undergoing portal vein ligation.

The insertion of an autogenous vein graft to bridge the defect in the portal vein (using the left common iliac vein, left renal vein, or a paneled saphenous vein graft) may be preferable to a portacaval shunt if the patient's condition is stable and the proximal and distal ends of the injured vein are suitable for the insertion of a graft. This procedure should prevent portal hypertension or hepatic deterioration that may occur if the vein is ligated. If, however, associated injuries are severe, then ligation of the portal vein may make it possible to save the patient. Even though portal vein ligation may cause portal hypertension, interruption of the vein is compatible with the patient's survival in about 80 percent of the cases. It should, of course, be emphasized that in those associated hepatic arterial injuries, a good repair of the hepatic artery must be achieved before accepting treatment of portal vein injuries by ligation.

Pancreas

Travers described the first pancreatic injury found in an intoxicated woman who was struck by a stage coach wheel in England in 1827. Although about two-thirds of pancreatic injuries are caused by penetrating trauma, recently there has been an increase in the incidence of blunt pancreatic trauma; most of this increase is caused by steering wheel injuries. Northrup and Simmons recently reviewed 734 cases of pancreatic trauma in the English literature. They describe three basic mechanisms of blunt pancreatic trauma: (1) when the blunt forces are concentrated to the right of the vertebral bodies, the head of the pancreas may be crushed, and, in addition, there may often be hepatic lacerations, avulsions of the common bile duct, and rupture of the duodenum; (2) when the blunt abdominal trauma is concentrated in the midline, where the pancreas normally crosses the vertebral bodies, the classic pancreatic transection injury is often produced, frequently without associated injuries; (3) if the impact forces are directed to the left of the vertebra, distal pancreatic contusions and lacerations, with associated splenic lacerations, may occur.

DIAGNOSIS. Diagnosis of pancreatic injuries is based upon a complete history, including the mechanism of injury, thorough physical examination, serum amylase level, and adequate visualization of the pancreas at surgical exploration. The history of trauma may be the only clue to the diagnosis of pancreatic injury. Signs and symptoms may initially be absent. In patients with isolated blunt pancreatic trauma, clinical manifestations of the injury typically appear slowly. Symptoms have been reported to be absent for as long as 5 days even after a complete pancreatic transection, and for up to 92 hours after avulsion of the pancreatic and biliary ductal systems from the duodenum. Moreover, symptoms following isolated blunt pancreatic trauma may even be delayed until a pseudocyst develops weeks, months, or years later. The delay in appearance of symptoms in patients with isolated pancreatic injuries may be caused either by an initial secretory inhibition of the pancreas after injury or by failure of pancreatic enzymes to be activated in the absence of other visceral injuries.

Not only are symptoms of isolated blunt pancreatic trauma often mild and delayed, but physical signs may also be absent or minimal. Usually, however, there is at least mild upper abdominal tenderness, but in the absence of a history of significant trauma or severe symptoms this sign may be overlooked. Injuries to retroperitoneal organs such as the pancreas may not produce clinical findings of loss of bowel sounds, tenderness, guarding, or spasm for several hours.

Serum Amylase Determination. Over 25 years ago Matthewson and Halter advocated routine serum amylase determinations in patients sustaining blunt trauma and emphasized that pancreatic injury was more common than had been previously appreciated. Serum amylase elevation alone has not been considered an indication for exploratory celiotomy. If signs of peritonitis are present (such as spasm, tenderness, and absent bowel sounds), then a celiotomy is performed. Unrecognized severe pancreatic injury can be a fatal lesion, particularly when it is accompanied by disruption of pancreatic tissue and leakage of pancreatic juice.

Many patients have been found to have an elevated serum amylase level but negative abdominal findings. These patients are closely observed for evidence of peritonitis or until the amylase level returns to normal. An amylase determination is performed on peritoneal lavage fluid, but the elevation is more often due to small-bowel injury than to pancreatic injury.

Recent studies by Olsen, Moretz and associates, and White and Benfield have indicated that improper interpretation of elevated amylase determinations may be misleading. Olsen stated that 33 percent of patients with hyperamylasemia had no significant intraabdominal trauma, and no patient in his series with hyperamylasemia had significant intraabdominal injury without other evidence of such trauma. He reemphasized that hyperamylasemia alone without any other evidence of visceral injury is not an indication for exploratory celiotomy. White and Benfield found that only 26 percent of the patients in their series who had significant blunt or penetrating pancreatic trauma had preoperative hyperamylasemia.

Though these various reports show that it is unwise to perform exploratory celiotomy on the basis of elevated amylase levels alone, nevertheless, the detection of hyperamylasemia in asymptomatic patients who have sustained abdominal trauma cannot simply be dismissed. These patients are admitted to the hospital and closely observed. Plain abdominal x-ray films may show evidence of retroperitoneal trauma. This is suspected when there is obliteration of the psoas margin, retroperitoneal air along a psoas margin or around the upper pole of the right kidney, or displacement of the stomach. Upper gastrointestinal studies with water-soluble media may show leakage of contrast media from the retroperitoneal duodenal area. Serial sonographic studies of the upper part of the abdomen, when strongly positive, may also indicate pancreatic or other retroperitoneal injuries and thus give sufficient reason for performing exploratory celiotomy in patients with blunt abdominal trauma who have asymptomatic hyperamylasemia.

Visceral arteriography may be helpful in these diagnostically challenging patients. It may clearly show vascular injuries in the region of the pancreas that definitely indicate the wisdom of exploratory celiotomy. As more experience is gained with endoscopic retrograde pancreatography it is quite possible that this technique may have a role in the diagnosis of pancreatic injury.

Surgical Exploration. When preoperative diagnostic studies indicate a probability of pancreatic injury, it is very important to visualize the entire pancreas. The head of the pancreas and the duodenum are completely mobilized to the midline by performing a Kocher maneuver. The gastrocolic omentum is also divided in order to enter the lesser sac and view the entire body of the pancreas. The tail of the gland is mobilized by freeing the spleen and retracting it medially, along with the tail of the pancreas, thus allowing direct visualization and palpation of both sides of the distal part of the gland. Cattell and Braasch described a technique that provides easy access to the third and fourth portions of the duodenum, the head and part of the uncinate process of the pancreas, and the superior mesenteric vessels where they cross the duodenum. This technique entails mobilization of the right region of the colon and its mesentery along with the small bowel and its mesentery from the retroperitoneal attachments.

Any retroperitoneal hematoma in the upper part of the abdomen or a peripancreatic hematoma should be considered presumptive evidence of pancreatic injury and should be explored.

ASSOCIATED INJURIES. Isolated pancreatic injury is rare and occurs in less than 10 percent of all patients with pancreatic trauma. Associated injuries are usually more obvious indications for surgical exploration than suspected pancreatic injury. Death and serious complications are frequent in pancreatic trauma but are only rarely caused by the pancreatic injury. Massive hemorrhage from associated vascular, hepatic, or splenic injury is the main cause of death.

Although the pancreas is a vascular organ, it is not often responsible for uncontrollable hemorrhage. When profuse bleeding occurs from the pancreatic area, the pancreas is mobilized and the superior mesenteric and the splenic vessels, the aorta, and the vena cava are inspected, since they are often the source of severe hemorrhage. Because of the location of the pancreas, injuries to the liver and the stomach are frequent. In a series of 175 patients with pancreatic injuries reported by Jones and Shires, 58 percent had an associated retroperitoneal injury in addition to the pancreatic injury.

MANAGEMENT OF PANCREATIC INJURIES. It is essential to control all bleeding at the time of initial exploration of pancreatic injuries. Bleeding vessels in the pancreas are exposed by carefully debriding surrounding devitalized tissue sufficiently to gain secure hemostasis by precise placement of shallow mattress sutures of fine nonabsorbable material. Complete mobilization of the injured pancreas permits temporary control of bleeding by anterior and posterior compression of the bleeding site with the fingers of one hand while hemostatic stitches are placed with the other hand. Nonabsorbable sutures must be used, since absorbable material is quickly digested away by the proteolytic enzymes from the pancreas. Suturing of the bleeding points should be done without preliminary application of hemostatic clamps, since such clamps cause more damage to the viable pancreas and often cause tearing and further bleeding from the fragile pancreatic vessels. Control of bleeding from the pancreas should not be attempted by blind clamping, by mass ligatures, or by deep sutures which may injure or obstruct major pancreatic or biliary ducts or major mesenteric blood vessels and thus cause further serious complications.

After bleeding from the pancreas or from adjacent major blood vessels is controlled, the extent of the pancreatic injury is determined. In general, pancreatic injuries may be classified as follows: (1) simple pancreatic contusion without rupture of the pancreatic capsule or significant hemorrhage; (2) more severe contusion and disruption of the pancreatic parenchyma with rupture of the capsule but without major ductal injury; (3) severe pancreatic injury with major ductal disruption; and (4) combined pancreatic and duodenal injury.

Simple Contusions without Capsular or Ductal Disruption. Simple pancreatic contusions without capsular or ductal disruption and without persistent hemorrhage require no suturing or debridement. These injuries should be drained with a sump and several large Penrose drains placed directly at the site of the pancreatic contusion and brought out along a short, direct tract. A properly functioning sump drain allows air to enter the tract, preventing the occurrence of a vacuum. It also allows measurement of the amount of pancreatic juice being lost and helps prevent skin digestion. These drains should exit through a stab wound in the upper part of the flank which is placed as dependently as possible and made sufficiently large to admit two fingers easily. The drains are left in place for 10 days to 2 weeks, since moderate drainage may not occur during the first week following injury. Drainage from the pancreas might not be expected with a simple contusion and an apparently intact pancreatic capsule; however, minor capsular disruptions might be easily missed during exploration of the pancreas. Lack of drainage to such areas of unrecognized capsular injury may lead to complications associated with intraabdominal collections of pancreatic secretions such as pseudocysts, pancreatic abscesses, lesser-sac abscesses, and subphrenic abscesses.

Capsular Laceration without Ductal Injury. Most surgeons agree that simple pancreatic penetration or lacerations with capsular disruptions without loss of tissue or major ductal injury are best treated by simple suture of the capsule with nonabsorbable material and extensive drainage. Such injuries with significant loss of pancreatic tissue that precludes suture repair to the capsule obviously can be treated only by direct suture of any bleeding points and extensive drainage. Extensive drainage to control leakage from a pancreatic injury is more important than attempting to prevent a fistula by capsular repair.

Injury with Ductal Disruption. Disruption of the main pancreatic duct is a much more serious injury than capsular disruption and requires especially careful management. Major ductal injury almost always causes a pseudocyst or abscess if not recognized and drained. If treated by drainage alone, these injuries usually produce a troublesome and persistent fistula.

Distal Pancreatectomy. An effective method of treatment for pancreatic injuries with disruption of the pancreatic duct in the body or tail of the gland is distal pancreatectomy. This is performed at the point where the main duct is injured, and allows removal of the traumatized and devitalized tissue.

When performing a distal pancreatectomy, suture stick ties are placed in the superior and inferior borders of the pancreas approximately 1.5 to 2 cm from the edge. This, along with isolation of the splenic vessels during distal pancreatectomy, prevents unnecessary blood loss and provides better visualization. In resecting the distal pancreas, the cut edge is beveled in a fishmouth fashion. This enables a better closure of the proximal end of the pancreas. The transected duct of Wirsung in the remaining proximal gland is ligated with a transfixion suture of fine monofilament, nonabsorbable material such as Prolene, to discourage fistula formation. The cut surface of the transected proximal pancreas is oversewn with interrupted, interlocking mattress sutures, which facilitate hemostasis. The stump of the pancreas is extensively drained with a sump and large Penrose drains.

Yellin and associates reported excellent results with distal pancreatectomy in 60 patients. In eight of their patients, the injury was located considerably to the right of the superior mesenteric vessels and as much as 13 to 15 cm of distal pancreas was resected. (The average normal pancreas has a length of 15 cm, is 3 cm thick, and weighs 60 to 125 Gm.) Only one patient (1.6 percent) developed diabetes mellitus after distal pancreatectomy; this percentage is similar to the result in the series from Parkland Memorial Hospital in which Jones and Shires reported no incidence of pancreatic insufficiency or diabetes following distal pancreatectomy.

Distal Pancreatectomy with Roux-en-Y Anastomosis. This technique has been utilized in patients undergoing primary distal pancreatectomy for trauma when there is much contusion and edema of the remaining pancreatic head. In these cases the surgeon may anticipate that there will be significant obstruction in the proximal ductal system, leading to persistent leakage of pancreatic secretions from the end of the transected pancreas, if the pancreatic duct and stump are simply oversewn and drained instead of being implanted in a defunctionalized Roux-en-Y limb of jejunum. This procedure is time-consuming and is not recommended in patients whose condition is tenuous because of hemorrhage and severe injuries to structures adjacent to the pancreas.

Roux-en-Y Pancreaticojejunostomy. Several methods of treating pancreatic transection have been described. For the pancreas completely transected over the superior mesenteric vessels and to the right of these vessels, a Roux-en-Y anastomosis suturing both ends of the pancreas to the defunctionalized limb has proved satisfactory (Fig. 6-14). This treatment has been recommended by Jones and Shires

Fig. 6-14. Technique of Roux-en-Y anastomosis of both ends of transected pancreas.

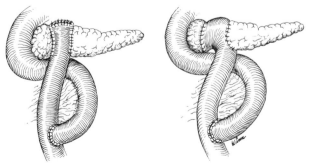

for treatment of injuries which require removal of 75 percent or more of the pancreas. Transections of less magnitude are treated by simple distal pancreatectomy. A Roux-en-Y anastomosis to both ends of the severed pancreas has eliminated the need to find a severed duct or to reanastomose it. This method leaves all functioning pancreatic tissue, thereby avoiding the possibility of pancreatic insufficiency or diabetes. The risk of injury to the underlying superior mesenteric vessels seems less with this mode of treatment than with resection. The possibility of fistula and pseudocyst formation is also minimized.

The easiest method of accomplishing the Roux-en-Y anastomosis to both ends of the severed pancreas is an end-to-end anastomosis of one end of the pancreas to the jejunum and of the remaining end of the pancreas to the side of the jejunum. This is accomplished using permanent sutures placed approximately 1 cm apart in a single-layer anastomosis. Once this anastomosis is accomplished, drainage tract is established with Penrose and sump drains.

Jordan and associates advocate complete transection of the pancreas with a Roux-en-Y anastomosis to the pancreatic fragment with oversewing of the proximal pancreas. The Roux-en-Y limb should be at least 30 cm in length and is usually passed through the transverse mesocolon to the site of injury. As long as the duodenum is intact and viable, there is little justification for a pancreaticoduodenectomy for this type of injury.

Unless the completely severed pancreatic duct is managed with definitive surgery, a pseudocyst or fistula will almost always result. A Roux-en-Y anastomosis to one fragment of the severed pancreas is little more time-consuming than resection of the distal fragment, which requires a splenectomy.

If location of the pancreatic injury suggests the possibility of injury to the intrapancreatic portion of the common bile duct, the common bile duct is opened in its supraduodenal position and a cholangiogram obtained. If a partial tear of the distal common duct has occurred but some ductal continuity remains, a T tube is inserted for decompression.

Repair and Stent of Pancreatic Duct. It is difficult to locate the pancreatic duct with considerable bleeding and hematoma, and even more difficult to suture it after it is found. Nevertheless, several reports have appeared in which the pancreatic duct has been identified, found to be completely transected in the region of the neck of the pancreas, and successfully repaired by stenting and suture repair. The stent may be inserted into the duct at the area of injury and threaded through the ampulla into the duodenum. The second method by which this has been accomplished is by duodenotomy and catheter cannulation of the pancreatic duct through the ampulla, with or without a sphincterotomy, with passage into the distal pancreatic duct past the point of transection. The pancreatic duct is then reapproximated with 6-0 or 7-0 nonabsorbable suture. This is not a preferred but an alternate method, which might be of some benefit in selected cases in which the injury would require radical resection of the pancreas in the critically ill patient. Although fistula, late stricture formation at the site of injury, or recurrent pancreatitis secondary to partial obstruction of the pancreatic duct is possible, these complications have not been reported.

Anterior Roux-en-Y Pancreaticojejunostomy. A Roux-en-Y pancreaticojejunostomy may be placed to the anterior surface of the pancreas over the injury in selected cases. This method of treatment has been satisfactory only if the posterior pancreatic capsule is intact. If the posterior pancreatic capsule is broken, drainage will continue into the retroperitoneal space rather than into the Roux-en-Y limb and result in abscess, pseudocyst, or fistula formation.

The most severe form of pancreatic injury is extensive laceration and shattering of the head of the pancreas, which leaves virtually none of the proximal pancreas or its main ductal system intact. Extensive injuries of the pancreatic head not involving the duodenum are preferably treated by either a Child 95 percent pancreatectomy or a Jones-Shires double pancreaticojejunostomy. Only rarely should pancreaticoduodenectomy be done for injuries of the pancreatic head alone.

Combined Duodenum and Pancreatic Injuries

Northrup and Simmons reported an overall mortality of duodenal injuries alone of 20 percent, which is equal to the overall mortality of pancreatic injuries alone. Combined pancreatic and duodenal injuries, however, increase the mortality rate to an average of 44 percent, with some reports exceeding 60 to 70 percent. Some 30 percent of duodenal injuries are associated with pancreatic trauma, and approximately 20 percent of pancreatic injuries are associated with duodenal trauma. The high mortality rate among patients with combined injuries is related not only to the intensity and severity of forces that cause injury to the pancreas and duodenum but also to the frequent involvement of the adjacent major blood vessels, with resultant immediate or early death from hemorrhage. A large amount of devitalized tissue and complicated pancreaticoduodenal fistulas also contribute to the high mortality rate.

Combined injuries of the pancreas and duodenum are treated by either a Berne duodenal "diverticulization" procedure (Fig. 6-6), as previously described under Duodenum, for relatively less severe combined injuries or a Whipple procedure for very severe combined pancreaticoduodenal injuries.

Pancreaticoduodenectomy. Prior to performing a pancreaticoduodenectomy the presence of a pancreatic ductal injury should be verified. This may be accomplished by duodenotomy, cannulation of the pancreatic duct, and pancreatogram. The common duct is identified and proved to be intact by operative cholangiogram. An alternate method of determining ductal injury is by mobilizing the tail of the pancreas and performing a pancreatogram through the distal pancreatic duct. Hemostatic sutures are placed 1.5 to 2 cm into the superior and inferior portions of the pancreas prior to incising the tail. If the common bile duct and major duct system are intact and the duodenal injury can be closed, then a pancreaticoduodenectomy is usually not indicated.

Indications for pancreaticoduodenectomy include rupture of the duodenum and head of the pancreas, avulsion of the common duct from the duodenum with avascular duodenal wall, and stellate fracture with bleeding from a crushing injury of the head of the pancreas. This procedure also is indicated for combined injuries to the head of the pancreas and duodenum with destruction of both, to control hemorrhage, remove devitalized tissue, and restore ductal continuity. The overall condition of the patient and associated injuries must be considered prior to submitting the patient to several more hours of surgery. There are times when this procedure is necessary, but they are rare, particularly if the duodenum is intact. Complications following pancreaticoduodenectomy are common. Thus, mortality rate of this procedure must be low to justify its use if any other form of management can be employed.

In addition to fistula formation and abscesses, marginal ulceration with upper gastrointestinal bleeding has occurred following pancreaticoduodenectomy in which a vagotomy or subtotal gastric resection was not performed. Symptoms of dumping, diabetes, and weight loss with diarrhea and semiformed bowel movements have occurred following pancreaticoduodenectomy for trauma. Foley and associates have reported a postoperative complication following pancreaticoduodenectomy with bleeding into the intestinal tract from the site of the pancreaticojejunostomy which was demonstrated by arteriographic studies and required reoperation to suture the bleeding point.

The average mortality rate for patients treated with the Whipple procedure continues to be about 35 percent, with some series reporting as high as 50 to 60 percent. This high mortality rate is frequently due to associated injuries, and it is probable that some of these patients would have died if a pancreaticoduodenectomy had not been done. Despite a very justifiable concern about the inappropriate use of the Whipple procedure in the treatment of less serious pancreatic and duodenal injuries, Yellin and Rosoff conclude that pancreaticoduodenectomy is an effective procedure for removing severely devitalized pancreas and duodenum when these organs are irreparably injured.

COMPLICATIONS. Complications following pancreatic trauma include fistula, pancreatic abscesses, vascular necrosis with hemorrhage from the drain site, pseudocyst formation, and duodenal fistula secondary to suture line breakdown from pancreatic juice activation.

Pancreatic enzymes liberated in an inactive form do not digest living tissue. In extensive injuries, duodenal and biliary enzymes are often released and the proteolytic pancreatic enzymes activated. Trypsinogen activated by enterokinase and hydrolyzed to trypsin breaks down protein. Mixtures of bile, gastric, and pancreatic juice are capable of digesting soft tissues with which they come in contact. As a result of digestion of surrounding tissues, any attempt at delayed definitive operation in this area becomes hazardous.

Fistula. Jordan et al. have reported the occurrence of pancreatic fistula as the most common complication following operative therapy, occurring in 35 percent of the cases and usually following blunt trauma. Most pancreatic fistulas are minor and close within a period of one month. Major pancreatic fistulas have been arbitrarily defined as those which drain longer than 1 month. The serum amylase level is frequently elevated while the fistula is present, probably because of transperitoneal absorption.

Almost all pancreatic fistulas will eventually close spontaneously; therefore treatment is mainly conservative. Attention must be given to preventing autodigestion of the surrounding skin. Dressings should never be applied to any fistula, since skin irritation will result from the fistula fluid in the dressings even in the presence of relatively bland pancreatic juice.

The use of Stomahesive provides an excellent method for managing the drainage from pancreatic or other types of gastrointestinal fistulas. An opening is made in the Stomahesive sheet just large enough to permit drains from the fistula tract to pass through. Stomahesive securely adheres to the skin for several days before it must be replaced and is virtually nonreactive and nonallergenic. A gas-sterilized polyethylene bag with adherent backing and a "drainable stoma" at the bottom is applied so that it adheres to the Stomahesive sheet rather than to the patient's skin. The Penrose drains, if these are still in place, are completely contained within the bag, and the suction catheter in the fistula tract exits through the "drainable stoma" in the bag. Leakage is prevented by placing rubber bands around the suction catheter and the polyethylene bag in order to make a tight seal where the catheter passes through the stoma. This method protects the skin, isolates the drains from outside infection, and permits accurate measurement of fluid loss from the fistula.

Vigorous fluid replacement with balanced salt solution to prevent volume deficit is indicated: the volume may be equal to that lost through the fistula. In order to minimize fluid and electrolyte losses, the pancreatic fluid from a fistula may be returned to the alimentary tract by way of a nasogastric tube, a gastrostomy tube, or a jejunostomy. However, except with very large-volume fistulas, refeeding of this fluid usually is unnecessary.

Many patients with pancreatic fistulas can continue oral intake of food, especially if the fistula drains less than 500 to 600 ml each day and the volume does not increase significantly when the patient eats. In the presence of large-volume pancreatic fistulas, it is preferable to institute intravenous hyperalimentation. Intravenous hyperalimentation has two beneficial effects on such patients: (1) it maintains excellent nutrition and nitrogen balance without stimulating the pancreas, as do oral feedings; and (2) intravenous hyperalimentation can significantly reduce the volume of pancreatic exocrine secretion (by one-half or more).

Baker and associates have advocated the use of atropine or other anticholinergics to reduce pancreatic secretion and decrease fistula drainage. These agents may cause discomfort to the patient by inducing dryness of the mouth, blurring of vision, urinary retention, and inspissation of pulmonary secretions.

With good supportive care of the patients who develop pancreatic fistulas following pancreatic trauma, surgical repair should be necessary in less than 5 percent. Although there are no rigid criteria indicating when conservative treatment should be abandoned, Baker and associates suggest that closure probably should be carried out in most patients who have fistulas that have persisted for more than 60 days and continue draining more than 1,000 ml/day. Internal drainage of these fistulas via a Roux-en-Y defunctionalized limb of jejunum is a very satisfactory method of management.

Pseudocyst. A pancreatic pseudocyst is a cyst whose wall of inflammatory fibrous tissue does not contain epithelium but is made of those structures surrounding the region of the pancreas in the retroperitoneum. The most frequent symptoms associated with a pancreatic pseudocyst are an abdominal mass, pain, nausea, and vomiting. The serum amylase level is usually elevated for a prolonged period of time during this illness. The pseudocyst rarely resolves spontaneously. Pancreatic pseudocyst is now a rare complication following pancreatic trauma if the pancreas has been explored and managed appropriately, such management including adequate drainage with a sump and numerous drains. The preferred method of draining pancreatic pseudocysts is internally by either cyst gastrostomy or Roux-en-Y cyst jejunostomy.

Sepsis. Intraabdominal abscess is a common complication following multiple abdominal trauma. Although pancreatic fistulas rarely cause death, they occasionally give rise to pseudocyst formation and lesser-sac abscesses requiring reoperation for drainage. A lesser-sac abscess may contribute to either sepsis or retroperitoneal bleeding and death. Cultures of the abscess grow a predominance of mixed gram-negative organisms; however, staphylococci and enterococci may often be present. The serum amylase level is not consistently elevated in patients with a pancreatic or lesser-sac abscess.

The method of management of pancreatic abscesses consists of adequate debridement and drainage plus insertion of gastrostomy and feeding jejunostomy tubes. Complications are often associated with a duodenal fistula. If such a condition is present, a Roux-en-Y jejunostomy is placed over the duodenal fistula wall when possible. Antibiotics are instituted in all cases.

MORTALITY. The mortality rate caused by pancreatic injury is quite variable and is chiefly related to hemorrhage from adjacent major blood vessels. Northrup and Simmons, in a review of 734 patients, found that the wounding agent was directly related to the mortality rate as follows: stab wounds—8 percent; gunshot wounds—25 percent; steering wheel injuries and other severe blunt trauma—up to 50 percent; and shotgun wounds—60 percent. Whatever the wounding agent, the average mortality rate of pancreatic head injuries was 28 percent, in contrast to the mortality rate of 16 percent from all types of injuries to the body or tail. This result is similar to that in the series reported by Jones and Shires (Table 6-6).

Early surgical intervention in both blunt and penetrating abdominal trauma, meticulous abdominal examination of all organs, and an aggressive approach to pancreatic injuries, including resection when indicated, are essential if the mortality rate is to be lowered. Jones and Shires reported a decrease in mortality due to blunt trauma to the pancreas from 37 percent in 1965 to an overall 16 percent in 1970. The mortality for isolated pancreatic injury was less than 5 percent.

Table 6-6. MORTALITY AND TYPE OF TRAUMA

	No. of patients	Died	Mortality, %
Penetrating . .	143	27	19
Stab	30	2	6
Gunshot . .	95	14	15
Shotgun . .	18	11	61
Blunt	32	5	16
Total	175	32	18

Spleen

The spleen is the abdominal organ most frequently injured by blunt trauma; such injuries to the spleen represent approximately one-quarter of all blunt injuries of the abdominal viscera. The spleen also is often injured by penetrating abdominal trauma and is frequently associated with blunt and penetrating thoracoabdominal injuries.

DIAGNOSIS. The diagnosis of splenic injury is usually easily made with penetrating trauma but is often more difficult in patients sustaining blunt trauma. The clinical manifestations are the systemic symptoms and signs of hemorrhage and local evidence of peritoneal irritation in the region of the spleen. Only about 30 to 40 percent of patients with splenic injury present with a systolic blood pressure below 100 mm Hg. However, many patients with splenic trauma may develop hypotension and tachycardia when assuming the sitting position. A tender abdomen with guarding and distension is apparent in only about 50 to 60 percent of those patients with splenic rupture.

A history of injury, which may be seemingly slight, followed by abdominal pain, predominantly in the left upper quadrant, left shoulder pain, and syncope is very significant. Often the left shoulder pain, or Kehr's sign, occurs only when the patient is in a supine or head-down position. This is caused by irritation of the inferior surface of the left side of the diaphragm by free blood or blood clots. Elevation of the foot of the bed or pressure in the left subcostal region may occasionally reproduce pain at the top of the left shoulder. Ballance's sign, which refers to fixed dullness to percussion in the left flank and dullness in the right flank that disappears on change of position of the patient, thus indicating large quantities of clot in the perisplenic region and free blood in the remainder of the peritoneal cavity, may be helpful in establishing the diagnosis. Whereas a decreased or falling hematocrit, leukocytosis of more than 15,000, x-ray findings such as fractures of the left lower ribs, gastric displacement, loss of splenic outline, and splinting or elevation of the left diaphragm are useful diagnostic findings, they are frequently absent. Abdominal paracentesis and diagnostic peritoneal lavage are extremely helpful in establishing the diagnosis in doubtful cases, particularly in patients whose sensibility is obtunded by other injuries. In patients with splenic trauma the incidence of false-negative diagnostic peritoneal lavage is reported in repeated series to be less than 1 percent.

Delayed rupture of the spleen was first described by Baudet in 1902, and the asymptomatic interval between abdominal injury and rupture of the spleen is known as the latent period of Baudet. It was postulated that bleeding appeared several days after injury because (1) a subcapsular splenic hematoma gradually increased in size until it caused a delayed rupture of the splenic capsule and intraperitoneal hemorrhage, or (2) there was initial bleeding from a splenic laceration which ceased spontaneously but began again in several days or weeks when the perisplenic hematoma became dislodged. This concept has recently been challenged by Olsen and Polley and by Benjamin and associates. These authors report a delayed rupture of the spleen of less than 1 percent in over 600 patients. They suggest that splenic rupture is an unusual occurrence and that the 15 percent incidence reported in older papers actually represents a delay in diagnosis rather than a delayed rupture in those patients.

TREATMENT. Splenectomy remains the only acceptable treatment for splenic injury. Even a slight nonbleeding tear of the splenic capsule may lead to recurrent fatal bleeding. Also, it is likely that a splenic hematoma will increase in size secondary to increasing osmotic pressure of the hematoma and imbibition of fluid, even though no further hemorrhage occurs. The splenic hematoma eventually reaches such size that the spleen ruptures, either spontaneously or following slight trauma, causing massive bleeding which may be rapidly fatal.

Nonoperative treatment was recognized very early to carry a high mortality rate; and when no operation is performed, the mortality rate is 90 to 95 percent. If an attempt is made to suture the spleen to stop bleeding or to tamponade it with omentum or other hemostatic agents, the estimated mortality rate ranges from 25 to 50 percent because of the high incidence of rebleeding.

Controversy surrounds the proper treatment of a minor nonbleeding splenic injury in the pediatric age group. Singer reported an incidence of fatal sepsis in children that was 58 times greater than that in the general population following splenectomies for trauma. Increasing experimental data and clinical evidence indicate that an intact spleen is required to produce important opsonic antibodies which are necessary for optimal function of the macrophage system in production of immunoglobulins.

Sepsis is a rather frequent occurrence following splenectomy for certain hematologic disorders, many of which have a diffuse reticuloendothelial abnormality. Many of these patients, however, receive various forms of therapy that alter immunity and response to infection.

There is no large series of carefully evaluated patients having had splenectomy for trauma in which overwhelming infection has developed. Without more proof that splenectomy in a patient with a normal reticuloendothelial system predisposes to infection, it is difficult to justify conservative management or partial splenectomy for splenic trauma, even in infants.

Another area of controversy is the issue of prophylactic antibiotics in the postsplenectomized patient, particularly in the pediatric age group. Most authors advocate prophylactic penicillin therapy until at least age five years, but it has been recommended that protection be extended into the teenage years, and isolated reports suggest indefinite protection. The use of long-term antibiotics is not without untoward effects, such as drug sensitivity, bacterial resistance, and suppression of natural immunologic defenses.

Operative Technique. Splenectomy is best performed through a long upper midline abdominal incision. The advantages of this incision are (1) it can be made very quickly; (2) it offers easy access not only to the spleen but also to other intraabdominal organs that may be injured; (3) it can be closed quickly and heals securely if closed with nonabsorbable, noninterrupted sutures of appropriate strength.

Good exposure can be obtained by downward retraction of the splenic flexure of the colon and the body of the stomach and by firm retraction on the left upper portion of the midline incision. The operator's right hand is then placed low and posterior to the spleen, and the spleen is grasped and delivered into the wound, either directly or after freeing the peritoneal reflection, which often attaches the lateral surface of the spleen to the diaphragm. Warm, moist sponges are packed into the splenic bed to aid in controlling bleeding from the bluntly divided ligaments and diaphragm and to maintain exposure of the spleen. Occasionally it is necessary to divide the splenorenal ligament by sharp dissection to obtain complete rotation of the spleen and optimum delivery through the incision. If there is considerable splenic hemorrhage, bleeding may be temporarily controlled by compressing the pedicle of the spleen between the index and middle fingers of the left hand or, if necessary, by placing a nontraumatic clamp such as a DeBakey vascular clamp or a Glassman clamp across the pedicle.

In some patients in whom the splenic pedicle cannot be quickly mobilized and compressed in order to control hemorrhage, the lesser sac can be rapidly entered by pulling the stomach inferiorly, opening the gastrohepatic omentum above the lesser curvature of the stomach, and then grasping and occluding the splenic artery and vein at the superior margin of the tail of the pancreas with the fingers of the left hand. This then permits rapid mobilization of the spleen and its pedicle by blunt dissection with the right hand, with much less blood loss during the mobilization.

Rotation of the spleen anteriorly and medially out through the midline abdominal incision in order to visualize the posterior aspect of the splenic pedicle is very important. This is necessary to avoid injury to the pancreas and to permit individual ligation of the hilar vessels of the spleen under direct vision. Whitesell in performing 50 anatomic dissections found the tail of the pancreas was either intimately applied to the spleen or within 1 cm of it in half the dissections, and in another 15 percent the tail approached to within 1.5 cm of the splenic hilum.

When the spleen is delivered, the pedicle is divided between long chest Péan clamps and ligated with heavy nonabsorbable suture. Suture ligatures should be used to control the portions of the pedicle containing the splenic artery and vein.

When delivering the spleen through the midline incision, care must be taken to avoid tearing the gastrosplenic ves-

sels. These must be carefully ligated in order to avoid injuring the wall of the stomach by including it in a mass ligature. Such injuries may cause necrosis of the stomach at this point and subsequent formation of a gastric fistula. After the spleen has been removed, the proximal greater curvature of the stomach should be carefully inspected; if there is any question about its integrity or viability the questionable area should be buttressed by imbricating the fundus on itself with several interrupted Lembert sutures.

Although drainage of the splenic bed following elective splenectomy is controversial, there is little question that drainage should be employed when splenectomy is performed under emergency conditions. The incidence of drain tract infections and subphrenic abscesses has been reported to be as high as 25 to 50 percent when drains were used, in contrast to 5 to 12 percent when drains were not employed. Many of these infections, however, were related to the presence of associated injuries, usually in the gastrointestinal tract, or to the immunologic defects often present in patients requiring splenectomies for conditions other than trauma, and not to the drains per se. The routine use of drains following splenectomy for trauma is supported by the series reported by Naylor and Shires. These authors reported an incidence of subphrenic abscess of only 3.4 percent in 408 patients undergoing splenectomy for trauma. Among the 72 patients who had splenectomy for trauma involving the spleen alone, there were no subphrenic abscesses and an incidence of drain tract infection of only 1.3 percent.

Thus, while it cannot be proved that drainage of the splenic bed after splenectomy for trauma reduces the incidence of subphrenic collections, it is most probable that drainage in such cases does not increase the incidence of subphrenic abscess. Also in those instances of splenic injury in which there is any question of associated pancreatic or gastric trauma, drainage of the splenic bed may prevent complications that could arise if such unrecognized injuries were not drained. Even those authors who incriminate the usage of splenic bed drains report no higher incidences of subphrenic abscess or other infections if the drains are removed before the sixth postsplenectomy day.

MORTALITY. Factors contributing to mortality following splenic injury include (1) associated injury; (2) mechanism of injury; (3) presence of shock on admission to hospital; and (4) advanced age. Naylor and associates reported an overall mortality rate of 11.2 percent in their series of 408 patients, which compares favorably with that in other reports.

Retroperitoneal Hematoma

The management of traumatic retroperitoneal hematoma is a controversial problem. The most common cause of retroperitoneal hemorrhage, according to Baylis et al. and according to the experience at Parkland Memorial Hospital, is pelvic fracture, which accounts for about 60 percent of all traumatic retroperitoneal hematomas. The diagnosis of retroperitoneal hematoma is most difficult following blunt, nonpenetrating trauma to the abdomen, and should be suspected in any patient following trauma who has signs and symptoms of hemorrhagic shock but no obvious source of hemorrhage. Hemorrhage within the retroperitoneal area may be massive and may exceed 2,000 ml of blood. Experimental data have shown that as much as 4,000 ml of fluid can extravasate into the retroperitoneal space under pressure equal to that in the pelvic vessels.

DIAGNOSIS. Abdominal pain occurs in approximately 60 percent of patients, and back pain in about 25 percent. The abdominal pain is usually vague and generalized but is occasionally localized over the hematoma. Local or generalized tenderness is present in about two-thirds of the patients, and shock occurs in approximately 40 percent. Occasionally, a tender mass is palpable through the abdomen or in the flanks, and in some cases, rectal examination will reveal a boggy mass anterior or posterior to the rectum. Dullness to percussion over the flanks or the abdomen which does not vary with changing positions of the patient has been recorded in some instances. At times, discoloration of the flanks from retroperitoneal hemorrhage has been noted after the lapse of a few hours (Grey Turner's sign). Progressive decrease in the hemoglobin and hematocrit is a consistent finding, and hematuria is found in 80 percent of patients. Hematuria may represent the first clue to the development of a retroperitoneal hematoma.

Somewhat more than half the patients produce free, nonclotting blood on diagnostic paracentesis or lavage of the abdomen; this blood is generally related to the presence of both retroperitoneal and intraabdominal hemorrhage. However, if the retroperitoneal hematoma which occurs without intraperitoneal hemorrhage is large enough to yield a so-called "false-positive" peritoneal tap or lavage from retroperitoneal hemorrhage alone, then the hematoma itself may require abdominal exploration to search for the persistent source of the retroperitoneal bleeding.

Roentgenography, according to Baylis et al., has been valuable in several respects; approximately two-thirds of the patients with peritoneal hematoma have had fractures of the pelvis, and other x-ray findings have included obliteration of the psoas shadow in 30 percent, abdominal mass in 5 percent, and paralytic ileus in 8 percent. Also, displaced bowel-gas shadows and fractured vertebrae have been noted. Baylis et al. also noted that in one patient a pelvic phlebolith was displaced by an expanding retroperitoneal hematoma. Intravenous pyelograms and/or retrograde cystograms are routinely obtained in all patients with suspected retroperitoneal hematomas, if the patient's condition is stable enough to have these studies performed. Arteriography has also been helpful in establishing the diagnosis of retroperitoneal injury. In the patient whose condition is deteriorating, however, immediate exploration is performed without obtaining such studies, in order to attempt rapid control of progressive bleeding. Most retroperitoneal hematomas from pelvic fractures will tamponade themselves within a short time, and the patient's condition will remain stable and the hematocrit normal, perhaps after transfusion of several units of blood.

TREATMENT. It has been recommended by some that retroperitoneal hematomas not be explored at the time of operation. This nonexploration is considered poor practice,

an opinion based on experience which indicates that nonoperative treatment of retroperitoneal hematomas (with the exception of retroperitoneal hematoma secondary to pelvic fracture) has led to an excessive mortality from continued or recurrent hemorrhage from injured retroperitoneal vessels such as the vena cava, aorta, lumbar veins, or renal veins. In addition, it is felt that nonexploration of retroperitoneal hematomas adjacent to partially extraperitoneal bowel is dangerous because of the possibility of missing a perforation in the bowel's extraperitoneal portion (e.g., duodenum). Consequently, it is recommended to explore all retroperitoneal hematomas discovered during celiotomy for the source of bleeding, as well as for associated injuries to the bowel, kidney, ureter, bladder, etc. This is done regardless of the size of the hematoma or whether or not it is increasing in size at the time of exploration. This policy has not been associated with any complications arising solely from such exploration.

Warnings have been made that if a small hematoma which is not enlarging is disturbed, uncontrollable bleeding may occur. However, it is felt that if such bleeding is to occur, it is best for it to take place at the time of the surgical procedure rather than postoperatively. If major vessels are not explored at the time that hematomas occur near them, major and sometimes fatal postoperative bleeding may occur. Present-day vascular surgical techniques obviate the fear of incurring massive hemorrhage as a contraindication to exploring retroperitoneal hematomas. This is with the sole exception of the treatment of large retroperitoneal hematomas due to pelvic fracture.

In massive retroperitoneal hematomas following pelvic fractures, it is often impossible adequately to control multiple small bleeding points. Consequently, it is advisable not to explore this type of massive pelvic hematoma (for fear of causing bleeding which may be very difficult to control) unless the hemorrhage from the fracture site fails spontaneously to tamponade itself and exsanguination threatens. However, spontaneous tamponade usually occurs. When not exploring these hematomas, it is important to be certain that there is no injury to the distal aorta, common iliac, or external iliac vessels.

Seavers et al. advise that the ligation in continuity of one or both hypogastric arteries may, at times, control persistent bleeding in the pelvic retroperitoneal space from pelvic fractures which cannot be controlled by any other means. This will often control the venous bleeding from this source, also. Certainly it is preferable to locate a single vessel which is bleeding and either ligate or repair it, than blindly to ligate the hypogastric arteries. Recent studies now indicate that infusion of vasospastic drugs or the embolization of autologous clots or hemostatic agents may be beneficial in controlling this type of hemorrhage. On rare occasions it may be necessary to pack the pelvis with large lap packs for 24 to 48 hours in order to achieve hemostasis.

Inferior Vena Cava

Inferior vena caval injuries associated with penetrating abdominal wounds are being seen with increasing frequency. It has been reported that one in every 50 gunshot wounds and one in every 300 knife wounds of the abdomen will injure the vena cava. These are serious injuries; one-third of the patients die before reaching the hospital, and up to half the remaining persons will die during hospitalization. Most deaths occur from bleeding because of the inherent difficulties in controlling injuries of large veins, but significant wounds of other structures, especially in the retroperitoneum, are common and often adversely affect therapeutic efforts.

ETIOLOGY AND DISTRIBUTION. Most injuries of the inferior vena cava are caused by gunshot wounds, but stab wounds or blunt trauma may also be involved (Table 6-7). Simple penetrating wounds produced by knives and low-velocity missiles are less lethal than those wounds caused by shotguns, high-velocity bullets, and especially blunt trauma. Widespread serious damage to other structures, particularly liver and major arteries and veins, are likely to result from shotgun wounds and blunt trauma to the abdomen and lower part of the chest.

The infrarenal vena cava is most susceptible and often injured (Table 6-8). The level of injury is a major determinant of survival, and injuries of the suprarenal, intrahepatic vena cava are extremely dangerous, especially when accompanied by wounds of hepatic and renal veins. Difficulties in exposure and control are invariably encountered, and adjunctive measures are often necessary.

DIAGNOSIS. Injuries of the inferior vena cava should be considered in all cases of penetrating wounds of the abdomen and lower part of the chest. Because of the vagaries of the trajectory of bullets, innocent-appearing small-caliber wounds may produce serious damage to retroperitoneal structures, without intraabdominal organ injury. Patients who have suffered stab wounds of the back or lower part of the chest may also harbor unsuspected caval injuries.

One of the major determinants of survival of these patients is the presence of hemorrhagic shock on admission. This is often a clue that despite the absence of identifying physical findings, major vascular injuries are present. Hemoperitoneum, hemothorax, subcutaneous blood staining from retroperitoneal bleeding, and evidence of distal vena caval obstruction may be helpful in diagnosis.

Except for direct venous studies with contrast media, radiographic examination is rarely specific. Routine x-ray studies, including anteroposterior and lateral films of the chest and abdomen, are useful and are recommended, but in a patient in unstable condition these should be obtained

Table 6-7. CAUSES OF INFERIOR VENA CAVAL INJURIES

	Total	Died	Mortality, %
Bullet	69	23	30
Shotgun	8	6	75
Stab	12	2	17
Blunt	12	11	84
Total	101	42	42

Table 6-8. LOCATION OF INFERIOR VENA CAVAL INJURY

	Total	Died	Mortality, %
Above renal veins	19	11	58
At renal vein level	21	13	62
Below renal veins	47	14	29
Bifurcation	14	4	27

in the operating room as preparations for surgery are in progress. It is usually best not to delay surgery for elaborate studies if firm indications for exploration exist.

TREATMENT. As alluded to in the discussion of other vascular injuries, associated injuries are common and are a major factor in survival of these patients (Table 6-9). Prior to exploration, resuscitation and attention to other problems often are important. An adequate airway must be obtained, volume and blood deficits repaired, and often fractures stabilized. Vena caval injuries may preclude the use of lower-extremity veins for fluid administration, and at least one large-bore catheter should be placed into the upper-extremity venous system. This line is best reserved for blood and fluid administration, and should not be used for primary anesthetic manipulations.

Thoracotomy may be required, especially in patients with suprarenal caval injuries. If transatrial intracaval shunts are needed, a median sternotomy offers good exposure for this maneuver as well as for control of associated hepatic injuries.

Abdominal exploration is performed through a midline incision which can be extended as required, and median sternotomy can be added if necessary. Rapid abdominal exploration will usually expose major injuries and establish priorities of repair. It is usually wise to control the bleeding, pause, and complete volume and blood restoration before definitive repairs are begun. Attempts to complete bowel repairs while bleeding persists from other injuries often extend the hypotensive episode and increase blood loss.

Centrally located retroperitoneal hematomas above the pelvis often harbor significant injuries, and usually are explored. Damage to other retroperitoneal structures is common (79 percent) and not always evident without formal exploration. The size or stability of the hematoma does not offer reliable evidence as to the presence or absence of significant injuries. Continued bleeding from the vena caval injury, however, is ominous. Patients actively bleeding at the time of operation have a very high mortality rate, especially if the vena caval injury is at or above the renal arteries and veins (Table 6-10).

Table 6-9. INJURIES ASSOCIATED WITH INFERIOR VENA CAVAL INJURY

Aorta, iliac artery ... 13	Kidney ... 21
Major splanchnic vessel ... 26	Pancreas ... 18
Renal artery or vein ... 20	Spleen ... 10
Liver ... 46	Colon ... 27
Duodenum ... 27	Other ... 21

Table 6-10. RELATIONSHIP OF BLEEDING
AND MORTALITY FROM
INFERIOR VENA CAVAL INJURIES

	Total	Died	Mortality, %
Active bleeding	41	32	79
Tamponade	57	9	16
Not specified	3	0	0

Initial control of bleeding can usually be obtained with pressure and packs. Occasionally temporary occlusion of the abdominal aorta at the diaphragmatic hiatus is useful in reducing blood loss from high caval injuries. Exposure of the inferior vena cava is obtained by reflecting medially the right colon, duodenum, and pancreas. Direct tamponade, manually or with sponge sticks, is usually effective in controlling bleeding. Simple lacerations or punctures are most common, but transections, avulsion, or multiple lacerations may be encountered, and control may be very difficult in the last group.

Simple lacerations can be controlled with gentle digital pressure and sutured by simply passing the needle under the occluding finger. In some cases the edge of the wound can be held gently in apposition with vascular forceps or blunt Allis clamps while repair is effected. Balloon catheter tamponade has also been employed for control of these wounds. Partial occlusion with vascular clamps is a useful technique and can be instituted after the initial use of other maneuvers (Fig. 6-15). These simple tangential wounds usually can be repaired without injury to lumbar veins, but occasionally ligation of gonadal and lumbar tributaries is required (Fig. 6-16).

Transections may be repaired by end-to-end vascular surgical techniques after mobilizing the vena cava. If there are multiple caval wounds requiring complicated repairs, or if repair poses an undue risk in a patient with multiple injuries, infrarenal ligation is preferable. In most cases construction of venous grafts is not required, and the time and effort necessary to perform these repairs may increase the operative morbidity and mortality.

Wounds at or above the renal veins are difficult to expose and repair. If bleeding from behind the liver is encountered and is not easily identified as coming from a laceration of the anterior cava wall below the caudate lobe, an intracaval shunt may be needed. The liver can be rotated medially after division of supporting ligaments, and if intrahepatic vena cava or combined hepatic vein lacerations are present, the shunt can be inserted as described by Blaisdell. The transatrial approach is easier than inserting the shunt from the intrarenal vena cava, and is very useful in managing these extremely dangerous wounds. A large chest tube (34 to 38 Fr) with a proximal side hole is inserted through the atrial appendage, and the tip is placed near the orifices of the renal veins. Umbilical tapes encircling the inferior vena cava within the pericardium and above the renal veins secure the catheter. The side hole in the catheter is placed at a level to permit the return of blood via the tube into the right atrium. This shunt, occa-

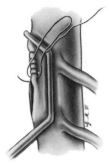

Simple Anterior Repair

Fig. 6-15. Repair of anterior laceration of the inferior vena cava. Note the use of a partially occlusive clamp.

sionally combined with temporary occlusion of the portal triad, will usually allow sufficient control of bleeding to effect repairs.

Unlike injuries of the infrarenal cava, all wounds above the renal veins should be repaired. Ligation of the inferior vena cava at this level produces serious complications. Few survivors have been reported, and those were in elective operations uncomplicated by hypotension, shock, or other injuries.

Those vascular procedures used in other areas are effective in repairing the suprarenal vena cava. Simple venorrhaphy often may suffice, but patch graft angioplasty or anastomosis may be needed (Fig. 6-17). If graft interposition is required, autogenous venous grafts obtained from the infrarenal cava or iliac vein are preferred (Figs. 6-18,

Fig. 6-16. Repair of through-and-through injury to the inferior vena cava. *A.* Anterior laceration is enlarged to permit closure of the posterior wall from within the lumen. *B.* Rotation of the posteroinferior vena cava.

Anterior and Posterior Rotation Repair Repair

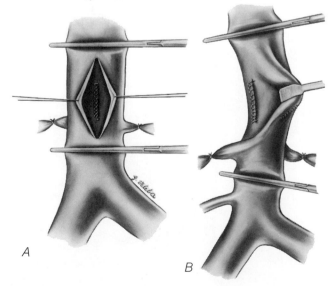

A   *B*

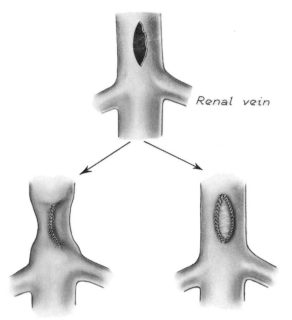

Fig. 6-17. Repair of the inferior vena cava using a patch graft to prevent stenosis.

6-19). Concomitant repair of hepatic vein injuries can be effected, but in some cases ligation may be preferable.

These repairs can usually be completed within 30 minutes, a period of ischemia well tolerated by the normothermic liver. Regional hypothermia may be induced with iced saline solution by irrigation techniques, thus conferring further protection of the liver during more prolonged ischemia.

Fig. 6-18. Construction of an inferior vena caval conduit from the saphenous vein.

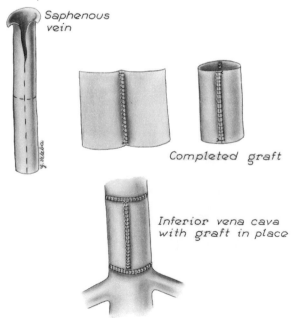

COMPLICATIONS. In patients with isolated wounds of the inferior vena cava, repair is usually effective and complications are few. In these patients, two episodes of ileofemoral venous thrombosis have been encountered, and an additional patient had a pulmonary embolus. Pancreatitis has also been encountered, and recurrent retroperitoneal bleeding occurred in one patient.

The mortality in patients with isolated inferior vena caval injuries was 11 percent in the present series, but 67 percent of the patients with one or more major vessel injuries died. All the patients with inferior vena caval wounds at or above the renal veins had significant associated injuries, usually liver and bowel, occasionally pancreas, stomach, and lung. The mortality is high in this group of patients, especially if the inferior vena cava is actively bleeding at surgery.

Female Reproductive Organs

Injuries to the female reproductive organs are infrequently seen following either blunt or penetrating trauma to the abdomen. A series reported by Quast and Jordan revealed only 27 patients with gynecologic injuries in a 16-year period at their hospital. Two of those injuries resulted from blunt trauma with rupture of the uterus in patients who were in the immediate postpartum period. These are apparently the only cases recorded of rupture of the nonpregnant uterus. The remaining injuries were penetrating wounds. An enlarged uterus was present in 10 of their patients. Six patients were pregnant, two had large uterine myomas, and two were in the postpartum period. No cases of rupture of an unenlarged uterus by blunt trauma have been recorded, however. Rupture of the pregnant uterus due to blunt trauma is rare, but has occurred in a number of instances. Of blunt and penetrating wounds to the female reproductive tract, 90 percent involve the uterine corpus, and 10 percent involve the remaining adnexa.

TREATMENT. The signs and symptoms from a ruptured pregnant uterus are those of abrupt and massive intraperitoneal hemorrhage. Associated with these findings are generalized abdominal pain and tenderness, abdominal distension, ileus, and the absence of fetal heart sounds and movements. If the patient arrives at the hospital alive (which is not often the case), immediate blood volume and extracellular fluid replacement must be instituted through several large-bore intravenous catheters, preferably placed in the upper extremities, since there may be an interference with venous return from lower extremities of these patients. Urgent celiotomy is necessary to control hemorrhage, even though the patient may still be in shock at the time, since the only means of controlling the shock is to stop the hemorrhage. Probably the only anesthesia which will be required is assisted respiration with 100 percent oxygen administered through an endotrachael tube. Other agents may be added if and when shock abates. The treatment of choice is evacuation of the uterus, closure of the disruption with large chromic catgut sutures, and thorough peritoneal toilet with removal of all blood and foreign tissue.

Wounds of the uterus and adnexa are repaired by figure-of-eight chromic catgut sutures without drainage in most instances, although in occasional patients hysterectomy is indicated, as in injury of the lower uterine segment and major uterine vessels caused by high-velocity missiles. In these instances, hysterectomy is preferable to an attempted suture repair, since repair may cause stenosis of the cervical canal with resultant hematometra and dystocia. Also, hysterectomy for lower-uterine-segment injuries is indicated to obtain proper control of bleeding vessels and to help rule out urethral injury at the point where the ureter and uterine artery are in juxtaposition.

It is wise to leave the vaginal cuff partially open following hysterectomy for trauma, because of the likelihood of vaginal cuff or cul-de-sac abscess formation, especially if there is appreciable blast injury or concomitant colon injury. If abscesses occur and the vaginal cuff has been left open, it is usually a relatively simple matter to drain the abscess with a finger inserted through the vagina into the open cuff. If gross fecal contamination is present from colon injury, the cuff should be left open and a Penrose drain led out of the vagina from the cul-de-sac. This drain may be secured to the vaginal cuff by a single small chromic catgut suture.

If massive uncontrollable or recurrent bleeding occurs following trauma to the female pelvic organs, it may be rapidly and adequately controlled by bilateral in-continuity ligations of the hypogastric arteries with nonabsorbable suture material. This will not often be required, but should be borne in mind as a very helpful and possibly lifesaving procedure.

Following injury to the pregnant uterus, the loss of the fetus is quite high. Quast and Jordan reported a salvage of only 1 of 10 pregnancies. One patient who was pregnant at the time of a tangential knife injury of the uterus had a uterine repair for penetrating trauma and subsequently delivered the child uneventfully per vagina.

Other instances have been reported in which penetrating uterine injury during pregnancy has been repaired with ensuing normal delivery. Quast and Jordan found that 81 percent of their patients with uterine injuries during pregnancy delivered subsequently per vagina with no difficulty. The cesarean section rate was 19 percent. Of the patients they followed after uterine injury, all who were in the childbearing age subsequently were able to conceive children. In this group, the abortion rate for these later pregnancies was 16 percent, with no apparent cause found.

By far the majority of pregnant patients with uterine injuries will abort shortly after the injury, frequently requiring curettage to control bleeding after spontaneous abortion. Others will require elective emptying of the uterine contents at the time of celiotomy in order to secure adequate hemostasis and uterine repair. Intravenous oxytocin should be given in such instances to aid in uterine contraction and hemostasis after hysterotomy.

Abdominal Wall

Injury to the abdominal wall without peritoneal injury is often difficult to diagnose. Muscular guarding and rigidity

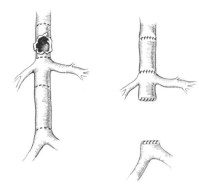

Fig. 6-19. Interposition of an excised segment of the infrarenal inferior vena cava to establish continuity of the suprarenal inferior vena cava.

are frequently present, and it may be impossible to rule out intraabdominal injury from a hematoma of the abdominal wall. Such hematomas are usually due to rupture of the rectus abdominis or the epigastric artery by direct trauma or severe muscular exertion. The epigastric artery may be injured also by penetrating trauma, so that a hemoperitoneum results. The patient may become hypotensive from such an injury because of the severe intraperitoneal bleeding which sometimes occurs.

The mass from the rectus abdominis hematoma is below the umbilicus in over 80 percent of the cases. To distinguish this mass from intraperitoneal masses, the patient should be requested to raise his head against resistance; the mass should disappear if it is intraperitoneal and remain the same if it is in the abdominal wall. This sign is not completely reliable, and if adjunctive diagnostic aids such as paracentesis and lavage are equivocal, then abdominal celiotomy should be performed.

References

General Considerations

Patman, R. D., Poulos, E., and Shires, G. T.: The Management of Civilian Arterial Injuries, *Surg Gynecol Obstet,* **118:**725, 1964.

Shires, G. T.: "Care of the Trauma Patient," McGraw-Hill Book Company, New York, 1966.

Metabolic Response to Trauma

Abbott, W. E., Krieger, H., Holden, W. D., Bradshaw, J., and Levey, S.: Effect of I.V. Administered Fat on Body Weight and Nitrogen Balance in Surgical Patients, *Metabolism,* **6:**691, 1957.

Cohn, I., Singleton, S., Harterj, Q. L., and Atile, M.: New I.V. Fat Emulsion, *JAMA,* **183:**755, 1963.

Coon, W. W.: Ascorbic Acid Metabolism in Postoperative Patients, *Surg Gynecol Obstet,* **114:**522, 1962.

Doolas, A.: Planning Intravenous Alimentation of Surgical Patients, *Surg Clin North Am,* **50:**103, 1970.

Elman, R.: Acute Starvation following Operation or Injury with

Special Reference to Caloric and Protein Needs, *Ann Surg,* **120:**350, 1944.

Hardy, J. D.: "Surgery and the Endocrine System: Physiologic Response to Surgical Trauma—Operative Management of Endocrine Dysfunction," W. B. Saunders Company, Philadelphia, 1952.

Krebs, H. A., and Lowenstein, J. M: "Tricarboxylic Acid Cycle: Metabolic Pathways," vol. 1, Academic Press, Inc., New York, 1960.

Lehr, H. B., Rhoads, J. E., Rosenthal, O., and Blakemore, W. S.: The Use of I.V. Fat Emulsion in Surgical Patients, *JAMA,* **181:**745, 1962.

Moore, F. D.: Hormones and Stress-Endocrine Changes after Anesthesia, Surgery, and Unanesthetized Trauma in Man, *Recent Prog Horm Res,* **13:**511, 1957.

———: Systemic Mediators of Surgical Injury, *Can Med Assoc J,* **78:**85, 1958.

———: "Metabolic Care of the Surgical Patient," W. B. Saunders Company, Philadelphia, 1959.

Olson, R. E.: The Two-Carbon Chain in Metabolism, *JAMA,* **183:**471, 1963.

Rea, W. J., Wyrick, W. J., Jr., McClelland, R. N., and Webb, W. R.: Intravenous Hyperosmolar Alimentation, *Arch Surg,* **100:**393, 1970.

Selye, H.: "Conditioning" vs. "Permissive" Actions of Hormones, *J Clin Endocrinol Metab,* **13:**122, 1954.

Shires, G. T., Williams, J., and Brown, F.: Acute Changes in Extracellular Fluids Associated with Major Surgical Procedures, *Ann Surg,* **154:**803, 1961.

Anesthesia

Bastron, R. D., and Hamilton, W. K.: Perils of Rapid Induction Techniques, *JAMA,* **201:**875, 1967.

Beck, G. P., and Neill, L. W.: Anesthesia for Associated Trauma in Patients with Head Injuries, *Anesth Anal (Cleve),* **42:**687, 1963.

Bowers, W. F.: Priority of Treatment in Multiple Injuries and Summation of Surgery for Acute Trauma, *Arch Surg,* **75:**743, 1957.

Clark, K.: The Incidence and Mechanisms of Shock in Head Injury, *South Med J,* **55:**513, 1962.

Crighton, H. C., and Giesecke, A. H.: One Year's Experience in the Anesthetic Management of Trauma—1964, *Anesth Anal (Cleve),* **45:**835, 1966.

Greene, N. M.: General Considerations in Anesthesia for Emergency Surgery, *Clin Anesth,* vol. 2, 1963.

Hamilton, W. K.: Atelectasis, Pneumothorax and Aspiration as Postoperative Complications, *Anesthesiology,* **22:**708, 1961.

Jacoby, J. J., Hamelberg, W., Ziegler, C., Flory, F. A., and Jones, J. R.: Transtracheal Resuscitation, *JAMA,* **162:**625, 1956.

Lee, J. F., Jenkins, M. D., and Giesecke, A. H.: The Anesthetic Management of Trauma: Influence of Alcohol Ingestion, *South Med J,* **60:**1240, 1967.

Nicholas, T. H., and Rumer, G. F.: Emergency Airway: A Plan of Action, *JAMA,* **174:**1930, 1960.

Sellick, B. A.: Cricoid Pressure to Control Regurgitation of Stomach Contents during Induction of Anesthesia, *Lancet,* **2:**404, 1961.

Walts, L. F.: Anesthesia of the Larynx in the Patient with a Full Stomach, *JAMA,* **192:**705, 1965.

Principles in the Management of Wounds

Alexander, J. W., Kaplan, J. Z., and Altemeier, W. A.: Role of Suture Materials in the Development of Wound Infection, *Ann Surg,* **165:**192, 1967.

Altemeier, W. A., and Wulsin, J. H.: Antimicrobial Therapy in Injured Patients, *JAMA,* **173:**527, 1960.

Artz, C. B., Barnett, W. O., and Grogan, J. B.: Further Studies concerning the Pathogenesis and Diagnosis of Peritonitis, *Ann Surg,* **155:**756, 1962.

Burke, J. F.: The Effective Period of Preventive Antibiotic Action in Experimental Incisions and Dermal Lesions, *Surgery,* **50:**161, 1961.

Cohn, I., Jr., and Kotler, A. N.: Intraperitoneal Kanamycin, *Ann Surg,* **155:**532, 1962.

Condie, J. P., and Ferguson, D. J.: Experimental Wound Infections: Contamination versus Surgical Technique, *Surgery,* **50:**367, 1961.

Crawford, D. T., and Ketcham, A. S.: Late Complications of Wire Sutures and Some Causative Factors, *Am J Surg,* **106:**898, 1963.

Douglas, D. M.: The Healing of Aponeurotic Incisions, *Br J Surg,* **40:**79, 1952.

Dunphy, J. E., and Jackson, D. S.: Practical Applications of Experimental Studies in the Care of the Primarily Closed Wounds, *Am J Surg,* **104:**273, 1962.

Elek, F. D., and Conen, P. E.: The Virulence of Staphylococcal Pyrogenes for Man: A Study of the Problems of Wound Infection, *Br J Exp Pathol,* **38:**573, 1957.

Houston, A. N., Roy, W. A., Faust, R. A., and Ewin, D. M.: Tetanus Prophylaxis in the Treatment of Puncture Wounds of Patients in the Deep South, *J Trauma,* **2:**439, 1962.

Jones, R. C.: "Care of the Trauma Patient," 2d ed., G. Thomas Shires (ed.), McGraw-Hill Book Company, New York, 1978.

Localio, S. A., Lowman, E. W., and Gibson, J.: Wound Healing in the Paraplegic Patient, *Surgery,* **44:**625, 1958.

Mann, L. S., and Levin, M. J.: Respiratory Depression with Intraperitoneal Neomycin, *Arch Surg,* **81:**690, 1960.

———, Spinazzola, A. J., Lindesmith, G. G., Levine, M. J., and Kuzerepa, W.: Disruption of Abdominal Wounds, *JAMA,* **180:**99, 1962.

McMullan, M. H., and Barnett, W. O.: Cephalothin—Effective Choice for Peritonitis, *Surgery,* **67:**432, 1970.

Ollodart, R., and Mansberger, A. R.: The Effect of Hypovolemic Shock and Bacterial Defense, *Am J Surg,* **110:**302, 1965.

Pissiotis, C. A., Nichols, R. L., and Condon, R. E.: Absorption and Excretion of Intraperitoneally Administered Kanamycin Sulfate, *Surg Gynecol Obstet,* **134:**995, 1972.

Pittinger, C. B., and Long, J. P.: Potential Dangers Associated with Antibiotic Administration during Anesthesia in Surgery, *Arch Surg,* **79:**207, 1959.

Rambo, W. M.: Irrigation of the Peritoneal Cavity with Cephalothin, *Am J Surg,* **123:**192, 1972.

Robertson, W. H.: Postoperative Wound Disruption, *Am Practitioner Dig Treat,* **9:**1615, 1958.

Rosen, R. G., and Enquist, I. F.: The Healing Wound in Experimental Diabetes, *Surgery,* **50:**525, 1961.

Singleton, A. O., and Julian, J.: An Experimental Evaluation of Methods Used to Prevent Infections in Wounds Which Have Been Contaminated with Feces, *Ann Surg,* **151:**912, 1960.

Sisson, R., Lang, S., Serkes, K., and Parevia, M. D.: Comparison of Wound Healing in Various Nutritional Deficiency States, *Surgery,* **44:**613, 1958.

Smith, P. S.: Management of Abdominal Incision: A Survey of Current Practices, *Arch Surg,* **88:**515, 1964.

Spencer, F. C., Sharp, E. H., and Jude, J. R.: Experiences with Wire Closure of Abdominal Incisions in 293 Selected Patients, *Surg Gynecol Obstet,* **117:**235, 1963.

Stanley, V. F., Giesecke, A. H., and Jenkins, M. T.: Neomycin-Curare Neuromuscular Block and Reversal in Cats, *Anesthesiology,* **31:**3, 1969.

Stone, H. H., Kolb, L. D., and Geheber, C. E.: Incidence and Significance of Intraperitoneal Anaerobic Bacteria, *Ann Surg,* **181:**705, 1975.

Thadepalli, H., Gorbach, S. L., Broido, P. W., Norsen, J., and Nyhus, L.: Abdominal Trauma, Anaerobes and Antibiotics, *Surg Gynecol Obstet,* **137:**270, 1973.

Thorngate, S., and Ferguson, D. J.: Effect of Tension on Healing of Aponeurotic Wounds, *Surgery,* **44:**619, 1958.

Wagner, D. H.: Errors in the Choice of Abdominal Wall Incisions and in Their Closure, *Surg Clin North Am,* **38:**175, 1958.

Bites and Stings of Animals and Insects

Auer, A. I., and Hershey, F. B.: Surgery for Necrotic Bites of the Brown Spider, *Arch Surg,* **108:**612, 1974.

Bitseff, E. L., Garoni, W. J., Hardison, C. D., and Thompson, J. M.: The Management of Stingray Injuries of the Extremities, *South Med J,* **63:**417, 1970.

Corey, L., Hattwick, M., Baer, G., and Smith, J.: Serum Neutralizing Antibody after Rabies Postexposure Prophylaxis, *Ann Int Med,* **85:**170, 1976.

Davidson, T.: Inside World of the Honeybee, *Natl Geograph,* **154:**188, 1959.

Dillaha, C. J., Jansen, G. T., Honeycutt, W. M., and Hayden, C. R.: North American Loxoscelism, *JAMA,* **188:**33, 1964.

Fardon, D. W., Wingo, C. W., Robinson, D. W., and Masters, F. W.: The Treatment of Brown Spider Bites, *Plast Reconstr Surg,* **40:**482, 1967.

Farrar, W. E., Warner, A. R., and Vivona, S.: Pre-exposure Immunization against Rabies Using Duck-Embryo Vaccine, *Milit Med,* **129:**960, 1964.

Gill, K. A.: The Evaluation of Cryotherapy in the Treatment of Snake Envenomization, *South Med J,* **63:**552, 1970.

Girard, K. F., Hitchcock, H. B., Edsall, G., and MacCready, R. A.: Rabies in Bats in Sourthern New England, *N Engl J Med,* **272:**75, 1965.

Hattwick, M. A. W., Weis, T. T., Stechschulte, C. J., Baer, G. M., and Gregg, M. B.: Recovery from Rabies: A Case Report, *Ann Intern Med,* **76:**931, 1972.

Hershey, F. B., and Aulenbacher, C. E.: Surgical Treatment of Brown Spider Bites, *Ann Surg,* **170:**300, 1969.

Hildreth, E. A.: Review: Prevention of Rabies, *Ann Intern Med,* **58:**833, 1963.

Huang, T. T., Lynch, J. B., Larson, D. L., and Lewis, S. R.: The Use of Excisional Therapy in the Management of Snakebite, *Ann Surg,* **179:**598, 1974.

Langlois, C.: Allergic Reaction to Insect Stings, *Postgrad Med,* **45:**190, May, 1969.

Levine, M. I.: Insect Stings, *JAMA,* **217:**964, 1971.

McQueen, J. L., Lewis, A. L., and Schneider, N. J.: Rabies Diagnosis by Fluorescent Antibody, *Am J Public Health,* **50:**1743, 1960.

Marr, J. J.: Portuguese Man-of-War Envenomization, *JAMA,* **199:**115, 1967.

Parrish, H. M.: Fatalities from Venomous Animals, *Am J Med Sci,* **245:**129, 1963.

———: Intravenous Antivenin in Clinical Snake Venom Poisoning, *Mo Med,* **60:**240, 1963.

———: Texas Snakebite Statistics, *Tex State J Med,* **60:**592, 1964.

———: Incidence of Treated Snakebites in the United States, *Public Health Rept (US),* **81:**269, 1966.

——— and Carr, C. A.: Bites by Copperheads in the United States, *JAMA,* **201:**927, 1967.

——— and Schwichtenberg, A. E.: Treatment of Venomous Snakebites: Fiction versus Fact, *Med Times,* **97:**153, 1969.

Paton, B. C.: Bites: Human, Dog, Spider and Snake, *Surg Clin North Am,* **43:**537, 1963.

Portuguese Man-of-War, *JAMA,* **192:**994, 1965. (Editorial.)

Russell, F. E.: Pharmacology of Animal Venoms, *Clin Pharmacol Ther,* **8:**849, 1967.

———, Carlson, R. W., Wainschel, J., and Osborn, A. H.: Snake Venom Poisoning in the United States—Experiences with 550 Cases, *JAMA,* **233:**341, 1975.

Shaffer, J. H.: Stinging Insects: A Threat to Life, *JAMA,* **177:**473, 1961.

Sikes, R. K.: Guidelines for the Control of Rabies, *Am J Public Health,* **60:**1133, 1970.

Snakebite Symposium, *J Fla Med Assoc,* **55:**307, 1968.

Snyder, C. C., and Knowles, R. P.: Snake Bite! *Consultant (SKF),* **3:**44, 1963.

Sparger, C. F.: Problems in the Management of Rattlesnake Bites, *Arch Surg,* **98:**13, 1969.

Strauss, M. B., and Orris, W. L.: Injuries to Divers by Marine Animals: A Simplified Approach to Recognition and Management, *Milit Med,* February, 1974.

Wood, J. T., Hoback, W. W., and Gran, T. W.: Treatment of Snake Venom Poisoning with ACTH and Cortisone, *Va Med Mon,* **82:**130, 1955.

Penetrating Wounds of the Neck and Thoracic Inlet

Ashworth, C., Williams, L. F., and Byrne, J. J.: Penetrating Wounds of the Neck, *Am J Surg,* **121:**387, 1971.

Brawley, R. K., Murray, G. F., Crisler, C., and Cameron, J. L.: Management of Wounds of the Innominate, Subclavian and Axillary Blood Vessels, *Surg Gynecol Obstet,* **130:**1130, 1970.

Bricker, D. L., Noon, G. P., Beall, A. C., Jr., and DeBakey, M. E.: Vascular Injuries of the Thoracic Outlet, *J Trauma,* **10:**1, 1970.

Fitchett, V. H., Pomerantz, M., Butsch, D. W., Simon, R., and Eiseman, B.: Penetrating Wounds of the Neck, *Arch Surg,* **99:**307, 1969.

Fogelman, M. J., and Stewart, R. D.: Penetrating Wounds of the Neck, *Am J Surg,* **91:**581, 1956.

Hubay, C. A.: Soft Tissue Injuries of the Cervical Region, *Surg Gynecol Obstet,* **111:**511, 1960.

Hunt, T. K., Blaisdell, F. W., and Okimoto, J.: Vascular Injuries of the Base of the Neck, *Arch Surg,* **98:**586, 1969.

Imamoglu, K., Read, R. C., and Huebl, H. C.: Cervicomediastinal Vascular Injury, *Surgery,* **61:**274, 1967.

Jones, R. F., Terrell, J. C., and Salyer, K. E.: Penetrating Wounds of the Neck: An Analysis of 274 Cases, *J Trauma,* **7**:228, 1967.

Shirkey, A. L., Beall, A. C., and DeBakey, M. E.: Surgical Management of Penetrating Wounds of the Neck, *Arch Surg,* **86**:955, 1963.

Steenburg, R. W., and Ravitch, M. M.: Cervico-thoracic Approach for Subclavian Vessel Injury from Compound Fracture of the Clavicle: Considerations of Subclavian-Axillary Exposures, *Ann Surg,* **157**:839, 1963.

Stone, H. H., and Callahan, G. S.: Soft Tissue Injuries of the Neck, *Surg Gynecol Obstet,* **117**:745, 1963.

Abdominal Trauma

Ahmad, W., and Polk, H. C., Jr.: Blunt Abdominal Trauma. A Prospective Study with Selective Peritoneal Lavage, *Arch Surg,* **111**:489, 1976.

Allen, R. E., and Blaisdell, F. W.: Injuries to the Inferior Vena Cava, *Surg Clin North Am,* **52**:699, 1972.

Awe, W. C., and Eidemiller, L.: Selective Angiography in Splenic Trauma, *Am J Surg,* **126**:171, 1973.

Anane-Sefah, J., Norton, L. W., and Eiseman, B.: Operative Choice and Technique following Pancreatic Injury, *Arch Surg,* **110**:161, 1975.

Anderson, C. B., Connors, J. P., Mejia, D. C., and Wise, L.: Drainage Methods in the Treatment of Pancreatic Injuries, *Surg Gynecol Obstet,* **138**:587, 1974.

Backwinkel, K.: Rupture of the Rectus Abdominis Muscle, *Arch Surg,* **90**:35, 1965.

Baker, R. J., Bass, R. T., Zajtchuk, R., and Strohl, E. L.: External Pancreatic Fistula following Abdominal Injury, *Arch Surg,* **95**:556, 1967.

Barnes, J. P., and Diamonon, J. S.: Traumatic Rupture of the Gallbladder Due to Nonpenetrating Injury, *Tex State J Med,* **59**:785, 1963.

Bartizal, J. F., Boyd, D. R., Folk, F. A., Smith, D., Lescher, T. C., and Freeark, R. J.: A Critical Review of Management of 392 Colonic and Rectal Injuries, *Dis Colon Rectum,* **17(3)**:313, 1974.

Bass, E. M., and Crosier, J. H.: Percutaneous Control of Posttraumatic Hepatic Hemorrhage by Gelfoam Embolization, *J Trauma,* **17(1)**:61, 1977.

Baudet, quoted by J. H. Terry, M. M. Self, and J. M. Howard: A Discussion of Injuries of the Spleen, *Surgery,* **40**:615, 1956.

Baylis, S. M., Lansing, E. H., and Glas, W. W.: Traumatic Retroperitoneal Hematoma, *Am J Surg,* **103**:477, 1962.

Beall, A. C., Bricker, D. L., Alessi, F. J., Whisennand, H. H., and DeBakey, M. E.: Surgical Considerations in the Management of Civilian Colon Injuries, *Ann Surg,* **173**:971, 1971.

Benjamin, C. I., Engrav, L. H., and Perry, J. F., Jr.: Delayed Rupture or Delayed Diagnosis of Rupture of the Spleen, *Surg Gynecol Obstet,* **142**:171, 1976.

Berman, J. K., Habeller, E. D., Fields, D. C., and Kilmer, W. L.: Blood Studies as an Aid in Differential Diagnosis of Abdominal Trauma, *JAMA,* **165**:1537, 1957.

Berne, C. J., Donovan, A. J., White, E. J., and Yellin, A. E.: Duodenal "Diverticulization" for Duodenal and Pancreatic Injury, *Am J Surg,* **127**:503, 1974.

Bollinger, J. A., and Fowler, C. F.: Traumatic Rupture of the Spleen with Special Reference to Delayed Splenic Rupture, *Am J Surg,* **91**:952, 1956.

Brawley, R. K., Cameron, J. L., and Zuidema, G. D.: Severe

Upper Abdominal Injuries Treated by Pancreaticoduodenectomy, *Surg Gynecol Obstet,* **126**:516, 1968.

Bricker, D. L., Morton, J. R., Okies, J. E., and Beall, A. C.: Surgical Management of Injuries to the Vena Cava: Changing Patterns of Injury and New Techniques of Repair, *J Trauma,* **11**:725, 1971.

Bull, J. C., Jr., and Mathewson, C., Jr.: Exploratory Laparotomy in Patients with Penetrating Wounds of the Abdomen, *Am J Surg,* **116**:223, 1968.

Burrington, J. D.: Surgical Repair of a Ruptured Spleen in Children: Report of Eight Cases, *Arch Surg,* **112**:417, 1977.

Burrus, G. R., Howell, J. F., and Jordan, G. L.: Traumatic Duodenal Injuries: An Analysis of 86 Cases, *J Trauma,* **1**:96, 1961.

Buscaglia, L. C., Blaisdell, W., and Lim, R. C.: Penetrating Abdominal Vascular Injuries, *Arch Surg* **99**:764, 1969.

Canizaro, P. C., Fitts, C. T., and Sawyer, R. B.: Diagnostic Abdominal Paracentesis: A Proposed Adjunctive Measure, *U.S. Army Surg Res Unit Annl Rept,* June, 1964.

Cassebaum, W. H., Bukanz, S. L., Baum, V., and Azzi, E.: Ligation of the Inferior Vena Cava above the Renal Vein of a Sole Kidney with Recovery, *Am J Surg,* **113**:667, 1967.

Cattell, R. B., and Braasch, J. W.: A Technique for the Exposure of the Third and Fourth Portions of the Duodenum, *Surg Gynecol Obstet,* **111**:379, 1960.

Cerise, E. J., and Scully, J. H., Jr.: Blunt Trauma to the Small Intestine, *J Trauma,* **10(1)**:46, 1970.

Chunn, C. F.: Wounds of the Rectum, *Surg Clin,* 1960, p. 1649.

Cleveland, H. C., and Waddell, W. R.: Retroperitoneal Rupture of the Duodenum Due to Nonpenetrating Trauma, *Surg Clin North Am,* **43**:413, 1963.

Cohn, I., Jr., Hawthorne, H. R., and Frabese, A. S.: Retroperitoneal Rupture of the Duodenum in Nonpenetrating Abdominal Trauma, *Am J Surg,* **84**:293, 1952.

Cornell, W. P., Ebert, P. A., Greenfield, L. J., and Zuidema, G. D.: A New Nonoperative Technique for the Diagnosis of Penetrating Injuries to the Abdomen, *J Trauma,* **7**:307, 1967.

Curtis, L. E., Simonian, S., Buerk, L. A., Hirsch, E. F., and Soroff, H. S.: Evaluation of the Effectiveness of Controlled pH in Management of Massive Upper Gastrointestinal Bleeding, *Am J Surg,* **125**:474, 1973.

Defore, W. W., Jr., Mattox, K. L., Jordan, G. L., Jr., Beall, A. C., Jr.: Management of 1,590 Consecutive Cases of Liver Trauma, *Arch Surg,* **111**:493, 1976.

Dickerman, J. D.: Bacterial Infection and the Asplenic Host: A Review, *J Trauma,* **16(8)**:662, 1976.

Drapanas, T., and McDonald, J.: Peritoneal Tap in Abdominal Trauma, *Surgery,* **100**:22, 1960.

Dudrick, S. J., Wilmore, D. W., Steiger, E., Mackie, J. A., and Fitts, W. T.: Spontaneous Closure of Traumatic Pancreatoduodenal Fistulas with Total Intravenous Nutrition, *J Trauma,* **10(7)**:542, 1970.

Duke, J. H., Jones, R. C., and Shires, G. T.: Management of Injuries to the Inferior Vena Cava, *Am J Surg,* **110**:759, 1965.

Edwards, J., and Gaspard, D. J.: Visceral Injury Due to Extraperitoneal Gunshot Wounds, *Arch Surg,* **108**:865, 1974.

Felson, B., and Levin, E. J.: Intramural Hematoma of the Duodenum: Diagnostic Roentgen Sign, *Radiology,* **63**:828, 1954.

Fish, J. C.: Reconstruction of the Portal Vein: Case Reports and Literature Review, *Am Surg,* **32**:472, 1966.

Fitzgerald, J. B., Crawford, E., and DeBakey, M. E.: Surgical

Considerations of Abdominal Injuries: Analysis of 200 Cases, *Am J Surg*, **100:**22, 1960.

Fogelman, M. F., and Robison, L. J.: Wounds of the Pancreas, *Am J Surg*, **101:**698, 1961.

Foley, W. J., Gaines, R. D., and Fry, W. J.: Pancreaticoduodenectomy for Severe Trauma to the Head of the Pancreas and the Associated Structures: Report of Three Cases, *Ann Surg*, **170:**759, 1969.

Forde, K. A., and Ganepola, A. P.: Is Mandatory Exploration for Penetrating Abdominal Trauma Extinct? The Morbidity and Mortality of Negative Exploration in a Large Municipal Hospital, *J Trauma*, **14(9):**764, 1974.

Freeark, R. J.: Role of Angiography in the Management of Multiple Injuries, *Surg Gynecol Obstet*, **128:**761, 1969.

Fullen, W. D., McDonough, J. J., Popp, M. J., and Altemeier, W. A.: Sternal Splitting Approach for Major Hepatic or Retrohepatic Vena Cava Injury, *J Trauma*, **14(11):**903, 1974.

———, Selle, J. G., Whitely, D. H., Martin, L. W., and Altemeier, W. A.: Intramural Duodenal Hematoma, *Ann Surg*, **179:**549, 1974.

Giddings, W. P., and McDaniel, J. R.: Wounds of the Jejunum and Ileum, in "Surgery of World War II," chap. 19, Office of the Surgeon General, Washington, 1955.

——— and Wolff, L. H.: Penetrating Wounds of the Stomach, Duodenum, and Small Intestine, *Surg Clin North Am*, **38:**1605, 1958.

Graham, A. S.: Penetrating Wounds of the Colon, *Surg Clin*, 1960, p. 1639.

Haddad, G. H., Pizzi, W. F., Fleishmann, E. P., and Moynahan, J. M.: Abdominal Signs and Sinograms as Dependable Criteria for the Selective Management of Stabwounds of the Abdomen, *Ann Surg*, **172:**61, 1970.

Hinshaw, D. B., Turner, G. R., and Carter, R.: Transection of the Common Bile Duct Caused by Nonpenetrating Trauma, *Am J Surg*, **104:**104, 1962.

Jones, R. C., and Shires, G. T.: The Management of Pancreatic Injuries, *Arch Surg*, **90:**502, 1965.

———, McClelland, R. N., Zedlitz, W. H., and Shires, G. T.: Difficult Closures of the Duodenal Stump, *Arch Surg*, **94:**696, 1967.

——— and Shires, G. T.: Pancreatic Trauma, *Arch Surg*, **102:**424, 1971.

Jordan, G. L., Burns, G. R., and Howell, J. F.: Surgical Management of Pancreatic Injuries, *Am J Trauma*, **1:**32, 1940.

King, J. C.: Trauma to the Abdominal and Retroperitoneal Viscera As It Concerns the Radiologist, *Southern Med J*, **49:**109, 1956.

Kobold, E. E., and Thal, A. P.: A Simple Method for the Management of Experimental Wounds of the Duodenum, *Surg Gynecol Obstet*, **116:**340, 1963.

Lauritzen, G. K.: Subcutaneous Retroperitoneal Duodenal Rupture, *Acta Chir Scand*, **96:**97, 1947.

Lavenson, G. S., and Cohen, A.: Management of Rectal Injuries, *Am J Surg*, **122:**226, 1971.

Ledgerwood, A. M., Kazmers, M., and Lucas, C. E.: The Role of Thoracic Aortic Occlusion for Massive Hemoperitoneum, *J Trauma*, **16(8):**610, 1976.

Letton, A. H., and Wilson, J. P.: Traumatic Severance of Pancreas Treated by Roux-y Anastomosis, *Surg Gynecol Obstet*, **109:**473, 1959.

Lim, R. C., Glickman, M. G., and Hunt, T. K.: Angiography in Patients with Blunt Trauma to the Chest and Abdomen, *Surg Clin North Am*, **52(3):**551, 1972.

LoCicero, J., III, Tajima, T., and Drapanas, T.: A Half-Century of Experience in the Management of Colon Injuries: Changing Concepts, *J Trauma*, **15(7):**575, 1975.

Lucas, C. E.: What Is the Role of Biliary Drainage in Liver Trauma? *Am J Surg*, **120:**509, 1970.

——— and Ledgerwood, A. M.: Factors Influencing Outcome after Blunt Duodenal Injury, *J Trauma*, **15(10):**839, 1975.

——— and ———: Prospective Evaluation of Hemostatic Techniques for Liver Injuries, *J Trauma*, **16(6):**442, 1976.

——— and Walt, A. J.: Analysis of Randomized Biliary Drainage for Liver Trauma in 189 Patients, *J Trauma*, **12(11):**925, 1972.

———, Canizaro, P. C., and Shires, G. T.: Repair of Hepatic Venous Intrahepatic Vena Caval and Portal Venous Injuries, in Madding, G. F. and Kennedy, P. A., "Trauma to the Liver," 2d ed., Saunders, Philadelphia, 1971, chap. 10, pp. 146–153.

McClelland, R. N., and Shires, T.: Management of Liver Trauma in 259 Consecutive Patients, *Ann Surg*, **161:**248, 1965.

———, ——— and Poulos, E.: Hepatic Resection for Massive Trauma, *J Trauma*, **4:**282, 1964.

McInnis, W. D., Aust, J. B., Cruz, A. B., and Root, H. D.: Traumatic Injuries of the Duodenum: A Comparison of 1° Closure and the Jejunal Patch, *J Trauma*, **15(10):**847, 1975.

Madding, G. F., Lawrence, K. B., and Kennedy, P. A.: War Wounds of the Liver, *Tex J Med*, **42:**267, 1946.

Mattox, K. L., Espada, R., and Beall, A. C., Jr.: Traumatic Injury to the Portal Vein, *Ann Surg*, **181:**519, 1975.

Maynard, A. L., and Oropeza, G.: Mandatory Operation for Penetrating Wounds of the Abdomen, *Am J Surg*, **115:**307, 1968.

Mays, E. T.: Lobar Dearterialization for Exsanguinating Wounds of the Liver, *J Trauma*, **12(5):**397, 1972.

Merendino, K. A., Dillard, D. H., and Cammock, E. E.: The Concept of Surgical Biliary Decompression in the Management of Liver Trauma, *Surg Gynecol Obstet*, **117:**285, 1963.

Miller, D. R.: Median Sternotomy Extension of Abdominal Incision for Hepatic Lobectomy, *Ann Surg*, **175:**193, 1972.

Moretz, J. A., III, Campbell, D. P., Parker, D. E., and Williams, G. R.: Significance of Serum Amylase Level in Evaluating Pancreatic Trauma, *Am J Surg*, **130:**739, 1975.

Morgenstern, L.: Microcrystalline Collagen Used in Experimental Splenic Injury: A New Surface Hemostatic Agent, *Arch Surg*, **109:**44, 1974.

Morton, J. R., and Jordan, G. L.: Traumatic Duodenal Injuries: Review of 131 Cases, *J Trauma*, **8(2):**127, 1968.

Naffziger, H. C., and McCorkle, H. J.: Recognition and Management of Acute Trauma to Pancreas with Particular Reference to Use of Serum Amylase Test, *Ann Surg*, **118:**594, 1943.

Nance, F. C., and Cohn, I., Jr.: Surgical Judgment in the Management of Stab Wounds of the Abdomen: A Retrospective and Prospective Analysis Based on a Study of 600 Stabbed Patients, *Ann Surg*, **170:**569, 1969.

———, Wennar, M. H., Johnson, L. W., Ingram, J. C., and Cohn, I., Jr.: Surgical Judgment in the Management of Penetrating Wounds of the Abdomen: Experience with 2212 Patients, *Ann Surg*, **179:**639, 1974.

Naylor, R., Coln, D., Shire, G. T.: Morbidity and Mortality from Injuries to the Spleen, *J Trauma*, **14(9):**773, 1974.

Northrup, W. F., III, and Simmons, R. L.: Pancreatic Trauma: A Review, *Surgery,* **71(1):**27, 1972.

Ochsner, J. L.: Discussion of Buscaglia, L. C., Blaisdell, W., and Lim, R. C.: Penetrating Abdominal Vascular Injuries, *Arch Surg,* **99:**764, 1969.

——, Crawford, E. S., and DeBakey, M. E.: Injuries of the Vena Cava Caused by External Trauma, *Surgery,* **49:**397, 1961.

Olsen, W. R.: The Serum Amylase in Blunt Abdominal Trauma, *J Trauma,* **13(3):**200, 1973.

—— and Polley, T. Z., Jr.: A Second Look at Delayed Splenic Rupture, *Arch Surg,* **112:**422, 1977.

——, Redman, H. C., and Hildreth, D. H.: Quantitative Peritoneal Lavage in Blunt Abdominal Trauma, *Arch Surg,* **104:**536, 1972.

O'Mara, R. E., Hall, R. C., and Dombroski, D. L.: Scintiscanning in the Diagnosis of Rupture of the Spleen, *Surg Gynecol Obstet,* **131:**1077, 1970.

Parvin, S., Smith, D. E., Asher, W. M., and Virgilio, R. W.: Effectiveness of Peritoneal Lavage in Blunt Abdominal Trauma, *Ann Surg,* **181:**255, 1975.

Pellegrini, J. N., and Stein, I. J.: Complete Severance of the Pancreas and Its Treatment with Repair of the Main Pancreatic Duct of Wirsung, *Am J Surg,* **101:**707, 1961.

Perry, J. F., Jr., DeMeules, J. E., and Root, H. D.: Diagnostic Peritoneal Lavage in Blunt Abdominal Trauma, *Surg Gynecol Obstet,* **131:**742–743, 1970.

—— and LaFave, J. W.: Biliary Decompression without Other External Drainage in Treatment of Liver Injuries, *Surgery,* **55:**351, 1964.

Perry, M. O., Thal, E. R., and Shires, G. T.: Management of Arterial Injuries, *Ann Surg,* **173:**403, 1971.

Pinkerton, J. A., Sawyers, J. L., and Foster, J. H.: A Study of the Postoperative Course after Hepatic Lobectomy, *Ann Surg,* **173:**800, 1971.

Printen, K. J., Freeark, R. J., and Shoemaker, W. C.: Conservative Management of Penetrating Abdominal Wounds, *Arch Surg,* **96:**899, 1968.

Quast, D. C., and Jordan, G. L.: Traumatic Wounds of the Female Reproductive Organs, *J Trauma,* **4:**839, 1964.

——, Shirkey, A. L., Fitzgerald, J. B., Beall, A. C., and DeBakey, M. E.: Surgical Correction of Injuries of the Vena Cava: An Analysis of Sixty-one Cases, *J Trauma,* **5:**3, 1965.

Reich, W. J., and Nechtow, M. J.: Ligation of the Internal Iliac (Hypogastric Arteries): A Life-saving Procedure for Uncontrollable Gynecologic and Obstetric Hemorrhage, *J Intern Coll Surg,* **36:**167, 1961.

Reinhardt, G. F., and Hubay, C. A.: Surgical Management of Traumatic Hemobilia, *Am J. Surg,* **121:**328, 1971.

Resnicoff, S. A., Morton, J. H., and Bloch, A. L.: Retroperitoneal Rupture of the Duodenum Due to Blunt Trauma, *Surg Gynecol Obstet,* **125:**77, 1967.

Richie, J. P., and Fonkalsrud, E. W.: Subcapsular Hematoma of the Liver, *Arch Surg,* **104:**781, 1972.

Roof, W. R., Morris, G. C., and DeBakey, M. E.: Management of Perforating Injuries to the Colon in Civilian Practice, *Am J Surg,* **99:**641, 1960.

Root, H. D., Hauser, C. W., McKinley C. R., LaFave, J. W., and Mendiola, R. P., Jr.: Diagnostic Peritoneal Lavage, *Surgery,* **57:**633, 1965.

Rosoff, L., Cohen, J. L., Telfer, N., and Halpern, M.: Injuries of the Spleen, *Surg Clin North Am,* **52(3):**667, 1972.

Rydell, W. B., Jr.: Complete Transection of the Common Bile Duct Due to Blunt Abdominal Trauma, *Arch Surg,* **100:**724, 1970.

Ryzoff, R. I., Shaftan, G. W., and Herbsman, H.: Selective Conservatism in Abdominal Trauma, *Surgery,* **59:**650, 1966.

Salyer, K., and McClelland, R. N.: Pancreaticoduodenectomy for Trauma, *Arch Surg,* **95:**636, 1967.

Schrock, T., Blaisdell, F. W., and Mathewson, C.: Management of Blunt Trauma to the Liver and Hepatic Veins, *Arch Surg,* **96:**698, 1968.

—— and Christensen, N.: Management of Perforating Injuries of the Colon, *Surg Gynecol Obstet,* **135:**65, 1972.

Schwartz, S. I., Adams, J. T., Cockett, A. T. K., and Morton, J. H.: Blunt Trauma to the Upper Abdomen, *Surg Annu,* **3:**273, 1971.

Seavers, R., Lynch, J., Ballard, R., Jernigan, S., and Johnson, J.: Hypogastric Artery Ligation for Uncontrollable Hemorrhage in Acute Pelvic Trauma, *Surgery,* **55:**516, 1964.

Shaftan, G. W.: Indications for Operation in Abdominal Trauma, *Am J Surg,* **99:**657, 1960.

Sheldon, G. F., Cohn, L., and Blaisdell, W.: Surgical Treatment of Pancreatic Trauma, *J Trauma,* **10:**795, 1970.

Shires, G. T., Jackson, D., and Williams, J.: Temporary Duodenal Decompression as an Adjunct to Gastric Resection for Duodenal Ulcer, *Am Surg,* **28:**709, 1962.

Singer, D. B.: Postsplenectomy Sepsis, in H. S. Rosenberg and R. P. Bolande (eds.), "Perspectives in Pediatric Pathology," vol. 1, pp. 285–3111, Year Book Medical Publishers, Inc., Chicago, 1973.

Smiley, K., and Perry, M. O.: Balloon Catheter Tamponade of Major Vascular Wounds, *Am J Surg,* **121:**326, 1971.

Smith, A. D., Jr., Woolverton, W. C., Weichert, R. F., and Drapanas, T.: Operative Management of Pancreatic and Duodenal Injuries, *J Trauma,* **11:**570, 1971.

Smithwick, W., III, Gertner, H. R., Jr., and Zuidema, G. D.: Injection of Hypaque (Sodium Diatrizoate) in the Management of Abdominal Stab Wounds, *Surg Gynecol Obstet,* **127:**1215, 1968.

Sparkman, R. S.: Massive Hemobilia following Traumatic Rupture of the Liver, *Ann Surg,* **138:**899, 1953.

Sperling, L., and Rigler, L. G.: Traumatic Retroperitoneal Rupture of Duodenum: Description of Valuable Roentgen Observation in Its Recognition, *Radiology,* **29:**521, 1937.

Starzl, T. E., Kaupp, H. A., Beheler, E. M., and Freeark, R. J.: Penetrating Injuries of the Inferior Vena Cava, *Surg Clin North Am,* **43:**387, 1963.

Sturmer, F. C., and Wilt, K. E.: Complete Division of the Common Duct from External Blunt Trauma, *Am J Surg,* **105:**781, 1963.

Thal, E. R.: Evaluation of Peritoneal Lavage and Local Exploration in Lower Chest and Abdominal Stabwounds, *J Trauma,* **17:**642, 1977.

—— and Saretsky, N.: Negative Laparotomy, Morbidity, Mortality and Rationale. (In preparation.)

—— and Shires, G. T.: Peritoneal Lavage in Blunt Abdominal Trauma, *Am J Surg,* **125:**64, 1973.

Travers, B.: Rupture of Pancreas, *Lancet,* **12:**384, 1827.

Trunkey, D., Hays, R. J., and Shires, G. T.: Management of Rectal Trauma, *J Trauma*, **13(5):**411, 1973.

————, Shires, G. T., and McClelland, R. N.: Management of Liver Trauma in 811 Consecutive Patients, *Ann Surg*, **179(5):**522, 1974.

Turpin, I., State, D., and Schwartz, A.: Injuries to the Inferior Vena Cava and Their Management, *Am J Surg*, **134:**25, 1977.

Vannix, R. S., Carter, R., Hinshaw, D. B., and Joergensen, E. J.: Surgical Management of Colon Trauma in Civilian Practice, *Am J Surg*, **106:**364, 1963.

Weckerson, E. C., and Putman, T. C.: Perforating Injuries of the Rectum and Sigmoid Colon, *J Trauma*, **2:**474, 1962.

Weichert, R. F., III, Hewitt, R. L., and Drapanas, T.: Blunt Injuries to Intrahepatic Vena Cava and Hepatic Veins with Survival, *Am J Surg*, **121:**322, 1971.

Werschky, L. R., and Jordan, G. L.: Surgical Management of Traumatic Injuries to the Pancreas, *Am J Surg*, **116:**768, 1968.

White, P. H., and Benfield, J. R.: Amylase in the Management of Pancreatic Trauma, *Arch Surg*, **105:**158, 1972.

Whitesell, F. B.: A Clinical and Surgical Anatomic Study of Rupture of the Spleen Due to Blunt Trauma, *Surg Gynecol Obstet*, **110:**750, 1960.

Wilder, J. R., Habermann, E. T., and Schachner, S. J.: Selective Surgical Intervention for Stab Wounds of the Abdomen, *Surgery*, **61:**231, 1967.

————, Lotfi, M. W., and Jurani, P.: Comparative Study of Mandatory and Selective Surgical Intervention in Stab Wounds of the Abdomen, *Surgery*, **69:**546, 1971.

Williams, R. D., and Sargent, F. T.: The Mechanism of Intestinal Injury in Trauma, *J Trauma*, **3:**288, 1963.

———— and Zollinger, R. M.: Diagnostic and Prognostic Factors in Abdominal Trauma, *Am J Surg*, **97:**575, 1959.

Witek, J. T., Spencer, R. P., Pearson, H. A., and Touloukian, R. J.: Diagnostic Spleen Scans in Occult Splenic Injury, *J Trauma*, **14:**197, 1974.

Yajko, R. D., Seydel, F., and Trimble, C.: Rupture of the Stomach from Blunt Abdominal Trauma, *J Trauma*, **15(3):**177, 1975.

Yellin, A. E., Chaffee, C. B., and Donovan, A. J.: Vascular Isolation in Treatment of Juxtahepatic Venous Injuries, *Arch Surg*, **102:**566, 1971.

———— and Rosoff, L., Sr.: Pancreatoduodenectomy for Combined Pancreatoduodenal Injuries, *Arch Surg*, **110:**1177, 1975.

————, Vecchione, T. R., and Donovan, A. J.: Distal Pancreatectomy for Pancreatic Trauma, *Am J Surg*, **124:**135, 1972.

Chapter 7

Burns

by P. William Curreri

Etiology of Burns

Immediate Therapy

Maintenance of Airway
Intravenous Resuscitation
Sedation
Antibiotics
Tetanus Prophylaxis
Escharotomy
Gastric Decompression
Medical Evacuation

Therapy of the Burn Wound

Debridement and Excision
Topical Chemotherapy
Bacteriologic Monitoring
Heterograft and Homograft
Autograft

General Therapeutic Considerations

Metabolism and Nutrition
Physical Therapy, Splinting, and Rehabilitation

Complications

Smoke Inhalation Syndrome
Burn Wound Sepsis
Distant Septic Complications
Gastrointestinal Complications

Special Problems

Long Bone Fractures
Burn Injury of Joints
Burns of the Face

Morbidity and Mortality

The complex pathophysiologic alterations which accompany major thermal injury present the surgeon with an extraordinary therapeutic challenge. During the past two decades, few areas of medical science have experienced more rapid development of new treatment modalities. As a result, marked improvement in the care of patients with major burn injury has been noted. Comprehensive treatment centers now utilize sophisticated, multidisciplinary teams to aid in the diagnosis of rapidly changing physiologic responses to the injury and to assist in providing the vast array of specialized therapeutic services which are necessary to minimize morbidity and mortality.

Burn injury constitutes a major national health problem. More than 2,000,000 persons suffer thermal injury annually, of whom 70,000 must be hospitalized. As in other types of trauma, thermal injury frequently afflicts children and young adults. Prolonged morbidity, as well as temporary or permanent disability, associated with thermal injury results in a staggering economic drain on social resources. Financial support is often required to defray expenses associated with prolonged hospitalization, loss of family income sources, and replacement of lost manpower within the working force.

ETIOLOGY OF BURNS

Burns are caused by the application of heat to the body. The depth of the resulting burn injury will be dependent on the intensity and duration of heat application and the conductivity of the tissues involved. The most common heat sources are an open flame and hot liquid. In addition, thermal injury is frequently observed in patients who have been exposed to direct contact with hot metal, toxic chemicals, or high-voltage electric current. Damage as a result of heat rarely occurs below 45°C. Between 45 and 50°C, gradations of cell injury may occur; and above 50°C, denaturation of protein elements of the cell becomes apparent.

Laboratory accidents, civilian assaults, industrial mishaps, and inexpert application of agents used for medical purposes account for most of the chemical burns in the civilian population. A principal difference between thermal and chemical injury is the length of time during which tissue destruction continues, since the chemical agent causes progressive damage until inactivated by reaction with tissue, while thermal injury ceases shortly after removal of the heat source. Tissue destruction associated with exposure to chemicals may be limited by the application of neutralizing agents or by dilution with water. When compared to thermal injury, the severe, full-thickness chemical burn may appear deceptively superficial, with only mild bronze discoloration of intact skin during the first few postburn days.

In contrast to both thermal and chemical burns, electrical injury usually results in minimal destruction of skin. The magnitude of the injury is directly related to the amount of current passing through tissue between the point of contact with the electrical source and the exit site at which the patient is grounded. The magnitude of current passing through various organs is indirectly related to the resistance of the tissue. Nerve, blood, and muscle offer the least resistance to electric current and thus sustain the maximum amount of tissue damage. As a result, cutaneous injury may be apparent only at the entrance and exit sites, although considerable deep tissue destruction of upper and lower extremity musculature may be present. The electrical resistance of skin is markedly reduced by moisture. Thus small burns in the antecubital space or the axilla often are observed in the patient with severe electrical injury of the upper extremity. These burns result from the arcing of current across the joint through skin moistened with perspiration. When arc burns are present, they are nearly always accompanied by extensive, deep muscular destruction. Thermal injury to musculature is frequently associated with release of hemachromagens into the bloodstream which are subsequently excreted via the urinary tract. Thus "port wine"–colored urine containing myoglobin is not unusual following major electrical injury.

IMMEDIATE THERAPY

Initial therapy of the patient with a major burn should be directed toward restoration of normal physiologic parameters and prevention of life-threatening complications. With the exception of chemical burns, in which the toxic agent must be diluted with water and physically removed as rapidly as possible to prevent further tissue destruction, the burn wound is of secondary importance during the first few hours after the injury.

Maintenance of Airway

Immediate pulmonary complications may become manifest in the thermally injured patient. Excessive exposure to smoke may result in carbon monoxide poisoning. Patients exhibit the signs and symptoms of hypoxia, which may range from pronounced tachypnea and agitation to respiratory arrest and coma. The diagnosis may be quickly confirmed by analyzing the concentration of carboxyhemoglobin in the blood. Treatment includes the administration of 100% oxygen, with ventilatory support if necessary, in order to displace the tightly bound carbon monoxide from the hemoglobin molecule. Since carbon monoxide is not toxic to lungs per se, the syndrome is entirely reversible, provided anoxic damage to distant tissues (e.g., the central nervous system) has not occurred. Although several decades ago few patients with severe carbon monoxide poisoning survived long enough to reach the emergency room, the development of sophisticated paramedical teams trained to insert endotracheal tubes and administer ventilatory support in the field has allowed greater salvage of such patients in the last several years.

Upper airway obstruction in patients with burns of the head and neck may occur during the first 48 hours after injury. The obstruction is related to soft tissue edema of the oral pharynx and vocal cords following exposure to hot gases. Direct thermal injury to the lower respiratory tract is exceedingly unusual, since the nose and oral pharynx are extremely efficient heat exchangers, allowing cooling of inhaled hot gas prior to its entrance into the trachea. Since it is more difficult to extract heat from liquid, direct thermal injury of the lower respiratory tract is occasionally noted in patients injured by superheated steam.

Upper airway obstruction is usually heralded by an increase in the respiratory rate and progressive hoarseness. In addition, a patient may exhibit increased difficulty in clearing bronchial secretions as the vocal cords become more edematous. Confirmation of impending obstruction is made by direct visualization of the posterior oral pharynx and cords, utilizing either direct laryngoscopy or fiberoptic endoscopy. The latter is usually preferred, since at the same time, assessment of smoke inhalation may be accomplished by visualizing the lower respiratory tract.

Impending upper airway obstruction is treated by the immediate insertion of an endotracheal tube. Soft tissue edema is maximal at between 24 and 48 hours. Therefore the endotracheal tube is usually not removed until the third postburn day, since reintubation often is technically difficult to perform.

Intravenous Resuscitation

Cardiovascular alterations occur almost immediately following burn injury. There is a massive shift of fluid and electrolytes from the intravascular and extracellular fluid space into the cells. Reversion of water and sodium from the intracellular fluid back into the extracellular fluid begins between 24 and 48 hours but is not complete until the tenth postburn day. In general, these changes are directly proportional to the extent and depth of burn. Therefore any consideration of fluid resuscitation to prevent hypovolemic shock requires an accurate estimation of the magnitude of burn injury. The burned wound is three-dimensional, therefore not only the depth but the surface area involved must be estimated.

Burns are classified as first, second, or third degree (Table 7-1). First-degree burns are characterized by simple erythema of the skin, with only microscopic destruction of superficial layers of the epidermis. A mild sunburn is characteristic of a first-degree injury. The first-degree injury is of little clinical significance, since the water barrier of the skin is not disturbed. Systemic cardiovascular disturbances are rarely observed following first-degree burn injury. The burns rapidly heal if the patient avoids further exposure to a heat source. First-degree burns are *not* considered when estimating the magnitude of burn injury for purposes of planning intravenous fluid replacement.

Second- and third-degree burns are of equal physiologic significance and may be summated in the estimate of total body surface burn injury. Second-degree burns extend through the epidermis into the dermis. By definition, viable epithelial elements from which epithelial regeneration can occur are retained in second-degree burn injury; thus the burn is often described as *partial-thickness*. Even when most of the epithelium is destroyed, regeneration may occur from epithelial cells surrounding hair follicles or sweat glands. On the other hand, third-degree burns are characterized by total irreversible destruction of all the

Table 7-1. CLASSIFICATION OF BURNS

Classification	Morphology	Clinical appearance	Cause
First degree	Only superficial layers of epidermis devitalized; dilatation and congestion of intradermal vessels.	Erythema only—blanches on pressure.	Ultraviolet exposure (ultraviolet light, sunburn), very short flash
Second degree	Destruction of varying depths of epidermis with coagulation necrosis; clefting of epidermis with fluid collection (blister formation); congestion and coagulation in subdermal plexus. Some skin elements remain viable (often only skin appendages), from which epithelial regeneration can occur.*	Erythematous, weeping, painful. Blisters and bullae often present. Superficial layers of skin can be readily wiped away. Remaining skin elements waxy white, soft, dry, insensitive.	Short flash, spill scald
Third degree	Destruction of all skin elements; coagulation of subdermal plexus.	Dry, hard, inelastic, translucent, with thrombosed vein visible.	Flame, immersion scald, chemical contact, electric current

*Initial injury may be partial-thickness, with only dermal appendages (hair follicles and glands) remaining, but these skin elements are readily destroyed by infection, with resulting conversion to full-thickness (third-degree) burn.

skin, dermal appendages, and epithelial elements. Spontaneous regeneration of epithelium is not possible, and the burns are described as *full-thickness*. Such burns require the application of skin grafts if the development of scar tissue is to be avoided.

Since skin varies in thickness in different parts of the body, application of the same intensity of heat for a given period of time will result in a burn which will vary in depth, depending on the thickness of the skin itself in the local area, as well as the existence and degree of development of the dermal appendages (sweat glands and hair follicles) and dermal papillae. In the very old person, in whom dermal papillae and appendages are atrophic, and in the very young, in whom they have not yet fully developed, deep burns result from the same heat intensity that produces a moderate second-degree burn in the middle-aged adult. Since the skin of the back is thicker than that on any other part of the body, full-thickness burns are less common in this area. On the other hand, skin covering the inner arm is extraordinarily thin, thus full-thickness injury is frequently observed in this area.

The length and width of the burn wound is expressed as a percentage of the total body surface area displaying either second- or third-degree burns. The extent of the body surface involved is most commonly estimated by the "rule of nines" (Table 7-2). The major anatomic portions of the adult may be divided into multiples of 9 percent of the body surface area. The proportion of each of these areas with second- or third-degree burns is estimated, and the summation of these estimates represents the percentage of the total body surface area burn. Because the surface area of the head and neck in childhood is significantly larger than 9 percent of the total body surface area and the surface area associated with the lower extremities is

smaller, the rule of nines may not be used to estimate total body surface area burns in children. For example, a one-year-old child has 19 percent of the total body surface area associated with the head, as compared to only 7 percent in the adult patient. In contrast, each lower extremity represents only 13 percent of the total body surface area in the year-old infant. Thus the total body surface area burn in children is best estimated by the utilization of charts which relate regional body surface to age.

Over the past 20 years, many resuscitation formulas have been developed as guides to initial resuscitation in hypovolemic shock following thermal injury. Most utilize various combinations of crystalloid and colloid solutions but differ widely in the ratio of colloid to crystalloid, as well as the rate of fluid administration. The ideal resuscitation formula would rapidly restore normal hemodynamic stability. However, such a response is dependent on the rate at which fluid is lost from the extracellular fluid compartment, the composition of the fluid lost, and the ability of various solutions to restore an effective circulating extra-

Table 7-2. "RULE OF NINES" FOR ESTIMATING PERCENTAGE OF BODY SURFACE INVOLVED IN BURNS

Anatomic area	Percent of body surface
Head	9
Right upper extremity	9
Left upper extremity	9
Right lower extremity	18
Left lower extremity	18
Anterior trunk	18
Posterior trunk	18
Neck	1

cellular volume. Unfortunately, most formulas have been derived empirically from clinical experience, in which the amount of fluid required to restore renal function was accepted as optimal replacement therapy.

Although much controversy still remains over "the solution" for resuscitation in burn shock, scientific investigation supports the need for both crystalloid and colloid solutions. *It is of relatively little consequence which formula is utilized to begin such therapy, as long as this is modified according to the patient's changing requirements.* The formula shown in Table 7-3 has been popularized by Baxter and is known as the "Parkland formula." This formula has been adopted in most burn centers and is currently the standard against which new formulas must be compared. Data from numerous studies now suggest that both volume and the sodium ion are critical to providing adequate resuscitation in hypovolemic burn shock. Administration of crystalloid solution results in early expansion of depleted plasma and extracellular fluid volumes and return of the cardiac output toward normal. After 24 hours, colloid remains the most effective solution to maintain plasma volume without further increasing edema formation. The Parkland formula was derived to provide specific replacement of known deficits measured by simultaneous determinations of red cell volume, plasma volume, extracellular fluid volume, and cardiac output during burn shock. The formula calls for the administration of 4 ml of lactated Ringer's solution/kg of body weight/percent of body surface area burn during the first 24 hours postinjury. Fluid therapy during the second 24 hours, according to this formula, consists in the administration of free water (5% dextrose in water) in quantities sufficient to maintain the serum sodium concentration at 140 mEq/L (approximately 4 to 5 liters in a 70-kg patient with a 50 percent burn) and plasma sufficient to return the plasma volume to normal and sustain adequate perfusion of peripheral organs and tissues (approximately 250 ml for each 10 percent total body surface area burn over 20 percent). Potassium replacement is required to replace increased urinary losses associated with both the resuscitation and the subsequent catabolic state.

During the first 24 hours, the rate of fluid administration is adjusted to correspond as closely as possible with the rate of extracellular fluid loss. Baxter's studies have confirmed that extracellular deficits occur rapidly within the first 6 to 12 hours postinjury. Therefore one-half of the total calculated fluid volume is delivered during the first 8 hours *from the time of injury* and the remaining fluids more slowly over the next 16 hours.

The adequacy of resuscitation can best be judged by frequent measurements of vital signs, central venous pressure, hourly urine output, and observation of general mental and physical response. Urine output (normal, 30 to 100 ml/hour in the adult) still remains one of the most reliable guides to adequacy of fluid therapy. Acute tubular necrosis, with resultant renal failure, is extremely rare in an adequately resuscitated patient, with the possible exception of a patient in whom there is extensive muscle damage (electrical burns) resulting in hemachromogen release and intratubular protein precipitation. Therefore oliguria during the early postburn period is most often an indication of inadequate resuscitation, and increased fluid administration is the treatment of choice. Restriction of fluid is almost never indicated, and the administration of diuretics should be reserved for those cases in which tubular damage from circulating pigments appears likely, and then only after a sufficient amount of resuscitation fluids has been administered.

Urinary outputs of 30 to 100 ml/hour should be maintained during the first 24 hours in the adult patient. In the absence of hypoxia related to respiratory dysfunction, the patient's sensorium accurately reflects cerebral circulation. Well-resuscitated patients with major thermal injury rarely display hysteria, acute anxiety, or hostility.

Sedation

One of the most frequent therapeutic errors in the treatment of patients with major burns is the overuse of sedation. An insignificant burn of a minute area incurred during a common household mishap may be quite painful. Projection of such an experience by medical and paramedical personnel has resulted in marked overestimation of the pain associated with a major burn. If there is full-thickness skin destruction, the intrinsic sensory nerve endings have also been destroyed and the wound itself is painless. In contrast, the second-degree burn can be quite painful initially. Therefore the requirement for sedation is inversely proportional to the depth of the initial thermal injury.

Sedation should be kept at an *absolute minimum* to prevent depression of cardiopulmonary function and to allow evaluation of the sensorium, an important indicator of the adequacy of fluid resuscitation. Decreased peripheral circulation to muscle and skin is often associated with the hypovolemic state, so any narcotics administered intramuscularly or subcutaneously are subject to erratic uptake. Therefore narcotics should always be administered in small doses by the intravenous route during the first 4 to 5 days. Administration by this route assures rapid and predictable concentrations of the drug in the central nervous system and prevents the narcosis which may result following fluid resuscitation if repeated doses of narcotics have been administered by the intramuscular route. After 48 hours, the requirements for sedation are markedly reduced, except

Table 7-3. FLUID RESUSCITATION OF BURNED PATIENTS: PARKLAND FORMULA

First 24 Hours:
Electrolyte solution (lactated Ringer's): 4 ml/kg body wt./% second- and third-degree burn
Administration rate: $\frac{1}{2}$ first 8 hours, $\frac{1}{4}$ second 8 hours, $\frac{1}{4}$ third 8 hours
Urine output: 30–70 ml/hr

Second 24 Hours:
Glucose in water (D_5W): To replace evaporative water loss, maintaining serum sodium concentration of 140 mEq/L
Colloid solution (plasma): To maintain plasma volume in patients with more than 40% second- and third-degree burns
Urine output: 30–100 ml/hr

during times when the wound is actively debrided during the waking state.

Antibiotics

Subsequent to thermal injury, microorganisms contaminating the surface of the wound and persisting in the depth of the hair follicles and sweat glands begin to proliferate rapidly if topical chemotherapeutic agents are not applied. In the absence of topical chemotherapy, the superficial areas of the burn wound contain up to 100 million organisms per gram of tissue within 48 hours following injury.

Characteristically, gram-positive organisms are responsible for this initial proliferation and colonization of the burn wound. Therefore most experienced clinicians prophylactically administer penicillin to patients with major burn injuries for a period of 3 to 4 days. Antibiotic treatment with penicillin prevents overgrowth of the gram-positive organisms and has virtually eliminated streptococcal infections, one of the most common causes of death following burn injury 30 years ago. The systemic administration of antibiotics after the fourth postburn day has not resulted in decreased morbidity from infection. Since the full-thickness burn is relatively avascular after 48 hours, the concentration of antibiotic which reaches the burn wound from the bloodstream is inadequate to prevent subsequent gram-negative bacterial colonization. Therefore systemic antibiotics are not usually administered after the fourth postburn day unless a specific distant bacterial infection (e.g., pneumonia) has complicated the burn.

Tetanus Prophylaxis

All burn injuries must be considered contaminated, and tetanus prophylaxis is mandatory except in those patients actively immunized within the preceding 12 months. If a booster was received within the preceding 10 years, the intramuscular administration of 0.5 ml of absorbed tetanus toxoid will usually provide adequate prophylaxis. In the absence of active immunization within 10 years prior to the burn injury, 250 to 500 units of tetanus immunogobulin (human) should be simultaneously administered at another site, utilizing a different syringe and needle so as to prevent inactivation of the immune globulin by toxoid.

Escharotomy

A principal characteristic of human skin is a remarkable degree of elasticity, which allows the skin to stretch with only minimum applied force. The elasticity of skin allows considerable edema of underlying soft tissues without increasing central limb pressure, which might impede either venous outflow or arterial inflow. If the skin were unyielding, a patient with a severely sprained ankle might lose blood flow to the distal foot as soft tissue edema occurred. Skin with second-degree injury retains its elastic properties. However, full-thickness injury (third degree) is characterized by almost complete loss of elasticity. Thus circumferential third-degree burns are frequently associated with decreased peripheral blood flow as fluid resuscitation, ac-

companied by soft tissue edema, progresses. Failure to recognize this situation may result in unnecessary loss of distal extremities.

The usual clinical signs associated with poor peripheral blood flow in the nonburned patient, that is, diminished peripheral pulses and decreased skin temperature, are unreliable in patients with severe thermal injury. Hypovolemia with peripheral vasoconstriction usually results in decreased temperature of distal extremities in all patients with major second- and third-degree burns, and distal pulses often may not be felt as a result of overlying soft tissue edema preventing palpation of the underlying artery. More reliable signs of decreased peripheral flow in patients with circumferential third-degree burns are slow capillary refill (observed in the nail beds) and the onset of neurologic deficits. The most accurate monitoring device for assessing distal blood flow to extremities is the ultrasonic Doppler, which allows repetitive evaluation of both venous and arterial flow in the digital arteries and veins.

Patients with circumferential third-degree burns of the extremities should be encouraged to actively exercise those extremities in order to maintain patency of the small venules. In addition, the extremities should be elevated in order to promote venous and lymphatic drainage and minimize soft tissue edema. However, should vascular impairment become apparent, escharotomies should immediately be performed. An escharotomy is simply an incision through the full depth of the skin, allowing the eschar to separate, thus relieving underlying pressure on the central arteries and veins. These incisions may be performed without anesthesia, since third-degree burns are anesthetic. Blood loss is minimal because of the extensive intracapillary coagulation which has occurred as a result of the thermal injury. The escharotomies are usually performed on the lateral and medial aspects of the extremity and must be carried across the joints, since the skin is most tightly adherent to the underlying fascia at these points and vascular obstruction is most likely to occur in these areas. In the upper extremity, the escharotomy should extend through all areas of third-degree burn down to and including the thenar and hypothenar spaces, in order to preserve the intrinsic muscles of the hand. Similarly, in the lower extremities, escharotomies should extend to the base of the large and small toes if the foot exhibits extensive third-degree burns.

Fasciotomy, that is, linear excision of the deep fascia surrounding the muscles, is rarely indicated in patients with severe burns. In rare instances of extensive incineration when burns involve not only the skin but the underlying fat and muscle, fasciotomy becomes necessary as a result of swelling within the muscle compartments. More frequently, fasciotomy is required in the treatment of electrical burns where there has been extensive muscle injury which appears potentially reversible.

Gastric Decompression

Most patients with more than 20 percent total body surface area burns will develop a reflex paralytic ileus some time during the first 24 hours. Although bowel sounds are usually active for 6 to 10 hours following the injury, intestinal motility is gradually lost for a short period of time during the latter half of the first 24 hours. Unfortunately, the development of ileus frequently occurs at the time when medical and nursing surveillance has relaxed and the patient is asleep following sedation and restoration of fluid volume. Vomiting in such a patient carries a high risk of pulmonary aspiration, a complication which is associated with severe morbidity and high mortality. For this reason, patients with major burns require placement of a nasogastric tube, in order that the stomach may be effectively decompressed until normal gastrointestinal motility has been demonstrated.

The insertion of a nasogastric tube will also serve to allow inspection of the gastric contents at periodic intervals. Patients with major burns are at risk of hemorrhagic gastritis as a result of increased stress. For this reason, gastric aspirates should be monitored frequently for the presence of frank blood or guaiac-positive material, and antacid should be instilled through the nasogastric tube at hourly intervals to prevent superficial erosions of the gastric mucosa.

Medical Evacuation

Although most hospitals are equipped to provide emergency therapy of the patient with a major burn, the majority of community hospitals have neither the nursing nor the paramedical expertise to comfortably care for a patient with massive burn injury. Furthermore, because of the special physical requirements necessary for optimal treatment of such patients, it is not uncommon for personnel in community hospitals to transfer such patients to special facilities as soon as appropriate arrangements can be made.

Extensive experience with medical evacuation of severely burned soldiers during the Korean and Vietnam wars has yielded valuable information which may assist in assuring safe transfer of burned patients. In general, such patients tolerate evacuation best if they are moved within the first 24 to 48 hours. Prior to transfer, a fluid resuscitation program should be started. Patients with a larger than 20 percent burn should have a Foley catheter inserted into the bladder, so that urinary output can be monitored during the evacuation and fluid administration appropriately adjusted. Pulmonary function should be assessed, and if impending upper airway obstruction or severe smoke inhalation is suspected, an endotracheal tube should be inserted prior to transfer. Extensive debridement or treatment of the burn wounds is unnecessary and is generally to be avoided, since it interferes with evaluation of the burn wound by the receiving hospital. Rather, the wounds should be temporarily wrapped in sterile dressings to provide maximal comfort during the transfer. If air evacuation is to be utilized, it is especially important to insert a nasogastric tube, since air within the stomach will expand at increased altitude, often inducing acute gastric distension and vomiting. This, in turn, could result in aspiration pneumonitis, which would be particularly compromising in a patient with the smoke inhalation syndrome.

THERAPY OF THE BURN WOUND

Debridement and Excision

Second-degree wounds (partial-thickness burn injury) usually present as vesicular lesions. Unless very small, the overlying blister should be punctured and the nonviable skin removed. This permits the direct application of topical chemotherapeutic agents to the underlying viable dermal remnants. Failure to prevent secondary bacterial infection of deep second-degree burn wounds may result in conversion of the partial-thickness injury to a full-thickness injury. Debridement can usually be accomplished without anesthesia, utilizing careful surgical technique and modest amounts of sedation prior to removing the nonviable superficial epithelium.

The nonviable skin of the third-degree burn is referred to as the "eschar." Usually the eschar remains tightly adherent to the underlying subcutaneous tissues and cannot be sharply debrided without severe hemorrhage and significant pain. Therefore, except in special circumstances, only loose eschar, which may be debrided without anesthesia or excessive blood loss, is removed initially. The remaining eschar is left intact, and efforts are made to prevent bacterial colonization and invasion by the use of topical chemotherapeutic agents. Topical chemotherapeutic agents do not sterilize the third-degree burn eschar, and eventually bacterial growth will occur. The topical agents are employed to control the rate of proliferation of bacteria within the burn wound, so as to prevent invasion of underlying viable tissue, with entrance of bacteria into the bloodstream. At about 18 to 24 days following burn injury, the third-degree burn eschar will separate from the underlying viable tissue as a result of the liberation of bacterial proteases. At this time, it is extraordinarily important that the eschar be promptly debrided, in order to prevent systemic sepsis as a result of localized abscess formation beneath the eschar. Normally, the patients are taken to a hydrotherapy area once or twice a day during the first 3 weeks in order to cleanse the surface of the eschar and to inspect the wound. Each day, the physician debrides any loose areas of eschar and carefully inspects the wound and unroofs any localized abscess pockets.

Modern surgical principles dictate the surgical debridement of nonviable tissue in the treatment of major injury. However, in the case of burn injury, immediate total debridement of nonviable eschar has not proved to be a safe procedure because of the extensive hemorrhage associated with major excision of eschar. Some investigators have advocated the use of topical enzyme preparations to more rapidly remove the eschar. The advantages of such an approach include debridement without anesthesia and limitation of associated hemorrhage. However, the efficacy of currently available enzymes has not been conclusively demonstrated. Furthermore, most enzyme preparations require the use of overlying wet dressings to maintain the activity of the enzyme. Such dressings promote wound infection, since they provide a warm, moist environment. In addition, some of the enzyme preparations inhibit the effectiveness of topical chemotherapeutic agents in controlling the rate of proliferation of bacterial growth. Therefore other authors have condemned the use of enzymatic debridement, maintaining that the risks of sepsis far outweigh the benefits of early debridement. In addition, some enzyme preparations do not effectively differentiate nonviable eschar from underlying normal tissues, and erosion of vessels in viable tissue occasionally induces unexpected bleeding from the wound.

Other surgeons have advocated tangential excision to rapidly and safely remove full-thickness eschar. The eschar is tangentially excised, utilizing either a specially designed knife or an air-driven dermatome, to sequentially remove layers of the eschar in sheets of approximately 0.015 inches in thickness until viable tissue, as evidenced by capillary bleeding, is encountered. This procedure can usually be accomplished without anesthesia, since the third-degree burn is anesthetic. The procedure is technically rather difficult after full-thickness removal of skin is accomplished, since the underlying subcutaneous fat does not debride easily at uniform thickness, and viability of the relatively avascular fat is often difficult to appreciate. The exposed subcutaneous fat must be covered with either heterograft or homograft to preserve its integrity, and, unfortunately, adherence of the physiologic dressing is nonuniform.

Several investigators have utilized the carbon dioxide laser to excise third-degree burn eschar. The CO_2 laser allows removal of tissue with relatively little blood loss, and the level of excision can be readily selected by the surgeon. However, the procedure is very slow, because of the limited power which can be generated by the CO_2 laser with safety for both the patient and the operating room personnel. Thus the procedure results in prolonged operating time. Furthermore, the required equipment is expensive and somewhat cumbersome to use. Since the laser beam may cause serious damage to the retina following exposure, operating room personnel must wear protective glasses. Finally, the laser energy is partially dissipated in the underlying viable tissue (the graft recipient site), and the resulting injury to superficial cells may prevent acceptance of heterograft, homograft, and autograft.

When third-degree burns are relatively limited in size (less than 5 percent), as may occur following contact with a hot piece of metal, the full-thickness eschar may be excised primarily under anesthesia without excessive hemorrhage. The wound should be covered immediately with autograft. This approach markedly decreases postburn morbidity and often results in a better cosmetic appearance. Others have now suggested that patients with massive burn injury, that is, more than 70 percent total body surface burns, of which at least 60 percent is third-degree, should undergo early, deep burn wound excision in order to reduce the burn size to a total body surface area which is more compatible with survival. Such procedures should be attempted only in major centers, since this approach is still unproved and requires enormous medical, paramedical, and nursing support. Prior to excision, the burn wound must be sterile or contain only a relatively low concentration of bacteria (less than 10^4 organisms per gram of tissue). Some authors advocate the preoperative infusion of antibiotics by subeschar clysis into the eschar which is to be excised. In this manner, maximum antibiotic concentration is achieved in the relatively avascular eschar, and the chances of seeding the bloodstream during the procedure are presumably reduced. Both the eschar and the underlying subcutaneous fat are excised. The exposed deep fascia must be immediately covered with homograft. Failure to provide immediate physiologic coverage results in desiccation of the fascia and subsequent secondary infection. Thus an unlimited bank of homograft, obtained from cadavers, must be maintained. Furthermore, excision of 20 percent of the total body surface is frequently associated with loss of the patient's complete blood volume. Therefore centers evaluating this approach must have blood banks capable of providing significant quantities of both stored and fresh blood. In some cases, the blood loss has been reduced by utilizing deliberate hypotensive anesthesia during the procedure. Obviously, the operative procedure inflicts great stress on the patient, who already will have evidenced marked pathophysiologic alterations. Extraordinary intensive care support by both physicians and specialized nursing personnel is therefore required postoperatively in the intensive care area.

While most patients are gradually debrided of full-thickness injury over a period of 2 to 3 weeks, patients with electrical injury require more aggressive therapy. Since these patients often have injury to the muscle compartments of the extremities, early surgical exploration, fasciotomy, and removal of nonviable muscle should be performed when motor dysfunction or massive edema of the extremity occurs. If possible, hemodynamic stability should be obtained by the intravenous administration of lactated Ringer's solution prior to operative exploration.

Cutaneous burns resulting from contact with hot tar or asphalt are not infrequently encountered. By the time the physician sees the patient, the tar has solidified on the burn wound as it has cooled. It may be removed by applying generous quantities of Neopolycin ointment to the burn wound, over which a large occlusive dressing is applied. The dressing may be removed 18 to 24 hours later. At this time most or all of the tar will be dissolved, and a water-soluble topical chemotherapeutic agent may be applied.

Topical Chemotherapy

Modern antibacterial topical therapy was advocated by Monafo and Moyer in the early 1960s. These investigators utilized aqueous silver nitrate (0.5%) solution as a continuous wet soak, in combination with large, bulky dressings. The mode of action of silver nitrate is not specifically known but probably depends on the free silver ion, which is active at relatively low concentrations. Silver nitrate is effective against most gram-positive organisms and most strains of *Pseudomonas,* although it has limited effectiveness against other gram-negative bacteria such as *Enterobacter* and *Klebsiella.* The agent sterilizes the surface of the wound but has limited penetration of deeper tissues. Therefore the eschar must be removed rapidly when deep bacterial colonization occurs, in order to prevent invasion of underlying viable tissue. The major complication associated with the use of silver nitrate solution is severe electrolyte depletion (primarily sodium and chloride), necessitating frequent monitoring of serum electrolytes, since specific replacement therapy is required. Silver nitrate therapy has been acclaimed as the most economical topical agent. The drug itself is inexpensive and available in most hospital pharmacies. However, the large quantities of dressings required, the increased nursing personnel requirements to effect the dressing changes, and the major housekeeping problems associated with discoloration caused on contact by precipitation of silver salts, significantly increase the cost of this form of treatment. In addition, the necessity for bulky dressings inhibits the early active movement of extremities and therefore encourages less than optimum joint function.

In the mid-1960s, Lindberg, Moncrief, and Mason introduced mafenide acetate (Sulfamylon), a topically applied cream that allowed open treatment of burn wounds. Mafenide acetate has proved effective against a wide range of gram-positive and gram-negative organisms, as well as most anaerobes. This drug actively diffuses through the eschar, thus providing protection in the depth of the eschar at the interface between the viable and nonviable tissue. Since the burns remain exposed, wounds can be more readily examined. In addition, the treatment does not interfere with intensive physical therapy and allows uninhibited treatment of associated soft tissue injuries. Unfortunately, the drug is a potent inhibitor of carbonic anhydrase and therefore may induce acid-base derangements. Acidosis may develop rapidly in the presence of pulmonary dysfunction. The use of the drug is associated with a pronounced reduction of the buffering capacity of the blood, as a result of increased bicarbonate excretion by the kidney, and simultaneous hypocapnea secondary to hyperventilation. Other disadvantages associated with the use of this drug include pain on application, an occasional hypersensitivity reaction (5 to 7 percent), delayed eschar separation due to improved bacterial control, and the emergence of opportunistic infections, including *Providencia, Serratia,* fungal, yeast, and viral infections.

Silver sulfadiazine (Silvadene), developed by Fox in the late 1960s, has essentially the same bacterial spectrum as mafenide acetate but is associated with fewer disadvantages. The major side effects are hypersensitivity reaction to sulfa (5 to 7 percent), delayed eschar separation, and emergence of opportunistic infections. The agent appears to desiccate the wound less than other topical drugs and consequently keeps the eschar soft, allowing for greater joint mobility. It does not inhibit carbonic anhydrase activity, and its application is soothing rather than painful.

Betadine, a water-soluble topical antiseptic complex of polyvinylpyrrolidone (povidone) iodine, is effective against a wide range of gram-positive and gram-negative organisms, as well as some fungi. The drug is manufactured as an ointment and as an aerosol cream. The drug readily diffuses through the eschar and is absorbed and excreted rapidly. Systemic toxicity is apparently rare. One major disadvantage of this agent is its propensity to cause rapid desiccation of the eschar, resulting in interference with progressive active physical therapy programs. In addition, its application to partial-thickness burns may be associated with mild to moderate pain. This agent has only recently been extensively utilized for the topical therapy of burns and, as in the case of other topical agents, emergence of opportunistic infections may be expected after more extensive experience.

The properties of each of the currently utilized topical chemotherapeutic agents are summarized in Table 7-4. Newer and even more effective topical agents are currently in clinical trial and may be expected to be marketed in the near future. It is important to emphasize that burn wounds treated with these topical agents are not sterilized; rather, the bacterial population is effectively suppressed and remains at levels below that associated with the development of invasive burn wound sepsis. Furthermore, the agents are effective in preventing bacterial conversion of second-degree burns to full-thickness injury, thus reducing the amount of skin grafting which might be required had the agents not been employed.

Table 7-4. PROPERTIES OF TOPICAL CHEMOTHERAPEUTIC AGENTS

Agent	Antibacterial spectrum	Dressings required?	Disadvantages
Sodium mafenide (Sulfamylon)	Gram-positive and gram-negative organisms and most anaerobes	No	Pain on application; skin allergy; carbonic anhydrase inhibition; resistant organisms
Silver nitrate 0.5%	Most gram-positive organisms and some strains of *Pseudomonas*	Yes	Hyponatremia; hypochloremia; failure to penetrate eschar; methemoglobinemia
Silver sulfadiazine (Silvadene)	Gram-positive and gram-negative organisms and *Candida albicans*	No	Skin allergy; resistant organisms
Povidone-iodine (Betadine)	Gram-positive organisms and fungi; possibly less effective vs. some gram-negative organisms	Yes (cream) No (aerosol)	Pain on application; excessive drying of eschar

Bacteriologic Monitoring

Despite the use of topical chemotherapeutic agents, some patients, particularly those with burns of more than 60 percent of the total body surface, will evidence progressive colonization of the burn wound, with subsequent invasion of viable tissue and bloodstream dissemination of the bacteria. Therefore clinical bacteriologic monitoring of the burn wound is imperative in order to diagnose incipient burn wound sepsis and effect immediate treatment.

In general, cultures of the burn wound surface have failed to accurately predict progressive bacterial colonization or incipient burn wound sepsis. Qualitative and quantitative correlation is poor between flora on the surface of the burn wound and bacterial colonization of the deep layers of the eschar. Blood cultures, although helpful if bacterial growth is demonstrated, have not proved particularly useful, since life-threatening sepsis may occur in the absence of bacteremia, and the presence of bacteria in the bloodstream is a relatively late phenomenon, often just preceding death. Bacterial growth in burn wounds is best monitored by semiquantitative burn wound biopsy cultures. Multiple full-thickness wound biopsies are obtained serially from representative areas of the burn wound. The tissue is weighed, homogenized, serially diluted, and inoculated on blood agar and eosin–methylene blue plates. In this manner, the precise number of viable organisms per gram of tissue can be calculated. When wound biopsy cultures reveal more than 10^5 organisms per gram of tissue or a hundredfold increase in the concentration of organisms per gram of tissue is observed within a 48-hour period, it may be assumed that the organisms have escaped effective control by the topical chemotherapeutic agent and that burn wound sepsis is incipient.

Heterograft and Homograft

Immediately following eschar separation, the wound is seldom ready to accept a cutaneous autograft. However, all terrestrial mammals require an intact epithelial covering in order to maintain water, electrolyte, and thermal homeostasis. During the time interval between eschar separation and definitive cutaneous autograft, the open wound of granulation tissue can be temporarily covered with a physiologic dressing. Either porcine heterograft or homograft obtained from cadavers is most commonly utilized. The application of these materials, providing early temporary wound closure, can contribute to the prevention and control of infection, the preservation of healthy granulation tissue, and maintenance of joint function. Specifically, the physiologic dressings decrease evaporative water loss and diminish heat loss secondary to evaporation; they cover exposed sensory nerves and therefore decrease pain associated with the open wound; and they protect neurovascular tissue and tendons which would otherwise be exposed. When the physiologic dressing adheres to the underlying granulation tissue, bacterial proliferation is readily inhibited, since the heterograft or homograft provides an acceptable surface against which neutrophils may entrap

bacteria. Until the wound is ready for definitive autograft, the granulation tissue is protected from desiccation. The physiologic dressings prevent the development of hypermature granulation tissue and promote a well-nourished recipient bed; and they act as an excellent test material to determine the optimal time for subsequent autograft. When adherence is observed, the granulation tissue may be assumed to be in optimal condition for autograft and postoperative loss of split-thickness skin grafts (autografts) will rarely occur.

Heterograft and homograft are most commonly used for temporary coverage of granulation tissue, as described above. The grafts are removed within 5 days and replaced with new physiologic dressing until autografting has been accomplished. These physiologic dressings may also be utilized to debride untidy wounds immediately after eschar separation. The heterograft or homograft hastens separation of very tiny pieces of eschar left behind at the time of debridement. It should be emphasized, however, that physiologic dressings may be used for this purpose with safety only if more than 95 percent of the eschar has been mechanically removed in the course of daily debridement.

Either heterograft or homograft may be utilized electively over reepithelializing deep second-degree burns, once superficial necrotic debris has been entirely removed (usually 7 to 10 days postburn). Adherent physiologic dressings at this time will promote the rate of reepithelialization and decrease pain in the wound, allowing decreased hospitalization time. Some clinicians utilize heterograft or homograft to immediately cover superficial second-degree burns. The advantages of such treatment include marked decrease in pain, decreased hospitalization, earlier return of joint function, and more rapid reepithelialization of the burn. However, utilization of physiologic dressings in this manner must be undertaken with caution. One must be certain that the wound is indeed partial thickness, since coverage of a full-thickness wound essentially closes an open abscess and may precipitate burn wound sepsis. In addition, the homograft or heterograft must be applied within hours after the burn injury, at the time of the initial debridement. It is important that the physiologic dressing and burn wound be inspected within 24 hours to assure continued adherence to the dermal remnants. Should the physiologic dressing become dislodged or should fluid accumulate beneath it, the material should be removed immediately and the wound treated with topical chemotherapeutic agents in the conventional manner. If the heterograft or homograft remains adherent, it is important that it not be removed but rather be allowed to separate spontaneously as reepithelialization occurs. Frequent changing of physiologic dressings applied to second-degree burns results in sequential removal of epithelial cells at the time of removal and may convert them to full-thickness burn wounds.

Autograft

Definitive closure of burn wounds as soon as possible after injury is the ultimate objective of all burn wound care. As soon as an area of full-thickness burn wound has been adequately prepared by the use of temporary physiologic dressings as described above, it should be covered with the patient's own skin. There are, however, priorities of coverage dictated by functional and cosmetic considerations. In general, the hands, feet, joints, and face should be covered prior to nonfunctional surfaces. Autografts may be applied as sheets of skin without the need of suture fixation or "pie-crusting" incisions to allow release of plasma, provided the wound has been preoperatively prepared by application of physiologic dressings. Fixation with bandaging is not required unless accidental dislodgement is likely, e.g., on circumferentially burned limbs or on burns of patients with uncontrollable motion. Exposure of the freshly applied autograft allows continuous graft inspection and early evacuation of any collections of blood or serum which may occur beneath the graft. When dressings are utilized, they should be removed 72 hours following grafting. If the grafts are adherent, active motion of the burned area may be begun.

Patients with extensive burns often present a serious disproportion between the area requiring autografting and available donor sites. Mesh or expanded grafts may be utilized to cover large areas from limited donor sites. After harvest of the skin grafts, the grafts are placed on plastic carriers and passed through a Tanner-Vanderput mesh dermatome. A series of parallel incisions is made in the sheet graft, allowing expansion of up to six times the area of the original donor site. The small interstices are rapidly filled by epithelialization (4 to 8 days), resulting in a somewhat thinner but physiologically functional skin cover. In general, mesh grafts are not used on the face, hands, feet, and flexion creases, since the healed grafts are not as cosmetically acceptable as intact autografts. In addition, mesh grafts are less able to withstand recurrent localized trauma.

GENERAL THERAPEUTIC CONSIDERATIONS

Metabolism and Nutrition

Hypermetabolism characterizes the human response to major injury. Several investigators have now shown a direct relationship between the magnitude and duration of the hypermetabolic response and the severity of the sustained trauma. Wilmore has demonstrated a curvilinear relationship between the resting metabolic expenditure and the magnitude of total body surface burn in human patients. Resting metabolic rate approached a maximum response of approximately twice normal in patients with burns of more than 60 percent of the total body surface. Both Reese and Wilmore have documented caloric expenditure in excess of 60 kcal/m²/hour in patients with major thermal injury. Total daily energy consumption during the nonresting state in severely burned patients approached 40 kcal for each percent of body surface burned, plus 25 kcal/kg body weight.

Previously, the hypermetabolic response was attributed

in part to obligatory energy losses in the form of heat associated with a marked increase in evaporative water loss. The increase in evaporative water loss results from destruction of the water barrier within the skin. However, if water evaporation is mechanically prevented, there is no significant decrease in the metabolic rate observed in the burn patient. Furthermore, one cannot reduce oxygen consumption in thermally injured patients to normal levels by manipulation of environmental temperature and humidity. This suggests that the hypermetabolic response is non-temperature-dependent. A close correlation has been demonstrated between oxygen consumption and urinary catecholamine excretion. In addition, hypermetabolic response has been partially blocked by the administration of alpha- and beta-adenergic blocking agents. The hypermetabolic response in human beings is associated with increased rectal and skin temperatures, and animal experiments have demonstrated that burn injury is associated with a true increase in critical temperature. These studies suggest that the hypermetabolic response to burn injury is mediated through the hypothalamic temperature center, which emits an efferent signal expressed via catecholamine excretion.

In addition to elevated energy requirements, a marked catabolic response accompanies severe burn injury. The postburn catabolism is associated with weight loss, retarded wound healing, and negative nitrogen, potassium, sulfur, and phosphorus balance. Again, the magnitude and duration of the catabolic response roughly parallels the severity of the burn injury. Up to 30 Gm of nitrogen/day may be recovered from the urine of severely burned patients. If extraordinary means to provide excessive dietary nitrogen are not pursued, negative nitrogen balance may be observed for up to 2 months following the thermal accident. However, protein catabolism does not proceed uniformly in all tissues. Structural and functional integrity of vital organs such as the heart and liver are maintained at the expense of muscle protein.

Posttraumatic negative nitrogen balance can be ameliorated if sufficient caloric and nitrogen intake is provided. More than 20 Gm of nitrogen/m² of body surface/day is required in patients with major burns during the first postburn month in order to maintain positive nitrogen balance. During the second postburn month, nitrogen intake of 13 to 16 Gm/m²/day will maintain nitrogen equilibrium. The catabolic response in burn patients is associated with increased levels of glucagon and catecholamine (catabolic hormones) in the plasma and depressed levels of insulin (anabolic hormone).

Total oxidation of a normal 70-kg male would yield approximately 166,000 endogenous kcal. It is estimated that healthy persons can tolerate acute losses of up to one-third of lean body weight before death ensues. Thus an extensively burned adult, with energy requirements of 5,000 kcal/day, becomes a severe nutritional risk within 2 weeks, assuming no oral or parenteral caloric intake. Since most of the kinetic energy requirements of the supine, bedridden patient are associated with maintenance of normal respiratory function, the most common cause of death in these patients is pulmonary sepsis. An ineffective respiratory effort results in progressive atelectasis and subsequent lung infection by opportunistic pathogens.

The clinical consequences of inadequate nutritional replacement include profound weight loss, development of superior mesenteric artery syndrome, decreased immunologic response, diminished leukocyte function (host resistance), impaired wound healing, and severe inhibition of cellular active transport, resulting in cellular dysfunction.

Current knowledge of the hypermetabolic response following injury allows more rational therapy aimed at preventing morbid consequences of acute malnutrition. Control of the environment by maintaining an externally warm temperature (31°C) will alleviate patient discomfort and shivering associated with a cold environment and prevent further increases in the metabolic rate subsequent to cold stress. Furthermore, apprehension and pain may be treated appropriately with narcotics and tranquilizers, since both these stresses are known to potentiate the release of catecholamines.

Effective prophylaxis against infection and timely closure of the burn wound will ameliorate both the catabolic and the hypermetabolic response to burn injury. A progressive physical therapy program will also enhance the deposition of protein into lean muscle mass, which allows performance of kinetic work required for maintenance of normal function.

However, the cornerstone of nutritional management of the burn patient is the provision of adequate exogenous calories and nitrogen to prevent prolonged catabolism. Whenever possible, the gastrointestinal tract should be utilized for the various dietary regimens designed to supply the nutritional needs of the patient. Maintenance of adequate nutrition is best monitored by accurate daily measurements of body weight. Postburn weight loss of less than 10 percent is usually well tolerated, provided the patient was not nutritionally depleted prior to his burn injury. Weight loss which exceeds 10 percent of the preburn weight is often associated with an increased incidence of morbidity.

When the voluntary food intake of the burned patient is insufficient to provide for positive energy balance, the physician must intervene with forced feedings, by either the parenteral or the enteral route. Enteral feedings may be accomplished by insertion of a small silastic nasogastric feeding tube through which nutrients are delivered 24 hours a day via a constant delivery pump. Usually patients with major burns tolerate a complete homogenized diet. Partially digested or elemental diets are usually contraindicated, since the higher osmolality associated with these diets often results in gastric distension, profuse diarrhea, or dehydration when large caloric intakes are administered. When positive energy balance is unobtainable by utilization of the gastrointestinal route alone, intravenous hyperalimentation should be employed simultaneously in order to avoid prolonged periods of malnutrition. The intravenous administration of fat emulsions and amino acid solutions by peripheral vein may also be used to supplement enteral caloric intake, if necessary.

Physical Therapy, Splinting, and Rehabilitation

Contractures associated with serious loss of joint function may complicate severe thermal injury. It has now been documented that a progressive physical therapy program implemented immediately after hospital admission is associated with preservation of range of motion in joints with overlying burn injury. It should be emphasized that the program must begin on the day of admission and be continued until the burn wounds are healed and normal range of joint motion can be maintained by the patient. Major burn centers have found it necessary to employ full-time physical therapists to supervise active physical therapy at the bedside during waking hours. Repetitive exercises are conducted in the direction opposite that of any anticipated deformity.

Prolonged immobilization must be avoided, and early motion following skin grafting should be encouraged. In addition, proper positioning during bed rest must be monitored, and splints must be manufactured to maintain anticontracture positions during sleep. When a carefully supervised program of physical therapy is an integral part of burn wound care, 85 percent of the joints underlying surface burns should have a normal range of motion at the completion of therapy. The upper extremities are more susceptible to the deleterious effects of prolonged immobilization than the lower extremities. The ideal position for the lower extremities (knees extended, feet in neutral position) is comfortable to the patient and relatively easy to maintain in either the prone or supine position. However, the shoulders are difficult to position or splint in patients with extensive burns. Elevation and abduction of the arm at the shoulder joint are often uncomfortable, and a patient with burns at the shoulder invariably assumes and maintains a position of adduction and extension if not carefully monitored by nursing personnel and therapists.

Many factors influence the success of a physical therapy program, including patient motivation, but no factor is more deleterious to the preservation of motion than delay of treatment. Daily range-of-motion evaluation and appropriate daily exercises to achieve maximum potential range of motion in joints underlying both second- and third-degree surface burns are of paramount importance. Goals should be established during the early postburn period, which must be rapidly achieved and thereafter maintained. The patient should be encouraged to pursue daily self-care activities as soon as possible. By the time of discharge, the patient should be as independent as possible and should have mastered a home physical therapy program to maintain function.

The development of hypertrophic scars may occur after hospital discharge. The resultant scar overgrowth may inhibit function and often causes severe disfigurement. Larson and his associates have reported reduction of hypertrophic scar formation following the application of conforming isoprene splints and/or elastic dressings (Jobst stockings) during the convalescent period. These devices exert pressure on the scar, causing better alignment of collagen fibrils and reduction of local interstitial edema.

Such splints and elastic dressings should be used following hospital discharge for at least 6 months to discourage delayed development of hypertrophic scar.

COMPLICATIONS

Smoke Inhalation Syndrome

Smoke inhalation syndrome is an acute pulmonary dysfunction related to lower respiratory tract pathophysiology occurring within 72 hours after exposure to gaseous products of incomplete combustion (primarily aldehydes). The severity of this syndrome is a function of the type of smoke inhaled, its amount, and the magnitude of the accompanying thermal injury. Patients with smoke inhalation syndrome frequently exhibit *no* physical signs or symptoms of injury during the first 24 hours after sustaining a major burn. Smoke inhalation should be highly suspected in patients burned within an enclosed space, patients injured while under the influence of alcohol or drugs, and patients who lost consciousness at the time of the accident. Such patients are most likely to have inhaled large amounts of smoke prior to being evacuated from the scene of the fire.

Diagnosis is dependent on a high index of suspicion and careful physical and laboratory examination (Table 7-5). At the time of initial examination, sputum should be obtained from the lower respiratory tract and examined for the presence of carbon. When carbonaceous sputum is noted, the patient should be hospitalized and observed for the development of severe respiratory dysfunction within 18 to 36 hours. Carboxyhemoglobin concentration should be measured as soon as the patient reaches the hospital. Normal carboxyhemoglobin levels are of relatively little value, since the patient may have been exposed to smoke containing low concentrations of carbon monoxide or may have been treated effectively with oxygen by paramedical personnel prior to arrival at the hospital. However, the presence of increased concentrations of carboxyhemoglobin suggests the inhalation of a significant amount of smoke, and the patient should be retained in the hospital for observation, since most such patients will later develop a pathophysiologic condition of the lower respiratory tract

following recovery from carbon monoxide poisoning. Within 6 to 12 hours after injury, the hospitalized patient should be subjected to fiberoptic bronchoscopy to assess the lower respiratory tract. Direct visualization of the trachea and bronchus provides approximately 86 percent accuracy in indicating significant smoke inhalation. Objective findings include the extramucosal appearance of carbonaceous material, bronchorrhea, mucosal edema, vesicles, erythema, hemorrhage, and ulceration.

The Pa_{O_2} while the patient is breathing 100 percent oxygen may also be utilized to monitor for the development of smoke inhalation syndrome. Patients with an initial Pa_{O_2} of less than 300 should be suspected of significant smoke inhalation. This test also has an accuracy of approximately 86 percent.

Other authors have utilized a [133]xenon scan to diagnose lower respiratory tract injury. An abnormal scan following the injection of [133]xenon into a peripheral vein is indicated by incomplete washout from the lungs within 90 seconds or the presence of local radioisotopic trapping. The test is 87 percent accurate but has been infrequently utilized, since it requires the movement of severely ill patients to special radioactivity-counting facilities.

Between 24 and 48 hours after injury, the patient exhibits progressive bronchospasm with expiratory wheezes, rales, tachypnea, and progressive respiratory failure. The subsequent development of bronchopneumonia secondary to bacterial growth distal to occluding plugs (consisting of inspissated mucus and sloughed bronchial epithelium) is a fairly constant feature. Radiographic changes are usually not noted until 72 hours after the injury.

The treatment of smoke inhalation syndrome can be divided into nonspecific and specific therapy. Nonspecific modalities include rapid fluid resuscitation of burn shock, performance of escharotomies of the chest and the abdomen, the provision of external dry heat, and frequent monitoring of respiratory function. Prompt intravenous fluid resuscitation and restoration of normal intravascular volume prevents exacerbation of central nervous system hypoxia. When circumferential third-degree burns of the chest and abdomen are present, chest wall and diaphragmatic excursion are inhibited unless escharotomies are performed. The provision of an externally warm environ-

Table 7-5. SMOKE INHALATION SYNDROME

History: Enclosed space, alcohol/drugs, unconsciousness
Physical Exam: Altered mental status, carbon in sputum, delayed symptoms

Diagnostic tests	Advantages	Disadvantages
Carboxyhemoglobin	Simple, rapid	Nonspecific, rapid disappearance
Fiberoptic bronchoscopy	Simple, rapid objective	
[133]Xenon scan	Objective	Complicated, expensive
AaD$_{O_2}$ gradient	Simple, rapid, ? objective	Unproved

ment minimizes oxygen demand associated with an increased metabolic rate. Most important, however, is the frequent assessment of respiratory function by repetitive physical examination, serial determinations of arterial P_{O_2}, and evaluation of the P_{O_2}/F_{IO_2} ratio, which often decreases prior to a significant fall in the arterial P_{O_2}.

Specific treatment includes the provision of humidified air and oxygen as required. If respiratory failure is incipient, endotracheal intubation should be performed and the patient supported with mechanical ventilation. Often it is necessary to institute positive end-expiratory pressure (PEEP) to prevent progressive respiratory failure. Intravenous administration of bronchodilators often alleviates the severe bronchospasm. When smoke inhalation syndrome is complicated by pneumonia, appropriate antibiotics should be administered by a parenteral route.

Burn Wound Sepsis

One of the principal causes of death following massive thermal injury is burn wound sepsis. Burn wound sepsis is characterized by the active invasion of microorganisms into viable subeschar tissue, with subsequent bacteremia. Third-degree burn wounds are essentially avascular, so systemic delivery of antibiotics via the bloodstream does not substantially affect microbiological growth within the burn wound. Moreover, host resistance to infection is now known to be markedly diminished in patients with major thermal injury. Complement abnormalities, hypogammagobulinemia, cell-mediated immunity, decreased neutrophil intracellular bacterial killing, and abnormalities in the inflammatory response within the burn wound have all been described. In addition, there is a marked decrease in neutrophil and monocyte chemotactic responsiveness. These two factors, markedly decreased perfusion of the eschar and severely compromised host resistance to infection, may result in rapid bacterial colonization if topical chemotherapeutic agents are not utilized. Although the topical agents have reduced the incidence of bacterial invasion of the viable subeschar tissue, bacterial proliferation may still escape the control of all currently used chemotherapeutic preparations. When bacterial escape is proved by quantitative wound biopsy, administration of antibiotics by needle clysis beneath the eschar has been employed with success. This therapy is most effective when initiated at the time wound colonization reaches 10^4 organisms per gram of tissue. Antibiotics administered by subeschar clysis should be selected after review of in vitro sensitivity of the offending organism. The entire daily "systemic" dose of the selected antibiotic should be dissolved in a solution of isotonic saline solution or half-strength saline solution of sufficient quantity to infuse each 44-cm^2 area of burn eschar with 25 ml of solution once daily.

Utilization of antibiotics administered by subeschar clysis has allowed recovery of children with documented *Pseudomonas* burn wound sepsis accompanied by ecthyma gangrenosum. Prior to the utilization of subeschar antibi-

otics, this complication of *Pseudomonas* septicemia was uniformly fatal in burn patients. Up to 50 percent survival was reported in such patients in 1974 by Loebl and his colleagues.

Distant Septic Complications

Because of decreased host resistance, distant septic complications are not unusual in patients with severe burn injury. Bronchopneumonia is the most common complicating infection. Sputum cultures from such patients usually reveal the same microorganism which has colonized the burn wound. Bacteria may be aerosolized from the burn wound and inhaled in large doses as the patient is manipulated during the course of daily wound care. In about one-third of burn patients with pneumonia the bacteria are seeded via the bloodstream (hematogenous pneumonia) as a complication of burn wound sepsis. Conventional treatment with systemic antibiotics and respiratory support is indicated when septic pulmonary infiltrates are diagnosed by physical examination or chest radiography.

Suppurative thrombophlebitis occurs more frequently in patients with massive thermal injury than in other hospitalized patients with severe illness. This complication follows prolonged venous cannulation with polyethylene catheters utilized for the delivery of intravenous fluid. In contrast to bland thrombophlebitis, this type often exhibits no abnormal physical signs. Calf tenderness and edema are only infrequently present. More commonly, the patient presents with bacteremia of unknown origin. Blood cultures often yield staphylococci. The diagnosis may be confirmed by surgical exploration of all peripheral veins which have been cannulated during hospitalization. The vein is opened and milked in a retrograde manner, and any effluent is observed. If pus can be identified, the diagnosis is confirmed. In the absence of liquefied suppurative material, the vein should be biopsied and subjected to frozen section. Bacterial colonization of the intima of the vein also strongly suggests the presence of suppurative thrombophlebitis. The incidence of suppurative thrombophlebitis may be markedly reduced in the burn population by limiting the duration of any single intravenous catheter to periods of 72 hours or less. Should the complication occur, the offending vein must be excised in its entirety. Failure to employ prompt surgical treatment usually results in fatal bacteremia.

Thermally injured cartilage is another common site of bacterial infection. Cartilage is relatively avascular, and local host resistance to established infection is diminished as a result. The cartilage of the external ear is covered only by cutaneous tissue and thus frequently is injured when full-thickness burns of the ear are sustained. The development of suppurative chondritis often may be prevented in patients with severe ear burns by minimizing external pressure upon the ear. Such patients should sleep without bed pillows and be prevented from assuming a lateral position with the burned ear down. When suppurative chondritis occurs, either in the cartilage of the external ear or in other cartilaginous structures, surgical excision of the involved cartilage is necessary to arrest progressive septic destruction.

Gastrointestinal Complications

Gastric and duodenal ulcers have been reported previously as a common complication of major thermal injury. These ulcers were first described by Curling in 1842 and have been reported to occur in as many as 25 percent of hospitalized burn cases. The incidence of Curling ulcers has been markedly reduced during recent years, and operative intervention for upper gastrointestinal bleeding following burn injury is only rarely necessary today. In the past, 85 percent of upper gastrointestinal hemorrhage was associated with bacteremia. The decreased incidence of Curling's ulcer is associated with the reduced frequency of major septic complications, the prophylactic introduction of antacids into the stomach via a gastrointestinal tube (maintenance of a neutral pH in gastric aspirates), and the improved provision of nutritional supplements, allowing more rapid healing of small acute mucosal erosions.

If major upper gastrointestinal hemorrhage should occur, the patient should be promptly treated with iced saline solution gavage and blood volume replacement begun. When hemorrhage cannot be controlled by conservative means, prompt surgical intervention is indicated, since these critically ill patients do not tolerate prolonged periods of hypovolemic shock. The abdominal cavity can be, and often must be, opened through the burn wound. At closure, the subcutaneous tissue and skin are left open to prevent soft tissue infection. Once the bleeding source is identified by gastrotomy or duodenotomy, hemostasis is obtained by oversewing the base of the ulcer. Blood volume replacement is continued until the patient's condition is stable, and then a vagotomy and hemigastrectomy should be performed. Lesser procedures are associated with an unacceptable incidence of rebleeding, and reoperation carries a prohibitive surgical risk.

SPECIAL PROBLEMS

Long Bone Fractures

Often physicians are confronted with a patient who has sustained a long bone fracture with overlying cutaneous burns. Such a patient cannot be treated with closed cylinder casts, since second-degree burns will rapidly convert to full-thickness injuries as a result of bacterial growth. Furthermore, bacterial growth will be unchecked in third-degree burns, resulting in subsequent burn wound sepsis. Open repair of the fracture is generally contraindicated in the presence of potentially infected soft tissue defects. The fracture should be immobilized by insertion of Steinman pins or Kirschner wires in order to effect suspension of the extremity in balanced skeletal traction. The burn wounds can then be left exposed and treatment with topical chemotherapeutic agents initiated. The wounds must be cleansed and inspected daily and the chemotherapeutic agent reapplied.

Following electrical burn, bone may be thermally injured at the entrance and exit sites. This is most likely to occur when the entrance or exit site is on the scalp, the sternum, or the anterior leg. In these locations the underlying bone is in close approximation to the overlying skin. The burn wound is debrided of nonviable soft tissue, and topical chemotherapeutic agents are applied to remaining soft tissue defects and the exposed nonviable bone. When granulation tissue has developed over the soft tissue, temporary coverage with physiologic dressings is instituted until the soft tissue is definitively grafted. After soft tissue wounds are closed, the devitalized bone is decorticated until bleeding bone is encountered. Granulation tissue will develop from the endothelium of the vessels and eventually cover the remaining viable bone. Split-thickness skin graft can then be successfully applied.

Burn Injury of Joints

Occasionally burn injury may extend down to and include the joint capsules. Such injuries are most likely to occur where the overlying skin and soft tissue are relatively thin. The interphalangeal joints of the dorsal surfaces of the fingers and toes are most commonly involved. When it is apparent that the joint capsule has been devitalized and the joint is open, the cartilage should be surgically removed and a formal arthrodesis performed to allow ankylosis of the joint in an optimal position. Interphalangeal joints should be fixed in the extended position or with just a few degrees of flexion. Crossed Kirschner wires are utilized to hold joint position until healing of adjacent bony surfaces has occurred at about 6 weeks. When arthrodesis of joints is necessary, it is particularly important to maintain maximal function of adjoining joints. Ankylosis of the interphalangeal joints results in little long-term disability as long as metacarpophalangeal and metatarsophalangeal joint function is maintained.

Occasionally patients with burns of the hand cannot be maintained in appropriate position by splints during the acute postburn period. This problem most frequently occurs in infants and young children, in whom the fingers are not long enough to allow application of appropriate pressure dressings to maintain optimal extremity position within the splint. In such patients the temporal insertion of a single axial wire through both interphalangeal joints of each finger prevents interphalangeal flexion contractures. The wires are removed at 3 weeks and aggressive active physical therapy is employed to regain finger flexion.

Burns of the Face

Because of its exposed position, the head, with its appendages and orifices, is an anatomic area frequently burned. The protective action of the lids and the constant moisture which surrounds the ocular structures prevents the eyes from being directly involved by thermal injury, except in cases of contact, chemical, or electrical burns.

Injury due to these agents often results in perforation of the cornea or opacification of the cornea, which may require later correction with a corneal graft. Moreover, third-degree burn injury of the lids may cause retraction of the lids, allowing the cornea to be constantly exposed to the drying action of air. Thus extreme care must be directed toward protecting the cornea of the eye. The instillation of artificial tears (methyl cellulose) and the use of antibiotic ointments are often required to prevent corneal desiccation. When such third-degree burn injuries are present, it is often beneficial to perform tarsorrhaphies shortly after the burn injury, limiting subsequent lid contraction deformity. The upper and lower tarsal plates are sewn together in such a fashion as to allow union of the two cartilaginous structures. The patient is able to see through a small peep-hole in the center of the eye, where the upper and lower lids are not joined. The tarsorrhaphies are not released until long after autografting has been accomplished and further lid contraction is not expected. Skin should be grafted over the lids as soon as eschar separation is complete. If subsequent lid retraction still occurs, reconstruction of the eyelids is accomplished by blepharorrhaphy.

Patients with second- or third-degree burn injury of the face may develop microstomia as a result of gradual fibrosis of the circumoral tissues. Prophylactic treatment to prevent this complication is particularly cumbersome and of only limited success. Surgical reconstruction of the mouth may be carried out one year after the burn injury.

Frequently patients become very self-conscious about major or minor postburn scarring on the face. Most scars should be treated initially by conservative management, utilizing elastic pressure masks for a period of 1 to 2 years. Attempts at early surgical reconstruction are often unsuccessful, since the tissue remains extraordinarily hyperactive for a year or more. Scar revision for cosmetic purposes should generally not be attempted for an interval of 1.5 to 2 years following the burn injury.

MORBIDITY AND MORTALITY

Whereas survival after burns of 30 percent of the total body surface area was infrequent 25 years ago, today very few patients with injuries of this magnitude die. In several series, 50 percent patient survival has been observed in patients between the ages of 8 and 45 with 75 percent total body surface burn. However, patients over the age of 65 with burns of more than 25 percent of the total body surface still have markedly reduced survival, and prognosis should be guarded. Chronic disease states in this group frequently interfere with appropriate physiologic response to major thermal injury.

More importantly, the development of multidisciplinary teams to ensure total care of the burn patient has markedly reduced the morbidity associated with this severe injury. At several centers, more than 90 percent of surviving patients have been able to return to an occupation as remunerative as their preinjury employment. Self-respect and independence are preserved, and the quality of life experienced by the patient usually approaches, or in some cases exceeds, the preinjury level.

References

General

Artz, C. P., Moncrief, J. A., and Pruitt, B. A., Jr.: "Burns: A Team Approach," W. B. Saunders Company, Philadelphia, 1978.

Baxter, C. R.: Burns, in G. T. Shires (ed.), "Care of the Trauma Patient," p. 197, McGraw-Hill Book Company, New York, 1966.

Curreri, P. W., and Marvin, J. A.: Advances in Clinical Care of Burn Patients, *West J Med,* **123:**275, 1975.

Krizek, T. J., Robson, M. C., and Wray, R. C., Jr.: Care of the Burned Patient, in W. F. Ballinger, R. B. Rutherford, and G. D. Zuidema (eds.), "The Management of Trauma," p. 650, W. B. Saunders Company, Philadelphia, 1973.

Monofo, W. W.: "The Treatment of Burns: Principles and Practice," W. A. Green, Inc., St. Louis, 1971.

Polk, H. S., and Stone, H. H.: "Contemporary Burn Management," Little, Brown and Company, Boston, 1971.

Shuck, J. M., and Moncrief, J. A.: The Management of Burns, *Curr Probl Surg* (Monograph), *February,* 1969.

Etiology of Burns

Baxter, C. R.: Present Concepts in the Management of Major Electrical Injury, *Surg Clin North Am,* **50:**1401, 1970.

Curreri, P. W., Asch, M. J., and Pruitt, B. A., Jr.: The Treatment of Chemical Burns: Specialized Diagnostic, Therapeutic, and Prognostic Considerations, *J Trauma,* **10:**634, 1970.

DiVincenti, F. C., Moncrief, J. A., and Pruitt, B. A., Jr.: Electrical Injuries: A Review of 65 Cases, *J Trauma,* **9:**497, 1969.

Gruber, R. P., Laub, D. R., and Vistnes, L. M.: The Effect of Hydrotherapy on the Clinical Course and pH of Experimental Cutaneous Chemical Burns, *Plast Reconstr Surg,* **55:**200, 1975.

Jelenko, C.: Chemicals That Burn, *J Trauma,* **14:**65, 1974.

MacArthur, J. D., and Moore, F. D.: Epidemiology of Burns: The Burn-prone Patient, *JAMA,* **231:**259, 1975.

Moncrief, J. A., and Pruitt, B. A., Jr.: Electrical Injury, *Postgrad Med,* **48:**189, 1970.

Immediate Therapy

Baxter, C. R.: Crystalloid Resuscitation of Burn Shock, in H. C. Polk and H. H. Stone (eds.), "Contemporary Burn Management," p. 7, Little, Brown and Company, Boston, 1971.

———, Marvin, J. A., and Curreri, P. W.: Fluid and Electrolyte Therapy of Burn Shock, *Heart and Lung,* **2:**707, 1973.

———, ———, and ———: Early Management of Thermal Burns, *Postgrad Med,* **55:**131, 1974.

——— and Shires, G. T.: Early Resuscitation of Patients with Burns, in C. E. Welch (ed.), "Advances in Surgery, Vol. IV," p. 308, Year Book Medical Publishers, Chicago, 1970.

Curreri, P. W., and Marvin, J. A.: Advances in the Clinical Care of Burn Patients, *West J Med,* **123:**275, 1975.

——— and Pruitt, B. A., Jr.: The Evaluation and Treatment of the Burn Patient, *Am J Occup Ther,* **24:**475, 1970.

———, Rayfield, D. L., Vaught, M., and Baxter, C. R.: Extravascular Fibrinogen Degradation in Experimental Burn Wounds: A Source of Fibrin Split Products, *Surgery,* **77:**86, 1975.

Hummel, R. P., MacMillan, G. B., and Altemeier, W. A.: Topical and Systemic Antibacterial Agents in the Treatment of Burns, *Ann Surg,* **172:**370, 1970.

Loebl, E. C., Baxter, C. R., and Curreri, P. W.: The Mechanism of Erythrocyte Destruction in the Early Post-burn Period, *Ann Surg,* **178:**681, 1973.

————, Marvin, J. A., Curreri, P. W., and Baxter, C. R.: Erythrocyte Survival Following Thermal Injury, *J Surg Res,* **16:**96, 1974.

Salisbury, R. E., McKeel, D. W., and Mason, A. D., Jr.: Ischemic Necrosis of the Intrinsic Muscles of the Hand after Thermal Injury, *J Bone Joint Surg [Am],* **56-A:**1701, 1974.

Simon, T. L., Curreri, P. W., and Harker, L. A.: Kinetic Characterization of Hemostasis in Thermal Injury, *J Lab Clin Med,* **89:**702, 1977.

Zikria, B. A., Weston, G. C., Chodoff, M., and Ferrer, J. M.: Smoke and Carbon Monoxide Poisoning in Fire Victims, *J Trauma,* **12:**641, 1972.

Therapy of the Burn Wound

Baxter, C. R.: Topical Use of 1.0% Silver Sulfadiazine, in H. C. Polk and H. H. Stone (eds.), "Contemporary Burn Management," p. 217, Little, Brown and Company, Boston, 1971.

Burke, J. F., Bondoc, C. C., and Quinby, W. C.: Primary Burn Excision and Immediate Grafting: A Method Shortening Illness, *J Trauma,* **14:**389, 1974.

————, Quinby, W. C., Bondoc, C. C., Cosimi, A. B., Russell, P. S., and Szyffibein, S. K.: Immunosuppression and Temporary Skin Transplantation in the Treatment of Massive Third Degree Burns, *Ann Surg,* **182:**183, 1975.

Bromberg, B. E., Song, I. C., and Mohn, M. P.: The Use of Pig Skin as a Temporary Biological Dressing, *Plast Reconstr Surg,* **36:**80, 1965.

DiVincenti, F. C., Curreri, P. W., and Pruitt, B. A., Jr.: Use of Mesh Skin Autografts in the Burn Patient, *Plast Reconstr Surg,* **44:**464, 1969.

Fox, C. L., Roppole, B. W., and Stanford, W.: Control of *Pseudomonas* Infection in Burns by Silver Sulfadiazine, *Surg Gynecol Obstet,* **128:**1021, 1969.

Hummel, R. P., Kautz, P. D., MacMillan, G. B., and Altemeier, W. A.: The Continuing Problem of Sepsis Following Enzymatic Debridement of Burns, *J Trauma,* **14:**572, 1974.

Lindberg, R. B., Moncrief, J. A., and Mason, A. D., Jr.: Control of Experimental and Clinical Burn Wound Sepsis by Topical Application of Sulfamylon Compounds, *Ann NY Acad Sci,* **150:**950, 1968.

MacMillan, B. G.: Deep Excision and Early Grafting, in H. C. Polk and H. H. Stone (eds.), "Contemporary Burn Management," p. 357, Little, Brown and Company, Boston, 1971.

Monofo, W. W., Aulenbacher, C. E., and Pappalardo, E.: Early Tangential Excision of the Eschars of Major Burns, *Arch Surg,* **104:**503, 1972.

———— and Moyer, C. A.: Effectiveness of Dilute Aqueous Silver Nitrate in the Treatment of Major Burns, *Arch Surg,* **91:**200, 1965.

Polk, H. C.: Treatment of Severe Burns with Aqueous Silver Nitrate (0.5%), *Ann Surg,* **164:**753, 1966.

Pruitt, B. A., Jr., and Curreri, P. W.: The Burn Wound and Its Care, *Arch Surg,* **103:**461, 1971.

———— and ————: The Use of Homograft and Heterograft Skin, in H. C. Polk and H. H. Stone (eds.), "Contemporary Burn Management," p. 397, Little, Brown and Company, Boston, 1971.

Salisbury, R. E., Hunt, J. L., Warden, G. D., and Pruitt, B. A., Jr.: Management of Electrical Burns of the Upper Extremities, *Plast Reconstr Surg,* **51:**648, 1973.

Silverstein, P., Ruzicka, F. J., Helmkamp, G. M., Jr., Lincoln, R. A., Jr., and Mason, A. D., Jr.: In Vitro Evaluation of Enzymatic Debridement of Burn Wound Eschar, *Surgery,* **73:**15, 1973.

Snyder, W. H., Bowles, B. M., and MacMillan, G. B.: The Use of Expansion Meshed Grafts in the Acute and Reconstructive Management of Thermal Injury: A Clinical Evaluation, *J Trauma,* **10:**740, 1970.

Stone, H. H.: Mesh Grafting, in H. C. Polk and H. H. Stone (eds.), "Contemporary Burn Management," p. 383, Little, Brown and Company, Boston, 1971.

General Therapeutic Considerations

Curreri, P. W.: Long-term Supranormal Dietary Programs in Extensively Burned Patients, in W. L. Sheets and G. S. M. Cowan, Jr. (eds.), "Intravenous Hyperalimentation," p. 136, Lea & Febiger, Philadelphia, 1972.

————: Metabolic and Nutritional Aspects of Thermal Injury, *Burns,* **2:**16, 1975.

————, Hicks, J. E., Aronoff, R. J., and Baxter, C. R.: Inhibition of Active Sodium Transport in Erythrocytes from Burn Patients, *Surg Gynecol Obstet,* **139:**538, 1974.

————, Richmond, D., Marvin, J. A., and Baxter, C. R.: Dietary Requirements of Patients with Major Burns, *J Am Diet Assoc,* **65:**415, 1974.

————, Wilmore, D. W., Mason, A. D., Jr., Newsome, T. W., Asch, M. J., and Pruitt, B. A., Jr.: Intracellular Cation Alterations Following Major Trauma: Effect of Supranormal Caloric Intake, *J Trauma,* **11:**390, 1971.

Dobbs, E. R., and Curreri, P. W.: Burns: Analysis of Results of Physical Therapy in 681 Patients, *J Trauma,* **12:**242, 1972.

Larson, D. L., Abston, S., and Evans, E. B.: Splints and Traction, in H. C. Polk and H. H. Stone (eds.), "Contemporary Burn Management," p. 419, Little, Brown and Company, Boston, 1971.

————, ————, ————, Dobrkovsky, M., and Linares, H. A.: Techniques for Decreasing Scar Formation and Contractures in the Burn Patient, *J Trauma* **11:**807, 1971.

Linares, H. A., Kischer, C. W., Dobrkovsky, M., and Larson, D. L.: On the Origin of the Hypertrophic Scar, *J Trauma,* **13:**70, 1973.

Reiss, E., Pearson, E., and Artz, C. P.: The Metabolic Response to Burns, *J Clin Invest,* **35:**62, 1956.

Rickler, J. M., Bruck, H. M., Munster, A. M., Curreri, P. W., and Pruitt, B. A., Jr.: Superior Mesenteric Artery Syndrome as a Consequence of Burn Injury, *J Trauma,* **12:**979, 1972.

Salisbury, R. E., and Palm, L.: Dynamic Splinting for Dorsal Burns of the Hand, *Plast Reconstr Surg,* **51:**226, 1973.

Soroff, H. S., Pearson, E., and Artz, C. P.: An Estimation of the Nitrogen Requirements for Equilibrium in Burned Patients, *Surg Gynecol Obstet,* **112:**263, 1961.

Willis, B. A., Larson, D. L., and Abston, S.: Positioning in Splinting the Burned Patient, *Heart and Lung,* **2:**696, 1973.

Wilmore, D. W.: Hormonal Responses and Their Effect on Metabolism, *Surg Clin North Am,* **56:**999, 1976.

————, Curreri, P. W., Spitzer, K. W., Spitzer, M. E., and Pruitt, B. A., Jr.: Supranormal Dietary Intake in Thermally Injured Metabolic Patients, *Surg Gynecol Obstet,* **132**:881, 1971.

————, Mason, A. D., Jr., Johnson, D. W., and Pruitt, B. A., Jr.: Effect of Ambient Temperature on Heat Production and Heat Loss in Burn Patients, *J Appl Physiol,* **38**:593, 1975.

————, ————, and Pruitt, B. A., Jr.: Insulin Response to Glucose in Hypermetabolic Burn Patients. *Ann Surg,* **183**:314, 1976.

————, Orcutt, T. W., Mason, A. D., Jr., and Pruitt, B. A., Jr.: Alterations in Hypothalamic Function Following Thermal Injury, *J Trauma,* **15**:697, 1975.

Zawacki, B. C., Spitzer, K. W., Mason, A. D., Jr., and Johns, L. A.: Does Increased Evaporative Water Loss Cause Hypermetabolism in Burn Patients? *Ann Surg,* **171**:236, 1970.

Special Problems

Achauer, B. M., Allyn, P. A., Furnas, D. W., and Bartlett, R. H.: Pulmonary Complications of Burns: The Major Threat to the Burn Patient, *Ann Surg,* **177**:311, 1972.

————, Bartlett, R. H., Furnas, D. W., Allyn, P. A., and Wingerson, E.: Internal Fixation in the Management of the Burned Hand, *Arch Surg,* **108**:814, 1974.

Agee, R. N., Long, J. M., III, Hunt, J. L., Petroff, P. A., Lull, R. J., Mason, A. D., Jr., and Pruitt, B. A., Jr.: Use of ^{133}Xenon in Early Diagnosis of Inhalation Injury, *J Trauma,* **16**:218, 1976.

Alexander, J. W.: Emerging Concepts in the Control of Surgical Infections, *Surgery,* **75**:934, 1974.

————: Host Defense Mechanism against Infection, *Surg Clin North Am,* **52**:1367, 1972.

————: Immunologic Considerations and the Role of Vaccination in Burn Injury, in H. C. Polk and H. H. Stone (eds.), "Contemporary Burn Management," p. 265, Little, Brown and Company, Boston, 1971.

————, Dionigi, R., and Meakins, J. L.: Periodic Variation in the Antibacterial Function of Human Neutrophil and Its Relationship to Sepsis, *Ann Surg,* **173**:206, 1971.

Altman, L. C., Klebanoff, S. J., and Curreri, P. W.: Abnormalities of Monocyte Hemotaxis Following Thermal Injury, *J Surg Res,* **22**:616, 1977.

Asch, M. J., Curreri, P. W., and Pruitt, B. A., Jr.: Thermal Injury Involving Bone: A Report of 32 Cases, *J Trauma,* **12**:135, 1972.

————, Moylan, J. A., Jr., Bruck, H. M., and Pruitt, B. A., Jr.: Ocular Complications Associated with Burns: Review of a Five-year Experience Including 104 Patients, *J Trauma,* **11**:857, 1971.

Bartlett, R. H., and Allyn, P. A.: Pulmonary Management of the Burned Patient, *Heart and Lung,* **2**:714, 1973.

Baxter, C. R., Curreri, P. W., and Marvin, J. A.: The Control of Burn Wound Sepsis by the Use of Quantitative Bacteriologic Studies and Subeschar Clysis with Antibiotics, *Surg Clin North Am,* **53**:1509, 1973.

Bruck, H. M., and Pruitt, B. A., Jr.: Curling's Ulcer in Children: A 12-year Review of 63 Cases, *J Trauma,* **12**:490, 1972.

Curreri, P. W., Bruck, H. M., Lindberg, R. B., Mason, A. D., Jr., and Pruitt, B. A., Jr.: *Providencia stuartii* Sepsis: A New Challenge in Treatment of Thermal Injury, *Ann Surg,* **177**:133, 1973.

————, Heck, E. L., Brown, L., and Baxter, C. R.: Stimulated Nitroblue Tetrazolium Test to Assess Neutrophil Antibacterial Function: Prediction of Wound Sepsis in Burned Patients, *Surgery,* **74**:6, 1973.

DiVincenti, F. C., Pruitt, B. A., Jr., and Reckler, J. M.: Inhalation Injuries, *J Trauma,* **11**:100, 1971.

Heck, E. L., Browne, L., Curreri, P. W., and Baxter, C. R.: Evaluation of Leukocyte Function in Burned Individuals by *in vitro* Oxygen Consumption, *J Trauma,* **15**:486, 1975.

Loebl, E. C., Marvin, J. A., Heck, E. L., Curreri, P. W., and Baxter, C. R.: The Method of Quantitative Burn-wound Biopsy Cultures and its Routine Use in the Care of the Burned Patient, *Am J Clin Pathol,* **61**:20, 1974.

————, ————, ————, ————, and ————: Survival with Ecthyma Gangrenosum, a Previously Fatal Complication of Burns, *J Trauma,* **14**:370, 1974.

————, ————, ————, ————, and ————: The Use of Quantitative Biopsy Cultures in Bacteriologic Monitoring of Burn Patients, *J Surg Res,* **16**:1, 1974.

Marvin, J. A., Heck, E. L., Loebl, E. C., Curreri, P. W., and Baxter, C. R.: Usefulness of Blood Cultures in Confirming Septic Complications in Burn Patients: Evaluation of a New Culture Method, *J Trauma,* **15**:657, 1975.

Moncrief, J. A.: Burns of Specific Areas, *J Trauma,* **5**:278, 1965.

Munster, A. M., and Artz, C. P.: A Neglected Aspect of Trauma Pathophysiology: The Immunologic Response to Injury, *South Med J,* **67**:935, 1974.

Petroff, P. A., Hander, E. W., Clayton, W. H., and Pruitt, B. A., Jr.: Pulmonary Function Studies after Smoke Inhalation, *Am J Surg,* **132**:346, 1976.

Pruitt, B. A., Jr., Erickson, D. R., and Morris, A.: Progressive Pulmonary Insufficiency and Other Pulmonary Complications of Thermal Injury, *J Trauma,* **15**:369, 1975.

———— and Foley, F. D.: The Use of Biopsies in Burn Patient Care, *Surgery,* **73**:887, 1973.

Reckler, J. M., Flemma, R. J., and Pruitt, B. A., Jr.: Costal Chondritis: An Unusual Complication in the Burned Patient, *J Trauma,* **13**:76, 1973.

Rosenthal, A., Czaja, A. J., and Pruitt, B. A., Jr.: Gastrin Levels and Gastric Acidity in the Pathogenesis of Acute Gastroduodenal Disease after Burns, *Surg Gynecol Obstet,* **144**:232, 1977.

Silverstein, P., and Peterson, H. D.: Treatment of Eyelid Deformities Due to Burns, *Plast Reconstr Surg,* **51**:38, 1973.

Teplitz, C., Davis, D., Mason, A. D., Jr., and Moncrief, J. A.: *Pseudomonas* Burn Wound Sepsis: I. Pathogenesis of Experimental *Pseudomonas* Burn Wound Sepsis, *J Surg Res,* **4**:200, 1964.

————, ————, Walker, H. L., Raulston, G. L., Mason, A. D., Jr., and Moncrief, J. A.: *Pseudomonas* Burn Wound Sepsis: II. Hematogenous Infection at the Junction of the Burn Wound and the Unburned Hypodermis, *J Surg Res,* **4**:217, 1964.

Voorhis, C. C., Law, E. J., and MacMillan, B. G.: Operative Treatment of Curling's Ulcer in Children: Report of 4 Cases with 3 Survivors, *J Trauma,* **14**:175, 1974.

Wanner, A., and Cutchavaree, A.: Early Recognition of Upper Airway Obstruction Following Smoke Inhalation, *Am Rev Respir Dis,* **180**:1421, 1973.

Warden, J. D., Mason, A. D., and Pruitt, B. A., Jr.: Suppression of Leukocyte Chemotaxis *in vitro* by Chemotherapeutic Agents Used in Management of Thermal Injuries, *Ann Surg,* **181**:363, 1975.

Chapter 8

Wound Healing and Wound Care

by Erle E. Peacock, Jr.

INTRODUCTION

During the course of man's evolution he lost a valuable defense mechanism—the ability to regenerate compound tissues—and accepted in its place a much less complicated and far less valuable process—the phenomenon of healing. Although the ability to heal has been of enormous importance in natural selection, restoration of physical integrity by synthesis of scar tissue can be regarded, at best, as only a method of preserving homeostasis and cannot be compared to the more pristine function of multi-germ-layer regeneration. Moreover, the fibrous tissue synthesis stage of healing can be detrimental even to the extent of destroying the organism which it sought to preserve. Examples are the potentially fatal deformity of valve leaflets incurred during healing of rheumatic fever valvulitis, development of posthepatic cirrhosis, and development of esophageal stenosis after swallowing a corrosive agent. The patient may survive the initial disease or injury only to succumb months or years later from complications of fibrous tissue synthesis during healing.

Posthepatitic cirrhosis is of special interest to students of the biology of wound healing, because the liver is probably the only example of a compound organ in human beings in which almost embryonic propensity for secondary regeneration appears to be retained. Under most circumstances, the liver can be counted upon to regenerate about four-fifths of its preinjury mass; in fact, the failure of regeneration to occur with normal rapidity in severe nodular cirrhosis gives the distinct impression that only overgrowth of fibrous tissue may have prevented hepatic regeneration. The significance of this hypothesis is based on the possibility that fibrous protein synthesis anywhere in the body chokes or overpowers cellular regeneration; from an evo-

lutionary standpoint, such a hypothesis has some factual basis. The hydrozoan *Tubularia* will sometimes regenerate an amputated hydranth without formation of a connective tissue scar; at other times the organism will merely heal the wound by formation of scar tissue. When scar tissue is found, only an abortive attempt at regeneration can be identified. There is a very critical time in the development of newts when the ability to regenerate is disappearing. If during this time connective tissue synthesis is blocked by pharmacologic methods, the power to regenerate a new limb will be slightly prolonged.

With the exception of the liver, regeneration in man is essentially limited to simple tissue such as epithelium; compound structures such as skin, deep organs, and nervous system can heal only by sealing the wound in a manner to be described. The sealing process varies, depending upon whether structural integrity is interrupted or tissue substance is removed. In both types of wounds, epithelization is the fundamental process which seals the wound, and fibrous tissue synthesis is the process which provides structural strength. When tissue is missing, an additional process—contraction—moves tissue edges into closer approximation so that epithelization and fibrous protein synthesis can accomplish their objectives. Simple as this description may sound, most of the mistakes made by physicians in treating wounds are attributable to failure to realize and understand the limitations and end results of each of these fundamental processes and how they differ from pristine regeneration. Thus optimal wound management requires detailed knowledge of epithelization, fibrous protein synthesis, and the biology of wound contraction. Study of these processes requires, in addition, some knowledge of the milieu in which they occur—the ground substance.

WOUND CONTRACTION

In 1793 John Hunter wrote, "In the amputation of the thick thigh (which is naturally 7, 8, or more inches in diameter) . . . the cicatrix shall be no broader than a crown piece." The essence of this quotation is that full-thickness wounds of organs (including skin) do not heal by synthesis of fibrous scar with the exact dimensions of the original defect. A crown piece in Hunter's time was $1\frac{1}{2}$ in. in diameter, thus over 90 percent of the amputation wound was closed by central movement of skin edges. This process is called *contraction*—a dynamic term denoting action, which should not be used interchangeably with "contracture," the term for the end result (Fig. 8-1*A* and *B*). Just as loss of

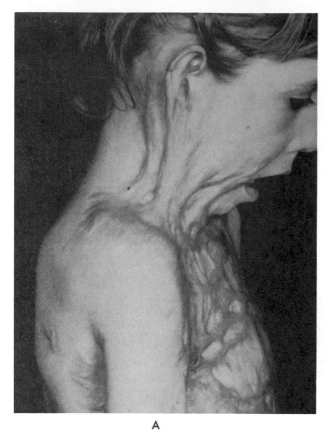

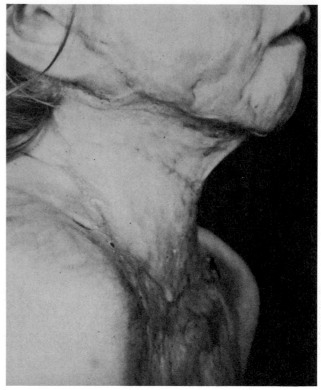

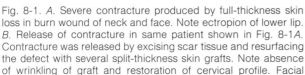

A   B

Fig. 8-1. *A.* Severe contracture produced by full-thickness skin
loss in burn wound of neck and face. Note ectropion of lower lip.
B. Release of contracture in same patient shown in Fig. 8-1*A.*
Contracture was released by excising scar tissue and resurfacing
the defect with several split-thickness skin grafts. Note absence
of wrinkling of graft and restoration of cervical profile. Facial
scars ultimately will be excised and resurfaced.

brain or stomach produces a permanent defect in man, loss
of skin also is permanent, and when a defect in the integument occurs, restoration of integrity is largely dependent
upon stretching surrounding skin to cover exposed subcutaneous tissue. Obviously, stretching skin will distort movable features such as lips, eyelids, breasts, or digits. The
fundamental process in contraction can be illustrated perfectly and the end result predicted positively by simply
grasping the edges of a gaping wound and manually co-
apting them. Such replication of the contraction process
produces the exact deformity that will result from natural
wound contraction over a longer period of time. If it is not
physically possible to coapt the edges of a wound by reasonable external force, one can be certain that natural
processes also will not be effective, as the amount of skin
present is all that will be available to be stretched over the
wound. The area which remains uncovered will either
remain as an open granulating wound or, if it is small
enough, be covered by epithelium, which is a poor substitute for normal skin and establishes a potentially dangerous area for the development of epidermoid carcinoma.

Thus the effectiveness of the contraction process in producing complete wound closure and the cosmetic and

functional deformity which closure by contraction will
produce are related to the amount of skin available in a
given area of the body. Because the hands and face of
a young person do not contain excess skin, closure of a
defect by contraction will cause distortion of facial features
or restriction of joint motion. In areas where there is
redundancy of skin, such as the cervical region or face of
old people, wound contraction can be extremely effective
in closing defects without producing cosmetic or functional
abnormalities. Where an excess of skin is not present but
flexion or extension of a joint will move wound edges
together, wound contraction inexorably results in movement of the joint into an extreme position. After healing
has occurred, the joint will be fixed because of lack of a
satisfactory envelope. When loss of skin occurs over an
area such as the malleolar area of the lower leg and ankle,
wound contraction simply cannot occur because there is
not enough skin to stretch over the defect. In this instance
the wound either becomes covered by a thin, almost gelatinous film of epithelium or remains open for an indefinite
length of time.

Three questions immediately arise about the contraction
process: What starts it? What stops it? What is the mechanism by which it occurs? On first consideration, the answer
to the first question appears obvious, in that interruption of
the integrity of skin always seems to be the initiating
stimulus. Close examination of the series of events which
occur following removal of a piece of full-thickness skin,
however, reveals that wound contraction does not begin

immediately and that about 4 days elapse before movement of the edges is measurable. The so-called "lag phase"
of healing seems to include the contraction phenomenon,
and it can only be surmised that a set of conditions must be
established or an assembly of cells or energy source completed before the actual work of mobilizing skin edges
begins. One might surmise also that reestablishment of
physical integrity is the stimulus which stops contraction;
but again, measurement of the timing of other events
reveals that contraction of a wound does not stop immediately with closure; indeed, wounds which were not caused
by a loss of tissue and which have their edges approximated immediately will sometimes undergo considerable
contraction. Even closure of a wound by the application of
a free split-thickness skin graft or pedicle graft does not
stop the contracting process once movement of wound
edges has begun (Fig. 8-2). An interesting observation is
that the rate of wound contraction is not the same for all
points on the circumference of a wound unless the wound
is a perfect circle. The ultimate configuration of the scar
produced by a contracting wound is the result of variations
in the rate of movement of different segments as well as the
firmness of attachment of different areas of the skin to both
movable and immovable structures. From a practical
standpoint, the surgeon may use such information to reduce the final extent of wound contraction. For example, a
wound created by bringing ileum through the abdominal
wall to form a permanent ileostomy can produce ileal
obstruction if the skin opening undergoes contraction. One
way to minimize skin wound contraction is to make the
skin incision a perfect circle.

The first step in studying the mechanism of wound
contraction is to try to define precisely where the fundamental process is located. In the crudest analysis it must
be determined whether centripetal movement occurs because an energy or power source located outside the defect
is pushing the skin edges in or whether a centrally located
power source is pulling the skin edges to the center of the
defect. Curiously, even after 15 years of intensive study, the
answer is not entirely clear. There is good evidence that
energy is being expended in both areas, and the question
becomes whether both processes are effective or whether
only one is effective and the other is either reacting to
wound contraction or is insufficient to produce effective
tissue movement.

Over the years most investigators have assumed either
that central granulation tissue in a contracting wound was
retracting and pulling the normal skin over the granulating
base or that contents of the wound were being absorbed as
the skin edges moved toward the center. In 1958, Grillo
et al. awakened interest in this question by reporting some
experiments designed to determine whether changes in the
central mass of wound tissue were pulling the skin edges
together or whether central wound tissue was merely adjusting to movement of wound edges propelled by peripheral force. The commonly held opinion that dehydration of
wound tissue was responsible for contraction was destroyed
by their measurements, which showed that water content
of central wound tissue at the beginning of wound contraction had not changed significantly at the end of contrac-

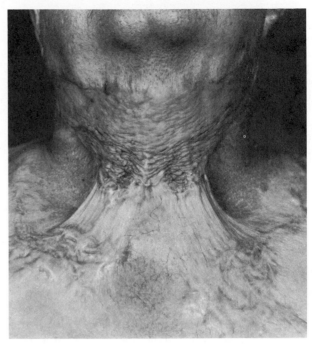

Fig. 8-2. Appearance of split-thickness skin graft applied to granulating wound while it was undergoing contraction. Note wrinkled
appearance of graft and effect of continued contraction on surrounding skin.

tion. The assumption that collagen synthesis and contraction might be responsible for drawing wound edges
together also was disproved by direct measurements of the
collagen content of wound tissue during the process of
contraction. Although collagen content increases markedly
between the fifth and eighth day of healing, total collagen
in the wound falls significantly after this period and cannot
be correlated with rate of wound contraction.

The result of these studies was that attention was focused
upon living cells as the motor units in the contraction
process. Wound contraction occurs only in living organisms, and the force producing migration of wound edges
is generated by living cells. As might be expected, cytochrome poisons, such as potassium cyanide, can be shown
to impair wound contraction although they do not abolish
it completely. Migration of mesodermal cells in tissue
culture also have been shown to be sharply restricted by
cytochrome poisons. These observations are readily reversible, which suggests an inverse relationship between inhibition of aerobic respiration and cell migration.

In an attempt to see if the cells responsible for wound
contraction were located in granulation tissue, Grillo excised all the central wound tissue from wounds in guinea
pigs every day during the contracting process. Curiously,
excision of central tissue did not affect rate of wound
contraction. Such data are not conclusive in localizing the
mechanism of wound contracture, however, because they
cannot be correlated with results produced by other manipulations of the central mass of wound tissue. For instance, if a square of granulation tissue in the center of a
healing wound is outlined by tattoo marks and then sepa-

rated from the rest of the wound tissue by circumferential incision during wound contraction, two interesting observations can be made: The centrally migrating wound edge will retract peripherally, and the centrally circumcised area of granulation tissue will contract centrally. This finding leads one to the inescapable conclusion that granulation tissue between two wound edges was not being compressed by peripheral skin moving inward but was under considerable tension between the advancing wound edges. Moreover, in other experiments, wounds which were splinted for several days and then released did not show marked acceleration of wound contraction following removal of the splint if any central granulation tissue was incised. Additional evidence that tension in granulation tissue is causally related to wound contraction is found in the ingenious experiments of James and Newcombe, who measured the contraction force of granulation tissue and plotted it against the length of tissue elements and the cross-sectional area of granulation tissue. No significant correlation between wound tension and overall wound area could be shown, but a highly significant correlation was found between cross-sectional area of granulation tissue and the tension which was developed during wound contraction. Such studies suggest that granulation tissue under tension resembles stretched elastic tissue, in that the amount of tension produced is related to cross-sectional area and not to overall length or surface area. These data, plus the demonstration that granulation tissue contains cells of a type which can exert migratory force of a magnitude necessary to mobilize skin edges, strongly suggest that the machinery for wound contraction is located in the central granulating mass. A recent discovery by Majno et al. of highly specialized cells (which he termed *myofibroblasts*) with smooth-muscle-like contracting powers lends additional support to this concept. Because myofibroblasts have been found ubiquitously in human beings, many investigators are uncertain about their specific role in wound contraction. Demonstration that topical application of Trosinate, a smooth-muscle antagonist, inhibits wound contraction supports the notion that contractile protein in living cells provides the energy necessary for movement of wound edges.

Grillo found that although wound contraction was not inhibited by excising the entire central mass of granulation tissue, it could be stopped decisively by excising a very limited zone of tissue just beneath the advancing dermal edge. He coined the term "picture frame area" to describe the strategic location of cells which appeared to constitute the machinery for wound contraction. Histologic examination of the "picture frame area" reveals a collection of large, stellate, pale-staining cells which have been thought to be the cells responsible for moving the overlying dermis.

Presently it can be said only that recent investigations have eliminated changes in nonliving materials as the cause of wound contraction and have established that the movement of wound edges requires a high order of energy transfer which is performed by living cells. No unifying hypothesis exists by which all the available data can be explained or the exact site or mechanism of action of wound contraction identified. The apparently incompatible findings of Grillo and of Abercrombie and James concerning the importance of the central granulation tissue can be explained in one of three ways. The first involves the contribution of the panniculus carnosus muscle, which is well developed in some animals and not as well developed in others. The excision of central or peripheral tissue could have vastly different effects on wound contraction depending upon the presence or absence of this structure and whether it was cut in either the primary wound or the secondary excision. The second explanation is that although central granulation tissue can and obviously does contract to some extent during wound contraction it may be contracting as the result of peripheral wound-edge movement and not actually producing it. The third, and in the opinion of the author the most likely, explanation for the seemingly incompatible data of Grillo and Abercrombie is that the wound margin makes its way over the surface of the movable granulation tissue, and as it does so, it forces it by counteraction in a centrifugal direction, thus putting central granulation tissue under enough tension to cause retraction when it is excised or divided. Whatever the mechanism, however, the phenomenon of wound contraction is one of the most predictable and powerful of all biologic reactions and must be positively reckoned with in the management of wounds where tissue has been lost.

EPITHELIZATION

An attempt to cover by regenerating epidermis any area of the body denuded of skin is the first irrefutable sign of wound repair and occurs long before any evidence of connective tissue synthesis can be detected. Factors which control the movement of epidermal cells and the mechanism by which they cover a denuded area are important to students of wound healing for two reasons. The first is that epithelization is necessary in the repair of all types of wounds if a watertight seal is to occur. Protection from fluid and particulate-matter contamination and maintenance of an internal milieu are dependent upon the physical characteristics of keratin. It should be pointed out, however, that just as the plastic liner of a home swimming pool contributes only a watertight seal while structural stability is maintained by concrete blocks, the epidermis provides very little structural strength for the wound. It is the surrounding fibrous protein framework which gives strength to the scar (Fig. 8-3). Actually, no cellular structure or globular protein can impart much strength in the repair of a wound. When structural strength is needed, fibrous protein must be synthesized. Thus highly cellular organs, such as liver, spleen, kidney, or brain, have almost no structural strength and cannot be sutured as effectively as fibrous tissue organs, such as dura, dermis, fascia, or peritoneum. A wound healed only by epithelium will stop "weeping" and be safe from bacterial invasion as long as the epithelium is intact, but the slightest trauma will literally wipe off what is hardly more than a gelatinous film; thus no degree of permanent protection has been achieved.

Second, epithelization is of great importance in the study

of wound healing because when certain variations in the control of cell division and cell movement occur, normal epithelization becomes uncontrolled growth, with awesome invasive potential. The recognized propensity to development of cancer in certain types of wound scars (radiant-energy-induced wounds particularly) and in all wounds which are prevented from healing emphasizes the close similarity between cancer and the healing process (Fig. 8-4A and 4B). Actually, a histologic section from a 5-day-old healing wound can be interpreted easily as fibrosarcoma if none of the historical details are available. Healing is dependent upon what may be thought of as a return to embryonic status; at certain times in the healing process the overall picture—characterized by mitosis, pleomorphism, disorganization, and loss of polarity— resembles the uncontrolled growth of a malignant neoplasm. A major difference exists, however: the factor of control. In a healing wound, the embryonic state is temporary and some controlling influence brings order out of disorder, a resting state to rapidly multiplying cells, and a remodeling of recently synthesized fibrous tissue to produce purposeful structural patterns. In the neoplasm, however, one may consider the situation as a healing wound in which the factor of control never reappears, so that healing continues without purpose or control until the entire organism is consumed by direct extension or metastasis of the products of regeneration. Considered in this way, there may be only a very fine distinction between healing and malignant growth; it may be that when we understand all the factors which influence cells to return to embryonic activity during healing, and even more important, the factors which control their growth and movement after healing has been accomplished, an important step will have been taken in solving the riddle of cancer. For now, however, it is important to remember that the stimulus following injury to overcome entropy and develop embryonic kinetics is one of the most powerful and predictable phenomena in biology.

Apparently cell division and ameboid movement cease only when cells are surrounded by other cells of their own type, and this characteristic behavior of individual cells has something to do with determining the direction in which a mass of cells will move. Weiss observed that when epithelial and mesenchymal cells are mixed and suspended in a proper medium, random movement of cells will occur, causing numerous collisions. Collisions of dissimilar cells (i.e., epidermal and mesenchymal) result in repulsion, whereas collision of similar cells results in the two cells sticking together and later developing protoplasmic bridges and protofibrils. Thus random movements and collisions over a sufficient period of time invariably result in all the cells of one type becoming agglutinated on one side of the medium and the remainder of the cells becoming agglutinated in a similar manner on the other side. As increasing portions of the circumference of a cell membrane become satisfied by attaching to cells of similar lineage, the remaining unsatisfied sides become the exploring or searching surface; thus some degree of polarity for the whole mass may be established. Failure to achieve complete surface contact with other cells results in a con-

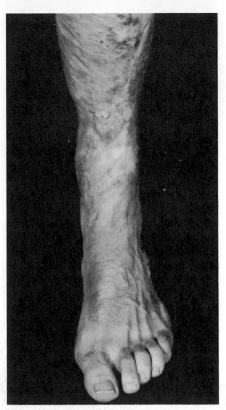

Fig. 8-3. Third-degree burn of lower leg following healing by epithelization. Absence of dermis accounts for shiny appearance and relative fragility of the surface.

tinued state of embryonic activity. One does not have to use much imagination to predict that as the cells continue to be driven by an insatiable desire to contact cells of their own types, the risk of loss of control over replication and locomotion increases with time. Until more is known about the factors involved in the control of cell growth and movement, however, one can only take cognizance of the fact that any wound which is prevented from healing is potentially a malignant neoplasm.

Wounds caused by certain agents such as radiant energy or specific chemicals have an unusual propensity for developing cancer in healed scars or unhealed wounds. In wounds induced by radiant energy, the length of time before cancer develops appears to be directly proportional to the wavelength of the damaging ray. Thus thermal burn wounds and scars may require 20 years for invasive cancer to develop, while in gamma- or x-ray wounds cancer may develop in a matter of a few months. Solar and cosmic radiation, a causative agent in most human skin cancer, is short-wavelength radiation, but because it is filtered by atmosphere and melanin, human development of epidermoid cancer from this source usually does not occur until late in life.

The development of cancer is more rare in surgical or traumatic wounds than in radiant-energy or chemical-induced wounds. No type of wound is exempt, however, when healing has been prevented by constant reinjury or inadequate skin replacement. Even in postphlebitic leg

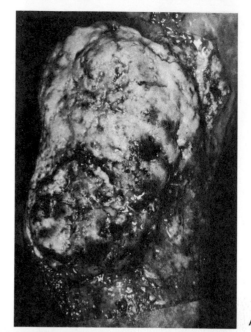

A

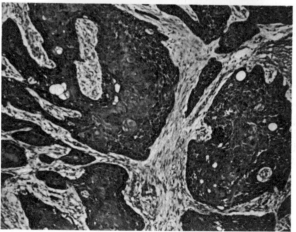

B

Fig. 8-4. *A.* Epidermoid carcinoma in open third-degree burn wound of thigh. Burn is 15 years old. *B.* Microscopic appearance of carcinoma shown in Fig. 8-5. Carcinoma developing in burn wounds metastasizes by vascular routes more frequently than other carcinomas.

ulcer (a common chronic ulcer) cancer may develop over a long period of time.

The mechanism by which epithelium attempts to close a wound has caused considerable speculation. Previous descriptions of the process, based on the assumption that mitosis was not a prominent occurrence, are not correct. Although it is difficult to find mitotic figures in the advancing margin of epithelium, the works of Bullough and of Gillman and Penn have shown conclusively that mitosis does occur in several layers of epithelium and that it is an important part of epithelization. Theoretically, it should be possible for a wound of any size to be epithelized, although there is a practical limit to the size of the area which can be covered. Mitosis is not an unlimited opera-

tion which assures that enough cells will always be present to cover any area.

Two important gross and histologic differences between normal epithelization in a healing wound and abnormal epithelial growth in epidermoid cancer are the size and the shape of the peripheral cell mass. A striking feature in a normally healing wound is the diminishing thickness to monolayer proportions of the advancing cell front (Fig. 8-5*A* and *B*). In carcinoma, cells pile up and tumble over one another to produce a grossly umbilicated appearance (Fig. 8-6*A* and *B*). Thus in normal epithelial regeneration, even though mitosis does occur, the most fundamental process is dedifferentiation and cell movement by development of ruffled membranes and pseudopods. The process begins early (within hours) and results in flat, thin, resting cells at the margin of the wound. These cells develop ruffled membranes and move across the center of the wound. When this occurs, the cell seems to adopt the characteristics of a typical basal cell; if it comes to rest in a more superficial position, it becomes a typical prickle cell.

In incised and sutured wounds, epithelization produces a watertight seal in 24 hours even though there is a dip where the cells have migrated into the crevice. Although the area of regeneration thickens with the addition of more cells, the center of the wound remains somewhat inverted until underlying connective tissue synthesis pushes the epithelium into an everted position. Gillman and Penn have pointed out that the cutaneous tract of a skin suture on either side of the scar is also a wound of the epithelium, and that the inverted contour of the epithelium over the main wound also occurs along the path of a suture to the extent that a completely epithelized tract may be produced or a small cyst formed after a suture is removed.

Epithelization of a surface wound (whether partial thickness of skin such as an abrasion, or split-thickness skin-graft donor site, or full-thickness wound such as postphlebitic ulcer of the ankle) involves similar movement of epithelial cells but over a much more hazardous terrain and greater distance than incised and sutured wounds. The early escape of blood and serum in open wounds produces a scab, and the regenerating epithelium moves beneath the scab, literally detaching it from the underlying surface as it seals the wound. Actually, epithelium does not move along the interface between dermis or fat and the scab but seems to prefer to infiltrate or actually cut through the fibrous tissue substrate by elaborating an enzyme which renders collagen soluble. This mysterious behavior has been somewhat clarified recently by identification of a collagenolytic enzyme found at the interface between epithelium and mesenchymal tissue. Confirmation of the observation that epithelium literally cuts its own path through fibrous tissue may be extremely important in understanding the remodeling of deep fibrous tissue to produce a new dermis.

The protective influence of a scab or other cover (eschar, surgical dressing, etc.) to prevent physical trauma, drying, hemorrhage, contact with caustic materials, and the like is the basis for medical care of secondarily healing wounds. In the final analysis, successful epithelization occurs only if the cumulative effect of physical manipulation, drying, bacterial enzymes, wound area, etc., does not exceed the finite capacity of available cells to divide, dedifferentiate, and move across the surface. Considered in the simplest analysis, it may be that interruption of epidermis merely allows the epidermis to do what it normally would do if it had room, since cell movement and cell division are to a large extent prevented in the intact epidermis by the compression effect of surrounding cells; to interrupt the integrity of an epithelium-lined surface may merely allow the cells to do what they would naturally do if they were not orderly and compactly arranged.

GROUND SUBSTANCE

Even as late as 1952, some treatises on wound healing made no mention of the role of ground substance. The mystery surrounding ground substance is nowhere better exemplified than in the name itself, a mistranslation of the German *grundsubstance,* which referred to a mysterious matrix from which all the formed elements of connective tissue were believed to originate. A similar connotation was expressed by the French *substance fondamentale.* Modern definitions have done little to clarify the true nature of this amorphous material, and the best that can be said, even now, is that the term "ground substance" usually refers to a continuous nonfibrillar matrix including water and electrolytes through which metabolites diffuse between blood vessels and cells. Histologically, ground substance is identified by a remarkable propensity to absorb certain dyes such as toluidine blue and to undergo characteristic reactions with periodic acid. By such staining reactions it can be seen that ground substance is relatively organized in some areas, such as basement membrane, and undergoes, during inflammation and healing, characteristic changes in staining reaction called *metachromasia.* Such histochemical reactions seem to be due to reactions with mucopolysaccharides, many of which contain hexosamine. Because of the characteristic staining reactions which they produce, attention has been focused on the acid mucopolysaccharides, even though it must be remembered that they account for only a small portion of ground substance. As a result, errors have been made by measuring hexosamine in connective tissues and drawing conclusions about the relative amount and importance of the ground substance on the basis of change in one small sugar moiety.

Meyer's division of the acid mucopolysaccharides into two major groups has been useful in the study of wound healing. These groups are nonsulfated mucopolysaccharides, of which hyaluronic acid and chondroitin can be easily identified, and sulfated mucopolysaccharides, of which chondroitin sulfate A, chondroitin sulfate B, chondroitin sulfate C, heparitin sulfate and keratosulfate have been identified. Presently it seems that the nonsulfated group is the main component of the structureless gel fraction of ground substance and that the sulfated group is most closely associated with the fibrillar elements of connective tissue. Thus changes in sulfated acid mucopolysaccharides are most likely to be of significance during the healing process, and, indeed, such substances are

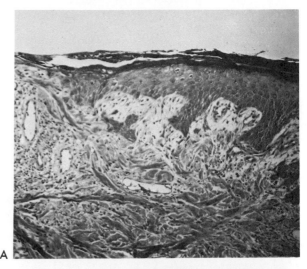

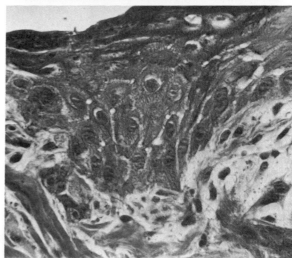

Fig. 8-5. *A.* Low-power view of epithelium advancing over granulating surface in a human wound. Note decreased thickness of advancing margin. *B.* High-power view of advancing epithelium in granulating human wound. Note dedifferentiation of cells, deep migratory activity suggesting subsurface enzyme activity at epithelial-mesenchymal tissue interface, and absence of mitotic activity.

found to be increased during early stages of wound healing. Determination of actual amounts of any of the components of ground substance may be misleading, however, as we are dealing with a very complex substance which involves polymerizing reactions and the formation of giant molecules with molecular weight varying between 10,000 and 10,000,000.

Because the healing process is characterized by polymerizing, cementing reactions, it is interesting to speculate upon the role of these complex substances. Discovery that acid-sulfated mucopolysaccharides accumulate during healing raises the question of whether linkages between fibrillar proteins and ground substance occur. The same question has been raised about normal tissues such as tendons, where chondroitin C is a prominent portion of

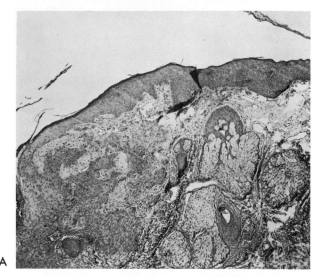

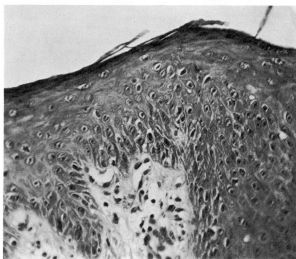

Fig. 8-6. *A.* Low-power view of epidermoid carcinoma of skin. Note accumulation of cells producing increased thickness of epithelium without purposeful migratory activity. *B.* High-power view of epidermoid carcinoma. Note numerous mitotic figures.

the ground substance; stabilization of tendon by cross linkages between collagen fibrils and chondroitin C has not been demonstrated conclusively. Chondroitin A protein complex seems important in stabilization of cartilage, and destruction of this complex by local injection of papain in a rabbit's ear will produce a lop-ear deformity which will return to normal as soon as the complex is reconstituted. It seems likely that ground substance is most important in the phenomenon of healing because of its relation to collagen synthesis and remodeling. Although chemical linkages between mucopolysaccharides and collagen have been extremely difficult to identify, chemical bonds are present which may be important in the development of strength or orientation of collagen fibers and fibrils. Certainly the assembly of collagen subunits into fibrils and fibers is dependent upon many environmental conditions, which ground substance provides. Variations in

the relative amounts of sulfated fractions are believed by many to be instrumental in determining the configurations of collagen fibrils, but how much this complicated substance actually participates in other aspects of the healing process awaits further investigation.

COLLAGEN

As far as the questions which patients ask their physicians following repair of wounds are concerned, fibrous protein synthesis is the essence of healing. Accurate answers to such questions as "When do the stitches come out?" "When can I go back to work?" "How bad will the scar be?" and others are dependent upon a thorough knowledge of collagen synthesis, collagen degradation, and the factors which influence the equilibrium between the two. Unfortunately, there are gaps in our knowledge about collagen metabolism; but enough is known so that the care of wounds does not have to be a mixture of craft and religion, as Paré expressed it, but can be, in most instances, a scientific exercise with a predictable outcome. Even such seeming trivia as the selection of a suture or dressing material can be the result of logical reasoning based upon factual knowledge.

Collagen is an extracellular secretion from specialized fibroblasts, and the monomeric particles or basic molecules which fibroblasts synthesize are frequently called *tropocollagen.* The tropocollagen molecule is one of the largest biologic macromolecules, with a molecular weight of about 300,000 and dimensions of 15 Å in width and 2800 Å in length. It is a stiff, elongated rod which can be visualized by an electron microscope and is soluble in cold salt solution. Thus tropocollagen is sometimes referred to as saline-extractable, or salt-soluble, collagen.

Recently it has become evident that genetic pleomorphism is expressed in subtypes of collagen molecules. Three types of collagens can be recognized by analyzing the composition of $\alpha 1$ and $\alpha 2$ chains. Type I collagen is the most prevalent type in the mature vertebrate organism. Type II collagen appears limited to cartilage and is found primarily in human articular and costal cartilages and in chick embryo bones. Type III collagen is found in association with Type I collagen and is most prevalent in tissue undergoing remodeling or fetal organogenesis. Type III collagen also appears to be an important component of tissues with an unusual degree of elasticity, such as those of the aorta, esophagus, and uterus.

The amino acids found only in collagen, and used to identify it in analytical procedures, are hydroxyproline and hydroxylysine. The amount of collagen in a specimen of tissue is determined by measuring the amount of hydroxyproline and multiplying the result by a factor of 7.8. Other fibrous tissues such as elastin do not contain significant amounts of hydroxyproline. Formerly it was believed that hydroxyproline in collagen had much to do with the formation of various intra- and intermolecular cross links which give collagen molecules, fibers, and fibrils their characteristic rigidity. The three-plane fixation of the triple helix structure results, teleologically speaking, in our being able to rely on collagen to transmit energy accurately in tendons or to support nonfibrous structures such as muscle. The supporting nonelastic properties of collagen can be destroyed by rupturing cross links within and between molecules, but fortunately, the destruction of cross links to this extent requires rather harsh treatment for mature collagen, such as temperatures over 70°C or exposure to strong acids or alkalies. Under these circumstances, what is produced is gelatin, which, of course, has no structural strength even though the essential amino acids are present. It seems evident now that hydroxylation of proline and lysine is most important in transport of the molecule across cell membranes.

Synthesis of collagen is an intracellular phenomenon which occurs on polysomes; a critical stage in construction of the molecule is the hydroxylation of proline to produce hydroxyproline. Externally administered hydroxyproline is rapidly excreted in the urine and apparently cannot be utilized by fibroblasts to synthesize collagen. Among other things, one of the metabolic defects which can be identified in collagen-deficiency diseases such as scurvy is the accumulation of proline-rich precursors and deficiency of hydroxyproline containing polypeptides. During active collagen synthesis the ergastoplasm of fibroblasts forms characteristic parallel lines, or canaliculi, and it appears that monomeric molecules are excreted into the extracellular milieu through these canaliculi. In ascorbic acid deficiency, the microsomes do not form parallel lines of canaliculi but are arranged, instead, in large cystic spaces. It is from these areas that proline-rich and hydroxyproline-poor amorphous material is found.

Before aggregation and normal assembly can occur, a specific enzyme, procollagen peptidase, is needed to remove nonhelical terminal extensions from both the N-terminal and C-terminal ends of the molecule. Recent evidence suggests that the terminal peptide extensions of the collagen molecule are registration peptides facilitating triple helix formation. They interfere with subsequent fibril aggregation, however, and failure to remove the registration peptides because of congenital absence of procollagen peptidase results in poorly assembled collagen with marked structural abnormalities. A type of Ehlers-Danlos syndrome has been found to be the result of persistent pro-αchains. A similar condition appears to be responsible for the structural malformations in a disease of Belgian cattle called dermatosparaxis.

Monomeric collagen particles exposed to proper pH, temperature, osmotic conditions, etc., in the intercellular milieu aggregate or polymerize rapidly by the formation of cross links of various types. The most important such cross links are covalent ester bonds such as a Schiff's base between an amino group of one molecule and an aldehyde group of another. Oxidative deamination of lysine by an important enzyme, lysyl oxidase, is a necessary first step to formation of covalent ester cross links. In addition, other types of cross links, such as oppositely charged electrostatic groups and Van der Waals interactions, are involved in assembling monomeric particles into polymerized aggregates.

The rodlike collagen molecules appear to lie in staggered, overlapping, parallel formation, with one-quarter-length overlap. It is this staggered one-quarter-overlap arrangement of tightly packed units which gives collagen its typical repeating axial periodicity of 640 Å. Whenever collagen molecules are assembled under physiologic conditions such as those provided by the extracellular ground substance, typical fibrils with 640 Å repeating periods are produced. In certain laboratory preparations, however, it is possible to alter the characteristic 640 Å periodicity by forcing the monomeric particles to line up exactly parallel or end-on. This can be accomplished by adding glycoprotein to the milieu or by charging the preparation with a high-energy system such as adenosine triphosphate. Under these conditions, fibrils with band widths of 2000 Å can be produced; such atypical fibers are called *segment long-spacing fibers,* or *fibrous long-spacing fibrils.* These preparations have been extremely valuable in the laboratory, as they have revealed much about the size and method of polymerization of collagen molecules; they are not of any physiologic importance, however, as far as is known.

Although the collagen molecule is basically a triple-helix molecule with a spiral configuration, heat-sensitive intramolecular cross links prevent it from having elastic or recoil properties. However, if a collagen fiber or fibril is placed in a water bath with a small weight suspended from one end and the temperature of the bath is elevated, a point will be reached when the heat-sensitive intramolecular cross links will be destroyed and recoil of the spiral polypeptide chain will occur. The temperature at which this phenomenon occurs is called the *thermal shrinkage temperature,* and the magnitude of this reaction is such that a fiber or fibril will shrink to one-third of its physiologic length. The thermal shrinkage temperature of collagen, therefore, is an excellent indicator of the strength and degree of inter- and intramolecular bonding. By measuring the thermal shrinkage temperature of various types of collagen, it has been possible to learn something about variations in bonding under physiologic conditions and, in some instances, to correlate the development of physical properties of collagen with the extent of cross linking. From such studies it has become clear that cross linking, among other factors, is a function of aging; the older a specimen of collagen becomes, the firmer and more numerous the cross links are. Thus, collagen gel which is only a few minutes old has relatively few cross links and a low thermal shrinkage temperature and is so flimsy that cold salt solution solubilizes it. If the gel is allowed to mature for 24 hours, the number and strength of the cross links increase to the extent that a weak acid may be needed to depolymerize even a portion of it and a higher temperature will be required to cause it to undergo thermal shrinkage. If the aggregate is allowed to polymerize for several weeks, the maximum number and firmness of cross links will be realized, with the result that a strong acid may be needed to get even a portion of the collagen into monomeric units and the thermal shrinkage temperature will be the highest yet. In summary, therefore, both solubility and thermal shrinkage temperatures can be used to measure the age of collagen as represented by the effectiveness of the cross-linking process.

In addition to naturally occurring cross links such as ester bonds, artificial cross links can be added to change the physical properties of collagen. Just as adding an agent which shares electrons easily, such as a sulfur molecule, will increase the stength of rubber (vulcanization) sevenfold, addition of a similar agent such as the methyl group in formaldehyde will increase the number and kinds of cross links in collagen. Just how much the addition and destruction of cross links has to do with the physical properties of wound-repair collagen in scar tissue is not known. It has been shown, however, that addition of methyl or amide cross links will increase the tensile strength of scar tissue in incised and sutured wounds in rats as much as threefold on the eighth postwound day. That variations in cross linking are partially responsible, however, for the final appearance, texture, or elasticity of human scars is becoming more certain for many investigators. Early studies suggested that apparent rapid acceleration of the rate of gain in tensile strength in dehisced and sutured wounds was the result of more efficient cross linking between collagen molecules. Recent data, however, strongly suggest that the phenomenon of secondary healing really is nothing more than briefly interrupted primary healing. Apparently brief physical disruption of coapted skin edges has little or no effect upon the fundamental biology and biochemistry involved in tensile strength gain of a healing wound.

At this point, other factors involved in tensile strength must be considered, for cross linking may have very little to do with tensile strength after fibrils and fibers have been formed. It is highly unlikely, in the opinion of the author, that fibrils and fibers are cross-linked very efficiently, because the average distance between fibrils is of the order of 1 μ. Chemical cross links are approximately 2.8 Å, which means that the distance is roughly 500 times too great for the usual types of cross links to span the distance between fibrils. However, because addition of cross links such as methyl or amide bonds definitely increases tensile strength in wet scar tissue, the inescapable conclusion seems to be that rupture of scar tissue must occur, to some extent, along inter- and intramolecular planes. There is not uniform agreement on this point, and the question of the importance of cross linking in the development of strength in scar tissue must be investigated further.

After a certain amount of collagen has been synthesized, the most important factor in gain of strength may be the physical weave of fibrils and fibers. Certainly it is possible to vary the physical properties of other fibrous materials by varying the weave of the small components exclusive of any chemical bonds. A good example of this principle is to be found in the physical weave of a nylon stocking. Nylon thread is nonelastic, yet a nylon stocking can be made elastic by properly weaving the fibers. Transposed to a biologic system, nonelastic tendon or fascia shows physical characteristics similar to nylon thread, while elasticity of the wall of the aorta is similar to that of a nylon stocking.

The old concept of collagen as a static, adynamic substance—the excelsior of the body—is erroneous. Actually, as will be shown later, collagen in wound scar is a relatively dynamic structure which, like other tissues, is undergoing constant remodeling and replacement. After the forty-second day of wound healing there is no measurable increase in the amount of collagen in a healing wound, yet the scar continues to gain strength for at least 2 years. Thus changes in collagen, such as increased cross linking and rearrangement of fibers and fibrils, must be occurring.

Before leaving the subject of remodeling, it is important to mention a disease, lathyrism, which has been useful in the study of collagen metabolism and which may have far-reaching implications for control of human scar tissue. The disease, recognized by Hippocrates, is caused by excessive ingestion of certain peas of the genus *Lathyrus*. Considerable differences exist between the human form of the disease, which is manifested by spastic paralysis, and the disease in laboratory animals, which is characterized by skeletal and cardiovascular abnormalities secondary to altered collagen metabolism. Curiously, attempts to produce neurolathyrism in rats have been unsuccessful; the *Lathyrus* species toxic to man and domestic animals are not toxic to rats, which thrive on them. The active and highly potent fraction which produces altered collagen metabolism is beta-aminopropionitrile. Considerable data are available on the effect of this substance on both developing and mature tissues. Most of these data support the hypothesis that the primary effect of beta-aminopropionitrile is to block the formation of inter- and intramolecular cross links during all stages of collagen aggregation. Thus beta-aminopropionitrile affects growing tissue more than adult tissue. Characteristically, beta-aminopropionitrile produces an enormous increase in the saline-extractable collagen, as it seems to block the assembly of monomeric collagen units into stable fibrils and fibers. There is some evidence to indicate that fibril formation is not stopped during lathyrism but that cross linking in fibrils is so unstable that cold saline will solubilize most of the collagen which was assembled during beta-aminopropionitrile poisoning. Growing embryos literally become saline-soluble under the effect of beta-aminopropionitrile, and mature animals will develop hernias or die suddenly of dissecting aneurysms. Wound healing, as might be predicted, is affected by beta-aminopropionitrile; there is a cessation of gain in tensile strength within hours after the agent is administered, while saline-extractable collagen increases approximately ten times. Clinical implications of the beta-aminopropionitrile effect are exciting, for it is a clear-cut demonstration that it is possible to alter the physical properties of collagen in dramatic fashion. Because some of the effects of fibrous tissue healing in specialized organs, such as the liver or heart, can be more ruinous to the health of the individual than the disease or injury which preceded healing, the demonstration that some control over deep scar formation is possible is an exciting one. If, in addition, mature recently synthesized collagen also could be solubilized selectively, a major breakthrough in many disease processes could evolve. Highly purified beta-aminopropionitrile has been administered to human beings with scleroderma, urethral stricture, and keloid. It can be given safely to human beings, and it is anticipated that clinical trials presently being performed will establish the effectiveness of induced controlled lathyrism as a therapeutic modality.

Several times in this chapter the term "remodeling" of scar tissue has been used. The thoughtful student is likely to be concerned over such a term, as it connotes not just synthesis of collagen but collagen breakdown as well. Because no enzyme able to lyse collagen had been identified in human beings until approximately 15 years ago, collagen turnover in either normal tissue or wound scar was suspect. Even though no such mechanism could be demonstrated, however, indirect evidence has been abundant that some enzyme or mechanism for solubilizing collagen must exist. There is always some extractable collagen in the skin of even the oldest and most depleted individuals. Obviously, if all tropocollagen were going into the skin, the dermis would soon be as thick as elephant hide. Some collagen must be coming out of the dermis, and the relatively constant thickness of skin only attests to an equilibrium which exists between collagen synthesis and degradation. Surface scars are raised above the surface 2 to 4 weeks after injury; yet they usually soften, become pliable, and decrease considerably in size with the passage of time. The loss of 50 percent of collagen from the gravid uterus 36 hours after parturition and the rapid disappearance of dermis when tetraplegic patients are allowed to lie unattended attest that man possesses an effective enzyme capable of degrading mature collagen. Search for such an enzyme previously has been unsuccessful because it was assumed that the enzyme could be extracted from tissues. In 1963, Gross, Lapiere, and Tanzer hypothesized that collagenolytic enzyme was the product of living cells and that contact with a living cell was necessary in order for collagenolysis to occur. In one of the most important experiments performed in the wound-healing field during the last decade, the hypothesis was tested by preparing culture plates of reconstituted collagen and amphibian Tyrode culture medium. Specimens of tissue from the rapidly absorbing tail of a metamorphosing tadpole (a structure containing mostly collagen which is absorbed and not broken off during metamorphosis) were placed on the collagen-Tyrode substrate, and the culture plates were incubated under suitable tissue culture conditions. After several days a clear zone appeared around each implant, and if the tissues were kept alive long enough, the entire substrate became lysed by collagenolytic activity. Failure of the cells to survive stops collagenolytic activity immediately; even after lysis has begun, it can be stopped by killing the cells. Thus Gross and Lapiere demonstrated that collagenolytic enzyme is a product of living cells and that cells which produce enzyme need to be in close contact with collagen fibers for lysis to occur. Grillo, using the same tissue-culture technique, cultured wound tissues from actively healing wounds in guinea pigs and found extremely active enzyme activity at the wound edge. Moreover, the most active lysis in a secondary healing wound appeared to be at the epidermis-dermis interface of an advancing wound margin. Riley and Peacock cultured a variety of normal and pathologic human tissues and found collagenolytic enzyme to be widely distributed, particularly in epithelium-containing structures.

The most uniformly positive tissue for collagenolytic enzyme in human beings is cutaneous scar. Scar tissue reveals positive lytic activity approximately 10 days after closure of a cutaneous laceration, and a high level of activity has been found in dermal scars as long as 30 years after injury. Granulation tissue is only slightly active; burn eschar does not show any activity for about 2 weeks. Between 2 and 3 weeks after a third-degree burn, however, cultures of separating dermal eschar are strongly positive for collagenolytic activity. These findings suggest that invasion of dead eschar by underlying connective tissue cells or undermining epidermal cells is necessary for contact between cells and heat-tanned collagen. Retarded wound healing may be the result of excessive collagenolysis. Serum, cysteine, and progesterone have been shown to inhibit tissue collagenase acting at neutral pH. Progesterone in ophthalmic concentrations may be the agent of choice in treating corneal injury, particularly alkali burns in which delayed tissue collagenase activity is the cause of rupture of the globe.

By measuring collagen synthesis and collagen breakdown, it is now possible to study healing from the standpoint of variations in metabolic equilibrium. Considered as such, scar tissue becomes a product of opposing forces of collagen synthesis and collagen destruction, and the result of such forces will vary according to the relative rate and effectiveness of each. The maximum amount of total collagen in a healing wound is found by the forty-second day. Although increased amounts of saline-extractable collagen (compared with nonwounded resting dermis) can be extracted from the scar for as long as 18 months, there is no further gain in insoluble (or mature) collagen. The conclusion would seem to be that, even though remodeling of the collagen continues, equilibrium has been established between collagen synthesis and collagen destruction. Recent demonstration by Cohen of accelerated collagen synthesis and deposition and collagenolytic activity in human keloids probably represents an abnormaility of such an equilibrium.

The concept that all collagen to some extent, and healing wound collagen particularly, is undergoing simultaneous construction and destruction can serve as a basis for speculation concerning some of the previously unexplainable findings in the healing process. One such enigma is the behavior of wounds during ascorbic acid depletion. In the classic descriptions of scurvy it is important to remember that sailors' wounds did not just fail to heal; they actually disrupted months after they had healed perfectly. This observation has been verified in animals and raises the question of whether collagen is dependent upon ascorbic acid for structural integrity. It is known that collagen can be repeatedly depolymerized and reconstituted in the laboratory without contact with ascorbic acid, and artificially reconstituted collagen does not lose tensile strength. Therefore, the notion that vitamin C has anything to do with strength of mature scar tissue is untenable. Because synthesis of new collagen is blocked during ascorbic acid deficiency, and because collagenolytic activity probably proceeds normally, a possible explanation for old scar dehiscence would seem to be that tissue previously in equilibrium becomes unbalanced by having synthesis knocked out and lysis continue. Inexorably, the scar will become weaker until a point is reached where normal tissue tension produces complete disruption.

Although to some extent hypothetical (actual quantitative measurements of lysis and synthesis are not sensitive enough now to prove or disprove the equilibrium hypothesis), the theory is important as it relates to the whole field of conditions erroneously referred to in the past as "collagen diseases." The collagen in these diseases is precipitated under physiologic conditions and, as might be predicted, is normal as far as can be determined by electron or light microscopy, x-ray defraction, or amino acid analysis. Thus all the evidence supports the idea that so-called "collagen diseases" represent abnormal amounts of collagen in abnormal places but are not specific diseases of the collagen molecule or fibril. Such an explanation is entirely logical, as one cannot have a disease of a nonliving structure. Collagen is a long-chain polymer in which the nearest thing that could be classified as a disease process is the abnormal construction of collagen during lathyrism. The collagen in such diseases as rheumatic fever, dermatomyositis, and scleroderma is probably much more accurately considered as the ash or scar from a burnt-out primary wound or inflammatory process. In the other direction, destruction of collagen in diseases such as rheumatoid arthritis is, at least partially, the result of excessive tissue collagenase activity. The concept of the collagen system as a dynamic, constantly remodeling one opens the door for investigation of a large number of diseases of unknown cause which are characterized by deficient or excessive collagen formation.

SEQUENCE OF EVENTS: SUMMARY

Once the basic processes in the healing phenomenon have been mastered, the student has only to relate them to one another in proper sequence to be ready to start the study of what physicians can do to aid healing. The most important concept in this regard is the understanding that healing is not a series of events but is a concert of simultaneously occurring processes, some of which continue for many years after physical integrity of wounded tissue has been reestablished. The most dramatic events, such as sealing the wound, regaining tensile strength sufficient to permit normal stress, and acquiring a scar which is cosmetically and functionally acceptable, occur in a relatively short period of time. Long-term processes, such as remodeling of collagen and development of cancer in scar tissue, fortunately are not processes which cause patients much concern. Although the basic processes are much the same in an incised and sutured wound properly coapted (healing by primary intention) and a wound in which tissue has been lost so that healing must occur by contraction and epithelization (secondary healing, or healing by secondary intention), the time required for secondary healing is so much longer and the area involved usually so much greater that it is convenient to study the secondary healing process

to see how the basic steps in wound healing relate to one another.

The first thing which happens after full-thickness skin loss is that normal elasticity of the skin and external tension produced in some areas by muscle pull enlarge the defect according to the amount of force exerted and the direction over which it acts. Thus the shape of a skin defect may have little relation to the size or shape of the fragment of tissue which was removed. If hemorrhage is not too severe, a clot forms quickly, then contracts and dehydrates to form a scab. Because a scab is essentially a dehydrated, fully contracted blood clot, it is less durable and effective in closing the wound than collagenous eschar. Nevertheless, a scab serves a useful purpose in providing limited protection from external contamination, satisfactory maintenance of internal hemostasis, and a surface beneath which cell migration and movement of the wound edges can occur. Classically, the beginning of wound healing is described as the "lag" phase—an inaccurate term which carries the connotation that there is a period when nothing of importance is happening. Actually, a great number of important things are happening even though they usually are not considered part of the healing process. One soon recognizes, however, that almost instantly following infliction of an injury the stage for healing is set, and the props and background for the events which are to follow are essentially those of controlled inflammation. Study of the biology of repair has emphasized that the most successful reparative processes occur against a background of inflammation and that, up to the point of necrosis, how well the wound heals is directly related to the amount of inflammation present. Specifically, the release of various amines from connective tissue mast cells, perfusion of capillaries surrounding the defect, change in permeability of capillary walls, release of enzymes, fluid, and protein into extracellular spaces, accumulation of white blood cells and connective tissue cells, and formation of thrombi in peripheral lymphatic channels are all well-known changes in general inflammation which are important in providing the best milieu for repair to proceed. It is only when bacteria, foreign bodies, medications, or accumulation of destructive enzymes cause necrosis of tissue that inflammation becomes a deterrent to healing. Therefore the author prefers to see the term "lag" phase replaced by strong emphasis on inflammation as an active part of the reparative process.

Approximately 12 hours after injury has occurred, and at a time when inflammation has been established, epithelial migration—the first clear-cut sign of rebuilding—occurs. In a primary wound, epithelization is complete in a few hours; in a secondary healing wound, migration of cells is rapid at first, but as the line of cells from the wound margin becomes extended and the epithelial probe dwindles to a monolayer, progress becomes slower, so that days or even weeks elapse before epithelization is complete. After 4 or 5 days, however, epithelization is assisted as the machinery of wound contraction begins, and the wound margins begin central movement.

A great amount of activity takes place in the center of the wound after a scar or eschar has been removed and before epithelium has covered the surface. Grossly, the surface which was once gray or yellow-brown and smooth becomes bright red and granular. The reason for this is an extravagant proliferation of richly perfused capillary loops. The knuckles or loops of blood vessels impart a granular appearance to the surface, and it is because of them that the wound is often described as granulating or showing granulation tissue. Granulation tissue provides a good defense against invasion by surface contaminants, but it is fragile and produces a difficult terrain for advancing epithelial cells. This is particularly true if surface infection, edema, or deep fibrous tissue interferes with return circulation. When this happens, the fiery red granular dots will change to a purple, soggy, gray-black cluster which may fill the entire wound cavity and spill over the wound edge, thus eliminating the possibility of epithelization.

Although no visible signs of collagen synthesis can be found until the fourth to sixth day, biochemical evidence of collagen synthesis can be found between the second and fourth days. The level of hydroxyproline in wound tissue rises rapidly, and the saline-extractable-collagen level becomes elevated shortly thereafter. Before signs of collagen synthesis occur, the ground substance changes, as evidenced by accumulation of sulfated mucopolysaccharides and development of metachromasia. On or about the seventh day wounds will show a delicate fine reticulum of young collagen fibrils. Actually, the gelation which is occurring at this time is so random that polymerization of new collagen fibrils is much like that of a new gel in a laboratory beaker—without purposeful orientation or polarity. There is a short period when young fibrils and fibers take silver stains selectively, and it is thought that this property reflects the presence of large numbers of unsatisfied bonding sites; mature collagen fibers do not stain selectively with silver. As fibrogenesis proceeds, purposefully oriented fibers seem to become thicker, presumably because they are accruing more collagen particles; nonpurposefully oriented fibers seem to disappear. The overall effect appears to be one of lacing the wound edges together by a three-dimensional weave. In secondary wounds the mass of scar tissue becomes dense, compact, and smaller in circumference but shows little in the way of purposeful organization. The overall direction is one of replacing granulation tissue, allowing the surface to become covered with epithelium, and filling in the remaining skin defect with scar tissue after contraction is complete. As far as filling the defect is concerned, contraction is the major influence; it exerts full potential before scar-tissue synthesis is complete. The central scar seems to remodel itself to fill the defect after contraction is over. Thus wounds surrounded by mobile and redundant skin will have a small central scar, while wounds surrounded with tight nonmovable skin will have relatively large central scars regardless of the size of the defect.

Development of tensile strength (strength per unit of scar tissue) and burst strength (strength of the entire wound) are the results initially of blood vessels growing across the wound, epithelization, and aggregation of globular protein. Later, collagen synthesis is important. The effect of vascularization and epithelization, although relatively small, is adequate on the fifth day to hold wound edges, if not under excessive tension, coapted without sutures. The really significant gain in tensile strength begins about the fifth day, however, when collagen synthesis becomes apparent; tensile strength measurements in laboratory animals usually are recorded from that day. Increase in strength is rapid for 17 days and slow for an additional 10 days; there is an almost imperceptible gain in tensile strength for at least 2 years. In spite of the measurable increase in tensile strength for such a long period, strength of scar in rat skin never quite reaches that of unwounded skin.

Collagen content of the wound tissue rises rapidly between the sixth and the seventeenth days but increases very little after the seventeenth day and none at all after the forty-second day. Gain in strength after the seventeenth day, therefore, is due primarily to remodeling of collagen and, hence, is not correlated with total collagen content except for a very short portion of the healing curve.

When a normally healing wound is disrupted mechanically after the fifth day and immediately resutured, the return of tensile strength is so rapid that within 2 days the burst strength is nearly what it would have been had the secondary wound not occurred. This phenomenon, commonly called the *secondary healing effect,* has been studied intensely to determine the exact mechanism of rapid gain of tensile strength following a secondary wound. Curiously, it is neither more rapid collagen synthesis nor more rapid assembly of collagen subunits; secondary wounds contain slightly less collagen than primary wounds of the same age. Because the thermal shrinkage temperature of secondary wound collagen is significantly higher than that of primary wounds of the same age, it has been suggested that more effective cross linking or better physical weave of collagen subunits is responsible for the rapid gain in strength of secondary wounds. The recent demonstration by Madden and Smith that secondary healing is really nothing more than continued primary healing (without a lag phase) invalidates previous cross-linking theories of secondary wound healing. Whatever the explanation, however, the machinery for producing rapid gain in tensile strength in secondary wounds is limited to an area of 7 mm around the first wound. Excision of skin edges more than 7 mm circumferential to the primary wound results in secondary wound healing at the same rate as in a primary wound.

WOUND CARE

From a treatment standpoint, there are essentially two types of wounds: those which are characterized by loss of tissue and those in which no tissue has been lost. Lacerations are an example of wounds without tissue loss, and avulsions or burns are examples of wounds which, in addition to interruption of surface continuity, result in destruction of tissue. A question which must be answered for both is whether immediate closure can be done safely.

Whether the wound can be closed by suturing the edges together or a graft of some sort is required, a decision must be reached about whether closure can be immediate or should be delayed until the danger of infection is past.

The history of wound surgery is, in large measure, the history of military surgery, and the decision of many surgeons about whether to close a wound primarily or to delay closure is based on principles and practices developed in military hospitals. The tendency of many surgeons to set a certain number of hours after a wound is sustained as the time during which primary closure can be performed safely probably dates back to World War I and a study of wound bacteriology made in French military hospitals. In an attempt to determine the number of hours within which immediate wound closure would be safe and beyond which closure should be delayed, many wounds were cultured and the growth of bacteria measured. It was determined that about 12 hours after wounding, the number of colonies on the wound surface doubled; this was interpreted as meaning that debridement and wound closure were safe before 12 hours had elapsed but likely to be dangerous after that time. It is interesting to follow the effect of this study through subsequent years and to note the difficulties that surgeons have encountered in performing primary wound closure in any predetermined length of time. As a result, the time set for closure has been shortened to the point where it is sometimes recommended that wounds should not be closed more than 2 hours after injury. Obviously, there is no fixed length of time within which primary closure is always safe and beyond which secondary closure must be done. The key to deciding when a wound should be closed is an understanding of the difference between contamination and infection; the trick to determining when one has become the other is the ability to recognize and interpret signs of inflammation. A contaminated wound can be converted by skillfully performed surgery into a clean wound which can then be closed safely; an infected wound cannot be surgically debrided without high risk of failure, including the potentially lethal complications of interfering with natural localizing processes. The history and physical examination contribute valuable information, because the length of time needed for contamination to become infection reflects, among other things, the strength of the bacterial inoculum and the ability of the substrate to combat invasion. A clean razor slice of highly vascular skin of the face might be closed safely 48 hours after injury, whereas a stable-floor-nail penetration of the foot of an elderly person might not be closed safely 1 minute after injury.

Once the decision has been made to close a laceration, the surrounding skin should be prepared with suitable antiseptic and local anesthetic injected. A guide to application of antiseptic is never to put anything in a wound that could not be tolerated comfortably in the conjunctival sac. Any caustic solution which is capable of sterilizing the surface of the skin will also destroy delicate cells on the surface of the wound. Therefore, harsh antiseptics should be applied only to the edge of a wound, never within it. Debridement of a wound can be done either hydrodynamically or mechanically. When the wound contains only surface contaminants not attached to wound tissues, a copious stream of saline solution will flush foreign bodies and undesirable organisms out of the wound cavity. When devitalized or contused tissue fragments are still attached to the wound tissues and external contaminants are partially driven into the tissues, however, surgical excision of affected tissues must be performed. When there is a redundancy of tissue and there are no important structures in the depth of the wound, such as nerve or tendon, the best type of debridement is excision of the entire wound to produce a new wound which is surgically clean. When there is a shortage of tissue or when a wound involves important structures which cannot be sacrificed without producing disability, damaged tissue must be carefully dissected until all dead tissue and extraneous material have been removed. In a wound of the hand involving numerous tendons and nerves, this type of debridement may be tedious and require several hours to perform.

After the wound has been debrided, proper suture materials must be selected for closure. There are two major types of sutures, absorbable and nonabsorbable, and selection of the proper suture should be based on what has been learned about the biology of the healing process. For the most part, absorbable sutures, which are made of sheep intestines or synthetic polymers, are used when infection is known to be present or when debridement has been difficult and thoroughness is in doubt.

Plain gut sutures will be solubilized by tissue collagenase in less than 10 days, while gut which has been tanned lightly with chromium salts will remain structurally intact for approximately 3 weeks. Absorbable sutures are usually not used when they can be avoided, because the reaction to a foreign animal protein is considerably greater than the reaction to such substances as cotton, silk, and nylon. Synthetic absorbable sutures may not be as locally irritating as animal proteins. Because the collagen-synthesis stage of wound healing is barely under way at 10 days and the scar tissue is far from mature even at 3 weeks, a more permanent material may be needed. Chromic gut sutures produce less soft tissue reaction than plain gut sutures, possibly because more available cross-linking sites have been satisfied by the tanning agent.

Nonabsorbable sutures are usually preferable because they produce less tissue reaction and can remain permanently below the surface of the integument. The major disadvantage of permanent sutures is that if they are placed in areas where infection develops, the suture material can harbor organisms; hence infection will not subside until the sutures are removed. A nonabsorbable suture of steel or some alloy may be mechanically irritating, and sometimes an inflammatory reaction develops around nonabsorbable sutures which resembles a local allergic phenomenon. Sutures are placed in different types of tissue for different reasons; before selecting and placing a suture in a wound, one should ask these questions: What is the suture being asked to do? and How long does it need to do it? Sutures which are placed in tissues to hold wound edges together under tension should be placed in fibrous tissue. Sutures placed in cellular tissues such as fat, epidermis, liver, or kidney provide little structural strength, as they tend to cut through the tissues, which have no appreciable strength. Sutures in weak tissues usually are used to obliterate a potential cavity (dead space), provide hemostasis, or act as a fine-adjustment leveling device on the surface of the skin. Objectives for such sutures are met in a few hours, thus absorbable sutures can be used satisfactorily if they are desirable.

A typical facial wound involving skin, subcutaneous fat, fascia, and superficial muscle might be repaired in the following way: After local anesthesia has been administered, the skin prepared, contaminants flushed out with saline solution, and any dead fragments of tissue excised, closure is performed. The muscle, being primarily cellular, would not support a suture, so the fibrous tissue surrounding it is closed with a permanent suture of silk or cotton. If hemorrhage has been significant in the muscle, a separate suture or ligature may be used to control it. If the skin is closed in a single layer, the retracted subcutaneous fat might not come together completely, thus producing a cavity which would become filled with blood and possibly infected. Another loosely tied stitch, which has no strength because it does not pass through fibrous tissue, may be utilized to obliterate a subcutaneous cavity and discourage hemorrhage. After the subcutaneous tissue has been closed, a decision should be made about the desired final appearance of the surface scar. The width of the wound following closure of the subcutaneous tissue will be a good indicator of how wide the final cutaneous scar will be if the next sutures merely approximate the skin edges and are tied on the outside. The reason is that, if suture marks are to be avoided, silk sutures should be removed in 6 to 8 days because of development of inflammatory reaction, epithelial lined tracts, or small stitch abscesses. Although the wound edges may be accurately coapted with only a hairline scar at the time that such sutures are removed, the wound is held together only by epithelium, blood vessels, and globular protein. Even though it usually will not dehisce before collagen production takes over, the scar will stretch and widen during the ensuing 21 days while collagen formation and remodeling are occurring. The result usually is that a 7-day-old 1-mm-wide scar may become a 1-cm-wide scar 3 weeks after the sutures have been removed. One way to reduce widening of a scar after skin sutures are removed is to place permanent sutures in the fibrous protein layers of the skin to bring the edges together. This is accomplished by a subcuticular or intradermal suture of fine silk or cotton. The overlying epidermis is gently retracted, and sutures are placed in the lower part of the dermis. The knot is sometimes placed deep in subcutaneous tissue but can be tied superficially provided that the ends of the suture are cut close and the knot and suture ends are covered by overlying epithelium. It is important to use a very fine suture that will not be palpable beneath the epithelium and a clear or light-colored suture material that will not show through translucent epithelium. It has been shown recently that permanent subcuticular sutures will not eliminate completely secondary widening of a scar; such sutures will reduce the extent of transverse remodeling in many wounds, however.

After subcuticular sutures have been placed, the skin edges will be as close together as it is possible to bring them, yet the overlying epithelial edges may be vertically uneven. A final row of sutures of fine silk or nylon which serve as a fine adjustment or leveler of the epithelial edges is frequently utilized to produce an even surface. Because these sutures are in cellular tissue, they contribute little to the strength of the wound and should not be placed more than 1 mm away from the wound edge. They should be tied loosely and removed before any epithelial reaction develops. Actually, external sutures in a wound closed in this manner probably can be removed in a few hours or as soon as the plasma clot seals the epithelial edges. For practical purposes, however, they are not removed until the first dressing, whenever that may be. In recent years the use of external cutaneous sutures has been partially eliminated by the development of various types of adhesive strips which can be used to hold skin edges together without producing epithelial sinuses or reaction.

When do you remove stitches? is a question frequently asked of surgeons. The answer is simple: when they have done the job they were put in to do, namely, hold the wound edges together until adequate tensile strength has developed. To set a finite period of time for removal of sutures is to imply that wounds heal at a standard rate; but the rate of healing is variable even in different parts of the body and under different conditions in a single individual. Instead of counting days until sutures can be removed, the wound must be examined; sometimes one or two sutures must be removed to see if the skin edges are sufficiently adherent to permit removal of all sutures. In wounds where a narrow scar is important and where some tension is unavoidable, it is advisable to splint the immature scar with adhesive strips for 2 or 3 weeks or until new collagen has attained sufficient strength and reliability.

The appearance of a linear scar is frequently worse between the third and fifth weeks after wound closure than it is at the time sutures are removed. The irregular, raised, purplish appearance of immature scar tissue can be a cause of great concern to young patients. Resorption of excess collagen, development of pliability, and the fading of undesirable color are called *maturation* of the scar, and maturation occurs more rapidly in older people than in the young. Children and teen-age patients, particularly, may have a distressing amount of red color in scars for several years. This condition is temporary, however, and redness should not be an indication for secondary surgical revision.

Scars should be revised secondarily only after they have undergone maximum maturation. Beefy, red, hypertrophic, immature scars usually recur after excision, and it is often amazing how much natural improvement will occur if sufficient time is allowed. It is seldom wise to attempt surgical improvement of a scar in less than 6 months; often natural improvement will continue for as long as 12 months.

Secondary revision should not be performed with the idea of changing the color of a scar or with the idea that a scar can be eliminated completely. All that secondary revision can accomplish is to take out a scar which resulted from unskilled closure or closure under unsatisfactory conditions and to close the defect as skillfully as possible under optimal conditions. Leveling uneven edges, changing the direction so that the scar does not cross lines of changing dimensions, and supporting a wide scar by the use of meticulously placed subcuticular sutures are the main improvements which can be accomplished. If scar tissue is elevated slightly above the level of surrounding skin, abrasion of that area by sandpaper or rotating brush will produce a smooth denuded surface over which new epithelium will spread in a more even sheet.

Wounds characterized by a loss of skin can be allowed to heal by contraction and epithelization if there is sufficient skin to be stretched across the defect. This is usually permitted only when infection prevents primary closure and when contraction does not produce a contracture which would interfere with function or produce a cosmetically unacceptable scar. In all other wounds, a skin graft should be performed to replace the skin which has been lost.

At the moment, there is no known catalyst to speed up wound healing; about all that a physician can do to aid normal healing is to protect the wound from physical, chemical, or bacteriologic complications which retard or prevent healing. One useful exception to this statement is the utilization of topical vitamin A to correct inhibition of epithelization caused by cortisone therapy. Vitamin A does not accelerate epithelization over normal expectation, it only corrects inhibition of epithelization caused by a specific drug effect. Protection usually means the use of an artificial dressing unless a natural dressing material, such as an eschar or scab, can serve the same purpose. Once the scab or eschar deteriorates, however, it, like any other dressing material, must be changed (debrided), and either definitive coverage provided or an artificial dressing applied. As in the selection of suture materials, choosing dressing materials involves a clear understanding of the objectives of each component of the dressing and the fundamental biologic processes that the dressing is supposed to protect. The first layer of a dressing is usually made of fine-mesh gauze, so that granulation tissue will not penetrate the interstices and cause hemorrhage when the dressing is removed. A long search for a pharmacologic substance to incorporate in the gauze to stimulate epithelial growth has been unsuccessful so far. Because certain by-products of the azo dye industry are carcinogenic, it was hoped that related dyes such as scarlet red might offer epithelial stimulation without being carcinogenic. All such substances have been disappointing, however, although most surgeons do use a gauze impregnated with some bland substance such as petroleum jelly or topical antibiotic in a water-soluble base. The main value of such medicated dressings is that there is less adherence of epithelium and vascular tissue to the dressing, hence less interference with wound healing when the dressing is changed. Dry gauze is a perfectly satisfactory dressing for most wound surfaces, however, and when carefully applied and removed, it can be as atraumatic as any other material. The usual coarse 4 × 4 hospital gauze sponge with its cotton-filled center is not a good material to place against open wounds; the interstices permit permeation by vascular tissue, and the cotton lint which is included becomes embedded in the wound. Sponges, mechanics' waste, cotton, and the like are used to give bulk to a dressing after the fine-mesh gauze has been applied to make the dressing conform to a desired shape and immobilize the wounded part. Nonstretchable, firm, roller gauze bandage and adhesive tape are used to complete the dressing in a typical occlusive (erroneously called "pressure") type of dressing. The nonstretchable gauze and adhesive tape provide a compact and stable immobilizing influence. A clean wound has very little drainage and no odor, and does not have to be dressed very often.

Infected wounds have considerable drainage and odor and, therefore, must be dressed often to provide suitable drainage and tolerable appearance. It is common practice to use a wet dressing on infected wounds, which means that the inside layers of the dressing are intentionally moistened with saline solution or some other substance. The realization that there is no catalytic effect upon healing or any control of infection from water and that maceration of skin or eschar produces favorable conditions for bacterial or fungus growth throws doubt upon the beneficial effects to be obtained by applying a wet dressing. The usual answer is that drainage is increased by capillary action or that debridement is accomplished as detritus sticks to the dressing. Such reasoning has never seemed logical to the author; a dry dressing will absorb more wound drainage than a saturated one, and debridement can usually be accomplished more efficiently by mechanical means. It often appears that wounds become cleaner more quickly with the use of wet dressings, but in the author's experience this is partly because wet dressings are changed more often. Of course, less pain may be associated with wet-dressing changes than with dry-dressing changes. However, when dry dressings are changed frequently and skillfully, surface detritus may be removed more effectively by dry dressings than by wet ones. One sound reason for using a wet dressing, however, is that wet heat is more penetrating than dry heat, and when additional warmth is desirable to increase the local inflammatory response, a warm moist dressing is effective. Failure to keep a moist dressing warm by the addition of external heat, however, results in a cold soggy dressing which has no particular virtue and which is definitely inferior to a frequently changed dry one.

SKIN GRAFTS

Skin grafts are classified as free grafts (meaning that they are separated completely from their donor sites before being transferred to recipient areas) and pedicle grafts (which maintain a vascular connection with the general circulation). Free grafts are full-thickness (which means that the entire thickness of the skin, including epidermis and dermis, is transferred) and split-thickness (which means that the entire epidermis and only a portion of the dermis are transferred). The remainder of the dermis after split-thickness skin grafting remains at the donor site.

The "take" of a free graft refers to the pink appearance of a graft which occurs between the third and fifth days after transfer, signifying that vascular connections have developed between the recipient bed and the transplant. Before this time, free grafts are white, unless microvascular surgery has provided instantaneous restoration of circulation, and do not show any change in color when pressed upon and released. It is a matter of considerable conjecture whether there is any diffusion of gases and nutrients between cells of the graft and underlying capillaries prior to development of actual vascular connections, and it has been assumed in the past that diffusion was necessary to keep cells nourished during the first few days. When grafts which include more than full thickness of the skin do not survive as free transplants, or when split-thickness grafts with pus or blood interposed between graft and capillary bed do not survive, it has been considered that diffusion could not occur through fat, pus, blood, etc. It seems more likely now, however, that diffusion is not important in the take of a graft and that mechanical barriers such as pus, blood, or fat prevent the take of a free graft by preventing vascular connections from occurring. Whatever the reason, the thicker the graft, the more likely will be the failure of take if mechanical or inflammatory conditions at the graft-wound interface are less than optimal. For this reason, thin grafts are used to cover less than ideally prepared wounds; full-thickness grafts are reserved for surgically produced wounds under optimal conditions.

In taking a full-thickness skin graft the surgeon will produce a wound which will have to be closed by suturing the edges together or by applying a split-thickness skin graft from another donor site. If this is not done, closing of the wound in one area with the graft will leave a wound of the same size and shape at the donor site. Full-thickness grafts are usually small grafts which can be taken from a place where there is an excess of thin skin, such as the inframammary fold or the groin, where the donor site can be closed by suturing the skin edges together.

It was once thought that split-thickness skin grafts must be taken through the level of the dermal-epidermal undulating interface so that small islands of stratum germinativum cells would remain to reepithelize the denuded surface. Because of this notion, surgeons were careful to take grafts as thin as possible, and the taking of a split-thickness skin graft was relegated to only a few highly skilled individuals (Fig. 8-7). It seems obvious now that if it were possible to take a graft through only the epithelium, a satisfactory take would be unlikely. Most of the cells would be dead, and the covered wound would be resurfaced by cells which would provide no better coverage than that which would have occurred from normal epithelization. The qualities of skin other than waterproofing (strength, flexibility, appearance, etc.) which are desired in a graft are qualities provided by the dermis. The final appearance of both the recipient and donor sites, therefore, reflects the amount of dermis which has been transferred and the amount of dermis which is left behind. Epithelial cells migrate out of deeply located glands and hair follicles, and donor sites which do not extend through the entire depth of the dermis will be reepithelized from these sources. Dermis, being a complex organ and not a simple tissue, does not regenerate, however, and if all the prop-

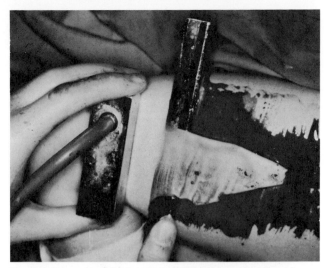

Fig. 8-7. Removal of thick split-thickness skin graft with a free-hand knife. The largest possible grafts can be taken by this method.

erties of normal dermis are desired in the recipient area, full-thickness dermis must be transferred; if less than the full thickness is transferred, the resulting graft will be abnormal in appearance and function.

In choosing the thickness of a free skin graft, qualities which are desired in the recipient area must be balanced against cost incurred in the donor site. How such factors influence selection of graft thickness can be illustrated by comparing two extremes in wound and donor-site conditions. In a large thermal burn, the recipient area is not optimal in that it is usually infected and edematous and involves a large area. The take of a graft is therefore uncertain, and revascularization is problematic. From the standpoint of the donor site, it may be necessary to procure several grafts from the same area to obtain enough skin for the entire wound; thus rapid healing, with a remaining dermis thick enough for subsequent grafts to be taken, is mandatory. In this case, both donor-site and recipient conditions require thin grafts. In contrast, a 2-cm-diameter wound caused by loss of skin from the cheek of a young person presents an entirely different set of requirements for an optimal graft. The recipient bed should be optimal if excised immediately or prepared later in the operating room. The need for full-thickness dermis is mandatory so that normal texture, color, and thickness will produce the most cosmetically acceptable result. The graft is small, so a variety of areas with a 2-cm redundancy of skin can be found for a donor site. Thus all factors point to the selection of a full-thickness graft. In other wounds the choice may not be quite so clear, but the principles involved in these two cases are the factors which must be considered in selection of any free graft (Fig. 8-8A and B).

Split-thickness skin grafts have a tendency to develop deep pigmentation after transfer. The thinner the graft, the more pronounced is postoperative pigmentation for 6 to 9 months following transfer. It is important to warn patients who have recently had split-thickness skin grafts placed on exposed areas of the body that protection from

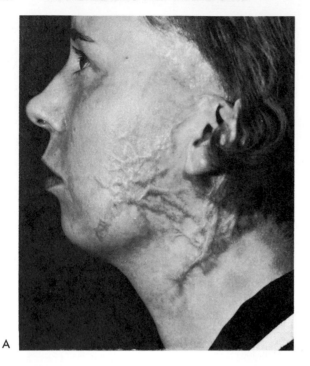

A

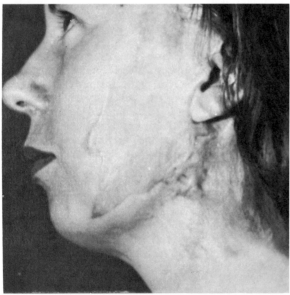

B

Fig. 8-8. *A.* Hypertrophic scar produced by deep second-degree burn. Although a significant amount of full-thickness skin has not been lost, overproduction of collagen has produced an unsightly scar. *B.* Patient shown in Fig. 8-8*A* following excision of facial portion of scar and application of a thick split-thickness skin graft. Cervical portion of scar will be resurfaced later. A single graft covering facial and cervical areas would obliterate submandibular groove. Note that scar at junction of graft and skin is most prominent near angle of mouth where motion and tension are unavoidable. Although different in texture, hue, and thickness from normal skin, the graft provides a smooth surface over which cosmetics can be applied more effectively than over previous scar.

solar radiation is mandatory for at least 6 months. Thick grafts have less tendency to develop undesirable pigment, and they will usually blend into their new surroundings more quickly than thin ones.

Finally, a word should be said about the concept of the "dressing graft." Split-thickness skin is the best possible dressing material for an open wound, and failure of many surgeons to take advantage of this fact in treating complicated wounds is usually based on the mistaken notion that placing a split-thickness skin graft on a wound is tantamount to closing the wound. Although the possibility that some portion or all of the graft may take and thus close the wound is the main advantage in using split-thickness skin grafts as a dressing material, placing the graft on a wound of questionable suitability for closure does not in itself produce a closed wound in the same manner as suturing two full-thickness skin edges together. Actually, a skin dressing does not close the wound any more than a petroleum jelly gauze dressing. If the wound has been inadequately debrided or infection is not yet controlled, the graft will slough in a few days and may disappear by the time of the first dressing. In such instances nothing will have been lost except a few square centimeters of split-thickness skin from the donor area. Dressing a questionable wound of relatively small size with split-thickness skin, therefore, is a sort of biologic test to determine suitability for closure, as well as providing some benefit if even a part of the graft survives. Xenografts of porcine skin and human allografts of split-thickness skin are useful also as biologic dressings and seem to improve various aspects of the healing process. Such grafts should be removed before take occurs and often are changed several times before optimum conditions for autograft application are obtained.

When more than the skin has been lost, and the skin plus some other tissue such as fat, tendon, muscle, or nerve must be replaced to restore function and appearance, transfer of skin by pedicle flap or direct vascular anastomosis is required (Fig. 8-9). As the name implies, pedicle transfers maintain vascular connection with the host, so that interruption of the capillary circulation never occurs. The vessels which are most important during transfer of tissue are the vessels in the subdermal plexus. These vessels are relatively large, frequently longitudinally oriented, and found on the undersurface of the dermis between it and the subcutaneous fat. One frequently hears that a pedicle flap has been made thicker than actually needed for cosmetic or functional purposes in order to provide a safe blood supply. Fat on the undersurface of a flap does not add any appreciable blood supply, and it may be removed safely to produce as thin a pedicle as needed, provided that surgical manipulation does not injure the important vessels lying on the undersurface of the dermis. The problem in transplanting tissue by the pedicle method is to design a pedicle so that the base is as narrow as possible in relation to the length needed to cover the deficient area. It becomes a matter of considerable judgment, therefore, to gauge the shape and dimensions of a flap so that blood supply through the intact pedicle will be adequate to nourish the distal end of the flap. A great deal depends upon the natural profuseness of vascular beds; thus it is possible to move a pedicle flap on the face or cervical region which is three times as long as it is wide, while it may not be possible (without performing preliminary procedures to increase the blood supply) to transfer a flap on the leg which is no longer than it is wide. The blood supply in the base of a contemplated flap can be improved by performing a procedure commonly referred to as delay of the flap. The principle of delay is to gradually reduce blood supply to small segments of the circumference of the flap and thus improve the remaining blood supply to the point where a pedicle which was of insufficient width before the flap was delayed becomes adequate to nourish the flap. The mechanism by which delay (gradual interruption of a portion of the blood supply to a flap) improves the circulation in the base is not completely clear. It seems doubtful that new blood vessels actually grow into the area, although casual observation of changes in the vessels at the base suggests that this is what may happen. The rapidity with which delay improves the circulation strongly suggests, however, that the release of various amines, probably in response to changes in pH secondary to increased anaerobic metabolism, causes a closure of normally open shunts that prevent perfusion of the entire capillary network. The effect is a substantial hyperemia at the base of the flap; over a period of several weeks and after several delaying procedures, the vessels in the pedicle base become racemose in appearance, and the amount of blood flow is increased to the extent that a relatively long flap can be transferred on a narrow pedicle. Following transfer of the flap, circulation must be observed carefully for the first 48 hours, as signs of impending circulatory embarrassment occur before irreversible thrombosis and cell death. It is not unusual for the distal end of a flap to be dusky following transfer; venous spasm secondary to the trauma of rotation may be all that is involved. Improvement usually occurs in a few hours, but during this time the danger of a venous thrombosis is increased; if there is any progression of cyanosis and edema, the possibility that tension on veins is interfering with return circulation must be investigated by removing a few sutures. Perhaps the most serious, but still reversible, sign of impending venous thrombosis is the development of a sharp line of color differentiation. A gradual change from normal pink to slight cyanosis is not so significant as a clear-cut line demarcating the area of circulatory deficiency from normal circulation. Even if all the sutures have to be removed and the flap returned to its original bed, the sign must be attended to, or an irreversible demarcation will soon develop, signifying complete thrombosis and certain distal necrosis. In sensibly planned and adequately prepared flaps, one does not have to be particularly concerned about arterial insufficiency; venous drainage is the function in which complications develop. Complications usually are the result of too much tension, poor dressing, hematoma, or infection. The use of heparin and low-molecular-weight dextran have seemed to be beneficial in dangerously compromised circulation. Hyperbaric oxygenation has been reported instrumental in saving flaps of laboratory animals, but is not practical for managing human flaps.

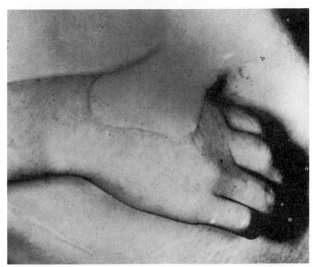

Fig. 8-9. Abdominal pedicle flap applied to dorsum of hand. Scar on hand has been turned back to resurface the raw side of pedicle and a portion of the donor site. Flap will be separated from the abdominal wall in 18 days.

Advancement flaps and rotation flaps are the simplest pedicle transfers. These are dependent upon a redundancy of soft tissue adjacent to a defect so that the donor defect can be closed by approximating the skin edges or applying split-thickness skin grafts. More complicated flaps require the use of an arm as a carrier to provide circulation during the period that skin is detached from the original donor site, such as abdominal wall, and transferred to a distant site, such as the lower leg. Because of similarity of tissue characteristics, safety in transfer, and expense and time involved, it is desirable to design flaps as close to the point where they are needed as possible. Widespread interest, perfecting of instruments and visual aids, and perfecting of technical procedures have made transfer of composite tissue grafts by direct small blood vessel anastomosis possible during recent years. As more experience is gained, microvascular anastomosis will circumvent the need for delays and carrier procedures in many patients.

One of the most sophisticated flaps is an island pedicle flap (Fig. 8-10), which combines the pedicle principle of intact blood and nerve supply with some of the advantages of a free graft. The principle of the island pedicle is that careful dissection of the artery and vein (and sometimes the nerve) to a piece of skin can be performed so that the skin is detached from surrounding skin and remains attached to the body only by essentials for survival—an artery, a vein, and sometimes a nerve. Depending on the length of these structures, it is possible to move a full-thickness skin and fat graft, or an intact finger, or a portion of a finger or toe, a surprising distance. Transfer of hair-bearing portions of the scalp on a temporal artery-and-vein supported flap to the supraorbital region for eyebrow reconstruction and transfer of a finger to replace a missing thumb are examples of island pedicle transfers which are useful.

Finally, it should be pointed out that, in the opinion

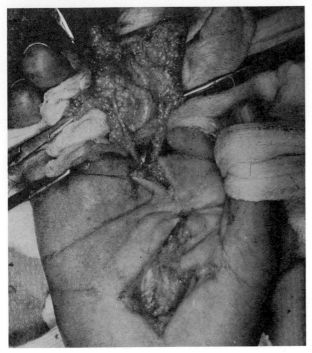

Fig. 8-10. Island pedicle flap developed during amputation of long finger. The flap is nourished by a single digital artery and nerve. Sensation is preserved by including a digital nerve in the vascular pedicle.

of many, maturity in restorative surgery can be measured, in part, by how often one thinks of a pedicle flap as the only means of rebuilding a damaged area and then devises a way to make a free graft do as well. Pedicles are dramatic, particularly as used by military surgeons to rebuild enormous tissue defects caused by high-explosive wounds; fortunately, however, civilian injuries are not often so devastating, and the practical points of expense, length of time away from work, shortage of hospital facilities, and the like have to be considered in each case where a pedicle could be used. In addition, although areas such as the face may appear in photographs to have been superbly restored by massive flaps, yet it must be remembered that flaps have no dynamic function; they are expressionless, and often look better in photographs than they do as part of the constantly moving facial features. When a pedicle flap is needed, nothing else will suffice, and pedicles are an extremely valuable part of restorative surgery. The high cost of donor-site mutilation, length of time required for transfer, and adynamic features, however, make the pedicle flap definitely second choice to a free graft if a free graft can be used as well.

References

General

Dunphy, J. E., and Van Winkle, W.: "Repair and Regeneration: The Scientific Basis for Surgical Practice," McGraw-Hill Book Company, New York, 1968.

Madden, J. W.: Wound Healing: Biologic and Clinical Features, in Sabiston, D. (ed.), "Textbook of Surgery," 10th ed., p. 249, W. B. Saunders Company, Philadelphia, 1972.

Montagna, W., and Billingham, R. E.: Advances in Biology of Skin, vol. V, "Wound Healing," *Proc Brown Univ Symp Biol Skin, 1963,* The Macmillan Company, New York, and Pergamon Press, New York, 1964.

Patterson, W. B.: Wound Healing and Tissue Repair, *Dev Biol Conf Ser Rept, 1956,* The University of Chicago Press, Chicago, 1959.

Peacock, E. E., Jr.: Wound Healing and Care of the Wound, in "Manual of Preoperative and Postoperative Care, A.C.S.," p. 3, W. B. Saunders Company, Philadelphia, 1971.

————, and Van Winkle, W.: "Wound Repair," 2d ed., W. B. Saunders Company, Philadelphia, 1976.

Wound Contraction

Abercrombie, M., Flint, M. H., and James, D. W.: Wound Contraction in Relation to Collagen Formation in Scorbutic Guinea-Pigs, *J Embryol Exp Morphol,* **4:**167, 1956.

————, James, D. W., and Newcombe, J. F.: Wound Contraction in Rabbit Skin, Studied by Splinting the Wound Margins, *J Anat,* **94:**170, 1960.

Billingham, R. E., and Russel, P. S.: Studies on Wound Healing with Special Reference to the Phenomenon of Contracture in Experimental Wounds in Rabbit's Skin, *Ann Surg,* **144:**961, 1956.

Danes, B., and Leinfelder, P. J.: Cytological and Respiratory Effects of Cyanide on Tissue Cultures, *J Cell Comp Physiol,* **37:**427, 1951.

Grillo, H. C., and Gross, J.: Studies in Wound Healing: III. Contraction in Vitamin C Deficiency, *Proc Soc Exp Biol Med,* **101:**268, 1959.

————, Watts, G. T., and Gross, J.: Studies in Wound Healing. I. Contraction and Wound Contents, *Ann Surg,* **148:**145, 1958.

James, D. W.: Intussusceptive Growth of Skin Islands within Wounds, *J Anat,* **93:**161, 1959.

————, and Newcombe, J. F.: Granulation Tissue Resorption during Free and Limited Contraction of Skin Wounds, *J Anat,* **95:**247, 1961.

Madden, J. W., Carlson, E. E., and Hines, J.: Presence of Modified Fibroblasts in Ischemic Contracture of the Intrinsic Musculature of the Hand, *Surg Gynecol Obstet,* **140:**509, 1975.

————, Morton, D., Jr., and Peacock, E. E., Jr.: Contraction of Experimental Wounds. I. Inhibiting Wound Contraction by Using a Topical Smoothe Muscle Antagonist, *Surgery,* **76:**18, 1974.

Majno, G., Babbiani, G., Hirschel, B. J., Ryan, G. B., and Statkov, P. R.: Contraction of Granulation Tissue *in vitro:* Similarity with Smooth Muscle, *Science,* **173:**548, 1971.

Phillips, J. L., and Peacock, E. E.: Importance of Horizontal Plane Cell Mass Integrity in Wound Contraction, *Proc Soc Exp Biol Med,* **117:**539, 1964.

Ryan, G. B., Cliff, W. J., Gabbiani, G., Iole, C., Montandon, D., Statkov, P. R., and Majno, G.: Myofibroblasts in Human Granulation Tissue, *Hum Pathol,* **5:**55, 1974.

Van den Brenk, H. A. S.: Studies in Restorative Growth Process in Mammalian Wound Healing, *Brit Surg,* **43:**525, 1956.

Watts, G. T., Grillo, H. C., and Gross, J.: Studies in Wound Healing: II. The Role of Granulation Tissue in Contraction, *Ann Surg,* **148:**153, 1958.

Epithelization

Abercrombie, M.: The Control of Growth and the Cell Surface, *Lect Sci Basis Med,* **8**(1958–1959):19, 1960.

Arey, L. B., and Covode, W. M.: The Method of Repair in Epithelial Wounds of the Cornea, *Anat Rec* **86:**75, 1943.

Brophy, D., and Lobitz, W. C.: Injury and Reinjury to Human Epidermis: II. Epidermal Basal Cell Response, *J Invest Dermatol,* **32:**495, 1959.

Bullough, W. S.: Mitotic and Functional Homeostasis, *Cancer Res,* **25:**1683, 1965.

——— and Lawrence, E. B.: The Control of Epidermal Mitotic Activity in the Mouse, *Proc R Soc Land [Biol],* **B151:**517, 1960.

Coman, D. R.: Decreased Mutual Adhesiveness: A Property of Cells from Squamous Cell Carcinomas, *Cancer Res,* **4:**625, 1944.

Gelfant, S.: Initiation of Mitosis in Relation to the Cell Division Cycle, *Exp Cell Res,* **26:**395, 1959.

Gillman, T., and Penn, J.: Studies on the Repair of Cutaneous Wounds, *Med Proc,* **2**(Suppl. 3):121, 1956.

Lobitz, W. C.: The Histochemical Response to Controlled Injury, *J Invest Dermatol,* **22:**189, 1954.

Medawar, P. B.: Biological Aspects of the Repair Process, *Br Med Bull,* **3:**70, 1945.

Meyer, K., Hoffman, P., and Linker, A.: Chemistry of Ground Substances, in I. Page (ed.), "Connective Tissue, Thrombosis and Atherosclerosis," p. 181, Academic Press, New York, 1959.

Needham, A. E.: "Regeneration and Wound Healing," Methuen & Co., Ltd, London, 1952.

Pace, D. M., and Layon, M. E.: Effect of Cell Density on Growth in HeLa Cells, *Growth,* **24:**355, 1960.

Sullivan, D. J., and Epstein, W. S.: Mitotic Activity of Wounded Human Epidermis, *J Invest Dermatol,* **41:**39, 1963.

Weiss, P.: The Biological Foundations of Wound Repair, *Harvey Lect,* **(55)**(1959–1960):13, 1961.

Winter, G. D.: Formation of the Scab and the Rate of Epithelialization of Superficial Wounds in the Skin of the Young Domestic Pig, *Nature (Lond),* **193:**293, 1962.

Collagen

Allgower, M., and Hulliger, L.: Origin of Fibroblasts from Mononuclear Blood Cells: A Study of *in vitro* Formation of the Collagen Precursor, Hydroxyproline, in Buffy Coat Cultures, *Surgery,* **47:**603, 1960.

Bornstein, P.: Disorders of Connective Tissue Function and the Aging Process: A Synthesis and Review of Current Concepts and Findings, *Mech Ageing Dev,* **5:**305, 1976.

Cohen, I. K., Keiser, H. R., and Sjoerdsma, A.: Collagen Synthesis in Human Keloid and Hypertrophic Scar, *Surg Forum,* **22:**488, 1971.

Dayer, J., Russell, R. G., and Krane, S. M.: Collagenase Production by Rheumatoid Synovial Cells: Stimulation by a Human Lymphocyte Factor, *Science,* **195:**181, 1977.

Duskin, D., and Bornstein, P.: Impaired Conversion of Procollagen to Collagen by Fibroblasts and Bone Treated with Tunicamycin, an Inhibitor of Protein Glycosylation. *J Biol Chem,* **252:**955, 1977.

Gould, B. S.: Ascorbic Acid and Collagen Fiber Formation, *Vitam Horm,* **8:**89, 1960.

Grillo, H. C.: Origin of Fibroblasts in Wound Healing: An Autoradiographic Study of Inhibition of Cellular Proliferation by Local X-irradiation, *Ann Surg,* **157:**453, 1963.

Gross, J.: On the Significance of the Soluble Collagens, in I. H. Page (ed.), "Connective Tissue, Thrombosis and Atherosclerosis," pp. 77–95, Academic Press, Inc., New York, 1959.

———, Highberger, J. H., and Schmitt, F. O.: Extraction of Collagen from Connective Tissue by Neutral Salt Solutions, *Proc Natl Acad Sci USA,* **41:**1, 1955.

——— and Lapiere, C. M.: Collagenolytic Activity in Amphibian Tissues: A Tissue Culture Assay, *Proc Natl Acad Sci USA,* **48:**1014, 1962.

Hance, A. J., and Crystal, R. G.: The Connective Tissue of Lung, *Am Rev Respir Dis,* **112:**657, 1975.

Hoffmann, H., Olsen, B., Chen, H., and Prockop, D. J.: Segment-long-spacing Aggregates and Isolation of COOH-Terminal Peptides from Type I Procollagen, *Proc Natl Acad Sci USA,* **73:**4304, 1976.

Leven, C. I., and Gross, J.: Alterations in State of Molecular Aggregation of Collagen Induced in Chick Embryos by Aminopropionitrile (lathyrus factor), *J Exp Med,* **110:**771, 1959.

Madden, J. W., and Peacock, E. E.: Studies on the Biology of Collagen during Wound Healing: III. Dynamic Metabolism of Scar Collagen and Remodeling of Dermal Wounds, *Ann Surg,* **174:**511,1971.

———, and Smith, H. C.: Studies on the Biology of Collagen during Wound Healing: II. Rate of Collagen Synthesis and Deposition in Dehisced and Resutured Wounds, *Surg Gynecol Obstet,* **130:**487, 1970.

———: Some Aspects of Fibrogenesis during the Healing of Primary and Secondary Wounds, *Surg Gynecol Obstet,* **115:**408, 1962.

——— and Biggers, P. W.: Measurement and Significance of Heat-labile and Urea-sensitive Cross Linking Mechanisms in Collagen of Healing Wounds, *Surgery,* **54:**144, 1963.

Miller, E. S.: Biochemical Characteristics and Biological Significance of the Genetically-Distinct Collagens, *Mol Cell Biochem,* **13:**165, 1976.

Olsen, B., Hoffmann, H., and Prockop, D. J.: Interchain Disulfide Bonds at the COOH-Terminal End of Procollagen Synthesized by Matrix-free Cells from Chick Embryonic Tendon and Cartilage, *Arch Biochem Biophys,* **175:**341, 1976.

Prockop, D. J., Peterkofsky, B., and Udenfriend, S.: Studies on the Intracellular Localization of Collagen Synthesis in the Intact Chick Embryo, *J Biol Chem,* **237:**1581, 1962.

Raju, D. R., Jindrak, K., Weiner, M., and Enquist, I.: A Study of the Critical Bacterial Inoculum to Cause a Stimulus to Wound Healing, *Surg Gynecol Obstet,* **144:**347, 1977.

Riley, W. B., Jr., and Peacock, E. E., Jr.: Identification, Distribution, and Significance of a Collagenolytic Enzyme in Human Tissue, *Proc Soc Biol Med,* **214:**207, 1967.

Ross, R., and Benditt, E. P.: Wound Healing and Collagen Formation: I. Sequential Changes in Components of Guinea Pig Wounds Observed in the Electron Microscope, *J Biophys Biochem Cytol,* **11:**677, 1961.

——— and ———: Wound Healing and Collagen Formation: III. A Quantitative Autoradiographic Study of the Utilization of Proline H³ in Wounds from Normal and Scorbutic Guinea Pigs, *J Cell Biol,* **15:**99, 1962.

Schiffman, E., and Martin, G. R.: Spontaneous Generation of Cross-Links in Aldehyde Containing Collagen, *Arch Biochem,* **138:**226, 1970.

Trelstad, R. L., Kimiko, H., and Gross, J.: Collagen Fibrillogenesis Intermediate Aggregates and Suprafibrillar Order, *Proc Natl Acad Sci USA,* **73:**4027, 1976.

Woessner, J. F.: Catabolism of Collagen and Non-collagen Protein in the Rat Uterus during Post-partum Involution, *Biochem J,* **83:**304, 1962.

Chapter 9

Oncology

by Donald L. Morton, Frank C. Sparks, and Charles M. Haskell

INTRODUCTION

Oncology (from the Greek *onkos,* mass, or tumor, and *logos,* study) is the study of neoplastic diseases. Neoplasms are an altered cell population characterized by an excessive, nonuseful proliferation of cells that have become unresponsive to normal control mechanisms and to the organizing influences of adjacent tissues. Malignant neoplasms are composed of cancer cells that exhibit uncontrolled proliferation and impair the function of normal organs by local tissue invasion and metastatic spread to distant anatomic sites. Benign neoplasms are composed of normal-appearing cells that are not locally invasive, or characterized by metastatic spread.

Cancer has plagued man since antiquity, and many of its clinical manifestations were described by Hippocrates (460–375 B.C.). Neoplasms have been identified in all species of animals including the lower vertebrates, such as amphibia and fish. The wide distribution of neoplasia in natural and human history suggests that cancer may be common to all multicellular organisms.

Neoplastic disease is the second most frequent cause of death in the United States. The magnitude of the cancer problem is exemplified by the fact that one of every four persons living today has or will develop cancer. An estimated 54 million Americans, one in four presently alive in the United States, will develop cancer sometime during their lifetime. Approximately one-third of those who get cancer will survive for at least 5 years after treatment. Until recently those facts caused many physicians and surgeons to approach the cancer patient with feelings of pessimism and despair that frequently interfered with adequate therapy. This aversion to the problems of cancer was reflected by the paucity of physicians willing to devote full time to its clinical studies. Furthermore, basic scientists were somewhat hesitant to investigate fundamental problems posed by the malignant state.

Fortunately, recent exciting developments in tumor immunology, viral oncology, and molecular biology and advances in the therapy of some neoplasms have led to a rebirth of interest in the basic biologic and clinical problems posed by cancer. The United States government has launched a massive Conquest of Cancer Program for cancer research. Specialty boards have been established in medical oncology and gynecologic oncology. A wide variety of scientists from many disciplines have been attracted to its study. As a result, it is probable that more advances will be made in cancer therapy during the next 10 years than in all previous times. This chapter is designed to introduce the student to general principles that can be used as the basis for acquiring further knowledge in this rapidly growing field.

EPIDEMIOLOGY

The changes in death rates caused by cancer by body site for males and females in the United States during the past 45 years are summarized in Figs. 9-1 and 9-2. Although there has been a decrease in mortality from certain neoplasms, the overall cancer death rates continue to show a slow, steady increase.

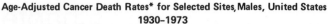

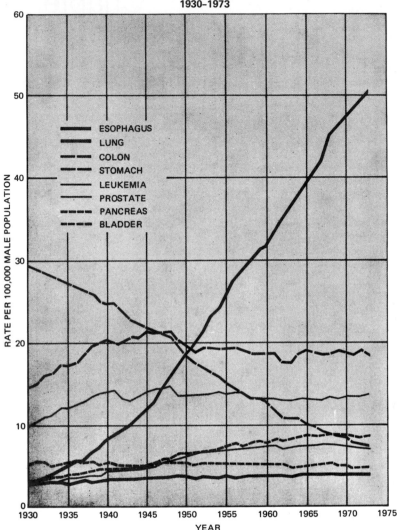

Fig. 9-1. Male cancer death rates by site, United States, 1930–1973 (standardized for age on the 1940 United States population). (*From National Vital Statistics Division and Bureau of the Census, United States.*)

Sources: U.S. National Center for Health Statistics and U.S. Bureau of the Census.
*Standardized on the age distribution of the 1940 U.S. Census Population.

The mortality rates from lung cancer have increased steadily and probably represent the most dramatic change for any cancer site. Compared with 40 years ago, the mortality is now eighteen times greater for men and six times greater for women. Lung cancer represents the leading cause of cancer death when both sexes are considered.

Pancreatic cancer death rates also have steadily increased through the years. Today, the rates are twice what they were in women and three times that in men when compared to 1930.

There has been a striking reduction during the past 40 years in death rates caused by cancers of the stomach and uterus. The stomach cancer death rate is now less than one-third the 1930 rate in men and less than one-fourth the 1930 rate in women, although there has been little improvement in the survival rates of stomach cancer. The

decreasing mortality is due to a decreased incidence of stomach cancer in both sexes. The reason for this declining incidence is unknown.

There has been a similar striking decline in death rates due to uterine cancer with mortality rates today only one-third what they were 40 years ago. In this case, the causes of the reduction are known to be earlier detection and improved treatment for cancer of the uterine cervix and corpus.

The incidences of cancer in different sites and the mortality rate in each sex are compared in Fig. 9-3. The sites most frequently causing cancer death in males, in order of decreasing frequency, are (1) lung, (2) colon and rectum, (3) prostate, (4) pancreas, and (5) stomach. The sites, in order of decreasing frequency in females, are (1) breast, (2) colon and rectum, (3) uterus, (4) lung, and (5) ovary.

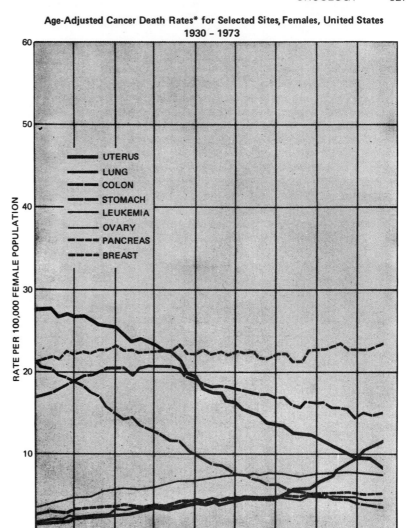

Age-Adjusted Cancer Death Rates* for Selected Sites, Females, United States 1930 – 1973

Fig. 9-2. Female cancer death rates by site, United States, 1930–1973 (standardized for age on the 1940 United States population). (*From National Vital Statistics Division and Bureau of the Census, United States.*)

Sources: U.S. National Center for Health Statistics and U.S. Bureau of the Census.
*Standardized on the age distribution of the 1940 U.S. Census Population.

It is obvious that there are differing incidences of kinds of cancer occurring in the male and female.

The incidence of various types of neoplasms differs from the death rates for the same neoplasms (Fig. 9-4) because different forms of cancer are not equally lethal. The most significant 5-year survival rates are achieved in patients with cancer of the skin (94 percent) and uterus (70 percent); the lowest survival occurs in patients with lung cancer (9 percent). Lung cancer is the leading cause of cancer death even though skin cancer occurs more commonly.

Females tend to have a greater number of 5-year survivals with cancers of any given primary site than males, although the reasons are unknown at this time. The overall 5-year survival for women with cancer is 50 percent, compared with only 31 percent for men. The overall 5-year cancer survival rates for common malignant tumors of selected sites are shown in Fig. 9-5.

ETIOLOGY

The primary etiologic factors responsible for most neoplasms in man are still unknown. In experimental animals, a wide variety of causative agents have been identified. These agents may be classified as chemical and physical, viral and genetic. There is no reason to doubt that a similar variety of factors is responsible for causing human cancer. Although the primary mechanisms by which these agents cause neoplastic transformation is unknown, it seems relatively certain that the inciting agents represent but one link in the chain of factors that leads to the development of

1977 ESTIMATES

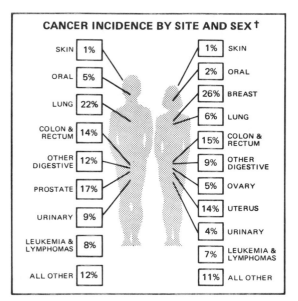

CANCER INCIDENCE BY SITE AND SEX †

	Male		Female	
SKIN	1%	1%	SKIN
ORAL	5%	2%	ORAL
		26%	BREAST
LUNG	22%	6%	LUNG
COLON & RECTUM	14%	15%	COLON & RECTUM
OTHER DIGESTIVE	12%	9%	OTHER DIGESTIVE
PROSTATE	17%	5%	OVARY
		14%	UTERUS
URINARY	9%	4%	URINARY
LEUKEMIA & LYMPHOMAS	8%	7%	LEUKEMIA & LYMPHOMAS
ALL OTHER	12%	11%	ALL OTHER

† Excluding non-melanoma skin cancer and carcinoma in situ of uterine cervix.

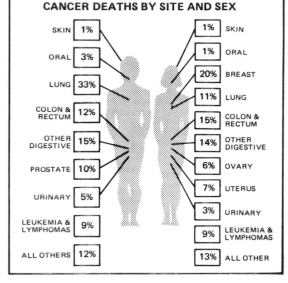

CANCER DEATHS BY SITE AND SEX

	Male		Female	
SKIN	1%	1%	SKIN
ORAL	3%	1%	ORAL
		20%	BREAST
LUNG	33%	11%	LUNG
COLON & RECTUM	12%	15%	COLON & RECTUM
OTHER DIGESTIVE	15%	14%	OTHER DIGESTIVE
PROSTATE	10%	6%	OVARY
		7%	UTERUS
URINARY	5%	3%	URINARY
LEUKEMIA & LYMPHOMAS	9%	9%	LEUKEMIA & LYMPHOMAS
ALL OTHERS	12%	13%	ALL OTHER

Fig. 9-3. Estimated cancer incidence and resultant deaths by site and sex. Incidence for major sites = 391,000 and deaths = 213,000. If carcinoma in situ is included in cancer of the uterus, incidence = 87,000; if nonmelanoma is included, incidence for skin = 300,000. (*From National Cancer Institute, Third National Cancer Survey, 1969–71.*)

cancer. Therefore, the identification of carcinogenic agents, although their mechanisms of action are unknown, can be extremely important in cancer prevention.

CHEMICAL CARCINOGENS. The first cause-and-effect relation between a carcinogenic stimulus and the development of cancer in man was described by Percival Pott, an English surgeon, in 1775, when he described a cancer of the scrotum frequently occurring in the chimney sweeps. However, Yamagiwa and Ichikawa, working from 1915 to 1918, identified the carcinogen when they experimentally produced cancers by painting the ears of rabbits with coal tar. Kennaway and Cook in studies from 1924 to 1932, demonstrated that pure hydrocarbons, such as 1, 2-dibenzanthracene and similar compounds isolated from coal tar,

were carcinogenic agents. Subsequently, a variety of chemical agents have been found that are capable of inducing neoplasms in experimental animals and in man. These chemicals are called *carcinogens*. There may be many years separating the time of exposure to a carcinogen and subse-

Fig. 9-4. *A.* Cancer death rates by sex, United States, 1900–1968 (standardized for age on the 1940 United States population). *B.* Forecast of cancer deaths based on present trends. (*From National Vital Statistics Division and Bureau of the Census, United States.*)

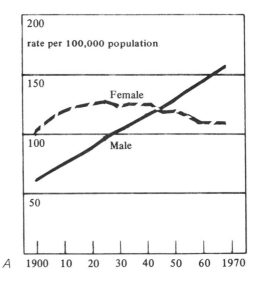

A

200

rate per 100,000 population

150 — Female

100 — Male

50

1900 10 20 30 40 50 60 1970

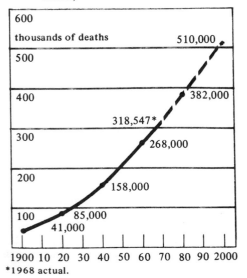

B

600

thousands of deaths   510,000

500

400   382,000

318,547*

300   268,000

200   158,000

100   85,000
    41,000

1900 10 20 30 40 50 60 70 80 90 2000

*1968 actual.

quent development of a neoplasm. Consequently, the present-day evaluation of the safety of food additives or other products for human consumption that are chronically ingested over long periods of time is a most difficult task.

A variety of chemicals which have been associated with different types of human neoplasms are summarized in Table 9-1. Aromatic amines are known to cause tumors of the urinary tract; workers in the dye industry have a higher incidence of this type of cancer. Benzene has been associated with acute leukemia, in shoe repairmen in Italy, solvent manufacturers, painters, and printers who use it as a solvent. Coal tar, pitch, creosote, and anthracene have been associated with cancer of the skin, larynx, and bronchus. A variety of paraffin oils, waxes, and tars are associated with cancer of the skin. Isopropyl oil has been associated with cancer of the sinuses, larynx, and bronchus in workers exposed to it. Mesotheliomas occur very frequently in miners and ship workers who have been exposed to asbestos. Certain metals have been associated with tumors, including chromium, nickel, and arsenic.

PHYSICAL CARCINOGENS. Ionizing radiation was found in the 1920s to be carcinogenic when subcutaneous sarcomas were induced by radium implants in experimental animals. The carcinogenic effects of radiation in man was recognized when radium dial painters who commonly licked brushes containing radioactive materials developed bone cancers. Since then, many examples of the carcinogenic effects of radiation in man have been recognized. In physicians and dentists who experience multiple x-ray exposures recurrent skin cancer has developed. Cancer of the thyroid in adults is frequently associated with neck irradiation in early childhood. The survivors of the atomic bomb detonations show an increased incidence of leukemia. Ultraviolet light on exposed areas may foster the development of skin cancer. Farmers and sailors have an increased incidence of skin cancers from excessive exposure to sunlight, as do fair-skinned people living in tropical regions.

Mechanical Irritation. Chronic mechanical irritation may be associated with the development of cancer, although the exact mechanisms are unknown. Examples include the malignant degeneration in old burn scars (the chronic ulcer of Marjolin), and cancer of the liver and bladder subsequent to parasitic infestation by schistosomes.

VIRUSES. These are carcinogenic in several animal species, and it is likely that some cancers in man are caused by viruses. Many animal-oncogenic viruses have been described since 1911 when Rous discovered a filterable agent which caused sarcoma in chickens. At least two distinct classes of viruses can cause tumors. Ribonucleic acid (RNA) viruses have been associated with sarcomas, lymphomas, leukemias, and mammary cancer in chickens, mice, rats, cats, monkeys, and gibbons. Deoxyribonucleic acid (DNA) viruses also are oncogenic. The polyoma virus can cause multiple tumors in mice, rats, and hamsters. Simian virus (SV-40) can cause a sarcoma in hamsters; papilloma virus causes papillomas in a variety of animals; adenoviruses have caused sarcomas in rodents. Pox viruses have been associated with fibromas in the rabbit and

FIVE YEAR CANCER SURVIVAL RATES*
FOR SELECTED SITES

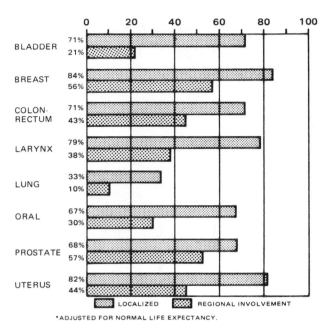

*ADJUSTED FOR NORMAL LIFE EXPECTANCY.

SOURCE; END RESULTS GROUP, NATIONAL CANCER INSTITUTE 1965-69.

Fig. 9-5. Five-year cancer survival rates for selected sites.

squirrel, and a tumor in the monkey. Herpes viruses cause neoplasms in frogs, chickens, and monkeys.

Despite clear-cut evidence for a viral cause of a variety of animal tumors, there has been no proof that viruses can cause human neoplasms. Yet, it would be surprising if man were not susceptible to some form of viral carcinogenesis because it is so common in all other animal species, and basic biologic phenomena are generally quite similar throughout nature. In fact, there is increasing evidence linking viruses with certain types of human neoplasms and suggesting a prominent role in etiology. The Epstein-Barr (EB) virus, probably the cause of infectious mononucleosis in man, is linked to the occurrences of Burkitt's lymphoma in Africa and to nasopharyngeal cancer in the Orient. RNA viruses of a characteristic type (type C) similar to those agents known to cause leukemias, and sarcomas in mice, have been associated with leukemias, sarcomas, and papillary urinary neoplasms in man. RNA viruses resembling the mammary tumor virus of mice have been found in the breast cancers and milk from women with this malignant disease.

Two modes of oncogenic viral transmission, vertical and horizontal, have been described. Vertical transmission involves passage of virus from parent to offspring. For example, the mouse mammary tumor virus is transmitted to progeny in the mother's milk, and the Gross leukemia virus is transmitted in the gametes of the parents to the offspring. Horizontal transmission is passage of virus to close contacts in excreta and airborne particles, as with the polyoma virus.

Table 9-1. CHEMICAL AND PHYSICAL CARCINOGENS IN HUMAN BEINGS

Carcinogen	Site of neoplasm	Site exposed	Persons at risk
Chemical agents:			
Aromatic amines, especially β-naphthylamine	Urinary tract	Cutaneous and respiratory	Chemical workers producing dye stuffs, rodenticides, laboratory reagents
Benzol or benzene	Blood, lymphatic organs	Cutaneous and respiratory	Coal tar refiners, solvent manufacturers, painters, printers, mechanics
Coal tar, pitch, creosote, anthracene, tobacco	Skin, larynx, bronchus	Cutaneous and respiratory	Coke oven workers, coal tar distillers, lumber industry workers, chemical workers, smokers
Petroleum, shale and paraffin oils, waxes, tars	Skin	Cutaneous	Workers in oil refineries, wax and asphalt producers, mechanics
Isopropyl oils	Sinus, larynx, bronchus	Respiratory	Producers of isopropyl alcohol
Asbestos	Bronchus, mesothelioma of pleura	Respiratory, generally > 2 years	Asbestos miners, shippers, millers
Chromium	Bronchus	Respiratory and cutaneous	Workers engaged in chromate ore reduction
Nickel	Nasal cavity, sinus, bronchus	Respiratory	Nickel miners, shippers, and refiners
Arsenic	Skin, bronchus, bladder	Respiratory	Smelters, pesticide manufacturers
Physical agents:			
Ionizing radiation	Skin, thyroid, tongue, tonsil, sinus, bone, blood	Local or systemic, therapeutic (e.g., treatment of spondylitic polycythemia)	Radium dial workers
	Bronchus	Respiratory	Pitchblend miners
Ultraviolet radiation	Skin	Cutaneous	Farmers, other outdoor workers, sailors, fishermen, and fair-skinned people in tropical climates

Experimental animals must be infected as newborn offspring with almost all oncogenic viruses to produce neoplastic change in adulthood. The immunologic immaturity of the neonate allows viral infection and induction of neoplastic transformation. Adult animals are resistant to infection with oncogenic viruses unless they are immunosuppressed.

Studies of viral oncogenesis can become quite complex in situations where multiple factors may interact to produce a situation which ultimately causes cancer. The development of mouse mammary cancer depends upon the cooperation of (1) genetic susceptibility, (2) proper hormonal stimuli, and (3) infection with the virus in the first 6 weeks of life. When all these conditions have been met, the breast cancer still requires 1 to 2 years to develop.

HEREDITARY FACTORS. Genetic factors have been demonstrated to be of major importance in determining the effectiveness of chemical, physical and viral carcinogens in animals.

Clear-cut examples of genetic factors playing a role in human cancer development are demonstrated when the same type of cancer occurs in identical twins, when colon cancer develops in persons with familial polyposis, and with the familial patterns associated with breast cancer. Cancer of the breast is about three times more common in the daughters of women with breast cancer and in women whose blood relatives have had at least two incidences of breast cancer. Furthermore, the daughters develop breast cancers at a younger age than did their mothers.

A more indirect genetic role was noted in certain families who seemed to have an increased incidence of neoplastic diseases. A clearly defined pattern of inheritance has been established for some of these tumors. It is often difficult to assess the importance of environmental factors in these cases. Substantiated examples include a pattern of dominant inheritance in some families for diseases such as retinoblastoma, lipomatosis, and colonic polyposis. In other families, there may be an association of multiple diseases that may include one or more neoplasms. An example of this is the association of pheochromocytoma with medullary (amyloid-producing) carcinoma of the thyroid, cerebellocortical hemangioblastoma, or neurofibromatosis. Other examples where tumors appear to be inherited in families as a dominant trait include some cases of polyendocrine adenomas (pituitary, parathyroid, pancreas), including the Zollinger-Ellison syndrome and hereditary adenocarcinomatosis (adenocarcinoma of the colon, stomach, uterus, and ovary occurring in different members of the same family). There are also several relatively rare heritable nonneoplastic diseases which have been associated with malignant tumors with great frequency. An example of this is the high incidence of skin cancer in patients with xeroderma pigmentosa. There also is an association between dermal inclusion cysts and multiple carcinomas of the colon, polyposis, multiple bony exostoses, and benign connective tissue tumors (Gardner's syndrome).

There are marked differences in the frequency of certain neoplastic diseases with respect to age, sex, and other constitutional factors suggesting that additional host determinants may be important. Acute lymphocytic leukemia is essentially a disease of childhood, whereas malignant melanoma is essentially a postpubertal disease. Testicular tumors and Hodgkin's disease are more frequent in young adults, and breast cancer is far more common in women than in men. In many other tumors, the frequency in both sexes increases markedly with increasing age.

GEOGRAPHIC FACTORS. Neoplasms may be found in all human populations, but there are some striking racial and regional differences in the occurrence of specific types of cancer. Although it is difficult to separate the genetic from the environmental factors, such as diet or habits, it is important to be aware of certain particularly strong differences. In a comparison study with the Caucasian population of the United States, Shimkin noted the following differences in cancer incidence:

1. High incidence of cancer of the stomach in Scandinavia, Iceland, and Japan
2. High incidence of primary cancer of the liver in South and West Africa
3. High incidence of cancer of the nasopharynx in China
4. High incidence of cancer of the urinary bladder in Egypt
5. Low incidence of cancer of the breast in Japan
6. Low incidence of cancer of the uterine cervix in Israel and in Jewish women in general
7. Low incidence of cancer of the skin in Negroes
8. Low incidence of cancer of the prostate in Japan and China

Custom and environment obviously play an important role in the development of cancer. It is almost certain that some of the geographic factors noted above are due more to environmental factors than to genetic ones. Migration of populations usually causes a shift toward the patterns of cancer incidence of the host country. For example, in Japan there is a very high incidence of stomach cancer and a relatively low incidence of lung cancer. However, a second generation Japanese-American has a low risk of stomach cancer, and if a heavy smoker, he has as high a risk of lung cancer as his smoking American counterpart.

For unknown reasons, socioeconomic factors may also influence cancer incidence. Cancer of the stomach and of the cervix are three to four times more frequent in lower economic groups than in middle and higher economic groups. On the other hand, cancer of the breast, leukemia, and multiple myeloma are more frequent in higher socioeconomic groups.

PRECANCEROUS CONDITIONS. Some clinical disorders are described as precancerous because they are so frequently followed by the development of cancer. It is particularly important that the physician be aware of these conditions in order to conduct careful follow-up of these patients. Some precancerous conditions are leukoplakia, actinic keratoses, polyps of the colon or rectum, neurofibromas, dysplasia of the cervix or bronchial mucosa, and chronic ulcerative colitis.

MULTIFACTORIAL ETIOLOGY. It is likely that in any given individual cancer is the result not of just one but of multiple factors. There may be an interaction of an oncogenic virus with a chemical or physical carcinogen. It is also possible that two chemical carcinogens may act synergistically to increase the incidence of cancer. A chemical may be a carcinogen only in those with a hereditary susceptibility. When condensations of smog or cigarette smoke are applied separately to the cheek pouch of the golden hamster, there is a low but definite incidence of tumor. However, a synergistic interaction is observed when they are applied together, with a markedly increased incidence of tumors. Similarly, viruses have enhanced the oncogenic effects of smog and cigarette smoke in tissue culture. It is very possible that such synergistic interactions also occur in man.

The possibility that multiple factors may be involved in the etiology of human neoplasia, although it makes the proof of any one factor as a causative agent more complex, may in itself increase the chances of ultimate cancer prevention by providing a larger number of factors to be manipulated. For example, in carcinoma of the lung, it may be that in addition to heavy cigarette smoking (perhaps only chronic irritation), one requires a specific genetic background (since not all heavy smokers develop cancer of the lung), suitable male hormonal factors (since males are more frequently affected), and a virus. In addition, the latent period between start of smoking and high incidence of lung cancer is roughly 35 years. Although cigarette smoking may not be the only cause of lung cancer, it is the only factor which is known at the present time that can be controlled. On the basis of present knowledge, lung cancer could be prevented by eliminating cigarette smoking altogether or by limiting cigarette smoking to a shorter period of time.

Custom and environment obviously play an important part in the etiology of cancer. Although cigarette smoking has been strongly implicated as a cause of squamous cell carcinoma of the lung, the habit is sufficiently ingrained in people in the United States to make its total elimination extremely difficult. Habits and customs in other parts of the world may be equally difficult to eliminate. The inhalation of snuff and the mastication of betel nuts have been associated with nasal and oral pharynx tumors, but the use of such materials continues despite their known carcinogenic effects. Nevertheless, efforts to identify the causative factors and to educate people regarding these factors must be continued.

BIOLOGY

Regardless of the etiologic agent, the cancer cell is a progeny of a normal cell that has lost its cellular mechanisms for controlling proliferation. The cancer cell differs from a normal cell in a variety of ways, but none of its new characteristics are absolutely indicative of malignancy. Cytogenetic studies of some cancer cells have revealed various abnormalities in chromosome number and appearance. However, these changes have not been shared by all cancer cells, and many cancer cells have normal chromosomal profiles.

Almost all malignant neoplasms seem to arise from a single cell that has undergone malignant transformation to form a malignant clone (group of cells); however, other human neoplasms such as the neurofibromas occurring in von Recklinghausen's disease may develop from multiple clones of cells. Simultaneously multifocal origins of carcinoma of the breast, oral pharynx, colon, and other organs also have been observed. Studies of breast carcinoma have demonstrated that at least 30 percent have other areas involved with in situ carcinoma. Nevertheless, the primary tumor mass which was the cause for clinical presentation arises from a single cell alone.

Although the proliferative rate of cancer cells is generally greater than the overall average of normal cells, the former do not divide more rapidly than some normal cells, such as leukocytes or cells of the intestinal mucosa. The proliferative rate of cancer cells generally decreases as the tumor mass grows. It has been shown that the proportion of cells undergoing mitosis is much greater when there are only a few cancer cells present than when there are many cells present in a large tumor mass. There are many rapid changes in the mitotic fraction of neoplasms during the initial growth phase, but after the tumor mass is 1 cm in diameter, the rate of division usually follows a predictable pattern.

After neoplastic transformation has occurred, the cancer cell differs from the normal cell not only in proliferative index but also in morphology, biochemistry, antigenetic expression, and many other aspects.

MORPHOLOGIC CHANGES. Malignant cells tend to revert to more primitive cell types, that is, to dedifferentiate. The normal orderly tissue patterns are lost or replaced by the random piling up of malignant cells without definite pattern. Other histologic changes may include cellular pleomorphism, a high index of mitoses, and hyperchromatism in the nucleus and nucleoli. Invasion of adjacent normal structures also may be seen microscopically. These morphologic changes are the basis for histopathologic or cytologic diagnoses of cancer and usually allow very accurate diagnosis of neoplastic diseases.

BIOCHEMICAL CHANGES. The biochemical activity of cancer cells is similar, though not identical, to that of normal cells. A great diversity exists in the biochemical characteristics of different tumor cells, usually correlating with rate of proliferation. Changes in DNA, RNA, and the chemical architecture of the cellular membrane of malignant cells are associated with the loss of contact inhibition to proliferation and intercellular adhesiveness. However, no single biochemical alteration has yet been defined that is absolutely characteristic of malignant transformation.

Reversion of the normal cellular biochemistry to that of the embryonal cells produces distinctive embryonal substances whose presence in the adult may be used to diagnose cancer. The carcinoembryonic antigen associated with gastrointestinal cancers, and α-fetoglobulin associated with hepatoma and embryonal cancers are thought to be examples of this type. The synthesis of these substances may be due to depression of fetal gene function that occurs during oncogenesis.

Malignant cells may also produce biologically active substances that are normally produced by the cells from which the neoplasm originated. The release of these substances may cause symptoms similar to hyperfunction of that particular organ, for example, hyperparathyroidism produced by parathyroid carcinomas. Neoplasms may also produce biologically active substances that are not normally produced by the cells of origin. Some bronchogenic carcinomas may produce parathyroidlike hormones, ACTH, antidiuretic hormones, and other hormones.

The mechanism of this ectopic hormone secretion is based upon the hypothesis of variable genetic activity or *selective derepression* of a specific gene. All cells contain the same genes; however, only about 10 percent of these genes are expressed in any one cell type; the remainder are repressed. Cancer cells are primitive cells; with the dedifferentiation, they acquire the ability to express some of these previously repressed genes. This new genetic expression is responsible for the production of a new specific-messenger RNA and the production of new polypeptides and hormones.

GROWTH RATES OF NEOPLASMS. Approximately two-thirds of the growth of human neoplasms occurs before they are clinically detectable. If one assumes that a cancer begins from a single cell, then it takes about 30 exponential divisions to produce a 1-cm nodule (1 billion cells). At 45 exponential divisions the patient is apt to be dead from the sheer bulk of the malignant tumor.

The growth rate of tumors can be expressed by the *tumor doubling time,* i.e., the time it takes for a tumor to double in volume. Tumor doubling times appear to be an accurate and precise method for comparing the biologic aggressiveness of neoplasms in different patients. This measurement is particularly applicable to metastatic pulmonary lesions, since these are usually peripheral in location and are discretely delineated on chest roentgenograms, so that accurate serial measurements are easily obtainable.

The method used in the measurement of the tumor doubling time is illustrated in Fig. 9-6. Briefly, the average of the greater and the lesser diameters of each metastatic nodule is determined from successive chest roentgenograms. The averages are plotted on semilogarithmic paper against the time in days between these points; the slope of this line represents the rate of tumor growth. Where this line crosses any two doubling lines, the horizontal distance between them represents the tumor doubling time in days. This measurement has been shown to be an accurate and reproducible method for the quantitation of the rate and pattern of tumor growth in individual patients.

The tumor doubling time of neoplasms varies from 8 to 600 days, most tumors doubling in 20 to 100 days. The measurement of tumor doubling times can be extremely helpful in determining prognosis, in evaluating response

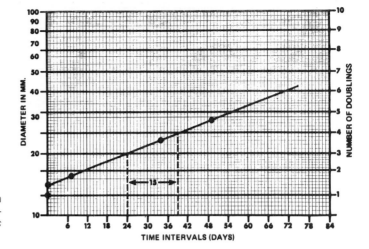

Fig. 9-6. Method of plotting tumor doubling time, based upon the direct measurement of the changing diameters of metastatic pulmonary nodules. (*From W. L. Joseph et al., J Thorac Cardiovasc Surg, 61:23, 1971.*)

to chemotherapeutic agents, and in comparing responses to different therapeutic regimens.

In one study the tumor doubling times of a large series of patients with pulmonary metastases from tumors of different histologic types were measured. Wide variations within particular types of neoplasms were found. The tumor doubling time correlated closely with the length of survival in three distinct groups of patients. This is illustrated in Fig. 9-7. This correlation might be expected, because the tumor doubling time represents the balance between the intrinsic proliferative rate of the tumor cell and the patient's inhibiting defense mechanisms.

Based on growth dynamics, most human tumors have been present in the body for at least 1 year and many for as long as 10 to 15 years prior to their clinical detection. Thus, it appears that there is a long period of time between the inception of neoplastic transformation and the development of clinical cancer. During this time, detection may be possible and surgical treatment might result in cure. Tests must be perfected to detect cancer earlier, thus shorten this preclinical interval, and make surgical treatment more successful.

Immunobiology

The concept that cancer patients may develop an immune response against their neoplasms is not new. This view became very popular at the turn of the century when

it was found that strong immunity could be induced against transplantable neoplasms in randomly bred laboratory rodents. A period of intense laboratory and clinical investigation followed, in anticipation that tumor immunity might lead to control of malignant disease. However, it soon became evident that the immunity was not directed against tumor-specific antigens (TSA), but instead against normal tissue antigens in the neoplasm due to genetic differences between tumor donor and recipient. Thereafter, interest in tumor immunology declined because no antigens other than the transplantation antigens could be demonstrated in neoplasms.

Interest in the immunology of neoplastic diseases was reawakened in the 1950s when tumor-specific antigens were conclusively demonstrated in methylcholanthrene-induced sarcomas of mice. In order to eliminate any histocompatibility factors the investigators used inbred strains of rodents that, after many years of inbreeding, had the genetic homogeneity of monozygotic twins. Specific tumor transplantation resistance was induced by presensitization with a transplant of tumor tissue which was allowed to grow for a time and then was excised. The immunized rodents were then resistant to challenge with further transplants of the same neoplasm (Fig. 9-8). However, the limitations of tumor immunity were evident by the fact that the immunity induced in these animals was relative, not absolute. Whereas a challenge with 100,000 tumor cells produced a growing tumor in control mice, it did not in

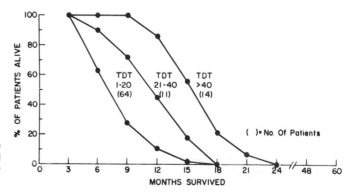

Fig. 9-7. Survival curves in 89 untreated patients following the onset of pulmonary metastases, showing three groups based upon tumor doubling time. (*From W. L. Joseph et al., J Thorac Cardiovasc Surg, 61:23, 1971.*)

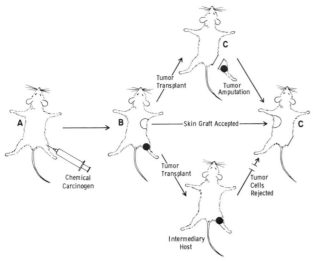

Fig. 9-8. Tumor induced with benzpyrene in mouse A is transplanted into mouse B. Mouse C, immunized by amputation of a tumor-bearing extremity, demonstrates tumor-specific immunity by rejecting tumor cells while accepting a normal skin graft from the same mouse.

Table 9-2. TUMOR-SPECIFIC ANTIGENS CAPABLE OF INDUCING REJECTION RESPONSES IN SYNGENEIC HOSTS

Inducing agent	*Antigenic specificity*
Chemical carcinogens:	
3-Methylcholanthrene	
1,2,5,6-Dibenzanthracene	
9,10-Dimethylbenzathracene	
3,4,9,10-Dibenzpyrene	Antigens distinct for
3,4-Benzpyrene-dimethylam-	each individual
inoazobenzene	neoplasm
Physical agents	
Films:	
Millipore filter	
Cellophane film	
Radiation:	
Ultraviolet	
^{90}Sr	
Virus:	
DNA:	
Polyoma	
SV-40	
Adenovirus 12,18	
Shope papilloma	
RNA:	Common antigens in
Mammary tumor agent	each neoplasm in-
Leukemia	duced by the same
Gross	virus
Moloney ⎫	
Rauscher ⎬ Shared common	
Friend ⎭ antigens	
Graffi	
Rich	
Rous (Schmidt-Ruppin)	

the immune mice. Challenge with larger numbers of cells (1 to 10 million), however, usually overwhelmed the immunologic defense, and progressive tumor growth was observed.

During the past 15 years there has been tremendous progress in tumor immunology. Tumor-specific antigens have been demonstrated in most viral, chemical, and physical-carcinogen-induced neoplasms, as well as in many spontaneous tumors. These tumor-specific antigens can elicit tumor-specific immunity against tumor transplantation in syngeneic animals; thus, they are known as *tumor-specific transplantation antigens* (TSTA).

ANTIGENIC SPECIFICITY OF ANIMAL NEOPLASMS. The wide variety of viral, chemical, and physical-carcinogen-induced neoplasms for which tumor-specific transplantation antigens have been demonstrated are summarized in Table 9-2. The antigenic specificity of these major types of carcinogenic agents have been found to be quite different.

Tumor-specific Antigens of Neoplasms Induced by Chemical and Physical Carcinogens. These are individually distinct for each tumor, even if induced by the same carcinogen, in the same strain, and of the identical histologic type (Fig. 9-9). For example, injection of a chemical carcinogen such as benzpyrene in two inbred mice of the same strain will result in two antigenically different tumors, t_1 and t_2. If mouse *A* is immunized with irradiated tumor cells from t_1, it will subsequently reject tumor cells from the same tumor transplanted into an intermediate host. However, the same animal, immune to t_1, will develop a tumor when injected with the same number of tumor cells from t_2.

Tumor-specific Antigens of Neoplasms Induced by Viral Carcinogens. In contrast to the unique tumor-specific antigens of chemical-carcinogen-induced tumors, the tumor-specific antigens of viral-induced neoplasms are common to all neoplasms induced by the same virus, but differ from those induced by other viruses (Fig. 9-10). For example, with inbred mice of the same strain, mouse *A* is immunized with SV-40 virus alone, mouse *B* is immunized with *irradiated* tumor cells from a SV-40 virus–induced mouse tumor, and mouse *C* is immunized with tumor cells from an SV-40 virus–induced rat tumor. All will reject challenge of tumor cells from SV-40 virus–induced tumor t. However, challenge with the same tumor cells in mice *D* and *E*, immunized with either polyoma virus alone or polyoma virus–induced tumor cells, leads to progressive tumor growth and death.

Although the generalization that virus-induced neoplasms contain common antigens and chemical-carcinogen-induced neoplasms contain individually distinct antigens is usually correct, more recent studies have demonstrated that this distinction is not as absolute as originally believed. Common antigens related to leukemia viral antigens have been found in chemical-carcinogen-induced sarcomas, and some carcinogen-induced neoplasms arising in the bladder have contained common antigens. Furthermore, spontaneous mouse mammary carcinomas induced by the mammary tumor virus contain individually distinct antigens in addition to the common antigens of the mammary tumor virus.

**MECHANISMS OF TUMOR-SPECIFIC IMMUNE REJEC-
TION.** The cellular immune response is thought to be more
important in controlling tumor rejection than the humoral
antibody response for several reasons: (1) tumor-specific
immunity can be adoptively transferred by lymphocytes
(Fig. 9-11) much more readily than by humoral antibody;
(2) immune lymphocytes or macrophages that kill tumor
cells in vitro can be demonstrated.

Many immune responses may be mediated by products
of stimulated macrophages or lymphocytes. These products
are collectively called *lymphokines* and may be important
for the modification and development of the cellular immune response. For example, macrophage inhibition factor and chemotactic factor are both produced by lymphocytes after antigenic stimulation and may control the
movement of macrophages or granulocytes in the development of delayed cutaneous hypersensitivity or inflammation. Many other such products have been described and
probably contribute to the interaction between different
cell types.

The lymphocyte may have a receptor site on its surface
that is specific for the tumor-associated antigen on the
tumor cell. Once contact is established, the lymphocyte
could mediate a cytotoxic event (perhaps via a toxic protein such as lymphotoxin) that causes disruption of the
tumor cell membrane and subsequent tumor cell death.

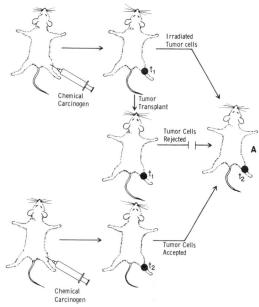

Fig. 9-9. Mouse A, immunized with benzpyrene-induced tumor t,
resists subsequent challenge with t tumor cells. Challenge with
cells from another benzpyrene-induced tumor, t_2, leads to progressive tumor growth and death of the mouse.

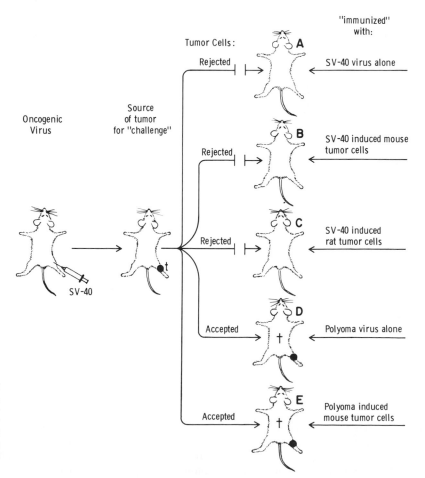

Fig. 9-10. Mice A, B, and C, immunized with
SV-40 virus or SV-40 virus–induced tumor cells,
reject challenge of tumor cells from SV-40 virus–
induced tumor t. Challenge with the same tumor
cells in mice D and E, immunized with polyoma
virus or polyoma virus–induced tumor cells, leads
to progressive tumor growth and death of the
mouse.

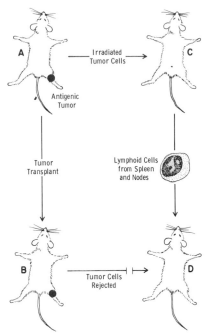

Fig. 9-11. Tumor induced in mouse A with benzpyrene is serially passed into another mouse, B, of the same strain. Mouse C is immunized with irradiated tumor cells of the same tumor. Immune lymphocytes transferred from mouse C to mouse D confer tumor-specific immunity to subsequent tumor challenge.

Thymus-derived lymphocytes have been credited as the main effector cells for tumor immunity. However, recent experiments have demonstrated the importance of macrophages and thymus-independent lymphocytes. Among the thymus-independent lymphocytes are cells known as *killer* or *K cells*. These K cells may or may not include B lymphocytes and are potentiated or armed by an antibody specific for antigens on the tumor cell in order to cause tumor cell destruction. This antibody-dependent cellular cytotoxicity (ADCC) is neither complement-dependent nor phagocytic, although monocytes can mediate ADCC. Antibody able to induce ADCC is usually of the IgG class.

Macrophages also play an important role in killing tumor cells. Two types of tumorocidal macrophages have been identified: the nonspecifically activated macrophage and the specifically armed macrophage. BCG and other microbes or microbial products can nonspecifically activate macrophages, which then are cytotoxic for tumor cells in vitro but not for normal cells. Sensitized lymphocytes specifically cytotoxic for a tumor or specific antisera can transmit their specificity to normal macrophages, which in turn become specifically cytotoxic to the sensitizing tumor.

Humoral antibodies can inhibit tumor growth in vivo and destroy tumor cells in vitro in the presence of complement. Usually, antibody must be given prior to or immediately after tumor transplantation in order to be effective. The sensitivity of various types of neoplasms to cytotoxic antibodies varies considerably. Leukemias and lymphomas are most sensitive, sarcomas and carcinomas more resist-

ant. There appears to be a correlation between the sensitivity of the tumor to cytotoxic antibodies in vitro and its response to antibodies in vivo. However, it is clear that the different classes of antibodies vary considerably in their ability to reduce tumor cell viability in vitro and inhibit tumor growth in vivo. Antibodies of the IgM class are generally more effective in inducing immunity by passive transfer.

In summary, T and B lymphocytes, K cells, macrophages, and antibody all have a role in controlling tumor growth. At best, they interreact to cause tumor cell destruction. At worst, they can lead to enhanced tumor growth both in vivo and in vitro. Much more research needs to be done before we can expect to understand how to manipulate the immune system for the maximum benefit of the patient.

IMMUNE SURVEILLANCE. The concept of immunologic surveillance is based upon the premise that carcinogenesis occurs frequently as a spontaneous mutation, from chemical carcinogens or from oncogenic viruses. Burnet postulated that the teleology of the immune system was to recognize the foreignness of tumor-specific antigens on the neoplastic cells and to mount an immune response capable of eliminating them. In this context, clinical cancer would represent a failure of the mechanisms for immunologic destruction, although it may be the exception rather than the rule.

Mechanisms for Evasion of Immune Surveillance. If neoplastic cells are capable of eliciting a host immune response that leads to their specific destruction, it is pertinent to ask why or how cancer develops. A variety of possible ways by which cancer cells evade the immune surveillance mechanisms have been described:

Insufficient antigenicity to evoke an immune response may account for the growth of some neoplasms. Tumor-specific antigens are usually weaker immunogens than transplantation antigens. Some neoplastic cells may have either an extremely weak tumor-specific antigen or an extremely low density of tumor-specific antigens on the cell surface. Thus, the tumor cell with the stronger tumor-specific antigen may be recognized and eliminated, whereas those cells with weak tumor-specific antigens may escape detection and destruction.

Antigenic modulation of a thymus leukemia (TL) antigen has been observed on a murine lymphoma cell. The TL antigen disappears when the cell is transplanted in immunized hosts or carried in tissue culture containing specific antibody, but it will reappear when the tumor cells are passed in tissue culture without antibody or transplanted in unimmunized hosts. Furthermore, antigenic shift may be another form of antigenic modulation whereby tumor cells escape control of immunologic surveillance. This phenomenon has been described with certain animal neoplasms in which the lung metastases are antigenically different from the primary tumor.

Immunologic indifference may explain the observation by Old and associates that small numbers of tumor cells having tumor-specific antigens develop into progressively growing tumors although larger numbers of cells are rejected. In this instance the small number of cells may not be immunogenic enough and can "sneak through" the host immune response.

Immunosuppression by irradiation, neonatal thymectomy, chemotherapy, or steroid or antilymphocyte globulin administration usually increases the frequency and growth rate, and shortens the latency period, for both virus- and carcinogen-induced neoplasms in experimental animals. The incidence of cancer in man increases significantly with advancing years as his immune response to a variety of antigens decreases. Furthermore, in human beings with congenital immunodeficiency diseases, the incidence of spontaneous cancer is 10,000 times that of the general age-matched population. In human organ transplant recipients on immunosuppressive drugs, the incidence of spontaneous cancer is more than seventy times that of the general age-matched population.

Immunologic tolerance that develops during the fetal or neonatal periods due to exposure to tumor-specific antigens or an oncogenic virus may account for tumor growth in some animals when the immunologic surveillance system would otherwise afford protection. Bittner discovered in 1936 that C3H female mice transmitted mammary tumor virus (MTV) through the milk to their nursing young which later induced mammary tumors in a high percentage of their adult female progeny. Morton demonstrated that mice infected as neonates subsequently became tolerant to the tumor-specific antigens of the MTV-induced neoplasms and consequently could not be immunized against them as adults. Newborn mice foster-nursed on non-MTV-carrying mothers from another strain were not tolerant to the virus and, when adult, could be effectively immunized against the MTV-induced mammary tumors. The incidence of mammary tumors in these foster-nursed mice was much lower than in those nursed on MTV infected mothers.

Low-dose immunologic tolerance similar to that seen with transplantation systems, but secondary to prolonged exposure to small amounts of weak tumor-specific antigens may account for the growth of some tumors. Low-dose tolerance may explain the development of metastases from breast cancer in immunocompetent patients many years after radical mastectomy.

Immunologic enhancement refers to the facilitated growth of some tumors in the presence of specific antibody against the tumor-specific antigen. The antibody may work on the afferent limb, the efferent limb, or the central portion of the immune response.

Afferent enhancement occurs when the antibody coats the antigen on the tumor cell and prevents processing of the tumor-specific antigen, either at the regional node or by a macrophage at the tumor cell. *Central enhancement* occurs when the antibody directly inhibits the reactivity of the immunocompetent cells. *Efferent enhancement* occurs when the antibody coats the antigenic site and prevents intimate contact between the immune cell and the tumor cell.

An important point to stress concerning the enhancement of tumor growth by specific antibody concerns the temporal relation between the transfer of antibody and tumor or organ allotransplantation. The antibody must be administered shortly before, at the same time as, or shortly after tumor or organ transplantation in order for enhancement to occur. If administration of the antibody is delayed for a week, the host cellular immune response has already been stimulated, and tumor rejection occurs in a normal fashion. Most animal and human neoplasms have a long latency period prior to clinical detection, and the host immune response is already sensitized to the tumor-specific antigens. Therefore, it is unlikely that immunologic enhancement by antibody is responsible for tumor enhancement or plays an important role in evasion of immunologic surveillance in naturally occurring neoplasms.

CLINICAL EVIDENCE FOR TUMOR IMMUNITY IN MAN

Until recently there was little evidence for the existence of tumor-specific antigens on human neoplasms. For obvious reasons the tumor transplantation techniques used to demonstrate these tumor-specific antigens of animal neoplasms were not applicable to the study of human tumors. Nevertheless, there are a number of well-documented clinical observations which suggest human host immune defenses against cancer. Although other physiologic, endocrinologic, and biologic explanations can be given for these observations, they are most easily explained on an immunologic basis:

1. Spontaneous regression of established tumors is a rare but well-documented phenomenon. Sometimes these regressions have followed a minor viral or bacterial infection. Although spontaneous regression has been observed in many different tumor types, it is most frequently seen in neuroblastomas of children, malignant melanoma, choriocarcinoma, adenocarcinoma of the kidney, and soft tissue sarcomas. However, spontaneous regression occurs less frequently than 0.5 percent in all types, except for neuroblastomas.

   Spontaneous regression of small pulmonary metastases following the surgical removal of the primary tumor has been observed and occurs most frequently in hypernephromas. Spontaneous regression also may account for the prolonged survival or cure of patients after incomplete surgical excision of the cancer.
2. Recurrence of tumor 10 years after successful treatment of the primary is often manifested by rapid tumor growth and death. Although endocrinologic changes may account for some of these observations in breast cancer, in other tumors this course suggests a host defense which inhibits the tumor growth during the disease-free interval.
3. Microscopic evidence of the histiocytic, plasmocytic, lymphocytic, and esosinophilic infiltration, which resembles that seen in an organ transplant or tumor transplant that is undergoing rejection in man, is associated with an improved prognosis. For example, in stomach cancer, these findings correlate better with survival than does adequate surgical removal of the tumor.
4. The presence of many tumor cells in the peripheral blood, lymphatics, pleural cavity, and operative wounds of patients who subsequently never develop metastases suggests host immune defense.
5. There is a low incidence of successful growth of tumor tissue, or autotransplants in patients with advanced disease. The resistance against tumor growth was relative rather than absolute, since challenge with greater numbers of cancer cells usually resulted in tumor growth. The immune nature of this resistance was suggested when autologous leukocytes or plasma was mixed with these tumor cells, and cancer growth decreased in approximately half the patients studied.

IMMUNOLOGIC EVIDENCE FOR TUMOR-SPECIFIC ANTI-GENS IN HUMAN NEOPLASMS. During the past decade, a variety of sensitive serologic techniques have demonstrated that every human neoplasm adequately studied contained specific antigens which elicited both cellular and humoral responses in cancer patients.

Humoral antibodies have been shown by the immuno-fluorescence, complement fixation, immunocytolosis, and immunodiffusion techniques. Cellular immunity has been demonstrated by lymphocyte-mediated cytotoxicity (the ability of lymphocytes to kill tumor cells in tissue culture), lymphocyte blastogenesis tests (the ability of lymphocytes to be stimulated to proliferate by tumor-specific antigens), and migration inhibition tests (macrophages or other blood leukocytes inhibited in their migration by tumor-specific antigens). Finally, it has been found that cancer patients develop delayed cutaneous hypersensitivity reactions to tumor-specific antigens. Thus, it has become increasingly apparent that tumor-specific antigens are capable of elicit-ing an immune response which can be monitored by the immunologic techniques used to study other types of im-mune reactions. The wide variety of human neoplasms in which tumor-specific antigens have been detected are listed in Table 9-3.

The antigenic pattern of most human neoplasms is simi-lar. Neoplasms of the same histologic type contain com-mon tumor-specific antigens which differ from tumor-specific antigens of other types of neoplasms. Thus, human sarcomas share a common antigen which is different from the antigens shared by bladder cancer.

In addition, some neoplasms such as malignant mela-noma have additional antigens with a pattern of more limited specificity, as well as the common melanoma-specific antigen. This pattern of both individually distinct and common antigens may be characteristic of other types of human neoplasms as well, although studies undertaken thus far have not demonstrated it. The discovery of the common antigen in neoplasms of the same histologic type may allow precise immunotherapeutic and immunopro-phylactic maneuvers based upon vaccines prepared for this common tumor antigen rather than from each patient's own tumor-specific antigens.

Carcinoembryonic, or Fetal, Antigens. Most of the tu-mor-associated antigens described above are located on the cell surface, where they are susceptible to immune attack by antibodies or lymphocytes. Thus, they are probably of

Table 9-3. HUMAN NEOPLASMS WITH
DEMONSTRATED TUMOR-ASSOCIATED
ANTIGENS

Burkitt's lymphoma
Malignant melanoma
Neuroblastoma
Osteosarcoma
Soft tissue sarcomas
Colon carcinoma
Breast carcinoma
Leukemia
Lung carcinoma
Bladder carcinoma
Renal carcinoma

considerable importance in the tumor-host relationship. However, there are other types of antigens which may not be located at the cell surface, although they are more or less specific for the neoplastic state. One such group is composed of the fetal, or carcinoembryonic, antigens.

Fetal antigens are produced by normal fetal organs during embryonic development. Their production is re-pressed shortly after birth, and they are not produced in significant quantities in normal adult organs. However, during neoplastic transformation, reversion of the cell to the embryonic state is accompanied by a renewed produc-tion of these fetal antigens. The fetal antigens are thought to represent the phenotypic expression of genes active during fetal life but not expressed during normal adult life. Their occurrence in tumors is thought to be secondary to alterations in the pattern of gene regulation as the result of the dedifferentiation and reversion of the cell to a primitive embryonic state.

The carcinoembryonic, or fetal, antigens may be a useful means of detecting malignant disease before other clinical evidence of disease is apparent or as a detector of recur-rence following therapy to provide a basis for further treatment. Fetal antigens that are common to many differ-ent histologic types of human neoplasms have been de-scribed, as have those that are restricted to the organ of origin.

α-Fetoglobulin. The α-fetoglobulin circulating in approx-imately 70 percent of patients with primary hepatomas is found in normal human fetal serum up to 1 year after birth. The fetal antigen also has been found occasionally in patients with gastric cancer, prostatic cancer, and primi-tive testicular tumors such as teratomas, although it ap-pears to be relatively specific for hepatomas. The specificity of the test was demonstrated when adult monkeys were given hepatic carcinogens; α-fetoglobulin appeared in the serum of a high percentage of these monkeys prior to any histologic evidence of neoplastic change.

The α-fetoglobulin test has been clinically evaluated and found to be useful in the diagnosis of hepatomas. It is not positive in patients with rapidly dividing cells due to he-patic regeneration following liver resection or in those with cirrhosis.

Carcinoembryonic Antigen. The carcinoembryonic anti-gen (CEA) reported in 1965 by Gold and Friedman is another tumor-associated antigen occurring in fetal gut, liver, and pancreas during the first two trimesters of gesta-tion. This antigen was originally thought to be specific for adenocarcinomas arising in the gastrointestinal tract and pancreas, but more recently it has been found in a variety of carcinomas, sarcomas, and lymphomas of many differ-ent histologic types.

Since the CEA appears in the bloodstream, it was ini-tially thought to be of great importance as a diagnostic tool for malignant disease prior to other clinical evidence of cancer. A radioimmunoassay capable of detecting nano-gram quantities of CEA in the blood was developed. How-ever, elevated CEA levels were found in patients with a variety of nonmalignant conditions including alcoholic cirrhosis, pancreatitis, cholecystitis, colonic diverticulitis, and ulcerative colitis. As a result, the incidence of elevated

CEA levels in mass screening of normal or hospitalized populations has been over 10 percent in some series. Therefore this test has not been useful as a serologic method for the diagnosis of malignant tumor.

The serum levels of CEA do appear to correlate with the extent of known carcinomas of the colon. Less than 20 percent of patients with early lesions (Dukes Stage A or B) have elevated CEA levels, whereas one-half of patients with Dukes C lesions and almost all patients with Dukes D lesions have elevated levels of CEA. Metastasis to the liver is frequently associated with the highest levels. These statistics suggest that CEA may have limited use in detecting early carcinoma of the bowel. It has been shown that the CEA level drops during the postoperative period in those patients who have successful resection of the tumor. Patients who develop tumor recurrence often show a rise in CEA titer to the preoperative levels. Thus, CEA may be extremely useful in following the clinical course of patients with known malignant disease in order to detect evidence of recurrence prior to its becoming clinically detectable.

GENERAL IMMUNE COMPETENCE OF CANCER PATIENTS. A number of studies have tested the general functional capacity of the cancer patient's immunologic system. Such studies can be grouped into two categories—those concerned with humoral antibody production and those dealing with cell-mediated immune reactions.

Formation of humoral antibody to known antigenic substances has been studied by many investigators, who have found most cancer patients have the ability to form humoral antibodies against a variety of antigenic substances, even in the presence of advanced disease. There is no evidence to implicate a defect in humoral antibody production in most cancer patients.

The cell-mediated immune reactions have been measured by the cancer patient's ability to manifest delayed cutaneous hypersensitivity to a variety of common skin test antigens to which most normal persons are reactive by virtue of previous exposure such as to mumps, tuberculin, streptokinase, or streptodornase. In addition, a primary immune response was tested against a new antigen by studying the survival of skin allografts and by sensitizing patients to an antigen, such as the contact sensitizer dinitrochlorobenzene (DNCB). DNCB reacts with proteins in the skin and forms a hapten which sensitizes the immunocompetent patient (Fig. 9-12). Cell-mediated immunity can

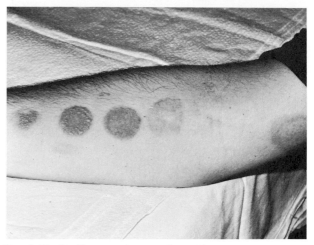

Fig. 9-12. Positive reaction to dintrochlorobenzene (DNCB), showing initial exposure and subsequent challenges.

be studied with an in vitro test which requires lymphocyte recognition and proliferation in response to foreign tissue antigens or mitogens such as phytohemagglutinin.

These immunologic studies revealed that cell-mediated immune reactions are significantly impaired in patients with lymphoreticular neoplasia. Since these diseases usually diffusely involve the immune effector system, this might be expected. However, a similar impediment in cell-mediated immune reactions was found in patients with localized or advanced solid neoplasms that did not involve the immune system. The explanation for this immunologic defect in cancer patients is unknown, but there does appear to be a strong correlation between an impaired cell-mediated response and the clinical course of the malignant disease.

This correlation becomes particularly evident when the postoperative course of cancer patients is compared with their ability to become sensitized to DNCB (Fig. 9-13). More than 95 percent of normal control volunteers, patients with benign neoplasms, patients free of disease 5 years or more following cancer surgery, and patients with a history of spontaneous regression of cancer could be sensitized to DNCB. On the other hand, only 65 percent of patients who presented for definitive cancer surgery could be sensitized to this chemical. Seventy-two percent of these immunocompetent patients had localized neo-

Patients	DNCB Positive	DNCB Negative
Control	19/20 = 95%	1/20 = 5%
Benign	10/10 = 100%	0/0 = 0%
Longterm survival (>5 yrs) .	16/16 = 100%	0/16 = 0%
Spontaneous regression. . .	8/8 = 100%	0/8 = 0%
All cancer patients	152/237 = 64%	85/237 = 35%
Free of disease (6 mo) . . .	110/152 = 72%	1/85 = 1%
Inoperable or early recurrence	42/152 = 28%	84/85 = 99%

Fig. 9-13. Correlation between delayed cutaneous hypersensitivity to DNCB and prognosis.

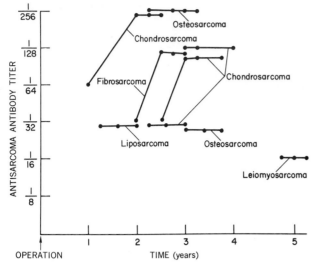

Fig. 9-14. Antisarcoma antibody titers determined by complement fixation against the HuSA-I liposarcoma antigen. Serial serum samples obtained from patients who remained free of disease up to 5 years after resection of the primary sarcoma. (*From D. L. Morton et al., Ann Intern Med, 74:587, 1971.*)

plasms that could be resected, and they subsequently remained free of disease for at least 6 months after surgery. However, those patients who were anergic had a poor prognosis following operation. Ninety-nine percent were inoperable because of local or metastatic spread of the disease or, when resected, had recurrence of disease within 6 months after surgery. Regardless of the histologic type of neoplasm, most patients who had severe impairment of their cell-mediated immune reactions apparent from cutaneous anergy to DNCB had a poor prognosis after operation.

There were considerable differences, however, in the pattern of DNCB reactivity in patients with different histologic types of solid neoplasms. Patients with epidermoid carcinoma of the cervix, mouth, pharynx, or larynx showed a very strong correlation between the positive DNCB response and a good prognosis after cancer surgery. Most of these patients who could be sensitized were operable and free of disease for at least 6 months, whereas those who were anergic had a poor prognosis. There was little correlation between a positive DNCB test and recurrence after surgery with the skeletal or soft tissue sarcomas and melanomas; many of these patients developed a recurrence even though they were immunologically competent. The explanation for the differences in cutaneous reactivity with various tumor types is unknown at the present time. It is possible that these patterns are indicative of some important variations in either the causes of or the response to the different types of human neoplasms. In some instances, it appears that the presence of a neoplasm is clearly related to the immunosuppression, because resection of the neoplasm results in return of immunologic competence. This is particularly true in patients with large, bulky skeletal and soft tissue sarcomas.

Some clarification of the immunosuppression that results

from malignant disease has come from recent studies. Patients who converted from anergic to positive during sequential skin testing with DNCB appeared to have gained control of their tumor just as often as those patients who were initially reactive to DNCB and who maintained their reactivity after surgical procedures. Conversely, those patients who converted from positive to an anergic response usually had progression of their disease. It would seem, therefore, that the defect in systemic immunity was the result of the neoplastic process and that the immunosuppression could be reversed by successful therapy. Other studies have shown that lymphocyte function is depressed in cancer patients when compared to normal controls and that this depression is directly related to the extent of tumor burden. Another investigation demonstrated serum factors in samples from cancer patients that inhibited function of lymphocytes from normal donors. These factors undoubtedly contribute to the immunosuppression observed in cancer patients.

Thus it appears that the immunosuppression seen in cancer patients could be the result of a humoral factor dispensed by the cancer cell or a complex physiologic response against the cancer cell that can depress normal cell-mediated immunity.

CORRELATIONS BETWEEN IMMUNE RESPONSE TO TUMOR-SPECIFIC ANTIGENS AND CLINICAL COURSE OF HUMAN CANCER. More sophisticated immunologic studies demonstrated a correlation between the cell-mediated and humoral immune responses and the clinical course of malignant disease. Such studies show that patients with a normal immune response to DNCB may have instead abnormalities in their response to the tumor-specific antigens of their neoplasms that can be detected by other immunologic techniques.

While the antibody role in controlling tumor growth is controversial at the present time, there is a marked correlation between the antibody titer detectable by immunofluorescence and complement fixation and the clinical course in patients with melanomas and sarcomas. This correlation was especially striking when sera from sarcoma patients were tested by complement fixation.

Analyses of sera from patients who enjoyed long-term survival from previous sarcomas showed a persistently elevated antisarcoma antibody titer (Fig. 9-14). Little variation was noted, and persistence of antibody was evident 3 to 4 years after removal of the primary tumor. When sequential antisera samples were obtained before and after surgery for primary sarcomas, it was found that all those patients who had primary surgery and continued to be free of disease had at least a fourfold rise in tumor antibody following removal of the tumor. These antibody titers remained elevated as long as those patients remained free of disease (Fig. 9-15). In contrast, most patients who had no antisarcoma antibody preoperatively with no increase in antibody titer following surgery developed recurrence within 6 months. Furthermore, of the several patients with low antibody titers preoperatively who had a transient rise in antibody titer following tumor removal, all who developed subsequent pulmonary metastases showed a progres-

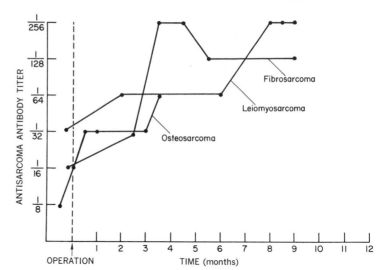

Fig. 9-15. Antisarcoma antibody titers determined by complement fixation against the HuSA-I liposarcoma antigen. Serial serum samples obtained following resection of the primary sarcoma in patients who remained free of disease. (*From D. L. Morton et al., Ann Surg, 172:740, 1970.*)

sive decline in antisarcoma antibody titers to nondetectable levels as the metastatic disease progressed (Fig. 9-16). In careful, frequent sampling of a few sarcoma patients, it appeared that the antibody titer fell 2 to 3 months prior to development of detectable pulmonary metastatic disease. Thus, careful monitoring of the sarcoma patient's complement fixing antibody titer in the postoperative period may be helpful in early detection of recurrence of disease.

The observation of Hellstrom and associates regarding the presence of blocking factors in the sera of sarcoma patients who have growing neoplasms or who subsequently will develop recurrent disease is probably of considerable importance in the tumor-host relationship. They found that lymphocytes specifically cytotoxic for tumor cells can be demonstrated throughout the course of malignant disease regardless of whether patients have been cured of their tumors or have growing neoplasms. However, the sera of those patients with growing tumors contained blocking factors that inhibited the cytotoxic action of the killer lymphocytes upon tumor cells in vitro. Further stud-

ies suggested that the blocking factors were probably circulating tumor antigen-antibody complexes or tumor antigen alone rather than simple enhancing antibodies. This blocking factor could be completely neutralized by admixture with serum that had the cytotoxic or deblocking antibodies from patients free of malignant disease. A most significant correlation to clinical course was found when these in vitro studies demonstrated the deblocking antibodies in patients free of disease but found the blocking serum factors in patients who had recurrence of the disease. Obviously such techniques can be useful in predicting in which patients the disease will recur. The day may come when the balance between antibody and cellular immunity may be manipulated to the patient's benefit through such studies as this.

In addition to the correlations of clinical course to specific humoral immunity, it does appear that delayed cutaneous hypersensitivity reactions to tumor-specific antigens extracted from various types of human neoplasms also correlate in a general way with clinical course. Patients with arrested melanomas, Burkitt's lymphoma, and leuke-

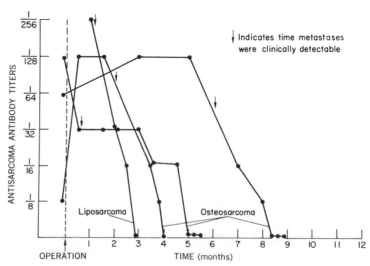

Fig. 9-16. Antisarcoma antibody titers determined by complement fixation against the HuSA-1 liposarcoma antigen. Serial serum samples obtained following resection of primary sarcoma in patients who developed recurrent disease with pulmonary metastases. The time at which pulmonary metastases were detected on the chest roentgenogram is indicated by an arrow. (*From D. L. Morton et al., Ann Intern Med, 74:587, 1971.*)

mia exhibit delayed skin reactions to antigens extracted from their tumor cells. These skin reactions become negative with relapse.

POSSIBLE APPLICATIONS OF IMMUNOBIOLOGY TO CANCER THERAPY. There are many possible applications of cancer immunobiology to cancer therapy besides those of the immunotherapy. Immunoprevention by vaccine prepared from the common tumor antigens or tumor viral antigens is theoretically possible. However, because of the long latency period of most human neoplasms, it would require several decades to evaluate such a vaccine even if it were already in hand.

Immunobiology has great potential as a guide to standard cancer therapy. Immunologic monitoring of cancer patients undergoing therapy for malignant disease could be extremely useful in determining choice of therapy, as well as determining the patient's response to the therapy. Immunologic testing also may be useful in following the patient's response to certain therapeutic modalities that are known to be immunosuppressive, such as chemotherapy or radiation therapy, so that therapeutic regimens that are nonimmunosuppressive may be devised. Furthermore, with multiphasic immune monitoring, it may become possible to carry out immunologic engineering in patients with defective immune responses. The deficiencies then might be corrected by appropriate adjunctive therapy once the site of the defect has been diagnosed.

PATHOLOGY

When confronted with a tumor mass, the clinician must first determine whether it is a neoplastic or inflammatory process and, if neoplastic, whether it is benign or malignant. This is usually accomplished by biopsy of the mass.

In general, biopsy of a neoplasm should always be obtained before therapy is instituted. The pathologist's interpretation of materials submitted for microscopic examination depends not only upon his experience and the quality of the material submitted but also upon the clinical history and findings on the patient and a review of any previous biopsy material. The features to which the pathologist must direct his attention are partly histologic, that is, the arrangement of the tumor cells and their relation to the surrounding tissue, and partly cytologic, namely, the nature of the tumor cells and, in particular, the appearance of the nucleus and nucleoli.

The characteristics of benign and malignant neoplasms are listed in Table 9-4. *Anaplasia* means lack of differentiation. *Polarity* is the normal orderly alignment of epithelial cells, which are arranged in sheets. One of the early signs of malignant change is the loss of this normal polarity, so that the cells may present as a disorderly arrangement in relation to the surface and to each other. *Nuclear changes* of the malignant cells are often seen as enlarged and hyperchromic nuclei. These three features may all be seen before invasion of the deeper tissues has occurred. This is known as *preinvasive carcinoma,* or *carcinoma in situ.*

One of the most characteristic features of malignant disease is *local infiltration of adjacent tissues,* i.e., malignant colonic epithelial cells invading the muscular or serosal layers of the colon. In contrast, a benign tumor grows by expansion, compressing the surrounding tissues to form a capsule.

Based upon these microscopic criteria, the pathologist usually has no difficulty in determining whether the neoplasm is malignant or benign. Sometimes the microscopic diagnosis is difficult and opinions are divided among the different pathologists examining the tissue. When this happens, several paths are open to the clinician: If the biopsy is not adequate, more material should be obtained. Special stains are sometimes helpful, such as oil red O, to show fat globules as in liposarcoma. Outside expert opinion may be useful, such as from the Armed Forces Institute of Pathology or the National Cancer Institute, which act as referral centers for patients with unusual malignant neoplasms.

The electron microscope has been helpful in diagnosing some undifferentiated tumors, such as malignant melanoma and soft tissue sarcomas. Tissue culture characteristics also may be useful in identifying some malignant

Table 9-4. GENERAL CHARACTERISTICS OF BENIGN AND MALIGNANT NEOPLASMS

Characteristic	Benign neoplasms	Malignant neoplasms
Nuclear structure	Normal size, staining and shape	Large, hyperchromatic with variation in size and shape
Mitotic figures	Usually rare	Frequent and perhaps atypical
Anaplasia	Absent	Varying degree
Polarity	Orderly arrangement	Disorderly arrangement
Local invasion or infiltration	Absent (except angioma)	Usually present
Capsule	Present	Absent or a pseudocapsule
Recurrence	Absent or rare	Frequent
Metastases	Absent	Frequent
Growth	Slow, self-limited	Often rapid
Systemic effects	Rare, except for neoplasms	Frequent

Table 9-5. SIMPLE CLASSIFICATION OF NEOPLASMS

Tissue of origin	Site of origin	Benign	Malignant
Epithelial origin (ectoderm or entoderm)	Skin, mouth, larynx, lung, esophagus, urinary tract, cervix	Papilloma	Squamous cell carcinoma
	Breast, stomach, colon pancreas, liver	Adenoma	Adenocarcinoma
Mesodermal origin	Fibrous tissue	Fibroma	Fibrosarcoma
	Muscular tissue	Leiomyoma, rhabdo-myoma	Leiomyosarcoma, rhabdo-myosarcoma
	Fatty tissue	Lipoma	Liposarcoma
	Vascular tissue	Angioma	Angiosarcoma
	Hemopoietic tissue		Leukemia, multiple myeloma, lymphoma
	Bone	Osteoma, chondroma	Osteogenic sarcoma, chondrosarcoma
Special types:			
Melanocytes	Skin, eye	Nevus	Malignant melanoma
Neural tissue	Brain, spinal cord nerve	Astrocytoma	Glioblastoma multiforme
		Ganglioneuroma	Neuroblastoma
Trophoblast	Placenta testis	Chorioepithelioma	Choriocarcinoma
Notochord	Spine	Chordoma	Chordoma
Blastoderm	Mediastinum, ovary, testis	Teratoma	Teratoma

neoplasms. Hormonal assay may be helpful, as in diagnosing a glucagon-producing alpha cell cancer of the pancreas. However, it is well to remember that sometimes tumors produce biologic substances that are not normally produced by the tissue from which they originated.

It may not be possible, in certain situations, to differentiate histologically between a benign and a malignant neoplasm, as with the parathyroid carcinomas, giant cell sarcomas of bone, and thymomas. In these cases, clinical characteristics of the lesions in terms of the development of recurrence, metastases, and progressive growth may be the only differentiating criteria available to the clinician.

CLASSIFICATION OF NEOPLASMS. Many different classifications of tumors exist, but the most useful one is based upon the cell type of tissue of origin. When the neoplasm is undifferentiated, the special methods discussed above may help to classify it.

Neoplasms arising from epithelial cells regardless of whether in the ectoderm or the entoderm are known as carcinomas. Sarcomas arise from connective tissue and include tumors of fibrous, muscular, fatty, vascular, and skeletal origin. Teratoma signifies a neoplasm in which anaplastic, immature somatic cells, comparable to blastoderm, are usually dominant; it exhibits varying degrees of differentiation into mature somatic cells of ectodermal, mesodermal, and entodermal types. Teratomas occur in the testis, ovary, and mediastinum. A simplified classification of benign and malignant neoplasms arising from different sites is given in Table 9-5.

GRADING OF MALIGNANCY. Broders classified carcinomas into four grades according to their degree of differentiation, the appearance of cells, their nuclei, and the number of mitotic figures. On this basis, the least malignant are classified as grade 1, and the most malignant are grade 4. In general, the lower-grade, more differentiated neoplasms are less malignant and tend to metastasize less frequently than the higher-grade, more anaplastic ones.

Although the grading of neoplasms is sometimes useful, growth rate and presence of metastasis may be more important in determining prognosis.

CARCINOMA IN SITU AND OTHER PREMALIGNANT LESIONS. Carcinoma in situ is a lesion with the cytologic characteristics of malignant tumors but with no detectable invasion into the surrounding tissue. It seems to develop into invasive cancer after variable delay periods. The interval between the detection of carcinoma in situ of the cervix and invasive carcinoma may be 10 to 15 years. Carcinoma in situ also occurs in the skin, bronchus, stomach, and pharynx. When these lesions are adequately treated, a complete cure is assured.

ROUTES FOR SPREAD OF NEOPLASMS. There are few subjects of greater importance to the oncologist than the spread of cancer. Much is known about the routes of spread but little about the conditions which determine that spread. Some cancers are metastatic at the time of their clinical discovery, while others of the same type and in the same organ tissue may remain localized for years.

Metastases may entirely dominate the clinical picture, while the primary tumor remains latent and asymptomatic. For example, neoplasms of the brain secondary to silent cancers in the bronchus or the gastrointestinal tract are often mistaken for primary brain tumors.

Knowledge of the particular manner in which different types of cancer spread is important in planning therapy. In general, a malignant tumor may spread by four routes: directly by infiltrating surrounding tissue; via lymphatics; by vascular invasion; or by implantation in serous cavities (Fig. 9-17). Knowledge of the patterns of neoplastic spread in different types of cancer is important in planning definitive therapy. Metastatic patterns of various types of human tumors are summarized in Table 9-6.

Direct Extension. Cancer cells may spread by direct extension through tissue spaces. Some neoplasms, such as soft tissue sarcomas and adenocarcinomas of the stomach

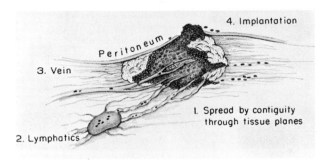

Fig. 9-17. Four mechanisms of the dissemination of cancer cells. This is a diagrammatic illustration; the original tumor could be one of many organs with cells disseminating by the four mechanisms. (*From W. H. Cole, et al., "Dissemination of Cancer," Appleton-Century-Crofts, Inc., New York, 1961.*)

or esophagus, may extend for considerable distances (10 to 15 cm) along tissue planes beyond the palpable tumor mass. Other neoplasms, such as basal cell carcinoma of skin, rarely extend for more than a few millimeters beyond the visible margin.

Lymphatic Spread. Tumor cells can readily enter lymphatics and extend along these channels by permeation or embolism through the regional lymphatics to lymph nodes. Permeation is the growth of a colony of tumor cells along the course of the lymph vessel. This occurs commonly in the skin lymphatics in carcinoma of the breast and in the perineural lymphatics in carcinoma of the prostate.

Spread along the lymphatics by embolism to the regional nodes or distant lymph nodes is of much greater importance. Lymph node metastases are first confined to the subcapsular space; at this stage the node is not enlarged and may appear normal to the naked eye. Gradually the tumor cells permeate the sinusoids and replace the parenchyma. There is little direct spread from node to node, because the capsule is not penetrated until a late stage. The tumor cells travel by anastomosing lymphatics, and the spread occurs in other nodes by way of collateral lymph channels. When a lymph node containing tumor is more than 3.0 cm in diameter, tumor has usually extended beyond the capsule into the perinodal fat.

The lymph from the abdominal organs and lower extremities drains into the cisterna chyli and then into the thoracic duct, which finally opens into the left jugular vein. Tumor cells pass from the lymph to the bloodstream by this route. Spread along the thoracic duct explains those cases in which cancer of the gastrointestinal tract is associated with pulmonary metastasis while the liver remains clear. Involvement of the supraclavicular lymph nodes is usually related to entrapment of tumor emboli from the thoracic duct behind the valves near the termination of the duct, followed by extension of these cells along the lymphatics to the node. Thus, lymphatic spread may eventually become vascular dissemination.

Lymphatic spread is extremely common in epithelial neoplasms of all types, except basal cell carcinoma of the skin, which does not metastasize to regional lymphatics. Sarcomas metastasize to lymph nodes in only a minority of cases, usually less than 10 percent.

VASCULAR SPREAD. Cancer cells may reach the bloodstream either by the thoracic duct, as just described, or by invasion of blood vessels. The veins are invaded frequently, the arteries rarely. The chief reason for the striking differences in invasion characteristics between arteries and veins appears to be that lymphatics frequently penetrate the walls of the large veins from without and form a plexus reaching to the subendothelial region, thus providing a portal of entry for tumor cells through the vein wall. When the vascular endothelium is destroyed, a

Table 9-6. ESTIMATED FREQUENCY* OF PATTERNS OF NEOPLASTIC SPREAD FOR COMMON HUMAN NEOPLASMS

Neoplasm	Hematogenous	Lymphatic	Local infiltration (expressed as local recurrence)
Adenocarcinoma			
Breast	4	3	2
Colon	3	3	1
Stomach	4	4	3
Pancreas	4	4	3
Epidermoid carcinoma			
Lung	4	3	2
Oral pharynx	1	3	3
Larynx	1	3	2
Cutaneous neoplasm			
Squamous cell carcinoma	1	2	1
Melanomas	3	3	2
Basal cell carcinomas	0	0	1
Sarcomas			
Bones	4	1	1
Soft tissue	4	1	3
Brain neoplasms	0	0	4

*0—Does not occur, 1—1 to 15 percent, 2—15 to 30 percent, 3—>30 percent, and 4—>50 percent.

thrombus forms that is quickly invaded by tumor. It is this combination of thrombus and tumor which detaches to form the emboli that result in metastases. Vascular invasion is commonly seen in both carcinomas and sarcomas and is frequently associated with a poor prognosis. Some types of neoplasms have a remarkable tendency to grow as a solid column along the course of veins, for example, renal carcinomas and sarcomas. Renal carcinomas have been known to grow out of the renal vein into the inferior vena cava and up the inferior vena cava to the right atrium.

Spread through Serous Cavities. Tumor cells occasionally gain entrance to serous cavities via direct growth of tumor through the wall of certain organs, or by growth on the surface of such potential spaces. Many tumor cells are capable of growth in suspension without a supporting matrix. In either case, it is common for tumor cells to spread widely when they encounter a space lined with a serous surface. Thus, widespread peritoneal seeding is commonly seen with gastrointestinal neoplasms and tumors of ovarian origin. A similar mechanism appears to operate in the case of malignant gliomas, which may spread widely within the central nervous system via cerebral spinal fluid.

CLINICAL MANIFESTATIONS OF CANCER

The manner in which neoplastic disease presents itself clinically is varied and inconstant. Current ability to define, detect, and quantify the neoplastic state is limited. Cancer may present as an asymptomatic lesion too small to be seen without magnification, as an asymptomatic lump, or as symptomatic disease. Often, symptoms are nonspecific and resemble those of nonmalignant diseases. The clinical abnormalities produced by advancing neoplastic diseases may be grouped into two categories—those abnormalities which stem directly from the presence of a tumor mass and those physiologic derangements which are produced indirectly. By including the possibility of neoplastic disease in every differential diagnosis and by teaching patients those key symptoms which require medical evaluation, one may be able to achieve earlier diagnosis and treatment, thereby improving the survival of cancer patients.

The onset of the neoplastic state is difficult to date in human beings. As previously discussed, a prolonged latent or induction period is likely before clinically detectable disease evolves. Therefore, the use of the word "early" in describing a cancer may lead to confusion. To avoid this, we will use the terms "early" and "late" in relation to the clinical stage of a neoplasm rather than to indicate its duration in the body. When viewed in this manner, the curable cancer may have been present a long time prior to its diagnosis and therapy. The term *early* usually means a neoplasm that can be effectively treated. These neoplasms are small rather than large, do not extend into essential organs, and have not metastasized. Some lesions that have been present for years still may be early, whereas other lesions with more rapid growth rates may be *late* even if present for only a few months.

The "Seven Danger Signals of Cancer," as formulated

Table 9-7. CANCER'S SEVEN WARNING SIGNALS

Change in bowel or bladder habits
A sore that does not heal
Unusual bleeding or discharge
Thickening or lump in breast or elsewhere
Indigestion or difficulty in swallowing
Obvious change in wart or mole
Nagging cough or hoarseness

by the American Cancer Society, are listed in Table 9-7. These may be helpful in the ongoing effort to educate people and increase the frequency of early diagnosis for certain major tumors. The more common patterns of clinical presentation, and some of the more common syndromes related to cancer will be discussed in detail in the paragraphs which follow.

Carcinoma in situ and other premalignant lesions were discussed earlier under pathology and will not be discussed further here.

SIGNS OF EXPANSILE GROWTH. The signs attributable to the expansile growth of a tumor depend upon its location. When the neoplasm is either on or near the surface of the body, it may present simply as a visible or palpable mass. In the gastrointestinal, biliary, respiratory, and urinary tracts, signs are frequently related to obstruction. Examples are vomiting, jaundice, cough, or urinary retention. Within the central nervous system, expansile growth may cause pain and paralysis.

Expansile growth of a tumor may also result in destruction of host tissues. Examples are pathologic fractures, hepatic insufficiency, and Addison's disease.

SIGNS OF INFILTRATIVE GROWTH. Pain and paralysis may result when tumor infiltrates nerves. Frequently, signs of nerve invasion are also signs of incurability. Examples are lumbosacral plexus pain in cancer of the cervix and rectum, dorsal and lumbar spine pain in cancer of the pancreas, and the shoulder and arm pain and palsy when carcinoma of the lung infiltrates the brachial plexus. Other signs of infiltration generally denoting incurability are thickening of the uterine ligaments in cancer of the cervix and fixation to the chest wall in breast cancer.

SIGNS OF TUMOR NECROSIS: BLEEDING AND INFECTION. Tumors may become necrotic, ulcerate, and bleed. Fatigue and weakness may be the only symptoms or signs in cancer of the stomach or right colon, because the tumor ulceration and bleeding have resulted in anemia. If gastric or colonic cancer becomes ulcerated and infected, the signs of inflammation include edema, pain, tenderness, and fever. The inflammation caused by cecal cancer can mimic the clinical symptoms of acute appendicitis or cholecystitis. Therefore, response of such inflammation to antibiotics or the healing of an ulcer does *not* necessarily indicate a nonneoplastic lesion.

Tumor necrosis at any site may produce fever, leukocytosis, elevation of sedimentation rate, anorexia, and malaise. Such necrosis constitutes one of the causes of the "fever of unknown origin." Keller and Williams, in studies of 46 patients with unexplained fever, found that in 19 who underwent exploratory laparotomy the cause of the fever was intraabdominal malignant disease.

UNKNOWN PRIMARY TUMORS PRESENTING AS METAS-TASES. Although the primary neoplasm often grows to considerable size before metastatic lesions are seen, in other cases the primary neoplasms may be so small as to be undetectable. The initial presentation of a tumor may be at a distance from its origin. In fact, the primary neoplasm giving rise to the metastases may have regressed completely and may never be detected in some neoplasms, such as malignant melanoma and carcinomas of the oral pharynx.

The most frequent sites of presentation of metastatic neoplasms are the cervical and supraclavicular lymph nodes, lungs, liver, bones, and brain. The most common metastatic sites for unknown primary neoplasms are listed in Table 9-8.

SYSTEMIC MANIFESTATION OF MALIGNANT DISEASE. Tumors may have a variety of remote and systemic effects that contribute to morbidity. Cancer patients frequently develop unusual symptoms and physiologic derangements which cannot be attributed to the mechanical presence of primary or metastatic disease, or to physiologic changes resulting from hormones normally secreted by the tissue of origin.

Some symptoms, such as the cachexia of carcinomatosis, may result from competition between the tumor and the host for basic components of the same metabolic pool. However, the pathogenesis of many of these disorders is unknown. Some of these nonmetastatic, systemic manifestations of malignant tumors are thought to result from (1) the ectopic production of known hormones; (2) the secretion of unidentified, physiologically active substances which do not resemble known hormones; (3) autoimmune phenomena in which the host is sensitized to an antigen

Table 9-8. UNKNOWN PRIMARY TUMORS
PRESENTING AS METASTASES

Site of metastasis	Primary neoplasm
Lymph nodes:	
Cervical nodes	Nasopharynx, pharynx, oral cavity, thyroid, larynx, lymphomas
Supraclavicular nodes	Bronchus, breast, stomach, esophagus, pancreas, colon, testis, ovary, cervix
Axillary nodes	Breast, melanoma, lymphoma
Inguinal nodes	Genitalia, anus, melanoma
Skin and subcutaneous tissues	Melanoma, breast, bronchus, stomach, kidney
Lung	Breast, colon, kidney, stomach, testis, melanoma, thyroid, sarcomas
Liver	Stomach, colon, breast, pancreas, bronchus
Ovary	Stomach, colon
Bones	Breast, bronchus, prostate, thyroid
Central nervous system	Breast, bronchus, kidney, colon
Serous cavities	Bronchus, breast, ovary, lymphoma

from the tumor; and/or (4) toxic substances secreted from the tumor.

The nonmetastatic clinical manifestations of malignant disease and the neoplasms with which they are associated are presented in Table 9-9. Sometimes palliative surgery is indicated to treat these systemic manifestations, for example, resection of metastases which are producing hormones that induce hypercalcemia, or of a pulmonary osteoarthropathy.

CANCER DIAGNOSIS AND STAGING EXTENT OF CANCER

Diagnosis

Diagnosis of cancer should proceed in an orderly fashion: careful history, thorough physical examination with examination of the blood and urine, and investigation of suspicious findings by appropriate radiologic examinations and radioisotope scans.

A history of any of the following is suspicious and should prompt a search for cancer: weight loss; loss of appetite; bleeding or a discharge from any body orifice or nipple; a sore that has not healed in 3 weeks; changing color or size of a mole; persistent cough or wheeze; change in voice; difficulty in swallowing; growing lump either in or under the skin, in the breast, in the abdomen, or in the muscles; and/or change of bowel habits.

Physical examination includes a thorough search of the entire skin surface for squamous cell and basal cell carcinomas, indurated lesions, ulcers, suspicious or irritated nevi, nodules, and other signs of malignant disease. Lymph nodes should be palpated for enlargement. Breasts should be palpated with the patient rotated to take the tension off the suspensory ligaments. All body orifices should be examined. A Papanicolaou smear from the cervix should be examined prior to a bimanual pelvic examination. Rectal examination should include proctoscopic examination of patients who have hemorrhoids or rectal symptoms. The oral pharynx should be examined with special attention to the floor of the mouth. Indirect laryngoscopy should be performed if the patient is hoarse or is suspected of having an intrathoracic neoplasm in cancer of the thyroid gland.

Laboratory examination should include complete blood cell count, urinalysis, examination of stool for occult blood, and chest roentgenogram. Other tests should be ordered where indicated by symptoms. Before operating on a patient for cure or palliation, a metastatic work-up should be done, directed by symptoms and the most likely site of metastases. Prior to extensive disfiguring or disabling procedures, tomograms of the lungs, bone marrow biopsy, scalene node biopsy, isotope scans, or arteriography may be useful in determining whether the neoplasm is still localized. Cytologic examination should be performed if a pleural effusion or ascites is present.

Diagnosis of solid tumors rests upon locating a space-occupying lesion and taking a portion of it for histologic

Table 9-9. SYSTEMIC MANIFESTATIONS OF MALIGNANT DISEASE

Clinical manifestations	Associated neoplasms
Cutaneous	
Acanthosis nigricans	Cancer of stomach, lung, and breast
Dermatomyositis	Cancer of stomach, breast, lung, and ovary
Erythema multiforme, exfoliative dermatitis, bullous phemphigoid	Allergic response to a variety of neoplasms, lymphoma, myeloma
Peutz-Jeghers syndrome	Intestinal polyposis
Hematologic	
Abnormal red cell mass	
Erythrocytosis (increased erythropoietin)	Renal cell carcinoma, hepatoma, uterine myoma, cerebellar tumors, pheochromocytoma
Anemia:	
Myelophthisic	All tumors
Hypoproliferative	Thymoma, renal cell carcinoma
Hemolytic	Hematopoietic neoplasm
Miscellaneous causes (infection, bleeding, radiation effects, uremia, etc.)	
Abnormal leukocyte or platelet mass	
Leukemoid reactions	Miscellaneous neoplasms
Leukopenia	Hemopoietic neoplasms, lung, pancreas
Thrombocytosis	
Coagulation and bleeding disorder	
Disseminated intravascular coagulation (DIC)	Mucin-secreting adenocarcinoma
Vascular	
Thrombophlebitis	Cancer of lung, reproductive tract, pancreas, and breast
Fibrinogen deficiency (increased fibrinolysin)	Cancer of prostate and lung
Flushing, vasodilatation, violaceous skin, asthma	Carcinoid tumor
Hormonal and metabolic effects of nonendocrine tumors	
Hypoglycemia (mechanism unknown)	Retroperitoneal or mediastinal mesenchymal tumors, hepatic tumors
Cushing's syndrome (increased ACTH)	Cancer of the lung, malignant thymoma, pancreatic cancer
Hypercalcemia (increased PTH, vitamin D–like substances or bone destruction)	Cancer of lung, kidney, breast, uterus, sarcomas, hemopoietic neoplasms
Hyponatremia (increased ADH)	Cancer of lung, intracranial tumors
Hyperthyroidism (increased TSH)	Choriocarcinoma, testicular embryonal carcinoma
Precocious puberty and/or gynecomastia (increased gonadotropin)	Hepatoma, lung, adrenal cancer, testicular tumors
Zollinger-Ellison syndrome (increased gastrin) or secretion	Pancreatic nonbeta islet cell adenomas
Elevated liver enzymes	Renal cell carcinoma
Anorexia and weight loss	Most neoplasms
Hyperuricemia	Hemopoietic neoplasms
Atypical carcinoid syndrome	Pancreatic duct, islet cell, gastric, thyroid, and oat cell cancer of lung
Nonmetastatic neuromuscular	
Multifocal leukoencephalopathy	Hemopoietic neoplasms
Subacute cerebellar degeneration	Multiple neoplasms, especially of lung, ovary, and breast
Polyneuropathy and/or myopathy	Multiple neoplasms, especially of lung, ovary, and breast
Myasthenia gravis	Thymoma

SOURCE: Modified from A. H. Owens, Jr., Neoplastic Diseases, in A. M. Harvey, et al., "The Principles and Practice of Medicine." Appleton-Century-Crofts, New York, 1972.

examination. This goal is most easily fulfilled when the tumor is near the body surface or involves one of the orifices of the body that can be examined with appropriate visual instruments, such as a bronchoscope, proctoscope, or cystoscope. Carcinomas of the breast, tongue, or rectum can be seen or palpated, and a portion can be excised for definitive diagnosis.

The most difficult cancers to diagnose, and unfortunately the most lethal ones, occur in the internal organs. Space-occupying lesions in the internal organs may grow quite large before causing symptoms. Techniques which may be useful in localizing such lesions include barium examinations of the stomach and colon, examination of the bronchial tree with soluble contrast media, selective arteriography of major vessels supplying internal organs, and the use of radioisotopes and radiopaque dyes that concentrate in various organs such as the liver, gallbladder, kidney, and lymph nodes. Despite the use of such indirect means of examination, major surgery is often required to confirm the diagnosis.

CANCER DETECTION EXAMINATION. Both physicians and patients have been rather slow to adopt the habit of regular examinations to detect asymptomatic neoplasms. The lack of popularity of cancer detection examinations is in direct relation to the low yield of cancers diagnosed. Any given individual stands approximately 1 chance in 4 of developing cancer during his lifetime. Therefore, in screening 1,000 persons for an entire life span, we will find cancer in 250 of them. Since a person can harbor more than one primary cancer and a second lesion will develop with increasing frequency as the number of people who have survived the first one increases, we might count on a very crude estimate of 350 cancers in our population of 1,000. Since we expect people to live an average of 72 years, we must carry out 72,000 annual examinations to discover 350 cancers, or less than 5 cancers per 1,000 examinations. By directing our search to the middle and late adult years when the incidence is highest, we might conceivably double the yield to 10 per 1,000. Thus, the chances of detecting cancer in a given annual examination are no more than 1 in 100 even under the most optimal circumstances.

The problem of cancer detection is further complicated by the relative insensitivity of our methods for clinical cancer detection. The earliest neoplasms must be at least 1 cm in size before they are detectable by physical examination, and often tumor masses up to 10 cm in diameter will go undetected if in the liver, retroperitoneum, or other "silent" areas.

Therefore, the best chance for early diagnosis will depend upon the development of biochemical or serologic methods for cancer diagnosis rather than on routine cancer examinations in asymptomatic patients.

BIOPSY. It is imperative that microscopic proof of malignant disease be obtained prior to institution of treatment, since significant morbidity and mortality may result from all forms of cancer therapy. Significant errors have been made when biopsies were not obtained; examples are radical mastectomies for fat necrosis and radiation therapy for renal cysts.

Even when biopsy reports from another hospital are available, the slides of the previous biopsy must be obtained and reviewed prior to the institution of therapy. This is essential because, not infrequently and particularly in rare neoplasms, an erroneous interpretation may have been made. *Definitive therapy cannot be planned rationally without knowing the nature of the neoplastic lesion.*

Three methods for biopsy of suspicious tissue are commonly used. They are the *needle,* the *incisional,* and the *excisional,* or open, biopsy; each has its advantages and disadvantages. Regardless of method used, the pathologic interpretation of the tumor mass can be valid only if a representative section of tumor is obtained. A problem of "sampling error" can occur with the needle and the incisional biopsies when only a small portion of the total tumor mass is submitted for pathologic examination.

Needle biopsy is the simplest method and may be used for biopsy of subcutaneous masses, muscular masses, and some internal organs, such as liver and kidney. Further, this method is inexpensive and causes minimal disturbance of the surrounding tissue. There is less chance of disrupting lymphatics and spreading cancer cells along tissue planes. The danger of implanting tumor cells in a needle track during aspiration biopsy is extremely small and can be avoided if the location of the needle track is such that it can be excised easily at the time of the definitive surgical procedure. Needle biopsy may be disadvantageous when the specimen is quite small and not representative of the total tumor, or the needle may miss the space-occupying lesion within the liver or kidney. Hence, a needle or aspiration biopsy does require experience to interpret. A negative report for malignant disease is always viewed with skepticism and should be followed by incisional or excisional biopsy if there is any doubt.

Incisional biopsy involves removal of only a portion of a tumor mass for pathologic examination. It is best performed under circumstances where, if tumor cells are spilled at the time of biopsy, the incisional wound can be encompassed and totally excised at the time of the definitive surgical procedure. Incisional biopsy includes removal of portions of tumor with forceps during endoscopic examination of the bronchus, esophagus, rectum, and bladder. Incisional biopsy is indicated for deeper subcutaneous or muscular tumor masses when needle biopsy fails to establish a diagnosis.

The incisional biopsy is also used when a tumor is so large that total local excision would prejudice any subsequent adequate, wide, locally curative resection because of the wide tissue planes that are necessarily exposed by biopsy. Such biopsy should take a deep section of tumor, as well as a margin of normal tissue, if possible. Incisional biopsy does suffer from the same hazard as the needle biopsy in that the removed portion may not be representative of all the involved tissue; hence, a negative biopsy does not preclude the presence of cancer in the remaining mass. Another theoretic objection to the incisional method is the possibility that the surgeon may seed cancer cells into the operative wound or that exposed open lymphatics may transport the cells to distant sites. Despite these dangers, one must keep in mind that definitive surgical procedures cannot be planned rationally without knowing the nature of the neoplastic lesion.

Excisional biopsy is total local removal of the tumor mass. This is used for small, discrete masses, 2 to 3 cm in diameter, when local removal will not interfere with the wider excision required for permanent local control. A major advantage of an excisional biopsy is that it gives the entire lesion to the pathologist. However, this method is contraindicated in large tumor masses because, again, the biopsy procedure often scatters tumor cells throughout a large biopsy incision that must be widely and totally encompassed by subsequent definitive surgical procedures. Therefore, excisional biopsy is usually contraindicated for skeletal and soft tissue sarcomas, although it is ideally suitable for superficial squamous or basal cell carcinomas and malignant melanomas. The surgeon should always mark the excisional biopsy margins with sutures so that if removal is incomplete, he will know where tumor margin was positive should further excision be indicated.

Biopsy incisions should be closed with meticulous hemostasis, since it may be possible for a collecting hematoma to extend tumor cell contamination by widespread infiltration of tissue planes. Contaminated instruments, gloves, gowns, and drapes should be discarded and replaced with noncontaminated substitutes when the definitive procedure is to follow immediately after the biopsy procedure.

The excisional method is principally used for polypoid lesions of the colon, for thyroid and breast nodules, for small skin lesions, and when the pathologist cannot make a definitive diagnosis from tissue removed by incisional biopsy. An unbiopsied lump is surgically removed when the suspicious character of the lesion, the need for its removal whatever the diagnosis, and the nonmutilating nature of the operation make such an approach reasonably definitive. Examples of such procedures include hemithyroidectomy for thyroid nodules, partial colectomy for lesions at any point beyond the reach of the sigmoidoscope, or a right colectomy for a cecal mass that might be inflammatory or neoplastic.

Lymph nodes should be carefully selected for biopsy. Cervical lymph nodes should not be biopsied until a careful search for a primary tumor has been made. Indirect laryngoscopy, pharyngoscopy, esophagoscopy, and bronchoscopy are included in the work-up. Enlargement of the upper cervical nodes is usually due to metastases from laryngeal, oropharyngeal, and nasopharyngeal neoplasms. Supraclavicular nodes are more frequently enlarged from metastases originating in the thoracic or abdominal cavity.

The specimen may be prepared for pathologic examination by either frozen or permanent sections. Frozen sections are made immediately, and pathologic diagnosis can be obtained within 10 to 20 minutes. Although frozen sections may be as adequate as permanent sections for diagnosis of some neoplasms, most pathologists would prefer to make a definitive diagnosis in questionable cases on permanent sections. Unfortunately, such sections require 1 to 2 days for processing. Therefore, frozen sections are used when the diagnosis is required at the time of major surgery and when it is in the patient's best interests to have the definitive resectional surgery carried out at that time. Examples in which the therapeutic decision will be based upon the results of frozen section examination include (1) deciding between a local or radical operation in carcinoma of the breast, (2) limiting the extent of excision in carcinomas of the lip or face, (3) determining the adequacy of surgical margins, and (4) identifying small structures such as parathyroid glands.

Occasionally, an exploratory thoracotomy or laparotomy will be necessary to obtain tissue for microscopic examination and confirmation of diagnosis. As a general rule, regardless of the clinical picture, the neoplastic nature of the disease process must be confirmed by frozen section examination prior to closure of the wound. This is critical because the permanent sections may fail to confirm the neoplastic nature of the pathologic process.

Exfoliative cytology constitutes one possible method for the early diagnosis of certain types of neoplasms. This technique is based upon the fact that cancer cells are shed from the surfaces of neoplasms arising in epithelial-lined body cavities and orifices, such as the vagina, bronchus, and stomach. These cells can be collected, stained, and recognized as malignant because of their individual morphologic changes.

Staging Extent of Cancer

The extent of the patient's tumor at a given point in time is expressed as its *clinical stage*. In addition to making an exact histologic diagnosis of cancer, it is essential that the clinical stage of the disease be determined prior to making a decision regarding therapy. This is especially important when the patient initially presents for treatment, but also it is often desirable to repeat some of the diagnostic procedures periodically during the patient's course in order to assess his true status. The recognized impor-

tance of this staging has led to a variety of international and national attempts to standardize the staging of the patient with cancer. To date, no single system has been universally accepted. However, Stage I usually indicates a neoplasm confined to its primary site of origin, Stage II indicates metastases to the regional lymph nodes, and Stages III and IV indicate distant metastatic spread.

The Union Internationale Contre Cancer (UICC) has attempted to standardize one system for all nations. This has been called the TNM system because it relies on a statement of tumor extent in terms of the primary tumor (T), presence or absence of node metastases (N), and the presence or absence of distant metastases (M). The system was developed following careful analysis of the results of treatment in patients with various constellations of clinical findings. It was found that patients with larger tumors did less well than those with smaller tumors; hence, the separation of various stages on the basis of tumor size. For different tumors size criteria vary, but in this system decreasing prognosis is indicated by increasing numbers after the T, such as T1, T2, T3, or T4 for lesions of increasing sizes. The presence or absence of regional spread is usually indicated by variations in the secondary category, under N for nodes. The absence of nodal metastasis is designated as N_0; the presence of nodal metastasis is N_1; for more extensive nodal involvement, additional numbers may be used. Finally, distant metastases are indicated by adding a subscript 1 following M for metastases, or a subscript 0 for their absence. Thus, a small lesion that has neither spread to regional nodes nor metastasized would be designated as a $T_1N_0M_0$ lesion. A lesion which was larger and involved regional nodes but without distant metastases might be identified as a $T_2N_1M_0$ lesion. A larger neoplasm with both regional and distant metastases would be designated a $T_3N_1M_1$ lesion.

Specific staging systems have been developed for Hodgkin's disease and other lymphomas. A distinction is made between the clinical stage, as defined by clinical tests, and the pathologic stage, as defined by biopsy or major operation. Stage I relates to diseases localized to one lymph node–bearing area. Stage II would be disease into adjacent regional areas, but on one side of the diaphragm and restricted to lymph node–bearing areas including the spleen and Waldeyer's ring (tonsilar area). Stage IV represents widespread metastases in organs, such as bone, bone marrow, liver, or lung.

Hodgkin's disease, which spreads from a localized region directly into an organ, in this classification scheme is identified as the respective stage plus the subscript E, for extension. Thus, a patient with disease in the mediastinum and neck, with extension into the pulmonary parenchyma adjacent to the mediastinal lesion, would have Stage II_E disease. For lymphomas, the importance of symptoms in prognosis is further identified by adding a designation for the absence or presence of symptoms. Patients with symptoms of night sweats, weight loss, or fever are identified as having Stage B disease, whereas patients lacking these symptoms are identified as having Stage A disease (for example, Stage II_EA). The tremendous importance of accurate staging is underlined by the fact that for many lymphomas an accurate decision regarding therapy may require pathologic staging of the presence or absence of disease below the diaphragm. Thus, patients with disease clinically limited to extensive areas above the diaphragm are commonly subjected to an abdominal exploratory operation in order to remove the spleen, examine the liver, and biopsy lymph nodes. This allows a much more precise designation of the extent of disease, and the findings frequently lead to a change in decision regarding a choice of therapy. Specifically, Hodgkin's disease in Stages I and II is curable by radiation therapy, while Stages IIIB and IV are generally treated with chemotherapy.

The importance of accurate staging when designating a therapeutic program for a patient with cancer cannot be overemphasized. It is an important consideration when comparing the results of therapy in different centers, and as therapeutic methods for cancer improve, it is only by careful staging that new forms of therapy can be appropriately evaluated.

Unfortunately, one of the great difficulties in the present staging methods is their inability to detect subclinical microscopic metastatic lesions. Many patients who are treated for apparently localized cancers already have disseminated metastases. For example, about one-half of those patients who have cancer of the breast and who undergo mastectomy have subclinical distant metastasis at the time of operation.

THERAPY

General Considerations

At present, approximately 55 percent of all cancer patients are treated by surgical resection (40 percent by surgery alone); 34 percent by radiation therapy (16 percent by radiation therapy alone); and 22 percent by chemotherapy alone or in combination with the other modalities. As the use of chemotherapy as an adjuvant to surgery increases, it is likely that a much larger percentage of patients will have chemotherapy as part of their cancer treatment. Fifteen percent of cancer patients receive no treatment.

Surgery and radiation therapy today represent the most successful means of dealing with cancer as long as it remains localized to the primary site and regional lymph nodes. Neither can be considered curative once the disease has metastasized beyond the local region, although both methods of therapy may be useful as palliative treatment. Chemotherapy and immunotherapy, unlike surgery and radiation therapy, represent systemic forms of treatment effective against tumor cells already metastatic to distant organ sites. These systemic therapeutic modalities have a greater chance of curing patients with a minimum number of tumor cells than those with clinically evident disease. Thus, though surgery and radiation therapy cannot be curative unless the tumor is confined locally or regionally, they can decrease the patient's tumor burden so that chemotherapy or immunotherapy may become more effective. During the past several years, enough evidence has

accumulated to suggest that treatment combining surgery, radiation therapy, chemotherapy, and, possibly, immunotherapy will significantly improve cure rates above those achieved with any single therapeutic modality.

Future cancer treatment, therefore, will be approached in an interdisciplinary manner. Just as oncology should be approached as a unique field of study, so cancer should be regarded as a single but complex disease requiring a multidisciplinary approach. The practice of assigning certain types of neoplasms to surgery, radiation therapy, or medicine with a further division into various anatomically oriented specialties should be discontinued.

GOALS OF THERAPY—CURE OR PALLIATION. Once the diagnosis of malignant disease has been made and the extent of disease determined, a decision must be made about the specific therapy. *Is the patient curable?* This is the foremost question that must be answered before the physician recommends aggressive therapy with its attendant complications. The goals of therapy vary with the extent of the cancer. If the cancer is localized without evidence of spread, the goal is to irradicate the cancer and cure the patient. However, when the cancer is spread beyond local cure, the goal is to control the patient's symptoms and to maintain his maximum activity for the longest possible period of time. Palliation should be measured in terms of useful life. Diabetes is not cured, but the manifestations of the disease are controlled so that a patient has many years of activity and useful life. Goals for the palliation of patients living with cancer are similar.

Patients are generally judged as incurable if they have distant metastases or evidence of extensive local infiltration of adjacent organs or structures. The most common criterion for incurability is distant metastases. However, some patients are potentially curable even if they have distant metastases. For example, patients with solitary pulmonary metastases may be curable by resection, and even those with widespread metastases who have choriocarcinoma may be curable with chemotherapy. Histologic proof of distant metastases should be obtained before the patient is assessed as incurable. Occasionally, an exploratory celiotomy or thoracotomy may be necessary to determine the nature of equivocal lesions in the lungs or liver. In some situations, e.g., multiple pulmonary metastases, the clinical situation may point so overwhelmingly to distant metastases that the patient may safely be considered incurable without biopsy.

Local extension may be a criterion of incurability. For each anatomic site, there are certain local criteria which place the patient unequivocally in an incurable status, while others imply a poor prognosis but are not absolutely indicative of incurability. In equivocal situations after extensive studies have failed to demonstrate metastatic or incurable local extension, the patient deserves the benefit of doubt and should be treated for cure.

CHOICE OF THERAPY. Surgery, radiation therapy, and chemotherapy are the most frequently used therapeutic modalities in the fight against cancer. Each may play a role in both curative and palliative therapy. Immunotherapy is a new modality that has a limited role in cancer therapy at the present time, but one which should become increasingly useful in the future. In choosing therapy, a variety of factors must be considered regardless of whether the aim is cure or palliation. The natural history of the disease and the results obtained from each type of therapy must be known prior to choosing a modality or combination of modalities.

The patient's general medical condition and the presence of any coexisting disease must be considered in planning therapy. Surgery may be contraindicated in a patient who has recently experienced a myocardial infarction. A patient with preexisting diabetes will be much more susceptible to the toxic effects of hormonal therapy with corticosteroids. Renal disease may increase the toxicity of some of the chemotherapeutic drugs, such as methotrexate. In addition, any evidence of infection or bleeding in a patient may make any form of cancer therapy dangerous, requiring vigorous treatment prior to the initiation of definitive therapy.

The psychologic makeup of the patient and the patient's life situation must be considered. A patient who is unable to accept the realities of a given treatment should be offered an alternative approach when possible. This is particularly true of any surgical procedures that significantly alter appearance or that involve change of organ function requiring the patient's daily care, such as colostomy. Experimental forms of therapy, such as intraarterial infusion of drugs, should also be avoided by some patients. Obviously, a patient who is going to be unwilling to tolerate the inconvenience of an intraarterial catheter and who might remove it without medical approval should not undergo such treatment.

Surgical Therapy

Surgical treatment represents the most frequently used and the most successful single method of cancer therapy currently available. More patients are cured of cancer by surgery than by any other therapeutic modality. However, only about one-third of cancer patients are cured by surgery alone, since surgical therapy, with few exceptions, is curative only in those patients in whom the disease is localized in the primary site and regional nodes.

Cancer surgery is based upon the concept that cancer begins as a local disease and spreads in an orderly fashion from the primary site to adjacent tissues by direct extension, to the regional lymph nodes by lymphatics, and through the blood vessels. The surgical procedure is designed to remove the primary neoplasms and the usual contiguous routes of spread with the aim of removing *every* cancer cell from the body.

Advances in surgical techniques, anesthesia, and supportive care (blood transfusion, antibiotics, and fluid and electrolyte management) have permitted the development of more radical and extensive operative procedures. This has resulted in significant improvements in the cure rates for certain human neoplasms. Ultraradical cancer surgery has extended operations to their anatomic limits, permitting the surgical removal of nearly all organs. Unfortunately, these more radical procedures have often failed to significantly increase cure rates.

There have been few significant improvements in the management of most human neoplasms by surgery alone during the past two decades. Furthermore, advances in cancer surgery techniques beyond those presently practiced are unlikely to significantly change the cure rates of most human neoplasms. It would appear, then, that any therapeutic advances must come from the combination of other modalities with cancer surgery.

PREOPERATIVE PREPARATION. Often, the physical condition of cancer patients is relatively poor. Many malignant tumors seem to have a toxic effect on the host disproportionate to the size of the lesion. Patients may have a poor nutritional status because of interference with normal alimentary function as with cancers of the oral pharynx, esophagus, and intestinal tract. Pain may contribute to anorexia and severe electrolyte disorder. Anemia, vitamin deficiencies, and defects in the coagulation mechanisms must be corrected before an operation can be safely performed.

Every effort should be made to correct nutritional deficiencies, restore depleted blood volumes, and correct hypoproteinemia prior to extensive surgical procedures. Otherwise the operative morbidity and mortality following extensive cancer operations will be excessive.

CANCER SURGERY

Once the decision has been made to proceed with surgical therapy, the operative procedure should be planned carefully. It is essential to realize that the best, and often the only, opportunity for cure is at the time of the first operation. If the neoplasm is incompletely excised at that time, tissue planes, lymphatics, and blood vessels are violated and tumor cells seeded throughout the wound. Any recurrence that follows may be difficult to separate from the inflammatory reaction and scarring that can distort tissue planes to a point where tumor margins are indistinct. Therefore, enucleation or incomplete excision of tumor masses is *never* indicated as a therapeutic measure.

PREVENTION OF CANCER CELL IMPLANTATION DURING SURGERY. Local recurrence of cancer following surgery may be due to incomplete removal or spillage of cancer cells into the operative area (Fig. 9-18). The cancer surgeon constantly must be aware of the possible danger of transferring cancer cells by inoculation into the surrounding tissues during the course of an operation. As soon as the incision is made, all edges of the wound should be protected with a plastic drape to prevent tumor cell contamination. This precaution is exemplified best when laparotomy or thoracotomy is performed for malignant disease within the abdomen or thorax.

Tumor cells may be inadvertently transplanted from the primary site to other sites during the surgical procedure. When preliminary biopsy has been done, the entire operative field should be reprepared after the biopsy incision is closed. The instruments and gloves used during the biopsy are not used again, because they may have been contaminated. Even the basin of saline solution in which the surgeon dips his gloved hand may be contaminated with cancer cells. The importance of this is illustrated by a patient with breast cancer who had a skin graft taken

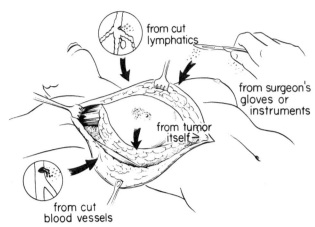

Fig. 9-18. During the operative procedure, cancer cells may be seeded in the wound by direct contact with the primary tumor, with lymph nodes containing metastatic tumor, or with contaminated gloves and instruments. Cancer cells may also enter the wound via cut lymphatics and divided blood vessels. (*From W. H. Cole et al., "Dissemination of Cancer," Appleton-Century-Crofts, Inc., New York, 1961.*)

from the thigh to close a skin defect after a mastectomy. Later, tumor nodules having the same histologic characteristics as the primary neoplasm developed on the thigh at the skin graft donor site.

If the tumor is entered during the operative procedure, the risk of implanting cancer cells into the wound is greatly increased. Should this happen, the operative field must be isolated; the cut surface of the tumor must be cauterized with the electrocautery and isolated from the remainder of the wound; and the contaminated knife, instruments, and gloves must be discarded. Then, and then only, can the operation continue through a new plane of dissection allowing a much wider margin around the tumor.

Many different cytotoxic solutions have been used to irrigate the wound following cancer surgery in an effort to sterilize the operative site. None have been very effective in decreasing the local recurrence rate, with the exception of 0.5% formaldehyde used to prevent local recurrence from carcinoma of the cervix. Sodium hypochlorite solution, nitrogen mustard, and thiotepa have all been tried, with little success.

The rate of local recurrence in the suture line following resection for carcinoma of the colon is about 10 percent. There has been some success with various techniques to prevent this local recurrence. Ligation of the bowel with umbilical tape proximal and distal to the tumor, or anastomosis, or irrigation of the cut ends of the colon with bichloride of mercury solution and then excision of the edge of each end of the bowel have been used and have decreased the recurrence rate to less than 2 percent. The use of closed anastomosis and iodized sutures has decreased the anastomotic recurrence rate in the laboratory.

PREVENTION OF VASCULAR DISSEMINATION AT SURGERY. Blood-borne metastases are a major factor in the death of patients with most tumors. Although cancer cells have been identified in the blood of many cancer patients, only a small number of these circulating cancer cells sur-

vive because of host resistance and other factors. Thus, tumor embolism and metastases are not synonymous. In fact, there appears to be little difference in the prognosis of patients with or without tumor cells in their blood preoperatively. However, there is a correlation between the presence of tumor cells seen in the blood during the operative procedure and prognosis. Furthermore, manipulation of the tumor at any time in the surgical procedure can greatly increase the number of cancer cells recovered from the blood.

Definite measures should be taken to prevent the dissemination of tumor cells during the operation. These can include (1) avoiding manipulation of the tumor ("no-touch" technique), (2) early ligation of the vascular pedicle, (3) the use of tourniquets on all extremity tumors.

Since any manipulation of the tumor mass may result in exfoliation of tumor cells into the lymphatics and blood, such manipulation must be kept to a minimum prior to the operative procedure, during preparation of the skin with antiseptic agents, as well as during the operative procedure. Furthermore, it is imperative to use an incision of proper size to minimize unnecessary manipulation of the tumor. One that is too small will not permit the necessary wide excision without excessive handling. Turnbull and associates have reported a significant higher survival in left colon cancer using the no-touch technique which combines minimal manipulation, early ligation of the vascular pedicle, and wide excision. However, the importance of early ligation of the vascular pedicle has been questioned by Stearns, who reported similar results without the early ligation.

TYPES OF CANCER OPERATIONS. Local Resection. Wide local resection in which an adequate margin of normal tissue is removed with the tumor mass may be adequate treatment for certain low-grade neoplasms that do not metastasize to regional nodes or widely infiltrate adjacent tissues. Basal cell carcinomas and the mixed tumors of the parotid gland are examples of such neoplasms.

Radical Local Resection. Some neoplasms may spread widely by infiltration into adjacent tissues. This is especially true for soft tissue sarcomas and esophageal and gastric carcinomas. For this reason, it is necessary to remove a wide margin of normal tissue with the neoplasm in these cases. The wide normal-tissue margin between the line of excision and the tumor mass also acts as a protective barrier against tumor cell spill into the severed lymphatics and vessels. The greater the thickness of normal tissue between the plane of dissection and the tumor, the greater likelihood of a complete local excision.

If the tumor was previously explored but not removed or if an incisional biopsy was performed, it is extremely important that a wide segment of skin and the underlying muscles, fat, and fascia be removed far beyond the limits of the original incision.

It must be constantly emphasized that malignant neoplasms are not well encapsulated. A pseudocapsule composed of a compression zone of neoplastic cells usually covers the tumor. This apparent encapsulation offers a great temptation for simple enucleation, because the tumor may be dislodged from its bed so easily. However, this temptation must be resisted. The surgeon must cut through normal tissue at all times and should never encounter the neoplasm during its removal. Dissection should proceed with meticulous care to avoid tumor cell spill. Retraction always should be away from, rather than toward, the tumor. It is important for the surgeon to remember that he must be as far as possible from the gross extent of the tumor on all sides including the deep aspect. He must be prepared to sacrifice important nerves, muscles, and blood vessels if necessary in order to encompass the tumor. Skin, subcutaneous fat and muscle usually can be sacrificed with impunity and little functional loss. However, involvement of major vessels, nerves, joints, or bones may require sacrifice of these structures and even amputation in order to obtain a curative result. During the surgical procedure, the extent of operation should be determined only by the concern for cure.

All deeply situated sarcomas lying between or within muscle groups require the removal of all muscle bundles from their origin to insertion within that particular fascial compartment; all surrounding or adjacent fascia, periosteum, vessels, nerves, and connective tissues; and all skin adjacent to the lesions. These procedures are imperative because sarcomas of the soft somatic tissues tend to infiltrate along fascial and muscle planes far beyond the palpable limits of the tumor. As the surgeon proceeds with the operation, he may be forced to alter his initial operative plan as he visualizes the extent of tumor and as the pathology reports of frozen section examinations of surgical margins are made available. These decisions as to extent of resection are difficult and require experienced judgment. In borderline situations, it is usually better to proceed with a potentially curative resection of the tumor mass unless there is histologic confirmation that the lesion has extended beyond the boundaries of possible surgical resection. Recent advances in the use of combined modality therapy for skeletal and soft tissue sarcomas have permitted the salvage of extremities rather than amputation in selected patients (see the section on Combined Modality Therapy).

Radical Resection with En Bloc Excision of Lymphatics. Since many neoplasms commonly metastasize by way of the lymphatics, operations have been designed to remove the primary neoplasms and the regional lymph nodes draining that area in continuity with all the tissues intervening between the primary neoplasm and regional nodes. Conditions are best for this type of operation when the collecting nodes of the lymphatic channels draining the neoplasm lie adjacent to the primary site or if there is a single avenue of lymphatic drainage which can be removed without sacrificing vital structures. The regional nodes farthest from the tumor should be dissected first, with dissection proceeding toward the tumor mass in order to prevent any exfoliation of tumor cells from the primary tumor into the regional lymphatics of the venous system.

This principle was applied to breast cancer by Meyer and by Halsted at the turn of the century and has formed the foundation of cancer surgery for many years. At the present time, it is generally agreed that such en bloc regional lymph node dissections should be performed in patients having clinical involvement of nodes by metastatic tumor. However, in many such cases, the tumor has already spread beyond the regional nodes, and the cure rates following such procedures may be quite low.

The high rate of local cancer recurrence following surgical removal when lymph nodes are grossly involved and the high error rate when trying to ascertain by palpation those nodes involved by tumor have led to routine dissection of regional nodes close to the primary tumor even though they are not clinically involved. Microscopic examination of the excised lymph nodes in these patients who have no clinical evidence of palpable enlargement reveals evidence of tumor spread in 20 to 40 percent of carcinomas. This concept is supported by comparison of the higher 5-year survival rate of patients showing microscopic involvement of lymph nodes with that of patients in whom lymph node involvement was clinically recognizable.

Recently, some surgeons have challenged the concept of elective or prophylactic resection in cases where the regional nodes are not obviously involved, because of the possibility that such removal may interfere with the patient's immune response to the tumor. This concept originated from experiments in laboratory animals in which removal of the regional nodes within 1 to 2 weeks after implantation of tumor transplants in an extremity interfered with the development of tumor immunity. The validity of these experiments must be challenged, however, because it has been demonstrated with other animal tumors that regional lymphadenectomy has little influence upon host immunity if the removal of the regional nodes is delayed 4 to 6 weeks until the immune response is already underway. The differences between these two sets of experiments depends upon the well-established observation that early excision of regional nodes will interfere with a primary immune response.

It is possible that the immune response against cancer in man is similar. Most human neoplasms have been present in the body for many months or years prior to clinical detection. Hence, cancer patients already have an active systemic immune response to their malignant condition, best demonstrated by the presence of killer lymphocytes in the blood and circulating antitumor antibodies. Thus, the importance of the regional lymph nodes as an immune barrier controlling tumor dissemination in man probably should not be considered an adequate argument against regional lymphadenectomy. In addition, when metastatic cancer cells are found in 20 to 40 percent of operative specimens, it seems likely that the regional nodes obviously are not doing an effective job of controlling the dissemination of cancer.

Nevertheless, this is a very controversial issue at the present time, with sufficiently numerous conflicting reports concerning the effectiveness of elective regional lymphadenectomy that a definite conclusion regarding its use cannot be made. We advocate regional lymphadenectomy in selected patients with clinically negative nodes who have neoplasms which frequently metastasize to lymph nodes because of data supporting higher 5-year survival rates with this technique. Furthermore, most studies comparing identical stages of primary disease have shown slightly improved survival when lymphadenectomy was done. There has been little evidence that removal of the regional nodes adversely affects the survival figures.

An important benefit of lymphadenectomy is the provision of more accurate staging in order to identify those patients at high risk for disease recurrence. Now that we have presumptive evidence for the effectiveness of adjuvant chemotherapy and immunotherapy in a variety of malignant diseases, it is particularly important to identify those patients who will benefit most from these therapies.

This controversy can be settled by a controlled clinical trial to demonstrate the effectiveness of elective or prophylactic lymph node dissections. Such studies are currently underway for several different types of neoplasms. Until more data are available, en bloc resection of regional nodes should continue as standard therapy for carcinoma of the mouth, pharynx and larynx, colon and rectum, breast, uterus and cervix, malignant melanoma, and testicular neoplasms.

Extensive Surgical Procedures. Some slow-growing primary tumors may reach enormous size and may locally infiltrate widely without developing distant metastasis. Supraradical operative procedures can be undertaken in these extensive, nearly inoperable tumors, with cure of occasional patients. Although surgical care, anesthesia, blood replacement, and physiologic monitoring are much improved over the past, these procedures should not be undertaken except by experienced surgeons who can select those patients most likely to benefit from such procedures. Since these extensive surgical procedures sometimes offer a chance for a cure that is not possible by other means, they are justified in selected situations when extensive laboratory work-up shows no evidence of distant metastases. However, the surgeon must be willing to accept the responsibility for the postoperative emotional rehabilitation of the patient before undertaking such extensive procedures as the pelvic exenteration, hemipelvectomy, forequarter amputation, or mutilating operations for head and neck carcinomas.

Pelvic exenteration is a well-conceived operation capable of curing patients with radiation-treated recurrent cancer of the cervix and certain well-differentiated and locally extensive adenocarcinomas of the rectum. This operation removes the pelvic organs (bladder, uterus, and rectum) and all soft tissues within the pelvis. Bowel function is restored with colostomy. Urinary tract drainage is established by anastomosis of ureters into a segment of bowel (ileum or sigmoid colon). The 5-year survival cure rate from pelvic exenteration is 25 percent in this situation.

Hemipelvectomy (resection of the lower extremity and iliac bone) can sometimes be curative for skeletal sarcomas limited to the head of the femur or acetabulum or to one-half of the pelvic structures, and in some slowly growing soft tissue sarcomas of the upper thigh and buttock which recur locally but metastasize slowly. Forequarter amputation (resection of the upper extremity and scapula) can offer similar cure when the neoplasm is limited to the bones of the scapula and upper humerus or to the soft tissues of the shoulder girdle.

SURGERY OF RECURRENT CANCER. There is a definite role for surgical resection of localized recurrent neoplasms of low-grade malignancy and slow growth where further resection may produce a long period of remission. Additional surgical procedures are frequently successful in controlling recurrent soft tissue sarcomas, anastomotic recurrences of colon cancer, and certain basal and squamous carcinomas of skin.

Gilbertsen and Wangensteen advocated routine "second look" operations over a scheduled period, perhaps 6 months after the original procedure, whether or not symptomatic or objective evidence of recurrence was evident. The results of these operations have not been impressive, although a few patients experienced an unexpected long-term control of their disease. However, many of these patients might have been salvaged anyway if reoperation and excision had been delayed until a symptomatic recurrence developed, since this is not uncommon. Thus, it is difficult to prove the second-look theory; for this reason, second-look operations have not become common practice.

RESECTION OF METASTASES. Although logic would suggest that once a neoplasm has metastasized to a distant site it should no longer be curable by surgical resection, removal of metastatic lesions in the lung, liver, or brain has occasionally resulted in a clinical cure. Therefore, in selected patients with slowly growing neoplasms, resections of the metastatic lesions may be indicated especially if the metastasis is solitary. Prior to undertaking resection, an extensive laboratory work-up should rule out metastatic spread to other body areas.

Most patients with diffuse liver metastases are candidates for systemic or intraarterial chemotherapy. Most will not survive beyond 2 years, and few, if any, will survive for 5 years. Therefore, prior to embarking on such therapy, it is important to remember that significant palliation and an occasional cure can be achieved by resecting hepatic metastases in selected patients. Resection can be recommended when the primary tumor is controlled and no other metastases are present and when the patient's condition, the location of the tumor, and the capability of the surgical team allows safe resection.

In a survey involving 126 patients who had resection of metastases from carcinoma of the colon and rectum, Foster and Berman reported an 18 percent 5-year survival. These patients were obviously chosen from a large group of patients and do not represent statistics that can be applied across the board to all patients with hepatic metastases. Nonetheless, it is advisable to consider resection prior to beginning systemic chemotherapy, since an occasional 5-year cure can be achieved (Fig. 9-19).

The results of resection of pulmonary metastatic lesions have been much more satisfactory than those of resection of liver or brain metastases. In fact, resection of solitary pulmonary metastases has given a higher rate of 5-year survival than has resection of primary bronchogenic carcinoma of the lung. Resection of pulmonary metastases may be indicated even when more than one metastatic lesion is present. Many patients die with pulmonary metastases and no other evidence of tumor at autopsy; resection of the pulmonary metastases could have resulted in cure.

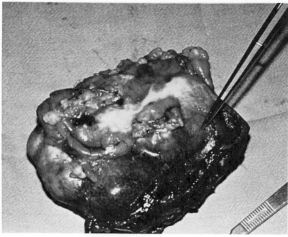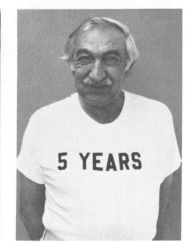

Fig. 9-19. Resected liver and smiling patient at 5-year anniversary of operation for hepatic metastases. (*From D. L. Morton, E. C. Holmes, and S. H. Golub, Chest, 71:640, 1977.*)

Our experience has shown measurement of the tumor doubling time to be useful in selecting those patients who will benefit most from resection of pulmonary metastases. Patients with tumor doubling times greater than 40 days received significant palliation from their pulmonary resections and remained free of disease for as long as 5 years. In contrast, patients with tumor doubling times of less than 20 days have not significantly benefited from resection of their metastatic lesions (Fig. 9-20).

Hepatic Dearterialization. Hepatic dearterialization has been advocated for the treatment of liver metastases, based upon the observation that metastases derive their blood supply predominantly from the hepatic artery whereas normal liver tissue receives blood from both the arterial and portal systems. In the absence of hypotension and sepsis, hepatic artery ligation is surprisingly well tolerated and results in selective necrosis of liver tumors. Because some tumor cells remain viable, postoperative chemotherapy is necessary to help control tumor growth. This procedure is not without risk and needs further evaluation to determine its role in managing patients with either primary hepatic carcinoma or hepatic metastases.

ADMINISTRATION OF CHEMOTHERAPY BY ARTERIAL INFUSION OR ISOLATED PERFUSION. The concentration of

chemotherapeutic drugs can be greatly increased when the drug is administered directly into the artery supplying the neoplastic lesion. Continuous infusion of chemotherapeutic drugs over a period of weeks can be carried out with portable infusion pumps attached to a catheter placed in the artery. Some striking remissions using this technique have been observed, although they usually have been of short duration. It appears logical to assume that this manner of administering chemotherapeutic agents would increase their effectiveness because of the greater concentrations obtainable. Patients with hepatoma have responded well to the intraarterial infusion of 5-FU. Hepatic artery ligation and 5-FU infusion have been combined with some success in treating patients with metastatic colon carcinoma.

One ingenious method of administering increased concentrations of chemotherapeutic drugs involves the isolated perfusion technique. The artery and veins supplying the tumor-bearing extremity are cannulated and isolated from the systemic circulation by connection to a pump-oxygenator. The tumor is then perfused for up to 90 minutes with oxygenated blood containing cancerocidal drugs in amounts that would be prohibitively poisonous if infused through the general circulation.

Recently it has been found that heating the blood with a heat exchanger similar to that used for cardiopulmonary

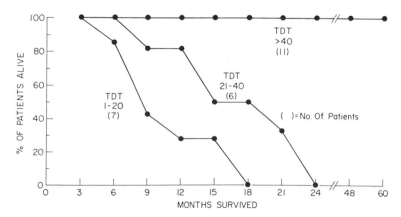

Fig. 9-20. Survival curves of 24 untreated patients following onset of pulmonary metastases. (*From W. L. Joseph et al., J Thorac Cardiovasc Surg, 61:23, 1971.*)

bypass appears to increase the effectiveness of the chemotherapeutic drugs. Hyperthermic perfusion with chemotherapeutic agents may be worthwhile in treating satellite or intransient metastasis from malignant melanoma and primary or recurrent sarcomas of the extremities. Some long-term survivors with malignant melanoma treated by this technique have been reported. Furthermore, Stehlin reports that hyperthermic perfusion of chemotherapeutic drugs, when combined with radiation therapy, may decrease the necessity of amputation in some primary or recurrent sarcomas which are bordering on vital structures of the extremity.

Despite a long experience with intraarterial infusion and regional perfusion for the administration of chemotherapeutic drugs, there is still no general agreement about their usefulness. Many chemotherapists believe systemic administration of drugs would be equally effective. However, we have observed more dramatic responses from the infusion/perfusion techniques than from systemic administration of chemotherapeutic drugs.

PALLIATIVE SURGERY. Surgical procedures are sometimes indicated to relieve symptoms, to reduce the severity of the patient's illness, or to prolong a useful comfortable life without attempting to cure the patient. Such an operation is justified to relieve pain, hemorrhage, obstruction, or infection when it can be done without great risk to the patient, and when it improves the quality of life even if it does not prolong it. Surgery that only prolongs a miserable existence certainly does not benefit the patient.

Some examples of palliative surgical procedures are (1) colostomy, enteroenterostomy, or gastrojejunostomy to relieve obstruction; (2) chordotomy to control pain; (3) cystectomy for infected, bleeding tumors of the bladder; (4) amputations for painful infected tumors in the extremities; (5) simple mastectomy for carcinoma of the breast, even in the presence of distant metastases, when the primary tumor is infected, large, ulcerated, and locally resectable; and (6) colon resection in the presence of hepatic metastases.

Radiation Therapy

Radiation therapy, like surgical therapy, can cure only localized cancer. The palliative effects of radiation therapy in treating symptoms of metastatic or recurrent cancer are well recognized. In fact, 40 percent of all cancer patients will receive radiation therapy at some time in the course of their disease. Irradiation can destroy neoplastic tissue with a minimum of damage to normal tissues surrounding the tumor and thus, when successful, leads to good functional and cosmetic results. Some neoplasms are best treated by this method, whereas other neoplasms can be managed equally well with surgery. Radiation therapy and surgery need not be competitive if specialists in each of the two areas understand the indications and limitations of each form of treatment. Often the two modalities can be used in combination to increase the cure rates for certain types of neoplasms.

MECHANISM OF ACTION. Regardless of the primary source of radiation energy, radiation penetrates and collides with the atoms in tissue, releasing energy that causes the ionization of water in cells. The hydroxy and peroxide radicals thus formed cause DNA and chromosome breaks in both tumor cells and normal cells. Thus, the mechanism of radiation damage relates to a direct effect on certain vital substrates within living cells. Although such effects occur in both normal and neoplastic cells, there are quantitative differences in toxicity, apparently related primarily to a more adequate mechanism for cellular repair in the normal cells, which can be translated into a useful therapeutic effect.

The cellular effects of radiation are both immediate and delayed. Changes in the appearance and behavior of individual cells are observed within a few minutes of exposure, whereas gross changes in irradiated tissue may not appear until weeks, months, or even years after exposure. Microscopic changes occur in both the cytoplasm and nucleus of the cell. Vacuoles often appear in the cytoplasm of the cell, which then becomes swollen. Nuclear chromatin may clump and shrink. The chromosomes may appear abnormal in the cell undergoing mitosis at the time of radiation exposure. Although the radiation may not cause immediate cell death, the cell may be unable to divide again.

The *rad* is the unit of measurement used to express the amount of radiation absorbed, whereas *roentgens* refer to the air dose. With unidirectional radiation therapy, the dose absorbed varies throughout the depth of the radiation field and is dependent upon the energy of the radiation source (Fig. 9-21). Since a tumor is three-dimensional, the dose varies across the tumor volume. There is a maximum and a minimum tumor dose. Without further qualification, a dose of 4,500 rads refers to the average tumor dose at the midpoint of the tumor.

By using various techniques such as multiple ports, rotational fields, lead shielding, and others, it is often possible to deliver larger doses of radiation to the tumor-bearing area than to the surrounding tissue.

Usually, patients tolerate radiation therapy much better when the total dose is fractionated over a number of days or when it is split into two treatment courses, allowing for a rest period between. The margin of safety between destruction of tumor and damage to surrounding tissue also is increased by these techniques.

Rets express the relation between the total dose delivered, the number of fractions, and the time it took to deliver the dose. The ret concept is a method of comparing dissimilar treatment schedules by reducing them to a similar unit of measurement.

There are three basic types of radiation: *alpha particles, beta, or electron, particles,* and *electromagnetic rays,* such as gamma rays and x-rays. Their qualitative effects upon tissue are similar. However, there is great variation in the distance to which these rays can penetrate tissues. Alpha particles penetrate only a few microns and are stopped by the epidermis. Beta particles penetrate tissue in proportion to their energy and in inverse proportion to the density of the tissue, but they do not usually penetrate tissues for more than a few millimeters. Gamma rays can penetrate several centimeters of metal, depending upon the energy and the distance from the target source. The penetration

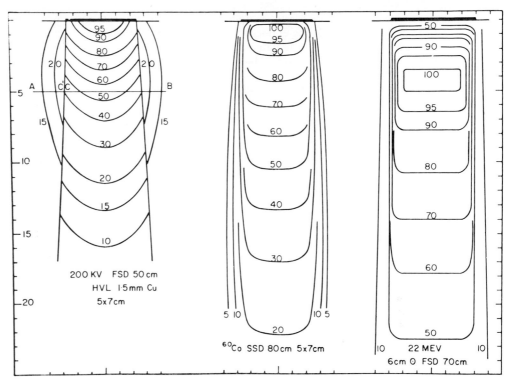

Fig. 9-21. Typical isodose distributions for low-energy (200 kv), high-energy (^{60}Co), and very high energy (22 Mev) radiation. The average patient is 20 cm thick. When treating a tumor situated midway through the patient, or at 10 cm, each of the three sources would deliver a different percentage of the maximum dose at that point—25 percent with 200 kv, 52 percent with ^{60}Co, and 83 percent with 22 Mev.

of x-rays depends upon the voltage of the machine used to produce the radiation and the distance from the source. Supervoltage machines producing 1,000 to 50,000 kv of energy are available. Such radiation can penetrate to greater depth and will cause less ionization, hence less skin damage, as it passes through the skin than the 250-kv machines used routinely in the past.

The relative biologic effectiveness of x-rays, gamma rays, and beta rays are approximately equal, although neutrons and alpha rays are ten to twenty times as effective, respectively. Therefore, it is possible that new types of neutron radiation may eventually prove very useful in reaching those deep-seated tumors which are relatively insensitive to the present forms of radiation treatment.

RADIOSENSITIVITY VERSUS RADIOCURABILITY OF TUMORS. Radiosensitivity and radiocurability are *not* synonymous terms. A tumor may be radiosensitive but not radiocurable, because of recurrence developing either locally or at a distant site. For instance, very few patients with Ewing's sarcoma, a very radiosensitive tumor, can be cured with radiation therapy, because they develop distant metastases. Some tumors, such as undifferentiated soft tissue sarcomas, initially may respond very rapidly, only to recur locally several months later. Other tumors, such as epidermoid carcinoma of the cervix or adenocarcinoma of the uterus, do not disappear immediately, but hyster-

ectomy several months later may reveal no evidence of tumor, and the patient may be cured.

Radiocurability depends upon radiosensitivity; however, tumors differ in their response to radiation therapy, as shown in Table 9-10. In general, tumor cells which are undifferentiated or in active mitosis are more sensitive to radiation. Furthermore, radiosensitivity of malignant tumors usually parallels the radiosensitivity of their cell of

Table 9-10 RELATIVE RADIOSENSITIVITY OF MALIGNANT TUMORS

(Listed in order of decreasing radiosensitivity)

Malignant tumors arising from hemopoietic organs (lymphosarcoma, myeloma)
Hodgkin's disease
Seminomas and dysgerminomas
Ewing's sarcoma of the bone
Basal cell carcinomas of the skin
Epidermoid carcinomas arising by metaplasia from columnar epithelium
Epidermoid carcinomas of the mucous membranes, mucocutaneous junctions, and skin
Adenocarcinomas of the endometrium, breast, gastrointestinal system, and endocrine glands.
Soft tissue sarcomas
Chondrosarcomas
Neurogenic sarcomas
Osteosarcomas
Malignant melanomas

SOURCE: From L. V. Ackerman and J. A. del Regato, "Cancer: Diagnosis, Treatment, and Prognosis," 4th ed., The C. V. Mosby Company, St. Louis, 1970.

origin. Hemopoietic cells, epidermoid cells, lymphocytes, germ cells of the gonads, and the lining epithelium of the alimentary tract are most sensitive to radiation. Usually tumors derived from these cells are also radiosensitive. However, there are exceptions, such as adenocarcinoma of the stomach and gonads. Tumor volume, tumor oxygenation, and the histology of the tumor are of equal importance in determining radiosensitivity and radiocurability.

COMPLICATIONS OF RADIATION THERAPY. Although usually associated with no immediate mortality, the morbidity, complications, and long-term effects of radiation therapy may be considerable. The complications of radiation therapy may limit the dose and the rate of delivery. Both systemic and local complications of radiation therapy may be seen, as well as the less frequent genetic and carcinogenic effects. The acute and chronic local effects of radiation on different organs are outlined in Table 9-11. The acute changes are caused by edema and inflammation, while the chronic changes are caused by scarring and fibrosis. Megavoltage radiation has largely obviated the skin changes seen in the past with lower-voltage radiation.

Many patients undergoing radiation therapy temporarily develop systemic symptoms associated with malaise, nausea, vomiting, weakness, and weight loss. These symptoms are directly related to dose, volume, and rate of delivery, and to type of tissue treated. Radiation sickness usually can be prevented, and the nausea and vomiting can be successfully treated with antiemetics such as Compazine.

The genetic and carcinogenic effects of radiation therapy are seen less frequently as these problems have become better understood. The genetic effects of radiation expressed as mutations and congenital abnormalities have been demonstrated in lower animals, but not conclusively in human beings. The late carcinogenic effects of radiation are manifested by lung tumors in uranium miners, skin cancer in radiologists, bone tumors in clock dial painters, leukemia in radiologists and atomic bomb survivors, and thyroid cancer in patients who have had radiation in childhood for an enlarged thymus, tonsils, or adenoids.

INDICATIONS FOR RADIATION THERAPY. A variety of localized neoplasms can be cured with radiation therapy.

Curative radiation therapy usually requires doses of 4,500 to 6,000 rads, delivered over 4 to 6 weeks. As most patients are unable to work during this time, the total time the patient is incapacitated is similar for both radiation therapy and surgery. The doses and complications for curative radiation therapy are significantly higher than those for palliative radiation therapy. To avoid unnecessary complications, it is vital that the stage of the tumor be carefully established in order to assure that the disease is still localized and therefore curable by radiation therapy. The best example of this is Hodgkin's disease, which is treated by aggressive and curative radiation therapy for Stages I, II, and possibly III without organ involvement other than the spleen. If other organs are involved, then systemic chemotherapy is indicated.

When the cure rate for a particular tumor appears equal by either radiation therapy or surgery, a variety of other factors must be considered by the surgical oncologist before making a decision on treatment. These include age, operative risk, cosmetic and functional deformity, and logistical problems such as distance and time. Squamous cell and basal cell carcinomas of the skin are good examples. Many of these tumors can be cured with a simple and quick diagnostic biopsy as an outpatient procedure. However, if these tumors are located in areas where surgery would lead to extensive cosmetic deformity, such as the nose or eyelid, then radiation therapy is usually the treatment of choice.

Some useful generalizations regarding choice between radiation therapy and surgery can be made. Usually surgery, rather than radiation therapy, should be used to treat radiation-induced (actinic) skin cancer in people with prolonged exposure to the sun. Radiation therapy may be the preferred treatment for recurrent carcinomas when the primary therapy was surgery, and vice versa. However, surgery is more likely to salvage a cure after a radiation failure, especially in the head and neck area.

Neoplasms in which radiation therapy is preferred to surgical therapy are lymphomas, Ewing's sarcoma, some malignant thymomas, locally unresectable carcinoma of the breast, oat cell carcinoma of the lung, locally advanced carcinoma of the prostate, and carcinomas of the skin

Table 9-11. LOCAL EFFECTS OF RADIATION

Organ	Acute changes	Chronic changes
Skin	Wet or dry epidermitis	Running
	Radiodermatitis	Ulceration
	Epilation	
Gastrointestinal tract	Edema, ulceration, infection, diarrhea, hepatitis	Stricture, ulceration, and perforation
Kidney		Nephritis, renal insufficiency
Bladder	Dysuria	Ulceration
Gonads	Sterility	Atrophy, menopause
Hemopoietic tissue	Lymphopenia	Pancytopenia
Bone	Cessation of epiphyseal growth	Necrosis
Lung	Pneumonitis	Pulmonary fibrosis
Heart	Acute pericarditis, myocarditis	Chronic pericarditis, myocarditis
Eye	Conjunctivitis	Cataracts
Nervous system	Cerebral edema	Radiation myelitis

Table 9-12. COMPARISON OF RADIATION THERAPY AND SURGERY IN TREATMENT OF MALIGNANT TUMORS

A. Cure rate higher with radiation therapy
   1. Lymphomas and Hodgkin's disease
   2. Ewing's sarcoma
   3. Certain malignant thymomas
   4. Carcinoma of the breast (locally unresectable)
   5. Certain basal and epidermoid carcinoma of the skin where surgery would lead to extensive cosmetic deformity
   6. Oat cell carcinoma of the lung
   7. Carcinoma of prostate (locally advanced)
   8. Nasopharynx
B. Cure rate higher with surgery
   1. Carcinoma
      a. Gastrointestinal tract [esophagus (distal one-third), stomach, pancreas, liver and biliary ducts, colon and rectum]
      b. Lung
      c. Breast (localized to breast and axilla)
      d. Urinary tract [kidney, renal pelvis, ureter, bladder, and prostate (early)]
      e. Genital tract (ovary, testis, penis, vulva, vagina, uterus, in situ cervix)
      f. Thyroid and parathyroid glands
      g. Salivary glands
      h. Adrenal gland
      i. Paranasal sinuses
      j. Carcinoma from any site with lymph node metastases (not bulky or mixed)
   2. Neuroblastoma
   3. Sarcomas (skeletal and soft tissue)
   4. Melanoma
   5. Cancer of the brain and spinal cord
C. Cure rate of radiation therapy and surgery approximately equal (choice depends on stage, size of tumor, and other factors—see text)
   1. Epidermoid carcinoma
      a. Skin
      b. Cervix
      c. Anus
      d. Lip
      e. Oral pharynx (tongue, floor of mouth, tonsil, gingiva)
      f. Hypopharynx
      g. Larynx
      h. Esophagus, upper two-thirds (low cure rate)

(basal or epidermoid) where surgery would lead to extensive cosmetic deformity. Table 9-12 compares the effectiveness of radiation therapy to surgery in the treatment of various types of neoplasms.

Palliative Radiation Therapy. Radiation therapy can relieve symptoms such as pain, hemorrhage, intractable cough, inability to swallow, intestinal obstruction from tumor, edema such as that produced by lung carcinomas with an associated superior vena cava syndrome, pathologic fractures, spinal cord compression, and varying degrees of paralysis secondary to brain metastases from a number of different tumors. In the presence of diffuse metastases, aggressive radiation therapy should not be given except for specific indications, because patients may be made more uncomfortable by the side effects of the radiation itself. An exception would be palliative radiation of metastases in weight-bearing bones such as the neck of the femur; this can prevent pathologic fractures and unnecessary hospitalization.

Even when a tumor is considered to be radioresistant, a trial of radiation therapy will sometimes result in unexpected palliation with regression or stabilization of the tumor. For instance, soft tissue sarcomas are not considered by many to be very radiosensitive or radiocurable. Yet, radiation therapy for palliation of soft tissue sarcomas often produces an objective response and relief of symptoms. However, radiation therapy should not be used for radioresistant tumors such as melanoma and osteogenic sarcoma unless it is clearly the best form of therapy or other methods of therapy are no longer available.

Combined Radiation Therapy and Surgery. Radiation therapy is a logical adjunct to surgery for treating many *locally advanced neoplasms.* Table 9-13 lists the tumors for which preoperative or postoperative radiation therapy has improved the cure rate or decreased the local recurrence rate.

Preoperative Radiation Therapy. Radiation therapy can sometimes convert an inoperable tumor into an operable one by decreasing both the size of the tumor and its fixation to surrounding tissues. In this manner, radiation therapy is a logical adjunct to surgery, because it is known that the cells at the periphery of a tumor are more radiosensitive because of their more rapid rate of growth and the availability of adequate oxygen. In contrast, tumor cells in the center of the tumor are often hypoxic and more slowly dividing, which makes them less sensitive to radiation therapy.

Preoperative radiation therapy may increase the cure rate or decrease the rate of local recurrence from tumor cells disseminated into the wound, lymphatics, or body cavities during surgery, either by killing the cells or by

Table 9-13. RADIATION THERAPY AS AN ADJUNCT TO SURGERY (LOCALLY ADVANCED CANCERS)

Preoperative radiation therapy
   Cure rate increased with these locally advanced carcinomas:
      Larynx
      Laryngopharynx
      Esophagus
      Bladder
      Uterus
      Retinoblastoma
      Paranasal sinuses
      Superior pulmonary sulcus
      Soft tissue sarcomas (liposarcomas)
      Bulky cervical node metastases from epidermoid carcinoma of the head and neck
   Local recurrence decreased with these locally advanced carcinomas:
      Rectum
      Endometrium
      Head and neck (epidermoid) with clinically positive lymph nodes
Postoperative radiation therapy
   Carcinoma of the lung for mediastinal node metastases
   Seminoma (periaortic and iliac node areas)
   Medulloblastoma (after biopsy)
   Wilms' tumor
   Bladder
   Ovary (dysgerminoma, granulosa cell, and cystadenocarcinoma)

destroying their ability to multiply. In experienced hands, preoperative radiation therapy usually can be given with little increased morbidity or mortality. Its usefulness needs to be further evaluated for a number of neoplasms, such as carcinomas of the breast, pancreas, and stomach. In cancer of the rectum, preoperative radiation therapy can convert an inoperable tumor into an operable tumor, decrease the local recurrence rate, and decrease the incidence of metastases seen in the regional nodes. As survival is usually determined by spread of cancer beyond the pelvis and regional nodes, it does not follow that decreasing the incidence of histologically positive nodes will increase survival. Nonetheless, a slight increase in survival has been reported in some studies. However, none of the prospective randomized studies have clearly demonstrated an increase in survival. Furthermore, one randomized study failed to substantiate a prior optimistic report from the same institution. Several prospective randomized trials of pre- and postoperative radiation therapy using higher doses are currently under way. One may hope that the results will clearly show whether adjunctive radiation therapy will increase the survival for patients with cancer of the rectum.

Preoperative radiation is not justified when a cancer is small and freely movable, and can be removed with a wide margin of normal tissue. With these tumors there is both a high cure rate and a very small chance of local recurrence.

Postoperative Radiation Therapy. Postoperative radiation therapy has some advantages over preoperative treatment. Once the histopathologic findings are available, those patients at high risk for local recurrence can be identified and treated. This approach saves those patients at low risk from the discomfort, expense, and potential long-term complications of radiation therapy. When the "tumor margin" of normal tissue surrounding the tumor is inadequate or when further surgery is either impossible or unacceptably deforming, postoperative radiation therapy is indicated. However, it should not be given in place of proper (adequate) surgery or when further "curative" surgery can be performed.

Postoperative radiation therapy is given routinely for Wilms' tumor, medulloblastoma, seminoma (to treat periaortic and iliac node-bearing areas), and in Stage II cancer of the ovary. For carcinoma of the bladder, both preoperative and postoperative radiation therapy appears to have some benefit in selected cases, though the data are not totally convincing.

Recent evidence suggests that postoperative radiation therapy may be useful in carcinoma of the lung for treating residual mediastinal node metastases. For breast cancer, radiation therapy can be effective in treating local recurrences and bone metastases. However, the routine use of postoperative radiation therapy, even in patients with positive nodes, has not been found to be of value in increasing the cure rate.

Chemotherapy

The treatment of cancer with drugs was initiated in 1941 by Huggins and Hodges, with the discovery that estrogens palliated prostatic cancer. Polyfunctional alkylating agents were developed in the later 1940s, as a result of experimental work performed during World War II. Since then there has been a tremendous increase in the number of chemotherapeutic drugs available; at present at least five major classes of drugs, plus an additional group of miscellaneous drugs, are available (Table 9-14). Although full elucidation of this complex field is beyond the scope of this chapter, certain general principles will be described regarding the use of chemotherapy. This section will consider the mechanisms of action of the major classes of chemotherapeutic drugs, the biologic and pharmacologic factors which are important in understanding drug therapy, and guidelines for the use of chemotherapy in patients with nonhematologic malignant conditions.

MECHANISMS OF ACTION. The majority of antineoplastic drugs appear to affect either enzymes, directly, or substrates of enzyme systems. In most cases the effects on enzymes or substrates relate to DNA synthesis or function, apparently by inhibiting cells which are undergoing DNA synthesis. Drugs which act by inhibiting the enzymes of nucleic acid synthesis are called *antimetabolites,* or *structural analogs.* Methotrexate, a structural analog of folinic acid, appears to act as a nearly irreversible inhibitor of the active site of the enzyme dihydrofolate reductase, which is necessary for DNA synthesis. Another commonly used antimetabolite is 5-fluorouracil, which appears to act as a reversible inhibitor of the enzyme thymidylate synthetase, which is necessary for the synthesis of thymidine, which is then used in DNA synthesis. This class of compounds acts directly on enzymes as either reversible or irreversible inhibitors, leading to the synthesis of abnormal DNA due to the incorporation of an abnormal building block or to disruption of DNA synthesis due to the lack of an essential building block.

Other major drugs appear to work primarily by affecting substrates. The usual substrate affected is the DNA macromolecule, although some of these agents will interfere with other substrates, such as proteins, and may have other diverse effects. Three major chemical classes of drugs appear to act by affecting specific substrates. The alkylating agents are extremely reactive compounds which can substitute an alkyl group (for example, $R-CH_2-CH_2^+$) for the hydrogen atoms of many organic compounds. The primary compounds affected appear to be the nucleic acids, especially DNA. Such alkylation produces breaks in the DNA molecule and cross linking of the twin strands of DNA, thus interfering with DNA replication and the transcription of RNA. Since these effects are somewhat similar to that seen with ionizing radiation, alkylating agents are sometimes called "radiomimetic." Another group of compounds which appear to work primarily on substrates are the *antibiotics.* These are natural products derived from certain soil fungi. They produce their antineoplastic effect by forming relatively stable complexes with DNA, thereby inhibiting the synthesis of DNA and RNA. The final class of drugs acting primarily on substrates is the *vinca alkaloids.* Although their total mechanism of action may not be completely defined, it is apparent that they can bind to microtubular proteins necessary for cell division. These proteins form the spindle apparatus which allows the chromosomes to separate to either end of the dividing cell; the vinca alkaloids appear to be able to dissolve this protein, leading to death of the cell during mitosis.

Other than these two known major mechanisms of drug action, the mechanisms of action for many drugs useful in the treatment of cancer are unknown. In some cases there may be combinations of activities, particularly for those steroid hormones which are active in treating cancer.

Table 9-14 lists representative examples of each group along with selected characteristics of their clinical importance.

BIOLOGIC AND PHARMACOLOGIC FACTORS IN CANCER THERAPY. A major theme in pharmacology has been the study of variations in drug absorption, distribution, metab-

olism, and excretion as related to a stable, invariant biologic receptor. In cancer chemotherapy, however, the biologic receptor, the cancer cell, is a variable and fluctuating target. Thus, the kinetics of tumor growth must be given as much attention as the kinetics of drug absorption or metabolism when considering cancer chemotherapy. Specifically, four general principles of tumor biology relevant to treatment appear to be extremely important. These include an understanding of (1) antineoplastic drug action as a function of the cell cycle, (2) tumor cell population growth, (3) the log–cell kill hypothesis, and (4) the critical role of drug scheduling in optimizing therapy.

Drug Action and the Cell Cycle. The life cycle of all cells, both normal and neoplastic, starts with mitosis, or cell division. This is followed by either differentiation or a

Table 9-14. DRUGS USED IN TREATMENT OF NONHEMATOLOGIC NEOPLASMS

Drugs	Route of administration	Cell cycle phase specificity*	Acute toxicity†	Principle delayed or cumulative toxicity†
Alkylating agents:		Nonspecific	N & V§	BM§; cyclophosphamide may cause alopecia, hemorrhagic
Nitrogen mustard	I.V.		N & V	cystitis.
Chlorambucil	P.O.§		None	
Phenylalanine mustard	P.O., I.V.‡, I.A.‡		None	
Cyclophosphamide	P.O., I.V.		N & V	
Thiotepa	I.V.		None	
Antimetabolites:				
Methotrexate	P.O., I.M., I.V.	Specific	None	BM, stomatitis, hepatitis.
5-Fluorouracil	I.V.	Nonspecific	N & V	BM, stomatitis, diarrhea, nausea, alopecia.
Hydroxyurea	P.O., I.V.‡	Specific	None	BM.
Cytosine arabinoside*	I.V.	Specific	N & V	BM.
Antibiotics:				
Actinomycin D	I.V.		N & V	BM, alopecia, stomatitis.
Mithramycin	I.V.		None	BM & hemorrhagic diathesis.
Adriamycin	I.V.		N & V, fever	BM, cardiac toxicity, stomatitis, alopecia.
Bleomycin	I.V., S.C., I.M.		Fever	Skin changes, pulmonary fibrosis.
Vinca alkaloids:				
Vincristine	I.V.	Specific	N & V, rare	Constipation, BM, peripheral neuropathy, alopecia.
Vinblastine				
Steroid hormones				
Adrenal corticoids	P.O., I.V., I.M.	(?) Nonspecific	None	Hypertension, peptic ulcer, diabetes, increased susceptibility to infection.
Androgens	P.O., I.M.	Unknown	None	Fluid retention, masculinization; may cause hypercalcemia in breast cancer.
Estrogens	P.O.	Unknown	N & V, occasional	Fluid retention, uterine bleeding; may cause hypercalcemia in breast cancer.
Progestins	P.O., I.M.	Unknown	None	May cause hypercalcemia in breast cancer.
Miscellaneous				
Nitrosoureas‡	I.V., P.O	Nonspecific	N & V	BM (may be delayed 4–6 weeks), liver dysfunction.
BCNU				
CCNU	I.V., I.A.‡			
Imidazole carboxamide		Nonspecific	N & V	BM, hepatotoxicity, fever.
Mitotane (o, p-DDD)	P.O.	Unknown	N & V	Skin eruptions, mental depression, muscle tremors.

*The distinction between a phase-specific and non-phase-specific drug may not be absolute. Some authorities distinguish additional categories or use different names for these categories, but these are not considered in this chapter since their clinical relevance remains to be defined.

†See manufacturer's package inserts for usual doses and for additional toxicity data.

‡Experimental drug or route of administration; not yet approved by the Federal Drug Administration or Division of Biological Standards; it may be available from the Cancer Chemotherapy National Service Center, Bethesda, Maryland.

§N & V = nausea and vomiting; BM = bone marrow depression; P.O. = orally (per os); I.A. = intraarterial.

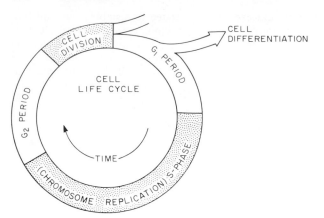

Fig. 9-22. Schematic diagram of the cell life cycle. G_1 is the first "gap" period, and G_2 is the second "gap" period. (*From R. Baserga (ed.), "The Cell Cycle and Cancer," Marcel Dekker, Inc., New York, 1971.*)

series of biochemically distinct phases known, in sequence, as G_1 (the first "gap" phase), S phase (DNA synthesis), G_2 (second "gap" phase), and mitosis (Fig. 9-22). Although these events are similar in neoplastic and normal cells, there appear to be some quantitative differences in the duration of the cycle and the sensitivity of cells to drugs during various phases of the cell cycle. Because of these differences, it has become apparent that one must differentiate between drugs which kill cells only during specific

phases of the cycle (*phase-specific*), and drugs which kill cells during all or most phases of the cell cycle (*phase-nonspecific*). The distinction between a phase-specific and phase-nonspecific drug may not be absolute. Some authorities distinguish additional categories or use different names for these categories. In particular, some workers separate the phase-nonspecific drugs into an additional two categories: *cycle-specific* and *non-cycle-specific*. For this discussion, drugs which can affect multiple phases of the cell cycle or which appear to be effective against nondividing cells are grouped together under the term *phase-nonspecific*, since the clinical usefulness of this group appears to be correlated with their lack of phase specificity.

Gompertz and Cell Population Growth. The human organism consists of communities of cells, many of which are capable of self-renewal through cell division. Generally these renewable populations grow rapidly when they are small in number and slowly when they are large. Thus, the fetus grows rapidly, but the adult organism remains constant in size, thanks to a balance between cell production and cell loss. This relation between size and growth rate may be expressed quantitatively in either of two ways: (1) as a function of volume doubling times (time for any given number of cells to double in number) or (2) as a function of the growth fraction (that fraction of cells undergoing division at any one time). Figure 9-23 presents a logarithmic plot of human fetal and childhood growth against time and includes specific data on the volume doubling times during growth. Growth in the early years

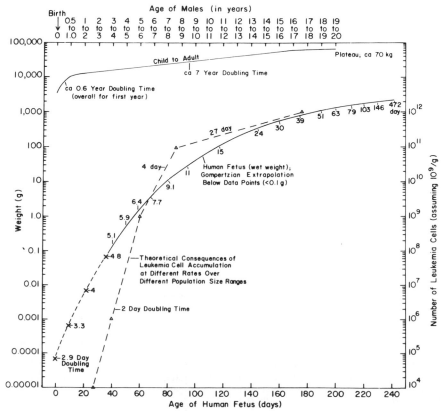

Fig. 9-23. Human fetal and childhood growth as a Gompertzian process, and the theoretic consequences of accumulation of leukemic cells at different rates over varying population ranges. (*From H. E. Skipper and S. Perry, Cancer Res, 30:1883, 1970.*)

is clearly exponential with a high growth fraction and very short volume doubling times. As time passes, the doubling time lengthens and the growth fraction decreases. The general slope of this curve can be expressed mathematically as an exponentially decreasing function. The specific equation describing this relationship was originally derived by the eighteenth-century mathematician Gompertz; therefore, biologic growth that conforms to this pattern is referred to as *Gompertzian growth.* Interestingly, evidence that not only normal cell growth but neoplastic cell growth follows a Gompertzian pattern is increasing. At least 18 different animal tumors conform to a Gompertzian growth curve, and Sullivan and Salmon have recent, preliminary evidence suggesting that human myeloma follows a Gompertzian growth pattern.

The Log–Cell Kill Hypothesis. Antineoplastic drugs are incapable of killing all cancer cells at any given exposure; rather, they will kill a variable fraction of cells from a very few up to a maximum of 99.99 percent. The fractional cell kill observed can usually be graphed as a line with a negative exponential slope, and so experimental chemotherapeutic data are usually expressed in logarithmic terms. Since the body burden of tumor cells in man with an advanced malignant tumor may be greater than 10^{12} cells, and since the best one can hope for with a single maximal exposure of tumor cells to a drug is 2 log cell kill, it is apparent that treatment must be repeated many times in order to achieve even partial control. Theoretically, this hypothesis also suggests that chemotherapeutic drugs may not be capable of totally eradicating any given population of tumor cells. There is good evidence that immunotherapy does not face this restriction, since it can completely eradicate small numbers of tumor cells; however, it may be totally ineffective against larger tumor cell masses (greater than 0.1 mg of tumor in most model systems).

DRUG SCHEDULING AND COMBINATION THERAPY. Studies with experimental animal tumors have conclusively demonstrated the critical importance of drug scheduling in therapy. Cytosine arabinoside, an antimetabolite which kills only cells in S phase, must be given frequently in order to assure contact with cancer cells during this critical period. When this drug is so employed, it is possible to "cure" some forms of murine leukemia, whereas maximally tolerated doses of the drug given at less frequent intervals fail to prolong survival. On the other hand, cyclophosphamide (Cytoxan), which is phase-nonspecific, achieves optimal suppression of most experimental neoplasms when given on an intermittent schedule.

A second factor related to drug scheduling is the growth status of any given tumor. In general, solid tumors with a large tumor mass will be growing slowly, and will have a small growth fraction (less than 10 percent) and a prolonged tumor volume doubling time. Since relatively few of these cells are dividing, these tumors are generally resistant to phase-specific drugs. Thus, the usual treatment for advanced nonhematologic tumors has been with phase-nonspecific drugs, such as the alkylating agents or 5-fluorouracil. However, successful treatment with such phase-nonspecific drugs may render the tumor more susceptible to phase-specific drugs, by converting the tumor from one with a low growth fraction with few of the cells in S phase to one with a higher growth fraction with many cells in S phase. Good experimental data exist supporting this concept. Schabel has shown that a hamster plasmacytoma, which grows with Gompertzian kinetics, can be "cured" with cyclophosphamide therapy when followed by cytosine arabinoside therapy. When either drug is used alone or in the reverse sequence, "cures" were not seen. These results are consistent with tumor conversion, i.e., by changing an insensitive tumor with a low growth fraction and few cells in S phase to one with a higher growth fraction and many cells in S phase and therefore sensitive to the phase-specific drug cytosine arabinoside.

Theoretic Model for Combination Chemotherapy. The practical application of these concepts in man remains to be accomplished, but studies are in progress. One approach (Fig. 9-24) is proposed by Schabel. The vertical axis gives the number of viable tumor cells in a patient, on a log scale, versus arbitrary time units on the horizontal axis. At the initial tumor mass of 100 Gm, a likely growth fraction of less than 10 percent can be predicted. The class of drug to be used initially will be phase-nonspecific because of the low growth fraction. A 2 log cell kill with such drugs is possible in many types of tumors. During the recovery time only those viable tumor cells that are in the cell division cycle will repopulate the tumor. A phase-specific drug might be capable of suppressing this process by a selective effect on dividing cells, although doses and scheduling would have to be carefully chosen to minimize toxicity to the vital normal cells of the patient. Alternating courses of the phase-nonspecific and phase-specific agents, provided cellular resistance or excessive host toxicity does not intervene, would be expected to result in progressively more successful killing of tumor cells. This prediction (Fig. 9-24*E* and *G*) relates to the decreasing tumor cell mass and the associated increase in tumor cell growth fraction. Specifically, as the tumor cell mass becomes smaller, the percentage of cells in S phase or mitosis will be greater, leading to increased cell killing by drugs specific for such phases. Finally, "cure" may be possible with continued chemotherapy, or possibly by appropriate immunotherapy.

Schabel's model is attractive but difficult to evaluate in man. Nevertheless, it is clear that the optimal way to use chemotherapy against human cancer is by using combinations of drugs. Since cancer chemotherapy usually involves the use of toxic drugs, one must design programs of combination chemotherapy with care in order to minimize dangerous toxicity. In general, the successful programs of combination chemotherapy have been designed with the following criteria in mind: (1) only drugs active against the tumor in question are included; (2) drugs included have different mechanisms of action, in order to minimize the possibility of drug resistance; and (3) drugs chosen generally have different spectra of clinical toxicity, thus allowing the administration of full or nearly full doses of each of the active agents. A final factor relates to the preference of most investigators for utilizing intermittent courses of intensive combination chemotherapy rather than continuous programs of drug administration. This approach tends to

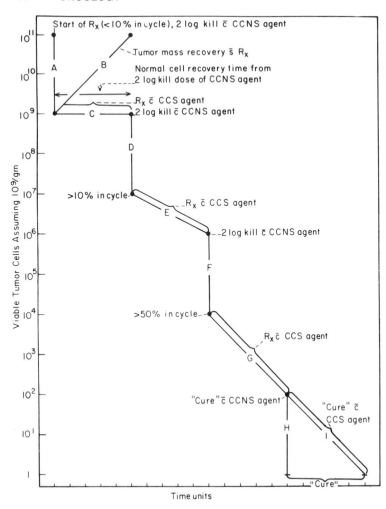

Fig. 9-24. Idealized approach to "curative" therapy of advanced tumors using a phase-nonspecific (CCNS) agent (for example, an alkylating agent) followed by a phase-specific (CCS) agent (for example, certain antimetabolites) in repeated courses. (*From F. M. Schabel, Jr., Cancer Res, 29:2384, 1969.*)

maximize tumor cell killing, is usually better tolerated by patients, and appears to cause less immunosuppression.

CHEMOTHERAPY AS AN ADJUVANT TO CANCER SURGERY. The proved ineffectiveness of surgical resection alone for many types of neoplasms has led many investigators to the use of cancer chemotherapeutic agents as adjunctive treatment. It was postulated that these agents might control microscopic foci of cancer already disseminated in the body. Controlled clinical trials have been carried out to determine the effectiveness of single chemotherapeutic agents when combined with surgical resection for carcinomas of the breast, lung, stomach, and colon. Very few significant benefits have been demonstrated thus far using single agents. However, the chemotherapeutic agents chosen for these studies, their dosage, and the duration of administration may not have been optimal for the desired result. It is likely that future applications of this concept using newer chemotherapeutic agents in combination for prolonged periods of time may well result in improved survival for these patients. This approach may be further enhanced by advances in immunotherapy and radiation therapy. An example of one approach to adjuvant

chemotherapy as applied to breast cancer appears later in this chapter.

CLINICAL PHARMACOLOGY. In addition to the principles relating to tumor biology described above, numerous pharmacologic principles must be considered in cancer chemotherapy. The first such consideration relates to the route of administration of a drug or a combination of drugs. A variety of routes can be chosen, such as oral, intravenous, intramuscular, intraarterial, or local application. By using a carefully selected parenteral route of administration, difficulties related to absorption of drugs are avoided. It also may be possible to improve the antitumor effect of a given drug. Particularly promising in this regard has been the use of intraarterial administrative drugs, such as when the primary tumor is in the liver or on an extremity. Using a portable infusion pump, drugs can be continuously infused over weeks or months. An extension of this approach has been with isolation-perfusion of an extremity with high doses of chemotherapy. As newer drugs are developed, particularly drugs with very short half-life periods, it is likely that the choice of the route of administration will become increasingly important.

A second consideration relates to transport mechanisms for the drug in question. If the drug is transported on serum proteins, it is possible that other drugs may alter significantly the proportion of the bound and free anticancer drug. An example of this is the ability of salicylates to displace methotrexate from its binding site on albumin. In this setting, high doses of salicylates may result in augmented host toxicity from methotrexate.

Another consideration is the possible effect of drug interactions when drugs are given in combinations. One well-established drug interaction involves allopurinol, a xanthine oxidase inhibitor, when it is used with 6-mercaptopurine (6-MP). Since degradation of 6-MP is catalyzed by xanthine oxidase, the use of allopurinol along with full doses of 6-MP has been shown in the past to be dangerous. Normal function of organs important in drug metabolism or degradation may be critical to the biologic fate of a drug. For example, serious liver disease may increase the toxicity of drugs which are cleared by that route, such as vincristine or adriamycin. Severe neurotoxicity has been observed in patients with concomitant liver disease when given otherwise clinically well-tolerated doses of vincristine.

The route of excretion of a drug may be critical. Methotrexate is primarily excreted by the kidney, and even modest elevation of the BUN (blood urea nitrogen) may be associated with major hematologic toxicity from the use of relatively low doses of methotrexate. For this reason the status of the kidneys must be observed very closely in all patients receiving methotrexate therapy. In fact, it is wise to observe renal function in all patients receiving cancer chemotherapeutic drugs, since nearly all of them have some extent of excretion by the renal route. In addition, it is not unusual for a brisk response to chemotherapy to result in elaboration of large amounts of uric acid, from the breakdown of the nucleic acids of the destroyed cancer cells. Uric acid nephropathy may result. Pretreatment with allopurinol may prevent this complication.

A final factor relates to the ability of a given drug to enter the cancer cell: many drugs require direct access to a specific biochemical pathway within the cell, and failure to gain entry will be associated with drug resistance. To some extent this effect may be overcome by giving very large doses of the drug; however, this is usually associated with unacceptable drug toxicity. An exception to this limitation may be the experimental use of large doses of methotrexate and its antidote, citrovorum factor. Cancer cells appear to lack this transport system. When normal and cancer cells are exposed to massive doses of methotrexate, a high intracellular drug concentration results. When the antidote is subsequently given in lower doses, the normal cells are "rescued" by virtue of the cell membrane transport system. Future work with this treatment and with others that rely on the transport of drugs across cell membranes may result in further improvements in drug therapy.

Ultimately, all factors which might alter either the concentration of the critical drug at its primary site of action or the duration of time available for such activity should be considered in the use of drugs. This may be expressed as a function of concentration times time, and because of its importance it is commonly referred to as the $C \times T$ function.

GUIDELINES FOR THE USE OF CHEMOTHERAPY IN PATIENTS WITH NONHEMATOLOGIC MALIGNANT TUMORS. The initial major question a physician must ask himself when considering chemotherapy for any patient with a neoplasm is whether benefit will result with tolerable toxicity. The physician must have all the facts regarding the patient, including the type, extent, and grade of the malignant tumor, its expected natural history, the results of current therapy, and the psychologic makeup of the patient. In addition, he must consider the following three principles:

1. The patient should have a histologic diagnosis of a malignant disease that is known to respond in a reasonable percentage of cases in a manner beneficial to the patient. Table 9-15 outlines the current status of cancer chemotherapy for a variety of nonhematologic neoplasms. Brief comments on specific drug-sensitive neoplasms will be presented subsequently. In general, patients in whom disease usually or often responds to chemotherapy should receive drug treatment, unless there is a specific contraindication. In addition, patients suspected of having minimal residual disease (micrometastases) after local therapy also may be candidates for adjuvant chemotherapy. Such therapy would be questionable for those patients with a tumor known to be minimally inhibited by commercially available drugs. Experimental therapy may be warranted for these patients.

2. It is absolutely essential that there be adequate facilities to monitor the potential toxicity outlined in Table 9-14, and a physician should not initiate therapy unless he is adequately trained in the use of drugs and committed to monitoring the patient for drug therapy. Chemotherapy is generally contraindicated for patients with nonhematologic malignant conditions if they have major bleeding or infection, although patients with leukemia and, in some cases, lymphomas may require treatment even during such episodes in order to control life-threatening bleeding or infection. Patients with major dysfunction of an organ system particularly susceptible to the toxicity of a cancer chemotherapeutic drug must be followed carefully and may be more suitably treated with an alternative drug. An example of this latter situation would be a patient with a severe neuromyopathy, who might be better treated with drugs other than vinca alkaloids, as these may exacerbate the condition. Patients in whom a rapid response to therapy is possible or who have preexisting renal disease should be treated with allopurinol to prevent the complication of uric acid nephropathy. Finally, patients who are under active chemotherapy and develop severe toxicity may require aggressive support with platelets, red blood cells, antibiotics, or in some cases, white blood cells for control of infection.

3. Cancer chemotherapeutic drugs are toxic. In order to minimize unwarranted toxicity, the physician should conduct a diligent search for disease markers to assist in monitoring treatment. Ideally, several parameters of tumor response should be followed in order to objectively assess the response to therapy. Some factors which can be considered in assessing response to treatment are described in more detail in Table 9-16. As a general rule, tumor size is of particular importance. Most oncologists require a 50 percent reduction in the product of the greater and lesser diameters of any given tumor to accept the change as a "partial response."

The specific choice of a drug or drugs for a given patient with

Table 9-15. CURRENT STATUS OF CANCER CHEMOTHERAPY FOR NONHEMATOLOGIC NEOPLASMS

Disease	Agent	Benefit
Highly Responsive Neoplasms:		
Trophoblastic tumors	Methotrexate, actinomycin-D, alkylating agents, vinca alkaloids	>80% response with permanent regression
Carcinoma of prostate	Estrogens	80% response; prolonged survival
Wilms' tumor, neuroblastoma	Actinomycin-D, vincristine	80% 2-year survival with combined surgery, radiation, and chemotherapy
Ewing's sarcoma	Cyclophosphamide, vincristine, actinomycin-D, adriamycin	>50% response; prolonged survival when combined with radiation therapy
Testicular carcinoma, germinal cell tumors	Actinomycin-D, vinca alkaloids, methotrexate, alkylating agents, mithramycin, Bleomycin, cis-platinum (experimental)	Clinical improvement in approximately 80%
Carcinoma of breast	Estrogens, androgens, 5-fluorouracil, alkylating agents, combination chemotherapy	25–75% response; prolonged survival for responders
Moderately Responsive Neoplasms:		
Sarcomas of bone and soft tissue (adult)	Actinomycin-D, vinca alkaloids, alkylating agents, adriamycin	15–50% objective response
Carcinoma of ovary	Alkylating agents	Clinical improvement in 30–50%
Adrenal carcinoma	*o,p'*-DDD	Occasional clinical improvement, sometimes prolonged
Carcinoma of bowel and stomach	5-Fluorouracil	Clinical improvement in 15–25%
Carcinoma of endometrium	Progestins	Clinical improvement in 25%
Minimally Responsive Neoplasms:		
Head and neck tumors	Bleomycin, methotrexate, adriamycin	10–30% objective response, usually of short duration
Hepatic and pancreatic tumors	5-Fluorouracil	10% objective response
Carcinoma of cervix	Alkylating agents	5% objective response
Lung cancer	Alkylating agents, adriamycin, nitrosoureas, 5-fluorouracil	25% objective response, usually of short duration
Melanoma	Imidazole carboxamide	20% objective response, but duration of response usually short

SOURCE: Modified and updated from M. J. Cline and C. M. Haskell, "Cancer Chemotherapy," 2d ed., pp. 10–11, W. B. Saunders Company, Philadelphia, 1975.

cancer and the precise choice of a dose and schedule for such single agent or combination therapy are best decided in the light of current therapeutic research. To some extent such choices can be determined by referring to Table 9-16 and the following section. Other useful sources of information include the *Medical Letter on Drugs and Therapeutics,* which periodically publishes information on the choice of therapy in the treatment of cancer (Dec. 17, 1976); monographs on cancer chemotherapy (such as that by Cline and Haskell); and the specialty journals of cancer (*Cancer; Cancer Treatment Reports; Seminars in Oncology*).

ILLUSTRATIVE NEOPLASMS HIGHLY RESPONSIVE TO CHEMOTHERAPY. Trophoblastic Tumors of the Uterus. Metastatic gestational choriocarcinoma is curable in 80 to 90 percent of women using chemotherapeutic drugs alone. The discovery by Li et al. in 1956 that methotrexate could control metastatic disease in women with choriocarcinoma represents a landmark in the history of cancer chemotherapy. Subsequent systematic study of this disease has markedly increased our understanding about cancer and its treatment. Certain points are worthy of special mention.

1. Methotrexate must be started as soon as possible after the diagnosis has been made. This relates to the finding that the

best prognosis, with cure rates of 95 to 100 percent, is seen in patients whose disease is treated within 4 months of onset, in whom metastases do not include the brain or liver, and in whom 24-hour urine quantities of human chorionic gonadotropins (HCG) are less than 100,000 I.U.
2. Combination chemotherapy should be used if the initial response to chemotherapy is suboptimal or if the patient presents with high titers of HCG, with liver or brain involvement, or with symptoms present longer than 4 months. Second-line drugs for this disease include actinomycin D, vincristine, alkylating agents, and adriamycin.
3. Therapy should be continued for 6 months after the chorionic gonadotropin titer has returned to normal. This is even more important than eliminating radiographic evidence of disease, since residual pulmonary lesions may be present despite cure of clinical growths. This is analogous to the residual changes of many nonneoplastic diseases, such as tuberculosis.

Carcinoma of the Prostate. The mainstays of therapy for disseminated cancer of the prostate are orchiectomy and estrogen therapy. These modalities have increased survival of these patients two- to threefold. Many different doses of the most commonly used estrogenic hormone have been employed. However, data from the Veterans Administration Cooperative Research Group have shown up to a

Table 9-16. CRITERIA FOR RESPONSES IN
PATIENTS WITH SOLID TUMORS

Tumor size	Palpation and measurement with calipers.
	Radiologic measurement.
	Radioisotope scans.
	Ultrasound.
Tumor products	Quantitative level of chorionic gonadotropin (choriocarcinoma and certain testicular tumors).
	Quantitative level of carcinoembryonic antigen (CEA) in bowel cancer.
	Quantitative level of α-fetoprotein in hepatoma.
	Serum or urine paraproteins in myeloma.
	Urinary adrenal hormone (adrenal carcinoma treated with *o,p'*-DDD).
Improvement in symptoms or sign of tumor	Improvement in hypercalcemia (particularly with carcinoma involving bone).
	Improvement in obstruction due to tumor (such as bowel obstruction or obstructed ureter).
	Disappearance of effusions from tumors involving pleura, peritoneum, or obstructing lymphatics.
	Subjective symptoms are important to patient but are generally poor indicators of anti-tumor response.

25 percent increased mortality from cardiovascular diseases in a group of patients treated with moderately high doses (5 mg daily) of diethylstilbestrol. A prospective study has since proved that a low dose of 1 mg daily results in good antitumor effects without significant cardiovascular toxicity.

Wilms' Tumor. Improvements in survival for patients with Wilms' tumor have developed steadily in recent years. Whereas this was once considered a hopeless tumor to treat, it is now possible to control the disease for substantial periods of time in 80 percent of children with the disease. This improvement involves the sequential use of optimal surgery, radiation therapy, and chemotherapy with actinomycin D and/or vincristine. A national study group is currently trying to resolve the optimal combination of these modalities; however, it is clear that the addition of effective chemotherapy has substantially improved the care of these patients.

Carcinoma of the Breast. Recent developments as a result of combination chemotherapy, estradiol receptor protein, competitive inhibitors of estrogen, medical adrenalectomy, and adjuvant chemotherapy have made breast cancer one of the most interesting tumors to treat.

Most physicians are currently treating advanced breast cancer with multiple combinations of drugs. One such combination includes 5-fluorouracil, cyclophosphamide, vincristine, methotrexate, and sometimes prednisone (CMFVP). Another combination includes adriamycin and cyclophosphamide (AC) or 5-fluorouracil, adriamycin, and cyclophosphamide (FAC). Response rates for these combinations have been generally 50 percent or greater, compared to 20 to 35 percent for the same drugs used as single agents. The median duration of response with combination chemotherapy has been in the range of 9 months.

Changing concepts of the biology of breast cancer have stimulated a number of clinical trials of adjuvant chemotherapy using single or multiple agents given intermittently over prolonged periods after operation. Many such studies are currently in progress, and most have demonstrated a reduced early recurrence rate for patients treated with adjuvant chemotherapy. One study has also shown an improved 3-year survival rate for patients treated after operation with cyclophosphamide, methotrexate, and 5-fluorouracil (CMF). If these exciting preliminary results are confirmed, they will mark the first real impact on the natural history of breast cancer since the Halsted radical mastectomy.

A number of interesting therapeutic options in breast cancer are being evaluated by studies currently in progress. These include investigations to determine (1) the optimal combination and sequence of drugs and/or hormonal agents; (2) the efficacy of adjuvant chemoimmunotherapy, chemohormonal therapy, or hormonal manipulation used alone in women with estradiol receptor–positive tumors; (3) whether surgical adrenalectomy and medical adrenalectomy using aminogluethimide are comparable; and (4) the usefulness of the estrogen antagonist or competitive inhibitors.

COMBINED MODALITY THERAPY. Pediatric oncologists pioneered the use of combined modality therapy—radiation in combination with chemotherapy and surgical therapy—to overcome childhood neoplasms. The cure rate for localized retinoblastoma and other sarcomas in children has been increased with radiation therapy and chemotherapy with cyclophosphamide. Wilms' tumor can be cured 75 percent of the time if surgical therapy is followed by radiation and chemotherapy with actinomycin, an increase of 40 percent over operation alone. Embryonal rhabdomyosarcoma responds best to combinations of radiation, chemotherapy, and operation.

Until recently, the effectiveness of multimodality therapy had been demonstrated only occasionally for adult neoplasms. A recent example illustrates the complexity of such combined therapy for skeletal and soft tissue sarcomas.

Surgical therapy, the accepted method for management of most skeletal and soft tissue sarcomas of the extremity, has been associated with frequent treatment failure. Even with amputation, approximately 50 percent of patients with soft tissue sarcomas and 80 percent of those with sarcomas of bone eventually developed and died from their distant metastases. In an attempt to improve results of treatment for the sarcomas, a regimen of combined pre- and postoperative therapy was developed. Preoperative continuous intraarterial infusion of adriamycin, radiation therapy followed by surgical resection, and postoperative adriamycin were found to result in improved short-term recurrence-free survival and preservation of a functional extremity in most patients. This regimen dramatically reduced the incidence of pulmonary metastases from both the osteosarcomas and the soft tissue sarcomas.

The preoperative therapy with intraarterial adriamycin followed by radiation was found to produce extensive tumor cell necrosis as high as 88 percent (Table 9-17 and

Table 9-17. SKELETAL AND SOFT TISSUE SARCOMAS:
HISTOLOGIC EFFECTS OF TREATMENT

		Percent necrosis*	
Treatment	*No. of cases*	*Pre-treatment*	*Post-treatment*
Surgical resection	67	. . .	9*
I-A Adriamycin	6	5	63
I-A Adriamycin & x-radiation	11	12	88†

*Average of the percent necrosis of specimens examined.
†Four of the eleven had no identifiable tumor.

Fig. 9-25*a*, *b*, *c*). The effectiveness of this preoperative therapy permitted local resection of the sarcoma and salvage. Diseased bone, in this instance, was replaced by cadaver allografts obtained from the National Naval Medical Center. The donor grafts were matched to the diseased bone for intercondylar width and for intramedullary diameter to facilitate fixation (Fig. 9-26). After operation, patients with femur replacement were placed in non-weight-bearing long leg casts for up to 8 weeks and then wore weight-bearing long leg braces. Subsequently, some of the patients used only a routine hinged knee brace (Fig. 9-27). Patients with homograft replacements in the upper extremity were placed in full arm casts and then in a supporting splint. Function of the extremity in both sets of patients has been excellent, even though knee motion is limited in those with leg homografts.

Although it is too early to tell whether these results represent merely a delay in recurrence of disease or possible cure, certainly for those patients who would have had to sacrifice an arm or an entire leg, the functional results are far superior to any achieved by prosthetic replacement.

Immunotherapy

One of the basic problems associated with all forms of cancer therapy is caused by the similarities in the biochemical and subcellular constituents of the cancer and normal cells. Although some cancer cells may have a rapid rate of cell division when compared to normal cells of the same organ, there are other normal cells in the body (e.g., those in the bone marrow and intestinal epithelium) that may grow even more rapidly. Hence, any therapy designed to inhibit the proliferation rate of cancer cells may also inhibit the function of these normal cells. Herein lies the fundamental deficiency of both radiation and chemotherapy. Similarly, cancer surgery often requires the sacrifice of normal tissues and organs to ensure an adequate margin around the cancer cells. In contrast, immunotherapy depends upon basic antigenic differences between neoplastic and normal cells for its therapeutic effect. Because the immune attack is directed only at those cells possessing tumor antigens, while sparing normal cells from damage, this treatment method can achieve a specific tumor cell kill greater than any other known therapeutic modality. At the

present time, however, immunotherapy has limited potency.

Immunity against cancer is relative rather than absolute. Host defenses are quite capable of destroying small numbers of tumor cells, 1 to 10 million, but 100 million tumor cells almost always result in progressive tumor growth. Since a neoplasm only 1 cm in diameter contains approximately 1 billion tumor cells, by the time most tumors are clinically detectable, they have already outgrown the patient's immune defenses. Therefore, it is unlikely that immunotherapy alone will ever bolster host offenses sufficiently to reverse tumor growth in patients with advanced disease.

In contrast, immunotherapy is a logical adjunct for the treatment of subclinical microscopic disease following definitive cancer surgery, radiation therapy, or chemotherapy, for the following reasons: (1) Patients who have only small foci of cancer cells remaining after destruction of the major tumor bulk are the most likely to benefit from immunotherapy, because the tumor mass that must be destroyed is smallest at that time. (2) The specificity of the immune response provides a possible therapeutic tool that has selectivity for small numbers of cancer cells not possible with any other therapeutic modality. (3) Patients with disease in earlier stages are more likely to respond to immunotherapeutic maneuvers, since the cancer patient's general immune competence is greatest when the disease is localized and is often impaired after metastasis. (4) Immunotherapy should complement rather than interfere with currently available methods of cancer therapy. However, since both irradiation and chemotherapy are immunosuppressive, the use of immunotherapy in combination with these therapeutic modalities must be carefully controlled. Because these treatment modalities can stimulate immune response when immunization is carried out under special conditions, the results of cancer therapy may improve when the influence of radiation therapy and chemotherapy upon the immune response is better understood.

Numerous attempts at immunotherapy of cancer have been undertaken since the turn of the century. Although an occasional striking regression was obtained, in most cases the results were neither impressive nor consistent, and interest in this treatment modality declined until re-

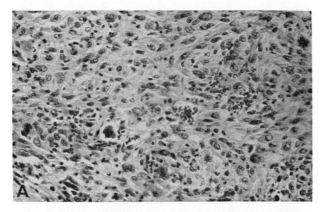

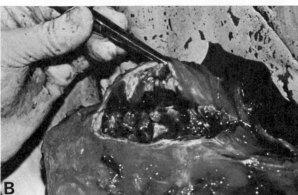

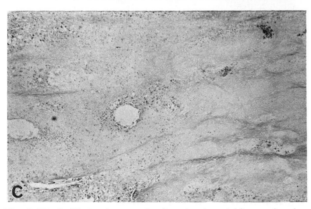

Fig. 9-25. *A.* Photomicrograph of pretreatment biopsy showing osteosarcoma with minimal necrosis. (×250.) *B.* Resected surgical specimen following preoperative treatment with intraarterial adriamycin and radiation therapy. Note gross tumor liquefaction and necrosis. *C.* Photomicrograph of posttreatment specimen showing 99 percent tumor necrosis with loss of nuclei. (×40.) (*From D. L. Morton et al., Ann Surg, 184:268, 1976.*)

responses and their influence upon the host's defense against cancer is somewhat controversial at the present time. Most approaches to immunotherapy do, in fact, stimulate both types of immune response. Three possible approaches to immunotherapy in man will be discussed—active; passive, or adoptive; and nonspecific.

ACTIVE IMMUNOTHERAPY

The greater effectiveness of active immunization over passive immunization in infectious diseases provided a

Fig. 9-26. Postoperative radiograph showing cadaver bone graft held in place by a Sampson rod and Stone staples used to reattach collateral ligaments. (*From D. L. Morton et al., Ann Surg, 184:268, 1976.*)

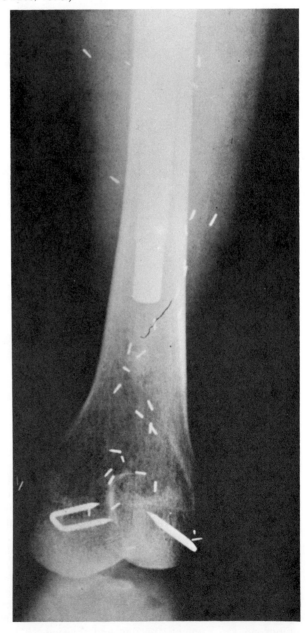

cently. A rational basis for cancer immunotherapy was provided only during the past 10 years as compelling evidence accumulated indicating the participation of immune responses in human cancer. It was found that cancer patients develop two types of immune response to the antigens of their neoplasms, *humoral antibodies* and *cell-mediated immune reactions.*

The relative importance of these two types of immune

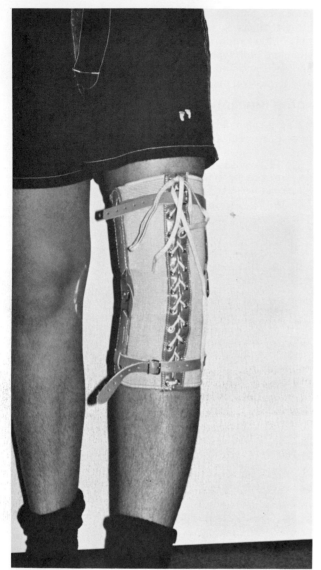

Fig. 9-27. Results 9 months after operation. Patient walks without crutches and can flex knee joint 20°. Brace is worn to assure stability of knee joint. (*From D. L. Morton et al., Ann Surg, 184:268, 1976.*)

strong stimulus for studies of active immunotherapy against cancer. The rationale for this approach is based upon animal studies demonstrating that a growing tumor does not induce a maximum immune response in the host (Fig. 9-28). In this method of treatment, efforts are made to increase the patient's tumor immunity by altering the tumor-specific antigen in such a way that it becomes more antigenic, or by stimulating the patient's lymphoreticular system with immunologic adjuvants.

Most attempts at immunotherapy in man have involved vaccines composed of whole tumor cells inactivated by a variety of different methods to render the cells incapable of proliferation. These methods have included radiation, mitomycin C treatment, freezing and thawing, or heat

treatment. Although such techniques have prevented progressive tumor growth, they may have inactivated the tumor-specific antigens as well. For example, the same freezing and thawing technique frequently used to prepare human tumor vaccines has often inactivated tumor-specific antigens of carcinogen-induced animal neoplasms.

Studies with animal neoplasms demonstrate that living tumor cells administered intradermally in numbers insufficient for progressive tumor growth generally are the most effective immunogens. The possibility that living tumor cells might result in tumor growth at the inoculation site has inhibited the use of such vaccines in man. However, it would seem that with certain tumors that share common tumor-specific antigens, such as skeletal and soft tissue sarcomas, one patient could be immunized with an allogenic vaccine of living tumor cells from another patient. An immune response could be induced against the foreign HLA transplantation antigens on the tumor cells, causing their rejection. Theoretically this immunization should induce a strong immune response against a common cross-reacting tumor-specific antigen as well.

Repeated attempts have been made to increase the antigenicity of tumor vaccines by modifying the tumor cells in a variety of ways. These have included coupling highly antigenic carrier proteins such as rabbit γ-globulin to the tumor cells, and chemical treatment by agents such as iodoacetate and, more recently, with neuraminidase and concanavalin A. Regression of established tumors has been observed in animals following active immunotherapy with such vaccines.

Many of these experiments have used immunological adjuvants as well, such as bacillus Calmette-Guérin (BCG) vaccine, *Corynebacterium parvum,* and Freund's adjuvant, in an attempt to enhance the host's immune response to the native or modified tumor antigens.

The ideal tumor vaccine in many respects, however, would be one composed of the isolated and purified tumor-specific transplantation antigens from the cell surface. Such vaccines would have the advantages of safety, stability, and ease of administration. Previous experience gained with guinea pig sarcomas from which isolated and partially purified tumor-specific antigen preparations induced good immunity to tumor challenge suggests that success can be anticipated for this approach. However, to date, there has been little progress along these lines with the human tumor-specific transplantation antigen.

In summary, active immunotherapy using vaccines prepared in a variety of ways combined with many different types of immunoadjuvants has been used in clinical trials. It can be demonstrated clearly that such autoimmunization procedures do enhance the patient's immune response to his own tumor (Fig. 9-29). Results to date, however, have not been impressive in patients with advanced disease where active immunization is used alone. Active immunotherapy has great potential when used in combination with other types of cancer therapy, such as surgery, chemotherapy, or radiation therapy. Preliminary experiences by Mathe with leukemia and Morton with melanomas and sarcomas would suggest that this potential will become increasingly evident in the future.

PASSIVE AND ADOPTIVE IMMUNOTHERAPY

Since patients with cancer develop two types of immune responses to their neoplasms—humoral antibodies and cell-mediated immune responses—passive immunotherapy is logically based upon the administration of either anti-tumor sera or lymphoid cells.

PASSIVE IMMUNOTHERAPY WITH ANTITUMOR SERA. In the past, antitumor sera produced in a foreign species proved to be very toxic to the recipient, because it contained antibodies against normal tissue antigens of the host. However, this problem may be resolved soon when successful isolation and purification of the tumor-specific transplantation antigens are achieved so that the antisera can be directed specifically against the tumor-specific transplantation antigens of the tumor cells. Another source of potential antisera may be from those patients cured of their malignant condition who demonstrate high titers of cytotoxic or deblocking antibodies.

An important concept of antisera therapy concerns the discovery of certain blocking factors that appear to inhibit the effectiveness of the lymphocytes. Thought to be circulating antigen or antibody-antigen complexes, these blocking factors may contribute to tumor growth by interfering with cellular immunity. In experiments using mouse and guinea pig sarcomas, as well as leukemias, tumor regression can be induced with antisera containing high titers of antitumor antibody. The mechanism for antitumor effectiveness is unclear. It could be due to a direct cytotoxic effect on tumor cells acting as cytophilic antibody that induces macrophages or lymphocytes to kill tumor cells or by neutralizing blocking factors. Nevertheless, these observations clearly indicate that antitumor sera can induce regression of established neoplasms and as such should receive serious consideration for immunotherapy of cancer.

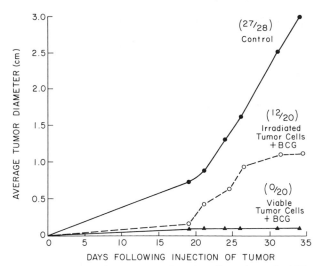

Fig. 9-28. Immunotherapy experiments with a transplantable liposarcoma in syngeneic strain 2 guinea pigs: 1×10^5 liposarcoma tumor cells were inoculated intramuscularly into the leg, and immunotherapy was initiated intradermally in four sites on the back with 1×10^6 living or 1×10^7 irradiated tumor cells mixed with bacillus Calmette-Guérin (BCG). (*From D. L. Morton et al., Ann Surg, 172:740, 1970.*)

IMMUNOTHERAPY WITH LYMPHOID CELLS. Adoptive immunotherapy with lymphoid cells from an immunized donor was accomplished with ease between inbred laboratory animals of the same strain and suggested that antitumor immunity was primarily cell-mediated. However, these animal experiments indicated that the transferred lymphocytes must persist in the host to have a significant immunotherapeutic effect. As studies were done in human cancer, the primary difficulty was with rejection of the transferred lymphocytes due to HLA dif-

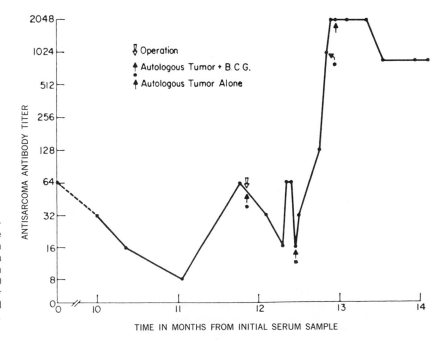

Fig. 9-29. Antisarcoma antibody titers determined by complement fixation against the HuSA-I liposarcoma antigen on serial serum samples from a sixteen-year-old boy with a primary osteosarcoma of the right femur in whom pulmonary metastases developed 10 months after resection of the primary, for which a left pneumonectomy was performed and immunotherapy initiated. (*From D. L. Morton et al., Ann Surg, 172:740, 1970.*)

ferences between host and donor. This problem was overcome when the lymphoid cells were obtained from family members who were identical by HLA matching or by bulk growth of the patient's own lymphocytes in tissue culture. The lymphocytes of the family members may be already sensitized to the tumor-specific antigens in certain neoplasms, such as human sarcomas, where our investigations have shown a high incidence of antibodies in close family members.

As with antisera, another source of lymphocytes may be those cancer patients who have been cured of their malignant disease. Sumner and Foraker reported one of the earliest successes by this means when they transfused a melanoma patient with whole blood from a second melanoma patient who had undergone complete remission. However, multiple attempts to repeat this transfer have been unsuccessful.

Moore and Gerner attempted to increase the lymphocyte ratio to tumor cells by growing a patient's lymphocytes in tissue culture and reinfusing them back to the patient. They reported significant regressions in two of three patients. However, the logistic problems of growing such large numbers of lymphocytes are considerable.

IMMUNOTHERAPY FOLLOWING IN VITRO ACTIVATION OF LYMPHOCYTES. Further studies of adoptive immunotherapy have concerned in vitro, nonspecific stimulation of lymphocytes with agents such as phytohemagglutinin. Some success has been reported when these treated autologous lymphocytes were reinfused into the patient or injected directly into tumor deposits. Another approach has involved specific sensitization of lymphocytes with tumor cells in vitro by incubation with mitomycin C-treated tissue culture tumor cells. The mitomycin C prevented replication of the tumor cells by eliminating their potential to form metastases. Though the results were not impressive in these human investigations, recent animal experiments suggest this means as a very effective way to induce an effective antitumor immunity. The ability to obtain large numbers of lymphocytes from any donor by continuous lymphophoresis using the NCI-IBM blood cell separator has considerably increased the feasibility of this approach.

IMMUNOTHERAPY WITH LYMPHOCYTES SENSITIZED BY TRANSPLANTATION OF TUMORS. Several investigators have attempted passive immunotherapy with cross immunization with tumor tissue followed by cross transfusions of lymphocytes or lymphocytes and serum. These studies have been undertaken in the following manner: Patients with incurable cancer were paired according to blood type and tumor types. Tumors from patients in group A were transplanted subcutaneously to patients in group B, and vice versa. Following sensitization to each other's tumors, the transfusions of lymphocytes from patients in group B to patients in group A, or vice versa, were begun and continued daily for variable periods of time. The response rate reported following this type of immunotherapy is from 15 to 20 percent. However, the criteria for therapeutic response have varied between investigators and in many cases have not met rigid specifications acceptable to many oncologists.

IMMUNOTHERAPY WITH EXTRACTS OF SENSITIZED LYMPHOID CELLS. One particularly appealing method of adoptive immunotherapy is the injection of informational molecules. These extracts of sensitized lymphoid cells are able to induce a specific immune response when injected into the host. Preliminary clinical investigations have been performed with two such substances, transfer factor and immune RNA.

Transfer factor, originally described by Lawrence, is of low molecular weight (4000 to 8000). Injections of this substance have induced immune reactions against fungal and bacterial antigens. Ongoing preliminary trials are using transfer factor in the immunotherapy of malignant tumors. There appears to be no toxicity, but therapeutic results are not definitive at this time.

Immune RNA, an RNA-rich extract of immune lymphoid cells, is the other means of transferring immunity by informational molecules. Immune RNA extracted from the lymphoid tissues of xenogeneic donors immunized with tumor tissue can induce immunity against that tumor in syngeneic recipients of the tumor transplants. The substance can stimulate normal human lymphocytes to react against human tumor cells in vitro. Ramming and deKernion recently reported a nonrandomized clinical trial of immune RNA in patients with metastatic renal cell carcinoma. There is a suggestion that such treatment may have clinical benefit, although these results must be subjected to a randomized, prospective clinical trial. Immune RNA is not antigenic, and there has been no toxicity associated with its use. Such a modality has significant theoretical advantages, since it is the only currently available system that uses the immunologic capacity of another species for the immunotherapy of humans.

NONSPECIFIC IMMUNOTHERAPY

The theoretic basis for nonspecific immunotherapy depends upon the observation that certain substances, such as mixed bacterial toxins and fractions of the tubercle bacillus, have the ability to nonspecifically enhance host resistance to most viral, fungal, and bacterial agents. Although the exact mechanism is unknown, these agents do appear to stimulate immune response to a wide variety of antigens, including tumor-specific antigens.

Historically, a type of nonspecific immunotherapy was described by Bradford Coley at the turn of the century in one of the first reports of a tumor regression possibly induced by immunologic means. Coley's interest in the possible value of such therapy was stimulated when he observed a recurrent inoperable sarcoma of the neck regress completely for 7 years after the patient had had attacks of erysipelas. This observation led to the development of Coley's toxins, a mixture of killed bacterial vaccines. Coley injected this admixture directly into tumor lesions or gave it intravenously. Some impressive regressions of tumors and long-term cures resulted from these agents. Because the responses were inconsistent, Coley's toxins never received widespread use, and interest in them died out. Recently a nonspecific immunotherapy of a similar type has been revived using attenuated bovine tuberculosis bacillus (BCG).

Our work with BCG began more than 10 years ago, when we injected BCG into metastatic nodules in the skin and subcutaneous tissues in patients with malignant melanoma. We observed that the intratumor injection of BCG caused 90 percent of the intradermal metastases to regress in patients who were immunologically competent as judged by their ability to develop delayed cutaneous hypersensitivity to DNCB and PPD. In addition, in about 20 percent of these patients, a few uninjected nodules were observed to regress. Satellite and in-transit metastases can be controlled in the extremity by this technique in two-thirds of patients. However, many of these patients still develop systemic metastases, as shown by our own experience in treating 24 patients with satellite and in-transit metastases in the leg. Ten of eighteen patients in whom local control was achieved later developed disseminated metastases, and seven of these ten patients have died. Although the intratumor injection of BCG may not control systemic disease, it is nonetheless a very useful method to control local disease that avoids the side effects of chemotherapy and can result in long-term survival.

There are several possible mechanisms to explain tumor regression following BCG injection; both specific and nonspecific immune reactions were probably involved. The tumor cells may be killed as "innocent bystanders" during the delayed cutaneous hypersensitivity reaction that occurs when lymphocytes and macrophages attack BCG dispersed throughout the tumor nodule. This is supported by the observation that the intratumor injection of BCG works only in patients who can be sensitized to BCG, as shown by their delayed cutaneous hypersensitivity reaction to PPD.

In addition to the nonspecific effect, a specific immune response to the melanoma tumor antigens also occurs in some patients because an associated rising titer of anti-melanoma antibody is observed following BCG immunotherapy. Sequential biopsies of tumor nodules following BCG inoculation reveals that the regression of these nodules is associated with a granulomatous infiltration of lymphocytes, monocytes, and fibroblasts surrounding and infiltrating the melanoma cells. Furthermore, the regression of melanoma nodules not given injection with BCG is accompanied by the appearance of lymphocyte infiltrates within the regressing melanoma tumor nodules (Fig. 9-30). The specific antitumor effect may result from more lymphocytes and macrophages coming into contact with the tumor cells so that the afferent limb of the immune response is increased. Conversely, it may work via the effector limb of the immune response by bringing greater numbers of both stimulated and unstimulated lymphocytes to the tumor.

Our results have now been confirmed by a number of investigators. The observation that the intratumor injection of BCG occasionally led to the regression of uninjected nodules suggested that BCG might be useful as an adjuvant to operation to control micrometastatic disease in man. BCG has been shown to prevent the growth of spontaneous metastases in some animal tumor models where the variables of tumor load and time of BCG vaccination can be carefully controlled. In man, a number of preliminary reports have suggested that intradermal BCG delays

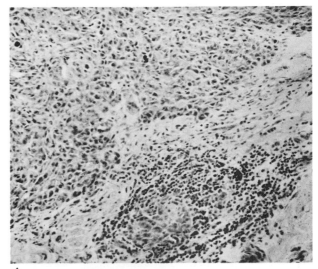

A

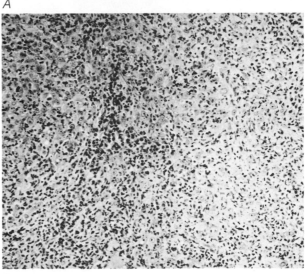

B

Fig. 9-30. *A.* Subcutaneous metastasis of malignant melanoma prior to immunotherapy with BCG. Note the absence of lymphocytic and monocytic infiltration among the tumor cells. *B.* Subcutaneous metastasis which had decreased in size from 10 to 5 mm during the 6-week period following immunotherapy with BCG injections into other melanoma nodules. BCG was *not* injected into this nodule. Note the marked lymphocytic and monocytic infiltration among the melanoma cells. (*From D. L. Morton, et al., Ann Surg, 172:740, 1970.*)

recurrence in patients with melanoma who are at high risk because of metastases to regional nodes (Fig. 9-31). However, the definitive answer on the usefulness of BCG in patients with melanoma will come from other prospective randomized controlled trials currently under way.

The most impressive results with BCG used as an adjuvant to operation for lung cancer have been reported by McKneally, who randomized patients to receive either BCG plus isoniazid or isoniazid alone administered as a single postoperative intrapleural dose following pulmonary resection. Patients with Stage I lung cancer who received

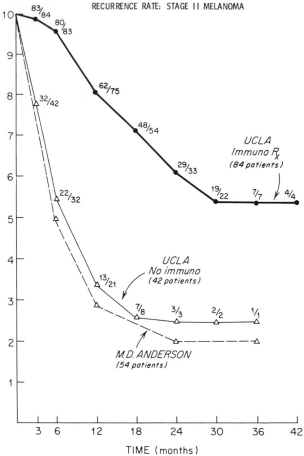

Fig. 9-31. Recurrence rate of Stage II melanoma showing the percentage of patients free of recurrent melanoma after regional lymphadenectomy alone or lymphadenectomy with postoperative immunotherapy. Numbers separated by a slash (/) indicate number of patients who remained free of disease over number of patients at risk of recurrence during that interval. P < 0.01 at each interval up to and including 30 months. Statistics on 54 patients from M. D. Anderson Hospital and Tumor Institute, University of Texas, Houston. (*From F. R. Eilber et al., N Engl J Med, 294:237, 1976.*)

Fig. 9-32. Schematic of cancer cell factory as it might function to enhance its growth by producing immunosuppression in the host. Theoretically, cancer surgery removes the cancer factory and its associated immunosuppressants, which allows the host immune responses to return to normal. (*From D. L. Morton et al., Chest, 71:640, 1977.*)

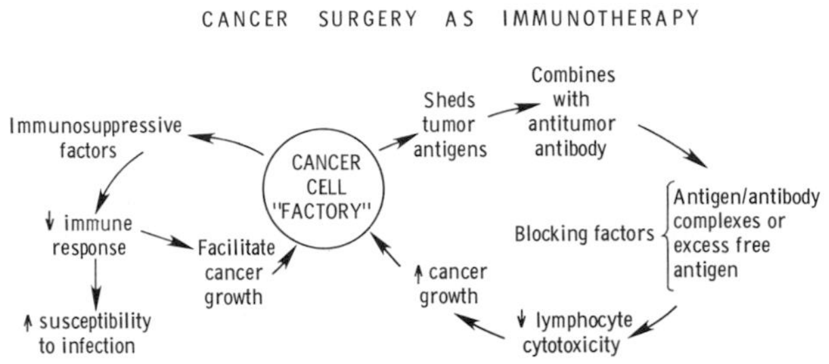

CANCER SURGERY AS IMMUNOTHERAPY

BCG had a significantly lower rate of recurrence and a correspondingly higher survival rate.

BCG is only one of a wide variety of agents that can nonspecifically stimulate the immune system's response to a variety of different types of antigens. Examples of other agents include *Corynebacterium parvum,* MER (methanol-extractable residue of BCG), bacterial antitoxins, and polynucleotides. We can anticipate that nonspecific immunotherapy will be tested in a wide variety of neoplasms and that new immunologic adjuvants will be developed.

Other impressive results with nonspecific immunotherapy come from the studies of Klein in patients with basal and squamous cell carcinomas of the skin. Here the induction of delayed hypersensitivity reactions to DNCB resulted in the resolution of more than 90 percent of superficial basal or squamous cell carcinomas. Klein observed that the mixture of multiple antigens such as PPD, mumps, and *Candida* increased the delayed hypersensitivity and effectiveness of this form of immunotherapy.

Another form of nonspecific immunotherapy involves the use of agents capable of restoring depressed immune responses. Several agents have been proposed in such a context, including thymic hormones such as thymosin and the antihelminthic drug levamisole, which is reported to increase host resistance to the benefit of patients with lung carcinoma.

The rational application of immunotherapy to human cancer will depend, to a large extent, on a better knowledge of tumor-associated antigens in human neoplasms and methods for increasing the immune response against these antigens. Specificity for cancer cells cannot be achieved by any other known therapeutic means; but the potency of immunotherapy is limited.

At the present time, the tumor immunologist is faced with a paradox in the clinical application of immunotherapy. Ideally, the patients who are most likely to respond to this therapeutic modality are those who are in the early stages of the disease and have minimal residual tumor burden following treatment with other therapeutic modalities. However, many of these patients may have been cured of their cancer by the primary treatment, so that immunotherapy can be evaluated only by controlled clinical trials of large numbers of patients. It should be emphasized, however, that the dosage indications, therapeutic results, and long-term toxicity of immunotherapy are largely unknown at the present time.

SURGERY AS IMMUNOTHERAPY

A tumor may promote its own growth by a number of immune mechanisms. The cancer cell may act as a "factory" that is constantly producing both immunosuppressive factors and tumor-associated antigens (Fig. 9-32). The specific and nonspecific immunosuppression decreases the patient's immune defenses and facilitates growth of the tumor.

The key to recovery of the balance in the host-tumor relationship depends on destruction or removal of the tumor cell "factory." Surgery appears to be the most efficient means of removing the factory. Once the mass of tumor is gone, the patient with cancer is more likely to be able to mount an immune response that may destroy any subclinical foci of tumor cells scattered through the body. However, if the recovery of the immune response is inadequate or if the number of tumor cells in any distant metastatic focus is too large, the patient may fail to regain control of the disease. Nonetheless, surgery for cancer becomes the first step in immunotherapy.

If this thesis is correct, it would follow that the approach to the surgical treatment for solid neoplasms must change dramatically. The future lies not in treating every patient with a solid neoplasm as one with localized disease but in assuming that the local disease is merely a manifestation of a systemic illness, whether or not the patient has overt metastatic disease. Not until we accept surgery as merely the first step in the treatment of cancer can we significantly improve our rates of cure. Therapeutic advances eventually must come from a multimethod combination of immunotherapy and chemotherapy with surgical therapy or radiotherapy. Unlike surgery and radiotherapy, both local treatments, the triple combinations represent a systemic treatment effective against tumor cells already metastatic to distant sites. However, at present, systemic therapeutic techniques have greater potential for curing those patients with a minimal number of tumor cells, rather than those with clinically evident disease. Thus, although surgery for cancer is not curative by itself, in most cases it can decrease the patient's burden of tumor cells and allow the immune response to normalize so that further chemoimmunotherapy has a chance to be more effective.

PROGNOSIS

Predicting the future course of a patient's malignant disease is one of the most difficult problems an oncologist faces. At the present time, it is impossible to predict the future course of a given patient except in general terms. However, a number of known factors are important in determining prognosis.

The *site of origin* of the primary tumor is one of the most important factors influencing prognosis. The propensity of a neoplasm to metastasize to distant sites varies according to its tissue of origin. Over 90 percent of carcinomas of the lung, pancreas, and esophagus spread beyond their primary site and cause death, whereas carcinomas of the skin, breast, and thyroid glands are frequently localized and curable, even when metastatic in some patients.

The *stage of disease* at the time of initial treatment is of considerable importance in determining survival for all types of neoplasms. The chance for cure is best when the neoplasm is confirmed to the organ of origin. The smaller the primary neoplasm, the better the prognosis, as well. Thus, in situ carcinoma of the cervix, carcinomas of the breast less than 1 cm in diameter, and small polypoid carcinomas of the colon are generally curable; larger neoplasms may not be curable. Direct extension into adjacent organs or metastases to regional nodes suggest a more guarded prognosis, although many patients are still curable at this stage of the disease. The spread of cancer by the bloodstream with metastases to distant sites portends a grave prognosis, and few patients are curable at this stage. As a general rule, lymph node involvement sharply reduces survival probability by about one-half that of patients without involved nodes. If only one node is involved, the prognosis is better than if the majority of lymph nodes are involved.

The *histopathologic features* of the neoplasm correlate in a general way to prognosis. The more undifferentiated, highly malignant-appearing neoplasms with frequent mitosis are more likely to develop early distant spread and local recurrence. However, some very malignant neoplasms still can be cured with adequate treatment. Venous invasion is a grave prognostic factor in all types of neoplasia.

Host immune factors, as previously discussed, may be the most important single factor in determining prognosis. Immunologic methods for monitoring immune responses are currently under development. It is already apparent that those patients who have spontaneous depression of their immune responses have a uniformly poor prognosis following therapy.

The *age of the patient* may be an important factor affecting prognosis. Some oncologists believe that neoplasms in younger patients carry a poorer prognosis than the same tumors in middle-aged or elderly patients, although elderly patients may have associated medical problems that do not permit adequate treatment of the cancer. While there may be some validity in this concept, it should not be overemphasized, because many young patients have a good prognosis. In fact, some have a much better prognosis than adults with the same neoplasms. Those neoplasms which occur prior to one year of age generally have a better prognosis than those which occur later in childhood. This can be determined in the following manner: The child is usually cured of the neoplasm if he is free of disease for 9 months after treatment, plus double the age at the time treatment was begun. This concept is based upon the supposition that if the earliest cancer cell started with conception and if the cancer grew at a constant rate, then it would reach a certain size at the time treatment was initiated. If treatment was successful in eliminating all cancer cells except one, then in a period equal to 9 months plus double the age of the child, the cancer size would again be equivalent to the original tumor mass. Therefore, if there is no recurrence after this time span, it can be assumed that the patient is cured.

The *adequacy of treatment* is most relevant to prognosis for certain types of neoplasms. The cure rate for some neoplasms, such as soft tissue sarcomas and certain childhood neoplasms, may be twice as high in sophisticated cancer centers when compared to cure rates in small community hospitals. Furthermore, some patients with seemingly hopeless prognoses may be cured with aggressive therapy by an experienced oncologist, whereas they might not be by the physician who only occasionally treats cancer patients and might be unwilling to undertake the aggressive therapy.

PSYCHOLOGIC MANAGEMENT OF THE CANCER PATIENT

The cancer patient's great fear of his disease usually can be decreased by understanding derived from free and open communication with the physician. Psychologic support and education to deal with any disability that may result from therapy are important. Examples include training in the care of a stoma following curative surgery for colonic and rectal cancer or referral to lay groups associated with the American Cancer Society for counseling the anxious patient with an altered body image resulting from mastectomy.

Despite the prognostic factors discussed previously, it is still impossible to predict the exact course of any malignant tumor. Patients with the most grim prognoses are occasionally cured by aggressive therapy, and spontaneous regressions are sometimes observed even in patients with metastases. In contrast, some patients with apparently localized disease may be dead of disseminated cancer in a few months. This uncertainty about the future is one of the most difficult adjustments faced by the cancer patient and his family. Most reassuring in this regard is to emphasize that for each month that passes following successful treatment of the primary neoplasm, the chances for cure improve. This is particularly correct for tumors such as squamous cell carcinoma of the lung or oral pharynx. Although other, more slowly growing neoplasms, such as carcinoma of the breast and malignant melanoma, may recur after disease-free intervals of 10 or 20 years, the chances of recurrence also decrease with time. Recognition that cancer is a chronic disease is an important aspect of management. Long-term, consistent follow-up provides opportunities for reassurance and usually can ensure detection of recurrence at an early stage.

Some patients do not want to know about their illness for fear of having their suspicions verified. Never lie to a patient, if possible, even if requested by the family. In general, gentle and optimistic truth is best. Untruths often create barriers between the patient and his family which can lead to psychologic isolation of the patient who is unable to discuss his fears and anxieties with those he needs most.

With the patient for whom primary cancer therapy has failed, one of the most difficult problems faced by the physician is "What should the patient be told?" Most oncologists who deal exclusively with cancer patients agree that the incurable patient also must be told the truth as gently and optimistically as possible. Hope and reassurance as to the physician's continuing concern are best sustained by continuing active treatment until it is certain that the patient can no longer benefit. Realistic and consistent support is actually more important to the patient and the family at this stage of the disease than earlier. There is increasing evidence that patients tolerate the process of dying much better when cared for in this manner.

Some incurable patients are unable to accept the realities of the situation. In this case, it is essential that a responsible family member be informed. The life duration of the incurable patient is so uncertain that predictions should be avoided. If, as frequently happens, the relatives insist upon some estimate, a combined minimum-maximum prognosis, such as from 6 months to 2 years, will help the family accept this uncertainty.

The basic aim in caring for the patient with advanced cancer is to prolong useful life, but not useless suffering. The patient should be permitted to die with dignity when active therapy can no longer benefit him.

References

Etiology

Barratt, R. W., and Tatum, E. L.: Carcinogenic Mutagens, *Ann NY Acad Sci,* **71:**1072, 1958.

Blum, H. F.: Sunlight as a Causal Factor in Cancer of the Skin, *Cancer Res,* **5:**592, 1945; **9:**247, 1948.

Buell, P., and Dunn, J. E., Jr.: Cancer Mortality among Japanese Issei and Nisei of California, *Cancer,* **18:**656, 1965.

Burdett, W. J.: "Viruses Inducing Cancer," University of Utah Press, Salt Lake City, 1966.

Cutler, S. J.: A Review of the Statistical Evidence on Association between Smoking and Lung Cancer, *J Am Statis Assoc,* **50:**267, 1955.

Gallo, R. C., and Todaro, G. J.: Oncogenic RNA Viruses, *Semin Oncol,* **3:**81, 1976.

Green, M., and Wold, W. S. M.: Oncogenic RNA Viruses: Replication, Tumor Gene Expression, and Role in Human Cancer, *Semin Oncol,* **3:**65, 1976.

Haenszel, W.: Cancer Mortality among the Foreign Born in the United States, *J Natl Cancer Inst,* **26:**37, 1961.

Hammond, E. C., and Horn, D.: The Relationship between Human Smoking Habits and Death Rates, *JAMA,* **155:**1316, 1954.

Heuper, W. C.: Environmental Cancer, in F. Homburger (ed.), "The Physiopathology of Cancer," p. 919, Harper & Row, Publishers, Incorporated, New York, 1959.

Kennaway, E. C.: The Formation of a Cancer Producing Substance from Isoprene (2-Methyl-Butadiene), *J Pathol Bacteriol,* **27:**233, 1924.

Khanolkar, V. R.: Oral Cancer in Bombay, India: A Review of 1,000 Consecutive Cases, *Cancer Res,* **4:**313, 1944.

Lorenz, E.: Radioactivity and Lung Cancer: A Critical Review of Lung Cancer in the Miners of Schneeburg and Joachimstall, *Cancer Res,* **5:**1, 1944.

Martland, H. S.: Occupational Poisoning in Manufacture of Luminous Watch Dials: General Review of Hazard Caused by Ingestion of Luminous Paint with Special Reference to the New Jersey Cases, *JAMA,* **92:**466, 1929.

Mayo, C. W., DeWeerd, J. H., and Jackman, R. J.: Diffuse Familial Polyposes of the Colon, *Surg Gynecol Obstet,* **93:**87, 1951.

Pifer, J. W., Toyooka, E. T., Murray, R. W., Ames, W. R., Hempelmann, L. H., Crump, S. L., and Dutton, A. M.: Neoplasms in Children Treated with X-rays for Thymic Enlargement: I. Neoplasms and Mortality; II. Tumor Incidence as a Function of Radiation Factors; III. Clinical Description of Cases, *J Natl Cancer Inst,* **31:**1333, 1357, 1379, 1963.

Porter, C. D., and White, C. J.: Multiple Carcinomata following Chronic X-ray Dermatitis, *Ann Surg,* **46:**649, 1970.

Prehn, R. T.: Specific Isoantigenicities among Chemically Induced Tumors, *Ann NY Acad Sci,* **101:**107, 1962.

Rapp, R.: Viruses as Etiologic Factors in Cancer, *Semin Oncol,* **3:**49, 1976.

Rous, P.: Transmission of a Malignant New Growth by Means of a Cell-free Filtrate, *JAMA,* **56:**198, 1911.

Shimkin, M. B.: Cancer Research, in L. V. Ackerman and J. A. Del Regato (eds.), "Cancer," pp. 35–57, The C. V. Mosby Company, St. Louis, 1962.

Biology and Immunobiology

Black, M. M., Opler, S. R., and Speer, F. D.: Structural Representations of Tumor-Host Relationships in Gastric Carcinoma, *Surg Gynecol Obstet,* **102:**599, 1956.

Burnet, F. M.: "Immunological Surveillance," Pergamon Press, New York, 1970.

DeVries, J. E., Cornain, S., and Rumke, P.: Cytotoxicity of Non-T versus T-Lymphocytes from Melanoma Patients and Healthy Donors on Short and Long Term Cultured Melanoma Cells, *Int J Cancer,* **14:**427, 1974.

Dhar, P., Moore, T. L., Zamcheck, N., and Kupchick, H.: Carcinoembryonic Antigen (CEA) in Colonic Cancer: Use in Pre- and Postoperative Diagnosis and Prognosis, *JAMA,* **221:**31, 1972.

Eilber, F. R., and Morton, D. L.: Impaired Immunologic Reactivity and Recurrence following Cancer Surgery, *Cancer,* **25:**362, 1970.

——, Nizze, A., and Morton, D. L.: Sequential Evaluation of General Immune Competence in Cancer Patients: Correlation with Clinical Course, *Cancer,* **35:**660, 1975.

Everson, T. C., and Cole, W. H.: "Spontaneous Regression of Cancer," W. B. Saunders Company, Philadelphia, 1966.

Fass, L., Ziegler, J. L., Heberman, R. B., and Kiryabwire, J. W. M.: Cutaneous Hypersensitivity Reactions to Autologous Extracts of Malignant Melanoma Cells, *Lancet,* **1:**116, 1970.

Fenyö, E. M., Klein, E., Klein, G., and Swiech, K.: Selection of an Immunoresistant Moloney Lymphoma Subline with Decreased Concentration of Tumor-specific Surface Antigens, *J Natl Cancer Inst,* **40:**69, 1968.

Foley, E. J.: Antigenic Properties of Methylcholanthrene-induced Tumors in Mice of the Strain or Origin, *Cancer Res,* **13:**835, 1953.

Gatti, R. A., and Good, R. A.: Occurrence of Malignancy in Immunodeficiency Diseases: A Literature Review, *Cancer,* **28:**89, 1971.

Gold, P., and Freedman, S. O.: Specific Carcinoembryonic Antigens of the Human Digestive System, *J Exp Med,* **122:**467, 1965.

Goodwin, W. E.: Regression of Hypernephromas, *JAMA,* **20:**609, 1968.

Griffiths, J. D., McKinna, J. A., Rawbotham, H. D., Tsolakidis, P., and Salsbury, A. J.: Carcinoma of the Colon and Rectum: Circulating Malignant Cells and 5-Year Survival, *Cancer,* **31:**226, 1973.

Haagensen, D. E., Jr., Mazoujian, G., Holder, W. D., Kister, S. J., and Wells, S. A., Jr.: Evaluation of a Breast Cyst Fluid Protein Detectable in the Plasma of Breast Carcinoma Patients, *Ann Surg,* **185:**279, 1977.

Hakala, T. R., and Lange, P. H.: Serum Induced Lymphoid Cell Mediated Cytotoxicity against Human Transitional Cell Carcinomas of the Urinary Tract, *Science,* **184:**795, 1974.

Hammond, W. G., Fisher, J. C., and Rolley, R. T.: Tumor Specific Transplantation Immunity to Spontaneous Mouse Tumors, *Surgery,* **62:**124, 1967.

Hellstrom, I., Sjogren, H. O., Warner, G., and Hellstrom, K. E.: Blocking of Cell Mediated Tumor Immunity by Sera from Patients with Growing Neoplasms, *Int J Cancer,* **7:**226, 1971.

Hellstrom, K. E., and Hellstrom, I.: Lymphocyte Mediated Cytotoxicity and Blocking Serum Activity to Tumor Antigens, *Adv Immunol,* **18:**209, 1974.

Hibbs, J. B., Lambert, L. J., and Remington, J. I.: Possible Role of Macrophage Mediated Nonspecific Cytotoxicity in Tumor Resistance, *Nature [New Biol],* **235:**48, 1972.

Klein, G.: Tumor Antigens, *Ann Rev Microbiol,* **20:**223, 1966.

Mach, J. P., Jaeger, P., Bertholet, M. M., Ruegsigger, C. H., Loosli, R. M., and Pettavel, J.: Detection of Recurrence of Large Bowel Carcinoma by Radioimmunoassay of Circulating Carcinoembryonic Antigen (CEA), *Lancet,* **2:**535, 1974.

Morton, D. L.: Acquired Immunological Tolerance and Carcinogenesis by the Mammary Tumor Virus. I. Influence of Neonatal Infection with the Mammary Tumor Virus on the Growth of Spontaneous Mammary Adencarcinomas, *J Natl Cancer Inst,* **42:**311, 1969.

——, Eilber, F. R., Joseph, W. L., Wood, W. C., Trahan, E., and Ketcham, A. S.: Immunological Factors in Human Sarcomas and Melanomas: A Rational Basis for Immunotherapy, *Ann Surg,* **172:**740, 1970.

——, Holmes, E. C., Eilber, F. R., and Wood, W. C.: Immunological Aspects of Neoplasia: A Rational Basis for Immunotherapy, *Ann Intern Med,* **74:**587, 1971.

Old, L. J., and Boyse, E. A.: Antigens of Tumors and Leukemias Induced by Virus, *Fed Proc,* **24:**1009, 1965.

——, ——, and Stockert, E.: Antigenic Properties of Experimental Leukemias: I. Serological Studies In Vitro with Spontaneous and Radiation-induced Leukemias, *J Natl Cancer Inst,* **31:**977, 1963.

——, Stockert, E., Boyse, E. A., and Kin, J. H.: Antigenic Modulation: Loss of TL Antigen from Cells Exposed to TL Antibody: Study of the Phenomenon In Vitro, *J Exp Med,* **127:**523, 1968.

O'Toole, C., Stejeka, V., Perlmann, P., Karlsson, M.: Lymphoid Cells Mediating Tumor-Specific Cytotoxicity to Carcinoma of the Urinary Bladder: Separation of the Effector Population Using a Surface Marker, *J Exp Med,* **139:**437, 1974.

Piessens, W. F.: Evidence of Human Cancer Immunity, *Cancer,* **26:**1212, 1970.

Pilch, Y. H., Meyers, G. H., Sparks, F. C., and Golub, S. H.: Prospects for the Immunotherapy of Cancer: Part I, Basic Concepts of Tumor Immunology, *Curr Probl Surg,* January 1975, p. 1.

Prehn, R. T., and Main, J. M.: Immunity to Methylcholanthrene-induced Sarcomas, *J Natl Cancer Inst,* **18:**769, 1957.

Shearer, W. T., and Parker, C. W.: Humoral Immunostimulation. V. Selection of Variant Cell Lines, *J Exp Med,* **142:**1133, 1975.

Sjogren, H. O.: Transplantation Methods as a Tool for Detection of Tumor-specific Antigens, *Prog Exp Tumor Res,* **6:**289, 1965.

Smith, R. T.: Tumor-specific Immune Mechanisms, *N Engl J Med,* **278:**1207, 1968.

Sophocles, A. M., and Nadler, S. H.: Immunologic Aspects of Cancer, *Surg Gynecol Obstet,* **133:**321, 1971.

Southam, C. M., Brunschwig, W., Levin, A. G., and Dixon, Q. S.:

The Effect of Leukocytes on Transplantability of Human Cancer, *Cancer,* **19:**1743, 1966.

Sparks, F. C., and Breeding, J. H.: Tumor Regression and Enhancement Resulting from Immunotherapy with Bacillus Calmette-Guérin and Neuraminidase, *Cancer Res,* **34:**3262, 1974.

———, O'Connell, T. X., Lee, Y-T., and Breeding, J. H.: BCG Therapy Given as an Adjuvant to Surgery: Prevention of Death from Metastases from Mammary Adenocarcinoma in Rats, *J Natl Cancer Inst,* **53:**1825, 1974.

Sugarbaker, E. V., and Cohen, A. M.: Altered Antigenicity in Spontaneous Pulmonary Metastases from an Antigenic Murine Sarcoma, *Surgery,* **72:**155, 1972.

Zamcheck, N. and Kupchic, H.: The Interdependence of Clinical Investigations and Methodological Development in Early Evaluation of Assays for Carcinoembryonic Antigen, *Cancer Res,* **34:**2131, 1974.

———, Moore, T. L., Dhar, P., and Kupchic, H.: Immunologic Diagnosis and Prognosis of Human Digestive Tract Cancer: Carcinoembryonic Antigens, *N Engl J Med,* **286:**83, 1972.

Pathology

Anderson, W.: The General Pathology of Tumors, in "Boyd's Pathology for the Surgeon," p. 92, W. B. Saunders Co., Philadelphia, 1967.

Bloom, H. J. G., Richardson, W. W., and Harries, E. J.: Natural History of Untreated Breast Cancer (1805–1933): Comparison of Untreated and Treated Cases according to Histological Grade of Malignancy, *Br Med J,* **2:**213, 1962.

Boyd, W.: "An Introduction to the Study of Disease," p. 210, Lea & Febiger, Philadelphia, 1971.

Cole, W. H., McDonald, G. O., Roberts, S. S., and Southwich, H. W.: "Dissemination of Cancer," Appleton-Century-Crofts, Inc., New York, 1961.

Collins, V. P., Leoffler, R. K., and Tivey, H.: Observations on Growth Rates of Human Tumors, *Am J Roentgenol Radium Ther Nucl Med,* **76:**988, 1956.

Cowan, D. R.: Mechanisms Responsible for the Origin and Distribution of Blood-borne Tumor Metastases, *Cancer Res,* **13:**397, 1953.

Everson, T. C.: Spontaneous Regression of Cancer, *Ann NY Acad Sci,* **114:**721, 1964.

Garland, L. H., Coulson, W., and Wollin, E.: The Rate of Growth and Apparent Duration of Untreated Primary Bronchial Carcinoma, *Cancer,* **16:**694, 1963.

Knox, L. C.: The Relationship of Massage to Metastases in Malignant Tumors, *Ann Surg,* **75:**129, 1922.

MacMahon, B., and Feng, M. A.: Prenatal Origin of Childhood Leukemia: Evidence from Twins, *N Engl J Med,* **270:**1082, 1964.

Moertel, C. G.: Incidence and Significance of Multiple Primary Malignant Neoplasms, *Ann NY Acad Sci,* **114:**886, 1964.

Pearson, H. A., Grello, F. W., and Cane, E. C., Jr.: Leukemia in Identical Twins, *N Engl J Med,* **268:**1151, 1963.

Pund, E. R., Nettles, T. B., Caldwell, T. D., and Nieburgs, H. E.: Preinvasive and Invasive Carcinoma of the Cervix Uteri: Pathogenesis, Detection, Differential Diagnosis, and Pathologic Basis for Management, *Am J Obstet Gynecol,* **55:**831, 1948.

Rigler, L. B.: Natural History of Untreated Lung Cancer, *Ann NY Acad Sci.* **114:**755, 1964.

Russell, W. O., Ibanex, M. L., Clark, R. L., and White, E. C.: Thyroid Carcinoma: Classification, Intraglandular Dissemination, and Clinicopathologic Study Based upon Whole Organ Sections of 80 Glands, *Cancer,* **16:**1425, 1963.

Slaughter, D. P.: Multicentric Origin of Intraoral Carcinoma, *Surgery,* **20:**133, 1946.

Clinical Manifestations

Barrie, J. G., Knapper, W. H., and Strong, E. W.: Cervical Nodal Metastases of Unknown Origin, *Am J Surg,* **120:**466, 1970.

Bhattacharya, S. K., and Sealy, W. C.: Paraneoplastic Syndromes Resulting from Elaboration of Ectopic Hormones, Antigens, and Bizarre Toxins, *Curr Probl Surg,* May, 1972.

Greenberg, B. E.: Cervical Lymph Node Metastases from Unknown Primary Sites, *Cancer,* **19:**1091, 1966.

Jesse, R. H., and Neff, L. F.: Metastatic Carcinoma in Cervical Nodes with an Unknown Primary Lesion, *Am J Surg,* **112:**547, 1966.

Keller, J. W., and Williams R. D.: Laparotomy for Unexplained Fever, *Arch Surg,* **90:**494, 1965.

Myers, W. P. L., Tashima, C. K., and Rothschild, E. O.: Endocrine Syndromes Associated with Non-endocrine Neoplasms, *Med Clin North Am,* **50:**763, 1966.

Owens, A. H., Jr.: Neoplastic Diseases, in A. M. Harvey, R. J. Johns, A. H. Owens, and R. S. Ross (eds.), "The Principles and Practice of Medicine," p. 641, Appleton-Century-Crofts, Inc., New York, 1972.

Smith, P. E., Krementz, E. T., and Chapman, W.: Metastatic Cancer without a Detectable Primary Site, *Am J Surg,* **113:**633, 1967.

Diagnosis and Staging

Commission on Clinical Oncology of the Union Internationale Contre Cancrum: "TNM Classification of Malignant Tumors," International Clinics against Cancer, Geneva, 1968.

Copeland, M. M.: American Joint Committee on Cancer Staging and End Results Reporting: Objectives and Progress, *Cancer,* **18:**1637, 1965.

Eilber, F. R., Holmes, E. C., and Morton, D. L.: Immunotherapy as an Adjunct to Surgery in Treatment of Cancer, *World J Surg,* **1:**547, 1977.

Glatstein, E., Guernsey, J. M., Rosenberg, S. A., and Kaplan, H. S.: The Value of Laparotomy and Splenectomy in the Staging of Hodgkin's Disease, *Cancer,* **24:**709, 1969.

Goldman, J. M.: Laparotomy for Staging of Hodgkin's Disease, *Lancet,* **1:**125, 1971.

Kennedy, W. B.: History and Physical Examination in the Diagnosis of Cancer, in T. F. Nealon, Jr. (ed.), "Management of the Patient with Cancer," p. 62, W. B. Saunders Co., Philadelphia, 1966.

Surgery

Ansfield, F. J., Ramirez, G., Skibba, J. L, Bryan, G. T., Davis, H. L. Jr., and Wirtanen, G. W.: Intrahepatic Arterial Infusion with 5-Fluorouracil, *Cancer,* **28:**1147, 1971.

Barnes, J. P.: Physiologic Resection of the Right Colon, *Surg Gynecol Obstet,* **94:**722, 1952.

Cole, W. H., Packard, D., and Southwich, H. W.: Carcinoma of the Colon with Special Reference to Prevention of Recurrence, *JAMA,* **155:**1549, 1954.

Deckers, P. J., Ketcham, A. S., Sugarbaker, E. V., Hoye, R. C., and Thomas, L. B.: Pelvic Exenteration for Primary Carcinoma of the Uterine Cervix, *Obstet Gynecol,* **37:**647, 1971.

Flanagan, L., and Foster, J. H.: Hepatic Resection for Metastatic Cancer, *Am J Surg,* **113:**551, 1967.

Foster, J. H., and Berman, M. M.: Solid Liver Tumors, Major Problems in Clinical Surgery, vol. 23, W. B. Saunders Company, Philadelphia, 1977.

Gilbertsen, V. A., and Wangensteen, O. H.: A Summary of Thirteen Years' Experience with the Second Look Program, *Surg Gynecol Obstet,* **114:**438, 1962.

Halsted, W. S.: The Results of Operations for the Cure of Cancer of the Breast Performed at the Johns Hopkins Hospital from June 1889 to January 1894, *Ann Surg,* **20:**297, 1894.

Huggins, C., and Bergenstal, D. M.: Inhibition of Human Mammary and Prostatic Cancer by Adrenalectomy, *Cancer Res,* **12:**134, 1952.

Kiselow, M., Butcher, H. R., and Bricker, E. M.: Results of the Radical Surgical Treatment of Advanced Pelvic Cancer: A Fifteen-Year Study, *Ann Surg,* **166:**436, 1967.

Krementz, E. T., and Ryan, R. E.: Chemotherapy of Melanoma of the Extremities by Perfusion: Fourteen Years Clinical Experience, *Ann Surg,* **175:**900, 1972.

Miles, W. E.: A Method of Performing Abdomino-perineal Excision for Carcinoma of the Rectum and the Terminal Portion of the Pelvic Colon, *Lancet,* **2:**1812, 1908.

Miller, D. R., and Albritten, F. F., Jr.: Principles of Surgery for Cancer, in T. F. Nealon Jr. (ed.), "Management of the Patient with Cancer," p. 154, W. B. Saunders Company, Philadelphia, 1966.

Mockman, S., Curreri, A. R., and Ansfield, F. J.: Second-Look Operation for Colon Carcinoma after Fluorouracil Therapy, *Arch Surg,* **100:**527, 1970.

Mueller, C. B., and Jeffries, W.: Cancer of the Breast: Its Outcome as Measured by the Rate of Dying and Causes of Death, *Ann Surg,* **182:**334, 1975.

Pierce, E. H., Clagett, O. T., McDonald, J. R., and Gage, R. P.: Biopsy of the Breast Followed by Delayed Radical Mastectomy, *Surg Gynecol Obstet,* **103:**559, 1956.

Ramming, K. P., Sparks, F. C., Eilber, F. R., Holmes, E. C., and Morton, D. L.: Hepatic Artery Ligation and 5-Fluorouracil Infusion for Metastatic Colon Carcinoma and Primary Hepatoma, *Am J Surg,* **132:**236, 1976.

———, ———, ———, and Morton, D. L.: Management of Hepatic Metastases, *Semin Oncol,* **4:**71, 1977.

Roberts, S. S., Hengesh, J. W., McGrath, R. G., Valaitis, J., McGrew, E. A., and Cole, W. H.: Prognostic Significance of Cancer Cells in the Circulating Blood: A Ten Year Evaluation, *Am J Surg,* **113:**757, 1967.

Sparks, F. C., Mosher, M. B., Hallauer, W. C., Silverstein, M. J., Rangel, D., Passaro, E., and Morton, D. L.: Hepatic Artery Ligation and Postoperative Chemotherapy for Hepatic Metastases: Clinical and Pathophysiological Results, *Cancer,* **35:**1074, 1975.

Stearns, M. W., and Schottenfeld, D.: Techniques for the Surgical Management of Colon Cancer, *Cancer,* **28:**165, 1971.

Stehlin, J. S.: Hyperthermic Perfusion with Chemotherapy for Cancer of the Extremities, *Surg Gynecol Obstet,* **129:**305, 1969.

Stehlin, J. S., Jr., Giovanella, B. C., Ipolyi, P. D., Muenz, L. R., and Anderson, R. F.: Results of Hyperthemic Perfusion for Melanoma of the Extremities, *Surg Gynecol Obstet,* **140:**339, 1975.

Turnbull, R. B., Kyle, K., Watson, F. R., and Spratt, J.: Cancer of the Colon: The Influence of the No-Touch Isolation Technic on Survival Rates, *Ann Surg,* **166:**420, 1967.

Watkins, E., Khazei, A. M., and Nabra, K. S.: Surgical Basis for Arterial Infusion Chemotherapy of Disseminated Carcinoma of the Liver, *Surg Gynecol Obstet,* **130:**581, 1970.

Wilkens, E. W., Jr.: The Surgical Management of Metastatic Neoplasms of the Lung, *J Thorac Cardiovasc Surg,* **42:**298, 1961.

Zike, W. L., Safaie-Sharazi, S., and Gulessarian, H. P.: Hepatic Artery Ligation and Cytotoxic Infusion for Treatment of Liver Neoplasms, *Arch Surg,* **110:**641, 1975.

Radiation Therapy

Higgins, G. S., Jr., Conn, J. H., Jordan, P. H., Jr., Humphrey, E. W., Roswit, B., and Keehn, R. J.: Preoperative Radiotherapy for Colo-Rectal Cancer, *Ann Surg,* **181:**624, 1974.

Johns, H. E., and Cunningham, J. R.: in "The Physics of Radiology," p. 345, Charles C Thomas, Publisher, Springfield, Ill., 1971.

Kligerman, M. M.: Radiotherapy and Rectal Cancer, *Cancer,* **39:**896, 1977.

Moss, W. T., and Brand, W. N.: "Therapeutic Radiology; Rationale, Technique, Results," 3d ed., The C. V. Mosby Company, St. Louis, 1969.

Paulson, D. L., Shaw, R. R., Kee, J. L., Mallams, J. T., and Collier, R. E.: Combined Preoperative Irradiation and Resection for Bronchogenic Carcinoma, *J Thorac Cardiovasc Surg,* **44:**281, 1962.

Powers, W. E., and Tolmach, L. J.: Preoperative Radiation Therapy: Biologic Basis and Experimental Investigation, *Nature,* **201:**272, 1964.

Stearns, M. W., Jr., Deddish, M. R., Quan, S. H. Q., and Leaming, R. H.: Preoperative Roentgen Therapy for Cancer of the Rectum and Rectosigmoid, *Surg Gynecol Obstet,* **138:**584, 1974.

Stevens, K. R., Jr., Allen, C. V., and Fletcher, W. S.: Preoperative Radiotherapy for Adenocarcinoma of the Rectosigmoid, *Cancer,* **37:**2866, 1976.

Chemotherapy

Bailor, J. C., and Byar, D. P.: Estrogen Treatment for Cancer of the Prostate, *Cancer,* **26:**257, 1970.

Baserga, R. (ed.): The Cell Cycle and Cancer, Marcel Dekker, Inc., New York, 1971.

Bonadonna, G., Brusamolino, E., Valagussa, B. S., Rossi, A., Brugnatelli, L., Brambilla, C., DeLena, M., Tancini, G., Bajetta, E., Musumeci, R., and Veronesi, U.: Combination Chemotherapy as an Adjuvant Treatment in Operable Breast Cancer, *N Engl J Med,* **294:**405, 1976.

Bruce, W. R.: The Action of Chemotherapeutic Agents at the Cellular Level and the Effects of These Agents on Hematopoietic and Lymphomatous Tissue, *Can Cancer Conf,* **7:**53, 1966.

Calabresi, P., and Parks, R. E., Jr.: Chemotherapy of Neoplastic Diseases, in L. S. Goodman and A. Gilman (eds.), "The Pharmacological Basis of Therapeutics," 5th ed., p. 1248, The MacMillan Company, New York, 1975.

Chabner, B. A., Myers, E. E., Coleman, C. N., and Johns, D. G.: The Clinical Pharmacology of Antineoplastic Agents, *N Engl J Med*, **292**:1107, 1159, 1975.

Cline, M. J., and Haskell, C. M.: Cancer Chemotherapy, 2d ed., W. B. Saunders Company, Philadelphia, 1975.

D'Angio, G. J., Evans, A. E., Breslow, N., Beckwith, B., Bishop, H., Feigl, P., Goodwin, W., Deape, L. L., Sinks, L. F., Sutow, W., Tefft, M., and Wolff, J.: The Treatment of Wilms' Tumor, *Cancer*, **38**:633, 1976.

Gilman, A.: The Initial Clinical Trial of Nitrogen Mustard, *Am J Surg*, **105**:574, 1963.

Haskell, C. M.: Immunologic Aspects of Cancer Chemotherapy, *Ann Rev Pharmacol Toxicol*, **17**:179, 1977.

———, Sparks, F. C., Graze, P. R., and Korenman, S. G.: Systemic Therapy for Metastatic Breast Cancer, *Ann Int Med*, **86**:68, 1977.

Huggins, C., and Hodges, C. V.: Studies on Prostatic Cancer. I. The Effect of Castration, of Estrogen and Androgen Injection on Serum Phosphatases in Metastatic Carcinoma of the Prostate, *Cancer Res*, **1**:293, 1941.

Laird, A. K.: Dynamics of Growth in Tumors and in Normal Organisms, *Natl Cancer Inst Monogr*, **30**:15, 1969.

Lewis, J. L.: Chemotherapy of Gestational Choriocarcinoma, *Cancer*, **30**:1517, 1972.

Li, M. C., Hertz, R., and Spencer, D. B.: Effect of Methotrexate Therapy upon Choriocarcinoma and Chorioadenoma, *Proc Soc Exp Biol Med*, **93**:361, 1956.

Mathe, G.: Immunotherapy in the Treatment of Acute Lymphoid Leukemia, *Hosp Prac*, **6**:43, 1971.

Schabel, F. M., Jr.: The Use of Tumor Growth Kinetics in Planning "Curative" Chemotherapy of Advanced Solid Tumors, *Cancer Res*, **29**:2384, 1969.

Skipper, H. E.: Cancer Chemotherapy Is Many Things: GHA Clowes Memorial Lecture, *Cancer Res*, **31**:1173, 1971.

——— and Perry, S.: Kinetics of Normal and Leukemic Leukocyte Populations and Relevance to Chemotherapy, *Cancer Res*, **30**:1883, 1970.

Strawitz, J. G.: Cancer Chemotherapy Using Isolation Perfusion, in I. Brodsky, S. B. Kahn, and J. H. Moyer (eds.), "Cancer Chemotherapy II," p. 443, Grune & Stratton, New York, 1972.

Sullivan, P. W., and Salmon, S. E.: Kinetics of Tumor Growth and Regression in IgG Multiple Myeloma, *J Clin Invest*, **51**:1697, 1972.

Sullivan, R. D., and Semel, C. J.: Arterial Infusion Cancer Chemotherapy for Solid Tumors, in I. Brodsky, S. B. Kahn, and J. H. Moyer (eds.), "Cancer Chemotherapy II," p. 453, Grune & Stratton, New York, 1972.

Combined Therapy

Ariel, I. M., and Briceno, M.: Rhabdomyosarcoma of the Extremities and Trunk: Analysis of 150 Patients Treated by Surgical Resection, *J Surg Oncol*, **7**:269, 1975.

Cortes, E. P., Holland, J. F., Wang, J. J., and Sinks, L. F.: Doxorubicin in Disseminated Osteosarcoma, *JAMA*, **221**:1132, 1972.

———, ———, ———, ———, Blom, J., Senn, H., Bank, A., and Glidewell, O.: Amputation and Adriamycin in Primary Osteosarcoma, *N Engl J Med*, **291**:998, 1974.

DiPietro, S., DePalo, G., Gennari, L., Molinari, R., and Domascelli, B.: Cancer Chemotherapy by Intra-arterial Infusion with Adriamycin, *J Surg Oncol* **5**:421, 1973.

Gerner, R. E., Moore, G. E., and Pickren, J. M.: Soft Tissue Sarcomas, *Ann Surg*, **181**:803, 1975.

Gilbert, H. A., Kagan, R. A., and Winkley, J.: Soft Tissue Sarcomas of the Extremities: Their Natural History, Treatment and Radiation Sensitivity, *J Surg Oncol*, **7**:303, 1975.

Haskell, C. M., Eilber, F. R., and Morton, D. L.: Adriamycin (NSC-12317) by Arterial Infusion, *Cancer Chemother Rep*, **6**:187, 1974.

———, Silverstein, M. J., Rangel, D., Hunt, J. S., Sparks, F. C., and Morton, D. L.: Multimodality Cancer Therapy in Man: A Pilot Study of Adriamycin by Arterial Infusion. *Cancer*, **33**:1485, 1974.

Jaffe, N., Frei, E., III, Traggis, D., and Bishop, Y.: Adjuvant Methotrexate and Citrovorum Factor Treatment of Osteogenic Sarcoma, *N Engl J Med*, **291**:994, 1974.

Lindberg, R. D.: The Role of Radiation Therapy in the Treatment of Soft Tissue Sarcoma in Adults, in "Proc. 7th Natl. Cancer Congress," J. B. Lippincott Company, Philadelphia, 1972.

Martin, R. G., Butler, J. J., and Albores, S. S.: Soft Tissue Tumors: Surgical Treatment and Results, in "Tumors of Bone and Soft Tissue," p. 333, Year Book Medical Publishers, Chicago, 1965.

Morton, D. L.: Soft Tissue Sarcomas, in J. F. Holland (ed.), "Cancer Medicine," p. 1845, Lea & Febiger, Philadelphia, 1974.

———, Eilber, F. R., Townsend, C. M., Jr., Grant, T. T., Mirra, J., and Weisenburger, T. H.: Limb Salvage from a Multidisciplinary Treatment Approach for Skeletal and Soft Tissue Sarcomas of the Extremity, *Ann Surg*, **184**:268, 1976.

McNeer, G. D., Cantin, J., Chu, F., and Nickson, J. T.: Effectiveness of Radiation Therapy in the Management of Sarcoma of the Soft Somatic Tissues, *Cancer*, **22**:391, 1968.

Murphy, W. T.: The Role of Radiation Therapy in the Management of Soft Somatic Tissue Sarcoma, *Proc. 6th Natl. Cancer Congress*, p. 775, 1968.

Rosen, G., Murphy, M. L., Huvas, A. G., Guitierrez, M., and Marcove, R. C.: Chemotherapy, En Bloc Resection and Prosthetic Bone Replacement in the Treatment of Osteogenic Sarcoma, *Cancer*, **37**:1, 1976.

———, Suwansirikal, S., Kwan, C., Tan, C., Wu, S. J., Beattie, E. J., and Murphy, M. L.: High Dose Methotrexate with Citrovorum Factor Rescue and Adriamycin in Childhood Osteosarcoma, *Cancer*, **33**:1151, 1974.

Suit, H. D., and Russell, W. O.: Radiation Therapy of Soft Tissue Sarcomas, *Cancer*, **36**:759, 1975.

———, ———, and Martin, R. G.: Sarcoma of Soft Tissue: Clinical and Histopathological Parameters and Response to Treatment, *Cancer*, **35**:1478, 1974.

Townsend, C. M., Jr., Eilber, F. R., and Morton, D. L.: Skeletal and Soft Tissue Sarcomas: Results of Treatment with Adjuvant Immunotherapy, *JAMA*, **236**:2187, 1976.

———, ———, and ———: Skeletal and Soft Tissue Sarcomas: Results of Surgical Adjuvant Chemotherapy, *Proc Am Soc Clin Oncol*, **17**:265, 1976.

Immunotherapy

Deckers, P. J., and Pilch, Y. H.: RNA-Mediated Transfer of Tumor Immunity: A New Model for Immunotherapy of Cancer, *Cancer,* **28:**1219, 1971.

Eilber, F. R., Morton, D. L., Holmes, E. C., Sparks, F. C., and Ramming, K. P.: Adjuvant Immunotherapy with BCG in Treatment of Regional Lymph Node Metastases from Malignant Melanoma, *N Engl J Med,* **294:**237, 1976.

Gutterman, J. U., Mavligit, G. M., and Hersh, E. M.: Chemoimmunotherapy of Human Solid Tumors, *Med Clin North Am,* **60:**441, 1976.

Halpern, B. N., Biozzi, G., Stiffel, C., and Mouton, D.: Correlation entre l'activitie phagocytaire du système reticulo-endothelial et la production d'anticorps antibacteriens, *C R Soc Biol (Paris),* **152:**758, 1958.

Holland, J. F., and Bekesi, J. G.: Immunotherapy of Human Leukemia with Neuraminidase-modified Cells, *Med Clin North Am,* **60:**539, 1976.

Israel, L., and Edelstein, R. L.: "Nonspecific Immunostimulation with *Corynebacterium parvum* in Human Cancer," The Williams & Wilkins Company, Baltimore, 1974.

Klein, E.: Hypersensitivity Reactions at Tumor Site, *Cancer Res,* **29:**2351, 1969.

————, Holterman, O., Milgrom, H., Case, R. W., Klein, D., Rosner, D., and Djerassi, I.: Immunotherapy for Accessible Tumors Utilizing Delayed Hypersensitivity Reactions and Separated Components of the Immune System, *Med Clin North Am,* **60:**389, 1976.

Lawrence, H. S.: Transfer Factor, *Adv Immunol,* **11:**195, 1969.

LoBuglio, A. F., and Neidhart, J. A.: Transfer Factor: A Potential Agent for Cancer Therapy, *Med Clin North Am,* **60:**585, 1976.

McKhann, C. F.: Immunobiology of Cancer, in J. S. Najarian and R. L. Simmons (eds.), "Transplantation," p. 297, Lea & Febiger, Philadelphia, 1972.

McKneally, M. F., Maver, C., and Kausel, H.: Regional Immunotherapy of Lung Cancer with Intrapleural BCG, *Lancet,* **1:**377, 1976.

Mathe, G., Schwarzenberg, L., and Amiel, J. L.: Bone Marrow, in J. S. Najarian and R. L. Simmons (eds.), "Transplantation," p. 588, Lea & Febiger, Philadelphia, 1972.

Moertel, C. G., Ritts, R. E., Jr., Schutt, A. J., and Hahn, R. G.: Clinical Studies of Methanol Extraction Residue Fraction of Bacillus Calmette-Guérin as an Immunostimulant in Patients with Advanced Cancer, *Cancer Res,* **35:**3075, 1975.

Moore, G. E., and Gerner, R. E.: Cancer Immunity: Hypothesis and Clinical Trial of Lymphocytotherapy for Malignant Diseases, *Ann Surg,* **172:**733, 1970.

Morton, D. L.: Cancer Immunotherapy: An Overview, *Semin Oncol,* **1:**297, 1974.

————: Immunotherapy of Cancer: Present Status and Future Potential, *Cancer,* **30:**1647, 1972.

————, Eilber, F. R., Holmes, E. C., Hunt, J. S., Ketcham, A. S., Silverstein, M. J., and Sparks, F. C.: BCG Immunotherapy of Malignant Melanoma: Summary of a Seven-Year Experience, *Ann Surg,* **180:**635, 1974.

————, ————, Joseph, W. L., Wood, W. C., Trahan, E., and Ketcham, A. S.: Immunological Factors in Human Sarcomas and Melanomas: A Rational Basis for Immunotherapy, *Ann Surg,* **172:**740, 1970.

————, Haskell, C. M., Pilch, Y. H., Sparks, F. C., and Winters, W. D.: Recent Advances in Oncology, *Ann Intern Med,* **77:**431, 1972.

————, Holmes, E. C., and Golub, S. H.: Immunologic Aspects of Lung Cancer, *Chest,* **71:**640, 1977.

Nathanson, L.: Use of BCG in Treatment of Human Neoplasms: A Review, *Semin Oncol,* **1:**337, 1974.

Oettgen, H. F., Pinsky, C. M., and Delmonte, L.: Treatment of Cancer with Immunomodulators: *Corynebacterium parvum* and Levamisole, *Med Clin North Am,* **60:**463, 1976.

Old, L. J., Benacerraf, B., Clark, D. A., Carswell, E. A., and Stockert, E.: The Role of the Reticuloendothelial System in the Host Reaction to Neoplasia, *Cancer Res,* **21:**1281, 1961.

Powles, R.: Immunologic Maneuvers in Management of Acute Leukemia, *Med Clin North Am,* **60:**463, 1976.

Ramming, K. P., and deKernion, J. B.: Immune RNA Therapy for Renal Cell Carcinoma: Survival and Immunologic Monitoring, *Ann Surg,* **186:**459, 1977.

Rojas, A. F., Feierstein, J. M., Mickiewicz, E., Glait, H., and Olivari, A. J.: Levamisole in Advanced Human Breast Cancer, *Lancet,* **1:**211, 1976.

Sparks, F. C.: Hazards and Complications of BCG Immunotherapy, *Med Clin North Am,* **60:**499, 1976.

————, and Ramming, K. P.: Immunotherapy of Gastrointestinal Cancer: The Potential, *Clin Gastroenterol,* **5:**855, 1976.

Stockert, E.: The Role of the Reticuloendothelial System in the Host Reaction to Neoplasia, *Cancer Res,* **21:**1281, 1961.

Sumner, W. C., and Foraker, A. C.: Spontaneous Regression of Human Melanoma: Clinical and Experimental Study, *Cancer,* **13:**79, 1960.

Prognosis

Berkson, J., and Gage, R. P.: Specific Methods of Calculating Survival Rates of Patients with Cancer, in G. T. Pack and I. M. Ariel (eds.), "Treatment of Cancer and Allied Diseases," Harper & Row, Publishers, Incorporated, New York, 1958.

Dunphy, J. E.: On Caring for the Patient with Cancer, *N Engl J Med,* **295:**313, 1976.

Kelly, W. D., and Friesen, S. R.: Do Cancer Patients Want to be Told? *Surgery,* **27:**822, 1950.

Wangensteen, O. H.: Should Patients Be Told They Have Cancer? *Surgery,* **27:**944, 1950.

Psychologic Management

Sherman, C. D., Jr., and Feasel, W. P.: "General Aspects of Cancer," University of Rochester School of Medicine and Dentistry, Rochester, N.Y., 1969–1970. (Syllabus.)

Silverberg, E., and Holleb, A. I.: "Cancer Statistics 1972," American Cancer Society, Inc., New York. (Reprinted from *CA,* **22:**2, 1972.)

Chapter 10

Transplantation

by Richard L. Simmons, John E. Foker, Richard R. Lower, and John S. Najarian

Man does not burst like a balloon—he falls apart, piece by piece. Clinical organ transplantation is designed to replace the exhausted parts as they fall. Because the immunologic barrier of allograft rejection stands in the way of attaining chimerism between host and graft, immunologists and surgeons have been working together since World War II to circumvent the rejection reaction. Unfortunately, the problems remain unsolved. Despite the clinical success of kidney transplantation, organs are still rejected, and attempts to prevent rejection can be fatal. The field of clinical transplantation, though no longer totally experimental, remains in flux, and many apparently well-founded principles are soon washed away. Much of the material presented in this chapter will not survive the decade.

The first part of this chapter discusses the immunobiology of the allograft, the rejection reaction, and the means for achieving immunosuppression. The current and incipient clinical applications of these biologic principles and techniques to the human patient are discussed in the second section.

IMMUNOBIOLOGY OF THE ALLOGRAFT

Tissue or organ grafts between individuals of the same species (allografts, or homografts) are rejected with a vigor proportional to the degree of the genetic disparity between them. Grafts between individuals of different species (xenografts, or heterografts) are rejected even more rapidly. Grafts between identical twins (isografts, isogeneic grafts, or syngeneic grafts), or from an individual to himself (autografts, or autogenous grafts) survive indefinitely once vascular supply has been reestablished.

Allografts normally survive surgical manipulation as well as isografts. If the recipient has not previously encountered the antigens present on the donor graft, the allograft is not morphologically or physiologically distinguishable from the isograft in the early posttransplant period—the rejection process normally takes several days. Medawar, in his classic demonstration of the immunologic nature of the allograft response, noted that skin grafts between randomly selected adult rabbits appeared normal until the fourth or fifth day. At that time inflammation appeared within the graft bed in the form of a dense leukocyte infiltrate which led to necrosis of the entire graft by about the tenth day. Medawar further demonstrated that the rejection process is the result of immunologic mechanisms. Whereas the "first-set rejection" takes place in 10 or 11 days, a second graft from the same rabbit resulted in an accelerated "second-set rejection." This process of first-set and second-set rejection of allogeneic graft takes place whether or not the graft is orthotopic (a graft placed in the anatomic position normally occupied by such tissue) or heterotopic (those grafts placed in abnormal recipient locations). The reaction is immunologically specific for the antigens involved, and the second-set rejections occur only when the recipient has previously encountered the antigens of the first graft.

Transplantation (Histocompatibility) Antigens

Tissue transplanted from one individual to another will be rejected if the new host can recognize that tissue as foreign. Foreignness is equated with the presence of antigens on the donor cells which the host does not possess and thereby recognizes as nonself. Foreign antigens on a tissue or organ graft are considered histocompatibility antigens if they can be related to graft rejection. Any histocompatibility antigen will lead to graft rejection if the antigen is present on donor tissue but absent from the host. In fact, some histocompatibility differences are probably present in all donor-recipient combinations with the exception of identical twins in human beings, and inbred strains in other animal species. The "strength" of different antigenic in-

compatibilities varies, however, and a "strong" mismatch can lead to graft rejection within 8 days, while "weaker" differences will permit graft survival of well over 100 days. The strongest antigens are xenogeneic antigens, i.e., those which elicit the rejection of grafts from animals of a different species. Xenograft rejection is often accomplished within minutes. In contrast, one of the weakest histocompatibility antigens is linked to the Y chromosome of male mice, so that female mice gradually reject grafts from male mice of the same inbred strain.

THE NATURE OF HISTOCOMPATIBILITY ANTIGENS

Antigens which stimulate the rejection of grafts are predominantly located on the cell surface. A group of strong histocompatibility antigens has been found in several species, including human beings, which are the products of a single chromosomal region. Although they have been given different names in different species, they are the major histocompatibility antigens. Mismatch of these antigens inevitably leads to graft rejection. The ABO system leaves the more complex and elusive major histocompatibility antigens as the main determinants of graft survival. Because of the ease of typing the ABO antigens they will not be further considered in this discussion of major histocompatibility antigens.

Tissues vary in the amount of the histocompatibility antigens present. In the mouse, for example, the strong histocompatibility antigens are found in high concentration in the liver, spleen, and lymphoid tissue. Intermediate amounts of the antigens are found on cells of the kidney, lung, adrenal gland, and gastrointestinal tract, while heart, muscle, and brain cells contain very little. The histocompatibility antigens appear on the cell surface very early in the development of the individual—Simmons and Russell found evidence that they are expressed on the fertilized egg. Age of the donor is, therefore, not a consideration in the antigenic strength of a potential organ graft.

The biochemical nature and the cell membrane relationships of the histocompatibility antigens are slowly yielding to investigation. Most of the studies have centered on the major antigens, and although they have not been completely characterized, much is known about them. They are proteins of approximately 45,000 mol wt and associated noncovalently in the membrane with B_2 microglobulins. Peptide mapping and amino acid analyses of tryptic digests of highly purified antigens indicate that the variability occurs in small discrete regions of the molecule. A constant framework of amino acids characterizes the remainder of these molecules. The large number of antigens results from changes in the amino acids at only a few locations. This phenomenon is not unique and has many counterparts in the biological world. Mutations may be acceptable at only a few locations; otherwise the functional capabilities of the molecule are destroyed. With antigens, as with other molecules, variety with preservation of activity is gained by amino acid changes at these few sites.

The complexities of the cell membrane are only beginning to be unraveled, but the membrane appears to be a bilayer of lipid molecules interspersed with globular protein islands (Fig. 10-1). The bilayer has a fluid character, and consequently the proteins, which provide the many membrane functions, have considerable mobility within the lipid shell. This fluid mosaic model of membrane structure has several important consequences. Some of the proteins may traverse the entire membrane, as those making up the transport sites would be expected to do. Other proteins seem to be related only to the inner or outer surface of the membrane and may be useful in receiving or sending various signals and providing communication with the cytoplasm. The fluid nature of the membrane also means that the density of the active protein sites can be varied as the cell requires.

The histocompatibility antigens are among the protein islands of the cell surface. Their function is not yet understood, but obviously they have not evolved to thwart graft rejection. More likely, they are important in recognition phenomena and cell-to-cell interactions, but the mechanisms are unknown. Susceptibility to certain diseases, including ankylosing spondylitis, acute uveitis, celiac disease, psoriasis, Hodgkin's disease, and several immune-based maladies, has been linked to the major histocompatibility locus and associated with certain antigens. These seemingly unrelated conditions may prove to have obvious connections when cell membrane function is better understood.

THE IMMUNOGENETICS OF HISTOCOMPATIBILITY

The strongest of the transplantation antigens is the expression of a single chromosomal region called the *major histocompatibility complex* (MHC). In human beings the MHC is located on chromosome 6. Several species commonly used in immunological studies have a similar MHC which governs the major transplantation antigens. These antigens, however, were discovered and named before much was known about their genetic origins, and so the nomenclature varies among species. In human beings, transplantation antigens were first investigated on leukocytes and were named human leukocyte antigens (HLA). Naturally, the first-discovered antigens would be likely to be the major determinants. In mice, the strongest antigens are called H-2 antigens, in rats AgB antigens, etc. All seem to originate from an MHC, suggesting that considerable similarity exists between species.

The HLA locus has begun to be dissected through immunogenetic analysis. The presence of HLA antigens on a cell surface is detected in one of two ways. The serological method uses antigen-specific antisera which either agglutinates or lyses cells carrying the antigen. This has identified the serologically defined (SD) HLA antigens, which had been expected to encompass all the major antigens. When this proposition was tested in cell culture by measuring the reactivity of host lymphocytes to lymphocytes from potential graft donors, it was found that certain SD identical combinations still provided considerable stimulation. The lymphocytes were reacting to other cellular transplantation antigens. By screening hundreds of potential donors and recipients by these mixed leukocyte cultures (MLC) it was found that another transplantation locus existed. The lymphocyte-defined (LD) locus was

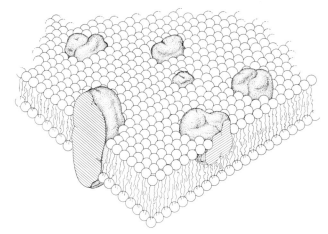

Fig. 10-1. Protein islands within the lipid bilayer of the cell membrane. Some proteins, such as those associated with transport, are thought to traverse the membrane; others are located only on the inner or outer surface. The transplantation antigens are complex proteins and are among the islands. Undoubtedly they are located on the outer portion of the membrane and perhaps extend to the inner surface as well. Their exposed position permits them to interact with immunocompetent cells and antibodies. (*From S. J. Singer and G. L. Nicolson, The Fluid Mosaic Model of the Structure of Cell Membranes, Science, 175:720, 1972.*)

found to be part also of the HLA complex but genetically distinct from the SD region. The two antigen testing methods, therefore, subdivided the HLA complex into SD and LD regions. Further genetic analysis has revealed the presence of additional components which do not code for cell antigens, and it is now clear that the human MHC consists of multiple genes—the number is not yet known but may be as large as several hundred.

At least three SD antigenic groups have now been found. The HLA-A and HLA-B antigens have formed the basis for transplantation tissue typing for many years, while HLA-C is a more recent discovery. Both the HLA-A and HLA-B loci have about 20 different alleles or antigens. Alleles are the alternative forms of a given gene locus, and, as noted, the allelic antigens may differ by only one or two amino acids. Less is known about the LD locus (now called HLA-D), but multiple alleles exist. Each individual inherits one chromosome and, hence, one set of HLA antigens from each parent. All the HLA antigens are expressed (codominant) on the cell surface, and thus, two A antigens, two B antigens, etc., are present.

The known loci of the HLA complex have been mapped on chromosome 6; their relative positions are shown in Fig. 10-2. The three SD loci (A, B, and C) are plotted, as is the LD locus (HLA-D). The site for complement factor C2 has also been found to be within the HLA complex. The relative positions of these five loci are known, but they are separated by a considerable amount of unidentified genetic material. Several other genes have been assigned to the HLA region, but their relative position is not known. The complement factors C4 and C8 are located somewhere within this region, and perhaps, as shown, a second LC locus is present. Recent evidence also suggests that the immune responsiveness of an individual is controlled by

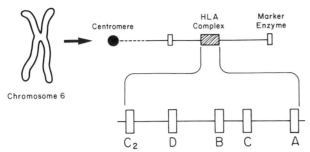

Fig. 10-2. Schematic representation of the HLA complex, the major histocompatibility determinants in human beings. The HLA complex is located on chromosome 6, although it is not known whether it is on the long or short arm. Many genes comprise the HLA complex; pictured are the relative positions of the HLA-A, -B, -C, and -D loci. Also shown is the location of the gene coding for the C2 component of the complement pathway. Many other genes, including that for the C4 component of complement, are probably found within the complex but are not yet well defined.

one or more genes within the HLA complex. How the products of these immune-response genes function is virtually unknown, but they may be of considerable importance in regulating the ability to react to antigens and thus to the immunological capabilities of the individual. Ultimately, the HLA region may be found to control a wide variety of membrane structures and functions.

The MHC loci have been found to be closely linked but

Fig. 10-3. Hypothetic examples of inheritance of serologically detectable HLA antigens of the A and B series. Four offspring of mating between parents with chromosomes labeled I-II and III-IV are shown, as well as one possible result of recombination within the HLA region and subsequent inheritance. The parental chromosomes are usually transmitted intact, and the offspring receive one chromosome containing an A and B pair from each parent. Occasionally, however, crossover occurs and the child receives a recombinant antigen pair from a parent. For simplicity, genes coding for the C and D series of antigens within the HLA complex are not shown. See Fig. 10-2 for the presumed location of the genes within the HLA complex.

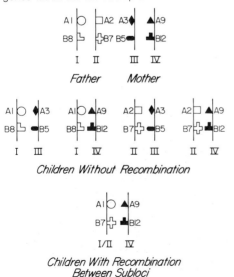

separable, and therefore genetic crossover between them, though rare, can occur. As shown in Fig. 10-3, the parental HLA-A and HLA-B pairs are usually inherited together, and the antigens originating from one chromosome are called an *HLA haplotype*. Almost always the haplotype the child receives from each parent corresponds to the haplotype of one of the parental chromosomes. When crossover occurs during meiosis, however, the child receives a recombinant haplotype from a parent. (In the example shown, recombination occurred between A and B antigens.)

Detection of the A and B alleles for tissue typing requires banks of monospecific sera. Typing is necessary because it seems clear that survival of transplanted organs correlates with the closeness of the A and B antigen match. The third SD locus, HLA-C, is presumably also a strong histocompatibility determinant, but the proof will come with greater use of HLA-C typing in transplantation studies. The role of the HLA-D sublocus (LD antigens) in transplantation is unclear. Lymphocytes in mixed leukocyte cultures respond to cells with different D antigens by proliferating. Even when the SD antigens are identical, lymphocytes with different LD antigens proliferate actively in MLC. The presence of proliferation in culture cannot be directly translated into antigraft activity, since the dividing lymphocytes acquire little cytotoxicity against the donor cells if only D differences are involved. Nevertheless, the proliferation induced by D antigens is essential for full development of cellular immunity against A and B antigens. Clinical tissue matching by mixed leukocyte culture to minimize HLA-D differences has proved to be valuable for bone marrow transplantation and may be valuable for kidney transplantation as well.

It is important to recognize that there are genes on other chromosomes outside the MHC which control weaker histocompatibility loci. In human beings, such antigens are not well understood, but a graft from a sibling identical at the HLA locus will be rejected if immunosuppressive drugs are not utilized. Such rejections are the natural consequence of these minor histocompatibility loci.

The Immune Apparatus

The presence of the histocompatibility antigens on the cells of transplanted organs triggers the rejection reaction. At birth, human beings are already immunologically competent and have undergone a complex developmental process. It is now agreed that there is a single hemopoietic stem cell, found in the extraembryonic yolk sac, which begins to proliferate. The resulting daughter stem cells migrate to various centers for further differentiation. Within these centers, progenitor cells for erythrocytes, eosinophils, basophils, neutrophils, and lymphoid cells arise, depending on the local microchemical environment. It is likely that further proliferation of these progenitor stem cells depends on the action of "poietins," which tend to expand the populations of specialized cells in the way that erythropoietin acts on the erythrocyte line (Fig. 10-4).

The lymphoid cell line first appears within two primary (or central) lymphoid tissues. The thymus governs the

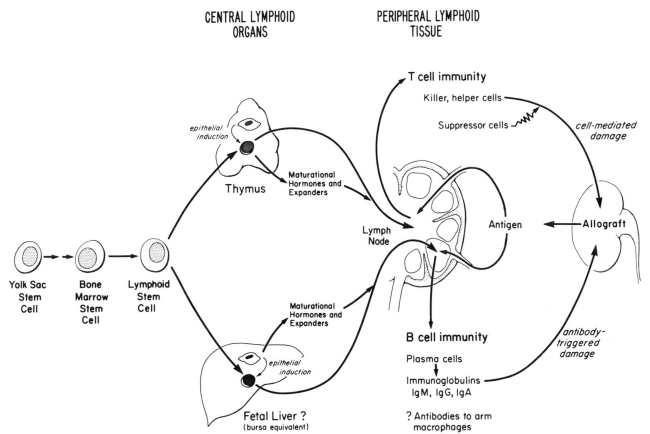

Fig. 10-4. Encapsulation of the extraordinarily complex developmental sequences of the immune system. Certain of the known inducers, expanders, growth factors, and sites of maturation needed to establish the T and B cell lines are presented. Much of this takes place before birth, so transplant recipients are fully competent with established peripheral lymphoid populations in the lymph nodes, Peyer's patches, and spleen. Therefore, clinical immunosuppression consists principally of lymphocyte depletion and inhibition of the activation of antigen-stimulated lymphocytes. [From J. E. Foker, R. L. Simmons, and J. S. Najarian, Principles of Immunosuppression, in D. C. Sabiston, Jr. (ed.), "Davis-Christopher Textbook of Surgery," p. 506, W. B. Saunders Company, Philadelphia, 1977.]

development of cellular immunity. In birds, the bursa of Fabricius governs the development of humoral immunity. The bursa exists as a clearly defined central lymphoid structure only in birds. The equivalent of the bursa of Fabricius has not been defined in mammals, but there is evidence that it exists—perhaps within the fetal liver. In human beings the characteristics of sex-linked agammaglobulinemia of the Bruton type—very low levels of immunoglobulins, with normal cellular immunity and thymus-derived lymphocytes—suggest that the bursa equivalent has failed to develop.

Both the thymus and the bursa (or its equivalent) are responsible for the further development of the peripheral lymphoid tissues, i.e., spleen, lymph nodes, Peyer's patches. Certain areas of the lymph node can be shown to be dependent on the functional presence of the thymus and bursa (Fig. 10-5). The paracortical regions between the

cortical germinal centers and the medulla are dependent on the thymus, while the germinal centers themselves and the medullary cord lymphoid tissue are under the developmental control of the bursal equivalent. Therefore, thymectomy early in the neonatal period or congenital thymic deficiency results in failure of development of the paracortical regions of the lymph nodes. In chickens, bursectomy leads to failure of development of germinal centers and medullary cord lymphoid tissues.

During ontogeny, the thymus is the site of a vigorous cell proliferation. Many of these cells migrate to the paracortical areas of lymph nodes. All such cells which were once dependent on the thymus for their development are called T cells. Among their several functions T cells represent the immunocompetent cell population responsible for the development of cellular immunity, rather than humoral immunity. These reactions include delayed hypersensitivity reactions, as well as many of the early reactions responsible for allograft rejection.

Once these cells have migrated from the thymus, they seldom return. There is some evidence that the thymus produces a "hormone" (thymosin), perhaps a poietin, that is necessary for the maintenance of the full functional capacity of the T-cell system. The thymus increases in size until puberty, at which time it begins to atrophy. The function of the T-cell system is maintained by T cells established in the bone marrow and peripheral lymphoid tissue.

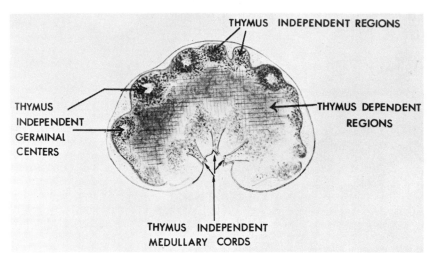

THYMUS INDEPENDENT REGIONS

THYMUS INDEPENDENT GERMINAL CENTERS

THYMUS DEPENDENT REGIONS

THYMUS INDEPENDENT MEDULLARY CORDS

Fig. 10-5. The thymus-dependent and thymus-independent areas are illustrated in this schematic representation of a lymph node. [*From R. A. Good and J. Finstad, Structure and Development of the Immune System, in J. S. Najarian and R. L. Simmons (eds.), "Transplantation," p. 26, Lea & Febiger, Philadelphia, 1972.*]

A humoral factor similar to that secreted by the thymus may also be at work here in maturing and maintaining the population of immunocompetent cells known as *B cells.* The B cells descend from stem cells in the bone marrow and become responsible for the manufacture of circulating immunoglobulins and thus for humoral immunity (Fig. 10-4).

It appears that the lymphoid system is the seat of the body's immunologic response and the small mature lymphocytes and the plasma cells are the immunocompetent cells. Once the lymphocytes (T or B cells) have migrated to the peripheral lymphoid tissue, they are fully immunocompetent. It is likely that Burnet's clonal selection theory holds true—i.e., a state of preparedness for a certain antigen or group of related antigens exists within a lymphoid cell so that it is capable of responding to only a narrow range of antigenic specificities. Whether this degree of specificity is "built in" or acquired during embryonic or early postnatal life is unknown. Nevertheless, only a small percentage of the lymphocytes in the body will respond to a specific antigen. Conversely, each cell can respond to only a narrow spectrum of antigens.

The B cells appear to be relatively sessile, but their end products, immunoglobulins and antibodies, can interact with foreign antigens at distant sites. The T cells responsible for cell-mediated immunity are of necessity more peripatetic and must migrate to the periphery in order to neutralize foreign antigens.

Immunologic Events in Allograft Rejection

INDUCTION OF IMMUNITY

ROLE OF THE SMALL LYMPHOCYTE. Mature lymphocytes appear to sit in a state of immunologic readiness. Whatever role other cells play in the development of immunity, there is little doubt that the small lymphocyte is the seat, and perhaps the only specific site, of immunologic recognition. The small lymphocyte has the capacity to recognize whether or not a molecule is foreign. Once

having reacted to an immunogen, the small lymphocyte, or its descendants, produces the molecules (antibodies or cellular receptor sites) that recognize and react with the antigenic determinants of the immunogen.

One of the major proofs in immunology was the demonstration of the ability of a virtually pure suspension of small lymphocytes from the thoracic duct of rats to cause a graft-versus-host (GVH) immune reaction in histoincompatible animals. Similarly, transfused small lymphocytes can bring about the adoptive destruction of long-tolerated skin allografts in rats. Gowans and associates observed that the small lymphocyte did not incorporate tritiated thymidine into deoxyribonucleic acid (DNA) until an appropriate immunogenic stimulus was encountered. When stimulated, the small lymphocyte transformed in the lymphoid tissue to large activated cells. This transformation heralds the onset of the lymphocyte response to an antigen.

Small lymphocytes not only initiate the immune response, they also carry immunologic memory. Gowans and Uhr showed that thoracic duct lymphocytes taken from rats immunized with phage particles would respond with high antibody titers after transfer to syngeneic irradiated recipients. These cells, or a portion thereof, have a life-span of many months in rats and many years in human beings. It is tempting to conclude that the small lymphocyte can carry out primary, secondary, and memory functions of the lymphoid system for allograft response, if not for all immunologic situations.

As stated above, the small lymphocyte recognizes the immunogenic determinants and translates that recognition into an immunologic response. The first phase of the immunologic response has been called the *afferent arc.* It involves the grafting process itself, the release of the immunogenic histocompatiblity antigens from the graft, the processing and recognition of the immunogens, and the stimulation of the responsive lymphoid cell population.

IMMUNOGEN RELEASE FROM THE GRAFT. The immunogens of a grafted organ, being surface components of the cell membrane, are readily available to the recipient's immune system. Most sensitization to allografts probably takes place within the peripheral lymphoid tissue of the host by antigens shed from the graft or on donor lymphocytes carried over in the transplanted organ. The remainder of the sensitization occurs in circulating host lymphocytes which migrate to the graft.

The route of administration of the immunogen is important in determining the onset of immunity, as well as its strength. The intravenous route will evoke the earliest response, but it is also the poorest immunogenic route and results in a less profound and less persistent state of immunity. The subcutaneous and the intraperitoneal avenues are more effective, and an intradermal route is the most efficient immunizing route. Thus permanent strong immunity follows intradermal injection of allogenic cells, and only weak immunity results from the intravenous infusion of dissociated cells. These findings may well account for the capacity of vascularized allografts (i.e., kidney, liver, heart) to withstand a graft rejection better than nonvascularized grafts (i.e., skin), which must develop a blood supply as they heal. Skin grafts appear to immunize primarily via the lymphatic system, whereas vascularized organ grafts immunize by the bloodstream, a far less immunogenic route.

PROCESSING OF THE IMMUNOGENS. The travels of microgram quantities of ^{125}I-labeled *Salmonella adelaide* flagella injected into rats were studied by Nossal and associates. Flagellar antigen was trapped in two locations in the lymph node. Antigen found in the medullary sinuses was overwhelmingly located inside macrophages. As will be discussed, the ingestion of antigen by macrophages may be the first step in the processing of antigens. In contrast to this, the immunogen in the follicular area of lymph nodes was retained in an extracellular location for as long as 3 weeks. It was most frequently found at or near the surface of fine processes of dendritic reticular cells, which in turn often interdigitated with the equally fine processes of lymphocytes (Fig. 10-6). Evidence for the development of immunity was the finding of transformed lymphocytes in the area that were identical morphologically to lympho-

cytes responding to antigens in vitro. When the rats had been previously sensitized to the flagellar antigen, the number of these responding cells greatly increased. The reticular cell may only facilitate contact between antigen and lymphocyte, or it may function in a more complex fashion as an inducer of lymphocyte transformation. Admittedly, these morphologic events are the response of an experimental animal to a bacterial flagellar immunogen, but nonetheless the events should be applicable to histocompatibility immunogens arriving at a lymph node (Fig. 10-7).

ROLE OF THE MACROPHAGE IN THE INDUCTION OF ALLOGRAFT IMMUNITY. The macrophage not only efficiently traps antigens but may also participate in the afferent arc as an antigen-processing cell. How the macrophage participates is not clear. It may simply partially digest the antigen to facilitate uptake by the lymphocyte. Others have proposed the macrophage processes the antigen more completely and transfers to the lymphocyte either an informative RNA (ribonucleic acid) molecule or an equally specific RNA-antigen complex (Fig. 10-7). The importance of the macrophage to transplantation immunity is not yet known. Considerable evidence obtained in cell culture indicates that the presence of macrophages is necessary to the development of immunity. Neither the subcellular mechanism, on one hand, nor the extension to the transplant patient, on the other, has been determined.

RECOGNITION OF THE IMMUNOGEN BY LYMPHOCYTES. The center of the immune response lies in the reaction of the lymphocyte to the immunogen. This most certainly requires direct interaction of the lymphocyte with the antigen or its products, since the most striking aspect of the immune response is its specificity. For each unique stimulus a distinctive population of antibodies or immune cells is elicited. The specificity of the immune response provides an important clue regarding the nature of the antigen receptors on the antigen recognition cells. The receptor

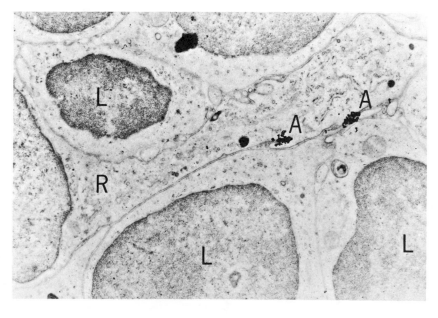

Fig. 10-6. An electron microscope radioautograph of a primary lymph node follicle which includes a reticular cell (R) and several lymphocytes (L). The labeled antigen (A) is located within or near surface invaginations of the reticular cell membrane and in close proximity to the lymphocytes. This relationship of lymphocytes, reticular cells, and antigens is appealing as a site of immunization. (*From G. J. V. Nossal, A. Abbot, J. Mitchell, and Z. Lummus, Antigens in Immunity: XV. Ultrastructural Features of Antigen Capture in Primary and Secondary Lymphoid Follicles, J Exp Med, 127:277, 1968.*)

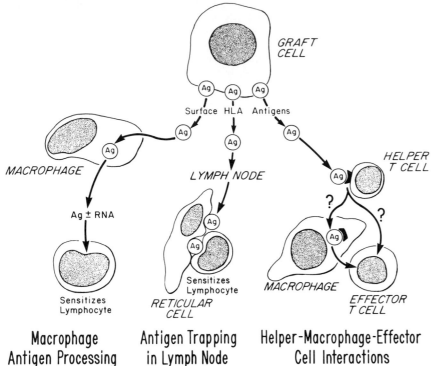

Macrophage
Antigen Processing

Antigen Trapping
in Lymph Node

Helper-Macrophage-Effector
Cell Interactions

Fig. 10-7. Three possible mechanisms of antigen processing and presentation. Macrophages may first need to process the histocompatibility antigens and pass them in more immunogenic form to lymphocytes. The processing may or may not require the attachment of an RNA molecule. The antigen may not need to be internalized, however, and may need to be presented only on the surface of the lymph node reticular cells. This may facilitate sensitization of the lymphocytes. More recently, it has been found that maximum sensitization may require an even more complex interaction. In this scheme the antigen is first recognized by a helper T cell, which in turn may pass it to a macrophage for processing or directly to an effector T cell to produce sensitization. Some of these helper-macrophage–effector cell studies have utilized transplantation antigens, and these conclusions may be applicable to allograft immunity. It is clear, however, from the extensive experimental data that the cell-cell interactions involved are complex and not yet understood.

sites must be at least as discriminatory as the antibody-combining sites or the cellular recognition sites on hypersensitive cells. The presence of recognition molecules has been shown by (1) the ability of radioactive antigens to interfere with lymphocyte activation, (2) inhibition of hapten-sensitive cells by the haptens themselves, and (3) the removal of specific lymphocytes by passage through antigen-coated columns.

It is probable that the receptors on B lymphocytes are antibodies because immunoglobulins have been demonstrated on the cell surface. Furthermore, antisera to immunoglobulins will stimulate B cells, suggesting that the antibody combining with the recognition site immunoglobulin mimics the signal generated by antigen-antibody combination. The antigen-recognizing molecule on T cells has been more difficult to demonstrate. There is no question that T cells possess specific antigen receptors; it is their nature that is unclear. Several investigators have demonstrated evidence that at least portions of immunoglobulins are located on these surfaces and presumably they may contain the recognition sites.

How recognition molecules on either T or B cells are induced during lymphocyte development is unknown. Burnet's clonal selection theory proposes that clones of lymphocytes specifically reactive to an antigen arise, probably by somatic mutation, prior to any actual experience with the antigen itself. Thus, the lymphocytes are precommitted and equipped with recognition molecules to the antigen before the initial encounter with it. An alternative, and currently less favored, theory would have an instructional role for the antigen in the first exposure with the

individual's lymphocytes, with the recognition sites and sensitivity resulting from the encounter.

LYMPHOCYTE TRANSFORMATION. When lymphocytes encounter foreign alloantigens, the clones of cells precoded to these antigens respond in two essential ways—they proliferate and they differentiate into specifically sensitized cells either actively manufacturing antibody (B cells) or capable of inflicting damage directly to the foreign graft (T cells). The activation of resting small lymphocytes was first described by Scothorne and McGregor, who noted the cellular changes which occurred in the regional lymph nodes and spleen following the placement of skin allografts in the rabbit. In these nodes, large lymphoid cells appeared which stained heavily for ribonucleic acid. The supposition was that lymphoid cells had enlarged and transformed in response to allograft stimulation, and that the transformation involved RNA synthesis. Further investigation has uncovered a myriad of subcellular and molecular events that accompany this transformation. This is not surprising, for small lymphocytes are very inactive—as they await antigenic stimulation. Whatever the subgroup of T or B lymphocytes and whatever their response to the antigen, this transformation from resting to large, active cells seems necessary to further events.

CELL-CELL INTERACTIONS. The lymphocytes do not act individually in graft rejection. A great deal of cellular cooperation is required, and such cooperation is not confined to the enlistment of immunologically nonspecific cells such as macrophages, neutrophils, and platelets into the inflammatory response. It is becoming more certain that extensive lymphocyte-lymphocyte interaction is needed for the development of maximum lymphocyte proliferative and cytotoxic activity. The cooperation occurs both between subpopulations of T cells and between T and B cells. Many studies of cell-cell cooperation have used histocompatibility antigens to provide the immunological stimulus, indicating these mechanisms are operating in graft rejection.

The requirement for cooperation between T and B cells was established by showing that neither cell population alone could mount an immune response to certain antigens, whereas mixtures of the two cell types resulted in the production of high levels of antibody. Because B cells are the precursors of antibody-forming cells, and T cells do not synthesize readily detectable amounts of immunoglobulin, the T cells must serve as "helper cells" which assist B cells to differentiate into producers of antibody. Response to the major histocompatibility antigens requires this cooperation, and suspensions of B cells alone or lymphocytes from athymic mice in tissue culture will not effectively produce antibodies to these antigens unless T cells are added. Therefore, T-cell recognition of at least a portion of the antigen is necessary for the production of specific antibody by the B cell. Not all T cells can function in this role, only the subgroup of helper T cells (T_H). Production of IgG, IgE, and probably IgA also seems to require aid from T_H cells for full efficiency.

Just as T_H cells are necessary for B-cell antibody responses, other T_H cells are needed for the development of lymphocyte-mediated cytotoxicity. The lymphocytes that produce direct cytotoxicity are also T cells; effector (T_E) or killer cells. The T_H cell is required for the T_E cell to develop fully the capacity to inflict cell damage. Cell-associated histocompatibility antigens are prominent among the antigens that require T_H–T_E cell cooperation for induction of maximum cytotoxicity.

There is evidence that yet another T-cell subgroup can inhibit either the development of antibody-producing B cells or the generation of T_E cells. These regulatory lymphocytes have been called *suppressor T (T_S) cells*. The functional presence of suppressor cells has been demonstrated in a variety of in vitro experimental preparations, but their role in modulating the immune response in general and allograft rejection in particular is incompletely understood. Nevertheless, suppressor cells offer considerable promise as a potential avenue to better immunosup-

pression. A schematic diagram of these several interactions is presented in Fig. 10-8.

The precise mechanisms by which cells interact are unknown but almost certainly quite complex. The collaboration could occur either (1) by direct contact and interaction of the involved cells in which the T_H cells focus and present antigen to either B cells or T_E cells of the appropriate specificity; or (2) by a mechanism in which the T_H cells release a molecule which can stimulate B cells or T_E cells. Among the uncertainties posed by these models are identifying which cells specifically recognize the antigen. Do the T_H, T_E, and B cells all precisely identify the same foreign antigen? Add to these interactions the apparent need for macrophages during the antigen-processing stage and the presence of one or more small molecules released by lymphocytes which either stimulate or suppress the reaction, and the complexity of the development of transplantation immunity is apparent.

One scheme for which there is good evidence has suggested that the T_H antigen receptors capture the antigens and both antigens and receptors are released for concentration on the surface of the macrophage. The concentrated antigen can then more efficiently stimulate either the B or T_E cells. In addition, soluble factors have been found released into the culture media which foster or hinder cellular cooperation and may serve as regulatory molecules. Much remains to be learned about these cell-cell interactions, and this scheme will certainly be heavily modified in the future. What is raised by this discussion are the roles of lymphocyte differentiation and proliferation in the development of allograft immunity.

LYMPHOCYTE DIFFERENTIATION AND PROLIFERATION. One of the most basic questions in cell biology is whether

Fig. 10-8. The development of specifically immune cells. The T-cell family is very active in these pathways, and helper T cells may be required to recognize the antigens for both B cells and other T cells. Following this recognition step and subsequent interaction with other lymphocytes, either cytotoxic killer T cells or antibody-producing B cells arise. The B-cell effect can be amplified by antibody attaching to other lymphocytes or macrophages. Specific immunity is thereby conferred on these antibody-directed cells. The development of immune cells is kept in check by either suppressor T cells or antibody providing feedback inhibition.

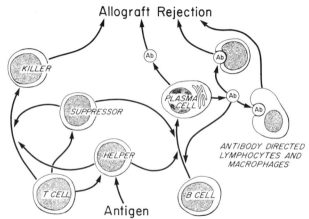

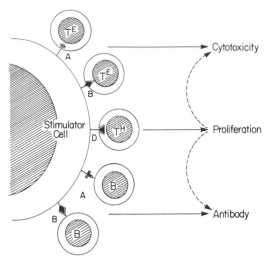

Fig. 10-9. The complexity of the antigen-cell relationships which occur during the development of allograft immunity. Helper T cells (T_H), which seem to be needed for maximal initial response to a foreign cell, respond to incompatible HLA-D antigens and begin to proliferate. The activated helper cells interact with other T cells or B cells to develop sensitized effector cells. Both the antibody-producing B cells or the cytotoxic T_E cells which result, however, develop their immunity against incompatible HLA-A or HLA-B antigens on the stimulator cell. Thus, lymphocytes proliferate in response to certain allogenic antigens and differentiate against other allogenic antigens on the graft cells. Effective immunity and graft rejection probably require both processes.

or not a cell must proliferate in order to differentiate further. Investigations into transplantation biology have not answered this question but have uncovered some surprising relationships between proliferation and differentiation in lymphocytes.

Dutton and Mishell have provided evidence that lymphoid differentiation to antibody-producing cells is accompanied by cellular proliferation. By combining assays indicative of DNA synthesis (uptake of tritiated thymidine) with an assay of antibody production by individual cells (Jerne plaque assay), they found virtually all the antibody-forming B cells had synthesized DNA. These results argue that production of antibodies, an example of cellular differentiation, also requires proliferation. At the end of the B-cell line is the plasma cell which has an abundance of rough endoplasmic reticulum engaged in the specialized production of antibody. Conversion from a transformed cell to a plasma cell is seen within a few days of grafting, in both organ allografts and the lymphoid tissues stimulated by these transplants. When the B cell proliferates, morphologic differentiation accompanies the proliferation, and the end result is a plasma cell busily engaged in making specific antibody.

The situation for T cells has proved to be a fascinating variation. The allogenic stimulation which occurs between two lymphocyte populations in MLC has become a standard model of the allo-immune response in vitro. The amount of immunogenic stimulation can be measured by the uptake of tritiated thymidine into DNA or by the

mitoses which soon follow. The ability of histocompatibility antigens on the surface of intact cells to stimulate lymphocyte proliferation is compelling evidence that similar cell activation occurs in vivo when an organ is allografted. Further investigation has yielded some surprising results, however. The T cell which proliferates most turns out to be the helper T cell (T_H), which recognizes the alloantigen but which develops little capacity to react against the foreign cells. The cell which differentiates and acquires the capability to inflict cytotoxic damage is the effector T cell (T_E), which undergoes relatively little proliferation. This has been best shown in mice, where the proliferating but noncytotoxic T_H cells bear one marker antigen (Ly 1) on their surface and the destructive but nondividing T_E cells have different (Ly 2,3) membrane antigens.

An analogous system almost certainly exists for human lymphocytes. Not only do the two cell types respond differently, but different antigens stimulate the T_H and T_E cells. The A and B loci of the HLA complex code for antigens which induce cytotoxicity, while the D antigens promote proliferation. It now appears that the precursor of the T_E cell has receptors for the A and B antigens, but when these antigens are mixed with a suspension of pure T_E cells proliferation of effector cells does not result. The helper T cell seems to be essential, but the T_H cell does not respond to A and B alloantigens; rather it requires a foreign D antigen to proliferate (Fig. 10-9). Thus T_E and T_H precursors respond to different alloantigens within the closely linked HLA complex, and different T-cell types appear to accomplish differentiation and proliferation. Differentiation requires proliferation, but quite unexpectedly they occur in different cells. In summary, lymphocyte differentiation and proliferation are complex subcellular events which are central to the development of transplantation immunity. Obviously, much remains to be learned about them, and the answers may be of considerable general biological importance.

EXPRESSION OF IMMUNITY: GRAFT DESTRUCTION

The recognition of antigens by sensitized cells or antibodies marks the beginning of the active effort of disposal of the foreign graft, but the reaction of an antibody, for example, with a graft antigen will not by itself destroy the graft. The recognition phase merely triggers the activation of several cascading enzyme systems, which include the complement, clotting, and probably the kinin pathways. In addition, a number of cellular mediators (macrophages, platelets, and polymorphonuclear leukocytes) are recruited, both as a consequence of the specific immunologic reaction itself and as a result of the subsequent enzymatic events. If the recognition molecule is on the surface of a cytotoxic T_E lymphocyte or an activated macrophage, destructive factors are released. Consequently, a variety of molecules and cells play an active role in disposing of the allograft. The efferent limb of the allograft reaction has both an immunologically specific (recognition) phase and an immunologically nonspecific (effector or amplification) phase.

ROLE OF SPECIFICALLY IMMUNIZED LYMPHOCYTES IN ALLOGRAFT REJECTION. The presence of inflammatory cells at the time and site of graft rejection has had a strong influence on immunobiologic thinking. The earliest and simplest explanation was that sensitized lymphocytes both recognized and destroyed the graft. Indeed, specifically sensitized T cells are present within most rejecting allografts and are capable of inflicting damage. It is only that their numbers do not seem capable of explaining the magnitude of the rejection reaction. It is more likely that a small number of specifically sensitized lymphoid cells initiate the rejection reaction but that the completion of the reaction requires many nonsensitized mononuclear cells, as well as PMNs, eosinophils, and plasma cells. Furthermore, there is convincing evidence that antibody can initiate graft destruction in the relative absence of a cellular reaction under appropriate circumstances.

In Vitro Lysis of Target Cells by Lymphocytes. The specifically sensitized lymphoid cells which collect at the site of an allograft have long been thought to damage the donor tissues directly. Recent in vitro studies support such a role for the specifically sensitized lymphocyte which can operate in the total absence of humoral antibody or complement. Direct contact between the sensitized lymphocyte and the target cell appears to be important. The ameboid lymphocyte contacts the target cells with its uropod and remains attached for 10 minutes. The lymphocyte then moves off, and 10 to 20 minutes later the target cells lyse.

Fig. 10-10. Activated (transformed) lymphocytes give off a variety of biologically active molecules (lymphokines). A number of properties have been ascribed to these lymphokines from cell culture experiments. These activities have obvious importance to allograft rejection. Chemotactic and migration inhibitory activity for macrophages and neutrophils, activating factors for lymphocytes, cytotoxicity for target cells, and vascular permeability factors all contribute to graft damage. What is not clear is how many kinds of molecules are involved; do a few have multiple properties?

The mechanism of cell membrane damage has not been identified, although several cytotoxic agents have been found which may be released by the lymphocytes. Such cytotoxic factors may well be the effector agents of cell-mediated immunity, but the specificity of the reaction in vitro favors the idea that interaction of cell surfaces is important to direct the damage of the target cell. The cytotoxic factors may be later released into the surroundings.

EFFECTOR MOLECULES (LYMPHOKINES) RELEASED BY ACTIVATED LYMPHOCYTES. The release of cytotoxic factors by lymphocytes infiltrating an allograft would be the most direct way to damage foreign cells, but probably not the most efficient since nonspecific cell killing would result. Several other kinds of molecules are released by specifically sensitized T cells, and these products or lymphokines serve to activate and enlist macrophages, polymorphonuclear leukocytes (PMNs), lymphocytes, etc., and thus amplify the initial cellular response. Several lymphokines have been identified, but it is not yet clear whether there is a small number of molecules with multiple functions or whether a different molecule is specific for each function. In Fig. 10-10 are depicted some of the best-studied lymphokines.

Macrophages seem to be very active participants in graft rejection; their role does not end with antigen processing. Two of the most investigated lymphokines, migration inhibitory factor (MIF) and chemotactic factor (CF), have similar properties and may be the same molecule. By attracting macrophages and then inhibiting their escape, the CF and MIF activities released by lymphocytes lead increased numbers of macrophages to the area. Another property of these factors, and perhaps of MIF itself, is macrophage activation. Macrophages resemble lymphocytes in that they have resting and activated states. In the later phase, the cytoplasm has the appearance of great activity, both morphologically and enzymatically. Phago-

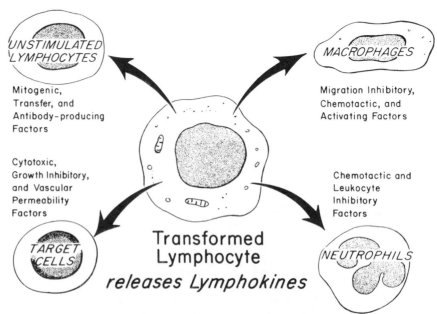

UNSTIMULATED LYMPHOCYTES

Mitogenic, Transfer, and Antibody-producing Factors

Cytotoxic, Growth Inhibitory, and Vascular Permeability Factors

TARGET CELLS

MACROPHAGES

Migration Inhibitory, Chemotactic, and Activating Factors

Chemotactic and Leukocyte Inhibitory Factors

NEUTROPHILS

Transformed Lymphocyte *releases Lymphokines*

cytosis, pinocytosis, bacteriostatic, and tumoricidal activities are increased. Many enzymes, including the digestive enzymes found in lysosomes, are markedly elevated. Macrophages found at the site of graft rejection appear to be in the activated state and thus better able to participate (Fig. 10-11).

A host of other activities has been ascribed to the lymphokines. Neutrophils, basophils, and eosinophils are attracted by them. Growth inhibitory and cytotoxic activities against target cells have been described in vitro. Several apparent lymphokines affect lymphocytes themselves and can be shown under suitable experimental conditions to stimulate mitoses and increase antibody production. Transformed lymphocytes also release a vascular permeability factor in addition to the cytotoxic lymphokines. Little is known about the permeability factor(s) and its possible effect on an allograft rejection. Tissue edema is, however, a prominent feature of graft rejection, and it may join the vascular permeability factors released by complement activation and neutrophil and platelet participation in the efferent arc of rejection.

It is apparent that the lymphokines are only beginning to be understood. How many and by what mechanisms these factors operate are unknown. To date what little information is available has been gathered from in vitro systems, and their role in allograft rejection has yet to be determined—it seems that both the number and the activities will increase with further investigation.

RECRUITMENT OF SPECIFICALLY SENSITIZED CELLS. It is apparent that the few specifically sensitized cells which migrate to the site of the allograft cannot be totally responsible for graft death. Their effect is amplified both by the nonspecific lymphokines and by expansion of the specifically sensitized cells.

It is likely that the specifically immune cell, upon encountering the antigen which elicited its maturation, can recruit specifically sensitized cells from unsensitized lymphocytes in their environment. Among the antibody-producing population there is evidence that the number of active cells is expanded in this way. When the kinetics of plaque-forming (antibody-producing) cells were looked at in one experiment, more cells arose than could be accounted for by cell division. Recruitment of lymphocytes producing cellular hypersensitivity may be accomplished in several ways: A recognition molecule manufactured and released by the specifically sensitized cell could be attached to the cell surfaces of adjacent cells. Such factors would quickly convert lymphoid cells into specific cells which on encountering the antigen could transform and become metabolically active. The impressment of the cells in this manner would allow quick amplification of the number of sensitized cells.

One recognition molecule that could be transferred from lymphocyte to lymphocyte is specific antibody. Clark and Weiss showed that immunoglobulin synthesis of cultured and stimulated lymphocytes appeared simultaneously with their ability to inflict cellular damage. Cell-bound or cytophilic antibody released in the presence of unsensitized lymphocytes does adhere to those lymphocytes. It has not yet been established, however, that cytophilic antibody can enlarge the lymphocyte population specifically sensitized to an allograft.

A second recognition molecule which may expand the sensitized cell population is the transfer factor described by Lawrence. Transfer factor is dialyzable material of less than 10,000 molecular weight which can be extracted from specifically sensitized lymphocytes, and will convert previously unsensitized lymphocytes to a specific antigen-responsive state both in vitro and in vivo. When the converted lymphocytes are subsequently exposed to the specific

Fig. 10-11. Macrophages are stimulated by products of an immune reaction, which include lymphokines, to participate actively in graft rejection. A variety of macrophage functions and cellular parameters have been shown to be increased by activation. Clearly the ability of these cells to contribute to allograft rejection is enhanced by these stimulatory factors.

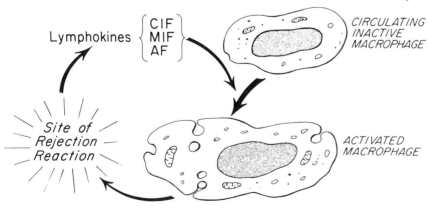

Increased Functions	Increased Cell Components
Phagocytosis	Metabolic Enzymes
Pinocytosis	Membrane Synthesis
Adherence	Lysosomal Enzymes
Cytotoxicity	Adenylate Cyclase

antigen, they will transform and proliferate. Transfer factor itself appears not to be an immunoglobulin but has a polypeptide-polynucleotide composition, although it is resistant to pancreatic ribonuclease (RNase). Transfer factor may act as a transmitter of immunologic information. Much controversy revolves around its presence and nature, however, and some writers regard it as transferred antigen or question its importance in allograft rejection.

Another potential mechanism for recruitment of specifically sensitized cells would be by transfer of the information needed to produce recognition molecules. In addition to the possible role of RNA in the transfer of processed antigenic information from macrophage to lymphocyte, RNA from sensitized cells may enlist other lymphocytes into specific immunity. Mannick and Egdahl were the first to extract RNA from the nodes of rabbits immunized to skin allografts. This RNA fraction conferred the capacity to produce transfer reactions on normal lymphoid cells when they were injected into the skin of the graft donor. In later experiments, they demonstrated that rabbit spleen cells exposed in vitro to RNA extracted from the lymph nodes of immune rabbits would sensitize isogenic rabbits to subsequent grafts from the skin donor. These RNA extracts would confer sensitivity to the immunizing antigen on lymph node cells as measured by the ability to inhibit the migration of macrophages or the production of delayed skin hypersensitivity.

The obvious conclusion has been that the transfer and incorporation of a messenger RNA (mRNA) will establish immunity in lymphoid cells. Although these experiments suggest such a conclusion, more understanding of the development of immunity at the molecular level will be needed before it can be established. In addition, it has not been shown that the RNA comes from lymphocytes. The RNA could be from macrophages.

The recruitment, or horizontal expansion, of sensitized cells is an appealing concept, and certain evidence suggests it may be true; however, it has not been established for

immunity in general, and its role in the allograft reaction is unknown.

ROLE OF ANTIBODY IN ALLOGRAFT REJECTION. Any discussion of the role of humoral antibody in the rejection of allografted tissues should take into consideration two recognized facts: First, circulating antibody is not an obligatory participant in the rejection of solid tissue allografts. In fact, the inability to make an immunoglobulin of any recognizable type does not preclude graft rejection. Animals incapable of making antibody (neonatally bursectomized chickens or bursectomized irradiated chickens) can still reject allografts. Agammaglobulinemic fetal sheep were also found to be capable of rejecting skin allografts even in the presence of heterologous antisheep immunoglobulins.

Second, humoral antibody provides only the recognition portion of graft rejection and tends to be obscured by the effector mechanisms it activates. Unlike cell-mediated immunity, where the recognition system is intimately associated with the destruction of the target, humoral antibody must activate other systems in order to effect cell death.

Even during the early days of organ transplantation it was known that antibodies are formed in concert with allograft rejection. It was initially concluded, however, that antibodies were formed in association with rejection but were not of great functional significance. There is now no doubt that rejection can be mediated by alloantibodies—especially the rejection of vascularized organ allografts.

Effector Pathways and Their Amplification: Antibody-induced Molecular Cascade Systems. Although antibodies bind to allografts, such binding is of no consequence by itself, and the antibody would probably be cleared during the course of normal cell membrane repair. The combination of antibody with the antigen produces an active complex, which triggers a number of nonspecific effector pathways (Fig. 10-12). Each effector pathway typically consists of a sequential activation of enzymes which attract and hold active cells, produce vascular permeability, release enzymes capable of degrading cell surfaces and other pro-

ANTIBODY STRUCTURE

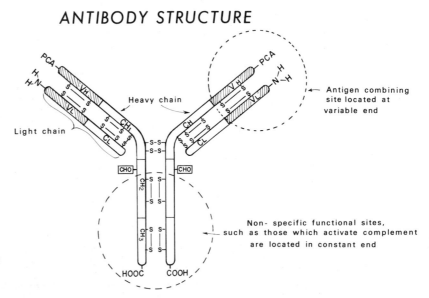

Fig. 10-12. Structure of the IgG antibody molecule. V_H and V_L are the variable portions of the heavy and light chains, respectively, and together they form the antigen-combining site. C_L is the constant portion of the light chain. CH_1, CH_2, and CH_3 are the subunits forming the invariable area of the heavy chain. The approximate positions of the inter- and intra-chain disulfide bridges are shown. [*From J. E. Foker, R. L. Simmons, and J. S. Najarian, Allograft Rejection: I. The Induction of Immunity: The Afferent Arc, in J. S. Najarian and R. L. Simmons (eds.), "Transplantation," p. 63, Lea & Febiger, Philadelphia, 1972.*]

teins, release factors causing smooth muscle contraction, and precipitate the formation of fibrin clots.

The immunologic response can be therefore both efficient and discriminatory. Relatively few specifically differentiated cells can produce molecules that will perform the recognition function. Since few cells are committed to each antigen, many more antigens can be discriminated. The antibodies in turn initiate a relatively general effector mechanism which can destroy the graft.

THE COMPLEMENT SYSTEM. The combination of antibody (of IgG_1, IgG_2, IgG_3, or IgM classes) with antigen changes the conformation of the antibody molecule. Included in this change is the activation of a site on the constant (Fc) end of the antibody molecule, which then triggers the complement pathway, is initiated by antigen-antibody complexes, and is presumably of greatest importance in rejection reactions. The alternate (properdin) pathway can be set off by the immunologically nonspecific serum proteins of the properdin system reacting with sugar structures found on bacterial surfaces and conceivably mammalian cells, or perhaps by combining with certain antibodies; its role in graft rejection, however, is unknown. The components of both pathways are circulating protein molecules which, when activated, react in a sequential fashion. At present, the system is known to be made up of at least 15 (11 classical, 4 alternate) chemically and immunologically distinct molecules which are capable of interacting with one another, with antibody, and with cell membranes, for the C1 to C5 components acquire enzymatic activity after interaction with the previous factor. Once activated they can act enzymatically on the next molecule in the sequence which serves as the inactive substrate. Components C6 to C9 are nonenzymatic and bind to the previous components, resulting in conformational and activity changes.

Most of the biologically significant activities of the complement system arise during activation of the last six react-

ing complement components, C3 and C5 through C9 (Fig. 10-13). The two parallel but entirely independent initial pathways—the classical and the alternate pathways—converge at the C3 component, and the remainder of the reaction sequence, involving the reactions of C5 through C9, is common to both pathways. Both lead to activation of the terminal, biologically important portion of the sequence. The terminal portion of the complement sequence may also be directly activated by certain noncomplement serum and cellular enzymes without participation of the early reaction factors. For example, fibrinolytic enzymes in plasma and certain lysosomal enzymes will activate the C3 and C5 stages.

The classical complement pathway (Fig. 10-13) appears to be the most important for immune reactions. Three biologic consequences of complement activation are most important in transplantation rejection. (1) Complement has been shown to be capable of mediating lytic destruction of many kinds of cells to which antibodies have bound. The active components are in the C8 and C9 complexes, but the mechanism of lysis is not clear; perhaps enzymatic activity of the complex damages the membrane directly. (2) Many kinds of cells possess receptors for the C3b or C4b (activated) components, including B lympho-

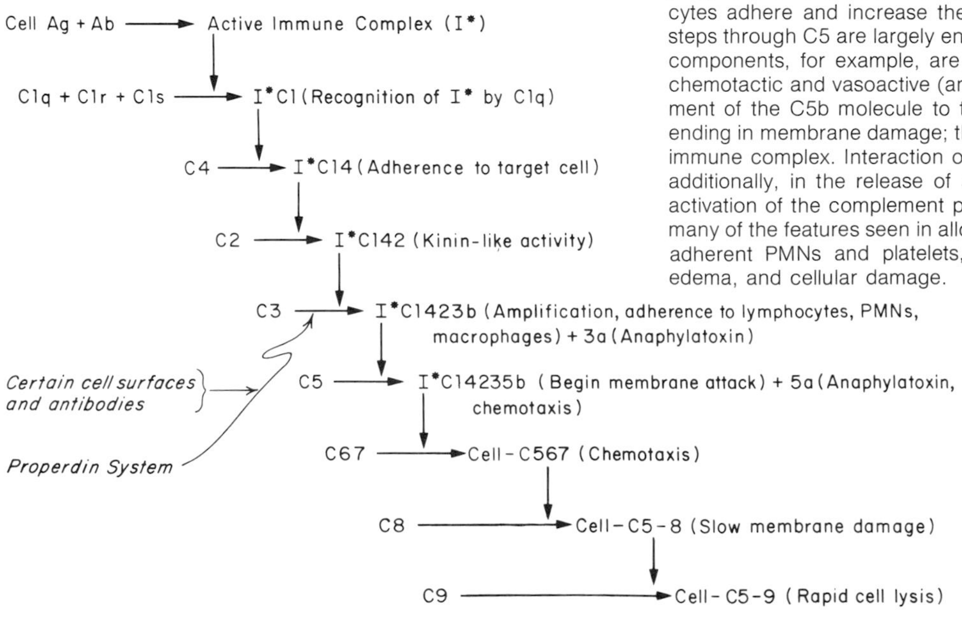

Fig. 10-13. The complement pathways and the biological activity released at each step. The classical pathway begins with a specific antigen-antibody reaction. The properdin pathway is triggered by a more nonspecific interaction between cell surfaces and the molecules which comprise the properdin systems. Both pathways, however, converge at the C3 step, where most of the biological activity associated with complement activation begins. Amplification also occurs at several steps, but it is greatest at C3. The subsequent steps lead to the molecular condensation on the target cell surface, which ultimately results in membrane damage and lysis. There are several other important consequences of complement activation. The presence of these molecules on the target cell surface makes them adherent to other cells. Macrophages, platelets, polymorphonuclear leukocytes, and lymphocytes adhere and increase the damage to the graft cells. The steps through C5 are largely enzymatic in nature; the C3 and C5 components, for example, are split during activation, releasing chemotactic and vasoactive (anaphylatoxins) molecules. Attachment of the C5b molecule to the cell begins the condensation ending in membrane damage; this seems to occur away from the immune complex. Interaction of the C6,C7 components results, additionally, in the release of another chemotactic factor. The activation of the complement pathway, therefore, contributes to many of the features seen in allograft rejection; cellular infiltrates, adherent PMNs and platelets, thrombosed vessels, interstitial edema, and cellular damage.

```
Cell Ag + Ab ─────────► Active Immune Complex (I*)
                                    │
                                    ▼
C1q + C1r + C1s ─────────► I*C1 (Recognition of I* by C1q)
                                    │
                                    ▼
        C4 ─────────► I*C14 (Adherence to target cell)
                                    │
                                    ▼
        C2 ─────────► I*C142 (Kinin-like activity)
                                    │
                                    ▼
        C3 ───────► I*C1423b (Amplification, adherence to lymphocytes, PMNs,
                                    macrophages) + 3a (Anaphylatoxin)
                                    │
Certain cell surfaces ┐            ▼
and antibodies        ├──►  C5 ─────────► I*C14235b (Begin membrane attack) + 5a (Anaphylatoxin,
                      ┘                              chemotaxis)
Properdin System ─────┘              │
                                     ▼
                   C67 ─────────► Cell-C567 (Chemotaxis)
                                     │
                                     ▼
                   C8 ─────────► Cell-C5-8 (Slow membrane damage)
                                     │
                                     ▼
                   C9 ─────────► Cell-C5-9 (Rapid cell lysis)
```

cytes, neutrophils, monocytes, and macrophages. If C3b or C4b attach to a damaged cell they may act as opsonins, bringing the target cells in contact with the phagocytic macrophages and monocytes or exposing the surface antigens of these cells to B lymphocytes. (3) Many of the complement cleavage products have biologic actions of their own. For example, C4a and C2b act as kinins. C3a has chemotactic activity for polymorphonuclear leukocytes, causes the release of histamine from mast cells (anaphylatoxin activity), has a kinin activity, and causes immune adherence. C5a is a very potent chemotactic factor, stimulates histamine release from mast cells, and liberates lysosomes from polymorphonuclear leukocytes. Therefore, the complement activation releases kinins which increase vascular permeability, leading to edema; attracts polymorphonuclear leukocytes which release other vasoactive compounds and lysosomal enzymes; encourages phagocytosis of damaged tissue; releases lysosomal enzymes from macrophages; opsonizes cells; binds cells to damaged cell surfaces (immune adherence); and leads to cell death.

An important biological characteristic of the complement system, as well as the other cascade systems discussed in this section, is that they are capable of self-amplification. Thus, in one study 450 C4 molecules were found fixed to each sensitized sheep red blood cell, but each erythrocyte had approximately 100,000 C3 components on its surface. In addition, the C3 components were distributed over the cell membrane surface, rather than confined to the site of the antigen-antibody combination, thus enlarging the area of effect. Although this step produces the greatest numerical amplification, other steps in the complement pathway also expand the number of active molecules.

THE CLOTTING SYSTEM. Theoretically the deposition of fibrin in the allografted organ may arise in two ways: The first, the so-called *extrinsic pathway* of thrombin formation, requires tissue thromboplastin to initiate the sequence of events. The release of this cellular substance may follow damage to the endothelial cell membranes either by antibody and complement or through the direct cytotoxic effect of lymphocytes. The activation of complement through C_3 would also promote the adherence of platelets which, in turn, would stimulate platelet retraction and release of platelet phospholipids. These phospholipids have been shown to promote clotting.

The second method of inducing clot formation, the *intrinsic pathway,* has the potential to be activated directly by immunologic reaction. In the intrinsic pathway, Hageman factor (factor XII) begins a sequence which proceeds through factors XI, IX, VII, and V to the activation of prothrombin factor to form thrombin with the eventual polymerization of fibrin. Antigen-antibody complexes will activate Hageman factor to trigger this cascade and produce clotting in vitro in the absence of platelets. Thus, an entry into the intrinsic pathway is present within the interactions of antigens and antibodies (Fig. 10-14).

As the reaction proceeds and tissue damage is produced, tissue thromboplastin is released, collagen fibers are exposed, and clotting is facilitated. It is now generally hypothesized that the progressive obliterative vascular reaction of a chronically rejecting allograft is a by-product of fibrin laid down along endothelium that has been damaged by immune mechanisms.

THE KININ SYSTEM. The kinin or killikrein system is initiated by activation of coagulation factor XII, leading eventually to the formation of kallikrein, which acts on kininogen, an alpha-globulin substrate in the plasma, and results in bradykinin. Bradykinin is one of the kinins, a group of active peptides which are rather rapidly inactivated, after formation, by kininases present in plasma. The kinins possess a variety of biological activities, including chemotaxis of PMNs, smooth muscle contraction, dilatation of peripheral arterioles, and increase of capillary permeability. The involvement of the kinin system in graft rejection is likely but is as yet unproved.

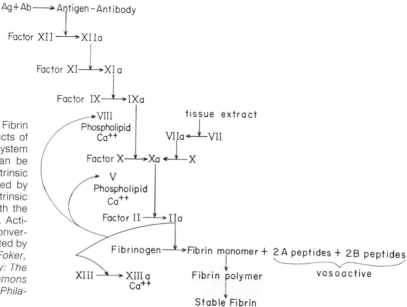

Fig. 10-14. The coagulation cascade system. Fibrin and two vasoactive peptides are the final products of the cascade. The two modes of activation of the system are diagrammed. Factor XII (Hageman factor) can be activated by immune complexes initiating the "intrinsic pathway." Tissue damage (presumably produced by immunologic damage) could precipitate the extrinsic system. In both systems, the factors shown, with the probable exceptions of V and VIII, are enzymes. Activation of the pathways involves the sequential conversions of these enzymes to active forms (represented by XIIa, XIa, etc). [*From J. S. Najarian and J. E. Foker, Allograft Rejection: II. The Expression of Immunity: The Efferent Arc, in J. S. Najarian and R. L. Simmons (eds.), "Transplantation," p. 94, Lea & Febiger, Philadelphia, 1972.*]

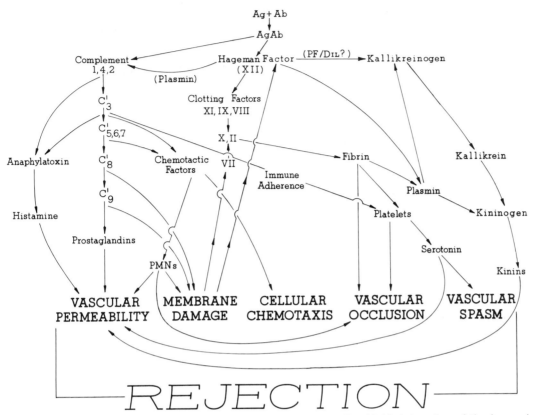

RECOGNITION

Ag + Ab

AgAb

Complement 1,4,2 ← Hageman Factor (XII) — (PF/DIL?) → Kallikreinogen

(Plasmin)

C'_3

Clotting Factors XI, IX, VIII

$C'_{5,6,7}$

X, II

Kallikrein

Anaphylatoxin

C'_8

Chemotactic Factors

VII

Fibrin

Immune Adherence

Plasmin

Histamine

Kininogen

C'_9

Platelets

Prostaglandins

Serotonin

PMNs

Kinins

VASCULAR PERMEABILITY **MEMBRANE DAMAGE** **CELLULAR CHEMOTAXIS** **VASCULAR OCCLUSION** **VASCULAR SPASM**

REJECTION

INTERRELATIONSHIPS OF THE MOLECULAR CASCADE SYSTEMS (Fig. 10-15). Antigen-antibody complexes activate complement and Hageman factor. Hageman factor in turn produces clotting, activates plasmin, and perhaps directly activates complement. Plasmin in turn can activate C_3 to produce, among other effects, chemotactic factors, immune adherence, and opsonization. Activation of Hageman factor also leads to kinin production. Activation of the complement system produces aggregation of platelets and, consequently, initiation of the clotting mechanism. Thrombin formation, in turn, stimulates the production of plasmin from plasminogen. Prostaglandin activity is released following complement activation, and may contribute to vascular permeability, although the significance of this in allograft rejection remains unclear.

Not only are the activators of these systems interrelated, but also the inhibitors are intertwined. The C_1 esterase inhibitor also decreases the activity of the kinin and plasmin systems. Neither activation nor inhibition of one system can occur without affecting the other pathways.

The complexity of the allograft reaction is just beginning to be understood. Not only does it involve a variety of recognition molecules (antibodies) and presumably a similar variety of specifically sensitized cells; there is much recent evidence that unsensitized lymphocytes can be specifically directed and actively lyse target allogenic cells by a coating with antibody. In addition, the main force of the reaction may be produced by a bewildering array of am-

Fig. 10-15. Integration of the humoral amplification system in graft rejection. This diagram suggests the complexity of allograft rejection. The three main cascade pathways—complement, clotting, and kinin—generate many active molecules, including the kinins, chemotactic factors, anaphylatoxins, histamine, and serotonin. These molecules, together with platelets and polymorphonuclear leukocytes (PMNs), produce the destructive effects on the graft. The most prominent consequences include increased vascular permeability (edema), spasm, and occlusion as well as cell and basement membrane damage and cellular chemotaxis (infiltration). It is clear that these systems do not operate singly but tend to activate each other. Not shown are the many interlocking inhibitory factors that keep these systems in check once they are activated. [*From J. S. Najarian and J. E. Foker, Allograft Rejection: II. The Expression of Immunity: The Efferent Arc, in J. S. Najarian and R. L. Simmons (eds.), "Transplantation," p. 94, Lea & Febiger, Philadelphia, 1972.*]

plifying chain reactions which include both molecular amplification schemes and cellular amplifiers. The activation of complement, the clotting system, kinin formation, and the stimulation of PMN, macrophages, and platelet assault produce a variety of damage to the transplanted organ. Included are occlusive phenomena within the graft vessels, induced permeability of these same vessels with interstitial edema accumulation, disruption of cellular basement membranes, and the infiltration of the graft with a profusion of cell types (Fig. 10-15).

AN INTEGRATED VIEW OF THE REJECTION OF ORGAN ALLOGRAFTS. Rejection morphology has two main components: The first component is the host response, and it is

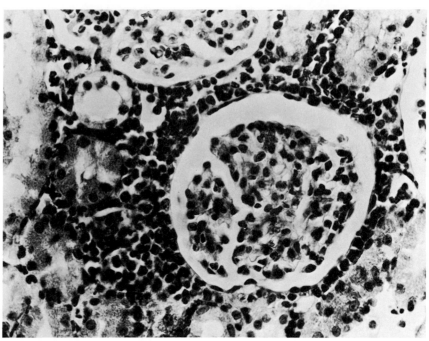

Fig. 10-16. Canine renal allograft 48 hours after transplantation into unmodified recipient. Round cell infiltration, usually the first overt sign of host activity against the allograft, is apparent within 6 to 12 hours after transplantation. By 48 hours the number of invading cells is substantial. The original perivascular infiltrate has surrounded a glomerulus and adjacent tubules. [*From J. E. Foker and J. S. Najarian, Allograft Rejection: III. The Pathobiology of Organ Rejection, in J. S. Najarian and R. L. Simmons (eds.), "Transplantation," p. 122, Lea & Febiger, Philadelphia, 1972.*]

composed of effector cells and molecules, both immunologically specific and nonspecific. In rapid rejections these comprise most, if not all, of the pathologic picture so that the speed of the reaction virtually precludes response by the organ cells. The second component becomes prominent only with longer survival of the transplanted organ and encompasses the various morphologic alterations of the organs. In fact, the responses of these cells can form an important part of the pathologic picture.

A predictable series of events ensues when an unsensitized patient is allografted. The first visible change is a perivascular infiltration of round cells accomplished by migration through the cytoplasm of the endothelial cells (Fig. 10-16). The accumulation of cells is not significant for several hours after transplantation but can reach considerable numbers within 24 hours. This delay suggests that although the immunogenicity of the graft may be a sufficient stimulus to transmigration by the lymphoid cells, transformation of the host cells or other cellular events must transpire before migration occurs. The confrontation between graft and host immunocompetent cells may be important in the development of this infiltrate.

The temporal aspects have been best worked out for the kidney, but the sequence appears to be the same for most organs. During the first 48 hours following grafting the number of infiltrating cells continues to increase. The original enclaves around small vessels spread, and the interstitial space is further infiltrated. A potpourri of cells accumulates: cells resembling small lymphocytes are seen, as well as large transformed lymphocytes with basophilic cytoplasm. Large histiocytes or macrophages are just beginning to arrive in numbers. Plasma cells are still relatively scarce: as a terminal product of cellular differentiation, they may require several cell divisions before they appear in the organ (Fig. 10-17).

Antibody and complement are deposited in the area of the capillaries, and some of the infiltrating lymphoid cells are producing immunoglobulins by the third day. Recognition molecules (antibody) as well as sensitized cells are therefore present early in the allograft reaction.

Sensitized lymphoid cells, upon recognizing the foreign tissue, release several mediators of inflammation and cell damage. The release of cytotoxic factors directly injures membranes of adjacent cells. Mitogenic products stimulate division of lymphoid cells, perhaps expanding the immunocompetent population. Activated, phagocytic macrophages are effectively concentrated in the area by migration inhibitory factor and other chemotactic factors. In addition vascular permeability agents are released.

Meanwhile, complement is fixed, thereby producing chemotactic factors, anaphylatoxins, and finally cellular damage when the terminal components are activated. Capillary permeability is increased by anaphylatoxins from the complement chain and probably by kinins. Interstitial edema becomes prominent. At the same time there are several additional inducements to cellular infiltration. The complement cascade generates molecules which produce immune adherence and others which have chemotactic activity. Damaged cells release additional compounds which contribute to infiltration by PMNs as well as other cells. PMNs in turn release vasoactive amines (including histamine or serotonin, depending on the species) and

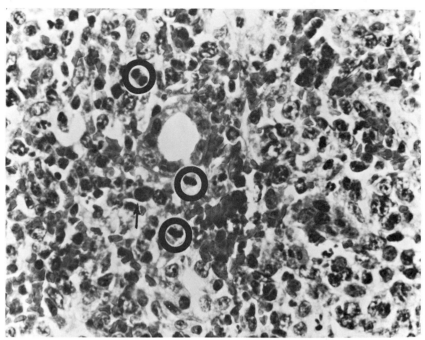

Fig. 10-17. Canine renal allograft 4 days after transplantation into an unmodified recipient. Invading cells all but obscure the architecture of the kidney. Numerous mitoses (circles) can be found, and this cellular proliferation may be producing immunologically competent cells within the graft. A plasma cell (arrow) is present, but most of the cells resemble lymphocytes and macrophages. [*From J. E. Foker and J. S. Najarian, Allograft Rejection: III. The Pathobiology of Organ Rejection, in J. S. Najarian and R. L. Simmons (eds.) "Transplantation," p. 122, Lea & Febiger, Philadelphia, 1972.*]

additional vascular permeability–promoting factors. The PMNs squeeze through the enlarged endothelial cell junctions and release proteolytic cathepsins D and E, causing basement membrane damage.

Fibrin, and α-macroglobulins, whose contribution is not understood, are deposited by 7 days. During this time, lymphoid cells have continued to accumulate and, joined by significant numbers of plasma cells and PMNs, obscure the normal architecture. The round cell population presumably contains many macrophages and other immunologic nonspecific cells at this point. Increasingly frequent mitoses may indicate the production of immunocompetent cells within the graft.

The small vessels become plugged with fibrin and platelets, diminishing the perfusion and preventing function. In this relatively rapid sequence of events the organ has little chance to respond, and the pathologic process is dominated by the host effector pathways.

Obviously, rejection modified by immunosuppressive agents is not a distinct morphologic classification but is only a continuation of the events comprising the rejection reaction. The morphologic features associated with this more chronic rejection become dominated by the response of the organ tissue itself. Here the normal response of tissue to injury predominates in the pathologic picture. A good deal of endothelial cell damage occurs in the allograft, and the responses of cellular repair, hypertrophy and hyperplasia, follow.

Endothelial cell damage also elicits repair processes. Aggregations of platelets within the intimal layer are resolved, and the dissolution of the thrombi is accompanied by the infiltration of macrophages and foam cells. The result is a thickened intimal layer with the loss of smooth endothelial lining and the presence of vacuolated cells. The lumen narrows as a result. Narrowing of the vessel lumen is also a consequence of the medial thickening. Studies using nonimmunologic disease models have shown that most of the cells proliferating in response to the stimulus of injury are smooth muscle cells. A reasonable extrapolation is that hyperplasia of these cells produces much of the lumenal narrowing in the allograft (Fig. 10-18).

Although the exposed position of the endothelial cells and the striking proliferation of the smooth muscle cells argue for their being an important target of the immune reaction, there is evidence that the basement and elastic membranes of the vessel absorb a major portion of immune-mediated damage. Either immune complexes or antibodies to the vascular basement membrane activate complement and attract polymorphonuclear cells. These nonspecific effector cells release at least four protein factors which increase the permeability of the vessel and in addition produce cathepsins D and E, which digest basement membranes. The PMNs are active in reaching the basement membrane and will lift the endothelial cells to gain this access.

Platelets may be of greater significance than PMNs in mediating damage. Immune complexes (which activate complement) will result in platelet adherence and the release of vasoactive substances. Platelet aggregation leads to the release of histamine, serotonin, and other capillary permeability factors which expose more basement membrane; the exposed collagen fibers of the basement mem-

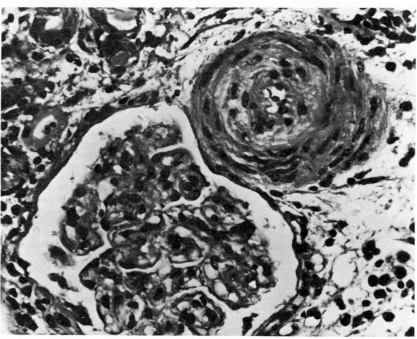

Fig. 10-18. A rejected human allograft removed 18 months post-transplant. The lumen of the arteriole has all but disappeared as a consequence of hyperplasia of the cells of the vessel. Most of the thickening of the wall is probably due to proliferation of smooth muscle cells, with spindle-shaped nuclei. Endothelial cells, with rounder nuclei, almost fill the lumen. [*From J. E. Foker and J. S. Najarian, Allograft Rejection: III. The Pathobiology of Organ Rejection, in J. S. Najarian and R. L. Simmons (eds.), "Transplantation," p. 122, Lea & Febiger, Philadelphia, 1972.*]

brane further enhance platelet aggregation. Platelets and PMNs drawn to these sites release cathepsins, elastases, and phosphatases which increase destruction and attract other nonspecific cellular effectors including macrophages.

The myocardial cell is the characteristic cell of the heart, the tubular cell of the kidney, the acinar and islet cell of the pancreas, etc. The differentiation and function of these cells demand an ample oxygen supply and if destroyed they cannot be replaced by further cellular division. Therefore, compromise of respiration by vascular endothelial and medial hypertrophy, intravascular aggregations of platelets, and interstitial accumulations of edema and mononuclear cells will have predictable consequences for these cells. They will atrophy, and death may be followed by replacement fibrosis (Fig. 10-19).

The interstitial area concomitantly increases in size. The interstitial area, however, has much activity in its own right. Repair of immunologic damage stimulates many fibroblastic cells to proliferate, and it attracts macrophages. The persisting immunogenic capacity of the allograft is indicated by the inevitable presence of infiltrating plasma cells and lymphoid cells.

It is impossible to determine what proportions of these effects result from ischemia produced by vascular occlusion, interstitial edema, or cellular infiltrates. Similarly, the contribution made by the direct cytotoxic action of specific and nonspecific effector cells and molecules is unknown.

CIRCUMVENTING REJECTION

Clinical Immunosuppression

Theoretically, there are nine methods by which the allograft rejection response can be suppressed: (1) destroying the immunocompetent cells prior to transplantation, (2) making the antigen unrecognizable or even toxic to the reactive lymphocyte clones, (3) interfering with antigen processing by the recipient cells, (4) inhibiting lymphocyte transformation and proliferation, (5) limiting lymphocyte differentiation into killer or antibody-synthesizing cells, (6) activating sufficient numbers of suppressor lymphocytes, (7) inhibiting destruction of graft cells by killer lymphocytes, (8) interfering with the combination of immunoglobulins with target antigens, or (9) preventing tissue damage by the nonspecific cells and molecules that are activated by sensitized cells or antigen-antibody complexes.

In practice, clinically useful immunosuppression largely depends on the destruction or elimination of the immunocompetent cells and on inhibiting the differentiation and proliferation of these cells. Methods of inducing specific immune tolerance by various antigen preparations prior to grafting, or by inhibiting sensitized cells and antibodies once they have been produced, have not been clinically successful. Furthermore, it is more difficult to inhibit the immune response after it is underway, and less clinical effect can be gained after sensitization has occurred. To be most effective, immunosuppression must be present at the time of transplantation, or even before. Nevertheless, some success can be achieved in reversing the exacerbations of the rejection reaction seen in clinical transplantation. Lesser, but still significant, benefits have also resulted from

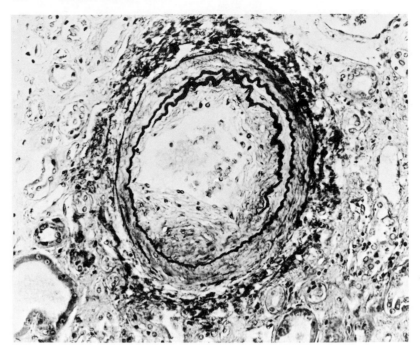

Fig. 10-19. Extensive damage to this small artery in a human renal allograft removed 14 months posttransplant is apparent. The elastic membranes are badly frayed, and the elastica interna has been destroyed entirely along half the circumference of the vessel. The intimal layer shows extensive disruption and loss of cells. The cells remaining are often vacuolated. The lumen is narrowed by tissue from several origins: proliferation of smooth muscle cells in the media, endothelial cell swelling and hyperplasia, and the presence of an organized thrombus. The adventitial area shows damage and edema formation. Note also that severe tubular atrophy and interstitial fibrosis are present. [*From J. E. Foker and J. S. Najarian, Allograft Rejection: III. The Pathobiology of Organ Rejection, in J. S. Najarian and R. L. Simmons (eds.), "Transplantation," p. 122, Lea & Febiger, Philadelphia, 1972.*]

inhibiting such immunologically nonspecific cells as platelets.

The true complexity of immune rejection is only beginning to be revealed, but many potential points for inhibition have already been exposed. At this time, however, a similar complexity does not exist in clinical immunosuppression. Virtually all clinical transplantation immunosuppression regimens include azathioprine, steroids, radiation, and antilymphocyte antibodies. Agents which are occasionally used or are purely experimental will be presented more briefly.

ANTIPROLIFERATIVE AGENTS

Most of the commonly used immunosuppressive agents, including antimetabolites, alkylating agents, toxic antibiotics, and x-rays, have been borrowed from cancer chemotherapy for their antiproliferative activity. They inhibit the full expression of the immune response by preventing the differentiation and division of the immunocompetent lymphocyte after it encounters the antigen. The plethora of investigational immunosuppressive drugs has been reduced to a few for clinical use. All of them, however, fall into one of two broad mechanistic categories. Either they structurally resemble needed metabolites or they combine with certain cellular components, such as DNA, and thereby interfere with cell function.

The former group, the antimetabolites, have a structural similarity to cell metabolites and either inhibit enzymes of that metabolic pathway or are incorporated during synthesis to produce faulty molecules. The antimetabolites include purine, pyrimidine, and folic acid analogs, which are most effective against proliferating and differentiating cells. They are given at the time of transplantation when the immunocompetent cells are first stimulated, and then

for the life of the graft to interfere with the continuing stimulus to the immune system.

Alkylating agents and certain antibiotics include those compounds which combine with DNA and other cellular components. Although these agents would be useful in the pretransplant period to reduce the number of effective immunocompetent cells in the recipients, and thereafter to prevent proliferation, they are so toxic that their use has been limited to bone marrow transplantation and as occasional substitutes for azathioprine.

PURINE ANALOGUES. The purine analogue azathioprine (AZ) (Imuran) is the most widely used immunosuppressive drug in clinical organ transplantation. Azathioprine is 6-mercaptopurine (6-MP) plus a side chain to protect the labile sulfhydryl group. In the liver, the side chain is split off to form the active compound, 6-MP. The mechanism of action would seem to be similar for these two compounds; however, azathioprine seems to enjoy the advantage of slightly lower toxicity.

Full metabolic activity comes in the cell with the addition of ribose 5-phosphate from phosphoribosyl pyrophosphate to form 6-MP ribonucleotide. The structural resemblance of this molecule to inosine monophosphate is obvious, and 6-MP ribonucleotide inhibits the enzymes that begin to convert inosine nucleotide to adenosine and guanosine monophosphate (Fig. 10-20). In addition, the presence of 6-MP ribonucleotides slows the entire purine biosynthetic pathway by fraudulent feedback inhibition of an early step. The steric similarity to either adenosine or guanine nucleotides is not great enough to allow significant incorporation into DNA or RNA and synthesis of faulty molecules. The result of inhibiting these several enzymes, however, is to block the synthesis of cellular RNA, DNA, certain cofactors, and other active nucleotides.

Fig. 10-20. Mechanism of antimetabolite action. 6-Mercaptopurine (6-MP) ribonucleotide resembles inosine monophosphate in its steric configuration. It thereby competes with inosine in its transformation into adenosine monophosphate and guanosine monophosphate and their subsequent incorporation into RNA and DNA. In addition, 6-MP inhibits the purine biosynthetic pathway, since it resembles a product of that biosynthetic pathway (feedback inhibition). [*From R. L. Simmons, J. E. Foker, and J. S. Najarian, Principles of Immunosuppression, in D. C. Sabiston, Jr. (ed.), "Davis-Christopher Textbook of Surgery," p. 471, W. B. Saunders Company, Philadelphia, 1972.*]

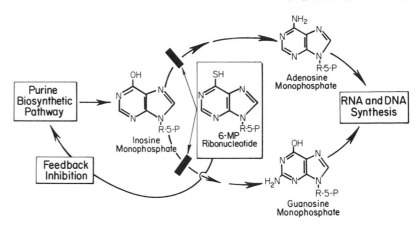

The biologic activity of azathioprine and 6-MP is greatest when nucleic acid synthesis is most required. They will inhibit the development of both humoral and cellular primary immunity by interfering with the differentiation and proliferation of the responding lymphocytes. The inhibition of nucleic acid synthesis by azathioprine is most effective in these rapidly replicating cells. Once expansion of fully immunocompetent cells has been completed, nucleic acid synthesis is less important and the drug is less effective. The benefit of azathioprine may also result from a reduction of neutrophil production and macrophage activation. This effect would reduce the nonspecific inflammatory aspect of the immune reaction.

The toxicity of azathioprine results from the same mechanisms. The primary toxic effect of azathioprine is bone marrow suppression, leading to leukopenia. Again, it is the antiproliferative effect of inhibiting nucleic acid synthesis that affects this rapidly dividing cell population. Liver toxicity can also result, possibly because of the high rate of RNA synthesis by these cells, but because hepatic dysfunction does not seem to be dose-related, the mechanism is unclear.

PYRIMIDINE ANALOGUES. Although pyrimidine analogues have been studied extensively as immunosuppressants in the laboratory, they have had only limited clinical use. The structure of 5-bromodeoxyuridine resembles thymidine, and it is incorporated into DNA (Fig. 10-21). Once incorporated, however, it does not have the precision in base pairing that thymidine has, and subsequent synthesis of DNA and RNA is defective. Although 5-bromodeoxyuridine will prolong animal skin grafts and act in synergy with antilymphocyte globulin, its clinical use is untested.

Another pyrimidine analogue, cytosine arabinoside, also inhibits DNA synthesis and, therefore, the proliferative phase of the immune response. This molecule has an altered sugar moiety and is confused with cytosine riboside. Experimentally, the immunosuppressive effect of cytosine arabinoside has been more easily demonstrated in primary humoral antibody responses than in cell-mediated reactions. Clinically it is used to prepare leukemic recipients for eventual bone marrow transplantation. With more experience this agent may become more widely employed.

FOLIC ACID ANTAGONISTS. The immunosuppressive effect of a diet deficient in pteroylglutamic acid was originally noted by Little, and set the stage for the use of the folic acid antagonists, aminopterin and methotrexate. Both drugs inhibit the enzyme dihydrofolate reductase, and prevent the conversion of folic acid to tetrahydrofolic acid. This step is necessary for the synthesis of DNA, RNA, and certain coenzymes, Again, proliferating cell systems are most affected.

Some of the toxicity of aminopterin and methotrexate can be abrogated by the administration of folinic acid some hours or even days after the use of the antagonist. Nevertheless, the ratio of immunosuppression to toxicity has not justified their use in clinical kidney transplantation.

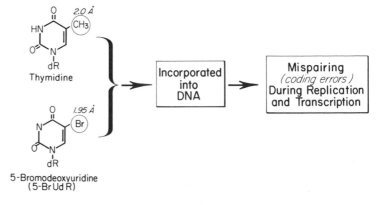

Fig. 10-21. Mechanism of antimetabolite action. 5-Bromodeoxyuridine (5BrUdR) strongly resembles thymidine in its steric configuration. Even the bromine molecule is similar in size to the methyl. 5-BrUdR thereby competes with thymidine incorporation into DNA. [*From R. L. Simmons, J. E. Foker, and J. S. Najarian, Principles of Immunosuppression, in D. C. Sabiston, Jr. (ed.), "Davis-Christopher Textbook of Surgery," p. 471, W. B. Saunders Company, Philadelphia, 1972.*]

The immune reactions that accompany bone marrow transplantation are more difficult to control, and methotrexate is used to both prevent and reverse the severe graft-versus-host reactions that occur. Since methotrexate is usually used with one or more other drugs, its toxic effects can be difficult to identify. Megaloblastic hemopoiesis, mucosal breakdown with severe gastrointestinal bleeding, and liver damage seem to be related to methotrexate therapy. These effects, even with high dosages of methotrexate, can usually be prevented by folinic acid (citrovorum rescue). Obviously, depression of the transplanted marrow may also result from the activity of methotrexate, although assigning the cause may be difficult in the complex clinical situation.

ALKYLATING AGENTS. The alkylating agents have highly reactive rings as part of the molecular structure. These unstable rings have electron-seeking points which combine with electron-rich nucleophilic groups such as the tertiary nitrogens in purines and pyrimidines, or with $-NH_2$, $-COOH$, $-SH$, and $-PO_3H_2$ groups on a variety of molecules. The high-energy rings of alkylating agents break and combine with these constituents to form stable covalent bonds. Obviously, many cell components have such groups, including DNA, RNA, and the enzymatic and structural proteins. Alkylation of DNA is probably the most detrimental. If the DNA strands are not repaired, chromosomal replication will be faulty in proliferating cells. Both DNA and RNA can be alkylated at several points, but a common site appears to be N-7 of the guanine ring (Fig. 10-22). Mispairing of DNA during replication may result from the presence of the alkylating agent itself, the clipping out of the alkylated guanine residue, or the cleavage of an alkylated guanine ring. Also chain breaks and cross-linkages frequently interfere with chain replication.

Since the damage to DNA can be repaired, these effects are apparently time-dependent. Consequently, the administration of alkylating agents just before and during stimulation by the antigen would most interfere with the ability of the immunocompetent cells to respond to that antigen. Continued use of the alkylating agents would also muffle the proliferative response of these cells in the face of a persistent stimulus. There are differences, however, in the response of T and B cells. The B cell seems to be more susceptible to cyclophosphamide than the T cell. This drug is a potent inhibitor of antibody formation, but its effect on skin or kidney rejection is much less spectacular. The reason for this apparent difference is unknown.

The usefulness of alkylating agents, which include nitrogen mustard, phenylalanine mustard, busulfan, and cyclophosphamide, is limited by their toxicity. Even so, cyclophosphamide has been used with good results in renal transplantation when liver toxicity prohibited the use of azathioprine. Cyclophosphamide is frequently used in clinical bone marrow transplantation, where it potentiates the effects of radiation and enhances the disruption of DNA. When cyclophosphamide is used, lower doses of radiation are required to deplete the recipient bone marrow population and provide space for donor cells. When leukemia is the indication for bone marrow transplantation, cyclophosphamide will aid in the destruction of these cells.

Toxicity is high, however, and predictable reactions occur, principally to rapidly replicating cell populations. Stomatitis, nausea, vomiting, diarrhea, skin rash, anemia, and alopecia are all common reactions. The more specific effects of cyclophosphamide administration are prompt fluid retention, occasionally severe hemorrhagic cystitis, and cardiac toxicity. The cardiac and edema problems suggest that even nonreplicating cell populations are adversely affected by this drug.

ANTIBIOTICS. The immunosuppressive antibiotics include the inhibitors of nucleic acid synthesis, and chloramphenicol and puromycin, which interfere with cellular protein synthesis. Actinomycin D binds to the guanine residue of DNA, thereby sterically interfering with RNA

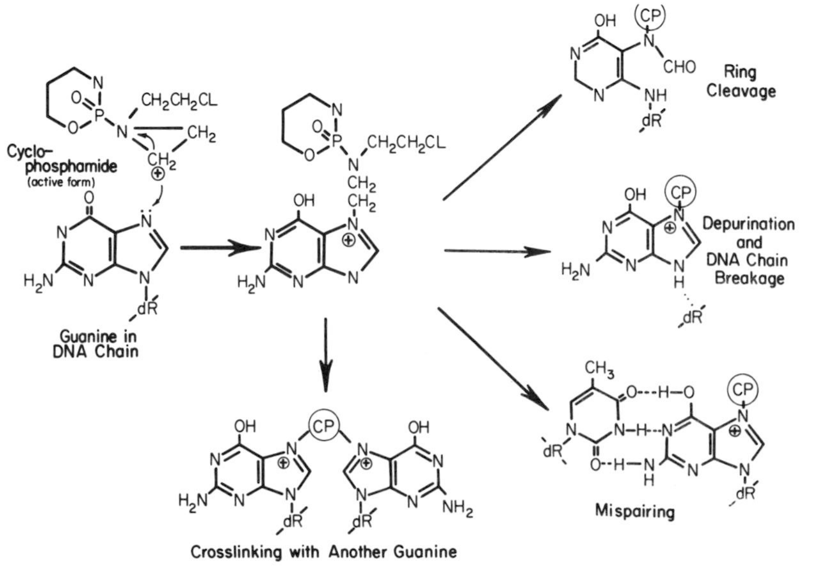

Fig. 10-22. Mechanism of the action of the alkylating agent cyclophosphamide (CP). CP binds to the guanine molecule within the DNA chain. The guanine-CP complex leads to further damage to the DNA molecule. Four examples of the damage to DNA are shown. [From R. L. Simmons, J. E. Foker, and J. S. Najarian, Principles of Immunosuppression, in D. C. Sabiston, Jr. (ed.), "Davis-Christopher Textbook of Surgery," p. 471, W. B. Saunders Company, Philadelphia, 1972.]

polymerase and, consequently, with DNA-directed RNA synthesis. This potentially effective means of suppressing the development of immunity led to its use in reversing acute rejection of kidney grafts. The toxicity of actinomycin D has limited the overall clinical benefit, however, and it has been used less and less frequently. Mitomycin C combines with cellular DNA and hinders replication. This compound would also be useful in inhibiting allograft immunity, but its toxicity has precluded clinical use.

Both puromycin and chloramphenicol inhibit protein synthesis, and both can be immunosuppressive. Puromycin structurally resembles an amino acid–charged transfer RNA molecule and is accepted into the ribosome. There is no amino acid to be donated, however, and the peptide chain is prematurely terminated. Although protein synthesis is obviously central to immunological expression, it is so general a requirement for other cells that inhibition, and hence toxicity, will be widespread. Chloramphenicol has also been investigated experimentally. It is most potent in prokaryotic (bacterial) cell systems, and its effects on mammalian cells may be due to inhibiting mitochondrial synthesis. Unfortunately, it is only weakly immunosup-

pressive, and its potentially severe bone marrow toxicity precludes its use.

In general, only the antibiotic agents which primarily affect DNA synthesis can be expected to be clinically successful. Inhibition would be concentrated on dividing cell populations, and generalized toxicity would be less likely. This would potentially allow a favorable benefit/toxicity ratio.

IMMUNOSUPPRESSION BY LYMPHOCYTE DEPLETION

ADRENAL CORTICOSTEROIDS. Adrenal corticosteroids are the immunosuppressive agents most commonly used in clinical practice. They are effective in a variety of situations, from transplantation to the treatment of lupus erythematosus, childhood nephrotic syndrome, and asthma. Why steroids are beneficial for patients is not clear in most clinical situations. Experimentally, many effects have been described in a variety of cells from numerous species. Consequently, much of the uncertainty of mechanism of action stems from the difficulty in relating the many isolated in vitro effects to the patient. This is compounded by the variation in species susceptibility to steroids, which makes extrapolation difficult. In fact, direct evidence for immunosuppression by corticosteroids in human beings is lacking, and their benefit may be due primarily to inhibition of the inflammatory response. Despite this uncertainty about the mechanism of action, steroids are necessary for successful human transplantation and are commonly used to produce immunosuppression in other types of patients.

Many effects of steroids are known (Fig. 10-23). The problem is deciding which are primary and which are secondary actions. Steroids cross the cell membrane and bind to specific receptors in the cytoplasm of most cells,

Fig. 10-23. Adrenocortical steroids play an important role in clinical allograft immunosuppression. Many apparent sites of action have been located experimentally. These compounds bind to cytoplasmic receptors, and this complex combines with DNA. How this relates to the many functional consequences of steroids presented in this diagram is unclear. In the complex clinical transplantation setting it is not possible to determine if the primary suppression of lymphocytes is more important than the anti-inflammatory effects on neutrophils and macrophages in the suppression of allograft rejection reactions. Nevertheless, they produce a significant portion of the immunosuppressive effect of current clinical therapy.

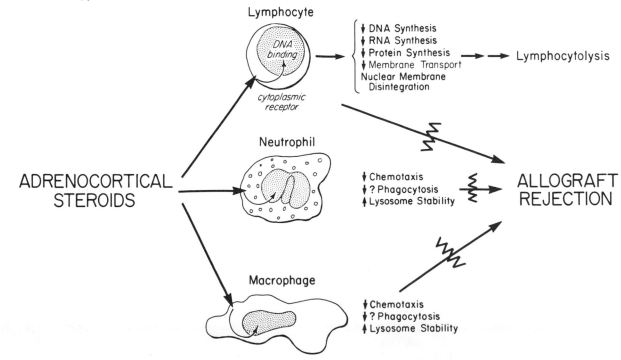

lymphocytes included. Many experiments have shown a corollation between binding affinity and steroid potency, specifically between binding and lymphocyte resistance or susceptibility. The steroid-receptor complex then enters the nucleus and interacts with DNA in an unknown way. Subsequently in lymphocytes DNA, RNA, and protein synthesis are inhibited, as are glucose and amino acid transport. At a sufficient dosage, lymphocyte degeneration and lysis occur. Cytolysis can readily be produced in vivo, and T cells appear to be most susceptible. In some experiments the disintegration of nuclear membranes takes place within hours of exposure to steroids. Depletion of small T lymphocytes occurs both in the peripheral and central lymphoid tissues. Although it is unclear why the resting small lymphocyte should be so susceptible, it would seem that the primary antilymphocyte action of steroids may be to deplete small lymphocytes before they are activated by antigen.

The functional effects of steroids are predictable, and all T-cell responses are depressed. Paradoxically, the steroid-resistant thymocytes that remain after an injection of steroids have increased activity, but the net immunological capability of the treated animal is reduced.

Although B-cell activity and antibody production are relatively unaffected by steroids, many other cell types which participate in graft rejection are damaged. Neutrophil chemotaxis is inhibited, but whether or not suppression of phagocytosis occurs remains controversial. Similar results and controversies surround the effects on macrophages. It seems certain, however, that the accumulation of neutrophils, macrophages, and monocytes at sites of immune and inflammatory activity is reduced when steroids are given. Steroids also increase the membrane stability of digestive lysosomal particles in these cells, which reduces their inflammatory activity. These observations provide a basis for understanding the anti-inflammatory action activity of steroids. Inflammation is so intertwined with any substantial immune reaction that the various effects are inseparable. The variety of immunologic activities that steroids will suppress means that their effectiveness against the rejection reaction is probably the sum of many influences. When these effects are understood at the molecular level, however, there may prove to be a common discrete point of inhibition.

The effectiveness of cortisone in suppressing the allograft reaction was first recognized by its prolongation of skin graft survival in rabbits. Increased skin graft survival was subsequently shown in mice and guinea pigs, but the results were not as conclusive in pigs, dogs, monkeys, and human beings when cortisone was used alone. In experimental kidney allografts, steroids have not been convincingly effective by themselves, but they are valuable in combination with such agents as azathioprine, nitrogen mustard, and antilymphocyte globulin. Similarly, steroids alone cannot prevent clinical allograft rejection but, together with other compounds, are potent in both preventing and reversing rejection reactions.

Steroid toxicity of some degree is frequent and commonly includes a Cushinoid appearance. Other characteristic problems from steroid therapy are hypertension, weight gain, peptic ulcers and gastrointestinal bleeding, euphoric personality changes, cataract formation, hyperglycemia which may progress to steroid diabetes, and osteoporosis with avascular necrosis of bone. The appearance and severity of these complications vary considerably, but all too frequently they are life threatening. Clinical transplantation will be improved tremendously when more specific means of immunosuppression are developed and present steroid dosages can be reduced.

ANTILYMPHOCYTE GLOBULIN. The use of antilymphocyte antibodies to suppress the immune response is an interesting aspect of the transplantation story. In experimental studies, antilymphocyte globulin is a potent immunosuppressive agent, yet evidence for its value in clinical transplantation is controversial. This apparent contradiction results more from the difficulties which surround analyzing a complex clinical situation than from the ineffectiveness of antilymphocyte globulin. Evidence for the benefit of antilymphocyte globulin exists, but better-designed studies will be needed to measure the effects accurately.

The ability of an antiserum to destroy white cells was noted as early as 1899 by Metchnikoff. After guinea pigs were stimulated with lymph node or spleen cells from either rats or rabbits, their serum would agglutinate and kill polymorphonuclear leukocytes of the donor species. In the same year, Flexner found that lymphoid depletion occurred in animals treated with anti-lymph node serum. It was only during the last decade, however, that the functional consequences of heterologous sera made against lymphoid tissue were investigated. Certain immunologic reactions, e.g., tuberculin sensitivity and allograft rejection, were found to be depressed. Monaco and Russell induced potent antisera that were very effective in prolonging skin graft with strong histocompatibility differences, even including xenografts. Starzl was the first to use antilymphocyte serum in clinical kidney transplantation, and subsequently these preparations have been widely used.

Antilymphocyte globulins (ALG) are produced when thoracic duct, peripheral blood, lymph nodes, thymus, or spleen lymphocytes are injected into animals of a different species. Cell membranes or cultured lymphocytes serve equally well to provide the antigenic stimulation. The addition of adjuvants, usually Freund's complete adjuvant, is used to enhance the immunogenicity of the foreign lymphocytes and produce sera that are consistently more immunosuppressive. The rabbit, goat, and horse are commonly used to produce antisera for clinical transplantation.

Most of the relatively specific antibody against human lymphocytes resides in the IgG fraction. Further purification of the sera by separating the globulin fraction can be achieved by Cohn fractionation, column chromatography, or forced-flow electrophoresis. The purified material can be administered intravenously, intramuscularly, or subcutaneously. Unlike the immunosuppressive drugs used clinically, the course of ALG is short—usually the first few days or weeks after transplantation.

The action of ALG seems to be directed mainly against the T cell. The suppression produced by ALG can be at least partially reversed by T cells, but not by bone marrow cells. Thymectomy will enhance the effect of ALG, and ALG decreases the number of circulating T cells. Even in vitro, ALG will reduce the number of T cells. As would be expected, ALG administration interferes most with the cell-mediated reactions—skin or renal allograft rejection, tuberculin sensitivity, and the graft-versus-host reaction. ALG can abolish preexisting delayed hypersensitivity reactions, and larger doses will prolong the survival of some xenografts. ALG has a definite, but lesser, effect on humoral reactivity, and this, too, is concentrated on T cell–dependent antibody production.

The net effect of the relatively selective antilymphocyte activity of ALG is to enhance the activity of steroids, alkylating agents, and azathioprine against graft rejection. Most simply, the background of lymphocyte depression provided by ALG potentiates the effect of these agents without adding to the toxicity against other rapidly dividing cell systems. The fact that ALG and the other immunosuppressive drugs reinforce one another means that large doses of ALG can be used as a priming agent, followed by small doses of the more toxic immunosuppressants for a more effective and safer clinical regimen.

Many theories have been used to explain why ALG is a powerful (at present the most potent) inhibitor of cell-mediated immunity but only weakly affects antibody formation. Most of the explanations can be discarded because the anti-T-cell activity is more a function of the structure of the immune system than of the specificity of ALG itself. The spectrum of in vitro ALG activity can be easily shifted from anti-T to anti-B cell by changing the cells used to stimulate antibody production. Antithymus sera are richer in anti-T antibodies, anti-bone marrow sera have more anti-B-cell activity, while anti-spleen and lymph node sera contain large amounts of both types of antibodies. When ALG is given to the transplant patient, however, there is poor penetration of the antilymphocyte antibodies in the lymphoid regions where most of the relatively sessile B cells reside. The circulating long-lived lymphocytes, which are overwhelmingly T cell in origin, therefore absorb the bulk of the antibody. Lymphocytes coated with ALG share the fate of erythrocytes coated with antibody. They are either lysed or cleared from the blood by reticuloendothelial cells in the liver and spleen. More prolonged administration of ALG will deplete the paracortical regions of the lymph nodes where T cells reside, but high doses will also reduce the B cells in the medullary regions and follicles of the nodes.

Antilymphocyte globulin is widely used in clinical transplantation, with apparently beneficial results. Absolute proof of the effect of ALG is lacking, but the weight of the evidence suggests it is of value. What the many studies show is that it is difficult to analyze one factor, here ALG, in a complex clinical situation. Several studies have shown an increased percentage and length of survival, and renal function was increased among cadaver allografts when high doses of ALG were given (Fig. 10-24). The studies were not randomized, however, and the treatment groups not strictly comparable. Many considerations must be balanced in such a study, including (1) the length of time on dialysis, (2) the presence of presensitization, (3) the number of patients with depressed immune response, (4) the condition of the recipient, and (5) the condition of the graft, if it is from a cadaver donor.

The factors influencing the results are so numerous that a broad randomized study may not be able to equalize them all. Such an attempt has been made, however, by the Medical Research Council of Canada, with interesting results. There was no apparent effect of horse antithymocyte globulin on the 1-year survival of either living related or cadaver kidney allografts. But these patients did show a decrease in the average number of acute rejection episodes, an improvement in renal function, and a decrease in the amount of steroids given. These results could be interpreted to mean that the effect of ALG is greatest on the early, cell-mediated rejection reactions and less on later, antibody-produced graft damage. Unanswerable at this time is how much ALG adds to the risk of infection in the immunosuppressed patient. The benefit of ALG may be offset by an increased susceptibility to infection, and this may account for the lack of improved survival of patients in the clinical studies.

Fig. 10-24. The effect of ALG on kidney allograft function in transplant patients at the University of Minnesota. All kidneys were from cadavers; graft losses due to technical difficulties and hyperacute rejection were excluded. Although this is not a randomized study, improved function seems to occur in patients treated with ALG. The results with high doses (> 25 mg/kg/day) and medium doses (10 to 25 mg/kg/day) of ALG given for 14 days after transplantation do not seem to be significantly different. An accurate dose-response analysis is not possible, however, because of the lack of a satisfactory assay for the potency of individual batches of ALG. [*From J. E. Foker, R. L. Simmons, and J. S. Najarian, Principles of Immunosuppression, in D. C. Sabiston (ed.), "Davis-Christopher Textbook of Surgery," W. B. Saunders Company, Philadelphia, 1977.*]

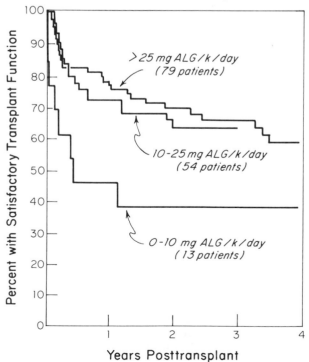

The use of ALG is not confined clinically to kidney transplantation, and beneficial results have also been reported in bone marrow transplantation. These studies have suggested that ALG pretreatment of the recipient is of value in suppressing the response to the donor cells and for enlarging the marrow space. Also in this situation, a potentiating effect with certain drugs, such as procarbizine, has been described. Furthermore, it seems that ALG may be useful in the treatment of the graft-versus-host reactions which arise in these patients.

The toxicity of any heterologous serum preparation prepared against human tissue depends on two factors, (1) its cross-reactivity with other tissue antigens, and (2) the ability of the patient to make antibodies against the protein itself. When administered intramuscularly, ALG produces an area of erythematous induration accompanied by high fever. This probably results from the combination of antibodies with cellular antigens at the injection site. The combination of anemia and thrombocytopenia can also occur and presumably results from a reaction between ALG and host erythrocytes and platelets. Although prior absorption with human platelets and red cell stroma reduces the severity, some cross-reactivity to these cells persists in most ALG preparations. Cross-reactivity to renal glomerular basement membranes has occasionally been found, but no evidence for functionally significant nephrotoxic serum nephritis has been presented. These cross-

Fig. 10-25. X-ray-induced damage of DNA molecule. Irradiation frequently induces single breaks in the deoxyribotide backbone of the DNA double helix. More rarely, irradiation induces double breaks within the backbone. [From R. L. Simmons, J. E. Foker, and J. S. Najarian, Principles of Immunosuppression, in D. C. Sabiston, Jr. (ed.), "Davis-Christopher Textbook of Surgery," p. 471, W. B. Saunders Company, Philadelphia, 1972.]

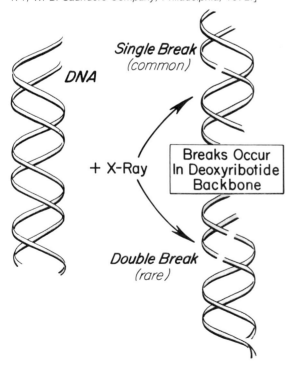

reactions can be reduced by using a purer lymphocyte suspension to stimulate ALG production. Either cultured lymphoblasts or thoracic duct lymphocytes will produce a more specific ALG than will the heterogeneous cell populations found in the spleen or bone marrow.

Allergic reactions to the antiserum itself were formerly the most common clinical problem associated with the use of ALG. Urticaria, anaphylactoid reactions, and serum sickness, including joint pain, fever, and malaise, all resulted from the patient developing immunity to the heterologous globulin. The incidence of these reactions has been reduced by inducing immunologic unresponsiveness to the foreign proteins in ALG by intravenous administration of a highly purified, deaggregated IgG fraction. This method has been used experimentally to produce tolerance to foreign proteins, and it is especially effective in the presence of the other immunosuppressive drugs used in renal transplantation.

The major problem in the production of a standardized antihuman ALG is the inability to develop a satisfactory method of assaying its in vitro immunosuppressive potency. Other immunosuppressive drugs are available in measurable quantities; therefore the response is more predictable. Unfortunately, individual laboratories make their own ALG preparations, and a standard method of assay has not been developed. Cytotoxic assays, the formation of cellular rosettes by antibody-coated cells, and animal assays for immunosuppressive activity have all been attempted, but their correlation with graft prolongation has been inconsistent. Standardization is important because two batches of ALG prepared by the same method will have varying degrees of immunosuppressive potency. A suitable assay is necessary to identify the better ALG preparations and make their use increasingly beneficial.

RADIATION. Radiation was probably the first agent used to produce immunosuppression. Ionizing radiation (x-rays, alpha rays, beta rays) affects both cellular proteins and nucleic acids. Despite the fact that relatively small doses of irradiation may disrupt the secondary protein structure formed by hydrogen bonding and the tertiary conformation that results, biologically significant alterations of protein function seem to require very high dosages. Consequently, most of the immunosuppressive effects of x-radiation are caused by changes produced in nucleic acids. DNA is particularly vulnerable, and therefore so is cellular replication. The most important of the several modes of damage is the production of scattered breaks in the deoxyribose-phosphate backbone of DNA (Fig. 10-25). Disruption of either the carbon-carbon bonds of the deoxyribotides or the bonds involving the phosphate groups produces breaks in one of the DNA strands. Occasionally both strands are broken at the same point. Other sites of damage, such as the bases themselves, are even less frequent.

Repair mechanisms exist to mend the breaks, but insufficient time may be available in the dividing cell. Therefore, the effectiveness of radiation is dependent upon the phase of the cell cycle in which the cell is found (Fig. 10-26). Cells in the M or G_2 phase are most sensitive to irradiation. Presumably, DNA breaks that occur during these phases cannot be repaired quickly enough, and the synthetic events and precise apportionment of cellular components which occur during mitosis may become scrambled. Conversely, the early G_1 phase and the latter part of the S phase are the most resistant portions of the cell cycle. Although irradiation is, in general, most effective just prior to or during mitosis, lymphocytes are a special case. For reasons that are not known, these cells are also sensitive in their resting, or G_0, phase.

Despite the complexity of the subcellular mechanisms, the effect of irradiation on the immune response is predictable and depends greatly on its timing with relation to antigen exposure. The possibilities are best seen when a relatively simple response, antibody production against a defined antigen, is measured. When the antigen is given soon after irradiation, the immune response will be inhibited because there is insufficient time for the immunocompetent cell population to recover before the antigen is encountered. If radiation is given during the time of maximal proliferation of the immunocompetent population to an antigen (soon after antigen administration), the response will be strongly inhibited. On the other hand, if antigenic stimulation is delayed long enough for the precursor cells to recover from the radiation, there will even be a slight augmentation of the response. Radiation is also ineffective if given long after the antigen, when a mature population of antibody-synthesizing cells has been formed. Fully differentiated plasma cells, and presumably cytotoxic lymphocytes, are radioresistant. Although radiation is relatively ineffective in blocking the secondary response of an immunized animal, paradoxically, an augmented antibody response may occur under certain circumstances. The timing of radiation must be carefully planned for the greatest immunosuppressive effect.

X-radiation has limited use in clinical transplantation. Effective suppression of the recipient's lymphoid tissues can be achieved, but the toxicity associated with the total body radiation is too great. Local irradiation of the graft, however, may provide some immunosuppressive effects. When given prior to transplantation, x-ray of the kidney may destroy the passenger leukocytes in the graft. These cells seem to be a potent source of antigen to the host, and thus the stimulus is somewhat diminished. After transplantation, radiation of the graft may damage invading cells, as well as produce nonspecific anti-inflammatory effects. Although proof of the benefit is lacking, some centers irradiate the kidney graft at the onset of a rejection reaction.

Other methods of using radiation have been tried. Selective irradiation of circulating lymphocytes has been done experimentally by diverting blood via a shunt through an extracorporeal radiation source. The circulating lymphocytes are depleted, and immunocompetence is reduced. Selective irradiation has the advantages that the neutrophils remain active in clearing infection, and protein loss is avoided. The inefficiencies of the system, however, and the need for nearly continuous irradiation make this technique impractical for clinical use.

Total body radiation does have one application at present in clinical transplantation. It is used to eliminate the immune reactivity of patients in preparation for bone

Lymphocyte Cell Cycle

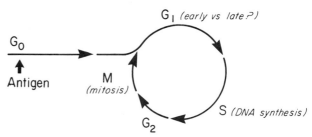

Fig. 10-26. The phases of the cell cycle. Following stimulation by an antigen, or other type of mitogen, small lymphocytes are activated. They are converted from the resting G_0 phase to the active G_1 phase. The G_1 phase lasts 10 hours or longer before DNA synthesis (S phase) begins. The S phase lasts about 10 hours and is followed by a short (2 to 4 hours) G_2 phase before mitosis (M phase). M phase is relatively brief, usually less than 2 to 3 hours, after which the cells are returned to the G_1 phase. The susceptibility of the cell to the immunosuppressive agents used in transplantation varies with the phase of the cycle. Periods of most intense nucleic acid synthesis, particularly S phase, are most vulnerable to the antimetabolites. As discussed in the text, the resting, G_0, lymphocyte is also susceptible to several of the clinically used immunosuppressive agents. [From J. E. Foker, R. L. Simmons, and J. S. Najarian, Principles of Immunosuppression, in D. C. Sabiston, Jr. (ed.), "Davis-Christopher Textbook of Surgery," p. 509, W. B. Saunders Company, Philadelphia, 1977.]

marrow transplantation. The toxicity is predictable. The rapidly replicating skin and gastrointestinal tract are universally affected, and nausea, vomiting, diarrhea, and skin changes occur. Late problems—growth retardation, vertebral deformities, sterility, cataracts, and a likely increased incidence of cancer—are also probably attributable to damage to the cellular genetic apparatus.

THYMECTOMY. There is some evidence that the adult mammalian thymus continues to play a role, albeit a diminished one, in maintaining the immunologic responsiveness of the animal. Its extirpation, therefore, may enhance the effects of immunosuppressive agents or irradiation. Unfortunately, although thymectomy can be performed rather simply through a cervical incision as well as by the classical transsternal route, it has not proved to be of use in clinical transplantation. In the early days of renal transplantation, Starzl tried thymectomy in a number of patients but had little improvement in results. It may be that a relatively small increment of benefit may be more apparent now when better results are regularly achieved. Perhaps thymectomy deserves another try. It must be conceded, however, that the thymus in an adult has largely completed its inductive functions and removal may have no measurable consequence. Furthermore, even if thymectomy could augment immunosuppression, it may not be desirable to produce greater general immunological incompetency in transplant recipients. In summary, it seems unlikely that the admittedly small potential gain will stimulate another clinical trial of thymectomy unless it is shown to be important to the production of tolerance.

LYMPHOID EXTIRPATION. Immunity becomes rapidly systemic. It is not confined for long to the regional lymph nodes or to a single major lymphoid organ like the spleen. Experimentally, the acquisition of immunity can be delayed for only brief periods by interrupting the lymphatic channels, by placing grafts in sites with poor lymphatic drainage, or by excising local lymphoid tissue. In one of the earliest clinical experiments, transplanted kidneys were placed in plastic bags after completion of the vascular anastomoses. This approach failed because vascularized organ grafts do not require lymphatic drainage to disseminate the antigen to awaiting lymphocytes. Excision of locally draining lymph nodes or the spleen is also ineffective as an immunosuppressive technique.

THORACIC DUCT DRAINAGE. Cannulation and drainage of the thoracic duct will successfully deplete the body of a large proportion of its circulating T lymphocytes. Such depletion will lead to prolongation of allograft survival, and to lesser, but real, decreases in the capacity for antibody synthesis. Thoracic duct cannulation and drainage have been used for clinical immunosuppression; although the technique seems to produce prolongation of allografts, it is cumbersome, the indwelling cannula can become plugged or infected, and protein depletion may result. There has been a recent resurgence of interest in this technique.

CONSEQUENCES OF CLINICAL IMMUNOSUPPRESSIVE THERAPY

The complications of immunosuppressive therapy in recipients of organ allografts are difficult to distinguish from the complications of recurrent rejection. Patients who do not have rejection episodes generally do not suffer major complications of immunosuppressive therapy. Conversely, the patient who requires repeated large doses of prednisone to avoid further rejection episodes or who suffer diminished renal function in the presence of high doses of azathioprine will have potentially lethal complications. The major complications all relate to a relative inability to respond effectively to a large variety of pathogenic, and even to normally saprophytic, organisms. There may be, moreover, a decrease in the normal capacity to destroy mutant, potentially neoplastic cells. This leads to a number of interesting and clinically important consequences of immunosuppression that must be considered.

PARAMETERS OF IMMUNOSUPPRESSION. Obviously the process of graft rejection can be prolonged, but are other parameters of immunocompetence concurrently depressed in the transplant patient? Can immunosuppression be measured in any other way than by the life of the graft? All methods of clinical immunological monitoring are restricted to measuring the specific or nonspecific responses in peripheral blood—the spleen, thymus, and lymph nodes not being readily available. With this restriction in mind, a number of studies have been performed. During the first two weeks after kidney transplantation an immunosuppressive effect can be detected. The response of the patient's circulating lymphocyte to either the mitogen phytohemagglutinin (PHA) or to foreign leukocytes is depressed. The loss of reactivity seems to be roughly proportional to the decrease in T cells among the peripheral lymphocytes and to the rise in null cells which occurs. The latter are

lymphocytes, coated with ALG and consequently inhibited.

Overall, the depressed lymphocyte reactivity probably results from a combination of acute destruction of T cells by ALG steroids, inactivation of other lymphocytes by masking with ALG, and inhibition of the lymphocyte proliferative response by azathioprine. Among these agents, ALG would seem to be the most responsible, because lymphocyte reactivity begins to return shortly after the ALG course is ended. Surprisingly, peripheral lymphocytes from kidney graft recipients show a normal response to PHA and foreign lymphocytes shortly thereafter. Because the kidney grafts continue to survive, an immunosuppressive effect which is not measured by these assays must persist. At the present time, there is no way to monitor the level of immunosuppression achieved after the effect of ALG has disappeared. Nor is it possible to predict incipient rejection accurately, although some success has been claimed for the detection of a rise in lymphocyte-dependent antibodies immediately prior to rejection. Because the degree of immunosuppression cannot yet be measured, the dosages of immunosuppressive agents are regulated instead by the toxicity produced.

BACTERIAL AND FUNGAL INFECTION. Immunosuppression understandably increases the risk of infection, but the consequences may offer some surprises. The routine post-transplant immunosuppression regimen does not necessarily result in a higher bacterial infection rate. With suitable precautions the postoperative wound infection incidence is very low. These patients seem to cope satisfactorily with inevitable contamination during the operation despite the increased immunosuppressive therapy used at the time. When there are no severe rejection reactions and the graft maintains good function, the day-to-day bacterial challenge to the recipient is handled. Although urinary tract infections are frequent, they are usually mild and easily controlled by antibiotics.

We do not mean to imply that bacterial infection is an insignificant problem for transplantation patients. On the contrary, infection is still the most common complication of immunosuppression, and overall it is the most common cause of death in transplant recipients. Even so, increasing experience has both lowered the incidence of serious infection and lengthened the time before it occurs.

The recent report of the American College of Surgeons/National Institute of Health Organ Transplant Registry stated that sepsis was the primary cause of death in 47 percent of all renal allografts recipients who died. Graft rejection not associated with sepsis accounted for less than 10 percent of deaths. Rejection of a kidney graft should not be fatal because the patient can be maintained on hemodialysis. The difficulties seem to arise with the treatment of rejection. Rejection causes decreased kidney function, which further potentiates the increased immunosuppression used to combat the rejection episode. The consequence is usually a severely immunodepressed patient, often with very few circulating polymorphonuclear leukocytes, who is highly susceptible to infection. In this setting, particularly if it is prolonged, severe bacterial infections and generalized sepsis can occur.

Most deaths, early in the history of kidney transplantation, occurred in the first few posttransplant months as a result of highly pathogenic bacterial infections. For example, pneumococcal pneumonia has been reported to be the most common type of pneumonia in kidney recipients. Since then, improved antibiotics and greater skill in immunosuppression therapy have shifted the spectrum of organisms. There has been a relative increase in lethal infection caused by organisms that are normally weakly pathogenic. Antibiotics will eradicate the more aggressive bacteria, but they leave opportunistic organisms free to colonize the susceptible transplant patient.

The opportunistic organisms, that are normally eliminated by cellular mechanisms, can now blossom in the face of the relative T-cell depression. Fungi are prominent opportunists, and they can cause urinary tract and pulmonary infections, skin lesions, and central nervous system involvement, as well as generalized sepsis. *Candida albicans* infections are probably the most common. The inevitable mucosal candidiasis can be satisfactorily prevented by oral mycostatin. Candida can become more deep-seated, and the pneumonia, usually part of a mixed infection, can be lethal. Characteristically, it produces soft, bulky, pulmonary infiltrates, although invasion of pulmonary arteries can lead to infarction and wedge-shaped peripheral infiltrates. Candida sepsis is most often associated with indwelling catheters, but it can take a more entrenched systemic form.

Aspergillus species are probably the second most common cause of fungal infection and typically produce upper lobe pulmonary cavities. *Rhizopus oryzae, Histoplasma capsulatum,* and *Cryptococcus neoformans* also invade the lung, and the latter occasionally causes meningitis. The indolent bacterium *Nocardia asteroides* occasionally infects, producing nodular pulmonary lesions. The protozoan *Pneumocystis carinii,* more commonly seen in patients undergoing cancer chemotherapy, usually causes an alveolar infiltrate with disproportionate dyspnea and cyanosis.

Standard patient isolation precautions are useless against these organisms, and prophylactic antibiotics are not available for most of them. Prevention is dependent upon avoiding excessive doses of immunosuppressive agents in a futile attempt to prolong the function of a rejected graft. An exception seems to be the protection against *P. carinii* provided by prophylactic trimethoprim and sulfamethoxazole.

VIRAL INFECTIONS. Viral infections seem to be almost ubiquitous among kidney transplant recipients. The herpes group of DNA viruses are most commonly present. Infection or antibody response to cytomegalovirus (CMV) is found in up to 90 percent of patients after renal transplantation. Herpes simplex infection occurs in about 25 percent and herpes zoster in 10 percent of graft recipients. Reports from England have shown that the Epstein-Barr virus commonly infects transplant patients, but the clinical significance of this is unclear. Antigenic evidence for hepatitis B virus infection can be detected in 15 percent of transplant patients. It seems almost certain that as detection methods improve, evidence will appear for other kinds of viral infections in these transplantation patients.

Several questions are raised by the recent appreciation of viral infections in kidney recipients. Are these infections of any consequence, or are they merely laboratory curiosities? The case of the hepatitis B virus is particularly interesting. Paradoxically, transplantation and hemodialysis patients who have circulating HB antigens usually have no symptoms of hepatitis. The intriguing question is why the disease is apparently much milder in these patients. It seems likely that liver cell damage results from an immune reaction against the viral antigens on the cell and that this may be reduced in these immunodepressed patients. The hepatitis virus does not seem directly cytotoxic for liver cells.

The situation with cytomegalovirus infection appears to be only slightly clearer and no less intriguing. Most evidence suggests that cytomegalovirus infection usually produces a clinical illness characterized by fever, neutropenia, and frequently a decrease in kidney function and apparent rejection. The virus may be newly acquired from blood transfusions or from foreign graft itself, but it is far more likely that apparently new infection is a reactivation of latent intracellular viruses. The finding that most normal adults have antibodies to CMV supports the latent virus hypothesis.

In transplant patients, does the infection cause the rejection or does the rejection encourage viral activation? Rejection reactions are accomplished by bursts of lymphocyte proliferation, cell division is known to activate latent viruses experimentally, and most immunosuppressive agents are mutagenic. Viral infections, on the other hand, can be associated with either an augmented or a depressed immune response. If the patient is able to produce antibody against virus, graft rejection is also enhanced. In preimmunized individuals, viruses seem to act as immunological adjuvants and enhance the response both to virus and to graft. When no antibody response accompanies the viral infection, a generalized immunodepression is usually present. At present it can be said only that viral infections and rejection reactions are clearly linked; which initiates and which follows is usually unknown.

A special case of CMV infection is worthy of note. The typical CMV infection is a mild febrile illness, followed by an antibody response and regression of viral symptoms. A rejection episode usually accompanies the viral infection and raises the controversy discussed in the previous paragraph. These patients remain asymptomatic but may continue to excrete CMV in urine or saliva despite the presence of antibodies to CMV. In certain patients, however, there is no antibody response or apparent rejection and the infection can be lethal. These severely immunodepressed patients are at the mercy of this usually trivial parasite. This would suggest that rejection is not essential for viral infection. Certainly the ability of the patient to respond to the virus is very important to his or her survival. Recently, surgical specimens taken from patients with bleeding gastric or cecal ulcers have shown heavy cellular infestation with CMV.

The other herpes viruses seem to behave in a similar manner. Transplant patients also have infections typical of herpes simplex and varicella zoster. The infections may be more severe than in normal patients, and although the lesions may be localized, the viruses are systemic and can be recovered in the urine. Fever, neutropenia, and allograft rejection may accompany the infection, and antibody response to the virus seems to be important for the patient.

We are not sure when the viral infections actually occur in relation to the clinical symptoms. With the exception of the hepatitis infection, these may represent activation of a normal intracellular viral flora, rather than recent infection. In transplant patients, studies suggest that cytomegalovirus "infection" takes place about the time of transplantation, when the mutagenic antirejection drugs are begun at high levels. This obviously may merely result from activation of latent intracellular viruses.

PREVENTION OF INFECTION. The incidence of severe, near-fatal infections can be reduced through a number of precautions: (1) The most important precaution is to eliminate all sources of infection prior to transplantation, especially those in the urinary tract and shunt site. Other sources of infection should be sought by routine preoperative cultures of nasopharynx, throat, sputum, urine, stool, and hemodialysis cannula sites. If any source is found, it should be eliminated by the appropriate use of surgical drainage or antibiotic therapy. (2) Technical problems clearly predispose to sepsis. Urinary extravasation frequently leads to wound infections. Abscesses deep to the transplant are difficult to drain, and mycotic aneurysms may develop at sites of anastomosis or in the iliac vessels. It is frequently necessary to remove the kidney to obtain control of the infection. (3) Organs from related and well-matched cadavers elicit less frequent and less vigorous rejection reactions. If repeated rejection can be avoided, the doses of immunosuppressive drugs can be minimized and the rate and severity of infection will diminish. (4) Many patients who die of infection develop leukopenia (especially neutropenia) at some time. Some bouts of leukopenia can be attributed to cytomegalovirus infections. Leukopenia can be prevented by careful reduction in azathioprine doses when the leukocyte count or platelet count falls and when renal function is lost for whatever reason. The use of other bone marrow depressants (chloramphenicol) should be scrupulously avoided in patients already on azathioprine therapy. (5) Gowns, masks, and gloves were formerly used to minimize infections in the initial postoperative care. Most transplant units have discontinued their use because they restrict access to the patients, impose psychologic stress, and are probably ineffective against viral, fungal, or endogenous bacteria.

MALIGNANCY. Cancer has been an unexpectedly frequent companion of clinical transplantation. The incidence of cancer is not high enough, however, to contraindicate the transplant procedure. Tumors in kidney recipients have come from two general sources. Some have been unfortunately transplanted from cadaver donors in whom the cancer was unsuspected. These tumors usually can be treated simply by halting immunosuppression therapy and allowing rejection of the tumor tissue, as well as the kidney, to occur. The more common cancers are the primary tumors which appear in the immunosuppressed recipient.

The data are still accumulating on these primary tumors, and precise frequencies are not yet available. It would seem, however, that the rate of development of malignancy in patients surviving renal transplantation may be as high as thirty times that of a similar, normal population.

Only certain tumors grow more readily in immunodepressed patients. Seventy-five percent of the spontaneous cancers are either lymphoid or epithelial in origin. Carcinoma in situ of the cervix, carcinoma of the lip, and squamous or basal cell carcinomas account for about half of this group, while lymphomas, predominantly reticulum cell carcinoma, make up the remainder. It has been estimated that the risks to the transplant recipient of developing skin cancer, lymphoma, or reticulum cell sarcoma are increased by 4, 40, and 350 times, respectively. The lymphomas are unusual both in their frequency and behavior. Almost 50 percent of the immunosuppressed patients with lymphomas have brain involvement, which occurs in only 1 percent of nontransplanted related cases of lymphoma. These lymphomas, moreover, are difficult to treat and have led to death in almost all cases.

Recent evidence suggests that the lymphomas are not true neoplasms. Immunological analysis has indicated that these tumors secrete several different types of immunoglobulins, i.e., they do not have the nomenclatural characteristics of cancer. Other evidence suggests that they may represent uncontrolled B cell proliferative responses to Epstein-Barr virus. The superficial malignant lesions of the lip, skin, and cervix are usually successfully treated by standard operative techniques. There is no need to jeopardize the allografts by reducing the immunosuppressive therapy.

We do not know why transplant patients have an increased risk for cancer in general and epithelial (and perhaps lymphoid) cancers in particular. It has been postulated that the surveillance and elimination of tumor cells as they arise by lymphocytes is an important natural defense of human beings against cancer. Certainly this function would be depressed in transplantation patients who are immunodepressed by antirejection therapy. Despite this, two observations argue that this explanation is incomplete: (1) only a few kinds of cancer are increased in these patients, and, perhaps more telling, (2) patients receiving hemodialysis have an increased risk of cancer, but tumors arise with the usual spectrum and frequency distribution. Dialysis patients have decreased immunological competence. Perhaps, the inhibition of a surveillance mechanism contributes to their increased risk.

Transplant patients, however, must have additional factors operating which contribute to the development of cancer. They are immunosuppressed, which may be important, but the presence of the mutagen azathioprine is a more certain factor. Azathioprine, theoretically, could either act as a primary mutagen on dividing lymphocytes and epithelial cells or contribute to the activation of viruses and their transformation of normal cells into tumors. It is unclear what consequences steroids and ALG have, but at least two reticulum cell sarcomas have sprung up at the site of ALG injections. It would seem possible that the most important effect the immunosuppressive agents have on tumor development is to encourage viral transformation of normal cells into cancer cells.

Cancers of the epithelium, for example, may be a consequence of herpes virus transformation. This group of viruses is carcinogenic in animals, and circumstantial evidence exists for a role in human cervical cancer. Herpes viruses are usually dormant, but the stress of transplantation or the action of antimetabolite may activate them. The viruses might then either proliferate and cause a clinical viral illness or produce cellular transformation into cancer cells. Similar possibilities exist for the lymphomas. Several animal lymphomas are produced by RNA viruses, and transformation by related viruses could be occurring in these patients. Perhaps a simpler explanation would do. Active lymphoid proliferation occurs after transplantation, and cell division in the presence of the mutagenic immunosuppressants may carry an increased risk of transformation of normal cells into cancer.

CUSHING'S DISEASE. Most transplant patients receiving steroid therapy undergo a series of changes that are referred to as iatrogenic Cushing's syndrome. The rate of its development is a result of the dose of steroid and number of rejection episodes. The appearance of the face is altered by rounding, puffiness, and plethora; fat tends to be redistributed from the extremities to the trunk and face. There is also an increased growth of fine hair over the thighs and trunk and sometimes over the face. Acne may increase or appear, and insomnia and increased appetite are noted; however, the underlying metabolic changes that accompany the obvious changes can be serious by the time the latter actually appear. The continuing breakdown of protein and diversion of amino acids to glucose increase the need for insulin and result in weight gain, fat deposition, muscle wasting, thinning of the skin with striae and bruising, hyperglycemia, growth suppression (in children), and sometimes the development of steroid diabetes, cataracts, and osteoporosis. In some patients a myopathy develops, the nature of which is unknown.

The cushingoid changes may on rare occasions represent such a psychologic problem that transplant nephrectomy will be necessary on that basis alone. Women and adolescents are more severely affected physically, and the psychologic problems are greater. These problems can be enormous in children, who grow less well, and most particularly in small girls on chronic steroid therapy, who seem to grow very little after age thirteen. The male psyche tolerates steroids better; the plethora and broad faces give many men a healthier look than they had while on dialysis.

STEROID DIABETES. Steroid diabetes is an occasional complication of chronic steroid administration, even when the steroid doses are not high. This may represent exacerbation of a prediabetic state. The diabetes is often mild, but its onset is frequently insidious, and the patient may have diabetic acidosis before the diabetic state is discovered.

GASTROINTESTINAL BLEEDING. Gastrointestinal bleeding due to reactivation of a preexisting ulcer or diffuse ulceration of the gastrointestinal tract is a frequently fatal

complication. The relative contribution of progressive uremia and repeated massive steroid administration in the pathogenesis of gastrointestinal hemorrhage is unknown, but when bleeding appears, it is severe and difficult to control by nonoperative means. Occasionally the use of cimetidine or the intramesenteric arterial infusion of vasopressin is effective.

During moderate doses of steroid therapy, episodes of gastrointestinal bleeding can be almost totally prevented by the use of antacids between meals. Magaldrate (Riopan) is a useful antacid, since it is required in only small doses. In patients with recurrent rejection who require many episodes of high steroid dosage, antacid therapy must be intensified with each increase in steroid administration. Magnesium-containing antacids, however, are contraindicated in patients with poor renal function, since hypermagnesemia will result.

OTHER INTESTINAL COMPLICATIONS. A number of colonic complications, including diverticulitis, bleeding, and ulceration, is associated with immunosuppressive treatment. A syndrome of acute cecal ulceration with gastrointestinal bleeding has also been reported in transplant patients.

CATARACTS. Cataracts are common in patients who require steroids. The cataracts, which develop slowly, appear to be independent of the absolute prednisone dosage.

THROMBOSIS AND THROMBOEMBOLIC PHENOMENA. Thrombophlebitis may occur in the transplant recipient, particularly on the side of the graft where the venous anastomosis may become partially or completely thrombosed. This complication has occurred in patients who previously had steroid-resistant nephrotic syndrome, and it has been speculated that this is related to recurrence of the original kidney disease. No reason is known for this possible association.

When attention is focused on immunologic and infectious phenomena, thrombophlebitis and pulmonary embolism may be overlooked. Swelling of the leg on the side of the transplant site is a frequent sign of rejection, associated with increases in weight, pulmonary infiltrates, and slight increases in serum creatinine level. When the differential diagnosis is difficult, a femoral venogram is indicated. The diagnosis of pulmonary embolisms may also be difficult, and multiple pulmonary infiltrates should not be treated as fungal pneumonia on the basis of sputum cultures alone.

HYPERTENSION. Many of the patients who come to renal transplantation are already hypertensive. Hypertension can usually be controlled with dialysis or, if more refractory, with nephrectomy. Hypertension in most patients will develop soon after transplantation, but posttransplant hypertension is mild and easily controlled with dietary salt restriction and drugs. The hypertension seems to be due not only to prednisone but also to failure to regulate the normal salt and water balance in the early posttransplant period and secretion of renin by the kidney. Nevertheless, antihypertensive drugs can usually be stopped as maintenance levels of prednisone are reached. Hypertension returns with rejection and may be a sign of this problem. It should be remembered, however, that significant hypertension may be due to renal arterial stenosis, and arteriography may be necessary for the differentiation.

DISORDERS OF CALCIUM METABOLISM. Patients frequently come to transplantation with renal osteodystrophy. Alterations in vitamin D metabolism and secondary hyperparathyroidism are prominent factors in the pathogenesis of skeletal disease. Long-standing acidosis may likewise be contributory. The resulting osteoporosis, osteomalacia, and osteitis fibrosa cystica in the child can lead to growth restriction, epiphysiolysis, skeletal deformities, and pathologic fractures. The bone disease in some cases can be arrested with pharmacologic doses of vitamin D or aluminum hydroxide, or by total or subtotal parathyroidectomy.

Hemodialysis can correct the uremic state, but the bone disease may actually progress if the stimulus to parathyroid hormone secretion is not effectively eliminated. Great attention should be directed toward keeping the dialysate calcium concentration at a level (6 to 7 mg/100 ml) that does not promote calcium loss from the blood. Again, parathyroidectomy may be indicated if osteitis fibrosa cystica is progressive and cannot be reversed by maintaining the calcium concentration in the serum at normal or slightly elevated levels.

Parathyroidectomy performed in the patient with renal failure or on hemodialysis may help to arrest progressive bone disease. Frequently, however, the calcium levels will remain high and will fall only after renal transplantation. Conversely, if prompt transplantation from a related donor is planned or if the cadaver list is short, transplantation by itself will usually lead to the reversal of the hyperparathyroid state. The hypercalcemia of the immediate post-transplant period can be managed with a high-phosphate diet, low calcium intake, and furosemide diuretics. Even patients with flagrant osteitis fibrosa cystica with metastatic calcification will respond to transplantation alone without parathyroidectomy. Parathyroidectomy seems primarily indicated for patients on chronic hemodialysis in whom transplantation is not planned.

The role of persistent (tertiary) hyperparathyroidism after successful renal transplantation has been difficult to assess. At the present, parathyroidectomy is rarely indicated after transplant.

MUSCULOSKELETAL COMPLICATIONS. A most disturbing complication of successful renal transplantation is avascular necrosis of the femoral heads and other bones. Its occurrence is most closely correlated with the dosage of steroid used. Transient rheumatoid symptoms precede changes visible by radiography by several months. The bone changes apparently occur secondarily to steroid osteopenia or osteonecrosis with resulting microfractures. Alterations in lipid metabolism caused by fluctuating high levels of steroids likewise appear to be important in explaining the pathogenesis. The treatment is for the most part symptomatic. It is doubtful that bone lesions can revascularize sufficiently to restore normal architecture in the presence of maintenance steroids. Should symptoms increase in the hip and bone destruction progress, replacement arthroplasty may be indicated.

Migratory arthralgis, myalgia, and tendonitis are common, but persistent joint pain and swelling are most often signs of intraarticular infection. Occasionally, an unexplained septic arthritis crops up in these patients.

PANCREATITIS. Pancreatitis may appear suddenly and unexpectedly in renal allograft recipients; it may occasionally be fatal. Its cause is obscure; it has been attributed variously to corticosteroid therapy, azathioprine, cytomegalovirus, or hepatitis virus. The clinical course is sometimes accompanied by increases in serum creatinine, which may or may not be related to rejection. Most cases subside with conventional therapy and do not recur.

ERYTHREMIA AND ANEMIA. The transplanted kidney is apparently fully capable of manufacturing and secreting erythropoietin. During rejection, the serum level may be increased. Erythremia also may appear, but apparently it is not related to elevated erythropoietin levels.

Anemia usually is not present except in association with uremia or immunodepression secondary to azathioprine toxicity. A microangiopathic hemolytic anemia has also been thought to be induced by the vascular changes within the chronically rejecting organ.

GROWTH. The antiproliferative effects of immunosuppressive drugs would seem to make satisfactory growth in children unlikely after transplantation. Since chronic renal failure itself is inhibitory to development, these children are usually far behind their peers in size. After successful transplantation their growth response is highly variable and may depend on age, previous growth rate, renal function, and immunosuppressive drug regimen. Many children return to a normal growth rate; unfortunately the growth that was lost during their original illness is not made up, so these children will always be smaller than their peers.

Wound healing, a specific case in this category, is to all outward appearances normal. It is apparent clinically, however, that wound healing is severely affected when debilitation, chronic renal failure, and high steroid levels are present.

PREGNANCY. Many arguments can be raised against the likelihood of a successful pregnancy and a normal child being born when a patient has received a kidney graft. Excessive steroid levels, the antigrowth and mutagenic effects of the immunosuppressive agents, and viral activation and infection all should be detrimental to the fetus. As usual, however, the story is complicated.

By 1975 the Human Transplant Registry had reported on 132 graft recipients who had become parents. The experience at the University of Minnesota has been examined in detail and seems to be representative. Of these patients, 17 became pregnant after transplantation, and 12 children were born. Only one spontaneous abortion occurred. The children had a normal size distribution, and no congenital defects were found. There is no doubt, however, that azathioprine, and probably steroids, are mutagenic and that the risk of congenital abnormalities is real. Multiple defects have been reported in the child of a male transplant recipient. From the overall experience, it would appear that the risk is not high, but the incidence is still unknown. Steroids also cause their own peculiar problems, and a few cases of severe neonatal adrenocortical insufficiency, as well as lymphopenia, have been reported.

Transplant recipients who are pregnant are often beset with medical problems. Toxemia has occurred in over half the pregnancies, and bacterial and viral infections, particularly of the urinary tract, are common. Both these factors may contribute to the higher incidence of premature labor that has been reported. Another important medical concern is the effect of the pregnancy on renal functions. Although the data are insufficient to judge whether or not pregnancy is deleterious to kidney function, each series has apparent examples that show it may be. An indication for the termination of pregnancy is the compromise of graft function. The increased risk of cancer, in particular of the cervix, in transplant patients has already been discussed. The effect of pregnancy on this tendency is unknown. Another important problem that must be faced is the decreased life expectancy of the transplant recipient. Parenthood is a long-term obligation, and counseling of these patients should include a discussion of these considerations.

TOLERANCE. Many kidneys survive for years in their new host. That this represents an acquired tolerance, a specific nonreactivity to the graft antigens, has been suggested in the literature and is hoped for in immunosuppressive therapy. The question of tolerance has been raised earlier in this chapter, and the possible means of achieving it will be discussed under Experimental Immunosuppression, below. It has been found that even after long accommodation of graft and host, cessation of immunosuppressive therapy almost invariably leads to rejection. Some adaptation must occur, however, and long-term graft survival can be achieved at immunosuppressive dosages which do not immunologically cripple the recipient or produce other severe toxic consequences.

EXPERIMENTAL IMMUNOSUPPRESSION

The complexity of the immune response gives rise to the hope that many potential points of vulnerability exist. New approaches are constantly being tried and old ones refined to produce better immunosuppressive therapy.

ANTIGEN RECOGNITION AND PROCESSING. An obvious, if difficult, approach to immunosuppression would be to alter or mask graft antigens. Evidence exists that by perfusing the organ, before transplantation, with concanavalin A (Con A) the host response to it may be reduced. Although the mechanism is not known, presumably, Con A aggregates on graft cell surfaces and interferes in some way with host recognition. Subsequently, the cell membrane is cleared by normal repair processes, but may no longer be as antigenic as before.

Many agents have been tried to generally blockade the reticuloendothelial systems. Talc and gold, to name a few, can depress particle uptake and presumably antigen processing, by these cells. The effect of talc and gold on graft survival, however, has been negligible.

IMMUNOSUPPRESSION BY SPECIFIC ANTIGENS. The complications of immunosuppression constantly reinforce the importance of developing modes of immunosuppression that will be specific for the incompatible graft anti-

gens. The immunosuppressive drugs and antilymphocyte globulin all act by suppressing the capacity of the immunocompetent cell to respond to any antigen. Thus, even ALG, with its predilection for cellular immunity, cannot select between T cells destined to reject an allograft and T cells necessary for immunity against viruses and tumors. The ability to produce a state of tolerance would obviously be of enormous benefit to the field of transplantation. Experimentally, a functional state of tolerance has been produced in two general ways—manipulation of the stimulating antigens, and infusion of specific antibodies; both have been successful.

A variety of conditions has been shown to predispose to the introduction of tolerance, rather than immunity, on exposure to antigen. The best example of antigen-directed immunologic unresponsiveness is the tolerance enjoyed by animals to their own body constituents. This apparently develops early, before or during maturation of the immune mechanism, and is usually maintained throughout life. Burnet, as part of his clonal selection hypothesis, considered this unresponsive state to result from direct contact between "self" antigens and the individual's own lymphocytes. The clones of lymphocytes reactive to "self" are eliminated, and tolerance ensues. He further predicted that specific unresponsiveness could be induced to foreign antigens if they were given very early in life. Experimental proof by Billingham, Brent, and Medawar followed and demonstrated tolerance to histocompatibility antigens after neonatal injection of replicating allogeneic cells.

Obviously this opportunity has passed for transplant patients, but under certain carefully controlled conditions, tolerance has been produced experimentally in adult animals. Thus, hope exists for future progress in this area, and several techniques have yielded limited but encouraging results. Repeated injection of small, subimmunogenic doses of antigen or the use of very large amounts of antigen preparations has produced unresponsiveness. When these preparations are cleared of aggregated material, the tendency to induced tolerance is greater. Certain antigens (e.g., serum proteins) are endowed with properties that are particularly favorable for the induction of immunologic unresponsiveness. These seem to be the ability to persist in the circulation and equilibrate within the extravascular spaces, thereby coming in contact with antigen-reactive cells in effective concentration. Whether or not this results in deletion of the antigen-reactive lymphocytes, however, is unknown. More likely suppressor cells are selectively or predominantly stimulated by such antigenic presentation.

Unfortunately, viral and bacterial antigens and transplantation antigens do not have these properties and, in addition, may possess multiple antigenic specificities. A diminished response to transplantation antigens can be induced in adult animals, but the antigen dose, physical state of the antigen, and route of injection all must be carefully chosen to avoid immunization. Tolerance is more easily produced to weak antigens; therefore, close histocompatibility matching is desirable. Irradiation, chemical immunosuppression, and antilymphocyte globulins have been used to inhibit the immune response and potentiate the emergence of a relatively unresponsive state. Although only modest successes have been achieved so far by these approaches, careful control of the conditions of antigen presentation may yet be important in the production of tolerance.

Recently, attempts to produce tolerance have utilized antigens tagged with radioactive compounds or alkylating agents. The purpose is to form a lethal combination with the specifically reactive lymphocyte clones and eliminate them. So far, only a hyporesponse state of short duration has been induced, but this approach may yet be fruitful.

In summary, the induction of tolerance by manipulating the presentation of the incompatible antigens is an attractive idea. So far, success for allografts has not been achieved, but it remains a promising pathway.

IMMUNOSUPPRESSION BY SPECIFIC ANTIBODIES. Tolerance can be easily defined. A conceptual understanding of tolerance is readily attained by considering the lack of reactivity toward self. Understanding the subcellular mechanisms involved is far more difficult, and they are unknown at this time. Tolerance may result from the absence of the reactive clone of lymphocytes or from the predominance of a suppressor clone. An alternative to these mechanisms is that tolerance is due to an antibody that interferes with the development of immunity. Certainly the immune system is regulated and subject to feedback control; the presence of an adequate level of antibody may block further activity. Experimentally, the immune response can be eliminated by the passive transfer of specific antibody prior to, or shortly after, giving the antigen.

Two general mechanisms for this phenomenon have been proposed. In the first the antibodies formed are inactive and do not trigger the effector mechanisms such as complement. These blocking antibodies have been best demonstrated in tumor immunology, where they have been shown to enhance the growth of transplanted tumors and prevent rejection. The second explanation is that these antibodies produce a negative feedback effect. The most striking example of this is the prevention of erythroblastosis fetalis in newborns by the administration of an Rh factor antiserum to the pregnant mother. The antiRh antibodies suppress the synthesis of antibodies in response to the foreign Rh antigens. Both these mechanisms for production of tolerance require the presence of antibody to the antigen. While the appropriate antibodies cannot always be detected in animals following the induction of "tolerance," they are often present. Furthermore, antibodies are frequently detected in patients with well-functioning, long-term kidney allografts. Graft function is thought to be prolonged by the presence of a specific antibody that inhibits the development of truly effective antigraft immunity. If immunosuppression is reduced, however, the balance is tipped and the common result of graft rejection is observed. Consequently, the apparently paradoxical hypothesis that tolerance to an antigen requires the presence of antibodies to that antigen may yet be valid.

When applied to transplantation, the application of this theory has yielded some success. The best results, however, for experimental kidney graft prolongation have been following the administration of both graft-specific antigens

and antibodies against them. Therefore, the distinction between antigen and antibody-induced tolerance is blurred, and they may meet at virtually the same point in the subcellular response.

IMMUNOSUPPRESSION BY CELLULAR MECHANISMS. Even more theoretical than the preceding are two recent proposals for inducing immunological unresponsiveness. As previously mentioned, the ability to induce a sufficient number of suppressor T cells could effectively block graft rejection. A further requirement, of course, would be that the suppressor cells are antigen-specific or general immunosuppression would result.

Additional leverage on the immune response may be gained by manipulating the genes which govern the response to histocompatibility antigens. Not all individuals respond in the same way to different histocompatibility antigens, and part of this difference may be ascribable to a specific genetic locus. Matching the immune response governing loci in a similar way to aligning histocompatibility antigens may yield improved results.

INHIBITION OF LYMPHOCYTE METABOLISM. Normal cell metabolism results in turnover of adenine and other purines and pyrimidines. Several enzymes, including adenosine deaminase and purine nucleoside phosphorylase, are necessary for purine salvage and are present in all tissues. Lymphocytes may be unique in that absence of either enzyme cripples cell function and clinically is associated with a severe immunodeficiency state. This has stimulated investigation of experimental production of immunosuppression using adenine analogues to inhibit these enzymes selectively. It is possible that this approach may become clinically useful because other tissues do not seem to require this pathway and toxicity is low. Part of the immunosuppressive activity of azathioprine may be due to this mechanism.

INTERFERENCE WITH NONSPECIFIC EFFECTORS. The combination of sensitized cells or antibodies with the foreign antigens marks the beginning of the active effort to dispose of the graft. The complex of sensitized cells or antibodies with the antigens triggers the recruitment of a multitude of effector systems. We have mentioned the cascading enzyme systems, the complement, clotting, and kinin pathways, as well as the cellular mediators, lymphocytes, macrophages, platelets, and polymorphonuclear leukocytes. These are enlisted both by the specific immunological reaction itself and as a result of subsequent events. All play an active role in disposing of the allograft.

It is conceivable that one could reduce the effect of an immune response by (1) interfering with the complement, clotting, and kinin cascades that are activated by antigen-antibody complexes; (2) destroying factors secreted by activated cells (migration-inhibiting factor, chemotactic factor, cytophilic antibody, transfer factor, mitogenic factor); or (3) neutralizing the vascular permeability factors, lysosomal enzymes, or lymphotoxins.

A number of agents or combination of agents that interfere with the expression of immunity have been tested. For example, anticomplementary drugs (vitamin A, cobra venom factor) are either ineffective or, if potent, are short-acting and not clinically useful. Antimacrophage globulin, carrageenin, and silica all destroy macrophages but are weak transplant immunosuppressants. Antibodies to lymphotoxins or migration-inhibitory factors and other effector molecules are still in very early experimental states of evaluation. Antihistamines and antiserotonin agents are also relatively weak immunosuppressant drugs. Anticoagulants (heparin), agents that interfere with platelet aggregation (dipyridamole, aspirin), and fibrinolytic agents have been employed to interfere with the thrombosis of graft vessels. The antiplatelet agents have been found to improve long-term clinical function in both kidney and cardiac grafts and will undoubtedly be more widely used in the future. More information is needed on the role platelets play in the production of arterial narrowing, which seems often to limit graft survival.

The limited success with these agents reinforces the difficulty in attempting to interfere with the immune response after antibody has been synthesized and large numbers of immunologically committed effector cells have been mobilized. In fact, it is difficult to inhibit the secondary or anamnestic response of any immune reaction. Successful interference with the effector mechanism of graft rejection is prohibited by both the complexity and the interdependence of the reaction. Many pathways and cellular participants need to be blocked. In addition, there are points of cross activation between these pathways which make it difficult effectively to inhibit any or all of them. If true immunosuppression is to be achieved, with respect to a certain antigen, interference must take place during the early phases of the primary immune response.

PRIVILEGED SITES FOR ALLOGRAFTS. First-set grafts need to develop either vascular or lymphatic connections to sensitize the host. Certain sites within the recipient, therefore, may permit extended graft survival of first-set grafts. A presensitized recipient can usually reject a second-set allograft before these connections are made, however.

The anterior chamber of the eye has been the most frequently used privileged space for allografts and xenografts of both normal and malignant tissues. Grafts at this site were originally thought to survive because of their inability to sensitize the host, not because they are protected from immunologic mediators of rejection. Tissues in the anterior chamber are rejected if the host is sensitized by conventional means. Therefore, the anterior chamber of the eye has been considered an excellent site for the study of the afferent arc of immunity. It is one of the rare locations in which lymphatic vessels are completely lacking, and the prolonged survival of grafts provides further evidence for the importance of lymphatic connections in host sensitization.

Absence of lymphatic connections may not be the only explanation. Raju and Grogan have presented evidence that grafts within the anterior chamber become vascularized rapidly and sensitize the recipient only slightly less rapidly than other grafts. Despite such sensitization, however, the grafts continue to survive unless sensitization is induced by more conventional techniques. Implants in unsensitized recipients become infiltrated by small round cells which somehow are *not* associated with graft destruction. The extended survival of grafts in the anterior chamber may represent a combination of both afferent arc delay and efferent arc blockade.

Other sites provide a special environment for allografts. It has been known for almost 50 years that the meninges of the brain shelter grafts. The implants must be within the meninges and without encroachment on the ventricles. The extended survival is dependent on a lack of vascular connections to the host, which in turn prevents sensitization. The immunologic insulation of the testis may relate to its circuitous lymphatic supply. Presentation of the antigens to the host may be inefficient. Cartilage, too, can be successfully allografted without immunosuppression. The mucoprotein matrix seems to shield the graft cells from host lymphocytes.

The cheek pouch of the hamster has been used as a location for a variety of foreign grafts. Once again, graft survival is due to reduced ability to sensitize the host, since grafts will not survive in the cheek pouches of hamsters previously sensitized to donor antigens. Even well-established grafts will be rejected promptly if the host is sensitized through conventional means. The immunologic arc seems to be interrupted on the afferent side because the mucopolysaccharide-containing connective tissue of the pouch acts as an immunologic insulator.

HISTOCOMPATIBILITY MATCHING

It is obvious that, other things being equal, the less antigenic the graft, the less the host will react against the graft. In human transplantation, when the donor and recipient are identical twins, there is no antigenic difference of any significance, and the tissues will be readily accepted. When the donor and recipient are siblings or when a parent donor is used for offspring, there is a greater statistical likelihood of antigen sharing between donor and recipient than when a cadaver or other unrelated donor is used.

Several methods have been developed for the purpose of demonstrating antigenic similarities between donor and recipient prior to transplantation, so that donor and recipient pairs may be selected which are relatively histocompatible. This should lessen the need for large doses of immunosuppressive drugs and increase the likelihood of an ultimately successful outcome. Although many methods have been tried, the currently most promising are leukocyte typing and MLC (mixed lymphocyte culture).

LEUKOCYTE TYPING. The rationale for leukocyte typing is based upon two observations: The first is that leukocytes are capable of immunizing animals to a subsequent skin or kidney graft and thus must share many important antigens with these and other tissues of the body. The second rationale is that antisera from certain patients who have received multiple transfusions will react with cells from some patients but not from others. Investigators observed that antisera of this type were also found in certain multiparous women. Subsequently, many antisera obtained from multiply transfused patients or from women with multiple pregnancies (and occasionally from other sources) have been assembled and tested for their ability to detect leukocyte antigens. Some of the antisera seem to recognize groups of antigens, and others recognize single antigens (monospecific antisera). Using the patient's leukocytes and a group of standard antisera it is thus possible to characterize many, if not all, of the strong HLA-A and -B histocompatibility antigens on the human lymphocyte membrane. This is done for both donor and recipient, and the two patterns are then compared to determine whether the donor is likely to be compatible with the recipient or not.

Antigens found less frequently have been identified which appear not to be at this locus; it is likely that other antigenic loci may be defined in the future. The inheritance of HLA antigens was discussed above. Weaker histocompatibility antigens at other loci have not been detected by serologic techniques in human beings.

Currently antigens are detected by isolating lymphocytes from the peripheral blood of potential donors or recipients. The cells are incubated with antisera of various specificities and rabbit serum as a source of complement. Cells which react with antibodies in the serum die in the presence of complement and can be stained with vital dyes. Typing sera is becoming increasingly standardized. A typical set of results from the University of Minnesota typing laboratories is illustrated in Table 10-1.

Histocompatibility typing is useful in determining the best match between donor and recipient when family donors are utilized. Siblings who share all four HL-A antigens in common and who have inherited identical HL-A haplotypes from their parents are the best possible donor-recipient pair. But several points about histocompatibility matching deserve emphasis: (1) Recipients receiving grafts even from donors who are "perfect" matches with them will still reject the graft (although more slowly) unless immunosuppressive drugs are utilized. Only an identical twin is truly a perfect match. In the context used here "perfect" simply means that there are no detectable antigenic differences between donor and host with the antisera employed and that the degree of compatibility is suffi-

ciently high so that, with the judicial use of immunosuppressive drugs, the outcome is likely to be good. (2) Even with poor histocompatibility matches between relatives, the results are frequently good. Those results probably indicate that, with the current immunosuppressive drugs, it is sometimes possible to suppress even great degrees of antigenic incompatibility. (3) Even in the presence of a good histocompatibility match, the graft may fail if the host happens to have preformed antibodies against a donor's tissues. These antibodies can be recognized if recipient serum is allowed to react with donor lymphocytes in a cytotoxicity test. This test, called *cross matching,* should be performed with fresh serum as a final test of compatibility prior to transplant. Preformed cytotoxic antibodies to donor tissue cannot be detected by the usual typing procedure itself. (4) The presence of ABH antibodies will lead to the prompt rejection of tissue bearing incompatible blood group substances. Transplants in the face of such barriers should not be performed. (5) Despite the results of tissue typing, a related donor will generally yield better transplant results than an unrelated (cadaver) donor. This statement is controversial, but the results of kidney transplantation strongly support it. (6) Tissue typing for unrelated cadaver donors is not as successful as typing for related donors, but increasing evidence supports the correlation between graft success and HLA-A and -B locus matching (Fig. 10-27).

MIXED LYMPHOCYTE CULTURE (MLC). The other method of detecting degrees of histocompatibility between donor and recipient is the MLC test, which detects differences principally at the HLA-D locus. Lymphocytes of the recipient are mixed with lymphocytes of the donor in tissue culture. If significant antigenic differences exist between the two, they will respond by transformation into blast cells, DNA synthesis, and mitosis. The incorporation of tritiated thymidine into DNA can be quantified to assess the degree of stimulation. As the test was originally de-

Table 10-1. LYMPHOCYTE ANTIGEN TYPING REPORT OF THEORETIC FAMILY*

Family member	ABO	Genotype	HL-A locus (LA)								HL-A 2d locus (four)														
			HL-A1	HL-A2	HL-A3	HL-A9	HL-A10	HL-A11	W19	W28	HL-A5	HL-A7	HL-A8	HL-A12	HL-A13	W5	W10	W14	W15	W16	W17	W18	W21	W22	W27
Father AB	A	AO	+	+	–	–	–	–	–	–	–	+	+	–	–	–	–	–	–	–	–	–	–	–	–
Mother CD	A	AO	–	–	+	+	+	–	–	–	+	–	–	+	–	–	–	–	–	–	–	–	–	–	–
Son AC (patient)	O	OO	+	–	+	–	–	–	–	–	+	–	+	–	–	–	–	–	–	–	–	–	–	–	–
Son AD	A	?	+	–	–	+	+	–	–	–	–	–	+	+	–	–	–	–	–	–	–	–	–	–	–
Daughter BC	O	OO	–	+	+	–	–	–	–	–	+	+	–	–	–	–	–	–	–	–	–	–	–	–	–
Daughter BD	A	?	–	+	–	+	+	–	–	–	–	+	–	+	–	–	–	–	–	–	–	–	–	–	–
Daughter AC	O	OO	+	–	+	–	–	–	–	–	+	–	+	–	–	–	–	–	–	–	–	–	–	–	–

*The specificities for the first and second loci are those currently used at the University of Minnesota.

Son AC is the prospective transplant recipient. Daughter AC is a perfect match for all four antigens; she shares the inheritance of both HL-A haplotypes and is the ideal donor. Both parents, son AD, and daughter BC share only one haplotype with the potential recipient and are theoretically not as good donors. Daughter BD shares no HL-A haplotypes with the recipient and is the poorest donor in the family.

More important than the HL-A type are the ABO blood types. The father, mother, son AD, and daughter BD *cannot* donate, because they are all blood group A and the recipient is blood group O and possesses anti-A antibodies in his serum.

vised, it was a two-way test—cells of the donor were capable of reacting against cells of the recipient and vice versa. In order to isolate the response of the recipient cells to the donor antigens, the donor lymphocytes can be inactivated by irradiation or exposure to mitomycin C. More and more evidence supports the usefulness of this test in predicting success in organ and bone marrow transplantation.

CLINICAL TISSUE AND ORGAN TRANSPLANTATION

Clinical allotransplants may be of several types: (1) temporary free grafts, such as skin allografts and blood transfusions; (2) partially inert struts which provide a framework for the ingrowth of host tissue, such as bone, cartilage, nerve, tendon, and fascial grafts; (3) permanent, partially privileged, structurally free grafts, such as cornea, blood vessels, and heart valves; (4) partially privileged functional free grafts such as parathyroid, ovary, and testes; (5) whole organ grafts, such as pancreas, kidney, liver, lung, and heart; and (6) bone marrow which acts as a functional replacement of the entire hemopoietic and lymphopoietic systems. Immunosuppression is warranted only for grafts essential for life. Tooth bud and thyroid grafts, which would require immunosuppression for any success, are trivial grafts and are easily replaced by prostheses or medication.

Clinical autotransplants have been carried out with hair, skin, teeth, kidney, legs, arms, veins, arteries, pericardium, valves, bone, cartilage, fascia, fat, tendons, nerves, stomach, bowel, parathyroid, thyroid, ovary, testis, adrenal, and hemopoietic tissue. Allotransplants have been carried out employing cornea, teeth, thyroid, parathyroid, adrenal, ovary, testis, pituitary, spleen, lymph node, bone marrow, skin, bone, cartilage, fascia, tendons, nerves, arteries, valves, veins, hemopoietic tissue, pancreas, duodenum, kidney, liver, lung, and heart. Xenografts of skin, heart valves, heart, kidney, testis, bone, and cartilage have been tried in the past.

Skin

Autotransplants of skin containing hair are used to reconstruct eyebrows or to replace the scalp after traumatic avulsion. Autotransplants of individual hair roots are sometimes used as a treatment for baldness. Skin autotransplants have been used to reconstruct the esophagus, urinary tract, vagina, and hernial weaknesses as well as the usual surface defects. The main use of skin autografts is to cover and replace areas destroyed by trauma, burn, or operation.

Skin allotransplants are also used quite extensively in burned patients. They are commonly used in three different ways: In the first they are applied as a dressing to the burned area and are removed after 3 or 4 days. At this time additional allografts are reapplied if the area does not appear to be clean enough to accept autografts. If the area does appear to be clean, autografts are applied. The theory behind this is that the skin allograft provides a better

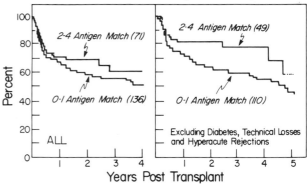

Fig. 10-27. The effect of tissue typing on the subsequent function of cadaver renal allografts at the University of Minnesota. If more (two to four) of the antigens are matched between graft and recipient, better kidney function is likely to result. If only zero to one of the four HLA-A and -B antigens on graft and recipient cells are the same, success is less likely. This difference is enhanced if diabetic recipients, technical kidney losses, and kidneys rejected by hyperacute reactions are excluded.

coverage than any other material, and during the period of time when it is taking, it prevents the continued spread of sepsis.

The second method is to place alternate thin strips of autografted and allografted skin side by side to cover large defects. As the allografted skin is gradually rejected, it is replaced by epithelial cells which grow in from the autografts.

In the last method the allograft is applied and allowed to take. When it begins to be rejected, it is removed, and autografts are applied. Prolongation up to 50 days of skin allograft survival can be achieved with immunosuppression. Massive burns can now be treated with excision and allografting within the first 10 days postburn. The allografts are then serially excised and replaced with autografts as the initially limited autograft donor sites regenerate. Bacterial complications of the burn and immunosuppression are minimized by temporarily housing the patient in protected "germ-free" environments.

Xenografts of skin are commonly used as temporary biologic dressings to be replaced at 2- to 4-day intervals. The commercial preparations of pig skin are nonviable and do not become vascularized. Similarly, chemically fixed grafts might be useful in the future as temporary covers to reduce burn mortality and morbidity.

Vascular Grafts

AUTOGRAFTS

Vein autografts have been used for over 50 years to replace segments of damaged arteries. This is still by far the best bypass graft for occluded vessels in the lower extremity below the level of the inguinal ligament. After a period of time in the arterial circuit the vein wall thickens, and the vein becomes somewhat arterialized. Although there are occasional instances in which vein grafts weaken and rupture, by and large they make very satisfactory arterial substitutes. The three most common usages at the present time are in femoro–popliteal artery–saphenous vein bypass grafts, aorto–renal artery–saphenous vein bypass grafts, and coronary artery bypass grafts. Pieces of autologous vein are also used as patch grafts either for small stenotic areas, such as the renal artery, or over long segments of endarterectomized artery. It is also possible to carry out successful autologous vein grafts to bridge defects in veins, although veins are less likely to stay open than arteries. Autologous vein grafts have also been used as tendon sheath and bile duct replacement without success.

Autografted arteries are also sometimes used as vascular replacements—most often the hypogastric artery is utilized. Pieces of pericardium are sometimes used to patch defects or divert flow in the repair of intracardiac defects.

ALLOGRAFTS

The use of allografted arteries had a considerable vogue a few years ago, but they are seldom used now. There are three reasons for this: (1) aneurysms sometimes occur, with rupture and a fatal outcome; (2) plastic prostheses have proved so suitable for the larger blood vessels; (3) for smaller blood vessels the use of the autologous saphenous vein has proved to be better than either prostheses or allografts. Arterial allografts, even if viable, do not survive but in part are replaced by host tissue and in part persist as semi-inert material.

When organs are transplanted, the artery supplying the organ becomes an arterial allograft. It has been shown that the epithelium of smaller blood vessels is antigenic and some degree of allograft rejection occurs.

Fresh, sterile aortic valve allografts have been used quite extensively. They appear to elicit a minimal antigenic response when compared with arterial allografts. Even so, gradual thickening, immobility, and calcification of these valves occur; their functional life expectancy in patients has not yet been determined.

Vein allografts have been used for a number of years in sporadic fashion, and umbilical vein allografts have become commercially available for arterial bypass. Allografts have always been, and will almost certainly continue to be, inferior to fresh autografts. There is, of course, no reason whatsoever for the inferiority of arterial and venous grafts to autografts of the same type *except* for the antigenicity of the allograft and the mild rejection reaction which these grafts elicit. For some reason there has been a great reluctance among surgeons and others to accept the fact that arterial and venous allografts are antigenic. It is true that the antigenicity is relatively mild and that the graft can provide structural function even in the face of the immunologic response, but it eventually limits the life of the graft.

Fascia

Fascial autografts, either free or attached at one end, are used as living sutures to repair inguinal hernias; for the repair of chest wall defects, torn ligaments and tendons, abdominal wall hernias, and defects in the pleura, dura, diaphragm, trachea, and esophagus; for wrapping aneurysms; in arthroplasty; for fascial slings to correct paralysis of the facial muscles; in the stabilization of fractures and joints; in the construction of flexor sheaths; and to correct urinary incontinence. Fascial autografts have been used most commonly because of their convenience and ready availability. Some freeze-dried, preserved (nonviable) allografts have been used, however, and these dead grafts have united with muscle nearly as quickly as living fascia. Such allografts lose much of their histoincompatibility and serve as strong lattice for the ingrowth of autologous tissue.

Tendon

Free tendon autografts are used every day in standard surgical procedures. By far the most common use is that of repairing severed flexor tendons to the fingers. Usually the palmaris longus or extensor tendons of the toes are used, and the graft is inserted from the level of the midpalm of the hand to the distal phalanx.

The only use of a tendon allograft is that suggested by Peacock and Madden, in which both flexor tendons and all surrounding tissue are removed from the hand and finger of a cadaver prior to transplantation into a recipient with loss of digital flexor mechanism. Under these circumstances, adhesions form only to the outer layer of the tissue, and the graft continues to glide against the inner surfaces which are normally against it. The advantage of this technique is to prevent adhesions from disrupting the function of the digital flexor mechanism. The cadaver allograft apparently works better and for longer periods of time than the more frequently utilized silastic rod to develop a nonadherent tunnel. The technique, however, is cumbersome, and cadavers are not readily available. Stored, freeze-dried, nonviable flexor tendons should serve as well, and the development of tissue banks may permit wider application of this technique.

Nerve

Nerve autotransplants are used to bridge defects in important motor nerves or sometimes to transfer the function of one nerve into the distal end of another, to repair a severed facial or recurrent laryngeal nerve, for instance. It has been nearly 100 years since it was demonstrated that a nerve autograft was capable of conducting impulses across a nerve defect. The autografts undergo wallerian degeneration with proliferation of Schwann cells and are penetrated by regenerating fibers of the host's nerve after a few weeks. When the nerve graft is thick, the center of the graft may develop a zone of avascular necrosis in which regeneration fails to occur, whereas this does not happen with thin grafts. As a consequence of this, some investigators have advocated the use of cable grafts consisting of several strands of smaller nerves to bridge defects in nerves of large caliber. Sensory recovery can occur as well as motor recovery.

When allografts are used, wallerian degeneration also

takes place but occurs a little more slowly than in autografts. The proliferation of Schwann cells is not as vigorous as in autografts, and after a few days the cells appear to become necrotic. Despite this fact, allografts are capable of penetration by the nerve fibers and have permitted return of nerve function across the defect. The rate and intensity of nerve fiber penetration is less in allografts than in autografts. The ultimate outcome of allografts is clearly far inferior to that obtained with autografts, and in general they should probably be used only when autografts cannot be obtained. Xenografts have been tried but appear to be of no value to man. It is likely that the inflammatory rejection response interferes with the passage of autologous nerve endings down the transplanted nerve sheath.

Cornea

Perhaps the most common clinical allotransplant is that of the cornea. The eye should be harvested from cadavers within at least 1 hour after death, although intervals up to 5 hours are permissible. Eyes removed more than 15 hours after death are unsuitable for corneal transplantation. The whole eye is generally preserved in sterile liquid paraffin at a temperature of 3 to 5°C, and the graft is cut from it at the time of use. The eye is suspended from a suture passed through the severed optic nerve to keep it from coming in contact with the sides of the vessel. Frozen corneas are not as good as those preserved this way, and freeze-dried corneas are completely unsatisfactory. Xenografts are useless.

Two types of corneal transplants are utilized; the full-thickness graft and the lamellar, or partial-thickness, graft. The full-thickness graft should give the best results, but complications such as secondary glaucoma, anterior synechiae, and a partial lifting off of the graft, causing astigmatism or opacification, are frequent. These complications are avoided in lamellar keratoplasty, which is the operation of choice when the corneal opacity does not involve the full thickness of the cornea. In order to achieve a successful graft there must be good apposition between the graft and the host, the graft must be in contact with healthy cornea at some point in the circumference if it is to remain transparent, and blood vessels must not invade the graft to any appreciable extent.

The best patients for grafting are those with central corneal scars and healthy surrounding cornea with no vascularization; keratoconus, especially if the apex of the cone is beginning to break down; corneal dystrophy; indolent corneal abscesses; and perforating ulcers of the cornea which have resulted in a descemetocele. The results are somewhat less good in acne rosacea and herpetic keratitis because of the danger of recurrence of the disease.

Corneal grafts are apparently so successful because they remain effectively isolated from the host's cells so long as the graft itself and the cornea directly around it remain avascular. Many corneal grafts remain clear indefinitely, although occasionally a graft which has remained clear for several weeks becomes opaque. Apparently the fibrous barrier which is formed at the junction between the host and the graft is almost impervious to blood vessels and helps to maintain the isolation of the graft even when vessels have entered the host's cornea. The clouding over of a previously clear graft is due to the allograft reaction, usually because of vascularization. It has been demonstrated experimentally that if a graft of skin from the donor of the cornea is put on 2 to 6 weeks after corneal transplantation, the graft becomes opaque, whereas if a skin homograft from another donor is applied, nothing happens. Skin from the original donor transplanted 6 weeks or more after the corneal transplantation is no longer capable of causing it to become opaque. This is presumably due to adaptation, the development of the scar tissue barrier between the host and the graft, or replacement of the cells of the graft by host's cells. Recently, short-term organ culture of corneas in order to reduce graft immunogenicity has been tried, but it is not yet known if this will improve the clinical results.

Bone

Bone implants are used for the following indications: (1) to hasten the healing of defects and cavities, e.g., the use of cancellous bone chips in the residual defect after curettage of a unicameral bone cyst; (2) to supplement the arthrodesis of joints, e.g., extraarticular arthrodesis of the tuberculous hip; (3) to achieve bony union in cases of delayed healing or pseudarthrosis arising after fracture, e.g., sliding or barrel stave grafts for nonunion of tibial shaft fractures; (4) to supplement the healing of certain fresh fractures for which open reduction and internal fixation are required, e.g., cancellous implants for fractures of both bones of the forearm in an adult; (5) to reconstruct major skeletal defects arising as a result of trauma, disease, or congenital malformation; (6) to reconstruct contour, e.g., replacement of calvarial defects after surgery for trauma by compact bone implants.

A variety of grafting techniques has been devised to meet the differing clinical requirements. The most frequent types of bone grafts are inlay grafts, onlay grafts and/or internal fixation, barrel stave grafts, sliding grafts, and application of cancellous chips. In addition, there are pedicled grafts of two types, those with a bony base and muscle pedicle grafts. The pedicle technique applies strictly to autografts and was devised to circumvent devitalization, thereby hastening healing.

Autografts are preferred for clinical use, since the cellular elements of bone allografts usually elicit a rejection response. Bone allografts do elicit new bone formation (osteoinduction) and serve as struts for the ingrowth of autologous bone (osteoconduction). As such, allografts are of great clinical use although they are always somewhat inferior to autografts.

For the most part stored or processed bone allografts are used in human beings. Preservation methods include (1) refrigeration, (2) freezing, (3) freeze-drying, (4) boiling or autoclaving, (5) deproteinization, (6) decalcification, (7) any one of the above plus irradiation for sterilization, and (8) removal of marrow elements and replacement by autologous marrow. Such nonviable grafts mainly serve to stimulate and conduct new autologous bone formation.

Cartilage

It has been long known that cartilage can be successfully transferred between individuals of different genetic backgrounds without the need for immunosuppression therapy. This immunologic privilege is attributable to the presence of the mucoprotein matrix, which acts as an insulation to prevent host lymphocytes from reaching the graft chondrocytes. Cartilage cells can elicit allograft responses, but cartilage grafts will survive even in highly immunized hosts.

Free autografts of cartilage have been used most extensively in plastic reconstructive surgery (1) to rebuild the contours of the nose after congenital or posttraumatic deformity, (2) to reconstruct the pinna, and (3) to fill out defects in the facial bones and the skull.

The fresh cartilage autograft comes closest to fulfilling the description of an ideal cartilage graft: it should maintain its structure, have the potential for growth and repair, provoke no untoward reaction, and form a firm union with host tissues, persisting without loss of viability or absorption.

The fresh cartilage allograft, however, has been a reasonable substitute for the autograft, particularly because of its greater ease of procurement. The major drawback of such grafts is that despite the immunologic privilege of cartilage, the bulk of experimental and clinical evidence suggests that the tendency for late deterioration and absorption is somewhat greater than that of autografts.

The preserved cartilaginous allograft has been used as a substitute for the fresh implant primarily because of the convenience that storage of such implants in cartilage banks provides. Boiled, refrigerated, frozen, and chemically preserved sections of cartilage have all been used with success.

The cartilage xenograft should be mentioned since it enjoys a prolonged survival and relative exemption from transplantation rejection unrivaled by any other tissue. Even so, the exemption is not complete, and some xenografts elicit strong inflammatory responses and are absorbed.

COMPOSITE GRAFTS OF BONE AND CARTILAGE

Composite grafts involve the surgical transfer of entire functional units rather than the implantation of bits and pieces of cartilage or bone.

EPIPHYSEAL GROWTH PLATES. The object of the transplantation of epiphyseal growth plates is to restore longitudinal growth in hypoplastic limbs, whether congenital or acquired. This type of procedure has been used in efforts to improve the function of children with congenital deficiency of the radius. In these cases, autotransplantation of the proximal fibula has been used as a substitute for the radial deficiency. Although, in some cases, enlargement of the transplant could be demonstrated, this was always inferior to the natural growth potential and has not been sufficient to justify incorporation of this procedure into the surgical armamentarium.

OSTEOCHONDRAL GRAFTS. The diseases that destroy the articular cartilage are common. The osteochondral or osteoarticular graft might be a useful substitute. Transplants of articular cartilage, in conjunction with a very thin shell of subchondral supporting bone, are still in the experimental stage. Such operations will require allografting.

TRANSPLANT OF HEMIJOINTS OR WHOLE JOINTS. The experimental transplantation of joints was initiated by Judet in 1908. Autografts tend to heal their osteosynthesis sites, revascularize the bony component, and in general maintain the articular surfaces in a fair state of preservation. On the other hand, both fresh and preserved allogenic transplants give unpredictable results, sometimes healing well with good function, and other times showing progressive deterioration. These latter changes in the allogenic groups are associated with delayed revascularization of the bony component, subchondral fracture and collapse, and the late development of degenerative arthritic change. Artificial hemijoints or whole joints have superseded transplantation, at least for the present.

Extremity Replantation

Autotransplants or replantation of extremities have been carried out with increasing frequency in recent years. This has usually involved the upper extremity, because the chances for nerve regeneration are far greater in the arm than in the leg. Satisfactory prostheses exist for the lower extremity, but they are much more complex and unsatisfactory for the upper. Shortening of the reimplanted extremity usually is necessary, and this produces much more incapacity in the leg than in the arm. Replantation of the leg might be considered when the opposite leg has been extensively damaged or lost or when the amputation has been so high that good prostheses are not available. Advances in microsurgery have permitted replantation of digits to become almost routine if adequate experience and appropriate instrumentation, including an operating microscope, are available.

The technique of limb replantation initially requires a general evaluation of the patient to assess other associated injuries. This should include roentgenography of the proximal stump as well as the amputated extremity itself, and particularly of the spine to be certain that the spinal roots to the extremity have not been avulsed. After securing hemostasis and being certain that no serious injury has been overlooked, the replantation can begin. During this initial phase the severed limb should be packed in ice. It should not be frozen, however, and dry ice should be avoided. If the facilities are available, the artery of the limb should be perfused with cold Ringer's lactate solution to which albumin and heparin have been added. The limb may be replanted even though several hours have elapsed between its severance and the start of replantation. The exact critical period has not definitely been established, but it appears that at least 6 hours and sometimes even more can elapse with successful results after replantation. Satisfactory hypothermia of the extremity increases this period. The more distal the amputation, the better the preservation of the extremity, and the more prolonged is the tolerance to ischemia.

When perfusion is completed and replantation is about

to begin, a limited debridement of grossly devitalized tissue is carried out. Questionably viable tissue is not removed. Then the bone is fixed so that the limb will be stabilized before beginning the repairs of the vessels and nerve supply. Larger bones may require slight shortening to freshen up the ends and to gain additional length for relaxation of the arteries and nerves. Intramedullary fixation is used whenever possible.

After proper fixation of the bones the blood vessels are joined. The largest vein is joined first, so that there will be an outflow tract at the moment when the blood is ready to flow through the artery.

If the nerve injury has been a crushing one, nerve repair is delayed until healing is complete. If the nerve has been cleanly severed with a sharp instrument, particularly if the injury has been at the level of the wrist, immediate primary repair is carried out. While the results of nerve allografts are still highly problematic, an autograft or allograft should be used to bridge any large defect in the nerve. A better result is obtained in distal nerve transections than in proximal ones, and in young people as compared with older ones. Motor recovery in the median nerve is much more common than in the ulnar nerve.

After completing the arterial and venous anastomoses and after either joining the ends of the nerves or deciding to perform nerve suture as a secondary procedure, attention is turned to the soft tissues. With the blood supply restored, viability of tissues is easier to ascertain, and debridement can be completed. The shortening of the bone makes it possible to join several muscles together with a particular view to covering the blood vessels with living tissues. If soft tissue loss is minimal, the covering can be achieved with the skin of the extremity, and other defects can be covered with split-thickness skin grafts. If the soft tissue defect is great and no covering is available, the defect must be covered by a pedicle flap.

In the postoperative period the patient's arm must be kept in an elevated position to minimize edema. It is important to do a fasciotomy at the end of the replantation to avoid severe ischemia from swelling if damage to the arm was severe. Heparin and dextran are not generally used postoperatively. Some degree of hypotension may occur as a consequence of leakage of plasma into the replanted extremity. This is particularly true of a lower extremity. The hypotension is counteracted by the administration of plasma. There may be an acute period of acidosis as a consequence of absorption of metabolic products from the ischemic extremity, and this is counteracted by the administration of bicarbonate. Both bicarbonate and mannitol are administered to protect against renal damage, and prophylactic antibiotics are also administered. If early severe sepsis supervenes, the extremity may have to be amputated. Low-grade late infection, usually consisting of osteomyelitis, is treated by drainage and irrigation, and the fixation materials are left in place until the bone heals even in the face of sepsis—because fixation must be achieved if possible.

Passive movement of all joints is begun immediately and continued throughout the course of treatment. Galvanic stimulation of the intrinsic muscles of the hand is utilized to maintain the tone of the muscles. Extensive physical therapy is instituted. If primary nerve suture has not been carried out, the nerves are reexplored 6 weeks or more after the injury, and repair is carried out then. In subsequent months and years many reconstructive but functional results have been surprisingly good.

Hemopoietic and Lymphoid Tissues

BONE MARROW

Bone marrow is easily destroyed by whole-body ionizing irradiation, drugs, or chemicals. The erythrocyte stem cell compartment is the most sensitive site. Its final products, the mature peripheral blood cells, are in most instances not sensitive to injury by irradiation or by chemical substances, but these cells have a relatively short life-span, and a regular supply of new cells is needed. In leukemia, the bone marrow is replaced by tumor cells, a situation effectively the same as that existing when marrow is destroyed by other means.

Injury to bone marrow by drugs, chemicals, and disease poses several clinical problems. Bone marrow transplants between identical twins have been successfully carried out in many cases of irradiation exposure, aplastic anemia, and leukemia. Autologous marrow transplantation has also been found useful in a few patients after planned treatment with toxic levels of alkylating agents.

Marrow allotransplants are far less successful. Marrow is highly immunogenic and will be readily rejected by the immunologically normal host. If, however, the marrow is allotransplanted into an immunologically crippled (irradiated, immunosuppressed) host, a chimera is produced. The problem then becomes, not destruction of the marrow by the host, but the maturation of donor marrow stem cells to total immunological competence and rejection of the host by the graft. This graft-versus-host (GVH) phenomenon is not seen with skin, kidney, heart, liver, grafts, etc., but it is a major, unsolved problem in the transplantation of foreign bone marrow, white blood cells, and lymphoid tissues. Theory predicts, and practice shows, that GVH disease does not occur in bone marrow transplants between identical human twins. An important additional point is the finding of reduced severity of the GVH reaction when the donor and host, even though not genetically identical, have been closely matched at the HLA locus.

The major sites of injury in GVH reactions are the lymphatic tissues, the skin, the intestine, and the liver of the host. Dermatitis, diarrhea, loss of weight, poor liver function, and infection associated with immunoincompetence are intrinsic parts of the reaction. The GVH reactions in bone marrow transplantation in human beings have been of overwhelming importance and are the major problem in this new clinical area. Congdon has summarized some of the experimental and clinical approaches to the problem of the control of GVH disease (Table 10-2). A combination of tissue typing and immunologic suppression is now utilized to control the GVH reaction in human beings.

A long-range goal in marrow transplantation is the use

Table 10-2. SOME APPROACHES TO THE
CONTROL OF GRAFT-VERSUS-HOST DISEASE

A. Immunologic compatibility: histocompatibility typing and
   matching of donor and recipient
B. Immunologic suppression
   1. Treatment of marrow recipient
      a. Methotrexate
      b. Cyclophosphamide
      c. Antilymphocyte serum
   2. Treatment of marrow donor: antilymphocyte serum
C. Removal of immunologically active cells
   1. Manipulation of the marrow in vitro
   2. Cell separation
D. Innate absence of immunocompetent cells: use of fetal and
   newborn blood-forming tissue as the donor source

of these grafts as a means of promoting acceptance of other organs, such as liver, heart, and kidney. Investigations in the mouse have shown that once the foreign marrow is established, a state of relative or complete specific nonreactivity against donor antigens is conferred, and other tissues taken from the same donor as the marrow can be successfully transplanted without further immunosuppression. The transplantation of foreign bone marrow in laboratory animals is an experiment in the production of tolerance and, as such, has potential wide application. The mechanism of adaptation by the graft to the host is not clear, but once such adaptation is accomplished, other grafts from the same donor will survive without immunosuppression.

In practice, human bone marrow allotransplantation has enjoyed increasing success. HLA identical marrow transplants (from matched siblings) are commonly used to treat aplastic anemias. Transplantation with HLA matched but nonidentical twin marrow usually produces a mild to moderate (but occasionally lethal) GVH reaction. Dramatic success has been achieved in the treatment of certain congenital immunodeficiency diseases, where no host-versus-graft reaction is possible, so that host immunosuppression is not required. In all other patients, marrow allotransplantation requires doses of immunosuppressive cytotoxic drugs much larger than those used to gain acceptance of kidney grafts, and the use of non-HLA matched donors has rarely been successful.

A few patients with leukemia have been helped by intensive chemotherapy followed by HLA matched marrow transplantation, but many die of GVH disease, recurrent leukemia, or infection. The hope, seldom realized thus far, is that the leukemia cells surviving chemotherapy will be killed by the GVH reaction.

THYMUS

The congenital absence of thymic tissue prevents the maturation of the entire T-cell system. Such patients are deficient in cell-mediated immune responses and those B-cell responses requiring T-cell interaction. Transplantation of an embryonic fresh or cultured thymus into such patients has resulted in considerable improvement in these normal defense mechanisms. The exact indications and

success rate have not been fully defined, but this is a promising field of investigation.

SPLEEN AND LYMPH NODE

Patients with agammaglobulinemia have been treated by free transplantation of lymph nodes or by transplantation of the spleen with vascular anastomoses. No success has been achieved, but, surprisingly, neither have any serious difficulties eventuated. If a patient with agammaglobulinemia were indeed able to accept allotransplants readily, it might be expected that the spleen or lymph node would react against the immunologically inadequate host.

Several splenic allografts have been carried out in human beings for a variety of indications. These include attempts (1) to transplant immunoglobulin-producing tissue for agammaglobulinemia, (2) to transplant enzyme-producing tissues to treat congenital enzymatic deficiencies (e.g., Gaucher's disease), and (3) to treat cancer with spleen immune to tumor antigens. None of these transplants were successful. Spleen transplants have also been proposed to treat hemophilia, since splenic tissue may be one source of antihemophilic globulin. Since the spleen and lymph nodes are highly antigenic tissues, their successful transplantation must require one of two circumstances: (1) either that the host have a severe type of congenital immunologic deficiency, thus permitting a successful allotransplant but subjecting the patient to the GVH disease, or (2) if the host has a somewhat greater degree of immunologic competence, that immunosuppressive drugs be administered, thus rendering the host even more vulnerable than before to serious infection. These transplants do not, therefore, hold out much hope of clinical success, and bone marrow transplantation may be a better solution which does not entail an operative procedure.

Endocrine Autografts

Most of the clinical experience with endocrine autografts is of only historical significance, because little scientific information has been acquired and there has been only doubtful benefit to the patient. At best such clinical attempts provided temporary indirect evidence of function. Claims of long-term success were never supported by histologic proof.

The placement of endocrine fragments as autografts into intramuscular pockets has proved successful in several clinical situations. For example, the indications for parathyroid autotransplantation have recently been listed by Wells et al. (Table 10-3). When it appears possible that a patient may have insufficient parathyroid tissue following removal of the thyroid gland, the implantation of small fragments into the exposed neck muscles has repeatedly proved worthwhile. Parathyroid glands excised during removal of thyroid mass should be diced and implanted into intramuscular pockets. When removal of the parathyroid tissue is planned, as in cases of secondary hyperparathyroidism, the volar forearm muscle is a useful site for autotransplantation. The parathyroids are readily available for subsequent excision if hyperparathyroidism recurs. Be-

Table 10-3. INDICATIONS FOR PARATHYROID TRANSPLANTATION

A. Autotransplantation
   1. Severe secondary hyperparathyroidism
   2. Primary generalized parathyroid hyperplasia
   3. Inadvertent removal of parathyroid tissue
B. Allotransplantation
   1. Congenital absence of parathyroid glands—DiGeorge's syndrome
   2. Iatrogenic aparathyroidism which is not controllable with a medical regimen

cause secondary hyperparathyroidism is common in chronic renal failure, and hemodialysis is now possible for many years, the indications for total parathyroidectomy and autotransplantation may increase in the years ahead.

Similar indications may exist for other endocrine organs: in a child with lingual thyroid, the tissue from the lingual mass may be the only functional thyroid. Perhaps it should be autotransplanted. Woodruff has made a similar plea for the autotransplantation of ovarian fragments into the rectus muscle in selected cases. Testicular slices have been successfully autotransplanted (albeit without histologic or functional documentation) to prevent the need for replacement therapy in case of accidental castration. Such a procedure should always be attempted when uncontaminated tissue is available, with placement of the implants in a readily accessible muscle. The fragments must not exceed 1 mm in thickness if function is to be expected.

In adrenal hyperplasia with Cushing's syndrome, the accepted surgical therapy has changed from subtotal adrenalectomy to total adrenalectomy with indefinite steroid replacement therapy, because of high incidence of recurrent disease after subtotal adrenalectomy. Autotransplantation of hyperplastic slices with functional and histologic success has been reported, with placement of the grafts at a site accessible for secondary removal. It may represent a reasonable surgical alternative in selected cases of Cushing's syndrome.

Endocrine Allografts (Other than the Pancreas)

The prognosis for endocrine allotransplants as a useful surgical procedure is in doubt. Replacement therapy for endocrine deficiency (aside from insulin deficiencies, to be discussed below) is efficient and generally adequate, and there is seldom an indication for the use of systemic immunosuppressive drugs to eliminate the need for endocrine replacement therapy. In the case of parathyroid allotransplants, there has been an insistent and recurrently hopeful effort. Parathyroid deficiency is not treated with specific hormone replacement, but rather with calcium and vitamin D, which give inadequate results. Groth et al. have reported a successful parathyroid allotransplant in a patient with a functioning renal allograft already receiving immunosuppressive drugs. Most other reports of parathyroid allotransplant success have been based on indirect evidence of decreased replacement therapy, and none has

been substantiated by histologic or functional evidence. There is no evidence that parathyroid tissue is immunologically privileged in human beings, and effective immunosuppressive therapy is probably not worthwhile.

Although endocrine allografts are of little clinical usefulness at present, two important experiments used endocrine transplantation to advance the field of endocrinology. Harris and Jacobsohn first illustrated the control of pituitary secretion by releasing factors from the hypothalamus traveling through the portal-hypophyseal vessels. Pituitary transplants functioned normally when returned to that location but did not function when transplanted to an area vascularized by temporal lobe vessels. Parathyroid physiology was advanced by Barnicot, who found that glands transplanted onto the surface of parietal bone resorbed directly. This observation is the cornerstone of the accepted hypothesis that parathyroid hormone acts directly on bone to raise the calcium in the blood, rather than indirectly by the phosphaturic effect on the kidney.

Pancreas

The discovery of insulin in 1921 was hailed as the cure of diabetes; it prevented death from diabetic coma, controlled the overt symptoms of diabetes, and provided an increased life expectancy. As diabetic patients lived longer, however, previously unseen complications developed. Diabetes was responsible for at least 30,000 deaths in 1974, and it is the leading cause of new cases of blindness in adults. Diabetics are 17 times more liable to kidney disease, five times more liable to gangrene of the extremities, and twice as likely to develop heart disease. Obviously, new approaches to treatment are required. Pancreas and islet transplantation offer the possibility that the development and progression of diabetic lesions will be prevented by precise regulation of carbohydrate metabolism—control not achieved by injected insulin.

An unresolved question is whether juvenile-onset diabetics suffer only from a lack of insulin or whether the absence of insulin reflects other subcellular derangements. Whether normalization of carbohydrate metabolism in these patients will prevent the development of systemic lesions is still unanswered. Several observations, however, support the hypothesis that angiopathic lesions associated with diabetes are secondary to abnormal metabolism: (1) Nephropathy and retinopathy occur in patients who develop diabetes as a result of other disease states (e.g., hemochromatosis) or after total pancreatectomy. (2) Numerous longitudinal, clinical studies have shown a relationship between duration of the disease, control of plasma glucose, and development of lesions. (3) Nephropathy and retinopathy occur in animals with induced diabetes. (4) Studies in animals have demonstrated that reduction of hyperglycemia by insulin therapy or by transplantation of whole pancreas or islets prevents or minimizes formation of diabetic lesions in the eye, kidney, and nerve. (5) Kidneys transplanted from normal to diabetic rats develop histologic lesions characteristic of diabetes in the rat, whereas kidneys transplanted from diabetic to normal rats

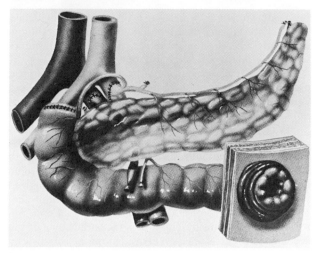

Fig. 10-28. Technique used for pancreaticoduodenal allotransplantation in the first four patients. The distal end of the duodenum was brought out as a cutaneous duodenostomy. [*From R. C. Lillehei and J. O. Ruiz, Pancreas, in J. S. Najarian and R. L. Simmons (eds.), "Transplantation," p. 627, Lea & Febiger, Philadelphia, 1972.*]

Fig. 10-29. Present technique of grafting donor duodenum to recipient small intestine. Both renal and pancreaticoduodenal allografts are illustrated. [*From R. C. Lillehei and J. O. Ruiz, Pancreas, in J. S. Najarian and R. L. Simmons (eds.), "Transplantation," p. 626, Lea & Febiger, Philadelphia, 1972.*]

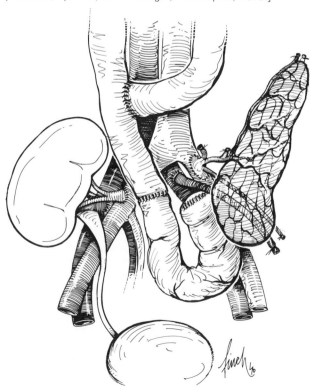

showed disappearance or lack of progression of these lesions. These observations suggest that it may be possible to prevent the systemic complications of diabetes by insulin released from transplanted pancreatic islets. Alternative methods to provide precise glucose homeostasis, such as an implantable glucose sensor coupled to an insulin pump are also possible, however.

EXPERIMENTAL TRANSPLANTATION OF THE WHOLE PANCREAS

The ability of pancreatic transplants to ameliorate diabetes has long been known. The major problems with the procedure include vascular thrombosis, difficulty in establishing drainage of the pancreatic duct, autodigestion of the pancreas, and graft rejection. Theoretically, ligation of the pancreatic duct results in atrophy of exocrine tissue without affecting endocrine tissue. But in practice a severe inflammatory reaction occurs and leads to a constricting fibrosis which damages even the islets. Therefore, transplantation of the duct-ligated pancreas has included attempts to decrease pancreatic exocrine activity by irradiation of the duct-ligated pancreas, administration of 5-fluorouracil, methylprednisolone, or glucagon. These measures have helped but not solved the problem.

The alternative approach, transplantation without ligation of the pancreatic duct, has many variations. Initial attempts used a combined pancreaticoduodenal approach, with the duodenum serving as a conduit for drainage of exocrine enzymes (Figs. 10-28 and 10-29). The transplanted duodenum, however, is particularly susceptible to rejection and to anastomotic leakage, bleeding, ulceration, or perforation, even when evidence of pancreatic graft rejection is minimal. These complications can be eliminated by direct anastomosis of the pancreatic duct to a drainage site. If a small rim of mucosa is left around the pancreatic papilla, a direct anastomosis of the duct to the jejunum can be made which maintains exocrine and endocrine function of the graft. The anastomosis of the main duct of a segmental pancreatic graft to the recipient ureter has also been reported in animals as well as several patients.

Successful whole-organ pancreatic transplants produce circulating insulin and normal plasma glucose levels. When the venous drainage of the pancreatic graft was hooked up to the systemic circulation, the circulating insulin levels were higher than when the venous anastomosis was made to the portal system, although the plasma glucose levels were similar. Animals given whole pancreas isogenic transplants soon after induction of diabetes do not develop the renal, eye, and neural lesions that develop in the nontransplanted diabetic animals. In allograft models, rejection is heralded by increasing serum amylase followed by return to the diabetic state.

CLINICAL TRANSPLANTATION OF THE WHOLE PANCREAS

Since 1966, 49 whole-pancreas transplants have been reported. Evidence from patients 10, 12, 22, and 47 months following transplantation have shown that a functioning vascularized pancreatic allograft will correct the metabolic deficiency in diabetes. The fact that only one of these recipients, however, is still alive with a functioning graft reflects the severe problems associated with pancreatic transplantation.

Of the first 20 pancreatic transplant procedures, 11 were pancreaticoduodenal grafts performed in conjunction with a kidney transplant. The eventual graft failure and subsequent death of the patient were frequently caused by sepsis as a consequence of duodenal rejection and associated complications. Duodenal rejection seemed to occur frequently while the pancreas was functioning, and gave the impression that pancreatic grafts were less immunogenic than duodenum or kidney grafts. This impression, however, has not been confirmed, and the pancreas seems to have an average amount of histocompatibility antigens on its surface.

Variations in clinical pancreatic transplantation have been tried in an attempt to improve the results. Staggering the pancreatic and kidney grafts for end-stage diabetic nephropathy has been done. One patient had a segmental pancreatic graft with anastomosis of the main pancreatic duct to the ureter so that exocrine pancreatic drainage was via the bladder, and then received a renal allograft 145 days later. This patient, the sole survivor with a long-term functioning pancreatic graft reported to the ACS/NIH Transplant Registry, had complete abolishment of insulin requirements, a normal insulin response to glucose, improvement in vision, and abatement of neuropathy 47 months later. Segmental pancreatic transplants have been tried with exocrine drainage into a retroperitoneal jejunal Roux-en-Y loop. In the two patients whose grafts functioned, an intravenous glucose load resulted in a rapid, although subnormal, rise in plasma proinsulin and insulin levels.

Clinical transplantation of the whole pancreas can produce normal glucose homeostasis and an excellent functional result. Unfortunately, technical problems are severe, rejection can be disastrous, and the morbidity and mortality rates are high at this time. The clinical results may improve, however, especially if the allograft rejection can be more effectively suppressed.

EXPERIMENTAL TRANSPLANTATION OF ISLET TISSUE

Immediate vascularization, in general, is not essential for endocrine tissue transplantation to be successful, and in the last several years it has been possible to cure experimental diabetes by transplantation of islet tissue. The transplantation of adult pancreatic fragments was unsuccessful because the associated exocrine enzymes autodigested the transplanted tissue or injured the host. When specific techniques to separate islets from the nonendocrine pancreas were developed, transplantation of isolated adult islets was successful. The current technique for isolation of adult islets from the pancreas involves mechanical disruption, enzymatic digestion, and density gradient separation. Isolated adult islets will produce long-lasting control of diabetes in rats. Transplantation via the portal vein is more effective than intraperitoneal transplantation, and more islets survive in the liver, either because of the immediate availability of the blood supply or because of a physiologic

advantage to this site. Furthermore, transplantation via the portal vein can be accomplished without deterioration of liver function.

The isolation of islets from the adult pancreas is a laborious process, and the yield is low. In contrast, the neonatal pancreas can be successfully transplanted without separation of the islets from exocrine components, since it possesses such an extraordinarily low exocrine enzyme content that damage to autologous islets or recipient tissues is minimal. The successful transplantation of dispersed neonatal pancreatic tissue suggested that the adult pancreas could be transplanted without islet isolation if the digestive enzyme content of the exocrine tissue could be reduced. New techniques designed to reduce the exocrine effect have included (1) the use of donors whose pancreatic duct had been previously ligated, (2) short-term tissue culture of pancreatic fragments, and (3) transplantation of fresh pancreatic fragments into the spleen, which is better able to tolerate the exocrine enzymes. The successful transplantation of adult pancreatic fragments by one of these methods may solve a major problem: the procurement of sufficient islet tissue from a single cadaver donor to cure one diabetic recipient, since an increased quantity of islet tissue is available when the islets are not separated.

An even more frustrating aspect of islet transplantation is the apparent increased susceptibility of islets to allograft rejection. Survival is difficult to achieve even when immunosuppression that will prolong skin, kidney, or heart allografts is used. The clinical application of islet transplantation will also require techniques such as cold storage or culture to preserve the cells.

Despite these formidable difficulties, the numerous experimental demonstrations that transplanted islet tissue can prevent, halt, and even improve the vascular and neurological lesions of diabetes provide a tremendous impetus to continue to attack these problems.

Gastrointestinal Transplants

Various segments of intestine have been experimentally and clinically autotransplanted by removal from the body and reimplantation. Stomach, small bowel, and colon can all be used to replace esophagus, with reimplantation of the vascular supply. Allotransplantation of the small bowel and stomach has been carried out experimentally (Fig. 10-30). These grafts are rejected in the usual fashion, and within the same general time period as those in kidneys and other organs. There is some evidence that the lymphoid tissue within the intestinal wall can initiate a graft-versus-host reaction.

Although there is little apparent clinical use for a gastric transplant, there is a definite need for transplantation of the small bowel. Infarction of the bowel sometimes requires excision of the entire small bowel, and this leads to a fatal nutritional deficiency. Patients with various nutritional and motility problems, as well as certain patients with Crohn's disease, might well benefit from safe and successful bowel transplantation. A few attempts in human beings have been successful for several months, but no long-term survival has been achieved.

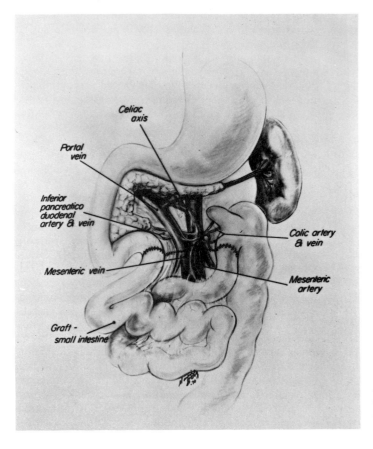

Fig. 10-30. Diagram showing the operative technique of orthotopic transplantation of the entire small intestine in a dog. [*From J. O. Ruiz, H. Uchida, and R. C. Lillehei, Intestine, in J. S. Najarian and R. L. Simmons (eds.), "Transplantation," p. 646, Lea & Febiger, Philadelphia, 1972.*]

Liver

EXPERIMENTAL TRANSPLANTATION IN ANIMALS

Two major surgical approaches to the transplantation of the liver are presently employed. The graft may be positioned in the normal anatomic location (orthotopic transplantation) following a recipient hepatectomy. Alternatively, the donor organ is placed in an ectopic site (heterotopic transplantation), generally with retention of the host's liver (auxiliary transplantation). Each of these techniques has unique inherent advantages, disadvantages, and requirements. The greatest success has been obtained with orthotopic transplantation, even though it is more technically difficult.

ORTHOTOPIC TRANSPLANTATION. The earliest studies evaluating orthotopic liver transplantation in the dog had an extremely high operative mortality rate. Initially, the inferior vena cava and portal vein of the anhepatic dog recipient were cross-clamped during total extirpation of the host's liver prior to receipt of the graft. Dogs subjected to this insult, without an adequate pathway for return of blood from the intestines and lower extremities, often died. To circumvent this dilemma, temporary shunts from the inferior vena cava and portal vein into the superior vena cava are necessary (Fig. 10-31). In human beings collateral venous networks usually develop as a consequence of existing liver disease, thereby eliminating the clinical need for shunts.

Experimentally, the graft is transplanted in its normal anatomical position by performing vena cava–to–vena cava and portal vein–to–portal vein anastomoses. An arterial anastomosis is created between the aorta of the graft and the aorta of the recipient. Biliary drainage is provided through construction of a cholecystoenterostomy (Fig. 10-32) after ligating the transected end of the graft's common duct.

With good surgical technique there is little early evidence of coagulation defects, severe acidosis, hypoglycemia, or biochemical derangements indicative of a significant hepatic injury pattern. But in the nonimmunosuppressed recipient, a pattern of rejection is almost invariably present by the fifth day. Elevations in the level of alkaline phosphatase, serum glutamic oxaloacetic transaminase (SGOT), and serum glutamic pyruvic transaminase (SGPT) develop at the same time as, or shortly prior to, the onset of jaundice. By the seventh day there are usually a progression of hyperbilirubinemia and other biochemical parameters reminiscent of biliary obstruction, as well as hepatic parenchymal cellular injury. A periportal mononuclear cell infiltrate, centrilobular necrosis, and intracanalicular bile stasis are present on microscopic examination. The recipient usually dies by the tenth postoperative day.

The pig appears to have inherent advantages as an experimental animal compared to the dog. In the pig there are fewer bacteria within the liver parenchyma and a greater

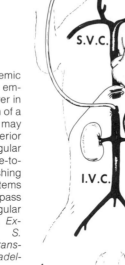

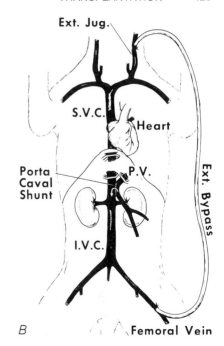

Fig. 10-31. Various splanchnic and systemic venous decompression techniques are employed during removal of the recipient liver in the healthy dog prior to revascularization of a hepatic graft. *A*. Two external shunts may provide for venous return from the inferior vena cava and portal vein into the jugular veins. *B*. Alternatively, a temporary side-to-side portacaval anastomosis establishing continuity between both venous systems permits the use of a single external bypass between the femoral and external jugular veins. [*From L. Brettschneider, Liver: I. Experimental (Transplantation), in J. S. Najarian, and R. L. Simmons (eds.), "Transplantation," p. 497, Lea & Febiger, Philadelphia, 1972.*]

resistance to problems caused by interrupting the portal circulation. Most remarkably, a number of liver transplant recipients have lived for many months, without much evidence of rejection. The cause of the absent or mild rejection pattern following transplantation of the pig liver is speculative. Most evidence supports the idea that the pig's reactions to vascularized organ grafts are less strong and the liver is a less immunogenic organ.

HETEROTOPIC TRANSPLANTATION. The theoretic advantages of auxiliary liver homotransplantation are great. The procedure is technically less arduous than orthotopic transplantation, retains the residual function of the host's liver, and avoids the necessity of removing the diseased organ from a critically ill recipient. These theoretic advantages have proved to be less useful in practice, however, because of complicating mechanical and physiologic factors.

The original technique (Fig. 10-33) placed the allograft outflow into the transected vena cava of the host below the renal vessels. The failure rate following auxiliary transplantation by this technique is extremely high. Even if survival can be obtained for several weeks in canine recipients of auxiliary grafts with immunosuppression (using azathioprine), the transplanted organ atrophies after 2 to 3 weeks.

The lack of hepatotrophic factors in splanchnic venous blood flow to the auxiliary transplant probably contributes to hepatic allograft atrophy. If splanchnic blood flow to the allograft is maintained, atrophy can be prevented. Splanchnic blood flow can be maintained by an anastomosis between the donor portal vein and recipient superior mesenteric vein, followed by ligation of the host's portal vein. This provides for retrograde flow of portal blood through the allograft, rather than through the host's own liver (Fig. 10-34).

Fig. 10-32. Orthotopic transplantation involves total substitution of the host's own liver with the donor organ placed in its normal location. The vena cava and portal vein are generally reestablished anatomically. In the earlier experiences, a segment of donor aorta in continuity with the celiac artery was sutured to the recipient's aorta. A cholecystoduodenostomy afforded biliary drainage. [*From L. Brettschneider, Liver: I. Experimental (Transplantation), in J. S. Najarian and R. L. Simmons (eds.), "Transplantation," p. 496, Lea & Febiger, Philadelphia, 1972.*]

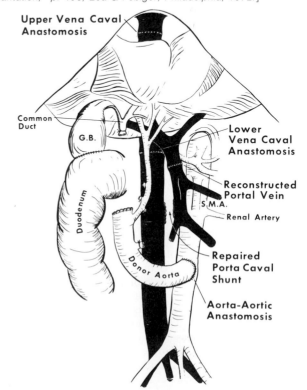

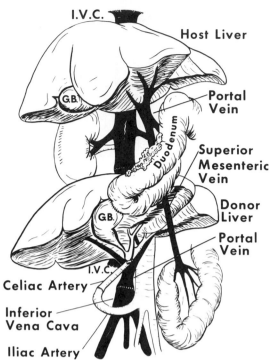

Fig. 10-33. Canine heterotopic transplantation as described by Welch. Anastomosis of the host's vena cava with the portal vein of the donor organ provides a systemic venous inflow. The hepatic artery is anastomosed to the transected iliac artery. Biliary drainage is afforded through a cholecystoduodenostomy. Graft atrophy is almost invariably noted following this procedure. [*From L. Brettschneider, Liver: I. Experimental (Transplantation), in J. S. Najarian and R. L. Simmons (eds.), "Transplantation," p. 496, Lea & Febiger, Philadelphia, 1972.*]

HEPATOCYTE TRANSPLANTATION. Over the past few years, orthotopic liver transplantation has been attempted in certain metabolic diseases with the hope that the grafted tissue would provide the enzyme or "factor" missing in the disease. An alternative approach has been proposed: viz., the transplantation of isolated hepatocytes. Several experimental investigations have demonstrated that intraportal and intramuscular transplantation of isolated hepatocytes in an enzyme-deficient animal can, at least partially, replace that enzyme. The advantages of such a rather simple surgical procedure compared with the more complex surgical procedures involved in whole-organ liver transplantation are obvious.

CLINICAL TRANSPLANTATION

Clinical hepatic transplantation is still experimental, and progress has been slow. Orthotopic transplants appear to be more successful than heterotopic grafts.

INDICATIONS. In the United States, approximately 15,000 persons, between the ages of five and sixty years, died in 1963 as a result of primary hepatic disease. Some patients with this disease will never be good candidates for liver transplantation, but others may benefit substantially.

Intrahepatic or extrahepatic congenital biliary atresia, if not surgically correctable, will generally lead to death before the age of two; few patients survive up to 5 years. Such a child is the ideal candidate for a liver transplant.

Patients with either primary hepatomas or cholangiocarcinomas are far less ideal candidates. If, however, it can be ascertained that the malignant condition is entirely confined to the liver, these patients should be considered for liver transplantation. Often the final diagnosis of disease confined to the liver may not be made until the operation.

The patient with cirrhosis raises additional problems. Rapid death is not as certain in these patients as in those with biliary atresia or primary malignant disease. On the other hand, the terminal stages of the cirrhosis make these patients extremely poor candidates for any operative procedure. Patients with postnecrotic cirrhosis without a history of alcoholism may be better risks, as will be the patient with primary biliary cirrhosis, Wilson's hepatolenticular degeneration, or hemochromatosis.

Acute liver failure may represent one of the best indications for liver transplantation, especially in those patients who have been exposed to hepatotoxins. Viral hepatitis, on the other hand, may or may not recur in the transplanted liver.

Each indication may require a different type of transplant. For example, acute liver failure may respond well to the temporary support of an auxiliary liver or the injection of isolated hepatocytes that will permit the host liver to recover. The child with biliary atresia will almost certainly require an orthotopic transplant with total hepatectomy, since the small child also has no abdominal space for an auxiliary liver. Patients with hepatic malignant disease will also require total hepatectomy and orthotopic transplantation.

In choosing a hepatic donor, the same guidelines should be followed as in choosing a donor for cadaver renal transplantation. Size is a more important criterion in liver transplantation than it is in renal transplantation, particularly when children with congenital biliary atresia are the potential recipients. Usually these children (weighing from 3 to 15 kg) cannot tolerate a liver larger than that from a child weighing 30 kg. Severe postoperative respiratory distress has occurred when donor livers from larger children were used.

PRECAUTIONS. The hepatic transplantation candidate is usually in severe preterminal hepatic failure. In addition, anemia, pulmonary insufficiency, myocardial fibrosis, inanition and protein depletion, and ascites may be present, singly or in combination. The anemia and hypoalbuminemia should be corrected with packed red blood cells and protein-containing solutions as soon as transplantation is contemplated.

Pulmonary insufficiency in hepatic failure can be traced to several causes: First, chronic abdominal ascites restricts the diaphragm and fosters compression atelectasis of the lower portions of the lungs. Also, extensive collateral circulation consequent to portal vein hypertension shunts blood from the portal system to the pulmonary veins via enlarged paraesophageal, mediastinal, and bronchial veins, resulting in venous admixture of systemic blood. Intrapulmonary shunts may also develop in cirrhotic patients, so that arterial hypoxemia is frequently encountered. These conditions make it more difficult for the anesthesiologist to provide adequate ventilation and oxygenation during surgery and require that he avoid techniques employing borderline oxygen concentration.

In cirrhotic patients, diffuse myocardial fibrosis frequently develops that reduces ventricular contractility, stroke volume, and work capacity.

The bedridden patient with hepatic failure invariably suffers from debilitation and poor nutrition, which make him vulnerable to hypotension following anesthesia, moderate hemorrhage, or positional change. Drugs which ordinarily produce mild vasodilation often evoke unusually severe and prolonged effects in the cirrhotic patient that are out of proportion to the dose administered. Most anesthetic drugs provoke such responses and must therefore be administered slowly in small increments. Sudden removal of ascitic fluid may also precipitate or exaggerate hypotension, but the mechanism of this response is obscure.

It is apparent from these considerations that in undertaking to provide anesthesia for the transplant patient, the anesthesiologist faces several difficult challenges. He must, on the one hand, provide conditions adequate for a massive intraperitoneal procedure; at the same time, he must keep in mind that his patient will probably not tolerate deep anesthesia and that the implanted liver may be slow to metabolize and detoxify anesthetic drugs. Most of all, intraoperative and postoperative respiratory distress must be anticipated and minimized. In addition, there is almost no time for proper preparation of the patient. Once a donor is available, the operation must commence promptly so that agonal ischemia of the donor organ may be as brief as possible. The recipient frequently comes to surgery unexpectedly, perhaps an hour or two after a meal. A full stomach is added to the already imposing list of preoperative problems.

The following preparatory procedures are carried out either before anesthesia is induced or immediately after: (1) A central venous pressure catheter is positioned in the right atrium or superior vena cava and a Swan-Ganz catheter for measurement of pulmonary wedge pressures is placed. (2) A second large-bore plastic needle is placed in an upper extremity vein for fluid and blood replacement; it is important to remember that intravenous input via the lower extremities is not adequate during the actual transplantation phase, since the inferior vena cava is clamped. (3) Another needle is placed in either the brachial or radial artery for direct blood pressure monitoring and arterial blood sampling. (4) A rubber warming blanket is placed under the patient and kept between 100 and 105°F. (5) An esophageal temperature probe is positioned so that its sensor lies directly behind the heart. (6) A catheter is placed in the urinary bladder and connected to a graduated collecting flask.

TECHNIQUE OF ORTHOTOPIC HEPATIC TRANSPLANTATION. A transverse abdominal incision with an extension into the thorax, if necessary, is the most common incision.

Recipient hepatectomy must be preceded by careful inspection to determine the feasibility of the procedure. This is particularly true of patients with primary hepatic

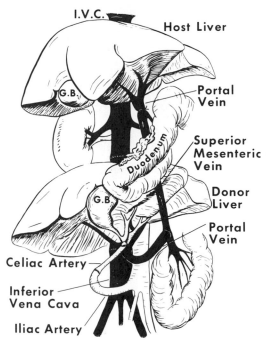

Fig. 10-34. Marchioro et al. modified the technique described in Fig. 10-33. By ligating the portal blood supply to the host's own liver and diverting the splanchnic blood to the homograft by creating an anastomosis between the graft's portal vein and the in situ superior mesenteric vein, homograft atrophy was prevented. [*From L. Brettschneider, Liver: I. Experimental (Transplantation), in J. S. Najarian and R. L. Simmons (eds.), "Transplantation," p. 496, Lea & Febiger, Philadelphia, 1972.*]

neoplasms to ensure that no extrahepatic spread of the tumor has occurred.

The allograft anastomoses are shown in Fig. 10-35. The suprahepatic caval anastomosis is the most difficult to perform. The second anastomosis is usually the hepatic artery but if visceral congestion is great, the portal vein anastomosis should be performed before the hepatic artery to relieve the venous congestion of the intestine. After the hepatic artery or portal vein anastomosis is completed, the inferior hepatic caval clamps should be briefly removed, leaving the suprahepatic vena cava clamped. The arterial or portal vein inflow should be opened to allow the liver to be perfused with warm blood. This sequence is useful to remove the cold perfusate from the liver and prevent systemic hypothermia and heparinization. As soon as the perfusate is washed from the liver and it becomes firm and pink, the intrahepatic vena cava is clamped, and the suprahepatic vena cava clamp is removed. The remaining vascular anastomoses can then be accomplished.

Following the vascular anastomoses, biliary drainage must be obtained. A Roux-en-Y cholecystojejunostomy is most often used, but occasionally a cholecystoduodenostomy is employed. No universally satisfactory technique has been devised, and obstruction, biliary leakage, and necrosis of the gallbladder are common complications. Biliary catastrophes may be the most common cause of death in these patients.

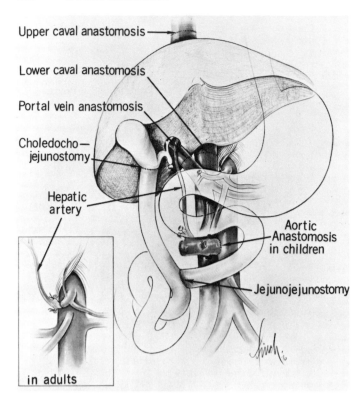

Upper caval anastomosis

Lower caval anastomosis

Portal vein anastomosis

Choledocho—
jejunostomy

Hepatic
artery

Aortic
Anastomosis
in children

Jejunojejunostomy

in adults

Fig. 10-35. Orthotopic liver transplantation in children and adults. In children an aortic cuff can be used for anastomosis; in adults (inset) a direct anastomosis of the hepatic artery and celiac axis can be used. [*From J. S. Najarian, Liver: III. Clinical (Transplantation), in J. S. Najarian and R. L. Simmons (eds.), "Transplantation," p. 522, Lea & Febiger, Philadelphia, 1972.*]

TECHNIQUE OF AUXILIARY LIVER TRANSPLANTATION. Auxiliary, or heterotopic, transplantation is the second alternative for patients with benign liver disease. The major disadvantage of this procedure is its requirement for abdominal volume in which to accommodate the second large organ. When auxiliary transplants are performed, the recipient's own liver is retained to offer some metabolic support during and after the operation. Thus, with the auxiliary liver transplant there is no urgent need for immediate function of the graft, and the operation is shorter and less traumatic.

As noted above, splanchnic blood should be supplied to the graft. This technique is illustrated in Fig. 10-36. The portal vein may be anastomosed to the side of the superior mesenteric vein or to the end of the splenic vein. The advantage of this technique is twofold. It allows for the decompression of the hypertensive recipient portal system, and it provides splanchnic blood flow through the auxiliary liver transplant.

OPERATIVE COMPLICATIONS. Technical Complications. Bleeding is the major technical problem during hepatic transplantation. Portal hypertension predisposes to an extensive collateral venous circulation, and laceration of any smaller vein precipitates extensive bleeding, especially during recipient hepatectomy. The failure of the diseased liver to produce a normal quota of coagulation factors compounds this problem.

It is important to remember that the cystic duct may not enter the common duct except in its terminal course. Therefore, during the donor operation one must be sure that the common duct is ligated distal to its anastomosis with the cystic duct, if bile is to be expected to flow down the common duct and into the gallbladder. As noted above, biliary leakage due to primary anastomotic breakdown or thrombosis of the cystic artery is a common postoperative problem. Late complications of the biliary drainage procedure may include obstruction of the anastomosis by biliary sludge.

As many as 30 to 40 percent of patients have double hepatic arteries, and one of them may arise from the superior mesenteric artery. Care must be taken during the donor operation to preserve this arterial supply.

A common complication is paralysis of the right side of the diaphragm, which apparently results from crushing of the right phrenic nerve by the vascular clamp applied to the suprahepatic inferior vena cava. Enough length must be preserved during total hepatectomy for the clamp to be applied without impinging on the diaphragm.

Metabolic Complications. Because pulmonary insufficiency is common following hepatic transplantation, a sterile nasotracheal tube should be placed at the outset of anesthesia, with the intention of maintaining intubation and mechanical ventilation until respiratory competence is reestablished.

Because of increased tissue uptake of glucose and reduced glycogen conversion, hypoglycemia develops insidiously in response to hepatic ischemia, hypotension, and acidosis. Hyperglycemia is a hazard of hypertonic glucose infusion. The blood sugar should be regularly measured, and glucose infusion should be modified according to the values obtained.

Precise measurement of blood loss and fluid sequestration is not possible, and evaluation and correlation of suction loss, weight loss, arterial blood pressure, cardiac rate, venous pressure, acid-base status, and urine volume must be made frequently by the anesthetist. At this point of the operative procedure, central venous pressure measurement is useful as a guide to the adequacy of the filling pressure of the right side of the heart, but manipulation of the liver and its great vein attachments may produce high-pressure artifacts and make an estimation of left atrial pressure more useful.

Hypotension is a particular danger during the anhepatic period, its severity depending upon the adequacy with which collateral venous circulation maintains venous return to the heart. If blood pressure is seriously depressed, the transfusion rate is increased, but often the hypotension cannot be fully overcome until the caval clamps are removed. This disturbance of cardiac output is the major cause of the progressive metabolic acidosis that characterizes this portion of the transplant operation.

When the anastomoses are completed, further dangerous metabolic and hemodynamic changes occur. The great veins draining the intestines and lower half of the body now discharge blood containing a heavy load of acid metabolites. At the same time, the vascular space within the liver takes up a considerable volume of blood and discharges additional products of ischemia as it again becomes an integral part of the circulation. Thus the metabolic acidosis suddenly worsens and is accompanied by hypovolemia. Severe hypotension, cardiac arrhythmias, bradycardia, and other bizarre configurations of the ECG pattern appear abruptly at this point. Blood loss from leaks in the vascular anastomoses frequently compounds the hemodynamic problems. Whole blood must be rapidly administered at this phase of the operation until the systolic arterial blood pressure stabilizes at 100 mm Hg or better. Simultaneously, blood-gas analyses are made every 5 minutes to provide guidance in adjustment of acid-base balance at this critical juncture.

Hypothermia is a concomitant hazard as the donor liver is revascularized. The whole transplantation procedure, with its extensive visceral exposure and heavy blood loss, tends to produce hypothermia. Furthermore, the donor liver is flushed with iced saline solution prior to transplantation into the host's circulation to increase its tolerance of ischemia. The *coup de grâce,* therefore, is the sudden inclusion of this ice-cold organ directly upstream of the heart. Consequently the core temperature usually falls 3 to 4°C within 2 minutes of release of the clamps. Such abrupt cardiac cooling fosters arrhythmias and poor myocardial function. Perfusion of the liver through the infrahepatic vena cava prior to opening the suprahepatic vena cava will warm the liver and work out the cold perfusate. In addition, irrigation of the abdominal cavity with warm saline solution (40°C) and transfusion with warm blood can also compensate for this problem.

Potassium disturbances impose an additional hazard during revascularization. Several factors (hepatocellular ischemia, massive blood replacement, and metabolic acidosis) favor hyperkalemia when hepatic circulation is restored. There may be a concomitant decrease in serum

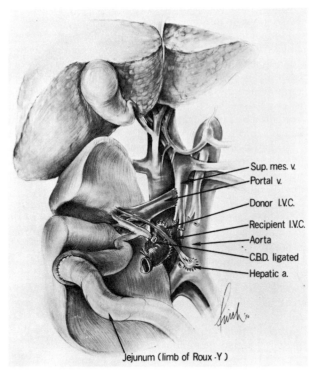

Fig. 10-36. The method of auxiliary liver transplantation utilizing splanchnic blood flow. The hepatic arterial supply comes directly from the aorta, and the portal vein supply to the liver is derived from the splanchnic circulation. The portal vein can be anastomosed either to the superior mesenteric vein, as shown, or to the portal vein, whichever is most convenient. The donor's inferior vena cava is anastomosed end to end to the inferior vena cava. In this method portal decompression is provided, as well as splanchnic circulation to the transplanted liver. [*From J. S. Najarian, Liver: III. Clinical (Transplantation), in J. S. Najarian, and R. L. Simmons (eds.), "Transplantation," p. 522, Lea & Febiger, Philadelphia, 1972.*]

calcium due to the heavy citrate load from the multiple transfusions and the impaired capacity of the new liver to metabolize that load. These cation shifts have not been systematically quantified, but the abrupt appearance of peaked T waves and conduction disturbances have been observed on the ECG as liver circulation is reestablished. Disturbance of the potassium/calcium ratio is known to depress myocardial function and cardiac output; when acidosis, hypothermia, and a sudden increase in the vascular bed add their own special depressant effects, severe hypotension and arrhythmias result. Prompt correction of hypovolemia and acidosis are the keys to success in negotiating this critical period. Then, if myocardial weakness still persists, one can assume that a potassium/calcium ratio disturbance is present and slowly inject 0.5 to 1.0 Gm of calcium chloride. The serum electrolyte determinations made every 15 minutes until the circulation stabilizes provide guidance in adjusting ionic balance. Hypokalemia is the most prominent electrolyte problem in the early postoperative period.

POSTOPERATIVE CARE. There is a high potential for postoperative respiratory insufficiency in most hepatic transplant patients, because (1) pulmonary dysfunction is always present in some degree, (2) the extensive upper abdominal incision causes abdominal muscle splinting and reduces vital capacity, and (3) the transplanted liver is often significantly larger than the organ it replaces, so that breathing is further compromised until abdominal wall accommodation takes place. The nasotracheal tube is therefore usually left in place after surgery. Mechanical ventilation is applied for at least 12 hours or until the patient's own respiratory competence is proved by normal blood gases. Strict adherence to sterile technique in respiratory care is essential because of the patient's immunosuppressed state. Sterile distilled water should be used to provide humidification of respiratory gases.

After operation, the transplant recipient is kept in a 30°-angle head-up position to reduce the pressure of the abdominal contents on the diaphragm. He is also turned from side to side each hour, and vibratory chest percussion is applied each time a positional change is made. Chest roentgenograms are made daily to detect atelectasis, which is dealt with by postural pummeling, directional tracheobronchial suction, and hyperinflation with a self-inflating bag.

Most of the remaining problems are related to metabolic changes that may be minimal if the quality of the new liver is good. If, however, the liver quality is impaired by prolonged ischemia or agonal changes in the donor, the liver will be unable to regulate blood sugar, and either hypoglycemia or hyperglycemic nonketotic coma may occur.

The coagulation changes that accompany the transplantation of the liver have been thoroughly discussed by the Denver group. Because most of the coagulation factors are hepatic in origin and the liver is involved in the clearing of substances active in coagulation and fibrinolysis, a damaged liver frequently fails to produce sufficient coagulation factors to prevent hemorrhage. The problem is compounded by the probability that intravascular coagulation accompanies the trauma and shock of the procedure, thereby consuming whatever factors are present. A rapid return of coagulation tests to normal in the early posttransplant period is a good indicator of satisfactory hepatic function.

Hepatic transplant recipients receive the same immunosuppressive drugs used in renal transplant recipients (azathioprine, prednisone, and ALG). The hepatotoxicity of azathioprine, however, requires that a reduced level be utilized (1 mg/kg), although the levels of prednisone and ALG remain the same. Cyclophosphamide has recently been used in place of azathioprine.

DIFFERENTIAL DIAGNOSIS OF HEPATIC MALFUNCTION. Many causes of hepatic malfunction other than rejection exist. Since there is evidence that rejection of the liver is less severe than that of other organs, technical complications should be ruled out prior to treating hepatic malfunction with more immunosuppression. The diagnosis may require surgical exploration.

While the milder rejection episodes may not be clinically apparent, severe rejection crises are accompanied by systemic signs that may mimic toxic hepatitis. Fever, malaise, anorexia, and hepatomegaly are present, and the patient generally appears quite ill. The laboratory findings reveal elevated serum bilirubin, alkaline phosphatase, and serum transaminase levels. The 99m technetium liver scan will reveal either a patchy or diffuse decrease in hepatic uptake and an increased uptake in the bone marrow and lungs. The serum bilirubin level is such a reliable indication that it should be tested two or three times weekly in the posttransplant period.

Septic infarcts within the liver are among the most severe problems encountered after liver transplants; they are usually fatal. This syndrome appears as a distinct clinical triad: (1) gram-negative septicemia, (2) evidence of massive liver necrosis with increased serum levels of liver enzymes, and (3) liver scans showing absence of isotope concentrations in one area of the liver allograft. Ischemic infarction then follows, and the liver can no longer deal with the enteric organisms normally traversing the portal venous system. The ischemic segment soon becomes abscessed. An increase in serum transaminase, a positive blood culture, and an area that fails to concentrate the isotope on liver scan are all positive indications of an abscessed ischemic segment. The cause is more likely to be technical problems of surgery than immunological rejection.

RESULTS. Of the 106 patients receiving orthotopic liver grafts in Denver prior to August, 1976, 27 were alive 1 year or more after grafting and 16 survived longer than 2 years. The longest survival period was 6.3 years. Of the 50 patients in the Cambridge/King series, 12 survived more than 6 months, four of these lived beyond a year, 10 were currently living, one was alive 2.5 years after transplantation. The longest survivor lived 5.2 years after orthotopic grafting. Younger patients seem to do better, and one-third of the recipients under age eighteen survived more than 1 year in the Denver series.

In all series, uncontrolled rejection reactions were the primary cause of death in about 10 percent of the patients. More commonly, the deaths were due to a wide variety of biliary tract problems and intraabdominal sepsis. The longest survivor of the Cambridge series lived for 5.2 years until calcified sludge blocked the anastomosis between the gallbladder and recipient common duct. Deaths were also caused by a variety of problems, including pneumonia, cerebrovascular accidents, and the recurrence of cancer in patients who had primary hepatomas or cholangiocarcinomas.

Heart

Cardiac transplantation is emerging as a truly therapeutic intervention for some patients with terminal or intractable heart disease for whom no alternative therapy is currently available. By July 1977, 346 cardiac transplants had been performed in human beings by 65 teams in various countries of the world. Though the overall survival rate has been disappointingly low, the potential for long-term survival has been established by 11 patients who are currently alive between 5 and 9 years after transplantation. Equally gratifying is their high degree of rehabilitation.

HISTORICAL BACKGROUND

Prior to the initiation of human trials, a number of fundamental areas required extensive laboratory investigation—development of a surgical technique, demonstration of adequate postoperative function of the acutely denervated heart, early detection and prevention of homograft rejection, and resuscitation and preservation of the cadaver heart. An encouraging degree of progress was made in each of these areas during the 10 years preceding the first clinical transplant in Cape Town, South Africa, in December of 1967.

Before the development of modern methods for cardiopulmonary bypass, studies of cardiac transplantation, of necessity, were confined to placement of the heart in an ectopic position, usually in the neck of a larger dog. As early as 1905, Carrel and Guthrie, using previously unknown suturing techniques, carried out heterotopic transplantation of the heart and of the heart and lungs and demonstrated the capacity of the transplanted heart to continue beating despite severance from its nerve supply. Subsequent studies by other investigators using various modifications of the original preparation added considerably to our knowledge of the transplanted heart. Much was learned about the susceptibility of the heart to the process of rejection; its vulnerability to hypoxia, thrombosis, and air embolism; and the protective effect of hypothermia against the metabolic abnormalities which occur with transplantation. In addition to these studies, the heterotopically transplanted heart has been investigated as a means of assisting circulation.

Subsequent to the development of techniques for generalized hypothermia and extracorporeal circulation, the possibility of complete cardiac replacement was investigated by several groups. Survival in the initial dog studies was limited to a few hours, but much was learned about the technical problems. In December of 1959, Lower and Shumway demonstrated that a dog could recover fully after orthotopic replacement of the heart with a homograft. In an initial series of 10 animals, 6 survived from 6 to 21 days without immunosuppression. Five days of survival was also achieved after orthotopic homotransplantation of the heart and both lungs as a unit.

Subsequent animal studies demonstrated that the ECG voltage was a useful means of monitoring the transplant in order to detect impending rejection episodes and that prolonged survival could be achieved in some animals by appropriate use of azathioprine and high doses of steroid to combat rejection crises. The feasibility of using cadaver hearts was also established, as was the successful hypothermic storage of the donor heart for several hours prior to transplantation.

Extensive physiologic studies of autotransplanted dog hearts confirmed the capacity of the denervated heart to function normally for several years under a variety of physiologic stresses and demonstrated that signs of autonomic reinnervation would frequently reappear within months to a year after transplantation. These laboratory investigations established the technical and physiologic feasibility of cardiac transplantation in man and set the stage for the clinical trials which were initiated in December of 1967 and carried out most extensively in 1968 in several centers. In subsequent years, because of the high rate of immunologic failure of the grafts, cardiac transplantation has been performed less frequently and only in a few centers as carefully studied clinical investigations.

SELECTION OF PATIENTS

Because of the relatively high risk of allograft failure from rejection or of death from complications of immunosuppression, patient selection for cardiac transplantation generally has been reserved for those under age fifty with terminal or intractable heart failure for whom no alternative therapy is available. The majority have had severe coronary disease with multiple infarctions and extensive or diffuse loss of left ventricular myocardium. Many of these patients have been failures of prior revascularization attempts, but these have proved to be an especially favorable group (see below). Another group for consideration includes patients with cardiomyopathy who do not respond satisfactorily to medical therapy. It has now been established in some long-term survivors that the cardiomyopathy is not likely to recur in the transplanted heart, and one such patient in our own series is alive after 4 years with normal cardiac function. Another group is composed of infants with the hypoplastic left-heart syndrome for whom transplantation from anencephalic donors might prove successful. Of particular interest is the high success rate reported by the Stanford University Medical Center group for patients who had prior cardiopulmonary bypass procedures, which suggest that, rather than the anticipated high rate of sensitization to donor antigens, some measure of graft enhancement may have occurred.

Up to the present time histocompatibility typing has provided no predictive value in matching donor and recipient, but to avoid the problem of accelerated rejection a lymphocyte cross match must establish that the recipient harbors no preformed antibodies against the potential donor. Otherwise, successful transplantation has required only the geographic and temporal proximity of recipient and donor with appropriate ABO compatibility. Cardiac donors have sustained brain death usually from trauma or from spontaneous intracerebral hemorrhage, and complete cessation of brain function has been certified by an independent team of neurologists and neurosurgeons.

TECHNIQUE

The operative approach (Fig. 10-37) for cardiac transplantation used by most groups follows with a few modifications the procedure which proved successful in the animal model. The recipient is prepared for cardiopulmonary bypass using a median sternotomy incision. Venous drainage catheters are placed through the right atrial wall in a posterior position, or they may be inserted through peripheral veins. Arterial cannulation is via the femoral artery or ascending aorta. The recipient's diseased heart is excised by appropriate incisions in the right and left atrial walls and atrial septum, retaining in the recipient the posterior portions of both atria. This residual atrial tissue not only facilitates anastomosis of the donor heart but

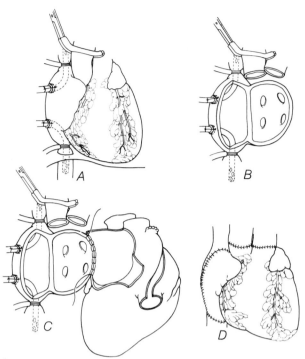

Fig. 10-37. *A.* The recipient has been prepared for cardiopulmonary bypass with insertion of caval catheters through the posterior portion of the right atrium. *B.* The recipient's heart has been excised leaving in place the posterior remnants of right and left atria. *C.* Suturing of the donor heart is begun with the left atrial wall, followed in sequence by the atrial septum, right atrium, pulmonary artery, and aorta. *D.* Suturing is complete, and coronary circulation is restored by removal of the aortic clamp. [*From R. R. Lower, Cardiac Transplantation, in J. C. Norman (ed.), "Cardiac Surgery," 2d ed., p. 599, Appleton Century Crofts, New York, 1972.*]

preserves some of the afferent innervation to the atria which may play a significant role in maintaining homeostatic fluid balance in the postoperative period. Blood supply to the retained atrial tissue is adequately provided by the bronchial circulation, but retention of excessive amounts, particularly the appendages, is avoided to minimize the risk of ischemia, stasis, and thrombosis. The aorta and pulmonary artery are transected at a convenient point distal to the semilunar valves.

Simultaneously, the donor is heparinized and the heart exposed by a second team. Removal of the donor heart is carried out by division of the venae cavae, the pulmonary veins, and the great arteries. The excised heart is then immersed in saline solution at 5 to 10°C to provide protective cooling of the myocardium during transport to the recipient, as well as during the remainder of the transplantation procedure. Further preparation of the donor heart includes suture ligation of the superior vena cava, incision of the lateral right atrial wall from the inferior vena cava to the atrial appendage avoiding the major internodal pathways, and preparation of the left atrium by incision between the pulmonary venous openings.

Implantation of the donor heart consists of suturing the left atrial wall, atrial septum, and right atrial wall in suc-

cession by continuous suture, followed by anastomosis of the pulmonary artery and ascending aorta. Prior to completing the final anastomosis, care is taken to evacuate all residual air from the cardiac chambers. With release of the aortic clamp and rewarming of the heart, cardiac rhythm often returns spontaneously, or ventricular fibrillation may require electrical cardioversion. In each of our cases, the transplanted heart has resumed vigorous contractions once coronary circulation has been restored, and cardiopulmonary bypass has been discontinued.

In 1977 we extended the procurement of donor hearts for urgent transplantation to include long-distance transportation of the hearts up to 900 miles by chartered jet. In four such cases ischemic times were from 1 hour 53 minutes to 3 hours 17 minutes, during which periods the hearts were protected by simple hypothermia. In each instance excellent cardiac function was restored in the recipient. Two patients later died, one of rejection, one of infection, and two recipients of the long-distance transplants remain alive.

POSTOPERATIVE CARE

The most immediate problem in the postoperative period is the capacity of the transplanted right ventricle to cope with the preexisting pulmonary hypertension which usually results from long-standing failure of the left side of the heart. Under these circumstances, the heart may temporarily require inotropic support for 1 or 2 days. The precise level of pulmonary hypertension which precludes a successful transplant has not yet been defined, but adequate cardiac function without prolonged pharmacologic support has been recovered in most instances despite the additional theoretic problems of acute denervation and interrupted cardiac lymphatics.

Once the posttransplant circulatory status is stable, the major emphasis in management shifts to the immunologic problem. The heart transplant recipient appears to be less immunologically depressed than a kidney transplant recipient with prolonged uremia and thus requires higher levels of immunosuppression in the early posttransplant weeks. Azathioprine is given in the maximally tolerated daily dose of 3 to 4 mg/kg, with careful observation for signs of hematologic toxicity. Prednisone is begun at a dose of 200 mg/day and tapered gradually to 60 mg/day by the end of 2 weeks. Further tapering of the dose is more gradual, reaching a level of 30 mg/day at 3 months, if the clinical condition permits. Antithymocyte globulin is administered over a 10-day period, although its importance and dosage are incompletely known at this time. To minimize the emergence of resistant microorganisms, antibiotics are administered only at the time of operation and for specific indications thereafter.

Monitoring for episodes of impending rejection depends almost entirely on daily or twice daily observation of the ECG. The majority of patients will have a rejection episode during the first 2 postoperative weeks, and the most significant ECG changes will include a stepwise decrease in voltage, rightward shift in the frontal plane axis, and the occasional occurrence of atrial arrhythmias or right bundle branch block (Fig. 10-38). An epicardial electrode implanted at operation serves to enhance the accuracy of voltage changes in the first few postoperative weeks.

Clinical signs of rejection may include the development of a protodiastolic gallop sound and the murmur of tricuspid insufficiency. Other signs and symptoms, such as pericardial friction rub, fever, and malaise, are rather nonspecific in the early postoperative period and therefore of little diagnostic value. Other confirmatory diagnostic maneuvers include fluoroscopy or ultrasound to demonstrate cardiac chamber enlargement, decreased amplitude of ventricular wall pulsations, and diminished ventricular compliance. A suspected rejection crisis may be further confirmed by transvenous endocardial muscle biopsy as described by the Stanford University Medical Center group (Fig. 10-39).

The treatment of a rejection episode requires a large intravenous dose of steroid, usually 1 Gm of methylprednisolone on the first day and 0.5 Gm on the second day, with subsequent return to maintenance levels if the clinical condition permits. The adjunctive value of graft irradiation and anticoagulant therapy is incompletely settled at the present time. Late postoperative management includes a vigorous exercise program to minimize the catabolic effects of steroid therapy. The likelihood of acute rejection diminishes after 4 months, and ECG studies are reduced to twice weekly.

The major late problem, aside from infectious complications, has been the development of vascular lesions characteristic of chronic rejection. Even small lesions may produce ischemic damage to the conduction system, and the occurrence of conduction defects may require transvenous pacing. The value of prolonged therapy with warfarin and dipyridamole is under investigation in the hope of minimizing the vascular complications. Control of hyperlipidemia is also carefully managed in the appropriate patients.

RESULTS

Survival data have been periodically compiled and published by the ACS/NIH Organ Transplant Registry. The majority of cardiac transplants from 1971 to 1977 were performed at the Stanford University Medical Center, and this group has also published several detailed analyses of their steadily improving results which currently indicate a 48 percent 1-year and 38 percent 2-year survival rate.

Seventy-seven patients are currently alive in the world experience, of whom 11 have survived more than 5 years, attesting to the therapeutic potential of this procedure. Late deaths occurring more than 3 months after operation have usually resulted from infectious complications or from the graft arteriosclerosis associated with chronic rejection (Fig. 10-40). Four patients have died of disseminated malignant disease.

The majority of patients surviving beyond 6 months have returned to an active and productive existence and have enjoyed an excellent exercise tolerance. Postoperative cardiac catheterization studies reported by the Stanford

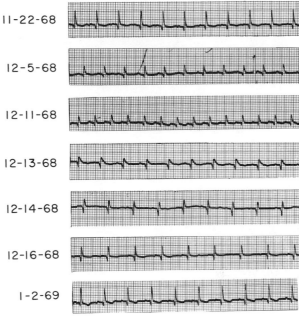

CARDIAC TRANSPLANT   L.R. ECG LEAD III

11-22-68

12-5-68

12-11-68

12-13-68

12-14-68

12-16-68

1-2-69

Fig. 10-38. ECG evidence of an acute rejection episode $3\frac{1}{2}$ months after cardiac transplantation. The significant changes include a decrease in voltage and the development of right bundle branch block; these changes were reversed with a temporary increase in the steroid dose, and the patient remains the longest surviving transplant 5 years after operation. [*From R. R. Lower, Cardiac Transplantation, in J. C. Norman (ed.), "Cardiac Surgery," 2d ed., p. 599, Appleton Century Crofts, New York, 1972.*]

group on seven patients 12 to 14 months after operation revealed normal resting pressures in the right and left sides of the heart and a fall in pulmonary vascular resistance from a preoperative average of 5.8 units to an average of 2.4 units in the postoperative study. There was no evidence in any patient of autonomic reinnervation, but the cardiac index increased from 2.5 liters/min/m² at rest to 4.8 liters/min/m² during moderate exercise with a concomitant increase in left ventricular end-diastolic pressure to an average of 21 mm Hg. It is thus concluded from the patient and animal studies that the denervated transplanted heart increases cardiac output during exercise by two sequential mechanisms: in the initial phase of 2 to 3 minutes there is predominantly an increase in stroke volume due to the Starling mechanism with little change in rate, followed later by a gradual increase in heart rate in response to peripherally produced catecholamines.

Additional considerations include retransplantation as employed successfully by the Stanford group for uncontrolled acute rejection or severe chronic rejection. Also, Barnard's group in Capetown has employed the donor heart as a heterotopic transplant, placing it in tandem with the recipient's heart to avoid the lethality of a severe rejection episode. The exact role of these two approaches in improving the results of cardiac transplantation remains to be defined.

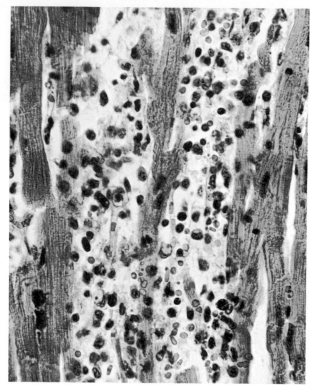

Fig. 10-39. Right atrial myocardium from a patient who died from acute rejection 7 days after cardiac transplantation. There are marked interstitial edema, hemorrhage, and an extensive mononuclear cell infiltration. [*From R. R. Lower, Cardiac Transplantation, in J. C. Norman (ed.), "Cardiac Surgery," 2d ed., p. 599, Appleton Century Crofts, New York, 1972.*]

Lung

Transplantation of the lung presents some rather unique problems: (1) for a long time it appeared that technical factors related to denervation of the transplanted lung would make it impossible to achieve normal or even adequate function of the transplant (this, however, no longer seems to be the case); (2) with the currently employed immunosuppressive agents, the lung is by far the most common site of infection in patients with kidney transplants. As an allotransplant, with the added hazard of immunosuppression, it is even more likely that the lung will become involved in bacterial, fungal, or viral infections which lead to its destruction and to the death of the host. Despite these formidable barriers to successful transplantation of the lung, some progress has been made in this field.

AUTOTRANSPLANTATION

EXPERIMENTAL STUDIES. Autotransplantation of the lung involves division of pulmonary and bronchial arteries, the pulmonary veins, the nerves, and the lymphatics. Each of these structures has a role in subsequent pulmonary events. Permanent division of the pulmonary artery results in fibrosis, but not necrosis, of the lung. Simple ligation of the bronchial arteries is without adverse effect upon the

function of the lung but probably contributes to the high incidence of disruption, leakage, and stenosis at the bronchial anastomosis after lung transplantation. Completion of the pulmonary venous anastomosis without residual stenosis has proved to be a common technical problem. If obstruction exists, pulmonary edema may result, especially if contralateral pneumonectomy or pulmonary artery ligation is carried out. Unilateral denervation of the lung by hilar stripping has sometimes been said to produce a decrease in ventilation, oxygen consumption, and compliance, while in other instances no alteration of pulmonary function has been observed. Bilateral denervation by hilar stripping reduces lung function but permits survival of the animal. In summary, the physiological effects of unilateral lung reimplantation are not life threatening in the absence of technical error.

The chief technical advance in transplantation of the lung has been the technique described by Metras and later by Neptune et al., in which a portion of the left atrium is removed along with the pulmonary veins. The venous anastomosis can be made using the wall of the left atrium instead of suturing the individual pulmonary veins (Fig. 10-41). This, in turn, reduces the likelihood of pulmonary venous obstruction. Bilateral autotransplantation has even been successfully carried out in dogs and baboons.

CLINICAL EXPERIENCE. Autotransplantation was once used in the treatment of severe bronchial asthma in human beings. A single lung was replaced in six patients, and in one additional patient bilateral staged autotransplantations were carried out. Two patients died ultimately of pulmonary hemorrhage from bronchovascular fistulae, while the other five patients, including the one with bilateral reimplantation, survived. The asthma was said to be improved. The procedure is not recommended.

ALLOTRANSPLANTATION

EXPERIMENTAL STUDIES. As with renal and hepatic transplantation, the function of the allotransplanted lung in the untreated recipient lasts for 6 to 8 days. Death of the recipient usually occurs within 2 weeks. A variety of drugs has been used in attempts to obtain prolonged survival of lung allotransplants. The function of the transplanted lung is often severely diminished even in those animals which survive for long periods of time. If the contralateral lung is removed or the contralateral pulmonary artery ligated in animals living for a long time with a lung allograft, only a few animals survive.

CLINICAL EXPERIENCE. More than 37 lung transplants have been performed in patients with end-stage pulmonary disease. Although one patient survived as long as 10 months, all efforts have ultimately failed. These failures have provided important information and have indicated areas for futher evaluation and study.

Certain technical considerations should be kept in mind. The transplanted lung must be capable of immediate function: there are no adequate artificial lungs available with which life can be maintained while waiting for the transplanted lung to function. Therefore, it is particularly important to perform a perfect venous anastomosis between the pulmonary veins and the left atrium. If this anastomosis is defective, thrombosis will occur in most cases, and even those patients with patency will demonstrate an increased vascular resistance and poor function. Other technical problems have frequently developed at the bronchial suture line because of the deficient blood supply of the transplanted bronchus, which must derive its blood supply from collaterals between the pulmonary and bronchial arteries. There is a high incidence of bronchial leakage and stenosis due to varying degrees of ischemic necrosis at the transplanted bronchus.

Lungs can be transplanted singly or along with the heart as a cardiopulmonary bilateral lung transplant. The latter procedure has been used on several patients and is preferred by some surgeons, since the anastomoses are rather simple. Bronchial anastomoses are eliminated, and a simpler tracheal anastomosis is substituted. In addition, cardiopulmonary transplantation circumvents the possibility that overexpansion of the emphysematous contralateral lung will compress the freshly transplanted lung causing immediate malfunction. This complication has been reported in several human unilateral transplants but has not proved to be a problem in most cases.

Lung transplantation in human beings has not been very successful and most patients have died within a few days. Veith has recently reviewed the difficulties which have led to this dismal state and found three groups of problems: First suitable donor lungs are extremely scarce. Even minimal ischemia of a donor lung produces transient malfunction after transplantation, and this cannot be tolerated by a recipient who is almost totally dependent on his transplanted lung. To minimize donor lung ischemia, donor and recipient must be located in the same institution, or new procedures for lung preservation must be developed. Infections other than pulmonary problems are common in prospective donors, most of whom have had long periods of tracheal intubation and controlled ventilation. Finally, the size of the donor lung, its hilar structures, and particularly its bronchus, must approximate those of the recipient to minimize technical problems.

The second major problem in lung transplantation consists of complications resulting from imperfect handling of the bronchial anastomosis, and include anastomotic disruption with air leakage, infection, bleeding, stenosis, or mucosal necrosis. The pathogenesis of these problems has been attributed to ischemia of the transplant bronchus, which must be nourished retrograde by collaterals from the pulmonary artery. Additional factors probably include rejection, high-dose corticosteroids, and size discrepancy between donor and recipient bronchi. A number of potential remedies have been suggested such as shortening the donor bronchial stump, reinforcing the anastomosis with surrounding vascularized tissue, or intussuscepting the donor bronchus within the recipient bronchus during anastomosis. Some investigators have also advocated revascularization of the transplant bronchial arteries by implanting a button of donor aorta containing their origin into the recipient aorta.

The final problem is lung allograft rejection, and Veith has postulated that this tends to take one of two forms. In one, an infiltrative rejection due to inflammatory cells

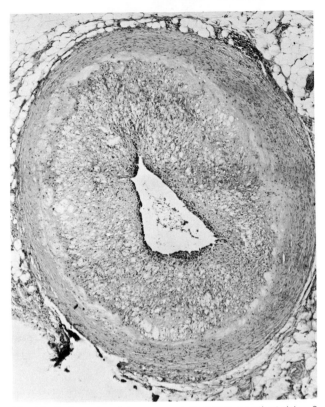

Fig. 10-40. An epicardial coronary artery from a patient dying 8 months after cardiac transplantation showing marked arteriosclerosis characteristic of chronic rejection. [*From R. R. Lower, Cardiac Transplantation, in J. C. Norman (ed.), "Cardiac Surgery," 2d ed., p. 599, Appleton Century Crofts, New York, 1972.*]

predominates; in the second, pulmonary edema is the major finding. Both are associated with opacification or infiltration of the transplanted lung on chest x-ray film and a decrease in arterial oxygen tension, fever, leukocytosis, and importantly, no change in sputum cultures. Obviously, better methods are needed for reliable differentiation of rejection from pneumonia; needle biopsy may prove helpful.

Kidney

The technical knowledge necessary to perform kidney transplants has been available since Carrel and Guthrie developed the techniques of vascular suture at the turn of the century.

Between the years 1951 and 1953 Hume performed nine cadaver kidney transplants. Function was adequate to maintain these patients for a limited period; one patient survived for 6 months. Steroids were used in some of these patients, but the doses were apparently inadequate. In 1954 Murray et al. successfully transplanted kidneys between identical twins, and the technical feasibility of routine human renal transplantation was confirmed. The discoveries by Schwartz and Dameshek that 6-mercaptopurine was immunosuppressive in rabbits, and the subsequent demonstrations by Calne and by Zukoski et al. that immuno-

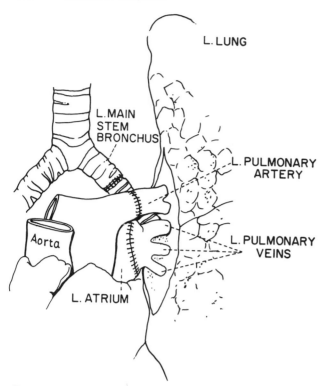

Fig. 10-41. Technique for lung transplantation (described by Metras). A portion of the left atrium is removed along with the pulmonary veins, so that the anastomosis can be made through the wall of the left atrium instead of through each individual pulmonary vein.

suppression would prolong renal allografts in dogs, led directly to the success of human renal allotransplantation. Renal transplantation is now the treatment of choice for most patients with renal failure, although hemodialysis can serve as an adequate substitute for certain patients.

RECIPIENT SELECTION AND INDICATIONS FOR TRANSPLANTATION

CRITERIA FOR SELECTION. Rigid criteria for the selection of recipients of renal allotransplants have never been defined. In general, irreversible renal failure in the patient less than sixty years of age with a normal urinary outflow tract, without active infection, severe malnutrition, disseminated malignancy, or incapacitating systemic disease should be considered for transplantation. We have found that most of the generally accepted contraindications to renal transplantation are unnecessarily exclusive. The only absolute contraindications are active infection or malignant disease that cannot be brought under control.

Renal transplantation has been carried out for almost every imaginable renal disease. Results of transplantation in most cases justify the indications, although certain precautions should be taken.

Congenital or hereditary diseases of the urinary tract are obvious indications without contraindication. Of particular note is the high degree of success with congenital obstruction and ureterovesical reflux and neurogenic bladders. It is possible to correct most such abnormalities or to substitute

intestinal conduits for bladders that cannot be repaired.

Among the acquired diseases, most transplants are carried out for either chronic glomerulonephritis or chronic pyelonephritis. In fact, many patients do not present a classic history of either disease, and the kidney disease is so far advanced by the time biopsy is performed that the pathogenesis is indeterminate. Rather than assign a definitive diagnosis suggesting a cause, it is best to regard such patients as having end-stage renal disease of unknown cause.

The more specific glomerulonephritides include Goodpasture's disease, in which antibodies to glomerular basement membrane can be detected by fluorescent techniques within the kidney. Such patients may or may not also have pulmonary hemorrhage, and they usually pursue a rather acute course of renal failure. It is generally agreed that serum titers of antiglomerular basement membranes should be performed and that the nephrectomy should precede transplantation in these patients. Transplantation should be delayed until the antiglomerular basement membrane antibody has reached a low level, and the patient should be maintained on dialysis for 6 months to 1 year following nephrectomy before transplantation.

The other glomerulonephritides are less well defined. One that is becoming increasingly well understood is related to low complement levels within the bloodstream and a proliferative membranoglomerulonephritis. Here, complement (β-C_1) can be detected in discrete fragments along the basement membrane without marked degrees of antibody deposition. Although the cause of this disease is not understood, it does not seem to be related to direct antikidney antibodies, so that delay in transplantation is not necessary. In the absence of well-defined disease, renal failure that follows an acute course complicated by a nonspecific glomerulonephritis should probably be treated by nephrectomy and delayed transplantation, although prompt transplants have been performed with success in such cases.

Most children with a nephrotic syndrome recover spontaneously or with steroid or immunosuppressive therapy. Other patients, however, develop the nephrotic syndrome and progress toward terminal renal failure despite the use of steroids. Following transplantation, some of these patients will develop recurrent nephrotic syndrome because of transmission of the disease to the fresh kidney—but most such patients will ultimately receive successful transplants.

Most patients with hypertensive nephrosclerosis present with gradual increase in hypertension and renal failure. A number of patients, however, have presented with sudden onset of malignant hypertension and renal failure. Emergency nephrectomy can occasionally be performed in such patients with resolution of the hypertension prior to transplantation.

Transplantation has been carried out in a number of patients with both benign and malignant tumors primarily arising within the kidney. Patients with benign tumors associated with tuberous sclerosis respond well to transplantation. If the tumor is malignant, it is best to maintain these patients on hemodialysis for several years prior to transplantation to avoid grafting patients with metastatic malignant disease. Diabetic end-stage renal disease was formally a contraindication to transplantation. Large series now confirm that more than half these patients will survive more than 5 years with transplants. Chronic hemodialysis is a poor second therapeutic choice.

Lupus erythematosus appears to produce an immune complex nephritis. Anti-DNA antibodies combine with systemic DNA and are filtered out in the kidney, leading to renal damage. There has not been much experience with transplantation for lupus erythematosus with renal disease, but is felt to be satisfactory if other manifestations of lupus erythematosus have been brought under control by immunosuppressive drugs.

A number of metabolic diseases (gout, oxalosis, cystinosis, hyperoxaluria, nephrocalcinosis, and amyloidosis) have very little in common except for the accumulation of abnormal deposits within the kidney leading to or associated with renal failure. Transplants in most of these diseases can be successful, although recurrence after oxalosis is common.

Patients with chronic obstructive pulmonary disease in addition to their renal disease require careful individual scrutiny. Such patients tolerate pulmonary infections poorly, and since pulmonary infections are a frequent cause of death in patients with renal transplantation, careful selection of these patients is required. Heavy smokers should be given a long period to discontinue smoking. Prolonged physical therapy for chronic pulmonary disease should also be done prior to transplantation. This is of particular importance in chronic granulomatous diseases, such as histoplasmosis, coccidioidomycosis, and tuberculosis. Such diseases may remain inactive prior to the institution of immunosuppression and be exacerbated in the presence of immunosuppressive drugs. Transplantation is not absolutely contraindicated—but the patient must be carefully followed for exacerbations.

The social and psychologic barriers to selection used by some groups seem capricious. It is extremely difficult to judge the psychologic and social stability of a patient who is dying of long-term renal disease. Similarly, one cannot exclude, out of hand, patients with coronary disease or cerebrovascular accidents. Patients with peptic ulceration do quite well if surgical correction of the peptic ulcer disease is carried out prior to transplantation. Patients with severe liver disease, however, may be more susceptible to azathioprine toxicity. Liver disease therefore remains a relative contraindication.

In short, all transplantation centers are now rapidly expanding their indications for transplantation and finding that the number of contraindications has greatly diminished.

CLINICAL EVALUATION OF POTENTIAL RECIPIENTS AND TIMING OF DIALYSIS. More important than the actual selection technique of the potential recipient is the choice of time for the institution of dialysis treatment. The conservative management of renal failure will not be discussed in detail here. In principle, homeostasis can be achieved by manipulation of the sodium, potassium, chloride, bicarbonate, water, and protein intake. An occasional dialysis may be necessary for exacerbations of renal failure secondary to infections in urinary tract or elsewhere. The protein-limited (high-quality) diets developed by Giodono and Giovanetti, and described by Anderson and associates, are essential. It is even possible to maintain patients in positive nitrogen balance over several months and even years on this diet. The main problem, however, has been motivation of the patient, and near-suicidal binges of eating are a constant problem over a long period.

Dialysis should always be instituted prior to the development of uremic complications. Once hypertension, pericarditis, cardiac failure, severe bone disease, bleeding, malnutrition, severe anemia, and neuropathy appear, management is markedly complicated and rehabilitation compromised. Ideally, the conservative management of patients treated for progressive renal functional deterioration should be carried out in conjunction with nephrologists associated with both dialysis and transplant centers. In this way, the complication of severe uremia can be rapidly prevented by dialysis without the delays inherent in the referral process.

The main indication for the institution of dialysis has been a serum creatinine level greater than 15 mg/100 ml or a creatinine clearance less than 3 ml/minute despite meticulous conservative care. It is obvious that there are exceptions to this rule. Some patients, particularly patients with polycystic kidney disease, with serum creatinine levels greater than 15 mg/100 ml can be maintained well for months on dietary management. In other patients, especially diabetic patients, severe complications of uremia will develop long before the serum creatinine level reaches that level. The most pernicious of these complications is peripheral neuropathy. If there are signs of motor involvement, the patient should have dialysis and transplantation without delay, since very rapid progression of the disease can make it impossible ever to rehabilitate such a patient. Another indication for early dialysis-transplantation is uncontrollable hypertension, or hypertension that can be controlled only at the expense of severe orthostatic hypotension and other side effects. Severe anemia with anemic symptoms (dyspnea at the mildest exertion), severe bone disease (especially in children), and the failure to maintain his diet or carry on his social and family obligations all should lead to early dialysis and transplantation. There is little to be gained by a delay of 3 to 6 months, and lives may be lost in futile attempts at conservative management.

Since some of the complications of uremia may appear suddenly during conservative management, it is extremely important that the patient be fully evaluated prior to the institution of dialysis, if possible. In addition to the medical evaluation, this preparation should include interviews with the patient and his family by the business office of the hospital, the rehabilitation clinic, and social service in order to ameliorate the financial and social difficulties that may accompany dialysis and transplantation. Rehabilitation of the patient can be actively pursued even prior to the institution of dialysis.

PREPARATION FOR HEMODIALYSIS AND TRANSPLANTATION. The pretransplantation studies are listed in Table 10-4. Most of these studies are used by many transplant

Table 10-4. WORK-UP OF POTENTIAL RECIPIENTS OF RENAL TRANSPLANTATION

1. General
   a. History and physical examination
   b. Chest x-ray
   c. ECG
   d. Electrophoresis
   e. Fasting blood sugar
2. Hematologic
   a. Hemoglobin
   b. Leukocyte count and differential count
   c. Platelet count
   d. Bleeding-clotting time
   e. Prothrombin time, partial thromboplastin time, thrombin time
3. "Allergic" potential for complications
   a. Serum electrophoresis
   b. LE test
   c. Antiglomerular basement antibodies
4. Renal
   a. Flat plate of abdomen (kidney size) (tomography)
   b. Creatinine clearance
   c. 24-hour protein excretion
   d. (Electrophoresis/urine, protein excretion selectivity)
   e. Electrolyte status in blood
   f. (Electrolyte status in urine)
   g. Urinalysis × 3
   h. Urine culture × 3
   i. (Renal biopsy)
5. Signs of hyperparathyroidism
   a. Bone x-ray (hands, skull, clavical, lamina dura)
   b. Ca, PO_4, Mg, alkaline phosphatase
6. Hypertensive work-up
   a. Chest x-ray (heart size)
   b. ECG
   c. Ophthalmic examination
   d. Serial blood pressure
7. Urologic evaluation
   a. Voiding cystogram
   b. (Retrograde pyelography)
   c. (Cystometrography)
   d. (Bladder biopsy)
   e. (Bladder stimulation)
8. Upper gastrointestinal x-ray
9. (Colon x-ray in older patients)
10. Typing
    a. ABO
    b. Blood pedigree
    c. Tissue typing including serial cytotoxic antibody determinations
11. (Pulmonary function studies)
12. Infectious work-up
    a. Chest x-ray
    b. Purified protein derivative (fungal skin tests)
    c. Urine culture
    d. Blood culture
    e. Skin-nose-throat culture
    f. Feces culture
    g. (Sinus-teeth x-ray-ear, nose, throat consultation)
13. Financial-social rehabilitation
    a. (Psychologic-psychiatric)

Note: The tests listed within parentheses are not administered routinely during the potential recipient work-up, but only when the circumstances so indicate.

groups and for patients on dialysis. A few deserve elaboration.

The urinary tract should be evaluated for patency of its outflow and absence of ureterovesical reflux. In general, a voiding cystogram suffices. That test makes it possible to determine that the urethra is unobstructed, that the bladder empties, that there are no abnormalities of the bladder wall, and that there is no ureteral reflux. Prostatic obstruction, urinary stricture, and bladder neck obstruction should be repaired prior to transplantation but only after the patient has been dialyzed for several weeks.

It is difficult or almost impossible to evaluate bladder emptying in the presence of ureterovesical reflux. Contraction of the bladder wall leads to reflux of the urine into the ureters, which then empty back into the bladder when the bladder wall is relaxed. It may be necessary to remove both ureters at the ureterovesical junction prior to evaluation of the bladder for competence.

The upper gastrointestinal tract should be evaluated for the possibility of a preexisting peptic ulceration. If significant disease is present, vagotomy and pyloroplasty or a comparable operation should be carried out at least several weeks prior to transplantation. Such precautions have almost completely eliminated upper gastrointestinal tract bleeding as a problem.

Electromyography may be useful for documenting the progress or improvement of peripheral neuropathy. Because so many patients with uremia also have hearing deficits, periodic audiograms should be carried out.

Obviously dialysis frequently must be instituted prior to the completion of these studies. Most of the studies listed are primarily designed to prepare for transplantation. Dialysis is both a definitive therapy and the most important part of the preparation for transplantation. It should not be delayed in order to complete other studies, the results of which no longer exclude the patient from treatment.

Tissue Typing and Cross Matching. The principles of transplantation immunogenetics have been presented in detail above. Prior to transplantation, tissue typing to match donor and recipient should be carried out—both for the selection of the most appropriate donor and for the determination of the prognostic implications of tissue matching. It is possible at present to type most patients completely at the HLA-A and HLA-B locus of the HLA major histocompatibility complex (Table 10-1). Typing at the HLA-D locus previously was thought to depend on mixed leukocyte reactivity of recipient against potential donor, but more recently antibodies have been developed which can detect antigenic differences at both C and D subloci of the HLA complex. What role matching at the C and D sublocus will have in prognosis is not yet known.

It is important to determine whether a putative recipient has antibodies against one or more A or B antigens by utilizing a panel of lymphocytes derived from persons bearing known HLA-A or -B specificities. Patients who have been presensitized by blood transfusion, pregnancy, or previous transplantation can then be identified; it may be possible actually to identify those A or B specificities to which the antibodies are directed. Some patients will have antibodies to the entire spectrum of A and B subloci. The detection of preformed antibodies against the C or D sublocus is far less advanced, but almost certainly such antibodies will be found.

There is strong evidence that typing for A and B sublocus antibodies and matching donor and recipient at those antigens will have beneficial consequences for the outcome of renal transplantation. Whether this is true for C and D subloci is as yet unknown.

Since patients who have preformed antibodies against the HLA-A and -B subloci might possibly have antibodies against a potential renal allograft donor, cross matching of the patient's serum to detect antibodies against donor leukocytes should be carried out immediately prior to the transplant. If these preformed antibody barriers are crossed, immediate (hyperacute) rejection almost always ensues. Varying cross-matching techniques have varying degrees of sensitivity, and the most sensitive method should be utilized, since organ preservation techniques currently permit prolonged storage of kidneys (up to 48 and frequently to 72 hours). Cross-matching techniques which take several hours should always precede transplantation.

Most transplant units draw serum samples monthly on all patients awaiting transplantation in order to detect the formation of anti-HLA-A and -B antibodies. The use of several of these sera for final cross matching should always be performed, since antibodies appear and disappear without apparent reason in recipients. Nevertheless, if a patient has previously made antibodies against the putative donor, it is likely that an accelerated rejection will occur and that that donor should not be utilized.

Principles of Hemodialysis

Dialysis removes toxic products of small molecular size from the blood and reinstitutes acid-base balance and electrolyte homeostasis. Although such treatment will not relieve all the complications of uremia, it will prevent death in a large percentage of cases. Blood is passed through a tubing composed of a semipermeable membrane, so that dialyzable substances within the blood pass into the dialysis bath and dialyzable materials within the bath pass into the blood. Fluid can be removed (ultrafiltration) (1) by increasing the osmolarity of the dialysate bath (by adding glucose), (2) by constricting the outflow of blood from the dialyzer, or (3) by running dialysate at negative pressure to raise the filtration pressure.

Transplant dialysis is not an end in itself. It merely maintains the patient while he awaits transplantation, prepares him for the operations required, and retrieves him if the transplant is temporarily or permanently unsuccessful. Three requirements are necessary to perform dialysis: (1) access to a flow of blood, (2) a semipermeable membrane tubing, and (3) a dialysate bath of appropriate composition.

Access to Blood Flow. *Indwelling Cannulae.* The Quinton-Scribner Silastic Teflon cannula was the instrument first widely used for access to blood in dialysis. The technique currently used for insertion is shown in Fig. 10-42A and B. A number of other devices similar in principle are also currently in use. Either upper or lower extremities can be used for cannulation, but the upper extremity is preferable in order not to immobilize the patient while the wounds are healing. The ideal vessels are the radial artery and the cephalic or basilic vein on the nondominant arm.

The persistence of the cannulae within the vessels and the subsequent passage through the skin have predictable consequences—the vessels may clot, the cutaneous fistulae may become infected, and the shunt is in danger of bleeding. The clotting problem looms especially large after major surgical procedures.

Infectious complications at the shunt site are particularly dangerous before transplantation. *Staphylococcus aureus* is the most common infecting agent. Long-term treatment with synthetic penicillinase-resistant penicillin plus intensive local treatment with heat and elevation can cure these infections in most instances. Systemic gram-negative infections have been rare when using disposable dialyzers. Infections are best prevented by handling all shunts with sterile technique. Mask and glove precautions should be enforced whenever the shunt is opened or manipulated. The shunt should be removed as soon as possible after function of the transplanted kidney has been established.

Arteriovenous Fistulae. Because the problems of shunt care increase with time, external shunts are most satisfactory when transplantation is scheduled within a few weeks or months. In patients being dialyzed for prolonged periods while awaiting a kidney from a cadaver, the subcutaneous arteriovenous fistula described by Brescia et al. and modified by many others has been a major advance. Here an arteriovenous anastomosis is performed, usually between the radial artery and the cephalic vein at the wrist (Fig. 10-43). The superficial veins become dilated, and blood can be obtained for passage through the dialyzer by the use of two large-bore needles inserted into the dilated venous system.

There are several advantages to this type of fistula: (1) no foreign bodies inviting infection pass through the skin except during dialysis; (2) the fistula has a lesser tendency to clot than does the Quinton-Scribner shunt; (3) the arteriovenous fistula can remain open in the posttransplant period, thereby facilitating dialysis if rejection occurs months or even years later; (4) the dilated veins are useful for the administration of any thrombogenic substance (e.g., antilymphoblast globulin) because of the rapid flow through the veins; and (5) it provides rapid access for the frequent blood samples required in the posttransplant period. Many modifications of these fistulas have been devised which utilize vascular or prosthetic grafts to bridge gaps between artery and vein; but all provide a dilated subcutaneous vessel for repeated puncture with large-bore needles.

SELECTION AND EVALUATION OF LIVING DONORS

The principles of histocompatibility typing and matching have been described above. From the recipient's point of view it is generally preferable that the donor be a biologic relative. It is still controversial whether or not histocompatibility typing can discern cadaver donors who will be more suitable than a relative. Even mismatched sibling and parent kidneys may survive with better function and for

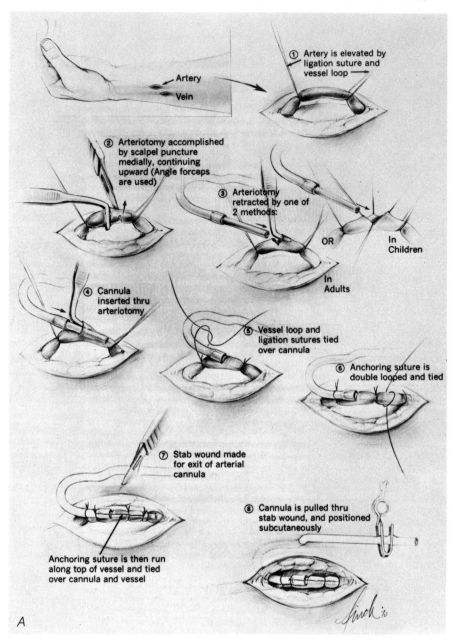

Fig. 10-42. Insertion of Scribner shunt (*A*) and connecting the two shunt limbs (*B*). [*From C. M. Kjellstrand, R. L. Simmons, T. J. Buselmeier, and J. S. Najarian, Kidney: I. Recipient Selection, Medical Management, and Dialysis, in J. S. Najarian and R. L. Simmons (eds.), "Transplantation," p. 418, Lea & Febiger, Philadelphia, 1972.*]

① Artery is elevated by ligation suture and vessel loop

② Arteriotomy accomplished by scalpel puncture medially, continuing upward (Angle forceps are used)

③ Arteriotomy retracted by one of 2 methods:

OR   In Children

In Adults

④ Cannula inserted thru arteriotomy

⑤ Vessel loop and ligation sutures tied over cannula

⑥ Anchoring suture is double looped and tied

⑦ Stab wound made for exit of arterial cannula

Anchoring suture is then run along top of vessel and tied over cannula and vessel

⑧ Cannula is pulled thru stab wound, and positioned subcutaneously

A

more prolonged periods than do closely matched cadaver kidneys. Before the advent of histocompatibility typing, it was shown that kidneys from sibling donors functioned better than kidneys from parental donors. Because the genes governing the expression of histocompatibility antigens are situated at one (complex) locus, there will always be one major allelic difference between the parent and the offspring, whereas one-fourth of siblings will be identical, one-half will have a one haplotype difference, and one-fourth will have both haplotypes different. Tissue typing can usually identify that sibling (if any) who shares all the serologically detectable antigens at the major histocompatibility complex (MHC). Such sibling grafts have a better than 90 percent chance for long-term success.

A living related donor offers other advantages to the recipient: the delay between renal failure and rehabilitation is shorter, posttransplant renal function is usually immediate, and there are fewer rejection episodes, so that smaller doses of immunosuppressive drugs are required.

The major blood group antigens (ABO) are strong transplantation antigens. Although a number of successful allotransplants have been carried out across isoantibody barriers, it is generally unwise to perform transplants into patients with known preformed isohemagglutinins against the donor blood type. The same rules apply to clinical transplantation that apply to transfusion: i.e., AB is the universal recipient and O the universal donor. When such blood type barriers are crossed, the most violent type of

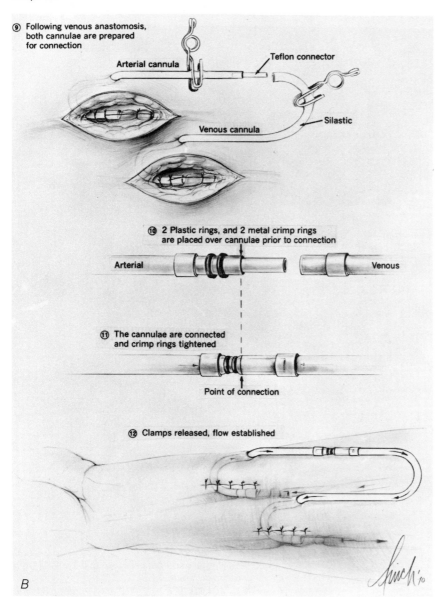

⑨ Following venous anastomosis, both cannulae are prepared for connection

Arterial cannula

Teflon connector

Silastic

Venous cannula

⑩ 2 Plastic rings, and 2 metal crimp rings are placed over cannulae prior to connection

Arterial

Venous

⑪ The cannulae are connected and crimp rings tightened

Point of connection

⑫ Clamps released, flow established

B

Fig. 10-42. Continued.
See legend on facing page.

hyperacute rejection reaction may occur. While there is no convincing evidence to suggest that minor blood group factors (Rh, Duffy, Kell) act as histocompatibility antigens, the possibility exists that they may make a minor contribution to graft antigenicity.

The living related donor should be in perfect health to minimize any risks inherent in an operation of this magnitude. A death following renal donation from a healthy person has been reported, and the utmost caution must be exerted not to harm or diminish the renal reserve of a healthy volunteer. Table 10-5 lists the examinations routinely carried out on volunteer related donors.

ETHICAL PROBLEMS. Selection of a related donor is made on the basis of histocompatibility testing when possible; often, however, there is only one volunteer. The ethical and social problems of donor selection have been extensively discussed elsewhere, but brief consideration is pertinent here.

In practice, the recipient is informed of the risks and benefits of receiving a kidney from a related donor. The recipient knows best which relatives he can approach and which he cannot. When a volunteer appears he is blood-typed and tissue-typed. If he is acceptable on these grounds, the risk of donor nephrectomy is explained to him. The risk to life in an otherwise perfectly healthy patient has been estimated to be 0.05 percent. The long-term risk has been estimated by actuarial statistics to that incurred by driving a car 16 miles every working day. Much evidence suggests that no long-term harm results from life with a single kidney. Although the risks are small, the pain, anxiety, and loss of work time are real.

It is difficult to conceive of a living related donor who is

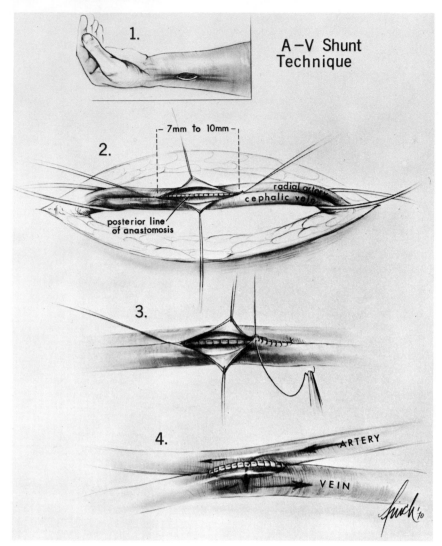

1.

A–V Shunt Technique

2.   – 7mm to 10mm –

radial artery
cephalic vein

posterior line
of anastomosis

3.

4.   ARTERY

VEIN

Fig. 10-43. Technique for constructing an arteriovenous anastomosis between radial artery and cephalic vein at the wrist. [*From C. M. Kjellstrand, R. L. Simmons, T. J. Buselmeier, and J. S. Najarian, Kidney: I. Recipient Selection, Medical Management, and Dialysis in J. S. Najarian and R. L. Simmons (eds.), "Transplantation," p. 418, Lea & Febiger, Philadelphia, 1972.*]

Table 10-5. PROTOCOL FOR LIVING RELATED
DONOR WORK-UP

1. History and physical examination
2. Hematology: hematocrit, leukocyte count, differential count, platelet count
3. Coagulation: prothrombin time, partial thromboplastin time, thrombin time
4. Chemistry: serum Na^+, K^+, Cl^-, $CO^=$, SGOT, bilirubin, uric acid, Ca^{++}, P, BUN, creatinine, fasting blood sugar, glucose tolerance test
5. Urine: urinalysis, 24-hour urine for creatinine clearance
6. Microbiology: clean-catch urine culture × 2
7. Immunology: blood type (major and minor), tissue typing, leukocyte cross match for recipient antidonor and leukocyte antibodies; VDRL; Australian antigen
8. X-ray: chest x-ray, posteroanterior and lateral; intravenous pyelogram (IVP), renal arteriograms
9. Isotope: bilateral renogram
10. Electrocardiogram

not subject to some family pressure to donate. That such pressures exist, however, is evidence that people have feelings of family and role obligations within the society. When a person freely volunteers to donate, both the benefits to the recipient and the risks to the donor are explained. No pressure is exerted to persuade or dissuade the potential donor. He is not subjected to extensive psychologic interviews or testing. Careful studies of actual donors indicate a remarkably favorable psychologic response in most donors, but some ambivalence and conflict within the family occur in a minority. On occasion, when the potential donor expresses anxiety concerning his donation, it is necessary to fabricate a medical excuse not to donate that can be used by the otherwise medically and immunologically compatible donor.

Sometimes it is necessary or advisable to use donors under the age of eighteen. This has frequently been necessary for identical-twin transplants. The use of such donors, however, should be restricted to those circumstances in which other donors are not available. A court of law will also find it difficult to decide whether an adolescent should donate to his parents or siblings when family pressure may exist. Teen-aged donors have been used when they insisted on donation and the court has agreed to it.

Unrelated persons are not generally encouraged to donate, since the results are no better than that achieved with cadaver donors. It is possible that a pool of living unrelated donors may exist that could be typed and matched against a similar recipient pool in order to obtain ideal donors within unrelated populations. Such a system was tried at the University of California but with results no better than if cadaver donors were used. Prisoners, mental defectives, and psychiatric patients are not generally used as donors for the obvious reason that undue pressure might be exerted on these persons against their own best interests. The purchase of organs, with its inevitable consequences, the selling of living unrelated organs, or even the selling of a cadaver organ must be discouraged.

SELECTION OF A CADAVER DONOR

The ideal cadaver kidney donor (1) is young, (2) has remained normotensive until a short time before death, (3) is free of transmissible infection and malignant disease, and (4) has died in the hospital after observation for a number of hours, during which time blood group and tissue type have been determined and urinary function has been assessed. Under these ideal conditions the donor kidneys can be removed within minutes to minimize the warm ischemia time. It is often necessary, however, to compromise with these ideal principles. The age of the donor is not of crucial importance. A donated kidney can recover from long periods of shock and anuria that occur while it is still in the donor. But not more than 1 hour of warm ischemia time should elapse during harvesting.

CRITERIA OF BRAIN DEATH. The procurement of cadaver organs for transplantation has raised some serious moral, ethical, legal, and psychologic problems. The first problem is to establish when death occurs. Since the decision is a clinical one, made by the physician in the interest of the patient (potential donor), it should be based primarily on clinical criteria of irreversible brain damage—fixed dilated pupils, absent reflexes, unresponsiveness to external stimuli, and the inability to maintain vital functions such as respiration, heartbeat, and blood pressure without artificial means. The decision should be made by physicians who are not associated with the potential recipient in any way, either as the referring physician or as a member of the transplant team. The exact criteria vary among institutions and have been fully discussed by Schwab, Potts and Bonazzi, the Harvard Committee, and Juul-Jensen. An increasing number of states have passed laws which permit the absence of brain function to be used to define death.

Juul-Jenson established four criteria of brain death: (1) The type of cerebral lesions must be established; the donors must therefore be selected among neurosurgical patients with severe trauma, vascular lesions, or tumors. Neuroradiologic studies, arteriography revealing the absence of cerebral blood flow, and surgical exploration assist in the diagnosis of irreversible brain damage. (2) The level of consciousness must be that of deep coma, in which the patient does not respond to any form of external stimulus. Neurologic examination must reveal dilated and reactionless pupils, absence of corneal and pharyngeal reflexes, no reaction to tracheal suction, absence of deep and plantar reflexes, and hypotonia. The patient must be without spontaneous respiration and must require controlled respiration. In this state, atropine will evidence no change in cardiac rhythm. These two criteria have generally been sufficient for most neurosurgeons to pronounce cerebral brain death after a period of observation and knowledge of the cerebral disease. A recent autopsy study confirmed that the brain damage in 24 consecutive cadaver donors was incompatible with recovery when these clinical criteria also were satisfied.

Despite this evidence, Juul-Jensen considers two more criteria, (3) a negative caloric test and (4) an isoelectric electroencephalogram (EEG), to be important. Juul-Jensen feels that the isoelectric EEG is essential, but points out that isoelectric EEGs have been described in anesthetized patients in hypothermia. He furthermore requires that the tests be repeated within a 24-hour interval where the EEG is recorded with normal amplification and double amplification with both a normal time constant and an increased time constant. These stringent EEG criteria are felt to be excessive by most physicians; vital signs will frequently fail before an isoelectric EEG will appear. A number of donors have been unnecessarily lost because of delay despite the presence of a destroyed brain.

In the past, a falling blood pressure has been used as a criterion of brain death, but it is frequently the result of dehydration due to diabetes insipidus. This is aggravated by loss of vasomotor tone, which produces hypotension. Almost all patients with total brain death can be maintained for prolonged periods with normal vital signs using plasma and vasopressors; cardiac stimulants are rarely required. Urinary output can likewise be maintained with hydration and diuretics. Even the head-injury patient who has been anuric and in shock for many hours can be restored to hemodynamic stability by restoration of a normal blood volume.

All decisions regarding the death of the potential donor must be made by physicians who understand the criteria of brain death and who have had no contact with the potential recipient. Various administrative techniques have been used; the best require the determination of brain death to be made by a team of neurologists and neurosurgeons.

The principles of organ preservation are described in a subsequent section. The advances in organ preservation have alleviated the urgency of cadaver transplantation. It is possible to harvest kidneys at the moment of death and preserve them in iced solutions for 24 hours until the transplant recipients are ready. Kidneys can now be routinely preserved by hypothermic perfusion for more than 48 hours (see subsequent section). The use of machines for this purpose has increased the availability of cadaver kidneys, because the kidneys can be transported for long distances. The development of preservation also allows for more careful typing, matching, shipping, and sharing of organs between various centers.

ORGAN HARVEST

RELATED LIVING DONOR. The actual technique of the donor operation is not as crucial as those factors that maintain urinary output in the donated kidney and in the remaining donor kidney. An active diuresis in the donor at the moment of renal artery occlusion favors prompt function in the recipient. Conversely, a soft cyanotic kidney in spasm after a difficult dissection frequently is slow to put out urine even if the period of ischemia has been short. For these reasons, the urine output is monitored throughout the donor operation and should not fall below 1 ml/minute/ kidney. The patient is hydrated during the night prior to operation, and both colloid (5 ml/kg/hour) and crystalloid solutions (5 ml/kg/hour) are administered during the operation, with constant attention to the central venous pressure and the urine output. Mannitol and furosemide

are given shortly before the kidney is removed. In addition, systemic heparinization is carried out 5 minutes before the renal artery is occluded. The heparin is then counteracted with protamine.

The technique of donor operation is described in Fig. 10-44. It is carried out through a flank incision. The peritoneum is retracted, the ureter identified, and a length of ureter is dissected free. The ureter is then transected (preserving its blood supply from the renal pelvis) so that the urinary output of the donor kidney can be observed throughout the operation. The remainder of the ureter is dissected free up to the renal vein. A large lumbar vein, the ovarian or testicular vein, and the adrenal branch of the renal vein are doubly ligated on the left side. There are no major branches of the renal vein on the right side. Dissection on the renal vein is carried down to the vena cava. The artery is not dissected free until the dissection of the renal

Fig. 10-44. Harvest of a kidney from a living related donor. [*From R. L. Simmons, C. M. Kjellstrand, and J. S. Najarian, Kidney: II. Technique, Complications, and Results, in J. S. Najarian and R. L. Simmons (eds.), "Transplantation," p. 445, Lea & Febiger, Philadelphia, 1972.*]

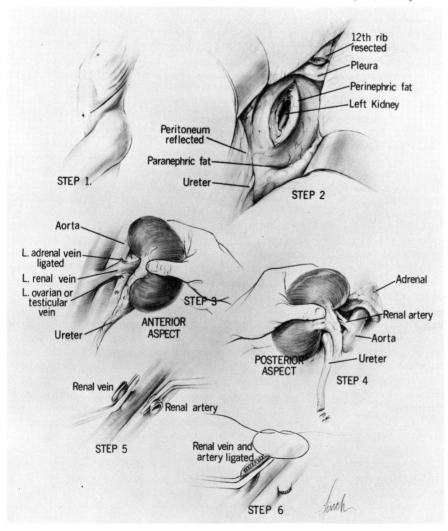

vein is complete. The kidney is not removed until urinary output from the donor kidney itself is excellent. At that time the renal artery and vein are sequentially clamped and divided.

Minor complications of nephrectomy in healthy related donors are common, but serious complications are quite rare. The function of the remaining kidney increases very quickly. Within the first hours after surgery, the renal clearance is 70 percent of the preoperative value. By 2 to 3 days cellular hypertrophy and hyperplasia have taken place and the kidney size has increased. Prolonged follow-ups indicate that the health and life expectancy of the donor are not adversely affected by donation.

CADAVER DONOR. The technique of kidney harvest from a cadaver donor depends to a large degree on the status of the donor's circulation. If the cadaver is brain-dead but with intact circulation and urine output, nephrectomy can be performed as in living donors, but by the transperitoneal route. The circulatory function of the cadaver can also be maintained by closed heart massage or artificial circulatory devices during the harvest procedure.

If the donor has a sudden irreversible circulatory collapse, the kidneys must be removed more rapidly to minimize ischemia time. The donor is heparinized, and both kidneys are removed together by clamping the aorta and vena cava above the origin of the renal arteries and veins and pulling the kidneys up together, prior to transection of the aorta and vena cava below the origin of the renal vessels and the ureters in the pelvis. Prompt cooling of the organs is required, and both kidneys can be perfused with iced crystalloid solution prior to storing them in the cold or perfusing them on preservation machines.

PREPARATION OF THE RECIPIENT FOR TRANSPLANTATION

NEPHRECTOMY. It is probably not necessary to remove the kidneys from most patients, but the decision should be carefully considered for all. Removal of the patient's diseased kidney may be desirable to (1) control hypertension, (2) eliminate a potential or real source of infection, (3) remove ureters from patients with ureterovesical reflux, and (4) eliminate the patient's diseased kidneys as potential pathogenetic agents in the recurrence of the primary disease. The latter reason is of theoretic importance only, since the recurrence of the glomerulonephritis in the transplanted kidney is not known to be aggravated by the presence of the diseased kidneys.

When indicated, many transplantation centers perform bilateral nephrectomy at the time of the transplantation. Others feel that it is better to stage the operations and perform the nephrectomy sometime prior to transplantation in order (1) to minimize the surgical stress at transplantation; (2) to minimize the surgical shock incurred, which might interfere with the function of the transplanted kidney; (3) to apply the minimal surgical stress when immunosuppressant drugs are utilized; (4) to eliminate completely urinary tract infection before immunosuppression is begun; and (5) to control hypertension prior to transplantation.

When two-stage transplantation is carried out (i.e., ne-

phrectomy preceding the transplantation by a week or 10 days), the postnephrectomy management is simple. Hyperkalemia is a recurrent postnephrectomy problem, but it can usually be prevented if a 20% glucose solution is administered prophylactically (with insulin if the patient has diabetes). Rectal ion-exchange resins may be required to control hyperkalemia. Dialysis can usually be postponed 2 or 3 days with these techniques. Delay in reinstituting dialysis is preferred because heparinization is required and although it is regional, systemic effects may occur and invite postoperative hemorrhage.

Splenectomy and/or thymectomy have also been performed in kidney recipients prior to transplantation. Thymectomy has fallen into disuse since its performance was associated with a high rate of morbidity without improvement of renal function survival. Most groups still debate whether splenectomy contributes to the well-being of the recipient. There is no evidence that splenectomy increases the functional survival of the graft, although excision of a large portion of the bodies of lymphoid mass was the original indication for splenectomy.

During preparation for transplantation, sepsis from any source must be scrupulously removed. Frequent sources of sepsis are (1) the hemodialysis cannulae, if present, (2) the bladder in patients with preexisting urinary tract infections, and (3) the skin of patients with uremic dermatitis. The bladder of the nephrectomized patient frequently becomes infected, and the bladder should be irrigated with appropriate antimicrobial agents several times weekly, prior to grafting.

Dialysis should be frequent and intense in the immediate pretransplantation period. Recipients of cadaver kidneys will have little preparation time prior to transplantation. Many patients will be maintained on systemic anticoagulants because of clotting problems in hemodialysis shunts; the anticoagulants must be discontinued, and vitamin K must be administered.

TECHNIQUE OF RENAL TRANSPLANTATION

The operative technique of renal transplantation used at the University of Minnesota is described in Figs. 10-45 and 10-46.

OPERATIVE MANAGEMENT. There must be no deficit in blood volume following the vascular anastomoses. Hypovolemia interferes with the rapid resumption of renal function. Urine usually appears within a few minutes of completion of the vascular anastomoses in related living donor kidneys; mannitol and furosemide may be helpful in hastening the appearance of urine, a useful sign that there are no serious technical deficiencies.

Three methods are generally available for establishing urinary tract continuity. The preferred method involves ureteroneocystostomy. Pyeloureterostomy and ureteroureterostomy have also been recommended, but the incidence of urinary extravasation is far more common with the latter techniques.

Renal biopsy at the time of transplantation can be useful where hyperacute rejection is suspected, but it is rarely necessary in a primary transplant from a living related donor.

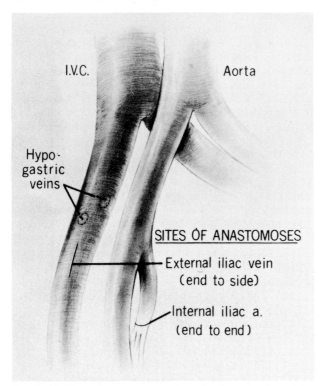

Fig. 10-45. Sites of anastomoses of renal vein to the side of the iliac vein. [*From R. L. Simmons, C. M. Kjellstrand, and J. S. Najarian, Kidney: II. Technique, Complications, and Results, in J. S. Najarian and R. L. Simmons (eds.), "Transplantation," p. 445, Lea & Febiger, Philadelphia, 1972.*]

Fig. 10-46. Anastomosis of hypogastric artery to renal artery. [*From R. L. Simmons, C. M. Kjellstrand, and J. S. Najarian, Kidney: II. Technique, Complications, and Results, in J. S. Najarian and R. L. Simmons (eds.), "Transplantation," p. 445, Lea & Febiger, Philadelphia, 1972.*]

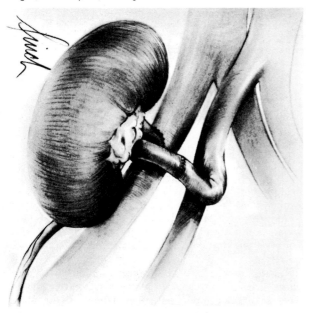

ANESTHESIA IN THE ANEPHRIC PATIENT. Certain precautions are necessary during any operation on an anephric patient. In particular, certain anesthetics are excreted almost exclusively by the kidney and should not be used. These include the muscle relaxant gallamine triethiodide. Both curare and succinylcholine are metabolized by the liver, but both may also be accompanied by prolonged paralysis in the postoperative period. In the case of succinylcholine, a number of investigators have found that serum cholinesterase is broken down during hemodialysis. In such patients, succinylcholine would be expected to have prolonged action. Conduction anesthesia has been used, but most anethesiologists prefer general anesthesia.

In the administration of anesthetics and fluids, it should always be assumed that the kidney will not function immediately after transplantation, even if dialysis is rarely required after transplantation. Similar thinking should be employed with regard to hyperkalemia in the uremic patient. Other concerns of the anesthesiologist are the loss of the hypertensive state after induction of anesthesia to normal levels, and the low hematocrit in patients with chronic uremia. The hematocrit should be raised to 30 prior to transplantation, and hypovolemia due to excessive ultrafiltration during hemodialysis should be avoided.

ROUTINE POSTTRANSPLANT CARE

The management of kidney allograft patients in the early posttransplant period does not differ radically from the management of other postoperative patients. Vital signs are monitored frequently for the first day, and the central venous pressure is utilized as a guide to blood volume. A Foley catheter is left in the bladder, and it is not irrigated unless clots are thought to be occluding the catheter. The urine output is measured at least every hour. The volume of urine should be replaced with intravenous fluids. A convenient replacement solution consists of one-half normal saline solution with 5% dextrose and water and 10 mEq of sodium bicarbonate per liter. Potassium need not be added to the intravenous fluids except in small children, whose urinary electrolytes should be replaced milliequivalent for milliequivalent.

The urinary output in the early postoperative period may be enormous, partly because of tubular dysfunction but primarily because of the overhydrated state of even the best-dialyzed patient. A creatinine clearance obtained on the evening of transplantation will be helpful in assessing renal function. So called high-output renal failure has an associated obligatory diuresis, so urine output is not an infallible guide. If the clearance is satisfactory, however, acute renal failure is not present. The lower the clearance, the greater the degree of failure. When high-output ischemic damage has been ruled out, fluid restriction can be practiced to keep from "chasing" the urinary output with intravenous fluids. The use of 1% dextrose and water with half-normal saline solution (as an intravenous infusion when urinary outputs are greater than 500 ml/hour) will diminish the osmotic diuresis due to glycosuria.

The Foley catheter can be removed almost any time after the first day. The tip of the catheter should be cultured at that time. Prophylactic antibiotics are used during the perioperative period. Thereafter oral antibiotics which are concentrated in the urine are used to prevent urinary tract infections. Moderate hypertension is frequently seen in the early posttransplant period, and a low-sodium diet and low doses of antihypertensive medication (α-methyldopa, hydrochlorothiazide, or hydralazine) are useful to counteract this tendency. Antacids appear to be useful in preventing the appearance of gastrointestinal ulceration of patients on immunosuppressive drugs.

The patient is allowed out of bed and oral fluids are begun on the first postoperative day.

ROUTINE POSTTRANSPLANT LABORATORY DETERMINATIONS. The creatinine clearance is determined for two 2-hour periods. The first is during the second to fourth postoperative hours, and once more in the sixth to eighth postoperative hours. These determinations are extremely useful in interpreting early oliguria. The hematocrit should be followed at 4-hour intervals, since rebleeding is a rare but severe complication which can produce oliguria and the onset of acute tubular necrosis (ATN).

A ^{131}I Hippuran renogram is usually performed soon after transplantation. Intravenous pyelography (IVP) is rarely necessary. Determinations of blood urea nitrogen (BUN), serum creatinine, and creatinine clearance suffice to estimate daily renal function. Serum electrolyte determinations can usually be discontinued after good renal function is established. Periodic leukocyte and platelet counts are necessary to assay the state of the bone marrow during immunosuppression. Rarely, hyperglycemia and hypercalcemia are complications, and therefore blood sugar and calcium levels should be determined from time to time. The diabetic patient will require frequent blood sugar determinations and adjustments of insulin dosage.

Prophylactic Immunosuppression. The principles of immunosuppression have been described above. Standard immunosuppressive management at most clinical transplant centers consists of azathioprine with or without prednisone or ALG. A number of centers also use prophylactic irradiation of the graft. So many factors are involved in the success or failure of the transplant that the differences in immunosuppression methods used at different centers cannot easily be evaluated. The present regimen used at the University of Minnesota is typical. It is summarized in Table 10-6.

COMPLICATIONS OF RENAL TRANSPLANTATION

RENAL FAILURE. The most serious complication of renal transplantation is the failure of the graft to initiate or maintain function. Although the causes of failure can easily be defined, the differential diagnosis may, at the time, be impossible. The functional failure of the kidney is best examined in relation to the time after transplantation: The kidney may (1) never function, (2) have delayed onset of function, (3) fail to function after a brief or prolonged time, or (4) gradually lose its function over a period of months or years. In each phase, four general diagnoses should be considered: (1) ischemic damage to the kidney; (2) rejection of the kidney by reactions directed against

Table 10-6. PROPHYLACTIC IMMUNOSUPPRESSION FOR RENAL TRANSPLANTATION AT THE UNIVERSITY OF MINNESOTA

A. Antilymphoblast globulin (ALG)
  1. 30 mg/kg intravenously daily for cadaver and mismatched related organ recipients for 2 weeks
  2. 10 mg/kg intravenously daily for related organ recipients for 2 weeks
B. Azathioprine (evening dose after checking leukocyte count)
  1. Preoperative dose is 5 mg/kg/day for 2 days
  2. First and second postoperative days: 5 mg/kg
  3. Third through sixth postoperative days: 4 mg/kg
  4. Seventh postoperative day: 3 mg/kg; maintain at 2 to 3 mg/kg
  5. Adjust at all times with respect to WBC, platelet count, and renal function
  6. Caution: Reduce dosage to 1.5 mg/kg for severe renal functional impairment
C. Prednisone
  1. Related kidney
    a. 0.25 mg/kg every 6 hr beginning 36 hr prior to transplant
    b. First and second postoperative days: 1 mg/kg/day
    c. Third through sixth postoperative days: 0.75 mg/kg/day
    d. Seventh through ninth postoperative days: 0.5 mg/kg/day
    e. Reduce level slowly to achieve a maintenance dose of 0.15 to 0.25 mg/kg/day
  2. Cadaver kidney
    a. 0.5 mg/kg every 6 hr on first 3 postoperative days (total dose 20 mg/kg)
    b. 1.5 mg/kg/day for the next 3 days
    c. 1.0 mg/kg/day for 3 days
    d. 0.75 mg/kg/day for 3 days
    e. 0.5 mg/kg/day until discharge
    f. Reduce dose slowly to achieve a maintenance dose of 0.3 to 0.4 mg/kg
D. Methylprednisone
  1. 20 mg/kg/day intravenously on evening of transplantation and on first 2 postoperative days

histocompatibility antigens on the kidney; (3) technical complications; and (4) the development of renal disease, either a new disease or recurrence of the original.

The simplest and best assay for decreased renal function is the frequent determination of BUN, serum creatinine, and the determination of creatinine clearance. Occasional renograms or intravenous pyelograms are also useful. The differential diagnosis of renal malfunction, however, may require echography, retrograde pyelography, arteriography, and renal biopsy.

Early Anuria and Oliguria

Early anuria or oliguria is a major diagnostic problem. The possibilities include (1) hypovolemia, (2) thrombosis of the renal artery or renal vein, (3) hyperacute rejection of the kidney, (4) ischemic renal damage (ATN), (5) compression of the kidney (by hematoma, seroma, or lymph), and (6) obstruction of the urinary flow.

Differential Diagnosis of Early Oliguria. The investigation of early posttransplant anuria should be rapidly performed in a strict sequence. The Foley catheter should first be irrigated and/or changed to remove any question of catheter obstruction. Unfortunately, whatever the cause of anuria, a clot can be obtained by bladder irrigation in the first posttransplant day. The clot may not be the primary cause of anuria, however, because blood will clot within the bladder if the urine is not copious enough to wash it out prior to coagulation. Therefore, even if a clot is present within the urinary catheter, the urine output should be monitored for the first 10 to 15 minutes after emptying the bladder to determine urine output adequacy.

If the obstructed catheter has not caused the oliguria, one must rule out hemorrhage and hypovolemia combined with compression or displacement of the kidney by the hematoma. If hypotension and tachycardia are present and the central venous pressure is low, hypovolemia is very likely. A roentgenogram of the abdomen will reveal displacement of the intraperitoneal contents by a massive hematoma. Echography and repeated hematocrit determinations will confirm the diagnosis. The normal degree of ischemic damage to the transplanted kidney plus hypovolemia and compression of the kidney and vessels by a hematoma all conspire to impair renal function. If anuria or severe oliguria is present, restoration of the blood volume will seldom suffice to restore renal function, even if furosemide or other diuretics are used. Many patients will require reexploration to control the bleeding point. After exploration, if the period of hypovolemia and renal compression has been relatively brief and diuretics have been used during ischemia, prompt restoration of renal function usually occurs.

The diagnosis of bleeding is frequently apparent and obviates the need for the next step in the investigation sequence—an ^{131}I Hippuran renogram (Fig. 10-47A and B). The renogram permits assessment of the blood flow to the kidney and the ability of the kidney to concentrate and excrete the Hippuran. The results are never diagnostic. If the vascular phase and concentration are near normal, however, the renal arterial and venous anastomoses are patent. If the Hippuran uptake by the kidney is severely depressed, a renal arteriogram should be done. Arteriography will assess the renal arterial anastomosis, and if it reveals the presence of intravascular thrombosis of the kidney the diagnosis of hyperacute rejection will be suggested.

Technical Complications Causing Early Oliguria. Thrombosis of the renal arterial anastomosis is rare. Partial obstruction due to torsion or kinking of the vessels is more common and should be promptly repaired. When the renogram demonstrates poor concentration of the ^{131}I Hippuran, an arteriogram should be performed to detect correctable technical complications (Fig. 10-48A and B). Thrombosis of the renal vein occurs even more rarely than thrombosis of the renal artery. When it does occur, thrombosis of the artery ensues because the collateral venous circulation of the kidney has been interrupted by the transplant procedure. Partial thrombosis of the renal and iliac veins has occurred. Usually, this is accompanied by swelling of the ipsilateral lower extremity, fever, and evidence of pulmonary embolism.

Formerly, one of the most common, and most frequently fatal, complications following renal transplantation was urinary extravasation due to distal ureteral necrosis. Rejection was seldom at fault. The problem can generally be avoided by (1) shortening the ureter as much as possible; (2) avoiding tension at the ureteroneocystostomy site; (3) avoiding hematomas within the wound, which put tension on the ureter and also interfere with the developing

Fig. 10-47. Function of a homotransplanted kidney. *A.* A radiorenogram showing a half-life of 6.3 minutes and a completely normal-appearing curve. *B.* A scan of the same transplant showing excellent uptake in the kidney and the appearance of the radioactive material in the bladder. This transplant continued to have excellent function 5½ years later. (*From D. M. Hume, "Advances in Surgery," vol. II, Year Book Medical Publishers, Inc., Chicago, 1966.*)

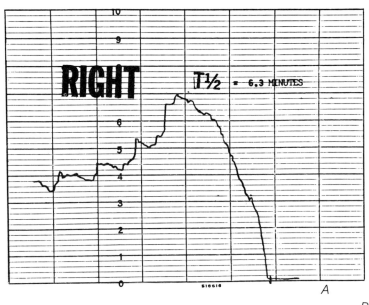

A

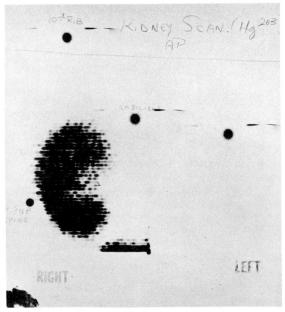

B

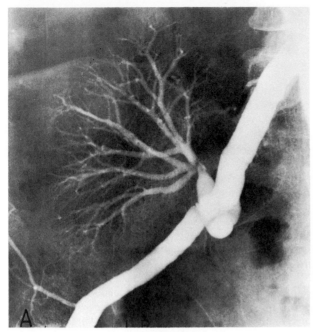

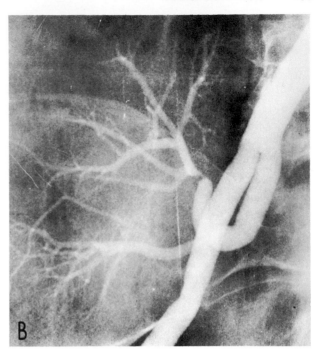

Fig. 10-48. Correctable arterial complications in the early post-transplant period. Oliguria was present in both patients. [131]I Hippuran revealed poor vascular phase. The arteriograms revealed (*A*) torsion distal to the renal arterial anastomosis, which was corrected by a reanastomosis, and (*B*) a suture that had caught the periadventitial tissues of the superior renal artery, kinking it. The defect was corrected by prompt lysis of the adventitial band. [*From R. L. Simmons, C. M. Kjellstrand, and J. S. Najarian, Kidney: II. Technique, Complications, and Results, in J. S. Najarian and R. L. Simmons (eds.), "Transplantation," p. 445, Lea & Febiger, Philadelphia, 1972.*]

collateral blood supply to the distal ureter; (4) avoiding transperitoneal "clotheslining" of the ureter by always placing the ureter in the retroperitoneal position where tension will be minimal and the collateral blood supply can develop. Urinary extravasation from ureteroureterostomies and from pyeloureterostomies occurs much more commonly than that from ureteroneocystostomies.

Urinary extravasation is a serious complication that leads to infection and frequently to death. It demands urgent reexploration with reimplantation of the ureter into the bladder, nephrostomy, or performance of a pyelo-ureterostomy to the host ureter. On occasion, the pelvis of the transplanted kidney may be involved, and nephrectomy may be required. Delay in definitive repair will frequently lead to infection, the development of mycotic aneurysms, loss of the kidney, and death.

Technical errors can become manifest long after the immediate posttransplant period. Arterial stenosis, venous thrombosis, and late ureteral leaks and strictures are frequently confused with rejection (see below). Prior to any antirejection treatment, technical problems should be ruled out by echography, arteriography, renography, or intravenous or retrograde pyelography.

Hyperacute Rejection Causing Early Oliguria. Hyperacute rejection of the kidney is almost always mediated by humoral antibody, with the subsequent participation of the

complement, coagulation, and kinin cascade systems. Platelets, PMNs, and vasospasm may also play a role. Hyperacute rejection occurs most frequently in patients who have demonstrable cytotoxic antibody directed against donor histocompatibility antigens. A lesser number of patients will reject renal allografts in the absence of demonstrable cytotoxic antibody, but a degree of subliminal sensitization that cannot be detected with current techniques may be present. Indeed, detectable cytotoxic antibody will appear and disappear at intervals in patients awaiting transplantation. The classic hyperacute rejection appears in patients who have received multiple transfusions or who have rejected a previous transplant. In these patients, the kidney will fail to regain its normal turgor and healthy pink color after anastomoses are established, despite patent anastomoses. Biopsy and histologic study at this time may reveal leukocytes in the glomerular capillaries, and intravascular renal thrombosis follows (Fig. 10-49). On rare occasions, the intravascular coagulation will be so severe that a consumptive coagulopathy with a bleeding diathesis is produced. Definite evidence of a hyperacute rejection should be treated by immediate nephrectomy. A less acute rejection may occur, however, and renal function may not fail until a day or two following transplantation. Such rapid rejection has been differentiated by the term "accelerated rejection."

Since the advent and improvement of in vitro cytotoxic cross-match tests, antibodies against donor leukocytes can be detected prior to operation. Careful cross matching is therefore essential to any transplant program (see above).

Acute Tubular Necrosis Causing Early Oliguria. The diagnosis of ischemic renal injury is one of exclusion. If all other causes of renal functional failure in the early post-transplant period have been ruled out, one must assume that the diagnosis is ATN. "Acute tubular necrosis" in

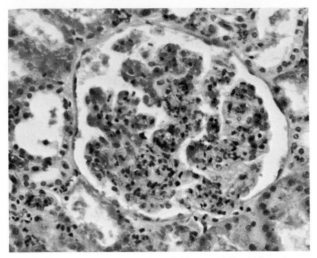

Fig. 10-49. Hyperacute rejection. A biopsy of the kidney transplant taken 90 minutes after transplantation. The glomerulus may be seen to be filled with polymorphonuclear leukocytes. These cells fill the small vessels of the cortex and aid in the rapid destruction of the endothelium.

clinical parlance refers to kidneys whose function is impaired from ischemia or a variety of other causes. If kidneys from this clinical spectrum are biopsied, they most frequently show only hydropic changes. The more severe the insult, the more likely will be the presence of tubular necrosis. The correlation between tubule pathology and function, however, is not always good and suggests the interplay with other mechanisms, including prolonged vasoconstriction and vascular endothelial cell swelling. Most kidneys will recover, but disruption is so severe that cellular repair is not possible.

ATN occurs most commonly in cadaver recipients when the donor had undergone long periods of stress and hypotensive insult to the kidney to be transplanted. Another cause of recipient ATN is a long period of warm ischemia preceding transplantation. Kidneys with warm ischemic intervals greater than 1 hour should not be utilized for transplantation, because function will seldom return to normal. Cold ischemia is much better tolerated, and preservation up to 48 hours is now very satisfactory.

Almost all transplanted kidneys have undergone some degree of damage secondary to trauma and ischemia. A second trauma (hypovolemia, hypoxemia, renal compression, bacteremia, allergic reactions to ALG) that normally might not result in ATN in normal kidneys may cause oliguria in transplanted kidneys. One must not diagnose rejection and institute massive steroid therapy in the early posttransplant period without ruling out the possibility that an additional insult to an already damaged kidney has occurred and that the diagnosis is not acute rejection but ATN. Renal biopsy may be necessary to make this differentiation.

The management of the patient with ATN is simple. Urinary flow will resume in almost all cases within 2 or 3 weeks, but anuria for as long as 6 weeks with total recovery has been observed. [131]I Hippuran renograms are useful in following improvement prior to resumption of urinary flow. Dialysis is maintained intermittently during the period of oliguria. A number of studies have shown that the long-term function of renal transplants is independent of the presence or absence of oliguria in the early posttransplant period.

Rejection

Technical errors may not become evident for several weeks post grafting, and any trauma can aggravate the degree of ATN in a previously damaged kidney. Nevertheless most renal failure appearing after the first posttransplant week can be attributed to rejection.

With better immunosuppression, the acute rejection episodes that formerly appeared in the first month following transplantation are seen less and less frequently. The majority of patients, however, will sustain at least one acute rejection episode during the first 3 to 4 months following transplantation. Clinical rejection is rarely an all-or-nothing reaction, and the first episode seldom progresses to complete renal destruction. The functional changes induced by rejection appear to be in large part reversible; therefore, the recognition and treatment of the rejection episode prior to the development of severe renal damage is of extreme importance. Usually the rejection reaction responds to increased prednisone doses and local irradiation. Even with prompt treatment the creatinine clearance may be permanently impaired, however slightly, following each clinical rejection episode.

Differential Diagnosis of Renal Allograft Rejection. The clinical picture of a rejection reaction may be distressingly similar to several other problems: ureter leak or obstruction, hemorrhage with consequent ATN infection, or stenosis or twist in the renal artery or vein. Classic renal rejection is characterized by oliguria, enlargement and tenderness of the graft, malaise, fever, leukocytosis, hypertension, weight gain, and peripheral edema. Laboratory studies have shown lymphocyturia, red cell casts, proteinuria, immunoglobulin fragments, fibrin fragments in the urine, complementuria, lysozymuria, decreased urine sodium excretion, renal tubular acidosis, and increased lactic dehydrogenase in the urine. The level of the blood urea nitrogen increases, as does serum creatinine and lactic dehydrogenase, while the serum complement level is unstable. Creatinine clearance is obviously decreased; renograms will show slow uptake of the Hippuran and slow urinary excretion. An intravenous pyelogram is usually normal. The renal cortical blood flow is also decreased during rejection, and an arteriogram may show narrowing of the cortical vessels with irregularity of the distal vessels.

The most important parameter to follow is the serum creatinine level. Unlike the BUN, which is sensitive to a number of changes (steroid administration, fever, and high-protein diet), serum creatinine levels are relatively stable for each patient. The creatinine clearance is more sensitive, but it depends on a carefully timed collection of urine. The most reliable confirmatory test of renal functional deterioration (whatever the cause) is the radiorenogram. When compared with previous renograms, the early signs of rejection are a decreased excretory rate and a slight

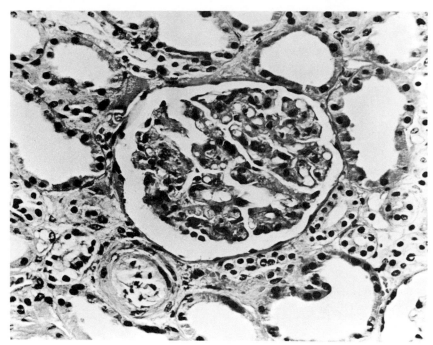

Fig. 10-50. Human allografted kidney 11 months posttransplant. The flattened, atrophic-appearing tubules are the most striking feature. The narrowed arteriole in the lower left quadrant of the picture suggests that the basis for the atrophy may be ischemia. The paucity of infiltrating host immune cells reflects both the patchy nature of the rejection reaction and the indolent pace imposed by relatively effective immunosuppression. [*From J. E. Foker, and J. S. Najarian, Allograft Rejection: III. The Pathobiology of Organ Rejection, in J. S. Najarian and R. L. Simmons (eds.), "Transplantation," p. 122, Lea & Febiger, Philadelphia, 1972.*]

delay in the vascular phase. These changes are probably related to decreased cortical blood flow and may appear prior to changes in serum creatinine. More sophisticated modes of evaluating the disturbances in renal blood flow that always occur in transplant rejection have been described, but they have not yet achieved widespread clinical acceptance.

The most reliable clinical signs of renal functional deterioration are a slight decrease in urinary output, slow weight gain, small increases in diastolic blood pressure, and edema of the lower extremity on the side of the graft. A peripheral leukocyte count and a serum creatinine level should be determined to confirm renal functional deterioration. A renogram and intravenous pyelogram should be promptly performed and compared with those obtained at the peak of renal function (usually prior to discharge from the hospital). In the face of poor renal function, tomograms during intravenous pyelography may outline a normal ureter. If ureteral obstruction cannot be ruled out, retrograde pyelography can be carried out, although it may be difficult to cannulate the ureteral orifice. Finally, arteriography may reveal (1) characteristic changes of decreased concentration of dye flowing into the kidney, (2) decreased nephrogram effect, (3) an irregularity of the cortical vasculature and intralobar vasculature characteristic of rejection, and (4) normal renal artery and anastomosis, eliminating the possibility of a technical problem.

Renal biopsy should be a definitive diagnostic tool. Both open biopsy and needle biopsy techniques have been described, and the histologic changes of rejection are characteristic (Figs. 10-18, 10-19, 10-49 through 10-52). A normal kidney biopsy is diagnostic, but a biopsy that reveals renal damage may merely reflect acute rejection, a chronic ongoing process, exacerbation of the preexisting renal disease, or damage due to infection or radiation. Nevertheless, needle biopsy of transplanted kidneys is a safe procedure in experienced hands and gives very useful additional information.

Infection and Rejection. Many apparent allograft rejection episodes are preceded or accompanied by rather mild bacterial or viral infections (Fig. 10-53). The cause-effect relationship here is unclear. The infectious agent may act as a nonspecific adjuvant, upsetting the delicate immunologic balance that exists between donor organ and host and stimulating the rejection reaction. Alternatively, the antigens on the bacteria or virus may cross-react with the histocompatibility antigens and exacerbate the host immune response. Whatever the cause, appearance of mild infection in a renal transplant recipient often precedes renal functional deterioration. Conversely, the appearance of a rejection episode should prompt a search for underlying infection.

Treatment of Rejection. Most institutions have developed a standard rejection regimen for allografted kidneys (Table 10-7). This standard regimen can be repeated as many as three times within a 2-month period in patients for whom rejection appears to be unremitting. If it is repeated more often than that, infection may appear and be lethal. The decision to stop immunosuppression and sacrifice the transplant frequently depends on subtle factors and is difficult to make, particularly in patients who have deterioration of renal function over a period of months and years.

Renal Failure Due to Recurrent Disease

Renal grafts between identical twins have been performed in human beings for 20 years. Even though such transplants do not encounter the severe immunologic barriers to success that allografts do, they have not been

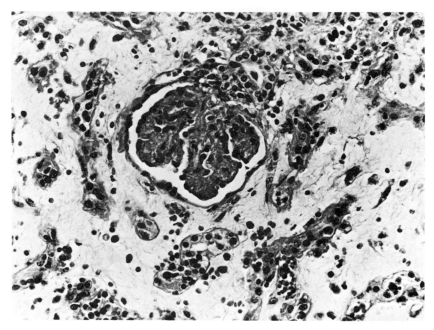

Fig. 10-51. Human renal allograft 27 months posttransplant. The interstitium dominates the morphologic features of this chronically rejected kidney. The area formerly occupied by tubule cells is largely replaced by ill-defined strands. The vacuolated appearance suggests the presence of edema. A modest round cell infiltrate, tubular atrophy, and occluded glomerular loops are also part of chronic rejection. [*From J. E. Foker, and J. S. Najarian, Allograft Rejection: III. The Pathobiology of Organ Rejection, in J. S. Najarian and R. L. Simmons (eds.), "Transplantation," p. 122, Lea & Febiger, Philadelphia, 1972.*]

uniformly successful. Recipients of renal isografts whose original disease was glomerulonephritis frequently develop a lesion in the graft identifiable as glomerulonephritis. An original disease of rapidly progressive glomerulonephritis is associated with the earlier and more frequent appearance of glomerular lesions on the isografts and subsequent progression to chronic renal failure. In contrast, a slowly

progressive glomerulonephritis is correlated with lower instances of glomerular lesions in isografts and a greater opportunity for survival. Glomerulonephritis of the isograft rarely appears in recipients whose primary disease was not categorized as glomerulonephritis.

The recurrent disease in the isografts in some respects resembles the late-onset glomerular lesion of the allo-

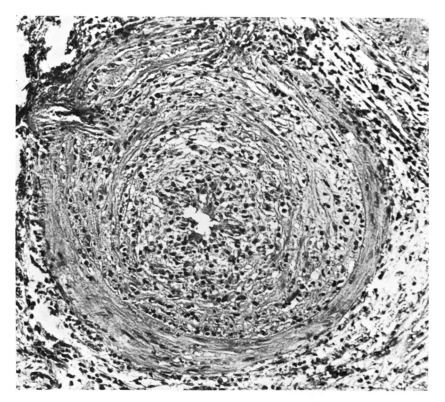

Fig. 10-52. Chronic rejection in a human renal allograft 11 months after transplantation. A small artery shows the result of endothelial cell damage and medial hypertrophy—a pinpoint lumen may be damaged endothelial cells. The bulk of the increase in vessel wall thickness, however, may be due to smooth muscle cell proliferation. The stimulus to cellular division among these cells may result from the immunologic activity on the elastic membranes of the vessel. [*From J. E. Foker and J. S. Najarian, Allograft Rejection: III. The Pathobiology of Organ Rejection, in J. S. Najarian and R. L. Simmons (eds.), "Transplantation" p. 122, Lea & Febiger, Philadelphia, 1972.*]

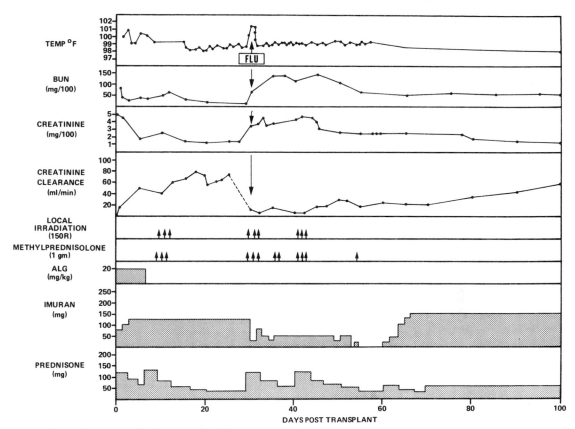

Fig. 10-53. The course of a patient whose "rejection episode" was preceded by an upper respiratory infection in both the patient and his wife. Despite prolonged and vigorous antirejection therapy, renal function returned to normal slowly. (*From R. L. Simmons, R. Weil III, M. B. Tallent, C. M. Kjellstrand, and J. S. Najarian, Do Mild Infections Stimulate Allograft Rejection? Transplant Proc, 2:419, 1970.*)

grafted kidney; the nephrotic syndrome may occur in either situation. The glomerulonephritis of isografts is associated with basement membrane and mesangial deposition of IgG, complement, and fibrinogen. The presence of preformed antiglomerular basement antibodies as well as immune complexes has been implicated in the pathogenesis of the recurrent disease. The high recurrence rate of glomerulonephritis in isografts and the apparent low rate in allografts is thought to be due to the relative universal use of immunosuppressive therapy in the latter group. Genetic predisposition to glomerulonephritis may also exist among the donor-recipient pairs in the isograft series.

Although experience is limited, prophylactic immunosuppression appears to have merit in the prevention and treatment of recurrent glomerulonephritis in isografts. Whether it is beneficial to remove the diseased host kidneys is not known. The general strategy is not to delay allotransplantation or isotransplantation after the nephrectomy of patients with proved glomerulonephritis unless the disease is of acute onset or there are high circulating titers of antiglomerular basement membrane (anti-GBM) antibody present. If the disease is of recent onset with rapid progression to failure, nephrectomy is performed and the titer of anti-GBM antibody follows until it falls to negligible quantities. At that time, transplantation should be carried out with immunosuppressive coverage in both isogeneic and allogeneic recipients.

Because so many of the changes that accompany chronic kidney disease are nonspecific, there is still active debate about the incidence of recurrent nephritis in renal allotransplants. In patients with complex nephritis, either of unknown cause or secondary to lupus erythematosus, it is possible that precipitation of complexes on the transplanted kidney GBM will reactivate the disease. It is also

Table 10-7. STANDARD ANTIREJECTION
THERAPY AT THE UNIVERSITY
OF MINNESOTA

1. Therapy
   a. Solumedrol: 20 mg/kg/day intravenously × 3.
   b. Prednisone: 2 mg/kg × 3 days; then 1.5 mg/kg × 3 days; then 1.0 mg/kg × 3 days; thereafter reduce prednisone slowly to a maintenance dose.
   c. Azathioprine: Regulate dose to prevent leukopenia; do not increase.
   d. Irradiate kidney transplant: 150 r every other day for three doses.
2. Adjuncts
   a. Reinstitute antacid therapy.
   b. Reinstitute oral nystatin (100,000 units twice daily) to prevent mucosal candidiasis.
   c. Reduce protein and fluid intake if renal function is significantly impaired.

possible that complexes of antibody will be filtered with streptococci, other bacteria, viruses, or ALG. Alternatively, direct binding of antibody with the GBM may take place, not only as a consequence of preexisting anti-GBM antibodies, but also secondary to GBM binding by ALG or by the development of Masugi nephritis. One or more mechanisms may be operating in a given patient, but, in general, most of the glomerular changes in allotransplants can be considered to be part of the rejection process.

RESULTS OF RENAL TRANSPLANTATION

TRANSPLANT REGISTRY RESULTS. The results presented here are the results of the "Thirteenth Report (1977) of the ACS/NIH Human Renal Transplant Registry" (Tables 10-8 and 10-9). All the data reported to the Registry are analyzed collectively. Although large numbers aid analysis, the reported results are neither as good as those of the most experienced centers nor as poor as those centers with the worst record. The report, therefore, should be thought of as an average of performance achieved by groups reported to the Registry.

The data for calculations in this report were derived from 19,631 transplants reported to the Registry. These include transplants performed in the United States, Europe, Australia, and Canada. It is clear from Tables 10-8 and 10-9, pooled from first transplants performed from around the world, that kidneys from living related donors survive much better than do those from cadaver donors. This has been a fairly consistent finding throughout all the years of renal transplantation. It is also clear that the improvements in results seen in the early days following transplantation have now leveled off and that the results of transplantation are not better than they were in 1968, although the mortality statistics continue to improve.

Other consistent findings from the Transplant Registry include the following: (1) Results of transplantation do not depend on the diagnosis of that disease which caused end-stage renal disease. There are several exceptions to this rule, i.e., patients with familial nephritis are usually children or adolescents and appear to have better survival, while poorer survival rates are seen in patients with malignant hypertension and cancer of the kidney. Similarly, diabetics have poorer survival, and patients with Fabry's disease and oxylosis have very poor results. (2) In general, when the results of transplantation in infants are excluded, the results of transplantation get worse with the age of the recipient. This is particularly striking after age forty or fifty. (3) The Registry has not been able to detect differences associated with splenectomy, although patients with splenectomy appear to do slightly better. (4) The Registry has not been able to detect differences associated with bilateral nephrectomy prior to transplantation.

Other registries and compilations of data from many centers have yielded slightly different data but have given indications that the following relations are also true: (1) Patients who receive blood transfusions prior to transplantation, i.e., transfusions at some time during their uremic anemia, appear to do better following transplantation than those who do not receive blood transfusions. This result is unexpected, since blood transfusions have been traditionally avoided by nephrologists for fear of sensitizing recipients to the HLA-A and -B antigens. Two factors may be at work here: (a) the patients who become sensitized, presumably from the blood transfusion, are excluded from transplantation, and this selects against the vigorous responders; and (b) patients who receive blood transfusions and who do not become sensitized may be a hypoimmunized group, i.e., have less immune capacity to respond against the graft as demonstrated by their failure to respond to the transfusion. (2) Certain registries have demonstrated poorer results in kidneys preserved by perfusion rather than ice-cold storage (see below). These results have not been confirmed by others, who show no difference in kidney survival regardless of the method of preservation. (3) Certain registries have found that patients who develop antibodies to the HLA-A and -B series of antigens reject donor kidneys more often than those who do not develop antibodies to the HLA-A and -B antigens prior to transplantation. Although sensitization is to be avoided at all costs, most investigators cannot confirm these findings and show only that if patients are transplanted with kidneys to which they have already developed cytotoxic antibodies, the results of transplantation are less favorable.

TRANSPLANTATION IN CHILDREN. Renal failure in children is a common cause of death. Traditionally, young children have not been considered ideal candidates for renal transplantation, although excellent results have been reported by a number of investigators. The small caliber of vessels and active social behavior of children make their management on hemodialysis extremely difficult. Long-term immunosuppressive therapy is also thought to interfere with normal growth with resultant social problems. Long-term hemodialysis is seldom satisfactory, and a parent is almost always willing to donate a kidney. The Human Renal Transplant Registry statistics reveal that patients above the age of five do extremely well posttransplant, confirming the impression of several large pediatric transplant groups. Several infants have had transplants, and at least one has survived for more than 1 year. The growth of children following transplantation has been the subject of several studies. Most children with allografts grow slightly slower than normal. The adolescent growth spurt is absent in children with transplants and adolescent growth is particularly depressed in girls.

This early cessation of growth causes the typical appearance of girls with transplants who are short and more cushingoid than the boys. Attempts to correlate the amount of first-year posttransplant growth with the kidney donor, renal function, or prednisone dosage have been unsuccessful. No such correlations can be made, even though it is generally felt that prednisone interferes with growth.

Sexual maturation in boys appears to be normal, although the period of observation has been short. Similarly, some girls have failed to menstruate at the usual age despite relatively normal renal function and only moderate doses of prednisone. Most girls have resumed menstruating if previously mature, or they undergo a normal menarche upon reaching age thirteen or fourteen.

MULTIPLE TRANSPLANTS. A number of studies have

Table 10-8. SURVIVAL OF PATIENTS: FIRST TRANSPLANT ONLY BY DONOR SOURCE AND YEAR OF TRANSPLANT

Donor source and year of transplant	Sample size	3 Months Percent functioning	± SE	6 Months Percent functioning	± SE	1 Year Percent functioning	± SE	2 Years Percent functioning	± SE	3 Years Percent functioning	± SE	4 Years Percent functioning	± SE	5 Years Percent functioning	± SE
Sibling															
1968	207	94.0	1.7	90.4	2.1	87.7	2.3	82.4	2.7	79.7	2.9	76.2	3.1	73.6	3.3
1969	226	90.5	2.0	85.3	2.4	82.4	2.6	78.6	2.8	77.1	2.9	72.8	3.1	71.6	3.2
1970	280	91.6	1.7	88.6	1.9	85.8	2.1	83.8	2.3	80.6	2.5	78.2	2.6	78.2	2.6
1971	420	94.2	1.2	91.0	1.5	85.5	1.8	82.0	2.0	81.0	2.1	78.9	2.3		
1972	484	94.2	1.1	91.7	1.3	89.8	1.4	85.5	1.7	82.2	1.7				
1973	449	92.2	1.3	89.7	1.5	88.1	1.6	84.6	2.0						
1974	395	92.6	1.4	88.6	1.7	84.8	2.2								
Parent															
1968	210	86.7	2.4	83.2	2.6	79.6	2.8	75.4	3.1	70.4	3.3	66.1	3.5	64.0	3.6
1969	242	89.3	2.0	85.7	2.3	77.4	2.8	72.2	3.0	68.1	3.2	63.7	3.3	61.2	3.4
1970	274	94.7	1.4	90.0	1.9	85.9	2.2	81.6	2.5	78.4	2.6	75.3	2.8	74.5	2.9
1971	340	91.7	1.5	89.1	1.7	86.8	1.9	82.1	2.2	78.1	2.4	76.8	2.6		
1972	402	91.2	1.5	88.4	1.7	86.0	1.8	81.5	2.1	77.3	2.4				
1973	424	92.6	1.3	88.7	1.6	84.2	1.9	81.1	2.2						
1974	315	93.7	1.4	91.8	1.7	88.2	2.4								
Cadaver															
1968	655	73.4	1.8	64.3	2.0	58.5	2.1	51.5	2.1	46.4	2.2	44.3	2.2	42.0	2.2
1969	862	78.7	1.4	71.3	1.6	64.5	1.7	58.5	1.8	54.2	1.8	50.8	1.9	49.0	1.9
1970	1,183	81.0	1.2	74.9	1.3	68.5	1.4	62.5	1.5	57.6	1.6	54.0	1.7	51.0	1.8
1971	1,617	80.9	1.0	74.5	1.2	68.7	1.3	62.7	1.3	59.6	1.4	55.0	1.5		
1972	1,877	82.1	.9	75.7	1.1	69.8	1.2	63.7	1.3	61.4	1.3				
1973	2,110	82.4	.9	76.6	1.0	71.2	1.1	65.4	1.3						
1974	1,836	84.6	.9	79.3	1.1	72.3	1.4								

SOURCE: Data from the "Thirteenth Report of the ACS/NIH Human Renal Transplant Registry."

Table 10-9. FUNCTION OF TRANSPLANTED KIDNEYS: FIRST TRANSPLANT ONLY BY DONOR SOURCE AND YEAR OF TRANSPLANT

Donor source and year of transplant	Sample size	3 Months		6 Months		1 Year		2 Years		3 Years		4 Years		5 Years	
		Percent functioning	± SE	Percent functioning	± SE	Percent functioning	± SE	Percent functioning	± SE	Percent functioning	± SE	Percent functioning	± SE	Percent functioning	± SE
Sibling															
1968	207	88.4	2.2	83.6	2.6	80.2	2.8	74.4	3.0	71.4	3.1	65.8	3.3	61.9	3.4
1969	226	86.3	2.3	79.6	2.7	76.5	2.8	72.1	3.0	69.3	3.1	65.0	3.2	62.4	3.3
1970	280	87.1	2.0	83.6	2.2	80.3	2.4	77.2	2.5	72.7	2.7	68.8	2.9	65.9	3.1
1971	420	84.3	1.8	80.0	2.0	73.9	2.1	69.7	2.3	68.3	2.3	66.1	2.4		
1972	484	86.8	1.5	82.2	1.7	78.6	1.9	72.9	2.0	68.8	2.2				
1973	449	83.4	1.8	79.1	1.9	75.7	2.0	70.2	2.3						
1974	395	83.8	1.9	77.7	2.2	72.5	2.5								
Parent															
1968	210	83.3	2.6	78.1	2.9	72.4	3.1	67.1	3.2	59.9	3.4	53.2	3.5	50.5	3.5
1969	242	83.5	2.4	78.1	2.7	69.0	3.0	62.3	3.1	56.7	3.2	50.4	3.3	45.1	3.3
1970	274	87.6	2.0	82.8	2.3	75.2	2.6	69.6	2.8	62.4	2.9	58.0	3.0	54.7	3.2
1971	340	84.4	2.0	80.0	2.2	74.7	2.4	67.4	2.6	61.1	2.7	56.9	2.9		
1972	402	80.8	2.0	76.1	2.1	72.1	2.2	64.7	2.4	57.5	2.7				
1973	424	80.1	1.9	74.7	2.1	68.7	2.3	62.2	2.6						
1974	315	80.0	2.3	74.5	2.6	66.2	3.2								
Cadaver															
1968	655	63.0	2.0	53.1	2.0	46.4	2.0	38.8	1.9	33.8	1.9	31.1	1.8	28.6	1.8
1969	862	69.5	1.6	61.4	1.7	53.7	1.7	46.8	1.7	41.7	1.7	37.7	1.7	35.4	1.7
1970	1,183	69.4	1.3	61.9	1.4	55.4	1.4	47.1	1.5	42.3	1.4	38.4	1.5	34.6	1.5
1971	1,617	67.0	1.2	60.0	1.2	53.0	1.2	45.9	1.2	42.0	1.2	37.1	1.3		
1972	1,877	66.5	1.1	58.3	1.1	50.8	1.2	43.8	1.2	40.0	1.2				
1973	2,110	64.3	1.0	56.3	1.1	49.5	1.1	41.1	1.2						
1974	1,836	62.2	1.2	53.9	1.2	46.3	1.3								

SOURCE: Data from the "Thirteenth Report of the ACS/NIH Human Renal Transplant Registry."

shown that second and third transplants are less successful than the first, if the first was rejected soon after transplantation. The rejection of one transplant may sensitize the patient to a number of weaker histocompatibility antigens that cannot be easily detected by sensitive cross-match techniques. In addition, such patients may have less compromised immune systems which permitted the rejection of the first transplant. In contrast, patients who have maintained a successful first transplant for several years will, after losing the first transplant, accept the second transplant more readily.

XENOGRAFTS

Xenografts between related species are rejected by the same immune mechanisms as are allografts. Xenografts between distant species are rejected by an additional mechanism—the reaction of the xenograft with preformed antibodies which then trigger the efficient complement and clotting cascades. In short, xenografts across distant species barriers are rejected like hyperacute rejections.

There is not much information about clinical xenografts, because, in general, they have not proved to be useful. Xenografts of calf skin have sometimes been used for burn dressings and appear to offer some advantage over other dressing material, although they are not as useful as allografts. Some xenograft calf heart valves have been placed in patients, although it seems likely that these will not be as successful as are allografts, and they might be expected to calcify and become incompetent over a period of years. One xenograft chimpanzee heart has been placed in a patient, but this functioned for only about an hour. Since allografted hearts are invariably rejected experimentally, it would be expected that cardiac xenotransplants would suffer the same fate even more quickly. Renal xenografts using both chimpanzee and baboon donors have been done in a number of human beings, but this procedure has been abandoned. Surprisingly enough a few relatively long-term survivors were achieved with chimpanzee transplants which were considerably better tolerated than baboon transplants. Some testicular xenografts have been carried out in man in the past but have long since been abandoned. Bone and cartilage xenografts are still used from time to time but seem to offer no advantage over allografts. The use of organs from nonhuman species for extracorporeal perfusion, both kidneys and livers, has been tried but currently is of little value.

ORGAN PRESERVATION

The viable preservation of whole organs is one of the essential components of any transplantation program. Only cadaver donors can be used for some organs (heart and liver), and even when the organ is expendable (as in one of a pair of kidneys), the use of cadaver donors avoids the risks inherent in surgical removal of the organ from living persons. If tissue typing and matching ever achieve their true potential, it may be necessary to store the organ until these matching procedures can be carried out. Even more time-consuming procedures, such as tolerance induction, may ultimately become available to pretreat the recipient and make him unresponsive to specific histocompatibility antigens. Table 10-10 lists some of those procedures which might be useful to carry out during organ preservation.

Methods of Viable Organ Preservation

The main problem associated with preservation of organs in a viable state seems to be hypoxia. When the organ is removed from its physiologic state, it is deprived of its normal oxygenation. The two major approaches to organ preservation have been what might be called metabolic inhibition and metabolic maintenance.

Metabolic inhibition seeks to prevent the normal catabolic processes from causing severe or irreversible damage to the tissues during the period of preservation. It is currently best achieved by hypothermia, which protects the organ by slowing metabolic activity and decreasing oxygen need. Two techniques of cooling are currently available: (1) simple cooling of a kidney by immersing it in, or flushing it with, a cold solution, which allows many hours of preservation and is almost always used for short periods of time, prior to transplantation of any organ, and (2) perfusion cooling, which allows longer periods of preservation.

Metabolic maintenance, the second approach to organ preservation, attempts to sustain a level of metabolic activity as close to physiologic normalcy as is feasible. Usually it implies perfusion of the organ in vitro with a carefully controlled fluid medium, although tissue oxygenation may be attempted. In practice metabolic maintenance is always best combined with perfusion cooling. The best system, at present, utilizes a pulsatile pump and pooled homologous plasma passed through a membrane oxygenator. Excellent transplantation results are obtained after perfusion as long as 72 hours. These moderately long preservation

Table 10-10. PROCEDURES DURING ORGAN STORAGE

A. Evaluation of the organ
  1. Typing and matching
    a. ABO typing
    b. Lymphocyte typing
    c. Organ cell typing
    d. Mixed lymphocyte culture with the recipient
  2. Diagnosis of disease in the donor or donor tissue
    a. Malignant tumors
    b. Infections
    c. Degenerative conditions
  3. Determination of functional state
  4. Restoration of normal function
B. Preparation of the recipient
  1. Induction of tolerance
  2. Immunosuppression
  3. Surgical procedures
C. Logistical procedures
  1. Stockpile various sizes and types
  2. Transport to a distant recipient
D. Modification of the immunogenicity of the organ

periods provide adequate time for accurate matching of donors and recipients.

Not all organs can be perfused equally well by the same approach. Certain precautions are necessary. It is necessary *to maintain optimal organ function* up to and beyond the moment of clinical death. For kidneys, adequate hydration and maintenance of systemic blood pressure are recommended. Manipulation of the organ also contributes to vasospasm, and so surgical dissection should be as rapid and efficient as possible. The *period of time* between the cessation of blood flow through the organ and the establishment of the organ in its new environment (warm ischemia time) is critical in preservation studies. *Temperature* is also important. Successful perfusion systems have incorporated hypothermia to reduce the need for oxygen and metabolic nutrients. *Oxygenation* is also critical. Oxygen dissolves in aqueous solution more readily at lower temperatures; a membrane oxygenator is incorporated into the system.

The *flow rate* necessary at 37°C can be substantially reduced when metabolic activity is lessened by hypothermia; flow rates of one-fifth to one-third of normal have been satisfactory. The *viscosity of the perfusion fluid* may have some influence on perfusion pressure and flow rate. The perfusion pressure is significant. If the flow rate is adequate to provide the nutrients and waste removal, then the absolute level of pressure is not critical, but excessive perfusion pressure invariably causes transudation of the perfusate, tissue edema, and, ultimately, obstruction to the flow. Another factor is *pulsation*. Perfusion results in less damage when the flow is pulsatile, particularly at normothermic temperatures. The necessity for pulsatile flow during hypothermic perfusion is less well documented. It is probably not necessary to maintain any *venous pressure gradient*. The *perfusate composition* has apparent significance. Whole plasma probably is the most physiologic perfusate and contains most of the nutrient ingredients, including fatty acids, which might be required for the metabolic activity of organs. Many other formulations have been successful, including dextran, albumin, other plasma expanders, tissue culture media, and balanced salt solutions. *Osmolarity* is important. Crystalloids are poor perfusates and lead to edema. The perfusate must be maintained at "normal" *pH* range of 7.35 to 7.45. CO_2 buffering may be necessary with the addition of 2.5 to 5 percent of this gas to the oxygenator. Extremes of alkalosis and acidosis can be prevented with the addition of HCl or $NaHCO_3$ as necessary. A number of *additives* to the perfusate have been tried. These include membrane stabilizers, vasodilators, and anticoagulants. *Hyperbaric oxygenation* has also been used to prolong the viability and storage time of organs in conjunction with hypothermia or a combination of hypothermia and perfusion. Hyperbaric oxygenations will probably play no significant role in organ preservation, or at least its effects may not prove to be additive to those of hypothermia and perfusion.

There is evidence that an adequate flow rate during perfusion is a good prognostic sign of the viability and transplantability of the organ. The most significant indication of inadequate flow rate is the swelling caused by fluid retention. This edema is usually the result of anoxia with subsequent lysosomal and cellular damage. Poor perfusion itself can produce anoxia, so that a vicious cycle of edema-anoxia-edema can be started. Other possible causes of interstitial edema are perfusate osmolarity and excessive perfusion pressure. Even hypothermia alone may cause cellular swelling. Another important factor in the obstruction of flow is simple blockage of the microvasculature. The many causes of this blockage have been described in detail and include bubbles in the perfusion system, fibrin, red cell agglutination, the adherence of platelets and leukocytes to endothelial cells, cell breakdown due to mechanically imperfect pumps, crystal formation, and even agglutination of bacteria. Some of this blockage can be prevented with adequate filtration, but even blood-derived perfusion media like whole plasma have been shown to contain aggregates that appear during hypothermic perfusion. This aggregated material has been identified as lipoprotein. Fortunately, these substances can be removed from plasma quite easily by freezing, which causes flocculation of the lipoprotein, and by subsequent filtration and/or ultracentrifugation to remove the aggregates.

When plasma or plasma products are used as perfusates, immunological damage is possible. This may be due to antibodies directed against organ antigens or to the precipitation of circulating antigen-antibody complexes within the organ. Although complement cannot be activated at hypothermic temperatures, bound antibody will activate complement within the recipient's body soon after transplantation. Although this has led to few recognized complications after renal transplantation, elimination of immunoglobulins from perfusates would be preferable.

One of the major problems in organ preservation research is the lack of methods to assay the functional state of organs in vitro and the consequent inability to measure the effectiveness of innovations in organ preservation techniques. Ultimately, of course, each preservation method must be tested by reimplantation of the organ. This is an all-or-none test which requires a large number of transplants in order to get statistically valid data. What is needed is an in vitro assay technique that can predict the transplantability of an organ and provide quantitative assessment of viability as the organ is subjected to the various preservation protocols. For practical purposes, such an assay should be utilized both before preservation (to determine whether postmortem changes have rendered the organ unfit for preservation) and immediately before transplantation (to determine whether the preservation efforts have been effective). As mentioned, the currently most popular technique involves the measurement of perfusate flow to the preserved kidney. Studies of enzymes or metabolites (like lactate) released from the graft appear promising.

Various pharmacologic agents have also been used as metabolic inhibitors. These include such drugs as magnesium sulfate, chlorpromazine, chloroquine, hydrocortisone, and diuretics such as mersalyl. Unfortunately, experiments utilizing such agents in addition to hypothermia show little additive effect. Most recently, however, allopurinol has been shown to protect against some of the anoxic damage to organs.

Organ Freezing

Since hypothermic storage is the mainstay of most preservation systems, it would seem logical to extend hypothermic to subfreezing temperatures in order to produce total inhibition of metabolic activity. It has long been possible successfully to store individual tissue cells bathed in cryoprotective agents and frozen at controlled rates. Bone marrow cells for transplantation and lymphocytes for immunologic typing and cross matching are stored by these techniques. Freeze preservation of intact solid organs presents several unique cryologic problems not present on homogeneous cell suspensions. (1) Solid organs are composed of a mixture of cell types that at least have the potential of having different optimal requirements for cryoprotective concentration and freezing and thawing rates. (2) The large volume-to-surface area ratio of solid organs leads to a lack of uniform heat distribution throughout the organ during freezing and thawing. Thus irregularity in both freezing and thawing are common. (3) Vascular patency is required for adequate perfusion of all organ parts, and the vascular integrity must be maintained for ultimate organ function. (4) An organ requires the integrated function of its many component tissues.

The best results utilizing frozen kidneys have required (1) gentle surgical technique harvested without warm ischemia while undergoing diuresis, (2) a quick, effective perfusion technique which will ensure the distribution of cryoprotectant uniformly throughout the kidney, (3) the proper choice of cryoprotective agent. Nondiffusible macromolecules or polymers are not satisfactory for solid organs since they have difficulty diffusing out of blood vessels to exert their cryoprotective effects on the cell membranes. The highly diffusible penetrating types of cryoprotectant, e.g., dimethylsulfoxide (DMSO), ethylene glycol, or glycerol, equilibrate rapidly (in 20 to 30 minutes) but exert a direct cellular toxicity and have a high osmotic effect. Therefore, the cryoprotectant must be added or removed in a gradual or stepwise fashion in order to prevent osmotic shock resulting in organ edema and vascular endothelial injury. Direct toxic effects of these agents are minimal in very cold temperatures. (4) The temperature of the kidney should be lowered to about $10°C$/minute to minimize both cold shock and mechanical cellular fracturing due to differential freezing rates of the core and surface layers of the organ. These rates also minimize damage from intracellular ice formation or osmotic effect. (5) Long-term storage of freeze-preserved organs requires consideration of the fact that there is continual biodegradation through enzymatic activity even at subfreezing temperatures. Therefore, storage at $-70°$ to $-100°C$ permits safe storage of bone marrow for weeks to months. The longest storage periods require temperatures of $-196°C$. Controlled freezing-cooling rates for these temperatures have not been thoroughly studied.

There seem to be two main components to the rewarming of frozen organs. The first aspect is rate of temperature increase and the second is the rate of thawing, i.e., the rate of solid to liquid phase transition. There is probably an optimal thaw rate, but the best rate for cells, tissues, and complex organs is not yet known. Some method for uniform thawing is necessary, and emersion will not work because of the difficulties in the large volume-to-surface areas of solid organs. Electromagnetic radiation appears promising, but this technique is not perfected yet. Finally, the reinstitution of hypothermic ex vivo perfusion is necessary to permit the gradual removal of cryoprotectant, which in turn reduces osmotic shock to the organ. Hypothermic perfusion also reduces the direct toxic effect of the cryoprotectant and permits evaluation of organ function. At this time, organ-freezing research is still in an empirical stage and even the general method is theoretical.

Storage of Nonviable Tissues by Freeze-Drying

Tissue grafts have been used in human reconstructive surgery for several decades. A majority of these grafts are from connective tissue and do not require that the graft be viable to function adequately. A major constituent of most of these tissues is collagen, which seems to maintain its integrity (or at least its strength) even after long-term storage by freezing or freeze-drying. Many thousands of patients each year receive bone, fascia, dura, tendon, heart valve, or skin grafts in treatment of traumatic or surgical defects. The architecture of these grafts is used as a framework for reconstruction as the host slowly replaces the tissue.

These tissues are probably best preserved by freeze-drying, which consists of rapid freezing of the tissue and the application of vacuum for removal of the water from the frozen state to the vapor state without permitting it to become liquid. Such a process usually results in maintenance of morphologic structure and therefore maintains the strength and structural integrity of the tissue. The rapidity of the initial freeze is important, as slow freezing can result in the formation of large ice crystals which can disrupt the tissue. This is apparently not a severe problem in tissues which consist largely of collagen. Other tissues, such as vascular grafts that contain elastic fibers, can show a disruption of these fibers due to crystal formation. In this instance, the most rapid freeze possible would be indicated to minimize crystal size. The graft is then dehydrated to a residual moisture of 5 percent. At this level it has been noted that tissues can subsequently be stored under vacuum at room temperature for years without further degradation or activation of metabolic processes. On reconstitution, it has been found preferable to inject water or saline solutions into a vacuum bottle containing tissue, so that the fluid can enter the tissue before it is exposed to air. Prior exposure to air apparently allows air molecules to enter the tissue and delays or prevents subsequent penetration of the water molecules necessary to rehydrate the tissue.

The usefulness of freeze-dried allografts is at least partly due to reduced antigenicity remaining in such grafts. The results of using freeze-dried allogeneic bone and autografting bone are not remarkably different. The dura has also been preserved by freeze-drying and functions extremely well when used to cover large cranial defects. Flexor tendon grafts of the hand have also been freeze-dried and used successfully, particularly when removed with their tendon sheaths intact. Many other freeze-dried tissues have been used with greater or lesser success. Cornea for nonpenetrating lamellar transplants, fascia, cartilage, heart valve, and nerve have all been tried.

Similarly, freeze-dried grafts have served as temporary biologic dressings to cover large burn wounds. In these instances the nonviable, freeze-dried graft "takes" and is even revascularized. It remains in place for several weeks or months, before it is finally sloughed. These grafts can be applied repeatedly without sensitization or acceleration of sloughing. Skin grafts have proved to be the best biologic dressing to prevent infection and to promote maximum granulation tissue formation in open skin wounds.

The usefulness of these techniques for the preservation of transplantable tissue has recently led to the organization of the American Association of Tissue Banks. The purpose of this organization will be to encourage research into and to standardize successful methods for the harvest, storage, and distribution of tissues and organs to needy patients.

References

General

Bloom, B. R., and David, J. R.: "In Vitro Methods in Cell-Mediated and Tumor Immunity," Academic Press, Inc., New York, 1976.

Calne, R. Y.: "Clinical Organ Transplantation," Blackwell Scientific Publications, Ltd., Oxford and Edinburgh, 1971.

Castro, J. E.: "Immunology for Surgeons," University Park Press, Baltimore, Md., 1976.

Fundenberg, H. H., Pink, J. R. L., Stites, D. P., and Wang, A. C.: "Basic Immunogenetics," Oxford University Press, New York, 1972.

Munster, A. M.: "Surgical Immunology," Grune & Stratton, Inc., New York, 1976.

Najarian, J. S., and Simmons, R. L.: "Transplantation," Lea & Febiger, Philadelphia, 1972.

Nelson, D. S.: "Immunobiology of the Macrophage," Academic Press, Inc., New York, 1976.

Peer, L. A.: "Transplantation of Tissues," The Williams & Wilkins Company, Baltimore, 1959.

Rapaport, F. T., and Dausset, J. (eds.): "Human Transplantation," Grune & Stratton, Inc., New York, 1968.

Russell, P. S., and Monaco, A. P.: "The Biology of Tissue Transplantation," Little, Brown and Company, Boston, 1965.

Snell, G. E., Dausset, J., and Nathenson, S.: "Histocompatibility," Academic Press, Inc., New York, 1976.

Starzl, T. E.: "Experience in Renal Transplantation," W. B. Saunders Company, Philadelphia, 1964.

———: "Experiences in Hepatic Transplantation," W. B. Saunders Company, Philadelphia, 1969.

Woodruff, M. F. A.: "The Transplantation of Tissues and Organs," Charles C Thomas, Publisher, Springfield, Ill., 1960.

Yunis, E. J., Gatti, R. A., and Amos, D. B. (eds.): "Tissue Typing and Organ Transplantation," Academic Press, Inc., New York, 1973.

Transplantation Immunology

Anderson, N. F., Delorme, E. J., and Woodruff, M. F. A.: Induction of Runt Disease in Rats by Injection of Thoracic Duct Lymphocytes at Birth, Transplant Bull, 7:93, 1960.

Anderson, R. E., and Warner, N. L.: Ionizing Radiation and the Immune Responses, Adv Immunol, 24:215, 1976.

Bach, F. H.: Genetic Control of Major Complex Histocompatibility Antigens, Genetics, 79:263, 1975.

——— and Carnaud, C.: Thymic Factors, Prog Allergy, 21:342, 1976.

——— and Kisken, W. A.: Predictive Value of Results of Mixed Leukocyte Cultures for Skin Allograft Survival in Man, Transplantation, 5:1046, 1967.

Becker, E. L., and Henson, P. M.: In Vitro Studies of Immunologically Induced Secretion of Mediators from Cells and Related Phenomena, Adv Immunol, 17:94, 1973.

Billingham, R. E., and Brent, L.: Further Attempts to Transfer Transplantation Immunity by Means of Serum, Br J Exp Pathol, 37:566, 1956.

——— and ———: Simple Method for Inducing Tolerance of Skin Homografts in Mice, Transplant Bull, 4:67, 1957.

———, ———, and Medawar, P. B.: "Actively Acquired Tolerance" of Foreign Cells, Nature (Lond), 172:603, 1953.

——— and Silvers, W. K.: Studies on Homografts of Foetal and Infant Skin and Further Observations on the Anomalous Properties of Pouch Skin Grafts in Hamsters, Proc R Soc Lond (Biol), 161:168, 1964.

Boak, J. L., Christie, G. H., Ford, W. L., and Howard, J. G.: Pathways in the Development of Liver Macrophages: Alternative Precursors Contained in Populations of Lymphocytes and Bone-Marrow Cells, Proc R Soc (Biol), 169:307, 1968.

Boyse, E. A., Old, L. J., and Thomas, G.: A Report on Some Observations with a Simplified Cytotoxic Test, Transplant Bull, 29:435, 1962.

Brent, L., Brown, J., and Medawar, P. B.: Skin Transplantation Immunity in Relation to Hypersensitivity, Lancet, 2:561, 1958.

——— and Medawar, P. B.: Quantitative Studies on Tissue Transplantation Immunity: V. Role of Antiserum in Enhancement and Desensitization, Proc R Soc Lond (Biol), 155:392, 1962.

Burnet, F. M.: "The Clonal Selection Theory of Acquired Immunity," Vanderbilt University Press, Nashville, Tenn., 1959.

——— and Fenner, F.: Genetics and Immunology, Heredity (Lond), 2:289, 1948.

Carpenter, C. B., d'Apice, A. J. F., and Abbas, A. K.: The Role of Antibodies in the Rejection and Enhancement of Organ Allografts, Adv Immunol, 22:1, 1976.

Cerottini, J.-C., and Brunner, K. T.: Cell-Mediated Cytotoxicity, Allograft Rejection, and Tumor Immunity, Adv Immunol, 18:67, 1974.

Claman, H. N., Chapman, E. A., and Triplett, R. F.: Thymus-Marrow Cell Combinations: Synergism in Antibody Production, Proc Soc Biol Exp Med, 122:1167, 1966.

——— and Mosier, D. E.: Cell-Cell Interactions and Antibody Production, Prog Allergy, 16:40, 1972.

Clark, D. S., Foker, J. E., Good, R. A., and Varco, R. L.: Humoral Factors in Canine Renal Allograft Rejection, Lancet, 1:8, 1968.

Cochrum, K. C., and Najarian, J. S.: Quantitation of Antigen Release from Renal Allografts, *Fed Proc*, **26**:572, 1967 (abstract).

David, J. R., and David, R. R.: Cellular Hypersensitivity and Immunity: Inhibition of Macrophage Migration and the Lymphocyte Mediators, *Prog Allergy*, **16**:300, 1972.

Dickler, H. B.: Lymphocyte Receptors for Immunoglobulin, *Adv Immunol*, **24**:167, 1976.

Diener, E., and Langman, R. E.: Antigen Recognition in Induction of Immunity, *Prog Allergy*, **18**:6, 1975.

Dupont, B., Hansen, J. A., and Yunis, E. J.: Human Mixed-Lymphocyte Culture Reaction: Genetics, Specificity, and Biological Implications, *Adv Immunol*, **23**:107, 1976.

Dutton, R. W., and Mishell, R. I.: Cellular Events in the Immune Response: The In Vitro Response of Normal Spleen Cells to Erythrocyte Antigens, in L. Frisch (ed.), "Cold Spring Harbor Symposia on Quantitative Biology (Vol. XXXII, Antibodies)," p. 407, Cold Spring Harbor Laboratory of Quantitative Biology, New York, 1967.

Egdahl, R. H., and Hume, D. M.: Immunologic Studies in Renal Homotransplantation, *Surg Gynecol Obstet*, **102**:450, 1956.

Feldman, J. D.: Ultrastructure of Immunologic Processes, *Adv Immunol*, **4**:175, 1964.

———: Immunological Enhancement: A Study of Blocking Antibodies, *Adv Immunol*, **15**:167, 1972.

Ferrone, S., Pellegrino, M. A., and Reisfeld, R. A.: The Major Histocompatibility Complex in Man: Biological and Molecular Approaches, *Prog Allergy*, **21**:114, 1976.

Fishman, M.: Induction of Antibodies In Vitro, *Annu Rev Microbiol*, **23**:199, 1969.

Foker, J. E., Clark, D. S., Pickering, R. J., Good, R. A., and Varco, R. L.: Mechanisms of Leukocyte Infiltration of Allografts: I. The Separation and Early Appearance of Two Components, *Surgery*, **66**:42, 1969.

George, M., and Vaughan, J. H.: In Vitro Cell Migration as a Model for Delayed Hypersensitivity, *Proc Soc Exp Biol Med*, **111**:415, 1962.

Globerson, A., and Auerbach, R.: Reactivation In Vitro of Immunocompetence in Irradiated Mouse Spleen, *J Exp Med*, **126**:223, 1967.

Goldstein, A. L., Asanuma, Y., Battisto, J. R., Hardy, M. A., Quint, J., and White, A.: Influence of Thymosin on Cell-Mediated and Humoral Immune Responses in Normal Immunologically Deficient Mice, *J Immunol*, **104**:359, 1970.

Gorer, P. A.: Some Recent Work on Tumor Immunity, *Cancer Res*, **4**:149, 1956.

Götze, O., and Müller-Eberhard, H. J. O.: The Alternative Pathway of Complement Activation, *Adv Immunol*, **24**:1, 1976.

Gowans, J. L.: The Fate of Parental Strain Small Lymphocytes in F1 Hybrid Rats, *Ann NY Acad Sci*, **99**:432, 1962.

———, McGregor, D. D., and Cown, D. M.: The Role of Small Lymphocytes in the Rejection of Homograft Skin, in G. E. Wolstenholme and J. Knight (eds.), "The Immunologically Competent Cell," p. 20, Little, Brown and Company, Boston, 1963.

——— and Uhr, J. W.: The Carriage of Immunological Memory by Small Lymphocytes in the Rat, *J Exp Med*, **124**:1017, 1966.

Grebe, S. C., and Streilein, J. W.: Graft-versus-host Reactions: A Review, *Adv Immunol*, **22**:119, 1976.

Greeves, M. F., Torrigiani, G., and Roitt, I. M.: Blocking of the Lymphocyte Receptors Site for Cell Mediated Hypersensitivity and Transplantation Reactions by Antilight Chain Sera, *Nature (Lond)*, **222**:885, 1969.

Häyry, P.: Problems and Prospects in Surgical Immunology, *Med Biol*, **54**:1–38, 73–107, 1976.

Howard, J. G., and Mitchinson, N. A.: Immunological Tolerance, *Prog Allergy*, **18**:43, 1975.

Hume, D. M., and Egdahl, R. H.: Progressive Destruction of Renal Homografts Isolated from the Regional Lymphatics of the Host, *Surgery*, **38**:194, 1955.

Interbitzen, T.: Histamine in Allergic Responses of the Skin, in J. G. Shaffer, G. A. LoGrippo, and M. W. Chase (eds.), "Mechanisms of Hypersensitivity," p. 493, Little, Brown, and Company, Boston, 1958.

Jureziz, R. E., Thor, D. E., and Dray, S.: Transfer with RNA Extracts of the Cell Migration Inhibition Correlate of Delayed Hypersensitivity in the Guinea Pig, *J Immunol*, **101**:823, 1968.

———, ———, and ———: Transfer of the Delayed Hypersensitivity Skin Reaction in the Guinea Pig Using RNA-Treated Lymphoid Cells, *J Immunol*, **105**:1313, 1970.

Kaliss, N.: Immunological Enhancement of Tumor Homografts in Mice: Review, *Cancer Res*, **18**:992, 1958.

Katz, D. H., and Benacerraf, B.: The Regulatory Influence of Activated T Cells on B Cell Responses to Antigen, *Adv Immunol*, **15**:1, 1972.

Lawrence, H. S.: Transfer Factor, in F. J. Dixon, Jr., and H. G. Kunel (eds.), "Advances in Immunology," vol. II, p. 195, Academic Press, Inc., New York, 1969.

Liacopoulos, P., and Ben-Efraim, S.: Antigenic Competition, *Prog Allergy*, **18**:97, 1975.

McClusky, R. T., Benacerraf, B., and McClusky, J. W.: Studies on the Specificity of the Cellular Infiltrate in Delayed Hypersensitivity Reactions, *J Immunol*, **90**:466, 1963.

Mannick, J. A., and Egdahl, R. H.: Transformation of Nonimmune Lymph Node Cells to State of Transplantation Immunity by RNA, *Ann Surg*, **156**:356, 1962.

Medawar, P. B.: Second Study of Behavior and Fate of Skin Homografts in Rabbits: Report to War Wounds Committee of Medical Research Council, *J Anat*, **79**:157, 1945.

Miller, J. F. A. P.: Immunological Function of Thymus, *Lancet*, **2**:748, 1961.

——— and Mitchell, G. F.: The Thymus and the Precursors of Antigen Reactive Cells, *Nature (Lond)*, **216**:659, 1967.

Mitchison, N. A.: Passive Transfer of Transplantation Immunity, *Proc R Soc Lond (Biol)*, **142**:72, 1954.

Monaco, A. P., Wood, M. L., and Russell, P. S.: Some Effects of Purified Heterologous Antihuman Lymphocyte Serum in Man, *Transplantation*, **5**:1106, 1967.

Murphy, J. B.: "Lymphocyte in Resistance to Tissue Grafting, Malignant Disease and Tuberculous Infection," Rockefeller Institute for Medical Research Monograph 21, p. 168, 1926.

Najarian, J. S., and Feldman, J. D.: Passive Transfer of Tuberculin Sensitivity by Tritiated Thymidine-Labeled Lymphoid Cells, *J Exp Med*, **114**:779, 1962.

——— and Ferguson, R. M.: Transplantation Immunology, in J. R. Schmidtke and R. M. Ferguson (eds.), "Immunology for the Practicing Physician," p. 113, Plenum Press, New York, 1977.

Nelson, D. S., and Gatti, R. A.: Humoral Factors Influencing Lymphocyte Transformation, *Prog Allergy*, **21**:261, 1976.

Nossal, G. J. V., Abbot, A., and Mitchell, J.: Antigens in Immunity: XIV. Electron Microscopic Radioautographic Studies of Antigen Capture in the Lymph Node Medulla, *J Exp Med,* **127:**263, 1968.

Parker, C. W.: Control of Lymphocyte Function, *N Engl J Med,* **295:**1180, 1976.

Perey, D. Y., Cooper, M. D., and Good, R. A.: Normal Second Set Wattle Homograft Rejection in Agammaglobulinemic Chickens, *Transplantation,* **5:**615, 1967.

Raju, S., and Grogan, J. B.: Immunology of the Anterior Chamber of the Eye, *Transplant Proc,* **3:**605, 1971.

Rapaport, F. T., Dausset, J., Hamburger, J., Hume, D. M., Kaho, K., Williams, G. M., and Milgram, F.: Serologic Factors in Human Transplantation, *Ann Surg,* **166:**596, 1967.

Riesfeld, R. A., Pellegrino, M. A., Ferrone, S., and Kahan, B. D.: Chemical and Molecular Nature of HL-A Antigens, *Transplant Proc,* **5:**447, 1973.

Ritzmann, S. E.: HLA Patterns and Disease Association, *JAMA,* **236:**2305, 1976.

Scothorne, R. J., and McGregor, I. A.: Cellular Changes in Lymph Nodes and Spleen following Skin Homografting in the Rabbit, *J Anat,* **89:**283, 1955.

Sercarz, E., and Coons, A. H.: The Exhaustion of Specific Antibody Producing Capacity during a Secondary Response, in M. Hašek, A. Lengerová, and M. Vojtíšková (eds.), "Mechanisms of Immunological Tolerance," p. 73, Academic Press, Inc., New York, 1962.

Shreffler, D. C., and Chella, S. D.: The H-2 Major Histocompatibility Complex and the I Immune Response Region: Genetic Variation, Function, and Organization, *Adv Immunol,* **20:**125, 1975.

Simmons, R. L., and Russell, P. S.: The Histocompatibility Antigens of Fertilized Mouse Eggs and Trophoblast, *Ann NY Acad Sci,* **129:**35, 1966.

Singer, S. J.: Molecular Biology of Cellular Membranes with Applications to Immunology, *Adv Immunol,* **19:**1, 1974.

Snell, G. D.: Histocompatibility Genes of Mouse: II. Production and Analysis of Isogenic Resistant Lines, *J Natl Cancer Inst,* **21:**843, 1958.

Spitler, L. E., Levin, A. S., and Fudenberg, H. H.: Transfer Factor, *Clin Immunobiol,* **2:**153, 1974.

Stuart, F. P., Saitoh, T., Fitch, F. W., and Spargo, B. H.: Immunological Enhancement of Renal Allografts in the Rat, *Surgery,* **64:**17, 1968.

Terasaki, P. I., and McClelland, J. D.: Microdroplet Assay of Human Serum Cytotoxins, *Nature (Lond),* **204:**998, 1964.

Unanue, E. R.: The Regulatory Role of Macrophages in Antigenic Stimulation, *Adv Immunol,* **15:**95, 1972.

Ward, P. A.: Chemotaxis of Mononuclear Cells, *J Exp Med,* **128:**1201, 1968.

Warner, N. L.: Membrane Immunoglobulins in Antigen Receptors on B and T Lymphocytes, *Adv Immunol,* **19:**67, 1974.

Weaver, J. M., Algire, G. H., and Prehn, R. T.: Growth of Cells In Vivo in Diffusion Chambers: II. Role of Cells in Destruction of Homografts in Mice, *J Natl Cancer Inst,* **15:**1737, 1955.

Weigle, W. O.: Immunological Unresponsiveness, *Adv Immunol,* **16:**61, 1973.

Wilson, D. B.: The Reaction of Immunologically Activated Lymphoid Cells against Homologous Target Tissue Cells In Vitro, *J Cell Comp Physiol,* **62:**273, 1963.

Woodruff, M. F. A., and Anderson, N. A.: Effect of Lymphocyte Depletion by Thoracic Duct Fistula and Administration of Anti-lymphocyte Serum on Survival of Skin Homografts in Rats, *Nature (Lond),* **200:**702, 1963.

Liver Transplantation

Brettschneider, L.: Liver: I. Experimental, in J. S. Najarian and R. L. Simmons (eds.), "Transplantation," p. 496, Lea & Febiger, Philadelphia, 1972.

Calne, R. Y.: Clinical and Experimental Liver Grafting, *Guys Hosp Rep,* **123:**1, 1974.

————: The Present Status of Liver Transplantation, *Transplant Proc,* **9:**209, 1977.

————, White, H. J. O., Binns, R. M., Herbertson, B. M., Milard, P. R., Pena, D. R., Samuel, J. R., and Davis, D. R.: Immunosuppressive Effects of the Orthotopically Transplanted Porcine Liver, *Transplant Proc,* **1:**321, 1969.

Daloze, P., Fourtanier, G., Beaudouin, M., Corman, J., Smeesters, C., and Saric, J.: Biliary Function after Liver Transplantation, *Transplant Proc,* **9:**309, 1977.

DuBois, R. S., Rodgerson, D. O., Martineau, G., Schroter, G., Giles, G., Lilly, J., Halgrimson, C. G., and Starzl, T. E., with Sternlieb, I., and Scheinberg, I. H.: Orthotopic Liver Transplantation for Wilson's Disease, *Lancet,* **1:**505, 1971.

Fortner, J. G., Beattie, E. J., Jr., Shiu, M. H., Kawano, N., and Howland, W. S.: Orthotopic and Heterotopic Liver Homografts in Man, *Ann Surg,* **172:**23, 1970.

————, Kim, D. K., Shiu, M. H., Yeh, S. D. J., Howland, W. S., and Beattie, E. J., Jr.: Heterotopic (Auxiliary) Liver Transplantation in Man, *Transplant Proc,* **9:**217, 1977.

Groth, C. G., Arborgh, B., Björkén, C., Sundberg, B. and Lundgren, G.: Correction of Hyperbilirubinemia in the Glucoronyltransferase-Deficient Rat by Intraportal Hepatocyte Transplantation, *Transplant Proc,* **9:**313, 1977.

————, Porter, K. A., Otte, J. B., Daloze, P. M., Marchioro, T. L., Brettschneider, L., and Starzl, T. E.: Studies of Blood Flow and Ultrastructural Changes in Rejecting and Non-rejecting Canine Orthotopic Liver Homografts, *Surgery,* **63:**658, 1968.

Halgrimson, C. G., Marchioro, T. L., Faris, T. D., Porter, K. A., Peters, G. N., and Starzl, T. E.: Auxiliary Liver Homotransplantation: Effect of Host Portacaval Shunt, *Arch Surg,* **93:**107, 1966.

Jonasson, O., Reynolds, W. A., Snyder, G., and Hoversten, G.: Experimental and Clinical Therapy of Diabetes by Transplantation, *Transplant Proc,* **9:**223, 1977.

Lilly, J. R., and Starzl, T. E.: Liver Transplantation in Children with Biliary Atresia and Vascular Anomalies, *J Pediatr Surg,* **9:**707, 1974.

Machado, M. C. C., Monteiro da Cunha, J. E., Margarido, N. F., Bacchella, T., Gonçalves, E. L., and Raia, A. A.: Hyperosmolar Coma Associated with Clinical Liver Transplantation, *Int Surg,* **61:**368, 1976.

Marchioro, T. L., Porter, K. A., Kickinson, T. C., Faris, T. D., and Starzl, T. E.: Physiologic Requirements for Auxiliary Liver Homotransplantation, *Surg Gynecol Obstet,* **121:**17, 1965.

Martineau, G., Porter, K. A., Corman, J., Launois, B., Schroter, G. T., Palmer, W., Putnam, C. W., Groth, C. G., Halgrimson, C. G., Penn, I., and Starzl, T. E.: Delayed Biliary Duct Obstruction after Orthotopic Liver Transplantation, *Surgery,* **72:**604, 1972.

Najarian, J. S.: Liver: III. Clinical Transplantation, in J. S. Najarian and R. L. Simmons (eds.), "Transplantation," p. 522, Lea & Febiger, Philadelphia, 1972.

——, Sutherland, D. E. R., Matas, A. J., Steffes, M. W., Simmons, R. L., and Goetz, F. C.: Human Islet Transplantation: A Preliminary Report, *Transplant Proc,* **9**:233, 1977.

Portmann, B., Schindler, A.-M., Murray-Lyon, I. M., and Williams, R.: Histological Sexing of a Reticulum Cell Sarcoma Arising after Liver Transplantation, *Gastroenterology,* **70**:82, 1976.

Putnam, C. W., Bell, R. H., Jr., Beart, R. W., Jr., and Starzl, T. E.: Hepatic Transplantation, 1975, *Postgrad Med J,* **52** (suppl 5): 104, 1976.

——, Porter, K. A., Weill, R., III, Reid, H. A. S., and Starzl, T. E.: Liver Transplantation for Budd-Chiari Syndrome, *JAMA,* **236**:1142, 1976.

Roddy, H., Putnam, C. W., and Fennell, R. H., Jr.: Pathology of Liver Transplantation, *Transplantation,* **22**:625, 1976.

Schröter, G. P. J., Hoelscher, M., Putnam, C. W., Porter, K. A., Hansbrough, J. F., and Starzl, T. E.: Infections Complicating Orthotopic Liver Transplantation: A Study Emphasizing Graft-Related Septicemia, *Arch Surg,* **111**:1337, 1976.

Starzl, T. E.: "Experience in Hepatic Transplantation," W. B. Saunders Company, Philadelphia, 1969.

——, Porter, K. A., Putnam, C. W., Schroter, G. P. J., Halgrimson, C. G., Weil, R., III, Hoelscher, M., and Reid, H. A. S.: Orthotopic Liver Transplantation in Ninety-Three Patients, *Surg Gynecol Obstet,* **142**:487, 1976.

Stuart, F. P., Torres, E., Hester, W. J., Dammin, G. J., and Moore, F. D.: Orthotopic Autotransplantation and Allotransplantation of the Liver: Functional and Structural Patterns in the Dog, *Ann Surg,* **165**:325, 1967.

Sutherland, D. E. R., Matas, A. J., Steffes, M. W., Simmons, R. L., and Najarian, J. S.: Transplantation of Liver Cells in an Animal Model of Congenital Enzyme Deficiency Disease: The Gunn Rat, *Transplant Proc,* **9**:317, 1977.

Welch, C. S.: A Note on the Transplantation of the Whole Liver in Dogs, *Transplant Bull,* **2**:54, 1955.

Cardiac Transplantation

Barnard, C. N.: A Human Cardiac Transplant, *S Afri Med J,* **41**:1271, 1967.

Campeau, L., Pospisil, L., Grondin, P., Dyrda, I., and Lepage, G.: Cardiac Catheterization Findings at Rest and after Exercise in Patients following Cardiac Transplantation, *Am J Cardiol,* **25**:523, 1970.

Childs, J. W., and Lower, R. R.: Preservation of the Heart, *Prog Cardiovasc Dis,* **12**:149, 1969.

Cooley, D. A., Bloodwell, R. D., Hallman, G. L., and Nora, J. J.: Transplantation of the Heart: A Report of Four Cases. *JAMA,* **205**:479, 1968.

DeBakey, M. E., Diethrich, E. B., Glick, G., Noon, G. P., Butler, W. T., Rossen, R. D., Liddicoat, J. E., and Brooks, D. K.: Human Cardiac Transplantation: Clinical Experience, *J Thorac Cardiovasc Surg,* **58**:303, 1969.

Ellis, R. J., Lillehei, C. W., and Zabriskie, J. B.: Detection of Circulating Heart-reactive antibody in Human Heart Transplants, *JAMA,* **211**:1505, 1970.

Griepp, R. B., Stinson, E. B., Bieber, C. P., Reitz, B. A., Copeland, J. G., Oyer, P. E., and Shumway, N. E.: Human Heart Transplantation: Current Status, *Ann Thorac Surg,* **22**:171, 1976.

Grinnan, G. L., Graham, W. H., Childs, J. W., and Lower, R. R.: Cardiopulmonary Homotransplantation, *J Thorac Cardiovasc Surg,* **60**:609, 1970.

Hardy, J. D., Chavez, C. M., Kurrus, F. D., Neely, W. A., Eraslan, S., Turner, M. D., Fabian, L. W., and Labeck, T. D.: Heart Transplantation in Man: Developmental Studies and Report of a Case, *JAMA,* **188**:1132, 1964.

Kahn, D. R., Reynolds, E. W., Jr., Walton, J. A., Kirsh, M. M., Vathayanon, S., and Sloan, H.: Human Heart Transplantation for Cardiomyopathy, *Surgery,* **67**:122, 1970.

Kosek, J. C., Bieber, C., and Lower, R. R.: Heart Graft Arteriosclerosis, *Transplant Proc,* **3**:512, 1971.

——, Hurley, E. J., and Lower, R. R.: Histopathology of Orthotopic Canine Cardiac Homografts, *Lab Invest,* **19**:97, 1968.

Lower, R. R.: Cardiac Transplantation without Complete Cardiac Denervation: The Role of the Afferent Receptors, *Am Heart J,* **72**:841, 1966.

——, Dong, E., Jr., and Shumway, N. E.: Long Term Survival of Cardiac Homografts, *Surgery,* **58**:100, 1965.

——, Stofer, R. C., and Shumway, N. E.: Homovital Transplantation of the Heart, *J Thorac Cardiovasc Surg,* **41**:196, 1961.

——, Szentpetery, S., Thomas, F. T., and Kemp, V. E.: Clinical Observation on Cardiac Transplantation, *Transplant Proc,* **8**:9, 1976.

Milan, J. D., Shipkey, F. H., Lind, C. J., Jr., Nora, J. J., Leachman, R. D., Rochelle, D. G., Bloodwell, R. D., Hallman, G. L., and Cooley, D. A.: Morphologic Findings in Human Cardiac Allografts, *Circulation,* **41**:519, 1970.

Schroeder, J. S., Popp, R. L., Stinson, E. B., Dong, E., Jr., Shumway, N. E., and Harrison, D. C.: Acute Rejection following Cardiac Transplantation: Phonocardiographic and Ultrasound Observations, *Circulation,* **40**:155, 1969.

Sewell, D. H., Kemp, V. E., and Lower, R. R.: The Epicardial ECG in Monitoring Cardiac Homograft Rejection, *Circulation,* **39** (*Suppl* 1):21, 1969.

Thomas, F., Kemp, V. E., Szentpetery, S., and Lower, R. R.: Monitoring and Modulation of Immune Reactivity in Cardiac Recipients, in J. Davila (ed.), "Second Henry Ford Hospital International Symposium on Cardiac Surgery," Appleton-Century-Crofts, Inc., New York, 1977.

Thomas, K. E., Linehan, J. D., and Lower, R. R.: Size Disparity in Dogs between Donor and Recipient in Cardiac Transplantation, *Surg Forum,* **21**:183, 1970.

Willman, V. L., Kaiser, G. C., Harades, Y., Cooper, T., and Hanlon, C. R.: Physiological Alterations following Transplantation of the Heart, *Adv Transplant Proc 1st Cong Transplant Soc,* 1968, p. 661.

Lung Transplantation

Arnar, O., Andersen, R. C., Hitchcock, C R., and Haglin, J. J.: Reimplantation of the Baboon Lung after Extended Ischemia, *Transplantation,* **5**:929, 1967.

Blumenstock, D. A.: Transplantation of the Lung, *Transplantation,* **5**:917, 1967.

—— and Veith, F. J.: Lung (Clinical Transplantation), in J. S. Najarian and R. L. Simmons (eds.), "Transplantation," p. 569, Lea & Febiger, Philadelphia, 1972.

Haglin, J. J., and Arnar, O.: Physiologic Studies of the Baboon

Living on Only the Reimplanted Lung, *Surg Forum,* **15:**175, 1964.

Veith, F. J.: Lung Transplantation, *Transplant Proc,* **9:**203, 1977.

Kidney Transplantation

Advisory Committee to the Renal Transplant Registry (Barnes, B. A., Bergan, J. J., Braun, W. E., Fraumeni, J. F., Jr., Kountz, S. L., Mickey, M. R., Rubin, A. L., Simmons, R. L., Stavens, L. E., and Wilson, R. E.): Renal Transplantation in Congenital and Metabolic Diseases, *JAMA,* **232:**148, 1975.

Advisory Committee to the Renal Transplant Registry: Twelfth Report of the Human Renal Transplant Registry, *JAMA,* **233:**787, 1975.

Aldrete, J. S., Sterling, W. A., Hathaway, B. M., Morgan, J. M., and Diethelm, A. G.: Gastrointestinal and Hepatic Complications Affecting Patients with Renal Allografts, *Am J Surg,* **129:**115, 1975.

Alfrey, A. C., Jenkins, D., Groth, C. G., Schorr, W. S., Gecelter, L., and Ogden, D. A.: Resolution of Hyperparathyroidism, Renal Osteodystrophy and Metastatic Calcification after Renal Homotransplantation, *N Engl J Med,* **279:**1349, 1968.

Anderson, C. B., Codd, J. E., Graff, R. J., Gregory, J. G., Gorce, M. A., and Newton, W. T.: Serum Lactic Dehydrogenase and Human Renal Allograft Failure, *Surgery,* **77:**674, 1975.

Anderson, C. F., Nelson, R. A., Margie, J. D., Johnson, W. J., and Hunt, J. C.: Nutritional Therapy for Adults with Renal Disease, *JAMA* **223:**68, 1973.

Asbury, A. K.: Recovery from Uremic Neuropathy, *N Engl J Med,* **281:**1211, 1971.

Astle, J. N., and Ellis, P. P.: Ocular Complications in Renal Transplant Patients, *Ann Ophthalmol,* **6:**1269, 1974.

Balch, C. M., Morgan, J. M., Sterling, W. A., Bradley, E. L., and Dietheim, A. G.: Kidney Transplantation in Patients with End Stage Congenital Renal Disease: Report of Eighteen Cases and Review of the Organ Transplant Registry, *Am J Surg,* **130:**303, 1975.

Bartrum, R. J., Jr., Smith, E. H., D'Orsi, C. J., and Tilney, N. L.: Evaluation of Renal Transplants with Ultrasound, *Radiology,* **118:**405, 1976.

Baxby, K., Taylor, R. M. R., Anderson, M., Johnson, R. W. G., and Swinney, J.: Assessment of Cadaveric Kidneys for Transplantation, *Lancet,* **2:**977, 1974.

Beecher, H. K.: After the "Definition of Irreversible Coma," *N Engl J Med,* **281:**1070, 1968.

Belzer, F. O., Ashby, B. S., Gulyassy, P. F., and Powell, M.: Successful Seventeen-Hour Preservation and Transplantation of Human-Cadaver Kidney, *N Engl J Med,* **278:**608, 1968.

———, Perkins, H. A., Fortmann, J. L., Kountz, S. L., Salvatierra, O., Cochrum, K. C., and Payne, R.: Is HL-A Typing of Clinical Significance in Cadaver Renal Transplantation?, *Lancet,* **1:**774, 1974.

Bernstein, W. C., Nivatvongs, S., and Tallent, M. B.: Colonic and Rectal Complications of Kidney Transplantation in Man, *Dis Colon Rectum,* **16:**255, 1973.

Blaufox, M. D., Birbari, A. E., Hickler, T. B., and Merrill, J. P.: Peripheral Plasma Renin Activity in Renal-Homotransplant Recipients, *N Engl J Med,* **275:**1165, 1966.

Bolton, C. F., Baltzan, M. A., and Baltzan, R. B.: Effects of Renal

Transplantation on Uremic Neuropathy: A Clinical and Electrophysiologic Study, *N Engl J Med,* **284:**1170, 1971.

Braun, W. E., Banowsky, L. H., Straffon, R. A., Nakamoto, S., Kiser, W. S., Popowniak, K. L., Hewitt, C. B., Stewart, B. H., Zelch, J. V., Magalhaes, R. L., Lachance, J.-G., and Manning, R. F.: Lymphoceles Associated with Renal Transplantation: Report of 15 Cases and Review of the Literature, *Am J Med,* **57:**714, 1974.

Brescia, M. J., Cimino, J. E., Appel, K., and Hurwich, B. J.: Chronic Hemodialysis Using Venipuncture and Surgically Created Arteriovenous Fistula, *N Engl J Med,* **275:**1089, 1966.

Butt, K. M. H., Friedman, E. A., and Kountz, S. L.: Angioaccess, *Curr Probl Surg,* **8:**1, 1976.

Callender, C. O., Simmons, R. L., Yunis, E. J., Toledo-Pereyra, L. H., DeShazo, M. T. M., and Najarian, J. S.: Anti-HL-A Antibodies: Failure to Correlate with Renal Allograft Rejection, *Surgery,* **76:**573, 1974.

Calne, R. Y.: Cadaveric Kidneys for Transplantation, *Br Med J,* **2:**565, 1969.

Casali, R., Simmons, R. L., Ferguson, R. M., Mauer, S. M., Kjellstrand, C. M., Buselmeier, T. J., and Najarian, J. S.: Factors Related to Success or Failure of Second Renal Transplants, *Ann Surg,* **184:**145, 1976.

Cosimi, A. B., Wortis, H. H., Delmonico, F. L., and Russell, P. S.: Randomized Clinical Trial of Antithymocyte Globulin in Cadaver Renal Allograft Recipients: Importance of T Cell Monitoring, *Surgery,* **80:**155, 1976.

Dausset, J., Hors, J., Busson, M., Festenstein, H., Oliver, R. T. D., Paris, A. M. I., and Sachs, J. A.: Serologically Defined HL-A Antigens and Long-Term Survival of Cadaver Kidney Transplants: Joint Analysis of 918 Cases Performed by France-Transplant and the London Transplant Group, *N Engl J Med,* **290:**979, 1974.

David, D. S., Sakai, S., Brennan, B. L., Riggio, R. A., Cheigh, J., Stenzel, K. H., Rubin, A. L., and Sherwood, L. M.: Hypercalcemia after Renal Transplantation: Long-Term Follow-Up Data, *N Engl J Med,* **289:**398, 1973.

Demling, R. H., Salvatierra, O., Jr., and Belzer, F. O.: Intestinal Necrosis and Perforation after Renal Transplantation, *Arch Surg,* **110:**251, 1975.

Dietzman, R. H., Rebelo, A. E., Graham, E. F., Crabo, B. G., and Lillehei, R. C.: Long-Term Functional Success following Freezing of Canine Kidneys, *Surgery,* **74:**181, 1973.

Dossetor, J. B., Zqeig, S. M., Treves, S., and Ross, W. M.: The [131]I Ortho-iodohippurate Photoscan in Human Renal Allografts, *Can Med Assoc J,* **102:**1373, 1970.

DeShazo, C. V., Simmons, R. L., Bernstein, D. M., DeShazo, M. M., Willmert, J., Kjellstrand, C. M., and Najarian, J. S.: Results of Renal Transplantation in 100 Children, *Surgery,* **76:**461, 1974.

Ettenger, R. B., Terasaki, P. I., Ting, A., Malekzadeh, M. H., Pennisi, A. J., Uittenbogaart, C., Garrison, R., and Fine, R. N.: Anti-B Lymphocytotoxins in Renal-Allograft Rejection, *N Engl J Med,* **295:**305, 1976.

Evans, D. B., and Calne, R. Y.: Renal Transplantation in Patients with Carcinoma, *Br Med J,* **4:**134, 1974.

Fellner, C. H., and Schwartz, S. H.: Altruism in Disrepute: Medical versus Public Attitudes toward the Living Organ Donor, *N Engl J Med,* **284:**583, 1971.

Ferguson, R. M., Schmidtke, J. R., Simmons, R. L., and Najarian, J. S.: Functional and Anatomic Lymphocyte Subpopulation Redistribution following Transplantation, *Transplant Proc,* **9:**55, 1977.

———, Simmons, R. L., Noreen, H., Yunis, E. J., and Najarian, J. S.: Host Presensitization and Renal Allograft Success at a Single Institution: First Transplants, *Surgery,* **81:**139, 1977.

Festenstein, H., Oliver, R. T. D., Hyams, A., Moorhead, J. R., Pirrie, A. J., Pegrum, G. C., and Balfour, I. C.: A Collaborative Scheme for Tissue Typing and Matching in Renal Transplantation, *Lancet,* **2:**389, 1969.

Franksson, C., Lundgren, G., Mangnusson, G., and Ringden, O.: Drainage of Thoracic Duct Lymph in Renal Transplant Patients, *Transplantation,* **21:**133, 1976.

Frich, M. P., Loken, M. K., Goldberg, M. E., and Simmons, R. L.: The Use of 99-M Technetium Sulfurcolloid in the Evaluation of the Function of Renal Transplants, *J Nucl Med,* **17:**181, 1976.

Glassock, R. J., Feldman, D., Reynolds, E. S., Dammin, G. J., and Merrill, J. P.: Human Renal Isografts: A Clinical and Pathologic Analysis, *Medicine (Baltimore),* **47:**411, 1968.

Greene, J. A., Jr., Vander, A. J., and Kowalczyk, R. S.: Plasma Renin Activity and Aldosterone Excretion after Renal Homotransplantation, *J Lab Clin Med,* **71:**586, 1968.

Griffiths, H. J., Ennis, J. T., and Bailey, G.: Skeletal Changes following Renal Transplantation, *Radiology,* **113:**621, 1974.

Gustafsson, A., Groth, C. G., Halgrimson, C. G., Penn, I., and Starzl, T. E.: Fate of Failed renal Homografts Retained after Retransplantation, *Surg Gynecol Obstet,* **137:**40, 1973.

Hall, M. C., Elmore, S. M., Bright, R. W., Pierce, J. C., and Hume, D. M.: Skeletal Complications in a Series of Human Renal Allografts, *JAMA,* **208:**1825, 1969.

Hamburger, J., and Crosnier, J.: Moral and Ethical Problems in Transplantation, in F. T. Rapaport and J. Dausset (eds.), "Human Transplantation," p. 37, Grune & Stratton, Inc., New York, 1968.

Hansen, H. E., and Sell, A.: Isotope Renography Combined with Recording Isotype Cystogram in Patients with Renal Transplants, *Acta Med Scand,* **188:**205, 1970.

Harvard Medical School Committee: A Definition of Irreversible Coma: Report of the Ad Hoc Committee of the Harvard Medical School to Examine the Definition of Brain Death, *JAMA,* **205:**337, 1968.

Hattler, B. G., Jr., Rocklin, R. E., Ward, P. A., and Rickles, F. R.: Functional Features of Lymphocytes Recovered from a Human Renal Allograft, *Cell Immunol,* **9:**289, 1973.

Hinman, F., Jr., and Belzer, F. O.: Urinary Tract Infections and Renal Homotransplantation: I. Effect of Antibacterial Irrigations on Defenses of the Defunctionalized Bladder, *Trans Am Assoc Genitourin Surg,* **60:**46, 1968.

Ho, M., Suwansirikul, S., Dowling, J. N., Youngblood, L. A., and Armstrong, J. A.: Transplanted Kidney as a Source of Cytomegalovirus Infection, *N Engl J Med,* **293:**1109, 1975.

Hoover, R., and Fraumeni, J. F., Jr.: Risk of Cancer in Renal Transplant Recipients, *Lancet,* **2:**55, 1973.

Hume, D. M.: Homotransplantation of Kidneys and of Fetal Liver and Spleen after Total Body Irradiation, *Ann Surg,* **152:**354, 1960.

Husberg, B. S., and Starzl, T. E.: Outcome of Kidney Retransplantation, *Arch Surg,* **108:**584, 1974.

Irby, R., and Hume, D. M.: Joint Changes Observed following Renal Transplants, *Clin Orthop,* **57:**101, 1968.

Ireland, P., Rashid, A., Von Lichtenberg, F., Cavallo, T., and Merrill, J. P.: Liver Disease in Kidney Transplant Patients Receiving Azathioprine, *Arch Intern Med,* **132:**29, 1973.

Jeannet, M., DeWeck, A., Frei, P. C., Grob, P., and Thiel, G.: Cooperative Kidney Typing and Exchange Program, *Helv Med Acta,* **35:**239, 1969–1970.

Juul-Jensen, P.: "Criteria of Brain Death: Selection of Donors for Transplantation," Munksgaard, Copenhagen, 1970.

Kauffman, H. M., Swanson, M. K., McGregor, W. R., Rodgers, R. E., and Fox, P. S.: Splenectomy in Renal Transplantation, *Surg Gynecol Obstet,* **139:**33, 1974.

Kincaid-Smith, P.: Histological Diagnosis of Rejection of Renal Homografts in Man, *Lancet,* **2:**849, 1967.

Kjellstrand, C. M., Casali, R. E., Simmons, R. L., Shideman, J. R., Buselmeier, T. J., and Najarian, J. S.: Etiology and Prognosis in Acute Post-transplant Renal Failure, *Am J Med,* **61:**190, 1976.

———, Shideman, J. R., Lynch, R. E., Buselmeier, T. J., Simmons, R. L., and Najarian, J. S.: Kidney Transplants in Patients over 50, *Geriatrics,* **31:**65, 1976.

———, Simmons, R. L., Buselmeier, T. J., and Najarian, J. S.: Kidney: I. Recipient Selection, Medical Management and Dialysis, in J. S. Najarian and R. L. Simmons (eds.), "Transplantation," p. 418, Lea & Febiger, Philadelphia, 1972.

Kohler, B.: The Prognosis after Nephrectomy: A Clinical Study of Early and Late Results, *Acta Chir Scand,* **91** (suppl 94):1, 1944.

Koranda, F. C., Dehmel, E. M., Kahn, G., and Penn, I.: Cutaneous Complications in Immunosuppressed Renal Homograft Recipients, *JAMA,* **229:**419, 1974.

Ku, G., Varghese, Z., Fernando, O. N., Baillod, R., Hopewell, J. P., and Moorhead, J. F.: Serum IgG and Renal Transplantation, *Br Med J,* **4:**702, 1973.

Kyriakides, G. K., Simmons, R. L., and Najarian, J. S.: Wound Infections in Renal Transplant Wounds: Pathogenetic and Prognostic Factors, *Ann Surg,* **182:**770, 1975.

———, ———, and ———: Mycotic Aneurysms in Transplant Patients, *Arch Surg,* **111:**472, 1976.

Lacombe, M.: Arterial Stenosis Complicating Renal Allotransplantation in Man: Study of 38 Cases, *Ann Surg,* **181:**283, 1975.

Lazarus, J. M., Birtch, A. G., Hampers, C. L., and Merrill, J. P.: Hemodialysis Duration and Renal Transplant Survival, *Transplantation,* **15:**508, 1973.

Light, J. A., Annable, C., Perloff, L. J., Sulkin, M. D., Hill, G. S., Etheredge, E. E., and Spees, E. K., Jr.: Immune Injury from Organ Preservation: Potential Cause of Hyperacute Rejection in Human Cadaver Kidney Transplantation, *Transplantation,* **19:**511, 1975.

Linn, B. S., Portal, P., and Snyder, G. B.: Complementuria in Renal Transplantation, *Life Sci,* **6:**1945, 1967.

Lucas, Z. J., Palmer, J. M., Payne, R., Kountz, S. L., and Cohn, R. B.: Renal Allotransplantation in Humans: I. Systemic Immunosuppressive Therapy, *Arch Surg,* **100:**113, 1970.

McLean, R. H., Geiger, H., Burke, B., Simmons, R., Najarian, J.,

Vernier, R. L., and Michael, A. F.: Recurrence of Membranoproliferative Glomerulonephritis following Kidney Transplantation: Serum Complement Component Studies, *Amer J Med,* **60:**60, 1976.

Matas, A. J., Hertel, B. F., Rosai, J., Simmons, R. L., and Najarian, J. S.: Post-transplant Malignant Lymphoma: Distinctive Morphologic Features Related to Its Pathogenesis, *Am J Med,* **61:**716, 1976.

———, Simmons, R. L., Buselmeier, T. J., Kjellstrand, C. M., and Najarian, J. S.: Successful Renal Transplantation in Patients with Prior History of Malignancy, *Am J Med,* **59:**791, 1975.

———, ———, ———, ———, and ———: The Fate of Patients Surviving Three Years after Renal Transplantation, *Surgery,* **80:**390, 1976.

———, ———, Kjellstrand, C. M., Buselmeier, T. J., Johnson, T. L., and Najarian, J. S.: Increased Incidence of Malignancy in Uremic Patients and Its Significance to Transplantation, *Transplant Proc,* **9:**1137, 1977.

———, ———, and Najarian, J. S.: Chronic Antigenic Stimulation, Herpes-Virus Infection, and Cancer in Transplant Patients—Hypothesis, *Lancet,* **1:**1277, 1975.

Mauer, S. M., Barbosa, J., Vernier, R. L., Kjellstrand, C. M., Buselmeier, T. J., Simmons, R. L., Najarian, J. S., and Goetz, F. C.: Development of Diabetic Vascular Lesions in Normal Kidneys Transplanted into Patients with Diabetes Mellitus, *N Engl J Med,* **295:**916, 1976.

Miller, J., Kyriakides, G., Ma, W. K., Masler, D., and Brown, D. C.: Factors Influencing Morbidity and Mortality of Renal Transplantation in a High-Risk Population, *Surg Gynecol Obstet,* **140:**1, 1975.

Mills, S. A., Siegler, H. F., and Wolfe, W. G.: Incidence and Management of Pulmonary Mycosis in Renal Allograft Patients, *Ann Surg,* **182:**617, 1975.

Mohandas, A., and Chu, S. N.: Brain Death: A Clinical and Pathological Study, *J Neurosurg,* **35:**211, 1971.

Moore, T. C.: Effective Use of Isoniazid and an Antihistamine in Clinical Renal Transplantation, *Surg Gynecol Obstet,* **133:**75, 1971.

Murphy, G. P., Mirand, E. A., and Grace, J. T.: Erythropoietin Activity in Anephric or Renal Allotransplanted Man, *Ann Surg,* **170:**581, 1969.

Murray, J. E., Merrill, J. P., and Harrison, J. H.: Renal Homotransplantation in Identical Twins, *Surg Forum,* **6:**432, 1955.

Myburgh, J. A., Maier, G., Smit, J. A., Shapiro, M., Meyers, A. M., Rabkin, R., Van Blerk, P. J. P., and Jersky, J.: Presensitization and Clinical Kidney Transplantation: I. Favorable Course of a Substantial Number of Patients, *Transplantation,* **18:**206, 1974.

Najarian, J. S., Kjellstrand, C. M., Simmons, R. L., Buselmeier, T. J., Von Hartitzsch, B., and Goetz, F. C.: Renal Transplantation for Diabetic Glomerulosclerosis, *Ann Surg,* **178:**477, 1973.

———, Simmons, R. L., Condie, R. M., Thompson, E. J., Fryd, D. S., Howard, R. J., Matas, A. J., Sutherland, D. E. R., Ferguson, R. M., and Schmidtke, J. R.: Seven Years' Experience with Antilymphoblast Globulin for Renal Transplantation from Cadaver Donors, *Ann Surg,* **184:**352, 1976.

———, ———, Kjellstrand, C. M., Vernier, R., and Michaels, A.: Renal Transplantation in Infants and Children, *Ann Surg,* **174:**583, 1971.

Olsson, C. A., Mannick, J. A., Schmitt, G. W., Idelson, B. A., Williams, L. F., Lemann, J., Harrington, J. T., and Nabseth, D. C.: Nephrostomy in Renal Transplantation, *Am J Surg,* **121:**467, 1971.

Opelz, G., and Terasaki, P. I.: Prolongation Effect of Blood Transfusions on Kidney Graft Survival, *Lancet,* **2:**696, 1974.

Pasternack, A.: Fine Needle Aspiration Biopsy of Human Renal Homografts, *Lancet,* **2:**82, 1968.

Penn, I., Halgrimson, C. G., Ogden, D., and Starzl, T.: Use of Living Donors in Kidney Transplantation in Man, *Arch Surg,* **101:**226, 1970.

——— and Starzl, T. E.: Immunosuppression and Cancer, *Transplant Proc,* **5:**943, 1973.

Perkins, H. A., Howell, E., Gantan, Z., Mims, M. C., Dickerson, T., and Senecal, I.: Variation in Cytotoxic Antibody Response to Transfusion in Prospective Renal Allograft Recipients, *Transplantation,* **17:**216, 1974.

Pien, F. D., Smith, T. F., Anderson, C. F., Webel, M. L., and Taswell, H. F.: Herpesviruses in Renal Transplant Patients, *Transplantation,* **16:**489, 1973.

Pierce, J. C., and Hume, D. M.: The Effect of Splenectomy on the Survival of First and Second Renal Homotransplants in Man, *Surg Gynecol Obstet,* **127:**1300, 1968.

Quinton, W. E., Dillard, P. H., Cole, I. J., and Scribner, B. H.: Eight Months Experience with Silastic-Teflon Bypass Cannulas, *Trans Am Soc Artif Intern Organs,* **8:**236, 1962.

Rapaport, F. T., McCluskey, R. T., Hanaoka, T., and Shimada, T.: Induction of Renal Disease with Antisera to Group A Streptococcal Membranes, *Transplant Proc,* **1:**981, 1969.

Rattazzi, L. D., Simmons, R. L., Spanos, P. K., Bradford, D. S., and Najarian, J. S.: Successful Management of Miliary Tuberculosis after Renal Transplantation, *Am J Surg,* **130:**359, 1975.

Rosenberg, J. C., Azcarate, J., Fleischmann, L. E., McDonald, F. D., Menendez, M., Pierce, J. M., Jr., and Whang, C. W.: Indications for Pretransplant Nephrectomy, *Arch Surg,* **107:**233, 1973.

Salvatierra, O., Potter, D., Cochrum, K. C., Amend, W. J. C., Duca, R., Sachs, B. L., Johnson, R. W. J., and Belzer, F. O.: Improved Patient Survival in Renal Transplantation, *Surgery,* **79:**166, 1976.

Schwab, R. S., Potts, F., and Bonazzi, A.: EEG as an Aid in Determining Death in the Presence of Cardiac Activity (Ethical, Legal and Medical Aspects), *Electroencephalogr Clin Neurophysiol,* **15:**147, 1963.

Schwartz, R. S., and Dameshek, W.: Drug Induced Immunological Tolerance, *Nature (Lond),* **183:**1682, 1959.

Sciarra, J. J., Toledo-Pereyra, L. H., Bendel, R. P., and Simmons, R. L.: Pregnancy following Renal Transplantation, *Am J Obstet Gynecol,* **123:**411, 1975.

Scott, D. F., Whiteside, D., Redhead, J., and Atkins, R. C.: Ice Storage versus Perfusion for Preservation of Kidneys before Transplantation, *Br Med J,* **4:**76, 1974.

Sheil, A. G. R., Boulas, J., Drummond, J. M., May, J., Rogers, J. H., and Storey, B. G.: Controlled Clinical Trial of Machine Perfusion of Cadaveric Donor Renal Allografts, *Lancet,* **2:**287, 1975.

Shillito, J., Jr.: The Organ Donor's Doctor: A New Role for the Neurosurgeon, *N Engl J Med,* **281:**1071, 1969.

Simmons, R. L., Kjellstrand, C. M., Buselmeier, T. J., and

Najarian, J. S.: Renal Transplantation in High Risk Patients, *Arch Surg,* **103:**290, 1971.

——, ——, and Najarian, J. S.: Kidney: II. Technique, Complications, and Results, in J. S. Najarian and R. L. Simmons (eds.), "Transplantation," p. 445, Lea & Febiger, Philadelphia, 1972.

——, Lopez, C., Balfour, H., Jr., Kalis, J., Rattazzi, L. C., and Najarian, J. S.: Cytomegalovirus: Clinical Virologic Correlations in Transplant Recipients, *Ann Surg,* **180:**623, 1974.

——, Ozerkis, A. J., and Hoehn, R. J.: Antiserum to Lymphocytes: Interactions with Chemical Immunosuppressants, *Science,* **160:**1127, 1968.

——, Thompson, E. J., Yunis, E. J., Noreen, H., Kjellstrand, C. M., Fryd, D. S., Condie, R. M., Mauer, S. M., Buselmeier, T. J., and Najarian, J. S.: 115 Patients with First Cadaver Kidney Transplants Followed Two to Seven and a Half Years: A Multifactorial Analysis, *Am J Med,* **62:**234, 1977.

——, Van Hook, E. J., Yunis, E. J., Noreen, H., Kjellstrand, C. M., Condie, R. M., Mauer, S. M., Buselmeier, T. J., and Najarian, J. S.: 100 Sibling Kidney Transplants Followed 2 to 7½ Years: A Multifactorial Analysis, *Ann Surg,* **185:**196, 1977.

——, Yunis, E. J., Noreen, H., Thompson, E. J., Fryd, D. S., and Najarian, J. S.: Effect of HLA Matching on Cadaver Kidney Function: Experience at a Single Large Center, *Transplant Proc,* **9:**491, 1977.

Starzl, T. E.: "Experience in Renal Transplantation," W. B. Saunders Company, Philadelphia, 1964.

——, Groth, C. G., Terasaki, P. I., Putnam, C. W., Brettschneider, L., and Marchioro, T. L.: Heterologous Antilymphocyte Globulin Histoincompatibility Matching, and Human Renal Homotransplantation, *Surg Gynecol Obstet,* **126:**1023, 1968.

——, Halgrimson, C. G., Penn, L., Martineau, G., Schroter, G., Amemiya, H., Putnam, C. W., and Groth, C. G.: Cyclophosphamide and Human Organ Transplantation, *Lancet,* **2:**70, 1971.

Stenzel, K. H., Stubenbord, W. T., Whitsell, J. C., Lewy, J. E., Riggio, R. R., Cheigh, J. S., Marshall, V. F., and Rubin, A. L.: Kidney Transplantation: Use of Intestinal Conduits, *JAMA,* **229:**534, 1974.

Stewart, J. H., Johnson, J. R., Sharp, A. M., Sheil, A. G. R., Wyatt, K. M., and Johnston, J. M.: Successful Renal Allotransplantation in Presence of Lymphocytotoxic Antibodies: Importance of Preoperative Cross-Matching, *Lancet,* **1:**176, 1969.

Strauch, B., Andrews, L.-L., Siegel, N., and Miller, G.: Oropharyngeal Excretion of Epstein-Barr Virus by Renal Transplant Recipients and Other Patients Treated with Immunosuppressive Drugs, *Lancet,* **1:**234, 1974.

Swales, J. D., and Evans, D. B.: Erythraemia in Renal Transplantation, *Br Med J,* **2:**80, 1969.

Tallent, M. B., Simmons, R. L., and Najarian, J. S.: Birth Defects in a Child of a Male Kidney Transplant Recipient, *JAMA,* **211:**1854, 1970.

Terasaki, P. J., Kreisler, M., and Mickey, M. R.: Presensitization and Kidney Transplant Failures: I, *Postgrad Med,* **47:**89, 1971.

Thomas, F. T., and Lee, H. M.: Factors in the Differential Rate of Arteriosclerosis (AS) between Long Surviving Renal Transplant Recipients and Dialysis Patients, *Ann Surg,* **184:**342, 1976.

Toledo-Pereyra, L. H., Simmons, R. L., Moberg, A. W., Olson,

L. C., and Najarian, J. S.: Organ Preservation in Success of Cadaver Transplants, *Arch Surg,* **110:**1031, 1975.

Tunner, W. S., Goldsmith, E. I., and Whitesell, J. C.: Human Homotransplantation of Normal and Neoplastic Tissue from the Same Organ, *J Urol,* **105:**18, 1971.

Weil, R., III, Simmons, R. L., Tallent, M. B., Lillehei, R. C., Kjellstrand, C. M., and Najarian, J. S.: Prevention of Urological Complications after Kidney Transplantation, *Ann Surg,* **174:**154, 1971.

West, T. H., Turcotte, J. G., and Vancer, A. J.: Plasma Renin Activity, Sodium Balance, and Hypertension in a Group of Renal Transplant Recipients, *J Lab Clin Med,* **73:**564, 1970.

Williams, G. M., dePlanque, B., Lower, R., and Hume, D. M.: Antibodies and Human Transplant Rejection, *Ann Surg,* **170:**603, 1969.

——, White, H. J., and Hume, D. M.: Factors Influencing the Long-Term Functional Success Rate of Human Renal Allografts, *Transplantation, Suppl.,* **51:**837, 1967.

Wilson, D. R., and Siddiqui, A. A.: Renal Tubular Acidosis after Kidney Transplantation: Natural History and Significance, *Ann Intern Med,* **79:**352, 1973.

Wood, R. F. M., Gray, A. C., Briggs, J. D., and Bell, P. R. F.: Prediction of Acute Rejection in Human Renal Transplantation Using Leukocyte Migration Test, *Transplantation,* **16:**41, 1973.

Zukoski, C. F., Lee, H. M., and Hume, D. M.: The Prolongation of Functional Survival of Canine Renal Homografts by 6-Mercaptopurine, *Surg Forum,* **11:**470, 1960.

Transplantation of Organs other than Kidney, Liver, Lung, and Heart

Advisory Committee of the Bone Marrow Transplant Registry: Bone Marrow Transplantation from Donors with Aplastic Anemia: A Report from the ACS/NIH Bone Marrow Transplant Registry, *JAMA,* **236:**1131, 1976.

Baird, R. N., and Abbott, W. M.: Vein Grafts: An Historical Perspective, *Am J Surg,* **134:**293, 1977.

Barnicot, N. A.: The Local Action of the Parathyroid and Other Tissues on Bone in Intracerebral Grafts, *J Anat,* **82:**233, 1948.

Bortin, M. M.: A Compendium of Reported Human Bone Marrow Transplants, *Transplantation,* **9:**571, 1970.

Burke, J. F., Quinby, W. C., Bondoc, C. C., Cosimi, A. B., Russell, P. S., and Szyfelbein, S. K.: Immunosuppression and Temporary Skin Transplantation in the Treatment of Massive Third Degree Burns, *Ann Surg,* **182:**183, 1975.

Burwell, R. G.: The Fate of Freeze-Dried Bone Allografts, *Transplant Proc,* **8**(suppl 1):77, 1976.

Calhoun, A. D., Bauer, G. M., Porter, J. M., Houghton, D. H., and Templeton, J. W.: Fresh and Cryopreserved Venous Allografts in Genetically Characterized Dogs, *J Surg Res,* **22:**687, 1977.

Cohen, Z., MacGregor, A. B., Moore, E. T. H., Falk, R. E., Langer, B., and Cullen, J. S.: Canine Small Bowel Transplantation, *Arch Surg,* **111:**248, 1976.

Congdon, C. C.: Bone Marrow Transplantation, *Science,* **171:**1116, 1971.

Corry, R. J., and Russell, P. S.: Replantation of Severed Fingers, *Ann Surg,* **179:**255, 1974.

Fefer, A., Einstein, A. B., Thomas, E. D., Buckner, C. D., Clift, R. A., Glucksberg, H., Neiman, P. E., and Storb, R.: Bone-

Marrow Transplantation for Hematologic Neoplasia in 16 Patients with Identical Twins, *N Engl J Med,* **290:**1389, 1974.

Flosdorf, E., and Hyatt, G. W.: The Preservation of Bone Grafts by Freeze Drying, *Surgery,* **31:**716, 1952.

Fortner, J. G., Sichuk, G., Litwin, S. D., and Bettie, E. J., Jr.: Immunological Responses to an Intestinal Allograft with HL-Al Identical Donor-Recipient, *Transplantation,* **14:**531, 1972.

Friedlaender, G. E.: The Antigenicity of Preserved Allografts, *Transplant Proc,* **8**(suppl)**1:**195, 1976.

Gittes, R. F.: Endocrine Tissues, in J. S. Najarian and R. L. Simmons (eds.), "Transplantation," p. 698, Lea & Febiger, Philadelphia, 1972.

Green, W. T., Sr.: Fascia Grafts, *Transplant Proc,* **8**(suppl)**1:**113, 1976.

Groth, C. G., Hammons, W. S., Iwatsuki, S., Popovtzer, M., Cascardo, S., Halgrimson, C. G., and Starzl, T. E.: Survival of a Homologous Parathyroid Implant in an Immunosuppressed Patient, *Lancet,* **1:**1082, 1973.

Hardy, J. D., and Langford, H. G.: Surgical Management of Cushing's Syndrome: Including Studies of Adrenal Autotransplants, Body Composition and Pseudotumor Cerebri, *Ann Surg,* **159:**711, 1964.

Harris, G. W., and Jacobsohn, D.: Functional Grafts of the Anterior Pituitary Glands, *Proc R Soc Lond (Biol),* **139:**263, 1952.

Harris, J. E., and Rathburn, W. B.: Ocular Tissues, in J. S. Najarian and R. L. Simmons (eds.), "Transplantation," p. 613, Lea & Febiger, Philadelphia, 1972.

Hickey, R. C., and Samaan, N. A.: Human Parathyroid Autotransplantation, *Arch Surg,* **110:**892, 1975.

Jaffe, S., Earle, A. S., Fleegler, E. J., and Husni, E. A.: Replantation of Amputated Extremities: Report of Five Cases, *Ohio State Med J,* **71:**381, 1975.

Kelly, W. D., Lillehei, R. C., Merkel, F. K., Idezuki, Y., and Goetz, F.: Renal and Pancreatic Allotransplantation in the Treatment of Diabetic Nephropathy in Man, in J. Dausset, J. Hamburger, and G. Mathé (eds.), "Advance in Transplantation," The Williams & Wilkins Company, Baltimore, 1968.

Koumans, R. K. J., and Burke, J. F.: Skin Allografts and Immunosuppression in the Treatment of Massive Thermal Injury, *Surgery,* **66:**89, 1969.

Lance, E. M.: Bone and Cartilage, in J. S. Najarian and R. L. Simmons (eds.), "Transplantation," p. 655, Lea & Febiger, Philadelphia, 1972.

Leapman, S. B., Deutsch, A. A., Grand, R. J., and Folkman, J.: Transplantation of Fetal Intestine: Survival and Function in a Subcutaneous Location in Adult Animals, *Ann Surg,* **179:**109, 1974.

Lillehei, R. C., and Ruiz, J. O.: Pancreas, in J. S. Najarian, and R. L. Simmons (eds.), "Transplantation," p. 627, Lea & Febiger, Philadelphia, 1972.

Lohrmann, H.-P., Niethammer, D., Kern, P., and Heimpel, H.: Identification of High-Risk Patients with Aplastic Anemia in Selection for Allogeneic Bone-Marrow Transplantation, *Lancet,* **2:**647, 1976.

Malt, R. A., and Harris, W. H.: Replantation of Limbs, in J. S. Najarian and R. L. Simmons (eds.), "Transplantation," p. 711, Lea & Febiger, Philadelphia, 1972.

———, Remensnyder, J. P., and Harris, W. H.: Long-Term Utility of Replanted Arms, *Ann Surg,* **176:**334, 1972.

Mankin, H. J., Fogelson, F. S., Thrasher, A. Z., and Jaffer, F.: Massive Resection and Allograft Transplantation in the Treatment of Malignant Bone Tumors, *N Engl J Med,* **294:**1247, 1976.

Matas, A. J., Sutherland, D. E. R., and Najarian, J. S.: Current Status of Islet and Pancreas Transplantation, *Diabetes,* **25:**785, 1976.

———, ———, Steffes, M. W., and Najarian, J. S.: Islet Transplantation, *Surg Gynecol Obstet,* **145:**757, 1977.

Mathe, G., Schwarzenberg, L., and Amiel, J. L.: Bone Marrow, in J. S. Najarian and R. L. Simmons (eds.), "Transplantation," p. 588, Lea & Febiger, Philadelphia, 1972.

Metras, H.: Note préliminaire sur la greffe totale du poumon chez le chien, *C R Acad Sci [D] (Paris),* **231:**1176, 1950.

Meuwissen, H. J., Rodey, G., McArthur, J., Pabst, H., Gattis, R., Childgren, R., Hong, R., Frommel, D., Coifman, R., and Good, R. A.: Bone Marrow Transplantation-Therapeutic Usefulness and Complications, *Am J Med,* **51:**513, 1971.

Nasseri, M., and Voss, H.: Late Results of Successful Replantation of Upper and Lower Extremities, *Ann Surg,* **177:**121, 1973.

Norman, J. C., Covelli, V. H., and Sise, H. S.: Transplantation of the Spleen: Experimental Cure of Hemophilia, *Surgery,* **66:**1, 1968.

Paloyan, E., Lawrence, A. M., Brooks, M. H., and Pickleman, J. R.: Total Thyroidectomy and Parathyroid Autotransplantation for Radiation-Associated Thyroid Cancer, *Surgery,* **80:**70, 1976.

Parrish, F. F.: Total and Partial Half-Joint Resection Followed by Allograft Replacement in Neoplasms Involving Ends of Long Bones, *Transplant Proc,* **8**(suppl 1):77, 1976.

Peacock, E. E., Jr.: A Review of Composite Tissue Allografts of the Digital Flexor Mechanism, *Transplant Proc,* **8**(suppl 1):119, 1976.

——— and Madden, J. W.: Human Composite Flexor Tendon Allografts, *Ann Surg,* **166:**624, 1967.

Rapaport, F. T., and Converse, J. M.: Skin Transplantation, in F. T. Rapaport and J. Dausset (eds.), "Human Transplantation," p. 304, Grune & Stratton, Inc., New York, 1968.

Rapaport, I., Pepino, A. T., and Dietrick, W.: Early Use of Xenografts as a Biologic Dressing in Burn Trauma, *Am J Surg,* **120:**144, 1970.

Ruiz, J. O., Uchida, H., and Lillehei, R. C.: Intestine (Clinical Transplantation), in J. S. Najarian and R. L. Simmons (eds.), "Transplantation," p. 646, Lea & Febiger, Philadelphia, 1972.

Schechter, I.: Prolonged Retention of Glutaraldehyde-Treated Skin Allografts and Xenografts: Immunological and Histological Studies, *Ann Surg,* **182:**699, 1975.

Schneider, J. R., and Bright, R. W.: Anterior Cervical Fusion Using Preserved Bone Allografts, *Transplant Proc,* **8**(suppl 1):73, 1976.

Slavin, R. E., and Santos, G. W.: The Graft Versus Host Reaction in Man after Bone Marrow Transplantation: Pathology, Pathogenesis, Clinical Features, and Implication, *Clin Immunol Immunopathol,* **1:**492, 1973.

Stamford, W. P., and Hardy, M. A.: Fatty Acid Absorption in Jejunal Autograft and Allograft, *Surgery,* **75:**496, 1974.

Sutherland, D. E. R., Matas, A. J., and Najarian, J. S.: Pancreas and Islet Transplantation, *World J Surg,* **1:**185, 1977.

Taylor, A. C.: Rates of Freezing, Drying and Rehydration of Nerves, *J Cell Comp Physiol,* **25:**161, 1945.

Thomas, E. D., Storb, R., Clift, R. A., Fefer, A., Johnson, F. L., Neiman, P. E., Lerner, K. G., Glucksberg, H., and Buckner, C. D.: Bone-Marrow Transplantation, Part 1, *N Engl J Med,* **292:**832, 1975; Part II, *N Engl J Med,* **292:**895, 1975.

Toledo-Pereyra, L. H., Raij, L., Simmons, R. L., and Najarian, J. S.: Role of Endotoxin and Bacteria in Long-Term Survival of Preserved Small-Bowel Allografts, *Surgery,* **73:**474, 1974.

———, Simmons, R. L., and Najarian, J. S.: Prolonged Survival of Canine Orthotopic Small Intestinal Allografts Preserved for 24 Hours by Hypothermic Bloodless Perfusion, *Surgery,* **75:**368, 1974.

Transplantation and Burns, *Lancet,* **1:**1017, 1975.

U.C.L.A.: Bone Marrow Transplant Team: Bone-Marrow Transplantation in Severe Aplastic Anaemia, *Lancet,* **2:**921, 1976.

Waksman, B. H., Arbouys, S., and Arnason, B. G.: The Use of Specific "Lymphocyte" Antisera to Inhibit Hypersensitive Reactions of the "Delayed" Type, *J Exp Med,* **114:**997, 1961.

Wells, S. A., Gunnells, J. C., Shelburne, J. D., Schneider, A. B., and Sherwood, L. M.: Transplantation of the Parathyroid Glands in Man: Clinical Indications and Results, *Surgery,* **78:**34, 1975.

White, R. J.: Experimental Transplantation of the Brain, in F. T. Rapaport and J. Dausset (eds.), "Human Transplantation," p. 692, Grune & Stratton, Inc., New York, 1968.

Organ Preservation

Filo, R. S., Bell, R. T., Small, A., and Sell, K. W.: Current Status of Kidney Freeze Preservation, *Transplant Proc,* **8**(suppl 1):215, 1976.

Sell, K. W., and Friedlaender, G. E. (eds.): Proceedings of the Tissue Bank Symposium, *Transplant Proc,* **8**(supplement 1): June, 1976.

Chapter 11

Anesthesia

by **Nicholas M. Greene**

GENERAL CONSIDERATIONS

Anesthesiology consists of two parts. One lies outside the operating (or delivery) room, the other within. The former centers about management of critically ill patients, especially their ventilatory care (Chaps. 12 and 13). It also involves diagnosis and treatment of chronic pain problems. The latter centers about operative anesthesia, that is, relief of pain, provision of operating conditions adequate for the surgery at hand, and supportive treatment with fluids, electrolytes, blood, and vasoactive drugs.

Surgical anesthesia inevitably entails risk. This is so because while each anesthetic has its advantages, each also has its disadvantages. But there is no anesthetic magic bullet that relieves pain without side effects. Each anesthetic, even the simplest, creates a state of physiologic trespass with attendant risk. The risk may be greater or smaller depending upon the circumstances, but it can never be eliminated.

Quantitation of anesthetic risk is difficult to achieve in terms of either morbidity or mortality. The problem lies in obtaining epidemiologically sound data. All deaths or complications associated with anesthesia are iatrogenic by definition. This immediately raises the specter of mediocolegal action if an anesthetic death is honestly recorded as such. Death certificates and discharge diagnoses become

completely unreliable indices of anesthetic mortality rates under such circumstances. Added to this is the fact that many anesthetic deaths are so subtly related to the anesthetic and so cryptic in origin that the true relation between the fatal outcome and the anesthetic may be missed. Spectacular deaths due to anesthetic explosions or to cardiac arrest during induction of anesthesia are relatively easily identified. Less obvious, though considerably more frequent, are the "quiet" anesthetic deaths due to effects of anesthetics on pulmonary ventilation, hepatic function, cerebral blood flow, coronary blood flow, and metabolism—effects which may linger far into the postoperative period and prove particularly inimical to the poor-risk patient but may be extremely difficult to identify under clinical conditions. Finally, anesthetic deaths appear, especially to the casual observer, to occur only very infrequently. Their true incidence can be determined only when statistically accurate data are gathered from many thousands of patients over long periods of time. This is seldom done. The expense in terms of time, effort, and money usually aborts efforts to obtain such data long before statistical validity can be achieved. The vagaries of human memory and clinical impression further compound the problem. An average surgeon performing 400 operations per year may not encounter an anesthetic death for several years at a time. If the surgeon fails to recognize such a death for what it is when it does occur or fails to remember a previous anesthetic death, he or she soon comes to believe that no problems exist insofar as the safety of anesthetics is concerned; anesthetics are seen as a necessary but not particularly important accompaniment of surgery. The same thing can occur with the anesthesiologist caring for 800 patients a year, even though the time span between exposures to anesthetic death may be shorter.

Despite the problems inherent in quantitating anesthetic death rates, several studies in the past have addressed themselves to the matter using adequate statistical techniques. The results of these studies, while varying in detail, are remarkably consistent in finding that of approximately every 1,600 patients given an anesthetic, one patient dies primarily as a result of having received the anesthetic. The figure of 1 in 1,600 is based on all types of operative anesthesia, from the most "minor" to the most major. There is no evidence to suggest that contemporary anesthetic death rates are materially lower than those determined 15 years or more ago; indeed, the opposite may even be true.

The consideration of anesthetic death is not merely an

academic exercise. Approximately 18,000,000 anesthetics are said to be administered annually in hospitals in the United States, although it is hard to obtain figures and the number is probably higher. If the anesthetic death rate of 1 in 1,600 applies nationally—and there is every reason to believe it does—then the annual number of deaths associated with anesthesia in the United States is in excess of 10,000. Furthermore, antibiotics and blood banks have decreased death rates associated with certain so-called "minor" procedures such as tonsillectomy, inguinal herniorrhaphy, and hemorrhoidectomy to the vanishing point. There has, however, been no parallel decrease in deaths associated with anesthesia. The result is that anesthetic risk now exceeds surgical risk in many operations. Anesthetic death rates remain a major, if hidden, public health problem.

Because of the magnitude of the risk involved, the patient's safety must always be the first and most important consideration in any discussion of surgical anesthesia. True patient safety based upon sound physiologic and pharmacologic principles is not synonymous with the ability to "get away with" a calculated risk a certain number of times.

Bearing in mind the primacy of patient safety and the fact that no anesthetic agent or technique is without its disadvantages and dangers, it may be said that the selection of anesthetic agents and techniques in an individual clinical case depends upon five factors:

1. The condition of the patient. The presence of concurrent conditions such as obesity, a full stomach, coronary artery disease, or chronic pulmonary disease may contraindicate certain anesthetics.

2. The physiologic and pharmacologic effects of the various anesthetic agents. It is this aspect of anesthetic management which will be emphasized in the present chapter, noting that these effects are not necessarily the result of the anesthetic agent itself. A major portion of the physiologic trespass associated with anesthesia is due to factors such as mechanical effects of the apparatus used to administer the anesthetic, changes in blood-gas tensions, changes in fluid and electrolyte balance resulting from blood loss, creation of a surgical third space, and administration of intravenous fluids.

3. The site and type of surgical procedure to be performed. The anesthetic requirements for inguinal herniorrhaphy are different from those for pneumonectomy. Failure to recognize that the anesthetic should be tailored to the type of operation has led to inaccurate and dangerous generalizations as to anesthetic selection based solely upon the patient's condition and the pharmacologic effects of the anesthetic agent.

4. The experience, training, and background of the person who is to administer the anesthetic. Not all persons who can administer an anesthetic are necessarily equally qualified to administer all types of anesthetics. It is frequently advisable for an anesthetist to administer the type of anesthetic with which he has had the most experience, hence that in which he has the most confidence, rather than to administer on rare occasions an anesthetic which theoretically may have certain advantages but with which he has had little experience.

5. The skill, training, and requirements of the surgeon. The anesthetic requirements for an appendectomy by an experienced surgeon who will accomplish the entire operation in 20 minutes are markedly different from those for a surgeon who is less experienced and who may require an hour and a half of anesthesia.

Selection of anesthetic agent and technique based upon the preceding five factors will result in maximal patient safety. Convenience, surgical or anesthetic, should not play a significant role in selecting anesthetic agents, especially convenience measured in terms of minutes saved during induction of anesthesia. Similarly, what is most pleasant for the patient or what is acceptable to the patient should not be a primary consideration in selection of anesthetic agent or technique. Patient acceptability and surgical or anesthetic convenience may coincide with selection of the anesthetic which is also safest for the patient, but this should be regarded as fortuitous rather than the goal of selection of anesthetic agent and technique.

GENERAL ANESTHESIA

General anesthesia is produced either by anesthetics directly injected into the blood via the intravenous route or by anesthetics absorbed into the blood from the alveoli following inhalation. The advantages and disadvantages of inhalation general anesthesia as opposed to intravenous anesthesia and the physiologic and pharmacologic effects of the two techniques are such that it is best to discuss the two methods separately. These methods, however, do have two things in common, the risk of overdosage and the risk of inadequate ventilation. The vast majority of cardiac arrests, if not all cardiac arrests due to general anesthesia, result from one or both of these two factors. Avoidance of overdosage may prove difficult under clinical conditions, especially in the hands of a novice, for two reasons: First, individual variations of patients' responses to general anesthetics are so great that reliable dose/response relationships do not exist. General anesthetics cannot be administered in a predetermined dosage based on milligrams of anesthetic per kilogram of patient's body weight without running the risk of serious overdosage in some patients and inadequate depth of anesthesia in others. Second, evaluation of depth of anesthesia is neither easy nor precise but instead highly subjective, clinical signs varying not only with each general anesthetic but also with each patient. Even electroencephalography, a technique perhaps suitable for research purposes, is of no use in judging depth of anesthesia under clinical conditions. Signs such as pupillary size, eye motion, and character of respirations, as described by Guedel, apply only to ether and then only under select circumstances. The signs of depth of anesthesia with the more widely used present-day anesthetics are less well defined. Many anesthetics are such potent respiratory depressants, even in barely anesthetic concentrations, that respirations become an inadequate guide to depth of surgical anesthesia. Pragmatically, overdosage, whether absolute or relative, can be said to exist when arterial hypotension or (less frequently) cardiac arrhythmias are produced by a general anesthetic and is best avoided by repeated measurements of blood pressure and heart rate and by continuous electrocardiographic monitoring.

There are three principal causes of inadequate ventilation during general anesthesia: obstruction of the airway, pharmacologic interference with normal respiratory mechanisms, and anesthetically induced abnormalities of gas exchange between alveoli and pulmonary capillary blood. Obstruction may occur at any level in the airway, from pharynx to bronchi, and may be caused by anything from the tongue falling back into the pharynx to laryngospasm, bronchospasm, or aspiration of blood, gastric contents, secretions, or foreign bodies. Airway obstruction must immediately be treated by correction of the cause, whether by manipulation of the soft tissues of the upper airway (elevation of the chin or entire mandible), by insertion of artificial pharyngeal or endotracheal airways, or by endotracheal suctioning. If left untreated, obstruction results in hypoxia and hypercapnia, i.e., asphyxia. *General anesthesia is contraindicated unless a patent airway can be assured at all times.*

Pharmacologic causes of inadequate ventilation include interference with the normal neural or muscular mechanisms of respiration. These, together with anesthetically induced inadequacies of respiratory gas exchange secondary to abnormal alveolar ventilation/perfusion ratios, are included in the subsequent discussion of the individual anesthetic agents. It must be emphasized that pharmacologic derangements of respiration are often subtle and difficult to recognize although they are potentially as dangerous as, or more dangerous than, the more obvious forms of inadequate ventilation due to obstruction. They are especially insidious because the classic signs and symptoms of hypoxia and carbon dioxide retention are notoriously unreliable during clinical anesthesia. Respiratory rate, tidal volume, blood pressure, pulse rate, and color of the skin are all inaccurate indices of potentially dangerous levels of hypoxia or hypercapnia in a patient who is under general anesthesia. The only method by which abnormal blood levels of oxygen or carbon dioxide can be verified is measurement of the tensions (i.e., partial pressures) of these gases in *arterial* blood. Because of the difficulties inherent in estimating the adequacy of pulmonary ventilation and because of the dangers of inadequate ventilation compared with only minor and rather hypothetic disadvantages of hyperventilation, it is better to overventilate patients artificially during general anesthesia than to permit possible underventilation to occur. Hyperventilation is readily accomplished by intermittent manual compression of the anesthesia reservoir bag. Mechanical ventilators are not required. Neither is an endotracheal tube invariably required. Although this may prove necessary or desirable, endotracheal intubation does not guarantee adequate alveolar ventilation or even airway patency.

Inhalation Anesthesia

The principal advantage of inhalation anesthetics is controllable reversibility. As what enters via the lungs exits via the lungs, the rate at which the inhalation anesthetic exits can be as readily controlled as the rate at which it enters. Therefore, the administrator of an inhalation anesthetic can control its duration of action. This control does not exist following the intravenous administration of anesthetics and muscle relaxants, which require biotransformation or excretion for termination of action, processes over which the anesthetist has no control. Even specific antagonists to narcotics and muscle relaxants are not invariably reliable means for reversal of intravenous anesthetics. The half-life of the antagonist often differs significantly from the half-life of the agonist it is given to reverse, a situation which can lead to recurarization or reanesthetization of the patient after leaving the operating room.

Controlled reversibility and the ability to depress excitability of neuronal tissues are the only pharmacologic properties common to all inhalation anesthetics. Their pharmacologic effects and the physiologic responses they induce are otherwise too diverse to allow generalization. For one thing, inhalation anesthetics vary widely in their potency. Potency of inhalation anesthetics is commonly measured in terms of minimum alveolar anesthetic concentration (MAC), that is, the alveolar concentration of an anesthetic which prevents somatic response to painful stimuli in 50 percent of subjects. Alveolar concentration is emphasized in this definition because at equilibrium the partial pressure of an anesthetic in the alveoli is the same as it is in arterial blood, which, in turn, is the same as the partial pressure of the anesthetic in the central nervous system. Partial pressure of an anesthetic, not concentration in blood or brain, determines anesthetic effect. Differences in molecular weight and in air/blood and blood/lipid coefficients of distribution mean that equal partial pressures of different anesthetics are associated with quite different concentrations in blood, tissues, and cell membranes. MAC is widely used as a standard of reference for comparisons of different inhalation anesthetics. The side effects of anesthetics on, for example, respiration or cardiovascular function are meaningful only when equieffective concentrations of the anesthetics are compared. This is most conveniently done by comparing similar MAC values.

The concept of MAC represents an important advance both clinically and in understanding the mechanism of action of inhalation anesthesia. It has, however, limitations which must be understood if its value is to be appreciated. For example, the MAC of an anesthetic often shows substantial differences depending upon the species in which it is determined, thereby making difficult the application to man of MAC values derived in experimental animals. Furthermore, since MAC is defined as the alveolar concentration of anesthetic which prevents response to a painful stimulus in 50 percent of subjects, it follows that at MAC the other 50 percent of subjects are not anesthetized. More meaningful than MAC under clinical circumstances is the alveolar concentration which anesthetizes all subjects, the EC_{100} or AC_{100}. This is difficult to determine, however. An AC_{100} cannot be differentiated from an AC_{110}. Also important is the fact that MAC refers to alveolar, not inspired, concentration of anesthetic. The difference between inhaled and alveolar concentrations depends upon the level of total body equilibration with the anesthetic. This, in turn, is a function of duration of administration, as well as solubility of the anesthetic in various body fluids and tissues. Furthermore, although 1.0 MAC values of different anesthetics represent equal levels of anesthesia, multiples of MAC may not represent equianesthetic levels. Dose-response curves of inhalation anesthetics are not identical. They are not even parallel. In addition, since MAC refers to alveolar concentration, not tension, MAC values vary with atmospheric pressure, i.e., with altitude. Finally, although alveolar and arterial tensions of anesthetics are usually identical, alveolar-arterial pressure gradients may exist, especially with the more highly soluble anesthetics and in the presence of abnormalities of distribution of ventilation and perfusion within the lung.

All inhalation anesthetics have the potential for contaminating the air within operating rooms with subanesthetic trace amounts of anesthetic which have either escaped from the anesthesia circuit or been exhaled by the patient. The resulting pollution of air in operating rooms has been shown to produce demonstrable if subtle impairment of higher cerebral cortical functions, including judgment, among those exposed to such atmospheres. Data also suggest that contamination of operating-room air with trace concentrations of inhalation anesthetics may be associated with an increased incidence of spontaneous abortion and perhaps even increased frequency of congenital birth defects in children born to mothers repeatedly exposed to such an atmosphere in early pregnancy. It has also been suggested, though not proved, that hepatic and renal diseases as well as malignant diseases may be more frequent in those working in an atmosphere contaminated by trace concentrations of inhalation anesthetics. The danger involves not only those who administer anesthetics but surgeons, nurses, and others who work in operating rooms. Trace concentrations of anesthetics can be effectively controlled by scavenging systems attached to each anesthesia machine. All operating rooms should be equipped with such devices.

NITROUS OXIDE

Nitrous oxide (N_2O) is an inhalation analgesic. Nitrous oxide 20% provides analgesia equal to that produced by 10 mg of morphine sulfate. Increasing the concentration of nitrous oxide increases the degree of analgesia, but the MAC for nitrous oxide is over 100, so true anesthesia cannot be achieved (at 1 atmosphere) without decreasing inspired oxygen to the point where hypoxia occurs.

The analgesia produced by nitrous oxide differs substantially from the analgesia produced by narcotics. It is not associated with the profound respiratory and cardiovascular side effects characteristic of narcotics. And it is rapidly, almost immediately, reversible. These properties of nitrous oxide, combined with the fact that it is nonexplosive and odorless (and therefore enjoys high patient acceptance), make nitrous oxide the most widely used drug in surgical anesthesia. It is rarely used alone because of its lack of anesthetic potency. Instead it is employed in conjunction with other, more powerful, agents to decrease the amounts

of them that are needed and thus to diminish the magnitude of adverse side effects with which the more potent anesthetics are associated. Nitrous oxide 70%, for example, decreases the MAC of halothane by 60 percent. Nitrous oxide is also employed for the same reason during intravenous anesthesia: when nitrous oxide is used, fewer narcotics and barbiturates are needed. Because of the effectiveness of nitrous oxide as a nondepressant analgesic, it has been used in low concentrations for the relief not only of postoperative pain but also of the pain of myocardial infarction. The utility of nitrous oxide for this purpose is limited by the difficulty in maintaining its concentration at a level adequate to relieve pain yet not great enough to cause the delirium characteristic of the excitement state of light levels of general anesthesia.

Nitrous oxide is not, however, devoid of side effects. It increases sympathetic activity, probably by direct action on medullary vasomotor centers, and thereby increases peripheral vascular resistance, blood pressure, and heart rate. It also appears to have a slight stimulatory effect on respiration, shifting the CO_2-ventilation response curve to the left. These subtle effects are usually obscured under clinical conditions by the cardiovascular and respiratory effects of other more potent anesthetics simultaneously being administered. Chronic exposure to nitrous oxide also produces leukopenia.

Two clinical situations exist in which nitrous oxide may have unexpected and potentially undesirable effects not because of its pharmacologic action but because of its physical properties. Both situations are due to the fact that nitrous oxide is 30 times more soluble than nitrogen in blood. The first situation, diffusion hypoxia, may occur when a patient who is equilibrated with 80% nitrous oxide–20% oxygen spontaneously starts to breathe room air (80% nitrogen in 20% oxygen). The blood solubility differences between nitrous oxide and nitrogen being such that at equal partial pressures approximately thirty times more nitrous oxide than nitrogen is dissolved, when the patient starts to inhale room air there will be thirty times greater diffusion of nitrous oxide out of the bloodstream than of nitrogen into the bloodstream at the alveolar level. The net result is an increase in gas volume within the alveoli. Since intraalveolar pressure equals ambient pressure, the increased gas volume displaces oxygen molecules from the alveoli, with resulting transient hypoxemia. The phenomenon of diffusion hypoxia is transitory, lasting only moments, and involves at the most a 40-torr decrease in alveolar (and arterial) oxygen tension. It may be prevented by increasing alveolar oxygen tension to 150 to 200 torr at the conclusion of anesthesia. All nitrous oxide need not be eliminated to avoid diffusion hypoxia, nor should it be eliminated if analgesia is required during extubation of the trachea at the end of anesthesia.

The opposite of diffusion hypoxia, hyperoxia, occurs during induction when a patient starts breathing 80% nitrous oxide in oxygen instead of 80% nitrogen in oxygen (room air). The greater solubility of nitrous oxide means that uptake of nitrous oxide exceeds excretion of nitrogen, a concentrating effect which increases alveolar oxygen tension. The same concentrating effect also causes a transitory increase in alveolar carbon dioxide tension. Alveolar concentration of an inhalation anesthetic such as halothane is additionally accelerated, so induction of anesthesia is more rapid when nitrous oxide is used for induction of anesthesia, in part because of the concentrating effect of nitrous oxide.

The second situation in which solubility of nitrous oxide may cause difficulties occurs in patients with gas pockets containing room air, as in pneumothorax, intestinal obstruction, pneumoencephalography. When such patients are anesthetized with nitrous oxide, the anesthetic enters the air pocket at a faster rate than the nitrogen exits from it. The result is that the volume of the gas pocket increases. This can produce a shift in the mediastinum or collapse of adjacent aerated lung in the case of penumothorax or an increase in intraabdominal or intracranial pressure in the case of intestinal obstruction or pneumoencephalography.

During the administration of nitrous oxide–oxygen, the degree of oxygenation of the arterial blood cannot be accurately estimated merely by observing the flows of oxygen and nitrous oxide being delivered by the anesthesia machine. The reasons for this are twofold: First, when nitrous oxide–oxygen is administered at a time when respirations are controlled by intermittent positive pressure, a progressive and significant decrease in arterial oxygen tension can take place even though oxygen tension in the inspired air remains constant. Reasons for this are discussed in the section dealing with muscle relaxants. Second, following equilibration with the anesthetic gases, the concentration of oxygen in the inspired air during nitrous oxide–oxygen anesthesia on a semiclosed system is influenced by the amount of oxygen being metabolically consumed. For example, if a patient consumes 250 ml of oxygen per minute and is anesthetized on a semiclosed circuit into which 1 liter each of oxygen and nitrous oxide are flowing per minute, after equilibration the patient will not be inhaling 50% oxygen, because over the period of 1 minute he will consume 250 ml of the 1,000 ml of oxygen being delivered in that minute. He will therefore be inhaling approximately 42% oxygen. The importance of the metabolic requirements for oxygen as a determinant of the concentration of oxygen in the inspired mixture on semiclosed systems is a function of the total flow of anesthetic gases. The 250 ml of oxygen being metabolized per minute has little significant effect if the total flow rate into the anesthesia circuit is 8 liters per minute, but the same 250 ml will have a major effect if the total flow rate into the semiclosed system is only 1 liter per minute, e.g., 500 ml each of nitrous oxide and oxygen per minute. The concentration of oxygen in the inspired air when nitrous oxide is being administered is related not only to the percentage of oxygen delivered to the anesthesia circuit but also to the total flow rates at which these gases are being delivered.

HALOTHANE

Halothane ($CF_3CHBrCl$) is an extremely potent inhalation anesthetic. The MAC for halothane is 0.75. Surgical levels of anesthesia can usually be obtained with alveolar concentrations of about 1.0 vol %. The advantages of halothane are that it is nonexplosive, that it is not unpleasant for the patient to breath, and that both onset of action and emergence are rapid. A potential advantage of halothane is that because it is so potent it can be administered with 98–99% oxygen. Such potency can also be a disadvantage. The difference between lethal and clinically effective concentrations of halothane in the inspired air is well below 1.0 vol %. Halothane should be administered only by experienced persons employing calibrated vaporizers, the accuracy of which must be independent of changes in temperature and changes in volume of gas flow through them. These specially designed vaporizers must be placed outside the anesthesia circuit to prevent accumulation of halothane within the circuit.

Cardiovascular depression is a frequent accompaniment of surgical levels of halothane anesthesia. It is the result of multiple actions of halothane on different parts of the cardiovascular system: direct depression of medullary vasomotor centers; inhibition of ganglionic transmission within sympathetic nerves innervating the heart and peripheral vasculature; alteration of threshold responses of baroreceptors within the carotid and aortic arch sinuses; and direct depression of both myocardial muscle fibers and peripheral vascular smooth muscle fibers. Hypotension and decreased cardiac output often occur during halothane anesthesia, especially in aged or hypovolemic patients and in patients with myocardial ischemia, valvular heart disease, or coronary artery insufficiency. Halothane also increases the sensitivity of ventricular pacemakers to arrhythmogenic stimuli, including epinephrine, probably because of anesthetically induced depression of conduction within the heart. It is for this reason that use of epinephrine must be restricted to less than 10 ml/70 kg body weight of a 1:100,000 solution every 10 minutes during halothane anesthesia.

Since the cardiovascular-depressant actions of halothane are dose-dependent (i.e., concentration-dependent), a frequent technique for decreasing the magnitude and frequency of such adverse side effects is to administer halothane with nitrous oxide. Nitrous oxide 70% decreases the anesthetic requirements of halothane by 60 percent. Since nitrous oxide has a slight stimulatory rather than a depressant effect on cardiovascular function, the combination of 70% nitrous oxide and 0.3% halothane produces less physiologic trespass against the cardiovascular system than does 0.7% halothane in 100% oxygen, yet depth of anesthesia is the same in each instance. Use of nitrous oxide to decrease halothane concentration diminishes the magnitude of the arterial hypotension and decreased cardiac output produced by the halothane, but it does so at the cost of decreasing arterial oxygen content below the level obtainable when 100% oxygen is given with the halothane. The increase in oxygen content of arterial blood associated with 100% oxygen is sufficient to maintain at normal levels the rate at which oxygen is delivered to peripheral tissues even if cardiac output decreases 15 percent. Decreasing the amount of halothane by using nitrous oxide and thus lowering inspired oxygen to 30% will be of little avail in terms of the rate at which oxygen is delivered to the periphery if the combination of N_2O and halothane is still associated with a 15 percent decrease in cardiac output. Addition of nitrous oxide in this situation may even be deleterious.

Halothane is a potent vasodilator. The vasodilation affects the circulation of almost all organs. Notable is the effect of halothane on the cerebral vasculature. Even when the respiratory-depressant effects of halothane are compensated for by artificial respiration to assure a normal arterial carbon dioxide tension of 40 torr, surgical levels of halothane anesthesia are associated with significant increases in cerebral blood flow due to the decrease in cerebrovascular resistance produced by the halothane. The resultant increase in intracranial pressure can be deleterious in patients with preexisting increase in pressure due to space-occupying lesions. This potential danger can be offset to a major extent by artificially hyperventilating the patient during halothane anesthesia to lower arterial carbon dioxide tension to 30 torr or less and thus restore cerebral blood flow and intracranial pressure to preanesthetic levels.

Halothane, like the majority of general anesthetics, decreases the sensitivity of the respiratory center to carbon dioxide. Spontaneous ventilation during surgical levels of halothane anesthesia is therefore inevitably associated with elevation of arterial carbon dioxide tension. The resultant respiratory acidosis can be only partially compensated for by assisting respirations. The increase in apneic threshold produced by halothane means that as long as any inspiratory effort remains, an inspiratory movement is needed to signal the exact moment when positive pressure must be applied to the anesthesia reservoir bag if inhalation is to be assisted, when carbon dioxide tension is above normal levels of 40 torr. When artificial ventilation succeeds in lowering carbon dioxide to 40 torr, apnea usually ensues and assisted ventilation becomes impossible. Eucapnia during halothane anesthesia can be assured only when respirations are controlled, not assisted.

Halothane, in common with other commonly used inhalation anesthetics, is metabolized by hepatic microsomal enzyme systems. The amount metabolized averages about 20 percent of that absorbed by the patient, but this varies from patient to patient and can be expected to be increased in patients in whom enzyme induction has been produced either by prior administration of drugs such as phenobarbital or by recent prior exposure (self-induction). The metabolism of halothane has no clinically significant effect on uptake, distribution, or MAC. The metabolites are pharmacologically largely inert. With prolonged exposure to high concentrations of halothane, however, enough inorganic bromine may be released to elevate serum bromine levels to the point where they may produce sedation. For this reason, prolonged (6 to 8 hours) administration of halothane may be inadvisable, especially in neurosurgical patients in whom rapid return of normal cerebral function postoperatively may be desirable. The possibility that the metabolites of halothane are toxic has been extensively studied. The consensus is that they are not, except possibly to the liver, as discussed below.

Because halothane is a highly halogenated hydrocarbon, the possibility that it might be a hepatotoxin has received considerable attention. Objective clinical data remain difficult to obtain, and the clinical significance of much of the data obtained from experimental animals remains obscure. Three things are, however, generally agreed upon. First, though rare and sporadic, instances of postoperative hepatic damage have been reported often enough in association with halothane to indicate that the matter deserves careful scrutiny and investigation. Second, halothane is not a true hepatotoxin in the sense that carbon tetrachloride is, for example. Halothane does not produce predictable dose/concentration–dependent hepatic damage in all species the way a true hepatotoxin does. And, third, the risk of an adverse hepatic response to halothane is not greater in the presence of preexisting liver disease. It may even be less in the case of cirrhosis. Halothane, furthermore, causes no greater exacerbation of preexisting liver disease than do other anesthetics. It is therefore not necessarily contraindicated in patients with liver disease.

Those who believe halothane is capable of producing hepatic damage describe a clinical picture in which a diffuse hepatitis develops 2 to 5 days following anesthesia. The onset of jaundice is preceded by high, unexplained fever for about 12 to 24 hours and is accompanied by eosinophilia. The syndrome is said to be more frequent in females than in males, more frequent following multiple exposures to halothane, and more frequent if a previous exposure to halothane was associated with unexplained fever. Biopsy specimens reveal a picture indistinguishable from that observed in infectious hepatitis. The damage to the liver may be mild and short-lived or it may progress to fatal liver failure.

"Halothane hepatitis" has been ascribed to an allergic or hypersensitivity reaction to halothane or its metabolites. This, it is said, agrees with its reported higher incidence among females and the associated eosinophilia and with the higher incidence of the syndrome following multiple exposures to halothane. Yet substantial series of cases have also been reported in patients who have been exposed on multiple occasions to halothane without adverse effects. The fact that "halothane hepatitis" has been reported in patients following a first exposure to halothane is explained on the basis of relatively nonspecific sensitization, comparable to the sensitivity of certain persons to horse serum even though they have not previously been exposed to it. The most compelling evidence that "halothane hepatitis" does indeed represent a sensitization phenomenon is a report of an anesthetist who developed hepatitis whenever he employed halothane as an anesthetic. When challenged with a trace concentration of halothane under controlled conditions at a time when the hepatitis had been quiescent for several months, there was prompt and immediate onset of fever and arthralgia and recrudescence of the hepatitis confirmed by biopsy.

The response of such a person to a challenge exposure to halothane is compatible with the hypothesis that the syndrome is a sensitization reaction. The response does not rule out, however, other possibilities. The trace concentrations of halothane or its metabolites may have been adequate to depress normal immune responses to a virus causing hepatitis and thereby cause a smoldering or incipient infection to become active enough to be clinically and histologically evident. The stress, both emotional and physical, of such a challenge test may also be sufficient to cause acute exacerbation of a previously quiescent condition. Finally, extensive in vitro immunologic tests have consistently failed to prove the existence of a sensitization reaction or an allergy to halothane in patients recovering from "halothane hepatitis."

Another explanation offered for "halothane hepatitis" is that certain persons are susceptible to halothane or its metabolites not on an immunologic or sensitivity basis but rather on the basis that they have an inherent abnormality of metabolism, either acquired or genetic in origin, which results in production of abnormal metabolites from halothane which are in themselves hepatotoxic. This view receives support from the demonstration that under the proper circumstances a small portion of the metabolites of halothane can produce damage to liver cells in vitro or in vivo in experimental animals. That this applies to man remains to be proved.

A major problem in determining the true incidence of "halothane hepatitis" lies in the fact that many other conditions encountered in surgical patients are capable of producing a similar picture. Chief amongst these is viral hepatitis. Making a differential diagnosis in an individual case between viral hepatitis and "halothane hepatitis" with absolute certainty is so difficult as to border on the impossible. Yet it is essential to do so. The natural incidence of viral hepatitis is such that the condition is bound to occur in a substantial number of the 18,000,000 persons anesthetized annually in this country, regardless of whether they had halothane or not. To complicate matters further, many drugs other than halothane administered to surgical patients are also capable of producing hepatic dysfunction; and shock, sepsis, and other complications of surgery can result in liver damage. Not all cases of hepatic damage following halothane are due to the halothane.

A fundamental question with regard to "halothane hepatitis" is the overall safety of halothane compared to other anesthetics. The massive National Halothane Study studied this insofar as deaths associated with postoperative liver failure are concerned. The results of this study conclusively demonstrated that the frequency of postoperative hepatic dysfunction not related to shock, sepsis, other forms of hepatitis, or the like is no greater following halothane than it is following any other anesthetic, and may even be less. The study also showed that otherwise inexplicable hepatic dysfunction was rare, occurring at most about once in 8,000 to 10,000 anesthesias, and not every case was fatal. But the safety of halothane as a clinical anesthetic cannot be judged solely by the incidence of associated hepatic damage. Substitution of another anesthetic for halothane in hope of avoiding a rare but perhaps possible case of "halothane hepatitis" may introduce risks greater than that of hepatitis. To replace halothane with an anesthetic associated with an incidence of ventricular fibrillation of 1 in 2,500 accomplishes little in terms of overall patient safety.

To summarize: Whether "halothane hepatitis" even exists as a clinical syndrome is debatable. If it does exist, the mechanism by which halothane causes hepatitis remains unproved. Even if it exists, the risk involved in the judicious use of halothane has not been proved to be greater than the risk of avoiding it in favor of other anesthetics; it may well be less. Halothane remains a safe and effective inhalation anesthetic when properly administered.

Finally, mention should be made of the fact that halothane is a potent depressant of uterine musculature. This property of halothane has been utilized for relaxing contraction rings and for performing internal versions. It is a property, however, which contraindicates use of halothane in most obstetric situations.

ENFLURANE

Enflurane (CHF_2OCF_2CHFCl) is representative of a group of recently synthesized compounds which combine an ether linkage (for anesthetic effect) with halogenation (F for nonflammability, Cl for anesthetic effect). About half as potent as halothane (the MAC of enflurane is 1.2), enflurane has nevertheless many of the properties of halothane. They are about equally rapid in onset of action. Recovery is also about equally rapid. Both depress respiration and the cardiovascular system to about the same extent when administered in equianesthetic concentrations.

Enflurane differs from halothane, however, in four respects. First, in a small percentage of normal patients it is associated with development of electroencephalographic patterns characteristic of epilepsy. This occurrence is markedly diminished in frequency and can perhaps even be eliminated if hyperventilation and hypocapnia are avoided. The clinical significance of these EEG patterns is dubious. Rarely are they associated with corresponding behavioral changes in the form of mild epileptiform movements. The appearance of these abnormal EEG patterns does not appear to be more frequent in epileptics.

Secondly, while enflurane does not protect against the arrythmogenic effects of epinephrine and similar compounds to the extent that a halogenated ether such as methoxyflurane does, it does not increase the irritability of ectopic ventricular pacemakers to the extent that halothane does. Enflurane is a particularly useful inhalation anesthetic when epinephrine is used by intravenous infusion for its inotropic effects or by injection for its vasoconstrictor effects to decrease operative blood loss. Enflurane is also useful in patients with pheochromocytomas when inhalation anesthesia is employed.

Thirdly, enflurane is metabolized, but the percentage of enflurane which undergoes biotransformation is but a fraction of that with other halogenated anesthetics, including halothane. This may be particularly advantageous during inhalation anesthesia of long duration. Enflurane avoids the problem of possible prolonged postoperative sedation due to increased bromine levels associated with lengthy halothane anesthetics.

Finally, cases of postoperative "hepatitis" have been reported following enflurane anesthesia, although less frequently than following halothane anesthesia. Since enflurane is metabolized less than halothane, this has been said to support the hypothesis that the metabolic products of halothane rather than halothane itself are responsible for sensitization reactions leading to "halothane hepatitis."

Equally possible is the alternative explanation, that enflurane and the few metabolites it produces are so immunologically inert that they are incapable of initiating a sensitization reaction. But whether "hepatitis" is in fact less frequent after enflurane than after halothane is in doubt. It has yet to be proved statistically. Perhaps the incidence of "hepatitis" associated with enflurane appears to be lower because enflurane has only recently been available for general clinical use, or perhaps there is a lower level of suspicion in regard to enflurane.

OTHER INHALATION ANESTHETICS

CYCLOPROPANE. Cyclopropane (C_3H_6) is a highly explosive, extremely rapidly acting inhalation anesthetic of intermediate potency (its MAC is 9.2). Anesthetic concentrations are associated with a pronounced centrally mediated increase in sympathetic activity. The blood pressure rises. The pulse slows, however, because of activation of baroreceptor reflexes the sensitivity of which is probably increased by the anesthetic. Blood levels of catecholamines, norepinephrine especially, rise as the rate of norepinephrine release from postganglionic sympathetic fibers exceeds the capacity for reuptake and local enzymatic breakdown. The elevated blood levels of catecholamines predispose to ventricular arrhythmias, including ventricular fibrillation, particularly if catecholamine levels are further increased by the exogenous administration of epinephrine or the endogenous release of still more catecholamines by hypoxia or carbon dioxide accumulation. Hypercapnia is particularly liable to occur in the absence of controlled ventilation because of the respiratory-depressant effects of cyclopropane. Because of the increase in sympathetic activity, cyclopropane is particularly advantageous in hypovolemic patients. Cyclopropane, however, is now infrequently used because of its explosiveness and the widespread use of electrocautery for surgical hemostasis.

DIETHYL ETHER. Ether ($CH_3CH_2OCH_2CH_3$) is an explosive, potent (its MAC is 1.9) inhalation anesthetic that differs from other general anesthetics in that respiration is not depressed by anesthetic concentrations. Like cyclopropane, it increases sympathetic activity, but to a somewhat lesser extent. Ether is rarely used today in the United States for three reasons: it is explosive; it is the most difficult of all general anesthetics to administer smoothly, principally because of its high solubility, especially in blood and other extracellular fluids; and finally, it is osmically offensive, an esthetic point—it smells bad. Ether remains, nevertheless, uniquely valuable in those rare instances in which surgical levels of anesthesia must be maintained with spontaneous respiration. Ether is also still widely employed in developing countries because it is the least expensive of all general anesthetics and because, being an easily handled and easily vaporized liquid that does not depress respiration, it can be administered with a minimum of equipment.

METHOXYFLURANE. Methoxyflurane ($CH_3OCF_2CHCl_2$) is another nonexplosive, halogenated ether. It is the most potent of all inhalation anesthetics, with a MAC of 0.16, and it has the lowest vapor pressure of all anesthetics, 20 torr at 18°C. Furthermore, it is the most highly soluble of all anesthetics in lipids: its oil/gas partition coefficient is about 1,000. The physical properties of methoxyflurane mean that induction of anesthesia may be prolonged. Recovery may also be prolonged, often for hours. Its pharmacologic properties are much like those of other halogenated inhalation anesthetics. It depresses respiration and the cardiovascular system about as much as equieffective concentrations of halothane or enflurane. It protects against epinephrine-induced arrhythmias, however. The major distinguishing characteristic of methoxyflurane is that it is extensively metabolized with release of inorganic fluoride. Fluoride is nephrotoxic when serum levels exceed a level of about 50 μm/liter. These levels are apt to be equaled or exceeded under clinical conditions, especially when methoxyflurane is administered for more than an hour or two and especially in an obese patient. The danger of high-output renal failure in the postoperative period is so real that today methoxyflurane is infrequently used. When it is employed, it is most often used for brief periods in low concentrations, often intermittently, as an inhalation analgesic, especially in labor.

Intravenous Anesthesia

General anesthesia is also produced by the intravenous injection of one or, more commonly, a combination of two or more depressants. Intravenous anesthesia almost always also includes the simultaneous administration of nitrous oxide. When a single drug is used intravenously, it is most often a thiobarbiturate. When combinations of drugs are used, they are usually of different types, including narcotics, ketamine, hypnotics, or neuroleptics. "Balanced anesthesia" means different things to different people but most often refers to a combination of drugs used intravenously to obtain amnesia, analgesia, sedation, and muscular relaxation. A thiobarbiturate and a narcotic are almost always included (along with nitrous oxide). Neuroleptics and sedative-tranquilizers such as diazepam (Valium) may also be used, as well as a muscle relaxant.

An advantage of intravenous anesthesia is agreeableness for the patient. The rapid onset of unconsciousness without exposure to odorous vapors and without the claustrophobic feeling of a mask applied to the face makes intravenous anesthesia popular with patients. Another advantage is convenience for the anesthetist. Rapid induction of anesthesia without the problems inherent in the somewhat longer and certainly more exacting induction of anesthesia by inhalation techniques has appealing aspects.

Against these advantages must be weighed the disadvantages of intravenous anesthesia. Chief among these is the fact that although intravenous anesthetics produce immediate and profound depression, true anesthesia—that is, absence of response to painful stimuli—may not be complete. This can lead to a situation, for instance, in which depression is great enough to cause obstruction of the upper airway as the tongue and other soft tissues fall back into the pharynx, yet the patient is not deeply enough anesthetized to permit instrumentation in the airway by insertion of an artificial airway or an endotracheal tube to remove the obstruction. The result can be a patient unable to breathe adequately because of airway obstruction yet not deeply enough anesthetized to allow the situation to be corrected. The dilemma can be solved by paralyzing the patient with a muscle relaxant and then immediately performing a laryngoscopy and placing an endotracheal tube in place for artificial ventilation. This solution to the problem is based on the assumption that endotracheal intubation can *always*—in *all* patients—be immediately accomplished. If this assumption proves incorrect, as it occasionally may even in the most skilled hands, the obstructed, semianesthetized patient who is at least trying to breathe past an obstruction is converted to an obstructed, semianesthetized patient who is apneic, not trying to breathe, and cannot be ventilated artificially. The result can be disastrous. Even if endotracheal intubation is accomplished, the patient is still not anesthetized, although this will not be evident because the lack of anesthesia is covered up by paralysis. A corollary of this situation can arise during intravenous anesthesia in which a muscle relaxant is administered during maintenance of anesthesia. Redistribution of the intravenously administered neuronal depressants may cause blood levels and hence brain levels of narcotics and hypnotics to decrease to the point where awareness is regained. When the patient is paralyzed the anesthetist may be unable to recognize the fact that the patient is aware of his surroundings and may even be experiencing pain. Changes in blood pressure and pulse rate in response to surgical stimulation are sufficiently blunted under these circumstances by the intravenous anesthetics so that they are no longer reliable indications of the depth of anesthesia. The difficulty in maintaining constant and predictable levels of anesthesia with intravenous anesthetics is reflected by the fact that MAC values for intravenous anesthetics cannot be determined. The pharmacokinetics of uptake, distribution, metabolism, and excretion are too complex to allow establishment of a pharmacologic state steady enough for such a determination.

Another disadvantage of intravenous anesthesia, as already mentioned, is that the duration of action of the drugs used is determined by factors the anesthetist has no control over, namely biotransformation and renal or biliary excretion. Specific antagonists to narcotics and relaxants are available for use at the conclusion of intravenous anesthesia and are often helpful, but antagonists are often only a partial answer to the problem of controlled reversibility. There are no specific antagonists to barbiturates, neuroleptics, and other hypnotics which may be used during intravenous anesthesia. Furthermore, the duration of action of the antagonist may be less than the duration of action of the agonist.

Finally, the polypharmacy involved in intravenous anesthesia holds the potential for drug interactions of such complexity that they are difficult to unravel even under controlled experimental conditions in laboratory animals, let alone in human beings under clinical conditions. Intravenous anesthesia commonly involves use of at least ten drugs, often more, including premedicants and antagonists in addition to the intravenous anesthetics. The theory behind such polypharmacy is that the desirable attributes of each drug in a combination of drugs supplement or potentiate one another. Less desirable attributes may also,

however, be supplemented or potentiated. A combination of neuronal depressants may produce a more satisfactory state of anesthesia, analgesia, and amnesia than would a single drug. At the same time, however, the adverse side effects of the drugs on cardiovascular function and on respiration may also be, and often are, greater.

Despite its disadvantages, intravenous anesthesia enjoys a well-deserved niche in the armamentarium of the anesthetist. Its apparent simplicity, however, belies the fact that intravenous anesthesia requires even more skill and experience than does inhalation anesthesia if it is to prove equally safe.

BARBITURATES

The intravenous agents most frequently used to produce surgical anesthesia are thiobarbiturates. Their popularity is based on the fact that they are "ultra-short-acting" barbiturates, i.e., rapid in onset and short in duration. Their pharmacologic actions, using thiopental (Pentothal) as a prototype, may be considered according to the cause of their "ultrashort action," with a brief comparison of their effects with those of inhalation anesthetics.

The rapid onset and apparently short duration of action of thiobarbiturates is a function primarily of increased lipoid solubility associated with the substitution of a sulfur atom for the oxygen atom in the barbituric acid ring. Thiopental is structurally similar to pentobarbital (Nembutal), except that a sulfur atom has been substituted for the oxygen atom in the latter. The increased lipoid solubility, plus a pK which makes thiopental only slightly dissociated at a pH of 7.40, cause the rapid onset of action. The rate at which drugs cross the so-called blood-brain barrier is directly related to their lipoid solubility and inversely related to their degree of ionization. These properties of thiopental combined with high cerebral blood flow result not only in an immediate onset of action (one circulation time) but also in an extremely short duration of action. Because the central nervous system has such a high flow compared to other areas of the body, more thiopental is delivered to it; this combined with high lipoid solubility produces a higher concentration in the central nervous system than elsewhere in the body immediately after administration of a single dose. With the passage of time other areas of the body with lesser blood flows gradually receive the barbiturate. In lean body mass, represented primarily by skeletal muscle, a concentration of thiopental develops after peak central nervous system concentrations have been achieved and in so doing produces a decrease in concentration of thiopental within the central nervous system. This hemodynamic redistribution of thiopental following a single intravenous injection is later followed by further redistribution to the areas of the body with the least blood flow, namely, adipose tissue. The buildup of thiopental in fatty depots throughout the body is relatively slow because of the low blood flow, but as time goes on the concentration in these areas becomes significant because of thiopental's high lipoid solubility in such tissues. As a result of this redistribution there is a relatively rapid reversal of the high central nervous system concentration following a single intravenous injection, and consciousness rapidly returns toward normal. This apparently ultrashort duration of action results not from a high rate of metabolism or excretion but from the dynamics of uptake and redistribution. The same sequence of events takes place, but to a less pronounced degree, following repeated intravenous injections of small amounts of the drug. The redistribution of thiopental within the body results in a regression of the state of central nervous system depression but does not result in its complete reversal until all the barbiturate has been metabolized or excreted.

The pharmacologic properties of thiopental are qualitatively comparable to those previously outlined for inhalation anesthetics, but with the additional disadvantage that when administered in equianesthetic doses thiopental is more depressant than true inhalation anesthetics. Thus thiopental is a cardiovascular and respiratory depressant. As a cardiovascular depressant, it acts directly on the myocardium to decrease the force of ventricular contraction. In addition it causes peripheral vasodilatation. The hypotension which may accompany thiopental administration may be extreme, especially in patients in or bordering on oligemic shock. But the hypotension of thiopental does not have the saving grace of being associated with a state of true surgical anesthesia, as is usual with an agent such as halothane. The respiratory depression of thiopental resulting in an elevated threshold response of the respiratory center to carbon dioxide is unassociated with the production of a truly anesthetic state and so is of completely different clinical significance from that produced by, for example, halothane.

Another major disadvantage of thiopental is that its depressant effects last longer than those observed with inhalation anesthetics. For example, the respiratory depression with enflurane is rapidly reversed moments after its administration has been terminated, while the effects of intravenous anesthetics such as thiopental may linger on for hours. The complete metabolism or excretion of thiopental occurs at an extremely slow rate. Thus, although the greater part of the thiopental-induced anesthesia may be reversed within moments following a single injection, a long-lasting and subclinical degree of central nervous system depression may persist for many hours until the barbiturate has been metabolized in the liver and removed not only from the brain but also from the lean body mass and the fatty depots. The prolonged but subtle central nervous system depression following thiopental anesthesia is exemplified by the electroencephalographic changes, which may be detected for 18 hours following a brief period of thiopental anesthesia.

Thiobarbiturates today are mainly used to supplement other relatively weak anesthetics such as nitrous oxide or other intravenous anesthetics or to induce general anesthesia prior to the administration of other more potent inhalation anesthetics. When employed as a means of inducing general anesthesia, thiobarbiturates are best administered in "sleep" or hypnotic doses of 150 to 200 mg/70 kg of body weight and not in anesthetic doses (500 to 600 mg). Thiopental is contraindicated (as is any general anesthetic) in the presence of a full stomach or in other situations in which the patency of the patient's airway cannot be assured at all times.

NARCOTICS

Narcotics are not anesthetics. Nevertheless they are employed frequently and advantageously enough as adjuncts to anesthesia to warrant discussion in this chapter. Narcotics are primarily used in two situations: during general anesthesia in combination with weak anesthetics such as nitrous oxide or intravenous anesthetics to provide more intense analgesia and during regional anesthesia to provide relief of pain or discomfort. In such instances narcotics should be administered only intravenously. Intramuscular and subcutaneous injections are so slowly and erratically absorbed and have such unpredictable onset and intensity of action that administration by such routes should be limited to premedication. When administered intravenously, narcotics must be given in repeated small doses rather than in a single therapeutic dose, to prevent development of transient dangerously high blood and brain levels.

The main disadvantage of narcotics as adjuvants to anesthesia is that some degree of respiratory depression is inevitably produced whenever narcotics are employed in therapeutic amounts. There is no significant difference in the degree of depression caused by the different narcotics *when administered in equianalgesic dosages.* Duration of action may, however, differ among the narcotics. Notable is the short duration of action of fentanyl (Sublimaze), the most potent narcotic presently available. With approximately fifty times the activity of morphine, fentanyl has a duration of action less than half that of morphine. Attempts to increase the usefulness of narcotics during anesthesia by administration of narcotic antagonists in the belief that respiratory depression will be alleviated without affecting analgesia have proved futile.

A completely different anesthetic use of narcotics involves their administration in amounts large enough to produce true anesthesia. Morphine is especially useful in this regard when given in doses of 2 to 3 mg/kg during cardiac surgery requiring cardiopulmonary bypass. Use of morphine in this manner is predicated on the assumption that respirations will be continuously controlled via an endotracheal tube in the immediate postoperative period, which is of considerable benefit to many cardiac patients.

Narcotics also are used during regional anesthesia, whether spinal, epidural, or nerve block, either to supplement inadequate sensory blocking or to relieve patient discomfort if the regional anesthesia wears off before the operation has been completed. The wisdom of using narcotics in either situation is often doubtful, because considerable depression is produced without real relief of pain. It is often wiser to give the patient a small amount of intravenous narcotic followed by a nondepressant, rapidly reversible analgesic such as nitrous oxide rather than try to provide true anesthesia with the narcotic alone. Intravenous narcotics in small amounts, however, are often of real value for patients undergoing lengthy procedures under regional anesthesia, as the immobile patient with spinal anesthesia on an uncomfortable operating table for 4 hours becomes restless because of the physical discomfort of the unanesthetized portions of the body.

OTHER INTRAVENOUS ANESTHETICS

Neuroleptic anesthesia (or analgesia) is an intravenous anesthetic technique in which a potent psychomotor sedative, the neuroleptic, is combined with a narcotic and a hypnotic. The most widely used neuroleptic is droperidol (Inapsine), which is supplied commercially either alone or in combination with the potent narcotic fentanyl in a ratio of 50:1 as Innovar. The combination of drugs in Innovar presupposes that when sedation is required a narcotic is required and vice versa, and furthermore that both are always needed in the same arbitrarily predetermined proportions. This may be true at times, but scarcely all the time. Innovar is best used in intravenous anesthesia to help establish a basic level of sedation and analgesia during induction of anesthesia. Subsequent analgesia is thereafter best maintained with nitrous oxide together with repeated injections of small amounts of fentanyl, while sedation is maintained either with further droperidol alone or with a thiobarbiturate.

Ketamine, although not a narcotic in the classic sense, produces profound analgesia combined with striking subjective dissociation from the environment. Administered intravenously or intramuscularly in the proper dosage, ketamine provides anesthesia adequate for superficial operations requiring no muscle relaxation without producing respiratory or cardiovascular depression. In fact, the arterial pressure frequently is elevated and the heart rate increased. Ketamine also has the important advantage of not relaxing muscles and soft tissue of the upper airway, as other narcotics and sedatives are prone to do. Therefore, airway obstruction is infrequent, though by no means impossible, during ketamine anesthesia. However, ketamine has the disadvantage of being occasionally associated with highly unpleasant hallucinations or subjective responses best described as nightmares. Since this adverse psychic response is particularly liable to occur in adults, ketamine is often restricted to children. As ketamine accentuates pharyngeal and laryngeal reflexes, it is usually contraindicated for operations on or about the mouth, lips, and nose because of the possibility of precipitating severe laryngospasm. It also rather sharply increases intracranial pressure and so is contraindicated in certain neurologic conditions.

RELAXANTS

Intravenously administered muscle relaxants allow profound muscular relaxation without deep levels of anesthesia. The avoidance of the adverse physiologic effects of deep general anesthesia by such means is not, however, without its disadvantages. These are related to the profound interference with normal respiration produced by all muscle relaxants when administered in amounts adequate to provide required degrees of muscular relaxation. The respiratory effects of muscle relaxants must be compensated for by artificial ventilation to maintain a normal

arterial oxygenation and a normal carbon dioxide excretion. This is not always readily achieved under clinical circumstances, and the clinical signs of respiratory acidosis or hypoxia are unreliable in the anesthetized patient.

An additional problem associated with the use of muscle relaxants is that their duration of action may exceed the duration of surgical procedures, with the result that a patient is apneic or hypoventilated after the operation and anesthesia have been completed. Although prolonged apnea following the use of muscle relaxants is not always due solely to their prolonged action, the apnea cannot always be reversed at will.

A third difficulty associated with the use of muscle relaxants is that the intermittent positive-pressure ventilation which their use necessitates may be associated with arterial hypoxemia even though alveolar ventilation adequate for removal of carbon dioxide is provided. Arterial hypoxemia may supervene despite amounts of oxygen in the inspired air adequate to maintain normal arterial oxygenation in the unanesthetized patient. The reason is that intermittent positive-pressure ventilation often is associated with derangements of normal alveolar ventilation/perfusion ratios, and certain alveoli are perfused with blood when they are not ventilated. The uneven alveolar ventilation, which to some extent inevitably follows the institution of positive-pressure respirations, results in an increased gradient in oxygen tension between alveoli and pulmonary venous (i.e., peripheral arterial) blood because of the continued perfusion of unventilated or underventilated areas. For this reason it is necessary to provide at least 33% oxygen in the inspired air when artificial respiration is being carried on for long periods of time, as during nitrous oxide–oxygen anesthesia with muscle relaxants or halothane. The same events can occur in patients on controlled respiration for long periods of time in the postoperative recovery room and in intensive care units.

Muscle relaxants may be divided into two major categories depending on the method by which they produce muscle paralysis: those such as curare and pancuronium (Pavulon), which interfere with transmission of the nerve impulse at the myoneural junction by competing with acetylcholine for the motor end plate (nondepolarizing muscle relaxants), and those such as succinylcholine, which interfere with myoneural transmission by producing depolarization of the motor end plate, rendering it unresponsive. Agents such as curare are, by and large, longer acting than depolarizing agents. Curare, for example, shows significant regression from its peak action approximately 20 minutes after administration, the greater part of its action disappearing within approximately 40 minutes. Although curare is to a large extent ultimately excreted by renal mechanisms, its action is terminated after about 45 minutes primarily because of its redistribution throughout the body. Therefore, curare, like thiopental, may have a subtle subclinical effect persisting beyond its peak effect. Thus, curare has a cumulative effect, and a subsequent dose to produce muscular relaxation equal to that produced initially will be considerably lower than the first.

Unlike curare, the depolarizing agent succinylcholine

has a short duration of action, because it is metabolized by the enzyme pseudocholinesterase in approximately 8 minutes. However, after prolonged periods of administration the method by which succinylcholine produces neuromuscular block becomes more complex; it no longer resembles a depolarizing type of block so much as a nondepolarizing or curare type of block. This nondepolarizing phase of myoneural block is especially liable to be encountered after prolonged intravenous administration of dilute concentrations of succinylcholine.

The initial depolarization produced by single injections of large amounts of succinylcholine frequently results in onset of brief fasciculation of skeletal muscles and often in equally brief uncoordinated myoclonic contractions gross enough to resemble seizures. One result of the depolarization is an increase in intraocular pressure due to fasciculations of extrinsic muscles of the eye. This is of no consequence in normal patients, but in a patient with an open orbit or with preexisting increased intraocular pressure due, for example, to glaucoma, this side effect of succinylcholine can prove highly deleterious. Succinylcholine is often also associated with an increase in intraabdominal pressure due to fasciculation of muscles of the anterior abdominal wall and, perhaps, the diaphragm. This also is of little consequence in normal patients. In a patient suffering from disruption of an abdominal incision, however, the increased intraabdominal pressure can make the dehiscence worse. Intragastric pressure also increases when intraabdominal pressure is elevated during fasciculations. This is particularly dangerous in a patient with a full stomach because of the possibility of massive regurgitation of gastric contents into the upper airway and mouth, with subsequent aspiration into the trachea and bronchi.

Depolarization of skeletal muscles induced by succinylcholine is accompanied by efflux of potassium from skeletal muscles. In normal subjects this results in minor and quite transitory elevations of serum potassium levels of no clinical significance. In other patients, however, the hyperkalemia may be so pronounced as to result in ventricular fibrillation. This is particularly liable to occur in patients suffering from burns, from crush injuries involving skeletal muscles, and from injuries involving denervation of skeletal muscles.

Finally, the depolarization of succinylcholine can result in severe and distressing postoperative muscle pains. Clinical impression to the contrary, these pains are not related to gross jactitations of muscles which occur as muscle masses undergo depolarization at different rates. Muscle pains are due to the depolarization per se and can be observed postoperatively in patients who exhibited no gross movements of muscles following succinylcholine.

Increases in intraocular and intraabdominal pressures, hyperkalemia, and postoperative muscle pains associated with succinylcholine can all be prevented if a small amount of a nondepolarizing relaxant (e.g., 3 mg of *d*-tubocurarine/70 kg) is administered 5 to 8 minutes prior to injection of succinylcholine. When this is done, the amount of succinylcholine subsequently administered must be increased, because a nondepolarizing relaxant shifts the dose-response curve of a depolarizing relaxant to the right.

Succinylcholine, along with halothane and other inhalation anesthetics, has been shown to be capable of triggering, in certain rare individuals, a potentially lethal and rapidly progressing condition referred to as *malignant pyrexia,* often (though not invariably) characterized by muscular rigidity instead of relaxation following succinylcholine. The body temperature is rapidly elevated to levels as high as 107°F within 30 minutes or less. Once established, the pyrexia often proves fatal because of associated neurologic damage, cardiovascular collapse, and profound metabolic derangements. The biochemical events responsible for the massive increase in body heat remain to be fully elucidated, though they obviously involve skeletal muscles. The syndrome has, however, been shown to represent a genetically transmitted susceptibility to succinylcholine and many inhalation anesthetics which, when encountered, is most likely to be seen in young, muscular males who are otherwise quite healthy. There is no accurate method of diagnosing the condition in advance except for sophisticated and complex metabolic studies performed on muscle biopsies from those suspected of being at risk. Most valuable is a detailed family history in all patients to detect a familial history of adverse responses to anesthetics. Malignant pyrexia in a patient at risk because of a positive family history can be avoided by use of anesthetic techniques which do not rely on muscle relaxants or halogenated inhalation anesthetics. Management of the condition once it has been triggered depends on prompt recognition based on a high level of suspicion when patients respond atypically to succinylcholine, plus routine monitoring of body temperature, followed by immediate and aggressive physical measures to lower temperature as rapidly as possible. Pharmacologic treatment of malignant hyperpyrexia previously rested upon the uncertain benefits of intravenous procainamide. More promising is dantrolene, a drug currently under investigation but not yet commercially available for this purpose in an intravenous form.

The duration of action of muscle relaxants is altered by a number of clinically important conditions. In the case of succinylcholine, duration may be prolonged when, following continuous infusion of dilute solutions of succinylcholine to maintain surgical relaxation for long periods of time, the block has changed from depolarizing to nondepolarizing in character. Prolonged apnea is also observed in rare patients suffering from a genetically transmitted abnormal form of pseudocholinesterase incapable of metabolizing succinylcholine and other esterases as rapidly as normal. Prolonged apnea due to lack of pseudocholinesterase may be diagnosed by determination of plasma pseudocholinesterase levels. This is a test so difficult to perform as to preclude its routine use to screen for susceptible patients and to preclude most routine laboratory measurement of pseudocholinesterase activity in cases of prolonged apnea suspected as being of this origin. Treatment of prolonged apnea due to pseudocholinesterase insufficiency is mainly expectant. Artificial ventilation, together with monitoring of blood-gas tensions and twitch responses of muscles to indirect electrical stimulation, should be maintained for hours if necessary until such amounts of pseudocholinesterase as are present have been able to metabolize the succinylcholine. Transfusions of plasma or whole blood containing normal amounts of pseudocholinesterase should be reserved for rare instances in which little or no metabolism is effected after many hours.

In the case of nondepolarizing relaxants, prolongation of action can be observed in patients suffering from water intoxication or other abnormalities of electrolyte balance, especially calcium, and in patients given certain antibiotics, e.g., neomycin. The most frequent causes of prolonged apnea following muscle relaxants remain, however, not lack of pseudocholinesterase, electrolyte abnormalities, or antibiotics, but rather residual effects of inhalation anesthetics or narcotics, especially when combined with hyperventilation to the point where arterial carbon dioxide tensions have been reduced to below the apneic threshold.

Since the duration of action of muscle relaxants can and usually does exceed the duration of an operation, even in normal patients, the question is frequently raised whether the relaxants should be pharmacologically reversed at the conclusion of anesthesia. Only neuromuscular blocks of the nondepolarizing type seen after curare or pancuronium are susceptible to reversal. They can be safely and effectively reversed by the intravenous administration of an anticholinesterase such as neostigmine (Prostigmin). Neostigmine administration must always be accompanied by injection of atropine or a similar compound in amounts adequate to block the muscarinic stimulation and profound bradycardia otherwise produced by anticholinesterases. Atropine in doses of 1.5 to 2.0 mg intravenously is required for this purpose. Neostigmine should not, however, be routinely given to all patients at the conclusion of anesthesia during which nondepolarizing relaxants have been administered. The magnitude of neuromuscular blockade must first be measured to ascertain whether prolonged apnea or relaxation is due to residual effects of relaxants or to other factors. If the existence of significant impairment of neuromuscular transmission is established, the susceptibility of the blockade to anticholinesterases must then be established. Persisting depolarizing block from succinylcholine, for example, must be proved absent. This requires that tests be performed to obtain objective data on the function of the patient's muscle. One such test involves evaluation of the ability of the patient to lift the head and to maintain his head off the pillow for at least 30 seconds. This test requires a level of cooperation and motivation often lacking in a patient recovering from anesthesia while still on the operating table. The ability to lift the head may furthermore not always give an accurate indication of the status of the muscles of respiration. Different muscle groups not only have different sensitivities to muscle relaxants but also recover from their effects at different rates. The same limitations apply to hand grip as a measure of normal muscle function. More reliable are measurements of tidal volume and maximum inspiratory capacity, using a ventilation meter attached to an endotracheal tube. Equally useful is measurement of the patient's ability to generate at least 20 cm negative pressure during inhalation when ventilation is momentarily obstructed.

The most reliable means for determining the magnitude of neuromuscular blockade following muscle relaxants, as well as for defining the type of blockade, is electrical stimulation of a peripheral motor nerve (often the ulnar) while observing the response of peripheral muscle(s). This not only gives information of value in determining when muscle relaxants should be reversed at the conclusion of anesthesia but also provides an important means of monitoring the degree of paralysis during the course of anesthesia and operation and thus contributing to maintenance of constant intraoperative levels of surgical relaxation, while avoiding the dangers of relaxant overdosage. Three responses to electrical stimuli are evaluated: the magnitude of response to a single electrical stimulus; the ability to maintain contraction during tetanic stimulation; and the presence or absence of posttetanic facilitation. The resulting information defines whether a neuromuscular blockade is present and, if it is, whether it can be reversed by neostigmine. To be most accurate, these measurements should include recorded tracings of muscle responses. This technique of nerve stimulation cannot, however, quantitate percentage of recovery of normal neuromuscular transmission unless control data have been recorded prior to administration of relaxants. The problem of control observations can be solved by use of train-of-four stimuli, a technique also of value for monitoring intraoperative relaxant requirements. The ratio between the magnitude of response to the fourth of four stimuli and the magnitude of response to the first stimulus gives perhaps the most accurate appraisal of return to normal function of previously paralyzed muscles. The major disadvantages of the train-of-four technique are that it, too, gives information on function of hand muscles, not muscles of respiration; that it involves paper write-out of motor twitches to measure the ratios involved; and that it requires precise positioning of the wrist and hand.

REGIONAL ANESTHESIA

Regional anesthesia has the advantage of producing nonexplosive maximal sensory anesthesia and profound muscular relaxation without profound physiologic effects, *provided that the extent of anesthesia is limited.* The disadvantages of regional anesthesia include the fact that if it is extensive, the resultant physiologic trespass may be greater than during well-administered general anesthesia. For example, the regional anesthesia necessary for a gastrectomy is associated with physiologic changes more profound and potentially more dangerous than the changes accompanying a well-administered general anesthetic for the same operation. On the other hand, the physiologic disturbance associated with regional anesthesia for an operation such as hemorrhoidectomy is considerably less than that associated with general anesthesia for this procedure. The difference between the effects of extensive regional anesthesia and regional anesthesia limited in area is frequently unrecognized or forgotten but is one of the major considerations in evaluating the usefulness of this method. The inherent limitations of regional anesthesia relate both to the anesthetist and to the surgeon. For regional anesthesia to be smooth and successful, the anesthetist must have extensive experience and be highly skilled. Errors of omission or commission during regional anesthesia not only are dangerous but are immediately (and painfully) apparent to all. The surgeon operating with regional anesthesia must be gentle and silent to realize its full benefits.

Spinal Anesthesia

Spinal anesthesia consists of the injection of a local anesthetic into the subarachnoid space. The resulting anesthesia of somatic motor and sensory fibers is its raison d'être, but from a physiologic point of view the most important result of spinal anesthesia is the concurrent blocking of preganglionic sympathetic fibers. Almost all the profound physiologic changes which may be associated with spinal anesthesia are due to the effects of the sympathetic denervation. The sensory denervation produced by spinal anesthesia has little or no physiologic effect. The somatic motor denervation also has little physiologic effect, despite theories that somatic motor paralysis causes venous pooling, with a decrease in cardiac output. Succinylcholine is not associated with such changes, though the muscle relaxation is as profound as with spinal anesthesia. The physiologic effects of spinal anesthesia are also not due to any hypothetic ascent of the local anesthetic agent intracranially into the ventricular system to cause a direct depression of the vasomotor or respiratory centers.

Since the sympathetic nervous system block of spinal anesthesia is such an important determinant of the physiologic response to anesthesia, there are three aspects which deserve special emphasis. The first is that different types of nerve fibers are blocked by different concentrations of local anesthetic, smaller nerve fibers being blocked by lower concentrations of local anesthetic than larger fibers. The largest fibers in the human subarachnoid space being somatic motor fibers, these are the most resistant to local anesthetics. The next smaller fibers are somatic sensory fibers. The smallest fibers are the preganglionic fibers. These are blocked by concentrations of local anesthetic which have no effect on either sensory or motor nerve roots. Because the concentration of local anesthetic within the subarachnoid space decreases as the distance from the site of injection increases, a point is reached at which the concentration of local anesthetic in spinal fluid is no longer adequate to block somatic sensory fibers even though it is adequate to block sympathetic fibers. As a result, the sympathetic denervation of spinal anesthesia extends an average of two spinal segments beyond the level made anesthetic to pinprick. The physiologic response to spinal anesthesia may therefore be more profound than indicated by the extent of sensory denervation, especially if, as is sometimes the case, the zone of differential block extends beyond the usual two spinal segments to as much as six spinal segments. For the same reason, the level of somatic motor block during spinal anesthesia extends approximately two spinal segments below (i.e., caudal to) the level made anesthetic to pinprick. This is one reason why it is possible to have sensory anesthesia adequate for skin incision during appendectomy performed under spinal anesthesia without adequate muscular relaxation. The zone of differential anesthesia involving sympathetic, sensory, and

motor nerves also explains why phrenic paralysis rarely occurs even during high spinal anesthesias, including those with cervical sensory levels.

The second factor concerning the sympathetic denervation associated with spinal anesthesia is related to the fact that the highest (i.e., most cephalad) preganglionic sympathetic fiber arises at the T_1 level. Because sympathetic block extends approximately two spinal segments higher than sensory block, complete sympathetic denervation will be present in patients who have spinal anesthesia with a sensory level at approximately T_3. In other words, spinal anesthesia with high sensory levels is associated with the physiologic changes inherent in total sympathetic denervation. As a corollary, since the vast majority of the physiologic effects of spinal anesthesia are due to the concurrent sympathetic block and since the sympathetic block is complete with sensory levels to T_3, the physiologic response to cervical levels of anesthesia is no greater than to high thoracic levels. A patient with a sensory block to the T_3 level has essentially the same physiologic response as a patient with a sensory level at C_5 or C_6.

The third important aspect of sympathetic block produced by spinal anesthesia relates to the fact that each preganglionic sympathetic fiber, after penetrating the dura and entering the paravertebral sympathetic chain, ascends and descends in the chain, synapsing with a number of postganglionic fibers which are distributed to the periphery in a nonsegmental fashion. A single preganglionic fiber may synapse with as many as 18 postganglionic fibers. Stimulation (or block) of a single preganglionic fiber accordingly produces a diffuse peripheral response extending over a large number of peripheral segmental dermatomes, a response which is not limited to the peripheral segmental dermatome corresponding to the spinal segmental level at which the sympathetic fiber was stimulated (or blocked). Therefore, the sympathetic response to spinal anesthesia may be surprisingly extensive peripherally.

Just as the sympathetic blocking of spinal anesthesia is the most important determinant of the physiologic response, the cardiovascular changes resulting from the sympathetic blocking represent the most important physiologic alteration during this type of anesthesia.

The sympathetic denervation produces peripheral arterial and arteriolar vasodilatation. In the presence of a fixed cardiac output, the resulting decrease in peripheral vascular resistance produces a decrease in mean arterial pressure. The decrease in resistance is, however, relatively modest, amounting to 12 to 15 percent even in the presence of a total sympathetic denervation. It also is limited because peripheral vascular resistance is not eliminated by the denervation. The major site of resistance is merely shifted more peripherally, and there is still resistance to flow through the postarteriolar capillary circulation. In the normal individual, approximately 60 percent of the total peripheral vascular resistance arises at the arteriolar level, approximately 40 percent arising at the postarteriolar level. Following sympathetic denervation, approximately 40 percent of the resistance is at the arteriolar level, and 60 percent at the postarteriolar level. Even maximal vasodilatation on the arterial side of the circulation does not eliminate resistance to flow at the tissue level. Since total peripheral vascular resistance decreases so modestly during even high levels of spinal anesthesia, arterial and arteriolar vasodilatation cannot be accepted as the cause of severe arterial hypotension during spinal anesthesia. A 10 to 15 percent decrease in systolic pressure during spinal anesthesia can be ascribed to a decrease in peripheral resistance, but the severe degrees of hypotension must be ascribed to another cause, a decreased cardiac output.

From a cardiovascular point of view the most important result of the sympathetic denervation of spinal anesthesia is the effect on venous circulation. Because veins are innervated by the sympathetic nervous system, spinal anesthesia also results in venodilatation in the denervated areas. There is, however, a major difference between the sympathetic denervation produced on the venous side of the circulation and that produced on the arterial side. Although vasodilatation is not maximal following denervation on the arterial side of the circulation, it can be and often is maximal on the venous side. The smooth muscle in the arterial side of the circulation and in the postarteriolar bed maintains a considerable degree of autonomous tone after removal of its sympathetic nervous supply, with the result that sympathectomy is rarely associated with maximal vasodilatation. There is little or no autonomous tone in veins, however, after their sympathetic denervation. Whether or not a vein is dilated following sympathetic denervation depends primarily upon the effects of gravity. If the sympathectomized vein is below the level of the right atrium, gravity causes the blood to pool in the dependent vein and venodilatation becomes maximal. On the other hand, if the sympathectomized vein is above the level of the right atrium, gravity causes the blood to drain out, and essentially no venodilatation occurs.

If a significant degree of peripheral venodilatation occurs during spinal anesthesia because the patient is in a position in which the greater part of the denervated peripheral circulation is below the level of the right side of the heart (e.g., in the head-up position), there will be a pronounced decrease in venous return to the right side of the heart and resultant decrease in cardiac output. This in turn will cause a severe arterial hypotension. Decreases in cardiac output, including those great enough to lead to cardiac arrest, during spinal anesthesia are almost always consequent to significant decreases in venous return to the right side of the heart.

The most frequent cause of impaired venous return to the heart during spinal anesthesia is the head-up position. The second most frequent cause is administration of spinal anesthetic to a patient with decreased blood volume. Since the safety of spinal anesthesia is related to maintenance of an adequate arterial blood pressure and cardiac output and since these are related to maintenance of normal venous return to the right side of the heart, the head-up position should be employed only very cautiously during high levels of anesthesia. Of course, this position should be employed to regulate the level of anesthesia when hyperbaric spinal solutions are being used, but if severe hypotension ensues or if an inadvertently high level of anesthesia is obtained, there should be no hesitation about putting the patient in the head-down position in order to assure adequate venous return and cardiac output. The head-down position may result in a higher level of anesthesia, but it will not result in cardiac arrest. Injudicious use of the head-up position during spinal anesthesia, under the misapprehension that limiting the spread of the anesthetic is the primary consideration, constitutes the major cause of cardiac arrest during spinal anesthesia.

Respiratory function during spinal anesthesia remains normal even during high levels of sensory block. The intercostal paralysis accompanying a high spinal anesthetic is compensated for by the diaphragm, especially in the presence of a relaxed abdominal musculature so that arterial carbon dioxide and oxygen tensions remain within normal limits. This occurs even during cervical sensory levels of anesthesia, because the phrenic nerves are highly resistant to the effects of local anesthetics. Respiratory arrest can occur during spinal anesthesia, but the most frequent cause is not phrenic paralysis but a centrally induced apnea consequent to decreases in cardiac output great enough to result in ischemic medullary paralysis. The association between respiratory arrest and cardiac output is exemplified by the fact that the vast majority of respiratory arrests during spinal anesthesia immediately precede or follow cardiac arrest. Furthermore, once resuscitation has restored cardiac output, the patient usually exhibits spontaneous respiration. Respiratory arrest due to phrenic paralysis during spinal anesthesia undoubtedly can occur, but it is infrequent and only exceptionally the cause of apnea. Misguided attempts to avoid respiratory arrest by use of the head-up position lead to more cardiac and respiratory arrests than does judicious use of the head-down position. Even if apnea due to phrenic paralysis were to occur during spinal anesthesia, artificial means of ventilation are today such a standard part of every anesthetist's armamentarium that no harm will result. The same cannot be said for artificial means of maintaining cardiac output.

It is apparent from the above that the physiologic effects of high levels of spinal anesthesia are inevitably greater than with low levels of anesthesia. The difference in physiologic responses to high and low levels of spinal anesthesia is so great that from a practical and clinical point of view the two techniques should not be considered together. The advantage of low levels of spinal anesthesia is that profound sensory and muscular denervation can be achieved with relatively little other physiologic change. This is especially advantageous in patients with concurrent disease involving the cardiovascular or respiratory systems. The same cannot be said for high levels of anesthesia. The patient for whom a low spinal anesthesia is indicated during repair of an inguinal hernia because of concurrent disease, for example, is often the one for whom spinal anesthesia during cholecystectomy or gastrectomy is contraindicated because of concurrent disease. In modern practice there are few indications for the use of spinal anesthesia for surgical procedures above the level of the umbilicus, as the resulting total or near-total sympathetic denervation is too great a price to pay.

One potential drawback to spinal anesthesia is the association of the technique with postoperative headaches.

So-called "spinal headaches" are especially frequent in the younger age groups and in females, the highest incidence being in obstetric patients. Although all the etiologic factors producing headaches following spinal anesthesia have not yet been completely defined, it has been demonstrated that the incidence of headache is related to the size of the needle used to perform the lumbar puncture. The use of 18-gauge needles is associated with postspinal headaches in as many as 20 percent of patients. On the other hand, the routine use of 24- or 25-gauge spinal needles is associated with postspinal headaches in less than 2 percent of patients. If a spinal headache does occur, it should be treated conservatively with hydration (by intravenous routes if necessary) plus mild analgesics. If the headache is severe or if imminent discharge from the hospital indicates more radical therapy, injection of 8 to 10 ml of the patient's own blood (freshly and aseptically obtained) into the lumbar epidural space will usually produce prompt and permanent relief of the headache.

In modern practice the risk of possible neurologic complications from spinal anesthesia is more potential than actual. It is now apparent that the vast majority of neurologic complications associated with spinal anesthesia are the result of chemical contamination of the material being injected into the subarachnoid space. If the contaminating material is injected in a high concentration or if it is a strongly neurolytic substance such as alcohol or phenol, the resulting neurologic damage may be a chemical transverse myelitis which appears immediately and is irreversible. This is most frequently due to mistaken identification of ampules used to produce spinal anesthesia. On the other hand, if the contaminating material is injected in low concentrations or is only weakly neurolytic, the resultant neurologic deficit is more often a chronic adhesive arachnoiditis which may not become apparent for days or even weeks after the anesthesia but which, once it appears, progresses inexorably as the arachnoiditis spreads cephalad from the site of the injection. Since chemical contamination constitutes the most frequent single cause of neurologic complications associated with spinal anesthesia, the spinal set and drugs used should be not only bacteriologically sterile—a condition readily achieved by autoclaving—but also chemically sterile and free of all pyrogens and other contaminating substances, a condition achieved only by meticulously detailed preparation techniques. Not all neurologic deficits following spinal anesthesia are due to the anesthetic techniques. While the risk of neurologic or other complications with spinal anesthetics is negligible, it does exist. However, the risk of neurologic deficits following spinal anesthesia for operations on the lower extremities and perineum may well be less in the long run than that involved in the use of general anesthesia for such procedures.

Efficiency and safety in spinal anesthesia are best achieved by relying upon one or two local anesthetics (one of long, one of short duration) and regulating their spread in the subarachnoid space solely by changing the position of the patient, keeping constant the specific gravity of the solution injected. A satisfactory local anesthetic of proved safety for spinal anesthesia is 1% tetracaine (Pontocaine).

When mixed with equal volumes of 10% dextrose, a hyperbaric solution is achieved. The dosage of tetracaine will vary with the size of the patient and the extent and duration of anesthesia required but should not exceed 18 mg. The duration of tetracaine spinal anesthesia may safely be approximately doubled by the addition of 0.3 to 0.5 mg epinephrine.

Epidural Anesthesia

The physiologic response produced by the injection of local anesthetic agent into the epidural space is similar to that associated with spinal anesthesia in that sympathetic denervation is produced. But differences exist in the responses to the two techniques: First, the large amounts of local anesthetic agent used to produce epidural anesthesia may be absorbed and produce systemic effects on the cardiovascular system which add to the effects of the sympathetic block. The small amounts of local anesthetic employed in spinal anesthesia, on the other hand, produce no systemic effects. The physiologic response to epidural anesthesia also may be altered if epinephrine is injected with the anesthetic into the epidural space to prolong the duration of anesthesia. Epinephrine, even when administered in the pharmacologically ideal concentration of 1:200,000, can have peripheral systemic effects, whereas vasoconstrictors used intrathecally during spinal anesthesia are unassociated with such systemic responses.

The clinical advantage of epidural (i.e., peridural) as opposed to spinal anesthesia is to a large extent a function of the degree of apprehension on the part of the patient, anesthetist, or surgeon regarding spinal anesthesia. The pharmacologic and actuarial basis of a psychologic advantage is dubious, and epidural anesthesia, like spinal anesthesia, can on rare occasions also be associated with neurologic complications. Moreover, epidural injection of local anesthetic involves transfer of the local anesthetic across the dura into the subarachnoid space. Therefore, since epidural anesthesia is essentially spinal anesthesia, it is not clear why one is pharmacologically superior to the other with regard to the dangers of neurotoxic reactions. Properly performed epidural anesthesia does have the advantage of being associated with a lower incidence of spinal headache. But epidural anesthesia in clinical practice does not eliminate the danger of spinal headache, since the needle sometimes inadvertently may penetrate the dura instead of stopping in the epidural space during induction of this anesthesia. In large series of unselected cases, the incidence of spinal headache following routine use of 24-gauge needles for spinal anesthesia has been essentially the same as the incidence following epidural anesthesia complicated by occasional inadvertent perforation of the dura by the larger needles employed in epidural anesthesia.

There are two situations in which epidural anesthesia appears to have significant advantages over spinal anesthesia, the first being when rectal surgery is to be performed in the prone, jackknife position. In such a position it is clinically more convenient to produce caudal anesthesia with minimal patient manipulation and minimal physiologic effects from the anesthesia than to rely on spinal anesthesia, hypobaric or hyperbaric. Second, continuous epidural anesthesia with use of catheters has more to recommend it than does continuous spinal anesthesia when regional anesthesia is to be continued for long periods of time.

Nerve Block

Nerve block, infiltration, and topical anesthesia are advantageous techniques but present technical complexities beyond the scope of the present chapter. The disadvantages of infiltration anesthesia arise from two sources: First, too much is expected of the anesthesia. A laparotomy cannot be performed under infiltration anesthesia alone. Second, the systemic toxicity of local anesthetics is often ignored when infiltration anesthesia is used. Toxic reactions to local anesthetics are the result of inadvertently high blood levels of local anesthetics. They are not the result of allergic reactions or hypersensitivity. The high blood levels may be the result of using total dosages exceeding the recognized safe limits, injection of the local anesthetic into highly vascular areas, or accidental intravenous injection.

Toxic reactions to local anesthetics may involve either the central nervous system, in which case they are characterized by twitching progressing to convulsions, or the cardiovascular system, in which case they are characterized by sudden hypotension. Treatment and prevention of the former consists in the intravenous injection of small amounts of diazepam (Valium). Treatment of cardiovascular depression due to absorption of local anesthetics consists of placing the patient in the head-down position, followed by use of intravenous vasopressors. Oxygen should be administered in both cases. Safe dosage levels of local anesthetics depend upon the age, weight, and physical status of the patient and the speed and site of injection. A healthy 70-kg adult should not receive over 1.0 Gm of procaine or over 500 mg of lidocaine (Xylocaine) within 20 minutes. Tetracaime as a topical anesthetic for mucous membranes should not be administered in doses exceeding 40 mg.

Although nerve blocks and infiltration anesthesia have a definite role in surgery, the physiologic and pharmacologic effects of large amounts of local anesthetic injected into the operative area are often more adverse than the physiologic and pharmacologic effects of a well-administered general anesthetic. Present anesthesia techniques are such that *major* surgery is generally more safely and efficiently performed with techniques other than infiltration anesthesia. This is especially true in the poor-risk patient, in whom the systemic toxicity of a local anesthetic may be unusually difficult to handle. Major intra-abdominal surgery under infiltration anesthesia is especially contraindicated if the surgical diagnosis is not definite. The initiation of an exploratory laparotomy in a poor-risk patient under infiltration anesthesia all too frequently results in the necessity of inducing general anesthesia under the most adverse circumstances possible: a poor-risk patient in pain, often with a full stomach, with the abdomen open, and suffering from the adverse systemic effects of local anesthetics.

PREMEDICATION

The objectives of preanesthetic medication are, in order of decreasing importance, alleviation of anxiety, decreased reflex irritability, and decreased requirement for general anesthetic agents. Mental relaxation and detachment, not coma or unconsciousness, are the goals. The establishment of rapport between the anesthetist and the patient is more predictably able to produce the desired state of tranquility than is the use of drugs affecting the central nervous system. Nevertheless, drugs will continue to be used for psychic premedication. When pharmacologic agents are to be relied upon, those agents should be employed which produce the maximal desired effect with the greatest predictability and the fewest side effects. Evidence indicates that in the absence of pain, therapeutic amounts of barbiturates most frequently achieve the desired state of mental relaxation. Barbiturates, when employed for such purposes, also have the advantage of producing no respiratory depression. This is in contrast with the respiratory depression produced by narcotics in the absence of pain. Since maintenance of adequate ventilation during and after anesthesia is a frequent concern, it is often inadvisable to administer drugs preanesthetically which will further depress respiration. Barbiturates used in therapeutic amounts as premedicants also do not undermine the stability of the cardiovascular system to the same extent that narcotics do. Finally, normal persons without pain do not find the administration of a narcotic a pleasant experience; in fact, they show a high incidence of dysphoria rather than euphoria following narcotic administration. Barbiturates, on the other hand, do not have this effect.

The role of narcotics as premedicants is best limited to two major areas: First, narcotics should be administered preanesthetically to those patients who are in pain or who will experience pain prior to the induction of anesthesia. Second, narcotics are useful premedication for patients without pain but whose anesthetic management is to include balanced anesthesia. In such cases, the preoperative narcotic is essentially part of the anesthetic.

Tranquilizers have been used as premedicants with varying degrees of success. The disadvantage of routine preoperative tranquilizers is that many have diverse and frequent side effects in addition to their tranquilizing effects. This is particularly true of phenothiazine tranquilizers, which have adrenolytic, antihistaminic, parasympatholytic, and other actions. While nonphenothiazine tranquilizers such as diazepam (Valium) and hydroxyzine (Vistaril, Atarax) may not have such high incidences of undesirable side effects, their effectiveness in producing tranquility without physiologic trespass has not been demonstrated to be superior to barbiturates. The pharmacologic shotgun effect characteristic of many tranquilizers often represents a major disadvantage during subsequent general anesthesia. Tranquilizers have also been employed preoperatively to decrease the incidence of postoperative nausea and vomiting. The antiemetic effect of tranquilizers in such cases is unquestioned, but the incidence and severity of side actions such as arterial hypotension and prolongation of unconsciousness postoperatively detracts considerably from their usefulness. Since it has been demonstrated that any agent, including pentobarbital, which prolongs "sleep time" following general anesthesia will decrease the incidence of nausea and vomiting, the use of barbiturates as antiemetics is often more effective because of their lower incidence of side effects.

Finally, drugs may be administered preoperatively to decrease adverse reflex activity. Since the reflexes causing most concern are parasympathetic reflexes, in particular vagal cardiac and laryngeal reflexes, parasympatholytic agents are the most widely used. When they are employed in proper dosage, the incidence of bradycardia during anesthesia is lessened by the use of parasympatholytic agents. Whether the incidence of laryngospasm is significantly decreased by these agents is difficult to determine, since it is affected by so many factors, including the skill and training of the person administering the anesthetic.

Whether atropine, glycopyrrolate, or scopolamine is employed as the parasympatholytic agent is a matter of personal preference. The theoretic advantage of scopolamine in producing amnesia is offset in practice by the increased incidence of postoperative delirium in patients who have received the drug. When scopolamine is employed it should be administered in doses equal to two-thirds the atropine dose. Glycopyrrolate has the advantage of being unable to cross the blood-brain barrier and so is devoid of central nervous system actions. Of all the drugs used for premedication, parasympatholytic drugs are perhaps the most misused, in that they are either administered in doses incapable of producing the degree of parasympathetic block which is intended or they are administered when parasympathetic denervation is not required.

References

General

Beecher, H. K., and Todd, D. P.: A Study of Deaths Associated with Anesthesia, *Ann Surg,* **140:**2, 1954.

Bodlander, F. M. S.: Deaths Associated with Anaesthesia, *Br J Anaesthiol,* **47:**36, 1975.

Cullen, S. C., and Larson, C. P., Jr.: "Essentials of Anesthetic Practice," Year Book Medical Publishers, Chicago, 1974.

Eger, E. I.: "Anesthetic Uptake and Action," The Williams & Wilkins Company, Baltimore, 1974.

Kaufman, R. D.: Biophysical Mechanisms of Anesthetic Action, *Anesthesiology,* **46:**49, 1977.

Taylor, G., Larson, C. P., Jr., and Prestwich, R.: Unexpected Cardiac Arrest during Anesthesia and Surgery, *JAMA,* **236:**2758, 1976.

Inhalation Anesthetics

Bruce, D. L., Bach, M. J., and Arbit, J.: Trace Anesthetic Effects on Perceptual, Cognitive, and Motor Skills, *Anesthesiology,* **40:**453, 1974.

Cohen, E. N., Brown, B. W., Bruce, D. L., et al.: Occupational Disease among Operating Room Personnel: A National Study: Report of an Ad Hoc Committee on the Effects of Trace Concentrations on the Health of Operating Room Personnel, *Anesthesiology,* **41:**321, 1974.

————, and Van Dyke, R. A.: "Metabolism of Volatile Anesthetics: Implications for Toxicity," Addison-Wesley Publishing Company, Inc., Menlo Park, Calif., 1977.

Cousins, M. J., and Mazze, R. I.: Methoxyflurane Nephrotoxicity: A Study of Dose-Response in Man, *JAMA,* **225:**1611, 1973.

Dykes, M. H. M.: Is Halothane Hepatitis Chronic Active Hepatitis? *Anesthesiology,* **46:**233, 1977.

Eger, E. I., and Saidman, L. J.: Hazards of Nitrous Oxide Anesthesia in Bowel Obstruction and Pneumothorax, *Anesthesiology,* **26:**61, 1965.

————, ————, and Brandstater, B.: Minimum Alveolar Anesthetic Concentration: A Standard of Anesthetic Potency, *Anesthesiology,* **26:**756, 1965.

Fukunaga, A. F., and Epstein, R. M.: Sympathetic Excitation during Nitrous Oxide–Halothane Anesthesia in the Cat, *Anesthesiology,* **39:**23, 1973.

Hornbein, T. F., Martin, W. E., Bonica, J. J., et al.: Nitrous Oxide Effects on the Circulatory and Ventilatory Responses to Halothane, *Anesthesiology,* **31:**250, 1969.

Klatskin, G., and Kimberg, D. V.: Recurrent Hepatitis Attributable to Halothane Sensitization in an Anesthetist, *N Engl J Med,* **280:**515, 1969.

Merin, R. G.: Inhalation Anesthetics and Myocardial Metabolism: Possible Mechanisms of Functional Effects, *Anesthesiology,* **39:**216, 1973.

Saidman, L. J., and Eger, E. I.: Effects of Nitrous Oxide and of Narcotic Premedication on the Alveolar Concentration of Halothane Required for Anesthesia, *Anesthesiology,* **25:**302, 1964.

Tinker, J. H., Gandolfi, A. J., and Van Dyke, R. A.: Elevation of Plasma Bromide Levels in Patient following Halothane Anesthesia: Time Correlation with Total Halothane Dosage, *Anesthesiology,* **44:**194, 1976.

Intravenous Anesthesia

Ali, H. H., and Savarese, J. J.: Monitoring of Neuromuscular Function, *Anesthesiology,* **45:**216, 1976.

Bendixen, H. H., Hedley-Whyte, J., and Laver, M. B.: Impaired Oxygenation in Surgical Patients during General Anesthesia with Controlled Ventilation: A Concept of Atelectasis, *N Engl J Med,* **269:**991, 1963.

Britt, B. A., and Kalow, W.: Malignant Hyperthermia: A Statistical Review, *Can Anaesth Soc J,* **17:**293, 1970.

Graves, C. L., Downs, N. H., and Browne, A. B.: Cardiovascular Effects of Minimal Analgesic of Innovar, Fentanyl, and Droperidol, *Anesth Analg (Paris),* **54:**15, 1975.

Gronert, G. A., and Theye, R. A.: Pathophysiology of Hyperkalemia Induced by Succinylcholine, *Anesthesiology,* **43:**89, 1975.

Katz, R. L. (ed.), "Muscle Relaxants," Excerpta Medica, Amsterdam, 1975.

Lee, C., Barnes, A., and Katz, R. L.: Neuromuscular Sensitivity to Tubocurarine: A Comparison of 10 Paramaters, *Br J Anaesthiol,* **48:**1045, 1976.

Lowenstein, E.: Morphine "Anesthesia": A Perspective, *Anesthesiology,* **35:**563, 1971.

Pender, J. W.: Dissociative Anesthesia, *JAMA,* **215:**1126, 1971.

Rehder, K., Marsh, M., et al.: Airway Closure, *Anesthesiology,* **47:**40, 1977.

Traber, D. L., and Wilson, R. D.: Involvement of the Sympathetic Nervous System in the Pressor Response to Ketamine, *Anesth Analg (Paris)*, **48:**248, 1969.

Regional Anesthesia

Bonica, J. J., Akamatsu, T. J., Berges, P. U., et al.: Circulatory Effect of Peridural Block: Effects of Epinephrine, *Anesthesiology,* **34:**514, 1971.

Bromage, P. R.: Physiology and Pharmacology of Epidural Anesthesia, *Anesthesiology,* **28:**592, 1967.

Covino, B. G., and Fassallo, H. G.: "Local Anesthetics: Mechanisms of Action and Clinical Use," Grune & Stratton, Inc., New York, 1975.

Dripps, R. D., and Vandam, L. D.: Long-Term Follow-up of Patients Who Received 10,098 Spinal Anesthetics, *JAMA,* **156:**1486, 1954.

Greene, N. M.: "Physiology of Spinal Anesthesia," 2d ed., The Williams & Wilkins Company, Baltimore, 1969. (Reprinted by R. E. Knieger Co., Huntington, N.Y., 1976.)

Sivarajan, M., Armory, D. W., and Lindbloom, L. E.: Systemic and Regional Blood Flow during Epidural Anesthesia without Epinephrine in the Rhesus Monkey, *Anesthesiology,* **45:**300, 1976.

Strichartz, G.: Molecular Mechanisms of Nerve Block by Local Anesthetics, *Anesthesiology,* **45:**421, 1976.

Premedication

Beecher, H. K.: "Measurement of Subjective Responses," Oxford University Press, New York, 1959.

Frumin, M. J., Herekar, V. R., and Jarvik, M. E.: Amnesic Actions of Diazepam and Scopolamine in Man, *Anesthesiology,* **45:**406, 1975.

Leighton, K. M., and Sanders, H. D.: Anticholinergic Premedication, *Can Anaesth Soc J,* **23:**563, 1976.

Lo, J. N., and Cumming, J. F.: Interaction between Sedative Premedicants and Ketamine in Man and in Isolated Perfused Rat Livers, *Anesthesiology,* **43:**307, 1975.

Ramamurthy, S., Ylagan, L. B., and Winnie, A. P.: Glycopyrrolate as a Substitute for Atropine, *Anesth Analg (Paris)*, **50:**732, 1971.

Chapter 12

Complications

by **Seymour I. Schwartz**

GENERAL CONSIDERATIONS

Surgical care must encompass an appreciation and anticipation of postoperative complications which may result from the disease process per se, errors of omission, or errors of commission in technique. In regarding the patient postoperatively, any deviation from the anticipated norm for clinical evaluation and/or diagnostic findings should alert one to focus on complications of the disease and also to retrace the operative procedure. It is unusual, although certainly possible, that clinical and laboratory abnormalities may be caused by the chance occurrence of an unrelated disease during the postoperative period. Acute cholecystitis and appendicitis are two examples of diseases which may become manifest during the postoperative course of the patient. Routine care of a patient following surgical treatment includes repeated evaluation of the vital signs, i.e., temperature, pulse, blood pressure, and respiration. The extent of pain in the region of the incision and generalized discomfort are assessed, anticipating progressive improvement. The chest is auscultated for pleural rubs, bronchial breathing, and rales, while the abdomen is auscultated to determine the return of intestinal activity. The lower extremities are palpated in order to detect physical signs of deep venous thrombosis. The hematocrit and white blood cell count are measured at appropriate intervals to assess blood loss and continued infection, respectively. These determinations plus appropriate clinical chemistry determinations should be carried out when they are pertinent, not routinely.

TEMPORAL CONSIDERATIONS. Fever which presents shortly after surgical treatment in a patient who was previously afebrile is generally related to atelectasis or aspiration. Fever may also appear early in the postoperative course secondary to urinary tract infection, particularly if the patient has been catheterized. Fever of wound infection and leakage of an intestinal anastomosis or closure more frequently become evident on the fourth to seventh postoperative day. Hypotension in the early postoperative phase may be due to continued hemorrhage or the effects of depressive drugs which have been administered during the recovery period. Hypotension later in the postoperative course in a patient with sepsis should alert one to the possibility of endotoxin shock. The incidence of deep venous thrombosis and pulmonary embolism increases with duration of bed rest. Wound dehiscence usually does not become manifest until the fifth postoperative day.

WOUND COMPLICATIONS

Wound Dehiscence

Wound disruption, or dehiscence, generally refers to a separation of an abdominal wound, involving the anterior fascial sheath and deeper layers. The inaccuracy of computing the frequency of wound disruption is notorious; the incidence in the literature ranges from 0.5 to 3 percent, averaging 2.6 percent when all abdominal operations are considered collectively. The incidence is definitely related to age and is reported to be 1.3 percent for patients under forty-five years in contrast to 5.4 percent for those over forty-five years. There is a higher incidence in elderly, debilitated patients with poor nutrition and in the presence of significant ascites. Carcinoma is also associated with an increased incidence. In a collective review by Hartzell and Winfield, 22 percent of disruptions occurred when cancer was present, and 38 percent of dehiscences in Wolff's series were in cancer patients. Over 5 percent of laparotomies in patients in whom cancer was found are reported to have wound disruption in contrast to a 2 percent incidence when laparotomy demonstrates a benign condition. Other general factors which have been implicated include hypoproteinemia and atelectasis with its associated coughing, which, along with retching and hiccuping, increases the intraabdominal pressure and puts a strain on the incision. A lack of correlation between anemia and wound disruption has been reported. Obesity is definitely associated with an increased incidence.

Local factors involved in wound disruption include hemorrhage, infection, excessive suture material, and poor technique. Prompt wound healing is facilitated by a minimum of necrotic residue, bacterial contamination, and foreign material. Sutures should not be tied too tightly but should be positioned so that there is minimal peritoneal defect, since several theories suggest that wound disruptions start with a tiny wedge of omentum or bowel finding its way through such a defect, which is then enlarged.

Several series have suggested that the incidence of wound dehiscence is increased with vertical incisions. This has been related to the relative holding power of the fascia. The rectus abdominis sheath fascia runs horizontally, and therefore a transverse incision is in line with the fascial fibers, while a vertical paramedian incision transects the fascial fibers which act as a distracting force on the incision. It has been demonstrated that the pull on the fascial edges of a vertical incision is thirty times greater than that exerted on a transverse incision. A midline incision represents an exception, since there is marked decussation of the fibers with varying lines of forces. In reference to incisions for cholecystectomy, Pemberton and Manax noted no difference in incidences of dehiscence when vertical and transverse incisions were compared in a thoroughly randomized series. When an intestinal stoma or a drain is brought out through any incision, the incidence of wound dehiscence increases.

CLINICAL MANIFESTATIONS. Most disruptions are concealed in the deeper layers of the wound and do not manifest themselves until the fifth postoperative day, although the separation may, in fact, occur in the operating room or recovery room. The presenting sign is serosanguineous drainage from the wound, and if this occurs subsequent to the first 24 postoperative hours, it is virtually pathognomonic. Frequently, wound dehiscence becomes manifest when the skin sutures are removed and evisceration of intraperitoneal contents, either intestine or omentum, occurs. In some instances, wound disruptions remain concealed beneath an intact cutaneous closure and go unrecognized initially, only to become manifest later in the form of a postoperative ventral hernia.

TREATMENT. The management depends on the patient's condition. If the patient can tolerate the procedure, a secondary operative closure is indicated. The author prefers through-and-through horizontal mattress sutures placed superficial to the peritoneum or buried figure-of-eight monofilament stainless steel sutures to approximate the muscle and fascial layers. In some instances, it is preferable to treat the patient conservatively with an occlusive wound dressing and binder and to accept the complication of a postoperative hernia. If evisceration occurs, sterile moist towels should be applied to cover the extruded intestine or omentum, and the patient should be taken directly to the operating room. After general irrigation, the abdomen is closed with one of the two previously mentioned techniques.

The mortality associated with wound disruption depends on the patient's age and original pathologic condition; reported incidences range from 11 to 85 percent. The incidence of postoperative hernia in one large series was 31 percent.

Wound Infection

Postoperative wound infection results when bacteria within the wound multiply, exciting a local reaction and, frequently, a systemic response. Most wounds become infected in the operating room while they are open, but the presence of bacteria in the wound at the end of the surgical procedure does not usually result in a wound infection. The bacterium most frequently implicated is *Staphylococcus aureus.* Enteric organisms are the causative agents when bowel operation has been performed, and hemolytic streptococci account for about 3 percent of infections. Other common pathogens include enterococci, *Pseudomonas, Proteus,* and *Klebsiella.*

The reported incidence of wound infection has a wide range. In 1963, Howe and Mozden reported 350 major and 117 minor wound infections following 15,658 major operations. Barnes et al., in reporting "standardized operations," noted rates ranging from 1.7 to 9.4 percent for various procedures. The Public Health Laboratory Service of England and Wales reported an overall wound infection rate of 9.7 percent. In a combined study conducted by the Division of Medical Sciences, National Academy of Science-National Research Council, and reported in 1964, the overall incidence of infection in five participating hospitals varied from 3 to 11.1 percent. Clean atraumatic and uninfected operative wounds in which neither the bronchi, nor the gastrointestinal tract, nor the genitourinary tract was entered and which were elective, primarily closed, and undrained had an overall incidence of definite infection of 3.3 percent, while similar wounds which were either not elective, or not primarily closed, or drained mechanically through the incision or via a stab wound had a 7.4 percent incidence of wound infection. Operative wounds in which the bronchus, gastrointestinal tract, or oropharyngeal cavity were entered but without unusual contamination had an overall incidence of infection of 10.8 percent. Open, fresh traumatic wounds, operations with a major break in sterile technique, and incisions encountering acute non-purulent inflammation were associated with an incidence of wound infections of 16.3 percent. Old traumatic wounds and those involving abscesses of perforated viscera had the highest rate of infection (28.6 percent).

A variety of factors other than the nature of the wound also influences the incidence of infection. Age is a definite factor; the rate of wound infection rises steadily from 4.7 percent in the fifteen- to twenty-four-year-old group to 10.7 percent in the sixty-five to seventy-four-year-old group. There is virtually no difference in sex and race. The presence of diabetes is associated with an increase in infection rate, but when this is adjusted for age, there is no statistical significance to this figure. Steroid therapy affects the wound infection rate adversely. An incidence of 16 percent for patients receiving steroids has been contrasted with 7 percent for those not on such drugs. Patients who are extremely obese also have a more than doubled rate of wound infection when compared with control groups. In the combined study, patients with severe malnutrition also displayed a markedly increased rate of wound infection, but this was distorted by other factors, which, if corrected, cast doubt on the widely held belief that malnourished patients are intrinsically more susceptible. Patients who harbor infections remote from the operative incision have an increased infection rate. The duration of operation exerts a profound influence on wound infection, the incidence rising steadily from 3.6 percent for procedures lasting less than 30 minutes to 18 percent for those lasting over 6 hours.

The urgency of operation only indirectly influences the wound infection rate. The type of closure also influences the rate indirectly. Although 7 percent of wounds primarily closed became infected, 15 percent of those not closed or incompletely closed became infected. The difference appears to result from the greater proportion of nonclean operations in the group without primary closure. When adjusted for wound classification, the infection rate of the two groups was essentially the same. Secondary wound closure, however, was associated with a 28 percent infection rate and skin graft closure with a 17 percent rate. The use of a drain was associated with an 11 percent infection rate, whereas undrained wounds had a rate of 5 percent, but it could not be concluded that the drains themselves were responsible for the infection. Patients hospitalized for fewer than 2 days preoperatively had an infection rate of 6 percent, whereas those hospitalized for periods greater than 3 weeks preoperatively had a rate of 14 percent, and this relationship could not be explained on the basis of other associated factors. The prophylactic use of antibiotics was paradoxically associated with a much higher wound infection rate in the combined series, and similar findings were reported by Schonholtz et al. for orthopedic cases. In contrast, Ketcham et al., in a double-blind study, reported a reduction of wound infection in patients with extensive cancer who were placed on prophylactic antibiotics. In addition, Polk and Lopez-Mayor noted that preoperative and early postoperative cephaloridine reduced the incidence of wound infection in patients in whom segments of stomach or intestine were opened.

The two factors of importance in the genesis of infection are breaks in surgical technique and the host parasite relationship. Two potential sources of contamination are the patient himself, particularly the gastrointestinal tract, and the environment of the operating room including the operating team. Carriers of *S. aureus* in the hospital population have become an increasing source. It has been demonstrated that patients who are nasal carriers of *S. aureus* have a higher incidence of wound infection than noncarriers.

CLINICAL MANIFESTATIONS. In a typical situation about 3 to 4 days following operation, there is some increase in pulse rate, and about the fourth postoperative day, a low-grade, intermittent fever is noted. Usually there is edema and redness of the wound, but the most important early sign is undue pain. In some types, marked thrombosis of surrounding blood vessels is an important feature. Wound dehiscence is usually not caused by infection per se unless the infection is neglected. The diagnosis is usually made on the fifth to seventh day, but this interval may be extended if the patient has been on antibiotics. At that time, the wound is commonly seen as a suppurative process, essentially an abscess. Systemic features of septicemia may be present.

TREATMENT. The most important prophylactic measure is excellent technique. In human volunteers, Elek and Conen have shown that the presence of suture material enhances the infective power of *S. aureus* 1,000 to 10,000 times. Therefore, fine sutures and accurate hemostasis should reduce the incidence. It is generally felt that prophylactic antibiotics do not contribute to a reduction in the incidence of wound infection.

Once diagnosed, the treatment consists of surgical drainage. The skin sutures should be removed and the wound irrigated with saline solution and lightly packed. As a general principle, antimicrobial drugs are not required unless the offending organism is *S. pyogenes* or hemolytic streptococci, which should be treated with penicillin for a period of at least 1 week. Also, patients with wound infections around the central area of the face should receive antimicrobial therapy to prevent intracranial extension. Finally, if the wound sepsis is associated with bacteremia or spreading cellulitis, antimicrobial therapy is also indicated.

See Chap. 5 for a discussion of specific infections, i.e., staphylococcal infections, streptococcal infections, anaero-

bic clostridial cellulitis, clostridial myonecrosis, streptococcal myositis, and tetanus.

Wound Hemorrhage, Hematoma, and Seroma (Accumulation of Serum)

Wound hemorrhage is generally related to an error in technique in which hemostasis is not accomplished. There is a higher incidence in patients with polycythemia vera, myeloproliferative disorders, or coagulation defects and in patients receiving anticoagulant therapy (see Chap. 3). Postoperative hemorrhage usually becomes manifest with a sensation of pressure or pain within the wound shortly after the patient awakes from anesthesia. There may be leakage of sanguineous or serosanguineous material at that time. To control bleeding from the wound edges, pressure may be applied initially, but if the bleeding continues, additional sutures or reexploration of the wound may be required.

The placement of drains in areas of anticipated wound bleeding is usually not indicated. If the bleeding is trivial, the drain is unnecessary, while if the bleeding is severe, it will not evacuate the material. Drains or catheters connected to closed suction are appropriately used to evacuate serous fluid from underneath skin flaps, such as that associated with radical mastectomy, in order to prevent the vicious cycle in which an expanding serous collection produces significant bleeding as it separates the wound. If a large skin flap has been raised, it should be anticipated that fluid will develop, and in order to facilitate apposition between the subcutaneous tissue and deep fascia, the drainage should be effected. This obviates formation of a serous accumulation, a seroma.

Once a seroma develops, it should be aspirated initially; if multiple aspirations are required, a polyethylene catheter may be inserted and attached to negative suction. Prompt treatment is indicated, since the presence of contained serous fluid increases the incidence of subcutaneous infection. The same situation pertains to a subcutaneous hematoma, and drainage is required, since the blood affords an excellent culture medium and also prevents apposition between the two surfaces.

POSTOPERATIVE PAROTITIS

Postoperative parotitis is a serious complication and is associated with a high mortality that is related to it and to the primary disease with which it is associated. Recent reviews indicate an incidence of 1:1,000 postoperative cases, and there is a real recrudescence which is related to the increasing age of the surgical population. The right and left glands are involved equally, and in 10 to 15 percent of cases, the disease presents bilaterally. Seventy-five percent of patients are seventy years or older, and the overwhelming majority have associated diseases. Patients having major abdominal surgical treatment, fractured hip, debilitating diseases, and severe injury are among the most commonly afflicted.

The factors which have been implicated in the etiology include poor oral hygiene, dehydration, and the use of anticholinergic drugs. In one large series, one-third of the patients with acute suppurative parotitis had carcinoma, and one-half had preexisting major infection elsewhere in the body. In only one-third of the cases in this series the acute suppurative process developed in the postoperative period.

The pathogenesis is thought to be a transductal inoculation of the parotid, and the majority of infections are due to staphylococci. The combination of poor oral hygiene and lack of oral intake predisposes to bacterial invasion of Stensen's duct. The inflammatory lesions of early parotitis are confined to an accumulation of cells within the larger ducts. The parenchyma of the smaller ducts are initially spared, but once penetration of the parenchyma occurs, multiple abscesses form and later coalesce. If the process continues, the purulent material penetrates the capsule and invades the surrounding tissue along one of three routes: downward into the deep fascial planes of the neck, backward into the external auditory canal, or outward into the skin of the face.

CLINICAL MANIFESTATIONS. The interval between operation and the onset of parotitis varies from a few hours to many weeks. The patient initially presents with pain in the parotid region. The pain is usually unilateral but may become bilateral in a short period of time. Initially, inspection shows the gland to be slightly swollen, and palpation demonstrates exquisite tenderness. The course of postoperative parotitis is rapid and fulminating with severe cellulitis developing on the affected side of the face and neck. The temperature and leukocyte count may be extremely high. Obstruction of the airway may necessitate tracheostomy, and the abscess may rupture into adjacent structures of the ear, mastoid, pharynx, or anterior and posterior triangles of the neck. Parotitis is to be differentiated from benign postoperative swelling of the parotids, which occurs more frequently in Negroes and may be related to straining, belladonna, and neuromuscular depolarizing drugs.

TREATMENT. Prophylactic therapy consists of adequate hydration and good oral hygiene which can be aided by allowing the patient to take ice chips and stimulating salivary flow. Prophylactic antibiotics are apparently of no value.

Once the diagnosis is entertained, pus should be expressed from Stensen's duct and culture and sensitivity tests performed. A broad-spectrum antibiotic which acts against the staphylococci should be started while awaiting results. In one series of 66 glands cultured, 64 contained staphylococci. In some cases, these were combined with streptococci, gram-negative bacilli, and pneumococci. If there is considerable pain and the disease is less than 24 hours old, irradiation of the gland in small doses is indicated. Irradiation may provide symptomatic relief by reducing the secretions of the obstructed gland, but this type of therapy does not affect the course of the disease as much as antibiotics or surgical drainage.

Frequent observation of the patient is essential. If the

disease persists or progresses, drainage should be considered as early as the third day. If there is moderate improvement, drainage may be delayed for a day or two, but in no circumstance should it be delayed beyond the fifth day. An incision is made anterior to the ear, extending down to the angle of the mandible, and flaps are reflected, exposing the gland. A hemostat is inserted through the capsule and opened in the direction of the course of the branches of the facial nerve. Multiple drainage sites are thus established, and the wound is packed lightly open. Deferring drainage until fluctuation is apparent is unwise. Stimulation of the salivary flow by massage of the gland or other means is contraindicated, once the inflammatory process is established.

PROGNOSIS. In a recent series, the mortality rate approximated 20 percent, but this was frequently related to the patient's basic disease. However, 36 percent of the patients who died demonstrated active parotitis. In 80 percent of patients treated with incision and drainage the parotitis was palliated or cured.

POSTOPERATIVE RESPIRATORY COMPLICATIONS

Respiratory Failure

The availability of techniques to measure the arterial P_{O_2} (Pa_{O_2}) has focused attention on respiratory failure in the postoperative period. Neely and associates, Moore et al., and Pontoppidan et al. have indicated that respiratory failure is a major cause in 25 percent of postoperative deaths and a major contributory factor in another 25 percent. Acute respiratory failure has been defined as a situation in which the Pa_{O_2} is below the predicted normal for the patient's age or the Pa_{CO_2} is above 50 mm Hg in the absence of metabolic acidosis. A broad spectrum of patients fall in this category; well over two-thirds have experienced surgery or trauma.

PATHOPHYSIOLOGY. Physiologic causes of acute respiratory insufficiency following surgery include (1) hypoventilation, (2) diffusion defects, (3) abnormalities in the ventilation/perfusion ratio, (4) shunting which is either anatomic or related to atelectasis, (5) reduction in cardiac output with concomitant persistent shunt, and (6) alteration in the hemoglobin level and/or dissociation curve.

A variety of measurements of ventilation and oxygenation have been applied, with multiple refinements. Those which are relatively routinely performed will be considered in this discussion. Ventilatory mechanics are evaluated by routine monitoring of the respiratory rate and determination of the vital capacity and inspiratory force. Ventilation, itself, is assessed by consideration of respiratory rate, tidal volume, and, more particularly, Pa_{CO_2}. A frequently employed refinement to assess CO_2 elimination is VD/VT, where VD is the physiologic dead space and VT is the tidal volume. This ratio is defined as that portion of the tidal volume which is ineffective in the removal of CO_2 from the blood. The technique involves collection of ex-

pired gas over several respiratory cycles for about 2 minutes and simultaneous measurements of Pa_{CO_2}. VD/VT is influenced by cardiac output, tidal volume, and the pattern of respiration.

The adequacy of intrapulmonary blood-gas exchange is determined by measuring the Pa_{CO_2} and the Pa_{O_2} in relation to the inspired P_{O_2}. The efficacy of oxygen exchange within the lung is expressed as the alveolar-arterial oxygen tension difference ($A - aDO_2$). Factors which influence the $A - aDO_2$ include the difference between the arterial and venous oxygen content; the mixed venous oxygen content, itself, which may reflect oxygen consumption; the cardiac output; the inspired oxygen concentration (Fi_{O_2}); the position of the oxygen hemoglobin dissociation curve; and the position of the Pa_{O_2} on the curve. Abnormalities in the ventilation/perfusion ratio ($\dot{Q}_S/\dot{Q}_T$) express right-to-left physiologic shunt. This ratio can be determined precisely by measuring the oxygen content of the pulmonary end-capillary arterial and mixed venous blood, but more frequently a nomogram can be used to define $\dot{Q}_S/\dot{Q}_T$ based on the measurement of Pa_{O_2} and pulmonary alveolar oxygen tension (PA_{O_2}), as shown in Fig. 12-1. As can be seen, small changes in the $\dot{Q}_S/\dot{Q}_T$ are more readily detected when the patient is breathing 100% oxygen for 20 or 30 minutes. Determinations are affected by alterations in the cardiac output and pH.

Fig. 12-1. Analog-computed relationship between percent right-to-left shunt ($\dot{Q}_S/\dot{Q}_T \times 100$), arterial P_{O_2}, and inspired oxygen or alveolar oxygen tension (PA_{O_2}). The alveolar-arterial oxygen tension gradient can be obtained by drawing a horizontal line from the ordinate (arterial P_{O_2}) to the appropriate PA_{O_2} line. For example, when $\dot{Q}_S/\dot{Q}_T \times 100 = 20$, and $PA_{O_2} \times 680$ mm Hg, then the arterial P_{O_2} is approximately 175 mm Hg and the $A - aDO_2 = 680 - 175 = 505$ mm Hg. Note that below a right-to-left shunt value of 30, small changes in $\dot{Q}_S/\dot{Q}_T \times 100$ can produce drastic alterations in arterial P_{O_2} particularly when the subject is breathing high concentrations of oxygen. The curves were drawn assuming a hemoglobin concentration of 15 Gm/100 ml, an arterial pH of 7.40, an $A - V_{O_2}$ difference of 6 ml/100 ml, and a standard oxyhemoglobin dissociation curve. *(From H. Pontoppidan et al., Adv Surg 4:163, 1970. Copyright 1970 by Year Book Medical Publishers, Inc., Chicago. Used by permission. Graphs kindly prepared by Dr. M. A. Duvelleroy.)*

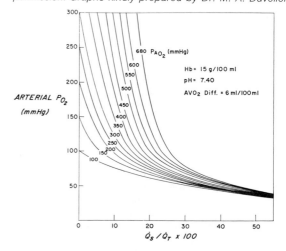

PATHOGENESIS. The major etiologic and contributory factors are conveniently considered under the categories listed in pathophysiology. Hypoventilation may be related to thoracic trauma; muscle weakness; and deleterious changes in the respiratory mechanics, which have been shown to exist for several days following thoracotomy and laparotomy. Diffusion defects may exist in patients who are chronic long-term smokers with consequent intraalveolar septal thickening. The defects also may be related to the aspiration of gastric content, which is now appreciated to occur more commonly; an incidence of 10 percent has been reported for intubated patients undergoing elective surgery, and a higher percentage for patients undergoing emergency surgery. There is no evidence that tracheostomy protects against such aspiration. Oxygen, itself, has intrinsic toxicity, and when Fi_{O_2} is over 60%, destruction of respiratory epithelium may occur. Therefore, it is preferable to maintain patients with congestive heart failure and emphysema at Pa_{O_2} of 70 mm Hg with Fi_{O_2} of 60% rather than expose the airway to 100% oxygen for a long period of time. If Pa_{O_2} remains low, mechanical measures such as positive end-expiratory pressure (PEEP) or constant positive airway pressure (CPAP) should be used in an intubated patient. Fluid overload with pulmonary edema initially decreases compliance and ultimately impairs gas exchange (see below). Other intrapulmonary lesions which may contribute to interference with diffusion include microemboli, fat emboli, and pulmonary infection. Abnormalities of the ventilation/perfusion ratio ($\dot{Q}_S/\dot{Q}_T$) result when areas which are well perfused with blood are underventilated. Maintaining the patient in a supine position accentuates this maldistribution, and the pathophysiologic consequence of atelectasis is a significant abnormality in $\dot{Q}_S/\dot{Q}_T$. Other factors which alter the ventilation/perfusion ratio are obesity and upper abdominal surgery with consequent collapse of the basal aveoli. Both atelectasis and reduced cardiac output result in intrapulmonary shunting. A shift in the oxygen-hemoglobin dissociation curve to the left decreases oxygen delivery to the tissues. This may be caused by respiratory alkalosis and also by deficiency in 2,3-diphosphoglycerate, which results from transfusion of banked blood more than 3 days old.

It is now felt that the term "shock lung" is inappropriate. Hemorrhagic shock unassociated with sepsis rarely causes acute pulmonary insufficiency. Davis and Pollack have shown that there is no distinct pathologic lung lesion in patients dying of hemorrhagic shock. $Na^+ - K^+$ transport and adenosine nucleotides in the lung are unchanged in hemorrhagic shock, indicating that cellular energy utilization or production in the lung is unchanged.

CLINICAL MANIFESTATIONS. Among the situations which should alert the observer to the development of the syndrome of postoperative pulmonary insufficiency are (1) congestive failure, (2) dyspnea, (3) cyanosis, (4) evidence of obstructive lung disease, and (5) pulmonary edema. Early in the evolution of the syndrome, the patient manifests hyperventilation associated with a reduction in Pa_{CO_2} below 35 mm Hg which precedes any significant reduction in Pa_{O_2}. Ultimately there is a reduction in Pa_{O_2} which becomes more significant when the patient does not respond to increases in Fi_{O_2}. Roentgenologic changes tend to occur late in the course of the condition and may represent the effects of therapy. These lesions are characteristically scattered, ill-defined, bilateral densities. A correlation exists between the extension of the densities and deterioration of pulmonary function.

TREATMENT. This should be mainly preventive and consists of ancillary measures and respiratory support. Antibiotics are indicated to treat established infections, and diuretics are useful in the management of pulmonary edema. Care is taken to avoid fluid overload of the patient, and the colloidal osmotic pressure of the plasma should be maintained at normal level. A difference of opinion regarding the use of albumin persists. There is concern as to whether administration of albumin will result in more substantial and longer-lasting interstitial pulmonary edema. Normal hemoglobin level is also important. Respiratory support includes physical therapy; the importance of moving the patient in order to avoid ventilation-perfusion abnormalities is emphasized.

The prophylactic use of artificial ventilation for respiratory support represents a major recent advance in the management of these patients. The indications for respiratory support have been categorized according to pathologic alterations (Table 12-1). Ventilatory support may be accomplished either through an endotracheal tube or a tracheostomy, since ventilation via a face mask or mouthpiece is rarely effective for more than short periods. Endotracheal intubation is considered the technique of choice when control of airway is urgently required.

The prolonged use of endotracheal intubation for ventilatory support is now gaining popularity as an alternative to tracheostomy. Although endotracheal tubes are not tolerated as well as tracheostomy tubes and it is appreciated that prolonged intubation is associated with laryngeal swelling, 6 days in adults and up to 3 weeks in children are regarded as reasonable periods of prolonged endotracheal intubation. In general, intubation via a nasotracheal route is tolerated better than via the orotracheal route, but insertion may be more difficult. The major advantage of endotracheal intubation is that the mortality is low, the complications are minimal, and the hazards associated with tracheostomy are avoided.

Tracheostomy is now generally reserved for the patient who requires prolonged ventilatory support and, as is pointed out in Chap. 19, may be associated with the complications of stenosis which are generally related to cuff pressure. The introduction of low-pressure cuffs may reduce the incidence of this complication.

In general, ventilatory support is first accomplished using intermittent positive-pressure breathing (IPPB) in which expiration is unobstructed and intrapulmonary pressure returns to atmospheric level. The patient's blood gases are monitored while on ventilatory support, and if necessary the Fi_{O_2} is increased up to 60% to maintain the Pa_{O_2} at normal levels. If IPPB is ineffectual, positive end-expiratory pressure ventilation (PEEP) is instituted. PEEP results in increased functional residual capacity, reduced normal negative intrathoracic pressure with, at times, conversion to positive values, increased venous pressure, and

Table 12-1. INDICATIONS FOR RESPIRATORY SUPPORT

		Acceptable range	Chest physical therapy, oxygen, close monitoring	Intubation, tracheostomy, ventilation
Mechanics	Respiratory rate	12–25	25–35	>35
	Vital capacity, ml/kg	70–30	30–15	<15
	Inspiratory force, cm H_2O	100–50	50–25	<25
Oxygenation . . .	$A - aDO_2$, mm Hg*	50–200	200–350	>350
	Pa_{O_2}, mm Hg	100–75 (Air)	200–70 (On mask O_2)	<70 (On mask O_2)
Ventilation	VD/VT	0.3–0.4	0.4–0.6	>0.6
	Pa_{CO_2}, mm Hg	35–45	45–60	>60†

* After 15 minutes of 100% O_2.
† Except in chronic hypercapnia.

decreased venous return to the heart. PEEP ventilation is particularly effective in causing a rise in Pa_{O_2} and a fall in physiologic shunt, and the greater amount of shunting across the lung, the greater the effect of this modality. PEEP ventilation is preferred for patients with profound hypoxemia, significant physiologic shunting, atelectasis, and high cardiac output. It is particularly appropriate for patients with massive chest wall injuries. PEEP is contraindicated for conditions characterized by normal oxygenation, hyperexpansion of the lung, and low cardiac output. In general, it is felt that the end-expiratory pressure should be maintained at 5 cm H_2O and should rarely be increased above 10 cm H_2O because of the danger of producing pneumothorax.

Prolonged artificial ventilation has been characterized by the formation of edema and deterioration of blood-gas interchange, which is generally manageable by water restriction and the administration of diuretic agents such as furosemide or ethacrynic acid. When there is objective evidence that lung function is adequate to permit transfer from artificial to spontaneous ventilation, a gradual weaning process is required. The patient on PEEP is initially converted to IPPB. Difficulty in weaning can be attributed to abnormalities in blood-gas exchange, pulmonary mechanics, reduction in cardiac output, and general muscle weakness. A more gradual weaning, employing intermittent mandatory ventilation (IMV), may expedite the process. Weaning should be accomplished only with careful monitoring of blood gas and exchange; the pulmonary mechanics are indicated in Table 12-1.

Atelectasis

Atelectasis comprises 90 percent of all postoperative pulmonary complications, but a lack of definition and difficulty in diagnosis has resulted in a wide range of reported incidences varying between 1 and 80 percent depending on the type of operation and the reporting institution. The term "atelectasis" is derived from the Greek meaning "incomplete expansion" but is generally applied to the situation in which there are airless alveoli. Although collapse of alveoli may occur within definite anatomic units such as segments, lobes, or an entire lung, the most commonly encountered variety is platelike and subsegmental. Moersch reported atelectasis in 10 percent of operations on the thorax or upper abdomen and 4 percent of operations on the lower abdomen. Clendon and Pygott found 38 percent in patients undergoing abdominal surgical treatment and only 2.7 percent when operations were performed in areas other than the abdomen or thorax. Kurzweg indicated that atelectasis occurred in 3 percent of all operations, 10 to 20 percent of cases with abdominal surgery, and 20 to 30 percent of cases involving upper abdominal surgery. Becker et al., who took roentgenograms in a series of patients postoperatively, demonstrated that 51 percent of patients with upper abdominal surgical treatment had atelectasis. Three percent were lobar, fourteen percent segmental, and thirty-one percent platelike in distribution. When pulmonary function studies were used to determine the diagnosis, Beecher found evidence of collapse in 83 percent of laparotomies.

ETIOLOGY. The two major factors which have been implicated as causes of atelectasis are bronchial obstruction with distal gas absorption and hypoventilation or ineffectual respiration. The loss of chemical elements which stabilize the lung at low volumes by reducing alveolar surface tension, i.e., *surfactants,* has been implicated.

Obstruction of the tracheobronchial airway occurs secondary to changes in bronchial secretion, defect in the expulsion mechanism, and reduction in bronchial caliber. Subsequent to tracheobronchial obstruction by secretion, vomitus, blood, or tumor material, there is a period during which a change occurs in the composition of gases within the alveolus, following which the gas composition in the obstructed alveoli remains constant until absorption is complete. The rate of absorption is a function of the pressure difference between the gas in the alveoli and the gas in the blood, the absorption coefficient of the gas, and the rate and quantity of blood flow.

Obstruction of a large conductive airway certainly leads

to atelectasis of the distal lung segment. However, there are many observations which cast doubt on bronchial obstruction as the sole or major causative factor in postoperative atelectasis. It is common to find atelectasis at autopsy with no obstructive plug. Conversely, it is uncommon for atelectasis to be accompanied by a definite plug, the removal of which leads to recovery. The excessive secretions associated with atelectasis might be a secondary effect rather than a cause. For atelectasis to occur on an obstructive basis, the obstruction must be complete; it seems unlikely that postoperative secretions could establish an obstruction in so short a time. Also, the fact that atelectasis can be prevented or relieved by hyperventilation suggests that the obstructive origin is improbable. Finally, Van Allen and Adams found that, in dogs breathing normally, bronchial occlusion did not result in atelectasis, and they felt that this was due to sufficient collateral respiration or circulation of gas to prevent collapse of the alveoli. Perhaps the strongest case against the etiologic necessity of airway obstruction is the demonstration by Griffo and Roos that the time course of atelectatic changes does not vary with the varying solubility of inspired gases.

Currently, many feel that atelectasis usually consists of small and diffuse lesions which are nonobstructive in origin and are due to inspiratory insufficiency. The concept of inspiratory failure was first demonstrated by Mead and Collier and subsequently expanded by several writers, particularly Bendixen and his associates. It has been shown that spontaneous or artificial ventilation at constant tidal volumes usually will result in decreased compliance, decreased lung volume, and increased shunting (venous admixture). These signs all suggest a decrease in the number of functioning alveoli and occur more rapidly than could be explained by the absorption of gases due to an obstructing lesion. The changes are almost completely reversible with pulmonary inflation beyond the tidal volume range or with intermittent deep breathing. Thus, atelectasis is thought to occur without airway obstruction as a result of a constant volume ventilation with volumes approximating normal tidal volume, and the process is reversible by hyperinflation. The validity of this etiologic concept is also debatable as evidenced by the findings of Brattstrom, who noted that before and after operation in patients with and without lung complications, the course of ventilation was essentially similar. There was no evidence of decreased effectivity of ventilation in the functioning alveoli nor of impaired pulmonary mixing.

The third major cause of alveolar collapse is related to the surface forces acting at the gas-liquid interface within the alveolar units. Normally, there is a film, surfactant, which has the property of reducing surface tension when the alveolar volume is decreased. Increased surface tension of this film encourages collapse or decrease in the size of the alveolus and makes it more difficult to inflate. Regional changes in the pulmonary circulation may alter the characteristics of surfactant. Clements postulates that deep breathing mobilizes surfactant from within the alveolar cell to augment or replace the aging surfactant on the alveolar surface, maintaining stability and preventing atelectasis.

Many factors predispose to the development of post-

operative atelectasis. There is an increasing incidence in patients who smoke and those who suffer from bronchitis, asthma, emphysema, or other chronic lung diseases. Anesthesia and postoperative narcotics depress the cough reflex, while chest pain, immobilization, and splinting with bandages reduce the effective nature of the cough. The incidence of atelectasis is related to the duration and depth of anesthesia, and although higher incidences have been reported with general anesthesia than with regional anesthesia, when the same postoperative care was applied to the two groups, the difference disappeared. Nasogastric tubes have been implicated because of the increased secretions and predisposition toward aspiration. Bronchospasm is a predisposing factor, but severe bronchospasm is rarely encountered during clinical anesthesia. Congestion of the bronchial walls due to edema represents another source of decrease in the bronchial lumen. As mentioned previously, there is a definite increase in atelectasis associated with upper abdominal as opposed to lower abdominal or extraabdominal surgical procedures. Transverse incisions are associated with a lower incidence of atelectasis when compared to vertical incisions in the same area.

CLINICAL MANIFESTATIONS. Atelectasis usually becomes manifest in the first 24 hours after an operation and rarely appears after 48 hours. There is usually a sudden onset of fever and tachycardia. Frequently, the pulmonary manifestations are so minor that they are not recognized. Early findings include rales located posteriorly in the bases, diminished breath sounds, and bronchial breathing. With massive involvement, there may be a shift of the trachea, mediastinum, and heart to the involved side, but this is not present with the more common subsegmental lesions. Pronounced dyspnea and/or cyanosis are relatively uncommon. Roentgenograms may demonstrate areas of consolidation, but in early cases bronchial breathing is detected more frequently than roentgenographic changes. Determination of blood gases indicating intrapulmonary shunting of blood provides the diagnosis. Characteristically with atelectasis and significant shunting, the arterial Pa_{O_2} is decreased while the arterial Pa_{CO_2} may be normal or decreased. The ventilation is normal or increased.

If atelectasis persists, the clinical manifestations are those generally associated with pneumonia. The temperature increases to a greater extent, and there is increasing tachycardia, dyspnea, and cyanosis. It is felt that the great majority of postoperative pneumonias begin as atelectasis, since atelectatic areas are poorly drained and represent good sites for infection. In some instances, however, pneumonia may result from the aspiration of infected material. Another consequence of atelectasis is the development of lung abscess, which also may be initiated by the aspiration of foreign material, such as teeth or blood during tonsillectomy and purulent material from putrid abscesses in the mouth. Aspiration of gastric contents also represents a possible cause of lung abscess.

TREATMENT. Prophylaxis begins preoperatively by having the patient cease smoking, if possible, for at least 2 weeks prior to operation and instructing the patient in deep abdominal breathing and productive coughing. Postoperative prophylaxis includes the minimal use of depressant drugs, the prevention of pain which may limit respiration, frequent changes of body position, deep breathing and coughing exercises, and early ambulation. Sustained maximal inspiration, which can be accomplished with the aid of a variety of devices, is the most important factor in the prevention and treatment of atelectasis. The usual IPPB units do not have the mechanism for instituting sighing or deep breathing, but manual inflation using an Ambu bag may accomplish this end. Becker et al. reported that the routine use of IPPB with bronchodilator and bronchodetergent drugs did not prevent the occurrence of atelectasis or accelerate its disappearance, once it was established.

Three groups of medications have been applied to the prophylaxis and therapy of atelectasis. These are (1) expectorants to provide more liquid and less viscous secretions, (2) detergents and mucolytic solutions to alter the surface tension of secretions and render their elimination more likely, and (3) bronchodilators used primarily by inhalation to provide increased size of the tracheobronchial tree and elimination of bronchospasm. The mucolytic agents, such as Mucomist or Alevaire, are indicated because inhaled air with a relative humidity lower than 70% inhibits ciliary activity and tends to desiccate secretions.

Once atelectasis becomes clinically manifest, coughing, clearing of secretions, and increase in depth of respiration may be stimulated by endotracheal suction with a soft rubber catheter or the instillation of 1 to 2 ml of saline solution directly into the trachea via an intracatheter polyethylene tube. If these measures are not successful, bronchoscopy may be required, and if multiple bronchoscopic aspirations are necessary, tracheostomy should be performed to facilitate subsequent aspiration.

Atelectasis, pneumonia, aspiration pneumonia, and lung abscesses are also discussed in Chap. 17.

Pulmonary Edema

Pulmonary edema may occur during or immediately after an operation. The increased use of massive blood transfusions, plasma expanders, and other fluids during operative procedures has resulted in an increased incidence of this complication. Circulatory overload represents the most common cause of pulmonary edema. Other factors which have been implicated include incomplete cardiac emptying, shift of blood from the peripheral to pulmonary vascular bed, negative pressure on the airway which increases the gradient between the transmural capillary pressure and the alveolar pressure favoring transudation, and injury to the alveolar membrane by noxious substances.

Although circulatory overload is most frequently due to infusion of fluid during operative procedure, it may also result from the absorption of solutions during irrigation of hollow viscera, such as the bladder, and is frequently associated with subclinical heart failure in those patients in whom pulmonary edema becomes manifest.

Incomplete cardiac emptying may be attributed to any anesthetic, narcotic, or hypnotic agent, since all are capable of decreasing myocardial contractility. Incomplete cardiac emptying may also be due to gross irregularities in rhythm.

Pulmonary edema is rarely the result of this single factor, and there is usually elevated atrial and pulmonary blood pressure associated with incomplete cardiac emptying. Similarly, the etiologic mechanism of shift of blood to the pulmonary vascular bed is usually associated with other factors. Peripheral vascular beds may vasoconstrict, causing blood to shift centrally and result in pulmonary edema. A reflex mechanism of neurogenic origin which causes redistribution of blood from the periphery to the pulmonary bed has been reported to occur during manipulation of the brain and following head trauma.

Pulmonary edema caused by injury to the alveolar membrane is associated with the inhalation of noxious gases or vapors and the aspiration of gastric contents or chemicals, particularly kerosene, which are pulmonary irritants.

CLINICAL MANIFESTATIONS. The initial disturbance of pulmonary edema is thickening of the capillary and alveolar membranes. In the early stage, the principal effect is a reduction in diffusion, and unless increased oxygen tension is present, hypoxemia results. A reduction in lung compliance precedes evidence of carbon dioxide retention in the blood. Bronchospasm usually occurs and contributes further to reducing the compliance. As frank edema develops, a frothy pink-stained fluid appears in the alveoli, bronchi, and trachea, and at this time the problem is one of airway obstruction rather than diffusion. Clinically, bronchospasm and marked reduction in lung compliance in a patient being ventilated should provide premonitory evidence and anticipate the development of dyspnea and cough. A few scattered rales may appear early, but as the process intensifies, bubbling rales and rhonchi are heard all over the chest. The systemic blood pressure is usually raised initially but may be normal or reduced, and characteristically there is a marked tachycardia. Shock may appear with signs of peripheral circulatory failure, and death may occur from asphyxia.

TREATMENT. Therapy is directed at (1) providing oxygen, (2) allowing oxygen access to the alveoli by removing obstructive fluid, and (3) correcting the circulatory overload. Oxygen saturation can be restored by increasing the concentration of oxygen in inspired air. An increase in alveolar oxygen tension of 50 mm Hg, which can be achieved by a 7 percent increase in inspired oxygen, is sufficient to restore arterial oxygen tension to normal, even in the presence of the more severe diffusion defects. Hypoxemia, however, will persist even if pure oxygen is breathed unless the fluid is removed from the alveoli.

Measures to reduce the pulmonary capillary pressure include venous occlusion tourniquets, placing the patient in a head-up or sitting position to reduce the flow of venous blood to the heart, and phlebotomy. Since systemic vasoconstriction has been shown to be a precipitating cause, therapy may be indicated to reverse this mechanism. Spinal anesthesia has been applied successfully in the treatment of pulmonary edema, as has the ganglionic blocking agent Arfonad.

In the intubated patient, IPPB with PEEP or CPAP can rapidly reverse the process. However these modalities must be used with caution, since they may impair the efficiency of an already failing circulation. Drug therapy includes furosemide or ethacrynic acid for rapid diuresis and digitalis glycosides for situations where myocardial failure and lower output coexist (particularly in mitral stenosis) or where there is arrhythmia such as flutter or fibrillation. Morphine has been shown to be of value, though its mode of action remains unclear.

CARDIAC COMPLICATIONS

This section considers cardiac arrhythmias and myocardial ischemia and infarction related to surgery. A discussion of cardiac arrest and the postcardiotomy syndrome is presented in Chap. 19.

Arrhythmias

Although cardiac arrhythmias are frequently associated with operative repair of congenital and acquired lesions of the heart (see Chaps. 18 and 19), they represent a potential complication of any surgical procedure. As the age of the surgical population increases, one should encounter an increasing incidence of these disturbances.

INCIDENCE. The incidence varies and is somewhat determined by whether sinus tachycardia is included in the series. In a recent review, Reinikainen and Pontinen report that the incidence of cardiac arrhythmias occurring during extrathoracic operative procedures ranged between 30 and 100 percent. During thoracotomies carried out under general anesthesia, incidences as high as 77 percent have been recorded. Heart diseases increased the incidence; in one series, in 51 percent of cardiac patients as contrasted with 20 percent of other patients, arrhythmia developed during anesthesia. Kuner and associates, monitoring continuous electrocardiographic signals on magnetic tape for prolonged periods of time, found the incidence of cardiac arrhythmia during anesthesia to be 61 percent. The arrhythmias which they noted most frequently were wandering pacemaker, atrioventricular (AV) dissociation, and nodal rhythm and premature ventricular systoles. Relating intraoperative arrhythmias to type of anesthesia, Reinikainen and Pontinen recorded arrhythmias in 24 percent of patients in whom operations were carried out under local anesthesia. The majority of these were of vagal origin and caused by the occulocardiac reflex. There were also ventricular systoles related to anxiety or fear. Under epidural anesthesia, the incidence was 23.5 percent, and this was frequently related to blood pressure reduction. When general anesthesia was established with halothane, arrhythmias occurred during intubation in 29 percent and during maintenance of anesthesia in 13 percent of patients.

A study of over 3,000 noncardiac cases revealed 2.4 percent had abnormal postoperative electrocardiograms. The majority of patients were asymptomatic, and most of the abnormalities were conduction disturbances. Taylor reported postoperative arrhythmias in about 5 percent of cyclopropane administrations. Buckley and Jackson studied 100 patients immediately after surgical treatment and noted sinus tachycardia in 32 percent, sinus bradycardia

in 2 percent, sinus arrhythmia in 3 percent, occasional ventricular contractions in 7 percent, and trigeminy in 1 percent. Arrhythmias occur much more frequently following thoracic surgical procedures, with paroxysmal fibrillation and atrial flutter or fibrillation representing the most common types. The time of onset is variable, 30 percent occurring on the first postoperative day and 60 percent with 72 hours of operation, though the onset has been noted as late as the eighteenth day. Wheat and Burford reported that 20 to 30 percent of patients recovering from thoracic operations exhibited cardiac arrhythmias. The site and extent of the procedure represented important factors. Arrhythmia occurred in 11 to 32 percent of cases following pneumonectomy and in only 5 percent following lobectomy or lesser resection procedures. When the thoracic lesions involved the vagus nerve, an increasing frequency was noted.

ETIOLOGY. Important predisposing factors include the patient's age and the presence of preexisting heart disease, arteriosclerosis, or hypertension. The highest incidence of arrhythmias occurs in patients over sixty, and it has been shown that the diseased heart is definitely more excitable. Other determining factors include the type of anesthetic, the duration of surgical procedures, the need for intubation, and hyperventilation. The anesthetic agents most frequently implicated are halothane and cyclopropane, though arrhythmias occur with all types of anesthesia. Halothane is usually associated with bradycardia and AV dissociation, and when vasopressors are used in combination with halothane, there is an increased incidence of paroxysmal arrhythmia. Atropine also has been noted to cause AV dissociation during anesthesia and in patients undergoing breast and perineal surgery. There is a high incidence of sinus bradycardia during Pentothal induction. Serum electrolyte abnormalities during the postoperative course are contributory factors, particularly acidosis and hypokalemia. Hypercalcemia following parathyroid manipulation or with inappropriate intravenous calcium therapy may precipitate rapid ectopic atrial arrhythmia. Thoracic surgery is associated with an increased incidence of arrhythmias. During the postoperative period, myocardial infarction and pulmonary complications are frequently associated with ventricular arrhythmias.

Postoperative cardiac arrhythmias frequently have their genesis in the preoperative period. Atrial arrhythmias are usually due to vagal stimulation. Other provoking factors are hypotension, hypoxia, and hypercapnia, all of which may cause inhibition of the sinus node and activation of a local pacemaker or reentrant atrial mechanisms. The most important reason for ventricular arrhythmia is increased excitability of the myocardium and specialized conduction pathways. This may be attributed to sympathomimetic drugs, such as epinephrine, and increase in blood pressure. It is generally held that some common anesthetic agents like halothane and cyclopropane produce sensitization of the myocardium, making it more responsive to the catecholamines, thus potentiating the development of arrhythmia. Muscle of the diseased heart is also more excitable, and hypercapnia provokes ectopic rhythm by decreasing pacemaker activity. Electrolyte disturbances, particularly alterations in potassium concentration, can cause ventricular arrhythmia. The vasovagal cardiac reflex has been implicated in arrhythmias which develop during intubation, surgical manipulation of the lung, and operations on the gallbladder and stomach. Positive-pressure breathing mechanisms may induce a high resistance in the pulmonary circulation, reduce venous return, and stimulate ventricular arrhythmia. Specific diseases which have been implicated as causes of arrhythmia during operative procedures are thyrotoxicosis and pheochromocytoma with its high catecholamine concentration in the plasma.

TREATMENT. In view of the high incidence of arrhythmia in elderly patients undergoing thoracic surgical procedures, some have suggested prophylactic digitalization, and others have employed quinidine and procaine amide therapy preoperatively. Digitalization is particularly applicable in patients with frequent atrial premature systoles, while withholding of digitalis is indicated in the presence of sustained or intermittent paroxysmal nodal rhythms. Many have advised discontinuing all myocardial depressant agents, including quinidine and procainamide preoperatively, and withholding all cardiac drugs in the operating room, unless an arrhythmia compromises cardiac output. A bipolar electrode may be inserted preoperatively into the apex of the right ventricle for emergency electronic pacing in patients with advanced second-degree heart block or third degree AV block.

Once an arrhythmia develops, if it is tolerated well by the patient, it may be simply observed, since a high percentage convert spontaneously. In general, therapy is directed at maintaining adequate cardiac output and coronary blood flow. Vasopressors may be administered to maintain the blood pressure while the definitive treatment is organized. If congestive failure threatens, digitalis is the treatment of choice. Digitalis is also the drug of choice in the presence of all supraventricular arrhythmias. For rapid digitalization, 1 mg of digoxin is administered in divided doses. However, paroxysmal and atrial tachycardia with block and nonparoxysmal nodal tachycardia may all be caused by inappropriate administration of digitalis. Although quinidine may convert atrial fibrillation to sinus rhythm, it does not represent the prime treatment in any real emergency. Cardioversion limits the applicability of quinidine to the prevention of arrhythmias. It is also unwise to administer calcium and depressant agents indiscriminately. If the arrhythmia is related to overdigitalization, potassium should be administered as 40 mEq of potassium chloride in 50 ml of solution, limiting the dose to 20 mEq/hour. Lidocaine, 1 mg/kg intravenously administered rapidly or as a continuous drip of 1 to 2 mg/minute, is preferred for ventricular arrhythmias. It has the advantage over procainamide that it is not associated with hypotension. Diphenylhydantoin (Dilantin) is effective as treatment for digitalis-induced supraventricular tachycardia and ventricular irritability. However, it may reduce myocardial contractility, increase AV block, and cause cardiac arrest. Propranolol, a beta-adrenergic blocker, is used for digitalis intoxication and for slowing ventricular rate in atrial flutter or fibrillation.

Sinus Tachycardia. By definition this disturbance in normal rhythm is not an arrhythmia. Sinus tachycardia is caused by increased sympathetic tone or decreased vagal tone frequently secondary to hypoxia, hypovolemia due to blood loss, and pain. Hypercapnia, dehydration, hyperthyroidism, and congestive heart failure are frequently associated with sinus tachycardia. A variety of drugs, including meperidine, atropine, and epinephrine, all increase the heart rate, as does digitalis intoxication. Treatment is directed at the cause.

Paroxysmal Supraventricular Tachycardia. This is usually characterized by the sudden onset of a regular heart rate ranging between 140 and 220 beats per minute. Rogers et al. reported an incidence of 0.2 percent during the postoperative period. The disturbance may be caused by digitalis or quinidine toxicity, myocardial infarction, congestive heart failure, thyrotoxicosis, and hypoxemia. The arrhythmia is more likely to occur in patients with a history of previous attacks.

The disturbance usually responds to carotid sinus stimulation, but immediate therapy is required only with extremely rapid ventricular rates. Depressive drugs may increase vagal tone via the carotid, and aortic sinus reflex stimulation associated with elevated blood pressure and phenylephrine hydrochloride is effective in about 80 percent of cases. Treatment includes cardioversion or rapid digitalization. Propanolol has also been effective in this situation.

Atrial Flutter. While the atrial rate resulting from ectopic stimuli ranges between 200 and 400 per minute, the ventricular rate is dependent upon the degree of heart block which characteristically occurs. The ventricular rate decreases with carotid sinus pressure only to increase again when the pressure is released, in contrast to the permanent conversion of an atrial nodal paroxysmal tachycardia to sinus rhythm. Atrial flutter occurs more frequently in elderly patients with cardiovascular disease and in patients undergoing intrathoracic surgical treatment. Vagal nerve stimulation, hypotension, and hypoxemia have all been considered as etiologic factors. Continued atrial flutter frequently causes congestive heart failure, particularly when the ventricular rate is rapid.

Digitalis is usually effective, and the flutter is usually converted to atrial fibrillation with a slower ventricular response. Quinidine also has been used therapeutically, but only after digitalization. However, cardioversion is now the treatment of choice.

Paroxysmal Ventricular Tachycardia. This is a rare disorder which has serious implications, since it is associated with a damaged myocardium. The pulse rate is usually between 140 and 180. There is no effect with carotid sinus pressure, and there may be some irregularities of rhythm. Ventricular tachycardia may represent one of the first findings in a patient with myocardial infarction. This disorder of rhythm has also been precipitated by hypercapnia and may progress rapidly to ventricular fibrillation.

Cardioversion or lidocaine given intravenously are the treatments of choice. If the disorder is related to digitalis intoxication, diphenylhydantoin and correction of hypokalemia may be therapeutic.

Sinus Bradycardia. This refers to irregular rhythm with

a rate less than 60 per minute. The low rate is normal in young athletic patients. The bradycardia may also be induced by drugs such as neostigmine, quinidine, procainamide, digitalis, methoxamine, and levarterenol. Arrhythmia usually does not require treatment unless there is evidence of reduced cardiac output, in which case atropine may be indicated.

AV Nodal Rhythm. This arrhythmia is usually a temporary disturbance caused by vagal inhibition of the sinus node and may be manifest only by a slow pulse, 40 to 50 per minute. Pronounced jugular venous cannon waves may be noted. The rhythm may be caused by carotid sinus pressure, endotracheal intubation, digitalis, and the vasopressor drugs. It usually corrects itself spontaneously, and no treatment is necessary.

AV Block. Incomplete block is an uncommon arrhythmia which is due to organic or surgically induced disturbance of the conduction pathway. Vagal stimulation, carotid sinus pressure, and vasovagal reflexes have also been implicated as have digitalis, quinidine, and morphine. The pulse is slow and regular, and the neck veins may demonstrate atrial pulsation. If the cause is reflex in origin, atropine is indicated, whereas if the condition is drug-induced, the drug should be withdrawn.

Complete AV block results in a ventricular rhythm of between 30 and 60 beats per minute and occasionally follows trauma to the conduction system during heart operation or intraoperative and postoperative septal infarction. Surgically induced blocks are best treated by a pacemaker.

Sinus Arrhythmia. This is more frequently noted in younger patients and children, and irregularity is characteristically associated with phases of respiration. It is occasionally seen in patients with digitalis toxicity. No treatment is required, though atropine will correct the abnormality, since it is related to vagal tone.

Sinoatrial Block. Either single beats drop out with regular sequence, or there are runs of two or three dropped beats. If the block is prolonged, nodal or ventricular escape occurs. The block is caused by increased vagal tone and depression of the sinus node impulse. It occurs during tracheobronchial suctioning, with carotid sinus pressure, and in hyperkalemia, and is associated with neostigmine administration. It may reverse itself spontaneously or with atropine administration.

Atrial Fibrillation. Atrial fibrillation with its characteristic irregular pulse most frequently appears postoperatively in arteriosclerotic patients subjected to thoracic surgical treatment. In early cases, the ventricular rate is usually rapid, but when digitalis has been given, a slow ventricular rate may be noted. In the absence of failure, no treatment is indicated, since spontaneous correction may occur. In the case of a paroxysmal atrial fibrillation, which may precipitate congesive heart failure, digitalis therapy is indicated. Quinidine or electric cardioversion may be used when there is no associated failure.

Premature Contractions. These represent the most common irregularities of the pulse, and they may originate from any portion of the conduction system. The premature beat characteristically occurs earlier than expected and is followed by a pause due to failure of the ventricle to respond to the next normal impulse. The abnormality occurs in 2 to 8 percent of postoperative patients. The occurrence has been associated with changes in posture, drug therapy with ephedrine and epinephrine, digitalis toxicity, and myocardial infarction. Usually premature contractions have no clinical significance and require no therapy, though if they occur with disturbing frequency, quinidine or lidocaine is recommended unless there is congestive failure, in which case digitalis is the drug of choice, provided it does not represent a possible cause.

Myocardial Infarction

The magnitude of the problem of postoperative coronary occlusion is evidenced by the fact that Master and associates, in 1938, reported that 5.6 percent of attacks of coronary occulsion in patients hospitalized during a given period of time occurred after an operative procedure. The majority of patients who died suddenly during the operative and immediate postoperative period demonstrated coronary artery thrombosis or myocardial infarction at autopsy in another series. The reported incidence for postoperative myocardial infarction ranges between 0.1 and 1.2 percent of all surgical patients, and between 0.9 and 4.4 percent of all surgical patients over the age of fifty. The incidence rose to 6 percent in a group of men over fifty with histories of previous coronary occlusion, and this relationship was more pronounced when the previous occlusion occurred within 2 years of surgical treatment. Eleven unsuspected acute myocardial infarctions were detected by routine postoperative electrocardiograms taken on 1,000 patients in the recovery room.

Tarhan et al. recently assessed the significance of operative procedures under general anesthesia performed in patients who had previous myocardial infarction; 6.6 percent had another infarct in the first week after operation, and 54 percent of these died. Reinfarction occurred most frequently after operations on the thorax or upper abdomen. In over one-third of patients operated on within 3 months of infarction, reinfarction occurred. This rate decreased to 16 percent in patients at 3 to 6 months postinfarction and to 4 to 5 percent when infarction occurred more than 6 months prior to surgery.

CLINICAL MANIFESTATIONS. The majority of cases occur on the operative day or during the first 3 postoperative days, and although infarction has been associated with all anesthetics, the incidence is higher after general anesthesia for abdominal or pelvic surgical treatment. The most important precipitating factor is shock, either during the operation or in the early postoperative phase. The more prolonged the shock, the greater the risk of coronary thrombosis and myocardial ischemia. The electrocardiogram may show ST depression and T-wave flattening with the loss of as little as 500 ml of blood in patients with previous coronary occlusion.

The diagnosis may be difficult, because chest pain is often absent or obscured by narcotics. It is appropriate to consider routinely monitoring patients with previous infarction in an intensive care unit. In the study of

Wroblewski and LaDue, chest pain occurred as a primary clinical manifestation in only 27 percent of patients, which is less than the 97 percent generally reported in patients in whom a coronary occlusion is not related to surgery. The sudden appearance of shock, dyspnea, cyanosis, tachycardia, arrhythmia, or congestive failure should alert one to the diagnosis. The triad of dyspnea, cyanosis, and arterial hypotension requires a differential diagnosis between cardiac and respiratory problems. The electrocardiogram may provide the diagnosis with a characteristic infarction pattern. However, this is not an unequivocal finding, since, in older patients, ST segment and T-wave changes may be associated with myocardial ischemia, and the same changes may be observed with postoperative shock. A study of arterial gases may provide a differential diagnosis in reference to respiratory problems. Left ventricular failure with pulmonary edema is not generally accompanied by carbon dioxide retention, and, in contrast to airway obstruction and alveolar hypoventilation, there is usually a reduction in arterial carbon dioxide tension (P_{CO_2}) and respiratory alkalosis when cardiac failure accompanies myocardial infarction. Increasing data indicate that the CPK-MB isoenzyme is the most precise method for detection of myocardial necrosis following operation. If myocardial infarction is suspected, serial studies, including ECG, SGOT, and CPK-MB, should be done daily.

TREATMENT (See Chap. 4). Preoperative preparation of patients with signs of cardiac insufficiency should include digitalization for patients with enlarged hearts or histories of previous cardiac failure. Anemia, if present, requires treatment, and attention should be directed toward the regulation of fluid and electrolyte balance and hypovolemia. Operation is contraindicated for a period of at least 6 weeks and preferably 6 months following myocardial ischemia or infarction, except in an emergency. During the operation, a broad spectrum of factors which precipitate myocardial infarction should be avoided. These include anoxia, hypotension, hemorrhage, dehydration, electrolyte disturbance, and arrhythmias. The regulation of blood pressure during anesthesia is probably the most important measure in the prevention of myocardial ischemia and infarction. When the blood pressure falls significantly, in the absence of blood loss, the prompt correction of anoxia by adequate ventilation with oxygen and the administration of vasopressors is indicated. Digitalization may be required when shock is combined with heart failure. The administration of blood or fluid is indicated to maintain blood volume.

Treatment of myocardial infarction itself consists of relief of pain and anxiety using morphine and sedation. Relief of anoxia is accomplished with 33 to 50 percent oxygen delivered via a BLB mask or nasal catheter. Suctioning of the tracheobronchial tree may be required to clear obstructing secretions. Shock is treated by vasopressor agents. Promptness in instituting vasopressor therapy will increase the chances of its being effective. Rapid digitalization is applicable in treatment of shock when the myocardial insufficiency may be responsible for the severe hypotension. Digitalization is also indicated for the treatment of heart failure, which is a frequent manifestation

of postoperative myocardial infarction. In addition to digitalization, parenteral diuretic therapy may be used in the treatment of cardiac failure. Some writers have advocated the use of anticoagulant therapy after the danger of excessive bleeding from an operative site ceases.

In 1952, Wroblewski and LaDue reported the mortality attributable to postoperative myocardial infarction to be 40 percent, which at the time was in keeping with the mortality rate for coronary occlusion unassociated with surgery. In contrast, Tarhan et al. and Mauney et al. reported that myocardial infarction after anesthesia and a major operation was more lethal than myocardial infarction alone.

DIABETES MELLITUS

Diabetes mellitus occurs in 2 to 3 percent of the general population with a higher rate among older people. In two series, the disease was discovered in the paraoperative period in 16 and 23 percent of patients. The most commonly associated operative procedures were complications of vascular disease, but in a high percentage of patients diabetes was discovered prior to an emergency procedure. Diabetic patients represent a special challenge during total surgical care, because the impairment of the homeostatic mechanism for glucose may result in ketoacidosis if untreated or hypoglycemia if overtreated and also because of the associated incidence of generalized vascular disease.

PATHOPHYSIOLOGY. Diabetes mellitus is characterized by hyperglycemia, usually accompanied by glycosuria. The basic defect is a lack of metabolically effective circulating insulin. The elevated blood sugar level is a result of deficient utilization on the part of peripheral tissues and an increased output of glucose by the liver. Excess glucose comes from dietary carbohydrates, liver glycogen, and glucose formed from protein and fat. In the course of metabolism, free fatty acids are released and metabolized in the liver to an end product of acetoacetate, which, by hydrogenation, is converted to β-hydroxybutyric acid or by decarboxylation to acetone. The three products are known collectively as *ketone bodies*. In diabetes, the breakdown of fatty acids is increased, and since the metabolism of the ketone bodies is limited, they accumulate in the bloodstream and are eliminated via the kidneys. Glycosuria itself produces an osmotic diuresis which is enhanced by the presence of ketone bodies and the associated loss of sodium and potassium. Evaluation of decompensated diabetes, therefore, includes not only measuring the blood glucose but also measuring acetone, electrolytes, and carbon dioxide–combining power of the serum.

The anesthetic agent may affect carbohydrate metabolism. Moderate elevation in blood glucose level occurs with cyclopropane and halothane; marked elevation occurs with ether, chloroform, and ethyl chloride; and only minor elevation is associated with nitrous oxide and trichloroethylene anesthesia. The hyperglycemia is related to an increased breakdown of liver glycogen and a concomitant catabolism of muscle glycogen with the formation of lactic acid. Also, the anesthetic agents affecting glucose catabolism cause an exaggerated hyperglycemic epinephrine response and an increased resistance to exogenously administered insulin. It has been suggested that these phenomena are related to activation of the sympathoadrenal system.

The stress of surgical treatment aggravates hyperglycemia because of the increased secretion of epinephrine and glucocorticoids. Increased epinephrine secretion results in an increased breakdown of liver glycogen to glucose, which is released into the general circulation. The glucocorticoids also increase hepatic glucose output via mobilized protein and exert an anti-insulin effect by stimulating a circulating insulin antagonist. The effects of both epinephrine and glucocorticoids are offset to some extent by an increased secretion of endogenous insulin in the normal person but may require the administration of larger doses of insulin in diabetic patients.

MANAGEMENT. In the diabetic patient, essential laboratory studies include hemoglobin determination, white cell count, urinalysis for sugar and acetone, fasting and timed postprandial blood glucose determination, blood urea nitrogen, and, in older patients, serum cholesterol determination and electrocardiography. Diabetic patients should have a preference for an early place on the operative schedule to minimize the effects of fasting and ketosis. Preoperative medication should be kept to a minimum, since diabetic patients, particularly elderly ones, are sensitive to narcotics and sedatives and there is a danger of hypercapnia and hypoxia. The choice of anesthesia should be determined by the operative procedure and the preference of the anesthesiologist. It should not be influenced by the presence of diabetes. It is true, however, that spinal anesthesia has little tendency to evoke hyperglycemia apart from the stress of the operation; among the inhalation anesthetics, nitrous oxide, trichloroethylene, and halothane have the least effect on carbohydrate metabolism. The degree of control is assessed by serial determination of the blood sugar and urinalysis for glycosuria and acetonuria. In general, it is safer to permit mild glycosuria and minimal elevation of the blood sugar level in the paraoperative periods, particularly in the elderly and cardiac patients. In the patient with postoperative hypotension, blood glucose determination should be obtained to rule out hypoglycemia as an etiologic factor.

Mild diabetics frequently do not require insulin, and dietary control is sufficient. The cornerstone of all diabetic management is the dietary or parenteral intake. The preoperative diabetic intake should contain 140 to 200 Gm of carbohydrates, 60 to 100 Gm of protein, and adequate vitamins and minerals, and should furnish 1200 to 2100 kcal daily. If parenteral fluids are required, there is a theoretical advantage to the use of fructose or sorbitol, which can be utilized in amounts up to 50 Gm daily in the diabetic patient. The goal of the dietary or parenteral fluid regimen is to keep the patient free of acetonuria and without excessive hyperglycemia. The patients in whom diabetes is well controlled with oral agents should continue the use of these drugs until the day prior to operation, particularly if the medication is tolbutamide or phenformin. With longer-acting agents, such as chlorpropamide, the drug should be discontinued 72 hours preopera-

tively if the administration of insulin is contemplated. Galloway and Shuman stated that patients who take tolbutamide preoperatively usually require insulin during and immediately after major surgical treatment whereas patients receiving chlorpropamide usually do not require insulin during the immediate paraoperative period.

Insulin Therapy. A variety of programs for the administration of insulin have been proposed. One of the popular methods of treatment employs a regimen in which the daily carbohydrate requirement is divided into four equal doses and given parenterally as 5 to 10% dextrose in water every 6 hours. This initiation of the parenteral glucose infusion is accompanied by the subcutaneous injection of unmodified regular insulin in doses equal to approximately one-fourth the dose of insulin which the patient required prior to operation. Urine is checked regularly, and supplementary doses of crystalline insulin are given as indicated. Based on the extent of glycosuria, 4 to 10 units of additional insulin is provided for each unit of positivity. Larger doses may be indicated when acetonuria, severe stress, infection, or marked hyperglycemia is present. The advantage of this method is that glucose and insulin are given at regular intervals permitting adjustment in the dose during the day. The major disadvantage is that inadvertent interruption of glucose infusion may result in hypoglycemia. With this regimen as with others, slight glycosuria is preferable provided there is no acetonuria.

For more labile diabetics and for patients in whom surgical treatment of great magnitude is anticipated, the use of short-term, unmodified insulin is preferable. In the case of the most labile patients, this regimen may be begun as early as 72 hours prior to operation and is sometimes continued well into the postoperative period. Although the caloric intake is generally less on the day of operation, the normal stress of anesthesia and the operative procedure usually more than compensate for the dietary deficiency. Some writers report having employed regular insulin directly in the intravenous glucose infusion, in doses ranging from 0.16 to 0.2 units/Gm of glucose, depending on the magnitude of the stress of surgical procedures and the fasting blood sugar level. Supplementary doses of 3 to 6 units of regular insulin are then given according to the glucose content of the urine. In general, however, the subcutaneous administration of insulin is preferred, since some of the insulin added to a solution may adhere to the walls of the bottle and tubing.

The second basic regimen is directed at patients who are under control with single-injection therapy employing long-acting insulin and in whom a complicated postoperative course is not anticipated. On the day of operation, the patient receives 50 Gm of glucose in 1,000 ml of solution, and at the time the intravenous solution is started, one-half the daily dose of insulin which previously was required is administered. Following operation and return to the recovery room or ward, the remainder of the usual daily dose of insulin is given subcutaneously. Thus, the amount of insulin given on the day of operation approximates that given the day before. On the day following operation, the usual dose of insulin is given in the morning prior to breakfast or at the time of starting an intravenous infusion. Modifications of this approach employ small doses of regular insulin subcutaneously during the post-operative period based on the extent of glycosuria. Supplementary doses of regular insulin are used if there is evidence of rapid deterioration of the metabolic status. In patients who have been treated with single daily injections and who are not under control prior to operation, conversion to a regimen of soluble insulin is indicated.

Management of Ketoacidosis. The preparation for surgical treatment of a patient with ketoacidosis is critical, and one should keep in mind that ketoacidosis itself may masquerade as a surgical emergency. The patient with frank diabetic coma is no candidate for surgical treatment regardless of the indication. Crystalline insulin should be used in all cases to establish control. Following the determination of the blood sugar level an appropriately large dose of crystalline insulin, occasionally higher than 200 units, is administered. A proportion of this may be given intravenously in an infusion of water and electrolytes. At this stage, the intravenous fluid should not contain glucose. Serial determinations of the blood glucose at 2-hour intervals are carried out, and additional doses of crystalline insulin are given as indicated. There is an associated deficiency of dehydration and electrolyte abnormality which must be corrected, and the ordinary patient with advanced coma will require an average of 2 to 4 or more liters of fluid to overcome the dehydration. The serum potassium should be determined at 6- to 8-hour intervals and potassium added to the fluid in quantities of 40 mEq/L administered at a rate of no greater than 25 mEq/hour. Usually the need for potassium does not exceed 80 mEq. There is generally no need to add glucose to intravenous fluid unless the blood glucose level falls below normal. Lactate solutions are contraindicated in acidosis with shock, since the excretion of lactate may be impaired and lactic acidosis may be potentiated. Gastric atony is a frequent accompaniment of diabetic ketoacidosis, and suction is frequently required to minimize pulmonary aspiration. It is usually possible to correct ketoacidosis in sufficient time so that the patient's surgical status is not compromised.

Nonketotic Hyperglycemic Hyperosmolar Coma. Hyperosmolar dehydration and coma is a relatively uncommon syndrome which usually occurs in elderly diabetic or nondiabetic obese patients and patients receiving total parenteral nutrition. The blood sugar level is frequently above 1,000 mg/100 ml, and ketone bodies are absent from the plasma and urine. Treatment consists of large amounts of hypotonic solutions plus insulin. Marked lowering of the blood sugar level may result with small doses of insulin, and it is recommended that a test dose of 10 units be given to determine responsiveness.

FAT EMBOLISM

Fat embolism is one of the important causes of increased morbidity and mortality in patients with fractures and extensive trauma. A distinction must be made between fat as a pathologically demonstrable phenomenon and fat embolism as a clinical entity. The presence of pulmonary fat embolism is a relatively common accompaniment of trauma, while the clinical entity is an infrequent occurrence. The pathologic entity of fat emboli in the pulmonary capillaries following trauma was described initially by Zenker in 1862. In World War I, Sutton estimated that 10 percent of the wounded suffered from fat embolism, and by 1931, 112 cases in which fat embolism was implicated as the cause of death had been reported. Mallory et al. reported that 65 percent of 60 patients who died of battle wounds in World War II had pulmonary fat embolism, and a similar finding was noted in 39 percent of 79 patients dying from war wounds in the Korean conflict. In 1962, Sevitt described 100 cases of fat embolism, 82 percent of which were related to long bone fractures.

There are two peaks of age distribution: the second and third decades, when fractures of the tibia and fibula are most frequent, and the sixth and seventh decades, at which time fractured hips are common. The occurrence of the pathologic entity of fat embolization is correlated with the degree of injury and survival time. In a study of 300 accident victims, 80 percent of those dying immediately had embolization of varying degrees. In those living up to 6 hours after accident, fat embolism was found in 96 percent of autopsies, and 12 hours after a fatal accident from mechanical trauma, there was not a single case without fat embolism. Massive fat embolism occurred in 26 percent of the cases with one fracture and 44 percent of those with multiple fractures.

In addition to fat embolization associated with extensive trauma, the clinical syndrome has been reported in blast concussion, with liver trauma, in burns, in severe infection (particularly that due to clostridia, which mediate alpha-toxins that disintegrate fat), in closed-chest cardiac massage, with the use of extracorporeal circulation, and following renal transplantation and high-altitude flights.

PATHOGENESIS AND PATHOPHYSIOLOGY. There is disagreement as to whether the embolized fat originates from bone marrow and soft tissue or from circulating blood lipids. The most popular theory, which implicates mechanical causes, proposes that with trauma there is a liberation of liquid fat and intravasation of fat into the vascular channels. Bone, with its high fat content, vascularity, and rigidity, provides an ideal setting. It is theorized that the thin-walled intraosseous veins are prevented from collapsing by their adherence to the bony framework and permit the pressure generated by trauma to force fat into the general circulation. Supporting this theory is the fact that most of the cases of fat embolism occur after fracture of major long bones with high fat content and also the occasional finding that hemopoietic marrow fragments have been found within the lung as an accompaniment of fat embolization.

The second theory is based on physicochemical changes in the circulating blood lipids. It is proposed that the normal emulsion of fat within the plasma is altered to allow coalescence of the chylomicrons into larger fat droplets with subsequent embolization. This is supported by the fact that emboli may be found in nontraumatic conditions and that the chemical makeup of the embolic fat more closely resembles circulating lipids than marrow or depot fat. Several contributing factors are important in the pathogenesis. These include shock, disseminated intravascular coagulation, sepsis, local pressure, and release of kinins.

Circulating fat macroglobules larger than 20 μ in diameter are the offending elements. The lung usually acts as a very effective filter, as evidenced by the observation of Kuhne and Kremser that 95 percent of patients dying of injury had pulmonary involvement while only 23 percent demonstrated systemic fat embolism. Thus, in approximately three-fourths of the patients with fat embolism the lesion is confined to the lung. The first stage is hypoperfusion due to the mechanical effects of the macroglobules and adherent platelets, red cells, and fibrin plus the chemical effects of released serotonin and kinins. Local lipolysis leads to the second stage, chemical pneumonitis. Damage to the alveolar wall interferes with lung surfactant activity. Pathophysiologically, early hyperpnea leads to a transitory respiratory alkalosis, but combined respiratory and metabolic acidosis evolves rapidly. The cardiac effects are related primarily to the increased pulmonary vascular resistance and, to a lesser degree, to diffuse fat embolism within the myocardium itself. If the fat emboli pass through the pulmonary filter to reach the circulation, they may lodge in the cerebral vessels, accounting for central nervous system manifestations, and in the skin, producing the characteristic petechial changes. Although the kidneys are involved quite regularly when there is systemic fat embolism, they are usually not severely damaged.

CLINICAL MANIFESTATIONS. Although pathologic pulmonary fat embolization is a common occurrence, the clinical manifestations are rare. Symptoms characteristically occur within 12 to 48 hours but have been noted as late as 10 days following injury. The main manifestations relate to pulmonary pathology. Before symptoms become apparent, blood gas determinations may define significant hypoxemia. Tachypnea and tachycardia are characteristic. Pulmonary infection may ensue and lead to augmented respiratory symptoms plus manifestations of sepsis. Rarely, massive pulmonary embolization of fat will result in the sudden onset of right heart failure.

Cerebral fat embolism usually does not occur without evidence of pulmonary involvement. Symptoms which suggest cerebral involvement include changes in personality, drowsiness leading to coma, muscle weakness, spasticity, or rigidity, diplopia or blindness, and, rarely, extreme pyrexia. The cerebral manifestations must be differentiated from delirium tremens, cerebral contusion, and epidural hematoma. The lucid interval with cerebral contusion is usually absent, whereas it characteristically lasts 6 to 10 hours with epidural hematoma and 24 hours with fat embolism. Coma may be present immediately with cerebral contusion and evolves rapidly with fat embolism and slowly with an epidural hematoma. Decerebrate rigidity occurs early in fat embolism and is a terminal event with epidural hematoma. Tachypnea and tachycardia are characteristic of fat embolism, whereas the pulse and respiratory rate are slow with epidural hematoma.

The classic physical finding of fat embolism is the appearance of petechial hemorrhages in the capillary plexus of the dermis. They occur in a distinctive pattern over the shoulders, chest, axilla, and, rarely, the abdominal wall and extremities. They may also be noted in the subconjunctival region and on the palate. Petechiae occur as early as the second or third day and as late as the ninth day after injury and are present in 20 percent of patients found at autopsy to have fat embolism. A counterpart to the petechial hemorrhages is evident on funduscopic examination as emboli within the retinal vessels, and there may be streaks of hemorrhage throughout the retina and macular edema. Renal involvement usually does not produce severe damage, and both gross hematuria and impaired function are rare occurrences. Recently, an association with acute peptic ulceration has been noted.

DIAGNOSTIC STUDIES. A sudden and precipitous drop in the hematocrit is frequently noted and has been related to trapping of red cells and occasionally an associated D.I.C. within the pulmonary parenchyma. It may occur as early as the second or third day following injury, just prior to the onset of dyspnea, disorientation, and the appearance of petechial hemorrhages. Thrombocytopenia occurs less frequently. Roentgenographic pulmonary changes are noted in about 36 percent of the cases, and when roentgenograms are taken at intervals following injury, they are helpful in establishing the diagnosis. The characteristic pattern is that of unevenly distributed areas of radiodensity, congestive hilar shadows, and increased bronchovascular markings with dilation of the right side of the heart (Fig. 12-2). Serial measurements of Pa_{O_2} offer a better index of the degree of pulmonary involvement. The electrocardiogram may reveal changes which reflect myocardial ischemia and right ventricular strain. These are usually noted 24 to 48 hours after injury. The important findings are the sudden appearance of a prominent S wave in lead I and prominent Q waves in lead III. Inversion of the T wave indicates severe overloading of the right ventricle. Depression of the RS-T segments suggests subendothelial ischemia. There may be a right bundle branch block. Arrhythmias are frequent. The electroencephalogram may indicate a diffuse slow wave pattern.

Detection of Fat. Lipuria occurs in the first few days following injury and is usually associated with a serious degree of fat embolism. Free fat in the urine has been demonstrated in over 57 percent of cases in one series. Examination of the urine is simple but must be precise. The collecting apparatus must be free of fat, and the bladder must be emptied completely, since the fat floats and the majority of globules remain in the bladder residue. The patient should be catheterized using a non-oily lubricant and the fluid collected in a volumetric flask. The meniscus may be skimmed, or, after centrifugation, the supranatant is smeared and stained with Sudan III. Deep-orange-colored droplets represent fat globules. Another method of demonstrating fat in the urine is the Scuderi "sizzle" test, which involves placing a wire loop containing the supranatant fluid over a flame and listening for a pop or sizzle produced by burning fat. The fat can be detected in concentrations as small as 1:1,000. The demonstration of fat in the sputum has little diagnostic value, since it is a common phenomenon following trauma. Biopsy of petechiae may establish the diagnosis, and frozen section is mandatory to determine the presence of fat. Needle biopsy of the kidney also has been applied to demonstrate fat globules.

Serum Lipase. A serum lipase level elevation occurs in about 50 percent of the cases, the rise usually beginning on the third day and reaching a maximum on the seventh or eighth day after injury. An elevation greater than 1 ml is significant, and this determination is considered by Peltier to be the best laboratory test between the third and seventh day. The serum lipase level can be suppressed by the administration of ethyl alcohol and augmented by heparinization. Once elevated, the level is thought to reflect the prognosis, and elevations greater than 2 ml are associated with a higher incidence of favorable outcome. In a patient with extensive trauma, an elevated serum lipase level in the first 48 hours is more suggestive of pancreatitis.

TREATMENT. Prophylaxis against potentiating fat embolization includes careful handling of the patient and early splinting of fractures. Vigorous applications of resuscitative measures are indicated to correct oligemic shock, since it has been demonstrated that fewer emboli may be lethal in the hypotensive than in the normotensive patient. There is some suggestion that Trasylol, which inhibits the effect of kinins and antagonizes hypercoagulability, may prevent or reduce the extent of the fat embolism syndrome. High doses of corticosteroids (1.0 to 1.5 Gm hydrocortisone) administered during the first 2 days may inhibit the pneumonitis or expedite its resolution. Pulmonary manifestations are treated with oxygen therapy, rapid digitalization, and intensive endotracheal suction to minimize the accumulation of secretions. IPPB or PEEP are frequently indicated. Pa_{O_2} should be monitored and maintained between 80 and 100 mm Hg. Endotracheal intubation is preferred over tracheostomy, since the latter has been associated with a high mortality rate in these patients. Cerebral manifestations are treated with sedation and anticonvulsive therapy.

Trasylol has been beneficial in several instances. Heparin in doses which do not have an anticoagulant effect will clear lipemic plasma and stimulate lipase activity. A dose of 5,000 units may be administered intravenously every 6 hours. In the presence of acute systemic toxicity or a rapidly rising lipase level, the drug should be discontinued, since the release of fatty acids is undesirable. Low-molecular-weight dextran (40,000) has been administered intravenously to counteract intravascular thrombosis. One thousand milliliters is administered per 24 hours for two days. Ethyl alcohol, which may decrease the rate of hydrolysis of neutral fat and slow the release of toxic free fatty acids, has been used. Presently, this applicability of alcohol is debatable.

PROGNOSIS. Old age, preexisting lung disease, and reduced cardiac reserve have adverse effects. The early appearance of marked hypoxemia and the requirement of persistently high Fi_{O_2} are bad prognostic signs, as is hypocalcemia resulting from ion binding by FFA, while a persistently high serum lipase level is a favorable sign. At the Birmingham Accident Hospital, a fatality rate of 12 per-

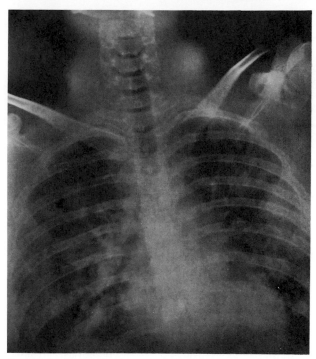

Fig. 12-2. Pulmonary fat emboli. Note bilateral extensive ill-defined nodular densities situated primarily in peripheral lung fields. Patient was in an automobile accident and fractured his femur and two metatarsals. Twenty-four hours after admission fever developed, and 3 days later hemoptysis and mental confusion. Changes were seen roentgenographically on the fourth day after trauma. There were lipid bodies in the urine, and the serum lipase level was elevated. The patient was treated with antibiotics, heparin, and dextran, and the symptoms subsided 7 days after therapy.

cent has been reported for 25 cases diagnosed according to strict criteria (all had petechial rash). While the "pure" cerebral form of the fat embolism syndrome generally has a better prognosis, the presence of coma is a poor sign. Acute respiratory disease usually is self-limiting.

PSYCHIATRIC COMPLICATIONS

Severe psychiatric disturbances may occur any time during an illness, but their appearance in the postoperative period is particularly significant. The first account of postoperative psychiatric disturbance presented by a surgeon was that of Dupuytren who, in 1834, wrote that "the brain itself may be overcome by pain, terror, or even joy and reason leaves the patient at the instant when it is most necessary to his welfare that he should remain calm and undisturbed." In 1910, Da Costa indicated that the anticipated frequency for such complications is as high as 1 in 250 laparotomies, while Lewis, more recently, suggested an incidence of 1 in 1,500. Scott described 11 cases in 2,000 surgical procedures. The validity of any of these figures, however, is open to question, since "postoperative psychosis" per se does not appear in the standard nomenclature and is frequently not coded on the patient's record, thus limiting the value of retrospective studies. Even more pertinent for surgical consideration is the study of Titchener et al., who evaluated 200 patients admitted to the surgical service of the Cincinnati General Hospital utilizing interview and the Minnesota Multiphasic Personality Inventory to substantiate a psychiatric diagnosis. Eighty-six percent of the sample had either distressing psychologic symptoms, disabling patterns of behavior, or both. The patients considered were in a municipal hospital and represented a lower socioeconomic group, but the figures of 21 percent having neuroses, 11 percent psychophysiologic reactions, 14 percent psychoses, 34 percent character behavior disorders, and 3 percent chronic brain syndrome are most impressive.

GENERAL CONSIDERATIONS. "Postoperative psychosis" cannot be considered as a distinct clinical entity. No single factor has been shown to be responsible, and the physical illness and operative procedure may merely bring to light a latent psychotic tendency. Both illness, particularly when prolonged, and surgical procedures represent threats to the integrity of the organism on somatic and psychologic grounds. In nearly every person informed of the need for a surgical procedure, some degree of anxiety arises. There may be fear of loss of life, of loss of body part, and of castration as with pelvic and hernia operations. The anxiety signal is assimilated and integrated by the patient in preparation for the surgical stress. Surgical intervention to cure, modify, or prevent illness is the beginning of a complicated and multifaceted process. The psychodynamic processes at work during the preoperative, postoperative, and convalescent periods may be classified as (1) psychophysiologic factors, (2) somatopsychic factors, and (3) psychosocial factors. Psychophysiologic factors represent processes originating from psychologic stress which act along neurogenic or humoral pathways to modify the healing process. A poorly functioning gastroenterostomy or marginal ulcer in a patient with emotional stress represents an example of this type. The somatopsychic factors have to do with the psychologic adaptation involved when the surgical procedure imposes a somatic defect, such as an ileostomy or colostomy. The psychosocial factors refer to the patient's concern with the effects of his physical illness or surgical procedure on his ultimate position in society. All these may interplay and contribute to anxiety, neurotic symptoms, severe depression, and frank psychosis.

CLINICAL MANIFESTATIONS. The time of occurrence of psychiatric derangement during illness is variable, and the duration of latent interval between surgical treatment and the psychologic disturbance may be days to weeks. Winkelstein and associates reported that, in the recovery room, patients who had been subjected to surgical procedures under general anesthesia exhibited a lack of concern about the operation and an absence of affective response, despite the fact that they were sufficiently oriented to be interviewed. After 24 hours the patients responded with these concerns and emotions which were so conspicuously absent in the immediate postoperative period. Both psychologic and pharmacologic factors are implicated in this response, since patients under spinal anesthesia exhibit immediate and overt emotional reaction.

The manifestations are extremely variable. Fear may be accompanied by depression or elation and overactivity. The clinical picture may be that of acute delirium with confusion and disorientation or merely a vague alteration in perception and mood. The manic type of reaction may incorporate psychomotor excitement, delirium, delusions, visual or auditory hallucinations, agitated depression, and feelings of persecution. The psychotic reactions which were observed in 44 of 200 patients in the Cincinnati series are indistinguishable from the range of psychoses observed under other circumstances. The acute brain syndrome, or delirium, was manifest in 20 patients.

Delirium may begin with an inappropriate remark or a dramatic agitated outburst and is frequently the first sign of continued mental deterioration leading to a chronic brain syndrome, particularly in an elderly patient. Therefore, delirium must be regarded as a potentially dangerous situation. It occurs most commonly in elderly patients who have lost closeness and support of family or friends and in patients who are immobilized for long periods of time.

Depressive reactions represented the second most important psychosis in surgical patients and occurred in 4.5 percent of patients in the Cincinnati series. The patient is characteristically uncooperative in an active way, or recovery may be impeded by listlessness, anorexia, and disinterest. The depressive reaction may be accompanied by physiologic changes; Moore et al. have demonstrated the effects of emotion on the pituitary-adrenal axis during the immediate and subsequent postoperative period. Suicide is a major risk in patients with depressive reaction.

Another category includes the paranoid psychotic disorder. Although it is not rare for schizophrenic reaction to have its onset in the surgical patient, no acute breaks of the schizophrenic type were noted among the 200 patients studied by Titchener et al. Generally, there is no contraindication to surgical treatment of patients with schizophrenia. Manic excitement is a particularly difficult problem in the management of surgical patients and requires the close cooperation of psychiatrist, surgeon, and anesthetist.

MANAGEMENT. The first step in the management of psychiatric disturbances occurring in the course of the surgical illness or following surgical procedures is that of anticipation. Although Knox has indicated that the incidence of postoperative psychosis was not related to the duration of preoperative hospital stay, the duration of illness, particularly when prolonged, does determine the patient's psychologic reaction to surgical experience. At the other end of the spectrum, sudden emergency operation often results in reactions marked by acute anxiety, nightmares, insomnia, irritability, and protective withdrawal from all stimuli. Age is an important factor, the highest incidence occurring in children under the age of two and in the elderly patients. In the latter group, this is particularly true of patients who have lost their proximity to and support of family and friends, and who have not developed a close relation with the hospital personnel. Knox has presented evidence of constitutional predisposition, and although 17 percent of his patients had had previous surgical treatment uncomplicated by psychiatric disturbances, 11 percent did have a previous psychiatric illness. Twenty-two percent of patients had a family history of mental illness of serious proportion. There is an increasing incidence of delirium in response to anesthesia and surgical treatment in patients who are alcoholic, while patients suffering from extensive trauma may have organic psychosis. Acidosis, acetonuria, hyperglycemia, and hepatic insufficiency may all cause postoperative mental aberrations, and cerebral hypoxia frequently results in behavioral changes. Medications, such as barbiturates, anticholinergics, and cortisone, also have been implicated.

There is an obvious need for integrating psychologic treatment with the management of surgical patients. As Titchener and Levine emphasize, it is not necessary, possible, or advisable for these needs to be turned over to psychiatrists, and it is frequently preferable that the measures be carried out by the surgeon in charge. Verbal communication between the surgeon and patient is the best means of overcoming emotional or mental difficulty. The anesthetist is regarded as an impersonal distant figure who carries out his task without emotional impact on the patient. The surgeon should become aware of the patient's feelings and attitudes and be appreciative of the effects of these factors on a patient's general well-being. Also, changes to increase the patient's positive adaptation to his illness should be constantly considered. The striking incidence of significant postoperative disturbance suggests the need for "mental check" to be incorporated into the usual postoperative surgical rounds. Efforts should be directed at removing toxic causes of the acute brain syndrome, removing undue stimuli without isolating the patient, and providing psychologic or pharmacologic tranquilization.

The physician's psychologic approach should include repeated reassurance of the patient. In some instances, specific counseling and directive treatment, which may require direct intervention in the patient's personal or family affairs and the assistance of the social service department, is indicated. The best prophylactic therapy, however, can be classified as supportive, in that the surgeon allows himself to be the object of dependency on the part of the patient. This relationship is fostered by interest on the part of the surgeon and trust on the part of the patient.

The provocative patient who emits anger or attempts to irritate others as a mechanism for covering fear or relieving guilt needs understanding of the emotional reason for the provocation and an attitude of firmness rather than anger from the physician. The attempt on the part of a patient to sign out against advice is a mechanism of expressing anger or fear and should be handled by the surgeon in such a way that the patient is allowed to change his mind without becoming embarrassed. In these and other situations, the patient may hide his real feeling behind an intellectual screen. For understanding himself, the patient must bring forth both the emotional and intellectual aspects of his personality.

Consultation with a psychiatrist is indicated in the case of any acute and severe emotional disturbance, and the referral should be candidly discussed between the surgeon and the patient. It is necessary for the patient to come to the conclusion that he requires expert help for his problems. Referral is also indicated for long-standing disturbances discovered during hospitalization and is frequently appropriate in patients with psychosomatic illness. Browning and Houseworth, in a study of patients with peptic ulcer, demonstrated that the removal of symptoms without altering the psychosomatic disorders led to the formation of a new spectrum of symptoms.

Special Surgical Situations

The very young and old patients are particularly vulnerable to the development of psychiatric complications following surgical treatment. Psychotic disturbances have been found in 2 to 3 percent of patients following cataract extraction. The combination of surgical procedure and the awareness of the implications of the illness is critical in the patient with cancer. Because of the high incidence of emotional disorders following surgical procedures, special consideration is indicated for mastectomy and gynecologic procedures, cardiac surgical treatment, dialysis and transplantation, and prolonged periods in an intensive care unit. The management of drug addicts is assuming greater importance.

PEDIATRIC SURGERY

In children, severe anxiety states may be precipitated by the shock of operation. Levy reported that of a group of 124 children who had operations, 20 percent showed residual emotional disturbances. This occurred most frequently in the one- to two-year-old group; after the age of three there was a sharp decrease with age. The age distribution was attributed to a greater dependence on home and mother, and Levy went so far as to suggest postponement of elective surgical treatment until the child could comprehend something about the situation. Postoperative reactions consisted of negativism, disobedience, tantrums, defiance, destructive behavior, and dependency, as manifested by clinging to the mother or attendant. The responses have been related to a feeling of betrayal and the consequent desire for revenge and rebellion. When a child is suffering from fears engendered by an operation, a second operation usually intensifies the earlier fears.

Prophylactic therapy is important. The maturity of the child's emotional adaptation is more a factor in the response than the operation per se. Parental absence is frequently associated with emotional difficulty. Prugh and associates compared two groups, one treated without organized consideration for emotional needs and another in which these needs were considered and ample opportunity for play was provided. Moderate or severe anxiety reactions, immediately after leaving the hospital, were observed in 92 percent of the control group and in 68 percent of the experimental group, with a peak incidence in children under three. Three months after discharge, the incidence of persisting anxiety had fallen to 58 percent for the control group and 44 percent for the experimental group. The youngest children reacted more severely with apprehension, feeding disturbances, and depression. The pattern for the four- to six-year-old group was a tendency toward obsessive worries, phobias, and accentuated aches and pains. The six- to ten-year-olds manifested conversion symptoms, compulsive behavior, and restlessness.

SURGERY IN THE AGED

Elderly patients are more prone to become emotionally disturbed when confronted with new situations, especially if they have inadequate comprehension and a generalized feeling of insecurity. The operative procedure also presents an obvious physical threat to the integrity of the nervous system. Titchener and associates reported a 25 percent incidence of significant and, at times, irreversible change in cerebral function in the patients in their group over the age of sixty-five. Some degree of depression was observed in 90 percent of the older patients, and this was of a disabling nature in about 50 percent. Indifference of the family, friends, and society contributed to the evolution of a paranoid cycle.

Attempts should be directed at limiting the physical insult to the brain, and postoperative mental evaluation is indicated on a routine basis in order to detect the early changes of the organic brain syndrome and delirium. Efforts should be made to familiarize the patients with the hospital and personnel, and visitors should be encouraged to maintain a human contact and prevent withdrawal. Collaboration with a social worker is frequently indicated for long-term rehabilitation.

GYNECOLOGIC SURGERY

Removal of the breast and a variety of gynecologic procedures are highly represented in most series of postoperative psychosis. Hysterectomy is associated with emotional disturbance more frequently than other gynecologic operations, and the more the procedure antedates the menopause, the more the likelihood of associated psychologic disturbance. The loss of menstrual function is perceived by the woman as a blow to normal feminine esteem. Hollender reported that of 203 women admitted to psychiatric hospital, 9 had pelvic surgical treatment as a precipitating event, and this was in contrast to a total of 5 women admitted following operations of all other kinds. Lindemann noted that the relative frequency of restlessness, insomnia, agitation, and preoccupation with depressive thoughts was greater after pelvic operations than after cholecystectomy.

CANCER PATIENTS

The cancer patient is exposed to two major threats, disease and extensive surgical treatment. He is concerned with death or injury during operation and disruption of his pattern of living as a result of the effects of cancer or the surgical procedure. Patients with emotional problems involving self-destruction are particularly vulnerable to preoperative anxiety concerning death and mutilation.

This may be manifest by anorexia, insomnia, tachycardia, fear, and panic. Acute depression with suicidal tendencies has been reported in anticipation of surgical procedures. Postoperatively, depression is related to an anticipated interference with valued activities. Sutherland and associates have demonstrated that colostomy imposed on almost all patients a new order of living, and the subjects were powerfully motivated to avoid social rejection. A rigid life arose from the fearful expectation of rejection because of the colostomy combined with the fear of death from cancer. There is a tendency toward seclusion, withdrawal, and nonparticipation. Spells of depression are frequent, and Sutherland and his associates are of the opinion that loss of an important bodily part or function is more depressing than the fear or expectation of death. The management of patients with carcinoma must be based on an appreciation that they frequently suffer a sense of isolation, guilt, and abandonment.

CARDIAC SURGERY

Serious psychiatric disturbances have been observed to occur with considerable frequency following mitral valvulotomy and open heart surgery. Fox and associates and Bliss et al. reported, respectively, a 19 and 16 percent incidence of serious emotional disturbance following mitral valve surgery. In contrast, Bolton and Bailey, in an evaluation of 1,500 consecutive patients, noted an incidence of psychosis of 3 percent with no relation to age, sex, severity of heart disease, duration of failure, or complications of surgical treatment. Egerton and Kay noted delirium in 25 of 60 adults following open heart surgery.

Manifestations generally occur after an initial lucid interval 3 to 5 days after operation and clear shortly after the patient is transferred from an intensive care unit to a standard hospital ward. Postoperative incapacitation and increased time on the heart-lung machine apparently are factors increasing the likelihood of delirium, while age and sex do not alter the incidence. Zaks has suggested that cardiac operation may produce organic brain damage, thus sensitizing patients and increasing the incidence of postoperative psychologic symptomatology. A prediction equation was successful in differentiating reactors from nonreactors. Using the ego strength variable of the Minnesota Multiphasic Personality Inventory, there is a significant inverse correlation between the reaction and the incidence of acute psychotic episodes following cardiac operation. The incidence of psychoses is greater in males, older patients, and those expressing minimal preoperative anxiety. A preoperative psychiatric interview reduces the incidence of postoperative psychosis by 50 percent.

Following operations on the heart, the patients with emotional disturbances manifest perceptual distortion, visual and auditory hallucinations, disorientation, and paranoia. Twenty-eight percent of adult patients subjected to open heart surgery, as reported by Egerton and Kay, had delirious states ranging in duration from several nights to several weeks, averaging 5 days. The delirious patients had no psychologic sequelae, and no relation could be established between the incidence of delirium and the duration of cardiac bypass, but open heart procedures were more likely to produce delirium than other intrathoracic operations. The writers felt that the precipitating factors for delirium included dehydration, hyponatremia, and the performance of a tracheostomy, while the predisposing factors included a familial history of psychosis, previous brain damage, overwhelming personal problems, and the presence of a rheumatic valvular lesion. Other psychiatric disturbances noted in patients following open heart surgery were disabling anxiety state, conversion hysteria, tension headaches, and, in a surprising 5 percent of the operative cases, exacerbation of peptic ulcer. The almost total absence of delirium and other emotional disorders in children is of particular interest and may be related to the fact that the concept of death as a permanent biologic process usually does not develop until the age of nine.

DIALYSIS AND TRANSPLANTATION

A variety of emotional disturbances has been observed in patients undergoing hemodialysis. The suicide rate is 300 times greater than for a comparable healthy population. Uremia, debilitating disease, and the repeated technical procedures which are performed all constitute etiologic factors. Wright et al. followed 11 patients on chronic dialysis and noted a number of stresses affecting them, such as unpredictability of well-being, tensions arising in the marital situation from guilt and anger, effects of separation on the families, and financial anxiety. Following each episode of dialysis, the main patient response was one of relief. Cramond and associates noted that their patients at first denied their illness and later realized that they had lost their health and independence and their futures were uncertain. This has been referred to as a "mourning reaction." From time to time the patients wished to be dead. They felt that life dependent on chronic dialysis was not worth living. Some patients passed from the mourning reaction to a state of active depression.

All patients undergoing dialysis become extremely dependent on the staff and emotionally attached to them. The patients often react emotionally to a sense of loss when any replacement of staff occurs. During the course of the dialysis program, regression occurs relatively frequently, and the patient becomes withdrawn and pretends to sleep. Insomnia and frightening dreams also occur, and the frequency with which emotional disturbances have been noted suggests that psychiatric assistance plays an important role in a dialysis program.

Two distinct groups of patients, the donors and recipients, must be considered in a renal homotransplantation program. Psychologic screening of the potential donors is indicated, and selection should be from individuals who are stable and who have mature judgment. Individuals with psychopathologic motives such as sacrifice or exhibitionism should be excluded, particularly when they are unrelated donors. It is to be emphasized that those who refuse to cooperate risk being rejected by the family and are frequently made to feel guilty. Therefore, when potential donors are rejected on psychiatric grounds, the rejection should be ascribed to a minor physical variation. In

four of five cases, Cramond noted an ambivalent relationship between the donor and recipient. The donor experienced emotional and physical investment in the patient and, at times, sought to overprotect the patient. He felt that his sacrificial gift was in jeopardy if the patient behaved in a manner with which he did not approve.

The recipient has been shown to be aware of his obligation to the donor and resents the dependency relationship. At times feelings of shame and guilt must be considered. Kemph, in a follow-up of recipients of renal homotransplants, has noted periods of severe depression and concern with bodily damage and sexual damage. After the operation the donors also experience depression. Many expressed the feeling that they were not attentively supported by the hospital personnel.

Some recipients regard the operation as symbolic of rebirth and may undergo a religious conviction. In some recipients, a graft from a donor of an opposite sex is considered a threat to sexual identity. All recipients demonstrate anxiety in reference to injury of the grafted kidney. Although severe depressions and emotional reactions are uncommon, psychologic adjustment takes longer than a year to accomplish. When given a choice, patients who have rejected their kidney transplants have almost uniformly chosen a second transplant over return to dialysis.

INTENSIVE CARE DELIRIUM

Delirium manifested by a wide variety of behavior patterns, ranging from apathy to restlessness and combativeness, is a common occurrence in intensive care units. Both environmental and metabolic factors have been implicated. The former can be corrected by transferring the patient to a regular hospital ward or room as soon as possible. Katz et al. indicated a physiologic abnormality, such as hypoxemia or electrolyte or acid-base abnormality, as the cause in the great majority of patients.

DRUG ABUSE

Beebe and Keats have shown that not all narcotic addicts require detoxification associated with an operation. Methadone is the drug of choice for treating withdrawal. Haloxone may be preferable in an emergency situation. For patients on methadone maintenance, this drug can be stopped temporarily and frequent doses of conventional narcotics substituted during the early postoperative period. Withdrawal from barbiturates prior to elective operation may take 2 to 3 weeks. There is no physiologic addiction requiring maintenance of amphetamines or hallucinogens.

COMPLICATIONS OF GASTROINTESTINAL SURGERY

The gastrointestinal complications considered in this section are divided into (1) vascular complications, including hemorrhage and gangrene; (2) mechanical problems of gastroenterostomy and enteroenterostomy, including stomal obstruction, the afferent, or blind, loop syndrome, extrinsic obstruction and internal hernia, and inadvertant gastroileostomy; (3) leakage of an anastomosis, including the duodenal stump blowout; (4) external fistulas and stomal problems; and (5) damage to adjacent organs, including postoperative pancreatitis and jaundice.

Vascular Complications

HEMORRHAGE

Gastrointestinal hemorrhage which occurs subsequent to a gastrointestinal anastomosis may become manifest postoperatively by hematemesis, melena, hematochezia, or, most frequently, the passage of bright blood via a nasogastric tube positioned in the stomach. Bleeding from the suture line is most commonly associated with gastric surgery, occurring in approximately 1 percent of patients following gastric resection, with a higher incidence in those patients in whom operation is performed for a duodenal ulcer. Bleeding from the suture line is apt to occur either immediately after the operation or on the first postoperative day, but a second minor peak in incidence has been noted between the seventh and tenth postoperative days. Bleeding arising from the suture line on the first postoperative day is usually minimal or moderate and requires no specific therapy, but if it is continuous, the stomach should be aspirated and irrigated with ice-cold saline solution. Hemorrhage which does not stop following conservative measures constitutes an indication for laparotomy, at which time the suture line should be inspected. It may be preferable to enter the stomach above the line of anastomosis and ligate vessels from within. Bleeding later in the course of convalescence is usually due to sloughing from the suture line and generally responds to iced saline lavage. Significant hemorrhage from the suture line of small intestinal and large intestinal anastomoses is extremely rare. Upper gastrointestinal bleeding following a surgical procedure in a patient who is debilitated or in whom sepsis develops frequently indicates a stress ulcer (see Chap. 26).

GANGRENE

Gangrene is a rare complication of resection of a segment of gastrointestinal tract, since the intestine is supplied with a rich network of arteries. Necrosis of the gastric remnant has been reported following a high subtotal gastrectomy, particularly if the procedure incorporates ligation of the left gastric artery and concomitant splenectomy. Devascularization of the areas to be anastomosed should not occur following small intestinal surgical procedures if attention is directed toward the vascular supply. A precautionary measure is to slant the lines of incision so that more intestine is resected on the antimesenteric aspect. Small intestinal gangrene is more frequently due to mechanical strangulation, obstruction secondary to postoperative adhesions, volvulus, internal hernias, or vascular thrombosis. Gangrene of the segment of intestine may be apparent in the case of a colostomy in which an inadequate vascular supply has been provided.

In each instance, the recognition of gangrene requires resection of the gangrenous segment of intestine or stom-

ach and reestablishment of intestinal continuity or a colostomy in bowel which is viable.

Mechanical Problems

STOMAL OBSTRUCTION

Although obstruction of the stoma may follow any intestinal anastomosis as a result of technical factors, postgastrectomy stomal obstruction represents the most common type and is frequently related to local edema. Factors which have been implicated in the etiology of edema include electrolyte depletion, hypochloremia, incomplete hemostasis, hypoproteinemia, leakage from the anastomosis, inadequate proximal decompression, and incorporation of too much tissue within the sutures. Other causes include rotation of the jejunum on its long axis, obstruction by the transverse mesocolon, particularly in an obese patient, obstruction by a fatty omentum, effect of vagotomy, and, rarely, jejunogastric intussusception, which has been reported as a complication in slightly over 100 cases of Billroth II procedures.

Postgastrectomy stomal obstruction is a most troublesome complication, and the reported incidence has ranged between 1 and 3 percent. Magnuson and associates indicated an almost identical incidence of 3 percent subsequent to gastrectomy for gastric ulcer as compared with gastrectomy for duodenal ulcer. Hibner and Richards, in a review of 648 partial gastrectomies, noted an incidence of 4.6 percent for patients requiring further operative therapy, 4.1 percent for Billroth II operations, and 3.5 percent for Billroth I types. In most instances in their series, the efferent loop was obstructed by the transverse mesocolon.

Symptoms usually occur on the third to fourth postoperative day, at which time there is abdominal fullness and increased return from the nasogastric suction. If the patient has been on oral intake, nausea followed by vomiting of large quantities of bile-colored gastric fluid occurs. Instillation of barium or Gastrografin via the nasogastric tube may reveal stomal obstruction or a patent stoma with distal loop obstruction. The symptoms usually persist for only short intervals and cause little disability, but occasionally they are prolonged and then have severe metabolic effects.

Prophylaxis is directed at avoiding the factors which have been implicated. Therapy of established stomal obstruction consists of adequate decompression and replacement of fluids and nutrients, while waiting for the obstruction to become relieved spontaneously. The course may be prolonged, extending over a period of several weeks. If there is not relief after extended conservative management or if the patient's condition is deteriorating, operative intervention is indicated. Rarely, a simple release of adhesions may be therapeutic, but more often the anastomotic site requires revision, a procedure which is frequently difficult in view of the extensive reaction around the stoma. It is generally preferable to transect the proximal and distal loops of intestine at their entrance to and exit from the indurated mass. These are then anastomosed to one another, and the short segment of intestine and a cuff of stomach are removed with the gastroenterostomy. Continuity is reestablished with a long antecolic gastrojejunostomy.

AFFERENT (BLIND) LOOP SYNDROME

The blind loop syndrome is a consequence of small intestinal surgical procedures and is presented in Chap. 27. The present discussion is concerned with the afferent loop syndrome which represents a complication of subtotal gastrectomy with Billroth II gastroenterostomy. The afferent loop consists of duodenum and a segment of jejunum of variable length. Acute or chronic obstruction can occur at any point proximal to the gastrojejunostomy. The incidence is difficult to estimate and is dependent upon the criteria for diagnosis. Quinn and Gifford reported five cases in 500 gastrectomies, while Blomstedt and Dahlgren reported an incidence of 18 percent with mild to moderate symptoms (type I and type II). The symptom complex of partial obstruction of the afferent loop was reported by Magnuson et al. to occur following gastrectomy in 4.2 percent of patients with gastric ulcer in contrast to 0.9 percent of patients with duodenal ulcer.

PATHOGENESIS. Normally after partial gastrectomy, biliary and pancreatic secretions enter the afferent loop, pass through the gastrojejunostomy to mix with gastric juice, and then pass through into the efferent loop. During a 24-hour period, approximately 1 to 1.5 liters of secretion enters the afferent loop. The afferent loop syndrome is caused by partial and, rarely, total obstruction of flow from the afferent loop. The pressure within the duodenum and segment of jejunum rises, and the loop becomes dilated by bile and pancreatic juice. After the ingestion of food, particularly a fatty meal, the duodenal contents increase rapidly, thus explaining the postcibal nature of the syndrome. With incomplete obstruction, pressure within the intestine eventually becomes sufficient to overcome resistance, and the contents are emptied into the stomach, causing variable amounts to be vomited. With total obstruction, the loop no longer has any communication with the stomach, and vomitus is free of bile.

CLINICAL MANIFESTATIONS. The symptoms of partial obstruction of the afferent loop occur most commonly in the early postoperative period. Two-thirds of the cases occur during the first week, but in some instances the syndrome becomes apparent months to years following gastrectomy. The symptoms vary in intensity and are characterized by postcibal vomiting. Mild symptoms consist of eructation of a mouthful of green biliary fluid within an hour and a half after a meal. Vomiting is generally preceded by the sensation of fullness and, at times, pain in the epigastrium. In some instances, the symptoms of chronic obstruction persist for several months, and the amount of biliary vomiting and antecedent epigastric pain are appreciable. With persistence of partial obstruction, the stools become bulky and gray, and contain much fat. Roentgenographic examination may show passage of contrast material into the efferent loop, while the afferent loop, as a rule, fails to fill. Chronic partial obstruction is associated with anemia, and the vitamin B_{12} absorption test may provide the diagnosis. Urinary excretion of B_{12} is reduced or absent and is unaffected by the administration of intrinsic factor, in contrast to pernicious anemia. However, following a course of 3 to 5 days of tetracycline, B_{12} urinary excretion returns to normal.

In the rare situation of the acute complete obstruction of the afferent loop, the patient becomes acutely ill with severe epigastric pain, and bile is characteristically absent from the vomitus. A mass may be felt in the upper abdomen. The patient's condition may deteriorate rapidly, and shock may occur as a result of compromise of the circulation of the duodenal wall and/or perforation with generalized peritonitis. Roentgenograms are of little diagnostic assistance. There may be delayed emptying of contrast material from the gastric remnant, and no barium enters the afferent loop. The amylase level may be markedly elevated.

TREATMENT. Incomplete obstruction generally subsides on a conservative regimen. Capper and Welbourn collected 44 cases requiring surgical intervention and reported that 36 of them had a good outcome. Surgical decompression of the afferent loop may be accomplished by anastomosis between the afferent and efferent loops, by employing a Roux en Y anastomosis or converting a gastrojejunostomy to a gastroduodenostomy. In the case of acute total obstruction, early operation with decompression of the afferent loop is mandatory.

INTESTINAL OBSTRUCTION

Intestinal obstruction in the immediate postoperative period is most frequently due to ileus or fibrinous adhesions; however, a variety of mechanical causes should be considered. Internal herniation represents a complication of subtotal gastrectomy, generally following a Billroth II antecolic anastomosis. Internal herniation of the small intestine may also take place through improperly closed mesenteric rents or when the mesentery of the ileum or colon is not tacked to the peritoneum in the course of an ileostomy or colostomy. Closed-loop obstruction generally results and may rapidly progress to compromise the vascular supply with ultimate perforation. Operative reduction and repair of an internal hernia are required. Adhesions and/or volvulus may occur in the postoperative hospitalization and require surgical intervention for relief of obstruction. The incidence is particularly high following resection for congenital atresia in infancy, especially when the proximal dilated bowel is not resected. Postoperative intussusception, generally involving the small intestine, is also to be considered in the pediatric age group.

INADVERTENT GASTROILEOSTOMY

The error of anastomosing the stomach to the ileum rather than the jejunum is fortunately uncommon. In 1949, Moretz indicated that 27 cases were recorded in the literature. The situation results in a malabsorption syndrome which begins as soon as the patient is allowed to eat solid food. Diarrhea, weight loss, and inanition in the absence of abdominal pain are characteristic. The stool contains a high percentage of undigested food and a large quantity of unabsorbed fat. Fecal vomiting and hemorrhage occasionally occur, and an ulcer may develop at the site of the ileum, in which case abdominal pain may be present. The diagnosis can be established roentgenographically by demonstrating a rapid transit and short distal intestine. The error should be avoided by using the ligament of Treitz as a landmark in establishing a gastroenterostomy; in the absence of a ligament of Treitz an anomaly of rotation should be suspected, and the loop of intestine for anastomosis should be selected by tracing the duodenum distad or the small bowel proximally from the cecum. The preoperative management of patients with gastroileostomy requires a vigorous preparation, and a preliminary feeding jejunostomy is of value in these cases. A block resection of the gastroileostomy is advocated for patients who have had subtotal gastric resection, while, in the absence of gastric resection, the ileostomy may be taken down directly. A gastrojejunostomy and reconstitution of intestinal continuity are then performed.

Anastomotic Leak

Suture line leakage represents a potential complication of any intestinal anastomosis. The three prime etiologic factors are (1) poor surgical technique, (2) distal obstruction, and (3) inadequate proximal decompression. Leak from an enteroenterostomy becomes manifest as localized or generalized peritonitis. Small leaks with localized response may be treated by proximal decompression and administration of appropriate antibiotics, while large leaks and diffuse peritonitis frequently require surgical intervention. Fistulization may develop as a tract becomes established between the point of leakage and the skin. A leak from the line of anastomosis is a relatively rare complication following gastroenterostomy. Such leakage occurs more frequently when there has been impairment of the blood supply of the residual gastric pouch and a concomitant splenectomy has been performed. A common point at which leaks develop has been referred to as the "angle du mort," where the residual gastric pouch of a Hofmeister closure meets the line of anastomosis of the small intestine.

Duodenal stump leakage (blowout) is a more frequent and critical complication of gastric resection. A review of gastrectomies performed at the Mayo Clinic in 1956 revealed that 4.5 percent of patients subjected to the procedure for gastric ulcer had some evidence of leak, while 5.6 percent of patients in whom the same procedure was carried out for duodenal ulcer revealed similar evidence. In that study, drains had been inserted into the stump region, and in many patients increased drainage represented the evidence of a leak. Edmunds et al. indicate that a review of gastrectomies performed at the Massachusetts General Hospital from 1946 to 1959 showed that an incidence of dehiscence of the stump was 1.1 percent and the mortality due to this cause was 0.6 percent.

Duodenal stump leakage occurs most commonly after operation for a duodenal ulcer and frequently when gastrectomy is performed as an emergency procedure to stop hemorrhage. In a great majority of cases, the leak arises as a result of a technical error and failure of the suture line. A scarred and edematous duodenum predisposes to the complication, as does obstruction of the afferent loop and local pancreatitis. Complications of duodenal leakage include peritonitis, subhepatic abscess, pancreatitis, sepsis, and establishment of an external fistula with fluid and electrolyte abnormalities.

Specific measures can be taken to avoid this complication. Before embarking on a gastric resection, the surgeon should be as sure as possible that the duodenal stump can be safely closed. In the face of marked inflammatory disease in the duodenal region, vagotomy and gastroenterostomy definitely represent safer procedures. When resection has been undertaken and duodenal closure is difficult, catheter duodenostomy may be used as an adjunct. Rodkey and Welch reported that in 51 cases with difficult duodenal stump closures in whom planned duodenostomy was carried out, there was only one death, and only five patients had drainage from the fistula that lasted more than 48 hours after the catheter was removed. As a compromise between primary closure and planned duodenostomy, some surgeons have advised drainage of the right upper quadrant with a Penrose drain placed in the region of the duodenal stump in the hope that if perforation occurs, the contents will discharge along the tract. However, this does not provide the safety factor of planned duodenostomy, since the drain tract may wall off from the stump before the perforation becomes established.

Duodenal blowout is a major catastrophe which is most likely to occur between the second and seventh postoperative day and becomes manifest by sudden pain, elevation in temperature and pulse rate, and general deterioration of the patient's condition. Adequate drainage must be instituted at once and is best accomplished by an incision below the right costal margin and insertion of a large sump catheter which is passed down to the duodenal stump area, with constant suction applied. Attention must be directed toward fluid and electrolyte therapy, and a high caloric and nitrogen intake should be maintained. Fistula closure can be anticipated within 2 to 3 weeks. Another area in which leaks are a major concern is low colon anastomoses; incidences of 5 to 51 percent have been reported. Recently Everett reported a randomized control trial in which it was shown that a single-layer technique is preferable for low colonic anastomoses. Pedicled omentum may be applied to seal the anastomosis. The mortality rate in patients with major colon leaks is extremely high, and this has led to a resurgence of enthusiasm for protective transverse colostomy if the anastomosis appears compromised.

External Fistulas and Stomal Complications

FISTULAS

External fistulas may arise from stomach, small intestine, or colon. In a review of the experiences at the Massachusetts General Hospital from 1946 to 1959, it was reported that in 157 patients with external fistulas, 55 fistulas originated from stomach, duodenum, or gastrojejunal anastomosis; 46 from jejunum or ileum, with drainage of over 100 ml of intestinal content daily; and 56 from the lower ileum and colon. Surgical complications were the direct cause of 67 percent of these fistulas.

Gastric and Duodenal Fistulas

The incidence of gastrojejunal or duodenal stump fistulas following subtotal gastrectomy has been reported to be 1 to 2 percent, approximately one-quarter of which originated from the gastrojejunostomy. Suture line failure accounted for 82 percent of all gastroduodenal fistulas. The causes of fistulas arising from the gastrojejunostomy may be related to the suture line containing tumor, ischemia of the gastric stump due to high ligation of the gastric artery and vasa brevia, stomal obstruction, and pancreatitis or tension on the suture line. The causes of duodenal stump fistula have been referred to in the previous section on stump leakage. The complications of an established gastric or duodenal fistula include electrolyte abnormalities and malnutrition, sepsis, intraperitoneal abscesses and wound infection, jaundice, and pancreatitis.

Treatment. Intensive fluid, electrolyte, and nutritional therapy is frequently required, and quantitative control of imbalance is critical. The amount of drainage should be measured and analyzed, and these determinations plus the base-line requirements should provide a formula for replacement therapy (see Chap. 2). Sump suction is the most efficient method of managing the drainage, and protection of the skin from autodigestion is usually required. The majority of fistulas which close spontaneously do so in less than 2 months. Surgical intervention may be indicated to drain abscesses or to establish a feeding jejunostomy. An established gastric fistula may require resection and correction of distal obstruction if the latter is present. Fistulas arising at the gastrojejunostomy stoma may require re-resection and establishment of a new gastroenterostomy. Fistulas arising from the duodenal stump are not generally amenable to direct closure. The literature reveals that definitive procedures rarely have been employed for fistulas in this segment of the gastrointestinal tract, and the mortality rate of 55 gastric and duodenal fistulas treated at the Massachusetts General Hospital was 65 percent. These fistulas are readily managed with parenteral hyperalimentation. In the report of MacFadyen et al., all duodenal fistulas closed spontaneously.

Small Bowel Fistulas (See Chap. 27)

Seventy-two percent of the 46 fistulas in this group reported by Edmunds et al. represented surgical complications secondary to dehiscence of anastomoses or inadvertent injury during dissection or closure of an abdominal incision. Although jejunal and proximal ileal fistulas are frequently characterized by profuse drainage, the fluid loss is generally less than that associated with duodenal fistulas, and therefore fluid and electrolyte abnormalities occur less frequently. Malnutrition develops in about three-quarters of these patients, and sepsis is a major complication. Twenty-two percent of the patients reported by Edmunds et al. died of generalized peritonitis, and a large number of intraperitoneal abscesses developed. Skin digestion is a frequent occurrence, and many of these patients eventually develop a ventral hernia due to wound complications.

Treatment. Supportive management of small bowel fistulas is similar to that outlined for gastroduodenal fistulas. This includes maintenance of fluid and electrolyte balance and nutrition. Hyperalimentation may be applicable. In the case of a proximal jejunal fistula, a distal feeding jejunostomy is frequently indicated to permit adequate fluid and nutritional intake. Oral feeding of low-residue diets is feasible with ileal fistulas. Control of fluid loss and diarrhea may be accomplished with the use of Lomotil, Kaopectate, and opiates plus nonabsorbable antibiotics when indicated. Drainage is best controlled by sump suction, and protection of the skin in the region of the fistula is indicated.

Of 46 patients reported by Edmunds et al., definitive procedures were carried out in 50 percent. The operative procedures include direct attack on a fistula with resection both of the fistula and the segment of intestine from which it arises or an indirect attack through a clean abdominal incision with a bypass operation or complete exclusion of the fistula by means of end-to-end anastomosis of the proximal and distal intestine. The excluded loop is then decompressed completely through a large fistula by exteriorizing the ends of the intestine to prevent later blowout. In general, and particularly in the face of peritonitis, early direct attack on the fistula is safer and more satisfactory than exclusion procedures, and most fistulas can be operated on within 3 weeks of onset. In the series reported by Edmunds et al., only 1 patient of 17 treated by resection died, while the mortality rate of patients treated conservatively was 80 percent. Using hyperalimentation, MacFadyen et al. reported that over 70 percent of small bowel fistulas closed spontaneously. An average of 40 days of hyperalimentation was required. By contrast, Aguirre et al. reported that gastrointestinal fistulas treated in part by total parenteral nutrition healed spontaneously in only 11 of 38 patients.

Colonic Fistulas (See Chaps. 27 and 28)

These are generally caused by anastomotic leaks or inadvertent trauma to the segment of intestine. Anastomosis in the region of tumor or inflammation and distal partial obstruction are predisposing factors. Fluid and electrolyte abnormalities are uncommon, while the incidence of infection is extremely high. This includes peritonitis, intraperitoneal abscesses, and wound infections. Significant skin digestion and irritation are rare.

Treatment. The patients can generally be managed on a low-residue diet, using enteric or parenteral antibiotics when indicated, and rarely require sump suction. Spontaneous healing of fistulas in these regions is the rule rather than the exception, but defunctionalizing colostomies for descending colon fistulas or ileal transverse colostomies for ascending colon and distal ileal fistulas may be indicated. Medical management is generally indicated for about 6 weeks to permit any active inflammation to subside. If the inflammation persists after this time, a defunctionalizing procedure is indicated. Definitive surgical treatment is indicated for fistulas which fail to progress satisfactorily after 6 weeks. If the fistula is accompanied by generalized peritonitis, early emergency resection is indicated and frequently should be accompanied by a proximal defunctionalizing procedure. Definitive operations include a turn-in procedure or resection which may be coupled with a temporary protective colostomy or bypass. Seventy-nine percent of the patients in the experience at the Massachusetts General Hospital were cured. Seventy-five percent of patients with no operation experienced spontaneous cure. Lichtman and McDonald reported that 74 percent of chronic fecal fistulas treated by turn-in or resection were cured.

EXTERNAL STOMAL COMPLICATIONS (See Chap. 28)

Ileostomy

Ileostomy performed for ulcerative colitis may be associated with complications related to technical factors, presence of disease, and the nature of the intestinal contents which are discharged. The location of ileostomy is critical to permit application of an effective collecting device, while the method of fixation of the ileal mesentery is important to prevent internal herniation. Formation of the ileostomy itself is important in reducing the incidence of complications. The technique of operative maturation by everting the mucosa reduces the incidence of serositis and peritonitis. Frozen section of the transected ileum is indicated, since ulcerative colitis may extend into the segment of ileum and result in improper function. The liquid nature of the ileostomy discharge requires that measures be taken to avoid excoriation of the skin, which is usually due to delayed application of the bag and a poor fit. When excoriation appears, it is generally wise to discontinue the use of cement and apply a soothing powder. The patient may be placed in a prone position on a frame so that the ileal contents are allowed to drain into a container and contact with the skin is avoided. The complication of prolapse, which requires revision, should be seen infrequently if the mesentery has been fixed. Fistulas which develop at or below the skin level are an indication for early revision of the ileostomy.

Cecostomy and Colostomy

Cecostomies generally demand more attention than colostomies, and frequent irrigation is indicated. Subsequent to removal of the cecostomy catheter, spontaneous closure is to be anticipated, but in unusual circumstances, surgical closure is required. Complications following colostomy include ischemia, gangrene, bleeding, wound abscesses, stenosis, or retraction of the stoma. In the case of a terminal colostomy, fixation during the operative procedure should prevent retraction. If either retraction or gangrene becomes evident, immediate operation is indicated to revise the colostomy using viable bowel of sufficient length.

References

General Considerations

Artz, C. P., and Hardy, J. D.: "Complications in Surgery and Their Management," W. B. Saunders Company, Philadelphia, 1967.

Wound Complications

Ad Hoc Committee of the Committee on Trauma, Division of Medical Sciences, National Academy of Sciences–National Research Council: Postoperative Wound Infections: The Influence of Ultraviolet Irradiation of the Operating Room and of Various Other Factors, Ann Surg [Suppl], vol. 160, 1964.

Alexander, H. C., and Prudden, J.: The Causes of Abdominal Wound Disruption, Surg Gynecol Obstet, 122:1223, 1966.

Barnes, J., Pace, W. G., Trump, D. S., and Ellison, E. H.: Prophylactic Postoperative Antibiotics: A Controlled Study of 1,007 Cases, Arch Surg, 79:190, 1959.

Dineen, P.: A Critical Study of 100 Consecutive Wound Infections, Surg Gynecol Obstet, 113:91, 1961.

———: Major Infections in the Postoperative Period, Surg Clin North Am, 44:553, 1964.

Elek, S. D., and Conen, P. E.: The Virulence of Staphylococcus pyogenes for Man: A Study of the Problems of Wound Infections, Br J Exp Pathol, 38:573, 1957.

Glenn, F., and Moore, S. W.: The Disruption of Abdominal Wounds, Surg Gynecol Obstet, 72:1041, 1941.

Halasz, N. A.: Dehiscence of Laparotomy Wounds, Am J Surg, 116:210, 1968.

Hartzell, J. B., and Winfield, J. M.: Disruption of Abdominal Wounds: Collective Review, Int Abstr Surg, 68:585, 1939.

Howe, C. W., and Mozden, P. J.: Postoperative Infections: Current Concepts, Surg Clin North Am, 43:859, 1963.

Ketcham, A. S., Lieberman, J. E., and West, J. T.: Antibiotic Prophylaxis in Cancer Surgery and Its Value in Staphylococcal Carrier Patients, Surg Gynecol Obstet, 117:1, 1963.

Pemberton, L. B., and Manax, W. G.: Complications after Vertical and Transverse Incisions for Cholecystectomy, Surg Gynecol Obstet, 132:892, 1971.

Polk, H. C., Jr., and Lopez-Mayor, J. F.: Postoperative Wound Infection: A Prospective Study of Determinant Factors and Prevention, Surgery, 66:97, 1969.

Rees, V. L., and Coller, F. A.: Anatomic and Clinical Study of Transverse Abdominal Incision, Arch Surg, 47:136, 1943.

Schonholtz, G. J., Borgia, C. A., and Blair, J. D.: Wound Sepsis in Orthopedic Surgery, J Bone Joint Surg [Am], 44A:1548, 1962.

Singleton, A. O., and Blocker, T. G., Jr.: The Problem of Disruption of Abdominal Wounds and Postoperative Hernia, JAMA, 112:122, 1939.

Thompson, W. D., Ravdin, I. S., and Frank, I. L.: Effect of Hypoproteinemia on Wound Disruption, Arch Surg, 36:500, 1938.

Thomsen, V. F., Larsen, S. O., and Jepsen, O. B.: Post-operative Wound Sepsis in General Surgery: IV. Sources and Routes of Infection, Acta Chir Scand, 136:251, 1970.

Wolff, W. I.: Disruption of Abdominal Wounds, Ann Surg, 131:534, 1950.

Postoperative Parotitis

Branson, B., Kugel, A. I., Stafford, C. E., and Morel, E. E.: The Re-emergence of Postoperative Parotitis, Western J Surg Obstet Gynecol, 67:38, 1959.

Carlson, R. G., and Glas, W. W.: Acute Suppurative Parotitis, Arch Surg, 86:659, 1963.

Hemenway, W. G., and English, G. M.: Surgical Treatment of Acute Bacterial Parotitis, Postgrad Med, 50:114, 1971.

Krippaehne, W. W., Hunt, T. K., and Dunphy, J. E.: Acute Suppurative Parotitis: A Study of 161 Cases, Ann Surg, 156:251, 1962.

Lary, B. G.: Postoperative Suppurative Parotitis, Arch Surg, 89:653, 1964.

Petersdorf, R. G., Forsyth, B. B., and Bernake, D.: Staphylococcal Parotitis, N Engl J Med, 259:1250, 1958.

Reilly, D. J.: Benign Transient Swelling of the Parotid Glands following General Anesthesia: "Anesthesia Mumps," Anesth Anal (Cleve), 49:560, 1970.

Postoperative Respiratory Complications

Adriani, J., Zepernick, R., Harmon, W., and Hiern, B.: Iatrogenic Pulmonary Edema in Surgical Patients, Surgery, 61:183, 1967.

Ashbaugh, D. G., and Petty, T. L.: Positive End-expiratory Pressure: Physiology, Indications, and Contraindications, J Thorac Cardiovasc Surg, 65:165, 1973.

Becker, A., Barak, S., Braun, E., and Meyers, M. P.: The Treatment of Postoperative Pulmonary Atelectasis with Intermittent Positive Pressure Breathing, Surg Gynecol Obstet, 111:517, 1960.

Beecher, H. K.: Measured Effect of Laparotomy on Respiration, J Clin Invest, 12:639, 1933.

Bendixen, H. H., and Bunker, J. P.: "Ventilation and Postoperative Period," paper presented at The Second World Congress of Anaesthesiologists, Toronto, Sept. 6, 1960.

———, Hedley-Shyte, J., and Laver, M. B.: Impaired Oxygenation in Surgical Patients during General Anesthesia with Controlled Ventilation: A Concept of Atelectasis, N Engl J Med, 269:991, 1963.

———, ———, and ———: Increased Physiologic Shunting during Anesthesia and Surgery, Anesthesiology, 24:122, 1963.

Brattstrom, S.: Postoperative Pulmonary Ventilation with Reference to Postoperative Pulmonary Complications, Acta Chir Scand Suppl 195, 1954.

Clements, J. A.: Surface Phenomena in Relation to Pulmonary Function (Sixth Bowditch Lecture), Physiologist, 5:11, 1962.

Clendon, D. R. T., and Pygott, F.: Analysis of Pulmonary Complications Occurring after 579 Consecutive Operations, Br J Anaesth, 19:62, 1944.

Collins, J. A.: The Causes of Progressive Pulmonary Insufficiency in Surgical Patients, J Surg Res, 9:685, 1969.

Davis, H. A., and Pollak, E. W.: Adult Respiratory Distress Syndrome in Postoperative Patients: Study of Pulmonary Pathology in "Shock Lung" with Prophylactic and Therapeutic Implications, Am Surg, 41:391, 1975.

Griffo, Z. J., and Roos, A.: Effect of O₂ Breathing on Pulmonary Compliance, J Appl Physiol, 17:233, 1962.

Hamilton, W. K.: Postoperative Respiratory Complications, chap. 10 in "Clinical Anesthesia," 1/1965.

Joffe, N.: Roentgenologic Findings in Post-shock and Postoperative Pulmonary Insufficiency, Radiology, 94:369, 1970.

Kurzweg, F. T.: Pulmonary Complications following Upper Abdominal Surgery, Am Surg, 19:967, 1953.

Laver, M. B., and Bendixen, H. H.: Atelectasis in the Surgical Patient: Recent Conceptual Advances, Prog Surg, 5:1, 1966.

Masson, A. H. B.: Pulmonary Edema during or after Surgery, pt. I, Anesth Anal Current Res, 43:440, 1964.

———: Pulmonary Edema during or after Surgery, pt. II, Anesth Anal Curr Res, 43:446, 1964.

Mead, J., and Collier, C.: Relation of Volume History of Lungs to Respiratory Mechanics in Anesthetized Dogs, J Appl Physiol, 14:669, 1959.

Moersch, H. J.: Bronchoscopy in Treatment of Postoperative Atelectasis, Surg Gynecol Obstet, 77:435, 1943.

Moore, F. D.: Postoperative Pulmonary Insufficiency: Anoxia, the Shunted Lung and Mechanical Assistance, in D. E. Harken (ed.), "Cardiac Surgery 2," Cardiovasc Clin, vol. 3, no. 3, F. A. Davis Company, Philadelphia, 1971.

———, Lyons, J. H., Pierce, E. C., Jr., Morgan, A. P., Jr., Drinker, P. A., MacArthur, J. D., and Dammin, G. J.: "Post-traumatic Pulmonary Insufficiency," W. B. Saunders Company, Philadelphia, 1969.

Neely, W. A., Robinson, T. W., McMullan, M. H., Bobo, W. O., Meadows, D. L., and Hardy, J. D.: Post-operative Respiratory Insufficiency, Ann Surg, 171:679, 1970.

Overfield, W., and Powers, S. R., Jr.: Arterial Oxygen Tension: Significance in the Surgical Patient, Surgery, 71:1, 1972.

Peters, R. M., Hilberman, M., Hogan, J. S., and Crawford, D. A.: Objective Indications for Respiratory Therapy in Post-trauma and Postoperative Patients, Am J Surg, 124:262, 1972.

Pontoppidan, H., Geffin, B., and Lowenstein, E.: Acute Respiratory Failure in the Adult: Trends in Treatment of Acute Respiratory Failure, N Engl J Med, 287:690, 1972.

———, ———, and ———: Acute Respiratory Failure in the Adult: Assessment of Respiratory Function, N Engl J Med, 287:743, 1972.

———, ———, and ———: Acute Respiratory Failure in the Adult: Effect of Mechanical Ventilation and Airway Pressures on Circulation and Blood Gas Exchange, N Engl J Med, 287:799, 1972.

———, Laver, M. B., and Geffin, B.: Acute Respiratory Failure in the Surgical Patient, Adv Surg, 4:163, 1970.

Sayeed, M. M., Chaudry, I. H., and Baue, A. E.: Na⁺-K⁺ Transport and Adenosine Nucleotides in the Lung in Hemorrhagic Shock, Surgery, 77:395, 1975.

Van Allen, C. M., and Adams, W. E.: The Mechanism of Obstructive Pulmonary Atelectasis, Surg Gynecol Obstet, 50:385, 1930.

Cardiac Complications

Buckley J. J., and Jackson, J. A.: Postoperative Cardiac Arrhythmias, Anesthesiology, 22:723, 1961.

Dack, S.: Postoperative Myocardial Infarction, Am J Cardiol, 12:423, 1963.

Dixon, S. H., Jr., Limbird, L. E., Roe, C. R., Wagner, G. S., Oldham, H. N., Jr., and Sabiston, D. C., Jr.: Recognition of Postoperative Acute Myocardial Infarction: Application of Isoenzyme Technics, Circulation [Suppl], 47 & 48:137, 1973.

Dreifus, L. S., Rabbino, M. D., Watanabe, Y., and Tabesh, E.: Arrhythmias in the Postoperative Period, Am J Cardiol, 12:431, 1963.

Krosnick, A., and Wassermann, F.: Cardiac Arrhythmias in Older Age Group following Thoracic Surgery, Am J Med Sci, 230:541, 1955.

Kuner, J., Enescu, V., Utsu, F., Boszormenyi, E., Bernstein, H., and Corday, E.: Cardiac Arrhythmias during Anesthesia, Dis Chest, 52:580, 1967.

Master, A. M., Dack, S., and Jaffe, H. L.: Postoperative Coronary Artery Occlusion, JAMA, 110:1415, 1938.

Mauney, F. M., Jr., Ebert, P. A., and Sabiston, D. C., Jr.: Postoperative Myocardial Infarction: A Study of Predisposing Factors, Diagnosis and Mortality in a High Risk Group of Surgical Patients, *Ann Surg,* **172:**497, 1970.

Merideth, J.: Cardiac Arrhythmias in the Postoperative Patient, *Surg Clin North Am,* **49:**1083, 1969.

Reinikainen, M., and Pontinen, P.: On Cardiac Arrhythmias during Anaesthesia and Surgery, *Acta Med Scand Suppl* 457, 1966.

Rogers, W. R., Wroblewski, F., and LaDue, J. S.: Supraventricular Tachycardia Complicating Surgical Procedures: Study of Contributing Causes, Course, and Treatment of This Complication in Fifty Patients, *Circulation,* **7:**192, 1953.

Sharnoff, J. G.: Postmortem Findings in 25 Cases of Sudden Heart Arrest in the Perioperative Period, *Lancet,* **2:**876, 1966.

Stein, I., and Caginalp, N.: The Postoperative Electrocardiogram, *Angiology,* **17:**323, 1966.

Tarhan, S., Moffitt, E. A., Taylor, W. F., and Giuliani, E. R.: Myocardial Infarction after General Anesthesia, *JAMA,* **220:**1451, 1972.

Taylor, I. B.: Cyclopropane Anesthesia: With Report of Results in 41,690 Administrations, *Anesthesiology,* **2:**641, 1941.

Wheat, M. W., Jr., and Burford, T. H.: Digitalis in Surgery: Extension of Classical Indications, *J Thorac Cardiovasc Surg,* **41:**162, 1961.

Wroblewski, F., and LaDue, J. S.: Myocardial Infarction as a Postoperative Complication of Major Surgery, *JAMA,* **150:**1212, 1952.

Diabetes Mellitus

Black, K.: Diabetes and the Surgical Patient, *Br J Clin Pract,* **20:**555, 1966.

Canary, J. J., Stoffer, R., Delawter, D. D., and Moss, J. M.: The Response of Tolbutamide-treated Patients to the Stress of Surgery, *Med Ann DC,* **28:**614, 1959.

Forsham, P. H.: Management of Diabetes during Stress and Surgery, in R. H. Williams (ed.), "Diabetes," chap. 36, Hoeber Medical Division, Harper & Row, Publishers, Incorporated, New York, 1960.

Galloway, J. A., and Shuman, C. R.: Diabetes and Surgery: A Study of 667 Cases, *Am J Med,* **34:**177, 1963.

Gastineau, C. F., and Molnar, G. D.: The Care of the Diabetic Patient During Emergency Surgery, *Surg Clin N Am,* **49:**1171, 1969.

Greenstein, A. J., and Dreiling, D. A.: Nonketotic Hyperosmolar Coma in the Postoperative Patient, *Am J Surg,* **121:**698, 1971.

Marble, A., and Steinke, J.: Physiology and Pharmacology in Diabetes Mellitus: Guiding the Diabetic Patient through the Surgical Period, *Anesthesiology,* **24:**442, 1963.

Packovich, M. J., Molnar, G. D., and Leonard, P. F.: Management of Diabetic patients during Surgery, *Surg Clin North Am,* **45:**975, 1965.

Weisenfeld, S., Podolsky, S., Goldsmith, L., and Ziff, L.: Adsorption of Insulin to Infusion Bottles and Tubing, *Diabetes,* **17:**766, 1968.

Fat Embolism

Ashbaugh, D. G., and Petty, T. L.: The Use of Corticosteroids in the Treatment of Respiratory Failure Associated with Massive Fat Embolism, *Surg Gynecol Obstet,* **123:**495, 1966.

Benoit, P. R., Hampson, L. G., and Burgess, J. H.: Value of

Arterial Hypoxemia in the Diagnosis of Pulmonary Fat Embolism, *Ann Surg,* **175:**128, 1972.

Collins, J. A., Hudson, T. L., Hamacher, W. R., Rokous, J., Williams, G., and Hardaway, R. M., III: Systemic Fat Embolism in Four Combat Casualties, *Ann Surg,* **167:**493, 1968.

Evarts, C. M.: The Fat Embolism Syndrome: A Review, *Surg Clin North Am,* **50:**493, 1970.

Greendyke, R. M.: Fat Embolism in Fatal Automobile Accidents, *J Forensic Sci,* **9:**201, 1964.

Henzel, J. H., Smith, J. L., Pories, W. J., and Burget, D. E.: Fat Embolism: Diagnostic Challenge of a Potentially Lethal Clinical Entity, *Am J Surg,* **113:**525, 1967.

Jackson, C. T., and Greendyke, R. M.: Pulmonary and Cerebral Fat Embolism after Closed Chest Cardiac Massage, *Surg Gynecol Obstet,* **120:**25, 1965.

Musselman, M. M., Glas, W. W., and Grekin, T. D.: Fat Embolism, *Arch Surg,* **65:**551, 1952.

Palmovic, V., and McCarroll, J. R.: Fat Embolism in Trauma, *Arch Pathol,* **80:**630, 1965.

Pazell, J. A., and Peltier, L. F.: Experience with Sixty-three Patients with Fat Embolism, *Surg Gynecol Obstet,* **135:**77, 1972.

Peltier, L. F.: The Diagnosis of Fat Embolism, *Surg Gynecol Obstet,* **121:**371, 1965.

Scuderi, C. S.: Fat Embolism: Clinical and Experimental Study, *Surg Gynecol Obstet,* **72:**732, 1941.

Sevitt, S.: "Fat Embolism," Butterworth Scientific Publications, London, 1962.

Sutton, G. E.: Pulmonary Fat Embolism, *Ann Surg,* **76:**581, 1922.

Weisz, G. M.: Fat Embolism, *Curr Probl Surg,* November 1974.

Psychiatric Complications

Altschule, M. D.: Postoperative Psychosis, *Surg Clin N Am,* **49:**677, 1969.

Bakwin, H.: Psychic Trauma of Operations, *J Pediatr,* **36:**262, 1950.

Beebe, H. G., and Keats, N. M.: Surgical Patients and Drug Abuse Syndrome, *Am Surg,* **39:**88, 1973.

Bliss, E. L., Rumel, W. R., and Branch, C. H.: Psychiatric Complications of Mitral Surgery: Report of a Death after Electroshock Therapy, *Arch Neurol,* **74:**249, 1955.

Bolton, H. E., and Bailey, C. P.: Surgical Aspects in Psychosomatic Aspects of Cardiovascular Surgery, in A. J. Cantor and A. N. Foxe (eds.), "Psychosomatic Aspects of Surgery," chap. 3, Grune & Stratton, Inc., New York, 1955.

Browning, J., and Houseworth, J.: Development of New Symptoms following Medical and Surgical Treatment for Duodenal Ulcer, *Psychosom Med,* **15:**328, 1953.

Cramond, W. A.: Renal Homotransplantation: Some Observations on Recipients and Donors, *Br J Psychiat,* **113:**1223, 1967.

———, Court, J. H., Higgins, B. A., Knight, P. R., and Lawrence, J. R.: Psychological Screening of Potential Donors in a Renal Homotransplantation Programme, *Br J Psychiat,* **113:**1213, 1967.

———, Knight, P. R., and Lawrence, J. R.: The psychiatric Contribution to a Renal Unit Undertaking Chronic Haemodialysis and Renal Homotransplantation, *Br J Psychiat,* **113:**1201, 1967.

Da Costa, J. C.: The Diagnosis of Postoperative Insanity, *Surg Gynecol Obstet,* **11:**577, 1910.

Deutsch, H.: Psychoanalytic Observations in Surgery, *Psychosom Med,* **4:**105, 1942.

Donovan, J. C.: Some Psychosomatic Aspects of Obstetrics and Gynecology, *Am J Obstet Gynecol,* **75:**72, 1958.

Egerton, N., and Kay, J. H.: Psychological Disturbances Associated with Open Heart Surgery, *Br J Psychiat,* **110:**433, 1964.

Fox, H. M., Rizzo, N. D., and Gifford, S.: Psychological Observations of Patients Undergoing Mitral Surgery: Study of Stress, *Psychosom Med,* **16:**186, 1954.

Hackett, T. P., and Weisman, A. D.: Psychiatric Management of Operative Syndromes. I. The Therapeutic Consultation and the Effect of Noninterpretive Intervention, *Psychosom Med,* **22:**267, 1960.

————, and ————: Psychiatric Management of Operative Syndromes. II. Psychodynamic Factors in Formulation and Management, *Psychosom Med,* **22:**356, 1960.

Halper, I. S.: Psychiatric Observations in a Chronic Hemodialysis Program, *Med Clin North Am,* **55:**177, 1971.

Hollender, M. H.: A Study of Patients Admitted to a Psychiatric Hospital after Pelvic Operations, *Am J Obstet Gynecol,* **79:**498, 1960.

Katz, N. M., Agle, D. P., DePalma, R. G., and DeCosse, J. J.: Delirium in Surgical Patients under Intensive Care: Utility of Mental Status Examination, *Arch Surg,* **104:**310, 1972.

Kemph, J. P.: Renal Failure, Artificial Kidney and Kidney Transplant, *Am J Psychiat,* **122:**1270, 1966.

Knox, S. J.: Severe Psychiatric Disturbances in the Postoperative Period: A Five-Year Survey of Belfast Hospitals, *J Ment Sci,* **107:**1078, 1961.

Kornfeld, D. S., Zimberg, S., and Malm, J. R.: Psychiatric Complications of Open-Heart Surgery, *N Engl J Med,* **273:**287, 1965.

Layne, O. L., Jr., and Yudofsky, S. C.: Postoperative Psychosis in Cardiotomy Patients: The Role of Organic and Psychiatric Factors, *N Engl J Med,* **284:**518, 1971.

Levy, D.: Psychic Trauma of Operations in Children and a Note on Combat Neurosis, *Am J Dis Child,* **69:**7, 1945.

Lewis, A.: "The Relation between Operative Risk and the Patient's General Condition," Report 16, Congrès International de Chirurgie, Copenhague, 1955.

Lindemann, E.: Observations on Psychiatric Sequelae to Surgical Operations in Women, *Am J Psychiat,* **98:**132, 1941.

Meyer, B. C.: Some Psychiatric Aspects of Surgical Practice, *Psychosom Med,* **20:**203, 1958.

————, Brown, F., and Levine, A.: Observations on the House-Tree-Person Drawing Test Before and After Surgery, *Psychosom Med,* **17:**428, 1955.

Moore, F., Steinberg, R., Bull, M., Wilson, G., and Myrden, J.: Studies in Surgical Endocrinology: I, *Ann Surg,* **141:**145, 1955.

Prugh, D., Staub, E., Sands, H., Kirschbaum, R., and Lenihan, R.: A Study of the Emotional Reactions of Children and Families to Hospitalization and Illness, *Am J Orthopsychiatry,* **22:**70, 1953.

Sand, P., Livingston, G., and Wright, R. G.: Psychological Assessment of Candidates for a Haemodialysis Program, *Ann Intern Med,* **64:**602, 1966.

Scott, J.: Postoperative Psychosis in the Aged, *Am J Surg,* **10:**38, 1960.

Shea, E. J., Bogdan, D. F., Freeman, R. B., and Schreiner, G. E.: Haemodialysis for Chronic Renal Failure: IV. Psychological Considerations, *Ann Intern Med,* **62:**558, 1965.

Sutherland, A.: Psychological Impact of Postoperative Cancer, *Bull NY Acad Med,* **33:**428, 1957.

————, and Ohrbach, C.: Psychological Impact of Cancer and Cancer Surgery: II. Depressive Reactions Associated with Surgery for Cancer, *Cancer,* **6:**958, 1953.

————, ————, Dyk, R., and Bard, M.: The Psychological Impact of Cancer and Cancer Surgery: I. Adaptation to the Dry Colostomy: Preliminary Report and Summary of Findings, *Cancer,* **5:**857, 1952.

Titchener, J. L., and Levine, M.: "Surgery as a Human Experience: The Psychodynamics of Surgical Practice," Oxford University Press, Fair Lawn, N.J., 1960.

————, Zwerling, I., Gottschalk, L., Levine, M., Culbertson, W., Cohen, S., and Silver, H.: Psychosis in Surgical Patients, *Surg Gynecol Obstet,* **102:**59, 1956.

Weisman, A. D., and Hackett, T. P.: Psychosis after Eye Surgery: Establishment of a Specific Doctor-Patient Relation in the Prevention and Treatment of "Black-patch Delirium," *N Engl J Med,* **258:**1284, 1958.

Weiss, S. M.: Psychological Adjustment following Open-Heart Surgery, *J Nerv Ment Dis,* **143:**363, 1966.

Winkelstein, C., Blacher, R. S., and Meyer, B. C.: Psychiatric Observations on Surgical Patients in Recovery Room: Pilot Study, *NY J Med,* **65:**865, 1965.

Wright, R. G., Sand, P., and Livingston, G.: Psychological Stress during Haemodialysis for Chronic Renal Failure, *Ann Intern Med,* **64:**611, 1966.

Zaks, M. S.: Disturbances in Physiologic Functions and Neuropsychiatric Complications in Heart Surgery, in A. A. Luisada (ed.), "Cardiology: An Encyclopedia of the Cardiovascular System," vol. 3, McGraw-Hill Book Company, New York, 1959.

Complications of Gastrointestinal Surgery

Aguirre, A., Fischer, J. E., and Welch, C. E.: Role of Surgery and Hyperalimentation in Therapy of Gastrointestinal-Cutaneous Fistulas, *Ann Surg,* **180:**393, 1974.

Beal, J. M., and Moody, F. G.: Postoperative Complications of Duodenal Surgery, *Surg Clin North Am,* **44:**379, 1964.

Blomstedt, B., and Dahlgren, S.: The Afferent Loop Syndrome, *Acta Chir Scand,* **120:**347, 1961.

Burnett, W. E., Rosemond, G. P., Caswell, H. T., Beauchamp, E. W., Jr., Tyson, R. R., and Wright, W. C.: Studies on So-called Postgastrectomy Pancreatitis, *Ann Surg,* **149:**737, 1959.

Capper, W. M., and Welbourn, R. B.: Early Postcibal Symptoms following Gastrectomy, *Br J Surg,* **43:**24, 1955.

Colcock, B. P.: Leakage from the Duodenal Stump following Gastric Resection, *Lahey Clin Bull,* **13:**190, 1964.

Edmunds, L. H., Jr., Williams, G. M., and Welch, C. E.: External Fistulas Arising from the Gastro-intestinal Tract, *Ann Surg,* **152:**445, 1960.

Everett, E. G.: Comparison of One-Layer and Two-Layer Technics for Colorectal Anastomosis, *Br J Surg,* **62:**135, 1975.

Habif, D. V.: Immediate Complications of Surgery of the Small Intestine, *Surg Clin North Am,* **44:**387, 1964.

Hibner, R., and Richards, V.: Stomal or Small Bowel Obstruction following Partial Gastrectomy, *Am J Surg,* **96:**309, 1958.

Hoffman, W. A., and Spiro, H. M.: Afferent Loop Problems, *Gastroenterology,* **40:**201, 1961.

Johnson, C. L., and McIlrath, D. C.: Management of Patients with Enterocutaneous Fistulas, *Surg Clin North Am,* **49:**967, 1969.

Lichtman, A. L., and McDonald, J. R.: Fecal Fistula, *Surg Gynecol Obstet,* **78:**449, 1944.

MacFadyen, B. V., Dudrick, S. J., and Ruberg, R. L.: The Management of Gastrointestinal Fistulae with Parenteral Hyperalimentation, *Surgery,* 1973. (To be published.)

McLachlin, A. D., and Denton, D. W.: Omental Protection of Intestinal Anastomes, *Am J Surg,* **125:**134, 1973.

Magnuson, F. K., Judd, E. S., and Dearing, W. H.: Comparison of Postgastrectomy Complications in Gastric and Duodenal Ulcer Patients, *Am Surg,* **32:**375, 1966.

Moretz, W. H.: Inadvertent Gastro-ileostomy, *Ann Surg,* **130:**124, 1949.

Morgenstern, L., Yamakawa, T., Ben-Shoshan, M., and Lippman, H.: Anastomotic Leakage after Low Colonic Anastomosis. Clinical and Experimental Aspects, *Am J Surg,* **123:**104, 1972.

Pettersson, S., and Wallensten, S.: Leakage at Suture Lines after Partial Gastrectomy for Peptic Ulcer, *Acta Chir Scand,* **135:**229, 1969.

Quinn, W. F., and Gifford, J. H.: Syndrome of Proximal Jejunal Loop Obstruction following Anterior Gastric Resection, *Calif Med,* **72:**18, 1950.

Rodkey, G. V., and Welch, C. E.: Duodenal Decompression in Gastrectomy, *N Engl J Med,* **262:**498, 1960.

Rousselot, L. M., and Slattery, J. R.: Immediate Complications of Surgery of the Large Intestine, *Surg Clin North Am,* **44:**397, 1964.

Spencer, F. C.: Ischemic Necrosis of Remaining Stomach following Subtotal Gastrectomy, *Arch Surg,* **73:**844, 1956.

State, D.: Immediate Complications of Gastric Surgery, *Surg Clin North Am,* **44:**371, 1964.

Turner, F. P.: Postoperative Complications following Gastric Resection, *Am J Surg,* **101:**711, 1961.

Chapter 13

Physiologic Monitoring of the Surgical Patient

by **Louis R. M. Del Guercio**

INTRODUCTION

Among the 14 definitions of the word "monitor" which appear in one dictionary, three appear applicable to medicine: "Something that serves to remind or give warning"; "A device or arrangement for observing or recording the operation of a machine or system, esp. an automatic control system"; and "To observe, record or detect an operation or condition with instruments that have no effect on the operation or condition."

This last definition offers the key to a basic problem of all patient monitoring, i.e., that the measuring system tends to change the measurements. The application of electrodes, cannulas, mouthpieces, and other paraphernalia definitely has psychologic and physiologic effects on the patient. From this it follows that the ideal monitoring system should be noninvasive and unobtrusive.

Another point to be stressed is that the most sophisticated and advanced electronic system can never substitute for close surveillance by an experienced and qualified health professional. Monitors in surgery are worthwhile only if they provide physiologic information about the patient which cannot be detected by the five senses of a physician or nurse. In addition, the transducers, signal processors, or readout devices should not so encumber the patient as to interfere with essential nursing care.

There is a tendency to think of monitoring in terms of complicated electronic devices and computers; in fact, the serial recordings of temperature, pulse, respiratory rate, and blood pressure are forms of clinical monitoring in common use for decades. This approach to monitoring had been observed by Harvey Cushing on a visit to Italy and, overcoming considerable resistance, he introduced routine blood pressure recording to the United States in 1903. These simple techniques served the surgeon fairly well until the advent of cardiopulmonary bypass and open heart surgery. At that point, it was recognized that optimum clinical care in the period following what could be considered at best a controlled physiologic insult, required a better assessment of the cardiovascular and respiratory status of the patient. Decisions regarding therapy had to be made rapidly on the basis of reasonably accurate measurements of physiologic variables.

This led in the early 1960s to the clinical use of central venous pressure and cardiac output determinations. The invention of the densitometer for the continuous recording of indicator dilution and of electrodes for the rapid determination of the partial pressures of oxygen and carbon dioxide in whole blood provided the technical impetus for the modern era of clinical monitoring.

Subsequently, many specialized diagnostic and treatment centers established within the hospital have included physiologic monitoring as an adjunct to patient care. Coronary care units, respiratory care centers, burn centers, neurosurgical intensive care units, pediatric and neonatal intensive care units, renal dialysis centers, and surgical intensive care units all utilize some forms of patient monitoring. Only in the coronary care unit, however, can it be statistically documented that lives are saved by monitoring. In this case, the electrocardiograph is an almost ideal monitor because it is safe, noninvasive, and specific for the physiologic aberration, cardiac arrhythmias, which kills most myocardial infarction victims.

The problem of monitoring for the surgical patient is much more complex, because there is as yet no known single physiologic variable which can be used to warn against impending disaster. And although there are many systems in daily operation which on the basis of cardiac output, arterial pressure, central venous pressure, and blood-gas tensions provide assessment of cardiorespiratory function and oxygen transport, these techniques are primarily used when it is already obvious that the patient is in serious trouble. Such systems at the present time are generally invasive and are used intermittently to assess the response of a desperately ill patient to specific modes of therapy. There are many models of these "shock carts" currently available commercially.

The second type of surgical monitoring involves the

continuous recording of one or two fundamental physiologic variables in order to show trends and changes which may warn of impending disaster. At the present time there is no system of this type in operation which has been proved to be practical for most surgical patients. Continuous rather than intermittent monitoring would be desirable for surgical patients if it could be performed inexpensively and noninvasively, because more information can be obtained from a variable which is measured in relation to time. Patterns and trends can be detected and compared with mathematical models obtained from studies of patients known to be in jeopardy. For example, it is believed by most experts that there is no such thing as cardiac arrest without antecedent events. Clinical studies have shown that long before cardiac standstill or ventricular fibrillation occurs, serious derangements of blood-gas tensions or hemodynamic variables can be demonstrated. Continuous monitoring of certain variables might reveal catastrophic trends.

But since cardiac arrest is a rare event, the need for surgical monitoring in the general population might be questioned, were it not for the National Halothane Study. That prospective statistical analysis of over 850,000 operations performed in 35 highly regarded hospitals revealed an overall 6-week mortality rate of 1.97 percent! This included ophthalmologic, plastic, and other low-death-rate operations. The overall need for surgical monitoring is mandated by that totally unacceptable mortality rate, which is higher than that for 1 year of combat service in World War II, Korea, or Vietnam!

PHYSIOLOGIC CONCEPTS AND MONITORING

One of the problems with patient monitoring today is that we tend to measure the variables which we *can* rather than the variables which we *should*. Thus far in the twentieth century, instruments have directed medicine rather than vice versa; we use the instruments which happen to be available. For example, the entire discipline of diagnostic cardiology developed around measurement of intracardiac pressure gradients and electric potentials rather than volume and flow relationships, because the strain gauge pressure transducer and electrocardiograph were the first instruments available. Monitoring to warn against surgical disaster or to record the proper operation of such a complex "automatic control system" as the human body must be based upon physiologic principles. Instruments and monitoring systems must be developed and designed to detect specific physiologic events known to be associated with surgical morbidity or mortality.

The overall physiology of oxygen transport, or the delivery of oxygen from the atmosphere to the mitochondria of the body cell mass, can be used as a model to assess the abilities of particular monitoring systems to detect critical events and trends. This process involves many organ systems and complicated feedback loops for regulation and compensation. It is imperative for the survival of the individual that the oxygen transport system continue in operation without interruption.

Even in the basal state, 4 ml of oxygen is required each minute for each kilogram of body weight. Human beings can store only a 4- or 5-minute supply in the lungs and blood cells. With cessation of oxygen transport anywhere along the line serious defects of oxygen tension gradient develop within 2 minutes. Even the highly trained pearl divers of Northern Australia dive for less than 2 minutes, and they still manifest markedly elevated blood lactate levels and frequent cardiac arrythmias. The best of the diving mammals, the whale, cannot store proportionately more than twice the amount of oxygen stored by nondiving mammals such as man.

The upper airways serve to humidify and warm or cool the air entering the tracheobronchial tree during spontaneous respiration. The difference in temperature between inspired and expired air provides a basis for monitoring the rate of respiration in patients. Simple thermistor probes have been developed which are fixed in front of the external nares to record the passage of warmed expired air. It is not possible by this means to evaluate the adequacy of ventilation, but a simple noninvasive means of monitoring the respiratory rate and signaling respiratory arrest could be of value. Respiratory rate is regulated by changes in arterial oxygen content through the carotid and aortic body reflexes, and by changes in pH and carbon dioxide tension through brainstem chemoreceptors. Hyperpnea can be a relatively nonspecific warning sign suggesting hypoxia, sepsis, increased metabolic demands, emotional excitement, or simply painful stimuli.

Table 13-1 traces the oxygen flow and partial pressure gradients from this point on. The critical importance of each stage is related to the oxygen stored beyond that point. For example, respiratory failure is tolerated far longer than circulatory arrest, because the circulatory system stores more than twice as much oxygen as the lungs. Cyanide kills quickly because it blocks the ability of the mitochondria to utilize oxygen. This is a point beyond which there is no oxygen reserve. Total body oxygen stores are about 1,500 ml. A monitoring system should detect a block of this most critical step, delivery of oxygen to the mitochondrion within the cell. At this point, oxygen stores are nil and the tension gradient is low.

The partial pressure of oxygen in the atmosphere is 159 mm Hg (20.84 percent of 760 mm Hg). As inspired air is rapidly humidified in the upper airways by the mucosa of the nasal turbinates, pharynx, and tracheobronchial tree, the partial pressure drops to 149 mm Hg due to the dilutional effect of the water vapor pressure at body temperature (47 mm Hg). As the alveoli are approached, the oxygen tension rapidly falls, because approximately 4 ml/kg of body mass of that gas is removed from the alveoli each minute. The 45 mm Hg fall in oxygen tension is replaced by a similar rise in carbon dioxide tension in the alveoli. It is the rapid removal of oxygen from the alveoli by the unsaturated blood entering the pulmonary capillary bed which establishes this gradient. This is why it is possible to maintain adequate oxygenation for several minutes by

Table 13-1. OXYGEN TRANSPORT AND MONITORING

Oxygen stores, ml	Oxygen tension gradient, mm Hg	Medium	Measurements
370	159 149 105	Atmosphere Airway Alveoli Interstitial fluid	Tidal volume, dead-space-to-tidal-volume ratio, lung compliance, work of breathing, functional residual capacity, end tidal CO_2, percent shunt, alveolar-arterial O_2 gradient, pulmonary transit time, blood gases
880	100 95 90	Pulmonary capillary Plasma Red cell membrane Hemoglobin Left side of heart Arteries Arteriole	Cardiac output, stroke volume, ejection fraction, ventricular function curves, systolic time intervals, central venous pressure, pulmonary wedge pressure, left ventricular end-diastolic pressure
	90–40	Capillary	Oxygen consumption, effective oxygen transport, mixed venous oxygen levels, P_{50}, blood lactate concentration, tissue oxygen tension, muscle surface pH
56	40 38 20 10	Endothelium Extracellular fluid Pericapillary tissue cylinder Cell membrane	
240	6	Myoglobin	
0	5	Mitochondrion	

Oxygen flow ←

Electron flow →

→ Oxygen + electrons + hydrogen ions ⟶ water

Cytochromes ⟶ 2 ATP
Ubiquinone
Flavoprotein ⟶ 1 ATP
Diphosphopyridine nucleotide (DPN)
Acetyl coenzyme A
Pyruvate
Glucose

flushing oxygen into a bronchoscope without any ventilation. Of course, the blood carbon dioxide level rises markedly. The energy cost of ventilation may represent a serious problem to some postoperative patients. Many physiologic variables associated with ventilation and lung mechanics can be measured at the bedside if necessary; among these are tidal volume, minute ventilation, dead-space-to-tidal-volume ratios, compliance, and functional residual capacity. All these give an assessment of the efficiency of the lung, chest, and diaphragm in exchanging air in the alveoli.

The next stage in oxygen transport is truly remarkable. In 5 seconds, the entire output of the right side of the heart is spread out over an area the size of a tennis court and sucked back up into the left atrium. The blood pressure differential across this system is only 6 mm Hg, and all of the blood, during the brief time which the red cells spend in the pulmonary capillaries, normally reaches equilibrium with the oxygen in the alveoli. Only 90 ml of blood is in the capillaries at one time. Moreover, this remarkably efficient manifold system can dynamically expand within seconds to handle three times the normal blood flow without any sacrifice in oxygenation. Roughton has estimated that at normal flow rates each red cell takes 0.8 second

to squeeze through two or three alveolar capillaries in succession. At high flow rates, during exercise or in hyperdynamic shock, the time spent in the capillary bed is reduced. When it is reduced below 0.35 second, there is insufficient time for the four heme positions of the hemoglobin molecule to take up oxygen, and unsaturation results because of this so-called "speed shunt." This situation can also occur when the cross-sectional area of pulmonary bed is reduced, as in pulmonary embolism, since a more rapid flow is forced past the remaining capillaries. Arterial hypoxemia is well known in pulmonary embolism.

It can be seen from Table 13-1 that oxygen flow from the alveoli to the hemoglobin within the red cell encounters a number of resistances: alveolar membrane, interstitial fluid, capillary membrane, plasma, red cell membrane, and the paracrystalline structure within the red cell. But since all these together are normally only a few microns thick, diffusion is rapid. Many things can go wrong with this efficient system, however, and opportunities for monitoring at this level have been recognized. The red cells normally leave the pulmonary capillaries with an oxygen tension of 100 mm Hg. When they arrive in the left side of the heart, the partial pressure has dropped to about 95 mm Hg because of the mixing effect of unsaturated blood from the bronchial and coronary circulation which empties into the left side of the heart. This shunted blood normally is 3 percent of the output of the right side of the heart.

The difference in the partial pressure of oxygen from the alveoli to the arterial blood is an important monitoring variable. It is called the *alveolar-arterial oxygen gradient* (A-aDO$_2$). It is most useful in assessing the efficiency of gas exchange in the lung and is an early indicator of incipient respiratory failure due to a variety of causes in surgical patients. The normal A-aDO$_2$ is 25 to 65 mm Hg when the inspired oxygen concentration is 100 percent.

When the arterial oxygen tension falls below 60 mm Hg in a surgical patient without previous lung disease or intra-cardiac defects, the diagnosis of acute respiratory failure is made. An arterial oxygen tension below 30 mm Hg is generally incompatible with survival for more than a few hours. Several factors, singly or in combination, can produce this severe hypoxemia. Abnormal distribution of blood to sections of the lung containing closed or non-ventilated airways or alveoli will result in so-called physiologic shunting of unsaturated blood into the arterial circulation. Injury to the pulmonary capillary endothelium or pulmonary vascular congestion frequently leads to increased interstitial lung water, which not only increases the diffusion distance for oxygen but causes collapse of alveoli. Pulmonary surfactant, which normally prevents alveolar collapse by reducing surface tension at low lung volumes, may be depleted by hypoxemia and lack of metabolic substrates in acute disease. Thus the collapse of more alveoli creates a vicious cycle of increasing hypoxemia. The reduced lung volume and loss of compliance, or distensibility, are characteristic of a group of nonspecific respiratory distress syndromes associated with shock, trauma, and other clinical problems. They all result in serious venous admixture, so that as much as 50 percent of the output of the right side of the heart may bypass ventilated alveoli. In this circumstance, the alveolar-arterial oxygen gradient may be more than 600 mm Hg, resulting in an arterial oxygen tension of only 60 mm Hg. It is important to detect such a problem early, before irreversible damage is done. The use of a respirator with continuous positive-pressure breathing (PEEP) reduces the cost of respiratory work and decreases shunting by ventilating more alveoli.

Thus far, in dissecting the oxygen transport system as a guide to physiologic monitoring, only oxygen loading has been considered. Other problems can occur downstream related to bloodflow, hemoglobin deficiency, hemoglobin affinity, or cellular defects. These more or less reflect the classic forms of hypoxia described by Barcroft and later appended by Van Slyke: anoxic, stagnant, anemic, and histotoxic hypoxia.

In considering the physiology of body blood flow, two important points must be made: the cardiac output alone is not an indicator of myocardial contractility, and arterial blood pressure alone is not an indicator of blood flow. Myocardial contractility refers to the state of health of the heart muscle and the rate at which the muscle fibers can shorten circumferentially around the bolus of blood within the ventricles. As will be seen later, myocardial contrac-

tility is intimately involved with myocardial oxygen transport.

Cardiac output, the actual amount of blood ejected by the heart, is related to three other factors besides contractility: preload, afterload, and pulse rate. The preload is the degree of muscle fiber stretch imposed by filling of the ventricles during diastole. According to Starling's law of the heart, this varies directly with cardiac output. The afterload is the impedance to cardiac ejection during systole imposed by vascular resistance, blood pressure, and blood viscosity. The stroke output of the heart varies inversely with the afterload. The cardiac output varies directly with the pulse rate up to a level of 160, at which point there is insufficient time for complete ventricular filling. Any monitoring system designed to assess the state of the myocardium must include these factors. The Sarnoff ventricular function curve is a plot of stroke work (the product of stroke volume and mean aortic blood pressure) against ventricular end-diastolic pressure or end-diastolic volume. It provides a good evaluation of myocardial contractility because it includes consideration of afterload and preload.

One manifestation of the human body as an automatic control system is the fact that a major determinant of cardiac output is increased metabolic activity which produces peripheral vasodilation and a reduced cardiac afterload. Increased metabolic activity also increases the venous return and thus slightly increases cardiac preload. The peripheral arterioles under control of the autonomic nervous system largely control the systemic vascular resistance. The systemic blood pressure varies with the product of the total vascular resistance and the cardiac output. This is why it is impossible to evaluate blood flow on the basis of the blood pressure alone. One seldom used clue to the level of total peripheral resistance is the pulse pressure or the difference between systolic and diastolic blood pressure. As total peripheral resistance increases, the pulse pressure narrows because of increased outflow impedance from the arterial tree.

The varying distribution of the cardiac output to the different organs and body tissues is the body's most important defense in oxygen transport deficiency. During resuscitation from cardiac arrest, the cardiac index is slightly over 1 liter/minute with open-chest cardiac massage. Closed-chest massage produces half of that. The normal cardiac index is 3 liters/minute/m^2 of body surface area. Yet these low flows are frequently enough to keep the brain alive, because flow to all other tissues except the myocardium is drastically curtailed.

The brain is particularly sensitive to hypoxia. It has no oxygen reserves and constantly requires 15 percent of the resting cardiac output and 20 percent of the total basal oxygen consumption just to maintain its structural and physiologic integrity. The reasons for this will be discussed later. However, irreversible brain damage occurs in man when cerebral oxygen consumption is 50 percent reduced, while the kidneys can tolerate one-third the normal flow for over an hour without damage although they normally receive 25 percent of the cardiac output. In general, organs with low oxygen extraction ratios tolerate decreased blood flow fairly well. The kidneys normally extract only 10 percent of the oxygen available in their arterial blood supply, the heart extracts 70 percent, and the body as a whole extracts 25 percent. An arm or a leg can survive total tourniquet occlusion of its blood supply for over an hour without permanent damage, and the cornea of the eye survives several hours after death of the individual.

During acute hypoxia or circulatory crises, blood is preferentially sent to the heart and brain. Since flow is curtailed to tissues with a low priority such as the skin, skeletal muscles, and corneas as soon as hypoxia or low flow threatens, monitoring flow or oxygen tension in these tissues would provide an early warning.

Organs other than the heart, which normally extracts most of the oxygen from coronary artery blood, can compensate for low blood flow by extracting more oxygen from their venous oxygen reserves. Thus, the arteriovenous oxygen difference of the body or of an individual organ is a measure of the extent to which blood flow matches the metabolic demand for oxygen. In the normal resting state, the entire body consumes only 25 percent of the oxygen transported to it by the cardiac output. This is confirmed from all the organs after it has been mixed in the right side of the heart. Normal mixed venous blood is found to be 75 percent saturated with a partial pressure of 40 mm Hg. Levels lower than this indicate increased oxygen demands which cannot be met because of decreased available arterial oxygen or decreased cardiac output. Since most surgeons would like to be warned of either of these circumstances, monitoring of mixed venous oxygen levels is becoming popular. Mixed venous oxygen tension during anesthesia responds to a fall in cardiac output before any change is noted in blood pressure, pulse rate, or central venous pressure. It would be useful to assess the oxygen supply to individual organs as well, particularly the brain. Cerebrospinal fluid from the cisterna magna of the brain responds promptly to hypoxemia or ischemia with a drop in oxygen tension, but this can hardly be considered a noninvasive approach.

Having considered the lungs, the heart, and major blood vessels, we now approach the business end of the oxygen transport system, where the partial pressure of oxygen rapidly drops from 90 to 40 mm Hg. The capillary bed of an organ is a rapidly changing dynamic system with precapillary sphincters under the control of tissue hypoxic feedback mechanisms as well as sympathetic and hemodynamic reflexes. When increased work, fever, inflammation, catecholamine stimulation, or increased thyroxine levels intensify the metabolic demands of an organ, precapillary sphincters relax and the capillary bed enlarges. A working skeletal muscle has ten to twenty times the number of functioning capillaries as a resting muscle. The myocardium has the most active set of sphincters and the most profuse capillary network of any organ. In the basal state, less than half the capillaries are open, but with increased demands the myocardial oxygen consumption can increase sixfold. Not only does more blood flow through the enlarged capillary bed, but the distance between open capillaries is reduced from 20 to 14 μ, so that oxygen has a shorter diffusion distance to the cells. This increased vascularity further reduces peripheral resistance and cardiac afterload in addition to that achieved by arteriolar dilatation. Up until this point, very little oxygen is lost from the arterial blood, but in the capillaries many factors combine to encourage oxygen unloading in the cylinder of tissue surrounding each capillary. The natural affinity of hemoglobin for oxygen is decreased by heat, hydrogen ions, carbon dioxide (Bohr effect), and red cell diphosphoglycerate (DPG). These agents act at a stereochemical level to help form a hemoglobin molecule which is more stable in its unsaturated state. The heat of working tissues, hypoxic acidosis, and carbon dioxide from cellular metabolism all tend to shift the oxyhemoglobin dissociation curve to the right where more oxygen is released at a higher tissue oxygen tension. The relative position of the oxyhemoglobin dissociation curve is identified by the P_{50} value, the partial pressure of oxygen at which the hemoglobin is half saturated at 37°C and pH 7.4. There is a biologic feedback mechanism which increases the red cell diphosphoglycerate in chronic hypoxic states, but like renal erythropoietin regulation, the mechanism is too slow to be of significance in clinical monitoring.

Red cell diphosphoglycerate may be of considerable clinical significance in patients requiring massive blood transfusions. Bank blood stored for more than 2 weeks is depleted of diphosphoglycerate, reducing the P_{50} value from 26 to 11 mm Hg. Adequate oxygen release in the capillary bed can occur only at lower oxygen tensions, thus reducing the oxygen diffusion gradient in the tissue cylinder surrounding the capillary. The cells at the venous end of the capillary, where the oxygen tension is normally lower, are the first to suffer. For this reason, the periphery of the pericapillary cylinder at the venous end is called the *todlische Ecke*, or "deadly corner." This effect is best seen in centrilobular necrosis of the liver, wherein hypoxic cell death first occurs near the central venule.

Another frequently overlooked problem of hemoglobin affinity is carbon monoxide poisoning. Patients who have been burned in closed spaces may have serious defects of oxygen transport caused by carbon monoxide displacing oxygen from hemoglobin and poisoning the mitochondrial cytochrome a_3 system. In addition, carbon monoxide lowers the P_{50}, which further reduces available oxygen (Fig. 13-7).

Since oxygen tension falls off with the square of the distance from the capillary, by the time oxygen diffuses through the pores of the cell membrane, the partial pressure of oxygen is about 6 mm Hg. Table 13-1 shows a value of 10 mm Hg outside the membrane. This does not mean that there is resistance to diffusion across the cell membrane but that, within the tissues, consumption of oxygen must occur in the cells in order to establish a gradient. Within the cell, myoglobin facilitates the passage of oxygen by serving as a sort of bucket brigade. As might be expected from what has been described in previous paragraphs, the cardiac muscle is richest in myoglobin. Myoglobin has a very high affinity for oxygen and releases it only at very low tensions, as needed. The actual utilization of oxygen occurs in complex intracellular organelles called *mitochondria*.

In the mitochondrion, an array of catalysts and cofactors comprising the Krebs cycle oxidize pyruvate produced by the anaerobic glycolysis of glucose. Anaerobic glycolysis of glucose yields only 50 kcal/mole, whereas the complete oxidation of glucose to carbon dioxide and water in the mitochondrion yields 686 kcal/mole of glucose. The higher animals cannot survive on the lower-energy-producing fermentative process alone. Some 1.2 billion years ago, organisms learned to protect themselves from the toxic oxygen molecules slowly building up in the primeval atmosphere by enzymatically catalyzing the reduction of oxygen to water while at the same time oxidizing the end products of cellular fermentation such as lactic acid. Trillions of generations later, the cells harnessed the extra energy thus released to the reconstitution of the high-energy phosphate bond of adenosine triphosphate (ATP). Vestiges of the earlier process are still found, even in human cells, in the form of other organelles called *peroxisomes*. Peroxisomes are believed to protect cells from excess oxygen by the enzymatic oxidation of amino acids and lactic acid. However, this oxidation is not coupled to energy storage.

Within the mitochondrion, the oxidation of pyruvate is carried out anaerobically by removal of electrons rather than the addition of oxygen. The electrons are passed along the respiratory chain, alternately oxidizing and reducing diphosphopyridine nucleotide (DPN), flavoproteins, ubiquinone, and cytochromes. At the final step cytochrome C passes two electrons to an oxygen atom, which combines with two hydrogen ions to form one molecule of water. An obligatory coupling of this process to the conversion of adenosine diphosphate (ADP) to ATP fulfills two functions. First, much of the high energy of the complete oxidation of glucose is stored for all forms of cellular work. Second, the rate of this oxidative phosphorylation is governed by the energy needs of the cell. The cell is protected from excess oxygen by the fact that only when ADP is present will oxygen be utilized to allow the establishment of an oxygen gradient across the cell membrane. As long as the intracellular oxygen tension is above 5 mm Hg, the rate-limiting factor of cellular respiration is the availability of ADP, not oxygen.

Certain agents, the best known of which is dinitrophenol, uncouple oxidation from phosphorylation permitting runaway oxidation without energy storage. This is a rapidly lethal process. Less well known is the uncoupling ability of certain bacterial endotoxins. Abnormally high oxygen consumption has been demonstrated just before death in patients with septic shock. Cyanide and carbon monoxide have the reverse effect on the cell; they block the transfer of electrons from cytochrome C to oxygen.

Britton Chance has defined three cellular respiratory states. First, in the resting state, oxidative phosphorylation is limited by low levels of ADP and phosphates. Second, in the working state, most of the ATP has been converted to ADP, establishing a relatively high oxygen gradient from the capillary to the mitochondrion. Third, ADP and phosphate are in excess; if oxygen is not available for diffusion from the capillary, critical pyridine nucleotide reduction

(CPNR) rapidly occurs. Critical levels of reduced DPN occur when oxygen tension in the mitochondrion falls to 0.1 mm Hg. This corresponds to a capillary oxygen tension of 4 mm Hg. The cell is forced to obtain energy from anaerobic glycolysis alone, thus building up an oxygen debt and conversion of pyruvate to lactic acid. Acidosis and elevated lactate levels can be detected in the peripheral circulation, but only if capillary perfusion is present to wash the cellular products into the venous circulation. This is why, in shock states, peripheral arterial pH may not accurately reflect intracellular pH. The autolytic washout products of critically hypoxic and injured cells have been monitored for decades on the false assumption that venous blood always equilibrates with ischemic tissue. A better approach would be to detect molecular signals at the cellular level.

Voluntary muscle can build up an oxygen debt of 40 ml/kg of cell mass, compared to a resting oxygen requirement of 4 ml/kg/minute. The 10 billion neuron units of the human brain can tolerate no oxygen debt. When the cerebral arterial oxygen tension falls to 20 mm Hg, that within the neurons is only 0.2 mm Hg. At this level of hypoxia, half of the electron carrier, DPN, is in the reduced state. When 90 percent of DPN is in the reduced state, even the respiratory center ceases to function, and irreversible damage occurs. As long as some circulatory flow exists, even with severe hypoxemia, there is a chance to maintain the critical 0.1 mm Hg tension within the neuron. With complete circulatory arrest, however, the oxygen is quickly used up, and the neuron dies. The brain requires constant energy supplies just to maintain the unsteady state of polarization for the transmission of the network of impulses which is an integral part of the cerebral life process. This peculiar and critical requirement of the brain is related to modern information theory, which explains the energy requirements of complex information systems. Long before the critical state of cerebral hypoxia is reached, other symptoms and signs occur, such as restlessness, unconsciousness, Cheyne-Stokes respiration, and EEG abnormalities. There is recent evidence by Safar's group that massive doses of short-acting barbiturates, given shortly after complete cerebral ischemia, provide protection for the brain and normalize its metabolism.

As other cells reach critical hypoxic states, they no longer have the energy to maintain important internal cell structures. One of these is the phospholipid lysosomal membrane which protects the cell from the necessary but potentially destructive enzymes contained within the lysosomes. When released into the cell, the powerful proteases, esterases, and phosphatases destroy the cell.

Britton Chance has led the way in developing methods to study cellular hypoxia. His fluorometric instrument makes it possible to measure intracellular oxygen tensions between 0.03 and 2 mm Hg. This is accomplished by measuring the fluorescence emission of the reduced state of DPN when it is stimulated by ultraviolet light. Other techniques of detecting molecular signals at a distance for monitoring purposes are possible, among them stimulated emission of oxygen in the microwave range, far infrared emission spectroscopy (chemiluminescence), and surface reflectance spectroscopy. Though exciting, all these are a long way from validation and routine clinical use in man.

INSTRUMENTATION AND CLINICAL TECHNIQUES

Physiologic Sensing

Rushmer has classified the methods used to obtain information from the human body for monitoring purposes. The most obvious is the analysis of samples of tissue, blood, respiratory gases, urine, cerebrospinal fluid, or other body fluids. Here the assumption is that the sample in question is a representative aliquot of the state of the entire organ system.

In surgical monitoring, the most useful aspects of this approach include continuous or intermittent analysis of arterial or mixed venous pH, blood gases (P_{O_2}, P_{CO_2}), and lactate. As pointed out earlier, the blood lactate level can be considered an indicator of the adequacy of oxygen transport to the Krebs cycle in the mitochondria. Elevated blood lactate levels indicate anaerobic metabolism as long as there is enough tissue perfusion to "wash out" the acid metabolites. Blood lactate, increased from above 1.5 mEq/L to levels above 10 mEq/L, is a grave prognostic sign unless the trend is promptly reversed.

The disadvantage of the tissue and fluid sampling approach to monitoring is that it is invasive and therefore carries some risk of infection or blood loss. An invasive technique is always more expensive than a noninvasive one, because it requires more highly trained personnel for insertion, sterilization of parts, and surveillance to prevent accidents. A corollary to this rule is that the more invasive a device, the less likely is its use before it is too late.

Rushmer's two other monitoring categories are (1) techniques which utilize intrinsic energy sources within the body of the patient and (2) methods which direct extrinsic energy probes at or into the body, with analysis of the emerging energy. Many physiologic processes are characterized by the generation of dynamic potentials, tensions, pressures, and electromagnetic emissions which constitute the intrinsic energy sources available for surgical monitoring. Examples of this approach include electrocardiography, electroencephalography, thermography, infrared emission spectroscopy, and muscle surface pH metering.

The energy used for interrogating beams in extrinsic energy probe monitoring can be ultrasound, mechanical stimuli, or photons originating at any point along the electromagnetic spectrum from gamma rays to microwaves. Examples include ultrasonic echography, videodensitometry, nuclear magnetic resonance flow probes, and impedance plethysmography.

Shannon and Weaver's classic work on information theory can be used to show that, in general, the higher the frequency of the interrogating beam or intrinsic energy source, the more information capacity (bits per second) it has. For example, a gamma ray probe could be expected to detect more physiologic information than an ultrasonic

probe. Other variables such as signal-to-noise ratio, of course, are important in determining the ultimate monitoring value of a particular system. A monitoring system employing extrinsic energy probes usually yields information with good spatial discrimination with regard to functional lesions, whereas devices which detect intrinsic energy usually provide an information-rich signal which often requires data processing for exploitation of its full information content.

The greatest need in the field of monitoring is for new sensors and transducers to detect critical states along the train of oxygen transport. Even very complicated occult signals from new sensing techniques can be made useful by modern spectral search systems. Computer programs are already available to examine and characterize more complex information in large amounts in order to analyze the fundamental properties of living systems.

Four guides to the development of new physiologic sensors are the following:

1. Detection of functional integrity of cells and cellular perfusion rather than the washout of autolytic products into the bloodstream.
2. A noninvasive mode; the device must not reduce the frequency of contact between the health professional and patient.
3. An information-rich signal originating from the desired organ system.
4. Extrinsic energy probes for spatial discrimination and intrinsic energy sources for a broader view of biologic activity.

A transducer is a device which converts energy from one form to another. A sensor is a device which detects an energy signal related to a particular state. In physiologic monitoring, a sensor is often a transducer, but not always. Electrocardiographic and electroencephalographic electrodes are sensors which do not convert energy from one form to another. The suitability of a sensing device for a particular clinical application is related to such factors as sensitivity, response time, linearity, and accuracy. The *sensitivity* is measured by the smallest change which is detectable by the device. The *response time* of an instrument is the period required to record a given change of input. *Linearity* refers to the constancy of the ratio of output signal to the measured variable. *Accuracy* is evaluated in terms of the ability to calibrate the instrument so that the output conforms precisely to the quantity of the measured variable. Accuracy is related to the error induced by unwanted variables such as temperature, pressure, and vibration.

Respiratory Monitoring

Respiratory monitoring can be very simple or extremely complex, depending on the trend or event to be warned against. The detection of a low-probability event such as respiratory arrest is easy compared to the on-line assessment of lung mechanics. Nevertheless, there is need for the former type of monitoring.

Next in complexity is the measurement of blood gases. The widespread use of pressure-cycled or volume-controlled respirators in the postoperative period would not be safe without blood-gas monitoring. In order to take over the work of breathing, when the patient's own respiratory reflexes and servo-control mechanisms are overridden or suppressed by respiratory depressants, it is essential to know if ventilation and gas exchange suit the patient's requirements. Were it not for the invention of the Clark polarographic oxygen electrode and the Severinghaus potentiometric carbon dioxide electrode in the 1950s, the task of monitoring blood gases by the classic manometric technique of Van Slyke and Neill would have imposed enormous difficulties. The Clark electrode depends on the diffusion of oxygen from the blood sample through a gas-permeable plastic membrane surrounding a platinum polarographic electrode. The electrode current is proportional to the number of oxygen molecules, but careful calibration with water of known oxygen concentration is necessary because of variations in membrane permeability and electrolyte characteristics. The Severinghaus potentiometric electrode is a glass pH electrode with bicarbonate buffer within the gas-permeable plastic membrane. Diffusion of carbon dioxide from the blood sample to the electrode produces a change in pH, which is recorded.

There are several commercial apparatus available which include thermostatically controlled water baths, calibration equipment, and digital readout. It is impossible to care properly for many surgical patients today without access to a blood-gas and pH analyzer of this sort. Unlike blood chemistries or electrolytes, these determinations require, for reliability, a rapid turnaround time and rigid quality control. For this reason, the blood-gas laboratory is often located in proximity to the intensive care unit, recovery room, and operating room.

Continuous methods of blood-gas monitoring have been developed for on-line applications, but problems of calibration, quality control, and expense reduce their utility over that of intermittent determinations. Mass spectrometry, which will be discussed later, shows promise as an accurate, rapid method for intermittent or continuous blood-gas monitoring.

Samples of arterial blood for these determinations can be obtained using an ordinary 20-gauge needle, by percutaneous puncture of the radial, brachial, or femoral arteries. The 5- or 10-ml glass or plastic syringe is first heparinized and then capped and placed in ice after the sample is drawn. Iced samples can be kept for 1 hour with a 1 percent drop in oxygen tension. Indwelling arterial and mixed venous lines can also be used as sampling sites, but the volume of blood contained in the catheter must first be discarded.

In assessing the process of gas exchange outlined in the upper part of Table 13-1, the decrement in oxygen tension from the alveolar level to the arterial blood is of considerable importance as a measure of the efficiency of oxygen exchange in the lungs. In normal man breathing room air, the alveolar-arterial oxygen tension gradient, abbreviated as $P(A\text{-a}DO_2)$, varies between 10 and 15 mm Hg. Half of this venoarterial admixture is caused by true shunting of desaturated blood into the left atrium, and the other half by ventilation-perfusion imbalance. When the patient with normal cardiorespiratory function breathes pure oxygen for 15 to 20 minutes, the alveolar-arterial gradient is between 25 and 65 mm Hg. Barometric pressure, less arterial carbon dioxide tension, less water vapor pressure, less the normal gradient yields a value of around 630 mm Hg for arterial oxygen tension while breathing pure oxygen. In this condition the gradient represents both anatomic shunting and perfusion of totally nonventilated alveoli. The effects of alveolar capillary diffusion barriers and ventilation-perfusion imbalance are eliminated by the high oxygen tension in all alveoli.

As mentioned earlier, an increased alveolar-arterial gradient on 100 percent oxygen is a very useful early warning sign for many postoperative pulmonary problems, among them atelectasis, pneumonia, interstitial pulmonary edema, septic shock lung, and posttraumatic pulmonary insufficiency. Although not very specific, it is very useful since an increase is easily determined at the bedside and occurs long before most radiologic changes are evident.

It is estimated that in normal resting man approximately 2 percent of total oxygen consumption is used to provide energy for breathing. In postoperative patients this may increase to 50 percent as a result of increased airway resistance and decreased compliance of the lung, chest wall, and diaphragm. Since much of this work can be taken over with proper use of a volume-cycled respirator, the clinical evaluation of respiratory resistance, compliance, and work has been the subject of much bioengineering research.

Patients with chronic obstructive lung disease, in whom the excess work of breathing is related primarily to expiratory rather than inspiratory effort, benefit little from respirator therapy alone. This situation generally should be detected in the preoperative state by standard pulmonary function testing, and the patient prepared for surgery by physiotherapy, bronchodilators, and antibiotics if infection is present.

Compliance is the change in pressure associated with each cubic centimeter increase in lung volume. When airway pressure is used, rather than the intrapleural pressure minus the intratracheal pressure, the compliance measurement includes that of the chest wall and diaphragm as well as the lungs. This is of little importance if the patient is entirely relaxed. However, in a postoperative patient, the difference between intraesophageal balloon or intrapleural pressure and aiway pressure must be used for meaningful results.

Volume is measured by integrating flow measured across a pneumotachograph at the airway. A *pneumotachograph* is a transducer which converts a pressure difference across a screen to an electric signal related to flow. Resistance is a function of the pressure necessary to overcome resistance at a given point in the respiratory cycle. Work per breath is the integral of the power expended during the respiratory cycle, where power is the transpulmonary pressure times flow.

The manual calculations for these variables of lung mechanics are much too tedious to be of clinical value, so a number of investigators have automated the procedures. Peters and coworkers have designed a mobile cart and digital computer programs for this purpose. Analog voltages are transmitted from an infrared carbon dioxide analyzer, a polarographic oxygen monitor, a Fleisch pneumotachograph, and a differential pressure transducer. The temperatures of inspired and mixed expired air are used for correction of gas volumes. The apparatus can be used with patients on respirators or breathing spontaneously.

The commercial version of this cardiopulmonary measurement cart also provides a channel for indicator-dilution determination of cardiac output. Measured variables include air flow, transpulmonary pressure, inspired oxygen concentration, and mean expired oxygen and carbon dioxide concentrations. From these a small, dedicated computer derives variables associated with respiratory mechanics and gas exchange. These include tidal volume, rate, compliance, resistance, work, oxygen consumption, carbon dioxide output, respiratory quotient, alveolar-arterial oxygen gradient, shunt fraction and dead-space ratio. The results can be viewed on a cathode ray tube or as teletype copy. The prototype device has been in clinical operation for several years. An analysis of patients studied thus far indicated that multiple variables of lung mechanics were better predictors of the need for a respirator than single tests. The commercial version permits telephone transmission of digitized data to a dedicated small computer or a larger time-shared system.

Osborn and associates have used a similar approach but with the transducers built in at the bedside and reliance on continuous monitoring with sophisticated trend analysis. The pneumotachygraph is specially modified with a warm air flush between sampling periods to minimize water condensation and base-line drift. The device can be left on line for as long as 48 hours. Continuous gas samples from a side tube at the expiratory end of the pneumotachygraph are analyzed with a special ceramic oxygen cell and an infrared carbon dioxide analyzer. A digital computer is used to calculate the derived variables and determine trends. Their studies of postoperative patients have revealed wide swings in the pH and blood gases related to the loss of respiratory control or changing ventilation requirements. Sudden fluctuations in carbon dioxide tensions often lead to cardiac arrhythmias or hypotension. The most useful variable in this regard is end-expiratory carbon dioxide tension. The gradient is usually less than 5 mm Hg from arterial blood to end-expiratory gas in patients, with relatively normal dead space. Such a system reduces the number of arterial blood-gas determinations necessary for the management of seriously ill patients. It has also been shown to reduce morbidity and mortality of postoperative patients requiring respirator support.

Kinney's group uses a different method for continuous spirometric determinations. A specially constructed clear plastic chamber covers the head with a snug fit at the neck. This permits the measurement of gas exchange and lung mechanics in spontaneously breathing patients with a minimum of cooperation. Several other centers employ custom-tailored computer-based respiratory monitoring systems, usually developed in cooperation with a major research-oriented corporation or an engineering school (Fig. 13-1). It is unlikely at the present time that the costs of such respiratory monitoring systems could be borne by even a large hospital on the basis of third-party payments. Nevertheless, the value of such systems for postoperative care of the high-risk patient has been proved.

Cardiovascular Monitoring

Most monitoring systems require access to arterial blood for sampling and direct pressure determinations. Monitoring, in many ways like politics, is the art of the possible. What is it possible to measure in the patient with consistent success and minimum risk? Maintaining an open arterial line without risk or discomfort requires skill and dedication to detail. The radial artery at the wrist is the site most frequently used because of safety and convenience. The presence of a functioning ulnar arterial arcade must be checked by pressure occlusion of both arteries at the wrist with subsequent release of the ulnar to produce a palmar flush (the Allen test). It is dangerous to perform even a radial arterial puncture unless such evidence of ulnar collateral flow is present. For percutaneous catheterization or a cutdown and cannulation of the radial artery, the wrist should be attached to an arm board and moderately extended. Strict glove, mask, and sterile drape technique should be used, as with all intravascular cannulations. The standards established by Dudrick and associates for indwelling central venous catheters should be followed for arterial catheters as well. Sterility should be maintained by removing the protective dressing every 3 days, rubbing off skin oil with acetone, and applying iodine tincture to the surrounding skin and antibiotic ointment to the catheter exit site. The occlusive dressing should be small and fixed carefully to the skin, using compound tincture of benzoin for better adherence. Unused stopcock sidearms should be capped with sterile rubber or plastic nipples to prevent contamination. Cannula sepsis is an iatrogenic disaster which can largely be avoided by good technique.

The type of cannula chosen is important. The long Becton-Dickenson Teflon cannula is easily inserted and can be plugged with a plastic stylet when not in use. Other polyvinyl or polyethylene cannulas are available commercially. Patency is best maintained with a constant slow infusion of 2 units of heparin diluted in 5 ml of saline solution delivered in 24 hours. This can be accomplished with either a Sage electrolytic (Fig. 13-2) or a disposable clockwork infusion pump. Both of these can be attached to the patient's arm to allow mobility.

Intermittent manual flushing to discharge clots is dangerous, since it has been demonstrated that as little as 3 ml may flush emboli back up into the cerebral circulation from a radial artery cannula. Other sites for indwelling arterial lines are the brachial or femoral artery, but these present the risk of distal ischemia and thrombophlebitis.

Catheterization of the central venous system or right side of the heart for manometry, injection of indicator, or mixed venous sampling is used as an integral part of many surgical monitoring systems. There are several routes of access to the central venous system (Fig. 13-3). In order of increasing risk these are the median basilic vein in the

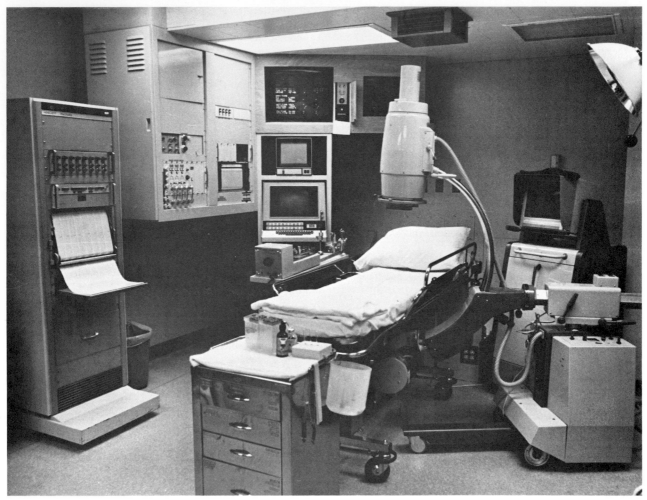

Fig. 13-1. Cardiorespiratory monitoring system based upon a central digital computer for physiologic data processing and storage. This is the equipment used by Weil and associates at the Center for the Critically III and the Shock Research Unit, University of Southern California School of Medicine.

antecubital fossa, the external jugular vein, the internal jugular vein, and the subclavian vein. The femoral vein is seldom used because of contamination and thrombophlebitis. The median basilic vein directs the catheter directly into the subclavian vein and superior vena cava if the arm is extended laterally during the procedure, whereas the cephalic vein is difficult to negotiate at the shoulder. The external jugular vein is best approached with the neck extended, turned to the opposite side and lower than heart level (to fill the vein and prevent air embolism). The vein can also be steadied and distended by proximal pressure at the neck. As with the antecubital approach, venisection is best done before the vein is ruined with multiple puncture attempts. If there is difficulty passing the jugular-subclavian junction, the catheter may pass if the shoulder is depressed. The internal jugular vein can be cannulated percutaneously above the clavicle. The puncture is made immediately lateral to the pulsation of the common carotid artery through the lateral head of the sternocleidomastoid muscle. The distance to the proper position in the superior vena cava requires a catheter 20 cm long.

Puncture and catheter introduction into the subclavian

vein involves a slightly greater risk of pneumothorax, but its ease of access makes it popular in emergency situations. As with the other sites, local anesthesia should be used as well as complete sterile precautions. Skin puncture is done just inferior to the clavicle at the junction of the middle and inner thirds, with the needle aimed at a point behind the manubrium. The catheter should not be threaded through or over the needle until venous blood is easily aspirated. When threaded through the needle, the catheter should never be withdrawn separately because of the danger of shearing if off with the sharp edge of the needle. Some commercial sets have protective sleeves which can be extended beyond the needle point to prevent cutting the catheter. A chest roentgenogram should always be obtained following central venous catheterization to check for pneumothorax and ascertain the position of the catheter tip. If a nonradiopaque catheter is used, it can be filled with contrast medium during the exposure. There are a number of commercial intravenous catheter sets available which are ingeniously designed to facilitate advancement of the catheter without contamination or kinking (Fig. 13-4). The Abbott set employs a reel device which is easily manipulated with one hand. The Sorenson catheter is housed in a longitudinally slit semirigid conduit with a sliding sleeve on the outside attached to the catheter inside through the slit. As the sleeve is advanced over the conduit, the catheter is pushed through the needle into the vein. These sets can also be used for arterial cannulations.

The proper interpretation of central venous pressure or pulmonary artery wedge pressure for monitoring surgical patients requires an understanding of *all* the factors which may cause elevated readings. Artifacts such as inaccurate zero level, blockage, or kinking should be excluded by observation of 1 to 2 cm pressure fluctuations with the respiratory cycle and careful sighting of the zero level at the midaxillary line. The zero level should correspond to the point of projection of the posterior leaflet of the tricuspid valve on the right chest wall. Noncardiac factors which increase central venous pressure are hypervolemia, vasoconstrictor drugs (metaraminol and mephentermine constrict the veins as well as arterioles), positive-pressure ventilation, pneumothorax, hydrothorax, flail chest, and mediastinal compression. If none of these factors exists, normal readings vary between 0 and 9 cm of water for central venous pressure and 5 to 12 mm Hg pulmonary artery wedge pressure ($\overline{PAw}$). Elevated values suggest the inability of either ventricle to handle its venous return. Filling pressure alone is not a measure of ventricular function or myocardial contractility, because afterload and ventricular work are unknown quantities. A high central venous pressure does serve as a warning that volume infusion should be continued with extreme caution. However, there are situations such as pericardial tamponade or pulmonary embolism where a high central venous pressure is essential to maintain an adequate cardiac output until definitive therapy is used to relieve the obstruction. The most logical use of central venous pressure or $\overline{PAw}$ as a guide to fluid replacement in seriously ill patients is the observation of the response to challenge with 100-ml increments of volume infusion. Infusion is stopped when a sharp rise in pressure occurs.

Fig. 13-3. Four routes of access to the central venous system. The direct line from the median antecubital vein to the superior vena cava makes this a safe approach, particularly with the arm extended. The cephalic vein empties into the subclavian vein at an acute angle, making central venous catheterization difficult. The external jugular vein is the next safest route. The arm should be at the side and the shoulder depressed to straighten the angle at which the external jugular enters the subclavian vein. The internal jugular vein can be cannulated by inserting the needle through the clavicular head of the sternocleidomastoid muscle, just lateral to the pulsation of the carotid artery. The subclavian cannulation over the first rib is shown. The danger of pneumothorax or hemothorax is greatest with this approach.

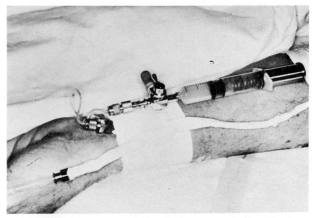

Fig. 13-2. Radial artery cannula with patency maintained by Sage electrolytic infusion pump. Note the sterile rubber nipple on the sidearm of the stopcock. A central venous catheter protected with adhesive tape is shown alongside the arm.

The distinction between right and left ventricular failure is not possible without some indication of left atrial or left ventricular end-diastolic pressure. For this reason, various techniques have been developed for bedside monitoring of pressures in the left side of the heart. Cohn et al. have

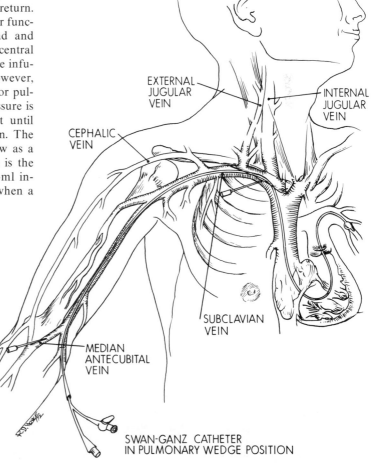

EXTERNAL JUGULAR VEIN

INTERNAL JUGULAR VEIN

CEPHALIC VEIN

SUBCLAVIAN VEIN

MEDIAN ANTECUBITAL VEIN

SWAN-GANZ CATHETER IN PULMONARY WEDGE POSITION

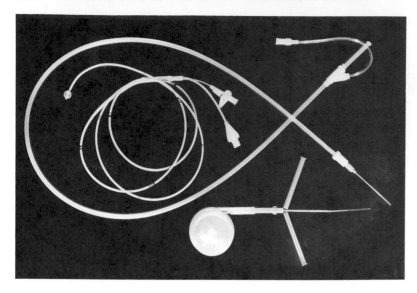

Fig. 13-4. Three popular types of monitoring catheters. The coiled Swan-Ganz balloon-tip catheter is designed to float into the pulmonary artery wedge position. The Sorenson catheter shown crossed in the photograph is contained in a conduit with a longitudinal slit to facilitate insertion into an artery or vein under sterile conditions. For similar purposes, the Abbott catheter is provided with a reellike device. The two halves of the sleeve which prevents shearing of the catheter are also shown.

used a precurved polyethylene catheter which is threaded over a wire guide from the femoral artery into the left ventricle. Fluoroscopic control is not used, but the electrocardiograph is observed for premature ventricular beats which signal entry into the ventricle and subside when the catheter is withdrawn a few centimeters. In shock associated with myocardial infarction, the left ventricular end-diastolic pressure is elevated in the 12 to 44 mm Hg range even though the central venous pressure may be normal. Such monitoring has permitted more precise fluid replacement and inotropic drug adjustment in patients with left ventricular failure.

The great majority of clinical physiologists prefer to approach the problem of bedside left ventricular dynamics from the right side of the heart. In 1959, Zohman and Williams described flow-guided pulmonary artery catheterization. The location of the catheter tip, as it floated along with the bloodstream through the right side of the heart, is determined by characteristic intracardiac electrocardiographic patterns conducted back through the soft catheter in a column of 7.5% sodium bicarbonate acting as a salt bridge. The pattern in the right atrium consists of a high, short inverted P wave, which becomes upright as the tricuspid valve is approached. The right ventricle pattern consists of a 7- to 9-mv downward QRS deflection. A standard low-voltage pattern is found in the pulmonary artery. The safety of flow-guided catheterization of the right side of the heart depends upon avoiding arrhythmias by careful observation of the intracardiac patterns. The hazard of ventricular fibrillation due to stray 60-cycle current should be minimized by careful appraisal of the electrocardiograph and the grounding capacity of its power supply. In 1966 Del Guercio et al. reported on a number of patients with suspected pulmonary embolism shock studied by a modification of this technique. Flow of the catheter was improved by a wind-sock effect created by heat curling the last 2 cm of catheter. The stylet kept it straight while it advanced through the veins.

More recently, a further advance of this approach was

the commercial development of the balloon-tipped Swan-Ganz catheter (Fig. 13-4). With the balloon inflated, the catheter sails through the right side of the heart into a wedge position in the pulmonary artery in less than 1 minute. In the absence of pulmonary vascular disease, pulmonary capillary wedge pressure ($\overline{PAw}$) is a reliable guide to left atrial and, in turn, left ventricular end-diastolic pressure. Without the wedge position, the pulmonary artery end-diastolic pressure is an acceptable indicator of mean left atrial pressure. Central venous pressure alone has been found to be an unreliable index of left ventricular function, since filling pressure in the left side of the heart may rise sharply and pulmonary edema occur without significant increases in right atrial pressures.

Right-sided catheterization with flow-guided catheters also can be monitored by intracardiac pressure changes or mobile radiologic image intensifiers. The catheter through the right side of the heart also can be used for obtaining mixed venous blood samples, injecting indicator, and infusion of medications. Extreme caution should be exercised when drugs are infused directly into the central circulation, because high myocardial concentrations are quickly achieved. These catheters also make it possible to obtain bedside pulmonary angiograms in cases of pulmonary embolism shock.

As pointed out earlier regarding physiologic concepts of monitoring, the mixed venous oxygen level reflects the extent to which the body must call upon the blood oxygen stores in states of cardiovascular stress. The value of right heart oxygen saturation monitoring during surgery has been demonstrated. Changes in cardiac output secondary to hemorrhage and other problems are reflected by early changes in right atrial oxygen saturations, usually before changes in arterial blood pressure, venous pressure, or heart rate. Changes in arterial oxygen content secondary to pulmonary shunting or decreased oxygen-carrying capacity also promptly affect mixed venous oxygen saturation. It was originally thought that pulmonary arterial samples would be necessary for this type of monitoring, but experience has shown that, in the stressed patient, right atrial or right ventricular samples correlate well with those from the pulmonary artery. Saturations below 50% from these sites are a bad prognostic sign and indicate either severe arterial hypoxemia or very significantly decreased cardiac output.

Border et al. originated a unique "no cost" bedside volumetric Van Slyke device for determining the volumes percent of unsaturation of mixed venous blood (Fig. 13-5). It is assembled from a heparinized 10-ml syringe, a stopcock, and the barrel of a 1-ml tuberculin syringe. Exactly 10 ml of mixed venous blood is drawn into the larger syringe followed by approximately 1 ml of pure oxygen. The smaller syringe, filled with saline solution, serves as a monometer to record the volume of the oxygen bubble used to saturate the blood. If the meniscus falls to the 0.5-ml mark, it indicates that the mixed venous blood required 5 vol % of oxygen for saturation. This is about normal. If the arterial blood is 100% saturated, this value would be equivalent to the arteriovenous oxygen difference. This device makes it possible for everyone to practice clinical physiology at the bedside, with little expense.

Cardiac Output Determinations

In spite of various questions regarding accuracy in high- or low-flow states, the description of indicator-dilution curves from central circulation remains the basic method for monitoring cardiac output. The technique, which goes back to 1897, involves the injection of an indicator into the right side of the heart and continuous determination of its concentration as it mixes with the cardiac output somewhere downstream. Any indicator can be used, as long as it does not affect hemodynamics or disappear from the blood before the concentration is measured. It can best be understood as a variation of the Fick principle, where the known amount of indicator is equivalent to a fixed amount of oxygen consumption, and the mean concentration of indicator after mixing is equivalent to the arteriovenous oxygen difference. It follows, then, that the faster the volume of blood flow, the lower the arteriovenous oxygen difference and mean concentration of indicator. All methods for the calculation of cardiac ouput from both continuous and single bolus injection of indicator use this principle in analyzing the time-concentration curves to obtain the mean concentration of indicator. The number of milligrams of indicator injected divided by the mean concentration of indicator gives the volume of flow during the time of the indicator-dilution curve. Thermal dilution curves are similar in principle, with use of cold saline solution as the indicator. They are popular because of their simplicity and the availability of bedside computers, but the required flow-directed balloon-tipped thermistor catheters are expensive. Since the cardiac output is usually expressed as flow per minute, the volume of flow during description of the curve is multiplied by 60 and divided by the number of seconds of duration of the curve.

It is convenient to mount the thermal dilution computer or the densitometer with its control box and motor-driven withdrawal syringe on a mobile cart, along with blood

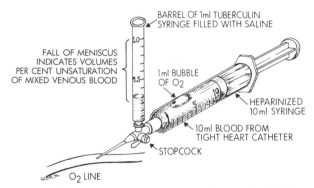

Fig. 13-5. Border's volumetric Van Slyke device for bedside determination of mixed venous unsaturation. Each 0.1-ml fall in the meniscus indicates 1 vol % unsaturation of blood. Normal is 4 to 5 vol %. When the arterial blood is fully saturated, this device indicates the arteriovenous oxygen difference. (*From J. R. Border et al., J Trauma, 6:176, 1966.*)

pressure transducers, an electrocardiograph, and a multichannel recording device. As noted earlier, this mobile apparatus has been called a shock cart; it can be used to bring fairly complete cardiovascular assessment to the bedside, operating room, or emergency room, rather than transport a critically ill patient to a clinical laboratory (Fig. 13-6). Intracardiac and arterial blood pressure tracings, indicator-dilution curves, and electrocardiograph tracings combined with arterial and mixed venous blood-gas data permit calculation of a number of derived cardiorespiratory variables of physiologic significance. Practical considerations in the design of a shock cart require a sturdy chassis with large wheels for mobility through elevator doors. There should be a waterproof work surface on top, since dilutions for calibration purposes are best done immediately. The instrument panel should be recessed out of harm's way, and the power cord should be long and mounted on a reel of some sort. The multichannel recorder should be of the direct write-out type that does not require developing. It is also more convenient to have positioning arms for the support and alignment of the pressure strain gauges and the densitometer cuvette. Some of these units can be provided with built-in computers for calculation of the cardiac output and other derived cardiovascular variables. Others provide space for a programmable calculator to serve the same purpose (Fig. 13-7).

Several hand-held calculators with program cards specifically made up for shock-cart calculating are available. The primary data obtained from the recorder and blood gas machines are entered on the keyboard, and the derived values are immediately computed. Civetta's and Shoemaker's groups have made available magnetic card programs for the rapid automatic calculation of up to 27 derived cardiorespiratory variables, using Hewlett-Packard and Texas Instrument calculators, respectively.

Data become information only in the brain of the beholder. The average physician is "turned off" by a column of numbers representing cardiac index, stroke index, right and left ventricular stroke work, pulmonary and systemic vascular resistance, ventricular function indices, intracardiac and systemic pressures, arteriovenous oxygen differ-

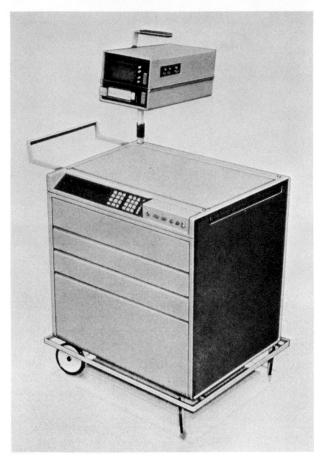

Fig. 13-6. The bedside "shock cart" approach to monitoring is shown by this model which represents the advanced state-of-the-art. By means of a balloon flotation catheter in the pulmonary artery and a radial artery cannula, cardiac output, pressures and blood gas measurements are taken from the patient and fed into a microprocessor computer to calculate derived physiologic variables which are printed out on a graphic profile (Fig. 13-7). This system is essentially a mobile, computerized cardiac catheterization laboratory as distinct from the built-in, hard-wired monitoring systems based upon a central computer.

ence, venoarterial admixture, oxygen consumption, P_{50}, serum lactate and arterial base excess or deficit. In an attempt to make dull data attractive, Cohn and Del Guercio devised a system for displaying these derived variables on an easily scanned, logically organized, bar-chart format. Arterial and mixed venous blood gas and saturation values along with cardiac output, temperature, height, weight and inspired oxygen concentration are entered on the keyboard of a minicomputer, and within seconds the derived variables are drawn on a preprinted sheet (Fig. 13-7) by an X-Y alpha-numeric recorder. This system, called the *automated physiologic profile*, is a compromise between the hand-held calculator approach and the very expensive built-in digital computer monitors. The profile serves as a useful permanent record of cardiorespiratory status before and after therapeutic interventions.

The example shown in Fig. 13-7 demonstrates a number of points regarding monitoring of the critically ill patient.

This was a study, with Swan-Ganz thermistor catheter and radial artery cannula, of a young man who suffered a 30 percent burn and smoke inhalation. The physiologic assessment was done 24 hours after injury and showed a "normal" cardiac index and blood pressure with an increase in oxygen consumption resulting from a widened arteriovenous oxygen difference. Why, then, was there evidence of anaerobic metabolism and hypoxic acidosis with twice normal serum lactate levels and a base deficit of 6 mEq/L? Because the patient's oxygen needs were even greater, and had the state of increasing oxygen debt continued, the patient surely would have died. The ventricular function curve in the lower right quadrant shows why the patient could not increase his cardiac output enough to supply his increased oxygen needs. The plot, representing the Starling-Frank relationship, is significantly below the zone of normal ventricular function. The cause for this cardiac failure could have been circulating myocardial depressant factors, known to be associated with burns, early sepsis, or poisoning of myocardial mitochondrial cytochromes by the high level of carbon monoxide (SCO), which probably had been much higher on admission. The high right atrial and pulmonary artery wedge pressures indicate that both ventricles had more than adequate preload. Since total peripheral vascular resistance was normal, that determinant of cardiac output (afterload) also was not the limiting factor. It was obvious from this physiologic profile (but not from the ECG, $\overline{PAw}$, or systemic BP) that the patient would not survive unless inotropic therapy could stimulate the myocardium to at least normal contractility. This was accomplished with digitalis, dopamine, and GIK (glucose, insulin, potassium).

At the same time, the profile also illustrated the need for a volume cycled respirator with PEEP to reduce the severe pulmonary shunting (venoarterial admixture) caused by the smoke inhalation. The most appropriate setting of end-expiratory pressure (optimum PEEP) was determined by performing automated physiologic profiles sequentially at increased levels of PEEP. Beyond a certain level, reduced cardiac output, resulting from restricted preload, produced a net decrease in oxygen transport, even though arterial oxygen content continued to improve. Had it not been for the information provided by the monitoring of these derived cardiorespiratory variables, it is unlikely that lifesaving therapeutic decisions could have been made in time.

The effect of the 15 percent carboxyhemoglobin concentration on the position of the oxyhemoglobin dissociation curve is also shown. The P_{50} STD value of 30.2 excludes the effect of carbon monoxide, and the P_{50} STDX value of 24.9 indicates the shift to the left caused by carboxyhemoglobin. The lines with the Xs on the bar-charts for "A-V Diff.," QO_2, and $\dot{Q}_A/\dot{Q}_T$ indicate those values at the patient's actual P_{50} compared with what they would have

Fig. 13-7. Graphic display of derived cardiorespiratory variables ▶ computed from arterial and mixed-venous blood gases, cardiac output, and other data obtained by means of a bedside "shock cart." For details of interpretation in this patient with 30 percent burns and smoke inhalation, see text.

NEW YORK MEDICAL COLLEGE
SURGICAL PHYSIOLOGY SERVICE

Automated Physiologic Profile

$Q_A : Q_T$

$Q_S : \dot{Q}_T$

$FIO_2 = .020$

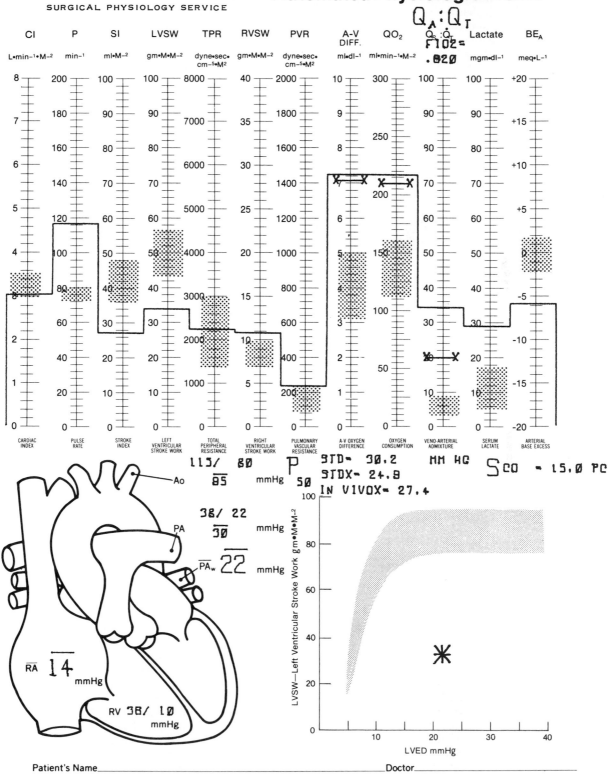

	CI	P	SI	LVSW	TPR	RVSW	PVR	A-V DIFF.	QO₂		Lactate	BE_A
units	L•min⁻¹•M⁻²	min⁻¹	ml•M⁻²	gm•M•M⁻²	dyne•sec•cm⁻⁵•M²	gm•M•M⁻²	dyne•sec•cm⁻⁵•M²	ml•dl⁻¹	ml•min⁻¹•M⁻²		mgm•dl⁻¹	meq•L⁻¹

CARDIAC INDEX · PULSE RATE · STROKE INDEX · LEFT VENTRICULAR STROKE WORK · TOTAL PERIPHERAL RESISTANCE · RIGHT VENTRICULAR STROKE WORK · PULMONARY VASCULAR RESISTANCE · A-V OXYGEN DIFFERENCE · OXYGEN CONSUMPTION · VENO-ARTERIAL ADMIXTURE · SERUM LACTATE · ARTERIAL BASE EXCESS

Ao 113/ 80 85 mmHg

PA 38/ 22 30 mmHg

$\overline{PA}_w$ 22 mmHg

$\overline{RA}$ 14 mmHg

RV 38/ 10 mmHg

P 50

STD= 30.2
STDX= 24.8
IN VIVOX= 27.4

SCO = 15.0 PC

LVSW—Left Ventricular Stroke Work gm•M•M⁻²

LVED mmHg

Patient's Name_____ Doctor_____

Lab. No._____ Rm._____ Date_____ Time_____

been had the P_{50} been normal (26 to 27 mm Hg). This type of calculation is of value clinically since it is possible to manipulate the P_{50} by pharmacologic means in order to improve oxygen transport. Harken's recent review of this aspect of monitoring emphasizes the importance of dissociation curve shifts in clinical syndromes.

The automated physiologic profile is in use in many institutions, including a number of community hospitals, where it has been proved cost-effective, particularly when used for preoperative assessment and physiologic fine tuning in the high-risk patient.

The technological goal in monitoring is to provide the maximum amount of cardiorespiratory and oxygen transport information with a minimum amount of blood sampling and trauma to the patient. In this regard thermal dilution techniques have become popular.

Another approach to this problem uses fiberoptic oximetry to record the concentration of green dye in the pulmonary artery after injection into the right atrium. A Swan-Ganz catheter was adapted with light-carrying glass fibers so that both oximetry for oxygen saturation measurement and densitometry for cardiac output determination could be carried out at the catheter tip. No arterial sampling is required when this technique is used.

There are other monitoring systems which involve the use of catheter-tip sensors. One measures pressure and electromagnetic flow velocity. When threaded retrograde into the left ventricle, this sensor permits the on-line recording of the left ventricular pressures, left ventricular pressure acceleration (dp/dt), intracardiac heart sounds, ascending aortic blood velocity, and ascending aortic blood acceleration. If the cross-sectional area of the aorta is known, total flow can be calculated. All these serve as very useful indices of left ventricular function, particularly following myocardial infarction. The problem of calibration of the electromagnetic flowmeter probe without a zero flow calibration point is a serious one, as it is for all clinical studies involving electromagnetic flowmeters.

A disposable, very thin polarographic oxygen-sensing electrode can be used for mixed venous oxygen tension monitoring. The miniature sensor is fabricated by dipcoating or painting the various insulators, diffusion membranes, and buffers directly onto the central wire electrode. Other similar devices are available complete with compact solid-state battery-powered recorders for use at the bedside.

The insertion of a long catheter from the radial artery up to the region of the aortic arch permits a detailed analysis of the aortic pulse contour. Warner has perfected this technique for clinical monitoring. Stroke volume is computed from the pulse contour on a beat-by-beat basis. This, combined with pressure variables, provides an almost instantaneous cardiovascular assessment. Unfortunately, McDonald et al. have pointed out, the method depends upon a stable vascular impedance, which is seldom the case in critically ill patients. For this reason, the technique is not in general use.

All the methods of estimating cardiac output described thus far are invasive to varying degrees and therefore present some risk and considerable expense because they require skilled personnel for their application. A number of promising noninvasive adaptations of the indicator-dilution principle are in clinical use. Included in this category are gamma densitometry (quantitative angiography), videodensitometry, isotope-dilution analysis, fluorescence excitation analysis, and magnetic fluid tracer dilution.

Information regarding flow rates, vascular volumes, distribution of pulmonary transit times, intracardiac and pulmonary shunting, and right or left ventricular ejection efficiency is theoretically contained in the shapes of indicator-dilution curves. With the conventional indocyanine green dye technique, sampling rates are too slow, and the injection and sampling sites are too far apart, for complete interpretation of the physiologic events that create the shape of the curve. Catheter lag between the sampling point and the densitometer cuvette also produces distortion of the curves and loss of potential information. Gamma densitometry, in which the indicator is a small bolus of radiopaque contrast medium and the blood vessels or cardiac chambers serve as the densitometer cuvettes, avoids these problems. Gamma rays or x-rays, projected through the cardiac silhouette, produce high-dynamic-response indicator time-concentration curves through the detection of changes in gamma photon density related, according to Beer's law, to the concentration of radiopaque indicator in the blood. In clinical practice, solid-state radiation detectors are placed behind the patient as in a portable x-ray unit. Five milliliters of Hypaque is then injected into the central venous catheter, and six simultaneous contrast dilution curves are recorded from the heart and great vessels. Analysis of these curves permits calculation of pulmonary circulation time, pulmonary blood volume, right and left ventricular ejection fraction, and other useful variables. More sophisticated interpretation requires electronic data processing for transfer function analysis.

Videodensitometry is similar in principle to gamma densitometry, except that an actual angiocardiogram is performed and recorded on magnetic tape. When played back on a television screen, the concentration of contrast medium is analyzed at any point in the heart and lungs by means of a movable electronic window. The advantages are that, at leisure, an infinite number of curves can be obtained from any point in the cardiac silhouette as the tape is played over and over. Disadvantages include great expense, lack of portability, and low signal-to-noise ratio requiring signal processing to obtain recognizable curves.

Isotope dilution analysis has made a great leap forward with the development of the Anger scintillation camera and other rapid-response isotope scanning devices. The ability to image and quantitate the distribution of a radioactive tracer second by second through the heart and lungs adds a new dimension of considerable value to surgical cardiovascular monitoring. High-photon-yield isotopes are injected intravenously and the gamma camera images recorded on magnetic tape. Later, specific areas can be analyzed to produce indicator-dilution curves which can be related to changes in size and position of the cardiac chambers. Jones et al. have produced good indicator-dilution curves for the right and left sides of the heart using an autofluoroscope. Spatial resolution and dynamic response, however, can never be as good as that obtained with the linear interrogating beams of radiation used in gamma densitometry. Furthermore, equipment for both isotope dilution and videodensitometry is expensive and bulky at present, and cannot be used for bedside studies.

Kaufman and associates have developed a highly innovative system for the bedside determination of cardiac output. Following the intravenous injection of a small amount of iodine containing radiographic contrast material, the iodine is caused to emit fluorescence in the gamma ray range by stimulation with an external gamma ray source. The stimulated emission of iodine is detected by a collimated silicon diode producing a characteristic indicator-dilution curve. The system is easily calibrated, and the radiation dose is low.

Another new method for the external noninvasive detection of indicator dilution has been described by Newbower. The indicator is a magnetic fluid tracer composed of fine ferromagnetic particles. The detection transducer is a simple set of air-core coils which easily measures the striking difference in magnetic susceptibility between the tracer and the background without the need for magnetic shielding. This novel approach has great potential because it does not involve ionizing radiation of any sort.

It is also possible to tag flowing blood in vivo by reversing the magnetic alignments of hydrogen nuclei in the water of the plasma by applying a powerful external magnetic field. These effects are detected further downstream by means of nuclear magnetic resonance. Nuclear magnetic resonance monitoring devices presently are under development. The technique is totally noninvasive.

It is obvious that noninvasive techniques for describing indicator-dilution curves will play a prominent role in surgical monitoring for years to come. Surgeons will be provided information regarding cardiac and circulatory function in their patients which will permit management of critical states on a firm physiologic basis.

The determination of systolic time intervals provides an external assessment of left ventricular function based entirely on intrinsic electrical and mechanical events. The methodology is gaining in popularity because it is physiologically sound and has been largely validated by extensive comparative clinical studies including catheterization of the left side of the heart.

Simultaneous recordings of the electrocardiogram, phonocardiogram, and external carotid pulse tracing are analyzed for the following time variables: total left ventricular systolic time (QRS complex to second heart sound), left ventricular ejection time (duration of carotid pulse upstroke), and preejection period (the difference between total left ventricular systolic and left ventricular ejection times). Although the calculations are straightforward, placement of the carotid pulse sensor and phonocardiogram microphone on the neck and chest is critical. With technical care in the performance of the recordings, remarkably good correlation with direct measures of the dynamics of the left side of the heart can be shown. Weissler et al. have found that the ratio of the preejection period to left ventricular ejection time (PEP/LVET) is relatively constant around 0.35 in patients with normal hearts. With failure of the left side of the heart, the PEP becomes longer and the LVET shorter, increasing the ratio. Serial studies reveal good correlation between the PEP/LVET ratio and left ventricular ejection fraction, end-diastolic volume, and end-diastolic pressure. This noninvasive approach, which requires inexpensive equipment, is useful for the continuous bedside monitoring of left ventricular function.

Alterations of left ventricular conduction, however, as in left bundle branch block, prolong the PEP selectively with no apparent change in LVET. Changes in peripheral impedance or vascular runoff, as occur in septic shock, may alter the relation between the PEP/LVET ratio and cardiac performance.

The application of ultrasound to clinical monitoring is undergoing a period of rapid growth. Both industrial and academic sectors are developing methods for cardiovascular assessment based on interrogating beams of high-frequency sound waves (less than 1 mm wavelength). Ultrasonic energy can penetrate all tissues except bone and air-filled structures and provide good spatial resolution for diagnostic studies. Thus far, at the levels of energy needed for clinical work, there has been no suggestion of injury to living tissue, not even the fetus. The lack of hazard and the reasonable cost of the equipment required has led to more clinical studies than with any other technique aside from electrocardiography.

There are two basic methods of operation of ultrasound for diagnostic purposes—the pulse-echo mode (sonar) and the backscatter frequency shift mode (Doppler effect). In the former, the distance between the emitter and any sound-reflecting interface deep within the body is measured in terms of the transit time of bursts of ultrasound to and from the tissue. An A-scan device is held stationary against the body and a recording of the depth of structures in the path of the beam made on the basis of the known speed of sound in tissue. The B scan is produced if the ultrasonic emitter is traversed across the body while echo-ranging, in order to produce a picture of the tissue cross section.

Not only is ultrasound less harmful than ionizing radiation, but it is capable of revealing internal surfaces which are invisible to roentgen rays. These include the internal structures of the heart and blood vessels. In addition, devices using the Doppler principle can detect rapid motions within the body. This makes them useful for studies of peripheral blood flow and cardiac valve function.

In echocardiography for ultrasonic determination of cardiac chamber size and stroke volume, a transducer is applied to the chest over the cardiac area. Sound in the 1- to 5-megacycle frequency is delivered through the chest in on-off bursts about 1,500 times per second. Echoes are detected during the off periods and recorded in terms of time lag (distance). The distances between the intraventricular septum and the posterior endocardial wall of the left ventricle are recorded at end diastole and end systole. The calculations of end-diastolic and end-systolic volumes are made on the assumption that the shape of the chamber is a prolate ellipse. The results from a number of investigators are remarkable. The left ventricular volumes measured by echocardiography and by biplane angiocardiography were very similar over a wide range of values (correlation coefficient .97). The problem with this technique for surgical monitoring is that the operator must be highly skilled and experienced in aiming the transducer and recognizing on the scan the exact structures he wishes to measure. The device cannot be simply strapped on and left alone for 24 hours to record left ventricular function. Some method will have to be devised for the ultrasonic beam to "lock on" to the left ventricular wall reflections. This will not be an easy task.

Fig. 13-8. Potentiometric electrode used to monitor muscle surface pH as an indicator of anaerobic metabolism related to inadequate perfusion. (*From N. P. Couch et al., Ann Surg, 173:173, 1971.*)

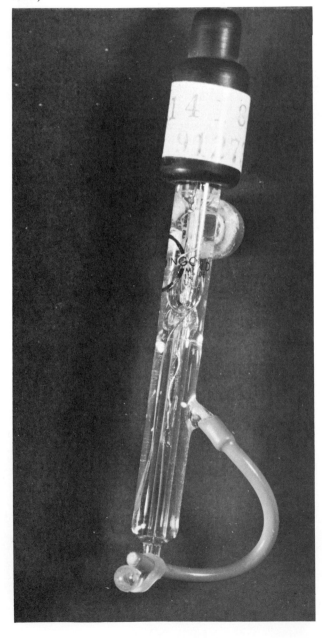

The Doppler flowmeter has achieved considerable sophistication as a clinical tool in the past few years. Readout varies from a simple audible signal related to pulse velocity to signals combining vessel cross section and velocity to provide actual flow measurements. These techniques cannot yet be applied to aortic flow determination, but the entire field of ultrasonics offers many possibilities for the evolution of the perfect cardiovascular monitor.

The concept of measuring pulse volume on the basis of the electric properties of blood goes back 40 years, but practical instruments for measuring electric impedance related to movement of electrolyte of the electromagnetic field have only recently been developed. In the instrument developed by Kubicek et al., two electrodes are placed around the neck and two around the abdomen just below the chest. The volume of blood between the electrodes decreases as the stroke volume flows up the carotids and down the aorta. This produces a decrease in electric impedance in the thorax. Since this cyclic change in impedance, compared to total chest impedance, is equivalent to less than one part in a thousand, considerable electronic sophistication is required for its detection. Alternating current is sent through the outer electrodes, and the change in voltage between the inner electrodes measured during cardiac systole indicates the impedance change due to left ventricular ejection. The problem, of course, is that venous inflow occurs more or less continuously, so that a net stroke volume during maximum ejection is measured. Great hopes were held for thoracic impedance plethysmography as a relatively inexpensive noninvasive means of monitoring cardiac output and ventricular function. Unfortunately, electrode motion artifacts and lack of correlation with other methods for the estimation of cardiac output in nonsteady states have dampened enthusiasm for this class of instruments.

There is no more consistently accurate method of measuring cardiac output than a properly calibrated electromagnetic flowmeter placed firmly around the ascending aorta. In fact, this approach is accepted as the standard against which other cardiac output monitoring equipment is evaluated for accuracy. Of course, electromagnetic flowmeters can be used only for assessing vascular operations.

Monitoring of Tissue Metabolism

It was pointed out early in the chapter that a systems approach to monitoring would direct most effort toward a study of tissue metabolism. Under certain conditions, such as hypoxemia or septic shock, a high cardiac output is no guarantee of adequate delivery of oxygen to the cells. Couch and colleagues have succeeded in developing a practical and simple solution to the problem of an early warning system for tissue hypoxia (Fig. 13-8). With an electrometer and right-angle pH electrode, skeletal muscle surface pH is continuously monitored. A 2-cm incision through skin, subcutaneous tissue, and fascia is required for placement of the electrode in gentle contact with the surface of the biceps muscle in adults and the quadriceps in children. Clinical monitoring by this technique has been continued for as long as 8 days.

The rationale for this approach is that with tissue deprivation of oxygen, oxidative phosphorylation ceases, and pyruvate is converted to lactic acid rather than carbon dioxide and water. Diffusion of the hydrogen ions and lactate across the cell membranes into the extracellular fluid is passive and rapid. Extracellular fluid acidosis related to anaerobic glycolysis precedes arterial pH depression because of a number of factors: in low flow states there is a delay of acid metabolite washout into the peripheral circulation; arterial pH will change only after the hemoglobin-, bicarbonate-, and phosphate-buffering capacity of the blood is exceeded; and metabolism of lactate by the heart and liver tend to reduce the peripheral lactate levels until late in shock. Skeletal muscle itself offers several advantages for surveillance of overall oxygen transport. Since it can tolerate hypoxia, its blood supply tends to get shut off early in critical states, and it tends to shift readily into anaerobic glycolysis and lactate production because of its high glycogen content. The surface of the muscle rather than the interior is monitored to avoid artifacts due to hematoma formation. Studies in man have shown that muscle surface pH is a sensitive indicator of muscle metabolism and as such is valuable as a practical monitoring instrument to alert against hypoxia of more vital tissues. The normal resting biceps pH is 7.38, slightly below arterial pH. When the normal oxygen gradient to the muscle cells is restored after the circulatory crisis is over, pH promptly returns to the normal resting level.

Couch's group has also done redox potential measurements of muscle as an indicator of balance between oxygen delivery and tissue needs. Redox potential of tissue reflects the overall balance of electron transfer which shifts toward the negative or reduced state with prolonged hypoxia. However, although the trends were found to be similar to the surface pH changes, absolute redox potential values were not as reliable indicators as pH changes. Muscle surface pH monitoring provides a good early warning of disaster during and after surgery. The small incision certainly can be justified in high-risk patients or those undergoing formidable operations.

Woldring et al. developed a mass spectrometer which accurately records partial pressures of oxygen, carbon dioxide, or other gases, sampled through plastic or rubber membranes mounted on a catheter tip. Using a mass spectrometer, Owens et al. measured intracerebral gas tensions continuously across a heparinized silastic membrane on a perforated cannula. Of course, the measurements represent the gas tensions in the extracellular fluid surrounding local tissue injury rather than intact cells. Other problems are related to changes in membrane permeability due to fibrin deposits and protein denaturation.

The quest for the perfect monitor of vital function is really just beginning, as investigators such as Chance learn about energy "spin-off" during bioenergetic exchange in the cells. More bioengineers are looking at the lower part of Table 13-1 to find noninvasive methods of scanning cellular bioenergetics. Huckabee has defined hypoxia as "the condition which exists when the supply of oxygen to the exterior of living cells is reduced to a rate insufficient for their current metabolic needs, with the result that various cellular oxidation-reduction systems must shift toward a more reduced state." Detection of this state by a safe external sensor is the ultimate goal.

A number of attempts in this direction are in progress. One involves the stimulation of intracellular oxygen molecules with modulated soft x-rays. The stimulated emission of oxygen is in the microwave area of the 0.5-cm band and can be detected externally with a suitable waveguide and amplifier system. This approach would offer some degree of spatial discrimination of tissue hypoxia in specific organs. Another experimental method is a cross between Chance's fluorescence emission technique and thermography. Energy transfers within living cells emit specific wavelengths of electromagnetic radiation according to quantum bioenergetic laws. Energy dissipation associated with inefficient anaerobic metabolism or uncoupling of oxidative phosphorylation should be detectable by suitable instrumentation. Such a system has been developed to detect and identify narrow band and line spectra associated with abnormal tissue states. These signals in a physiologic situation are superimposed on the broad band (black body) radiation of the skin or organ surface along with the far infrared spectral pattern of cellular water and carbon dioxide. The desired signals are somewhat analogous to the Fraunhofer lines of the solar spectrum due to absorption in the sun's mantle. The approach differs from conventional infrared thermography in that the strategy is to analyze the spectral pattern rather than to determine the energy level within a specified wavelength. A Fourier interferometer, which is about the size of a bread box, is used to scan the patient at the bedside. The recorded interferogram is then transmitted by a time-shared system over telephone lines to a computer for Fourier transform and signature analysis. Emission power spectral density tracings have been obtained from human limbs as well as other tissues and superficial carcinomas. Cross-correlation techniques have been used to establish significant differences. Alterations in infrared emission spectra reflect changes in tissue metabolism from analysis of the frequencies of radiation corresponding to molecular vibrations and rotations. Although highly experimental, this is a good example of monitoring at the business end of the oxygen transport chain.

References

Physiologic Concepts and Monitoring

Barcroft, J.: "The Respiratory Functions of the Blood," Cambridge University Press, London, 1925.

Brown, J. H. U. and Dickson, J. F., III: Instrumentation and the Delivery of Health Services, *Science,* **166:**334, 1969.

Bunker, J. P., Forrest, W. H., Jr., Mosteller, F., and Vandam, L. D. (eds.): "The National Halothane Study," National Institute of General Medical Sciences, Bethesda, 1969.

Chance, B.: Regulation of Intracellular Oxygen, *Proc Int Union Physiol Sci,* **6:**13, 1968.

Clark, L. C., Jr. and Lyons, C.: Electrode Systems for Continuous Monitoring in Cardiovascular Surgery, *Ann NY Acad Sci,* **102:**19, 1962.

Cohn, J. D. and Del Guercio, L. R. M.: Cardiorespiratory Analysis of Cardiac Arrest and Resuscitation, *Surg Gynecol Obstet,* **123:**1066, 1966.

Cushing, H.: On Routine Determinations of Arterial Tension in Operating Room and Clinic, *Boston Med Surg J,* **148:**250, 1903.

Dammann, J. F.: Assessment of Continuous Monitoring in the Critically Ill Patient, *Dis Chest,* **55:**240, 1969.

Del Guercio, L. R. M., Feins, N. R., Cohn, J. D., Coomaraswamy, R. P., Wollman, S. B., and State, D.: A Comparison of Blood Flow during External and Internal Cardiac Massage in Man, *Circulation,* **32**(*Suppl* 1):171, 1965.

Dickens, F., and Neil, E.: "Oxygen in the Animal Organism," The Macmillan Company, New York, 1964.

Harken, A. H.: Lactic Acidosis, *Surg Gynecol Obstet,* **142:**593, 1976.

Hershey, S. G., Del Guercio, L. R. M., and McConn, R.: "Septic Shock in Man," Little, Brown and Company, Boston, 1971.

Huckabee, W. E.: Relationships of Pyruvate and Lactate during Anaerobic Metabolism: II. Exercise and Formation of O_2 Debt, *J Clin Invest,* **37:**255, 1958.

Irving, L.: Respiration in Diving Mammals, *Physiol Rev,* **19:**112, 1939.

Maloney, J. V., Jr.: The Trouble with Patient Monitoring, *Ann Surg,* **168:**605, 1968.

Pontoppidan, H., Geffin, B., and Lowenstein, E.: Acute Respiratory Failure in the Adult. *N Engl J Med,* **287:**690, 1972.

Roughton, F. J. W.: The Average Time Spent by the Blood in the Human Lung Capillary and Its Relation to the Rates of CO Uptake and Elimination in Man, *Am J Physiol,* **143:**621, 1945.

Safar, P., Myers, D., Snyder, J., et al.: Clinical Trial Protocols for Brain Resuscitation, *Intensive Care Med,* **3:**165, 1977.

Sarnoff, S. J., and Mitchell, J. H.: The Control of the Function of the Heart, in "Handbook of Physiology," vol. 1, The Williams & Wilkins Company, Baltimore, 1962.

Van Slyke, D. D.: The Carbon Dioxide Carriers of the Blood, *Physiol Rev,* **1:**141, 1921.

Weil, M. H., and Shubin, H.: "Critical Care Medicine, Current Principles and Practices," Harper & Row, Publishers, Incorporated, New York, 1976.

Physiologic Sensing

Collins, J. A., and Ballinger, W. F., II: "The Surgical Intensive Care Unit," *Surgery,* **66:**614, 1969.

Giles, A. F.: "Electronic Sensing Devices," William Clowes and Sons, London, 1966.

Johnson, H. A., Information Theory in Biology after 18 Years. *Science,* **168:**1545, 1970.

Rushmer, R. F. (ed.): "Medical Engineering: Projections for Health Care Delivery," Academic Press, Inc., New York, 1972.

Shannon, C. E., and Weaver, W.: "The Mathematical Theory of Communication," The University of Illinois Press, Urbana, 1959.

Respiratory Monitoring

Kinney, J. M., Morgan, A. P., Dominguous, F. G., and Gilder, K. J.: A Method for Continuous Measurement of Gas Exchange and Expired Radioactivity in Acutely Ill Patients, *Metabolism,* **13:**205, 1964.

Lewis, F. J., Shimizu, T., Scofield, A. L., and Rosi, P. S.: Analysis of Respiration by an On-Line Digital Computer System: Clinical Data following Thoraco Abdominal Surgery, *Ann Surg,* **164:**547, 1966.

————, Deller, S., Yokochi, H., Rosi, P. S., Quinn, M. L., Kite, M., and Rabin, S.: Automatic Monitoring in the Postoperative Recovery Room, *Surg Gynecol Obstet,* **130:**333, 1970.

Osborn, J. J., Badia, W., and Gerbode, F.: Respiratory or Cardiac Work and Other Analogue Computer Techniques, *J Thorac Surg,* **45:**500, 1963.

————, Beaumont, J. O., Raison, J. C. A., Russell, J., and Gerbode, F.: Measurement and Monitoring of Acutely Ill Patients by Digital Computer, *Surgery,* **64:**1057, 1968.

Peters, R. M.: Work of Breathing following Trauma, *J Trauma,* **8:**915, 1968.

———— and Hilberman, M.: Respiratory Insufficiency Diagnosis and Control of Therapy, *Surgery,* **70:**280, 1971.

———— and Stacy, R. W.: Automatized Clinical Measurement of Respiratory Parameters, *Surgery,* **56:**44, 1964.

Powers, S. R., et al.: Physiologic Consequences of Positive End-expiratory Pressure (PEEP) Ventilation, *Ann Surg,* **178:**265, 1973.

Rosi, P. S., Yokochi, H., Deller, S., Quinn, M., Greenberg, A. G., Rabin, S., Blatt, S., Lewis, F. J., and Jacobs, J. E.: Noninvasive Automatic Patient Monitoring, *Surg Forum,* **20:**234, 1969.

Cardiovascular Monitoring

Bondurant, S. (ed.): Research on Acute Myocardial Infarction, *Circulation,* vol. 40, Suppl 4, 1969.

Border, J. R., Gallo, E., and Shenk, W. G.: Alterations in Cardiovascular and Pulmonary Physiology in the Severely Stressed Patient: A Rational Plan for the Management of Hypotension, *J Trauma,* **6:**176, 1966.

Cohn, J. N., Khatri, I. M., and Hamosh, P.: Diagnostic and Therapeutic Value of Bedside Monitoring of Left Ventricular Pressure, *Am J Cardiol,* **23:**107, 1969.

Dalton, B., and Laver, M. B.: Vasospasm with an Indwelling Radial Artery Cannula, *Anesthesiology,* **34:**194, 1971.

Del Guercio, L. R. M.: Cardiogenic Shock, in J. D. Hardy (ed.), "Rhoads Textbook of Surgery," 5th ed., pp. 78–84, Lippincott Company, Philadelphia, 1977.

————, Cohn, J. D., Feins, N. R., Coomaraswamy, R. P., and Mantel, L.: Pulmonary Embolism Shock: The Physiologic Basis of a Bedside Screening Test, *JAMA,* **196:**751, 1966.

Dudrick, S. J., Wilmore, D. W., Vars, H. M., and Rhoads, J. E.: Can Intravenous Feeding as the Sole Means of Nutrition Support Growth in the Child and Restore Weight Loss in an Adult? An Affirmative Answer, *Ann Surg,* **169:**974, 1969.

Ganz, W., and Swan, H. J. C.: Measurement of Blood Flow by Thermodilution, *Am J Cardiol,* **29:**241, 1972.

Garcia, E., Michenfelder, J. D., and Theye, R. A.: Right Atrial Oxygen Saturation Levels during Anesthesia and Surgery, *J Can Anaesth Soc,* **15:**593, 1968.

Kazamias, T. M., Gander, M. P., Ross, J., Jr., and Braunwald, E.: Detection of Left-Ventricular-Wall Motion Disorders in Coronary Artery Disease by Radarkymography, *N Engl J Med,* **285:**63, 1971.

Krauss, X. H., Verdouw, P. D., Hugenholtz, P. G., Hagemijer, F., and Polanyi, M. L.: Continuous Monitoring of O_2 Saturation in the Intensive Care Unit, *Circulation,* **45**(*Suppl* 2):178, 1972.

Lee, J., Wright, F., Barber, R., and Stanley, L.: Central Venous Oxygen Saturation in Shock: A Study in Man, *Anesthesiology,* **36:**472, 1972.

Lowenstein, E., Little, J. W., III, and Lo, H. H.: Prevention of Cerebral Embolization from Flushing Radial-Artery Cannulas, *N Engl J Med.* **285:**1415, 1971.

Owens, G., Belmusto, L., and Woldring, S.: Experimental Intracerebral PO_2 and PCO_2 Monitoring by Mass Spectrography, *J Neurosurg,* **30:**110, 1969.

Sheppard, L. C., Kouchoukos, N. T., Kurtis, M., and Kirklin, J. W.: Automated Treatment of Critically Ill Patients, *Ann Surg,* **168:**596, 1968.

Shubin, H., and Weil, M. H.: Efficient Monitoring with a Digital Computer of Cardiovascular Function in Seriously Ill Patients, *Ann Intern Med,* **65:**453, 1966.

Weinberg, D. I., Artley, J. L., Whalen, R., and McIntosh, H. D.: Electric Shock Hazards in Cardiac Catheterization, *Circ Res,* **9:**1004, 1962.

Woldring, S., Owens, G., and Woolford, D.: Blood Gases: Continuous In Vivo Recording of Partial Pressure by Mass Spectroscopy, *Science,* **153:**887, 1967.

Zohman, L. R., and Williams, M. H., Jr.: Percutaneous Right Heart Catheterization Using Polyethylene Tubing, *Am J Cardiol,* **4:**373, 1959.

Cardiac Output Determinations

Ashburn, W., L., Moser, K. M., and Guisan, M.: Digital and Analog Processing of Anger Camera Data and a Dedicated Computer Controlled System, *J Nucl Med,* **11:**680, 1970.

Bender, M. A., and Blau, M.: The Autofluoroscope, *Nucleonics,* **21:**52, 1963.

Civetta, J. M.: Cardiopulmonary Calculations: A Rapid, Simple and Inexpensive Technique, *Intensive Care Med,* **3:**209, 1977.

Cohn, J. D.: A Pump System for Performing Indicator-Dilution Curves without Blood Loss, *J Appl Physiol,* **26:**841, 1969.

———, Engler, P. E., and Del Guercio, L. R. M.: The Automated Physiologic Profile, *Critical Care Med,* **3:**51, 1975.

Del Guercio, L. R. M.: Contrast Dilution Analysis, *Trans NY Acad Sci,* **33:**387, 1971.

———, and Cohn, J. D.: Monitoring: Methods and Significance, *Surg Clin North Am,* **56:**977, 1976.

Feigenbaum, H., Zaky, A., and Nasser, W. K.: Use of Ultrasound to Measure Left Ventricular Stroke Volume, *Circulation,* **35:**1092, 1967.

Franklin, D. L., Schlegel, W., and Rushmer, R. F.: Blood Flow Measured by Doppler Frequency Shift of Back-scattered Ultrasound, *Science,* **134:**564, 1961.

Ganz, W., and Swan, H. J. C.: Measurement of Blood Flow by Thermal Dilution, *Am J Cardiol,* **29:**241, 1972.

Harken, A. H.: The Surgical Significance of the Oxyhemoglobin Dissociation Curve, *Surg Gynecol Obstet,* **144:**935, 1977.

Hillenbrand, W. I.: Desk-top Computers and Electronic Calculators for Engineers, *Electronic Products,* June 1966, pp. 50–53.

Jones, R. H., Klaphaak, R. B., and Sabiston, D. C., Jr.: Anatomic Resolution in Dynamic Radionuclide Studies by Computer Identification or Radioactivity Fluctuation with Time, Proc 2d Symp Sharing Computer Programs Technology Nucl Med (*AEC Conf-720430*), 1972, p. 151.

Kaufman, L.: Clinical Applications of Silicon Lithium Radiation Detectors, *Proc IEEE Nucl Sci Symp,* December 1972.

Kubicek, W. G., Patterson, R. P., and Witsoe, D. A.: Impedance Cardiography as a Non-invasive Method of Monitoring Cardiac Function and Other Parameters of the Cardiovascular System, *Ann NY Acad Sci,* **170:**724, 1970.

McDonald, D. A., Kouchoukos, N. T., Shepard, L. C., and Kirklin, J. W.: Estimation of Stroke Volume and Cardiac Output from the Central Arterial Pulse Contour in Postoperative Patients, *Circulation,* **38**(*Suppl* 6):118, 1968.

Newbower, R. S.: Blood Flow Measurements with Magnetic Tracers, *Proc Conf Engineering Med Biol,* **14:**147, 1972.

Papp, R. L., and Harrison, D. C.: Ultrasonic Cardiac Echography for Determining Stroke Volume and Valvular Regurgitation, *Circulation,* **41:**493, 1970.

Pombo, J. F., Troy, B. L., and Russell, R. O., Jr.: Left Ventricular Volumes and Ejection Fraction by Echocardiography, *Circulation,* **43:**480, 1971.

Shabot, M. M., Shoemaker, W. C., and State, D.: Rapid Bedside Computation of Cardiorespiratory Variables with a Programmable Calculator, *Critical Care Med,* **5:**105, 1977.

Siegel, J. H., Fabian, M., Lankau, C., Levine, M., Cole, A., and Nahmad, M.: Clinical and Experimental Use of Thoracic Impedance Plethysmography in Quantifying Myocardial Contractility, *Surgery,* **67:**907, 1970.

———, Greenspan, M., Cohn, J. D., and Del Guercio, L. R. M.: A Bedside Computer and Physiologic Nomograms: Guides to the Management of the Patient in Shock, *Arch Surg,* **97:**480, 1968.

Warner, H.: The Role of Computers in Medical Research, *JAMA,* **196:**944, 1966.

Weissler, A. M., Harris, W. S., and Schoenfeld, C. D.: Bedside Techniques for the Evaluation of Ventricular Function in Man, *Am J Cardiol,* **23:**577, 1969.

Wood, E. H., Sturm, R. E., and Sanders, J. J.: Data Processing in Cardiovascular Physiology with Particular Reference to Roentgen Videodensitometry, *Mayo Clin Proc,* **39:**849, 1964.

Monitoring of Tissue Metabolism

Cohn, J. D., Del Guercio, L. R. M., Ito, K., Pan, C. H. T., and Moross, G.: Infrared Emission Spectroscopy from Human Limbs, *Proc 25th Conf Engineering Med Biol,* 1972, p. 55.

———, ———, ———, ———, and ———: Infrared Spectral Analysis of Metabolic Function, *Fed Proc,* **31:**350, 1972.

Del Guercio, L. R. M., Cohn, J. D., Ito, K., Moross, G. G., and Pan, C. H. T.: Non-invasive Assessment of Cellular Function and Organ Perfusion, in "Advances in Automated Analysis; Diagnostic Medicine, Biomedical Profiling," vol 2, Mediad Incorporated, Tarrytown, N.Y., 1973.

Laks, H., Dmochowski, J. R., and Couch, N. P.: The Relationship between Muscle Surface pH and Oxygen Transport, *Ann Surg,* **183:**193, 1976.

Owens, G., Belmusto, L., and Woldring, S.: Experimental Intracerebral PO_2 and PCO_2 Monitoring by Mass Spectroscopy, *J Neurosurg,* **30:**110, 1969.

Woldring, S., Owens, G., and Woolford, D. C.: Blood Gases: Continuous In Vivo Recording of Partial Pressures by Mass Spectroscopy, *Science,* **153:**885, 1966.

Chapter 14

Skin and Subcutaneous Tissue

by **Seymour I. Schwartz**

PHYSIOLOGY

The skin, which is the largest organ in the body, represents more than a structure covering vital organs and separating them from the environment. It is a complex organ that possesses unique physical properties and physiologic functions.

Physical Properties

Both *tension* and *elasticity* are physical properties which are related to elastic fibers within the skin. Tension is the characteristic which accounts for the fact that the skin resists stretching by weak forces; the maximal deforming force which is resisted by the skin, expressed in dynes per centimeter, is a measurement of tension. Tension varies in different areas and is most marked where the skin contains dense elastic fibers, particularly in regions where the skin is thin. The direction of the tension also varies anatomically and forms the basis of the line system described by Langer in 1861. The tension of skin is greater in young than in elderly patients. Elasticity refers to the skin's ability to resume its original shape after an external force has been applied to cause deformation. This also varies with age, being less in the elderly and also in patients with edema.

Quantification of the physical properties of the skin has been made by determining the *tensile strength,* or the resistance of skin to tearing under tension. The average tensile strength of the adult skin, without fat, is approximately 1.8 kg/m². This is significantly reduced in infants up to three months of age, and the lowest values are found in the Ehlers-Danlos syndrome, which is characterized by a reduction of elastic fibers. In patients with Cushing's syndrome or those taking high doses of cortisone for prolonged periods of time, the tensile strength of skin is significantly less than normal, and there is also a low modulus of elasticity.

The electrical behavior of skin has been the subject of much investigation. The skin generates polarization currents which provide great resistance to external electric forces. The intensity of imposed current passing through the skin is therefore very low. The skin also offers a resistance to alternating currents by its property of impedence.

Functions of Skin

Important physiologic functions of skin include (1) percutaneous absorption, (2) an important role in the circulatory system, (3) serving as an organ of senses, (4) secretion of sweat, (5) providing an avenue for the insensible loss of water, and (6) contributing to thermal regulation.

PERCUTANEOUS ABSORPTION. This refers to the penetration of substances through the skin, permitting them to enter the bloodstream. It has been shown that radioactive water, applied either as a vapor or as a solution, appears both in the circulation and the urine. If the skin is warmed after exposure, the concentration in the urine increases rapidly. Electrolytes applied to the skin in aqueous solution either do not penetrate or may enter in small amounts via the appendages. The skin is impermeable to sodium and calcium when these are applied to the skin in the form of a chloride solution. However, there is some evidence that the iodide ion may enter the skin either because it increases the negative electric charge of skin or because it penetrates via appendages. When radioactive electrolytes are rubbed onto the skin, they are absorbed, and the absorption is increased if the skin is abraded or has been shaved.

Lipid-soluble substances are fairly rapidly and completely absorbed through the skin, and absorption appears to be faster if the substances are also soluble in water to some degree. In the latter instance, the penetration is so rapid that the rate of absorption is comparable to gastro-intestinal absorption and even absorption of the material injected subcutaneously. The percutaneous absorption of phenol has been recognized for many years, and fatal poisoning may be associated with the application of carbolic acid to large areas of skin. Salicylic acid also penetrates with great ease from alcoholic and aqueous solutions as well as from ointments. Estrogenic hormones, testosterone, progesterone, and desoxycorticosterone all penetrate the intact skin rapidly. Hydrocortisone may be therapeutically effective by percutaneous application, while cortisone acetate applied locally is poorly absorbed. Water-soluble hormones, such as insulin, are not absorbed. Lipid-soluble vitamins are absorbed with ease, while water-soluble vitamins do not penetrate the skin. Heavy metals may be absorbed to some extent, and their absorption is dependent upon the formation of compounds in combination with the fatty acid of the sebum. This is particularly true of mercury.

Substances in the gaseous form, with the exception of carbon monoxide, penetrate the skin easily. Oxygen, nitrogen, and carbon dioxide are examples of gases which perfuse readily. Carbon tetrachloride is also readily absorbed through the skin, as demonstrated by experiments with ^{14}C-labeled compound. Recently, the absorption of pharmaceutic agents through the skin has been employed by using dimethyl sulfoxide as a vehicle. The applicability of this technique has not been totally defined.

CIRCULATION AND VASCULAR REACTIONS. The cutaneous vascular system is extremely complex and contributes significantly to the general circulation and vascular reactions. Direct visualization of flow in minute vessels can be carried out by observing the capillary circulation of the base of the nail. The color of the skin is dependent upon the quantity of blood in the subpapillary plexus of vessels, particularly in the Caucasian, while the skin temperature depends chiefly on the rate of flow through the whole skin. The range of pressure in human skin capillaries is between 12 and 45 mm Hg, and the average capillary pressure is equivalent to the colloid osmotic pressure of plasma proteins. Arteriovenous anastomoses of digital skin play an important role in temperature regulation and are implicated in the formation of the glomus tumor.

Local vascular responses may result from direct action on the vessel wall or its contractile elements. Local vasoconstriction follows gentle stroking. However, if the mechanical stimulus is of greater intensity than that which causes constriction, a red local reaction may develop secondary to dilatation of small vessels. Circumscribed superficial edema of the skin in areas responsive to stimuli is referred to as a "wheal" and is due to leakage of plasma from dilated blood vessels into the extracellular space. There are two distinct steps in the formation of the wheal: (1) local dilatation and (2) increased capillary permeability. Stimulation of the sympathetic fibers supplying the skin causes vasoconstriction of the cutaneous vessels, while interruption of these fibers results in dilatation of the small arteries and arterioles. The cutaneous circulatory system also responds to chemical agents. Acetylcholine causes vasodilatation, while norepinephrine and epinephrine are important vasoconstricting drugs. Vasopressin is also an active vasoconstrictor. Nicotinic acid and nitrites cause flushing and warmth, increased temperature, and increased blood flow. Ergot alkaloids act as vasodilators by their sympatholytic action, but the drugs also directly constrict the muscles of the peripheral arterioles, and the net effect is a decrease in blood flow.

SENSORY FUNCTION. The skin's sensory functions pertain to the modalities of pain (including itching), touch, and temperature. Skin consists of a mosaic of multiple sensitive spots, the relative density of which varies with the region of body. Cold sensitivity is probably mediated by Krause's end bulbs, whereas Ruffini's endings are probably receptors for warmth. Meissner's corpuscles and Merkel's discs are implicated in the tactile sensation, and the Pacinian corpuscles are involved in the sensation of pressure. Pain is mediated by free nonmyelinated endings, which are in a plexiform arrangement. Following injury to the skin, there is a widespread area of hyperalgesia which radiates from the point of injury. After traumatic injury of a peripheral nerve, causalgia, in which there is increased pain accompanied by cutaneous vasodilatation, may occur. Sympathectomy at the appropriate level in this case brings about almost complete relief.

SWEAT SECRETION. The skin contains two types of sweat glands, eccrine glands, which are small sweat glands, and apocrine, or large, sweat glands. The eccrine glands are distributed all over the body and are the true secretory glands which produce clear, aqueous sweat responsible for heat regulation. The apocrine glands in the human being are almost rudimentary structures. If the environmental temperature rises above 31 or 32°C (90°F), there is a sudden outbreak of visible sweating over the entire body. At lower environmental temperatures, the sweat glands secrete microscopically visible droplets in a periodic fashion. The insensible sweat secretion constitutes one part of the total insensible water loss.

The distribution of sweat glands is such that the highest number per square inch are located in the palms and soles and are also more dense on the dorsum of the hand, forehead, and trunk. There are fewer glands in the lower extremity than in the upper extremity. In most instances, sweating is almost exclusively the result of nervous impulses, but the glands are able to respond directly to application of heat if it is sufficiently intense. The nonnervous sweat response is strictly limited to the local area of stimulation. The nervous response is almost entirely mediated over sympathetic nerves and results from the pharmacologic action of parasympathetic substances. The nerve fibers to the sweat glands liberate acetylcholine at their endings upon stimulation. Atropine and other anticholinergics block the receptor sites so that they are unable to respond and thus interfere with secretion. Hyperhidrosis (increased sweating) may result from an abnormal increase in nerve impulses as in central nervous system lesions or emotional states. Increased tonicity of the sweat fibers may intensify the sweat response to normal nervous and nonnervous stimuli.

Primary hyperhidrosis usually presents as excessive sweating noted early in life. Mild cases can be managed with anticholinergic drugs and antiperspirant creams. Sympathectomy at T_2 to T_4 or T_5 abolishes eccrine sweating in the involved areas of the upper extremity. A modified Hurley-Shelley operation is used for axillary hyperhidrosis. The hair-bearing axillary skin is excised, and the ganglia at T_2 and T_3 are removed for accompanying hand sweating.

Eccrine sweat is a clear aqueous solution containing 99 percent water and 1 percent solids, half of which are inorganic salts and half organic compounds. Under normal circumstances, it is hypotonic, but at high rates of sweating it may approach isotonic concentration. Although the composition of sweat depends on material within the bloodstream, it is not a simple ultrafiltrate of plasma but represents an active secretion. The concentration of sodium and chloride is lower than that in plasma, while the concentration of potassium is somewhat higher. The concentration of chloride depends on many factors and is usually in the range of 15 to 60 mEq/L. The sodium concentration is almost always entirely equivalent to that of chloride and varies in a parallel fashion. Chloride and sodium concentrations rise with prolongation of sweating and with the rate of sweating and temperature of the skin. The chloride content of palmar sweat is greater than that from other parts of the body. The salt concentration of sweat also depends on the intake, and an adequate supply of drinking water depresses the concentration. The loss of potassium through the skin ranges between 2.7 and 3.1 mEq/L.

Nitrogen compounds are also lost transdermally, and the concentration of urea in sweat is twice as high as that in the blood. Creatinine is present in sweat in only a minute amount, and amino acids have also been noted. Ammonia is a primary constituent of sweat, and it can be concentrated by the sweat glands with nearly the same efficiency as the renal excreting unit. Large amounts of lactic acid and lactate have been demonstrated in sweat, particularly during heavy muscular exercise and in association with thermogenic sweat. The concentrations are ten to twenty times higher than that in the blood, and it is felt that the lactic acid originates from breakdown of glycogen within the sweat glands.

Sweat provides the skin with an "acid mantle." The average pH of freshly secreted sweat is 5.7 to 6.4. As the sweating progresses, the acidity decreases, but considerable amounts of acid are still lost with profuse thermal sweating. There is increasing acidity with evaporation of water from the sweat. The acidity retards the growth of many bacteria which reside in the keratin layer, glands, and hair follicles.

In contrast to the eccrine glands, which develop from the upper dermis, the apocrine glands are formed from follicular epithelium, as are sebaceous glands. Like sebaceous glands and hair follicles, the apocrine glands have major development during puberty. They are greater in number in females and respond to autonomic nervous stimulation rather than thermal stimulation. They function by producing a somewhat viscous milklike droplet.

INSENSIBLE WATER LOSS. Sweat secretion provides but one of two separate mechanisms contributing to insensible loss of water through continuous evaporation which occurs at all environmental temperatures. The other mechanism is that of loss through the epidermis which, unlike sweat secretion, is not affected by atropinization. Water loss through the epidermis is contrasted with sweat in that it does not contain salts or other solutes. The total insensible water loss through skin and lungs is constant under basal conditions and amounts to about 200 $Gm/m^2/24$ hours, 60 percent of which is cutaneous loss. Total cutaneous water loss in the adult man at rest without visible sweating is about 500 to 700 ml daily. The insensible loss from both the skin and the lungs shows a linear relationship to the basal metabolic rate. Water intake has no effect on cutaneous loss in the adult but does increase it in children. In hypothyroidism, the water loss is conspicuously low, whereas in thyrotoxicosis, total insensible perspiration is greatly increased.

THERMOREGULATION. The skin plays an important role in the regulation of body temperature. Heat is lost through the skin under the processes of radiation, convection, conduction, and evaporation. Sweating is a useful process only when the sweat can evaporate. It is therefore very efficient as a regulatory mechanism in a dry, hot environment, but with increased humidity the efficiency decreases markedly. Humidity begins to be of importance between 30 and 31°C (86 to 88°F) air temperature, at which point the difference between 50 and 100 percent relative humidity decides whether the person will be comfortable or hyperthermic. If heat production is raised or atmospheric temperature is raised, there is a shift of blood flow from the interior to the skin. The converse is also true, and this process is carried out reflexly.

Cold stimuli of a moderate degree result in the production of pallor. After the stimulus has ceased, there is reactive arterial vasodilatation. Cold stimuli of long duration are associated with livid discoloration as a result of paresis in the venous limbs of the capillaries. With extreme stimuli, there may be a reddish discoloration due to dilatation of the arterioles. The condition, however, is not associated with increased blood flow, and skin temperature does not rise. The reduction in temperature is also accompanied by interference with the utilization of oxyhemoglobin. Emersion foot, or "trench foot," occurs when the skin is exposed for long periods of time to cold water. There is vasoconstriction and capillary damage, and if the skin's temperature is returned to normal rapidly, reactive hyperemia and blistering result. Thrombosis may complicate the situation. It is therefore felt that exposure to the cold should be treated by gradual increase in temperature. The role of sympathectomy early in the course of frostbite has been debated, but there is some real evidence to indicate that it is applicable if carried out within 24 hours.

Heat exhaustion refers to a syndrome characterized by excessive loss of salt and water when people are exposed to high temperatures. A sweat retention syndrome has been recognized among troops in hot, humid climates, in which situation the personnel lose their ability to sweat and become moderately hyperthermic. Exhaustion, headache, palpitation, and dizziness are the characteristic manifestations.

PRESSURE SORES

Pressure on an area of skin for 2 or more hours, particularly in patients with impaired nutritional status, may result in sufficient ischemia to cause a decubitus ulcer. The ulceration usually occurs over bony prominences. Supportive therapy includes a nutritive diet, correction of anemia, and relief of pressure over the area. Routinely turning the patient and using special mattresses are effective. Surgical therapy requires sharp debridement to excise the ulcer and underlying fascia and necrotic material. The bony prominence frequently requires excision, with care to achieve hemostasis. The bone should be covered with muscle, and a large rotation flap of skin and fat provides the best skin coverage.

HIDRADENITIS SUPPURATIVA

This is a chronic acneform infection of the cutaneous apocrine glands, subcutaneous tissue, and fascia. It is generally confined to areas in which these glands are found, namely the axilla, areola of the nipple, groin, perineum, and circumanal and periumbilical regions. The disease was first described by Velpeau in 1839, and clinical manifestations vary with the duration of the lesion. At first, there is a slight subcutaneous induration, and as the tumor enlarges, the process advances to the skin, which becomes inflamed and adherent. Suppuration eventually develops, and cellulitis surrounds the abscess. At this stage, pain is often severe. Incision and drainage at this point result in a few drops of thick, viscous, purulent material. The process may subside after 2 or 3 days, only to recur. In the chronic stage, the patient presents with multiple painful cutaneous nodules which coalesce and are surrounded by fibrous reaction. The pathologic picture is similar to that seen in any acute pyogenic infection of the skin, but involvement of the apocrine glands establishes the diagnosis. Culture of the pus yields a variety of saprophytic and pathogenic bacteria with a preponderance of staphylococci and streptococci.

Treatment consists of excision of the involved area or x-ray therapy for early cases. Cures can be achieved early in the course of the disease by improved hygiene and incision and drainage. In chronic cases, however, radical excision of all the pathologic tissue with split-thickness skin grafts for coverage affords the best opportunity for cure.

CYSTS

Epidermal Inclusion Cyst

When the epithelium of the skin is trapped subcutaneously, as a result of trauma or for other reasons, it may continue to grow and desquamate. This creates a cyst lined by epidermal cells and filled with keratin and desquamated cells. The lesions occur most frequently on the hand and are characterized by continued enlargement. Cure is effected by removal of the entire cyst and all its epithelial elements.

Ganglia

Ganglia are areas of mucoid degeneration of retinacular structures. They are tense, subcutaneous cystic masses occurring most commonly over the wrist and over tendon sheaths of the hands and feet. They grow very slowly and are usually associated with only minimal discomfort. The lesions consist of a wall of collagenous tissue which may or may not have synovial cells and contain thin clear collagenous material. They have been related to trauma, either accidental or occupational.

Treatment is by surgical excision which is usually performed after a tourniquet is applied to permit precise dissection. The ganglia which are closely adherent to a tendon sheath are relatively easy to remove, but those which communicate with the synovium of a joint require excision of the neck and base plate to protect against recurrence. Trauma to established ganglia usually results in rupture, but this is generally followed by recurrence.

Sebaceous Cyst

The ducts of ceruminous skin glands may be plugged or blocked for a variety of reasons. Sebaceous glands are most numerous on the face and in the midline of the trunk, and they are generally associated with hair follicles. They produce sebum, an oily material, which serves as a natural dressing for the hair and skin. If the exit of sebum is blocked, the material accumulates and a cyst is formed.

The lesions, which are lined with glandular epithelium and surrounded by an area of compression fibrosis, gradually increase in size. They are usually painless and nontender but may become secondarily infected.

If infection is present, incision and drainage should be performed followed by planned excision of the cyst as a second stage after the infection has totally disappeared. In the case of noninfected cysts, surgical excision of the entire cyst is indicated to prevent recurrence.

Dermoid Cyst

This is usually a congenital lesion which does not manifest itself until later in life. The dermoid cyst can be differentiated clinically from the sebaceous cyst in that it is cystic on palpation and does not exhibit a dimple or scar in the overlying skin. Dermoid cysts generally occur in the midline of the body, on the scalp over the occiput, on the nose, and in the abdominal and sacral regions. They are considered to be occlusion cysts, taking their origin from an embryonic process. Although it has been suggested that malignant degeneration may occur, Conway indicates that no authentic case has been reported. Surgical excision is the treatment of choice.

Pilonidal Cyst and Sinus

These are common malformations which occur over the sacrococcygeal region. Their origin is associated with the neurenteric canal, and it is thought that their development is related to blockage of a congenital coccygeal sinus which is a vestige of this canal. This is substantiated by evidence that some of the pilonidal cysts and sinuses result from penetration of local skin by growing hairs. The ingrowth of such hairs sets the stage for cyst formation and repeated infection. The lesions may often be present from birth but are usually not manifest until the late adolescent or early adult years. The disease has been referred to as "jeep-driver's disease," and it is thought that the bumpy driving merely aggravates a congenital condition. Histologically, both the cysts and sinuses are lined with the stratified squamous epithelium.

The clinical manifestations vary from a barely perceptible dimple at the superior end of the buttock crease to an obvious sinus tract or cyst at this site. The sinus may chronically drain or become infected. The cyst also gradually increases in size and is susceptible to secondary infection. There have been rare reports of escape of cerebrospinal fluid from the pilonidal sinuses and equally rare instances of meningitis resulting.

TREATMENT. If the cyst is acutely infected, tender, and erythematous, incision and drainage are indicated. Secondary removal of the cyst or sinus is then planned after the infection has subsided. Elective surgical removal must be complete, and methylene blue may be injected as a guide to determine the extent of arborization of the sinus tract. Following excision of the sinus, closure may be accomplished either primarily or by granulation. If there is any infection, it is preferable to leave the wound open, unroofing all the tracts and allowing it to heal by secondary

intention. Primary closure incorporates fascial flaps, and a great variety of techniques are directed at moving the scar from the midline. In some instances, a very thin split-thickness graft (0.005 to 0.008 in.) may be used to achieve early closure and still permit the desirable contracture of the wound which accompanies the open technique.

BENIGN TUMORS

Warts

The common wart, or verruca vulgaris, is caused by a filterable virus and is both contagious and autoinoculable. Lesions may occur on any part of the body but are most common on the hand and the soles of the feet. They appear as circumscribed intraepidermal tumors which may be elevated or flat. Verruca plantaris (plantar wart) is the most troublesome variety and is located on the soles of the feet in the region of the metatarsal heads or over the os calcis. These warts may become quite tender and painful.

Verruca vulgaris may be treated by a variety of simple methods including freezing with liquid nitrogen, caustic agents, and x-ray therapy. In general, however, electrodesiccation under local anesthesia is the best primary treatment. Surgical treatment has been somewhat disappointing in view of the infectious nature of the lesion and the incidence of recurrence. The symptoms of plantar warts may be relieved by using pads to remove direct weight bearing from the wart area. Chemotherapy and surgical paring have also been used, and injection of local anesthesia into the base of the wart has achieved some success. Hyfercation has been very effective. It is difficult to evaluate therapy of these lesions, since the clinical course is extremely variable and spontaneous disappearance, formation of daughter warts, and recurrence challenge conclusions.

Keratosis

This represents hypertrophy of the epidermis and is considered a precancerous lesion. Clinical classification includes senile keratosis, arsenical keratosis, and seborrheic keratosis.

Senile keratosis develops most commonly in individuals with fair complexion and characteristically presents as multiple lesions in the sixth, seventh, and eighth decades. Lesions suspected of being malignant should be treated by surgical excision, since other methods of therapy which may be applied, including trichloracetic acid, electrodesiccation, and x-ray, all deny microscopic evaluation.

Seborrheic keratosis (Fig. 14-1) develops in middle-aged or older people as multiple lesions occurring chiefly on the trunk. They appear as thickened areas and may be yellow, gray, brown, or black. They are often great in number and may be confluent. The darker lesions have been mistaken for melanotic tumors. Histologically, they may be differentiated from senile keratoses, and they generally remain benign, though occasionally they may de-

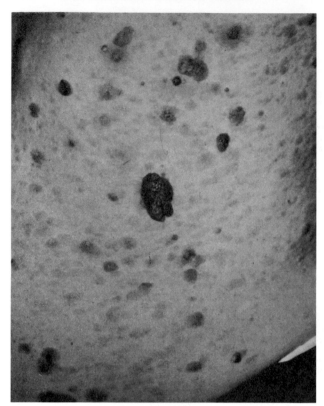

Fig. 14-1. Seborrheic keratosis: pigmented, greasy lesions which, when solitary, may be mistaken for melanotic tumors.

velop into basal cell carcinoma or, more rarely, squamous cell carcinoma. Treatment is usually conservative, employing electrocoagulation and curettage, but any rapid increase in size is indication for surgical excision.

Keloid

The term is derived from the Greek work meaning "crab's claw" and refers to a dense accumulation of fibrous tissue which extends above the surface of the skin and also circumferentially beyond areas which were originally traumatized or incised and sutured. The color may vary from red to pink to white, and the lesion is notorious for its recurrence following surgical excision. There is an increased incidence in Negroes and dark-haired Caucasians and a predilection for the lesions to occur on the face, neck, and skin over the sternum.

Treatment consists of excision with closure. In order to reduce the amount of foreign body reaction, sutures should not be left buried. Postoperative low-dose radiation has been applied with some success, and corticotropins also have been effective.

Vascular Tumors

CAPILLARY (PORT WINE) HEMANGIOMA

The lesion is made up of closely packed, dilated abnormal capillaries in the subpapillary, dermal, or subdermal region of the skin. Clinically, there is no elevation or contour change but rather a reddish or purplish patch of staining. Growth parallels that of the involved area. If the lesion is small, it may be treated by excision and closure with excellent results. Larger lesions, however, are most difficult to treat, since the entire dermis is involved and excision results in a contour defect and scar. The discoloration may be modified by tattooing, but repeated procedures are necessary, since the pigment is absorbed. Tattooing followed by the application of cosmetic preparations achieves the best approximation of normal skin color.

IMMATURE HEMANGIOMA (STRAWBERRY MARK) (Fig. 14-2)

This appears in infancy and undergoes a remarkable change with the growth of the child. The lesion generally enlarges, sometimes quite dramatically, during the first several months to 1 year, subsequent to which spontaneous regression usually occurs. Clinically, immature hemangiomas are raised and irregular, with some bright-red areas. They are compressible and may show superficial areas of opacity suggesting the beginning of regression. Regression takes the form of increasing opacity and whitening of the surface with progressive thickening and flattening. The hemangioma may become ulcerated if it is in an area subjected to trauma, but hemorrhage from these lesions is not common and is generally readily controlled by pressure. Such episodes of ulceration, minor hemorrhage, or superficial infection may actually hasten spontaneous resolution. Treatment in large part consists of reassuring the parents. Indications for surgical treatment, radiation, sclerosing agents, and local freezing are diminishing.

CAVERNOUS HEMANGIOMA

The lesions are full-sized in proportion to the child at birth and do not undergo changes with rapid growth or spontaneous regression. They consist of mature vessels and may include multiple arteriovenous communications. Cavernous hemangiomas frequently involve deep tissues, such as muscles and even the central nervous system. They may also be combined with lymphangiomatous elements. Rapidly growing tumors in childhood stop expanding or regress on a prednisone regimen. Treatment of established lesions is by wide surgical excision depending on the area of location.

SCLEROSING HEMANGIOMA

This is actually a subepidermal nodular fibrosis which occurs chiefly on the extremities and is related to trauma. It presents as a small nonpainful nodule, and the overlying epidermis may be pigmented in such a manner that the lesion is often mistaken for malignant melanoma. The treatment is surgical excision.

GLOMUS TUMOR

The glomus tumor is a benign, rare, and exquisitely painful small neoplasm of the skin and subcutaneous tissue occurring usually on the extremities and particularly in the nail beds of the hands and feet. The tumor is derived from the glomic end organ apparatus consisting of arteriovenous anastomoses which function normally to regulate the blood flow in the extremity. The organ contributes to the regulation of local and general body temperature through the dissipation or conservation of heat.

The tumors vary in structure but resemble the normal glomus unit and have often been referred to as *angiomyoneuroma*. The layers of circular muscle of the vessels may be separated from the endothelium by collagenous membrane, or the endothelium may be bordered directly by the so-called "glomus epithelioid" cells. In some tumors, the blood vessels are so enlarged that they resemble true angiomas. The glomus cells are supplied by nonmyelinated nerve fibers, which account for the painful nature of the lesion. Although the tumor per se is benign, a malignant counterpart exists and is referred to as a *hemangiopericytoma*.

The lesion is usually single, but multicentric origin has been reported. The color varies from deep red to purple or blue, and there is variation in color with changes in temperature. The patients usually present in the fifth decade, but the tumor has been reported at all ages. The pain associated with the lesion is the most prominent symptom and may occur either spontaneously, with pressure, or in association with trauma. The pain, which is described as stabbing, lancinating, and radiating from the tumor, may be intermittent in character or may occur only when the lesion is touched. The glomus tumor is radioresistant. Encapsulated tumors may be shelled out, but when an obvious capsule is not seen, wide excision is indicated.

LYMPHANGIOMA

Lymphangiomas, like hemangiomas, are congenital in origin. The most common type is deep and cavernous, consisting of lymph-filled spaces with thin-walled septums and some areas of fibrosis. A superficial variant presents as circumscribed lesions which appear as small blisters and slightly elevated skin patches. When deep lesions are present in the neck, mediastinum, and axilla, they are referred to as *cystic hygroma* (see Chap. 39). The treatment is surgical excision which, although frequently incomplete, is rarely associated with recurrence.

Fat Tumors

LIPOMA

This is an extremely common subcutaneous lesion which is composed of fat and is, at times, difficult to distinguish from the normal subcutaneous adipose tissue. Usually, however, there is a thin, fibrous capsule, and the lesion can be enucleated from surrounding normal fat. Benign lipomas occur more frequently over the back, between the shoulders, and on the back of the neck, and liposarcomatous transformation is extremely uncommon. Treatment is surgical excision.

WEBER-CHRISTIAN DISEASE

This is an uncommon inflammatory lesion of the subcutaneous fat characterized by painful reddened areas

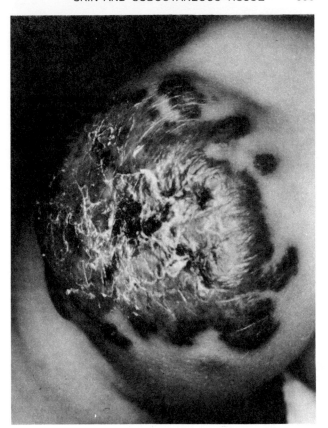

Fig. 14-2. Immature hemangioma (strawberry mark). Note opacification in the center. Lesion is undergoing spontaneous resolution.

involving the panniculus. The diagnosis is made by biopsy and is based on the presence of inflammatory cells in the adipose tissue. Recently, it has been demonstrated that many of the lesions which were so classified represented facticial dermatitis or skin manifestations of fat necrosis associated with pancreatitis.

Neuromas

These benign tumors involving the nerve tissue may be classified as neurilemmomas when the lesion arises from the sheath cell of Schwann or neurofibroma in which there are subcutaneous masses of neurofibromatous tissue. Neurilemmomas frequently arise from relatively small nerves and do not produce much pain. Treatment is surgical excision. Neurofibromas may be multiple and may be associated with von Recklinghausen's disease, including café au lait spots and scoliosis. Patients with neurofibromatosis are prone to develop meningiomas, gliomas, and pheochromocytomas, and eventual sarcomatous degeneration occurs in approximately 10 percent.

MALIGNANT TUMORS

Carcinoma of the skin occurs predominantly in exposed areas, most frequently in the weather-beaten skin of the aging sailor or farmer. It is generally a low-grade malignant tumor which may metastasize late, in which case the metastasis is usually to regional lymph nodes, so that curability is high compared with that of other tumors.

Basal Cell Carcinoma

This is a localized malignancy which grows slowly, at times taking 1 or more years to double in area. Basal cell carcinoma is more common than the squamous cell tumor, accounting for at least three-fourths of all cases in most clinical series. Lesions may be found over most areas of the body and are waxy, grayish yellow, or pink, often with telangiectasia below the surface. There is a predilection for the head and neck. In some instances, the tumors are darkly pigmented and difficult to distinguish from melanoma (Fig. 14-3). The lesions are firm but not indurated, and there is little sign of inflammation. As growth progresses, the skin is stretched, and the center of the lesion tends to necrose, resulting eventually in a flat ulcer. Basal carcinoma may extend deeper subcutaneously than is initially apparent, and extensive ulceration into the deep tissue without marked induration or infiltration has been referred to as *rodent ulcer*. If the tumor is not treated, it may erode into the deep structures including the skull, orbit, or brain. Less commonly, basal cell carcinoma may appear fungoid and grow large externally.

Squamous Cell Carcinoma

Squamous cell carcinoma tends to be more clearly defined than basal cell carcinoma. It grows more rapidly and may achieve in weeks the same size that the basal cell carcinoma reaches in months or years. Differential diagnosis between basal cell and squamous cell carcinoma can usually be made on the basis of site, appearance, history, type of skin, and presence of scars. However, only biopsy provides an accurate diagnosis.

The primary lesion of the squamous cell carcinoma is frequently surrounded by satellite nodules, and central ulceration may occur. The degree of induration around the

Fig. 14-3. Pigmented basal cell carcinoma. Note characteristics of melanotic tumor.

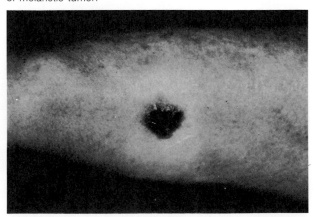

lesion is significant. The center gradually deepens into a crater with an irregular base which is covered by crust. Small pearls may be expressed from the ulcer, and rolled margins surrounding the ulcer contribute to the lesion's resembling a small volcanic crater. Growth may be superficial, or the lesion may burrow into deeper tissue with minimal effect on the cutaneous surface. Squamous cell carcinoma is more malignant than the basal cell variety and will metastasize to regional glands more rapidly.

Squamous cell carcinoma is particularly common in the lip at the vermillion border and in the folds of the paranasal area or in the axilla. Lesions occur more frequently in blond individuals with thin dry skin which is subjected to frequent irritation by rubbing or shaving. Squamous cell carcinoma is also particularly likely to originate in papillomas, senile warts, or cutaneous horns and develops at the site of postradiation dermatitis and ulcerations in old burn scars (Marjolin's ulcer). The incidence is also higher in people exposed to arsenicals, nitrates, and hydrocarbons.

Sweat Gland Carcinoma

This rare tumor usually occurs in the sixth and seventh decades of life, but it has been reported in adolescents. Characteristically, a soft tissue mass has been present for many years. Therapy consists of wide local excision with consideration of lymphadenectomy, since regional lymph nodes are involved in about half the cases. Following treatment, the reported 5-year survival is 38 percent for all patients and 24 percent for those with lymph node involvement.

TREATMENT OF CARCINOMA. Both electrodesiccation and electrocoagulation have been used but are to be condemned, since they destroy more tissue than is needed, result in retardation of healing, and do not provide a diagnosis. Radiation therapy may afford good results in the treatment of basal cell carcinoma, whereas squamous cell carcinomas are generally more resistant. Resolution of superficial basal cell carcinomas has been achieved with topical dinitrochlorobenzene (DNCB).

Although there is wide disagreement, surgical excision generally shows rates of cure which are higher than those for radiation. The results of radiation are certainly not as good for basal cell carcinomas over 2 cm in diameter as those achieved with surgical excision. Radiation therapy is contraindicated for any lesion which has recurred following unsuccessful radiation or for lesions which have developed in tissue which has been scarred following burns, keratoses, or xeroderma pigmentosum.

Mohs has used an escharotic preparation which is applied to the surface of the skin; 24 hours later the area fixed by the preparation is removed and examined microscopically. From this evidence, decision is made as to the requirements for additional application. The procedure is repeated until marginal biopsy shows only healthy tissue. The advantage of this method is the possibility of eradicating small extensions of the central lesion with certainty, and the granulation tissue below the lesion heals rapidly. Mohs has achieved 93 percent cures for carcinoma of the skin in all locations on the surface of the body and 87.5 percent cures for carcinoma of the lip. Few surgeons have utilized this technique.

Surgical treatment for carcinoma of the skin should include complete excision of all malignant tissue and a sufficient margin of normal tissue. For smaller tumors, a margin of 0.5 cm laterally and in depth is usually sufficient, whereas for larger lesions, the margins must be significantly greater. Many of the larger lesions require planned reconstructive surgical procedures, frequently employing skin grafts. Prophylactic dissection of regional nodes is not practical and should be performed only if there is evidence of clinical involvement.

PROGNOSIS. This is difficult to evaluate, but recurrence rates are very low. Overall 5-year survival rates of 96 percent for basal cell carcinoma and 80 percent for squamous cell carcinoma have been reported. Sharp and Binkley reported on 983 cutaneous carcinomas of all types and found that a 14 percent recurrence rate followed surgical treatment, while 10 percent recurred following roentgen therapy and 17 percent following radium therapy. In contrast, Conway reported only one recurrence in 168 cases of basal cell carcinoma treated surgically as compared with a 7.2 percent recurrence rate following roentgen therapy.

Other Malignant Tumors

Since the skin has a mesodermal origin, it is logical that sarcomas should develop, and the skin represents the site of origin of 6 percent of all cases of sarcoma. Primary sarcomas vary in degree of malignancy and in histologic characteristics. Excision is associated with an overall incidence of recurrence of 61 percent.

FIBROSARCOMA

This occurs most commonly in women in the buttocks, thigh, and inguinal regions and particularly frequently in scars. The tumors are usually of relatively low-grade malignancy and are radioresistant. Wide surgical excision is the treatment of choice, but it is followed by a high incidence of recurrence. In one series, 56 percent survived 10 years without recurrence. Distant spread occurs in 25 percent.

HEMANGIOPERICYTOMA

This is a malignant tumor of angioplastic origin and is considered a malignant variant of the glomus tumor. The lesions are extremely malignant, and the prognosis is poor, with only 27 percent surviving 5 years without evidence of disease. Surgical excision has proved unsatisfactory for larger tumors, and x-ray therapy is considered the treatment of choice.

KAPOSI'S SARCOMA

The etiology and pathogenesis of this lesion have not been resolved. It occurs more commonly in men. In Western countries there is a predilection for Jews, Italians, and Prussians. The tumor is prevalent in equatorial Africa and constitutes 9 percent of malignant tumors in Uganda. The

tumor usually starts in the hands or feet as multiple plaques which are reddish to purple and may be flat, ulcerated, or polypoid. The lymph nodes may be involved and obstruction of the lymph nodes may result in lymphedema.

X-ray may retard the growth of the lesion, but wide surgical excision and, at times, amputation offer more promise. Patients with florid lesions respond well to actinomycin D (dactinomycin). The prognosis is poor, although some cases have survived for prolonged periods of time. In the terminal stages, the tumor extends to the mucous membranes and portions of the gastrointestinal tract.

OTHER SARCOMAS

A wide variety of other tumors having origin in different cells have been described. Dermatrofibrosarcoma protuberans represents one tumor with relatively low-grade malignancy which generally occurs on the trunk. The tumors are radioresistant but respond to surgical excision, and 70 percent have been reported to be free of the disease for at least 5 years. Widespread dissemination is rare, but local recurrence may occur repeatedly.

Lymphangiosarcoma is almost always associated with chronic lymphedema. A recent review included 186 cases; 162 cases occurred postmastectomy an average of 10 years after surgery, with a range of 1 to 26 years. All patients had had radical mastectomy, and the overwhelming majority had received postoperative irradiation. Only 9 percent of the patients survived 5 or more years, and only 2 of 24 patients with nonpostmastectomy lymphangiosarcoma were alive at 5-year follow-up. Amputation gave significantly better results than radiation therapy.

MISCELLANEOUS LESIONS

Bowen's disease is a slowly growing cutaneous carcinoma in situ for which excision is recommended. *Adenoacanthoma,* which frequently develops on the face or ear, is characterized grossly by a verrucous appearance and microscopically by desquamated cells. Local excision is indicated, since it rarely metastasizes. *Keratoacanthoma* is an elevated, friable red lesion which may be of viral origin and is best managed by simple excision.

MELANOMA AND OTHER PIGMENTED LESIONS

General Considerations

Since melanoma is a relatively uncommon disease, occurring in 0.0018 percent of the general population, while the average Caucasian adult has 15 to 20 nevi, it is obvious that removal of all moles is not advisable. On the other hand, about 25 percent of patients who have malignant melanoma recall having had a "mole" at the site of origin of the malignant lesion. Therefore, in dealing with pigmented lesions, the surgeon must be aware of characteristics which should arouse suspicion of malignancy or premalignancy.

Several pertinent facts regarding the predilection for malignant melanoma aid in the evaluation of pigmented lesions of the skin. Melanoma is rare before puberty. Females and males are affected with equal frequency. The lesions tend to occur in people with fair skin. The type of mole is important in assessing the likelihood of development of melanoma. The junctional nevus, either alone or as part of a compound nevus, has been implicated more frequently than the pure intradermal nevus. The blue nevus is rarely the source of melanoma, and the development of malignancy in the small congenital hairy nevus is even more unusual. The incidence of malignant melanoma in giant pigmented nevi has been reported as 10 to 17.5 percent. Nevi of the palms, soles, nail beds, genitalia, and mucous membranes retain functional elements that are more prone to be the source of melanoma than moles at other sites. The ratio of the number of moles at this site to melanoma substantiates this notion. There is probably a genetic predilection for the development of melanoma as evidenced by the studies of Harnly, who has created a strain of flies in which melanotic tumors develop spontaneously. Kassel et al. have also induced melanotic cancer in *Drosophila,* using an extract of human tumors.

Many theories concerning pigmented lesions that enjoyed acceptance in the past have recently proved to be unfounded. MacDonald has shown that there is probably no difference in incidence among races. It is also untrue that melanoma occurs more frequently in areas of highest total sunlight. Although endocrine dysfunction is related to pigmentation in Addison's disease, Cushing's syndrome, thyrotoxicosis, and diabetes, there is no relationship to the development of malignant melanoma. Castration, adrenalectomy, hypophysectomy, and hormone therapy have all failed to alter the course of metastatic melanoma. White and George et al. have recently refuted the notion that pregnancy adversely affects survival in women with melanoma. Repeated trauma and its role in malignant transformation of moles remains theoretic and unproved.

Fig. 14-4. Typical malignant melanoma. Note central darkly pigmented elevation and surrounding halo of superficial satellite extensions. Sudden change in appearance and growth brought the patient to his physician.

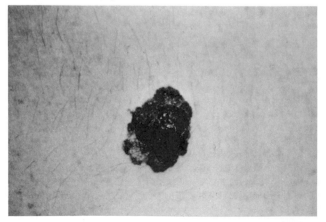

Benign Pigmented Lesions

These include the intradermal nevus, or common mole, the junctional nevus, compound nevus, juvenile melanoma, and freckles. The *intradermal nevus* is characterized by nests of melanoblasts which are confined to the dermis. The lesions are smooth or papillary and rarely occur on the soles or palms. The presence of hair is strong presumptive evidence of the diagnosis. In the case of the *junctional nevus,* the proliferation of melanoblasts originates in the basal layer of the epidermis and extends down into the dermis. The lesions are smooth, flat, or slightly raised. They occur on the genitalia, soles, palms, nail beds, and mucous membranes. The *compound nevus* is formed from junctional and intradermal elements. It is smooth, elevated, occasionally papillary, and hairless. *Juvenile melanomas* are nevi which occur prior to puberty, and although the microscopic picture is similar to that of melanoma, the lesions are clinically benign. They may be purplish red, brown, or black; they are generally smooth and hairless with irregular edges. The majority occur on the face and enlarge slowly. *Freckles* occur most commonly in blond and red-headed people on exposed portions of their bodies and represent pigment in the basal layer and upper dermis. They are not of clinical significance.

DIFFERENTIAL DIAGNOSIS. Although the classic mole has a characteristic appearance, the differential between benign pigmented skin lesions and melanoma may be quite difficult. Other lesions which cause particular confusion are (1) seborrheic and senile keratoses (Fig. 14-1) and (2) pigmented basal cell tumors (Fig. 14-3). Small intradermal hematomas may have an appearance similar to melanomas, and subungual hematomas have been mistaken for melanomas. High-speed dental drills may force silver fillings into the buccal mucosa, and the appearance mimics that of melanoma.

TREATMENT. If the pigmented lesion is considered to be a junctional nevus, excision is advisable. Various characteristics of any pigmented lesions are indications for excision. These include change in color or pigment distribution; development of erythema; change in size or consistency; change in the surface characteristic, i.e., scaling, oozing, bleeding, crustings or erosion; subjective symptoms such as pain, numbness, burning, itching, diffusion of pigment into normal skin; satellite nodules; and regional lymphadenopathy.

The *Hutchinson freckle* (lentigo maligna) is worthy of special note. This is a circumscribed precancerous melanosis of the face, generally occurring in elderly people. There are two stages of disease: In the macular stage, the lesion is smooth and light brown with irregular borders and uneven color. About one-third of the lesions then evolve into a tumor stage characterized by induration and all the histologic features of melanoma, but the behavior is not like melanoma. The prognosis is excellent when the lesion is excised from the face, but it is guarded when the lesion is found in other body areas, in which case it should be treated as a melanoma.

Excision of any suspicious lesion should be complete and should include a margin of normal skin.

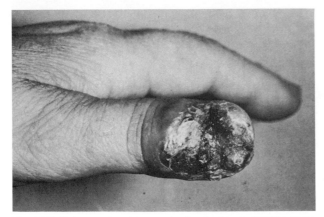

Fig. 14-5. Subungual melanoma. Lesion had been treated as an infection for nearly 1 year. Note pigmentation and replacement of nail. X-rays showed destruction of the distal phalanx. Axillary metastases were evident by this time.

Melanoma

The term, by definition, refers to a malignant lesion originating in the melanoblast of the skin, and therefore "malignant melanoma" represents a redundancy. The tumor may develop in any area of the skin or in the pigmented region of the eye. There is an almost equal distribution between the head and neck, lower extremity, and trunk, each accounting for approximately 25 percent of the cases. About 11 percent occur in the upper extremity, and the remainder involve the genitalia or represent cases in which the primary lesion is never determined. The typical skin lesion (Fig. 14-4) is darkly pigmented, smooth, firm, and nonhairy. Subungual melanomas are more frequent than pigmented nevi in the nail beds and may present difficulty in reference to differentiation from subungual hematoma and chronic paronychial infection (Fig. 14-5). All melanomas originate from the melanoblast at the dermal-epidermal junction, but the cell does not contain melanin at all times; therefore some lesions may be amelanotic. The cells are characterized by a dopa-positive reaction.

Microstaging has been determined by direct measurement or according to Clark's levels of invasion (Fig. 14-6). Level I (in situ) applies when all tumor cells are above the basement membrane. Level II has tumor extension into the papillary but not the reticular dermis. Level III refers to tumor cells in the ill-defined interface between the papillary and reticular dermis. Level IV is characterized by tumor cells in the reticular dermis. Level V has invasion into the subcutaneous fat. Clinically, Stage I relates to isolated skin involvement, Stage II to involvement of regional lymph nodes, and Stage III to distant metastases.

TREATMENT. Incisional biopsy is performed only when the lesion is extremely large. Biopsy provides the definitive diagnosis and should indicate the depth of involvement.

When invasion does not extend beyond the papillary dermis, simple excision is generally sufficient. When the tumor extends below the papillary dermis, a 5-cm margin beyond the lesion is indicated. Inadequate excision has

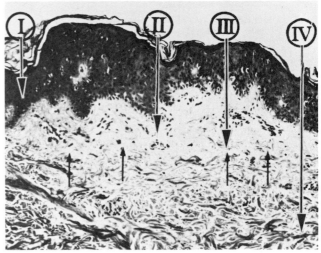

Fig. 14-6. Clark's levels of invasion. Papillary and reticular dermis of normal skin of the right upper arm; hematoxylin and eosin stain. The tissue just below the epidermis is pale and delicate, without obvious collagen bundles. Deep to this, collagen is organized into bundles, and the upper part of this zone forms an almost straight line with the papillary dermis (small arrows). Piling up of cells at this interface constitutes level III invasion. The arrows and their respective roman numerals indicate invasion levels. Level V (not shown) is into fat. (*From Cancer Res., 29:725, 1969.*)

been associated with the development of satellite nodules (Fig. 14-7).

The major argument in therapy centers around removal of the regional lymph nodes. Some advocate removing these nodes only when they are involved clinically, since

Fig. 14-7. Recurrent satellite nodules. These followed inadequate excision of a malignant melanoma which was thought to be a simple nevus. Note the characteristic deep-black color and emergence of lesions from the subcutaneous tissues to and through the skin.

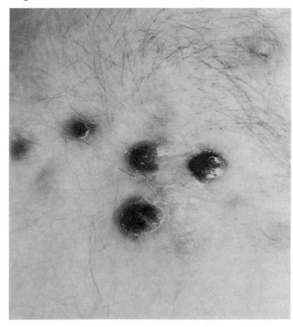

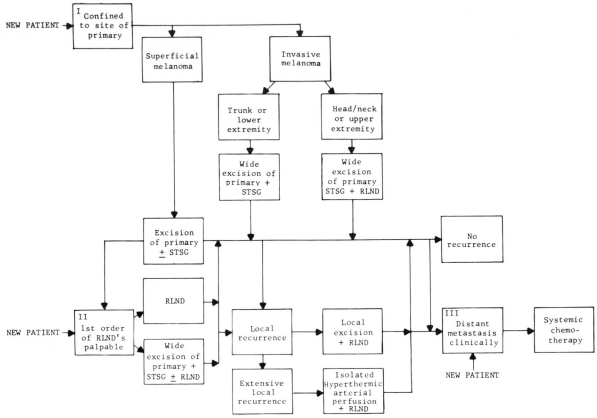

Fig. 14-8. Schematic diagram illustrating a treatment approach to melanoma patients. STSG, split-thickness skin graft; RLND, regional lymph node. (*From C. O. Knutson et al., Melanoma, Curr Probl Surg, The Year Book Medical Publishers, Inc., Chicago, December 1971.*)

there is significant morbidity associated with the procedure and statistical data do not demonstrate benefit. Others champion routine removal regardless of the clinical status in view of the accepted inaccuracy of clinical evaluation.

As a compromise, Knutson et al. recommend elective cervicofacial or axillary node dissection, in the absence of clinical involvement, for invasive lesions of the head and neck or upper extremity, since the consequent morbidity is minimal. Invasive melanomas of the trunk are treated with wide excision, and nodes are removed only if they are involved clinically, since lymphatic drainage is unpredictable. "Prophylactic" lymph node dissections generally are not advised for lower extremity lesions, since necrosis of skin flaps, delayed healing, infection, thrombophlebitis, edema, and satellitosis all contribute to a significant morbidity. Chronic lymphedema occurs in 6 percent of extremities following inguinal node dissection and 46 percent following ilioinguinal node dissection. The exception is a lesion which permits removal of the inguinal lymph nodes in continuity. Clinically palpable nodes should be excised (Fig. 14-8).

The appreciation of intermediate metastases between the primary tumor and regional nodes has led some writers to suggest aggressive amputation or, more recently, integumentectomy with removal of skin, subcutaneous tissue, and deep fascia from the foot to the inguinal ligament. In general, amputation is reserved for palliation of bulky, ulcerating, or painful lesions.

Groin Dissection (Fig. 14-9). The skin incision may be

oblique and parallel to the inguinal ligament, vertical, or S-shaped with an oblique limb running parallel to the inguinal ligament and the vertical limbs running parallel to the lateral margin of the rectus femoris muscles craniad and to the medial portion of the femoral triangle caudad. If the primary lesion is close to the line of incision or if the proposed skin incision is overlying a large lymph node which might be attached to the subcutaneous tissue, a wide ellipse can be removed beginning medial to the anterior superior iliac spine and continuing over the femoral triangle. On the abdominal wall, the subcutaneous and fatty tissue is dissected cleanly from the aponeurosis of the external oblique down to the inguinal ligament. With genital primary melanomas, the presymphysial lymphatics and areolar tissue of the spermatic cord or round ligament must be included in the dissection. The lower flaps are retracted, the lateral margin is exposed first, and the superficial fascia and fascia lata are dissected off the bare sartorius muscle to the lateral margin of the femoral triangle. The femoral sheath is entered, and the femoral artery and vein are dissected clean of fatty tissue. The greater saphenous vein is transected at two levels, first at the medial inferior portion of the transected tissue and second where the vein enters the femoral vein. Since the deep inguinal

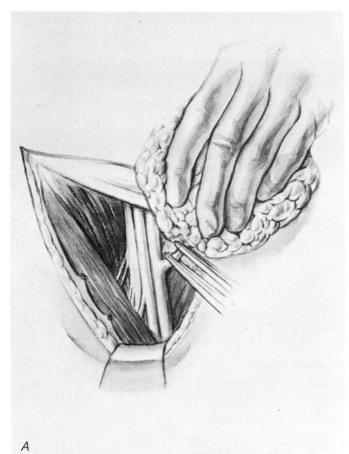

A

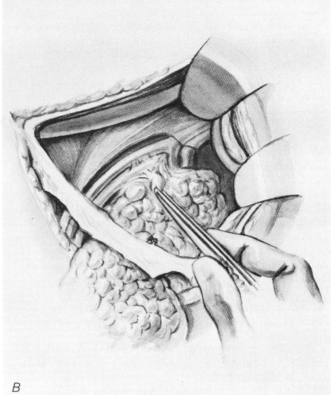

B

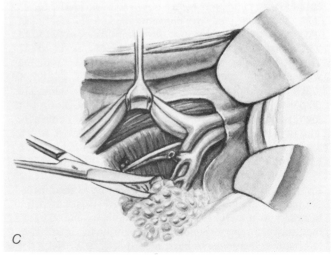

C

Fig. 14-9. Groin dissection. *A*. Dissection of upper thigh and sheath of femoral triangle. *B*. Dissection of inguinal region including excision of endopelvic fascia. Note exposure of iliac vessels. *C*. Dissection of obturator fossa containing medial chain of obturator lymph nodes. Note that external iliac vein is elevated and obturator nerve is isolated from the fascia. *(From J. S. Spratt, Jr., "Anatomy and Surgical Technique of Groin Dissection," The C. V. Mosby Company, St. Louis, 1965.)*

nodes lie in the areolar tissue about the femoral vessels, carrying the dissection down to the adventitial surface of the femoral artery and vein will include them in the dissected material. Mediad, the tissue is incised over the pectineus muscle, and eventually the specimen remains attached only by tissue passing into the femoral space medial to the femoral vein.

The iliac dissection represents a continuum of the inguinal dissection. The external oblique aponeurosis is incised, and a flap is established caudad down to the inguinal ligament. The fibers of the transversus abdominis and internal oblique muscles are separated from the inguinal ligament. The ligamentous attachment of the transversalis fascia to the inguinal ligament is divided, and the epigastric artery and vein are ligated and transected at the level of the inguinal ligament. Following the division of muscle and fascial fibers along the inguinal ligament to the anterior superior iliac spine, the peritoneum is exposed and reflected from the lateral pelvic wall by blunt dissection. This per-

mits visualization of the ureter and the iliac vessels. The endopelvic fascia is incised medial to the genitofemoral nerve from the inguinal ligament to above the bifurcation of the common iliac artery; the external iliac artery is rotated mediad, and the space between the artery and the muscle is dissected clear. The dissection then continues by reflecting the vascular sheath away from the external iliac artery and vein. The origin of the inferior epigastric arteries and veins will be exposed, and these are then transected. All the areolar tissue is swept down in a medial fashion. The medial chain of iliac lymph nodes is removed by dissection of the obturator fossa, retracting the external iliac vein laterally. In this dissection the bare muscle fibers of the internal obturator muscle are exposed, and the obturator veins must be transected. After the iliac dissection has been mobilized and freed from the margin of the inguinal-pectineal triangle, the inguinal ligament is elevated, and the iliac alveolar tissue and lymph nodes are delivered into the femoral triangle for completion of the en bloc dissection.

The lower abdominal wall is carefully reconstructed to avoid hernia formation, and the sartorius muscle transected and reflected mediad to cover the femoral artery and vein. Prior to closure of the subcutaneous tissue and skin, drainage is achieved with suction catheters.

Adjunctive Therapy. Systemic chemotherapy is used when there is recurrent or metastatic disease which precludes excision. Disseminated melanoma is one of the most chemoresistant cancers. Objective regression has been noted in about one-quarter of the patients receiving vinblastine or cyclophosphamide. Other effective agents include vincristine, hydroxyurea, and 1-phenylalanine mustard (melphalan), BCNU (1,3-bis[2-chloroethyl]-1-nitrosourea), and DTIC (dimethyl-triazeno-imidazole-carboxamine).

Isolated regional artery perfusion with L-phenylalanine mustard or a combination of drugs has had striking results as treatment for multiple local metastases or inoperable satellitosis of an extremity. Some writers have applied perfusion as an adjunct to patients without clinical subcutaneous or cutaneous metastases. Recurrence rates lower than those associated with conventional surgical treatment have been reported. However, the complications of arterial perfusion therapy are of such magnitude as to argue against this approach, with suggestion that perfusion be withheld until recurrences are noted.

Recent attention has been directed to the host immune response. A correlation between a patient's prognosis and his immune response to melanoma has been established. This response accounts for spontaneous regressions, which have been noted, and immunity to the tumor has been enhanced by active immunization with BCG (bacillus Calmette-Guérin) or autologous tumor cells. Dermal scarification has been associated with better results than intradermal vaccination. The best results have been noted for intradermal metastases, while subcutaneous and visceral metastases rarely respond. BCG therapy has toxic side effects, and deaths have been reported.

PROGNOSIS. In a recent review by Wanebo and associates, the 5-year cure rate was 100 percent for levels I and II, 88 percent for level III, 60 percent for level IV, and 15 percent for level V. In patients with level IV melanoma, the 5-year cure rate was 82 percent in those with negative nodes and 27 percent in those with nodal metastases after elective node dissection. In the same study the measured depth of invasion added significant clinical pathologic information. The incidence of nodal metastases at elective node dissection was 5 to 9 percent for melanomas showing 0.6 to 2.0 mm of invasion, 22 percent for melanomas measuring 2.1 to 3.0 mm, and 39 percent for melanomas invading beyond 3 mm. The cure rate was 100 percent for melanomas measuring less than 1 mm, 83 percent for melanomas invading 1.1 to 2.0 mm, 58 percent for lesions measuring 2.1 to 3.0 mm, and 55 percent for melanomas invading over 3.0 mm. In another review, Cady et al. reported that the depth-of-invasion criteria of Clark were no more accurate in predicting survival than careful measurement of maximal diameter. Melanomas of the lower extremity offer a slightly better survival rate than those of the upper extremity and a markedly higher survival rate than lesions of the trunk.

References

Physiology

Allen, A. C.: "The Skin: A Clinicopathological Treatise," 2d ed., Grune & Stratton, Inc., New York, 1967.

Ellis, H., and Morgan, M. N.: Surgical Treatment of Severe Hyperidrosis, *Proc Roy Soc Med,* **64:**768, 1971.

Hartfall, W. G., and Jochimsen, P. R.: Hyperhidrosis of Upper Extremity and Its Treatment, *Surg Gynec Obst,* **135:**586, 1972.

Rothman, S.: "Physiology and Biochemistry of the Skin," The University of Chicago Press, Chicago, 1954.

Pressure Sores

Herceg, S. J., and Harding, R. L.: Surgical Treatment of Pressure Sores, *Pa Med,* **74:**45, 1971.

Hidradenitis Suppurativa

Conway, H., Stark, R. B., Climo, S., Weeter, J. C., and Garcia, F. A.: The Surgical Treatment of Chronic Hidradenitis Suppurativa, *Surg Gynecol Obstet,* **95:**455, 1952.

Knaysi, G. A., Jr., Cosman, B., and Crikelair, G. F.: Hidradenitis Suppurativa, *JAMA,* **203:**19, 1968.

Cysts and Benign Tumors

Brasfield, R. D., and Das Gupta, T. K.: Von Recklinghausen's Disease: A Clinicopathological Study, *Ann Surg,* **175:**86, 1972.

Brown, S. H., Jr., Neerhout, R. C., and Fonkalsrud, E. W.: Prednisone Therapy in Management of Large Hemangiomas in Infants and Children, *Surgery,* **71:**168, 1972.

Conway, H.: "Tumors of the Skin," Charles C Thomas, Publisher, Springfield, Ill., 1956.

Dwight, R. W., and Maloy, J. K.: Pilonidal Sinus: Experience with 449 Cases, *N Engl J Med,* **249:**926, 1953.

Hvid-Hansen, O.: Treatment of Ganglions, *Acta Chir Scand,* **136:**471, 1970.

Mandel, S. R., and Thomas, C. C., Jr.: Management of Pilonidal Sinus by Excision and Primary Closure, *Surg Gynecol Obstet,* **134:**448, 1972.

Riveros, M., and Pack, G. T.: The Glomus Tumor: Report of Twenty Cases, *Ann Surg,* **133:**394, 1951.

Strahan, J., and Bailie, H. W. C.: Glomus Tumor: A Review of 15 Clinical Cases, *Br J Surg,* **59:**91, 1972.

Malignant Tumors

Ackerman, L. V.: "Surgical Pathology," The C. V. Mosby Company, St. Louis, 1964.

Castro, El B., Hajdu, S. I., and Fortner, J. G.: Surgical Therapy of

Fibrosarcoma of Extremities: A Reappraisal, *Arch Surg,* **107:**284, 1973.

Conway, H.: "Tumors of the Skin," Charles C Thomas, Publisher, Springfield, Ill., 1956.

De Cholnoky, T.: Cancer of the Face: A Clinical and Statistical Study of 1062 Cases, *Ann Surg,* **122:**88, 1945.

El-Domeiri, A. A., Brasfield, R. D., Huvos, A. G., and Strong, E. W.: Sweat Gland Carcinoma, *Ann Surg,* **173:**270, 1971.

Epstein, E.: Sarcoma Involving the Skin, *Arch Dermatol,* **60:**1130, 1949.

Futrell, J. W., Krueger, G. R., Morton, D. L., and Ketcham, A. S.: Carcinoma of Sweat Glands in Adolescents, *Am J Surg,* **123:**594, 1972.

Levis, W. R., Kraemer, K. H., Klingler, W. G., Peck, G. L., and Terry, W. D.: Topical Immunotherapy of Basal Cell Carcinomas with Dinitrochlorobenzene, *Cancer Res,* **33:**3036, 1973.

Mohs, F. E.: "Chemosurgery in Cancer, Gangrene and Infections," Charles C Thomas Publisher, Springfield, Ill., 1956.

Sharp, G. S., and Binkley, F. C.: The Treatment of Carcinoma of the Skin, *Am J Roentgenol Radium Ther Nucl Med,* **67:**606, 1952.

Vogel, C. L., Templeton, C. J., Templeton, A. C., Taylor, J. F., and Kyalwazi, S. K.: Treatment of Kaposi's Sarcoma with Actinomycin-D and Cyclophosphamide: Results of a Randomized Clinical Trial, *Int J Cancer,* **8:**136, 1971.

Woodward, A. H., Ivins, J. C., and Soule, E. H.: Lymphangiosarcoma Arising in Chronic Lymphedematous Extremities, *Cancer,* **30:**562, 1972.

Melanoma and Other Pigmented Lesions

Bluming, A. Z., Vogel, C. L., Ziegler, J. L., Mody, N., and Kamya, G.: Immunologic Effects of BCG in Malignant Melanoma: Two Modes of Administration Compared, *Ann Int Med,* **76:**405, 1972.

Cady, B., Legg, M. A., and Redfern, A. B.: Contemporary Treatment of Malignant Melanoma, *Am J Surg,* **129:**472, 1975.

Clark, W. J., Jr., From, L., Bernardino, E. A., and Mihm, M.C.: The Histogenesis and Biologic Behavior of Primary Human Malignant Melanomas of the Skin, *Cancer Res,* **29:**497, 1969.

Davis, N. C.: Cutaneous Melanoma: The Queensland Experience, *Curr Probl Surg,* vol. XII, No. 5, 1976.

George, P. A., Fortner, J. G., and Pack, G. T.: Melanoma with Pregnancy: A Report of 115 Cases, *Cancer,* **13:**854, 1960.

Goldsmith, H. S., Shah, J. P., Kim, D. H.: Prognostic Significance of Lymph Node Dissection in Treatment of Malignant Melanoma, *Cancer,* **26:**606, 1970.

Greeley, P. W., Middleton, A. G., and Curtin, J. W.: Incidence of Malignancy in Giant Pigmented Nevi, *Plastic Reconstr Surg,* **36:**26, 1965.

Harris, M. N., Gumport, S. L., and Maiwandi, H.: Axillary Lymph Node Dissection for Melanoma, *Surg Gynec Obst,* **135:**936, 1972.

Hueston, J. T.: Integumentectomy for Malignant Melanoma of the Limbs, *Aust NZ J Surg,* **40:**114, 1970.

Knutson, C. O., Hori, J. M., and Spratt, J. S., Jr.: Melanoma, *Curr Probl Surg,* December, 1971.

Krementz, E. T., Creech, O., Ryan, R., and Reemtsma, K.: An Appraisal of Cancer Chemotherapy by Regional Perfusion, *Ann Surg,* **156:**417, 1962.

McBride, C. M.: Advanced Melanoma of the Extremities, *Arch Surg,* **101:**122, 1970.

MacDonald, E. J.: Epidemiology of Melanoma, *Ann NY Acad Sci* **100:**4, 1963.

McKhann, C. F., Hendrickson, C. G., Spitler, L. E., Gunnarsson, A., Banerjee, D., and Nelson, W. R.: Immunotherapy of Melanoma with BCG: Two Fatalities Following Intralesion Injection, *Cancer,* **35:**514, 1975.

Morton, D. L., Eilber, F. R., Holmes, E. C., Hunt, J. S., Ketcham, A. S., Silverstein, M. J., and Sparks, F. C.: BCG Immunotherapy of Malignant Melanoma: Summary of 7-Year Experience, *Ann Surg,* **180:**635, 1974.

Polk, H. C., Cohn, J. D., and Clarkson, J. G.: An Appraisal of Elective Regional Lymphadenectomy for Melanoma, in G. D. Zuidema and D. B. Skinner (eds.), "Current Topics in Surgical Research," vol. 1, Academic Press, Inc., New York, 1969.

Raven, R. W.: The Clinicopathological Aspects of Malignant Melanoma, *Ann NY Acad Sci,* **100:**142, 1963.

Spratt, J. S., Jr., Shieber, W., and Dillard, B. M.: "Anatomy and Surgical Technique of Groin Dissection," The C. V. Mosby Company, St. Louis, 1965.

Wanebo, H. J., Woodruff, J., and Fortner, J. G.: Malignant Melanoma of the Extremities: A Clinicopathologic Study Using Levels of Invasion (Microstage), *Cancer,* **35:**666, 1975.

White, L. P.: The Role of Natural Resistance in the Prognosis of Human Melanoma, *Ann NY Acad Sci,* **100:**115, 1963.

Chapter 15

Breast

by Benjamin F. Rush, Jr.

The breast is man's insignia of membership in the class Mammalia. It is somewhat humbling to reflect that this badge of status had its origin as a modified sweat gland. In the male the breast is, with few exceptions, a dormant structure. In the female, from puberty to death, the breast is subjected to a constant dynamic role of physical changes related to the menstrual cycle, pregnancy, lactation, and the menopause. Associated with this active role are numerous malformations and dysfunctions which make diseases of the breast common clinical problems.

EMBRYOLOGY

The human breast makes its first appearance in the sixth week of embryonic development as an ectodermal thickening extending from the axilla to the groin, a distinct linear elevation called the *mammary ridge,* or *milk line.* Lens-shaped thickenings appear along the milk line, presaging the sites of developing breasts. In man the caudal two-thirds of the line disappears rapidly, and the pectoral thickening progresses with the ultimate formation of a breast primordium. Man shares this pectoral location of the breasts with other primates and with the elephant and sea cow, in contrast to the multiple breasts of the dog and pig and the inguinal location in the cow, goat, and whale.

In the fifth month of embryonic development the human primordial breast develops 15 to 20 solid cords which fan out beneath the skin in the underlying connective tissue. These primary milk ducts branch, and the ends develop club-shaped dilatations. During the seventh or eighth month the ducts hollow to develop lumina. During this same period the point in the skin corresponding to the nipple develops a small depression. At birth the breast is represented by a slight pit pierced by 15 to 20 openings into the primary milk ducts. The areola is a slight thickening in the skin which contains a few glands (of Montgomery). Shortly after birth the nipples become everted, and the areola is distinguished by a slight increase in pigmentation.

A few days after birth, bilateral or unilateral enlargement of the breast occurs in 70 percent of infants. In half the infants the swelling is accompanied by the secretion of a cloudy fluid similar to colostrum, the "witch's milk" of folklore. Histologically, these changes are associated with hypertrophy of the duct system, the appearance of acini, and an increased vascularity of the stroma. These alterations are considered an indirect effect of the high level of maternal estrogens in the infant's circulating blood. Following birth the falling estrogen level stimulates the hypophysis to produce prolactin, resulting in the mammary changes. These changes occur equally in male and female infants and regress spontaneously by the second or third week of life. Attempts to strip the breasts of their milk, as advocated by some superstitions, provoke the breasts to remain in the secretory state. Hyperplasia of the infant breast persisting over many months with persistent secretions has resulted from such manipulations.

CLINICAL CORRELATIONS. A number of developmental errors of the breast are of clinical importance. Most often observed is the persistence of one or more of the additional nipples in the milk line. These are commonly mistaken for moles. A rare anomaly is the occurrence of extramammary breast tissue, usually seen in the axilla or over the upper abdomen (Fig. 15-1), often not appearing until the tissue is stimulated by pregnancy and lactation. Excision of these supernumerary structures is the treatment of choice. Absence of one or both nipples or of one or both breasts also occurs, though rarely. While these conditions are serious cosmetic and functional defects, a more important functional deficiency is the often associated absence of the underlying pectoralis muscles and chest wall.

Occasionally the nipple fails to evert following birth and remains retracted or inverted throughout life. This is a

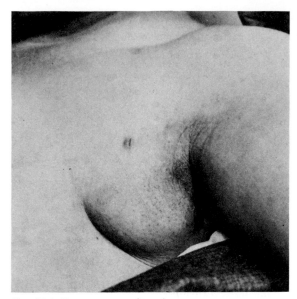

Fig. 15-1. Supernumerary breast.

serious functional problem when the patient attempts to nurse a child.

In some infants the collecting ducts fail to open onto the apex of the nipple, opening onto the areola instead. In a few instances collecting ducts are observed to empty onto the skin of the breast, failing entirely to traverse the nipple. These nippleless collecting ducts recapitulate the normal anatomy of the nippleless breast of the duckbill platypus.

ANATOMY AND DEVELOPMENT

Except for the neonatal period of hypertrophy and a period of slight hypertrophy occurring at puberty, the male breast undergoes little change throughout life. The female breast shows little change through infancy and childhood, but in the prepubertal period and throughout the remainder of life the breasts undergo numerous gross and microscopic changes (Fig. 15-2).

ADOLESCENCE. During the prepubertal period (from eleven to fifteen years) growth of the breast begins with the development of the prepubertal "bud." The areola becomes elevated and forms with the nipple a small conical protuberance. Histologically, the rudimentary primary ducts begin a rapid process of elongation and terminal branching, pushing down through the subcutaneous tissue toward the pectoral fascia and carrying with them sheaths of periductal connective tissue. A firm plaque of fibrous breast tissue forms as the lobes of the breasts develop, crowding out the subcutaneous fat. Roentgenograms of the breast at this period show a featureless, fibrous mass without trabeculae. Lobules do not form, however, until ovulation begins. Following ovulation at age fourteen to fifteen the breasts mature into their normal nulliparous form.

THE YOUNG ADULT. Anatomic Limits. The breast is suspended from the anterior chest wall, extending from the

second to the sixth rib. The medial boundary is at the lateral border of the sternum, and the lateral border stretches to the anterior axillary line (Fig. 15-3).

Areola and Nipple. The areola in the young female is convex and lens-shaped, surmounted at its center by the nipple. The areola gains a slight amount of pigmentation during adolescence, and although its surface is hairless, a few hairs may appear at the skin of the periphery. Both the subareolar area and the nipple contain much smooth muscle. The fibers of the areola are arranged in concentric rings as well as radially and are inserted into the base of the dermis. They function to contract the areola and to compress the base of the nipple. The bulk of the nipple is made up of smooth muscle fibers arranged both circularly and longitudinally. The nipple is made erect, smaller, and firmer by contraction of these fibers, and this involuntary action serves to aid in emptying the intrapapillary ducts. This response is evoked by suckling or by tactile stimuli. Sir Astley Cooper, a pioneer in describing the anatomy and diseases of the breast, first pointed out that the nipple lies to the lateral side of the center line of the breast and that its axis points upward and outward. The teleologic assumption is that this arrangement is for the convenience of the suckling child.

Glandular Tissue. The functional portion of the breast is a modified cutaneous gland, an appendage of the skin. It is enclosed between the superficial and deep layers of the superficial fascia. The glandular portion of the breast spreads out widely as a layer over the chest wall beneath the integument. It is roughly circular in outline except at the upper outer quadrant, where the axillary tail of Spence extends toward the axilla (Fig. 15-3). The tip of the axillary tail intrudes through an opening in the deep fascia of the axilla, Langer's foramen, to lie well up within the axilla. Neoplasms or deformities in this tail are sometimes mistaken for enlarged axillary nodes.

Portions of the fibrous tissue of the breast parenchyma extend from the surface of the glandular breast anteriorly to intermingle with the superficial layer of the superficial fascia. Similar processes arise from the deep surface of the gland to cross the retromammary space and fuse with the pectoral fascia. The anterior ligaments were described by Cooper, who noted, "The breast is slung upon the fore part of the chest, for [the ligaments] form a movable but very firm connection with the skin so that the breast has sufficient motion."

Blood Supply and Venous Drainage. Three major arteries generously supply the breast with blood. The perforating branches of the internal mammary artery pass through the first, second, third, and fourth intercostal spaces just lateral to the sternum to penetrate and pass through the origin of the pectoralis major muscle and enter the medial edge of the breast, supplying more than 50 percent of the blood to this organ. The lateral thoracic artery arises from the axillary artery and courses down along the lateral border of the pectoralis minor muscle. Its external mammary branches provide the second largest source of blood to the breast. The third artery of importance is the pectoral branch of the acromiothoracic artery, also a branch of the axillary artery. The pectoral artery is given off by the acromiothoracic at the medial edge of the pectoralis minor muscle. In its course between the pectoralis major and minor muscles, the pectoralis artery gives off branches to the posterior surface of the breast. The superior branch of the axillary artery, the lateral perforating branches of the intercostal arteries, and branches of the subscapular artery also contribute minor amounts to the blood supply.

The mammary glands have a rich, anastomosing network of superficial subcutaneous veins. These veins become markedly dilated during pregnancy and may sometimes become quite prominent over an area of underlying neoplasm. The majority of the superficial veins drain to the internal mammary vein. In some individuals these veins drain into the superficial veins of the lower neck.

The deep veins of the mammary gland drain along routes roughly corresponding to the arterial blood supply. Thus one major route is through the anterior intercostal perforating veins to the internal mammary veins. Another is by way of multiple branches to the axillary vein. A third route is by way of posterior branches anastomosing with the intercostal veins. This last route has special significance, since the intercostal veins communicate with the vertebral veins. This anastomosis with the vertebral veins is offered by Batson as the explanation for the often capricious metastasis of mammary cancer to the vertebral bodies or even the sacrum or pelvis without the presence of metastatic deposits in the lung. He holds that the wide variation in pressure within the thoracic cavity induced by straining or coughing may change the flow patterns within the valveless anastomosing veins so that blood from the breast draining through the lateral perforators to the intercostal vessels is forced down along the vertebral plexus.

The Lymphatics. A generous lymphatic plexus drains the skin and glandular tissues of the breast (Fig. 15-4). The lymphatic vessels empty into two main depots represented by the axillary and the internal mammary lymph nodes. There are an average of 53 lymph nodes in the axillary fossa, arranged along the course of the arteries and veins. Lymph from the lower outer quadrant of the breast drains to the lateral and inferior axillary nodes, while lymph from the areola, the upper outer quadrant of the breast, and the axillary tail drains to the medial superior axillary nodes. Within the axilla, lymph passes from the lateral inferior to the medial superior nodes at the apex of the axilla. Lymph then courses through lymphatic channels under the clavicle to the supraclavicular lymph nodes and by major lymphatic trunks to the junction of the subclavian and jugular veins. On the right, lymph enters the blood directly through these lymphatic trunks as they join the veins. On the left these trunks may first join with the thoracic duct, which shortly communicates with the venous system.

The internal mammary lymph nodes are much fewer in number than the axillary nodes, averaging but three or four nodes on each side lying along the internal mammary vessels, usually in the first, second, and third interspaces. Despite the scarcity and tiny size of these lymph nodes, most of the lymph from the upper and lower inner quadrants of the breast drains by this channel. Lymph from the nipple and areola may drain to both the internal mam-

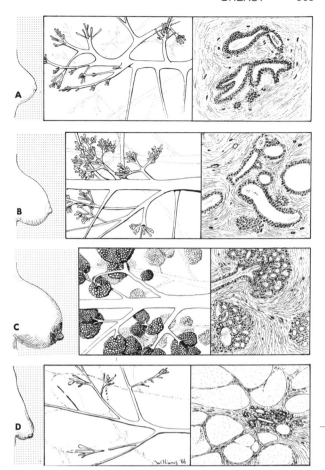

Fig. 15-2. Gross and microscopic appearance of breast at different stages of development. Central pictures show three-dimensional projection of microscopic structure. *A.* Adolescence. *B.* Pregnancy. *C.* Lactation. *D.* Postmenopausal period.

mary and the axillary nodes. The internal mammary lymphatic trunks eventually empty into the great veins of the neck, usually by way of the thoracic duct or of the right lymphatic duct.

Histology of the Resting Mammary Gland. Each lobe of the mammary gland is an independent compound alveolar gland. The mammary gland is a conglomeration of a variable number of such independent glands, each with its own excretory duct which has its separate opening on the surface of the nipple. The excretory ducts measure from 0.4 to 0.7 mm in diameter at the nipple surface and run perpendicularly through the nipple to turn and radiate out toward the periphery of the breast. Beneath the areola they dilate into a short fusiform area called the *milk sinus.* Beyond the milk sinus the excretory ducts begin to subdivide into smaller and smaller branches forming the lobules of the lobe. Within the lobules the ducts subdivide further, forming terminal, elongated tubes, the alveolar ducts, which are covered by round evaginations, the alveolae. Lobules are peripheral and scanty in the nulliparous breast (Fig. 15-2*A*).

There is mild controversy as to whether alveolae are present in the resting mammary gland. Some claim that

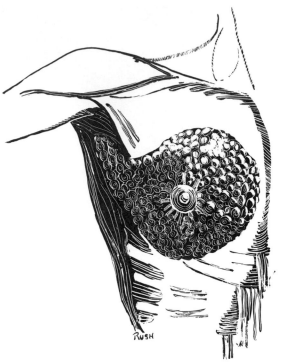

Fig. 15-3. Normal distribution of mammary tissue of adult female breast. Note long tail of Spence extending into axilla.

Fig. 15-4. Lymphatic drainage of breast. Nipple drains both laterally and medially. Medial side of breast drains to small internal mammary lymph nodes.

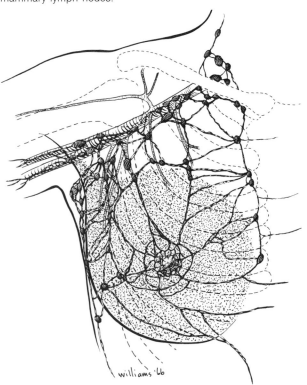

the resting gland is entirely a tubular structure and becomes tuboalveolar only during pregnancy. The majority opinion is that a few alveolae are scattered through the lobules in the resting state.

The walls of the alveolae and the alveolar ducts consist of a prominent basement membrane surrounding a layer of myoepithelial cells, which in turn lie beneath a layer of low columnar glandular cells. The myoepithelial layer is thin and difficult to identify in the acini and the alveolar ducts but becomes more prominent in the more major lobular ducts. These cells take a spiral course about the larger ducts and probably play a role in propelling milk from the acini to the nipple during lactation.

The collecting ducts are lined with a double layer of cuboidal to columnar epithelium until the milk sinus is reached. Here the lining changes to squamous epithelium. This continues through the milk sinus to the surface of the nipple.

Each lobule is surrounded by a coating of dense, firm, interlobular connective tissue, which is an intimate part of the breast parenchyma. The lobules are separated by a looser coating of less dense fibrous tissue, the interlobular connective tissue. This layer represents the supporting stroma of the breast. These layers are easily recognized histologically, but grossly the various lobules are intimately and firmly bound together and cannot be dissected apart.

Cyclic Changes of the Breast. Beginning about the eighth day of the menstrual cycle the female breast gradually increases in size, the volume often increasing by 50 percent by the immediate premenstrual period. At this point the breast is tense and may be somewhat tender. Part of the increase in size is due to interlobular edema and increasing congestion of the vasculature. Ingleby and Gershon-Cohen state that there is also a proliferation of the parenchyma, with the appearance of new lobules. These lobules then regress and fibrose during menstruation. Congestion and edema subside, and the breast again reaches its smallest size on about the eighth day after the onset of menstruation.

PREGNANCY AND LACTATION. Implantation of the ovum initiates a profound change in the gross and histologic structures of the breast. Grossly there is a pronounced enlargement of the breast, progressing throughout pregnancy. The normal size may be increased as much as two or three times. The nipple and areola become more prominent and more deeply pigmented. The openings of Montgomery's glands on the areola become prominent and are called *Montgomery's tubercles.* Pigmentation may spread beyond the areola onto the skin, forming a "secondary areola." The veins are engorged, and striae are frequently visible in the skin.

Histologically, the epithelium of the lobular ducts and alveolar ducts proliferates, and new ducts covered with multiple alveolar outpouchings are generated. The total number of lobules increases greatly. By the end of the sixth month the glandular cells of the acini produce small amounts of a secretion, colostrum, which increases toward the end of pregnancy (Fig. 15-2C).

Two or three days after delivery, globules appear in the supranuclear cytoplasm of the acinar cells. These push toward the cell lumen, increasing in size. The cell becomes tall and more columnar. Finally the globule is extruded into the lumen, and the cell shrinks to a cuboidal form, to begin the process again. The acini become distended with milk, which is propelled to the nipple during nursing. This process continues as long as suckling continues. When lactation ends, the extralobular tissue involutes, leaving small areas of fibrosis, and the breast gradually returns to the resting state. It never returns to the nulliparous form, however, but has the contour of maturity. The areola recedes into the breast tissue, with only the nipple projecting. Some of the darker pigmentation of the nipple and areola and residual skin striae persist.

MENOPAUSAL CHANGES. Following menopause the mammary gland gradually involutes (Fig. 15-2D). This change is slow and progressive, with gradual disappearance of lobules. Senile involution does not lead to complete extinction of mammary tissue; some lobules always remain, but they are scattered and small. In many areas only the larger lobular and collecting ducts may be found. The parenchyma and stromal fibrous tissue gradually blend together into a homogeneous mass, and the original lobular structure is almost completely lost. As the glandular tissues recede, there is a gradual invasion of fat, which aids in maintaining the breast outline, although in very thin women the breasts may become quite flabby as glandular tissue is lost.

CLINICAL CORRELATION. Both breasts of the adolescent girl usually develop at the same pace. Occasionally development is out of phase, and one breast will develop much more rapidly than the other, leading to distressing asymmetry (Fig. 15-5). The difference in size is usually repaired with time but occasionally persists. Patients complaining of asymmetric breasts during the adolescent period are advised to wait until maturation is complete. If asymmetry persists, a plastic surgical procedure may be required to adjust the difference.

A slight swelling of the breasts is often seen in adolescent boys. This is called *gynecomastia* and is a physiologic response to the change in the hormonal milieu in the pubertal male (Fig. 15-6). This slight hypertrophy normally subsides spontaneously but occasionally persists, either unilaterally or bilaterally. Persisting gynecomastia in young manhood requires an evaluation to exclude the possibility of abnormal endocrine secretion. If no abnormalities are found, the small button of hypertrophied breast tissue may be removed surgically to repair an embarrassing cosmetic defect in a young man.

Occasionally the growth of the female breast at puberty fails to cease and the breasts become huge—so-called virginal hypertrophy (Fig. 15-7). Breasts weighing 40 to 50 lb and descending to the level of the genitalia are described. Spontaneous regression does not occur, and the only solution is plastic surgical repair. This rare defect is seen in pregnant females as well and requires the same treatment.

EXAMINATION

INSPECTION. Physical examination of the breasts should begin with the patient erect, usually sitting on the edge

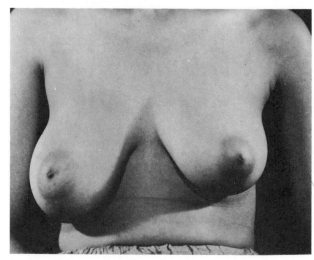

Fig. 15-5. Asymmetric breasts.

of the examining table. The breasts are observed for symmetry, dimpling of the skin, edema, deformity of outline, retraction of the nipple, or inflammation. Underlying masses will produce deformity or skin retraction, which is much more easily detected when the patient is erect and the breasts dependent. Haagensen suggests that the patient be allowed to lean forward to increase the breast dependency and further accentuate areas of deformity or dimpling.

PALPATION. Examination of the axillary and supraclavicular area is always part of a complete breast examination and is best done when the patient is erect. The axilla is examined with the humerus slightly abducted and the pectoralis muscle relaxed (Fig. 15-8B). The contents of the axilla are pressed gently against the rib cage, and the axilla is progressively palpated from apex to base. The apex of the axilla does not lie under the humeral head but anteriorly under the clavicle, where the axillary vein and artery

Fig. 15-6. Gynecomastia.

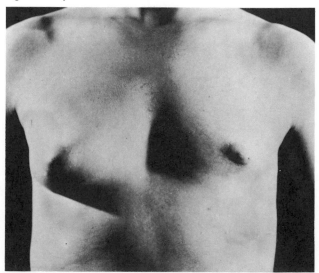

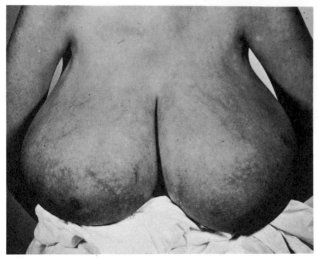

Fig. 15-7. Virginal hypertrophy. This growth occurred during 1 year in fifteen-year-old white girl and required plastic surgery for repair. (*Courtesy of Paul Weeks, M.D.*)

pass under the clavicle to become the subclavian vessels. Palpation of lymph nodes at this level is of great importance in predicting the prognosis in a patient with cancer.

The supraclavicular area is palpated with the tips of the fingers, making sure that the fingers are pressed down well behind the clavicle to roll the supraclavicular structures against the scalene muscles. In a thin neck the transverse fibers of the posterior belly of the omohyoid are sometimes mistaken for an enlarged lymph node. This can be differentiated by observing that a medial and lateral margin to

Fig. 15-8. Examination of breast. *A.* Observation with arms at side. *B.* Palpation of axilla. *C.* With arms raised. *D.* Palpation with patient supine.

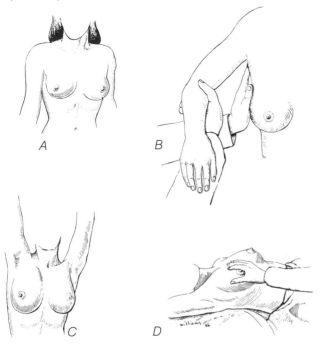

the supposed node cannot be felt, although an upper and lower border are easily detected. Following palpation of the axilla and supraclavicular area, the breasts are also palpated, although masses in the breasts are best felt when the patient is supine.

After inspection and palpation with the patient erect, the entire mammary gland is palpated carefully with the tips of the fingers with the patient in the supine position, with the arm first over the head and then at the side (Fig. 15-8). This should be done systematically and in the same way in each examination so that the examiner follows a definite pattern. One may begin at the upper inner quadrant, gradually inspecting the breast tissue from above downward until the medial portion of the breast has been examined. The areolar area is then palpated. If the patient has complained of secretions or blood from the nipple, the areola should be stroked toward the nipple to see if this symptom can be reproduced. The lateral portion of the breast is palpated starting at the upper outer quadrant and completing the examination at the lower outer quadrant. The tail of the breast should also be examined as it extends into the axilla.

By self-examination a woman can usually detect a smaller mass in her own breasts than can a physician if she knows the proper methods to use. Since cancer of the breast is one of the major neoplasms in females, instruction in self-examination is a valuable addition to the physician's examination of the breast. A patient is instructed to emulate the physician's pattern of inspection and examination. She carries this out upon herself in both the erect and supine positions. Women thirty-five years of age and older should conduct such an examination at home once monthly.

MAMMOGRAPHY. Mammography is an x-ray examination of the breast. It requires special techniques and film, and a radiologist skilled in interpretation.

This technique is not a substitute for biopsy, which still provides definitive confirmation, but is a helpful adjunct in diagnosis. Mammography is especially useful in (1) follow-up examinations of the contralateral breast following radical mastectomy; (2) examination of an indeterminate mass which cannot be considered a dominant nodule, especially when there are multiple cysts or several vague masses and the indication for biopsy is uncertain; and (3) the large, fatty breast, when the patient has complaints but no nodules are palpated. Tumors cannot be easily felt in such breasts, but the mammogram is most accurate in the fatty breast.

A skilled radiologist can detect cancer of the breast with a false-positive rate of 11 percent and a false-negative rate of 6 percent. A fine stippling of calcium on the radiogram in the area of the lesion is very suggestive of cancer. There is also a characteristic infiltration of the surrounding tissues; a typical skin thickening may be seen, and the density of the lesion itself is often helpful in interpretation (Fig. 15-9).

Radiography of the breast can detect some cancers which cannot be found in any other way. It has been estimated that the lead time for treatment of lesions discovered at this small size is 1 or 2 years compared to

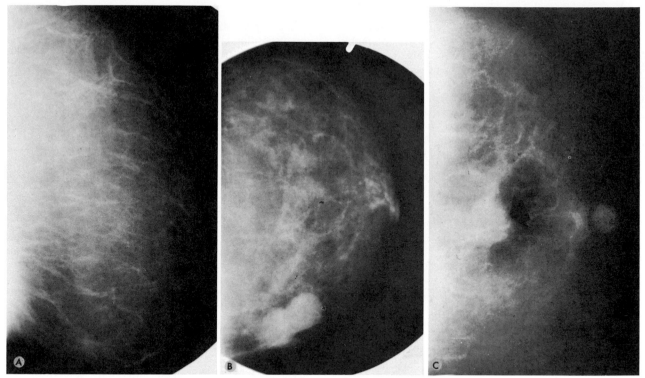

Fig. 15-9. Mammography of breast. *A.* Normal postmenopausal patient with atrophy of lobular tissue and ducts and predominance of fatty supporting tissue. *B.* Multiloculated cyst in menopausal patient. *C.* Scirrhous carcinoma in menopausal patient, demonstrating sunburst pattern; characteristic calcifications not present in this case.

cancers discovered by conventional palpation of the breast. Axillary nodal involvement is very rare in these early lesions, and preliminary results of follow-up indicate that 5-year survival rates for such tumors may exceed 90 percent. This data led to considerable activity in developing pilot mass screening programs for cancer of the breast which include mammography, careful physical examination, and thermography.

Recently increasing resistance has developed to the use of mammography for breast screening. If data obtained from women who had exposure of their breasts to 500 to 1500 rads is considered, the risk of breast cancer is increased markedly by radiation. Extrapolation of this data back to the low doses received from mammography indicates that the lifetime risk of breast cancer may be increased 1 percent for each rad absorbed, i.e., from 7.0 percent for the average American woman to 7.07 percent. Past studies of screening show that mammography in women over fifty years of age will save far more lives than might be threatened by the radiation used. Under fifty years of age there is no such evidence. Current guidelines of the National Institute of Health forbid screening women under fifty with mammography. The situation is very fluid, however, since much of the data being used to make these decisions are highly speculative. The situation is in flux, since the x-ray exposure produced by mammography has been decreased substantially to as low as 0.4 rads per examination, and newer techniques appear to be increasing the number of cancers found in younger women, so that the risk-benefit ratio may be shifting in this age group. It is likely that extended clinical trials will be necessary to solve this dilemma.

Xeroradiography of the breast is basically a radiographic technique which is carried out in exactly the same way as mammography, except that the image is recorded on a xerographic plate instead of the conventional x-ray transparency. The image is positive rather than negative and appears easier to read to the untrained eye. Unfortunately, a badly exposed xeroradiograph, too poor for proper interpretation, is harder to recognize than a poor radiomammograph and may fool the unwary physician.

THERMOGRAPHY. The skin over malignant tumors of the breast is usually warmer than the surrounding areas. Using special heat scanners it is possible to delineate these "hot spots" on film. This method may help to differentiate malignant and benign tumors. Infection may be associated with a false positive, and, conversely, not all cancers are "hot," so false negatives may occur. The method is still too new to have a definite place in the diagnostic armamentarium but may find a role in mass screening programs.

DISEASES OF THE BREAST

Neoplasms

From the standpoint of morbidity and mortality, cancer is by far the most important clinical problem that concerns the breast today. Most benign neoplasms of the breast would have little clinical importance if it were not for the difficulty in differentiating them from cancer. To emphasize this relationship, benign neoplasms are discussed in the section on differential diagnosis of cancer.

In recent years four major controversies have surfaced concerning breast cancer, concerning (1) the relation of treatment to the natural history of the disease; (2) the role of mammography in diagnosis, and especially in screening programs; (3) the appropriate operation for treatment; and (4) the use of postoperative chemotherapy as an adjuvant to primary therapy.

INCIDENCE

Cancer of the breast is the commonest form of cancer in females. Almost 6 percent of all women will develop cancer of the breast in their lifetime. The lifetime incidence of cancer of all types in females is 27 percent; thus one out of every four women with cancer will have cancer of the breast. In the United States, 50,000 to 70,000 new cases of breast cancer occur annually, and about 20,000 women die of the disease each year. According to the excellent cancer registry systems in Connecticut and upper New York State, the age-adjusted incidence of new cases has been increasing steadily since the middle 1940s.

Worldwide figures show that the Dutch have the highest national mortality of cancer of the breast, with 24.19 patients per 100,000 population. The United States ranks ninth, with 21.38 cases per 100,000 population. The Japanese rank lowest among all nations with reliable statistics, with an incidence of 3.76 per 100,000 population. The factors leading to this wide range of incidence are unknown, although studies seeking an answer are in progress.

ETIOLOGY

Sex is certainly an important contributing factor in this disease, since it is very rare in males. Maleness is not a complete protection, however; there is 1 carcinoma of the breast in men for every 100 carcinomas of the breast in women.

The age of the patient is also important (Fig. 15-10). Breast cancer is almost unknown in the prepubertal female and is very rare under the age of twenty. From the age of twenty onward there is a gradually increasing incidence, which reaches a plateau between the ages of forty-five and fifty-five at about 125 new cases each year for every 100,000 females of that age range. After fifty-five the incidence begins to rise again quite sharply, so that the annual risk of developing breast cancer for women eighty to eighty-five is twice as high as for women sixty to sixty-five (312 versus 153 new cases per 100,000 women per year). Some suggest that the plateau of incidence during the menopausal age period reflects the effects of a changing hormonal pattern in women at this time.

Genetic factors play a role in the development of this cancer, though the genetic effect does not seem to be strong and more than one allelic gene must be involved. When the mother has had a breast cancer, the chance of cancer of the breast developing in the daughter is two to three times greater than would be expected in the general popu-

lation, but no specific pattern of inheritance is evident. Some hypothesize that there is a genotype which has a predisposition to the formation of cancer but which must interact with some nongenetic agent before cancer develops.

Patients in whom breast cancer develops and who have positive family histories for the disease are generally younger and have a higher frequency of bilaterality than breast cancer patients with negative family histories. Blood type O, benign breast disease, and ovarian cysts and tumors also tend to be more common in patients with early diagnoses of breast cancer. Blood type A, diabetes, hypertension, and uterine disorders are more common in those who are older at the time of diagnosis.

Interlinked with factors of age, sex, national origin, and inheritance in the development of breast cancer is the important role played by hormonal environment. Some breast cancers are highly susceptible to changes in the patient's hormonal pattern and will regress for a time when hormones of various types are given. Mammary cancer can be induced in the mouse and rat by repeated injections of estrogens and in the rat by a combination of estrogen and progesterone. There is a vast literature concerning both experimental and clinical induction and extinction of tumors with hormonal agents. The exact role of hormones in human cancer still remains elusive. It is not known whether hormonal maladjustment is responsible for human breast cancer or what predisposing causes may be required to produce a susceptibility to hormonal change.

Breast cancer may well be multifactorial. Other interesting correlations with breast cancer include the incidence of coronary artery disease, which has a positive correlation with breast cancer death rates in 24 parts of the world. Hems has concluded that "early" breast cancer (age group forty to forty-four) appears to be genetically influenced, while "late" breast cancer (age group sixty-five to sixty-nine) is more closely associated with environmental factors, such as diet. Among younger women, higher risk is associated with late first pregnancy, while among women over fifty years of age the risk appears to increase with weight and the relation of weight to height. Zippin and Petrakis have reported an association between wet cerumen, or earwax, and breast cancer rates in diverse population groups, and breast cancer mortality is closely associated with wet cerumen. Such an association is plausible since the mammary and ceruminous glands are histologically of the apocrine type and have many similarities in their secretions. Cerumen exists in two phenotypic forms, wet and dry, which are controlled by a pair of genes in which the allele for the wet type is dominant over that of the dry type. The dry is homozygous recessive and is highly prevalent in the mongoloid population of Asia and in American Indians. The wet type predominates in Western Europeans, Caucasian Americans, and Negro Americans. These findings support the hypothesis that genetic variations in the apocrine system may influence susceptibility to breast cancer.

It has long been known that breast cancer in mice is related to a viral factor transmitted in the milk. Considerable excitement has attended the discovery of particles in human milk with the same morphologic characteristics as those found to be associated with breast cancer in mice. Antigens to these viral particles have been identified in human plasma. These particles have been found in the milk from the breasts of 60 percent of American women with family histories of breast cancer compared to 5 percent of women without positive family histories. The milk of thirty-nine percent of Parsi women in India also were found to contain these particles. The group of Parsi women is of particular interest because of their endogamous history over the centuries, resulting in an inbred population. Breast cancer accounts for approximately half of the cancers among Parsi women in contrast with Connecticut women, for example, in whom breast cancer represents one-fourth of all cancers.

NATURAL HISTORY

A typical carcinoma of the breast is a scirrhous adenocarcinoma beginning in the ducts and invading the parenchyma (80 percent). Beginning in the upper outer quadrant (40 to 50 percent), it grows slowly, doubling its volume every 2 to 9 months in 70 percent of patients. Starting from a single cell, it takes 30 doubling times for a tumor to attain a size of 1 cm—the smallest tumor of the breast normally found on physical diagnosis. Thus even the fastest-growing tumor of the more common type may require 5 years before it becomes clinically palpable. The use of doubling times to calculate the preclinical course of tumors of the breast is subject to many errors, the most obvious being that growth rates are not always constant, varying with areas of necrosis within the tumor and hormonal changes in the patient. Laboratory and clinical observations indicate, however, that growth rates are more consistent than is usually appreciated. The concept of the origin of these tumors in a single cell with increase in size by doubling is a useful model and suggests the long occult period which probably is present in many tumors before they are diagnosed and treated. Cancers of the breast are often multicentric (15 to 40 percent), but each tumor is assumed to have started from its own individual cell.

As the tumor increases in size and invades the surrounding glandular tissue, the accompanying fibrosis tends to shorten Cooper's ligaments, producing the characteristic dimpling in the skin (Fig. 15-11). Cords of tumor cells grow out along lymphatics, ultimately invading the skin itself. This invasion is preceded by localized edema of the skin as many lymphatic avenues are blocked and drainage of fluid from the skin is impeded. Eventually tumor cells replace the skin, which breaks down to form an ulcer. The tumor increases in size, and new areas of skin invasion may occur, indicated by small satellite nodules adjacent to the ulcer crater. As involvement and destruction of the skin progresses, blood vessels are invaded, and tumor cells seed into the circulation, passing into axillary or intercostal veins to be scattered through the pulmonary circuit into the lungs or by way of the vertebral veins up and down the vertebral column. When this seeding is early and small in amount, the majority if not all of these cells may fail to implant and are destroyed by an unknown mechanism, perhaps immunity. Eventually, perhaps as the number of

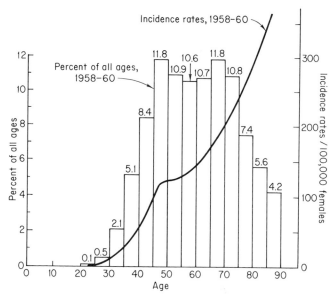

Fig. 15-10. Newly diagnosed breast cancer among women, 1958–1960: percentage distribution and incidence rates by age. Note plateau in incidence between ages forty-five and fifty-five.

cells seeded into the circulation begins to rise, they implant and grow in favorable locations. These implants may occur in the vertebral bodies, pelvis, lungs, liver, or brain.

As the breast tumor extends toward the skin, tumor cells simultaneously pass along the lymphatic vessels from the upper outer quadrant to the axillary nodes, where they implant and grow. As the axillary nodes enlarge, they are

Fig. 15-11. Dimpling of skin over primary carcinoma of breast in upper outer quadrant. Slowly growing lesion in seventy-year-old patient; dimpling had been present for 2 years.

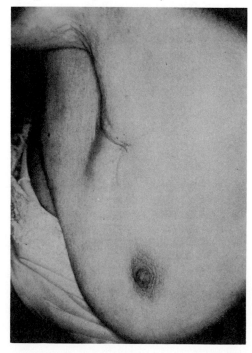

at first shotty and fairly soft, then firm and hard as they are increasingly replaced by tumor. Eventually the nodes adhere to one another in a large conglomerate mass, and as the tumor breaks out of the lymphatic capsule the mass of nodes become fixed to the medial wall of the axilla. As the axillary nodes become choked with tumor, cells are passed along the chain to the supraclavicular nodes, which also enlarge. Other cancer cells pass by way of the right lymphatic trunk or the thoracic duct into the bloodstream, heart, and lungs. Systemic spread is the rule, and 95 percent of patients who die of uncontrolled breast cancer have distant metastases. Lung (65 percent), liver (56 percent), and bones (56 percent) are the commonest sites for these deposits.

Patients today are rarely allowed to proceed through all stages of carcinoma without some therapeutic intervention. Data are available, however, from the latter half of the 1800s and the first few years of this century indicating the normal course of events in untreated tumors. The excellent report in 1962 by Bloom and associates summarizes much of the data. They cite the experience of the Middlesex Hospital in London, where in 1791 a cancer charity was founded to which patients were admitted to "remain an unlimited time, until either relieved by art or released by death." From the well-preserved records of this charity it was possible to collect a series of 250 advanced cases of untreated breast cancer seen between 1805 and 1933 (Fig. 15-12). All the patients reported died in the hospital, and in every case an autopsy was performed. In the last 86 cases, histologic sections were available. The mean survival in this series and for over 1,000 untreated cases collected from the literature was 38.7 months, with a range from 30.2 to 39.8 months. It must be noted that in all reports of untreated patients survival is calculated from the onset of the first symptom. Fifty percent of the patients died in 2.7 years (median survival); 18 percent survived 5 years,

3.6 percent 10 years, and 10.8 percent 15 years. The longest survivor in the group died in the nineteenth year after onset of symptoms. Histologic grading indicated that for 23 patients with grade 1 tumors the mean survival was 47 months. Autopsies indicated that 95 percent of the women died of their carcinoma, only 5 percent of intercurrent disease. Nearly three-fourths of the patients had ulceration of the breast at death, and in 21 percent this was very extensive, sometimes destroying the entire breast and excavating the chest wall. Bloom concluded that treatment of patients with breast cancer appeared to increase the length and improve the quality of survival.

DIAGNOSIS AND STAGING

The normal breast is a nodular structure by virtue of its lobular architecture, and this lobularity may be accentuated during the later portion of the menstrual cycle, pregnancy, or lactation. To the inexperienced examiner the normal nodularity may feel faintly suspicious throughout, although no obvious lesion can be felt. Palpation of the typical carcinoma of the breast normally leaves little doubt in the examiner's mind: the lesion is hard, almost cartilaginous; the edges are distinct, serrated, and irregular. This is true for the 75 to 80 percent of breast tumors associated with productive fibrosis. It is the remaining 20 to 25 percent of tumors, those associated with little fibrosis and those with a medullary or a colloid element or other less typical lesions, which form the spectrum of neoplasms most difficult to distinguish from benign lesions.

Physicians would prefer to have only the clues provided by the local mass to make the physical diagnosis of carcinoma, for it is only when the mass is localized to the breast that one can assume an "early" lesion and expect the best possible chance of long survival. Too often the later signs of breast cancer are present to confirm the diagnosis. As indicated previously, these are skin dimpling or nipple retraction, satellite skin lesions, edema or ulceration, and ipsilateral enlarged axillary or supraclavicular nodes. Signs of even wider spread may be present such as a history of back or leg pain, an enlarged and nodular liver, or perhaps a complaint of dyspnea associated with physical findings or fluid in the chest.

The physical examination of a patient with breast cancer should include an attempt on the part of the examiner to classify and record the stage of the patient's disease specifically. Only consistent classification can make possible clear conclusions concerning prognosis and type of treatment. The problem of comparing the results of treatment from institution to institution and among different operators has been impaired for years by a lack of adequate classification or by varying standards of classification. At present a strong effort is being made to promote the adoption of a standard system devised by the American Joint Committee on Cancer Staging and End Results Reporting, based on a system proposed by the International Union against Cancer in 1958. This system of classification is called the T.N.M. Classification, the T standing for "tumor," the N for "nodes," and the M for "metastasis." The general outline used in breast cancer is as follows:

Fig. 15-12. Survival of patients with untreated cancer of breast compared with natural survival. (*From H. J. G. Bloom, W. W. Richardson, and E. J. Harries, Br Med J, 5299:213, 1962, by permission.*)

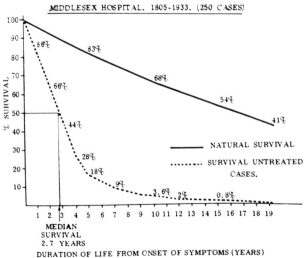

MIDDLESEX HOSPITAL. 1805-1933. (250 CASES)

T—Primary tumor

TX   Cannot classify (e.g., prior therapy)
T1S   Carcinoma in situ, lobular, ductal, Paget's (not a clinical classification)
T0   No tumor in breast (e.g., axillary mass; x-ray finding)
T1   Primary tumor freely movable, no fixation
T1a   Clinical classification not applicable (e.g., detected by mammography)
T1b   <1.9 cm
T1c   2–5 cm
T1d   >5 cm
T2a   Primary tumor <2 cm with fixation to skin, pectoral fascia, or muscle. *No* ulceration or edema (*peau d'orange*)
T2b   Primary tumor >2 cm with fixation to skin, pectoral fascia, or muscle. *No* ulceration or edema (*peau d'orange*)
T3   Primary tumor, any size, with skin edema (*peau d'orange*) and/or ulceration
T4   Primary tumor, any size, with fixation to chest wall (serratus, intercostals, ribs, or pectorals)
T5   Inflammatory carcinoma

N—Regional Axillary Nodes
(Infraclavicular are included as apical axillary)

NX   Cannot be evaluated (e.g., previous excision)
N0   Axillary nodes not involved by metastasis
N1   Clinical homolateral axillary nodes involved, 1–3 in number, less than 2 cm diameter; not fixed
N2   Clinical homolateral axillary nodes involved, >4 in number; any number fixed to one another but to no other structures, and/or any involved node >2 cm
N3   Homolateral axillary nodes involved fixed to neurovascular structures of axilla or chest wall (intercostals, serratus, ribs, *not* pectorals)
N4   Homolateral supraclavicular lymph node involved by metastasis

M—Distant metastasis

M0   No evidence of distant metastases
M1   Distant metastases, including skin beyond the breast area

Summary of clinical staging

In situ cancer (in situ lobular, pure intraductal, and Paget's disease of nipple without palpable mass):

Stage T1S   T1S, N0, M0

Invasive cancer:

Stage I   T1a, b, or c, N0, M0
Stage II   T0, N1, M0; T1d, N0, M0; T1a, b, c, or d, N1, M0; T2a, N0 or N1, M0
Stage III   T0, T1a, b, c, d, N2, M0; T2B, N0, M0; T3, N1 or N2, M0
Stage IV   T4, T5, and any N, M0; N3, 4, or 5 and any T, M0; M1 with any T and any N

DIFFERENTIAL DIAGNOSIS (BENIGN LESIONS)

CHRONIC CYSTIC MASTITIS. Chronic cystic mastitis was first described in the medical literature in the last two decades of the nineteenth century, by Reclus (1883), Brissaud (1884), Schimmelbusch (1890), and König (1893). For a time the disease was known as either Reclus' or Schimmelbusch's disease, but use of these eponyms dwindled following the introduction of the term *chronic cystic mastitis* by König. He chose this term to describe a group of pathologic lesions found in the breast because he thought

they were due to a "vicious cycle of secretion and irritation." While the disease is indeed chronic, it may not be cystic and is certainly not inflammatory, so this old name is at least two-thirds in error. Nonetheless, attempts to introduce more accurate or at least other nomenclatures have failed. Fibrocystic disease, fibroadenosis, mastopathy, nodular hyperplasia, cyclomastopathy, adenofibromatosis, mazoplasia, cystiphorous epithelial hyperplasia, adenocystic disease, and mammary dysplasia have all been offered, but chronic cystic mastitis is still the most widely used designation.

The term chronic cystic mastitis describes a family of lesions found in the breast. Pathologists disagree as to which lesions are legitimate family relations, so the morphology of the disease, like the terminology, appears rather fuzzy to the casual observer. Foote and Stewart have named 10 lesions often described as members of this group: cysts, papillomatosis, blunt duct adenosis, sclerosing adenosis, apocrine metaplasia, stasis and distension of ducts, periductal mastitis, fat necrosis, hyperplasia of duct epithelium, and fibroadenoma. These writers accept, however, only the first five of this group as being related lesions and forming part of chronic cystic mastitis; the others are held to represent different disease entities. They refer to the first five as the cystic and proliferative group, assuming that the proliferative lesions are responsible for the subsequent formation of cysts. A majority of pathologists accept this list, though some have argued for the inclusion of fibroadenoma. In addition, epithelial hyperplasia is usually accepted as part of the complex, with papillomas representing an advanced manifestation of hyperplasia.

The lesions of chronic cystic mastitis begin to appear in the breasts of a few women in their late twenties. The incidence is greater in the thirties and forties. Originally it was thought that the incidence of these lesions decreased after the menopause, but careful autopsy studies indicate that the lesions are common in the older age groups and may continue to increase in frequency with age. Frantz et al. found a 71 percent incidence of cystic and proliferative lesions in women over seventy years of age. Sandison noted epithelial hyperplasia of the ducts in 7 percent of women in their twenties and in 33 percent of women in their eighties. Rush and Kramer in 1963 reviewed step sections from the breasts of 20 women over seventy years of age. Approximately 100 sections were reviewed per patient, and with this close scrutiny two or more lesions of cystic mastitis were found in all the patients. Moderately severe epithelial hyperplasia was found in 14 of the 20 (Fig. 15-13). A case may be made for considering the lesions of cystic mastitis somewhat as one considers arteriosclerosis: a pathologic process which varies in degree and in time of onset but which is found to some degree in all adult females as they age.

Most of the lesions making up the complex of chronic cystic mastitis are proliferative, and almost from the first recognition of this disease there has been a suspicion that these lesions may represent a premalignant condition. Follow-up studies of patients shown by biopsy to have chronic cystic mastitis uniformly indicate that cancer sub-

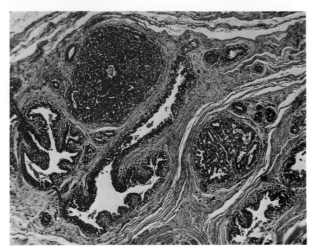

Fig. 15-13. Benign marked intraductal hyperplasia in eighty-eight-year-old female. (Hematoxylin and eosin; ×32). (*From B. F. Rush, Jr., and W. M. Kramer, Surg Gynec Obstet, 117:425, 1963.*)

sequently occurs three to five times more often in these patients than in the general population.

If one assumes that all women eventually develop some degree of chronic cystic mastitis, how can one conclude that the finding of chronic cystic mastitis on biopsy is associated with an increase in the incidence of cancer of the female breast compared to patients in the general population? A reasonable hypothesis is that patients in whom this complex develops early enough or severely enough to warrant biopsy do indeed represent a special group with a greater hazard of eventual cancer.

The lesions of chronic cystic mastitis which are most likely to present a problem in differential diagnosis and to require biopsy are cysts, fibroadenoma, ductal papilloma, and sclerosing adenosis.

CYSTS. The cystic component of chronic cystic mastitis

Fig. 15-14. Cystic disease with apocrine metaplasia in seventy-three-year-old female. (Hematoxylin and eosin; ×32.) (*From B. F. Rush, Jr., and W. M. Kramer, Surg Gynec Obstet, 117:425, 1963.*)

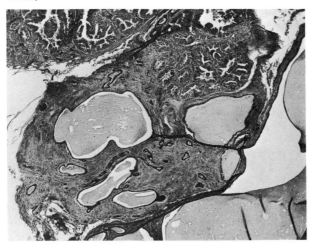

is most prominent in patients in their thirties and forties. The cysts may vary in size from microcysts of 1 to 2 mm to large masses several centimeters in diameter (Fig. 15-14). They are felt in the breast substance as firm, round, fairly distinct masses, often with a rubbery feeling indicative of their cystic nature. Lesions in the anterior and dependent portions of the breast may be transilluminated. They are sometimes tender and, like many of the other lesions of this complex, may increase in size toward the end of the menstrual period.

If a lesion in a patient's breast is clearly suggestive of a cyst, aspiration is a good method for confirming the diagnosis. This technique should not be used unless the rules for its employment are clearly understood. The fluid obtained should be the characteristic clear, brown-green fluid of a cyst. When the cyst is aspirated dry, no underlying mass should be palpable. If a residual mass remains after aspiration or if the fluid is bloody, biopsy must be done. The patient should be followed at intervals for a month or two after aspiration; if the cyst reappears, biopsy is also indicated. Approximately half the cysts treated by aspiration will disappear, and fluid will not reaccumulate.

FIBROADENOMAS. These lesions are most common in the twenties and early thirties. They present as lobular but not serrated masses with a firm, rubbery consistency. Their edges are sharply defined. Most commonly solitary, they may occasionally be multiple. They are differentiated from cancer by the smooth rather than irregular lobulations and by the age group in which they occur. Although a skilled examiner can probably detect a fibroadenoma with an accuracy of 80 to 85 percent, biopsy is mandatory.

DUCTAL PAPILLOMA. The hallmark of the ductal papilloma is abnormal secretion from the nipple, which is often blood-stained. In 30 percent a small nodule, 3 or 4 mm in diameter, will be palpated in the major ducts underlying the areola. In the absence of a palpable nodule the papilloma's general position can often be detected by stroking the areola toward the nipple with the tips of the fingers, carefully working around the areola in a clockwise direction until an area is discovered which on pressure results in secretion from the nipple. A bloody nipple discharge may also be indicative of an intraductal carcinoma or even a deeper-lying infiltrating ductal carcinoma. The incidence of malignancy in the presence of this physical finding is 20 to 30 percent. Diagnosis is confirmed and treatment accomplished by excision of that portion of the collecting duct system shown on physical examination to be responsible for the secretion. Urban and Baker propose that the entire collecting duct system should be excised en bloc, since these lesions are often multiple and a partial excision of the duct system will often result in the retention of other lesions which will lead to further bloody secretions later.

SCLEROSING ADENOSIS. These lesions can sometimes result in an area of fibrosis within the mammary tissue which is firm and irregular and impossible to differentiate clinically from an ordinary scirrhous carcinoma. Biopsy is required to make the differential diagnosis.

OTHER BENIGN LESIONS. Fat necrosis, thrombophlebitis of the breast, and granular cell myoblastoma are three benign lesions of the breast which can be confused on physical examination with malignant growths. All three are uncommon. Fat necrosis is the most common of the group and is probably due to trauma, although only half the patients who have this lesion recall a trauma of the breast. The breasts are in an exposed position, however, and may be hurt at the time of a larger accident when the injury to the breast is overshadowed by more serious injuries. The lesions are always superficial and often near the areola. In 40 to 50 percent of patients with this lesion, accompanying ecchymoses are lingering stigmata of previous trauma. In one-third of the patients there is a history of pain or tenderness. Retraction of the skin over the lesion is seen in 50 to 60 percent. Retraction is due to the fibrosis and scarring in the fatty lobules which involve Cooper's ligaments. As the scarring progresses and matures, skin retraction, which may first be seen within two weeks of the original injury, becomes more prominent. The mass of subcutaneous scar tissue that forms is distinct, irregular, and often very firm. It is easy to understand how such a mass associated with skin retraction may be mistaken for carcinoma, and in every instance a biopsy specimen of the lesion must be examined histologically. In decades past, many unnecessary radical mastectomies were done in patients with fat necrosis. Today, the practice of routinely examining frozen sections of biopsy material prevents this tragedy.

Granular cell myoblastomas occur most commonly in the tongue but may also occur in the breast. The clinical importance of this rare tumor is that it can produce all the clinical signs of early cancer of the breast. The lesion is hard and relatively fixed to the breast tissue surrounding it. It sometimes causes dimpling of the overlying skin. Moreover, on gross examination of the specimen at operation the lesion looks and cuts like a scirrhous carcinoma of the breast. Only frozen sections can confirm that one is dealing with a benign rather than a malignant lesion.

Thrombophlebitis of a superficial vein of the breast, called *Mondor's disease,* may rarely be mistaken for a tumor because of the dimpling of the skin it produces. The tubular shape of the thrombosed vein and the accompanying tenderness usually indicate the diagnosis, but biopsy is often required for confirmation.

BREAST BIOPSY

Breast biopsy is a procedure with little risk and can be done under local anesthesia. It is still the general custom to do the biopsy under general anesthesia and proceed to a definitive cancer operation if the frozen section of the lesion indicates malignancy. However, there is an increasing trend to do the biopsy under local anesthesia, often in an outpatient setting, and to continue with the larger operation, if indicated, a few days later. This delay in definitive operation has no effect on the recurrence or survival rates. A curvilinear incision in the direction of the skin lines is made over the supicious mass. If the lesion is small, total excision is preferred, but if a large lesion is encountered, a small excisional biopsy of the main mass is done.

Needle biopsy of breast masses is done in some institutions and is very satisfactory if the pathologist is familiar with this type of material. Negative needle biopsies have no significance, however, since an adequate sample may not be obtained.

HISTOPATHOLOGY

Malignant neoplasms of the breast, with few exceptions, are adenocarcinomas. The histologic features of these lesions vary considerably, and a number of classifications are available. The following was proposed by Foote and Stewart:

HISTOLOGIC CLASSIFICATION OF CANCER OF THE BREAST

A. Paget's disease of the nipple
B. Carcinomas of mammary ducts
   1. Noninfiltrating
   2. Infiltrating
      a. Papillary carcinoma
      b. Comedocarcinoma
      c. Carcinoma with productive fibrosis
      d. Medullary carcinoma with lymphoid infiltrate
      e. Colloid carcinoma
C. Carcinomas of mammary lobules
   1. Noninfiltrating
   2. Infiltrating
D. Relatively rare carcinomas
E. Sarcoma of the breast

PAGET'S DISEASE OF THE NIPPLE. This constitutes 1 percent of all breast carcinomas but has attracted an inordinate amount of attention and speculation, since for many years there was confusion as to whether this lesion arose primarily in the skin or in the mammary ducts. It is now generally accepted that this is a primary carcinoma of the mammary ducts of the nipple which has subsequently invaded the skin. The lesion presents as a scaling, eczematoid, and quite innocent-appearing lesion of the nipple (Fig. 15-15). In most instances it has a slow natural

Fig. 15-15. Typical scaling eczematoid lesion of Paget's disease; frequently misdiagnosed and treated by salves and ointments, with long delay in proper diagnosis.

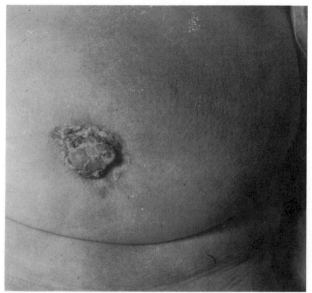

history, and the skin lesion may be the only evidence of neoplasm for many years. Ultimately an underlying mass will develop if the lesion is untreated. Any eczematoid lesion of the nipple in a postmenopausal female which persists for more than a few weeks should be biopsied to exclude the possibility of Paget's disease. Adequate histologic studies of surgical specimens almost always reveal underlying carcinomas of the mammary ducts. Invasion of the skin by these cells produces the interesting Paget's cell, a large cell with clear cytoplasm and commonly with binucleation. This is associated with evidence of chronic inflammation and a surface crust. Robbins and Berg's study of 89 cases indicated that one-third of the patients showed noninfiltrating carcinoma, and in this group the survival rate was 100 percent at 5 years. The remaining patients had infiltrating carcinoma. The overall survival rate for the group was 64 percent, indicating a better prognosis for this lesion than for the average carcinoma of the breast.

NONINFILTRATING CARCINOMAS OF THE MAMMARY DUCTS. These constitute 1 percent of carcinomas of the breast. It is unfortunate that more cancers are not seen at the noninfiltrating stage, since these lesions are carcinomas in situ and operation should result in 100 percent 5-year survival. That this is not the case, 5-year survival being about 90 percent, reflects the fact that the breast is a large organ and that lesions which appear to be noninfiltrating may in fact be infiltrating at some area which the pathologist has not examined. Foote and Stewart report that they have traced progression of intraductal carcinoma from benign papillary hyperplasia through atypism to noninfiltrating intraductal carcinoma and ultimately to infiltrating carcinoma throughout a breast specimen. They state that while this may be one route for the development of cancer of the breast, cancer may arise from normal intraductal cells directly. The differentiation of a noninfiltrating intraductal carcinoma from a benign hyperplasia may be difficult; areas of atypism can blend gradually from one state into the other. Histologically, the duct

Fig. 15-16. Intraductal carcinoma with stromal invasion in eighty-three-year-old female. Field shows almost entire extent of this very early lesion. (Hematoxylin and eosin; ×32.)

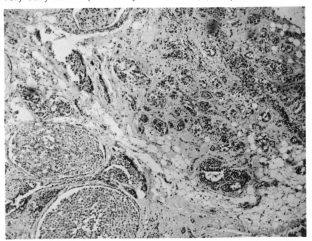

epithelium is usually seen to be thrown up into papillae which show a loss of cohesiveness and disorientation of cells, with pleomorphism and occasionally mitotic figures but without evidence of invasion of the basement membrane. A more dramatic form is the noninfiltrating comedocarcinoma, in which hyperplasia is more extreme, choking the entire duct for long distances with masses of cells. These lesions commonly develop central necrosis of the cells. A gross section of such a lesion will extrude small cores of tissue from the ducts very much as the core is extruded from a comedo when it is squeezed, thus giving rise to the term comedocarcinoma.

INFILTRATING PAPILLARY CARCINOMA. Presumably a later stage or a more aggressive form of the noninfiltrating papillary lesion, these carcinomas still tend to evolve slowly and have a better 5-year survival rate than the average carcinoma of the breast. They produce a mass rather soft to palpation compared with the typical hard, fibrous lesion usually associated with breast cancer. They may reach large size before metastasizing to the axilla. Dimpling and skin edema are less commonly seen, another index of the late infiltration of the lymphatics and of the failure to stimulate a fibrous response. Noninfiltrating papillary carcinomas are often seen in association with the infiltrating form.

Infiltrating comedocarcinomas comprise approximately 5 percent of all breast cancers. They are often found in association with other forms of adenocarcinoma that result in productive fibrosis, and the presence of comedocarcinoma together with other elements of carcinoma of the breast does not significantly alter the prognosis from the average.

INFILTRATING DUCT CARCINOMA WITH PRODUCTIVE FIBROSIS. This is the commonest form of breast cancer, constituting 78 percent of the specimens seen. There is a tremendous variation in the amount of fibrosis. The lesion has been termed *scirrhous carcinoma, fibrocarcinoma,* and *sclerosing carcinoma.* The desmoplastic response to the invading cancer cells accounts for the remarkable hardness of the average breast cancer. Grossly the lesions have uneven serrated edges. They cut with great resistance and often with a rather gritty feeling as the knife edge passes through them. Histologically the lesions may vary from scattered, well-differentiated adenomatous clusters and a massive amount of fibrostroma to dense cellular aggregates with only minor amounts of fibroplasia (Fig. 15-16). Electron microscopic examination of these tumors indicates that they originate in the myoepithelial cells of the mammary duct.

MEDULLARY CARCINOMAS. Five percent of carcinomas of the breast assume this pattern, and the diagnosis indicates a favorable prognosis for the patient. Even in the presence of metastatic disease the prognosis remains favorable; the 5-year overall survival rate for the lesion is 85 to 90 percent. These lesions are soft, bulky, and often large. Necrotic areas of varying size are usually present. Occasionally one finds a lesion which is almost totally infarcted. On physical examination these tumors are freely movable, and smaller tumors are likely to be diagnosed clinically as cysts or fibroadenomas. Histologically the tumors are made up of large rounded or polygonal cells with an abundant cytoplasm arranged in broad or narrow plexiform masses anastomosing with one another. Electron microscopic and histochemical evidence suggests that these cells originate in the ductal epithelium. There is an abundant lymphoid infiltrate. Plasma cells are often seen and are sometimes very prominent. Axillary metastases occur less frequently than in the ordinary carcinoma of the breast but are not uncommon, occurring in about 40 percent. Metastasis frequently involves only a single node.

COLLOID CARCINOMA. This is an infrequent mammary cancer constituting about 1 percent of all breast cancers. The lesions contain a much greater amount of mucin than the usual adenocarcinoma and may be frankly gelatinous on cut section. Clinically these lesions are soft and ill defined and, like the medullary lesions, may be quite bulky before detection. Histologically the predominant picture is of large mucinous lakes in which epithelial aggregates float. Patients with these lesions have a better-than-average survival rate.

CARCINOMA OF THE MAMMARY LOBULES. This lesion arises in the mammary lobules from the cells of the acini and the terminal ducts. Most of the acini of a lobule are involved. Lobules may be of normal size or enlarged, with an unsystematic hyperplasia of the lining cells until the lumen is plugged. At the in situ stage of development these are the only changes, and simple mastectomy at this point should produce cure. The lesion subsequently becomes infiltrative and ultimately may give rise to regular scirrhous carcinoma.

Multicentricity and bilaterality are important features of lobular carcinoma. Eighty-eight percent of breast specimens removed for in situ lobular carcinoma show other in situ lesions scattered throughout the specimen. Examination of the contralateral breast has demonstrated in situ lesions in from 35 to 59 percent of specimens.

SARCOMA OF THE BREAST. Sarcomas of the breast are very rare. The commonest sarcoma seen is cystosarcoma phylloides, but only one in ten of these is truly malignant, the great majority being a benign variant of fibroadenoma. Great confusion is created because both the benign and malignant form are called "cystosarcoma." When Müller first described and named the lesion in 1838 he was aware of its predominantly benign nature. At that time "sarcoma" meant simply a fleshy tumor and did not carry the meaning of malignancy that it does today. Modern synonyms for the benign lesion are *giant intracanalicular or pericanalicular fibroadenoma* and *intracanalicular myxoma.* The malignant variant has been called *adenocarcinoma.*

Cystosarcoma phylloides occurs at an older average age (forty), is larger, and has a more cellular stroma than fibroadenoma. When first seen clinically these tumors average 5 to 10 cm, have a firm and rubbery consistency, and may have a bosselated surface. In cut section the tumors have a discrete capsule. Small lesions present leaflike intracanalicular protrusions, and larger lesions have cystic spaces into which project densely packed polypoid masses.

The malignant variant metastasizes most commonly to the lungs, bones, and subcutaneous tissues. Axillary metas-tasis is so uncommon that simple mastectomy is an adequate procedure for both the benign and the malignant forms.

PRIMARY TREATMENT

The first historical reference to cancer of the breast appears in the Edwin Smith Surgical Papyrus (3000 to 2500 B.C.). The patient described is a man, but the description suggests most of the clinical features of breast cancer. The author concludes that "there is no treatment." References to cancer of the breast are scattered and brief over the following 2,500 years. Even in that large body of writings concerning Greek and Roman medicine, the Corpus Hippocraticum, direct reference to the treatment of breast cancer is absent, although it is clear that the condition was recognized.

Celsus, a Roman of the first century, spoke of operation and advised limiting it to early lesions: "None of these can be removed but the cacoethes [early lesion], the rest are irritated by every method of cure. The more violent the operations are, the more angry they grow." Galen, in the second century, inscribed one of the classic clinical observations:

We have often seen in the breast a tumor exactly resembling the animal the crab. Just as the crab has legs on both sides of his body, so in this disease the veins extending out from the unnatural growth take the shape of a crab's legs. We have often cured this disease in its early stages, but after it has reached a large size no one has cured it without operation. In all operations we attempt to excise a pathological tumor in a circle in the region where it borders on the healthy tissue.

Although Galen spoke of operations for tumors, his system of medicine ascribed the disease to an excess of black bile, and logically excision of a local outbreak could not cure the systemic imbalance. The Galenic theories dominated medicine until the Renaissance. Most established physicians looked down on attempts at operative treatment as misdirected and futile. Only when it was again established that a cancer could arise in a part as a local disorder quite separate from a systemic imbalance could excision of the tumor be recognized as rational therapy. Morgagni's definitive study of gross pathology, appropriately entitled *The Seats and Causes of Disease,* supplied this new rationale. Radical mastectomy until recently was the standard treatment for operable cancer of the breast in the United States. This operation involves the removal of the entire breast with a generous portion of overlying skin, all the underlying pectoralis major and minor muscles, and the entire lymphatic and fibrofatty contents of the axilla (Fig. 15-17).

This procedure evolved slowly from simple amputation of the breast. LeDran in the eighteenth century repudiated Galen's humoral theory and stated that cancer of the breast was a local disease which spread by way of the lymphatics to the regional nodes. He removed enlarged axillary nodes in his operations on patients with breast cancer. In the nineteenth century, Moore of Middlesex Hospital, England, emphasized wide removal of the breast and felt that when there was neoplasm in the axilla, the axillary con-

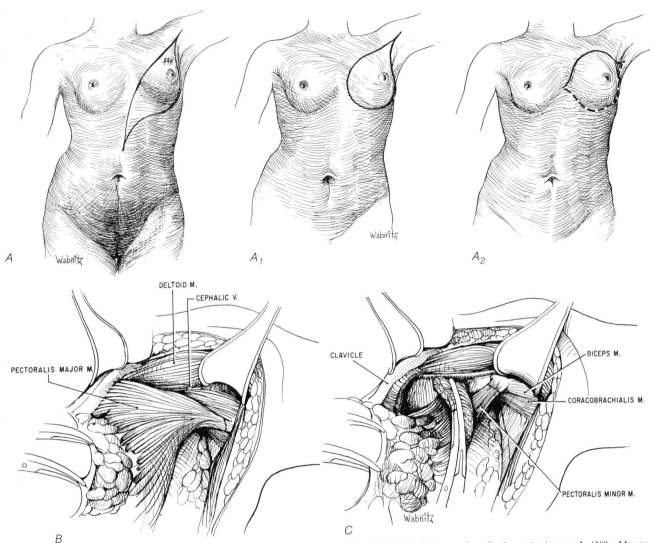

Fig. 15-17. Technique of radical mastectomy. *A.* Willy Meyer elliptical incision. *A₁* and *A₂.* Variations of mastectomy incision. *B.* Skin flaps developed and cephalic vein identified in order to delineate deltopectoral groove; tendinous insertion of pectoralis major muscle into humerus identified for transection. *C.* After transection of pectoralis major muscle, pectoralis minor insertion into coracoid process is defined. *D.* Pectoralis minor muscle transected and axilla being cleared of fatty tissue. *E.* Axillary vein cleared and all tributaries coursing caudad transected; long thoracic and thoracodorsal nerves identified and preserved; pectoralis major and minor muscle dissected with axillary fat and lymph nodes in medial direction. *F.* Dissection complete, showing chest wall including ribs and intercostal muscles cleared of pectoralis fascia, with sternum as medial limit of dissection. *G.* Incision closed and suction applied to obliterate dead space; with this technique, pressure dressing not needed.

tents should be removed in one block together with the breast. In a presentation before the British Medical Association in 1877, Banks supported Moore's concepts and advocated that axillary nodes should always be removed in one block with the breast tissue whether there were palpable nodes present or not, since occult involvement of the axillary nodes was so often present.

As Lewison notes, it remained for Halsted, the new professor of surgery at a young school called The Johns Hopkins Medical School, to "culminate the operation and germinate the present modern method." Halsted proposed a standard procedure, removing all the structures in one block. His first operation was performed about 1882, and he reported 13 cases in 1890. The procedure was almost exactly as it is today except that the pectoralis minor muscle was not removed. In 1894 he reported more than 50 cases over the preceding 12 years. In the same year Herbert Willy Meyer of New York reported six patients operated upon by a technique he had evolved independently. This procedure, almost a duplicate of the Hal-

sted mastectomy, added the removal of the pectoralis minor muscle. Halsted subsequently accepted this addition, and the modern radical mastectomy is often attributed to both these men. This procedure and the wide-block excision that it incorporated was soon adopted widely and for the following 50 years was the only operation used by the well-trained surgeon for treatment of breast cancer.

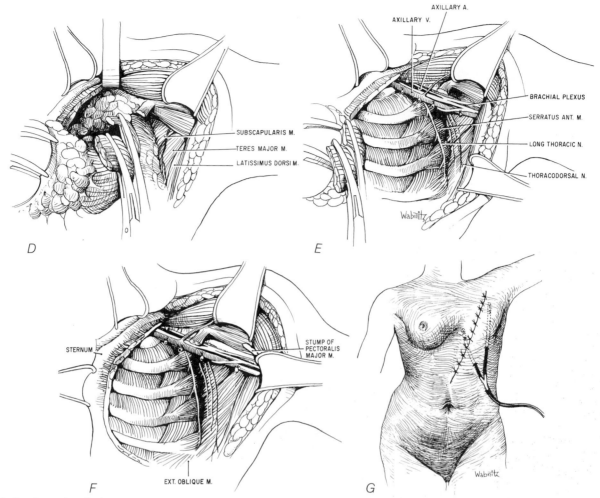

Fig. 15-17. See legend on facing page.

SELECTION OF PATIENTS. Operative treatment of breast cancer cannot be effective if disease has spread beyond the area removed by the operation. Distant spread to supraclavicular lymph nodes, lung, liver, or other sites is thus an absolute contraindication to the radical operation. Certain characteristics of the local lesion also indicate a high likelihood that operation would be futile. These generally accepted "criteria of inoperability" include fixation of the local breast lesion to the chest wall, fixation of the involved lymph nodes in the axilla, and inflammatory carcinoma of the breast. Haagensen compiled the following detailed list of criteria:

1. Extensive edema of the skin over the breast (Fig. 15-18)
2. Satellite nodules in the skin over the breast
3. Carcinoma of the inflammatory type (Fig. 15-19)
4. Parasternal tumor nodules
5. Proved supraclavicular metastases
6. Edema of the arm
7. Distant metastases
8. Any two or more of the following grave signs of locally advanced carcinoma:
   a. Ulceration of the skin
   b. Edema of the skin of limited extent (less than one-third of breast skin involved)

c. Solid fixation of tumor to the chest wall
d. Axillary lymph nodes measuring 2.5 cm or more in transverse diameter
e. Fixation of the axillary nodes to the skin or deep structures of the axilla

If these criteria are strictly applied, 75 percent of breast cancers seen will be operable. Figures from Connecticut indicate that from 1940 to 1959 ninety-five percent of all new patients there under sixty-five were treated by operation. This suggests that these clinical criteria are not observed in many institutions.

Haagensen has proposed an even stricter method of evaluation, called the *triple biopsy.* The object is "to exclude all patients who have no chance of cure." Patients who would otherwise be eligible for radical mastectomy are selected for triple biopsy if they have palpable axillary lymph nodes, primary lesions larger than 3 cm, or tumors in the center or the inner quadrants of the breast. Biopsy of the breast lesion, highest axillary nodes, and internal mammary nodes is done. If occult cancer is found in any of these areas, the patient is treated by radiation. This procedure reduces the number of patients eligible for operation to 50 percent of those seen.

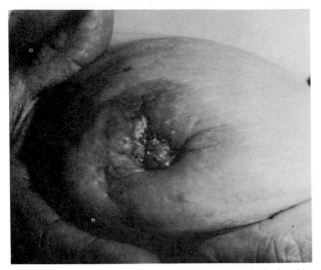

Fig. 15-18. Large cancer of breast with retraction of nipple, skin edema, and several satellite skin nodules.

MacDonald introduced the term *biological determinism* into the consideration of cancer, meaning that the biologic nature of the tumor primarily determines the response to therapy. Concerning the breast he suggests that one-third of the lesions do not develop the propensity to metastasize, and while excision removes a disagreeable local growth, the procedure is not lifesaving since such a tumor would never be life-threatening. One-third of the lesions, he estimates, are incurable almost from inception, since they become generalized early, before they are clinically detectable, and no matter how early or how widely the tumor is excised, the procedure will not change the course of the disease. Finally, he assumes that in the remaining one-

Fig. 15-19. Inflammatory carcinoma of breast. Bright pink to red suffuses area of skin involvement, reflecting inflammatory response to extensive scattering of tumor cells in subcutaneous tissues. Large skin lesion above nipple is congenital pigmented nevus unrelated to the cancer.

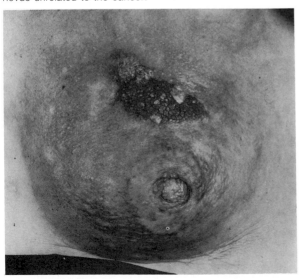

third of patients the systemic spread of the tumor is preceded by a long latent period in which the tumor reaches clinically detectable size before beginning to spread. In such patients early detection and excision of the tumor would be important, and treatment would have value in altering the course of the cancer. If this thesis is correct, a test to distinguish the different tumors, confining radical treatment to those of the last group only, would have great value. Such a test, as well as proof of this theory, remains to be provided.

The concept of biologic determinism would also explain much of the confusion that surrounds attempts to evaluate techniques of treatment by statistical methods. Butcher compares this effort to attempting to evaluate a remedy for snakebite in a series of patients who fell into a pit of vipers, some poisonous, some benign, and some moderately toxic, with no way of knowing which patients were bitten by which snakes.

Every effort should be made to identify patients with distant metastasis. Search for metastatic lesions preoperatively should include a chest film and liver and skeletal scintiscans. These tests, combined with urinary hydroxyproline, bone-derived alkaline phosphatase, and γ-glutamyl transpeptidase, have demonstrated a 40 to 45 percent incidence of distant metastasis in Stages I and II patients who were otherwise asymptomatic.

SELECTION OF THE OPERATION. For the past 20 years a controversy has been raging as to the appropriate operation for patients with operable breast cancer. Initially the debate was between radical mastectomy and total ("simple") mastectomy plus radiation therapy; then between radical mastectomy and total mastectomy alone; and finally between radical mastectomy alone and partial mastectomy with or without radiation therapy. While these have been the major themes, some minor variations of radical mastectomy have also appeared: either a little less than the radical mastectomy, sparing the pectoralis minor (Patey's operation) or both pectoral muscles (Madden's operation); or a little more than the radical mastectomy, taking the internal mammary lymph nodes and adjacent chest wall (Urban's operation).

The arguments for the various procedures have become remarkably bitter at times, with charges of bias, the citing of incomplete data, and irrationality being hurled not only in the scientific but in the lay press as well. Nonparticipants in this battle have been regarded darkly as agnostics who have failed to embrace either "true faith." American surgeons have remained reasonably level-headed during this period. At first they adhered to the traditional radical mastectomy. After all, the advantages of doing lesser operations were functional and cosmetic, while the penalty of being wrong was the life of a patient. A survey of New Jersey surgeons in 1971 showed that 75 percent would do a radical breast dissection and 15 percent a modified radical operation for a 2-cm lesion in the upper outer quadrant of a fifty-year old woman. Opinion is changing, however: in 1977, surgeons in the same state indicated that approximately 40 percent would do a radical mastectomy, 40 percent a modified radical mastectomy, 15 percent a total mastectomy, and 5 percent some other procedure.

My own rationale for selecting an operation involves the following considerations: Of the three major anatomic components in radical mastectomy—the breast, the axillary contents, and the muscles—current evidence strongly supports removal of at least the first two. Removal of all, rather than part, of the involved breast is required because of the high incidence of multicentricity of these malignant lesions. The risk of another tumor focus left in the remaining breast tissue following a segmental excision exceeds 50 percent.

The value of removing axillary contents has been defended in the past on the claim of improved survival. The results of controlled cooperative clinical trials indicate that treatment of the axilla does not change survival in patients with clinical Stage I tumors. Data from such trials are still accumulating concerning treatment of the axilla in clinical Stage II patients, and figures currently available are in conflict. On the other hand, the added information gained by knowing whether or not axillary nodes are histologically involved by malignancy is of enormous value to surgeons and patients, both in rendering an accurate prognosis and in influencing the trend of future therapy.

Hodgkin's disease, in which a major operation, exploratory laparotomy and splenectomy, is now felt justified for diagnostic and "staging" purposes, is an irresistible parallel. The addition of axillary dissection to breast resection adds very little in risk or morbidity, and the dividend in "staging" the extent of the disease is well worth the price whether survival is improved or not.

Should the muscles be removed as well, and if so, how much? In view of the enormous effort required to accumulate properly controlled series, this question may never be subject to scientific resolution. Pragmatically, muscle resection seems especially indicated for large or deep tumors which approach or invade fascia and muscle. This was the type of lesion most commonly seen in the late nineteenth century, for which the classic radical mastectomy was originally designed. Such large and often ulcerated tumors require the larger operations, often combined with radiation, to obtain proper local control of tumor. The object is to prevent recurrent uncontrollable local disease and improve the quality of survival, even though the eventual outcome will be death from distant metastasis.

Subcutaneous Mastectomy. The advent of mammography has led to an increasing diagnosis of in situ (T1S) and very small microinvasive cancers (T1a). This has coincided with the introduction of subcutaneous mastectomy, a technique in which most of the mammary tissue is removed but the skin of the breast is preserved. Contour is restored by inserting a silastic prosthesis into the subcutaneous pocket left by the excision of breast tissue. It is impossible to remove all breast tissue by this method, and 1 or 2 percent remains in the subcutaneous layer near the skin even if the nipple is sacrificed. Development of cancer in this residual mammary tissue has been reported, and in view of the multifocal nature of breast cancer, it is expected that some of the foci may be left behind. The risk/benefit ratio of this approach remains to be established and, while it is a very attractive alternative for women with in situ cancer of the breast, the accepted procedure for such lesions in the United States is still total mastectomy.

The Problem of Bilateral Mastectomy. Foote and Stewart have observed that "the most frequent precancerous lesion of the breast is a cancer of the opposite breast." Berg and Robbins noted that the incidence of occurrence of cancer in the contralateral breast following radical mastectomy was approximately 1 percent per year, so that the cumulative risk of cancer in the remaining breast among patients surviving radical mastectomy for 20 years was as high as 20 percent. As long ago as 1951, Pack published a plea for routine simple mastectomy of the remaining breast at the time of mastectomy for cancer. Presumably because of the psychologic blow to a woman who is asked to lose both her breasts, this approach has rarely been advocated by surgeons, and the usual routine after mastectomy has been to follow the contralateral breast with special care in the ensuing years. The recognition of the high risk of contralateral cancer in patients with in situ lobular carcinoma has caused a change in attitude toward this particular form of the disease. Currently recommended treatment for patients with either in situ or invasive lobular cancer of the breast is total mastectomy of the contralateral breast. Should this recommendation be refused, the patient is requested at least to permit a biopsy of the remaining breast in an area which represents a mirror image of the area of cancer in the involved breast. If this biopsy reveals in situ lobular cancer, a total mastectomy is carried out. If invasive lobular cancer is found, a radical or modified radical mastectomy is done. If the biopsy is negative, a very careful follow-up is recommended, with mammography and careful breast examination at least twice yearly.

A minority of physicians recommend a "watch" policy for in situ lobular carcinoma. They reason that only one-third of these lesions ultimately become invasive, and that even the invasive lesions of this tumor have a better prognosis than the usual invasive ductal lesion. Close follow-up would thus preserve a substantial number of women from what might be an unnecessary mastectomy. This view of therapy has not proved popular among patients and surgeons. Most women are uneasy about harboring a malignant breast lesion even if it is preinvasive, and most surgeons share this feeling. Moreover, the transition from preinvasive to invasive may go undetected for long periods, since it is not necessarily accompanied by any clinical signs.

ADJUVANT THERAPY FOLLOWING OPERATIONS FOR BREAST CANCER. Traditionally, patients who were discovered at operation for breast cancer to have metastatic tumor in the axillary nodes were subjected to radiation therapy given over the axilla and the parasternal and supraclavicular areas. This treatment was given in the hope of increasing the chance for survival in this high-risk group of patients. A number of cooperative clinical trials testing this hypothesis were launched in the 1950s and 1960s and have shown that such therapy has no effect on recurrence rate or survival. The National Surgical Adjuvant Breast Project (NSABP) conducted such a study starting in 1961 and found that at 5 years 50.6 percent of treated patients were disease-free, compared with 50.2 percent of patients who received no radiotherapy. Local recurrence of disease was affected, however, being twice as common (15.4 percent) when radiotherapy was not given as when it was (7.8 percent). Distant metastasis seemed to occur sooner in the radiated group. Current thinking is that adjuvant radiotherapy should be used only in breast cancer patients who are at very high risk of local recurrence.

It may be that cancer chemotherapy will provide an effective adjuvant to operative therapy where radiation has failed. In some of the early NSABP trials it was noted that a brief course of triethylene ethiophosphoramide (thiotepa), a nitrogen mustard analogue given at the time of operation, resulted in a decrease in recurrence rates in a special subset of the population treated. This special group comprised those premenopausal women with four or more axillary lymph nodes involved by tumor. This is a high-risk group with a recurrence rate of at least 90 percent in 5 years from operation. Long-term follow-up of these patients showed significantly improved survival at 5 and 10 years.

Subsequent cooperative clinical trials of adjuvant therapy with L-phenylalanine mustard (L-Pam, melphalan) were initiated. In the light of more modern concepts of cancer chemotherapy, the drug was given over a much longer period. Initial results again demonstrated significant improvement in the disease-free interval in the same subset of women up to 3 years after operation. More recent trials of a three-drug regimen suggest even more effective results in premenopausal women with four or more positive axillary lymph nodes (Fig. 15-20) and possible improvements in the disease-free period for women with similar advanced disease in the postmenopausal period as well. These are exciting results and seem to promise a real increase in survival in certain high-risk groups. However, another several years must elapse before final conclusions on these

Fig. 15-20. Early results of adjuvant therapy with a three-drug regimen (Cytoxan, methotrexate, and 5-fluorouracil) in women with four or more axillary lymph nodes involved by metastatic cancer. Major difference in recurrence rate is obvious. (*From U. Veronesi et al., World J Surg, 1:337, 1977, by permission.*)

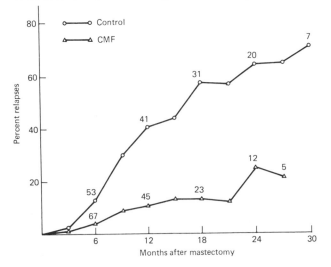

questions can be drawn. In the meantime, adjuvant chemotherapy of patients with Stage 1 lesions is not recommended, since the mortality due to cancer in this group is less than 15 percent at 5 and 10 years, and long-term hazards of chemotherapeutic drugs, especially the alkylating agents, have not been fully determined. There is some evidence that these are carcinogenic and may themselves induce some cancers.

Operative mortality is very low for all the various types of mastectomy. Kennedy and Miller reported no deaths following 212 simple mastectomies. Handley and Thackray reported no deaths following 143 modified radical mastectomies. Butcher reported 0.7 percent mortality in 425 radical mastectomies. Haagensen, Cooley, and their associates had no deaths in 556 radical mastectomies. In all the series cited above, any death of a patient up to 3 months after operation was considered an operative death. Even among patients with extended mastectomy, mortality is low: Sugarbaker reported 1 postoperative death in 250 patients with this procedure.

PROGNOSIS

The arguments for and against different forms of therapy in breast cancer are mainly statistical and are chiefly based on survival figures. Before an observer can appreciate this debate, a clear understanding of the data is required. The accurate comparison of results in different series demands that there be a common denominator. There is great variation in the base line of many published series, and astute investigation is often necessary to determine whether two sets of figures are truly comparable.

An older method of standard reporting required that all patients seen at an institution be reported in the final results, whether they were treated or not. This was called the "absolute," or "crude," survival figure. It had the advantage of indicating the effect of patient selection on the surgical, or "definitive," survival figures. Its disadvantage was that the total experience at different institutions varied greatly. Private hospitals and clinics have a much greater number of early and operable cases compared with cancer hospitals and charity institutions.

Favorable attention has been given to methods of clinical evaluation of the stage of the tumor. By this method the results in patients at an equal stage of disease can be compared among institutions. An advantage of this approach is that since the evaluation is based on pretreatment clinical findings, it is possible to compare the results in patients treated by radiation, radical mastectomy, simple mastectomy, or extended radical mastectomy even though microscopic evaluation of lymph node involvement is available with some forms of treatment and not with others. Disadvantages are that judgment of the extent of involvement is subjective and classification depends greatly on the skill and consistency of the examiner. The system of staging recommended by the American Joint Committee on Cancer Staging and End Results Reporting is most widely accepted; in addition there are the Columbia classification, the Manchester classification, and the Steinthal classification (Table 15-1).

Table 15-1. CLINICAL CLASSIFICATIONS OF CANCER OF THE BREAST

Manchester	Steinthal	Columbia
Stage I: Growth confined to breast, skin involvement over and in direct continuity with tumor and small in relation to breast	*Stage I:* Cancer limited to breast	*Stage A:* No skin edema, ulceration, or solid fixation of tumor to chest wall; axillary nodes not involved
Stage II: As Stage I but with palpable mobile axillary lymph nodes	*Stage II:* Limited to breast and axillary nodes	*Stage B:* As Stage A but axillary nodes present, not larger than 2.5 cm and without fixation to skin or deeper structures
Stage III: Growth extending beyond body of breast: a. Skin invaded or fixed over large area b. Tumor fixed to underlying muscle; nodes may be present but are mobile	*Stage III:* Adjacent structures involved, e.g., pectoral muscle skin (if ulcerated), opposite breast, cervical lymph nodes, viscera, skeletal tissue	*Stage C:* Any *one* of five grave signs present: 1. Edema of skin of limited extent (less than one-third) 2. Skin ulceration 3. Solid fixation to chest wall 4. Massive involvement of axillary nodes 5. Fixation of axillary nodes
Stage IV: Growth spread beyond breast: a. Fixation of axillary nodes b. Tumor fixed to chest wall (not just muscle) c. Supraclavicular nodes involved d. Satellite metastasis to skin beyond area of tumor e. Secondary deposits in opposite breast f. Distant metastasis		*Stage D:* All other more advanced cancer of breast

New diagnostic methods, especially mammography, have provided a new group of lesions not previously considered by any of the staging methods. Termed by some "minimal breast cancer," these are in situ and microinvasive lesions so small that they are not detectable by conventional palpation of the breast. Current data indicate that 5-year survivals in this group may exceed 90 percent.

The best way to evaluate methods of treatment is by cooperative programs among many institutions in which all factors are governed by the same rules and in which random selection of patients for the different methods of therapy is used. Even these trials are not an easy solution to the problem. Such trials tend to be biased toward false-negative results. Only in the largest of the cooperative trials is the chance of error in a negative result reduced to under 10 percent.

NO TREATMENT. In 1951 Park and Lees in a statistical analysis of 5-year survival figures for breast carcinoma tried to show that the course of the disease was not affected by operation. They regarded the improvement in 5-year survival seen following operation as an artifact introduced by operating upon patients earlier in the natural course of the disease. There are now available a number of studies of large groups of patients with untreated breast cancer. Survival computed from the onset of symptoms averages 19 percent at 5 years, 2.5 percent at 10 years. If one computes survival from onset of diagnosis, a figure more comparable to the situation in surgical series, the 5- and 10-year survivals average 8.6 percent and 1.2 percent, respectively. Bloom et al. found that untreated patients with histologically low-grade (grade 1 of 3) neoplasms had survivals of 22 percent, 9 percent, and 0 at 5, 10, and 15 years, respectively. They compared these to survivals of 82, 56, and 37 percent at the same time intervals for lesions of comparable histologic grade in their own treated series (Fig. 15-12).

RADICAL MASTECTOMY. If survival data following radical mastectomy between 1915 and 1958 are examined, one may wonder why the procedure has received so much criticism. The absolute survival gradually increased from 30 to over 50 percent (Fig. 15-21). In California the incidence of patients with localized disease in different age groups has increased from 14–27 percent to 27–39 percent in county hospitals and from 39–44 percent to 43–48 percent in private hospitals. The end-result group of the National Cancer Institute and a number of state tumor registries have reported small but steady increases in 5-year survivals in patients with both regional and localized disease since about 1950. Epidemiologic reports from Connecticut and from Saskatchewan, Canada, establish a significant increase in the incidence of breast cancer in the last several decades accompanied by a decrease in mortality, thus implying an increase in survival (Fig. 15-22).

Survival for 5 years following radical mastectomy does not provide the same assurance against recurrence that it does for some other cancers. The risk of death continues higher than for the general population for at least 25 years after the operation, although this risk gradually diminishes with time (Fig. 15-23). According to Berg and Robbins, change in risk over the postoperative period follows a log-log curve. From this model it can be predicted that after operation the risk of recurrence and death will continue to decrease but will always be present, being about 1 percent in the decade from 30 to 40 years after operation and 0.5 percent from 40 to 50 years after operation. The 20-year survival rate after operation for patients without axillary lymph node involvement is 65 percent, and that for all patients with radical mastectomy is 41 percent [Berg

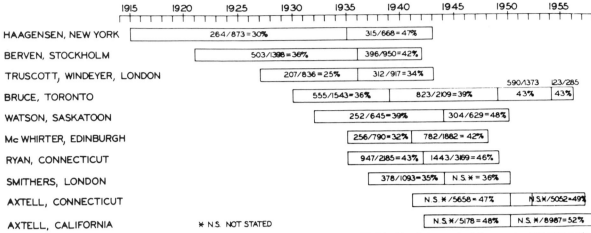

Fig. 15-21. Absolute survival figures in different series following treatment by radical mastectomy. Note improvement in survival from original observations to 1955. (*From H. Vermund, Trends in Radiotherapy in Breast Cancer, Proc 5th Natl Cancer Conf, Philadelphia, 1965, by permission.*)

Fig. 15-22. Contrary to past reports data from large population groups now indicate an increasing incidence and a decreasing mortality rate for breast cancer. (*From S. J. Cutler, B. Christine, and T. H. C. Barcley, Cancer, 28:1376, 1971.*)

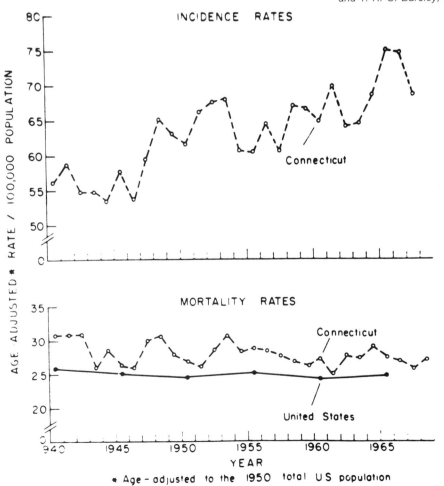

and Robbins]. If patients are considered who have node involvement at the apex of the axilla, the middle, and the lower portion, the 20-year survival is 11, 30, and 39 percent, respectively. These figures illustrate how important the absence or the extent of lymph node involvement is in determining patient survival. The increasing number of patients with primary lesions of the breast without lymph node involvement is the most important factor in the improving survival rates today compared with 25 years ago.

Our attitudes concerning survival and prognosis continue to be conditioned by our beliefs concerning the natural history of the disease. Mueller has reported data indicating that survival following treatment of breast cancer follows a log-normal curve, that is, that the annual risk of recurrence and death remains constant and if patients lived long enough all would eventually die of their tumor. If true, this would imply that all tumors have disseminated before clinical detection and treatment. In this circumstance treatment is effective only by altering the slope of the curve and delaying the ultimate death due to the cancer, long enough, it may be hoped, so that the patient dies of other "more natural" causes. This hypothesis is in conflict with the data of Berg and Robbins cited above and those of Blackwood and Rush, who indicated that the hazard function or risk of annual recurrence decreases significantly over time, following a well-known survival curve called the Wiebull distribution. Duncan and Kerr have examined a large series of patients treated in the 1940s with a follow-up of 20 or more years. Their data indicate that the "curability" of Stages I and II patients is 30.5 percent (Fig. 15-24).

Radical mastectomy is no longer the routine treatment for all patients with cancer of the breast, and even its stoutest defenders agree that there is a group of smaller cancers that can be treated by lesser procedures. It is still, however, the reference procedure, the operation with which we have the most experience over the greatest period of time. Defenders of radical mastectomy continue to be troubled by the fact that comparisons of survival with alternate procedures seem to favor the radical operation by 5 to 10 percent (Table 15-2). Such comparisons between institutional series have little or no statistical validity at this level of discrimination, and one must turn to the rapidly accumulating data from controlled cooperative clinical trials (Table 15-3).

RADICAL MASTECTOMY VS. OTHER SURGERY AND RADIATION THERAPY. There have been seven trials comparing total mastectomy plus immediate radiation therapy with radical mastectomy either with or without radiation since 1951 (Table 15-3). In every instance the results for survival and recurrence for Stage I tumors have been the same. For Stage II tumors the results were likewise similar except for the trial at Guy's, in which wide excision was done instead of total mastectomy. Stage II patients in this study had a significant increase in local recurrence and a significantly decreased survival at 5 years. Most such recurrences were in the axilla, and it has been noted that x-ray to the axilla in this series was considerably less than in other groups. By 10 years the survival rate in both groups was the same.

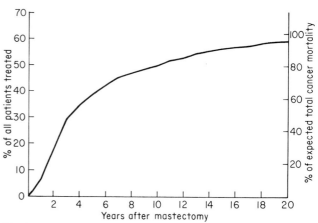

Fig. 15-23. Mortality 20 years after treatment by radical mastectomy; 95 percent of expected mortality has been realized, and over 40 percent of treated patients are still surviving. (*From J. W. Berg and G. F. Robbins, Surg Gynecol Obstet, 122:1311, 1966, by permission.*)

RADICAL MASTECTOMY VS. TOTAL MASTECTOMY. These trials are unique in that no radiation is used and that treatment to the axilla is omitted in one arm. Both the American and the Cardiff trials deal with Stage I disease. Early results in both trials show no difference in recurrence rate or survival. The Cape Town trial is the only one in this group in which axillary Stage II disease was observed and not treated. By the second year of the study, local recurrence rate (or continued growth of axillary nodes) was so great that the trial was stopped after entry of only 95 patients.

TOTAL MASTECTOMY AND RADIATION VS. TOTAL MASTECTOMY. Like the immediately previous trials, the effect of treating the axillary nodes versus watching them was being tested. In this case the primary treatment of the axilla was radiation. The three trials in this group differ in that the Edinburgh group and the NSABP-4 include only Stage I tumors—staged by histology in the former instance and clinically in the latter. In both groups early and thus

Fig. 15-24. "Curability" of breast cancer as determined in a group of patients treated 20 or more years. Survival rate in Stages I and II patients parallels the normal population at 20 years, and projection to the base line indicates that 30.5 percent of such patients are curable. (*From D. Brinkley and J. L. Haybittle, World J Surg, 1:287, 1977, by permission.*)

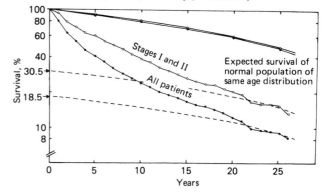

Table 15-2. METHODS OF TREATMENT COMPARED BY COLUMBIA CLASSIFICATION STAGES

Author	No. of patients		Method	5-yr survival, %	
	A	B		A	B
Kennedy and Miller	115	34	Simple mastectomy	62	41
Handley and Thackray	77	58	Limited radical mastectomy	75	57
Butcher	216	135	Classic radical mastectomy	76	48
Haagensen I	228	122	Classic radical mastectomy	82.5	59
Haagensen II	116	16	Classic radical mastectomy	87.9	62.5
Dahl-Iversen and Tobiassen	277	61	Extended radical mastectomy	77	48
Williams and Curwen	68	57	Limited radical mastectomy and radiation	72	60
Kaae and Johansen	159	28	Simple mastectomy and radiation	70	50
Baclesse	50	86	Radiation only	54	67

incomplete results show no differences. In the British Cancer Research Campaign trial, both clinical Stage I and Stage II lesions were included. In this trial, radiation significantly reduced the incidence of local recurrence or residual axillary disease. However, radiated patients with histologically positive axillary nodes had a 10 percent greater mortality in the first year of observation and a significantly higher incidence of distant metastasis.

RADICAL MASTECTOMY VS. EXTENDED RADICAL MASTECTOMY. A single cooperative trial has been conducted comparing these operative techniques. A total of 1,453 evaluable patients were admitted from 1963 to 1968 at several international hospitals. Five-year results indicate the same mortality and recurrence rate in both arms. But an interesting subset of patients, those with tumor in the axillary nodes with inner quadrant breast cancer, had a significantly better survival with the extended procedure, one of the rare reports in which removal of lymph nodes had any effect on prognosis.

SUMMARY. After a period of great confusion as to the proper treatment for breast cancer, during which surgeons continued to employ radical mastectomy because they were unsure what else to use, hard data are beginning to emerge from international cooperative clinical trials upon which we can base our future therapy: (1) Total mastectomy is as effective a treatment for clinical Stage I tumors as any other alternative tested, including radical mastectomy with or without radiation, total mastectomy with radiation, or extended radical mastectomy. (2) In Stage II breast cancer, the results of "watching" the axilla instead of treating it are still fairly early in controlled trials. On the basis of these early data, it appears that survival in the first 5 years of follow-up is unchanged. However, the local recurrence rate or continued growth of axillary nodes has proved unacceptable to one group of investigators and acceptable to another. Until such trials have matured further, physicians should continue to treat the axilla in Stage II patients by radiation or operation. (3) There is a

Table 15-3. SUMMARY OF INTERNATIONAL COOPERATIVE TRIALS

	Stage	Years	Patients
Radical and radiation vs. total and radiation			
Cambridge	II	1958–65	204
Cardiff/St. Mary's (part)	II	1967–73	139
Hammersmith			
Guy's (wide excision instead of total)	I,II	1961–71	370
Radical vs. total and radiation			
Denmark (superradical)	I,II,III	1951–57	400
Edinburgh I	I,II,III	1964–69	395
NSABP-4 (part)	I,II	1971–74	1226
Radical vs. total			
Cardiff/St. Mary's (part)	I	1967–73	154
Cape Town	I,II	1968–71	95
NSABP-4 (part)	I	1971–74	690
Total and radiation vs. total			
Cancer Research Campaign	I,II	1970–75	2268
NSABP-4 (part)	I	1971–74	689
Edinburgh II	I (histol.)	1974–	Still open

strong suspicion from several trials that radiation therapy increases the incidence of distant metastasis, and from one trial that early morbidity is significantly greater in patients with histologically positive axillary nodes. (4) No good data are available on the role of partial mastectomy in the treatment of breast cancer, and this procedure is contraindicated, used either alone or with radiation therapy, except as part of a controlled clinical trial.

As noted previously, this author believes that a prudent procedure for the treatment of Stages I and II breast cancer includes surgical removal of the breast and axillary contents. In more advanced malignant lesions of the breast, more extended operations such as radical mastectomy may be required, either with or without radiation therapy, to control local and regional disease and improve the quality if not the length of survival in such patients.

REHABILITATION. Most women require instruction in exercising the arm on the side of operation following radical mastectomy. Proper physical therapy in the immediate postoperative period should ensure complete return to normal function. Following operations which spare the pectoral muscles, full function of the arm usually returns promptly with little or no special help. Psychological support is also important in restoring the patient's self-image and her confidence that she is still desirable to a present or future husband. The Reach to Recovery program of the American Cancer Society has been most successful in providing advisors to the recent mastectomy patient from the ranks of women who have previously had the same operation.

Many women are interested in the possibility of subsequent reconstruction of the excised breast. If the previous operation was radical mastectomy, reconstruction is too complex a task to be worthwhile in most instances. In patients who have had a modified or total mastectomy, especially if the operation was performed through a transverse incision, reconstruction with a silastic implant is a relatively simple and feasible technique. The result is never a perfect match for the remaining breast, and decisions as to which patients will find these reconstructions worthwhile must be individualized.

TREATMENT OF RECURRENT CANCER

Prior to the 1950s recurrent cancer of the breast was treated either with radiation or operation or not at all. Radiation remains an extremely useful agent for painful osseous metastases and small subcutaneous lesions. Operation also may be useful for small local lesions. The basic problem in the patient with recurrent cancer is most often wide dissemination, and the new systemic agents of hormone therapy and chemotherapy are the treatments of choice.

Selection of hormonal therapy or chemotherapy as the initial treatment of recurrent disease depends on whether the patient's tumor is hormonally sensitive. For decades the only index of hormonal sensitivity was the patient's response to a trial of hormonal treatment. We now know that the response of breast cancers to hormones is dependent on the presence of hormone receptors in the substance of cancer cells. Hormonal receptors for estrogens, prolac-

tin, progesterone, and corticosteroids have been identified. Dependable clinical tests for estrogen receptors (ER) are now widely available, and all primary cancers should be submitted for testing when first removed; 50 percent of these tumors will prove to be ER-positive. Progesterone receptors (PR) also appear to have a predictive value. Eighty percent of patients with breast cancers which have both ER and PR will respond to hormonal manipulation. However, tests for PR are not widely available. A schema for treatment of patients tested for both ER and PR is shown in Fig. 15-25.

TREATMENT OF ESTROGEN RECEPTOR–POSITIVE RECURRENT TUMORS. Removal of estrogen-generating tissue in these patients will produce a remission in 60 percent. The major source of estrogens in the menstruating patient are the ovaries, and oophorectomy will result in an effective reduction in the estrogen level. In the postmenopausal patient some or most estrogen production has been assumed by the adrenals, thus bilateral adrenalectomy plus oophorectomy is required or, alternatively, hypophysectomy. Paradoxically, the postmenopausal woman also responds well to administration of estrogens in large doses, a far simpler procedure than the major operative procedures otherwise required.

Recently antiestrogen compounds have become available. These apparently block estrogen receptors at the cell. At best these may offer a useful substitute for ablative therapy, and at worst they offer a nonoperative test of which patients fall within the 60 percent who will respond to operative ablation.

TREATMENT OF ESTROGEN RECEPTOR–NEGATIVE RECURRENT TUMORS. Patients who have tumors which are estrogen receptor–negative rarely respond to estrogen ab-

Fig. 15-25. Schema for the treatment of patients with recurrent breast cancer when determinations for estrogen receptors and progesterone receptors are available. Patients who are estrogen receptor–positive (ERP) and progesterone receptor–positive (PRP) have an 80 percent response rate to surgical ablation. (*From G. A. Degenshein et al., Breast, 3:29, 1977, by permission.*)

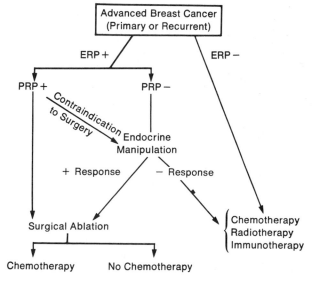

lative therapy (10 percent or less). Such patients, together with the 40 percent who fail to respond to a therapeutic trial of estrogen ablation or antiestrogens, are candidates for cancer chemotherapy. Multiple-drug regimens spaced at much longer intervals than the older single-drug programs are the current mode and have produced a doubling and even tripling of the improvement in the old results with single drugs. Arrest of tumor growth, partial remission, and even complete remissions can be expected in 65 percent of patients so treated. Because of the rapid improvement in the results of chemotherapy, there is now some controversy as to whether hormonal therapy should precede or follow chemotherapy. Wilson and Moore, among several clinicians, have combined total operative estrogen ablation with almost simultaneous cancer chemotherapy in patients with recurrent breast cancer. They suggest that the two forms of therapy work synergistically, with a better response for combination than for sequential use of these techniques when compared with historical controls. No controlled clinical trials are available to confirm this observation, and hormonal therapy remains the first treatment of recurrence at the present. Both therapies are palliative and not curative measures, and most patients will eventually receive most or all of the agents currently available. The aim of therapy is to improve the quality of life and the length of survival, but not as yet to provide cure.

Infection

ACUTE INFECTION

Bacterial infections almost always occur in the lactating breast in the first month or two following delivery. The portal of entry is an abrasion or fissure in the nipple. The best treatment is prevention, with the nursing mother carefully cleaning and drying her nipples after nursing. Because cleanliness is so important, infection more commonly occurs in patients from a lower socioeconomic stratum. It is also seasonal, being more common in the hot summer months.

The milk-containing ducts and acini of the lactating breast are a perfect culture medium, and infection, having gained access, often progresses rapidly through inflammation to suppuration. This is accompanied by extreme pain in the breast, and a good diagnostic sign of abscess is the patient's rapid withdrawal when the physician attempts to palpate the involved breast. The breast is red and the area of abscess indurated and firm. The tendency is to underestimate the size of the abscess on physical examination.

An abscess may be aborted by the use of systemic antibiotics given in the presuppurative period. Treatment of abscess, once it forms, is by surgical drainage. Antibiotics will suppress the process for a time, but it will flare up again when they are discontinued. A curvilinear transverse incision is made in the dependent portion of the breast and the gloved finger or a clamp used to break up the many septa which separate the cavity into loculations. A rubber drain is left in the wound. Culture of the pus usually demonstrates *Staphylococcus aureus*. Pain is relieved promptly by drainage, and the surrounding inflammation subsides rapidly.

CHRONIC INFECTION

Chronic infection of the breast is now rare. Tuberculosis is the major cause, and as the incidence of this disease has decreased, so have breast lesions caused by it. The genesis of breast tuberculosis is either pleural or, more commonly, the breaking down of a mediastinal node to involve one of the costal cartilages. Infection simmers in the cartilage for long periods, giving rise to lesions in the breast, which eventually form one or several fistulas to the skin. Antituberculosis drugs are now the primary treatment for this disease, but care of the breast lesion usually requires excision of the affected costal cartilage.

References

General

Geschickter, C. F.: "Diseases of the Breast," J. B. Lippincott Company, Philadelphia, 1943.
Haagensen, C. D.: "Diseases of the Breast," 2d ed., W. B. Saunders Company, Philadelphia, 1971.

Anatomy and Development

Batson, O. V.: The Function of the Vertebral Veins and Their Role in the Spread of Metastasis, *Ann Surg,* **112:**138, 1940.
Cooper, Sir A. P.: "The Anatomy and Diseases of the Breast," Lea and Blanchard, Philadelphia, 1845.
Ingleby, H., and Gershon-Cohen, J.: "Cooperative Anatomy: Pathology and Roentgenology of the Breast," University of Pennsylvania Press, Philadelphia, 1960.
Taylor, G. T.: Anatomy of the Breast with Particular Reference to Lymphatic Drainage, in W. H. Parson, "Cancer of the Breast," Charles C Thomas, Publisher, Springfield, Ill., 1959.

Examination of the Breast

Berger, S. M., and Gershon-Cohen, J.: Mammography of Breast Sarcoma, *Am J Roentgenol Radium Ther Nucl Med,* **87:**76, 1962.
Clark, R. L., Copeland, M. M., Egan, R. L., Gallagher, H. S., Geller, H., Lindsay, J. P., Robbins, L. C., and White, E. C.: Reproducibility of the Technic of Mammography (Egan) for Cancer of the Breast, *Am J Surg,* **109:**127, 1965.
Gershon-Cohen, J., and Berger, S. M.: Detection of Breast Cancer by Periodic X-ray Examinations: A Five-year Survey, *JAMA,* **176:**1114, 1961.
———, ———, and Klickstein, H. S.: Roentgenography of Breast Cancer Moderating Concept of "Biologic Predeterminism," *Cancer,* **16:**961, 1963.
——— and Ingleby, H.: Roentgenography of Unsuspected Carcinoma of Breast, *JAMA,* **166:**869, 1958.
Ingleby, H., Moore, L., and Gershon-Cohen, J.: A Roentgenographic Study of the Growth Rate of Six "Early" Cancers of the Breast, *Cancer,* **11:**726, 1958.
Snyder, R. E.: Mammography and Lobular Carcinoma In Situ, *Surg Gynecol Obstet,* **122:**255, 1966.
Treves, N., and Holleb, A. I.: Cancer of the Male Breast: A Report of 146 Cases, *Cancer,* **8:**1239, 1955.

Neoplasms

Abramson, D. J.: Delayed Mastectomy after Outpatient Breast Biopsy, *Am J Surg,* **132:**596, 1976.

Adair, F., Berg, J., Joubert, L. and Robbins, G. F.: Long-term Follow-up of Breast Cancer Patients: The 30-Year Report, *Cancer,* **33:**1145, 1974.

Anglem, T. J.: Management of Breast Cancer: Radical Mastectomy, *JAMA,* **230:**99, 1974.

Baclesse, F.: Five-year Results in 431 Breast Cancers Treated Solely by Roentgen Rays, *Ann Surg,* **161:**103, 1965.

Berg, J. W., and Robbins, G. F.: Factors Influencing Short and Long-Term Survival of Breast Cancer Patients, *Surg Gynecol Obstet,* **122:**1311, 1966.

—— and ——: Selection of Treatment Regimens for Women with Potentially Curable Breast Carcinoma, *Am Surg,* **43:**86, 1977.

Blackwood, J. M., Seelig, R. F., Hutter, R. V. P., and Rush, B. F., Jr.: Survival Distribution in Breast Cancer, *Surgery,* **82:**443, 1977.

Bloom, H. J. G., Richardson, W. W., and Harries, E. J.: Natural History of Untreated Breast Cancer (1805-1933): Comparison of Untreated and Treated Cases According to Histological Grade of Malignancy, *Br Med J,* **5299:**213, 1962.

Bonadonna, G., Brusamolino, E., Valagussa, P., Rossi, A., Brugnatelli, L., Brambilla, C., DeLena, M., Tancini, G., Bajetta, E., Musumeci, R., and Veronesi, U.: Combination Chemotherapy as an Adjuvant Treatment in Operable Breast Cancer, *N Engl J Med.,* **294:**405, 1976.

Branfield, J. R., Fingerhut, A. G., and Warner, N. E.: Lobular Carcinoma of the Breast—1969: A Therapeutic Proposal, *Arch Surg,* **99:**129, 1969.

Breslow, L.: Epidemiologic Considerations in Breast Cancer, *Proc 5th Natl Cancer Conf,* Philadelphia, 1965.

Brinkley, D., and Haybittle, J. L.: The Curability of Breast Cancer, *World J Surg,* **1:**287, 1977.

Butcher, H. R., Jr.: Effectiveness of Radical Mastectomy for Mammary Cancer: An Analysis of Mortalities by the Method of Probits, *Ann Surg,* **154:**383, 1961.

——: Radical Mastectomy for Mammary Carcinoma, *Ann Surg,* **157:**165, 1963.

Caceres, E., Lingan, M., and Delgado, P.: Evaluation of Dissection of the Axilla in Modified Radical Mastectomy, *Surg Gynecol Obstet,* **143:**395, 1976.

Cancer Research Campaign Trial: Management of Early Cancer of the Breast, *Br Med J,* **1:**1035, 1976.

Cant, E. L., Smith, A. F., Summerling, M. D., and Forrest, A. P. M.: "Superstaging" in Breast Cancer: A Correlation of Lymph Node Histology and Investigations Designed to Detect Occult Metastic Disease, *World J Surg,* **1:**303, 1977.

Crile, G., Jr.: Management of Breast Cancer: Limited Mastectomy, *JAMA,* **230:**95, 1974.

—— and Hoerr, S. O.: Results of Treatment of Carcinoma of the Breast by Local Excision, *Surg Gynecol Obstet,* **132:**780, 1971.

Cronin, T. D., Upton, J., and McDonough, J. M.: Reconstruction of the Breast after Mastectomy, *Plast Reconstr Surg,* **59:**1, 1977.

Cukier, D. S., Lopez, F. A., and Maravilla, R. B., Jr.: One-View Follow-Up Mammogram: Efficacy in Screening for Breast Cancer, *JAMA,* **237:**661, 1977.

Dahl-Iversen, E., and Tobiassen, T.: Radical Mastectomy with Parasternal and Supraclavicular Dissection for Mammary Carcinoma, *Ann Surg,* **157:**170, 1963.

Degenshein, G. A., Bloom, N., Ceccarelli, F., Daluvoy, R., and Tobin, E.: Estrogen and Progesterone Receptor Site Studies as Guides to the Management of Advanced Breast Cancer, *Breast,* **3:**29, 1977.

Duncan, W., Forrest, A. P. M., Gray, N., Hamilton, T., Langlands, A. O., Prescott, R. J., Shivas, A. A., and Stewart, H. J.: New Edinburgh Primary Breast Cancer Trials: Report By Co-ordinating Committee, *Br J Cancer,* **32:**628, 1975.

—— and Kerr, G. R.: The Curability of Breast Cancer, *Br Med J,* **2:**781, 1976.

Fisher, B.: Cooperative Clinical Trials in Primary Breast Cancer: A Critical Appraisal, *Cancer,* **31:**127, 1973.

——: United States Trials of Conservative Surgery, *World J Surg,* **1:**327, 1977.

——, Carbone, P., Economou, S. G., Frelick, R., Glass, A., Lerner, H., Redmond, C., Zelen, M., Band, P., Katrych, D. L., Wolmark, N., Fisher, E. R. (and Other Co-operating Investigators): 1-Phenylalanine Mustard (L-PAM) in The Management of Primary Breast Cancer: A Report of Early Findings, *N Engl J Med,* **292:**117, 1975.

—— and Fisher, B.: Lobular Carcinoma of the Breast: An Overview, *Ann Surg,* **185:**377, 1977.

——, Ravdin, R. G., Ausman, R. K., Slack, N. H., Moore, G. E., and Noer, R. J.: Surgical Adjuvant Chemotherapy in Cancer of the Breast: Results of a Decade of Cooperative Investigation, *Ann Surg,* **168:**337, 1968.

——, Slack, N. H., Cavanaugh, P. J., Gardner, B., and Ravdin, R. G.: Postoperative Radiotherapy in the Treatment of Breast Cancer: Results of the NSABP Clinical Trial, *Ann Surg,* **172:**711, 1970.

——, ——, ——, ——, and ——: Postoperative Radiotherapy in the Treatment of Breast Cancer: Results of the NSABP Clinical Trial, *Ann Surg,* **172:**711, 1970.

——, ——, Katrych, D. and Wolmark, N.: Ten Year Follow-Up Results of Patients with Carcinoma of the Breast in a Co-operative Clinical Trial Evaluating Surgical Adjuvant Chemotherapy, *Surg Gynecol Obstet,* **140:**528, 1975.

Fletcher, G. H., Montague, E., and White, E. C.: Evaluation of Preoperative Irradiation for Carcinoma for the Breast, *Proc 5th Natl Cancer Conf,* Philadelphia, 1964, 1965.

Foote, F. W., and Stewart, F. W.: Comparative Studies of Cancerous versus Noncancerous Breasts: I. Basic Morphology Characteristics, *Ann Surg,* **121:**6, 1945.

—— and ——: Comparative Studies of Cancerous versus Noncancerous Breasts: II. Mammary Carcinogenesis: Influence of Certain Hormones on Human Breast Structure, *Ann Surg,* **121:**197, 1945.

Forrest, A. P. M., Roberts, M. M., Cant, E., and Shivas, A. A.: Simple Mastectomy and Pectoral Node Biopsy, *Br J Surg,* **63:**569, 1976.

Gardner, B: Cancer Revisited, *JAMA,* **232:**742, 1975. (Editorial.)

Gibson, E. W.: Reconstruction of the Breast after Mastectomy for Cancer, *Clin Plast Surg,* **3:**371, 1976.

Goldenberg, I. S.: Hormones and Breast Cancer: Historical Perspectives, *Surgery,* **53:**285, 1963.

Green, R. B., Sethi, R. S., and Lindner, H. H.: Treatment of Advanced Carcinoma of the Breast, *Am J Surg,* **108:**107, 1964.

Guttman, R.: Radiotherapy in the Treatment of Primary Operable Carcinoma of the Breast with Proved Lymph Node Metastases: Approach and Results, *Am J Roentgenol Radium Ther Nucl Med,* **89:**58, 1963.

Haagensen, C. D.: The Choice of Treatment for Operable Carcinoma of the Breast, *Surgery,* **76:**685, 1974.

———, Cooley, E., Kennedy, C. S., Miller, E., Handley, R. S., Thackray, A. C., Butcher, H. R., Jr., Dahl-Iversen, E., Tobiassen, T., Williams, I. G., Curwen, M. P., Kaae, S., and Johansen, H.: Treatment of Early Mammary Carcinoma: A Co-operative International Study, *Ann Surg,* **157:**157, 1963.

Handley, R. S.: The Conservative Radical Mastectomy of Patey: 10-Year Results in 425 Patients, *Breast,* **2:**16, 1976.

——— and Thackray, A. C.: The Internal Mammary Lymph Chain in Carcinoma of the Breast: Study of 50 Cases, *Lancet,* **257:**276, 1949.

——— and ———: Conservative Radical Mastectomy (Patey's Operation), *Ann Surg,* **157:**162, 1963.

Hayward, J. L.: The Guy's Trial of Treatments of "Early" Breast Cancer, *World J Surg,* **1:**314, 1977.

Hems, G.: Epidemiological Characteristics of Breast Cancer in Middle and Late Age, *Br J Cancer,* **24:**226, 1970.

Hoge, A. F., Bottomley, R. H., Shaw, M. T., and Asal, N. R.: Adrenalectomy and Oophorectomy plus Limited-Term Chemotherapy in the Treatment of Breast Cancer, *Cancer Treat Rep,* **60:**857, 1976.

Holleb, A. I., Montgomery, R., and Farrow, J. H.: The Hazard of Incomplete Simple Mastectomy, *Surg Gynecol Obstet,* **121:**819, 1965.

James, F., James, V. H. T., Carter, A. E., and Irvine, W. T.: A Comparison of in Vivo and in Vitro Uptake of Estradiol by Human Breast Tumors and the Relationship of Steroid Excretion, *Cancer Res,* **31:**1268, 1971.

Kaae, S., and Johansen, H.: Breast Cancer: A Comparison of Simple Mastectomy with Postoperative Roentgen Irradiation by the McWhirter Method with Those of Extended Radical Mastectomy, *Acta Radiol [Suppl] (Stockh),* **155:**185, 1959.

——— and ———: Simple Mastectomy plus Postoperative Irradiation by the Method of McWhirter for Mammary Carcinoma, *Ann Surg,* **157:**175, 1963.

Karpas, C. M., Leis, H. P., Oppenheim, A., and Mersheimer, W. L.: Relationship of Fibrocystic Disease to Carcinoma of the Breast, *Ann Surg,* **162:**1, 1965.

Kaufman, R. J.: Medical Management of Breast Cancer, *Clin Bull Mem Hosp,* **2:**21, 1972.

Kay, S., and Poulos, N.G.: Evaluation of the Criteria of Operability of Carcinoma of the Breast, *Surg Gynecol Obstet,* **113:**562, 1961.

Kennedy, B. J.: The Role of Castration in Breast Cancer, *Arch Surg,* **88:**743, 1964.

———, Meilke, P. W., Jr., and Fortuny, I. E.: Therapeutic Castration versus Prophylactic Castration in Breast Cancer, *Surg Gynecol Obstet,* **118:**524, 1964.

Kennedy, C. S., and Miller, E.: Simple Mastectomy for Mammary Carcinoma, *Ann Surg,* **157:**161, 1963.

Kleinfeld, G., Haagensen, C. D., and Cooley, E.: Age and Menstrual Status as Prognostic Factors in Carcinoma of the Breast, *Ann Surg,* **157:**600, 1963.

Kraft, R. O., and Block, G. E.: Mammary Carcinoma in the Aged Patient, *Ann Surg,* **156:**981, 1962.

Kramer, W. M., and Rush, B. F., Jr.: Mammary Duct Proliferation in the Elderly: A Histopathologic Study, *Cancer,* **31:**130, 1973.

Kusama, S., Spratt, J. S., Jr., Donegan, W. L., Watson, F. R., and Cunningham, C.: The Gross Rates of Growth of Human Mammary Carcinoma, *Cancer,* **30:**594, 1972.

Lacour, J., Bucalossi, P., Cacers, E., Jacobelli, G., Koszarowski, T., Le, M., Rumeau-Rouquette, C., and Veronesi, U.: Radical Mastectomy Versus Radical Mastectomy Plus Internal Mammary Dissection: Five-Year Results of an International Co-operative Study, *Cancer,* **37:**206, 1976.

Legha, S. S., and Carter, S. K.: Antiestrogens in the Treatment of Breast Cancer, *Cancer Treat Rev,* **3:**205, 1976.

Leung, B. S., Krippaehne, W. W., and Fletcher, W. S.: Prognostic Value of Estrogen Receptor to Endocrine Ablation in Cancer of the Breast, *Surg Gynecol Obstet,* **139:**525, 1974.

Levitt, S. H., and McHugh, R. B.: Radiotherapy in the Postoperative Treatment of Operable Cancer of the Breast: Part I. Critique of the Clinical and Biometric Aspects of the Trials, *Cancer,* **39:**924, 1977.

———, ———, and Song, C. W.: Radiotherapy in the Postoperative Treatment of Operable Cancer of the Breast: Part II. A Re-Examination of Stjernsward's Application of the Mantel-Haenszel Statistical Method: Evaluation of the Effect of the Radiation on Immune Response and Suggestions for Postoperative Radiotherapy, *Cancer,* **39:**933, 1976.

Lewison, E. F.: "Breast Cancer and Its Diagnosis and Treatment," The Williams & Wilkins Company, Baltimore, 1955.

———: The Problem of Prognosis in Cancer of the Breast, *Surgery,* **37:**479, 1955.

———: The Results of Treatment of Breast Cancer at the Johns Hopkins Hospital 1941-1945, with a Discussion, *Surg Gynecol Obstet,* **107:**313, 1958.

———: An Appraisal of Long-Term Results in Surgical Treatment of Breast Cancer, *JAMA,* **186:**975, 1963.

———, and Lyons, J. G., Jr.: Relationship between Benign Breast Disease and Cancer, *Arch Surg,* **66:**94, 1953.

——— and Neto, A. S.: Bilateral Breast Cancer at the Johns Hopkins Hospital: A Discussion of the Dilemma of Contralateral Breast Cancer, **28:**1297, 1971.

Linden, G., Cline, J. W., Wood, D. A., Guiss, L. W., and Breslow, L.: Validity of Pathological Diagnosis of Breast Cancer, *JAMA,* **173:**143, 1960.

MacDonald, I.: The Natural History of Mammary Carcinoma, *Am J Surg,* **111:**435, 1966.

Madden, J. L.: Modified Radical Mastectomy, *Surg Gynecol Obstet,* **121:**1221, 1965.

McWhirter, R.: Treatment of Cancer of the Breast by Simple Mastectomy and Roentgenotherapy, *Arch Surg,* **59:**830, 1949.

Missakian, M. M., Witten, D. M., and Harrison, E. G., Jr.: Mammography after Mastectomy: Usefulness in Search for Recurrent Carcinoma of the Breast, *JAMA,* **191:**1045, 1965.

Moore, D. H., Sarkar, N. H., Kramarksy, B., Lasfargues, E. Y., and Charney, J.: Some Aspects of the Search for a Human Mammary Tumor Virus, *Cancer,* **28:**1415, 1971.

Moore, F. D., Van Devanter, S. B., Boyden, C. M., Lokish, J., and Wilson, R. E.: Adrenalectomy with Chemotherapy in the Treatment of Advanced Breast Cancer: Objective and Subjective Response Rates; Duration and Quality of Life, *Surgery,* **76:**376, 1974.

———, Woodrow, S. I., Aliapoulios, M. A., and Wilson,

R. E.: Carcinoma of the Breast: A Decade of New Results with Old Concepts, *N Engl J Med,* **277:**293, 1967.

Moore, S. W., and Lewis, R. J.: Carcinoma of the Breast in Women 30 Years of Age and Under, *Surg Gynecol Obstet,* **119:**1253, 1964.

Mouridsen, H. T., Palshof, T., Brahm, M., and Rahbek, I.: Evaluation of Single-Drug Versus Multiple-Drug Chemotherapy in the Treatment of Advanced Breast Cancer, *Cancer Treat Rep,* **61:**47, 1977.

Mueller, C. B., and Jeffries, W.: Cancer of the Breast: Its Outcome as Measured by the Rate of Dying and Causes of Pain, *Ann Surg,* **182:**334, 1975.

Murad, T. M.: A Proposed Histochemical and Electron Microscopic Classification of Human Breast Cancer According to Cell of Origin, *Cancer,* **27:**288, 1971.

Murray, J. G., MacIntyre, J., Simpson, J. S., and McDonald, A. M.: Cancer Research Campaign Study of the Management of "Early" Breast Cancer, *World J Surg,* **1:**317, 1977.

Nissen-Myer, R., Kjellgren, K., and Mansson, B.: Preliminary Report from the Scandinavian Adjuvant Chemotherapy Study Group, *Cancer Chemother Rep,* **55:**561, 1971.

Norris, H. J., and Taylor, H. B.: Carcinoma of the Breast in Women Less than Thirty Years Old, *Cancer,* **26:**953, 1970.

Oberman, H. A.: Sarcomas of the Breast, *Cancer,* **18:**1233, 1965.

Owen, H. W., Dockerty, M. B., and Gray, H. K.: Occult Carcinoma of the Breast, *Surg Gynecol Obstet,* **98:**302, 1954.

Pack, G. T.: Argument for Bilateral Mastectomy, *Surgery,* **29:**929, 1951. (Editorial.)

Papaioannou, A. N., and Urban, J. A.: Scalene Node Biopsy in Locally Advanced Primary Breast Cancer of Questionable Operability, *Cancer,* **17:**1006, 1964.

Papdrianos, E., Cooley, E., and Haagensen, C. D.: Mammary Carcinoma in Old Age, *Ann Surg.,* **161:**189, 1965.

Park, W. W., and Lees, J. C.: Absolute Curability of Cancer of the Breast, *Surg Gynecol Obstet,* **93:**129, 1951.

Parson, W. H.: "Cancer of the Breast," Charles C Thomas, Publisher, Springfield, Ill., 1959.

Pennisi, V. R., Capozzi, A., and Perez, F. M.: Subcutaneous Mastectomy Data, *Plast Reconstr Surg,* **59:**53, 1977.

Pichon, M. F., and Milgrom, E.: Characterization and Assay of Progesterone Receptor in Human Mammary Carcinoma, *Cancer Res,* **37:**464, 1977.

Priestman, T., Baum, M., Jones, V., and Forbes, J.: Comparative Trial of Endocrine Versus Cytotoxic Treatment in Advanced Breast Cancer, *Br Med J,* **1:**1248, 1977.

Prohaska, J. V., Houttuin, E., and Kocandrle, V.: Mammary Carcinoma Metastes: Response to Bilateral Adrenalectomy and Oophorectomy, *Arch Surg,* **92:**530, 1966.

Prosnitz, L. R., Goldenberg, I. S., Packard, R. A., Levene, M. B., Harris, J., Hellman, S., Wallner, P. E., Brady, L. W., Mansfield, C. M., and Kramer, S.: Radiation Therapy as Initial Treatment for Early Stage Cancer of the Breast without Mastectomy, *Cancer,* **39:**917, 1977.

Richards, G. J., Jr., and Lewison, E. F.: Inflammatory Carcinoma of the Breast, *Surg Gynecol Obstet,* **113:**729, 1961.

Robbins, G. F., and Berg, J. W.: Bilateral Primary Breast Cancers, *Cancer,* **17:**1501, 1964.

——— and ———: Curability of Patients with Invasive Breast Carcinoma Based on a 30-Year Study, *World J Surg,* **1:**284, 1977.

———, Brothers, J. H., III, Eberhart, W. F., and Quan, S.: Is Aspiration Biopsy of Breast Cancer Dangerous to the Patient? *Cancer,* **7:**774, 1954.

Rosato, F. E., Fink, P. J., Horton, C. E., and Payne, R. L., Jr.: Immediate Postmastectomy Reconstruction, *J Surg Oncolol,* **8:**277, 1976.

Rosen, P. P., Fracchia, A. A., Urban, J. A., Schottenfeld, D., and Robbins, G. F.: "Residual" Mammary Carcinoma Following Simulated Partial Mastectomy, *Cancer,* **35:**739, 1975.

———, Snyder, R. E., Foote, F. W., and Wallace, T.: Detection of Occult Carcinoma in the Apparently Benign Breast Biopsy through Specimen Radiography, *Cancer,* **26:**944, 1970.

Rubin, P.: "Carcinoma of the Breast," American Cancer Society, New York, 1967.

Rush, B. F., Jr.: Axillary Dissection in Breast Cancer: A Staging Procedure, *Surgery,* **77:**478, 1975.

——— and Kramer, W. M.: Proliferative Histological Changes and Occult Carcinoma in the Breast of the Aging Female, *Surg Gynecol Obstet,* **117:**425, 1963.

Sandison, A. T.: An Autopsy Study of the Adult Human Breast, with Special Reference to Proliferative Epithelial Changes of Importance in the Pathology of the Breast, *Natl Cancer Inst Monogr* 8, June 1962.

Sanger, G.: An Aspect of Internal Mammary Metastases from Carcinoma of the Breast, *Ann Surg,* **157:**180, 1963.

Schmidt, M. L., Nemoto, T., and Bross, I. D. J.: Prognostic Factors Affecting Adrenalectomy in Patients with Metastatic Cancer of the Breast, *Cancer,* **27:**1106, 1971.

Schottenfeld, D., Nash, A. G., Robbins, G. F., and Beattie, E. J., Jr.: Ten-Year Results of the Treatment of Primary Operable Breast Carcinoma: A Summary of 304 Patients Evaluated by the TNM System, *Cancer,* **38:**1001, 1976.

Schwartz, H. M., and Reichling, B. A.: The Risks of Mammograms, *JAMA,* **237:**965, 1977.

Seidman, H.: Screening for Breast Cancer in Younger Women: Life Expectancy Gains and Losses: An Analysis According to Risk Indicator Groups, *Ca,* **27:**66, 1977.

Sherlock, P., and Hartmann, W. H.: Adrenal Steroids and the Pattern of Metastases of Breast Cancer, *JAMA,* **181:**103, 1962.

Shimkin, M. B.: Cancer of the Breast: Some Old Facts and New Perspectives, *JAMA,* **183:**358, 1963.

———, Koppel, M., Connelly, R. R., and Cutler, S. J.: Simple and Radical Mastectomy for Breast Cancer: A Re-analysis of Smith and Meyer's Report from Rockford, Illinois, *J Natl Cancer Inst,* **27:**1197, 1961.

Shingleton, W. W., Sedransk, N., and Johnson, R. O.: Systemic Chemotherapy for Mammary Carcinoma, *Ann Surg,* **173:**913, 1971.

Silverstrini, R., Sanfilippo, O., and Tedesco, G.: Kinetics of Human Mammary Carcinomas and Their Correlations with the Cancer and the Host Characteristics, *Cancer,* **34:**1252, 1974.

Strax, P.: New Techniques in Mass Screening for Breast Cancer, *Cancer,* **28:**1563, 1971.

Sugarbaker, E. D.: Extended Radical Mastectomy: Its Superiority in the Treatment of Breast Cancer, *JAMA,* **187:**95, 1964.

Surgical Adjuvant Chemotherapy Breast Group: Breast Adjuvant Chemotherapy: Effectiveness of Thio-tepa (Triethylenethiophosphoramide) as Adjuvant to Radical Mastectomy for Breast Cancer, *Ann Surg,* **154:**629, 1961.

Tellem, M., Prive, L., and Meranze, D. R.: Four-quadrant Study of Breast Removed for Carcinoma, *Cancer,* **15:**10, 1962.

Treves, N., and Holleb, A. I.: Cancer of the Male Breast: A Report of 46 Cases, *Cancer,* **8:**1239, 1955.

Urban, J. A.: Bilaterality of Cancer of the Breast: Biopsy of the Opposite Breast, *Cancer,* **20:**1867, 1971.

——— and Baker, H. W.: Radical Mastectomy in Continuity with En Bloc Resection of the Internal Mammary Lymph-Node Chain: A New Procedure for Primary Operable Cancer of the Breast, *Cancer,* **5:**992, 1952.

Veronesi, U., Rossi, A., and Bonadonna, G.: Adjuvant Combination Chemotherapy with CMF in Primary Mammary Carcinoma, *World J Surg,* **1:**337, 1977.

Wanebo, H. J., Huvos, A. G., and Urban, J. A.: Treatment of Minimal Breast Cancer, *Cancer,* **33:**349, 1974.

Watts, G. T.: Restorative Prosthetic Mammaplasty in Mastectomy for Carcinoma and Benign Lesions, *Clin Plast Surg,* **3:**177, 1976.

Williams, I. G., and Curwen, M. P.: Total Mastectomy with Axillary Dissection and Irradiation for Mammary Carcinoma, *Ann Surg,* **157:**174, 1963.

Willis, K. J., London, D. R., Ward, H. W. C., Butt, W. R., Lynch, S. S., and Rudd, B. T.: Recurrent Breast Cancer Treated with the Antiestrogen Tamoxifen: Correlation between Hormonal Changes and Clinical Course, *Br Med J,* **1:**425, 1977.

Zippin, C., and Petrakis, N. L.: Identification of High Risk Groups in Breast Cancer, *Cancer,* **28:**1381, 1971.

Benign Lesions

Davis, H. H., Simons, M., and Davis, J. B.: Cystic Disease of the Breast: Relationship to Carcinoma, *Cancer,* **17:**957, 1964.

Frantz, V. K., Pickren, J. W., Melcher, G. W., and Auchincloss, H., Jr.: Incidence of Chronic Cystic Disease in So-called "Normal Breasts": A Study Based on 225 Postmortem Examinations, *Cancer,* **4:**762, 1951.

Grow, J. L., and Lewison, E. F.: Superficial Thrombophlebitis of the Breast, *Surg Gynecol Obstet,* **116:**180, 1963.

Urban, J. A.: Excision of Major Ducts of the Breast, *Cancer,* **16:**516, 1963.

Chapter 16

Tumors of the Head and Neck

by Benjamin F. Rush, Jr.

HISTORICAL BACKGROUND

The head and neck are such public regions of the anatomy that one would expect ancient medical manuscripts to give considerable attention to tumors affecting these parts. Strangely, the ancient writers rarely mention such lesions. The Smith Papyrus (2300 B.C.) mentions wounds of the head frequently, but not a single tumor of the area is discussed. The Ebers Papyrus (1500 B.C.) contains references to "eating ulcer" of the gums and "illness of the tongue," but the descriptions are too brief to be adequately interpreted. Celsus (A.D. 178) is often credited with devising an operation for cancer of the lower lip. Martin notes that Celsus recognized and described cancer of the skin of the face, but his operation on the lower lip was for repair of a "mutilation," probably a war wound.

A perusal of *The Surgery of Theodoric* (A.D. 1267) in the translation of Campbell and Colton gives an interesting perspective of the personal experiences of a master surgeon of the era who had a profound knowledge of the writings of preceding centuries. Theodoric describes numerous lesions about the head and neck, mostly of minor significance, i.e., wens, "white pustules or spots which appear by the nose and over the cheeks," "lumps or swellings occurring on the head called horns," "nodes or wens which are formed on the eyelids," lipoma, pustules on the face, freckles, brown patches, wrinkles, and black and blue spots on the face. There is a lengthy section on "the scrofula." He had a much clearer concept of cancer than most of his contemporaries, but in his entire writing he does not mention the treatment of a single lesion of the lip or intraoral area.

This frequent failure to single out cancerous lesions in this area reflects the inability of our medical ancestors to differentiate grossly between chronic infections and cancer. Certainly some miraculous cures were achieved by ointments and spells applied to hard, round ulcers which, in fact, were chronic infections. An early, operable lesion was certain to be treated at length with salves and potions, and when it was evident beyond doubt that the treatment had failed, it was too late to do anything else.

Galen had established firmly the concept that cancer was a systemic disease, an oversupply of black bile. It made more sense by this concept to treat the systemic cause of the affliction by "proper balancing of the constitution" with bleeding or purging or hot and cold baths than it did to attack directly a symptom of the internal problem which happened to occur on the face or in the mouth. The beginnings of rational operations for cancer awaited the discovery of cancer's primary origin in the various organs and the ability to differentiate cancer grossly and microscopically from other confusingly similar diseases.

In addition to the problems of diagnosis, extensive cancer operations were impossible without anesthesia. Even minor operations about the head and neck were few when the patient had to be conscious to witness them. The gruesome habit of excising the tongue for torture and punishment is as old as man, but the first such excision for cancer is attributed to Marchette in 1664. Avicenna (980–1037) described excision of tumors of the lip, the wound being left open to heal by secondary intention, but the classic V excision for cancer of the lip was not described until the first part of the nineteenth century. Tracheotomy to relieve laryngeal obstruction was described by Galen and through the ages was occasionally used to prolong somewhat the lives of those with carcinoma of the larynx, but laryngectomy was not accomplished until the late nineteenth century.

With the advent of anesthesia and microscopic pathology in the mid-1800s, operative attack upon cancer in all areas moved swiftly forward. This was especially true of tumors of the head and neck, since they involved easily seen structures and were so readily diagnosed and the suffering of the untreated patients was so apparent. Surgeons of the German school introduced an array of new techniques for operations upon the tongue, gingiva, mandible, maxilla, and larynx. Partial laryngectomy was introduced by Gurdon Buck in 1853, and total laryngectomy for cancer was first accomplished by Billroth in 1873.

In general, the results of these new procedures were more horrifying than gratifying. Operations in a septic field and without antibiotics produced a postoperative complication rate close to 100 percent with cellulitis, sepsis, abscess, pneumonia, and death the common results. Mortality rates exceeded 50 percent. Moreover, the results of many of the early and unsophisticated operations were not much better than if the cancer had not been treated. Billroth's famous first laryngectomy left the patient with an open pharyngostome and esophagostome, so that he constantly drooled saliva over his neck and had to feed himself with a rubber tube during the entire 8 months that he survived operation.

Operative excision was usually confined to the primary lesion, and in many of the patients fortunate enough to survive the initial operation metastatic disease subsequently developed in cervical nodes. Kocher and Butlin recognized this problem early and recommended excision of the lymphatic contents of the anterior triangle of the neck together with the removal of the primary lesion in the mouth.

At the turn of the century Crile devised radical neck dissection, removing all lymphatic tissue in both the anterior and posterior triangles of the neck together with the jugular vein and the sternocleidomastoid muscle. The basic elements of his classic procedure remain valid to the present.

Patients were willing to risk the high morbidity and mortality of operations in this region because the relentless progress of untreated disease offered a slow death by asphyxia, malnutrition, and eventual hemorrhage. Even the slimmest chance of avoiding this terrible triad seemed worthwhile.

As Crile was developing his operation for treating the cervical lymph nodes, radiation therapy for cancer was introduced. This, it was quickly apparent, offered a preferable alternative to operation, especially for primary lesions of the skin and oral cavity. Until the end of the 1930s most radical operations for cancers of the head and neck were abandoned, and the primary therapy was radiation. Techniques of radiation therapy became more refined and more successful. External radiation replaced radium as the treatment of choice, and fractionated therapy replaced the use of single applications of radium or a single dose of external therapy. With each refinement the percentage of patients who were cured increased. It was soon found that metastatic deposits in the neck did not respond as well to radiation as to operation, and radical neck dissection remained in use. Occasionally, patients who failed to respond to radiation or who had recurrent cancers were submitted to one or another of the old radical procedures. But when these operations were performed in a heavily irradiated fibrotic field, wound breakdown and complications often resembled the results of surgical treatment of the prior century.

In the 1940s, the introduction of endotracheal anesthesia, liberal use of blood transfusions, and antibiotics markedly changed the ability of surgeons to operate in and about the oral cavity. Postoperative morbidity and mortality dropped to a reasonable level. Radiation therapy, so long dominant in the treatment of oral lesions, seemed at a plateau with much dissatisfaction concerning the morbidity of overtreatment. These factors led to a reevaluation of operation. Grant Ward of The Johns Hopkins Hospital and Hayes Martin of the Memorial Center for Cancer led in devising combined operations whereby the primary lesions and the cervical contents were removed in a single block.

Application of this principle improved substantially the prognosis of patients with head and neck carcinomas, especially large lesions involving the oral cavity, hypopharynx, and larynx. In some institutions the pendulum swung from almost exclusive use of radiotherapy to almost exclusive use of operation. Increasing application of these combined operations during the 1950s made possible an evaluation of their mortality, morbidity, and effectiveness. By the end of the decade the place for surgical control of head and neck lesions was much more clearly defined and accepted.

Because of the late development of operative therapy after the long period of dormancy during the radiation era, this field of surgery is still something of a frontier with rapid developments of new techniques and the evolution of new ideas and approaches.

In the meantime, radiation therapy also acquired new techniques. Supervoltage radiation, originally with cobalt 60 and later with linear accelerators, delivered higher doses of therapy with a decreased morbidity, especially sparing the patient's skin and leaving a field more suitable for operation when this was required. Radiotherapists and surgeons who previously tended to disparage the results of each other's methods and to advance their own techniques as the primary treatment for tumors suddenly found that there was considerable common ground for the two methods and that there were patients who frequently could benefit from both operation and radiation as a planned course of integrated treatment.

Detection of most lesions of the head and neck is relatively easy, since the majority are readily available to the eye and the examining finger. Even so, it is tragic to find how often malignant lesions of this area are overlooked, not only lesions more difficult to diagnose, as in the maxillary sinuses and hypopharynx, but lesions readily visualized, such as tumors of the floor of the mouth, tongue, and tonsil.

DIAGNOSIS

Physical Examination

SKIN. The skin (see Chap. 14) of the face and neck should be closely scrutinized, keeping in mind that basal and squamous carcinomas of the skin are the most common of all cancers and that the most common site for such lesions is the area of the head and neck. Seborrheic keratosis, senile keratosis, and patches of atrophic skin often appear side by side with skin neoplasms. Differential diagnosis may be difficult, and biopsy is often required. Pigmented lesions must be examined closely to determine the presence of bleeding ulceration or satellitosis indicating melanoma. All lumps should be palpated to observe their firmness, whether they have a cystic or solid quality and whether they are fixed to the underlying tissues.

ORAL CAVITY. The oral cavity is often neglected in the course of a complete physical examination. It is said that the internist looks at the top of the tongue depressor, the otolaryngologist looks at the tonsils, and the general surgeon may not look at all. There is no excuse for this neglect, since the oral cavity is a rich source of pathologic processes, not only of local lesions, but often of lesions reflecting pathologic conditions elsewhere in the body.

Proper examination requires the use of a tongue depressor, finger cot or glove, and good lighting. If the examiner is skilled with the use of a head mirror, this will provide ideal illumination. However, there are numerous electric headlights which work equally well and which can be used at different points in the office or at the bedside without requiring an elaborate setup.

With the patient's mouth open, the light is directed into the oral cavity. If the patient has dentures of any sort, they should be removed. The examiner begins by looking at the anterior floor of the mouth and the openings of Wharton's ducts. Then the floor of the mouth is observed, progressing posteriorly along the gingivolingual gutter to the tonsillar pillars on either side. The undersurface of the anterior and lateral tongue can also be observed. This is a good place to detect early jaundice.

The lower gingiva and teeth are examined next. The condition of the teeth and the presence or absence of sepsis are considered. The gingivobuccal gutters are often the hiding place of small malignant lesions and should be inspected thoroughly.

The buccal mucosa can be examined next. Patches of hyperkeratosis are often seen here. The examiner looks for the nipple indicating the opening of Stensen's duct. Pressure on the parotid should express saliva from the orifice. The position and mobility of the tongue are observed. A deviated tongue may indicate injury to the hypoglossal nerve or a previous stroke. Numerous longitudinal fissures reflect previous syphilis, a condition now rarely seen. Malignant lesions are normally found on the edges or at the tip of the tongue.

Occasionally, a patch of dirty fibers will occupy the surface of the tongue. This condition, called "hairy tongue," often occurs in a dry mouth with impaired sali-

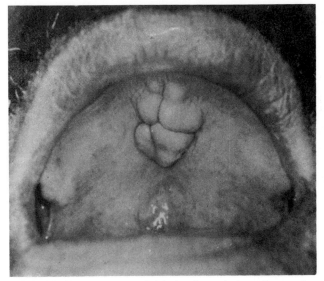

Fig. 16-1. Torus, a congenital lesion formed along the median raphe where the palatine processes of the maxilla join. These protuberances are normally smooth; the lobulation seen here is unusual.

vary secretion. Vitamin deficiencies are reflected by an atrophy of the taste buds with a flat, smooth, erythematous mucosa.

The tonsils and soft palate are considered next. The presence or absence of the tonsils or tonsillar tags should be noted. If the patient gags, the posterior tonsillar pillars rotate toward the midline, better exposing the tonsillar fossa itself. The anterior tonsillar pillar is a common site for patches of hyperkeratosis, or sometimes for very early carcinomas. Inappropriate hypertrophy of one tonsil may reflect a lymphoma. Paralysis of one side of the soft palate is often seen in patients who have had a cerebrovascular accident. Large tumors in the nasopharynx may push the soft palate forward and down.

The examiner can complete his observations with inspection of the hard palate. A smooth or occasionally lobular elevation running down the midline of the palate is usually a torus, a harmless, congenital deformity (Fig. 16-1). Tori of the mandible also occur, projecting into the mouth bilaterally at the level of the canine tooth. They have no particular importance except to the frightened patient who may notice them for the first time in adulthood and mistake them for new growths. Occasionally, patients with atrophied lower alveoli following total loss of the lower teeth will have a spur which projects backward from the midline into the floor of the mouth. This represents a prominence of the symphysis made detectable by the absorption of the surrounding bone.

Palpation is equal in importance to inspection. Many early lesions of the oral cavity cannot be detected except by the sense of touch. This is especially true of lesions buried within the substance of the tongue or in the salivary glands. The gloved finger is passed over the tongue, the floor of the mouth, and the gingivobuccal gutters. Any mass encountered can be made more prominent by bimanual or bidigital palpation, pressing the mass inward from the cheek or submental area toward the oral cavity. If the patient can tolerate it, palpation of the lateral pharyngeal wall may reveal masses in the deep lobe of the parotid. If the index of suspicion is high concerning lesions in the nasopharynx or base of tongue, these areas should be palpated as well.

NECK. Inspection and palpation of the cervical area are done methodically, keeping in mind a distinct list of structures to be felt. These should include the larynx, thyroid, trachea, sternocleidomastoid muscle, lymph node–bearing areas, and salivary glands. The submental area is examined for the presence of enlarged lymph nodes and the size and consistency of the submaxillary glands. In the older patient they may hang low in the anterior cervical triangle as the enveloping fascia becomes lax with age. In this location they often are mistaken initially for enlarged lymph nodes. The presence of any enlarged or firm lymph nodes incorporated within the substance of the submaxillary gland should be noted. Bimanual palpation through the floor of the mouth helps greatly.

The angle of the jaw is a common site for enlarged lymph nodes or not infrequently of a tumor in the tail of the parotid gland. The anterior border of the sternocleidomastoid may overlap a cystic mass representing a branchial cleft cyst. Cystic or fluctuant masses in the posterior cervical triangle may represent a lipoma or a cystic lymphangioma.

The most important consideration in the adult is the presence of enlarged lymph nodes. A number of structures in the neck deceive the novice and at first appear to be enlarged lymph nodes when in fact they are normal structures. The carotid bulb is commonly so mistaken, especially in older patients in whom arteriosclerosis has diminished or obliterated the pulse at the bulb. The tip of the hyoid bone adjacent to the carotid bulb sometimes fools the unwary, unless they are clever enough to palpate for this structure bilaterally. The posterior belly of the omohyoid muscle as it crosses the posterior triangle in the thin patient can mimic a fusiform node until the examiner realizes that the ends of the apparent node cannot be felt. Also in thin patients the tips of the transverse process of the second cervical vertebra are felt posterior to the ascending ramus of the mandible and may seem like a lymph node until it is realized that the structures are bony in consistency and bilateral.

Masses in the thyroid are best felt if the examiner stands behind the patient and palpates the lobes of the gland between thumb and forefinger. A midline mass just above the isthmus of the thyroid may represent an enlarged lymph node, a pyramidal lobe of thyroid, or a thyroglossal duct cyst.

PARANASAL SINUSES. The paranasal sinuses are relatively inaccessible to physical examination. Neoplastic lesions often hide within these recesses and are not manifest until quite late. Bulging, particularly asymmetric bulging of one maxillary sinus, can best be appreciated by observing the cheeks from above either by having the patient lean toward the examiner or by standing above the patient and looking down (Fig. 16-2). Palpation of the maxillary, ethmoid, or temporal areas may elicit tenderness or a sense of fullness. Transillumination of the sinuses by a bright light placed within the oral cavity of a patient in a dark room may reveal opacification of one or more of the sinuses. This is a relatively crude method of examination compared to x-ray examination.

INDIRECT LARYNGOSCOPY. There is a common misconception that indirect laryngoscopy is an examination to be performed only by specialists. Hoarseness and throat pain are such common symptoms and cancer of the pharynx and larynx so frequent that indirect laryngoscopy should be part of the armamentarium of any physician and part of the routine general physical examination.

The patient is seated in a chair slightly higher than the chair or stool of the examiner. The examiner sits opposite him with his right thigh and knee parallel and immediately adjacent to the right thigh and knee of the patient. The patient should extend his neck, thrusting his chin straight forward, as though he had just finished sneezing. The patient's tongue is wrapped in a gauze sponge, and the examiner, if he is right-handed, grasps the tip of the tongue between the thumb and second finger of the left hand, using the first finger to elevate the patient's upper lip. The tongue is drawn forward, and the patient is instructed to breathe rapidly in short, quick breaths, to "pant like a dog." As long as the patient continues to breathe in this fashion, gagging is inhibited. The examiner inserts a medium to large laryngeal mirror, previously flamed to keep it from fogging, into the oropharynx and shines his headlight on the mirror, reflecting a spot of light down into the hypopharynx (Fig. 16-3).

If one is a novice with the head mirror, an electric head lamp should be used. With the mirror in the oropharynx and directed downward, the posterior third of the tongue, the lateral pharyngeal wall, the posterior pharyngeal wall, the epiglottis, the valleculae, and the pyriform sinuses can all be examined thoroughly. The epiglottis will usually hide most of the glottic opening, and only the posterior portions of the arytenoids may be seen at first. The patient is told to breathe deeply several times. This often throws the uvula forward until more of the glottic opening and a little of the subglottic space is seen. The patient is asked to attempt to enunciate an "ee" sound. This throws the epiglottis even farther forward and usually brings the entire glottis, including the anterior commissure, into view.

The false cords, aryepiglottic folds, and posterior epiglottis can now be examined. The movement of the cords is considered, to determine whether both are moving adequately and whether they meet in the midline. Paralysis of one cord may indicate a malignant lesion in the mediastinum or cervical area or may be related to previous operation or cerebrovascular accident. If nodules in the pharynx or posterior tongue are noted, they should subsequently be palpated. As the examiner acquires skill in this procedure, most of these examinations can be accomplished without local anesthesia. Topical anesthesia with lidocaine 1% (preferably) or Pontocaine 1% should be used by the beginner.

In one or two patients out of every twenty, examination is incomplete or impossible because of a hypersensitive gag reflex or an acquired or congenital malformation of the

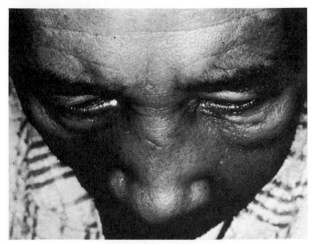

Fig. 16-2. Early swelling of the maxilla, seen best from above, as shown here. The patient had a space-occupying lesion within the sinus which was not as well appreciated in the frontal view.

epiglottis which makes visualization of the glottis impossible. In such instances, direct laryngoscopy must be used. While direct laryngoscopy is the more sophisticated and complex procedure, indirect laryngoscopy actually gives a

Fig. 16-3. Laryngeal mirror examination of the larynx. Cross section of the oral cavity illustrates the relation of the mirror to the larynx. Insert: View seen by the examiner. Note the epiglottis hiding the anterior portion of the cords.

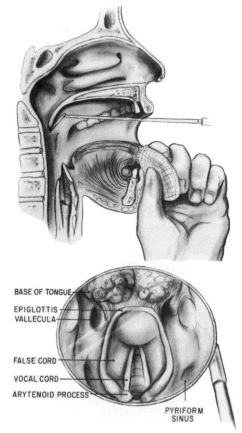

BASE OF TONGUE
EPIGLOTTIS
VALLECULA
FALSE CORD
VOCAL CORD
ARYTENOID PROCESS
PYRIFORM SINUS

better overall picture of the larynx and pharynx. The chief reason for resorting to direct laryngoscopy other than the above is the necessity of biopsy of lesions deep in the larynx. Direct laryngoscopy is sometimes performed using a *suspension laryngoscope,* which, once the cords are visualized, can be fixed in place so that the operator does not have to use his hands to hold the laryngoscope. This technique can be combined with the use of an optical device which greatly magnifies the cords so that small irregularities and tiny lesions may be examined. Occasionally in patients with unexplained hoarseness this approach will reveal very early any localized benign and malignant changes.

NASOPHARYNGOSCOPY. The mirror used for indirect laryngoscopy may be turned over and directed upward. The examiner, standing at the patient's shoulder and depressing the tongue with a tongue blade, may shine his headlight on the mirror and gain a fairly spacious view of the nasopharynx. In most instances the space between the soft palate and posterior pharyngeal wall is too small for the nasopharynx to be adequately visualized in this fashion. If physical findings or the history so indicate, complete examination of the nasopharynx is done by inserting a soft rubber #10 French catheter through either nasal passage, drawing its tip out through the mouth and retracting the soft palate forward, revealing the entire nasopharynx for indirect examination by the mirror (Fig. 16-4). The torus tubarius, the openings of the eustachian tubes, the posterior surface of the soft palate, the posterior aspect of the nasal septum arching back toward the sphe-

Fig. 16-4. Mirror view of the nasopharynx. Soft palate is drawn forward, and the mirror in the oropharynx is directed upward. Insert: View seen in the mirror.

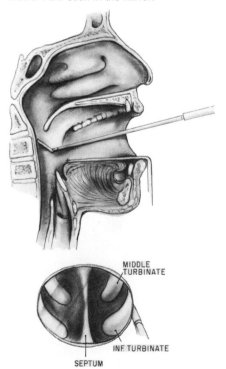

MIDDLE TURBINATE

INF. TURBINATE

SEPTUM

noid sinus, and the posterior tips of the turbinates are seen. The normal lymphatic tissue of the adenoids may lend a granular appearance to some of the posterior and superior mucosal surfaces.

The direct nasopharyngoscope is an instrument which can be used in the office. It is a small instrument like a miniature cystoscope and has a Foroblique or right-angled lens. The diameter of the tube is 5 to 8 mm, and the visual field is quite small and easily obscured by mucus or blood. Use of this instrument is a valuable adjunct to indirect inspection of the nasopharynx and is particularly helpful in searching for small neoplasms.

Diagnostic Studies

RADIOGRAPHY. Most of the bones of the face and neck are adjacent to air-filled cavities or are air-containing, creating an excellent situation for diagnostic roentgenograms. Lesions of the paranasal sinuses, nasal cavity, orbit, mandible, and larynx are readily revealed.

Arteriography. Injection of contrast medium into the vessels is a useful maneuver for evaluating tumors within the cranium or evaluating the arterial tree but has only rare indications for the evaluation of tumors in this region. The rare carotid body tumor can be nicely outlined by the use of radiopaque medium injected into the appropriate common carotid artery, and its appearance when examined in this fashion is pathognomonic. At times, arteriography is useful to outline the extent of a hemangioma of the face or oral cavity (Fig. 16-5).

Laminography. This technique is of great usefulness in examinations of the head and neck, especially for minute examination of the bony walls of the paranasal sinuses. Usually, the clouding of a paranasal sinus by tumor and by infection cannot be differentiated by x-ray unless obvious evidence of bone erosion is seen. Early detection of such erosions is best seen in laminographs. Tumors of the larynx are easily seen from above by indirect laryngoscopy, but their inferior extent is hidden from view unless the lesion is very small. Laminograms and lateral soft tissue views of the larynx play a useful role in revealing the extent of subglottic extension and often the degree of involvement of the pyriform sinuses, which may not otherwise be detectable (Fig. 16-6). Details of retropharyngeal and esophageal tumor spread can be seen on the lateral soft tissue view. Laryngograms are performed by the application of barium to the back of the tongue, cords, epiglottis, and all of the intrinsic larynx. A very clear examination of laryngeal structures can be obtained which offers excellent correlation with other diagnostic methods available.

BIOPSY. The vast majority of head and neck lesions can be easily biopsied in the office or clinic. The tools required are simple, and the procedure is short and uncomplicated. Lesions of the lip, skin, gingiva, floor of the mouth, tongue, and buccal mucosa can quickly be biopsied with a 4-mm dermatologist's skin punch. The area to be biopsied is cleansed with an antiseptic agent infiltrated with a small amount of local anesthesia, and the skin punch is pressed into the lesion to a depth of 4 to 6 mm, cutting a small disk of the tumor, and is withdrawn. The core of tissue which is still connected at its base is grasped with forceps, pulled up until the base is flush with the surface tissues, and cut off with a small pair of scissors. A silver nitrate stick thrust into the depth of the remaining cavity and mild pressure for a minute or two control bleeding in almost all instances. Lesions of the soft palate, tonsillar pillar, or posterior tongue which cannot be reached with a skin punch can often be biopsied easily and quickly with a cervical biopsy forcep; the techniques of anesthesia and hemostasis are essentially the same as described above.

If skill is obtained with indirect laryngoscopy, lesions of the lateral pharyngeal wall, pyriform sinus, epiglottis, and aryepiglottic folds can often be quickly biopsied in the office. While similar biopsies of the true and false cords sometimes can be achieved with skillful manipulation of the indirect mirror, such procedures are best carried out under direct laryngoscopy. Manipulation of biopsy forceps immediately above the cords is much more difficult for the patient to tolerate and may stimulate laryngeal spasm and bleeding at a site where aspiration of blood into the trachea is likely.

Biopsy of the primary lesion is always preferable, but sometimes although cervical nodes are enlarged, no primary tumor can be found. If so, needle biopsy of cervical nodes is indicated and is a rewarding procedure when the node contains metastatic squamous carcinoma. This neoplasm is easily diagnosed even with the smallest fragments of tissue. Nodes involved by lymphoma, on the other hand, are virtually impossible to diagnose by needle biopsy. Positive results of needle biopsy are useful and timesaving; the negative result of a needle biopsy has no significance and must be followed by open biopsy.

There has been much controversy concerning the tendency to spread tumor cells with the use of needle biopsies, and certainly it seems likely that tumor cells are spread into the needle tract by this manipulation. However, this is of greater theoretical than practical importance. Long experience with this technique at a number of major centers has not produced any gross difference in survival rates on long-term follow-up either in the head and neck or elsewhere. Open biopsy of a lymph node seems just as likely to scatter tumor cells, and even more widely.

VITAL DYES. Many cancers of the oral mucosa in their early stages are soft and superficial. They may have an erythematous appearance rather than a white color as usually thought and can easily escape detection even in a careful examination. If suspicion is aroused by a vaguely erythematous patch, the application of toluidine blue will aid in making the diagnosis. This technique will distinguish areas of dysplasia and carcinoma in situ as well as frank carcinoma of the mucosa. The method has its chief use in mapping out the full extent of dysplastic areas or areas of intraepithelial carcinoma.

CYTOLOGY. As used in the oral cavity exfoliative cytology is a superficial biopsy, since it does not reflect collection of fluid from the entire oral cavity but involves scraping a specific lesion with a spatula and spreading this scraping on a slide. Such cytologic examinations, therefore,

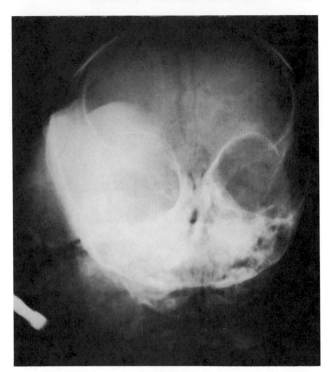

Fig. 16-5. Arteriographic demonstration of hemangioma of the oral cavity. On physical examination, only the cheek appeared involved. In the x-ray view, involvement of the lateral pharyngeal wall and oral cavity is noted. (*From B. F. Rush, Jr., Ann Surg, 164:921, 1966.*)

require a specific area of suspicion compared to sampling of an entire anatomic area such as in the cervix or bronchial tree. If a specific lesion is present, it is best evaluated by an actual biopsy. The chief virtue of oral cytology is that the physician who cannot bring himself to use office biopsy techniques or who feels they are beyond his competence can still have the opportunity to obtain a histologic specimen from the lesion in question. Unlike biopsy, cytology has no significance when it is negative. Thus, cytology will establish the presence of a lesion but cannot be relied on to rule that a questionable lesion is not malignant.

LIP

Squamous cell carcinomas of the lip are one of the common malignant tumors of the oral cavity, constituting 15 percent of all such lesions and 2.2 percent of all cancers. Basal cell carcinoma is much less frequent; only about 3 are seen for every 100 squamous cell carcinomas of the lip. Benign lesions which are occasionally seen in the lips include mucous cysts, tumors of the minor salivary glands, hemangiomas, lymphangiomas, venous lakes, fibromas, fissures, and hyperkeratosis.

ETIOLOGY. Like tumors of the skin, there is an important relationship between tumors of the lip and exposure to sunlight. About one-third of patients have a history of working outdoors, and the incidence of malignant squa-

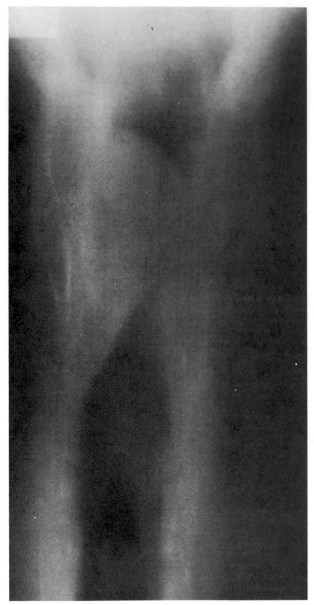

Fig. 16-6. Laminogram of the pharynx. Indirect laryngoscopy would show only the supraglottic portion of the tumor. The laminographic view indicates the large transglottic and subglottic component of the lesion. [*From B. F. Rush and R. H. Greenlaw (eds)., "Integrated Radiation and Operation in Cancer Therapy: A Symposium," Charles C Thomas, Publisher, Springfield, Ill., 1968.*]

mous cancers of the lip increases progressively the farther south the latitude of the patient population being considered. Thus, in the United States the highest incidence is in Florida and Texas. Actinic rays are stronger at higher altitudes and in dryer air, and in areas having these features the incidence of lip (and skin) cancer is increased. Fishermen, sailors, and farmers are among the occupational groups with an increased incidence.

Complexion also plays a role. Susceptible types are fair-skinned, light, blond or ginger-haired, and blue-eyed, with the kind of complexion that freckles and burns rather than tans on exposure to the sun. Resistant people have the opposite characteristics: they are brunet and dark-skinned; blacks are rarely affected.

While there is a relation between lip cancer and tobacco, the exact cause for this is less apparent than in patients with lesions of the intraoral area, larynx, or lungs. The average cigarette smoker receives almost no carcinogen from his tobacco directly to the lips, since the smoke is drawn into the oral cavity and tracheobraonchial tree without passing over the mucosa of the lips themselves. Some feel that the inmates of nursing homes and institutions are more prone to have carcinoma of the lip from cigarette smoking. Smokers in this population usually treasure their cigarettes, smoking them down to the smallest possible butt. Macerated, moist tobacco and heat are directly applied to the lips.

Reports in the literature implicating pipe smoking as a cause of lip cancer have been appearing since 1795, and the Advisory Committee to the Surgeon General on Smoking and Health has accepted the causal relationship as established. Pipestems of wood and clay which soak up tobacco tars directly and apply a "tar poultice" to the lips have been viewed with special suspicion. In any case, such stems are little used now, and indeed the incidence of cancer of the lip in the United States has been gradually decreasing over the past 30 years. One may speculate whether this reflects the decrease in pipe smoking, outdoor work, use of wood and clay pipestems, or a combination of these and other factors.

Cancer of the lip in women is very rare, occurring in only 1 woman for every 20 to 30 men.

Benign Tumors

The mucosa of the inner surface of the upper and lower lips is subject to the same benign lesions as those throughout the mucosa of the oral cavity. These are discussed in greater detail in the following section, Oral Cavity, and include such lesions as mucous cysts, hemangiomas, tumors of the minor salivary glands, hyperkeratosis, and inflammatory hyperplasia. Specific benign lesions that involve the exposed borders of the lips include venous lakes, pigmented spots, hemangiomas, and very rarely neuromas. Venous lakes are a telangiectasis, usually of the lower lip, occurring in older individuals as a small bluish spot. They appear to have no pathologic significance. The other three lesions all have interesting systemic correlations. Multiple pigmented spots of the lips may be associated with Peutz-Jeghers syndrome and denote the presence of multiple small intestinal polyps, which sometimes lead to bleeding and intussusception but are rarely malignant. Scattered small hemangiomas of the lip may be associated with similar lesions elsewhere in the oral cavity and gastrointestinal tract, those of Rendu-Osler-Weber disease. Neuromas of the lips, particularly at the commissures, suggest a neuroendocrine dysplasia, a fascinating syndrome associated with pheochromocytomas, medullary carcinoma of the thyroid, hyperparathyroidism, and hypertrophy of the gastrointestinal myenteric plexus.

Hyperkeratosis

This is a premalignant condition of the lips, usually associated with long exposure to sunlight. It typically occurs in a fair-skinned individual in his sixties or seventies who has a long history of outdoor employment. The normal distinct line marking the mucocutaneous border becomes indistinct and gradually retreats, indicating a metaplasia of the outer portion of the mucosa to a keratosquamous epithelium. The mucosa of the lip becomes paler, thinner, and more fragile. There may be perpendicular cracks and fissures. On this base, a white film indicative of early hyperkeratosis appears. This may grow gradually thicker and more exophytic as the condition progresses (Fig. 16-7) or may remain stationary for many years. Gradually, a small area of scabbing and ulceration occurs. This breakdown within the hyperkeratotic tissue represents a failure of the less resistant areas of hyperkeratosis to tolerate normal wear and tear. When such areas of ulceration appear, they continue to break down and heal and often give rise to carcinoma in situ and eventually invasive carcinoma. Persistent hyperkeratosis is a distinct premalignant lesion, and 35 to 40 percent of all carcinomas of the lip are preceded by this condition. Cancers arising on such a base can be prevented by excising the entire exposed mucosa of the lip, elevating the protected mucosa of the inner lip, and advancing it over the bed of the excised mucosa to form a new lining for the lip. This procedure is called a *lip stripping and resurfacing.*

Carcinoma of the Lip

Most cancers of the lip are squamous carcinomas. When basal cell carcinomas appear, they usually involve the skin of the lip beyond the vermillion border and probably should be considered with the cancers of the skin of the face. Ninety-three percent of the squamous cancers occur on the lower lip. These are usually low-grade, well-differentiated lesions, 80 percent being grade 1 or grade 2. The lesions most frequently start on the outer edge of the mucosa at the vermillion border and seem to favor the middle two-thirds of the lip somewhat more frequently than the commissures (Fig. 16-8).

The natural history of these lesions is of slow but relentless growth. Some grow to great size, destroying the entire lip without ever metastasizing, but the incidence of metastasis gradually increases with the increasing size of the tumors (Fig. 16-9). About 5 to 10 percent of all patients with lip cancer have cervical lymph node metastasis, and in half of these patients only one lymph node is involved. The normal spread of cancer from the lower lip is by way of lymphatics to the submental node on the side of the lesion. Metastases do not involve the opposite submental node unless the primary lesion crosses the midline. Lesions of the upper lip drain to lymph nodes in the anterior portion of the submaxillary gland.

An ulcer of the lip which fails to heal is soon detected by the patient or his friends, and in most urban populations such lesions quickly come to the attention of physi-

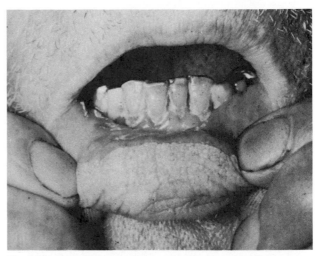

Fig. 16-7. Hyperkeratosis of lower lip. This degree of hyperkeratosis merits serious concern. The entire lower lip is involved and should be treated by excision (lip stripping) and advancement of the mucosa of the inner lip to cover the defect.

cians. In rural populations it is surprising how long patients will carry these ulcerations before seeking medical aid.

Treatment for carcinoma of the lip has remained a topic of controversy between radiotherapists and surgeons for many decades. Recent controlled series comparing treatment by both modalities in randomly selected patients indicate that there is no statistical difference between the two methods in terms of cure rate. The choice for therapy must be made on other grounds. Small lesions of the lip can usually be excised under local anesthesia with little or no hospitalization time. Good radiation therapy producing maximal regression with minimal residual scarring requires 2 to 4 weeks of outpatient therapy. Medium-sized lesions require the use of flaps from the upper lip or elsewhere for closure, and for these lesions radiotherapy often requires the same or less time and less morbidity.

Fig. 16-8. Squamous carcinoma of lip. Any patient with a chronic ulcer of this sort should seek medical advice. The chance of cure at this early stage approaches 100 percent.

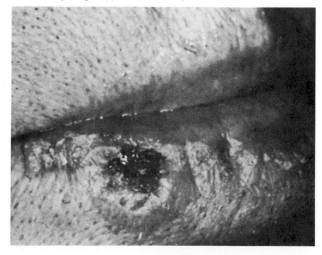

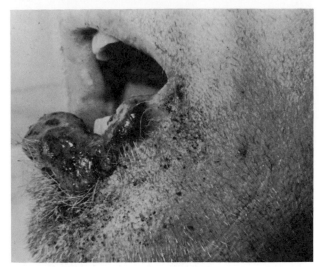

Fig. 16-9. Neglected carcinoma of the lip. A metastatic node is present along the line of the mandible. The chance of cure for this type of lesion is 50 percent or less.

For very large lesions which have destroyed most of the lip and are associated with metastasis to the neck, subsequent repair of the lip will be required under any circumstance as well as probable radical neck dissection for removal of cervical nodes; for these major lesions an integration of radiation and surgical therapy may be used to improve cure rates, which are relatively low for either radiation or operation alone. A final consideration is that most carcinomas of the lip are related to solar radiation. Since radiotherapy increases the sensitivity of tissues to such exposure, it is best to avoid radiotherapy in patients who expect to return to outdoor occupations.

Prognosis for lip cancers of 1 cm or less is excellent, ranging from an 87 to 95 percent 5-year survival rate without recurrence. Neglected lesions, especially with associated cervical metastasis, do much more poorly, with a 5-year survival of 50 percent.

ORAL CAVITY

The oral cavity includes the buccal mucosa, upper and lower gingivae, anterior two-thirds of the tongue (that portion anterior to the circumvallate papillae), floor of the mouth, and hard palate.

INCIDENCE. Eight percent of all malignant tumors occur in this area, 95 percent of such tumors being squamous carcinomas. The risk of carcinomas developing here in a male is approximately 1 percent in a lifetime. The risk in females is far less: oral cancer develops in about 1 woman for every 10 males. Benign tumors of the oral cavity are common in both sexes.

ETIOLOGY. Some benign lesions have a specific cause, which will be discussed with the descriptions of the lesions below. Contributing causes to squamous carcinoma are smoking, a heavy intake of alcohol, poor oral hygiene, and syphilis. While cancer often occurs without the presence of any of these factors, they are associated with a majority of the lesions seen.

The *Report on Smoking and Health* by the Advisory Committee to the Surgeon General notes a suggestive relationship between smoking and oral carcinoma. This is especially true in pipe and cigar smokers, where oral cancer has the highest mortality ratio, 3.3,* of all causes of death compared with the nonsmoking population. There are a number of exotic cancers of the oral cavity which serve to indicate the relationship of tobacco to cancer. In Andhra Pradesh, a state in India, the habit of smoking a cigar (i.e., *chutta*) with the burning end inside the mouth is widespread. Carcinoma of the palate, called *chutta cancer,* is common. Presumably, repeated thermal trauma and/or tobacco smoke provide the carcinogenic agents.

In Uttar Pradesh and Bihar, a mixture of tobacco and slaked lime is habitually sucked by men of the districts. The quid is kept in the lower gingivolabial fornix for many hours during the day; a high incidence of carcinoma is found at this site. This has come to be called *khaini cancer,* from the name of the tobacco-lime mixture.

Betel-nut chewing is a common habit among the Indians, Javanese, and Malayans. The chew is made of a mixture of ground betel nut, slaked lime, and spices, such as ginger or pepper. These are wrapped in a betel leaf and chewed. The Indians add tobacco to their betel preparations and have a high incidence of oral cancer, whereas the incidence is low among the Javanese and Malayans, who consume their betel nut without benefit of the tobacco additive. Among betel nut–tobacco chewers, oral cancer comprises 36 percent of all cancers.

Alcoholism has a highly suggestive role in oral cancer. As many as 42 percent of all patients so afflicted have a history of alcoholism. As a corollary, cirrhosis of the liver is a common finding in patients with oral cancer, 20 percent having cirrhosis as compared to 9 percent in a control population. It has been proposed that alcohol acts as an adjuvant to the use of tobacco in producing oral cancer. This is a difficult point to prove, since finding a control population of patients who drink heavily but do not smoke is virtually impossible.

The roles of poor oral hygiene and oral sepsis, mentioned for decades as etiologic agents for oral cancers, are also difficult to evaluate. These conditions are seen most commonly in patients at the lower end of the social scale and in the ward population rather than in private practice. Oral hygiene is poor in this group, but it cannot be said whether poor hygiene or social level or other correlated factors are responsible.

Syphilis has a direct relation to cancer of one specific site in the oral cavity, the tongue. When syphilitic glossitis, a lesion of late syphilis, heals, it often leaves the tongue fibrotic and scarred with longitudinal fissures and thick hyperkeratotic plaques. It is on this base that lingual cancer develops (Fig. 16-10). In the days of Bloodgood (1921) 21

*That is, 3.3 times as many pipe and cigar smokers died of oral cancer as did nonsmokers in the same age group. The mortality ratio for cancer of the lung in pipe smokers was 1:1, no different from that of the nonsmokers.

percent of American men with lingual cancer had syphilis. Willis still calls this condition "the most clearly established causative factor in European males."

Benign Lesions

Common benign tumors of the oral cavity are inflammatory hyperplasias and cysts. Less commonly seen are giant cell granulomas, salivary tumors, granular cell myoblastomas, dermoids, and hemangiomas.

INFLAMMATORY HYPERPLASIA

The oral mucosa is subject to a number of irritating conditions producing tumorlike projections which are not true neoplasms. Patients develop the nervous habit of sucking a portion of mucosa from the cheek, tongue, or lip between the teeth or through an interdental or edentulous space. The traumatized mucosa becomes edematous and prominent, and the irritation may be compounded by the patient who bites as well as sucks on the offending mucosal fold. Initially, the overlying mucosa is swollen, and eventually this undergoes metaplasia to squamous epithelium. The tissue underlying the elevated mucosa changes from edematous connective tissue to a denser and more fibrotic collection of collagen. At this stage the lesion may be termed a *fibroepithelial polyp* (Fig. 16-11). Similar lesions are often seen in the gingivobuccal gutter and on the palate in patients with ill-fitting dentures. Those lesions which occur along the vestibular mucosa next to the gingiva in this relation are sometimes called *epulis fissurata*. Another appropriate term, more descriptive of the later stages of these lesions when the fibrosis and scarring has advanced, is *irritation fibroma*. In the early inflammatory phase of these lesions, the overlying mucosa is friable and bleeds easily.

The chief responsibility of the examiner who has recognized the lesion is to reassure the patient that it is not malignant. Although these lesions are usually not ulcerated and are easily recognized, diagnosis should be confirmed by biopsy. Treatment is by correction of the causative factor, either by the design of new dentures or by discouraging the patient from manipulating and traumatizing the area involved. Excision may be necessary, but if the basic problem is not abolished, recurrence is prompt.

CYSTS

Mucous cysts are a common oral lesion occurring on the posterior surface of the lip, floor of the mouth, tongue, and buccal mucosa. These cysts arise from the salivary gland–bearing areas of the oral mucosa and were thought to be due to obstruction of the excretory duct of minor salivary glands. It has been found, however, that these cysts have no epithelial lining and that they result from a rupture of the excretory duct. Saliva spills from the defect in the duct and begins to collect in the tissues. At first it forms a diffuse lesion, but soon a circumscribed cyst with a wall of granulation tissue develops. These mucoceles measure from 1 or 2 mm to 1 or 2 cm in diameter and appear as elevated, translucent, bluish lesions of the

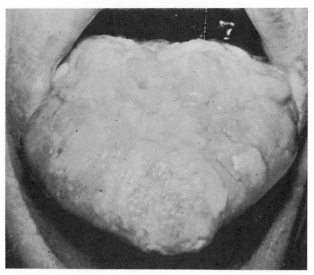

Fig. 16-10. Syphilis of the tongue. The dense, white patches are sometimes mistaken for "geographic tongue." Cancers of the dorsal surface often follow this condition.

mucosa (Fig. 16-12). They frequently rupture, discharging sticky mucoid material, and then recur as the laceration in the overlying mucosa heals. Treatment consists of wide surgical unroofing of the lesion.

A somewhat larger and more dramatic mucocele may result from obstruction and rupture of the major excretory ducts in the floor of the mouth, ducts of the lingual or submaxillary glands. Except for size, these lesions resemble in every way the lesions which result from obstruction of the minor salivary glands but have received the special name of *ranula*.

Fig. 16-11. Irritation fibroma. The lesion seen here was caused by persistent sucking and irritation of mucosa through the edentulous space, which can be seen adjacent to this polyp. (*Courtesy of Sheldon Rovin, D.D.S.*)

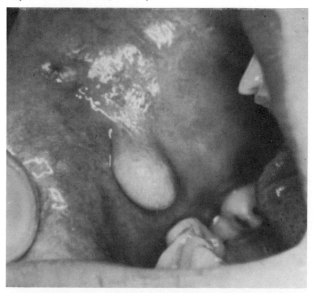

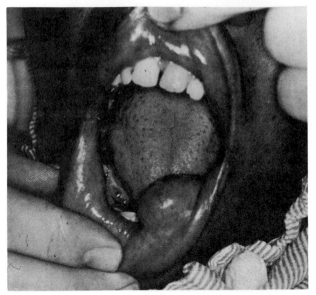

Fig. 16-12. Mucous cyst of the lip, the most common location for this lesion. This mucocele has resulted from rupture of a minor salivary gland duct with spillage of mucus into the surrounding tissue.

Dermoids may develop in the floor of the mouth and the base of the tongue along the midline. If neglected, these lesions grow slowly as they accumulate the sloughed-off cells, secretion, and hair of the epidermal lining. They present both as a swelling in the submental triangle and an elevation of the floor of the mouth (Fig. 16-13). They will eventually elevate the floor of the mouth and tongue until it touches the palate and interferes with speech. Treatment consists of operative excision of the cyst, which may be done either intraorally or extraorally. The lesion has a definite, thick capsule and can be shelled out with ease from its relatively avascular midline location.

Fig. 16-13. Dermoid of the mouth. This huge dermoid has elevated the floor of the mouth until the tongue is forced against the hard palate and in this illustration is out of sight behind the cyst.

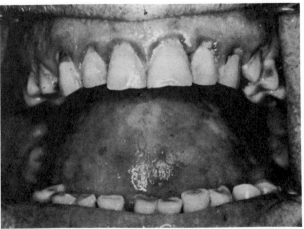

PERIPHERAL GIANT CELL REPARATIVE GRANULOMA

These benign tumors occur on the gingivae, affecting the maxillary or mandibular gingiva with equal frequency. Grossly, they appear as a slow-growing, reddish, smooth sessile tumor which bleeds easily. They often occur at an area of an interdental papilla (Fig. 16-14) but may also arise in edentulous patients. Histologically, the lesion is covered by stratified squamous epithelium. Endothelial and fibroblastic proliferations, multinucleated giant cells, and extracellular and intracellular hemosiderin are diagnostic microscopic criteria. Multinucleated giant cells are distributed unevenly throughout an area of rich fibroblastic proliferation. Some lesions show spicules of bone tissue. In general, the lesion closely resembles the giant cell tumor of bone seen in hyperparathyroidism. The descriptive term "peripheral" indicates that the lesion is of soft tissue, while the so-called "central" giant cell reparative granuloma is an intraosseous form found in the mandible or maxilla.

When these lesions arise in the mandible or maxilla, they may be confused with the giant cell tumors of long bones. The distinction between the two lesions must be made, since the oral lesions have no propensity for malignant transformation, as have the lesions seen elsewhere. Treatment of the soft tissue lesions is by complete excision. Inadequate removal may result in recurrence.

PERIPHERAL FIBROMA

These are also lesions of the gingiva and are in many respects similar grossly to the giant cell granuloma. They are usually firmer and under the microscope are made up of dense connective tissue. They may also contain bone spicules and may be calcified. One can speculate as to the relation of these lesions to the giant cell granuloma. They may represent a later stage of this lesion or may be a late stage of inflammatory hyperplasia. Excision is usually curative.

GRANULOMA PYOGENICUM

This is an elevated pedunculated or sessile lesion which may occur on the lips, tongue, buccal mucosa, or gingiva. It bleeds readily on being traumatized. Histologically it is made up of edematous, fibrous connective tissue with a prominent endothelial component arranged in lobules of varying sizes separated by bands of collagen. Numerous blood vessels are scattered throughout the tumor. No cause is known for the lesions of the lips, buccal mucosa, and tongue, but lesions of the gingiva are often associated with pregnancy. Thirty to forty percent of pregnant women show some degree of gingival enlargement. Of these, about 1 percent will have an isolated "tumor." These lesions in the pregnant female have been called "granuloma gravidarum." They appear about the third month of pregnancy and increase in size throughout the growth of the child in utero. They usually diminish in size and disappear following delivery, although with a subsequent pregnancy they may appear again in the same location. Lesions unassociated with pregnancy may be treated by excision. It is usually advisable to wait until the end of pregnancy to treat granuloma gravidarum.

SALIVARY TUMORS

Pleomorphic adenomas (mixed tumors) occasionally arise from any of the 400 to 700 minor salivary glands. Occurring most commonly on the lips, tongue, and palate, they can be found anywhere in the oral cavity where minor salivary glands are found. They are usually slow-growing, round masses of a rather rubbery consistency (Fig. 16-15). They have the potential of becoming malignant and if simply enucleated without adequate excision have a marked propensity for local recurrence. Treatment, therefore, is by wide local excision.

HEMANGIOMA

Capillary hemangiomas, not unlike the strawberry hemangioma of the skin, are sometimes seen in the mucous membranes of the oral cavity in infants. Like the lesions of the skin these lesions regress spontaneously, and unless they are so large that they interfere with function, they should be left to regress at their own pace. In most instances they will undergo involution by the end of the fifth year. Unlike the skin lesions they do not disappear completely and may still be seen as a small, dark lesion underneath the mucosa (Fig. 16-16). It is likely that the transparent nature of the mucosa reveals the sclerosed remnant in a manner that is not seen if the lesion is under the more opaque skin. The sclerosed hemangioma will remain visible throughout life but has no significance and does not require treatment. Rarely, large regional vascular malformations will involve the entire side of the mouth, including the tongue, gingiva, and buccal mucosa. Such lesions do not regress spontaneously. Their treatment is difficult, often requiring multiple plastic procedures to excise the hemangiomatous tissue and to return the contours of the mouth and oral cavity to normal.

GRANULAR CELL MYOBLASTOMA

This is a rare and interesting lesion which occurs most commonly within the muscle of the tongue, presenting as a small, firm spheroid mass detected best by manual palpation. These lesions have no malignant potential but may gradually increase in size with functional impairment. Treatment is by simple excision.

Hyperkeratosis

The gross finding of white patches on the oral mucosa elicits the diagnosis of leukoplakia from the clinician. "Leukoplakia" roughly translated means "white patches," so the physician need not feel too proud of his accomplishment; he has only managed to translate English into Latin. To some "leukoplakia" means a specific premalignant lesion. This meaning is not inherent in the original use of this term. Most pathologists adhere to a more rigid description of such lesions and describe the underlying microscopic changes: hyperplasia, keratosis, and dyskeratosis. White patches in the oral cavity may be associated with any of or all these basic changes (Fig. 16-17). Inflammation in this area often stimulates marked hyperplasia of cells, sometimes to the point where they resemble

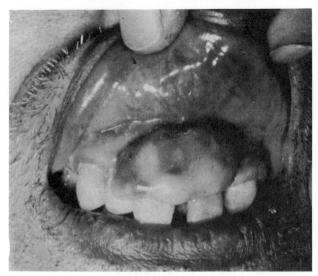

Fig. 16-14. Peripheral giant cell tumor. These often arise in interdental spaces as seen in photograph.

epidermoid tumors and are spoken of as *pseudoepitheliomatous hyperplasia.* Keratosis is a common response of the buccal mucosa and may appear in the presence of lichen planus, chronic dyscoid lupus, and Darier's disease, as well as be a possible forerunner of malignant change.

Dyskeratosis, the loss of normal stratification or orientation of cells together with irregularity in the size and shape of cells and abnormal staining characteristics, is a much more treacherous lesion and much more likely to precede malignant disease.

Hyperkeratosis is announced by the gradual development of whitened patches of the mucosa which appear first as a thin, white, translucent or opalescent film in the normal mucous membrane. No malignant or premalignant changes will be found at this point but only evidences of

Fig. 16-15. Mixed tumor of palate. This is a benign lesion. Adequate removal to ensure prevention of recurrences includes resection of the underlying hard palate and gingiva.

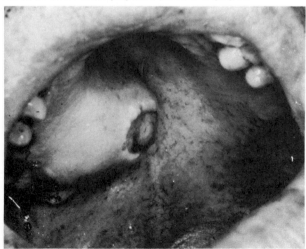

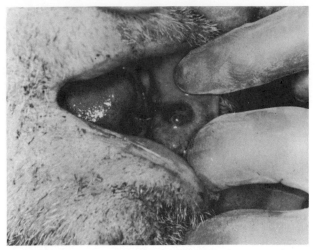

Fig. 16-16. Fibrosing hemangioma. Lesions in the mucosal area remain visible under the buccal mucosa, whereas similar lesions may not be discernible under the skin.

hyperplasia or keratosis. Later these lesions can become thickened and rougher; the white patches are now quite opaque. Palpation will reveal a definite change in the consistency of the mucosa. Microscopic examination may still show advanced hyperkeratosis and hyperplasia, but now areas of mild to marked dyskeratosis may be present as well. Eventually, areas of distinct carcinoma in situ will appear, and this can be followed in rapid order by microinvasion or the frank invasion of a well-developed cancer.

Obviously, the early appearance of hyperplasia and hyperkeratosis may or may not foreshadow malignant disease. Since there is no way of telling which is the case, patients with such lesions should be warned to avoid smoking or heavy intake of alcohol and should embark on a campaign of improvement of oral hygiene. Cancer

Fig. 16-17. Hyperkeratosis of mucosa. The white mucosa in the gingivobuccal gutter of the patient is due to an ill-fitting denture causing hyperkeratosis, a normal response of the oral mucosa to irritation. (*Courtesy of Sheldon Rovin, D.D.S.*)

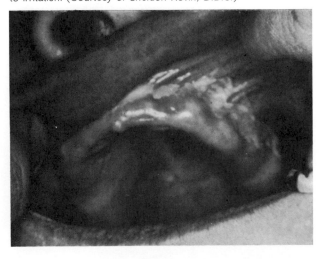

will ultimately develop in 5 percent of such patients, and it is significant that about 50 percent of all oral cancers develop in patients with associated areas of hyperkeratosis and dyskeratosis. The thin, early lesions require only a warning, and a biopsy is not necessary, but thickened lesions may already contain carcinoma in situ and should be biopsied in every instance and perhaps checked, as well, with vital dyes.

If a patch of dyskeratosis appears on biopsy to be particularly threatening and is limited in extent, local excision may be useful. More often, the extent of the lesion is so widespread that complete excision of the involved mucosa is impossible. Radiation therapy is contraindicated in these premalignant lesions. While the majority are associated with hyperkeratosis, which gives the whitish aspect to the surface, occasionally dyskeratosis and carcinoma in situ are the major elements. Such lesions may have a velvety erythematous appearance only slightly redder than the surrounding mucosa. These areas are difficult to detect, and toluidine blue may be very useful in mapping their true area.

Malignant Tumors

PATHOLOGY. Low-grade epidermoid carcinomas make up the overwhelming majority of all carcinomas of the oral cavity, varying from highly differentiated tumors, difficult to tell histologically from inflammatory hyperplasia, to less well-organized but still obvious epidermoid tumors usually with associated squamous pearls. Highly undifferentiated and anaplastic lesions are rare. The few adenocarcinomas found are derived from minor salivary glands. The occasional adenoid cystic carcinomas and mucoepidermoid carcinomas seen also arise from salivary tissues.

In the Southern United States a very low-grade cancer, verrucous carcinoma, is occasionally seen. This is an exophytic, shaggy white lesion usually found in the gingivobuccal gutter of patients who are tobacco chewers or "snuff dippers." Unless treated by radiation, the lesion never metastasizes, although it frequently invades surrounding tissues, including the mandible.

In general, lesions of the oral cavity are better differentiated and less malignant than lesions occurring in the oropharynx.

TONGUE

Carcinoma of the tongue commonly begins at the tip or along the free borders. It often starts in an area of hyperkeratosis and gradually develops as an ulcerated lesion with a moderately exophytic undermined border. The area of ulceration is related to the rest of the tumor as the tip of an iceberg is to its main mass, and palpation of the tongue may indicate that invasion has occurred deeply throughout underlying muscle (Fig. 16-18). Carcinomas beginning in an area of syphilitic glossitis are exceptions to the normal pattern and occur on the dorsal glossal surface.

Cancer of the tip of the tongue (Fig. 16-19) metastasizes to submental nodes, often bilaterally, while lesions along the borders of the tongue metastasize to ipsilateral submandibular nodes and occasionally to nodes at the angle of the mandible.

These lesions are quick to metastasize, and 40 percent of patients have nodes in the neck when first seen. In another 40 percent nodes develop at some point during therapy or during follow-up. For this reason therapy is designed to attack not only the primary lesion but also the nodes of the ipsilateral neck, as well. Combined operation including wide resection of the oral lesion together with radical neck dissection has been our treatment of choice in the past. More recently we have been inclined to treat all larger lesions of the oral cavity with radiation therapy, following this with radical neck dissection and in continuity excision of any residual cancer. The horizontal ramus of the mandible must be resected together with the tumor if the oral cancer has come in contact with the periosteum of the mandible at any point. Such contact seeds the periosteal lymphatics with tumor cells and makes resection of bone mandatory. The determinate 5-year survival for cancer of the tongue is 32 to 40 percent. If no palpable lymph nodes are present, the 5-year survival rate is 53 percent.

FLOOR OF THE MOUTH

The floor of the mouth is that portion of the oral cavity between the tongue and the inner surface of the mandible. This crescentic area of the mucosa lies over the sublingual and submaxillary salivary glands and contains their excretory ducts. It is divided into two halves by the frenulum, a fold of mucosa lying in the midline and extending to the tongue.

Squamous carcinomas developing in this area tend to develop a "run-around" extending anteriorly and posteriorly around the rim of the mandible, and if they are neglected long enough, the entire floor of the mouth becomes involved. This pattern of growth results in common bilateral involvement at the anterior floor of the mouth (Fig. 16-20) with frequent bilateral cervical metastases. These lesions tend to be less well differentiated than lesions of the tongue or gingiva and rapidly invade the surrounding structures, especially the periosteum of the adjacent mandible and the tissues of the submaxillary space. Metastases occur first to the submaxillary lymph nodes and are frequent. Taylor and Nathanson observed that 60 percent of these patients had palpable cervical metastases on admission, and in 90 percent cervical lymph node involvement had developed within a year of diagnosis.

The primary symptoms of these neoplasms are often neglected for some time, since they are quite minimal. Eventually the patient complains of pain, swelling of the tongue, and difficulty in eating and speaking. Early lesions are usually discovered by the patient himself while inspecting his mouth or have been noticed by an alert dentist or physician. Rarely, very early lesions may be seen involving only the superficial mucosa.

Large lesions of the floor of the mouth require wide excision in continuity with resection of a portion of the mandible and radical neck dissection. The neck dissection is done whether lymph nodes are palpable or not, in view

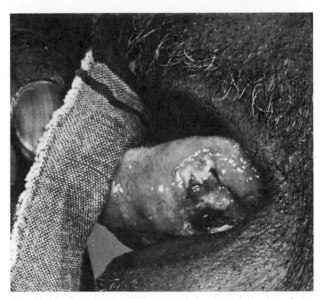

Fig. 16-18. Squamous carcinoma of the lateral border of the middle third of the tongue. The lesion is deeply invasive and much larger than the area of ulceration would indicate. The curled raised border is characteristic.

of the high incidence of positive cervical nodes. Operative therapy may be integrated with preoperative radiation in the larger lesions. The much less common superficial and in situ lesions can be treated by local excision only. The 5-year survival rates for cancers in this site are comparable with those for cancer of the tongue. James reports an average determinate survival of 37 percent, and the Tumor Registry of the Memorial Center for Cancer reports a 5-year survival rate of 39 percent.

GINGIVAE

Cancer of the gums is better differentiated and slower in its pattern of growth than lesions of the tongue and

Fig. 16-19. Squamous carcinoma of the tip of the tongue. An exophytic, fairly superficial lesion which histologically shows a well-differentiated structure. The prognosis for such a lesion is excellent.

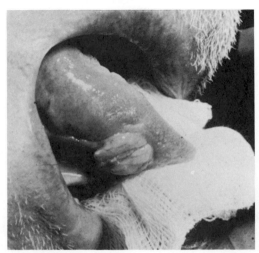

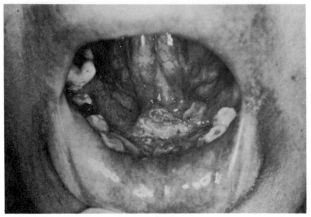

Fig. 16-20. Squamous carcinoma of the floor of the mouth. This lesion is in a typical location in the midline with spread in both directions around the curve of the mandible. It has invaded deeply into underlying structures.

floor of the mouth. Patients first note a mass (Fig. 16-21) or slight tenderness of the gum, sometimes with loosening of teeth in the area of the tumor. This often leads them to consult their dentist, who, if he is not alert to the problem, may extract the teeth under the mistaken impression that the patient has an underlying abcess or cyst. As the lesion progresses, it ulcerates, bleeds, and interferes with mastication. As a neoplasm invades the underlying bone, it can involve the mandibular nerve with the appearance of numbness in the mental and submental areas. Extraction of a tooth often accelerates the invasion of the mandible.

Treatment of cancer of the lower gingiva requires resection of the involved mandible and overlying gum together with a radical neck dissection. Metastases from cancers at this site are usually to the submaxillary lymph nodes and are present in about half the patients at their first visit. Epidermoid cancers of the upper gingiva are less

Fig. 16-21. Carcinoma of the gingiva. The adjacent teeth are loose and easily removed. The underlying mandible is already invaded.

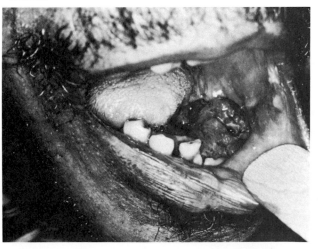

common and better differentiated than cancers of the lower gingiva. Metastases to cervical nodes are much less common. Therefore, treatment is restricted to local excision. Radical neck dissection is deferred until there is evidence of palpable cervical node involvement.

The definitive 5-year survival rate following treatment for carcinoma of the gingiva averages 45 percent.

HARD PALATE

The hard palate is the U-shaped area enclosed by the upper gingiva and bounded posteriorly by the attachments of the soft palate. It consists of the palatine processes of the maxillary bones in its anterior two-thirds and of the horizontal portions of the palatine bones in its posterior third.

The most common malignant lesions of the hard palate are tumors of the minor salivary glands. Adenoid cystic carcinomas (Fig. 16-22) and adenocarcinomas occur in almost equal number; malignant mixed tumors are somewhat less frequent. Epidermoid carcinomas primary in the hard palate are rare, although carcinomas primary in the maxillary sinus will occasionally invade the hard palate and perforate into the oral cavity.

The primary symptom is a mass usually noted first by the patient himself. There is no tenderness or other associated symptom until fairly late in the course of the tumor. As in most salivary malignant tumors, growth is very slow and metastases occur quite late, so that involved cervical lymph nodes are not found initially. Salivary neoplasms respond poorly to radiation therapy, and primary treatment is excision. The chief fault in treatment is underestimation of the extent and potential of these lesions. They are usually fixed to the underlying periosteum, and adequate excision must include resection of the hard palate together with the tumor mass. An attempt to enucleate the tumor from the underlying bone almost ensures a local recurrence. Excision with a wide margin including the bony palate leaves a substantial palatal defect requiring repair either by surgical reconstruction or the use of an upper plate constructed by a prosthodontist with an obturator which will plug the defect.

Despite the phlegmatic nature of these tumors, complete excision and complete eradication of the lesions are often elusive. The lesions tend to be of a higher grade than malignant lesions of the major salivary glands. Five-year survival rates between 30 and 40 percent are reported, but the incidence of new disease between the fifth and fifteenth year is frequent.

BUCCAL MUCOSA

The lateral walls of the oral cavity are formed by the cheeks, which consist of the buccinator muscle covered on its inner surface by a layer of mucosa extending from the upper to the lower gingivobuccal gutters and from the lateral commissure of the lips anteriorly to the ascending ramus of the mandible posteriorly. Lymphatics from this area pass through the buccinator muscle and follow the facial vein to end in the submaxillary and upper cervical lymph nodes.

The natural evolution of epidermoid carcinoma of the

buccal mucosa varies according to the grade of the tumor. About half of the lesions are rather undifferentiated and associated with ulceration, rapid invasion of the cheek, and sometimes even perforation of the skin and formation of an orocutaneous salivary fistula (Fig. 16-23). The majority of such lesions are accompanied by enlarged submaxillary lymph nodes when first seen.

A less aggressive form of buccal cancer is also encountered, especially in patients who are tobacco chewers and "snuff dippers." This is the so-called "verrucous carcinoma," which tends to occur in the gingivobuccal gutter and progresses very slowly, sometimes over a period of years. The tumor is locally invasive, but metastases have never been reported except in patients who have received previous irradiation. Verrucous lesions are easily recognized by their exophytic form and shaggy white appearance (Fig. 16-24). They may cover a wide area, sometimes the entire buccal surface, and have a propensity for bony invasion, often involving a large portion of the mandible or occasionally the maxilla.

Treatment of buccal carcinoma is dictated by the type of lesion encountered. External radiation therapy alone does not eradicate the less well-differentiated lesions, although it has been combined with interstitial therapy with some success. The highly differentiated verrucous carcinomas are fairly radiosensitive but have a marked tendency to recur following an early gratifying regression. In addition, the distressing propensity of these lesions for developing a higher grade of malignancy with metastases after being exposed to radiation is a unique characteristic which has discouraged many from using radiation in treatment. Therefore, the initial therapy for verrucous lesions is wide excision. Since cervical metastases are not ordinarily found, an accompanying radical neck dissection is not done.

For the high-grade lesions, block dissection of the cheek with radical neck resection is the operative treatment of choice. Additional benefit may be derived from combining this with preoperative radiotherapy; this type of combined treatment is still undergoing evaluation. James reported 5-year survival rates in 181 patients with carcinoma of the buccal mucosa of all types as 54.4 percent. The prognosis for the well-differentiated lesions, such as the verrucous carcinoma, should be much better than this.

OROPHARYNX

The oropharynx is the region of the mouth posterior to the anterior tonsillar pillars and the circumvallate papillae of the tongue (Fig. 16-25). It contains the soft palate, tonsil and tonsillar fossa, posterior third of the tongue, anterior surface of the epiglottis, and surrounding pharyngeal walls. The most common site for malignant tumors in this area is the tonsil.

TONSIL

The most common benign lesion of the tonsil is, as every layman knows, inflammatory swelling. This can lead to confusion in diagnosing nonulcerated tumors of these

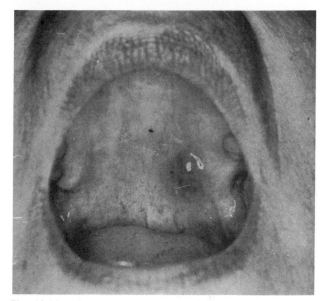

Fig. 16-22. Adenoid cystic carcinoma of the hard palate. Although this lesion is much smaller than the mixed tumor in Fig. 16-15, it is malignant. Treatment is by wide excision, including the underlying bone.

organs. Common malignant lesions are high-grade epidermoid carcinomas (78 percent) and lymphosarcomas (16 percent). A large group of miscellaneous tumors are found, including hemangiomas, neurofibromas, and salivary gland tumors. High-grade epidermoid carcinomas in this area are often described as lymphoepitheliomas and transitional cell carcinomas. It is our feeling that these are simply microscopic variants of highly undifferentiated epidermoid carcinomas.

The frequent first symptom of carcinoma of the tonsil is a slight feeling of tenderness in the area, a typical sore throat. This is easily ignored by the patient for long periods until its persistence finally forces a consultation with the

Fig. 16-23. Carcinoma of buccal mucosa. A well-differentiated and slowly growing lesion which was neglected and mismanaged for many years. (*From B. F. Rush, Jr., Curr Probl Surg, May, 1967.*)

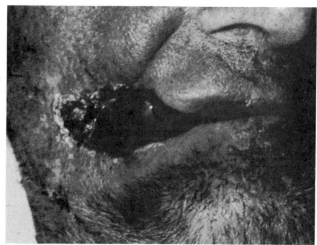

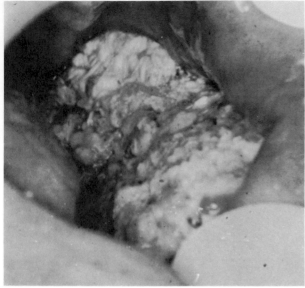

Fig. 16-24. Verrucous carcinoma. The shaggy white plaque along the gingivobuccal gutter is typical. The patient is seventy-five years old and has chewed tobacco for over 50 years.

physician. Even then the evidence of a growing tumor may be overlooked and the patient treated for some time with mouthwashes and antibiotics. The lesion will appear grossly as a swelling of the tonsil with a central ulcer. Palpation reveals firmness and induration spreading well beyond the area of ulceration. Trismus and pain in the ear are common complaints. The metastatic spread from this area is to the tonsillar node at the angle of the mandible, so often enlarged in children who have tonsillitis. The tonsil is a common site for very tiny "occult" carcinomas, which lead to large cervical masses and must be inspected minutely when one is searching for a primary

Fig. 16-25. Oropharynx. The shaded area delineates the oropharynx. The nasopharynx is located above, and the hypopharynx and larynx are located below.

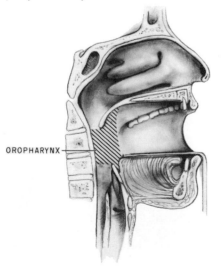

OROPHARYNX

site for cervical metastases (Fig. 16-26). Lymphosarcomas of the tonsil usually present with a more bulky primary lesion and are not as inclined to ulceration. The primary lesions may be bilateral with involvement of both tonsils.

Treatment of tonsillar carcinoma either by radiation or operation has never been very satisfactory. Lymphosarcomas are quite radiosensitive and should be treated primarily by radiation. Carcinoma, on the other hand, yields poorly to either form of therapy. Still under evaluation, integrated therapy with preoperative radiation to the tonsil followed by resection in continuity with a radical neck dissection may prove to produce the best results. The definitive 5-year survival following treatment of cancer of the tonsil is 25 percent.

POSTERIOR THIRD OF THE TONGUE

Tumors in the posterior third of the tongue differ markedly in their natural history from those in the anterior two-thirds. Whereas the anterior lesions tend to be well differentiated, remain confined to the primary site, or involve only high cervical nodes for long periods, lesions in the posterior third are of much higher grade, often being classified as *lymphoepitheliomas,* or *transitional cell tumors.* They spread rapidly to the cervical nodes and often beyond to distant sites. A frequent initial symptom of carcinoma of the posterior third of the tongue is a large cervical lymph node accompanied by the complaint of pain on swallowing. Unfortunately, this is a fairly silent area, and lesions may attain considerable size before causing pain or dysfunction. Wide ulceration causes a malodorous breath and dysphasia. Weight loss is prominent. Treatment has been highly unsatisfactory in the past. Radiation therapy infrequently controls the primary lesion. Operation often results in total loss of the tongue, an overwhelming psychologic and functional deficit. Since these lesions are often across the midline, bilateral neck dissection must be combined with resection of the tongue. Initial experience with combined radiation and operation indicates that occasionally the lesions can be reduced in size sufficiently by preoperative radiation to permit a more conservative resection of the posterior tongue, leaving a functional anterior tongue behind.

SOFT PALATE

Malignant tumors of the soft palate are almost always epidermoid carcinomas. These tend to be well differentiated, slow-growing, and late to metastasize. They are generally superficial lesions spreading over the anterior surface of the soft palate and down the tonsillar pillars. Often it is difficult to determine whether the lesions arose in the tonsil or in the soft palate. Spread may be extensive, covering much of the soft palate, the tonsillar fossa, and the tongue. Pain and dysphagia are the usual first symptoms. Diagnosis by inspection and palpation is a simple matter, and biopsy is easily accomplished.

Response to radiation therapy is only fair. Resection is more likely to produce a cure but often leads to a difficult functional defect, since the patient is unable to close the nasopharynx and will tend to regurgitate food through the nose on swallowing. This is a situation where the clever prosthodontist can help greatly by installing an adequate extension on an upper plate which extends backward into the pharynx to seal the palatal defect. An even more convenient method of closing the palatal defect is to raise a flap from the posterior pharynx and swing it forward to close the defect at the time of the original operation. Prognosis is difficult to determine, since these tumors are usually classed in the literature with tumors of the tonsil or of the hard palate.

EPIGLOTTIS

Malignant tumors of the anterior surface of the epiglottis are usually exophytic and well differentiated and have a slow, natural evolution. Dysphagia and aspiration are early symptoms. Treatment by radiation therapy is quite successful. Hemilaryngectomy of the upper larynx above the cords has also produced good results. Patients who have had resection of the epiglottis must relearn swallowing, and this requires a reasonable level of intelligence. Senile patients or those with poor learning ability should be treated either by radiation or total laryngectomy.

LARYNX

When describing the site of tumors of the larynx, the terminology can be confusing and frustrating. According to current usage, the larynx is made up of those structures lying both above and below the true vocal cords. Thus, the mucosa of the larynx extends along the posterior surface of the epiglottis including its tip, along the aryepiglottic folds, and over the arytenoid cartilages posteriorly. It covers the inner surface of the aryepiglottic folds, the false vocal cords, and the ventricles. All of the larynx thus far described constitutes the supraglottic larynx, i.e., that which is above the true vocal cords. The glottic portion of the larynx is that portion made up of the true cords themselves. The mucosa lining the area underneath the true cords down to the lower border of the cricoid cartilage covers the infraglottic portion of the larynx.

In the past the area just described was called the "endolarynx," or the "intrinsic larynx," although the latter term gradually came to mean the true cords alone. Tumors taking their origin on the outside of the larynx for many years were designated as arising from the "extrinsic larynx." However, this term came to be used for supraglottic lesions as well, so this usage has now been abandoned. Lesions involving any portion of the exterior of the larynx are now spoken of as "hypopharyngeal" or, by some, "laryngopharyngeal."

INCIDENCE AND ETIOLOGY. Cancer of the larynx accounts for 1.62 percent of all cancers in men and only 0.14 percent of all cancers in woman; thus the ratio of incidence favors the male sex by over 11:1. The report of the Advisory Committee to the Surgeon General on Smoking and Health reviewed 10 retrospective studies and 7 prospective studies on the relationship of smoking to carcinoma of the larynx. There was a statistically positive relationship in every study. In the prospective studies the mortality ratios for smokers averaged 5.4 times greater for cigarette smok-

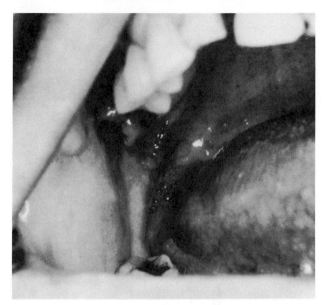

Fig. 16-26. Carcinoma of the anterior tonsillar pillar. These tiny lesions are invasive areas of carcinoma. Despite their size, the patient already had metastatic disease in the ipsilateral neck.

ers than for nonsmokers and 2.8 times greater for cigar and pipe smokers than for nonsmokers. Laryngeal cancer mortality has increased somewhat over the past three decades, but the increase has been much less than that for lung cancer. It appears that the induction of carcinoma of the larynx cannot occur solely as a result of tobacco tars but that a further agent, or cocarcinogen, is needed. One such agent may be alcohol, since a high percentage (30 to 40 percent) of patients with carcinoma of the larynx are alcoholics and come from population groups where the risk of alcoholism is great, such as bartenders and entertainers. Cirrhosis of the liver is a common complaint among patients with carcinoma of the larynx; this may be a secondary relationship due to the frequency of alcoholism in this group.

CLASSIFICATION. As it has for other cancers, the American Joint Committee on Cancer Staging and End Results Reporting has developed a "TNM system" for carcinomas of the larynx. Because of differences in prognosis at different sites the committee has divided the larynx into its three major areas: the supraglottic (posterior surface of the epiglottis, aryepiglottic folds, arytenoids, false cords, ventricles); the glottic (right and left vocal cords and anterior glottic commissure), and the subglottic (subglottic region exclusive of the undersurface of the true cords and down to the lower margin of the cricoid cartilage). About 56 percent of squamous epidermoid cancers of the larynx occur in the glottic region, 42 percent occur in the supraglottic region, and the remaining 2 percent are subglottic. The combination of topographic spread (T), nodal involvement (N), and distant metastasis (M) in a description of three separate anatomic sites results in a complex system, yet it is the most precise method whereby lesions can be classified and comparisons between institutions adequately made as to the results of treatment.

PATHOLOGY. Polyps, papillomas, granulomas, cysts, and areas of hyperkeratosis make up the common benign lesions of the cords. Rarely hemangiomas and chondromas of the laryngeal cartilages are seen. Ninety-nine percent of the malignant lesions of the larynx are epidermoid carcinomas, and most of these are of the ordinary cornifying (squamous cell) type. These lesions arise from the squamous epithelium of the cords themselves or from areas of metaplasia in the mucosa of the endolarynx. On the cord, carcinoma may be preceded by hyperkeratosis and stages of transition from hyperkeratosis to dyskeratosis, carcinoma in situ, and microinvasive carcinoma. Glottic cancers are usually very well differentiated, slow-growing, and late to metastasize. Supraglottic and infraglottic cancers are less well differentiated and more likely to have spread to lymph nodes when first seen.

DIAGNOSIS. Space-occupying lesions of the larynx produce initial symptoms through interference with phonation and respiration. Hoarseness, the usual first symptom, may be slight and intermittent but gradually becomes constant. What begins as a slight huskiness gradually progresses, until sounds are produced with difficulty. Respiratory obstruction is a later sign, although small lesions on the true cords will produce a greater degree of obstruction than somewhat larger lesions in supraglottic or infraglottic area. Obstruction progresses in severity until the patient may respire with visible effort, using his accessory muscles to force air through the cords, sometimes with audible stridor. At this point the patient's life is in jeopardy. At any moment the slightest additional swelling or edema can cut off breathing completely. The use of sedatives in patients at this phase of obstruction is fraught with danger. Under sedation the patient's tired muscles may fail, with a rapid shallowing of respiration, progressive anoxia, and cardiac arrest. The finding of a tumor on the cord associated with stridor, retraction, or the use of accessory muscles to

breathe indicates immediate tracheostomy. It is far better to elect a tracheostomy done in the operating room than to be forced into an emergency tracheostomy on the ward or in the emergency room under much less favorable circumstances.

Late signs of malignant lesions of the larynx are a malodorous breath, pain on swallowing, weight loss, and hemoptysis.

Any patient who has persistent hoarseness for more than three or four weeks should have a careful inspection of his vocal cords by indirect laryngoscopy. If this reveals no pathologic conditions but hoarseness persists, then direct laryngoscopy should be used to examine the cords even more closely.

Benign Tumors

POLYPS

According to Holinger, 43 percent of all benign lesions of the larynx are simple polyps. These arise on the phonating edge of the cord at the junction between the anterior one-third and the posterior two-thirds (Fig. 16-27). Their cause is obscure. Treatment is by removal with a cupped forceps at direct laryngoscopy.

VOCAL NODULES

The second most common benign tumor of the larynx, these are usually bilateral and, like polyps, occur at the junction of the anterior one-third with the posterior two-thirds of the cords. They are often called "singer's nodules" but certainly are not confined to singers and can occur in any occupational group. Treatment is by removal with the biopsy forceps.

Fig. 16-27. Pedunculated polyp of the right vocal cord arising at the junction of the anterior and middle thirds. (*From P. H. Holinger et al., Ann Otol Rhinol Laryngol, 56:583, 1947.*)

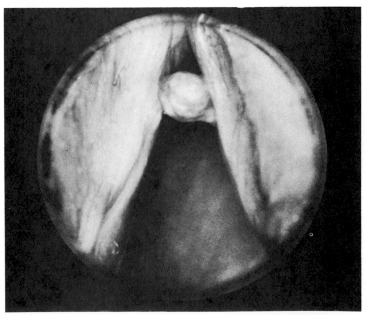
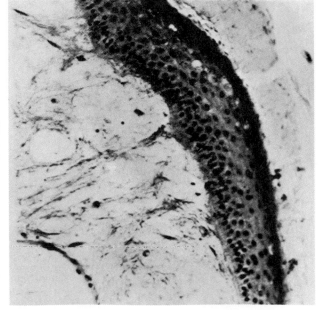

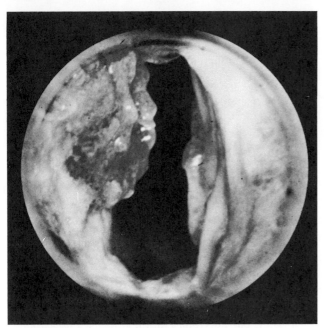

Fig. 16-28. Carcinoma involving the left side of the larynx and anterior commissure. (*From P. H. Holinger et al., Ann Otol Rhinol Laryngol, 56:583, 1947.*)

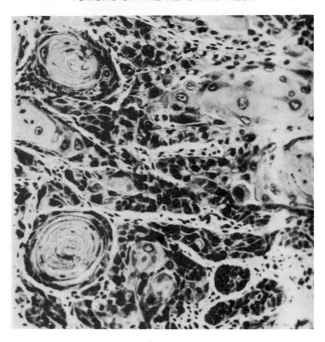

RETENTION CYSTS

About half of these occur on the vocal cords, the remainder being found in the aryepiglottic folds, arytenoids, or epiglottis. They appear to occur as a result of the obstruction of small mucous glands. These lesions can reach considerable size and offer marked embarrassment to respiration.

HYPERKERATOSIS

Hyperkeratosis can affect the vocal cords as it does any of the mucosal areas of the lips, oral cavity, or pharynx. These lesions are evidence of a premalignant change and should be stripped off the cord with the use of the biopsy forceps. Patients who have developed hyperkeratosis should be followed at twice yearly intervals to guard against recurrence or the appearance of a frank carcinoma.

PAPILLOMAS

These multiple lesions are found most often on the true cords but may appear on any portion of the larynx or pharynx and even on the soft palate. While they are most commonly reported in children prior to adolescence, some adults are also affected. Like warts, these tumors appear to be caused by viruses. Frequently the growths cover the mucosa of the cords in great profusion, causing severe respiratory embarrassment and requiring tracheostomy. They can persist for many years; during this period the patient often must continue to wear a tracheostomy tube while papillomas are cleared from his airway by frequent excisions through the laryngoscope. Repeated excision is the only effective treatment to date. The large number of other forms of therapy attempted indicates the generally unsatisfactory state of therapy. Eventually, after a period

of months or years of repeated excisions, the lesions gradually disappear.

Malignant Lesions

Carcinoma of the true cords (Fig. 16-28) is a lesion which should be easily detected. It gives warning of its presence at an early stage through hoarseness and grows slowly enough so that early therapy should be rewarded by a 90 percent or better 5-year survival rate. In many urban areas over half of the lesions of the true cords are stage 1 lesions confined entirely to the cord. In contrast, some rural areas report that in only 5 percent of patients reaching the physician the lesions are still in stage 1. As the tumor grows, it extends off the cord, either up into the supraglottic area or less commonly inferiorly into the infraglottic region. Invasion occurs slowly but relentlessly, eventually with perforation of the thyroid cartilage and direct invasion of the soft tissues of the thyroid gland and of the neck.

If cancer remains confined to the true cords, a high percentage of 5-year survivals can be obtained following treatment by radiotherapy alone. Holinger noted that in a series of 102 patients with cordal lesions treated with cobalt irradiation, only 9 patients had residual or recurrent cancer which required subsequent laryngectomy. None of the patients in this series died of carcinoma. Loss of the larynx is such a major functional and psychologic disability that if excellent results can be obtained by irradiation, this should be the treatment of choice.

Cancers which have invaded areas beyond the cord have a much different outlook. Involvement of cervical nodes becomes an important problem, and the ability to eradicate the disease by radiation alone is greatly decreased. For stage 2, 3, and 4 cancers, laryngectomy is mandatory. In addition, a radical neck dissection on the side of the lesion is usually performed, even though palpable nodes are not present. Using this approach, Norris has reported a 70 to 75 percent 5-year survival rate for stage 2 and 3 lesions of glottic and supraglottic origin. The very large stage 4 lesions do very poorly, with a 5-year survival rate of only 21 percent. Goldman et al. have combined radiation therapy and operation in treatment of advanced cancers of the larynx, and although the experience is still small, they feel that integration of the two modalities improves the long-term survival rate.

The major problem for the patient after laryngectomy is to regain a useful voice. About half of all such patients will learn to use effective esophageal speech, meaning they can communicate understandably with strangers and casual acquaintances. An additional 25 percent can make themselves understood to members of their family but find that their esophageal speech is too distorted to be useful in the general community. The remaining 25 percent of patients will be unable to conquer the technical problems of learning this method of conversation.

Esophageal speech is by far the most useful technique for speaking after laryngectomy, since it requires no additional paraphernalia and can be refined to the point where it very closely resembles the tone and expression of ordinary speech. It is produced by swallowing air and regurgitating it, creating a vibration in the pharynx—probably at the level of the cricothyroid muscle. The oral cavity modulates this tone just as it would a tone from the larynx.

For the 50 percent of patients who are partly or completely unable to learn esophageal speech, electric vibrating devices can be used to provide a tone in the oral cavity which is modulated by the patient's oral structures, giving a fairly reasonable method of communication.

HYPOPHARYNX

The hypopharynx is that area of the throat which surrounds the larynx. It is made up of the piriform sinuses on either side, the exterior portions of the aryepiglottic fold, and the lateral and posterior pharyngeal walls. It includes the mucosa overlying the posterior portions of the cricoid cartilage.

INCIDENCE. Cancer of the hypopharynx is three to four times as common as cancer of the larynx and constitutes 4.05 percent of all cancers in males. It is three times more common in men than in women. These tumors appear to be related to smoking. The correlation is stronger with pipe and cigar smoking than with cigarette smoking. Another etiologic factor is the Plummer-Vinson syndrome, found most commonly in Scandinavian women. This deficiency syndrome, now gradually disappearing, is clearly related to carcinoma of the hypopharynx and posterior tongue. At the Radiumhemmet in Stockholm carcinomas of the hypopharynx are seen more frequently in women than in men, and most of these cases are associated with a Plummer-Vinson syndrome.

PATHOLOGY. The great majority of these tumors are epidermoid carcinomas and compared with the oral cavity and endolarynx tend to be of a higher grade with a pre-

ponderance of grade 3 and 4 lesions. Better-differentiated forms are seen, however, most commonly on the exterior portions of the aryepiglottic folds and in the postcricoid area. Spread of the tumor occurs promptly and usually by way of the lymphatic channels which drain the hypopharynx, exiting between the lateral portion of the hyoid bone and the upper edge of the thyroid cartilage to travel with the superior thyroid artery to the midjugular chain of lymph nodes. Unlike most head and neck cancers, distant metastases are common with involvement of mediastinal nodes, lung, liver, and other distant viscera.

DIAGNOSIS. Since these lesions arise outside the endolarynx away from major paths of respiration and speech, hoarseness or dyspnea are uncommon findings until late in the growth of the tumor. Interference with swallowing, on the other hand, is the most common early symptom and is associated with choking and aspiration. Aspiration pneumonia may be the illness which first brings the patient to the physician. The lesions seem to have a long silent period and can grow to considerable size in the depths of the piriform sinus or on the pharyngeal walls before the first definite symptoms appear. Not uncommonly, the first sign is the appearance of a midjugular cervical node. The better-differentiated lesions invade and ulcerate widely, so that a malodorous breath is a common associated finding. Diagnosis is confirmed by indirect laryngoscopy and biopsy through a laryngoscope.

TREATMENT. Until recent years this was a highly lethal tumor with few cures either by operation or by irradiation. The introduction of wide radical excision with removal of the larynx and hypopharynx and en bloc radical neck dissection increased the cure rate perceptibly. This may be another area where judicious combination of irradiation and operation can improve the cure rate even more. Five-year survival rates with the older form of therapy were no more than 10 to 15 percent. With more aggressive operative approaches, cure rates in the vicinity of 30 percent have been reported.

NASOPHARYNX

The nasopharynx is at the top of the pharynx, just underneath the base of the skull. The body of the sphenoid bone forms a roof for this cavity, while its floor is formed by the soft palate. There is no anterior wall as such except for the posterior openings of the nasal passage together with the posterior aspects of the nasal septum and the turbinates. The roof of the cavity slopes into the posterior wall made up of the basiocciput and the atlas and the overlying covering of muscle and mucosa. Each lateral wall contains the opening of a eustachian tube guarded by a small prominence, the torus tubarius. The only structure lying within the nasopharynx is the lymphoid tissue of the adenoids scattered on the posterior and superior walls.

INCIDENCE. These tumors are uncommon but not rare, constituting about $\frac{1}{2}$ percent of all cancers. They are somewhat more common in males than in females (2.4:1). There is an interesting relation to race. This is a frequent tumor in the Near East, among the Filipinos, Malays, and

Dayaks, and especially among the Chinese. This cancer accounts for 30.4 percent of all cancers in males in Formosa. The incidence among the Chinese born in the Far East is more than thirty times greater than in this country, while the incidence among American-born Chinese is about six times as common as the incidence among the other racial groups here. This shift in pattern would suggest that both genetic and environmental causative factors are operating.

Benign Lesions

These include hypetrophied lymphatic tissue, juvenile nasopharyngeal hemangiofibroma, Rathke's pouch cyst, dermoids, and mixed tumors. Of these, hypertrophied adenoids occur commonly, and hemangiofibroma and Rathke's pouch cyst have a special predilection for this site.

Any enlarging, space-occupying lesion of the nasopharynx calls attention to itself by respiratory obstruction and nasal stuffiness. Obstruction to the eustachian tubes provokes earaches and often chronic ear infection. As the lesion encroaches on the soft palate, deglutition is disturbed with pain on swallowing or regurgitation of food and fluids into the nasopharynx and out of the nose.

HYPERTROPHIED ADENOIDS

The adenoids represent a portion of the large circle of lymphatic tissue surrounding the oral respiratory passageway at the level of the posterior tongue and tonsils. Chronic upper respiratory tract infections in infants and children often cause marked and persistent hypertrophy of some of this rim of tissue. In past decades resection of the adenoids and tonsils was one of the most common of operations in children. With the advent of the antibiotics the need for these procedures has diminished markedly. Nonetheless, in an occasional child a persistent hypertrophy of the adenoids will develop which disturbs his breathing pattern, causing mouth breathing, or more importantly will obstruct the eustachian tubes, leading to chronic ear infections with a threat to the child's hearing. These symptoms are adequate indication for operative excision.

JUVENILE NASOPHARYNGEAL HEMANGIOFIBROMA

Made up of a hard stroma of fibrous tissue, richly interlaced with capillaries and cavernous sinuses, this rare and interesting tumor appears to originate on the roof of the nasopharynx perhaps from the periosteum of the sphenoid bone (Fig. 16-29). It increases in size slowly but relentlessly and eventually begins to erode the anterior structures, obstruct the nasal passages and enter the maxillary sinus on one or both sides. The first symptom may be nasal obstruction but is usually epistaxis, which can be very profuse and even life-threatening.

This lesion is found exclusively in males, usually in the preadolescent or adolescent age groups. In some instances as the boy matures, the lesion appears to regress spontaneously. Just as often it persists, and hemangiofibromas of the nasopharynx have been described in males in their

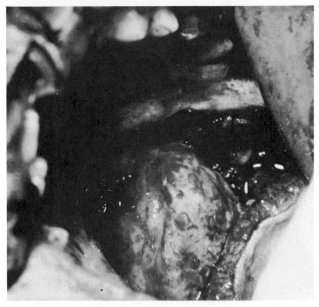

Fig. 16-29. Juvenile nasopharyngeal hemangiofibroma. A fibrous, highly vascular lesion on the posterior wall of the nasopharynx. This was first noted because of epistaxis. Exposure was obtained by an incision between the hard and soft palate with retraction of the soft palate downward.

twenties and thirties, either persisting from childhood or appearing for the first time.

The progressive destruction of surrounding bone by pressure and the continuing threat of major hemorrhage require prompt treatment, preferably before the lesions grow too large. Radiation therapy is ineffective, and operative excision appears the only mode of treatment. There is a tendency toward local recurrence following excision, and these patients must be followed carefully for some years after operation.

Malignant Lesions

These are epidermoid carcinoma, lymphosarcoma, adenoid cystic carcinoma, cervical chordoma, sarcoma, and myeloma. The only lesions occurring with any frequency are epidermoid carcinoma and lymphosarcoma.

EPIDERMOID CARCINOMA

These develop from areas of metaplasia in the respiratory epithelium of the nasopharynx and are moderately to highly undifferentiated. There is a liberal amount of lymphoid tissue in the nasopharynx, and frequently malignant epithelial cells are seen mixed with a prominent lymphoid stroma. This mixture of epidermoid and lymphoid cells gave rise to the term "lymphoepithelioma" introduced by Regaud and Schmincke. Many pathologists feel there is no place for this special term, since these tumors are probably highly anaplastic epidermoid carcinomas and the lymphoid element may not constitute an actual malignant part of the growth. Some feel that a large percentage of lymphoid intermixing indicates a more radiosensitive and more radiocurable tumor.

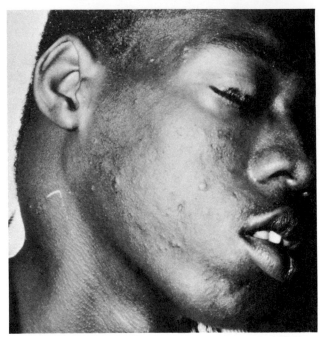

Fig. 16-30. Metastatic lymph nodes in the neck from lymphosarcoma of the nasopharynx. Note the characteristic location behind and inferior to the ear.

In addition to the obstructive symptoms described for benign tumors, the invasive qualities of malignant lesions produce a number of characteristic signs and symptoms. These lesions invade the roof of the nasopharynx entering the cavernous sinus with paralysis of the IIId, IVth, Vth, and VIth cranial nerves. The VIth nerve is usually paralyzed first; this is frequently accompanied by pain in the distribution of the supraorbital and infraorbital branches of the Vth nerve. The tumor reaches these nerves by spreading along the eustachian tube into the space between the pharynx and the maxilla, then extending upward through the suture line between the petrous portion of the temporal bone and the lateral wing of the sphenoid. Thus, the symptom complex is called the *petrosphenoidal syndrome*. Metastatic nodes in the retropharyngeal space tend to spread into the area along the base of the skull medial to the parotid gland, where they compress the IXth, Xth, XIth, and XIIth cranial nerves. This causes difficulties with deglutition from hemiparesis of the superior constrictor muscle, a perversion of the sense of taste in the posterior third of the tongue, and hypesthesia of the mucous membranes of the soft palate, pharynx, and larynx. Paralysis of the trapezius muscle, the sternocleidomastoid, the soft palate, and one side of the tongue may also occur. These signs may be associated with Horner's syndrome from compression of the cervical sympathetic chain. Invasion of the orbit and displacement of the globe will cause double vision and proptosis.

Unfortunately, the nasopharynx is a silent area, and tumors here can reach considerable size before any symptoms are evident. The early signs of nasal obstruction or brief episodes of epistaxis are easily ignored. In two-thirds of the patients, by the time diagnosis is made, invasion of the sphenoid bone and base of the skull or nerve paralysis is present. Not infrequently, the primary growth will remain small, even microscopic, and is announced by its cervical metastases. These occur in a characteristic location, high in the neck behind the lower portion of the ear with additional involved nodes scattered along the path of the spinal accessory nerve as it courses down the trapezius muscle (Fig. 16-30). Cervical metastases are found in 50 percent of patients when first seen and are the presenting symptom in one-third.

There is no acceptable way of obtaining an adequate margin of resection when operating upon lesions of the nasopharynx, and the only operative procedure used is biopsy. Treatment of the primary lesion and usually of the metastases is by radiation therapy. Considering the advanced state of most of these lesions when first seen, the 5-year survival rate as a result of therapy is remarkably good, with an overall absolute survival of 28 percent. For the occasional patient who does not have evidence of cervical node metastasis at the beginning of treatment the 5-year survival rate is 55 percent.

LYMPHOSARCOMA

Lymphosarcomas of the nasopharynx tend to occur at the extremes of age in childhood and in the seventh and eighth decades. The majority of these lesions announce their presence by the occurrence of cervical node metastases, which are usually bulky with a rubbery consistency; the nodes mat together but are less inclined to be invasive and fixed than nodes involved by carcinoma. While lymphosarcoma may mimic all the symptoms produced by epidermoid carcinomas, they invade bone infrequently, and paralysis of nerves is much less common. If there is no evidence of spread beyond the area of the head and neck, the radiotherapist usually administers a high level of therapy in the vicinity of 6,000 rads of cobalt to both the nasopharynx and the cervical lymphatic tissues bilaterally. Five-year survival in these highly radiosensitive tumors is slightly better than for epidermoid carcinoma, averaging 35 to 40 percent.

NASAL CAVITY AND PARANASAL SINUSES

The position of the eight nasal sinuses surrounding the nasal cavity is often poorly appreciated. The maxillary sinuses lateral to the nasal cavities and beneath the orbits are the largest and most important of the sinus structures. The ethmoid air cells occupying the space between the orbit and the upper nasal cavity are much smaller and are less commonly involved by tumors. The frontal sinuses bilaterally above the orbits are the second largest set of sinuses. The paired sphenoid sinuses divided by a thin septum just below the pituitary and over the roof of the nasopharynx are the most remote of the sinuses. The frontal and sphenoid sinuses are rare primary sites for tumors.

INCIDENCE. Tumors of the nasal cavity and paranasal

sinuses represent about 1 percent of all cancer seen. Malignant lesions are found here three times as commonly in men as in women. With the exception of the esthesioneuroblastoma no specific cause is known for lesions arising here.

Benign Tumors

Polyps of the nasal cavity and maxillary sinus are the most common growths seen. These are usually associated with chronic inflammation or, occasionally, allergy. Sometimes the underlying infection may be due to a tumor, so that the discovery of polyps should not be considered an adequate diagnosis until the possibility of an underlying tumor has been ruled out. While polyps can be eradicated by simple excision, they will usually re-form unless the basic pathologic condition leading to their growth has been determined and corrected. This may be allergy, septal deviation, or other factors which obstruct adequate drainage and promote infection.

Malignant Tumors

Of 293 patients with neoplasms of the nasal cavity and paranasal sinus examined at the Mayo Clinic approximately 50 percent had epidermoid carcinomas, 10 percent had lymphomas, and 20 percent had tumors which probably arose from minor salivary tissue. The remaining 20 percent had various soft tissue sarcomas such as fibrosarcoma, chondrosarcoma, neurofibrosarcoma, and osteogenic sarcoma. Among 648 patients seen in Sweden with epidermoid carcinomas arising from the paranasal sinuses, the average age ranged from fifty to seventy years, and the vast majority of the lesions arose in the maxillary sinus (Fig. 16-31). None of these tumors occurred in the sphenoid sinus and only one in the frontal sinus.

Tumors, whether benign or malignant, are announced by pain, nasal obstruction, and persistent nasal secretion. Fifty percent of the patients present with one or more of these three symptoms. Unfortunately, these are also the presenting symptoms of sinusitis; patients may be treated with antibiotics and other measures for long periods before the more serious nature of the disease is realized. Repeated epistaxis is more likely to suggest the presence of tumor but occurs in only 10 percent as a presenting symptom. Swelling or ulceration of the hard palate or gingiva, swelling of the cheek, or ocular symptoms are evidences of a much more advanced stage of tumor growth yet constitute the presenting symptom in 25 to 30 percent of patients (Fig. 16-32). Bone destruction seen on roentgenographic examination is almost certain evidence of a tumor and unfortunately is also a late sign. Absence of bone destruction does not rule out a malignant tumor. All tissue removed when polyps of the nose or maxillary sinus are treated or when the maxillary sinus is drained should be submitted for histologic examination. Not infrequently this is the first evidence of the presence of an underlying carcinoma and may be the only opportunity for diagnosis of such lesions at an early state.

TREATMENT. Electrosurgical therapy, radiation therapy,

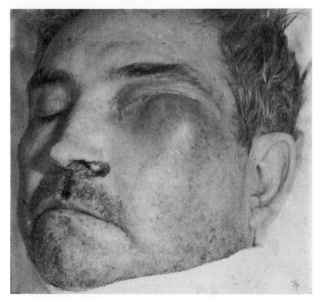

Fig. 16-31. Squamous carcinoma of the maxilla. The lesion had its origin in the upper portion of the maxillary sinus and invaded the floor of the orbit.

Fig. 16-32. Squamous carcinoma of the ethmoid sinuses. This lesion began in the left ethmoid and invaded the nasal cavity and right ethmoid sinus.

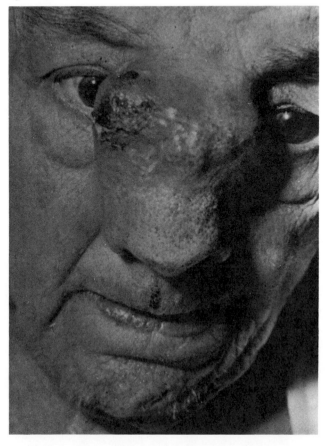

and operative excision have all been used to treat these tumors. Lymphomas are ordinarily treated by radiation alone. Epidermoid carcinomas of this site are refractory to either irradiation or operation. Integration of irradiation preoperatively with operative excision has been used for many years and has gained wide acceptance. This approach yields a 5-year survival rate of 30 to 35 percent for lesions of the maxillary sinuses. Cervical lymph nodes are involved late, and radical neck dissections are not done unless palpable nodes are present.

MANDIBLE

Tumors of the mandible arise from two main sources, from the tooth-forming (odontogenic) tissue and from bone.

Odontogenic Tumors

These neoplasms arise from ectodermal odontogenic tissue, mesodermal odontogenic tissue, or a mixture of both. They are invariably benign. The lesions most commonly seen are ectodermal odontogenic cysts: the follicular and radicular cysts. A rare and intriguing tumor is the ameloblastoma. Other odontogenic tumors are too rare to merit consideration here.

FOLLICULAR CYST

Some cysts are derived from the dental lamina and outer enamel epithelium of developing teeth. Remnants of this tissue sequestered during development may undergo proliferation and cystic change. Microscopically, they have fibrous walls usually lined by squamous epithelium. Occasionally remnants of odontogenic epithelium are present from which ameloblastomas may develop. Often the cyst

Fig. 16-33. Roentgenogram of a radicular cyst. Note the root of the tooth from which the cyst took origin. (*Courtesy of Sheldon Rovin, D.D.S.*)

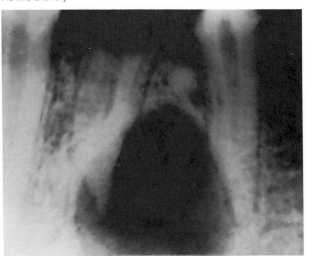

envelops an unerupted tooth. A pathognomonic x-ray finding is the appearance of a smooth symmetric cyst in the mandible containing an unerupted tooth in its cavity. Clinically the tumor is found as a mass causing enlargement of the ramus of the mandible or the rim of the gingiva. Treatment is by intraoral excision, removing the top of the cyst and excising its entire lining membrane.

RADICULAR CYST

Infection of the dental pulp is the most common cause of this frequent cyst. A dental granuloma forms when epithelial remnants of the sheath about the tooth root are entrapped. Nests of epithelial tissue proliferate to line a central lumen usually at the apex of the infected tooth (Fig. 16-33). Cysts may vary in size from 1 to several centimeters. Microscopically, there is a dense, fibrous connective tissue lining covered internally by squamous epithelium. Frequently, a generalized inflammatory reaction in the cyst wall is seen. Treatment is by extraction of the tooth involved and excision of the cyst with its lining.

AMELOBLASTOMA

Although very uncommon, this is the most frequent solid tumor of the mandible. It usually appears in the body of the mandible at its junction with the ramus. Growth is slow, and the lesion is relatively asymptomatic, although it may expand the bone about it and eventually attain enormous size, encroaching on soft tissues of the face and neck (Fig. 16-34). Microscopically, the tumor presents interlacing strands and nests of odontogenic epithelium enmeshed in a connective tissue stroma with numerous areas of cystic degeneration. Treatment is by segmental resection of the portion of the mandible affected by the tumor including a centimeter or two of normal bone on either side. Unless the wide excision is accomplished, recurrence is common. The adjacent soft tissues need not be resected, and a good bed is usually left for reconstruction of the mandible.

Osteogenic Tumors

The mandible is affected by the same group of benign and malignant tumors which affect other bones in the body. Benign lesions include exostosis (torus mandibularis), fibrous dysplasia, Paget's disease, and giant cell tumor. Primary malignant lesions are multiple myeloma, Ewing's sarcoma, osteogenic sarcoma, chondrosarcoma (Fig. 16-35), and periosteal fibrosarcoma.

Giant cell tumors of the mandible are often referred to as *central* reparative giant cell tumors and are equivalent to the peripheral giant cell tumors of the gingiva. Although this lesion grows slowly and expands the surrounding bone, it never appears to have the malignant potential of giant cell tumors seen elsewhere in the skeleton and may have a different histogenesis. Microscopically, no distinction can be made between mandibular giant cell tumors and giant cell lesions of other bones. Treatment is usually by unroofing the tumor and curetting its tissue from the bony cavity.

SALIVARY GLANDS

Salivary tissue is found in the parotid gland, the submaxillary gland, the lingual gland, and the numerous salivary glands. The parotid gland is a unilobular structure which is bent in a U shape about the posterior portion of the mandible in such a way that the larger external portion of the gland is often called the *superficial lobe* and the smaller internal portion lying on the internal surface of the ascending ramus is called the *deep lobe*. The VIIth nerve exiting from the skull by way of the stylohyoid foramen crosses the space between the mastoid and the ascending ramus of the mandible and plunges into the parotid gland at the point where it turns the corner around the posterior edge of the ascending ramus. The VIIth nerve usually bifurcates within the substance of the parotid. Each bifurcation further subdivides, and the branches eventually lie between the parotid gland and the underlying masseter muscle. The relationship of the VIIth nerve to the parotid gland is of clinical importance, since tumors of the parotid lie most commonly in the external portion of the gland; on excising such tumors great care must be taken not to cut the branches or the main trunk of this nerve.

The submaxillary gland is an ovoid structure lying in the submaxillary fossa beneath the horizontal ramus of the mandible. It is bounded by the anterior and posterior portions of the digastric muscle, thus occupying most of the digastric triangle in the neck. The important relationships of this gland are to the ramus mandibularis, the lowest branch of the VIIth nerve which courses over the upper portion of the gland. Injury to this nerve blocks innervation of the inferior quarter of the orbicularis oris on the side of the nerve and deprives the patient of the ability to pucker his lips normally. The lingual nerve, deep to the upper inferior surface of the submaxillary gland, provides the gland with some small branches. In addition, the lingual nerve parallels the course of Wharton's duct, which conducts saliva from the submaxillary gland to the mouth. When the gland is removed, injury to the lingual nerve can occur either when Wharton's duct is clamped or when the gland is pulled down into the neck dragging the lingual nerve along by its nerve attachments.

The lingual gland is the smallest of the three major salivary glands. It lies beneath the mucosa of the anterior floor of the mouth.

The minor salivary glands are small deposits of salivary tissue which are scattered throughout the mucosa of the oral cavity, maxilla, and nasopharynx. The term "ectopic salivary tissue" is sometimes used but carries an incorrect connotation, since this salivary tissue is a normal finding in all individuals and is not the result of an error in development.

INCIDENCE. About $\frac{1}{3}$ percent of all malignant tumors occurs in the salivary tissues. These tumors are equally common in men and women. About 60 percent of these lesions occur in the parotid glands, which is not surprising, since this is the largest single collection of salivary tissues. The second largest concentration of tumors is found in the submaxillary gland and the third largest in the minor

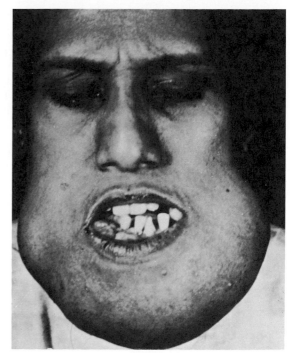

Fig. 16-34. Ameloblastoma. These lesions can grow to fantastic size, as shown here. Aside from the mass and functional disability, they are painless and never become malignant. (*Courtesy of Sheldon Rovin, D.D.S.*)

salivary glands. Tumors of the lingual glands are rare. No specific cause is known for any of the benign or malignant tumors of the salivary glands other than the occasional congenital or obstructive cyst. Women with malignant tumors of the salivary glands are known to have a higher incidence of cancer of the breast.

Benign Lesions. A variety of lesions may arise in salivary tissue.

Fig. 16-35. Chondrosarcoma of the mandible. This is a slowly developing lesion and was present in this patient for 9 years before medical aid was sought. The pressure of the upper gingiva has caused the groove which is seen in the dorsal surface of the tumor. Even at this late date, the tumor had not metastasized, and the patient was still alive and well 5 years after resection. (*From B. F. Rush, Jr., and K. Trinkle, South Med J, 60:714, 1967.*)

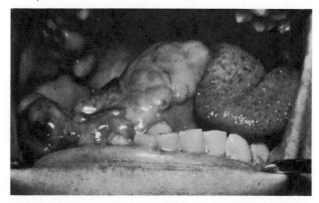

Mixed Tumors. The most common lesion of the salivary glands is the mixed tumor (pleomorphic adenoma). Fifty percent of all tumors of the salivary glands and over eighty percent of all benign tumors are mixed tumors. These probably originate from adult glandular epithelium and, as their name implies, have an extremely diverse structural pattern. In 90 percent of the tumors one finds areas where the tumor grows in a network of strands made up of spindle and stellate cells not always connecting and sometimes lying entirely detached. In about a third of all cases this loose myxoid pattern predominates but is by no means the sole structural component. Half the tumors have pseudocartilaginous structures. Twenty percent show tissue closely resembling hyaline cartilage. Well-formed tubular structures are common and present a wide variety of patterns. The lining epithelium may be single-layered, conspicuously double-layered, stratified, or pseudostratified. Some areas of metaplasia into squamous epithelium may be seen, and well-differentiated squamous epithelium can be found in about a fourth of the cases.

Papillary Cystadenoma Lymphomatosum (Warthin's Tumor). These curious lesions occur only in parotid salivary tissue and almost exclusively (95 percent) in males. About 10 percent of them are bilateral. Characteristically they are made up of a papillary epithelial component intermingled with well-developed lymphoid tissue commonly containing germinal centers. Their histogenesis is uncertain, but many feel they represent parotid duct tissue sequestered in lymph nodes within the parotid gland. They represent the second most common benign tumor of salivary tissue but are a poor second to mixed tumors, which are at least eight times more common.

Mikulicz's Disease. This disease is characterized by a dense infiltration of lymphocytes occasionally arranged in follicles throughout the salivary tissue. This is accompanied by atrophy and disappearance of acinar tissue. Scattered throughout the lymphoid tissue are foci of epithelial and myloepithelial cells in close relationship to distal structures. The more popular modern term for this lesion is *benign lymphoepithelial lesion,* and many feel it represents a phase of the larger disease complex *Sjögren's syndrome.* The diffuse lymphocytic infiltrate, much as one sees in lymphomatous thyroiditis, suggests the possibility of an autoimmune disease. While several of or all the major salivary glands may be involved, a single parotid gland is the most frequent site (80 percent). The highest incidence of the disease is in patients between thirty-one and forty years of age.

Asymptomatic Enlargement of Salivary Tissue. This affection is usually observed in both parotid glands but may involve all the major salivary glands. The characteristic microscopic findings are an increase in size of the glandular acini due to swelling of the individual acinar cells. There is an increase of the secretory granules, a fatty infiltration, and a moderate fibrosis. These changes seem associated with nutritional deficiencies and have been found in patients suffering from cirrhosis of the liver, kwashiorkor, and diabetes mellitus. It also has been found in whole populations suffering from malnutrition in India, in Greece during the occupation of World War II, and in the inmates of German concentration camps. Katsilambros believes that this is a fundamental response to a deficiency of vitamin A and has duplicated his findings in vitamin A–deficient rats.

Other Lesions. Cysts of the parotid glands are seen quite rarely and in some instances may represent cysts of the first branchial cleft. Hemangiomas in children have a predilection for the area of the parotid gland and sometimes persist into adulthood. Neurofibromas and lipomas of the parotid gland have been described.

Malignant Lesions. About 75 percent of all malignant salivary tumors arise from the parotid gland, and 25 percent of all parotid tumors are malignant. Ten percent of malignant salivary lesions arise in the submaxillary gland and an additional twelve percent in the minor salivary glands. The incidence of malignant lesions in the submaxillary and minor salivary glands compared to benign lesions is somewhat higher than in the parotid gland, averaging one-third to one-half of all lesions seen. Roughly one-third of the malignant lesions of salivary tissue arise from the acinar epithelium and are adenocarcinomas. Another third arise from the ductal epithelium as various forms of epidermoid carcinomas. The remaining third appear either as highly anaplastic and unclassified lesions or as malignant mixed tumors.

Epidermoid Carcinoma. The most frequent of these are the mucoepidermoid carcinomas originally identified as a special group by Stewart et al. in 1945. These interesting tumors are made up, as the name indicates, of epidermoid cells and mucus-containing cells. The name falls short of being completely descriptive, since there is a third cell called an "intermediate" cell, smaller than either of the other two, which closely resembles certain cells of the salivary gland duct. They are commonly seen in stratifications lining dilated ductlike structures. Stewart et al. suggest that this intermediate cell is capable of differentiation into mucinous cells or into epidermoid and even squamous cells.

Mucoepidermoid carcinomas are usually divided on the basis of the microscopic appearance into low-grade and high-grade tumors. Low-grade tumors contain a large portion of mucus-secreting cells, often with the presence of microcysts and large amounts of mucoid material which may leak diffusely through the tissues, generating variable degrees of inflammatory reaction. In the highly malignant tumors epidermoid and intermediate cells dominate the picture. Pseudoglandular formation is fairly frequent, and the growth pattern is commonly sheetlike or in coarse plugs.

Squamous cell carcinomas like mucoepidermoid carcinomas must certainly originate in the ductal epithelium, and the ability of salivary duct epithelium to undergo squamous metaplasia is well known. Stewart et al. suggest that most squamous cell carcinomas represent diffuse squamous cell overgrowth of tumors that were fundamentally mucoepidermoid. Microscopically, these lesions share the usual features of squamous cell carcinomas seen in the skin, oral cavity, and elsewhere. In this location, however, they are usually more malignant, and local and regional metastases are common.

Adenocarcinoma. *Adenoid Cystic Carcinoma (Cylindroma).* The chief histologic feature of these lesions is the arrangement of rather small, darkly staining cells with relatively low cytoplasm in anastomosing cords between which are acellular areas which may contain mucous, hyaline, or mucohyaline material. The cystic components of an adenoid cystic carcinoma usually stain positively with mucicarmine, indicating the presence of mucin. While the lesions are of sluggish evolution, metastases to cervical lymph nodes develop in 30 percent of the cases.

Acinar Cell Adenocarcinoma. These histologically distinct tumors are of low-grade clinical malignancy and fairly rare. They appear to arise from the acinar cells of salivary tissue and to be limited to the parotid gland. In the usual microscopic arrangement rounded or polygonal cells with a dark eccentric nucleus and a finely granular basophilic cytoplasm are packed closely together, sometimes in crude, acinar groups. While low-grade, these lesions are capable of metastasis both regionally and to distant locations.

Miscellaneous Adenocarcinomas. Adenocarcinomas may have a trabecular pattern and may be anaplastic or resemble adenocarcinomas of the gastrointestinal tract. These are usually highly malignant with a high degree of local invasiveness and regional and distant metastases.

Malignant Mixed Tumors. It is usually assumed that malignant mixed tumors arise from a neoplastic transformation of a previously benign mixed tumor. Patients who demonstrate these lesions are generally older than those with benign mixed tumors and have had a mass in the parotid for a longer period. Moreover, the malignant lesions are usually larger than the benign. In general, the microscopic picture is of a definite mixed tumor which contains within it malignant elements which may be adenocarcinomas, squamous cell carcinomas, or a malignant spindle cell alteration. The malignant component of a mixed tumor may so greatly overgrow the area of origin that it is extremely difficult to identify the previous benign mixed tumor.

NATURAL HISTORY. With the exception of the mixed tumor the common benign lesions of salivary tissue have no malignant potential. While the mixed tumor may have a very long history without malignant transformation and may grow for 20 to 30 years at a slow pace (Fig. 16-36), a rapidly growing and even anaplastic component can suddenly develop which markedly changes its course. On rare occasions mixed tumors have been found which have metastasized to local nodes without apparent histologic change and in their new location have pursued a slow course of growth. The most common pattern, however, is the development of a squamous cell carcinoma, adenocarcinoma, or other tumor which rapidly overgrows the original mixed tumor. Some very slowly evolving "chronic" carcinomas are known to develop from salivary tissue. Notable among these are the adenoid cystic carcinomas, which may develop their metastases 10, 15, and even 20 years after treatment of the primary tumor.

Many such tumors have been reported in which metastatic nodules in the lungs have been observed growing very slowly, at times appearing almost stationary for 10 and 15 years. The mucoepidermoid carcinoma, while not as

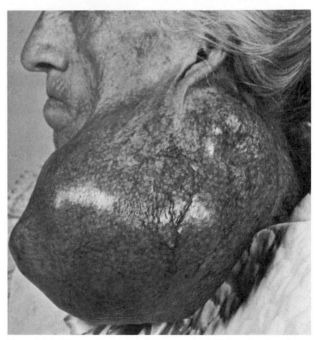

Fig. 16-36. Giant mixed tumor of the parotid. This lesion had been present for 29 years. It was still benign and was excised without evidence of recurrence in a 5-year follow-up. (*From B. F. Rush, Jr., and K. Trinkle, South Med J, 60:714, 1967.*)

slow-growing as the adenoid cystic carcinoma, is rather slowly progressive; however, this trait is offset by its great degree of local invasiveness, especially by perineural invasion. The chances for local recurrence are great even after wide local excision. Squamous cell carcinomas and adenocarcinomas of the salivary glands are almost always highly malignant, quick to invade and metastasize, and fatal in a high percentage of the patients affected.

DIFFERENTIAL DIAGNOSIS. Most tumors of the salivary glands appear as painless, slowly growing nodules (Fig. 16-37). Lesions of the parotid are bound by the heavy

Fig. 16-37. Multilobulated mixed tumor of the parotid. The lesion presents in the upper pole of the superficial portion of the gland.

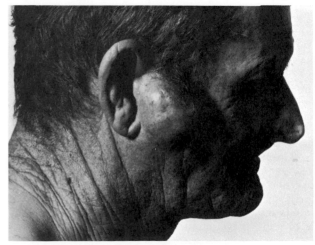

cervical fascia which splits on either side of the gland and invests it with a strong capsule. This dense covering obscures the actual size of the underlying tumor, and the surgeon may be surprised by the size and extent of a lesion at operation. Paralysis of the VIIth nerve is indicative of a malignant tumor and usually of a highly malignant lesion such as squamous carcinoma or adenocarcinoma. Mucoepidermoid carcinomas of the low-grade type or adenoid cystic carcinomas frequently spare the nerve until quite late in their course. Fixation of the gland to underlying structures and palpable nodes in the neck are also more commonly seen with the tumors of higher grade. Since there is nothing that can distinguish the benign mass in the salivary gland from an early malignant tumor, excision of the mass and histologic examination are indicated in every case.

TREATMENT. Benign mixed tumors, the most common solid tumors of salivary gland origin, are so easily disseminated that incisional biopsy is never indicated. In earlier decades the technique of choice for removal was enucleation. Follow-up of patients so treated indicated that local recurrence was late and slow to develop and occurred in as many as 50 percent. Attempt at excision of these lesions with a cuff of surrounding normal tissue was accompanied by a high rate of injury to one or more branches of the VIIth nerve.

Through these painful experiences the present method of therapy was developed. After isolation of the VIIth nerve, the superficial portion of the parotid gland is dissected from the underlying tissues and removed with the tumor contained within it, assuring against injury of branches of the facial nerve and against dissemination and local recurrence of the tumor.

Frozen section of the lesion should be done at operation. If a low-grade malignant lesion such as an acinar cell adenocarcinoma, a low-grade mucoepidermoid carcinoma, or an adenoid cystic carcinoma is identified, the remainder of the gland and probably the VIIth nerve should be removed. If a high-grade lesion such as an anaplastic adenocarcinoma or squamous carcinoma is identified, a radical neck dissection should accompany the procedure. Aside from the problem of dealing with the VIIth nerve, the same general rules apply for lesions in the submaxillary gland.

Most of the tumors of salivary glands have a reputation for being poorly radiosensitive; however, the more malignant the lesion, the less likely this is to be true. Many high-grade mucoepidermoid carcinomas, squamous carcinomas, and even an occasional adenocarcinoma will demonstrate considerable sensitivity to x-ray therapy.

PROGNOSIS. Benign mixed tumors will recur in 40 to 50 percent of patients if improperly excised. If excision is by superficial lobectomy, the recurrence rate should be 5 percent or less. Five-year survival rates tend to be misleading, particularly in the chronic, slow-growing tumors. Adenoid cystic carcinoma has an 86 percent 5-year survival rate but a 57 percent 10-year survival. Malignant mixed tumor may have a 5-year survival of 87 to 90 percent and a 10-year survival of 60 to 70 percent.

TUMORS OF THE NECK

Palpable or visible cervical swellings are a common complaint. Two to three percent of all admissions to hospital surgical services are for this condition. About half of these lesions occur in the thyroid gland; the remainder are due to a wide range of malignant, congenital, or inflammatory swellings.

Inflammation

Inflammatory swelling in the adult neck is now a rare hospital problem. Skandalakis and coworkers, in reviewing 1,616 nonthyroid masses of the neck, found that only 3.2 percent were inflammatory, whereas 84 percent were neoplastic and 12 percent congenital or miscellaneous. The inflammatory lesions requiring hospitalization of adults are largely acute, often resulting from drainage from infection elsewhere. A common source is an infected tooth draining to the nodes in the submandibular area and causing an abscess. Only two patients in Skandalakis' entire series had tuberculous adenitis (scrofula). This was once the most common cause of neck masses, but with the tuberculin testing of cows and the pasteurization of milk, bovine tuberculosis has virtually disappeared in this country.

Malignant Tumors

The vast majority of cervical masses in adults are due to neoplasms. About 80 percent of these are metastatic from some other site, while the remainder occur from primary lesions in the neck. Primary cervical neoplasms occur either in the major salivary glands (40 percent) or are lymphomas primary in the cervical lymph nodes (60 percent). At one time it was proposed the squamous carcinomas arose primarily in the neck from the lining of branchial cleft cysts. This diagnosis was often made only to discover at a later date that the lesion was actually a metastasis from the oral cavity, nasopharynx, or laryngeal area. While there is some evidence that branchiogenic cysts become malignant, the reported, provable cases number only a handful.

A knowledge of the statistics quickly indicates that a clinician's first suspicion concerning any nonthyroid, cervical mass in adults is of a malignant tumor. He may also suspect that it is metastatic and from a site at some point above the clavicle, since 85 percent of all metastatic cervical lesions come from a supraclavicular site.

When a firm to hard cervical node which suggests malignancy is found, the first responsibility of clinicians is a thorough exploration of possible sites of origin. Cervical tumors appearing below and behind the ear and along the cervical chain are more likely to come from the nasopharynx or lateral pharyngeal walls. Swollen lymph nodes at the angle of the mandible or in the area of the submaxillary gland are most commonly from lesions in the tonsillar area, buccal mucosa, floor of the mouth, and gingiva. Swelling of the lymph nodes in the submental area should provoke a thorough examination of the tip of the tongue, lower lip, and anterior gingivobuccal gutter. Lymph nodes involved by neoplasm which appear in the middle third of the neck should cast suspicion first on the hypopharynx, piriform sinus, larynx, or thyroid.

Only when enlarged lymph nodes appear in the supraclavicular area does metastasis from below the clavicle become a major possibility. These may stem from carcinoma of the upper lobes of the lung or mediastinum or, in women, from carcinoma of the breast. The left supraclavicular nodes are frequently involved by malignant tumors metastatic from the abdomen (Virchow's node). Advanced adenocarcinoma of the stomach, pancreas, biliary tree, and even large bowel metastasize to this site.

If a thorough search of all sites reveals no possible source of a primary lesion, biopsy of the cervical node is usually carried out. If this confirms the clinical impression of malignancy, further attempts to find the primary lesion are indicated. This can include surgical exploration of the maxillary sinuses. If all avenues have been searched thoroughly and no primary lesion has been found, the problem of local treatment still remains. The best course is to treat the lesion to achieve cure. If operation is chosen, it should be a radical neck dissection; if radiation therapy is used, it should be a full course of therapy. Since lymph nodes involved by metastatic disease respond poorly to radiation, the treatment of choice is normally operation. In the presence of advanced lesions a combination of radiation and operation may be used.

If a group of these patients treated without a known primary lesion is followed for 5 years, 80 percent of the patients will ultimately manifest the primary lesion. In some instances this may subsequently be resected for cure. A few patients may die over this period without ever demonstrating the source for the metastatic lesion, and even at postmortem examination it may not be found. Even more interesting, about 20 percent of the patients survive 5 or more years with apparent "cure" of their metastatic lesion even though the presumed primary lesion has not been found or treated. In those patients who received radiation therapy, either together with operation or alone, it may be that the port included the primary lesion as well. In those patients who are treated by operation alone, the fate of the primary lesion remains a mystery. A few of these patients may represent true branchiogenic carcinoma, or possibly the primary lesion regresses spontaneously.

Other Lesions

A host of other tumors, found infrequently in the area of the neck, present problems in differential diagnosis. Dermoids occur in the midline, most commonly in the submental area and sometimes along the line of the clavicle. Sebaceous cysts are common, especially in men, and probably are related to the trauma of shaving.

Carotid body tumors (chemodectomas) are rare tumors of the paraganglionic tissue found at the carotid bifurcation. Another lesion with a slow evolution, it gradually increases in size over many years, enveloping the bifurca-

tion and slowly compressing the adjacent nerves including the hypoglossal, vagus, and sympathetic chain. For many periods, the only symptom is the mass in the neck. Eventually nerve paralysis, dysphagia, and pain appear. Malignant transformation is rare, but early removal is indicated to avoid the late symptoms. Small lesions can be removed easily (Fig. 16-38), but advanced large tumors require resection of the carotid artery with the risk of subsequent hemiparesis.

TUMORS OF THE NECK IN CHILDREN

The order of frequency of masses in the neck in children differs markedly from that found in adults. Inflammatory lesions are by far the most common, often coming from related infections of the tonsils. The most common malignant lesion is the lymphoma, and the second most common is carcinoma of the thyroid. Congenital lesions, of course, are much more common in children than in adults.

CHEMOTHERAPY AND IMMUNOTHERAPY

In the past decade it has been discovered that certain types of neoplasms commonly found in the head and neck area can be cured by chemotherapy. Burkitt's lymphoma, a rare neoplasm in the United States but common in some parts of Africa, was the first such cancer. It became apparent that a predictable and consistent percentage of patients with this disease could be cured by the use of *systemic* chemotherapy alone. Recently we have also learned that squamous cancer of facial skin and of the lips, while in the in situ or microinvasive and superficial stages, can be

Fig. 16-38. Carotid body tumor of moderate size. The lesion lies between the internal and external branches of the carotid arteries; the adventitial layer binding it to the carotid bulb has been removed. (*From B. F. Rush, Jr., Ann Surg, 157:633, 1963.*)

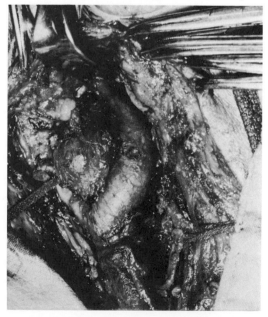

cured by the topical application of 5-fluorouracil used as a cream or paste. These lesions are multiple and often tedious to eradicate by operation or radiation. A third head and neck lesion in which chemotherapy has become important is embryonal rhabdomyosarcoma, an uncommon lesion found in infants and children. Cure of this lesion occasionally has been obtained by combining radiation, chemotherapy, and operation.

Epidermoid cancers of the head and neck respond transiently to a number of single agents. Methotrexate has been the most extensively used. Response rates range from 15 to 57 percent. Bleomycin has also been found to have significant activity, comparable to methotrexate, with reported responses ranging from 15 to 50 percent. Other, less effective, single agents are cyclophosphomide (36 percent), vinblastine (29 percent), hydroxyurea (39 percent), 5-fluorouracil (15 percent) and procarbazine (10 percent). Reports of many of these latter drugs are based on small series and represent, at best, rough estimates. The most recent drug to excite interest in treatment of these tumors is cis-dichlorodiammine platinum (II) (DDP or cis-platinum), which appears to match or exceed methotrexate and bleomycin in activity, especially when used in high doses with mannitol-induced diuresis to avoid renal injury.

Arterial infusion for the treatment of cancer in the head and neck area has received much attention. This involves the introduction of chemotherapy, usually methotrexate or 5-fluorouracil, into the external carotid artery via a catheter. The agents are administered either continuously or intermittently over 1 to several weeks. At present, this technique is known to produce a substantial to complete regression of the lesions in a large percentage of patients—as high as 50 percent in some series. Unfortunately, the response is usually transient, and the cancers return to continued growth within 2 to 3 months after treatment is discontinued. Long-term regression is uncommonly seen, and the period of regression obtained is rarely worth the morbidity and complications of the treatment itself. Nonetheless, these observations continue to tantalize clinical investigators seeking a clue which will lead to longer or even permanent remissions.

The growing body of knowledge concerning the interrelationships between cancer and the body's immune system has touched the field of head and neck cancer through the work of Chretian and others. At least half the patients with epidermoid cancer of the oral cavity, hypopharynx, and larynx show some degree of immune incompetence. Moreover, this incompetence is correlated with treatment failure following either radiation or operation. Immune competence can be restored in a number of these patients by improving nutrition, by the use of immunostimulant agents such as BCG or c-Parvum, and by "reconstitution" agents such as Levamisole, thymosin, and transfer factor. Trials to determine the effectiveness of manipulations of the immune system in the immune-incompetent patient are being developed.

Combined forms of treatment for head and neck cancers, which include chemotherapy and immunotherapy as well as radiation and operation, have enjoyed marked clinical and investigative interest in the past several years. The more our knowledge of the natural history of tumor growth develops, the more rational and logical it appears to combine available treatment methods. In the next decade clinical research will be devoted to determining the best dose schedules and the best combinations of drugs and techniques.

OPERATIONS OF THE HEAD AND NECK

The most commonly performed major operation for cancer of the head and neck is radical neck dissection. This procedure was originally designed by Crile to eradicate the cervical lymphatic network, thereby eliminating sites of metastasis from cancer of the oral cavity, pharynx, paranasal sinuses, or other areas of the head and neck. In the early days of head and neck surgery radical neck dissections were usually performed after the primary lesion had been controlled through the use of radiation therapy. Today, we are more inclined to combine radical neck dissection with a simultaneous resection of the primary lesion. This is sometimes preceded by a course of radiation therapy to the primary area as part of a planned program of tumor treatment. Combined operations have been called by a number of terms including *composite resections* and *commando operations*. Other common operations in this area are superficial resection of the parotid gland, V excision of carcinoma of the lip, and resection of the maxillary antrum.

Fig. 16-39. Common operative incisions for radical neck dissections. (*From B. F. Rush, Jr., Curr Probl Surg, May, 1966.*)

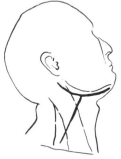

CRILE (T-INCISION)

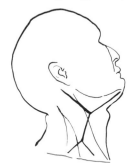

MARTIN (DOUBLE-Y INCISION)

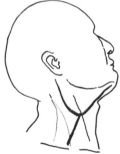

WARD (Y-INCISION)

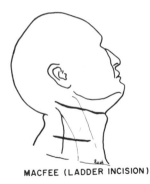

MACFEE (LADDER INCISION)

Radical Neck Dissection

Incisions for radical neck dissection are numerous and include a T-shaped incision originally used by Crile, a Y incision described by Ward, and a double Y incision described by Martin (Fig. 16-39). We prefer a hockey-stick-shaped incision with the ascending limb along the posterior border of the sternocleidomastoid muscle and the horizontal portion crossing the neck about 2 or 3 cm above the clavicle (Fig. 16-40). This last approach has the advantage of being outside areas of radiation when the neck has had previous exposure to radiation therapy and of being a simple linear incision avoiding small triangular-shaped flaps, which have a tendency to slough. The skin flap is reflected mediad, including the underlying platysma muscle, and dissection of neck structures begins in the posterior triangle, dissecting the fibroareolar tissue of this space away from the trapezius muscle and the underlying brachial plexus and scalene fibers. This portion of the dissection is carried mediad until the phrenic nerve lying on the anterior scalene muscle is identified.

The lower end of the sternocleidomastoid muscle is transected and the jugular vein identified and ligated. The accompanying vagus nerve next to the jugular vein in the carotid sheath is identified and spared. Dissection is then carried up the neck, gradually dissecting the lymph node chain free from underlying fascia and beneath the carotid artery. Just above the level of the carotid bulb the hypoglossal nerve is identified. In the upper portion of the neck the sternocleidomastoid muscle is again transected at the level of the mastoid together with the tip of the parotid gland. The submaxillary gland is dissected free from the digastric fossa and included with the specimen. The lingual nerve and artery in the depths of the submaxillary fossa are visualized and left intact. Care is taken to identify the ramus mandibularis, the tiny fiber of the VIIth nerve which innervates the lower lip, and to reflect this above the submaxillary gland so that its continuity is maintained. The spinal accessory nerve is usually sacrificed, being cut in the lower neck where it enters the trapezius muscle and in the upper neck where it enters the sternocleidomastoid muscle. The operation is completed with the transection of the jugular vein at the point where it leaves the base of the skull (Fig. 16-41). If a radical neck dissection alone is performed, the operation is ended at this point by closing the skin flaps. Multiperforated catheters are left underneath the flaps and are connected to suction. This helps to draw the flap firmly to the structures of the neck and eliminates the problem of fluid collecting under the flap.

COMBINED OPERATION

If a radical neck dissection is to be combined with the removal of structures within the oral cavity or tonsillar area, the contents of the neck dissection are left attached to the horizontal ramus of the mandible. The mandible is frequently divided. If the lesion is in the floor of the mouth or tongue, the horizontal ramus of the mandible may be resected. If the lesion is in the tonsillar fossa, the ascending ramus of the mandible is removed. If the lesion in the oral cavity is quite large, total removal of the hemi-

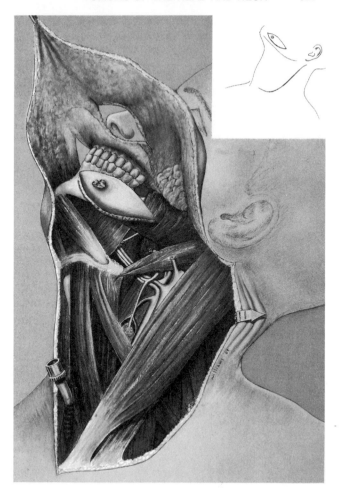

Fig. 16-40. Radical neck dissection through a hockey-stick incision (shown in insert) combined with an exposure of the mandible. The tumor has grown through the mandible and presented on the cheek so that a portion of the skin of the cheek has been left on the specimen. Structures of the neck are shown exposed and intact prior to the start of radical neck dissection. (*From B. F. Rush, Jr., Surg Gynecol Obstet, 121:353, 1965.*)

mandible on the side of the lesion may be necessary. Resection of the mandible is done to remove bone involved by tumor and sometimes to obtain a closure of the oral cavity which would not be feasible without removing a portion of the bony framework. Mandibular resection can be done with the acceptable cosmetic and functional result, especially when the anterior portion of the mandible is preserved (Fig. 16-42). The more anteriorly the mandible is resected, the more likely there is to be facial deformity. If the primary site of the tumor is in the larynx or thyroid, then these structures may also be removed with the radical neck dissection. The mortality for radical neck dissection alone is less than 1 percent. If neck dissection is combined with en bloc excision of a primary lesion, then mortality rates range from 2 to 5 percent.

BILATERAL RADICAL NECK DISSECTION

Lesions that are in the midline of the oral cavity often spread bilaterally, and it is necessary to remove lymph

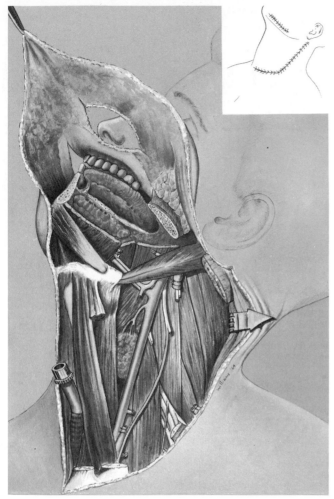

Fig. 16-41. Radical neck dissection completed, combined with excision of the horizontal ramus of the mandible. The jugular vein and sternocledomastoid muscle have been removed. The phrenic nerve and the common carotid artery are seen coursing across the operative field. The closure of the neck incision is seen in the insert. (*From B. F. Rush, Jr., Surg Gynecol Obstet, 121:353, 1965.*)

nodes on both sides of the neck. Simultaneous bilateral neck dissections are feasible with an acceptable mortality; however, the postoperative course is likely to be prolonged, since there is a period of marked facial edema following this extensive resection which can persist for several weeks. Some operators will spare the jugular vein on one side when a bilateral neck dissection is done in order to decrease the amount of postoperative edema. Others stage the dissection, allowing a delay of several weeks before operating on the second side.

Parotidectomy

Most lesions in the superficial lobe of the parotid gland are removed by superficial parotidectomy. This operation is designed to give maximal safety in operating about the branches of the VIIth nerve (Fig. 16-43). The VIIth nerve pierces the parotid gland at its posterior margin and lies underneath the gland on the muscles of the face. A Y-shaped incision is made with the lower limb lying behind the angle of the mandible and the arms of the Y on either side of the lobe of the ear. Dissection is carried down to identify the main trunk of the VIIth nerve, which lies in the space between the mandible and the mastoid bone approximately one fingerbreadth below the external auditory meatus. Once the main trunk is identified, dissection is carried along the external surface of the nerve and its branches, gradually separating away the overlying portion of the parotid gland. Stensen's duct is identified at the most medial portion of the midpoint of the parotid gland and is ligated. This technique sometimes causes temporary weakness in the fibers of the VIIth nerve but prevents transecting any of the major trunks of the nerve. Recovery of function in all branches is ensured by the knowledge that they are intact and usually occurs within a week or two following completion of the operation.

V Excision of the Lip

Most cancers of the lower lip are removed with the use of V excision (see Chap. 51). Between one-fourth and one-third of the lower lip can be easily resected by simple excision without resulting in residual deformity or interference with function. While we refer to this excision as a V, a much better cosmetic result is obtained if the outline of the incision resembles that of a shield. A true V excision results in some flattening of the lower lip with a loss of normal eversion. If a shield-shaped incision is used, the lip will evert normally.

If the tumor involves more area than can be excised with a V excision, a flap is migrated from the upper lip. This involves outlining a V-shaped flap in the upper lip which is left attached at its lower medial corner and is then rotated into the defect in the lower lip. Using this type of closure excision of up to two-thirds of the lower lip can be accomplished without difficulty.

Maxillectomy

Cancer of the hard palate or the lower maxilla requires subtotal excision of the maxillary sinus. Cancer in the upper maxilla involving the orbital plate requires total excision of the maxillary sinus together with an exenteration of the orbital contents. While these excisions are basically mutilating, they can be accomplished with little visible external deformity. The Weber-Fergusson incision is used. This begins at the midpoint of the upper lip, extends to the columella of the nose, and is carried around the edge of the nose and up to the corner of the eye. A horizontal portion continues laterally from the inner canthus to a point just beyond the outer canthus and about 2 or 3 mm below the palpebral fissure. The skin and muscles of the cheek are undermined laterally, so that the entire cheek is turned outward, opening a door to the maxillary sinus. The bony attachments of the maxillary sinus are divided, including the midline of the hard palate, the zygoma, the pterygoid plates; if the orbital plate is to be removed, the bony walls of the medial and lateral orbit are also transected. When this is accomplished, the entire maxillary sinus can be lifted like a small box from its normal position. The inner surface of the Weber-Fergusson flap is covered with a split-thickness skin graft, and the incision is closed. Because it falls in the normal skin lines and about the normal structures of the face, this incision is often difficult to detect after it has healed as long as the structures have been replaced precisely and in good apposition. This operation leaves a large defect in the hard palate on the side of the procedure. This is occasionally closed by subsequent operations, but more commonly a

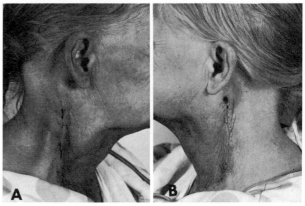

Fig. 16-42. Mandibular resection, 8 days after bilateral neck dissection and partial mandibulectomy on the left, with resection of a portion of the floor of the mouth and the anterior half of the tongue for carcinoma of the tongue. The portion of the jaw was replaced with a Steinmann pin. At 3 years postoperatively there still was no recurrence. Note that it is difficult to determine on which side the mandible was resected. (*From B. F. Rush, Jr., Curr Probl Surg, May, 1966.*)

Fig. 16-43. Superficial parotidectomy. *A.* Incision. *B.* Skin flaps established and fascia incised; greater auricular nerve transected and external jugular vein identified. *C.* External jugular vein transected; superficial lobe is being reflected anteriorly, and facial nerve with its mandibular and cervical branches are shown. *D.* Dissection continued anteriorly, demonstrating temporal, zygomatic, and buccal branches. *E.* Superficial lobe removed; if excision of the deep lobe is indicated, the facial nerve can be retracted craniad and the remaining parotid removed. *F.* Relationship of facial nerve and parotid gland. The nerve branches lie between the deep and superficial lobes of the parotid. (*Courtesy of Robert Chase, M.D.*)

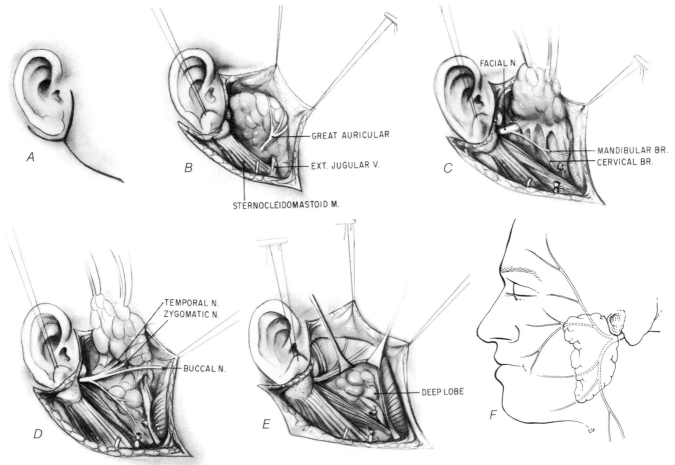

dental prosthesis with a large obturator which fits into the defect is constructed by the prosthodontist. This restores normal speech and relatively normal mastication for the patient.

Total Laryngectomy

Total laryngectomy is traditionally accomplished through a midline longitudinal incision. We have found definite advantages in accomplishing this procedure through a transverse incision in the lower neck very much like the typical thyroidectomy incision. The incision is made 4 cm above the clavicles and approximately 4 cm beyond the edge of the sternocleidomastoid muscles on either side; it is carried down through the platysma muscle, and the upper flap is then developed. The upper limit of dissection is approximately 1 cm above the hyoid, and at this point the entire group of strap muscles and the midportion of the hyoid are exposed. In cancer operations for glottic tumors of any size, all the anterior strap muscles are removed. Occasionally at the election of the operator in the presence of somewhat smaller lesions, the strap muscles on the side contralateral to the lesion may be preserved, or, rarely, the larynx is skeletonized with the preservation of strap muscles on both sides. In the ordinary instance, however, the sternothyroid and sternohyoid muscles are transected at the level of the cricoid, the digastric and mylohyoid muscles are separated from the hyoid above, and the body of the hyoid bone is cut at the junction of the attachments to the lateral wings on either side. The larynx is rocked laterally exposing the pharyngeal constrictors, which are cut at the lateral edge of the thyroid cartilages bilaterally. One can now enter the pharynx laterally, usually on the side opposite the tumor, so that proper visualization of the area can be obtained, and an adequate margin of excision of pharyngeal mucosa will be developed around the tumor. Once the pharynx is entered, it is possible for the surgeon to operate both outside and inside the pharynx. The remaining muscles of the tongue are severed from the hyoid, and the larynx is pulled forward. The vascular pedicles containing the laryngeal arteries and the superior laryngeal nerves are ligated bilaterally. An incision is made in the pharyngeal mucosa just posterior to the arytenoids, entirely circumscribing the point at which the larynx projects into the pharynx. As all pharyngeal mucosa is now separated from the larynx, the larynx is pulled forward, and a plane of dissection is developed between the larynx and the anterior esophageal wall. This dissection is carried inferiorly until the only remaining structure holding the larynx in place is the trachea. This is then divided obliquely around the site of the tracheostomy (if one has been done previous to the operation), or if an endotracheal tube has been used in anesthesia, this is now removed, and a tube is placed in the severed trachea so that anesthesia can be continued. After the larynx has been removed, the defect in the pharynx is closed transversely with an inverting Connell stitch. This is reinforced by interrupted sutures of 4-0 silk which are used to imbricate the constrictor muscles up and around the pharyngeal closure. This closure may further be reinforced by stitches which catch the platysma muscle and draw it down snugly along with the overlying skin. A generous circular portion of skin is removed in the lower midline; this measures about 3 to 4 cm in diameter with three-quarters of the circle lying above the transverse skin incision and one-quarter of the circle lying below. The beveled end of the trachea is then drawn up to the skin by interrupted sutures of nylon. Every attempt is made to obtain a delicate mucosa to skin closure, since the smaller the size of the scar at the junction between mucosa and skin, the less likely there is to be subsequent stenosis of the tracheal opening. The generous amount of skin excised tends to evert the trachea in a slightly "trumpet-like" manner, and this too ensures against subsequent stenosis. This type of trachea skin closure can be maintained without the use of an indwelling tracheostomy tube except for the first 24 hours or so postoperatively. The remainder of the wound is closed with interrupted sutures to the platysma muscle and skin. Two suction catheters are left in place on either side of the neck and are usually removed in 24 to 36 hours. The patient is maintained on postoperative feedings through a nasal tube made up of a #18 whistle-tip red rubber catheter inserted at the time of operation through the nose and into the esophagus before the pharyngeal defect is closed. This tube is sutured to the nasal columella. The patient is maintained on nasal tube feedings for about 10 days. A liquid diet is usually begun on the fifth or sixth day, and the patient may take solid food on the ninth or tenth day. The nasal tube is removed as soon as it is apparent that the patient can well maintain his own nutrition.

Partial Laryngectomy and the Neolarynx

In the past all lesions extending beyond the true cords have been treated by total laryngectomy. The functional importance of the voice and the great benefit of preserving it for the patient has led to an evaluation of cancer operations which do not remove the entire larynx. Ogura and Biller have led this effort and have proposed a number of new operations which involve removal of most or all of the larynx above the cords (supraglottic laryngectomy) or excision of most of one side of the larynx (hemilaryngectomy) for lesions which are confined enough in their growth to be suitable for this technique. This approach requires careful selection of patients who are young and flexible enough to overcome some of the swallowing and aspiration difficulties that often arise postoperatively. Since the resected margin around the tumor may be very limited, careful diagnostic techniques must be used to identify the outer margins. This technique is almost always combined with preoperative radiation therapy to ensure a lesser threat from residual cells at the periphery of the tumor which may be left by the surgeon. Using these techniques in patients with tumors advanced enough to cause fixation of the cord, Ogura and Biller have reported a 77 percent 3-year survival.

An alternative method for preserving the voice, especially in patients with lesions not amenable to partial laryngectomy, is creation of a pseudolarynx. This is done by suturing the trachea, usually after preserving the lower cricoid, to the hyoid bone. The tracheal stoma is covered by a flap of mucosa and a new glottis is formed by a small incision in the mucosal flap. Following this procedure patients usually must wear a tracheostomy tube and speak by occluding the tube, diverting air through the new glottis. Aspiration of swallowed fluids is often an early problem, but patients usually learn to avoid this in time. This procedure was introduced by Serafini in Italy in 1970 and further refined by Vega of Spain. It has only recently been introduced in the United States and is still undergoing refinement. It may offer a good method of preserving the voice in patients with larger lesions.

POSTOPERATIVE CARE FOLLOWING HEAD AND NECK OPERATIONS

Tracheostomy is performed at the time of operation in any patient in whom a portion of the mandible is removed or when there is extensive removal of oral structures. Postoperative edema plus the tendency for the larynx to shift position following sacrifice of many of its suspensory muscles predispose to aspiration and obstruction. Catastrophic anoxia may supervene rapidly, with little apparent warning. The tracheostomy tube must be aspirated frequently. This requires the presence of well-trained nursing personnel. If a patient appears to be accumulating unusual amounts of tracheal secretions, it is probable that saliva is being aspirated through an incompetent larynx. This can be controlled by diligent suctioning. In extreme instances, a cuffed tracheostomy may be required temporarily.

The patient with a tracheostomy has lost the usual humidifying effects of the nasal and pharyngeal passageways. The best way to provide humidity for the patient's trachea is to tie an umbilical tape about the neck above the tracheostomy and to hang a moistened 4 by 4 sponge over this tape very much in the manner that a towel is hung over a rail. The sponge must frequently be moistened, and after the first day or two the patient can be taught to moisten his own sponge and arrange it for himself.

There is no need to leave the tracheostomy in place for prolonged periods. As soon as the patient is found to be maintaining a dry, unobstructed airway and the skin flaps are sealed, the tracheostomy tube is covered with a piece of adhesive tape. This is done about 5 days postoperatively. If the patient tolerates the covering of the tracheostomy tube for 24 hours, it can be removed. This tube should always be removed in the morning, so that the patient can be observed during the daylight hours following removal.

Patients who have undergone combined resections have had extensive superficial operation, but the body cavities have been undisturbed, and the normal function of the gastrointestinal tract resumes almost immediately. A nasoesophageal tube consisting of a #16 French urethral catheter is left in place at the end of the operative procedure. The tip of the standard urethral catheter reaches to the lower third of the esophagus but does not traverse the esophagocardiac junction. Such tubes can be left in place for long periods without the risk of acid regurgitation and

peptic esophagitis. The patient receives fluids intravenously on the day of operation, but on the first postoperative day nasal feedings of half-strength milk are given. On the second postoperative day a nasal formula consisting of a blenderized regular diet diluted with milk is begun. This is continued until the fifth or sixth postoperative day or until the patient shows evidence that he can tolerate an adequate diet by mouth.

Except for the different flora encountered, there is little difference in the principles of operating on the mouth and other areas in the gastrointestinal tract. This is a contaminated area, and numerous tissue planes are open to this contamination. All patients should be placed on appropriate antibiotics postoperatively. Ketcham et al. demonstrated in a controlled study the advantages of prophylactic antibiotics in these patients.

The mental stress in a patient undergoing an oral operation of any magnitude is considerable. He awakens unable to speak because of his tracheostomy. He is unable to control his saliva and finds that he is constantly aspirating small amounts of mucus. His neck and shoulder are completely numb and boardlike because of the section of all cervical sensory nerves on the side of the lesion, and while he has little or no sharp pain, he has a pounding and persistent headache due to the ligation of the jugular vein and concomitant rise of spinal fluid pressure. In a day or two he looks into the mirror and may not recognize the swollen, edematous, and possibly deformed face which stares back at him. It would be abnormal if he were not

Fig. 16-44. Construction of a pseudolarynx by covering the tracheal stoma left after laryngectomy with a flap of mucosa and constructing a new glottis by an incision in the mucosa as shown here is another attempt to obtain immediate functional reconstruction in the head and neck patient. (*From A. Swaminathan, K. Jefferies, and B. F. Rush, Jr., Am J Surg, in press.*)

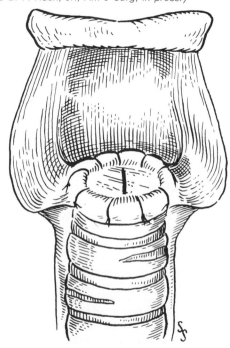

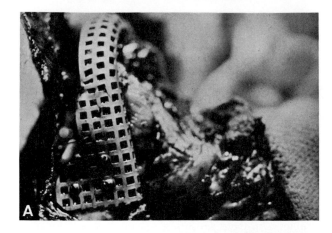

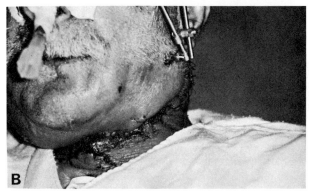

Fig. 16-45. *A*. Resection of the entire anterior mandible is one of the most devastating procedures for patients both cosmetically and functionally. Attempts at immediate reconstruction include use of a tantalum tray as shown here filled with cancellous bone chips. *B*. The tray is concorporated in a flap of cervical skin from the anterior neck, which also is used to line the residual tongue and floor of the mouth. The remaining mandible is immobilized with external pins. Immediate appearance and function are very acceptable.

depressed under these circumstances. Support for the patient depends on good preoperative preparation. The patient must understand clearly what to expect in the postoperative period. Patients do not panic if they understand their problems and realize that most of their deficiencies are reversible as edema subsides and the tracheostomy tube is removed.

REHABILITATION

As Shedd has pointed out, progress in medicine often brings new problems. In head and neck oncology the successful control of major cancers may leave a considerable number of patients whose posttreatment life involves a significant degree of disability. Major impairment in appearance, swallowing, taste, and speech all reduce the quality of life and the effectiveness of treatment. While the field of rehabilitation of these patients is too broad to detail here, the major thrust of recent years has been to accomplish as much of the rehabilitation as possible on the

operating table at the primary procedure. Techniques such as the construction of a pseudolarynx (Fig. 16-44) or primary implantation of a new mandible at the initial procedure (Fig. 16-45*A* and *B*) produce immediate cosmetic and functional results much more gratifying to the patient and the surgeon than multistaged reconstructions done secondarily, which often take months to accomplish. If primary reconstruction is still unobtainable, then the surgeon must be certain to guide his patient to the appropriate speech therapy, prosthetic substitution, or secondary reconstruction required.

References

General

Advisory Committee to the Surgeon General on Smoking and Health, "Report on Smoking and Health," *Public Health Serv Publ,* 1103, 1964.

Arons, M. S., and Smith, R. R.: Distant Metastases and Local Recurrence in Head and Neck Cancer, *Ann Surg,* **154:**235, 1961.

Baker, H.: Oral Cancer: A Six Part Series, *CA,* pt. I: January–February, 1972; pt. II: March–April, 1972; pt. III: May–June, 1972; pt. IV: July–August, 1972; pt. V: September–October, 1972; pt. VI: January–February, 1973.

Conley, J. (ed.),: "Cancer of the Head and Neck," Butterworth Inc., Washington, 1967.

Gowen, G. F., and deSuto-Nagy, G.: The Incidence and Sites of Distant Metastases in Head and Neck Carcinoma, *Surg Gynecol Obstet,* **116:**603, 1963.

James, A. G.: "Cancer Prognosis Manual," American Cancer Society, Inc., New York, 1967.

Kark, W.: "A Synopsis of Cancer: Genesis and Biology," The Williams & Wilkins Company, Baltimore, 1966.

MacComb, W. S.: Treatment of Head and Neck Cancer, Janeway Lecture, 1960, *Am J Roentgenol Radium Ther Nucl Med,* **84:**589, 1960.

Moore, C.: Smoking and Cancer of the Mouth, Pharynx and Larynx, *JAMA,* **191:**107, 1965.

Rubin, P.: Current Concepts in Cancer: Cancer of the Head and Neck, *JAMA,* **221:**68, 1972. (First of a continuing series of articles.)

Rush, B. F., Jr., Chambers, R. G., and Ravitch, M. M.: Cancer of the Head and Neck in Children, *Surgery,* **53:**270, 1963.

————, Horie, N., and Klein, N. W.: Intra-arterial Infusion of the Head and Neck: Anatomical and Distributional Problems, *Am J Surg,* **110:**510, 1965.

———— and Trinkle, K.: The Management of Low-Grade, Neglected Neoplasms, *South Med J,* **60:**714, 1967.

Schottenfeld, D.: Cancer of the Buccal Cavity and Pharynx: A Review of End Results of Primary Treatment in 2877 Cases 1949-1964, *Clin Bull Memorial Hosp,* **2:**51, 1972.

Serafini, I.: Larengectomia totale con mantenimento della respirazione per via naturale (resoconto sul primo case recentemente operato con technica personale), *Min Otorinolarin,* **20:**73, 1970.

Shedd, D. P.: Rehabilitation Problems in Head and Neck Patients, *J Surg Oncology,* **8:**11, 1976.

Taylor, G. W., and Nathanson, I. T.: "Lymph Node Metastases:

Incidence and Surgical Treatment in Neoplastic Disease," Oxford University Press, London, 1942.

Vega, M. F.: Larynx Reconstruction Surgery. A Study of Three-Year Findings: A Modified Surgical Technique, *Laryngoscope,* **85:**866, 1975.

Willis, R. A.: "Pathology of Tumors," Butterworth & Co. (Publishers), Ltd., London, 1960.

Historical Background

Absolon, K. B., Rogers, W., and Aust, J. B.: Some Historical Developments of the Surgical Therapy of Tongue Cancer from the Seventeenth to the Nineteenth Century, *Am J Surg,* **104:**686, 1962.

Campbell, E., and Colton, J.: "The Surgery of Theodoric," Appleton-Century Crofts, Inc., New York, 1955.

Fletcher, G. H., and Jesse, R. H., Jr.: The Contribution of Super-voltage Roentgenotherapy to the Integration of Radiation and Surgery in Head and Neck Squamous Cell Carcinomas, *Cancer,* **15:**566, 1962.

Lip

Ashley, F. L., McConnell, D. V., Machida, R., Sterling, H. E., Galloway, D., and Grazer, F.: Carcinoma of the Lip: A Comparison of Five Year Results after Irradiation and Surgical Therapy, *Am J Surg,* **110:**549, 1965.

Blackerby, J. N., and Hamilton, J. E.: Carcinoma of the Lip, *Surgery,* **51:**591, 1962.

Ward, G. E.: Carcinoma of the Lips, *Md Med J,* **5:**23, 1956.

Oral Cavity

Fayos, J. V. and Lampe, I.: Treatment of Squamous Cell Carcinoma of the Oral Cavity, *Am J Surg,* **124:**493, 1972.

Helfrich, G. B., Nickels, M. E., El-Doomeiri, A., and DasGupta, T.: Management of Cancer of the Floor of the Mouth, *Am J Surg,* **124:**559, 1972.

Kraus, F. T., and Perez-Mesa, C.: Verrucous Carcinoma: Clinical and Pathologic Study of 105 Cases Involving Oral Cavity, Larynx, and Genitalia, *Cancer,* **19:**26, 1966.

Lash, H., Erich, J. B., and Dockerty, M. B.: Pathologic Study of 217 Cases of Epithelioma of the Tongue, *Am J Surg,* **102:**620, 1961.

Marchetta, F. C., Sako, K., and Murph, J. B.: The Periosteum of the Mandible and Intraoral Carcinoma, *Am J Surg,* **122:** 711, 1971.

Martin, H. E.: The History of Lingual Cancer, *Am J Surg,* **48:**703, 1940.

Niebel, H. H., and Chomet, B.: In Vivo Staining Test for Delineation of Oral Intraepithelial Neoplastic Change: Preliminary Report, *J Am Dent Assoc,* **68:**801, 1964.

O'Brien, P. H., and Catlin, D.: Cancer of the Cheek (Mucosa), *Cancer,* **18:**1392, 1965.

Rush, B. F., Jr.: Combined Procedures in the Treatment of Oral Carcinoma, *Curr Prob Surg,* May, 1966.

——— and Humphrey, L.: Primary Repair of Full Thickness Excision of the Cheek, *Am J Surg,* **114:**592, 1967.

Sandler, H. C.: Oral Cytology, *CA,* **16:**97, 1966.

Shedd, D. P., Hukill, P. B., Bahn, S., and Ferraro, R. H.: Further Appraisal of In Vivo Staining Properties of Oral Cancer, *Arch Surg,* **95:**16, 1967.

———, Von Essen, C. F., Bevin, A. G., and Greenberg, R. A.:

Ten Year Survey of Oral Cancer in a General Hospital, *Am J Surg,* **114:**844, 1967.

Southwick, H. W., Slaughter, D. P., and Trevino, E. T.: Elective Neck Dissection for Intraoral Cancer, *Arch Surg,* **80:**905, 1960.

Stecker, R. H., Devine, K. D., and Harrison, E. G., Jr.: Verrucose "Snuff Dipper's" Carcinoma of the Oral Cavity: A Case of Self-induced Carcinogenesis, *JAMA,* **189:**144, 1964.

Thoma, K. H.: "Oral Surgery," The C. V. Mosby Company, St. Louis, 1963.

Yonemoto, R. H., Ching, P. T., Bryon, R. L., and Riihimaki, D. U.: The Composite Operation in Cancer of the Head and Neck (Commando Procedure), *Arch Surg,* **104:**809, 1972.

Oropharynx

Baker, R. R., and Weiner, S.: The Clinical Management of Tonsillar Carcinoma, *Surg Gynecol Obstet,* **121:**1035, 1965.

Barkley, H. T., Fletcher, G. H., Jesse, R. H., and Lindberg, R. D.: Management of Cervical Lymph Node Metastasis in Squamous Cell Carcinoma of the Tonsillar Fossa, Base of Tongue, Supraglottic Larynx and Hypopharynx, *Am J Surg,* **124:**464, 1972.

Keller, A. Z.: Cirrhosis of the Liver, Alcoholism and Heavy Smoking Associated with Cancer of the Mouth and Pharynx, *Cancer,* **20:**1015, 1967.

McIlrath, D. C., ReMine, W. H., Devine, K. D., and Dockerty, M. B.: Tumors of the Parapharyngeal Region, *Surg Gynecol Obstet,* **116:**88, 1963.

Perez, C. A., Ackerman, L. V., and Mill, W. B.: Malignant Tumors of the Tonsil: Analysis of Failures and Factors affecting Prognosis, *Am J Roentgenol, Radium Ther Nucl Med,* **114:**43, 1972.

Rush, B. F., Jr., Reynolds, G., and Greenlaw, R.: Integrated Irradiation and Operation in Treatment of Cancer of the Larynx and Hypopharynx: A Preliminary Report, *Am J Roentgenol Radium Ther Nucl Med,* **102:**129, 1968.

Larynx

Baker, R. R., and Cherry, J.: Carcinoma of the Larynx: Results of Therapy in 209 Cases, *Arch Surg,* **90:**449, 1965.

Carveth, S. W., Devine, K. D., and ReMine, W. H.: Laryngectomy with Radical Neck Dissection in Extensive Cancer of the Larynx, *Am J Surg,* **104:**705, 1962.

Clinical Staging System for Cancer of the Larynx, American Joint Committee on Cancer Staging and End Results Reporting, June, 1962.

Donegan, W. L.: An Early History of Total Laryngectomy, *Surgery,* **57:**902, 1965.

Flynn, M. B., Jesse, R. H., and Lindberg, R. D.: Surgery and Irradiation in the Treatment of Squamous Cell Cancer of the Supraglottic Larynx, *Am J Surg,* **124:**477, 1972.

Goldman, J. L., Cheren, R. V., Silverstone, S. M., and Zak, F. G.: Combined Irradiation and Surgery for Cancer of the Larynx and Laryngopharynx, in J. Conley (ed.), "Cancer of the Head and Neck," Butterworth Inc., Washington, 1967.

Holinger, P. H.: Cancer of the Larynx: Classification and Partial Laryngectomy, in J. Conley (ed.), "Cancer of the Head and Neck," Butterworth Inc., Washington, 1967.

Krause, L. G.: Clinical Review of Carcinoma of the Larynx: Experience of a Large Cancer Hospital, *Am J Surg,* **111:**206, 1966.

Norris, C. M.: Treatment of Cancer of the Larynx and the Hypopharynx, *Proc Natl Cancer Conf,* **5:**265, 1964.

Ogura, J. W., and Biller, H. F.: Preoperative Irradiation for Laryngeal and Laryngopharyngeal Cancer, *Laryngoscope,* **80:**802, 1970.

Ono, J., and Shigejo, S.: Endoscopic Microsurgery of the Larynx, *Ann Otol Rhinol Laryngol,* **80:**479, 1971.

Powell, R. W., Redd, B. L., and Wilkins, S. A., Jr.: An Evaluation of Treatment of Cancer of the Larynx, *Am J Surg,* **110:**635, 1965.

Shahrokh, D. K., Devine, K. D., and Harrison, E. G., Jr.: Statistical Evaluation of 115 Cases of Carcinoma of the Epiglottis (1943 to 1952), *Am J Surg,* **102:**781, 1961.

Shedd, D. P.: Role of Surgical Measures in Voice Restoration after Laryngectomy, "Symposium on Malignancies of The Head and Neck," The C. V. Mosby Company, St. Louis, Mo., 1975.

Smith, R. R., Caulk, R. M., Russell, W. O., and Jackson, C. L.: End Results in 600 Laryngeal Cancers Using the American Joint Committee's Proposed Method of Stage Classification and End Results Reporting, *Surg Gynecol Obstet,* **113,** 435, 1961.

Spalt, L., Greenlaw, R., and Rush, B. F., Jr.: Integrated Therapy for Carcinoma of the Larynx, in B. F. Rush, Jr. and R. H. Greenlaw (eds.), "Integrated Radiation and Operation in Cancer Therapy: A Symposium," Charles C Thomas, Publisher, Springfield, Ill., 1968.

Nasopharynx

Jesse, R. H.: Preoperative versus Postoperative Radiation in the Treatment of Squamous Carcinoma of the Paranasal Sinuses, *Am J Surg,* **110:**552, 1965.

Moench, H. C. and Phillips, T. L.: Carcinoma of the Nasopharynx: Review of 146 Patients with Emphasis on Radiation Dose and Time Factors, *Am J Surg,* **124:**515, 1971.

Thomas, J. E., and Waltz, A. G.: Neurological Manifestations of Nasopharyngeal Malignant Tumors, *JAMA,* **192:**103, 1965.

Nasal Cavity and Paranasal Sinuses

Kurohara, S. S., Ellis, F., Fitzgerald, J. P., Webster, J. H., Shedd, D. P., and Badib, A. O.: Role of Radiation Therapy and of Surgery in the Management of Localized Epidermoid Carcinoma of the Maxillary Sinus, *Am J Roentgenol Radium Ther Nucl Med,* **114:**35, 1972.

Rush, B. F., Jr., Knightly, J. J., and Jewell, W.: Transoral and Transverse Incision for Excision of the Maxillary Sinus, *J Surg Oncol,* **3:**53, 1971.

Tabah, E. J.: Cancer of the Paranasal Sinuses: A Study of the Results of Various Methods of Treatment in Fifty-four Patients, *Am J Surg,* **104:**741, 1962.

Mandible

Bernier, J. L.: "Tumors of the Odontogenic Apparatus and Jaws," Armed Forces Institute of Pathology, Washington, 1960.

Cramer, L. M., Culf, N. K., Hulnick, S. J., and Kodsi, M. S.: Reconstruction Management of the Mandible in the Treatment of Head and Neck, "Symposium on Malignancies of The Head and Neck," The C. V. Mosby Company, St. Louis, Mo., 1975.

Salivary Glands

Beahrs, O. H., Woolner, L. B., Caveth, S. W., and Devine, K. D.: Surgical Management of Parotid Lesions, *Arch Surg,* **80:**890, 1960.

Bhaskar, S. N., and Bernier, J. L.: Mikulicz's Disease, *Oral Surg,* **13:**1387, 1960.

Connell, H. C. and Evans, J. C.: Mucoepidermoid Carcinoma of the Salivary Glands, *Am J Surg,* **124:**519, 1972.

Foote, F. W., and Frazell, E. L.: "Tumors of the Major Salivary Glands," Armed Forces Institute of Pathology, Washington, 1954.

Grage, T. B., and Lober, P. H.: Benign Lymphoepithelial Lesion of the Salivary Glands, *Am J Surg,* **108:**495, 1964.

————, ————, and Shahon, D. B.: Benign Tumors of the Major Salivary Glands, *Surgery,* **50:**625, 1961.

Katsilambros, L.: Asymptomatic Enlargement of the Parotid Glands, *JAMA,* **178:**513, 1961.

Reynolds, C. T., McAuley, R. L., and Rogers, W. P., Jr.: Experience with Tumors of Minor Salivary Glands, *Am J Surg,* **111:**168, 1966.

Rosenfeld, L., Sessions, D. G., McSwain, B., and Graves, H., Jr.: Malignant Tumors of Salivary Gland Origin: 37-year Review of 184 Cases, *Ann Surg,* **163:**726, 1966.

Stewart, F. W., Foote, F. W., and Becker, W. F.: Mucoepidermoid Tumors of Salivary Glands, *Ann Surg,* **122:**820, 1945.

Stuteville, O. H., and Corley, R. D.: Surgical Management of Tumors of Intraoral Minor Salivary Glands: Report of Eighty Cases, *Cancer,* **20:**1578, 1967.

Winsten, J., and Ward, G. E.: The Parotid Gland: An Anatomic Study, *Surgery,* **40:**585, 1956.

Tumors of the Neck

Albers, G. D.: Branchial Anomalies, *JAMA,* **183:**399, 1963.

Hoffman, E.: Branchial Cysts within the Parotid Gland, *Ann Surg,* **152:**290, 1960.

Jesse, R. H., and Neff, L. E.: Metastatic Carcinoma in Cervical Nodes with an Unknown Primary Lesion, *Am J Surg,* **112:**547, 1966.

MacComb, W. S.: Diagnosis and Treatment of Metastatic Cervical Cancerous Nodes from an Unknown Primary Site, *Am J Surg,* **124:**441, 1972.

Marchetta, F. C., Murphy, W. T., and Kovaric, J. J.: Carcinoma of the Neck, *Am J Surg,* **106:**974, 1963.

Mooney, C. S., Jewell, W., Greenlaw, R., and Rush, B. F., Jr.: Simultaneous Bilateral Radical Neck Dissection following High Level Radiation Therapy, *J Surg Oncol,* **1:**335, 1969.

Rush, B. F., Jr.: Current Concepts in the Treatment of Carotid Body Tumors, *Surgery,* **52:**679, 1962.

————: Familial Bilateral Carotid Body Tumors, *Ann Surg,* **157:**633, 1963.

Skandalakis, J. E., Gray, S. W., Takakis, N. C., Godwin, J. T., and Poer, D. H.: Tumors of the Neck, *Surgery,* **48:**375, 1960.

Chemotherapy and Immunotherapy

Adams, G. L., Berlinger, N. T., Good, R. A., Pollak, K., Tsakraklides, V., and Yang, M.: Immunologic Assessment of Regional Lymph Node Histology in Relation to Survival in Head and Neck Carcinoma, *Cancer,* **37:**697, 1976.

Alexander, J. C., Jr., Chretien, P. B., Henson, D. E., Silverman,

N. A., and Smith, H. G.: Viral-Specific Humoral Immunity to Herpes Simplex-Induced Antigens in Patients with Squamous Carcinoma of the Head and Neck, *Am J Surg,* **132:**541, 1976.

Couture, J., and Deschenes, L.: Intra-arterial Infusion: An Adjuvant to the Treatment of Oral Carcinoma, *Cancer,* **29:**1632, 1972.

Cvitkovic, E., Gerold, F. P., Shah, J., Strong, E. W., and Wittes, R. E.: cis-Dichlorodiammineplatinum (II) in the Treatment of Epidermoid Carcinoma of the Head and Neck, *Cancer Treat Rep,* **61:**359, 1977.

Donaldson, R. C.: Methotrexate plus Bacillus Calmette-Guerin and Isoniazid in the Treatment of Cancer of the Head and Neck, *Am J Surg,* **124:**527, 1972.

Freckman, H. A.: Results in 169 Patients with Cancer of the Head and Neck Treated by Intra-arterial Infusion Therapy, *Am J Surg,* **124:**501, 1972.

Ohnuma, T., Selawry, O. S., Holland, J. F., DeVita, V. T., Shedd, D. P., Hansen, H. H., and Muggia, F. M.: Clinical Study with Bleomycin: Tolerance to Twice Weekly Dosage, *Cancer,* **30:**914, 1972.

Williams, A. C.: Topical 5 FU: A New Approach to Skin Cancer, *Ann Surg,* **173:**864, 1971.

Woods, J. E.: Current Status of Chemotherapy in the Treatment of Head and Neck Cancer, *Arch Surg,* **111:**1055, 1976.

———: The Influence of Immunologic Responsiveness on Head and Neck Cancer, *Plast Reconstr Surg,* **56:**77, 1975.

Operations of the Head and Neck

Frazell, E. L., and Moore, O. S.: Bilateral Radical Neck Dissection Performed in Stages: Experience with 467 Patients, *Am J Surg,* **102:**809, 1961.

Ketcham, A. S., Liebermann, J. E., and West, J. T.: Antibiotic Prophylaxis in Cancer Surgery and Its Value in Staphylococcal Carrier Patients, *Surg Gynecol Obstet,* **117:**1, 1963.

Lore, J. M.: "An Atlas of Head and Neck Surgery," W. B. Saunders Company, Philadelphia, 1962.

Madan, S. C., Rosenthal, S. P. and Bochetto, J. F.: Pneumomediastinum and Pneumothorax following Lower Neck Surgery, *Arch Surg,* **98:**153, 1969.

Martin, H., Del Valle, B., Ehrlich, H., and Cahan, W. G.: Neck Dissection, *Cancer,* **4:**441, 1951.

Moore, O. S., and Frazell, E. L.: Simultaneous Bilateral Neck Dissection: Experience with 151 Patients, *Am J Surg,* **107:**565, 1964.

Norris, C. M.: Composite Resections of Laryngeal and Supralaryngeal Cancer, in J. Conley (ed.), "Cancer of the Head and Neck," Butterworth Inc., Washington, 1967.

Royster, H. P., Noone, R. B., Graham, W. P., and Theogaraj, S. D.: Cervical Pharyngostomy for Feeding after Maxillofacial Surgery, *Am J Surg,* **116:**610, 1968.

Rush, B. F., Jr.: A Standard Technique for In-Continuity Incisions of the Head and Neck, *Surg Gynecol Obstet,* **121:**353, 1965.

———, Swaminathan, A. P., and Jefferies, K.: The Use of Cervical Flaps from Radiated Necks in Immediate Reconstruction, *Am J Surg.* (in press.)

Swaminathan, A. P., Jefferies, K. R., and Rush, B. F., Jr.: Construction of a Pseudolarynx following Laryngectomy and Radical Neck Dissection: A Preliminary Report, *Am J Surg.* (in press.)

Ward, G. E., Edgerton, M. T., Chambers, R. G., and McKee, D. M.: Cancer of the Oral Cavity and Pharynx and Results of Treatment by Means of the Composite Operation (in Continuity with Radical Neck Dissection), *Ann Surg,* **150:**202, 1959.

Wise, R. A., and Baker, H. W.: "Surgery of the Head and Neck," The Year Book Medical Publishers, Inc., Chicago, 1962.

Chapter 17

Chest Wall, Pleura, Lung, and Mediastinum

by **Lester R. Bryant and Calvin Morgan**

INTRODUCTION

The existence of life from moment to moment depends primarily on adequate function of the heart and lungs. Surgical procedures for the treatment of thoracic diseases or injury must be performed under circumstances which can guarantee continuing cardiopulmonary function during operative manipulations. Preexisting impairment of pulmonary function, operative removal of tissue from the chest wall or lungs, and postoperative pain are routine hazards to the patient's ability to continue adequate respiratory exchange following operation. From these considerations it is apparent that the development of thoracic surgery has necessarily followed the development of techniques for tracheal intubation with positive-pressure ventilation. This is not to imply that surgeons were unable to operate on the thorax until recent times. Attempts to manage chest wounds received in battle were recorded in very ancient writings, including the Iliad (about 950 B.C.). Galen described a patient who recovered after partial excision of the sternum and pericardium for recurrent abscess due to an injury. Writing about chest wounds in the thirteenth century, Theodoric noted that "the stitches should be placed in accordance with the size of the wound so that the natural heat cannot escape in any way nor the air outside be able to enter."

The introduction of firearms in the fourteenth century complicated the management of chest wounds because of uncertainty about the extent of damage inside the thorax and whether or not wounds should be closed when an open pneumothorax had been produced. Many surgeons held the view that the wound must be kept open to allow the drainage of blood. In recording the opposite view, Napoleon's surgeon, Baron Larrey, confirmed the sporadic observations of other surgeons about the lifesaving value of closing an open wound of the thorax. His description of the cardiopulmonary effects of an open chest wound can hardly be improved upon:

A soldier was brought to the hospital of the Fortress of Ibrahyn Bey, immediately after a wound penetrated the thorax, between the fifth and sixth true ribs. It was about 8 cm in extent. A large quantity of frothy and vermilion blood escaped from it with a hissing noise at each inspiration. His extremities were cold, pulse scarcely perceptible, countenance discolored, and respiration short and laborious; in short, he was every moment threatened with a fatal suffocation. After having examined the wound, the divided edges of the part, I immediately approximated the two lips of the wound, and retained them by means of adhesive plaster and a suitable bandage around the body. In adopting this plan, I intended only to hide from the sight of the patient and his comrades, the distressing spectacle of a hemorrhage, which would soon prove fatal; and I, therefore, thought that the effusion of blood into the cavity of the thorax, could not increase the danger. But the wound was scarcely closed, when he breathed more freely, and felt easier. The heat of the body

soon returned, and the pulse rose. In a few hours he became quite calm, and to my great surprise grew better. He was cured in a very few days, and without difficulty.

Drainage of lung abscesses and amputation of lung which has herniated through traumatic wounds in the chest wall have been performed for centuries. In the late 1800s successful transthoracic pulmonary resections were performed in animals, and methods for the control of respiration during operation were evaluated. On the basis of experiments that suggested a superiority of negative pressure over positive airway pressure, Sauerbruch developed a negative pressure chamber in 1904 in which the operating team and the patient could be housed during operation. Under these conditions, the lung would not collapse when the chest was open. The animal experiments gave some success, but the operations on patients were not so rewarding. Techniques of tracheal intubation and anesthesia were developing in parallel with the increasing desire to make surgery of the thorax an achievable reality at the close of the nineteenth century. Orotracheal intubation with metal tubes for the treatment of croup and for the prevention of aspiration during oral surgical procedures provided the early experience that led to endotracheal anesthesia for thoracic surgery. An artificial respiration device consisting of a hand bellows and a tracheostomy tube were introduced by Fell in 1893, and modified by O'Dywer in 1896. The latter substituted an orotracheal tube and a foot bellows with a greater volume capacity. Rudolph Matas in New Orleans advocated the use of the Fell-O'Dywer apparatus to allow a more general availability of thoracic surgical techniques, and he introduced his own modification of the equipment in 1900. The use of these early techniques to prevent lung collapse and ineffectual ventilation during thoracotomy were associated with hazards of their own. It is not surprising then to find that surgeons were still devising makeshift techniques to control the open pneumothorax associated with chest-wall resections as late as the first several decades of this century. These included various packing techniques, preoperative pneumothorax for "conditioning," and suturing the lung to the parietal pleura. It

Fig. 17-1. The relationship of the thoracic cage to the upper abdominal viscera must be remembered to avoid overlooking concomitant abdominal injuries in patients with thoracic trauma.

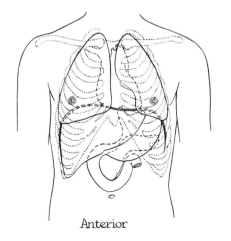

Anterior

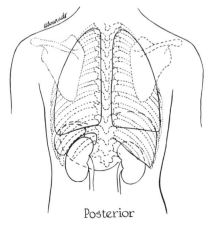

Posterior

was inevitable that refinements in laryngotracheal intubation, in design and materials of tracheal tubes, and in techniques of anesthesia would displace the local improvisations of a handful of surgeons. During the 1930s and the 1940s the majority of thoracic surgical techniques in use today for noncardiac disease were either developed or refined for widespread use.

Although the developments in cardiac surgery have overshadowed the progress being made in other areas of thoracic disease, the practice of thoracic surgery has nonetheless become more exciting as advances in technology are brought into clinical use. Though the flexible fiberscopes have transferred a major responsibility for endoscopic diagnosis to internists, these instruments have allowed the recognition of bronchopulmonary and esophageal neoplasms at an early stage. Surgical resection of the tumors in the "occult" stage has yielded cure rates previously considered to be unobtainable. Isotope methodology and computerized tomography for detection of systemic metastases have supplemented mediastinal exploration techniques, sharply reducing the percentage of unproductive thoracotomies in patients with incurable bronchogenic cancer. The early results of several methods to enhance immunocompetence in patients with pulmonary neoplasms strengthen the concept that surgical treatment of most neoplasms should be combined with continuing postoperative systemic therapy.

The current management of thoracic injuries has become more sophisticated, partly through the improvements and understanding of trauma pathophysiology and support techniques that can be attributed to the research-funded trauma centers. Lung transplantation remains out of reach for the present, but it seems inevitable that some limited success will be achieved in the near future.

ANATOMY OF THE THORAX AND PLEURA

Because of the palpable bony structures of the thoracic cage and the transmission of cardiac and breath sounds through the chest wall, the physician is aided in relating thoracic anatomy to principles of diagnosis. On the other hand, the overlap of the upper part of the abdomen by the lower ribs and the extension of the lung apices above the level of the clavicles can lead to serious errors, especially in patients with blunt trauma (Fig. 17-1). The lower ribs and costal margin overlap the liver, spleen, stomach, the upper pole of both kidneys, and the distal part of the pancreas. By providing support for the upper extremity, the thorax acquires the additional anatomic elements of the shoulder girdle. Because the skeletal and muscular components of the shoulder participate in several functions and diseases of the thorax, it is necessary to review the relations of these structures in any detailed study of thoracic anatomy.

The framework of the thoracic cage consists of the sternum, twelve thoracic vertebrae, ten pairs of ribs that end anteriorly in segments of cartilage, and two pairs of floating ribs (Fig. 17-2). The thoracic inlet is characterized by having a rigid structural ring formed by the sternal manubrium, the short, semicircular first ribs, and the vertebral column. As a result of its articulation with the manubrium and the attachment of the costoclavicular ligament, the clavicle participates in providing protection for the underlying vascular and neural structures which traverse the thoracic inlet. The same rigidity that provides protection from trauma, however, leaves little room for pathologic swelling, enlarging masses, or postural adjustments with age.

The cartilages of the first six ribs have separate articulations with the sternum; the cartilages of the seventh through the tenth ribs fuse to form the costal margin before attaching to the lower margin of the sternum. In children, significant flexibility is made possible by the vertebral joints and the elasticity of the costal cartilages. Although flexibility of the chest wall decreases progressively with age, serious trauma can be transmitted to the intrathoracic structures with little injury to the bony framework, even in adults.

The pectoralis major and minor muscles constitute the principal muscular covering of the anterior thorax, and the lower margin of the pectoralis major forms the *anterior axillary fold*. Auscultation of the chest in the axilla often allows the best determination of breath sounds, because the thoracic cage is covered only by the origins of the serratus anterior muscle in that location. The long thoracic nerve passes vertically on the axillary surface of that muscle—a point to be remembered when doing a thoracentesis or tube thoracostomy. A convergence of the latissimus dorsi and teres major muscles forms the *posterior axillary fold* on each side. The triangle of auscultation can often be palpated near the inferior medial border of the scapula, but the latissimus, trapezius, rhomboid, and other shoulder girdle muscles form a strong muscular coat for the posterior thorax. A disadvantage of the heavy muscle coat is the difficulty in accurately identifying specific ribs by palpation of the posterior chest wall.

Fig. 17-2. The radiolucent costal cartilages and the poor projection of the sternum on anteroposterior chest x-rays make it difficult to demonstrate major injuries or abnormalities of the anterior part of the chest wall.

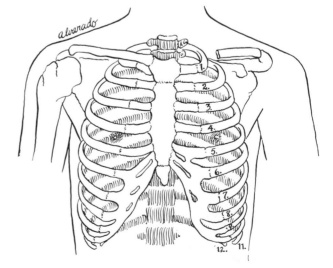

The sternal angle is almost always palpable, and this allows quick identification of the second rib because of its articulation with the sternum at this location. A plane that is parallel to the floor and passes through the sternal angle of an upright patient will also pass through the fourth or fifth thoracic vertebra. The tracheal bifurcation lies in this same plane, while the apex of the aortic arch is located slightly higher. There is a gradual increase in the length of ribs from the first to the seventh and a progressive lateral displacement of the rib-costal cartilage junctions. Because of the radiolucency of the cartilages, standard anteroposterior chest x-rays may fail to document injury to the thoracic cage even though a severe blunt injury to the chest has disarticulated and fractured multiple costal cartilages.

The *pleura* is a serous membrane of flat mesothelial cells overlying a thin layer of connective tissue in which a vascular and lymphatic network is distributed. That part covering the lungs is referred to as the *visceral* pleura, and it is continuous over the pulmonary hilum and the mediastinum with the *parietal* pleura, which covers the inside of the chest wall and the diaphragm. The pleura thereby forms a closed sac around the pleural cavity. With normal lung expansion the pleural cavity is completely filled and only a potential space exists. As shown in Fig. 17-3, the line of pleural reflection extends slightly beyond the lung border in each direction. This is expected because of the dynamic process of respiration and the need for the pleural sac to accommodate maximum lung expansion with deep inspiration. Conversely, with acute decreases in lung volume, such as that with lobar atelectasis, there is a limit to

Fig. 17-3. The relation of the pulmonary lobes and pleural sinuses to the chest wall.

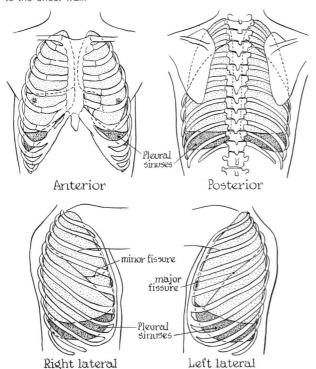

Anterior   Posterior

minor fissure

major fissure

Pleural sinuses

Right lateral   Left lateral

the pleural accommodation and fluid may be drawn into the pleural cavity to replace partially the lost lung volume.

There is no communication between the pleural cavity of each hemithorax, but the anteromedial borders of the two pleural sacs come nearly into apposition behind the sternum. A lateral divergence of the left pleural border between the fourth and sixth costal cartilages forms a cardiac notch which makes it possible to perform transthoracic aspiration of fluid from the pericardial cavity without entering the pleural cavity. The possibility of lacerating the internal thoracic artery as it descends just beyond the lateral sternal border must be remembered; aspiration through this approach should be attempted only when there is almost a certainty that significant pericardial fluid or blood is present. The inferior border of each pleural cavity is located at the ninth rib in the midaxillary line, and the borders continue posteriorly in the eleventh intercostal space. Occasionally the pleural sac extends as low as the twelfth rib. Posteriorly, the margins of the two pleural sacs lie on the anterolateral surfaces of the vertebrae, separated by the esophagus. A retroesophageal recess is occasionally formed when the pleural margins are in near-apposition. At the inferior margin of the lung hilum on each side, a double layer of mediastinal pleura is formed, the *inferior pulmonary ligament.*

The structures which occupy the *intercostal spaces* have considerable significance in relation to thoracic function, disease, and diagnostic procedures. The parietal pleura, for example, is well supplied with nerve endings for pain, while the visceral pleura is insensitive. Only when pulmonary disease extends to involve the parietal pleura or chest wall is pain produced. Figure 17-4 shows the structures in an intercostal space and emphasizes the layering effect of the muscles and fascia. Three layers of intercostal muscles are present in a major part of the thoracic wall, but some anatomists consider the innermost and the internal intercostals to be a single muscle entity. With quiet respiration the ribs are elevated by synchronous contraction of the intercostal muscles. Because the ribs of each side move as a unit in respiration, a localized painful lesion may eliminate effective function of the entire side. During quiet respiration, however, movements of the diaphragm provide approximately 75 percent of pulmonary ventilation and temporary loss of unilateral intercostal muscle function is not a threat to breathing. With labored breathing, the muscles of the upper extremity and those cervical muscles that attach to the chest wall assist in elevation and expansion of the thorax.

The *endothoracic fascia* is a layer of light areolar tissue subjacent to the parietal pleura. At the apex of each hemithorax it is thickened into a more substantial layer referred to as *Sibson's fascia.*

The vein, artery, and nerve of each interspace are located deep to the external and internal intercostal muscles and lie just behind the lower margin of the rib. For most interspaces a smaller collateral artery runs along the top border of the rib below. There is significant overlap of neural supply by adjacent nerves, and complete anesthesia in an interspace will generally not occur unless the intercostal nerve of the adjacent space above and below and the space in question are anesthetized. To minimize the risk of lacerating the intercostal artery, a thoracentesis needle or a clamp used to perforate the pleura for insertion of a catheter should be passed across the top of the lower rib of the selected interspace.

The lymphatic drainage of the chest wall extends in both anterior and posterior directions. Lymph draining from the anterior region of the first four or five intercostal spaces passes to lymph nodes along the internal thoracic arteries. These nodes may be connected by cross anastomoses before draining into a single or double trunk that joins the thoracic duct, a right lymphatic duct, or a bronchomediastinal trunk. Lymphatics that drain the posterior and lateral regions of the intercostal spaces are tributary to lymph nodes that lie near the vertebral ends of each interspace. In the lower part of the thorax these nodes join the drainage from the posterior mediastinum to contribute to the *cisterna chyli*. The posterior lymph nodes of the upper thorax drain into the thoracic duct or a right lymphatic duct.

A musculofibrous floor is provided for the thorax by the *diaphragm*. The peripheral muscular portions of the diaphragm arise from the lower six ribs and costal cartilages, from the lumbar vertebrae (right and left crus), and from the lumbocostal arches. Additional fibers arise from the xiphoid cartilage, and all the muscular elements converge into the central tendon. The central part of the tendon underlies the pericardium, while the right and left divisions extend posteriorly. Some of the lower intercostal nerves are thought to contribute to the sensory innervation of the diaphragm, but motor innervation is supplied by the phrenic nerve on each side.

Of the three major openings in the diaphragm the aortic hiatus is most posterior. The aorta, azygos vein, and thoracic duct pass through this opening. The esophageal hiatus transmits the esophagus and vagus nerves, and only the inferior vena cava goes through the foramen of that name.

Thoracic Incisions

A basic knowledge of the incisions used to perform thoracic operations is helpful in understanding the postoperative course of patients and the management of complications. Because of the rigidity of the thoracic cage, the incisions for major procedures must be relatively large and must disrupt the integrity of muscles and bone, or cartilage. The extensive division of tissues and the distortion or stretching associated with the use of strong mechanical retractors often result in severe postoperative pain.

There are two principal incisions: (1) *lateral thoracotomy,* performed either as an anterolateral or posterolateral incision, and (2) *median sternotomy,* performed as a vertical, sternal splitting incision. Other incisions are infrequently used, either because experience has shown them to be inferior, or because they are used in unusual circumstances. The *thoracoabdominal incision* combines an upper abdominal incision with an incision in a lower intercostal space (sixth, seventh, or eighth) that may be carried as far posteriorly as the posterior axillary line. The costal margin and diaphragm are divided to provide an extensive exposure of the upper part of the abdomen and the retroperitoneal and posterior thoracic structures. Prolonged pain associated with incomplete healing of the costal margin, as well as complicated wound management involving two body cavities if infection occurs, has reduced the enthusiasm for this incision. It still finds usefulness for certain operations involving retroperitoneal structures (kidney, thoracoabdominal aorta), and it may be the best incision to use for hepatic or thoracoabdominal trauma under emergency conditions.

A *bilateral transverse thoracotomy incision* with transection of the sternum is rarely used at present but was employed for routine operative approach to the heart and mediastinum before confidence was gained in the median sternotomy incision. The incision generally extends from

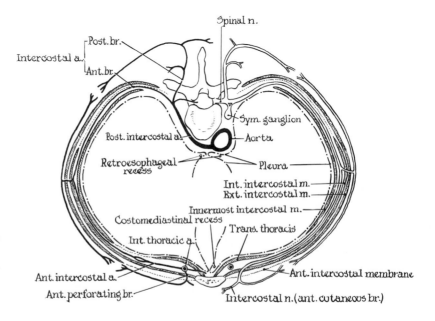

Fig. 17-4. An illustration of the structures within an intercostal space. [*Modified from C. E. Blevins, Anatomy of the Thorax and Pleura, in T. W. Shields (ed.), "General Thoracic Surgery," Lea & Febiger, Philadelphia, 1972, by permission of the author and publisher.*]

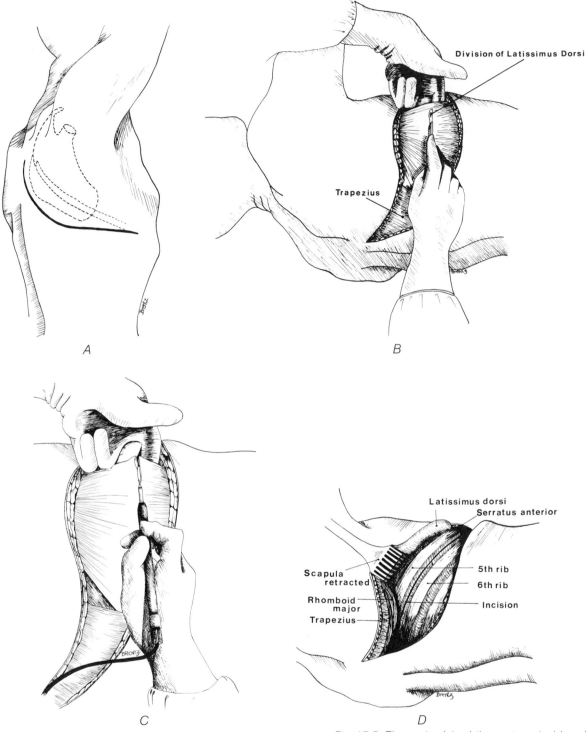

Fig. 17-5. The posterolateral thoracotomy incision. *A*. The skin incision begins near the anterior axillary line and curves posteriorly around the vertebral border of the scapula. *B*. The skin and muscle incisions are located in approximately the same position, whether the pleural cavity is entered in the fourth, fifth, or sixth intercostal space. *C*. Division of the shoulder-girdle muscles with the electrocautery may reduce blood loss and operating time. *D*. The pleural cavity is entered by dividing the intercostal muscles along the lower margin of the interspace.

one anterior axillary line to the other, either in the third or the fourth intercostal space. For reduced exposure needs the incision may be started on the side where the principal dissection will be done and extended only a short distance into the opposite hemithorax after transection of the sternum. The disadvantages of this incision include the longer time required to make the incision and to close the chest, compared to the median sternotomy incision. Both pleural cavities are usually entered with the transverse incision, but this may be avoided with the median sternotomy approach. In unusual circumstances, where the instruments necessary to perform median sternotomy are not available and there is urgent need to have access to both sides of the mediastinum, this incision may still be quite useful.

The *anterolateral and posterolateral* thoracotomy incisions are used most frequently for general thoracic operations. Each one requires division of one or more major shoulder girdle muscles, and this results in voluntary restriction of shoulder motion in the early postoperative period. Because they function as accessory muscles of respiration, it is possible that the selection and placement of the incision to minimize muscle injury could be important in an occasional patient with need for maximal muscle preservation. All patients must be encouraged to begin active shoulder and arm motion after operation, but elderly patients are especially likely to develop a restricted range of shoulder motion if not supervised carefully. The distal parts of the transected muscles lose their nerve supply and atrophy to a significant degree postoperatively. Commonly, patients note a zone of reduced sensation in the skin on the caudal side of the incision for months after operation.

The *posterolateral thoracotomy* is used for the majority of pulmonary resections (except lung biopsy), for esophageal operations, and for the approach to the posterior mediastinum and the vertebral column (Fig. 17-5). When the intent is to enter the pleural cavity in the fifth intercostal space, the most common selection, the skin incision is begun at the anterior axillary line just below the nipple level in the male, and at the corresponding position in the female. The incision extends posteriorly below the tip of the scapula and ascends midway between the vertebral border of the scapula and the spinous processes of the vertebrae. To expose the thoracic cage it is necessary to divide part of the serratus anterior, latissimus dorsi, trapezius, and rhomboid major muscles. The pleural cavity may be entered by dividing the intercostal muscles in the chosen interspace, or by resecting the posterior two-thirds of the corresponding rib. Only in circumstances where the rib is needed for bone grafting or when broad exposure is needed in a patient with a rigid thoracic cage is it necessary to resect the rib. The division of the rib posteriorly before the mechanical rib spreader is put in place may avoid accidental fracture of one or more ribs, or a costochondral separation by the instrument. The injury to the rib or cartilage may increase postoperative incisional pain and prolong the restricted motion of the chest cage.

Two advantages of the *anterolateral thoracotomy* may be important in trauma victims and in patients with an unstable cardiovascular system. The incision can allow rapid entry into the chest, and the patient may be placed in the supine position on the operating table. This is tolerated better than the lateral decubitus position, and it gives the anesthesiologist the maximum control over the patient's cardiorespiratory system. The incision may be used for mediastinal operations, for some cardiac procedures, and for wedge resections of the upper and middle lobes of the lung. It is preferable to make a submammary skin incision starting at the sternal border overlying the fourth intercostal space and extending to the midaxillary line. The pectoralis major muscle and part of the pectoralis minor are divided at the level of the fourth or fifth intercostal space, and the incision is extended into the serratus anterior. By extending the chosen intercostal muscle incision posteriorly along the top of the subjacent rib it is possible to obtain a wider opening in the chest than the length of the skin incision would suggest. Still further exposure may be obtained by transecting the sternum.

An *axillary thoracotomy incision* may be used in selected circumstances where only limited exposure of the upper hemithorax is needed. It is satisfactory for biopsy of an upper lobe, for resection of small apical pulmonary blebs and pleural abrasion in patients with recurrent pneumothorax, for upper thoracic sympathectomy, and for biopsy of upper mediastinal lymph nodes or masses. The skin incision parallels the course of the third rib in the axilla and extends from the anterior to the posterior axillary folds (Fig. 17-6). Retraction of the pectoralis major or latissimus dorsi muscles often makes it possible to enter the pleural cavity by dividing only the second or third intercostal muscles.

A hazard that is common to all the lateral thoracotomy incisions is the potential for injury to the brachial plexus and the axillary neurovascular structures from excessive displacement of the shoulder in positioning the patient on the operating table after anesthesia has been induced. By preventing posterior displacement of the shoulder this complication can be minimized.

The *median sternotomy incision* provides optimum exposure for anterior mediastinal lesions, and it is the principal incision used for cardiac operations. Either pleural cavity may be entered, or incision into the pleural cavities may be avoided if it is unnecessary. Disadvantages of the incision include an increased risk of infection if it is necessary to do a tracheostomy within a few days after operation, and the protracted course that occurs with infection because of involvement of the sternal fragments. An occasional patient who develops an acute wound infection also develops a severe mediastinitis associated with dehiscence of the sternal wound. The mortality rate for this complication is high but has decreased with the evolution of effective treatment.

The skin incision extends from just below the suprasternal notch to a point several centimeters below the xiphoid process (Fig. 17-7). Either an oscillating saw or a Lebsche knife and mallet may be used to split the sternum. A mechanical retractor is used to spread the incision, but the retractor blades may fracture the sternal halves with excessive pressure. After operation, patients who have had a sternotomy have less pain and less interference with pul-

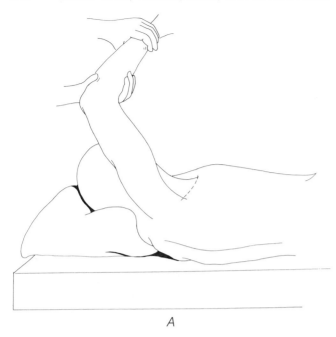

A

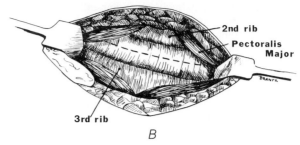

B

Fig. 17-6. *A.* An axillary thoracotomy incision requires minimal muscle division for entrance into the pleural cavity. *B.* The exposure is limited to the upper hemithorax, but postoperative recovery is more rapid than after a standard thoracotomy.

monary function than those who have had a lateral thoracotomy.

The pleural cavity is usually drained with one or two chest tubes connected to an underwater seal system at the conclusion of the intrathoracic portion of the operation. Each chest tube should be brought through a separate stab wound in the chest wall at least two interspaces away from the incision. If the pleural cavity is not entered in operations through a median sternotomy, it is advisable to drain the retrosternal space for 24 hours with an intercostal tube that is brought out through a stab wound in the epigastrium.

EVALUATION OF THE THORACIC SURGICAL PATIENT

At the same time that specific diagnostic procedures are being completed in the patient with a thoracic lesion, it is

pertinent to assess the ability of the patient to undergo operative treatment. In the first instance, the surgical lesion should be evaluated with all possible techniques that will allow the soundest and most effective operative procedure. For many patients the effective operation may require a removal or alteration of tissues with immediate loss of function. This consideration is the tie that binds the thoracic lesion to the several components of the patient's overall state of health.

An experienced surgeon will make a preliminary decision that incorporates his evaluation of the patient's health, the operation that would be required, the patient's age, and the complications or disability that may occur postoperatively. Obviously the potential benefit from operation must be weighed against the involved risk. Increasingly, it has become possible to evaluate patients in terms of the morphologic and functional effects of their thoracic disease, and to control the intraoperative and postoperative events that could threaten the desired result.

The history and physical examination, done with the consideration of a thoracotomy in mind, constitute the

Fig. 17-7. *A.* The median sternotomy incision is outlined. *B.* Exposure of the anterior mediastinum is optimum with the use of a mechanical retractor.

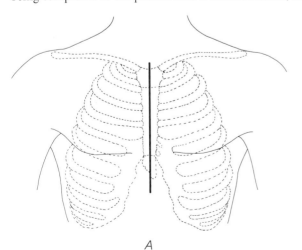

A

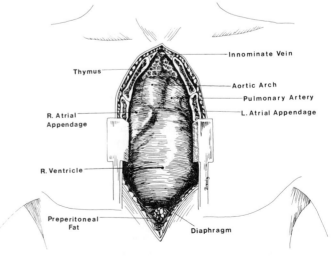

B

foundation of each patient's evaluation. If the patient is found to be in good health, is young, and has normal values for the hospital admission blood tests and urinalysis, no further evaluation may be necessary in some instances. Excision of a benign tumor of a rib, transthoracic sympathectomy for hyperhydrosis or causalgia, and resection of small apical pulmonary blebs are examples of operative procedures that may be performed with nothing more than clinical assessment of the patient's health.

More often the candidate for operation has a pulmonary or esophageal neoplasm or is a cigarette smoker with symptoms of chronic bronchitis and is at least middle-aged. If the person proves to be a satisfactory candidate for operation, a major procedure will be required that will almost certainly interfere with cardiopulmonary function. During an operation in one side of the thorax the corresponding lung will be either retracted or displaced in such a way that it can contribute little, if any, to respiratory gas exchange. Further, it may be necessary to retract intermittently against the pericardium in a way that either interferes with venous return to the atria or precipitates brief arrhythmias. Therefore, the functional status of the contralateral lung and the presence of preexisting cardiac disease are major determinants of the safety of the operation.

Following operation, the pain of a thoracotomy incision, whether or not the chest wall or pulmonary tissue has been resected, restricts the patient's ventilatory ability. A normally functioning lung on the side operated upon does not guarantee that the patient will recover without pulmonary complications, but there is a greater likelihood of recovery without major difficulty. If preexisting pulmonary disease is present, a significant effort will be necessary to prevent or reduce pulmonary complications. The additional factors of obesity, advanced age, abdominal distension, or infection can add to the risk of morbidity or mortality.

An assessment of the patient's nutritional state is always warranted, since thoracic operations result in severe degrees of surgical stress. A catabolic state is the expected result, and it may be important to plan for intensive preoperative and postoperative nutritional support. Though the relationship between infection and nutritional status is not objectively defined, there is a significant body of opinion that a catabolic state increases susceptibility to infection.

The need for preoperative cardiac evaluation is based on the expected postoperative demand for increased cardiac output, the frequency of coincidental cardiac disease, and the known frequency of cardiopulmonary complications. Any evidence of preexisting cardiac disease in a patient who is being prepared for a thoracic operation demands an adequate diagnosis, including cardiac catheterization if necessary. The development of even mild pulmonary edema can result in critical hypoxemia during or after operation. It is important to evaluate renal function as well, since fluid accumulation in the lungs or fluid and electrolyte imbalance may occur on the basis of renal insufficiency. The primary symptoms of the thoracic lesion may obscure any evidence of cardiorenal dysfunction, but the latter must be sought by screening examination.

A major consideration in recommending surgical treatment for a thoracic disease is whether the patient has adequate pulmonary function to tolerate the operation and the handicaps of the postoperative period. When the planned operation will result in a loss of functioning pulmonary tissue (lobectomy, pneumonectomy) there is a significant hazard of postoperative respiratory failure if the patient's preoperative pulmonary function is already compromised. Despite the common use of last-minute estimates of pulmonary function (such as the patient's ability to walk rapidly up two flights of stairs), it is better to measure function by objective techniques. This allows the most accurate interpretation of data and provides a permanent record for comparison with subsequent measurements.

No single test is yet available which provides an overall evaluation of lung function that would be adequate for surgical patients. The specific measurements that are of greatest value include lung volumes, mechanics of breathing, and arterial blood gases. Carefully performed spirometry forms the basis of the pulmonary function data most used in the evaluation of patients with thoracic lesions. Although most patients undergo pulmonary function testing in the hospital, the recent development of accurate electronic spirometers for office use makes it possible to perform satisfactory screening tests during an initial office visit. For the patient with compromised function, it is possible to institute a plan of management before hospitalization.

Figure 17-8 illustrates the subdivisions of lung volume in relation to a spirograph tracing. Functional residual capacity (FRC) and residual volume (RV) may be measured either by gas dilution techniques or by body plethysmography. FRC and RV are not routinely determined for surgical patients, but a broader use of these tests would be helpful. Body plethysmography has the additional advantage of permitting measurements of airway resistance and compliance.

Vital capacity, the amount of air that can be forcefully expelled from a maximally inflated lung position, can be a

Fig. 17-8. The lung volumes and their subdivisions related to a spirograph tracing. Functional residual capacity and residual volume must be measured by other techniques.

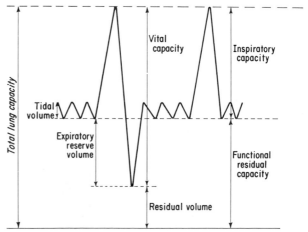

useful determination if its limitations are accepted. The predicted value decreases with age, and its measurement requires understanding as well as full cooperation from the patient.

The *mechanics of breathing* permits dynamic measurements of a patient's ability to move volumes of air during units of time. Individual laboratories vary in the panel of function tests that are performed, sometimes on the basis of an interest in a specific part of the expiratory flow curve of the spirogram. The *forced expiratory volume* in 1 second (FEV_1) is the commonest flow measurement, and it seems unlikely that measurements of an earlier portion of the curve, i.e., $FEV_{0.5}$, offer any advantage over FEV_1. Petty believes that the FEV_3 may be useful for detecting abnormalities in airflow that are not detected by the FEV_1. For example, small-airway disease is not generally detected at high lung volume flow, which is that part specifically measured by the FEV_1. In practice the FEV_1 is usually reported as a percentage of the VC (FEV_1/VC) as well as an actual volume. It is important to note its value both ways. If the VC is significantly reduced, the ratio FEV_1/VC may be satisfactory while the actual volume exhaled is markedly abnormal.

The *maximal midexpiratory flow* (MMEF) is derived from the midportion of the spirogram curve and is considered to be relatively *effort-independent*. It is not included in the report from many laboratories, but for surgical patients any flow rates below 1 liter/second suggest caution in advising a thoracotomy without an effort to improve pulmonary function.

Fig. 17-9. A fixed obstruction in the trachea markedly alters the maximum expiratory flow-volume curve (MEFV). The normal MEFV is shown by the interrupted line. (*Reproduced from R. E. Hyatt, Evaluation of Major Airway Lesions Using the Flow-Volume Loop, Ann Otol Rhinol Laryngol, 84:635, 1975, by permission of the author and publisher.*)

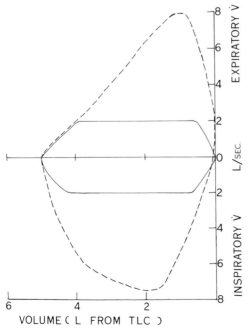

A test which is *effort-dependent* is the *maximal voluntary ventilation* (MVV—previously called the maximal breathing capacity), performed by having the patient inhale as deeply and rapidly as possible for 15 seconds. The MVV usually correlates well with the FEV_1, and in Petty's laboratory the expected relationship is $FEV_1 \times 34$ for males, $FEV_1 \times 40$ for females. If the actual measured value fails to correlate with the calculated value it suggests a poor effort or a fatigued patient. In most laboratories the patient is given an aerosol of a sympathomimetic amine bronchodilator and the spirometry is repeated. An improvement, sometimes significant, in flow rates and in VC may occur. A failure of severely decreased function values to improve does not mean that the patient has irreversible pulmonary disease. Aggressive therapy with the patient's cooperation can often improve pulmonary function, a benefit both to the patient's comfort and to the operative procedure.

The significance of early small-airway disease that is not demonstrated by standard spirometry has not been defined for thoracic surgical patients. Nevertheless, there is increasing interest in two tests of recent development that deserve evaluation. The *maximal expiratory flow-volume curve* (MEFV) is inscribed from a plot of airflow against the volume of vital capacity. This relationship of the data may provide information not given by a spirogram. Major airway lesions may distort the MEFV curve; Fig. 17-9 shows the abnormality seen with a fixed obstruction of the trachea. The *closing volume* (CV) depends on the fact that gravity results in a greater negative pressure at the apex of the lung than at the base in an upright person. That lung volume at which lung units in the dependent regions of the lung cease to ventilate, presumably because of airway closure, is referred to as the CV. The measurement can be made by monitoring the concentration of nitrogen in the exhaled gas during a vital-capacity maneuver after inspiration of a bolus of 100% oxygen. ^{133}Xenon or another gas may be used as the marker. An abrupt increase in the marker concentration in the terminal portion of the vital-capacity curve is the CV, and the value is expressed as a percentage of the vital capacity.

A measurement of the arterial blood gases and pH should be routine in the preoperative evaluation of a candidate for thoracic surgery. It would be an unusual situation in which the decision to advise operation depended solely on a single measurement of arterial oxygen or carbon dioxide tension. Even so, an occasional patient is discovered to have hypoxemia or CO_2 retention that was not suspected on the basis of clinical examination or spirometry. A measurement of the Pa_{CO_2} provides an immediate indication of the patient's alveolar ventilation; any value above 46 torr means that there is hypoventilation. There are multiple causes for this, and the specific reason should be sought in each patient. The ability of the lungs to excrete CO_2 is remarkable, and any persistent elevation of Pa_{CO_2} in a patient who might otherwise be considered a candidate for a major thoracotomy suggests serious abnormalities in distribution of ventilation and perfusion. Most operations will temporarily increase the ventilation-perfusion abnormality. A mild elevation of the Pa_{CO_2} in a patient with chronic lung disease may be treated aggressively to improve pulmonary function and allow the patient to be considered for operation. If pulmonary resection is contemplated in such an individual, the risk of postoperative respiratory failure is high and the decision to operate may depend on whether functioning pulmonary tissue would be removed.

The measurement of arterial P_{O_2} is valuable in the preoperative assessment of pulmonary function, but the number reported must be viewed with a consideration of the possibilities for error in its measurement. At sea level the normal Pa_{O_2} is above 85 torr. It is remarkable, however, how seldom one sees a patient with even minimal pulmonary disease who has an arterial oxygen tension in the normal range. The majority of patients considered by a thoracic surgeon have a Pa_{O_2} of 80 torr or below, and values in the range of 70 to 80 torr do not suggest unusual risk in the absence of other signals of caution. If the Pa_{O_2} is below 70 torr, an attempt should be made to determine the cause and to improve the patient's respiratory exchange. The possibilities include right-to-left shunting as a result of the thoracic disease for which the patient is being considered, uneven distribution of ventilation and perfusion, or diffusion barrier. More sophisticated pulmonary function tests may be indicated, including determination of alveolar-arterial oxygen difference, calculation of right-to-left shunt fraction, and split pulmonary function.

The pulmonary-function values obtained with spirometry in the individual patient must be compared with those obtained from other individuals of the same sex, age, and height who are known to be free of pulmonary disease. Data obtained from the spirometric studies in hundreds of normal males and females form the basis for *prediction nomograms* which facilitate that comparison. Figure 17-10 shows a prediction nomogram developed from studies of 422 normal adult males in a Veterans Administration–Army Cooperative Study of Pulmonary Function. To demonstrate the considerable information that may be accumulated about the individual patient's pulmonary function, Table 17-1 lists the values for a healthy young male breathing air at sea level. The panel of studies shown is adequate for most surgical patients, but it is possible that measurements of inspired gas distribution, diffusing capacity, pulmonary capillary blood volume, and the work of breathing could be determinants in the decision to operate on a patient with marginal pulmonary function.

Of the standard function tests, surgeons have come to place the greatest reliance on the expiratory flow rates and MVV as the critical determinants of operability for the patient with reduced function from respiratory disease, advanced age, or chronic illness. Mittman reported a 9 percent cardiopulmonary mortality rate in patients with a maximum breathing capacity (MBC) greater than 50 percent of the predicted value. By contrast, those patients whose MBC was less than 50 percent had a 45 percent cardiopulmonary mortality rate following thoracotomy. Similar results were reported by Miller for patients who underwent pneumonectomy, with a slightly lower mortality for those who had a lobectomy. Other studies have failed to support a precise correlation between a given level of reduced pulmonary function and an expected mortality

risk. In the last decade improvements in the facilities and tools (respiratory care units, arterial blood-gas measurements, volume-controlled respirators) for postoperative care have influenced many surgeons to become more aggressive in advising thoracotomy for patients with compromised pulmonary function. For example, a patient with a suspected bronchogenic carcinoma would be considered a high risk for pulmonary resection if the routine pulmonary function tests showed the VC, FEV_1, and MVV to be less than 50 percent of the predicted values. If operation would require right pneumonectomy, many surgeons would advise against surgical treatment. Others would insist on attempting to determine the contribution to pulmonary function of each lung.

Table 17-1. TYPICAL VALUES IN PULMONARY FUNCTION TESTS*

Lung volumes

Inspiratory capacity, ml	3,600
Expiratory reserve volume, ml	1,200
Vital capacity, ml	4,800
Residual volume (RV), ml	1,200
Functional residual capacity, ml	2,400
Thoracic gas volume, ml	2,400
Total lung capacity (TLC), ml	6,000
RV/TLC × 100, %	20

Ventilation

Tidal volume, ml	500
Respiratory dead space, ml	150
Respirations/min	12
Minute volume, ml/min	6,000
Alveolar ventilation, ml	4,200

Mechanics of breathing

Maximal voluntary ventilation, L/min	125–170
Forced expiratory volume, % in 1 sec	83
Forced expiratory volume, % in 3 sec	97
Maximal expiratory flow rate (for 1 L), L/min	400
Maximal inspiration flow rate (for 1 L), L/min	300
Compliance of lungs and thoracic cage, L/cm H_2O	0.1
Compliance of lungs, L/cm H_2O	0.2
Airway resistance, cm H_2O/L/sec	1.6

Alveolar ventilation/pulmonary capillary blood flow

Alveolar ventilation, L/min/blood flow, L/min	0.8
Physiologic shunt/cardiac output × 100, %	<7
Physiologic dead space/tidal volume × 100, %	<30

Arterial blood

Oxygen tension, torr	100
Carbon dioxide tension, torr	40
Oxygen tension (100% inhaled oxygen), torr	640
Alveolar-arterial P_{O_2} difference (100% inhaled oxygen), torr	33
Oxygen saturation (% saturation of hemoglobin)	97.1
pH	7.4

*The values shown are those of a resting young male, 1.7 m² body surface area, breathing room air at sea level, except where specified otherwise.

SOURCE: Modified from J. H. Comroe, Jr., "The Lung," 2d ed., Yearbook Medical Publishers, Inc., Chicago, 1962, with permission of the author and publisher.

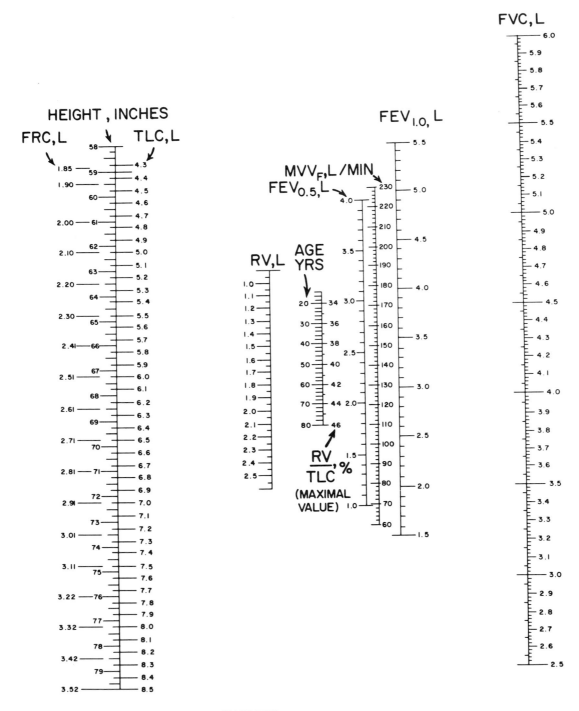

INCHES

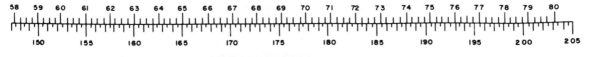

CENTIMETERS

It has been established that a centrally located neoplasm may sharply reduce the function of the ipsilateral lung even though the routine chest x-ray does not suggest this. Split lung function may be determined by bronchospirometry, but the difficulty in accurate placement of the double endotracheal tube (Carlen) has discouraged use of that technique. Radioisotope lung scintiscanning can be used more simply to suggest the relative contribution of each lung to total pulmonary function. Olsen has refined the radioisotope split-function test by measuring pulmonary artery pressure and calculating the predicted postpneumonectomy FEV_1 in a prospective study of patients considered at high risk for pulmonary resection. Although the cardiorespiratory mortality rate of nearly 18 percent for pneumonectomy in that series is impressive, it is likely that some of the surviving lung cancer patients would have been excluded from operation by standard function studies.

The interest in providing a satisfactory evaluation of the patient before thoracic operation must not obscure the ultimate purpose of the evaluation—to provide the patient with whatever physical and mental preparation is needed. Many patients are smokers, and every effort should be made to persuade them to stop smoking before operation, preferably for 2 weeks or more. The etiology of pulmonary infection should be identified and treated intensively, using respiratory therapy, physical therapy, or appropriate techniques. Thoracic operations often are associated with prolonged stays in intensive care units, with multiple chest tubes, with invasive catheters of several types, and with considerable pain. All patients deserve a full explanation of what to expect from the operation, presented in a way that assures them of excellence in their medical care and concern for their well-being.

THORACIC INJURIES

General Considerations

Increasing crime rates with deliberate attempts to kill the victims and a highly mobile population that rushes from one form of violent recreation to another provide a continuing high incidence of thoracic injuries. The spectrum of injury is especially broad and varies from a simple rib fracture or costochondral separation to fatal rupture of the heart from a crushing deceleration against an automobile steering wheel. When one realizes that chest trauma is the cause of approximately 25 percent of all accidental deaths, the need for accurate diagnosis and prompt treatment becomes obvious. Fundamental to the approach to any patient who has suffered a thoracic injury is a consideration of the preinjury cardiopulmonary functional status. The rib fracture or modest pneumothorax that is well tolerated without hospitalization in a healthy young man may lead to pneumonia, empyema, and even death in an older patient with chronic airways disease. Similarly, the patient with preexisting cardiac disease is particularly vulnerable to the development of pulmonary edema and hypoxia that may occur with the rapid administration of salt-containing intravenous fluids typically used for resuscitation of injured patients.

A rapid but perceptive overall evaluation of the patient is always indicated, whether the injury is thought to be serious or not. Chest trauma is often accompanied by other injuries, and the overlap of the upper part of the abdomen by the thoracic cage provides a border zone that is often the site of combination injuries. The young man who is complaining only of chest-wall pain because of one or two rib fractures received in a street fight may have a rapid pulse rate and vasoconstriction that are out of proportion to a broken rib. A consideration of the general region where the rib fracture is located may lead to a correct complete diagnosis that includes a rupture of the spleen or liver. Particularly challenging are those patients who cannot describe their chest pain, or their difficulty in breathing, because of associated head injuries or profound shock. From extensive experience Naclerio has recommended that patients with chest injuries should be approached on the basis of (1) physiologic, (2) etiologic, and (3) anatomic considerations. Since the primary aim of treatment is the prompt restoration of normal cardiopulmonary function, first consideration is given to the patient's physiologic status. Fundamental to this approach is an ability to detect physical abnormalities and relate them to the pathologic processes that are frequently associated with chest injuries. The classification of pathologic processes derived by Naclerio for clinical use is the following:

Group I	*Those peculiar to the outer region of the chest*
	1. Subcutaneous emphysema
	2. Paradoxical respiration (flail chest)
	3. Open pneumothorax
Group II	*Those peculiar to the inner region of the chest*
	1. Closed pneumothorax
	2. Hemothorax
	3. Secretional obstruction of lower airways (pulmonary contusion, "wet lung," aspiration pneumonitis)
Group III	*Those peculiar to the innermost region of the chest*
	1. Mediastinal emphysema
	2. Cardiac tamponade
	3. Compression atelectasis (traumatic diaphragmatic hernia)

Fig. 17-10. A prediction nomogram for pulmonary function in men. *FRC*, functional residual capacity; *TLC*, total lung capacity; *RV*, residual volume; $FEV_{0.5}$, 0.5-second forced expiratory volume; MVV_F, maximal voluntary ventilation (free); FEV_1, 1-second forced expiratory volume; *FVC*, forced vital capacity. The predicted values for *FRC* and *TLC* can be read directly from the left-hand scale, based on the patient's height. The scale at the bottom is for convenience in converting centimeters to inches. *RV/TLC* (%) may be read directly from the age scale. For the other predicted values, lay a straight edge between the patient's height and his age. Predicted normal values can be read directly from the points where the straight edge crosses the *RV*, $FEV_{0.5}$, MVV_F, FEV_1, and *FVC* scales. (*Reproduced from H. C. Boren, R. C. Kory, and J. C. Syner, The Veterans Administration–Army Cooperative Study of Pulmonary Function: II. The Lung Volume and Its Subdivisions in Normal Men, Am J Med, 41:96, 1966, by permission of the authors and publishers.*)

Regardless of whether a classification of pathologic processes is used as a reference, the physician who manages thoracic trauma must know what specific injuries are possible (Fig. 17-11). It is traditional to classify thoracic injuries on the basis of whether the thoracic cage was penetrated by the wounding object. *Nonpenetrating* or *blunt* injuries result from application of force to the chest wall or from sudden deceleration of the chest against a relatively unyielding structure, such as a steering wheel.

Fig. 17-11. The approach to diagnosis and emergency treatment of patients with major thoracic trauma is facilitated by a sound knowledge of the specific injuries that can occur. (*Reproduced from E. A. Naclerio, "Chest Injuries," Grune & Stratton, Inc., New York, 1971, with permission of the author and publishers.*)

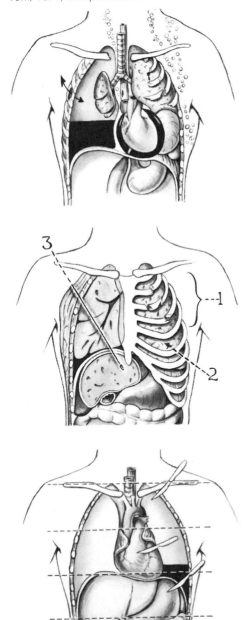

Minor impacts on the chest wall allow the dissipation of applied force with simple contusion of the soft tissues or the bony cage. With a blunt force of greater energy the chest wall transmits some of the wounding force to the intrathoracic structures. Because the lungs and heart present their surfaces to the inner chest wall, it can be expected that those organs are most likely to be injured by transmitted force. In some instances more complex relationships have to be considered to explain a laceration of the esophagus, a tear in the wall of a major bronchus, or a disruption of the thoracic aorta. For many such injuries the explanation is thought to lie in a difference of deceleration rates for adjacent regions of the same organ or structure, related to the degree of fixation of the adjacent regions.

The mortality rate of major blunt injuries has been reduced steadily during the past quarter century, but complications and death associated with pulmonary contusion, posttraumatic pulmonary insufficiency, and trauma to the heart and great vessels are still impressive. It is especially characteristic of blunt injuries that the maximal extent of cardiopulmonary functional loss and often the complete diagnosis require several days for development.

Penetrating injuries are those in which the wounding agent has at least entered the chest wall and generally has penetrated interior structures. In some classifications of wounds an additional category of perforating injuries is used to designate those penetrating wounds in which the wounding object passes through the body region and produces a wound of exit. The latter wound may be more ragged and larger than the wound of entrance. It is often possible to predict which tissue or organs have been damaged by estimating the direction from which the wounding object came and its apparent course. However, the bony structures of the thoracic cage can so markedly alter the course of a knife or small-caliber bullet that relatively little damage may be associated with an entrance wound that appears ominous because of its proximity to the mediastinum (Fig. 17-12). In general, the management of penetrating wounds depends on the same techniques for assessment and diagnosis that are applied in patients with nonpenetrating injuries. A greater utilization of emergency thoracotomy is required in those hospitals where the bulk of thoracic trauma consists of patients with penetrating injuries.

The penetrating injuries that produce a major disruption of the chest wall may result in an open wound—free communication between the pleural cavity and the outside. Because of the noise that is made by passage of air in and out of the wound with respiratory efforts, the open wounds are often referred to as "sucking wounds" of the chest. Shotgun blasts at close range, industrial accidents in which the victim's chest wall is impaled by motorized equipment, and high-speed car wrecks are examples of situations in which open chest wounds may be produced.

Naclerio's *anatomic* approach to chest injuries is especially useful for considering the management of knife wounds. When a stab wound has been made in the *upper part of the thorax* and there is no subcutaneous emphysema, it can be assumed that there is no injury to the trachea. If examination of the chest suggests only a minimal hemothorax, it sharply reduces the possibility that a major artery has been injured, either in the thoracic inlet or the superior mediastinum. But if a major hemothorax is present, injury to a large vessel is likely, and a decision must be made either to do an exploratory operation or to obtain immediate angiography. A patient whose esophagus has been penetrated by the stab wound may have some slight discomfort with swallowing, accompanied by mediastinal and subcutaneous emphysema. A contrast esophagogram is necessary to determine the level of an esophageal penetration and to help with the choice of procedure for its management.

If a patient has been stabbed in the *midthoracic region* the primary concern is whether the heart has been penetrated. When the entrance wound overlies the large central area occupied by the heart, and the patient is in shock, an immediate pericardiocentesis should be done to relieve any possible tamponade while preparations are made for emergency thoracotomy. A parasternal stab wound with evidence of hemothorax often requires operation for ligation of severed internal thoracic vessels, sometimes accompanied by cardiac injury. Stab wounds of the lung generally stop bleeding spontaneously, and the majority of patients who are stabbed in the lateral and posterior regions of the chest do not require thoracotomy. A moderate hemothorax resulting from penetration of the lung parenchyma may be managed by tube thoracostomy. However, if bleeding continues after the chest tube is put in, it is more likely to be due to an injured intercostal artery, and an exploratory thoracotomy will be required.

For stab wounds in the *lower thoracic region* the type of management is dominated by a consideration that the diaphragm may have been penetrated. Therefore, some surgeons believe that a stab wound of the left lower part of the chest mandates early abdominal exploration on the basis that the knife may have gone through the diaphragm to injure the spleen, stomach, or colon. An alternate approach, and the one generally used for patients with stab wounds of the right lower part of the chest, is to observe the patient carefully for evidence of peritoneal irritation, free air, or signs of bleeding in excess of the amount of blood drained by an intercostal catheter. Contrast radiologic studies of the stomach and colon may be done early if the patient's condition is good, or following the initial period of observation. Because the liver is generally the only abdominal structure injured by right-sided stab wounds that penetrate the diaphragm, it is reasonable to observe such patients for a period of some hours. Abdominal exploration is indicated if there is evidence of continuing blood loss, and additional thought must be given to possible late complications of delayed hemorrhage, bile peritonitis, or subphrenic abscess.

Rib Fractures

The most common injury of the chest is a fracture of one or more ribs, including fracture at the costochondral junction ("separation"). Children seem less liable to rib fractures, but chest x-rays are made less frequently in those young age groups with minor trauma. Fractures occur most

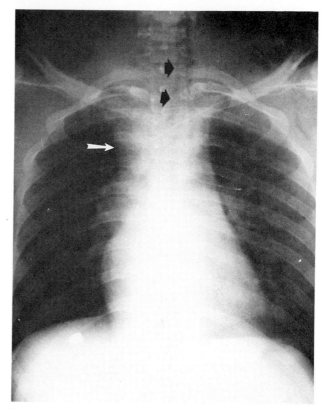

Fig. 17-12. This chest x-ray was taken less than 1 hour after the patient was shot in the left side of the chest with a .44-caliber pistol. The film shows mediastinal widening, greater on the right, with deviation of the trachea to the left (*upper arrows*). Coughing and pain were the only symptoms, but the patient underwent emergency mediastinal exploration with an expectation of finding major vascular injury. A hematoma was found in the mediastinum, but no major vascular structures were damaged. The bullet was lying free in the right pleural cavity in the location where it is seen on the x-ray.

commonly in the middle and lower ribs with blunt trauma, but the distribution with penetrating wounds varies with the distribution of the penetrating objects. The first rib is rarely fractured unless one or more upper ribs are also broken. There is inconclusive evidence that a direct relationship exists between first and second rib fractures and trauma to major vessels at the apex of the hemithorax (Fig. 17-13).

An inward displacement of the fracture fragments at the time of injury may lacerate the lung parenchyma and produce a pneumothorax with bleeding into the pleural cavity. With a single rib fracture the incidence of pneumothorax is not high, but there is an increasing likelihood of this complication as the number of fractured ribs increases. The occurrence of pneumothorax may be delayed for some hours or even days after the injury has occurred. Hemothorax of a significant degree occurring with rib fractures is usually due to laceration of an intercostal artery rather than to bleeding from the lung. Again, bleeding may be delayed in onset or it may recur after an interval of several days. Especially in the patient who has multiple rib fractures with segmental fractures of one or more ribs, a de-

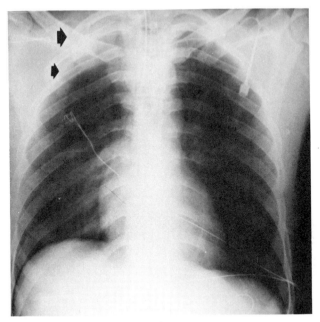

A

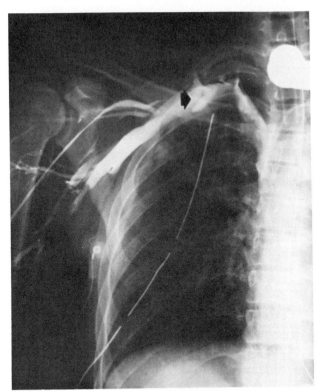

B

Fig. 17-13. *A*. The first chest x-ray of a twenty-five-year-old man who was injured in a motorcycle accident shows a fracture of the right first rib (*upper arrow*) and a small extrapleural hematoma at the right apex (*lower arrow*). *B*. A subclavian arteriogram and venogram were done 3 days after admission because of the sudden development of a massive hemothorax (2,000 ml blood) on the right side. Bleeding stopped spontaneously, and the venogram shows a tear in the subclavian vein at the rib fracture site.

layed pneumothorax or hemothorax may coincide with some shift of the rib fragments demonstrated in serial chest x-rays. In elderly or chronically ill patients rib fractures may occur with severe coughing or hard straining. The occurrence of a spontaneous fracture in any patient should alert the physician to the possibility of a bone abnormality such as metastatic neoplasm or hyperparathyroidism. Pneumothorax and hemothorax are infrequent with rib fractures that do not result from external trauma.

The diagnosis of a rib fracture may be implied from the pleuritic type of pain and marked tenderness over the fracture area. A sharply localized contusion of the chest-wall structures may mimic the findings, including shallow respirations with chest-wall splinting. Green-stick fractures are those not associated with separation of the fragments, and they may not be demonstrated by the initial chest x-ray examination. Several weeks may elapse before a suspected fracture is confirmed. However, when the patient has two or more adjacent fractured ribs, especially if the ribs are broken in more than one place (segmental fractures), the diagnosis is made with greater certainty by examination alone. Cartilage fractures and separation from either the rib or sternum are not demonstrated by chest x-rays.

The acute complications of rib fracture are pneumothorax, hemothorax, and interstitial emphysema. These will be discussed as separate items because of their frequent association with multiple types of chest trauma. Atelectasis and pneumonia may develop as complications because of re-

stricted chest-wall motion, bed rest, and preexisting respiratory disease.

The principal goal of treatment for patients without serious injury is relief of pain. If this is accomplished, patients may resume their normal activities except those that require a vigorous work effort. Adhesive strapping of the chest or chest binders to splint the fracture area may be used to diminish pain in young or middle-aged persons. These techniques are not good for the elderly and for patients with chronic lung disease. The adhesive strapping must be done carefully to avoid blistering and excessive skin traction. A disadvantage that many patients find inconvenient is the inability to shower or to bathe adequately while the adhesive tape is in place. For the majority of patients an adequate oral analgesic or an intercostal nerve block plus oral analgesics provides reasonable pain relief with minimal risk of side effects (Fig. 17-14). The nerve block may need to be repeated once daily for several days, but a single injection may suffice for individuals whose injury does not require hospitalization. A patient whose rib fracture is accompanied by minimal pneumothorax (less than 1.5-cm separation between the lung and the inner

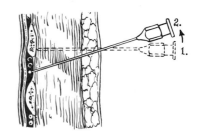

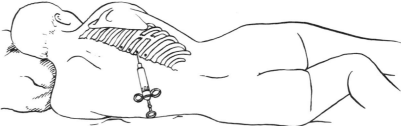

Fig. 17-14. Intercostal nerve blocks may be very effective in relieving the pain of rib fractures. The nerves above and below the fractured ribs must be blocked, in addition to those corresponding to the ribs fractured.

chest wall by x-ray), may be treated as an outpatient under ideal conditions of observation and follow-up. The management of more significant complications will be described below.

Sternal Fractures

Fractures of the sternum are generally the result of slamming against the steering wheel in car accidents. A fracture may occur with any type of blunt trauma to the anterior part of the chest, or occasionally may be produced by a penetrating missile. The fractures are usually transverse and most often occur in the body of the sternum at or near the junction with the manubrium (Fig. 17-15). Displacement of the fragments is not unusual, and when it occurs the upper fragment is behind the lower segment. There may be comminution of the sternal fracture as well as associated fractures of the costal cartilages and separation from the sternal borders. The term *crushed chest* refers to a constellation of blunt chest injuries in which there is extensive disruption of chest-wall structures, including sternal and rib fractures, associated with pulmonary and/or cardiac contusion. The instability of the chest wall is referred to as "flail chest," but fractures of the sternum are not a necessary component of all flail-chest injuries.

Sternal fractures should always signal the possibility of myocardial injury, rupture of the aorta or brachiocephalic vessels, or major tracheobronchial laceration. The pain of a sternal fracture may persist for a long time; when this occurs a nonunion should be suspected. This is usually the result of persistent displacement of the proximal fragment, and a closed reduction may be attempted under general anesthesia by hyperextension of the spine with the arms above the head. Occasionally, open reduction and wiring of the fragments are required.

Traumatic Pneumothorax

Pneumothorax due to penetrating or nonpenetrating trauma is usually the result of injury to the lung or the tracheobronchial tree. An occasional instance of esophageal perforation may be followed by a pneumomediastinum

Fig. 17-15. A lateral chest x-ray demonstrates the type of sternal fracture that occurs when the driver of a car is thrown against the steering wheel.

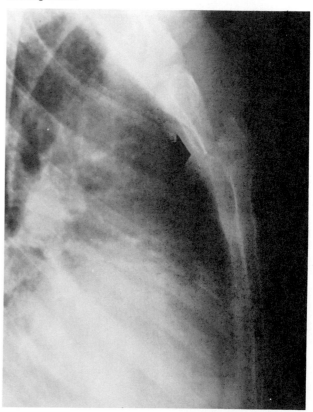

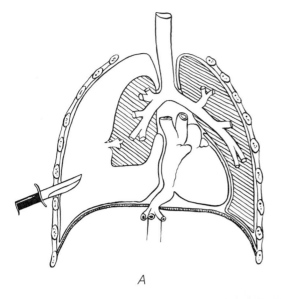

A

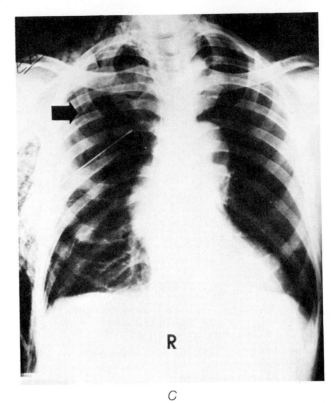

C

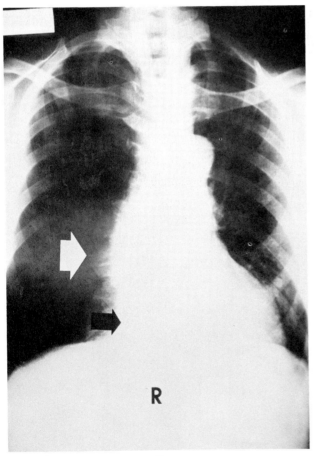

B

Fig. 17-16. *A.* In a tension pneumothorax there is compression of the contralateral lung and a displacement of the mediastinum that may sharply reduce venous return to the atria. *B.* If the diagnosis is strongly suspected, needle aspiration of the pleural space should be done without waiting for the chest x-ray. In this patient, the tension pneumothorax developed slowly and became symptomatic shortly after this film was taken. The lower arrow points to the displacement of the right heart border, and the lung is completely collapsed (*upper arrow*). *C.* Following needle aspiration a large intercostal tube was put in place, but a major air leak continued for several days and eventually required insertion of an additional chest catheter. The arrow points to the visceral pleura, showing incomplete expansion of the lung.

that ruptures into the pleural cavity. In addition, it is possible for a sucking wound of the chest to produce pneumothorax without pulmonary parenchymal injury. The term *closed pneumothorax* is sometimes used to distinguish a pneumothorax that is not in direct communication with the outside air from the type associated with sucking wounds of the chest. Whether the pneumothorax is associated with blunt injury and fractured ribs or is due to a penetrating wound, there is a variable amount of bleeding into the pleural cavity. The decision to use the term *hemopneumothorax* depends on the amount of blood in the pleural cavity and the likely consequences. If sufficient blood is present to require a concerted effort to assure its removal, or if its loss from the circulating volume requires transfusion replacement, it seems proper to use the double term.

Pneumothorax varies from that which is so slight that it may be missed on the initial x-ray examination to a massive, continuing air leak that displaces the mediastinum, depresses the diaphragm, and compresses the opposite lung—*tension pneumothorax* (Fig. 17-16). A pneumothorax due to a parenchymal lung injury tends to be self-limited because the developing lung collapse combines with blood clotting in the wound for a sealing effect. For some patients extensive adhesions already present between the visceral and parietal pleura may localize the pleural air and prevent a collapse of the lung (Fig. 17-17).

The mechanics of a developing tension pneumothorax may not be obvious when the patient is first seen. Pain may be the primary complaint, with no evidence of respiratory distress. But if the lung wound is behaving as a check valve, some air will escape into the pleural cavity with each inspiration or with each cough. Gradually, intrapleural pressure will build up, the lung collapses, and a tension pneumothorax may develop. A shift of the mediastinum and compression of the large veins result in a decreased cardiac output that may lead to sudden death.

With any chest injury it is wisest to presume that a pneumothorax is present until proved otherwise. Because of pain and limited chest motion on the injured side,

Fig. 17-17. A free pleural space will allow the development of a complete pneumothorax or a massive hemothorax. These potentially fatal complications cannot occur in patients with an obliterated pleural space. (*Reproduced from E. A. Naclerio, "Chest Injuries," Grune & Stratton, Inc., New York, 1971, with permission of the author and publisher.*)

physical examination may be inadequate for diagnosis of a minimal pneumothorax. When there is no respiratory distress it is proper to base the diagnosis on the results of an upright or lateral decubitus chest x-ray. With tension pneumothorax of rapid development the patient's life depends on rapid decompression of the pleural space, without waiting to confirm the suspected diagnosis by chest x-ray. In addition to dyspnea, with or without cyanosis, the patient may show distended neck veins, a hyperresonant percussion note over the injured hemithorax, absent or distant breath sounds, and a shift of the heart sounds and trachea toward the opposite side. To accomplish rapid decompression, a large-gauge needle with a stopcock and syringe may be passed into the pleural cavity through the second intercostal space in the midclavicular line. After initial decompression the needle should be replaced with an intercostal catheter attached to an underwater seal. Subsequent treatment depends on whether the lung reexpands and whether the air leak is associated with a parenchymal injury versus a major bronchial disruption.

Treatment of the more usual pneumothorax depends on symptoms of respiratory insufficiency, the extent of the pneumothorax, and the presence of significant hemothorax. There is a tendency to think of pneumothorax in terms of a two-dimensional concept that is conveyed by the anteroposterior chest x-ray. Instead, the hemithorax must

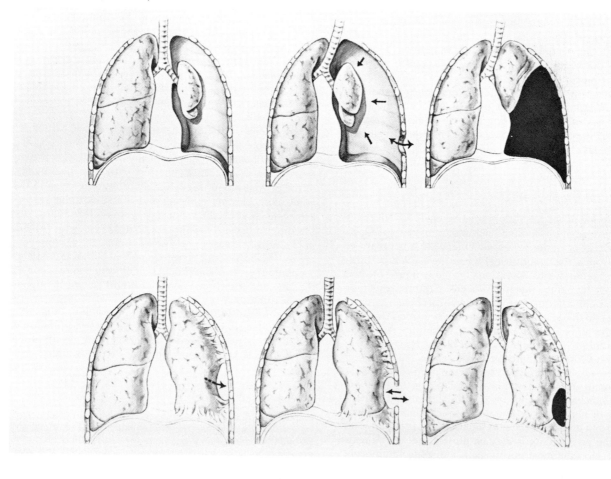

be considered a modified cylinder, and when the lung surface is separated from the chest wall by 3 cm or more the patient may have a 50 percent lung collapse (by volume) rather than the 25 or 30 percent collapse that the chest x-ray suggests. With a pneumothorax that is less than this amount, due to a nonpenetrating injury (theoretically, no contamination of the pleural space) and not accompanied by significant blood or fluid in the pleural cavity, no treatment may be required. A decision not to remove the pleural air implies that the patient has had a simple injury and that conditions for observation are ideal. Approximately 1.25 percent of the air will be absorbed each day, with full expansion expected in 3 to 6 weeks.

Aspiration of the air with a needle and insertion of an intercostal catheter only if lung collapse recurs is a reasonable method of treatment advocated by some physicians when the pneumothorax amounts to as much as 50 percent. In all cases with greater than 50 percent collapse, in those with hemopneumothorax, and in patients whose pneumothorax is the result of penetrating trauma, an intercostal catheter should be inserted and attached to a water seal with 10 to 25 cm H_2O negative pressure. In the majority of patients, lung reexpansion and cessation of the air leak will occur within a few hours or a few days. If not, a major bronchial injury may be present, and a thoracotomy may be required after appropriate diagnostic procedures.

There are three essential steps in the management of the open pneumothorax associated with sucking wounds. A watertight dressing should be used to cover the wound, and an intercostal catheter should be inserted in the pleural cavity. As soon as the patient's condition permits, debridement of the wound should be done, followed by wound closure if possible.

The use of prophylactic systemic antibiotics in patients with chest trauma is a subject of current debate, but their use in cases of nonpenetrating trauma seems unjustified. Certainly, the simple insertion of an intercostal catheter cannot be used as the justification for prescribing an antibiotic.

Interstitial Emphysema

Disruption of the respiratory tract at any level will result in the passage of air into the surrounding tissues. *Mediastinal emphysema* occurs when air enters the areolar tissue planes from a tracheobronchial wound or from a perforation of the esophagus. Occasionally, blunt injuries to the chest may disrupt the integrity of a group of bronchioles or alveolar units without disrupting the visceral pleura. As air escapes into the pulmonary interstitium it dissects centrally along the bronchi and pulmonary vessels to reach the mediastinum. When the mediastinal pleura remains intact, progressive loss of air into the tissue carries the dissection into the neck, where the air escapes the deep-tissue planes and spreads in the subcutaneous tissue (Fig. 17-18).

Subcutaneous emphysema may also be produced by penetrating or blunt injuries that disrupt the lung and parietal pleura so that air is forced into the tissues of the chest wall. An initial pneumothorax may be present, but the patients who develop the most massive subcutaneous emphysema often have delayed onset of pneumothorax. The progressive development of subcutaneous emphysema causes marked distortion of the patient's appearance and significant discomfort. However, there is seldom any reason to "treat" the condition by making a cervical incision to provide a point of air escape. Instead, attention should be directed at confirming the presumed source of the air leak so that an esophageal perforation or major bronchial injury is not delayed in its recognition.

Traumatic Hemothorax

Intrathoracic bleeding occurs with any form of chest injury that disrupts the tissues. In most instances of either penetrating or nonpenetrating trauma the blood is shed into the pleural cavity, often with some degree of pneumothorax. Although hemothorax develops at the time of injury in most patients, the bleeding may be delayed for several days. Occasionally an extrapleural hematoma will break into the pleural cavity and give the impression of delayed hemorrhage.

Bleeding from the lung as the result of rib fractures or small-missile wounds will generally stop before a sufficient volume has been lost to mandate an emergency thoracotomy. From accumulated military and civilian experience it can be estimated that slightly more than 10 percent of patients with traumatic hemothorax will require thoracotomy for control of bleeding or determination of the extent of injury. A progressive hemothorax or continued bleeding at the rate of more than 100 ml/hour beyond a few hours after placement of an intercostal catheter suggests bleeding from an intercostal artery, the internal thoracic artery, or a source that will require operative control. In particular, a major pulmonary laceration due to blunt trauma is generally characterized by continued major blood loss and a large air leak.

Movement of the diaphragm and thoracic structures causes partial defibrination of blood that is shed into the pleural cavity, and clotting is usually incomplete. Sufficient coagulation does occur to interfere with efficient drainage of the pleural blood through intercostal catheters, and the latter often become plugged with blood clot. Pleural enzymes begin to produce clot lysis within a few hours after bleeding stops, and the process of hemolysis with protein breakdown increases the osmotic pressure. Unless the pleural space is drained adequately the transudation of fluid into the space can produce significant compression of the lung and a shift of the mediastinum toward the opposite hemithorax.

The diagnosis of hemothorax with chest injuries is not a matter of determining whether it is present. The question is how much is present, and whether bleeding is still going on. A consideration of the type and extent of injury, gen-

Fig. 17-18. *A* and *B*. A patient with extensive subcutaneous emphysema due to a laceration of the right lung from a rib fracture. *C*. There is massive involvement of the face, trunk, and scrotum. A tracheostomy was done for harassing cough due to chronic bronchitis. *D*. Note the face of the patient 10 days later.

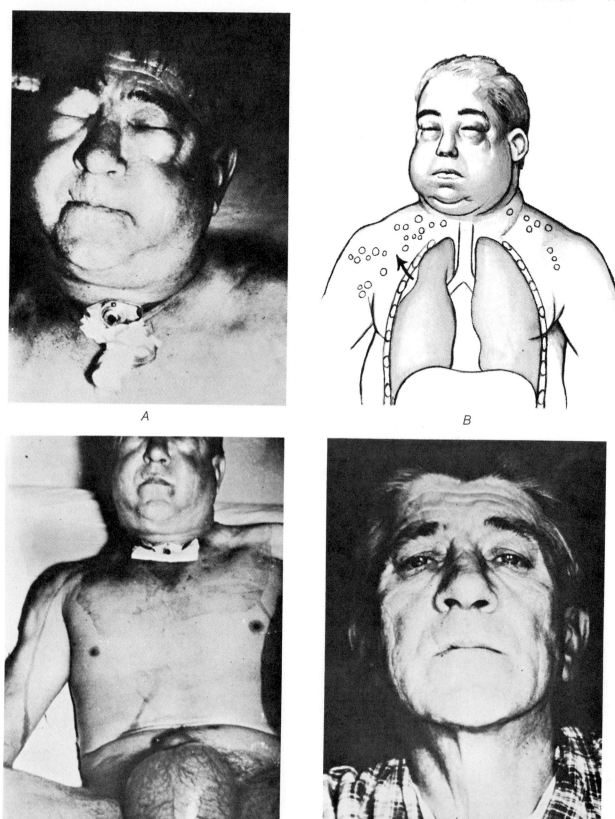

A

B

C

D

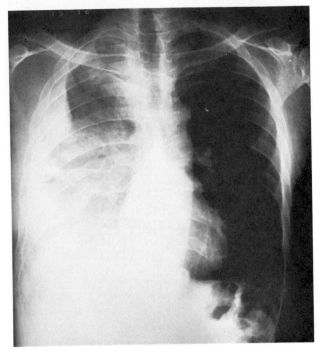

A

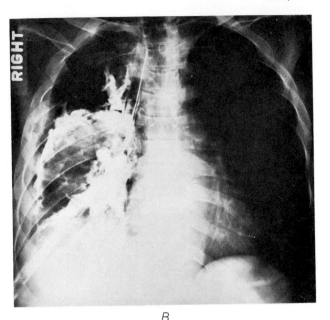

B

Fig. 17-19. *A.* A major hemothorax resulted from a gunshot wound in the right side of the chest of the fifty-year-old man whose chest x-ray is shown here. *B.* This film was taken several weeks later with injection of contrast material through the chest tube. The contrast material outlines a large, irregular cavity in the pleural space, representing an empyema cavity that had developed because of inadequate drainage of the hemothorax by chest catheters. *C.* After decortication there is complete expansion of the right lung, but considerable exudate and fluid are still present in the costophrenic sulcus.

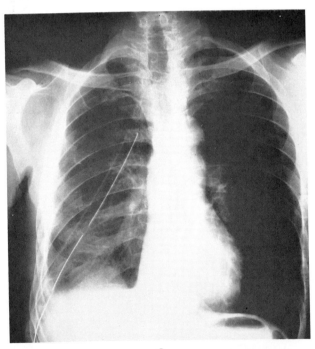

C

eral signs of blood loss, physical signs of fluid in the pleural cavity, and chest x-ray findings may all be needed to assess the extent of hemothorax. It should be remembered that as much as 400 to 500 ml of blood may be hidden by the dome of the diaphragm on the upright chest x-ray, and only the liquid part will be demonstrated by the lateral decubitus film.

A small hemothorax that produces little more than

blunting of the costophrenic angle on the chest x-ray does not require initial treatment. Instead, follow-up x-rays should be made at intervals of a few days to assist with the decision to drain the pleural cavity if there is a progressive accumulation. When the hemothorax exceeds an amount that fills the costophrenic sulcus, or when there is associated pneumothorax, one or more large catheters should be placed in the pleural cavity through the seventh, eighth, or ninth intercostal space in the posterior axillary line. Underwater drainage alone may be sufficient, but low suction applied to the catheters is often helpful when combined with active efforts at stripping the tubes of blood clot. If the initial drainage of blood is followed by continued bleeding in the absence of a clotting defect, a decision to operate must be made, with a broad consideration of the possible sources of the bleeding.

With a major hemothorax the success of tube drainage is often frustrated by extensive clot that obstructs the tubes (Fig. 17-19). An attitude should be adopted that a nonfunctioning chest tube represents a *liability* to the patient because of discomfort and the risk of carrying infection from the skin wound into the pleural clot. Patency of the intercostal tubes may be assured by careful irrigation with normal saline solution and by daily instillations of topical Varidase for lysis and drainage of remaining clotted blood.

Especially with penetrating trauma, a hemothorax that fails to drain adequately through intercostal catheters may develop into empyema. An additional hazard is the organization of residual clot to form a fibrothorax. Although the incidence of these complications is not high, the consequences are severe, and it is wiser to proceed with thoracotomy and evacuation of the hemothorax before an extensive decortication becomes necessary.

Pulmonary Injury

The lungs have a remarkable ability to tolerate penetrating injuries and blunt trauma without long-term residual effects. Civilian gunshot wounds of the chest penetrate a lung more frequently than any other structure, but the majority of patients with no other significant injury can be treated without a thoracotomy. Any penetrating object produces an air leak with a variable degree of pneumothorax. The disruption of tissue along the missile track causes bleeding, which usually ceases as the damaged parenchyma becomes swollen and filled with blood clot. With small-calibre and low-velocity bullet wounds that pass through the lung periphery, the amount of tissue damage produced may be sufficiently small that late follow-up chest x-rays fail to demonstrate the area of injury. With high-velocity bullets, the tissue destruction extends more widely, and even a peripheral bullet pathway may result in irreversible damage to a lobar or lung hilus. The occurrence of arterial air embolism as a cause of morbidity or death in patients with penetrating lung trauma has recently been emphasized by Thomas. The symptoms are related to involvement of either the cerebral or coronary circulation. A failure to produce systemic air embolism under experimental conditions and lack of clinical experience with the condition on a large trauma service have caused others to challenge the occurrence of this complication.

The immediate management of the patient with a penetrating injury is the insertion of at least one intercostal catheter for evacuation of the associated hemopneumothorax. Serial arterial blood gases and frequent evaluation of the patient's ventilatory ability allow an overall estimate of the effect of the injury on respiratory exchange. Civilian penetrating wounds do not require ventilatory assistance very frequently, but the effect of the injury may be underestimated. In some patients, the likelihood of injury to the heart or great vessels, a likely penetration of the diaphragm, or major bleeding may mandate immediate thoracotomy or abdominal exploration. More often, the need for thoracotomy to control bleeding or to perform pulmonary resection for an irreversibly injured lung becomes apparent only over a period of hours, or several days. A massive continuous air leak through the chest tube suggests a major bronchial laceration, but a similar air leak can occur with a peripheral lung wound that transects a number of small airways. A point of differentiation that can be helpful is the difficulty in achieving complete lung expansion and maintaining the expansion in the presence of a major bronchial injury.

Pulmonary contusion is the contemporary term used to indicate the consequences of blunt trauma to the lung. The frequent causes of contusion include rapid deceleration of the chest against an automobile steering wheel, falls from a height, and blast injuries. Particularly in young persons, severe pulmonary contusion can occur by transmission of force through the chest wall with minimal fractures of the ribs or sternum. In middle-aged or elderly persons significant pulmonary contusion is usually accompanied by multiple fractures of the thoracic cage.

The contused lung is characterized by capillary disruption that results in intraalveolar and interstitial hemorrhage, edema, protein and fluid obstruction of small airways, and leukocyte infiltration. Serial chest x-rays begun right after injury show a fluffy infiltrate that progresses in extent and in density over a period of 24 to 48 hours. Although the maximum lung injury is directly related to that region of the chest wall that receives the trauma, a "contrecoup" effect may be responsible for a wider distribution of the pulmonary damage. Unless the contusion involves only a small region of one lung, it may result in serious loss of respiratory function. The associated injury to the chest wall is aggravated by the loss of pulmonary compliance, increasing the work of breathing. Small areas of atelectasis become confluent, and progressive hypoxia further diminishes the patient's ability to compensate for the loss of function.

Pulmonary contusion is often part of a major chest injury that includes one or more fractures of the thoracic cage, pneumothorax, and hemothorax. If not present initially, a pneumothorax may subsequently develop from actual disruption of the contused pulmonary parenchyma. Although it is infrequent in patients who survive to reach the hospital, a major pulmonary laceration may represent the maximum extent of pulmonary contusion. In some instances the tissue disruption is the result of extensive penetration by rib fragments, but in others the causative factor is probably a severe shearing force. The clinical and x-ray findings suggest a serious chest injury but do not differentiate the patient with a major lung laceration from those with pulmonary contusion and associated hemopneumothorax. Continued or uncontrolled hemorrhage and massive air leak generally mandate an early thoracotomy. A major pulmonary resection is often necessary, and the mortality rate is high.

Treatment of pulmonary contusion must include an accurate clinical assessment of the patient's respiratory exchange and careful monitoring by serial measurements of the arterial blood gases. Unfortunately, the techniques of large-volume intravenous fluid administration commonly used to resuscitate patients with multiple injuries may worsen the pulmonary edema that accompanies pulmonary contusion. To reduce this likelihood, the rate of intravenous fluid administration should not exceed 50 to 75 ml/hour if this is at all possible. In addition, 20- to 40-mg doses of intravenous furosemide at intervals of 4 to 6 hours should aid the mobilization of edema fluid from the lung.

A high percentage of patients require temporary assisted ventilation, and it may be evident at the time of admission that endotracheal or nasatracheal intubation should be performed. Without question, aggressive respiratory therapy, including ventilatory support, should be initiated before cardiopulmonary decompensation requires treatment measures that add additional risks. Criteria for insti-

Table 17-2. CRITERIA FOR ASSISTED VENTILATION

Function	Normal values	Ventilate
Pulmonary mechanics		
Respiratory rate	12–20	>35
Vital capacity, ml/kg	65–75	<15
Maximum inspiratory force, cm H_2O (negative values)	75–100	<25–35
Gas exchange		
Pa_{O_2}, torr	76–100 (room air)	<65–70 (added oxygen)
Alveolar-arterial oxygen difference, torr (100% oxygen)	30–70	>350
Pa_{CO_2}, torr	35–45	>50
Dead space/tidal volume ratio	0.25–0.40	>0.6

tuting assisted ventilation are shown in Table 17-2. For most patients the need for assisted ventilation does not extend beyond 48 to 72 hours unless there is major injury to the chest wall or to other body regions.

Tracheobronchial Injury

Penetrating wounds of the thoracic trachea and the stem bronchi are especially serious because of concomitant damage to the major intrathoracic vascular structures. Rapid assessment of the likely course taken by a bullet or knife that entered the patient's mediastinum and prompt evaluation of respiratory distress, hemoptysis, and interstitial emphysema may allow successful treatment. The patients often have an associated pneumothorax, which may rapidly develop into a tension pneumothorax. Shock is not uncommon because of associated bleeding into the mediastinum and one or both pleural cavities. The alert patient often has coughing, and this causes the subcutaneous emphysema to develop more rapidly. Chest x-rays generally show mediastinal emphysema, and if bilateral pneumothorax is also present, it suggests a lacerated trachea.

Early insertion of a large intercostal catheter for pneumothorax may fail to result in expansion of the lung despite a large air flow produced by high-suction drainage. As soon as the patient's respiratory exchange is under control, bronchoscopy should be done to confirm a suspected tracheal or bronchial injury. At the same time, esophagoscopy should be done because of the frequency of associated esophageal injury.

For small penetrating injuries of the intrathoracic trachea and major bronchi, tracheostomy and effective pleural decompression may provide satisfactory definitive treatment. Those injuries which are associated with an actual defect in the tracheobronchial wall, including partial disruption, require operative exploration and repair. Tracheostomy will frequently be necessary to prevent high intratracheal pressures and to allow tracheal care postoperatively.

Penetrating injuries of lobar or segmental bronchi may produce a similar clinical picture to proximal tracheobronchial injuries. Bilateral pneumothorax is rare, and the principal immediate problem is to begin management of the major air leak and confirm the presence of a major

bronchial injury. Hemoptysis may not be detected, and the bronchial air leak may stop soon after an intercostal catheter is put in place. The definitive diagnosis may be delayed if the bronchus becomes obstructed by blood clot or mucus and the air leak ceases. Under these conditions the pulmonary lobe or segment becomes atelectatic and resists conservative methods to produce reexpansion. If infection does not occur, the injured bronchus may heal with significant distortion and obstruction, or the atelectasis may persist and lead subsequently to a correct diagnosis. Operative repair of the disrupted bronchus can be achieved even years after injury. If infection occurs at the site of the bronchial injury the patient may develop pneumonia, distal bronchiectasis, and empyema. Resection of the bronchus and the involved pulmonary lobe is then required.

Severe blunt chest trauma may result in tracheobronchial tears or complete disruption. The most common intrathoracic location is in a main-stem bronchus, the left being more frequently injured than the right. Respiratory distress is generally present, and death may occur from progressive obstruction of the respiratory tract by secretions and blood. Again, an injury may seal itself off, fail to be recognized, and heal with severe stenosis.

The diagnosis and successful management of tracheobronchial injuries depend on a high index of suspicion. Unfortunately, a significant number of tracheal injuries in trauma patients are the result of faulty techniques of endotracheal intubation or tracheostomy when these are performed under emergency circumstances, particularly with head and neck injuries. Improved tracheostomy tubes and better tracheostomy care based on an understanding of the pathophysiology of tube-related tracheal damage have reduced the incidence of tracheal stenosis. Nevertheless, tracheal damage due to overinflated balloon cuffs still occurs, and the patient whose chest x-ray is shown in Fig. 17-20 developed a tracheoesophageal fistula.

Flail Chest

The terms *crushed chest* and *flail chest* have often been used interchangeably, although they are not synonymous. A crushed-chest injury indicates the general cause and implies a disruption of tissue integrity that would be likely to result in flail-like motion of a chest-wall region and a varying degree of crushing (contusion) of any or all under-lying structures. It is better to restrict the use of *crushed chest* to indicate the mechanism of injury, rather than trying to have the term imply the several possible conse-quences of pulmonary contusion, myocardial injury, pneu-mothorax, hemothorax, and so on. Similarly, a diagnosis of flail chest should be accompanied by the tabulation of the specific associated injuries.

The diagnosis of flail chest is based on the presence of paradoxical respiratory movement in a segment of the chest wall. This generally requires at least two segmental fractures in each of three adjacent ribs or costal cartilages. Multiple combinations of rib or sternal fractures with costochondral or chondrosternal separations can result in the paradoxical respiratory motion that characterizes a flail chest. Figure 17-21 demonstrates the three major types of flail chest based on the location of the flail segment. The posterior type is rare, and in the absence of disrupted intrathoracic structures is the easiest to manage because of the strong muscular and scapular support, and because of the patient's natural tendency to lie with his back against the mattress.

Theoretically, the paradoxical motion markedly reduces respiratory efficiency and allows a back-and-forth move-ment of dead-space air across the carina between the two lungs during each respiratory cycle. This has been referred to as *Pendulluft* (pendulum-like movement of air), but it has been discounted experimentally.

Mediastinal motion away from the injured side with inspiration and toward the flail segment during expiration may reduce venous return and cardiac output if the flail area is large and if the patient's respiratory efforts are labored.

Emphasis on the chest-wall injury in patients with a flail chest may divert the physician's attention from the under-lying pulmonary and/or myocardial injury. Pulmonary contusion is an important feature of the great majority of flail-chest injuries, and early treatment should be directed toward minimizing the evolution of that lesion. In some patients, the paradoxical motion of the injured chest wall

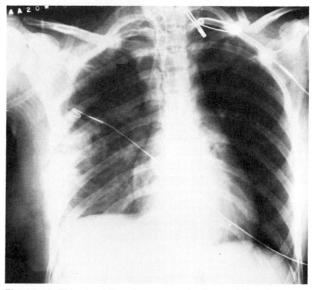

Fig. 17-20. This chest film shows a markedly overinflated trache-ostomy balloon cuff in a patient who required assisted ventilation for multiple injuries. The cuff was one of the current "low-pres-sure" types, but the patient developed a tracheoesophageal fistula.

may become apparent only after the associated lung injury has produced a sharp reduction in pulmonary compliance and a corresponding increase in respiratory effort. Pneu-mothorax or hemothorax is often present with severe flail injuries, and rapid placement of an intercostal catheter may partially relieve the respiratory distress. Especially with anterior chest injuries that include sternal fractures or disruption of costal cartilages, the probability of myocar-dial contusion must be considered. Serial electrocardio-grams, cardiac isoenzyme determinations, and radioisotope delineation of injured myocardium may be appropriate for correlation with clinical evidence of cardiac failure or pericardial friction rubs.

Chest-wall stabilization and reduction of respiratory dead space are major goals of treatment. For many years early tracheostomy has been considered routine in the management of patients with flail chest, because it allows

Fig. 17-21. The three major types of flail chest. (*Reproduced from E. A. Naclerio, "Chest Injuries," Grune & Stratton, Inc., New York, 1971, with permission of the author and publisher.*)

TYPES OF FLAIL CHEST

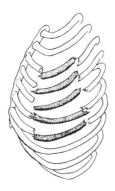

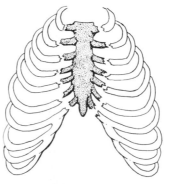

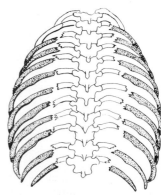

Lateral type   Anterior type   Posterior type

easy access for tracheobronchial suctioning, it reduces dead space, and it facilitates internal stabilization of the chest wall through mechanical ventilation. Other techniques for stabilizing the flail segment, such as the use of external compression dressings or the application of traction by encircling the fractured ribs with towel clips or wire, have largely been displaced by mechanical ventilation. For some patients with a small flail area and minimal pulmonary injury an intubation followed by tracheostomy may allow satisfactory recovery without the use of assisted ventilation. The improvements in respiratory therapy, including bed-side measurements of pulmonary mechanics and the wide-spread availability of arterial blood-gas determinations, have allowed greater individualization in the treatment of patients with flail-chest injuries (Fig. 17-22).

Tracheostomy and mechanical ventilation are associated with significant complications, the incidence of which varies directly with the duration of ventilatory assistance. These modalities are still the basis of management for those patients with the more severe forms of flail chest and for those with associated head injuries or multiple trauma. In those patients with a minimal or moderate chest-wall injury treatment should be directed at the respiratory dysfunction rather than at stabilizing the area of paradoxical motion. If respiratory support is required it should be initiated with nasotracheal intubation and discontinued when the patient can maintain satisfactory gas exchange. A rare patient presents with localized chest-wall fractures that can be stabilized by direct operative approach. Surgical stabilization of the fractures considerably shortens the convalescence of these individuals.

Traumatic Rupture of the Diaphragm

The diaphragm may be ruptured either by blunt thoracoabdominal trauma or by penetrating injuries. Auto-mobile accidents are the most frequent cause of blunt trauma, and the left hemidiaphragm is ruptured more frequently than the right, in a ratio of about 9:1. Bilateral rupture is rare, but the actual incidence may be higher than the present reports indicate. The right hemidiaphragm is said to be protected from rupture by the liver, and when rupture of the right side does occur the liver is usually the only abdominal structure that herniates into the chest. With lacerations of the left hemidiaphragm, the stomach, spleen, left transverse colon, and omentum in any combination may enter the left pleural cavity. When the diagnosis is delayed for several days or longer, there is often a progressive displacement of the abdominal viscera into the chest, or a progressive gaseous distension of the herniated stomach. The latter may occur despite an indwelling naso-gastric tube, and it may precipitate respiratory distress (Fig. 17-23).

This does not imply a casual approach to the diagnosis. Many patients with diaphragmatic rupture due to blunt trauma have associated injuries that demand first attention and prevent a detailed initial evaluation. The first chest x-ray after rupture of either hemidiaphragm may show nothing more than a blurring of the diaphragm with or without evidence of a small hemothorax. In some patients the diagnosis is made very early because the nasogastric tube is seen to lie within the confines of the left pleural cavity. Injection of air through the nasogastric tube during auscultation of the left side of the chest may add support to the diagnosis.

An occasional patient has minimal herniation and no symptoms to suggest the diagnosis. After several months or years, gastrointestinal obstruction may develop and lead to strangulation of herniated viscera. Penetrating diaphragmatic injuries rarely produce symptoms except those related to the other structures that are injured. The hole in the diaphragm is small, and herniation occurs slowly. At

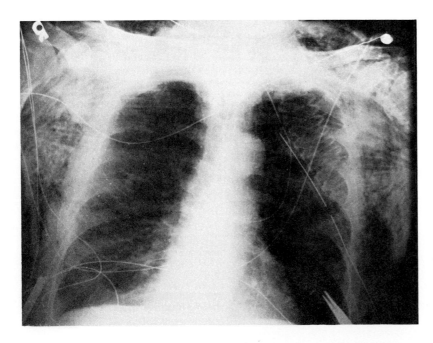

Fig. 17-22. This chest x-ray demonstrates extensive subcutaneous emphysema and multiple segmental rib fractures on the right side. The patient had a severe flail chest and a left pneumothorax, requiring nasotracheal intubation for 6 days and assisted ventilation for 5 days. Tracheostomy was not required.

the time of injury an effort should be made to confirm the diagnosis by contrast studies, by the use of pneumoperitoneum, and by radioisotope liver and spleen scans. Early transabdominal operation is indicated when the diagnosis is confirmed, and associated intraabdominal injuries may be repaired at the same time. The wound in the hemidiaphragm may vary from a simple radial tear to an extensive and complex laceration. Repair can usually be accomplished by direct suture, but a prosthetic patch is occasionally required. If the diagnosis is delayed for months or years a transthoracic approach is more appropriate.

Posttraumatic Pulmonary Insufficiency

The development of acute respiratory failure can be expected in a high percentage of patients who suffer major thoracic trauma. Preexisting pulmonary status will influence the severity of respiratory insufficiency, and the extent of actual pulmonary damage will determine whether the patient survives. An initial evaluation of respiratory exchange and ventilatory ability, confirmed by measurement of pulmonary mechanics and arterial blood gases, should be followed by serial reevaluations.

Especially in patients who have suffered multiple trauma, a respiratory distress syndrome may develop that is out of proportion to the extent of thoracic injury. A series of terms has evolved over the years to designate several forms of respiratory insufficiency that follow trauma and may be associated with a constellation of causative factors. Such terms as "wet lung," "shock lung," "congestive atelectasis," and "adult respiratory-distress syndrome" reflect some principal features that seemed to be characteristic of the cases that came to the attention of those who coined the terms. There is certainly some overlap in the causation of the several forms of respiratory failure that follow major trauma, and it is important to determine the specific causes in individual patients. Blaisdell and Lewis have presented a thorough discussion of posttraumatic pulmonary insufficiency, choosing the term *respiratory-distress syndrome of shock and trauma* for those cases not due to a specific cause. They suggest that eight different explanations for respiratory failure other than the respiratory-distress syndrome occur with reasonable frequency in patients who suffer major injury. These include aspiration, simple atelectasis, lung contusion, fat embolism, pneumonia, pneumothorax, pulmonary edema, and pulmonary embolism.

On the basis of their experience with a large number of cases, Blaisdell and Lewis have concluded that the respiratory-distress syndrome (RDS) is one and the same as the fat-embolism syndrome. Originally thought to result from fat embolism from fracture of long bones, the syndrome consists of pulmonary, neurologic, and systemic manifestations. The pulmonary manifestations appear first, generally within 24 to 36 hours after injury, and consist of dyspnea, tachycardia, fever, and cyanosis. Documentation that much of the fat which appears in the blood following injury represents a mobilization of free fatty acids from body neutral fat as a result of shock and increased levels of catecholamines has helped in understanding the mecha-

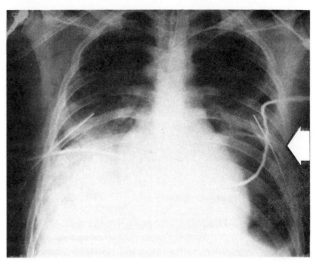

Fig. 17-23. Bilateral traumatic rupture of the diaphragm occurred in this eighteen-year-old student when he was thrown from the passenger's seat in a car wreck. The arrow points to the top of the distended intrathoracic stomach. Subsequent staged repairs of the diaphragm allowed him to return to college.

nism of this condition. Because some degree of intravascular coagulation can be demonstrated in all cases, this is almost certainly a factor in development of the syndrome.

For patients who suffer major chest injury it may be impossible to define what part of their respiratory failure is a result of direct trauma and how much is a consequence of the RDS. Treatment must be based on correction of the direct results of injury and on the anticipation or early recognition of respiratory insufficiency. The radiologic changes of RDS, consisting of diffuse lung infiltrates that progress to become confluent, may be superimposed on the effects of pulmonary contusion and atelectasis. Changes observed on serial chest x-rays lag behind the changes in pulmonary function, and a patient may be in critical respiratory failure before the films suggest a progressive pulmonary lesion.

Management of the RDS requires maintenance of good cardiovascular function and prompt institution of ventilatory support. An adequate volume replacement for external fluid and blood losses is complicated by the internal fluid losses due to increased capillary permeability in the lung, in all areas of direct tissue trauma, and to a varying degree throughout the body. Monitoring central venous pressure is the minimum for guidance of fluid and diuretic therapy in these patients, but placement of a Swan-Ganz catheter to allow left atrial and pulmonary artery pressures is superior. The need for inotropic myocardial support can be detected earlier by this access to left-sided heart pressures.

Ventilatory support techniques have advanced to allow a wider selection of ventilators and methods of assisted respiration. Attention to detail can offer the patient a maximum chance of survival with a minimum risk of complications. An unanswered question is the place of steroid therapy. The experience with these agents has been variable, and their employment is generally delayed until the patient appears to be nearing an irreversible state of progressive respiratory failure. This is probably too late for a reasonable drug effect, and on the basis of accumulating data it seems appropriate to advocate a broad trial of repeated pharmacologic doses of methylprednisolone as described by Sladen. By using a regimen of 30 mg/kg of that agent, given intravenously every 6 hours for 48 hours in combination with ventilatory support, Sladen demonstrated a significant reduction in mortality rate.

CHEST WALL

Congenital Deformities

Developmental abnormalities of the thoracic wall have become more important in the recent era because of widespread participation in competitive school athletics and because of the evolution in clothing styles that uncover more of the individual's chest. Because no obvious handicap appears to accompany the more common abnormalities, the subjects are expected to participate in sports, in physical education classes, and in other activities that require some exposure of their deformity to public view. The chest deformities seem not to evoke the sympathy engendered by limb or head and neck anomalies, and the child with a thoracic deformity is often viewed as a curiosity by his classmates. Fortunately, the abnormality is mild is many instances, and the children without an actual functional limitation often learn to cope with the stares or teasing remarks until growth and maturity of their peers make it unnecessary to consider operation.

Except for the more severe sternal deformities, it is generally not possible to predict whether a given deformity will progress during early childhood. Therefore, children who have mild abnormalities can be observed during the first 2 to 5 years and be considered for operative correction on the basis of the cosmetic and physiologic effects which evolve.

Vertebral abnormalities such as scoliosis may result in secondary deformities of the thoracic cage, with significant physiologic effects. The primary approach to treatment involves the vertebral column, and attempts at surgical improvement of the chest-wall deformity are seldom performed.

PECTUS EXCAVATUM

The most common deformity of clinical importance is the sternal depression called *pectus excavatum* (Fig. 17-24). Additional terms that have been used include *schusterbrust, funnel chest,* and *thorax en embudo.* The body of the sternum is displaced posteriorly from its expected position, resulting in a concavity from above downward and from side to side. The costal cartilages participate in the deformity, and their configuration determines whether the concavity is deep and central or broad and shallow. Though the sternal depression most commonly begins at a variable point below the angle of Louis, the posterior displacement can involve the manubrium in the most severe cases. Whether or not the depression begins at the

sternal angle, the lower end of the sternum may approximate the vertebra or project laterally into the vertebral gutter in the extreme deformities.

Mild asymmetry is not uncommon, and it always is associated with greater depression of the right costal cartilages as well as rotation of the sternum to the right. Breast asymmetry is relatively frequent and results in a less well developed right breast in girls. In infants and young children the deep deformities are often accentuated by a potbelly. As growth occurs the older children often present a characteristic posture, with rounded and forward-thrust shoulders. The neck may also project forward, and there is often a dorsal kyphos of the spine.

The deformity results in a variable displacement of the heart to the left, sometimes associated with significant rotation in that direction. Associated systolic murmurs at the cardiac base are not uncommon, but the chest x-ray appearance of the heart has limited diagnostic value because of the displacement. Operative correction of the deformity usually is followed by disappearance of the murmurs, but angiocardiography and cardiac catheterization are occasionally required to decide whether an intracardiac defect is responsible for the murmur.

Pectus excavatum is present at birth, but the milder forms may not be recognized for some months. The cause of the condition is a matter for speculation, and the factors which determine whether the sternal depression deepens in relation to the development of the thoracic cage as the child grows have not been identified. A familial tendency has been noted, but this seems to be expressed by its occurrence in two or more siblings of the same generation more often than in parent and child. This anomaly occurs frequently in patients with Marfan's syndrome, and it is one of several chest-wall deformities that show an increased frequency in children with congenital heart disease.

There is strong difference of opinion about the physiologic effects of pectus excavatum with relatively little evidence of cardiopulmonary dysfunction. Some physicians have contended that no physiologic defect is associated with the deformity and that a corrective operation is indicated only for psychologic or cosmetic reasons. This is strongly disputed by the majority of surgeons who have had extensive experience with this anomaly. The latter contend that exercise tolerance and maximal physical activity are sharply limited in patients with a severe deformity and that operative correction allows the patient to develop toward a normal capacity for cardiopulmonary function. Many individual patients have been reported with specific cardiac problems that were relieved by correction of the depressed sternum. This includes individuals with supraventricular tachycardias and recurrent heart failure.

Fig. 17-24. A two-year-old child with moderate pectus excavatum. *A.* The posterior displacement of the sternum appears to start at the level of the third chondrosternal junction. *B.* The potbelly that accompanies pectus excavatum in the young child is accentuated in the sitting position. *C.* The postoperative photograph shows an excellent cosmetic result. (*Photographs courtesy of Dr. Harold A. Albert.*)

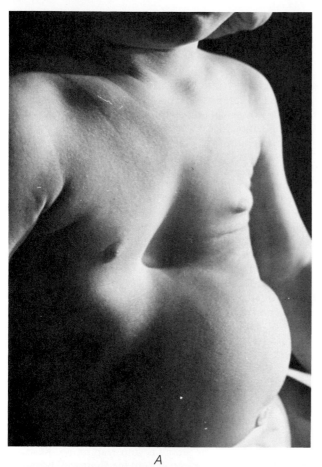

A

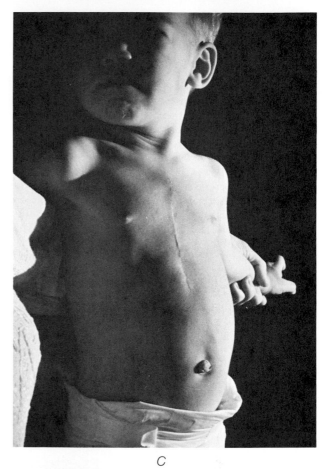

C

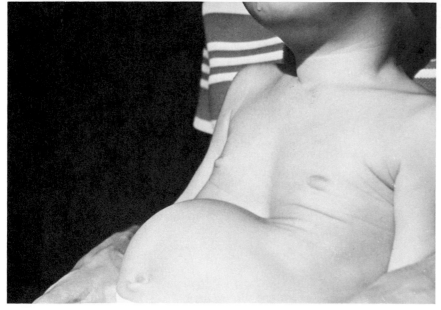

B

The spectrum of depression deformities is wide, and the remarkable ability of individuals to develop physiologic compensation for mild deviations from normal structure should not be surprising. Most studies of cardiac and respiratory function have shown either normal values or results that were in the lower range of normal. The shortcoming in attempts to provide objective corroboration of the clinical improvement experienced by patients who have operative correction has probably been due to inadequate testing methods. More recently, Weg has demonstrated a decrease in maximum voluntary ventilation and forced expiratory flow in a group of Air Force trainees who complained of exercise intolerance associated with pectus excavatum. An especially significant study was done by Beiser in which cardiac output response to exercise was measured in both supine and upright positions, before and after correction of the deformity. The results indicated that a mild to moderate deformity interfered significantly with cardiac function, primarily when exercise was performed in the upright position. The effects on the heart were

Fig. 17-25. Operative correction of pectus excavatum. The distorted medial portions of the costal cartilages have been resected and a steel bar has been placed behind the lower end of the sternum to decrease the possibility of late posterior sagging of the bone. From 9 to 12 months after operation the steel bar is removed through a small incision at the lateral ends. (*From G. W. Holcomb, Jr., Surgical Correction of Pectus Excavatum, J Pediatr Surg, 12:295, 1977, with permission of author and publisher.*)

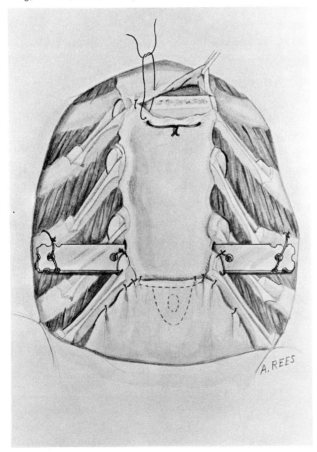

considered due to diminished space in the lower part of the thorax which interfered with optimal filling of the right side of the heart. In a completely asymptomatic patient, however, there is no reason to assume that such studies will show impairment of cardiac performance.

OPERATIVE TREATMENT. Though operation is rarely indicated in infants with pectus excavatum, Ravitch has noted an occasional infant with stridor who was relieved by early operation. Most surgeons prefer to observe children with this deformity until they are beyond two years of age. Because of the detrimental effect of the deformity on posture, however, operation should be performed between two and five years of age. There is no cause to wait until the child with a significant defect has developed a regressive personality or become a nonparticipator because of fear of exposing his chest. Although several operations have been described for correction of pectus excavatum; the procedure developed by Ravitch has been increasingly accepted. This includes excision of all the deformed costal cartilages, disarticulation of the xiphisternal joint, division of the intercostal muscle bundles from the sternum, and transverse posterior osteotomy of the sternum above the point of depression. The osteotomy is combined with a forward fracture of the sternum and insertion of a wedge of bone in the osteotomy site to provide an overcorrection of the deformity. Internal fixation of the sternum with metal pins or struts is usually not required, but in some instances the likelihood of recurrence can be minimized by use of temporary retrosternal support (Fig. 17-25).

At the end of the operation the loss in rigid support of the anterior part of the chest usually results in mild paradoxical motion of the sternum with respiration. Respiratory difficulty is rare, however, and the chest wall begins to be firm by 10 to 14 days postoperatively. Whether the indication for operation was exercise intolerance or to provide a more normal appearance of the chest, the results are so satisfying to the patient and his family that it is difficult to understand the opposition to treatment that is still seen with significant frequency.

PECTUS CARINATUM

The protrusion deformities of the sternum are much less frequent in occurrence than pectus excavatum. There is significant variation in the features of pectus carinatum from patient to patient, but Ravitch has pointed out that two principal types can be identified. In the chicken-breast type, a deep depression of the costal cartilages along each side of the sternum accentuates a mild protrusion of the sternum and creates an illusion of greater anterior projection. The deformity is usually developed maximally below the nipple level, involving the fourth through the seventh or eighth costal cartilages. There may be an asymmetry of the deformity with mild rotation of the sternum, most often to the right. Symptoms of exertional dyspnea or exercise intolerance may occur, but this is difficult to predict, and a teenage athlete with a severe deformity may have no symptoms.

In the second form of sternal protrusion, called "pouter-pigeon" variety by Ravitch, a double angle is formed in the sternum. The manubrium and upper costal cartilages project forward while the body of the sternum first angulates posteriorly for a variable distance and then sharply reverses to project anteriorly. This has the effect of creating a depression in the lower part of the sternum.

As with pectus excavatum, there is a range of severity in the deformity, and patients may be referred for operative treatment as infants or at any age. Operation may be performed at a time of convenience, but it should be done by five years of age to reduce secondary effects of the deformity on posture, thoracic development, and the child's personality. Operative correction of the chicken-breast deformity is done through a curved submammary incision that allows broad exposure of the deformed costal cartilages and costochondral junctions (Fig. 17-26). Subperichondral and subperiosteal resection of all the deformed cartilages and ribs is performed throughout the extent of their deformity. Reefing sutures are used to obliterate the excessive length of each perichondral bed, and a transverse osteotomy is used to adjust the contour of the distal sternum if it still projects forward. Correction of the pouter-pigeon deformity does not require a wide lateral dissection, but a cuneiform osteotomy of the sternum must be done at each of the two angulations in the bone.

The results of operative repair of pectus carinatum are usually excellent, with little likelihood of recurrence when the deformity is properly corrected.

STERNAL DEFECTS

The sternum is formed in embryologic life by the midline fusion of two lateral bars. Formation of the manubrium is contributed to from the developing ventral ends of the clavicles, and the process is generally complete by the tenth week. While the specific cause is yet unexplained, a partial or complete failure of fusion is responsible for the three types of congenital sternal defects that occur. Cardiac pulsations are quite prominent with each type of cleft sternum, giving rise to the visible suggestion that the heart is partially outside the chest wall (ectopia cordis). Fortunately, this is generally not the case, but in true examples of anterior ectopia cordis the sternum is partially cleft and the heart projects well beyond the chest wall. Associated cardiac defects and multiple anomalies in other body regions usually preclude survival.

Superior Sternal Cleft

In this type of sternal defect the cleft commonly extends inferiorly to the level of the fourth costal cartilage. The external appearance is that of a complete absence of the upper part of the sternum even though the unfused lateral halves are present. Because of the prominent pulsations of the heart, which is covered only by thoracic fascia and skin, there is an illusion that partial cardiac displacement into the neck accompanies the bony defect. Therefore, cervico-thoracic ectopia cordis is occasionally used in reference to superior sternal cleft.

The anatomic defect may be either U shaped or V shaped, and some patients have been reported in whom the sternal cleft extended down to the xiphoid. If operative repair is done in early infancy it may be possible to suture the two sternal halves together without extensive relaxing incisions in either the costal cartilages or the intact part of the sternum. Repair may be done at any age, but there are obvious disadvantages to leaving the heart unprotected from external trauma. As the child grows, the heart may shift forward and direct repair may become impossible because of intolerance of the heart for the reduced space available for it. At that stage the defect must be closed with use of a prosthetic graft such as Marlex mesh or Teflon felt. Autogenous bone or cartilage grafts can supplement the prosthetic material for additional firmness.

Distal Sternal Cleft

A defect in distal closure of the sternum is usually part of a syndrome of cardiac and parietal anomalies. Commonly, the syndrome is referred to as a pentalogy with the following components: (1) a cleft distal sternum, (2) a ventral abdominal defect that may be a true omphalocele, (3) an inferior pericardial defect with pericardiopleural communication, (4) a deficiency of the anterior diaphragm, and (5) congenital heart disease, commonly in the form of tetralogy of Fallot and sometimes with a left ventricular diverticulum. The sternal cleft may occur without the full syndrome, but the reported cases include several types of midline lesions that have the appearance of keloids or surgical scars.

Operative correction of the cleft sternum and the associated defects may require a staged approach, depending on the priority of the several defects. The presence of an omphalocele would most likely mandate primary attention to that anomaly, with delay of treatment for the cardiac defect. Early repair offers the best opportunity for direct closure of the sternal defect with attachment of the diaphragm.

Complete Sternal Cleft

A cleft of the entire sternum is the rarest of the three forms of failed fusion of the sternal halves. The external appearance of the anterior part of the chest and abdomen is striking, whether or not there is an associated defect in the anterior abdominal wall. When a defect of the musculofascial structures of the abdominal wall is present, there may be communication between the pericardium and the peritoneal cavity, with herniation of bowel into the pericardial cavity. The reported cases have shown variations in the defects involving the diaphragm as well as the pericardium and heart. Operative repair in early infancy is highly desirable, and it may be possible to close the sternum directly if no other defects are present. In other instances a prosthetic graft may be required to bridge over the gap in the anterior part of the chest wall.

ABNORMALITIES OF RIBS AND COSTAL CARTILAGES

Even though the costal cartilages and ribs are involved in the pectus deformities, it is the sternal deformity that forms the basis for the pectus classification. A complete classification of rib and cartilage anomalies is not yet available, although Ravitch has suggested a grouping of costal abnormalities that are associated with soft tissue defects. In the simplest form of abnormality a patient may have a

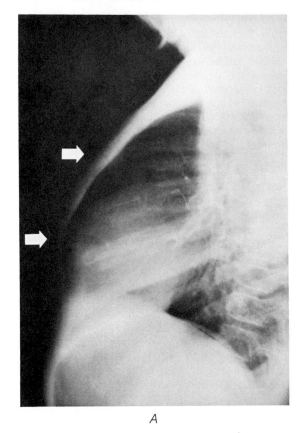

A

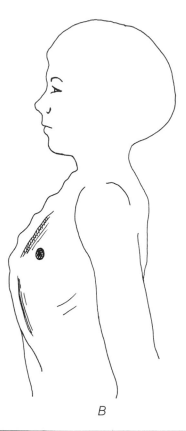

B

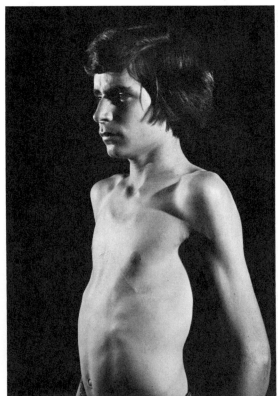

C

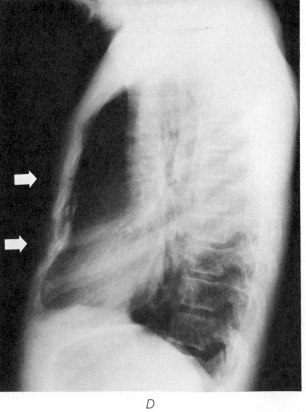

D

deformed, deficient, or enlarged cartilage or rib that is asymptomatic. With more complex anomalies there may be absence of one or more lower ribs, sometimes associated with hemivertebra, fused bony paravertebral bars, and progressive scoliosis. An absence of ribs or a costal deformity associated with divergence of adjacent ribs may result in regional paradoxical respiratory motion of the chest wall with a lung hernia through the bony defect. Bridging of bone between adjacent ribs posteriorly may be seen as part of the Klippel-Feil type of syndromes as well as of more bizarre abnormalities. In most instances the vertebral anomaly, rather than the costal defect, requires treatment, but the surgeon may need to apply individual innovation in providing the best possible correction.

Absence of the pectoralis major, absence or hypoplasia of the pectoralis minor, hypoplasia of the breast, and partial absence of the upper costal cartilages on one side of the chest constitute an unusual syndrome that may be recognized at birth. Depending on the extent of cartilage deficiency there may be an impressive lung hernia, paradoxical respiratory motion, or simple flattening of the anterolateral part of the chest wall. The breast and nipple are underdeveloped, and the deficiency in subcutaneous tissue accentuates the absence of the costosternal portions of the pectoral muscles.

When the anomaly is left-sided there is significant vulnerability of the underlying lung and heart, since only the skin, fascia, and pleura form a protective covering for these structures. Regardless of which side the defect is on, the concavity becomes relatively more severe as the child grows. Operative repair is indicated for cosmetic reasons, to eliminate paradoxical motion, and to provide protection for the intrathoracic structures. Split rib grafts to bridge the cartilage defect may be combined with Teflon felt to cover the area of muscular deficiency. The repair does not correct the soft tissue defect, but plastic surgery techniques may be utilized later to improve the cosmetic result.

Poland's syndrome is a spectrum of chest-wall defects like that just described along with a complex of hand anomalies including syndactylism, brachydactyly, or ectrodactyly. Those patients least affected have a unilateral absence of the costosternal portion of the pectoral muscles, hypoplasia of the breast, and intact costal cartilages. Severe involvement includes an absence of the second, third, and fourth, or fifth costal cartilages, the deficiency of the pectoral muscles and breast, and the hand anomalies. Surgical treatment is based on the desired correction of the chest-wall defects and the need for reconstruction of the digital anomalies.

◀ Fig. 17-26. A fourteen-year-old boy with pectus carinatum. *A.* The preoperative lateral chest x-ray shows remarkable anterior projection of the sternum. *B.* A line drawing demonstrates the forward projection of the sternum that is accentuated by the prominence of the knoblike costal cartilages. *C.* The postoperative photograph of the patient demonstrates a very satisfactory result. *D.* The postoperative lateral chest x-ray contrasts sharply with the preoperative film.

Cervical Ribs and Thoracic-outlet Syndrome

Cervical ribs are present in approximately 1 percent of the population, but symptoms attributable to the extra ribs are said to occur in only 10 percent of those who have the anomaly. The ribs are bilateral in 80 percent of cases, and they are characterized by their significant anatomic variation, including variation between the two sides in the same person (Fig. 17-27). In the simplest form, the rib is a short bar of bone that extends a few millimeters beyond the transverse process of C_7 vertebra and is completely enveloped in cervical and scalene muscles. Rarely, a complete rib is formed that articulates by a costal cartilage with the sternum. Between these two extremes are the majority that produce symptoms, and they vary in length, with occasional articulation with the superior surface of the first rib by a synchondrosis. The incompletely developed ribs often have a fascial condensation that extends as a ligament from the anterior tip to the superior surface of the first rib.

The lowest trunk of the brachial plexus (C_8 and T_1 nerve roots), the subclavian artery, and occasionally the subclavian vein course over the superior surface of the cervical rib, or over the ligament from the tip of the rib to the first thoracic rib. In symptomatic individuals it is most often the pressure on the lowest trunk of the plexus, particularly those fibers giving rise to the ulnar nerve, that causes progressive discomfort. Symptoms vary from vague and minor aching in the upper arm or shoulder to severe paresthesias down the medial side of the arm, forearm, and

Fig. 17-27. This patient's x-rays show a greater asymmetry in the cervical ribs than is usually seen. The right cervical rib is well developed (*arrows*), but the left one is represented only by a short bar of bone.

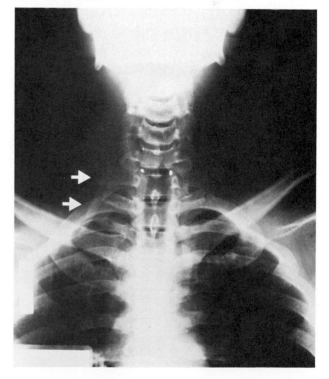

hand. Intermittent weakness in grip may cause the patient to drop things or to develop hand and forearm fatigue quickly when doing manual work. Neurologic symptoms are far more frequent than vascular symptoms, but the majority of patients demonstrate little objective evidence of nerve compression on physical examination. If compression of the brachial plexus has been progressive, the patient will begin to demonstrate atrophy and weakness of the intrinsic muscles of the hand, and eventually weakness of the forearm. Symptoms of arterial compression include numbness of the hand, pallor, fatigue, ischemic diffuse discomfort, coolness, occasionally a sensitivity to cold, and aggravation by postural elevation of the extremity. When venous compression occurs the patient notices intermittent swelling and a bluish discoloration of the extremity.

It has long been recognized that the symptoms of neurovascular compression at the thoracic outlet may occur whether or not a cervical rib is present. The compression is due to the small space between the first thoracic rib and the clavicle (Fig. 17-28). When a cervical rib is present it may be responsible for precipitating the symptoms by further reducing the space. Over the years several terms have been applied to the complex of symptoms that is now generally referred to as the *thoracic-outlet syndrome*. This includes hyperabduction syndrome, costoclavicular compression, and scalenus anticus syndrome. Symptoms are much more frequent in women, and the onset is rarely before the early adult years.

Many individuals with intermittent symptoms of shoulder or arm discomfort may consult a physician for relief. In the absence of other explanations for their symptoms a cervical rib that is discovered by x-ray examination is usually assigned the causative role. Whether or not the extra ribs are present, however, it is often difficult or impossible to distinguish symptoms representing brachial plexus compression from those caused by cervical nerve

root pressure or a herniated cervical disc. For that reason the work-up of the patient should include cervical spine films and a neurosurgical evaluation if there is suspicion of an abnormality affecting the cervical nerve roots or spinal canal.

A lack of conclusive evidence by physical examination that neurovascular compression at the thoracic outlet is responsible for a patient's symptoms has been characteristic. In slender patients a large cervical rib may be palpable and there may be distinct supraclavicular tenderness. A vascular bruit is occasionally heard over the subclavian artery, but this may be affected by the position of the arm. Rarely, a subclavian aneurysm may be suspected from the presence of a pulsating mass, or the patient may have serious ischemia of the arm and hand because of distal embolism or thrombosis of the aneurysm itself. Arterial compression tests, such as the Adson maneuver, have been found to be unreliable for diagnosis, since many asymptomatic persons show a positive response and the majority of symptomatic patients have intermittent neural compression rather than vascular obstruction. Selective subclavian arteriography or venography may be helpful by demonstrating vascular compression or by showing poststenotic dilatation of the subclavian artery (Fig. 17-29). Importantly, symptomatic neural compression can exist without a positive arteriogram, and many surgeons do not recommend arteriography in the absence of vascular symptoms.

Ulnar nerve conduction velocity has been proposed as an objective test to confirm a clinical diagnosis of thoracic-outlet syndrome with primary neural compression. An average normal value of 72 m/second across the thoracic

Fig. 17-28. The chest x-ray shows fusion of multiple cervical and thoracic vertebrae as well as posterior bridging of several upper ribs in this patient with Klippel-Feil syndrome. She had severe neurovascular compression at the right thoracic outlet because of encroachment on the space between the clavicle and the first rib.

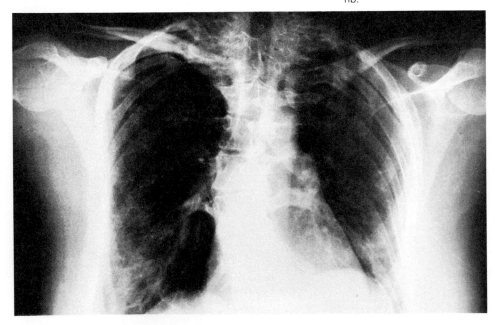

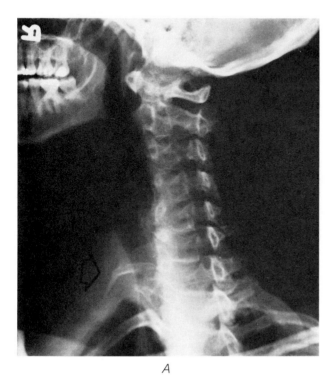

A

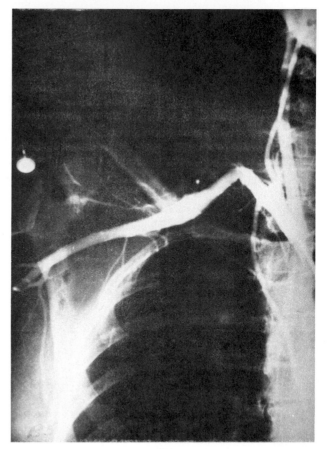

B

Fig. 17-29. This patient had recurrence of arm pain and numbness and tingling in her right hand several years after a transaxillary resection of the right first rib. *A*. The x-ray shows a right cervical rib that was incompletely removed through the axillary incision. *B*. A right subclavian arteriogram shows kinking of the artery as it courses over the cervical rib and poststenotic dilatation. Removal of the cervical rib and neurolysis of the brachial plexus through a parascapular approach relieved her symptoms.

outlet has been reported by Urschel, with an average of 53 m/second in the patients with outlet compression. Other groups have not found the nerve conduction velocity to be an accurate discriminator because some patients with a normal conduction velocity have received an excellent result from surgical treatment. A difference in techniques of electromyography may be partly responsible for the differing results.

The treatment of thoracic-outlet syndrome depends on the severity of symptoms, the apparent cause, and the presence of complications such as subclavian artery aneurysm. Even in the presence of a small cervical rib, patients who have nothing more than mild symptoms of numbness and tingling or fatigue in the arm may require no treatment. Instruction in posture improvement may be adequate, but professional physiotherapy may give better relief. Urschel suggests that nerve conduction velocity may be used as a guide for treatment with operation not advised unless the velocity is below 60 m/second. For persistent or

progressive symptoms a resection of the first rib along with any cervical rib or abnormal congenital bands gives the best result in the experience of many surgeons. An axillary incision can be used to resect the first rib in most patients, but considerable skill is required to do an adequate resection of a cervical rib through this approach. An alternate surgical approach is provided by a posterior parascapular incision which allows a better exposure of the brachial plexus and is especially helpful for reoperation. The presence of a significant aneurysm requires an anterior incision, often with partial resection of the clavicle.

Approximately 90 percent of patients have excellent relief of symptoms following operation, although they may have occasional discomfort at the time of increased work activity.

Tumors

Primary neoplasms of the chest wall are uncommon; even large medical centers require long periods of time to acquire useful experience with their treatment. Metastatic tumors, especially to the ribs, and direct invasion of the chest wall from primary lung and breast carcinomas easily outnumber the tumors arising from the chest wall. Soft tissue tumors that occur in other body areas such as cavernous hemangiomas, hemangiopericytoma, rhabdomyosarcoma, and so on have a special significance when they develop in the chest wall, because treatment may require extensive resection of the thoracic cage. A classification of chest-wall tumors would be convenient for study, but the number of cases is sufficiently small that anything other than a division into benign and malignant and by tissue of origin is not practical. Table 17-3 shows the types of primary tumors and their relative frequency in Adkins' experience during the years 1954–1970. It is apparent that the majority of patients in his practice were in younger age groups. This should not mislead, however, since there is a wide age spread in other reports, and in this author's experience the majority of patients have been older than 30 years.

The clinical manifestation of a chest-wall neoplasm is most often either pain, a palpable mass, or an abnormality detected on a chest x-ray. Surprisingly, with either benign or malignant lesions the discomfort is relatively mild, and patients often present with tumors that have been enlarging for months or years. Many patients will attribute the tumor origin to some episode of localized trauma, or they will state that they discovered the mass while rubbing their chest after a minor injury. A differential diagnosis will include the less frequent pulmonary infections that invade the chest wall, such as actinomycosis and nocardiosis, tuberculous chondritis, costochondral separation, and Tietze's syndrome (nonspecific chondritis). A suspicion of fluctuation in the mass and a corresponding pulmonary lesion may suggest that a diagnostic aspiration should be done in instances of probable infection. A true history of trauma and the ability to reproduce a clicking sensation with local pressure may reinforce the diagnosis of a suspected costochondral separation.

The most important aspect of diagnosis is the correlation of physical findings with adequate radiographic examination. The latter often requires the help of the radiologist by having him examine the lesion and determine what special views or techniques will allow maximum information about the extent of the lesion, its possible relationship to intrathoracic structures, and the presence of characteristics that may suggest malignancy. Radioisotope studies may be indicated to look for other areas of neoplastic involvement, and pulmonary function tests should be performed as a screening examination to determine the likelihood that chest-wall resection would be tolerated. Because the majority of tumors involving the costal cartilages and the sternum are malignant, the anterior location of a neoplasm will often suggest the need to plan for resection and extensive reconstruction.

BENIGN TUMORS

Fibrous Dysplasia

The ribs are the most common site of solitary fibrous dysplasia (osteofibroma, bone cyst), and this lesion constitutes 20 to 35 percent of the benign tumors of the thoracic cage. Located most frequently in the posterior or lateral portion of a rib, it usually presents as a slowly enlarging nonpainful mass. Diagnostic radiographs show expansion and thinning of the bony cortex, with a central trabeculated appearance. Histologic examination often shows fine calcification in a matrix of fibrous tissue, osteoid tissue, and occasional cysts. There may be involvement of more than one rib, suggesting metastatic malignancy. Fibrous dysplasia in ribs as well as other bones forms part of Albright's syndrome, a condition that includes skin pigmentation and precocious puberty in girls.

The lesion should be excised to establish the diagnosis and to prevent progressive enlargement that would eventually encroach on other structures.

Chondroma

According to Adkins, chondromas constitute 15 to 20 percent of benign tumors in the ribs. They occur at the costochondral junction, primarily in children or young people, and may be difficult to differentiate from chondritis or the sequela of a traumatic costochondral separation. Chest and rib x-rays show an expansion of bone with thinned but intact cortex. It is not possible to distinguish between a chondroma and chondrosarcoma by clinical examination, but the onset of pain and rapid growth in a preexisting lesion suggest a malignant change.

Chondromas slowly expand into the surrounding tissues without fixation, but adequate removal requires resection of a block of the chest wall to achieve an adequate margin. If the patient is operated upon when the lesion is small, no special techniques are required to close the defect that results from resection.

Osteochondroma

Osteochondromas generally arise from the cortex of a rib and slowly expand over a long period of time. They occur more frequently in men, but they are also seen in children. Pain is infrequent, but once the lesion has become palpable the patient is likely to complain of intermittent discomfort. As with other neoplasms, the occurrence of pain may signal accelerated growth, which produces concern over the possibility of malignant change.

Table 17-3. PRIMARY CHEST-WALL TUMORS

Benign (average age of patients, 21 years)

Fibrous dysplasia	8
Chondroma	4
Osteochondroma	4
Eosinophilic granuloma	2
Hemangioma	3
Total	21

Malignant (average age of patients, 25 years)

Chondrosarcoma	9
Osteogenic sarcoma	3
Myeloma	3
Ewing's tumor	2
Fibrosarcoma	3
Reticulum cell sarcoma	2
Liposarcoma	1
Undifferentiated	2
Total	25

SOURCE: Reproduced with permission from T. W. Shields, "General Thoracic Surgery," p. 445, Lea & Febiger, Philadelphia, 1972.

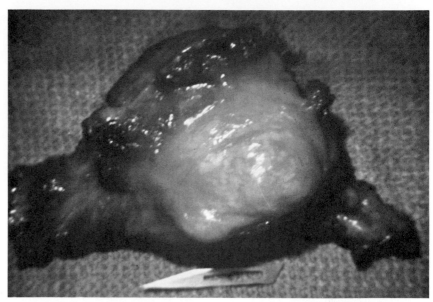

Fig. 17-30. This operating-room photograph of a resected segment of rib and attached tumor shows the typical appearance of an osteochondroma.

The roentgenographic appearance is often that of a distorted rib cortex with an overlying mass that has a thin rim of calcification (Fig. 17-30).

The lesion should be removed by a block resection with a margin of normal tissue.

Eosinophilic Granuloma

The lesions of eosinophilic granuloma are sometimes part of a disease that includes pulmonary lesions called *histiocytosis X* or *eosinophilic granuloma of the lung*. When it occurs in a rib, the granuloma is a solitary destructive process, often associated with pain and localized tenderness. Roentgenograms reveal a punched-out osteolytic lesion, which, when subjected to excision and microscopic examination, is found to consist of a chronic granuloma. Healing may occur spontaneously, or a pathologic fracture may develop through the area of osteolysis. Resection is primarily advised for the purpose of diagnosis. If only a biopsy is done the granuloma may be observed and attention diverted to a survey for additional lesions in the lung, the reticuloendothelial system, and the other bones.

Other less frequent benign tumors may occur in the chest wall, including soft tissue neoplasms that arise in the muscular, fibrous, vascular, or other tissues that are normally there (Fig. 17-31). Because of the frequency of malignancy in soft tissue neoplasms, these tumors must be approached bearing in mind the possibility that extensive resection may be required.

MALIGNANT TUMORS

Chondrosarcoma

Chondroma and chondrosarcoma are the most frequently occurring primary tumors of the chest wall, with the question of whether chondromas undergo malignant transformation still unanswered. Some investigators believe that all chondrosarcomas arise as malignant lesions. Either way, chondrosarcomas comprise between 45 and 60 percent of all malignant tumors of the bony thorax. The tumors occur most commonly in the anterior part of the thorax, and the incidence is greatest between the ages of twenty and forty years. Growth is often relatively slow, and the neoplasm may extend either internally or outwardly into the soft tissue of the chest wall. The overwhelming majority of sternal tumors are malignant, with chondrosarcoma and osteogenic sarcoma comprising the greatest percentage.

The chest x-ray generally shows a lobulated mass that appears to destroy cortical bone, with or without fine calcification. Because of a varied histologic picture that often fails to provide proof of malignancy, a simple biopsy of a chondrosarcoma may not be used to guide treatment. Though the decision to do so may be difficult, the performance of a wide excision of the tumor with a block of surrounding tissue is the proper treatment for chondrosarcoma.

Osteogenic Sarcoma

Osteogenic sarcoma is more malignant than chondrosarcoma but less frequent in occurrence. A pleural effusion tends to develop early, and the tumor may have rapid growth, particularly in young people (Fig. 17-32). Pain is mild at first but may become severe when the tumor has reached a stage where resection is unlikely. The predominant component may be cartilaginous, bony, or fibrous, and the lesion may result in both bone destruction and bone production.

There is often an early development of pulmonary metastases in osteogenic sarcoma, and in occasional instances it may be proper to resect the metastases at the same time

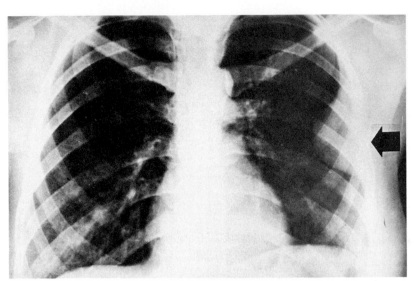

A

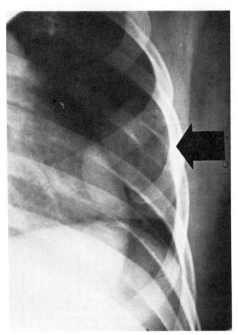

B

Fig. 17-31. An aneurysmal bone cyst. *A*. The posteroanterior chest x-ray shows a mass extending into the thoracic cavity and elevating the pleura on the posterolateral chest wall. *B*. A film for rib detail demonstrates the origin of the tumor from the left fifth rib. (*X-rays furnished by Dr. Arthur Lieber.*)

Fig. 17-32. An osteogenic sarcoma arising from the right tenth rib in this middle-aged man resulted in early pleural invasion with massive pleural effusion. Chemotherapy failed to affect rapid tumor growth, and he died with widespread metastases.

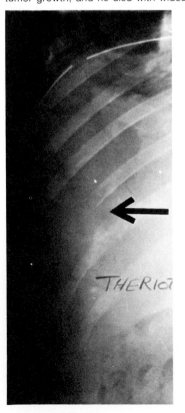

that the primary tumor is treated. For patients with a well-localized neoplasm the only form of adequate treatment is wide excision of the adjacent bony structures and soft tissue. When the sternum is involved, a complete resection must be done although 5-year survivals are unusual.

Ewing's Sarcoma

Occurrence during the first two decades of life, with a much reduced incidence beyond twenty years of age, characterizes Ewing's tumor. The tumor occurs more frequently in boys than in girls and is generally manifested by a painful mass that enlarges rapidly. Fever and malaise are common systemic symptoms.

Roentgenograms often show a characteristic onion-skin appearance that is due to elevation of the periosteum as the tumor enlarges. Spread to other bones occurs early in a high percentage of patients, but the tumor is generally radiosensitive. If the diagnosis is made by biopsy, the choice of treatment may be irradiation alone or radical excision combined with the irradiation. Unfortunately, the prognosis is poor regardless of the treatment chosen.

Myeloma

Plasma cell myeloma is more frequently a generalized disease than a solitary tumor affecting a single rib. When a solitary plasmacytoma does occur in the thoracic cage, the serum proteins are generally normal and Bence-Jones proteins are not found in the urine. Chest x-rays show the solitary lesion as a punched-out defect in the rib, with expansion and thinning of the cortex.

The clinical course of patients with a solitary myeloma is markedly different from that of patients who first appear with multiple lesions. The latter are almost always dead within 2 years after the diagnosis is made, but those who

have a solitary lesion initially may live for many years without evidence of other disease. A careful survey for other sites of disease should be made in patients who present with a solitary lesion, and if none is found the involved rib should be resected.

SURGICAL TREATMENT OF MALIGNANT CHEST-WALL TUMORS. Particularly with the cartilaginous tumors, an excisional biopsy may not be adequate to determine whether a lesion is malignant (Fig. 17-33). The surgeon must often make a judgment on the basis of the history, the roentgenograms, and the gross appearance of the neoplasm. Because most chest-wall tumors are not radiosensitive the best chance for cure is related to the adequacy of the initial resection. When malignancy is suspected, preliminary plans must be made for chest-wall reconstruction that will allow resection of a generous margin of normal

Fig. 17-33. A giant-cell tumor of the right clavicle. *A.* The preoperative photograph of the upper part of the chest and neck shows a tumor at the right sternoclavicular junction in this elderly man. A biopsy suggested the diagnosis but did not indicate the degree of malignancy. *B.* A chest x-ray indicates the origin of the tumor from the medial end of the clavicle, and the arrows suggest the extent of the mass. *C.* An operating-room photograph shows the completely resected clavicle with an en-bloc resection of the upper sternum and the anterior end of the first rib. The rounded tumor mass which projects toward the knife handle is covered with intact pleura.

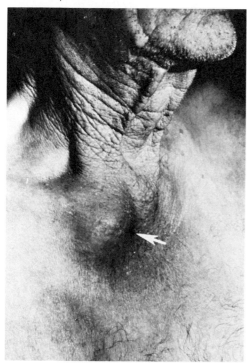

A

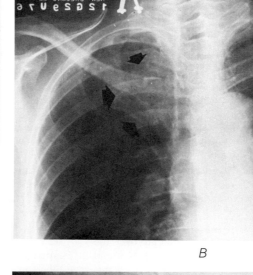

B

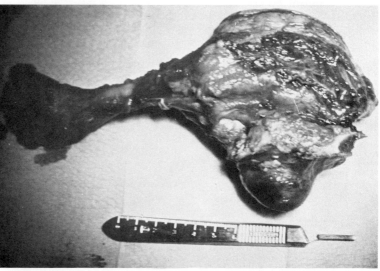

C

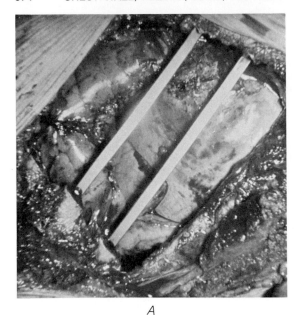

A

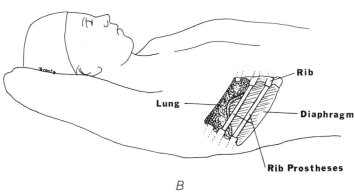

B

Fig. 17-34. A reoperation for chondrosarcoma. *A.* Two years earlier the patient had a localized resection of one rib for an apparent chondroma. The recurrence of a mass suggested the likelihood that chondrosarcoma was the correct diagnosis, and this operative photograph shows the extensive chest-wall resection that was done in continuity with a large wedge of the right lower pulmonary lobe. Two metal rib struts were used to provide stability to the anterolateral chest wall. *B.* The line drawing is intended to clarify the structures in the photograph.

tissue around the neoplasm. The resection should include at least one adjacent normal rib above and below the tumor, with all intervening intercostal muscles and pleura. When the lung periphery is involved in the neoplasm, it is proper to resect the adjacent part of the pulmonary lobe in continuity (Fig. 17-34). Presently available techniques for respiratory support are sufficiently good that a resection should not be compromised by a concern that the patient will not be able to ventilate satisfactorily during the immediate postoperative period.

Because the anatomy of the thorax appears to offer few, if any, natural limits to the spread of a neoplasm, and because of the sharply limited long-term survival with surgical treatment, there is a reasonable debate over the value of chest-wall resection. There is little to recommend radical treatment once a neoplasm has reached an advanced stage of musculoskeletal destruction with invasion of the pleural cavity. With selection of patients who have either slowly growing tumors or limited chest-wall involvement, extensive resection can provide excellent relief of pain and prolonged survival. In a series of 68 patients

Table 17-4. ORIGIN OF MALIGNANT TUMORS RESECTED FROM CHEST WALL

Type of tumor	No. of patients	
Primary chest-wall sarcoma..........	25	
Sarcoma metastatic to chest wall ...	7	
Carcinoma of lung....................	30	
Epidermoid carcinoma		17
Adenocarcinoma		7
Bronchiolar carcinoma		3
Miscellaneous.....................		3
Metastatic carcinoma.................	6	
Kidney............................		4
Miscellaneous.....................		2

who had chest-wall resections for malignant disease at the Memorial Sloan-Kettering Cancer Center, the cumulative 5-year survival rate was 34 percent. Table 17-4 shows that primary lung carcinoma with chest-wall invasion was slightly more frequent than thoracic sarcomas in that series. Of the 68 patients, 43 had a concomitant pulmonary resection, including 20 wedge resections and 20 lobectomies.

Reconstruction of a large defect in the chest wall requires the use of some type of material to avoid lung herniation or paradoxical respiratory motion. Marlex or prolene mesh, fascia lata, and metal struts are among the most frequently used materials for this purpose. When a loss of skin and subcutaneous tissue accompanies the musculoskeletal defect, reconstruction becomes more complicated because of the need to use skin flaps or a transposition flap of the omentum, covered by a skin graft.

PLEURA

Because primary diseases of the pleura are infrequent, it is easy to think of this tissue as a "membrane highway" for transport of infectious agents or neoplastic cells throughout the hemithorax, or as a reservoir for containing air, blood, or transudative fluids. A completely passive role for the pleura like that implied by the previous statement is obviously not correct. But from the surgeon's viewpoint it is a close description of pleural function as it affects surgical procedures. With few exceptions, most notably, the pleural tumors, the pathologic processes involving the pleura take origin from other sources. Symptoms and signs of pleural disturbance, therefore, may be first evidence of a disease process that has been developing in a relatively silent area such as the mediastinum or lung periphery.

The anatomy of the pleural space is altered by the disease processes that affect the space and the structures that form its boundaries. An injury to the phrenic nerve, for example, with paralysis of the diaphragm results in a reduced volume of the hemithorax. This could be significant if a thoracentesis were planned with an attempt to place the needle in the lowest part of the pleural cavity. Inflammation, trauma with hemothorax, or thoracic operative procedures often produce partial obliteration of the pleural space. A subsequent collection of pleural fluid, for whatever cause, may take an unusual appearance, including an isolated location in a fissure between pulmonary lobes, or confinement between the diaphragmatic surface of a lower lobe and the diaphragm. A more significant result of fibrosis in the pleural cavity is the occasional development of *fibrothorax,* in which the lung becomes encased in a layer of fibrous tissue. This generally results from incompletely treated hemothorax or empyema, and the lung is said to be "trapped." In addition to its restrictive effect on ventilation, fibrothorax may result in a mild scoliosis of the thoracic region of the spine. An age difference in the capability of the pleura to remove massive exudates without excessive fibrosis is suggested by the fact that decortication is required much less frequently in small children than in adults.

Pleural Effusion

The presence of fluid within the pleural space can have a variety of causes, a partial list of which is shown in Table 17-5. Additional rare causes have been reported, and in a few patients no cause is ever identified. The so-called "idiopathic effusions" are thought to have a viral causation in many instances, but careful skin testing for tuberculosis is always indicated, along with follow-up examination for at least a year.

Traditionally, effusions are classified as either transudates or exudates. Transudates have a specific gravity of less than 1.015 and a protein content of less than 3 Gm/100 ml. Most often a transudate is clear with a faint yellow tinge and no odor. Among the more common causes of transudates are the conditions associated with salt and water retention (e.g., congestive heart failure, nephrotic syndrome), ascites, and atelectasis. Pleural exudates vary greatly depending on the cause, but pleural inflammation is usually present. Infectious diseases, pulmonary infarction, and tumors are the common causes of pleural exudates. A hemorrhagic effusion is not easily classified as a transudate or exudate but may have properties of either. Neoplastic invasion of the pleura is the most frequent cause of bloody effusions, but pulmonary infarction, tuberculosis, and unrevealed trauma are additional causes that must be considered for individual patients.

A compromise of lung volume by fluid within the pleu-

Table 17-5. CAUSES OF PLEURAL EFFUSION

Relative frequency	Cause
Frequent	Congestive heart failure
	Infection: bacterial pneumonia, tuberculosis
	Neoplasm: bronchogenic carcinoma, pleural metastases, lymphoma
Common	Trauma
	Plumonary infarction
	Cirrhosis
Occasional	Viral pulmonary and pericardial infections
	Atelectasis
	Pneumothorax
Rare	Meigs's syndrome
	Intraabdominal infection: pancreatitis, subphrenic abscess: mycotic infection; systemic bacterial infection; rheumatoid arthritis
	Fluid retention: nephrotic syndrome

ral space is usually manifested by dyspnea and tachycardia. If the effusion is massive, the mediastinum can be shifted to the contralateral side, causing compression of the opposite lung (Fig. 17-35). Severe cardiorespiratory embarrassment with cyanosis may result, and if unrelieved, may precipitate a fatal cardiac arrhythmia.

A diagnostic thoracentesis is indicated in most patients with a pleural effusion unless the cause is either without question or of no relevance in the patient's management. The technique of thoracentesis and the method for insertion of an intercostal tube are shown in Fig. 17-36. In many circumstances, even if the patient is suffering mild respiratory embarrassment from a large pleural effusion, the first step is a simple needle or needle-catheter aspiration of the fluid. This may relieve the patient's symptoms temporarily and allow a diagnosis to be made from examination of the fluid. The decision to insert an intercostal tube for continuous drainage depends on the rapidity of its reaccumulation and the cause. Because the placement of an intercostal tube results in continuous discomfort for the patient and a restriction of activities, it is not indicated unless the fluid is associated with empyema or requires aspiration as often as every other day.

Thorough examination of the aspirated fluid includes determination of specific gravity and total protein content, and chemical measurement of sugar, fat, lactic acid dehydrogenase, and, occasionally, amylase content. In addition, cultures for bacteria, fungi, and mycobacteria may be indicated, along with cytologic examination for malignant cells. If a diagnosis is not obtained from fluid examination, a pleural biopsy by needle technique is often indicated. Satisfactory tissue for examination can be obtained in 60 to 80 percent of patients for whom a closed biopsy appears

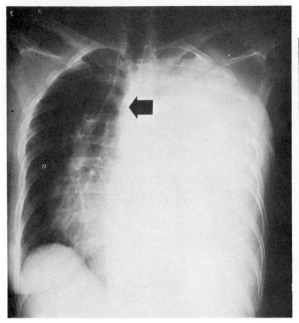

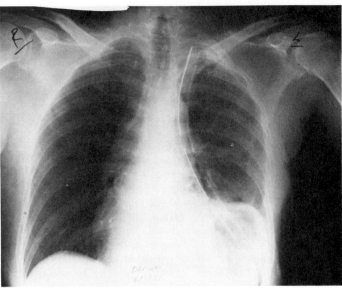

A

B

Fig. 17-35. A massive pleural effusion due to metastases from carcinoma of the left breast (previously excised by mastectomy). *A.* The arrow shows the tracheal displacement to the opposite side. *B.* After drainage of the malignant effusion by insertion of an intercostal tube, the trachea and mediastinum have shifted back toward a normal position. Paralysis of the left side of the diaphragm, presumably due to phrenic nerve involvement by the pleural metastases, was confirmed by fluoroscopy.

warranted. Open pleural biopsy is rarely done unless a concomitant lung biopsy has been suggested. However, there are patients who should have a definitive diagnosis made, and the technique of thoracoscopy described in the following section deserves wider application for this purpose.

THORACOSCOPY. In the past, visual inspection of the pleural surfaces by thoracoscopy was done primarily in association with induced pneumothorax therapy for patients with pulmonary tuberculosis. The technique has enjoyed somewhat of a revival in the United States and has been in constant use in Europe for many years. It has been reported highly successful in patients with pleural disease in whom a diagnosis could not be made by bronchoscopy, thoracentesis with closed pleural needle biopsy, or mediastinoscopy.

The one prerequisite for successful thoracoscopy is a reasonably free, nonadherent pleural space to permit adequate visualization of the pleura as well as manipulation of the thoracoscope and the biopsy forceps. Instruments such as the mediastinoscope and the flexible bronchoscope have been used for the examination in addition to the rigid thoracoscope.

If recurrent pleural effusion has been a problem and malignant pleuritis has been diagnosed, cytotoxic or pleurodytic agents can be introduced at the time of thoracoscopy. This has also been helpful in patients who are too ill for open thoracotomy, in children, and in cases of suspected traumatic rupture of the diaphragm.

Empyema

Empyema thoracis is the term generally applied to pyogenic infections of the pleural cavity, associated with purulent effusions. Bacterial pneumonia is the most frequent cause of empyema, but trauma, pulmonary infarction, septic pulmonary emboli, and spread of infection from intraabdominal sepsis are additional major causes. Empyema may develop as a complication of thoracic surgical procedures, with or without infection of the incision.

When the pleura is invaded by infection there is an outpouring of pleural exudates that may have a localized or generalized distribution. If infection continues, the effects of gravity lead to a volume concentration of the effusion in the posterior and inferior areas of the pleural cavity. As the leukocyte and fibrin content increase, the pleurae may become fused around the margins of the fluid accumulation. This localization may be thought of as an abscess, but it is generally referred to as a loculated empyema (Fig. 17-37).

The management of a pyogenic empyema depends on the stage at which the diagnosis is made. If the condition is diagnosed early, when the fluid is still thin, intensive treatment by needle aspiration and appropriate antibiotics may suffice. In a well-established empyema, a continuous form of drainage by one or more large intercostal catheters is necessary to keep the pleura free of an accumulation that would promote pulmonary collapse. With empyema not accompanied by an air leak from the lung (bronchopleural fistula), the volume of drainage seems to be unaffected by the addition of negative pressure to the underwater seal. In the presence of a bronchopleural fistula, every effort

CHEST WALL, PLEURA, LUNG, AND MEDIASTINUM

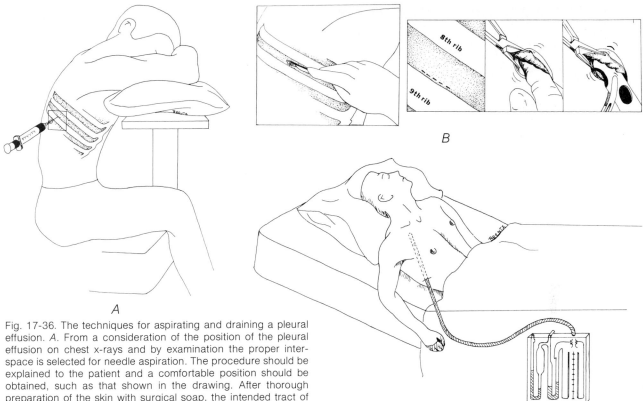

A

B

C

Fig. 17-36. The techniques for aspirating and draining a pleural effusion. *A*. From a consideration of the position of the pleural effusion on chest x-rays and by examination the proper interspace is selected for needle aspiration. The procedure should be explained to the patient and a comfortable position should be obtained, such as that shown in the drawing. After thorough preparation of the skin with surgical soap, the intended tract of the aspirating needle is anesthetized with 2 percent lidocaine. If a tube is to be inserted, the primary purpose of the aspiration is to confirm the locations and character of the effusion. *B*. For insertion of an intercostal catheter a short skin incision is made and the wound deepened by knife or scissors down to the rib level. After puncture of the intercostal muscles and pleura with a hemostat, the gloved finger is used to enlarge the intercostal opening and assess the character of the pleural lining. If loculations can be easily separated, this should be done. A large intercostal catheter (32 to 36F) should be inserted in the direction and distance suggested by the chest x-ray. *C*. Whether a simple underwater seal is adequate for drainage depends on the presence or absence of a bronchopleural fistula. If the patient has a continuous or an intermittent air leak, negative pressure should be utilized in the range of −10 to 50 cm of water.

should be made to keep the pulmonary lobes expanded. This requires the use of 10 to 50 cm of water negative pressure; if it is successful the need for open thoracotomy with decortication of the pleura may be avoided.

Unfortunately, patients are often referred to the surgeon for empyema management after the acute phase has been treated by antibiotics but without adequate drainage. Tube drainage may show that the lung is partially collapsed with no significant reexpansion after 48 to 96 hours of high-suction drainage. Although an excessive delay in the decision to perform decortication is frequent in these cases, Bryant showed that the need for operation could generally be determined within a few days after the drainage was initiated. Previous antibiotic treatment results in negative cultures of the aspirated fluid in more than half the patients who are seen at this stage, but the management is primarily a mechanical problem of draining the empyema

cavity or excising the inflammatory membrane that has trapped the lung and lines the chest wall.

Several complications of empyema thoracis may occur. Chronicity or persistence of a localized pleural infection with continuous or intermittent purulent drainage is not uncommon. This may be caused by premature removal of a drainage tube or failure to establish drainage at the dependent position of the empyema cavity. Inadequate drainage, particularly of a localized empyema, may be handled by converting to open drainage by rib resection (Fig. 17-38). When chronicity is the result of lung disease, especially in the presence of a bronchopleural fistula, decortication must be combined with pulmonary resection to effect a cure. When this is not possible, either because of the extent of lung disease or the failure of other methods, the pleural space may be obliterated by collapsing the chest wall down to meet the lung through performance of a thoracoplasty. Under special circumstances, such as chronic empyema following a pneumonectomy, techniques for long-term drainage by creating a defect in the chest wall (Eloesser flap) may be indicated.

Another complication of chronic empyema is *empyema necessitatis*. In this condition a neglected or unrecognized pleural abscess may provide its own drainage by breaking through either the visceral or parietal wall. Perforation into the lung and communication with a bronchus is indicated by the sudden expectoration of large amounts of purulent material. Prompt evacuation of the pleura and intensive bronchopulmonary toilet are urgent. Proper treatment of

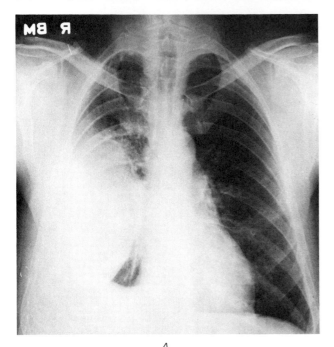

A

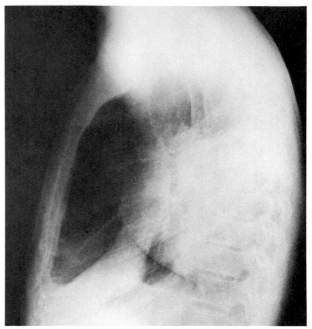

B

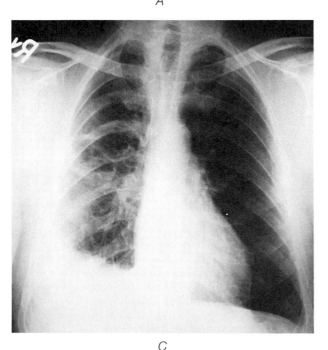

C

Fig. 17-37. A loculated pyogenic empyema. *A.* The posteroanterior chest x-ray shows a large opacity in the right hemithorax of a patient who was not recovering satisfactorily despite antibiotic treatment for an apparent pneumonia. *B.* The lateral x-ray shows that the opacity extends far posteriorly. The smooth, rounded borders suggested that the mass was fluid, and an empyema was confirmed by thoracentesis. *C.* Following aspiration the chest x-ray suggests significant pleural reaction and persistence of fibrinopurulent exudate in the costophrenic sulcus. A tube thoracostomy would probably need to be done to provide continuing drainage.

the empyema will often permit closure of the bronchial fistula. Penetration of the chest wall is less dramatic and usually presents as an enlarging local abscess. Appropriate treatment includes drainage of the abscess, including the underlying chronic pleural infection.

Tuberculosis

It is generally considered that pleural tuberculosis is the result of extension of tuberculosis to the pleura from a subjacent pulmonary lesion. The most common form is fibrinous pleurisy that causes localized pleural adhesions. Serofibrinous pleurisy develops in approximately 5 percent of all cases of pulmonary tuberculosis. In some patients the parenchymal lesion may be obscured by the overlying pleural involvement. Malaise and fever may be the presenting symptoms, and if the effusion is large the patient may have dyspnea.

It is important to recognize tuberculous empyema because the treatment differs from that for pyogenic empyema. Therefore, there is an increasing tendency to obtain a pleural biopsy to provide greater accuracy in diagnosis. Open drainage is necessary only when there is a bronchopleural fistula. Prior to the advent of effective chemotherapy for tuberculosis, a high mortality rate was associated with open drainage of tuberculous empyema. In selected instances pleural decortication is indicated, along with intensive chemotherapy, as an attempt to produce pulmonary reexpansion.

Pleural Calcification

Pleural calcification is occasionally seen in patients with chronic pleuritis. In most instances, there is considerable thickening of the parietal pleura, with plaques of calcium deeply embedded. Calcification of the pleura per se is usually not the cause of symptoms, and it rarely requires treatment even though the appearance of the chest x-ray may be impressive. The chief clinical importance lies in the association with a chronic empyema, of either tuberculous or nontuberculous origin. Almost certainly, the presence of the calcification makes the empyema more intractable.

Chylothorax

An accumulation of chyle in the pleural space may occur after trauma, or it may be spontaneous. Spontaneous chylothorax is frequently caused by a primary malignancy such as lymphosarcoma or a metastatic carcinoma which invades or compresses the thoracic duct. Rarely, a benign cystic lesion of the duct or its tributaries may be an etiologic factor. There is a low incidence of chylothorax after operative procedures such as thoracic sympathectomy, esophagectomy, aneurysmectomy, and cardiac procedures. Rupture of a normal duct has been seen as a result of blunt trauma, especially when accompanied by hyperextension of the spine.

The first indication of an injury to the thoracic duct may be a rapidly accumulating pleural effusion associated with tightness in the chest, dyspnea, and tachycardia. A specific diagnosis is made only when thoracentesis yields an opalescent or milky fluid which shows fat globules by microscopic examination. Chyle has a specific gravity which ranges between 1.010 and 1.020. The total lipid content varies from 1 to 4 percent, and the total protein content averages 3.5 to 4.5 Gm/100 ml. Normal chyle is sterile. The erythrocyte count may vary, and the lymphocyte count may be 6,000 per cubic millimeter or higher. After trauma, there is frequently an admixture of blood that can obscure the true nature of the effusion. Patients with large leaks can drain as much as 2,500 ml in 24 hours, and a prolonged loss of chyle can lead to dehydration, depletion of electrolytes and serum proteins, lymphocytopenia, low levels of blood lipids, and deficiencies of fat-soluble vitamins.

If an injury to the thoracic duct is recognized during an operative procedure, the structure should be mobilized only enough to permit double ligation. Reconstruction or repair of the injured duct is unnecessary. When a chylothorax is diagnosed several days after the causative event, the initial treatment should consist of repeated thoracentesis or tube drainage. Healing frequently occurs, especially if the patient is given a low-fat or elemental diet. Total parenteral alimentation is also helpful. If the chyle drainage does not respond in 7 to 10 days, operative exploration will frequently be necessary, especially if the injury involves the major thoracic duct on the right side.

Tumors

PRIMARY TUMORS

Primary pleural tumors are uncommon, and because of their origin in the thorax they are usually mistaken for pulmonary neoplasms on the initial chest x-ray. Since

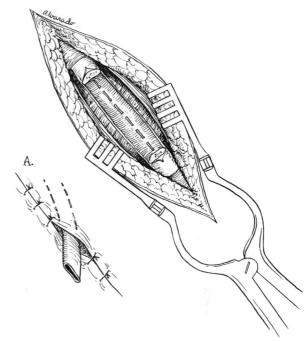

Fig. 17-38. Open drainage of a localized chronic empyema by rib resection. This technique is good for relatively small empyema cavities where a 5- to 10-cm length of rib can be resected over the dependent area of the cavity. An incision is made through the bed of the rib to unroof the cavity partially. A plastic tube is maintained in the cavity to prevent closure of the skin opening as the cavity gradually heals.

tumors of mesothelial origin may closely resemble adenocarcinomas, there may be difficulty in establishing the correct diagnosis even with biopsy material. The most widely used classification of primary pleural tumors is an anatomic one which divides them into localized and diffuse types. Almost all diffuse mesotheliomas are malignant, but so are a significant number of the localized tumors.

Evidence of a relationship between asbestos exposure and malignant pleural tumors now seems as convincing as the relationship between the mineral and carcinoma of the lung. The great majority of patients with asbestos exposure who develop a mesothelioma (asbestos miners, insulation workers) are also cigarette smokers, and their asbestos exposure has taken place over a long period of time.

Localized mesotheliomas most frequently arise from the visceral pleura, and the chest x-ray may simply show a solitary pulmonary nodule (Fig. 17-39). This lesion is often referred to as "benign fibrous mesothelioma" because of its excellent prognosis if resected with a margin of normal tissue. On occasion the tumor may arise from the parietal, mediastinal, or diaphragmatic pleura, and it may grow to become a very large solitary mass. These tumors are generally asymptomatic unless they reach a size that is sufficient to produce pulmonary compression and dyspnea. Chest pain, fever, and painful osteoarthropathy have been reported with the larger localized mesotheliomas, and the symptoms disappear after the tumor is removed. A pleural effusion may accompany the larger fibrous lesions, and the presence of significant red blood cells in the fluid does not

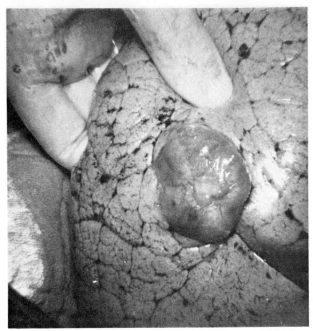

Fig. 17-39. A localized benign mesothelioma. This operative photograph shows a fibrous mesothelioma arising from the visceral pleura just at the juncture of the patient's lower and upper lobes of the right lung. The tumor was removed with a margin of normal tissue by wedge resection.

necessarily indicate a malignant state or inoperability. Hypoglycemia with convulsions has been reported; it is presumably due to the production of an insulin-like substance by the tumor.

A less frequent form of the localized mesothelioma is one that involves the subjacent lung without seeding the pleural cavity or producing metastases (Fig. 17-40). It must be considered a malignant tumor, but its slow growth and the fact that it is curable by pneumonectomy put it in sharp distinction to the diffuse form of mesothelioma.

A *diffuse mesothelioma* may arise from any region of the pleura and may spread along the pleural surface to encase the ipsilateral lung completely. Direct extension over the pericardial surface to the pleural cavity on the opposite side occasionally occurs. The histologic appearance is often that of erratic spindle cells resembling sarcoma in combination with elements that appear to have epithelial origin. There is often some uncertainty about the true origin of a diffuse malignant lesion that is considered to be a mesothelioma. This is because it may be impossible to say that such a lesion, examined either at operation or autopsy, actually arose from the pleura rather than from the lung or chest wall. In true mesotheliomas, metastases to regional lymph nodes or distant sites are said to be unusual.

A serous or serosanguineous pleural effusion accompanies a diffuse mesothelioma, and the tumor is associated with significant chest pain. Cytologic study of the aspirated fluid is often negative for cells that a pathologist can associate with malignant mesothelioma. Chest x-rays generally show an effusion with pleural thickening and a contracted or fibrotic lung. A closed-needle biopsy may yield satisfac-

tory tissue for diagnosis, and the identification of hyaluronic acid in the pleural fluid may be used as presumptive evidence for mesothelioma.

The treatment for a diffuse mesothelioma must be considered palliative. Even extensive resection involving the chest wall with pneumonectomy has generally failed to produce long-term survival. Radiation therapy, with systemic chemotherapy, may reduce the patient's chest pain. The prognosis is bad; the majority of patients live less than 1 year after the diagnosis is made.

METASTATIC TUMORS

The pleura may be the site of metastases from neoplasms in other body regions. There is often concomitant involvement of the lungs, but it is the pleural effusion that produces symptoms by lung compression. In addition to metastatic involvement of the pleural surface, obstruction of the lymphatic channels by neoplastic cells may result in massive accumulation of pleural fluid. An occasional patient first presents because of pleural and respiratory symptoms before the primary tumor is known. Pleural needle biopsy may need to be combined with examination of the aspirated fluid to develop an accurate diagnosis.

The treatment of a malignant pleural effusion depends on the symptoms produced and the sensitivity of the primary tumor to radiation therapy or chemotherapy. If respiratory symptoms are significant, it is satisfactory to insert an intercostal tube and drain the effusion. If the pleural cavity is kept drained for several days the lung is given a chance to reexpand and radiation or chemotherapy may be started (Fig. 17-41). A direct instillation of nitrogen mustard (0.2 to 0.4 mg/kg in 100 ml sterile water) through the intercostal catheter is very effective in reducing the reaccumulation of pleural fluid.

LUNG

Anatomy

The respiratory system arises as an outpouching from the primitive gut during the third week of embryonic life and undergoes a bifurcation of the distal end of the pouch into right and left primitive bronchial buds. Growth and secondary outpouching of each primary bud provides an early indication of the lobar development of each lung by the fourth week. Progressive branching then accompanies histologic differentiation from the cuboidal epithelium that lines the terminal buds during the first four fetal months to the flattened epithelium present at birth. Whether the lungs grow by additional branching of respiratory units after birth has been debated. On the basis of studies earlier in this century it was stated that the newborn infant's lung had 18 generations of branching. Comparison of this number with a reported 25 branchings in the adult middle lobe suggested that maturation continued by additional branching at least through early childhood. More recently, Boyden and Tomsett identified 23 to 27 branching generations in infants, adolescents, and adults, to support the concept that the lungs are completely developed at birth.

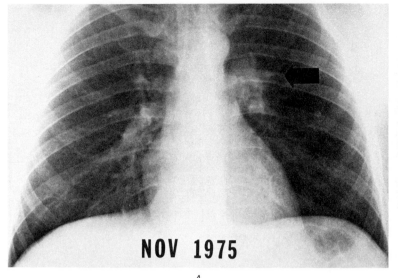

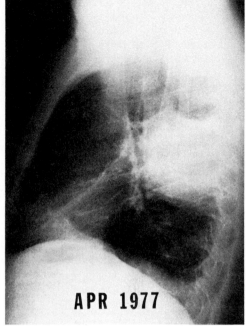

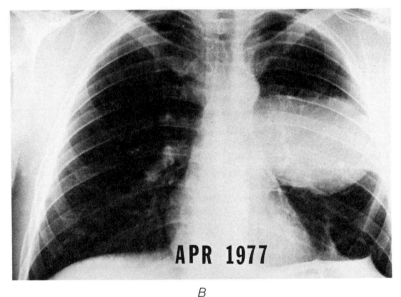

Fig. 17-40. A localized malignant mesothelioma. *A.* A chest x-ray in 1975 showed a small left hilar mass (*arrow*) in a twenty-six-year-old white male with pleuritic-type chest pain. He declined a recommended thoracotomy. *B.* By April 1977, the mass had become very large and was associated with pleural changes above the diaphragm. *C.* The lateral chest x-ray shows the posterior extent of the mass. Because of continued chest pain the patient accepted operation, and a left pneumonectomy was done. He has recovered satisfactorily without evidence of recurrence. (*Chest x-ray and case history courtesy of Jacqueline Coalson, Ph.D.*)

Although the number of respiratory units may not increase after birth, it does seem apparent that the newborn's lung is structurally immature. In place of alveoli, the lungs are made up of primitive air sacs that differentiate into alveolar ducts and sacs. Alveoli develop by outpouching and compartmentalization, so that by eight years of age the adult number of approximately 300 million alveoli is at-

tained. The fully developed alveoli give a surface area of 70 to 80 m² at three-fourths maximal inflation of the adult lung.

The segmental anatomy of the lungs and bronchial tree is illustrated in Fig. 17-42. Although there is continuity of the pulmonary parenchyma between adjacent segments of each lobe, the separation of the bronchial and vascular stalks allows subsegmental and segmental resections rather than lobectomy for certain localized lesions. The object of performing lesser resections is to preserve the maximum amount of pulmonary tissue. Inflammatory diseases such as tuberculosis and bronchiectasis characteristically involve segmental units of the upper and lower lobes, respectively, but often do so in a way that leaves one or more segments of the same lobe unaffected. Both these diseases, as well as metastatic pulmonary neoplasms, may involve more than one pulmonary lobe, either synchronously or metachronously. The advantages of a segmental concept of surgical

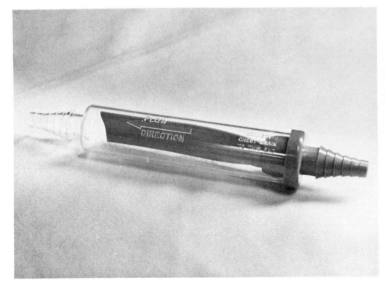

A

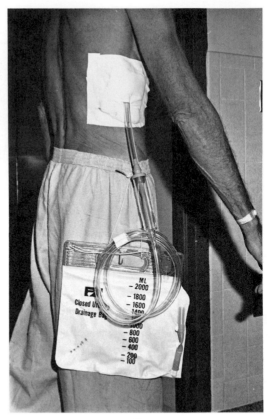

B

Fig. 17-41. Use of a one-way drainage valve to permit mobility of patients with a chest tube. *A*. The Heimlich one-way valve can be attached to an intercostal tube and eliminates the need for an underwater seal in some patients with either an air leak or drainage from the pleural cavity. *B*. By attaching the one-way valve to a collection bag the patient with a continuously draining pleural effusion can be completely ambulatory.

treatment are most apparent under these circumstances.

Abundant lymphatic vessels are located beneath the visceral pleura of each lung, in the interlobular septums, in the submucosa of the bronchi, and in the perivascular and peribronchial connective tissue. The lymph nodes which drain the lungs are divided into two large groups, the *pulmonary lymph nodes* and the *mediastinal nodes.* In turn, the pulmonary lymph nodes consist of (1) the intrapulmonary nodes, which lie at points of division of segmental bronchi or in the bifurcations of the pulmonary artery; (2) hilar nodes located along the main bronchi; and (3) interlobar nodes, situated in the angles formed by the bifurcation of the main bronchi into lobar bronchi.

The interlobar lymph nodes lie in the depths of the interlobar fissure on each side and have special surgical significance because they constitute a lymphatic sump for each lung. This designation results from the fact that all the pulmonary lobes of the corresponding lung drain into that group of nodes. On the right side the nodes of the lymphatic sump lie around the bronchus intermedius, bounded above by the right-upper-lobe bronchus, and below by the middle lobe and superior segmental bronchi. The lymphatic sump on the left side is confined to the interlobar fissure, with the lymph nodes disposed in the angle between the lingular and lower-lobe bronchi, and in apposition to the pulmonary artery branches.

The mediastinal lymph nodes consist of four principal groups: (1) anterior mediastinal, (2) posterior mediastinal, (3) tracheobronchial, and (4) paratracheal. The anterior mediastinal nodes are located in association with the upper surface of the pericardium, the phrenic nerves, the ligamentum arteriosum, and the left innominate vein. Within the inferior pulmonary ligament on each side are found the paraesophageal lymph nodes that constitute a major part of the posterior mediastinal group. Additional paraesophageal nodes may be located more superiorly between the esophagus and trachea in the region of the arch of the azygos vein.

The tracheobronchial lymph nodes are made up of three subgroups that are located about the bifurcation of the trachea. Included are the subcarinal nodes, the lymph nodes lying in the obtuse angle between the trachea and each main-stem bronchus, and a few nodes that lie anterior to the lower end of the trachea. The paratracheal lymph nodes are located in proximity to the trachea in the superior mediastinum. Those on the right side form a chain with the tracheobronchial nodes inferiorly and with some of the deep cervical nodes above. A few of the latter are referred to as the *scalene lymph nodes* because they lie on the anterior scalene muscle.

The high incidence of bronchial carcinoma is partly responsible for a continuing interest in identifying the precise patterns of lymphatic drainage of the lungs to the mediastinum. Previous studies suggested that drainage from the left lung was mainly contralateral and that from the right lung was ipsilateral. The development of mediastinoscopy and its extensive use in patients with bronchogenic carcinoma has allowed a slight modification of this concept. Lymphatic drainage of the right lung is ipsilateral except for an occasional incidence in which drainage to the

RIGHT LUNG AND BRONCHI

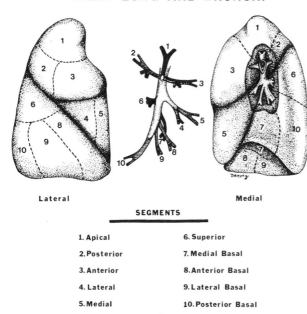

Lateral   Medial

SEGMENTS

1. Apical	6. Superior
2. Posterior	7. Medial Basal
3. Anterior	8. Anterior Basal
4. Lateral	9. Lateral Basal
5. Medial	10. Posterior Basal

A

LEFT LUNG AND BRONCHI

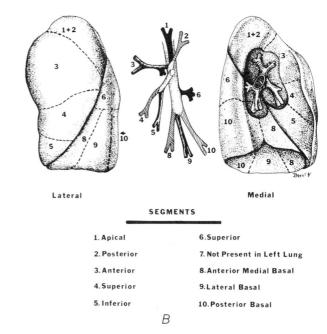

Lateral   Medial

SEGMENTS

1. Apical	6. Superior
2. Posterior	7. Not Present in Left Lung
3. Anterior	8. Anterior Medial Basal
4. Superior	9. Lateral Basal
5. Inferior	10. Posterior Basal

B

Fig. 17-42. *A* and *B*. The segmental anatomy of the lungs. An appreciation of these anatomic divisions often makes it possible to preserve pulmonary tissue by performing segmental resections for localized disease.

superior mediastinum is bilateral. Drainage from the left lung to the superior mediastinum is as frequently ipsilateral as it is to the opposite side.

Diagnostic Techniques

Despite their great variety, respiratory diseases, including congenital anomalies, have only a limited group of signs and symptoms, and there is considerable overlap in their clinical presentation. Notwithstanding the remarkable advances in roentgenographic techniques, it is often impossible to differentiate pulmonary inflammatory disorders from primary or secondary neoplastic diseases on the basis of chest x-rays. In addition, pulmonary lesions are sometimes found on a standard screening chest x-ray with a complete absence of symptoms. At least two factors may be considered conducive to continuing developments in pulmonary diagnostic techniques. The first is the free communication of the interior of the respiratory system with the oropharynx. This facilitates collection of secretions, infectious agents, and desquamated cells that may provide a definitive diagnosis. Second, roentgenograms and fluoroscopic techniques provide a "window" into the thoracic cavity for serial observations and for precise guidance of biopsy needles and forceps. Pulmonary angiography has been disappointing as a general diagnostic technique, but it can be important in defining congenital abnormalities.

In most acquired pulmonary diseases sputum collection and examination is indicated as an initial diagnostic procedure. The specific etiologic agent of infections is sought by examination of smears and by culture techniques. The flora of the upper part of the respiratory tract stops abruptly at the level of the larynx, and the tracheobronchial tree is normally sterile. Not infrequently, either the patient's sputum is scant or, because it is mixed with saliva and an oral bacterial flora, its diagnostic usefulness is reduced. To bypass these problems, percutaneous transtracheal aspiration may be performed through the cricothyroid membrane. A 16-gauge or 14-gauge intracatheter needle is used for the procedure after preparation of the skin with soap or iodine solution and local infiltration anesthesia with lidocaine. Coughing may be induced by injecting 5 to 10 ml sterile saline solution without preservative into the trachea. Aspiration of the diluted secretions into a 10- or 20-ml syringe should be followed by immediate delivery of the material to the laboratory.

This same technique may be used to collect material for cytologic examination in patients with a suspected pulmonary neoplasm, but because bronchoscopy is always indicated in these patients, it may suffice to collect secretions and saline irrigations (bronchial washings) through the bronchoscope. The sputum coughed up immediately after bronchoscopy is especially valuable for cytologic examinations. Chest physical therapy and intermittent positive-pressure breathing with saline solution and bronchodilators are additional techniques to facilitate the collection of sputum. Unfortunately, too little effort is spent in obtaining adequate samples of sputum in many hospitals, and the patient's diagnosis is often delayed while additional and more complicated procedures are done.

BRONCHOSCOPY. The visual examination of the tracheobronchial tree can be both diagnostic and therapeutic. Information can be gained from this procedure that is available from no other source: cell type of bronchial neoplasms by direct biopsy, mobility of surrounding structures, extent of endobronchial involvement in neoplasms and inflammatory disease, and on occasion, source of bleeding. In addition, the therapeutic aspects of bronchoscopy should not be overlooked. The removal of thick, inspissated secretions from the postoperative patient can be lifesaving. The benefit of foreign body extraction by endoscopic means is obvious.

The introduction of the flexible bronchoscope in 1967 by Ikeda greatly extended the benefits of this procedure. With this instrument examination of the tracheobronchial tree to the subsegmental level became possible. Brush biopsy and transbronchial lung biopsy also became practical.

Bronchoscopy may be performed under general or topical anesthesia, on conscious or unconscious patients, and under circumstances of spontaneous ventilation or with respirator support. Topical anesthesia is the preferred method under most circumstances.

BRONCHIAL BRUSHING. Bronchial-brush biopsy of pulmonary endobronchial lesions may be performed through the flexible fiberoptic bronchoscope, or it may be done as an independent procedure under fluoroscopic control. With the latter technique the patient is studied in the x-ray department and a catheter is guided into the appropriate segmental bronchus under topical anesthesia. After withdrawal of the guide wire, the special nylon brush is inserted through the catheter and advanced into the lesion. As the brush is passed back and forth through the lesion, the bristles entrap material that is scraped from its surface. As soon as the brush is removed from the catheter it is smeared on glass slides and the latter are placed in fixative solution according to the Papanicolaou technique. The brush may be cut off the guide wire and placed in any desired type of culture media.

Bronchial brushing has been very effective in the diagnosis of bronchogenic carcinoma, but less so with metastatic pulmonary neoplasms. Tuberculosis and fungal diseases have been diagnosed by this method, but the increasing performance of fiberoptic bronchoscopy by physicians in pulmonary medicine seems to have stopped the development of brush biopsy as an independent procedure.

MEDIASTINOSCOPY-MEDIASTINOTOMY. Since its introduction in 1959 mediastinoscopy has gained increasing use as a technique for exploring the routes of mediastinal spread of pulmonary neoplasms. The procedure is usually performed under general endotracheal anesthesia and utilizes a small transverse incision in the suprasternal notch. Digital exploration is carried inferiorly in the plane between the anterior surface of the trachea and the posterior surface of the innominate artery and the aorta. The paratracheal, tracheobronchial, and subcarinal lymph nodes are accessible to visualization and biopsy through the mediastinoscope, and tumor masses such as thymomas or thyroid lesions may be biopsied directly. The decision to perform thoracotomy in a patient with proved or suspected bronchogenic carcinoma may be supported when mediastinoscopy fails to show evidence of mediastinal spread. In some circumstances, the procedure is used as a means of obtaining tissue for confirmation of a suspected diagnosis of bronchial neoplasm when other methods such as bronchoscopy have failed. The technique provides a positive diagnosis in almost all patients with lymphoma who have radiographic evidence of enlarged mediastinal lymph nodes, and the yield is similarly very high for patients with infectious granulomatous disease. Mediastinoscopy is considered the procedure of choice for diagnosis of sarcoidosis in most institutions, and it has largely replaced scalene lymph-node and fat-pad biopsy for both benign and malignant lesions (Fig. 17-43).

Unfortunately, a metastasis to lymph nodes between the trachea and esophagus and to posterior mediastinal lymph nodes cannot be determined by mediastinoscopy. In addition, direct mediastinal extension to an extent that makes it impossible to perform curative resection is not detectable by this procedure. Additional methods for exploring the mediastinum have been developed, and the procedure referred to as anterior mediastinotomy has been used most frequently. Through either a transverse or vertical parasternal incision the second costal cartilage is removed on the side of the lesion. An effort is made to avoid opening the pleural cavity as the mediastinal pleura is freed from the undersurface of the sternum and dissected away from the mediastinum. By additional removal of the third costal cartilage a wider exploration can be performed, the object being to sample mediastinal lymph nodes and determine the extent of mediastinal spread of a centrally located bronchial neoplasm. If it is pertinent to the confirmation of the diagnosis, the mediastinal pleura can be opened to allow direct lung or pleural biopsy. The pleura may be opened also during a mediastinoscopy for the same purposes, but most surgeons are reluctant to use this technique with the sharply limited exposure of the mediastinoscopy incision.

On the right side, mediastinotomy allows exploration along the superior vena cava and the trachea. The left

Fig. 17-43. This chest x-ray of a twenty-four-year-old black woman shows bilateral hilar masses that could be lymphoma or sarcoidosis. Mediastinoscopy was performed to obtain tissue that confirmed the diagnosis of sarcoidosis.

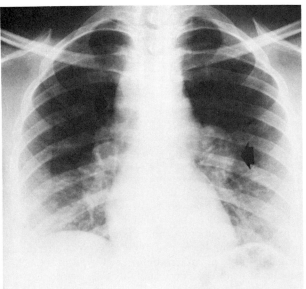

pulmonary hilum may be evaluated, and the possibility of neoplastic extension to involve the aorta may be partly determined by left mediastinotomy.

More recently, Arom and his colleagues have described a subxiphoid approach for anterior mediastinal exploration in which a short incision over the xiphoid process is used to allow entrance into the inferior aspect of the anterior mediastinum. Digital exploration is combined with the use of a mediastinoscope to provide an access to the entire anterior mediastinal compartment (Fig. 17-44). Biopsy of tumor masses or lymph nodes may be performed through this approach in the same fashion as with conventional mediastinoscopy.

LUNG BIOPSY. An accurate diagnosis is fundamental in the management of pulmonary and bronchial disease, whether localized or diffuse. Bronchial lesions may be biopsied during bronchoscopy or by bronchial brushing. It is also possible to perform lung biopsy via the broncho-scope, but the number of individuals using the transbron-chial technique was limited until development of the flexi-ble fiberscope. An increasing number of endoscoptists are utilizing transbronchoscopic lung biopsy for obtaining sufficient tissue samples to allow diagnosis of diffuse pul-monary diseases such as sarcoidosis, pulmonary alveolar proteinosis, and *Pneumocystis carinii* pneumonia. It is also possible to obtain tissue for diagnosis of localized lung disease by the transbronchial technique, but this requires good cooperation from the x-ray department to provide bi-plane image intensification. The morbidity rate of transbronchial lung biopsy has been low, with pneumotho-rax as the principal complication. Though the incidence of pneumothorax has varied from 5 to 20 percent, few pa-tients require active treatment.

Percutaneous needle biopsy and open lung biopsy through a limited anterolateral or transaxillary thoracot-omy are the more established methods for obtaining a tissue diagnosis in those patients who are not candidates for primary surgical treatment. Whether the patient has a diffuse lung disease or a presumed bronchial cancer that is inoperable, needle biopsy is preferable to open thoracot-omy. Both aspirating and cutting needles are available, but the disposable Tru-Cut needles have gained in popularity during the past few years. Contraindications to needle biopsy include (1) pulmonary hypertension, (2) suspected or proved bleeding diathesis, (3) an uncooperative patient, (4) a patient receiving continuous or frequent positive-pressure breathing, and (5) respiratory failure.

An occasional patient is encountered for whom thora-cotomy represents a high risk, but operation would be recommended if the localized lesion were known to be malignant. Some surgeons would argue against needle biopsy on the basis of the rare but documented occurrence of seeding the needle tract with malignant cells. In this special circumstance needle biopsy does appear warranted.

Needle biopsy is performed under local anesthesia, preferably with fluoroscopic control. Aspirated material must be immediately smeared or cultured, but pathology departments vary somewhat in their preference for the handling of tissue removed with cutting needles. The com-plications include hemoptysis, pneumothorax, and rarely

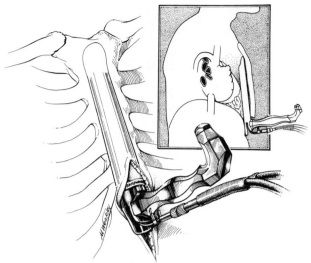

Fig. 17-44. A modification of mediastinoscopy is the technique of subxiphoid anterior mediastinal exploration recently described by Arom and colleagues. (*Courtesy of Kit V. Arom, M.D.*)

hemothorax. Although an incidence of pneumothorax as high as 30 percent has been reported, only an occasional patient requires tube thoracotomy for treatment. A special form of trephine needle biopsy using a high-speed turbine drill has been used in a few medical centers, but the method has not gained widespread interest.

The chief indications for open lung biopsy are failure of closed methods for diagnosis, including needle biopsy, and presence of a small localized lesion that should be totally removed by the biopsy. An example of the latter circum-stance is presented by the patient with a solitary pulmonary nodule and a previously controlled malignancy in another body region. Occasionally there is a need to remove a larger amount of tissue than can be obtained by needle biopsy in patients with either diffuse or localized disease.

Open lung biopsy is performed as a formal operation under general anesthesia, and the patient should be made to understand that it is not a minor procedure. One or more wedges of pulmonary tissue are removed with an automatic stapler or a careful suture technique to reduce the likelihood of postoperative air leak from the lung (Fig. 17-45). Since a leak does occur in a few patients, an inter-costal tube is placed at the time of operation and removed the next day if possible. The morbidity of open lung biopsy is minimal, and patients can often be discharged from the hospital in 48 to 72 hours if they require no further in-hospital procedures. The need for close follow-up must be emphasized to the patient when early discharge is allowed.

Congenital Disorders

Abnormalities in development of the lung and tracheo-bronchial tree may occur at any stage of intrauterine life, with clinical manifestations immediately after birth or at any subsequent age. Under normal circumstances the lungs are considered immature at the time of birth, but immatu-rity to even a greater degree is associated with respiratory-

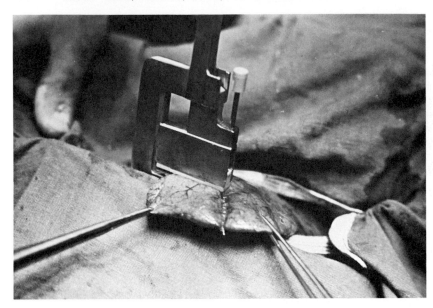

Fig. 17-45. Open lung biopsy is performed by delivering a margin of a pulmonary lobe through the small thoracic incision and applying the automatic stapler across the parenchyma, as shown here. The first line of staples has been applied, and the stapler is in place for the second line. A wedge of pulmonary parenchyma can then be amputated for appropriate studies.

distress syndromes, including hyaline membrane disease.

The most fundamental abnormality is bilateral *pulmonary agenesis,* in which there is failure of the primitive respiratory outpouching to develop. Unilateral pulmonary agenesis represents a failure of development of the right or left primary bronchial bud; its occurrence is twice as often on the left side. Unilateral agenesis is compatible with relatively normal physical growth and development if the child has no other major abnormalities. The lung that is present fills both hemithoraces. Lobar agenesis is probably more frequent than reported, because it produces no characteristic clinical picture and is most often found during examination for other conditions.

Congenital *tracheoesophageal fistulas* of several types are among the more serious abnormalities of pulmonary development. Esophageal atresia is present in the great majority of cases; these conditions are considered in detail in the chapter on diseases of the esophagus.

Small *diverticula* of the trachea or bronchi with a predilection for the distal trachea are occasionally seen. They are usually in free communication with the airway lumen, and symptoms are absent. Aberrant origin of a normal major bronchus is seen infrequently, but it can have major significance when pulmonary resection is indicated for another reason. The commonest example is origin of the right-upper-lobe bronchus or the apical segmental bronchus from the lateral wall of the trachea. In the *scimitar syndrome,* anomalous drainage of the right pulmonary veins into the inferior vena cava is associated with underdevelopment of the right lung, several bronchovascular abnormalities, and aberrant systemic arterialization of the right lung. A principal concern of management is redirection of the pulmonary venous flow into the left atrium and simultaneous repair of any intracardiac defects.

A *bronchocele* is a localized cystic structure filled with mucus and located immediately distal to an area of stenosis or atresia in the bronchial tree. Presumably, the lesion can be produced either by a congenital obstruction in the bronchial tree or subsequent to an acquired stenosis. It is generally asymptomatic in the absence of infection and presents as a density several centimeters in length on a routine chest x-ray. Most often, diagnosis is made by examination of the specimen following a segmental or subsegmental resection.

An interesting and rare pulmonary abnormality that may require urgent resection is the *cystic adenomatoid malformation.* Prematurity and stillbirth are frequent characteristics of this condition, and infants that survive may develop respiratory distress soon after birth. Mediastinal shift toward the normal side is common, and the chest x-ray shows a large mass in the lower part of the chest with depression of the hemidiaphragm. Emergency thoracotomy reveals replacement of the lower lobe by a greatly enlarged mass that may be studded with cysts. Some evidence of partial aeration may be present, but there is no suggestion of ventilatory function. A systemic arterial supply such as that which occurs with pulmonary sequestration is usually absent. A lobectomy is generally required, but pneumonectomy has been necessary in a few instances. If survival occurs without early operation, subsequent infection of the malformed lobe is likely to result in a diagnosis of congenital cystic bronchiectasis.

Microscopic examination of the resected tissue shows tubules lined with cuboidal or columnar epithelium, bronchial mucous glands, and occasionally bits of cartilage or smooth muscle. The presence of the multiple components of respiratory tissue has caused some authors to refer to this abnormality as a diffuse hamartoma.

An *accessory lung* or *lobe* occasionally develops in association with a supernumerary bronchus that communicates with the trachea or a major bronchial branch. Left-sided occurrence is more frequent, and the blood supply may come from either the pulmonary or systemic circuits. This lesion is distinguished from *pulmonary sequestration* by the lack of a bronchial communication in the latter condition. In addition, a pulmonary sequestration receives its blood

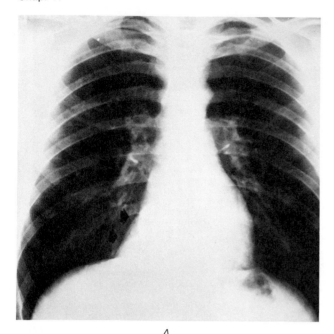

A

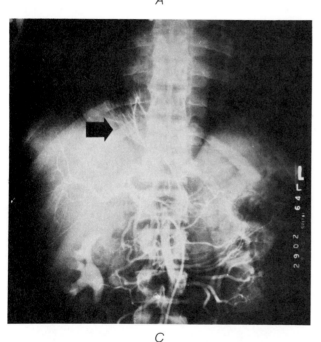

C

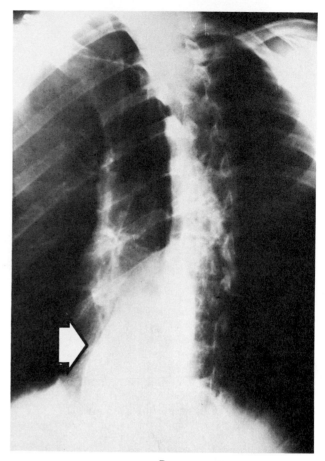

B

Fig. 17-46. An extrapulmonary sequestration discovered on a routine chest x-ray in a twenty-year-old male. *A.* The posteroanterior chest x-ray shows a triangular density adjacent to the right heart border and based on the diaphragm. *B.* An oblique view shows the density to be a large mass with sharp borders. *C.* An aortogram shows several arteries passing retrograde from the infradiaphragmatic aorta to supply the sequestration.

supply from an ectopic systemic artery, often arising from the aorta at a point below the diaphragm (Fig. 17-46). The sequestration may be located in a lower lobe of the lung (intrapulmonary) or as a cystic mass in the inferior mediastinum (extrapulmonary). Rarely, a sequestration may be intraperitoneal, or it may develop a fistulous communication with the distal esophagus.

Intrapulmonary sequestration is the commonest type, and it may remain without symptoms for years. The development of symptoms is usually the result of infection, even though no apparent communication exists between the lower-lobe bronchi and the cystic lumina of the sequestration (Fig. 17-47). Treatment requires surgical resection of the involved lower lobe for the intrapulmonary forms, and excision of the mass for the extrapulmonary lesions.

Several forms of *congenital cystic abnormalities* may occur in the lung. Unilateral absence of a pulmonary artery may be associated with hypoplastic development of the lung and a cystic transformation. Intrapulmonary bronchogenic cysts may occur that are thought to represent a pinching off of the developing bronchial buds well beyond the subsegmental level. They may be single or multiple, confined to a segment or a lobe, and histologically similar to the large bronchogenic cysts that are located in the mediastinum alongside the major bronchi. The cysts are typically lined with ciliated, pseudostratified epithelium, and they contain a viscid opaque fluid. Small communications with the bronchial tree can develop, and the cysts become partially air-filled. If infection occurs and resection is required, it may be difficult to distinguish a congenital cyst from a chronic pulmonary abscess or cystic bronchiec-

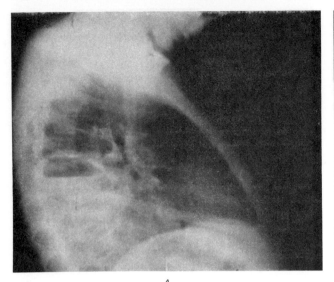

A

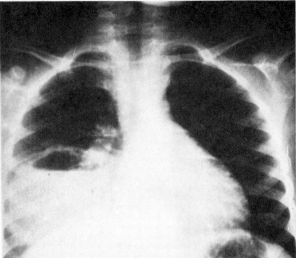

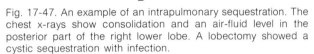

B

tasis. Other organs such as the kidney, liver, and pancreas may be the site of cystic changes in these patients.

Pulmonary arteriovenous aneurysms consist of fistulas between the branches of the pulmonary arteries and veins (Fig. 17-48). They vary in size from 1 or 2 mm up to lesions that may occupy a major portion of a pulmonary lobe. The occurrence of a single fistula is less common than the presence of multiple fistulas involving more than one lobe, especially in those patients with hereditary hemorrhagic telangiectasia (Osler-Rendu-Weber disease). More than one arterial branch and more than one vein are generally involved in a single aneurysm. The aneurysms are often subpleural in location, and spontaneous hemothorax occasionally occurs. Even when their individual size is small, a sufficient number of aneurysms may be present to produce

Fig. 17-47. An example of an intrapulmonary sequestration. The chest x-rays show consolidation and an air-fluid level in the posterior part of the right lower lobe. A lobectomy showed a cystic sequestration with infection.

massive right-to-left shunting, cyanosis, clubbing, polycythemia, and congestive heart failure in the first few years of life. In other patients the development of cyanosis may not occur until adult life, but cerebral symptoms may result from cerebral thrombosis or subacute bacterial endarteritis. Hemoptysis is unusual in young patients, but it may be life-threatening in the adult. Fluoroscopic examination

Fig. 17-48. *A.* The plain chest x-ray in this eight-year-old boy shows three lesions thought to be compatible with pulmonary arteriovenous aneurysms. *B.* The pulmonary arteriogram confirms the aneurysms, which were subsequently removed by staged bilateral thoracotomies.

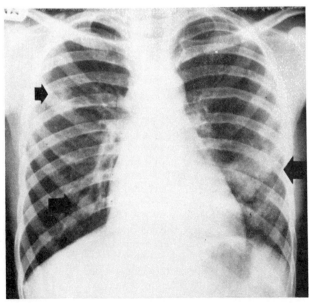

A

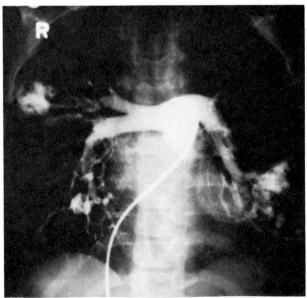

B

during the Valsalva and Müller maneuvers may show changes in the size of lesions that are suspected to be arteriovenous fistulas on plain chest x-rays. Pulmonary angiography is necessary to confirm the diagnosis and allow proper planning for surgical treatment. Ordinarily, the confirmation of the presence of one or more fistulas is adequate indication for operation, because of the risk of eventual serious complications. Conservative segmental and subsegmental resections rather than lobectomy are the procedures of choice.

Multiple chest-wall *systemic-to-pulmonary arterial fistulas* may present as a localized lesion associated with hemic murmurs and changes such as unilateral rib notching on the chest x-ray. The internal thoracic or several intercostal arteries may give origin to the systemic arterial components, and the fistulous connections may be formed with branches of the pulmonary arteries rather than with the veins. Angiography is required to determine the extent of the lesion, and the decision for resection must be carefully planned because of the danger of intraoperative hemorrhage.

INFANTILE LOBAR EMPHYSEMA

Michelson has stressed the need to use the term *infantile* lobar emphysema rather than *congenital* because the condition is not necessarily congenital in origin. There is characteristically a mild to marked overdistension of an upper or middle lobe, with compression of the remaining ipsilateral pulmonary tissue and mediastinal shift to the opposite side. Progressive distension results in herniation across the anterior mediastinum and atelectasis of the contralateral upper lobe (Fig. 17-49).

Lobar emphysema affects newborn as well as older infants and produces varying degrees of respiratory distress. Those with limited experience often think of it as an acute irreversible condition, but chronic forms as well as acute reversible emphysema may occur. It is especially important to understand that deficiency of the bronchial cartilage with resulting obstruction to expiratory air flow is only one of several causes of the disease. For example, lobar emphysema may develop as a result of acute bronchial infection with obstruction due to inflammatory secretions and mucosal edema. Proper management under these circumstances requires intensive treatment of the infection and close observation of the overdistended lobe or lobes. Evidence that the emphysema is reversible is provided by stabilization of the infant's respiratory distress and beginning reversal of the radiographic evidence of pulmonary overdistension.

In a significant number of the studied cases there has been dissatisfaction with the attempt to explain lobar emphysema on the basis of bronchial obstruction. An interesting mechanism that may produce upper-lobe overdistension in any age group is related to the concept that there is a relatively positive intrapleural pressure at the lung base compared to a relatively negative pressure at the apex. In the supine position the anterior portion of the lung is better ventilated than the posterior portion. Since the infant has a pliable chest wall and a spacious anterior mediastinum, it seems possible that increased ventilation would promote an overexpansion of the anterior segment, especially in the presence of any resistance to expiratory air flow.

Asymptomatic lobar emphysema may be found by chest x-rays in the newborn. Clearing of the emphysema within a day or two and failure to develop symptoms have suggested that bronchial obstruction was due to aspiration of amniotic fluid or mucus. Lobar emphysema resulting from extrabronchial compression due to bronchogenic or mediastinal neuroenteric cysts may be especially difficult to diagnose. The structure responsible for compression may not be seen on the chest x-rays, and a confusing clinical picture may result. An esophagogram will generally suggest the presence of a mediastinal mass, and this procedure should be performed when the infant's condition permits it. The presence of thoracic hemivertebrae may suggest the likelihood that a neuroenteric cyst can be present. Anomalous location of vascular structures such as the left pulmonary artery and the ductus arteriosus has been reported as an extrinsic cause of lobar emphysema.

Typical irreversible lobar emphysema is a disease of the newborn. Approximately 50 percent of the reported cases have occurred during the first 4 weeks of life, and symptoms of respiratory distress may begin shortly after birth. Chest x-ray evidence of overdistension of an upper or middle lobe may be subtle at first, but progressive symptoms are accompanied by mediastinal shift and compression of the opposite lung. Overinflation is often confined to the anterior segment of either upper lobe or the middle lobe, but the lower lobes are rarely involved.

The treatment of severe, acutely symptomatic lobar emphysema is immediate operation if the likelihood that primary bronchial infection is not the cause. Nonoperative treatment may result in a mortality rate as high as 50 percent. Congenital heart disease is associated with approximately 15 percent of infants with lobar emphysema, and occasionally it is appropriate to treat both conditions at the same time. Exploration of the emphysematous lobe and the mediastinum is done through a standard posterolateral thoracotomy incision. If a clear-cut cause of extrinsic bronchial compression is found, this is dealt with and a decision is made about removal of the distended lobe. Generally, a lobectomy will be required, and satisfactory expansion of the remaining lung can be expected.

EMPHYSEMATOUS BLEBS AND BULLAE

Infrequent air-containing spaces that are located in apparently normal lung parenchyma may represent a form of congenital blebs. These spaces may also be referred to as congenital air cysts, and they are characterized by an epithelial lining of the respiratory type. The incidence is unknown and the relationship between the very occasional infant or child with pulmonary blebs and the more frequently seen teenager or young adult with recurrent spontaneous pneumothorax is unclear. Similarly, the occurrence of giant bullae in the lungs of young adults who have no evidence of obstructive airway disease suggests a congenital defect in the integrity of the pulmonary parenchyma (Fig. 17-50).

The congenital air cyst may enlarge to produce pressure on adjacent lung, and such cysts may become infected.

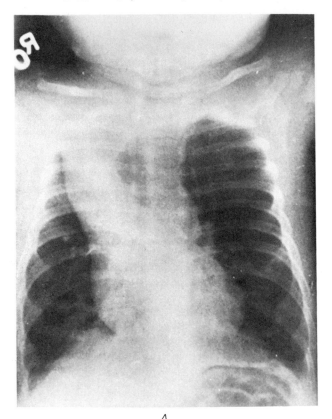

A

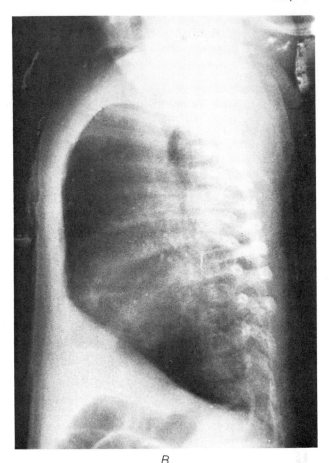

B

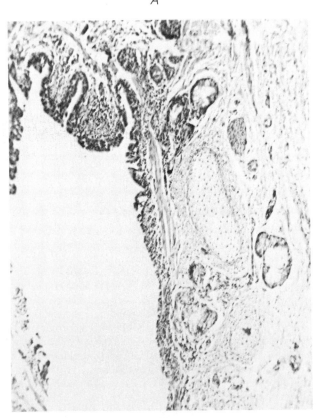

C

Fig. 17-49. Infantile lobar emphysema. *A*. The anteroposterior chest x-ray shows marked overinflation of the left upper lobe, with mediastinal shift to the right and compression of the right upper lobe. *B*. The lateral x-ray shows that most of the hyperinflation is anterior. *C*. Histologic examination of the resected left upper lobe bronchus shows incomplete cartilage development. (*From E. Michelson, Clinical Spectrum of Infantile Lobar Emphysema, Ann Thorac Surg, 24:182, 1977.*)

With infection, purulent fluid develops in the cyst (pyocyst), and treatment similar to that for lung abscess is required. The preferred treatment is surgical resection before infection occurs.

Emphysematous blebs and bullae are so much a part of the overall condition of pulmonary emphysema that it is difficult or impossible to consider their surgical significance without a consideration of the pathogenesis of emphysema. From the strict anatomic definition, pulmonary emphysema means enlargement of distal air spaces, often accompanied by destruction of septums. At least four processes are operative in the production of emphysema, but the relative role of each and the precise combinations that may be determinative in the individual patient are often uncertain. The processes are (1) traction, (2) airway obstruction, (3) destruction of interalveolar septums, and (4) loss of elasticity.

In the process of traction, overdistension of focal groups of alveoli occurs as an attempt to compensate for volume

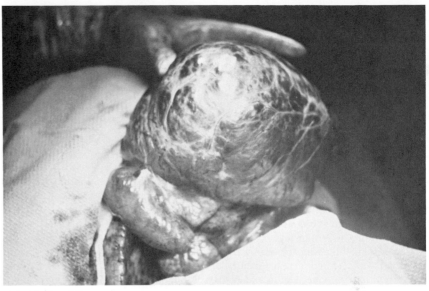

Fig. 17-50. An operative photograph showing a giant bulla arising from the upper lobe of an eighteen-year-old man with no symptoms of obstructive airway disease.

loss due to multiple areas of microatelectasis or pulmonary fibrosis. The obstructive processes vary in location from the lobar bronchi to the bronchioles, with a varied etiologic picture that encompasses both extrinsic and intrinsic causes of bronchial obstruction. With focal obstructive emphysema, air trapping occurs in isolated alveolar units, and

Fig. 17-51. *A.* Multiple pulmonary bullae are shown arising in the right upper lobe of a thirty-one-year-old salesman who had three episodes of spontaneous pneumothorax over a 2-year period. *B.* The bullae have been opened to show the netlike interior resulting from progressive parenchymal destruction as the bullae evolved.

overexpansion leads to the formation of bullae. Diffuse obstructive emphysema involves all the air spaces to a limited degree, but there may be an intermix with focal areas of greater distension and resulting bullae. In the presence of bullous emphysema a self-perpetuating cycle may be established. An enlarging bulla can produce partial obstruction of adjacent bronchioles with further air trapping and progressive distension of the bulla.

A process of tissue destruction almost certainly plays a key role in the development of bullae, because the interalveolar septums must give way as recruitment of increasing volume occurs (Fig. 17-51). Through this process the

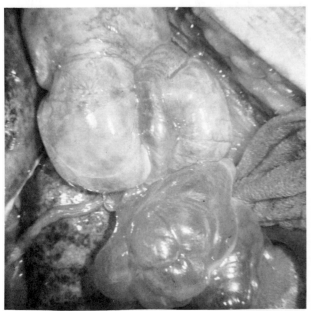

A

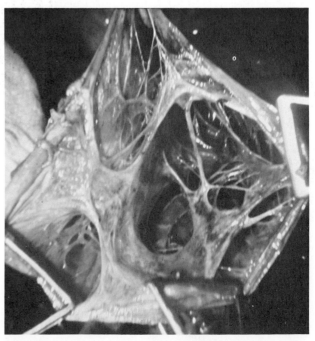

B

relatively simple air chamber of the bulla is formed from the complex of respiratory units that originally existed. The bulla communicates with a progressive number of bronchioles or bronchi as it enlarges. A loss of elasticity in the parenchymal structure accompanies the destruction of septums.

The surgical significance of pulmonary blebs and bullae is related to the complications that they may produce and to the implications of their presence when a patient is being considered for surgical treatment of another pulmonary lesion. Radiographic demonstration of bullae indicates the presence of emphysema and suggests (1) caution in the decision to offer a thoracic operation for treatment of the patient's primary problems, and (2) conservative resection when pulmonary tissue must be excised. Among the usual complications are (1) recurrent pneumothorax, often with prolonged air leak, (2) infection (pyocysts), and (3) occasional bleeding, (4) compression of adjacent parenchyma, and (5) respiratory insufficiency.

Giant bullae may be seen in all age groups, but decisions regarding surgical management seem to gather more attention and controversy in young adults and middle-aged persons. There are often minimal symptoms in the former, and any debate over surgical excision revolves around the question of whether the removal of the bullae will allow improved pulmonary function through reexpansion of the compressed parenchyma. Middle-aged and older patients with giant bullae often have symptoms of obstructive airway disease and evidence of generalized emphysema. The advocates of a nonoperative approach insist that data are lacking to support a significant improvement in pulmonary function due to removal of the bullae.

The apical region of the upper lobes and the superior segment of the lower lobes give rise to the greatest number of bullae (Fig. 17-52). While the walls of bullae may be

Fig. 17-52. This operative photograph shows multiple thick-walled blebs arising from the left upper lobe. Numerous adhesions were probably the result of many episodes of pneumothorax treated by tube thoracostomy.

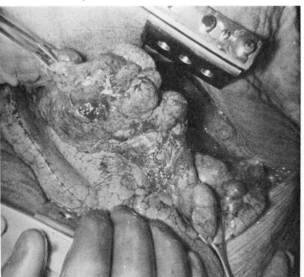

extremely thin, it is surprising how often they may be opaque and collagenous in consistency. Microscopically, there is often smooth muscle that is said to derive from the walls of bronchioles, bronchial vessels, and lymphatics.

Dyspnea with exercise is characteristic in patients with giant bullae, but the results of pulmonary-function testing will depend on the stage of the disease and associated pulmonary abnormalities. The residual volume and the functional residual capacity are generally increased while the maximum voluntary ventilation is decreased. Arterial oxygen tension is usually normal at rest, but graded exercise often produces desaturation. Routine chest x-rays and laminograms may be supplemented by radioisotope lung scans and pulmonary angiography in completing the evaluation of a patient to be considered for excision of bullae. These tests show the distribution of functioning lung tissue and indicate the degree of compression of the adjacent pulmonary parenchyma.

For the young patient without evidence of generalized respiratory disease, the bullae are simply resected either through a lateral thoracotomy, or in some cases with bilateral giant bullae, through a median sternotomy incision. The older patient with chronic bronchitis and evidence of airways obstruction requires careful preparation for operation. All measures are taken to improve pulmonary function and eliminate chronic bronchial infection. At operation the guiding principle is that of conserving the maximum functional pulmonary tissue. Only if a lobe is largely replaced by bullae should lobectomy be performed. Otherwise the bullae should be resected individually and attention devoted to closing all possible communicating bronchi.

SPONTANEOUS PNEUMOTHORAX

Pneumothorax is one of the common complications, or manifestations, of pulmonary diseases and injuries. In addition, however, there are many patients who have episodes of pneumothorax in which there appears to be no apparent cause for the leak of air from the lung parenchyma into the pleural space. These episodes of "spontaneous" pneumothorax are almost always the result of rupture of subpleural blebs that are located at the apex of the upper lobe or in the superior segment of the lower lobe. The cause of the blebs continues to be unknown, and the patients do not have obstructive airway disease. Since typically the episodes occur in young men of college age, the condition is common at universities and military bases. Spontaneous pneumothorax occurs much less frequently in women, but a rare woman will have episodes that seem to coincide with her menses (catamenial pneumothorax).

The peak age incidence is between twenty and forty years, but episodes can occur at the extremes of age. Patients who have had several episodes commonly indicate that symptoms have occurred on both sides, but rarely at the same time. Tension pneumothorax can occur and, less frequently, hemopneumothorax. There is no consistent history of exertion preceding the onset of pneumothorax, and many patients relate symptoms that suggest very mild episodes that did not cause them to seek medical attention. In other instances, the onset of pneumothorax may be

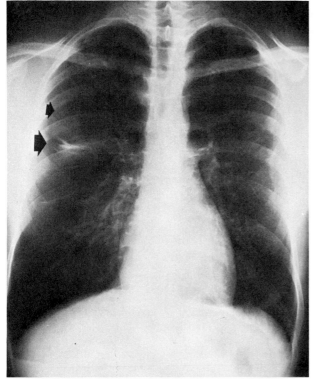

A

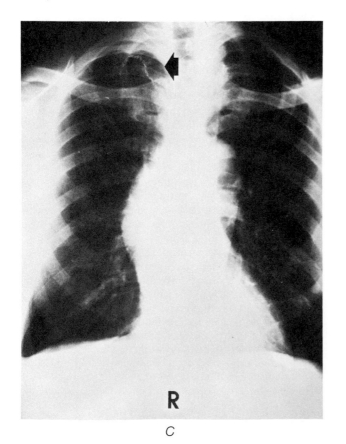

C

B

Fig. 17-53. Spontaneous pneumothorax. *A.* The arrows point to the lung margin. Occasionally a partial pneumothorax is missed during a rapid examination of an emergency chest x-ray. *B.* The right lung was easily reexpanded by placement of a large intercostal tube and initiation of pleural suction. *C.* Another patient who had multiple episodes of pneumothorax underwent right thoracotomy and obliteration of apical blebs with a row of metal staples (*arrow*).

associated with significant chest or shoulder pain and dyspnea. The findings on examination may suggest a major collapse of the lung with tracheal shift, or there may be nothing more than reduced breath sounds.

The chest x-ray usually confirms the suspected diagnosis and shows the extent of pneumothorax. Occasionally, when only a small pneumothorax is present, it is possible to misread the roentgenogram and conclude that a pneumothorax is not present (Fig. 17-53). From the x-ray, an estimate of lung collapse should be made, remembering that the lung is a modified cylinder. The x-ray badly underindicates the degree (percent) of collapse because it is only two-dimensional.

When there is minimal pneumothorax in a patient without significant symptoms, it is reasonable simply to observe the course of the pneumothorax without attempting to aspirate air from the pleural cavity. This conservative approach applies only when the patient can be observed and when sufficient hours have passed from the occurrence of symptoms to the time when the x-ray was made to presume that the air leak has stopped. When the pneumothorax exceeds 25 percent, or when the patient is symptomatic, placement of a tube thoracostomy in the second intercostal space anteriorly or in the fifth, sixth, or seventh intercostal space laterally will ordinarily allow prompt reexpansion of the lung when pleural suction is applied. Prophylactic antibiotics are not needed simply because a tube thoracostomy has been performed.

For the majority of patients, 24 to 72 hours of pleural suction is adequate to ensure reexpansion and sealing of the air leak. An occasional patient continues to leak air for many days, and it may be necessary to adjust or replace the thoracotomy tube. A persistent air leak beyond 7 to 10 days requires open thoracotomy for excision of the blebs or adhesions that are responsible for the continued leak. At the same procedure pleural abrasion should be performed with sterile gauze pads to encourage obliteration of the pleural space by adhesions.

Patients who have had a single episode of pneumothorax stand about a 30 percent chance of having a second episode. After a second episode the chances are 50-50 that a third and further episodes will occur. Therefore, it is prudent to recommend open thoracotomy after the second episode, and certainly after the third pneumothorax, regardless of whether the episodes have occurred on one side or the other. Operation can generally be performed through a transaxillary third interspace incision, with wedge resection, oversewing, or stapling of any blebs. Pleural abrasion should be done at the same time.

Pulmonary Infections

Though thoracic surgeons must still concern themselves with active participation in the treatment of patients with serious pulmonary infections, it is strikingly apparent that their role has progressively decreased. As recently as the early 1960s thousands of patients in the United States required pulmonary resection for lung abscess, bronchiectasis, and chronic granulomatous disease each year. In some areas of the world where adequate diagnostic techniques and chemotherapy are still far below regional needs these diseases continue to progress to those stages that can yield only to surgical management. Effective antibiotics, aggressive methods for accurate diagnosis, an increased standard of living, and public health programs are among the factors that have reduced the need to remove chronically infected or destroyed pulmonary tissue.

LUNG ABSCESS

Necrosis of pulmonary tissue with associated infection is the principal distinction between a lung abscess and an infected bulla (pyocyst) or an infected bronchogenic cyst. Table 17-6 shows a classification of pulmonary abscesses based on the precipitating event.

Although it is uncommon, primary pneumonias with bacterial species that are noted for their necrotizing ability may proceed to abscess formation. Postpneumonic abscesses of this type are frequently located in the upper lobes and may simulate tuberculous cavities in a chronic phase. In infants and young children the *Staphylococcus aureus* is most frequently associated with an acute course that rapidly proceeds to abscess formation and pleural empyema. Aspiration of gastric contents followed by

Table 17-6. CLASSIFICATION OF
LUNG ABSCESSES

A. Infection by specific necrotizing organisms
   1. Aerobic infection
      a. *Staphylococcus aureus*
      b. *Klebsiella pneumoniae*
      c. *Mycobacterium tuberculosis*
   2. Anaerobic infection
      a. *Bacteroides fragilis*
      b. *Bacteroides melaninogenicus*
      c. *Fusobacterium fusiformis*
      d. *Actinomyces*
B. Abscess following aspiration pneumonia
C. Abscess following pulmonary embolism
   1. Septic pulmonary emboli
   2. Infection of pulmonary infarct
D. Abscess following pulmonary trauma
   1. Infected hematoma
   2. Contaminated foreign body
E. Abscess due to bronchial obstruction
   1. Neoplasm
   2. Foreign body
F. Abscess due to extension from hepatic, subphrenic, or mediastinal abscess

pneumonia is probably the commonest mechanism of lung abscess at present, and the association with alcoholism is well-known (Fig. 17-54). An overdosage of drugs, general anesthesia, and vomiting associated with trauma are alternate items that may be significant in the patient's history. Abscesses that follow aspiration are usually located posteriorly and in the lower lobes. Retained foreign material (undigested food) is infrequent, but occasionally the endoscopist or the pathologist examining a resected lobe is surprised to find material that seemingly could have been expelled by coughing.

Lung abscesses due to septic emboli do not have a characteristic location but are distinguished by their association with septic pelvic, peritoneal, or musculoskeletal disorders. These abscesses are typically small, multiple, and bilateral. Infection developing in a pulmonary infarct is likely to lead to empyema as often as it produces a pulmonary abscess.

Rarely a pulmonary abscess will develop about a retained metallic fragment or other foreign material carried into the lung by a penetrating injury. The presence of foreign material is not necessary, however, if a parenchymal hematoma has been produced by the trauma, either penetrating or nonpenetrating.

Partial or complete bronchial obstruction is associated with pulmonary abscess frequently enough to make it mandatory that patients have bronchoscopy soon after management has begun. The cause of obstruction may be a bronchial neoplasm, bronchial stenosis from previous inflammatory disease, or trauma, and rarely, a foreign body. A question of the relationship between infected gums and teeth and the occasional development of an otherwise unexplained lung abscess remains unanswered. Such patients are usually found to have a generally accepted cause of their pulmonary infection if the history is sufficiently detailed.

A lung abscess usually forms communications with multiple bronchi as it develops, and the necrotic, purulent

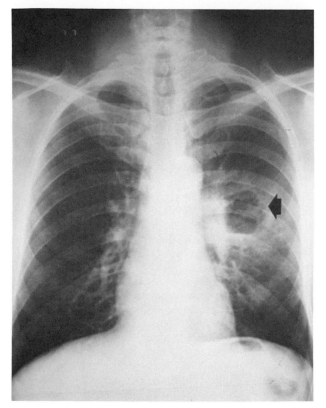

A

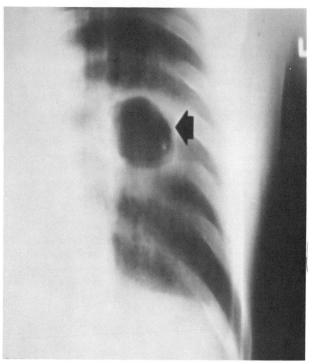

B

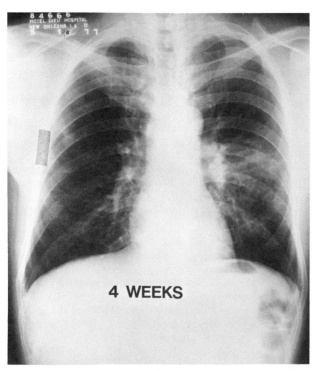

C

Fig. 17-54. Lung abscess due to vomiting and aspiration after an alcoholic binge. *A.* The posteroanterior chest x-ray shows an abscess cavity in the superior segment of the left lower lobe. *B.* A tomogram confirms the thin wall of the abscess and reduces the likelihood that the lesion could be a cavitated carcinoma. *C.* After 4 weeks of antibiotic therapy the abscess appears to be healing.

contents are intermittently discharged in the sputum. A zone of inflammatory consolidation continues to surround the abscess cavity as it passes to a chronic stage. Unfortunately, an abscess ignores the vague segmental boundaries within a lobe, and slow parenchymal destruction can necessitate complete lobectomy if operative resection is required. The diagnosis is usually made on the basis of clinical manifestations of pulmonary infection, foul or putrid sputum, and the roentgenographic demonstration of a lesion with an air-fluid level. If the latter is absent and the patient is a smoker beyond thirty-five years of age the pressure may mount to differentiate the lesion from a bronchogenic tumor. Even when an air-fluid level is shown on the chest x-ray, the abscess can be difficult to distinguish from a cavitated epidermoid carcinoma. Occasionally, a cavitated pulmonary mycosis can mimic lung abscess, as can infected congenital lesions such as bronchogenic cysts and intralobar sequestration.

The treatment of lung abscess is based on intense antibiotic therapy combined with techniques to promote bronchial drainage of the abscess cavity. As mentioned, diagnostic bronchoscopy should be done early. Formerly, repeated bronchoscopy at intervals of several days to a week was advocated to promote bronchial drainage. Postural drainage, chest physical therapy, appropriate use of bronchodilators, and, occasionally, special procedures such as the endotracheal placement of an aspirating catheter in children should be adequate for 80 to 90 percent of patients. Occasionally a surgical emergency is created when a patient's abscess ruptures into the pleural cavity to form a pyopneumothorax. Tube thoracostomy for drainage of the pleural cavity is required initially, but the formation of a chronic bronchopleural fistula may necessitate pulmonary resection.

Failure of the patient to respond to medical management by loss of systemic signs of infection, and lack of beginning resolution of the abscess are the principal indications for surgical intervention. If the patient is not critically ill, several weeks may be allowed for a determination of the response. Surgical treatment may consist either of *pneumonotomy,* for drainage of the abscess, or *pulmonary resection.* Pneumonotomy is a technique of direct drainage of the abscess through the chest wall after subperiosteal resection of a short rib segment overlying the abscess. Although performed infrequently, pneumonotomy is especially valuable for debilitated or elderly patients for whom lobectomy would seem to have a high risk. The result may be excellent, with subsequent rapid reduction in the ab-

Fig. 17-55. An oblique view of a left-sided bronchogram shows bronchiectasis of the basal segmental bronchi.

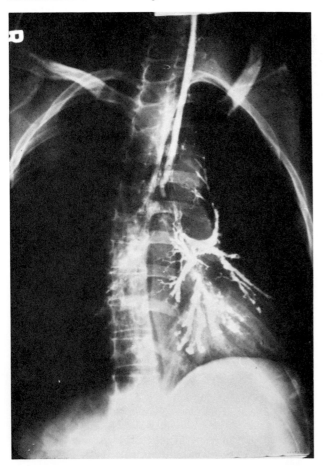

scess cavity. Healing of the track through the chest wall generally requires several months as the drainage tubes are gradually shortened.

Resection of a pulmonary abscess generally requires lobectomy, and care must be taken with the induction of anesthesia or positioning of the patient to prevent a spill of the abscess contents into the contralateral lung. Because an abscess can extend across an interlobar fissure to involve the adjacent lobe, it is important to recognize the need for surgical treatment before a more extensive resection might be required.

BRONCHIECTASIS

Bronchiectasis is a complex of pulmonary and bronchial infection characterized by bronchial dilatation. It encompasses a spectrum of disease with involvement of bronchi at several levels, primarily the segmental and subsegmental bronchi and their branches (Fig. 17-55). The basal segments of the lower lobes, the lingula, and the right middle lobe are the principal areas of involvement. Upper-lobe involvement (other than the lingula) is unusual except as a complication of preceding conditions such as tuberculosis. Bronchiectasis may follow partial obstruction of any bronchus due to a variety of causes, i.e., foreign body, neoplasm, extrinsic pressure. An example of this variation is the so-called *middle-lobe syndrome,* in which compression of the middle-lobe bronchus by enlarged peribronchial lymph nodes leads to destructive infection of the segmental bronchi. Lobar atelectasis and peribronchial fibrosis accompany the chronic infection, with resultant destruction of the lobe if the process is not reversed by early reexpansion (Fig. 17-56).

There has been a wealth of literature on the pathogenesis of bronchiectasis, but the singular fact remains that the cause of the average case is unknown. For each patient who presents with the disease it is pertinent to look for features that may signal the likelihood of a special variation such as bronchial obstruction or Kartagener's syndrome (situs inversus, pansinusitis, and bronchiectasis).

The bronchial changes may vary in severity from a mild tubular or cylindrical dilatation to cystic or saccular structures that are no longer recognizable as bronchi. The cystic dilatations almost always contain residual mucus with varying amounts of debris or purulent material, depending on the infection status. Broncholiths are occasionally found in the destroyed bronchi, and they may be associated with active ulceration. Fibrosis surrounding the diseased bronchi along with retained secretions may lead to a progressive loss of volume in the involved pulmonary segment.

Bronchiectasis is diagnosed in both sexes throughout the entire age spectrum from infancy to old age. Its highest incidence seems to range from late childhood through the fourth decade in varying regions of the world. The complications of recurrent pneumonia, hemoptysis, and metastatic infection such as cerebral abscess often precipitate an effort to confirm the suspected diagnosis. Retarded physical development, digital clubbing, and voluminous sputum production are sometimes allowed to progress for remarkable periods before medical attention is sought.

Although the diagnosis may be strongly suspected on the

basis of the clinical history and changes seen in the standard posteroanterior and lateral chest x-ray, bronchography is the definitive diagnostic procedure. Bronchoscopy should precede the contrast study to determine the presence of bronchial obstruction or foreign bodies and to obtain material for cultures. If the patient has a large sputum production it is appropriate to gain control of the infection and reduce the volume of secretions before attempting bronchography. Excessive secretions will interfere with an accurate mapping of the bronchial tree, the most critical feature of the diagnostic work-up.

The initial treatment of bronchiectasis consists of medical management with a goal of assessing the severity of the disease, the extent of pulmonary involvement, and the response to antibiotic therapy combined with postural drainage (Fig. 17-57). Especially in children there are often a generalized bronchitis and an evolving development of the bronchiectasis which are best handled by avoiding a premature decision for operation. An ideal candidate for surgical resection is the older child or adult whose disease is localized to one lobe or to one lobe on each side. Patients with simple cylindrical bronchiectasis can often be managed satisfactorily without surgical treatment. With advanced bronchial destruction to the stages of saccular or cystic disease, the involved pulmonary segments cannot function normally and represent greater liabilities than assets to the patient (Fig. 17-58). If the disease is sufficiently localized, these anatomic changes alone are adequate indications for operation. Recurrent pneumonia, hemoptysis, sputum production that interferes with the patient's ability to enjoy normal activities, and the general debilitating effects of chronic infection are the principal indications for pulmonary resection.

A maximum effort should be made to reduce sputum volume and infection prior to operation. Segmental resections are the procedures of choice, especially when more than one lobe is involved and bilateral disease is present. Postoperative care must be meticulous to reduce problems of atelectasis, pneumonia, and empyema. The results of a well-planned medical and surgical program should be satisfactory in more than 75 percent of patients.

TUBERCULOSIS

The development of effective chemotherapy and its influence on the course of pulmonary tuberculosis have to be

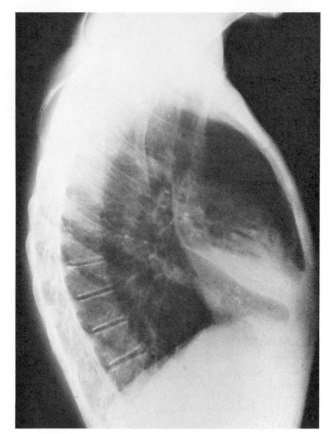

Fig. 17-56. This lateral chest x-ray shows a wedge-shaped density overlying the cardiac shadow and corresponding to a collapsed middle lobe. Resection of the fibrotic lobe showed marked bronchiectasis of the segmental bronchi (middle-lobe syndrome).

counted among the remarkable accomplishments of the past quarter-century. As evidence that the disease is still with us is the fact that more than 30,000 new cases of active tuberculosis were reported in 1975. The surgical significance of this new case rate is a great deal different, however, than it would have been in 1955. During that era the

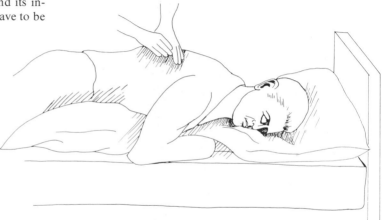

Fig. 17-57. Postural drainage combined with chest physical therapy is important in the medical management of bronchiectasis and in the preoperative care of patients who require pulmonary resection.

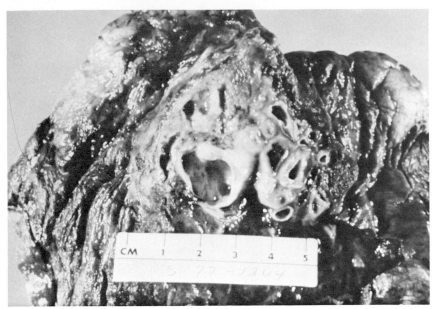

Fig. 17-58. The cut section of this right lower lobe shows one of several cystic bronchiectatic cavities with surrounding localized pneumonia.

surgical treatment of pulmonary tuberculosis required a significant amount of the available thoracic surgical manpower. In fact, the development of thoracic surgery was inseparably linked with the development of effective surgical techniques for the management of tuberculosis. Presently, the relatively few patients that are considered for operative treatment are insufficient to assure adequate experience with the disease for many thoracic surgery training programs.

Surgical techniques are rarely required in the treatment of first-infection ("childhood") tuberculosis. When there is a need, it is generally directed at complications such as massive pleural effusion or compression of mediastinal structures by enlarged lymph nodes (i.e., middle-lobe syndrome). Among patients with reinfection tuberculosis it is estimated that pulmonary resection will be indicated in about 1 percent of those undergoing first treatment with drug therapy, and in 5 percent of individuals receiving retreatment.

Fig. 17-59. Pulmonary tuberculosis, active. A. The posteroanterior chest x-ray shows an infiltrative lesion with pleural thickening at the left apex. B. A tomogram suggests cavitation in the lesion.

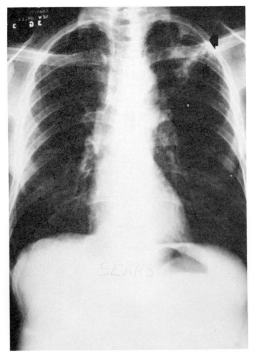

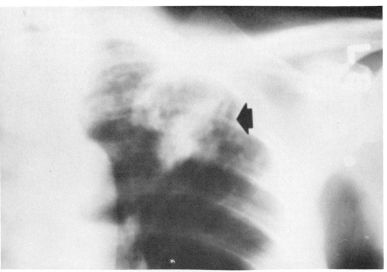

A   B

The typical lesion of reinfection tuberculosis begins as a bronchopneumonia in the apical or posterior segments of an upper lobe, less frequently in the superior segment of a lower lobe. Caseous necrosis occurs to a variable extent, along with an exudative reaction. A successful response by the patient, with or without drug therapy, may lead to resolution with predominant scar formation and some communication with bronchi (Fig. 17-59). If caseation is extensive, fibrous tissue is formed at the periphery and in multiple locules, producing a cavity in communication with the bronchi that provide its drainage. According to the patient's resistance to the continued growth of the *Mycobacterium tuberculosis* and the antibiotic effect of the chemotherapy regimen, the cavity may stabilize or continue to enlarge. Occasionally, a cavity undergoes rapid expansion as the result of air entrapment by stenotic bronchi (tension cavity).

With control of the organism and stabilization of the cavity an ingrowth of epithelium may occur. Thickening of the fibrous tissue follows, with eventual contraction and partial or complete obliteration of the cavity. In some patients, however, little contraction occurs and the cavity remains open—the so-called "open-negative" cavity that formerly was the subject of much debate over its validity as an indication for pulmonary resection.

Though bronchial artery branches in the walls of a cavity may be the source of significant hemoptysis, the life-threatening hemorrhages of tuberculosis are more often from the pulmonary arteries. The latter may become involved by the necrotizing process in the formation and expansion of tuberculous cavities, and fistulas may develop between bronchi and major pulmonary arterial branches. A dilated pulmonary artery branch which protrudes into the lumen of a cavity is referred to as a Rasmussen aneurysm.

In some patients a tuberculous bronchitis develops in the bronchi draining an active parenchymal lesion. The response to chemotherapy is usually good, but the destruction of tissue may result in bronchial stenosis. Another bronchial sequela, tuberculous bronchiectasis, is thought by many to be the result of traction on the bronchial wall during the healing of extensive parenchymal lesions. In these circumstances it is not necessary that the wall of the bronchus be involved by the actual tuberculous process.

It is important to remember that pulmonary tuberculosis can produce a variety of lesions in the lungs and that the lesions may vary in their location (Fig. 17-60). In the absence of cavitation, and without acid-fast bacilli in the sputum smears, a parenchymal lesion may be indistinguishable from bronchogenic carcinoma by x-ray studies. This is particularly the case with tuberculomas, and the latter are often removed because they present as solitary undiagnosed lesions. Improvements in diagnosis by bronchial brushing, flexible bronchoscopy, and percutaneous needle biopsy have reduced the number of patients who undergo thoracotomy and resection for diagnostic pur-

Fig. 17-60. Pulmonary tuberculosis, active. *A* and *B*. A large mass in the left upper lobe that was associated with marked atypia of cells obtained by bronchoscopy, and negative sputum smears for acid-fast bacilli. The resected lobe showed active tuberculosis without cavitation.

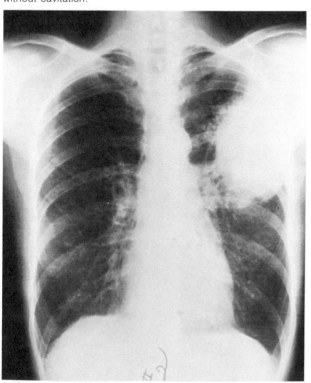

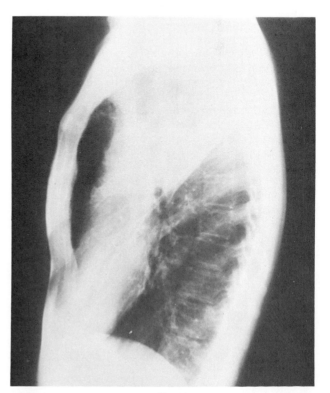

A   *B*

poses. Skin testing for tuberculosis can be helpful in the diagnosis, but only if the patient's previous status is known. A high percentage of patients with bronchogenic carcinoma have a positive tuberculin skin test, but no more than 5 percent of individuals with active pulmonary tuberculosis have a negative test if the procedure is done properly.

The deliberate, planned surgical treatment of tuberculosis is based on pulmonary resection after a period of drug therapy. In most instances lobectomy or segmentectomy is the procedure of choice. Pulmonary destruction is so extensive in an occasional patient that only pneumonectomy will suffice. The principal indications for resection are (1) extensive pulmonary destruction with bronchopleural fistula and empyema, (2) persistently active disease with drug-resistant organisms, (3) open-negative cavitary disease in selected irresponsible patients, (4) posttuberculous bronchostenosis with recurrent nontuberculous infections, (5) pulmonary hemorrhage, and (6) suspected (or proved) concomitant bronchogenic carcinoma.

Collapse therapy, consisting either of thoracoplasty or pneumonolysis, preceded pulmonary resection as a practical surgical approach to the treatment of tuberculosis. These techniques are inferior to resection, but an occasional patient with significant loss of pulmonary function and persistently positive sputum may not be a proper risk for removal of pulmonary tissue. In these circumstances thoracoplasty may be appropriate. An extrapleural removal of the necessary number of ribs may be done in two stages.

Pulmonary disease produced by acid-fast bacilli that are referred to as *atypical mycobacteria* has gained relative prominence in recent years. The two groups that are primarily responsible for pulmonary lesions are listed in Table 17-7, along with two additional groups that are principally associated with nonthoracic disease. Although the atypical mycobacteria are easily confused with *M. tuberculosis* in smears, they can be differentiated by their specific cultural and biological characteristics. *Mycobacterium kansasii* infections are seen predominantly in the Middle West, the Southwest, and California, while patients with disease due to the Battey bacillus are mostly located in the Southeast.

The pulmonary lesions caused by the atypical mycobacteria may be clinically and radiographically indistinguishable from those due to *M. tuberculosis*. Histologic studies of resected tissue may show characteristics suggesting the atypical causation, or the lesions may resemble straightforward tuberculosis.

The important difference is due to the resistance of the atypical mycobacteria to antituberculous drugs, and to their different skin test characteristics. Chemotherapy must be based on the results of sensitivity studies of the cultured mycobacteria, and three or four drugs are commonly used for initial treatment. Prolonged therapy of 2 to 4 years is generally anticipated. The indications for surgical treatment are approximately the same as for patients with infection due to *M. tuberculosis,* but a higher percentage will require resection because of drug failure.

ACTINOMYCOSIS AND NOCARDIOSIS

Clinical infection due to the actinomycetes occurs infrequently despite the wide and abundant distribution of the organisms. The *Actinomyces* are anaerobic or microaerophilic organisms; the *Nocardia* are obligate aerobes that show an acid-fast characteristic in sputum or tissue smears.

Actinomycosis is characterized by seemingly indolent, burrowing tissue invasion that leads to the formation of sinus tracts, abscesses, and fistulas. Considerable care may be required to identify the *Actinomyces israelii* by anaerobic cultures, and there is presently no serologic or skin test to allow confirmation of a suspected diagnosis. The oftenmentioned "sulfur granules" consist of colonies of the organism in which the filaments are coated with proteinaceous material.

The bulk of cases involve the craniofacial tissues or the abdomen, and only 15 percent of patients have pulmonary actinomycosis. Because the organism is so often found in the tonsillar crypts or other areas of the mouth it is assumed that the usual portal of entry is by bronchial aspiration. Embolic spread from other areas is also possible, as well as direct extension into the thorax. From an initial lesion of pneumonic consolidation the disease can extend to involve the pleura, mediastinum, and chest wall, with eventual discharge of an abscess through a cutaneous sinus if not treated. The chest x-ray generally shows a nonspecific pulmonary consolidation, sometimes with cavitation (Fig. 17-61).

Penicillin in doses in 6 to 12 million units daily forms the basis of treatment, but erythromycin may be used for those patients who cannot take penicillin. Pulmonary resection is not usually required, although an occasional patient undergoes operation because the lesion is an undiagnosed infiltrate compatible with neoplasm. Drainage of empyema or chest-wall abscesses may be needed, and sinus tracts may be biopsied to establish the diagnosis.

Nocardiosis occurs predominantly in males, and the majority have thoracic involvement. A pulmonary infiltrate or consolidation is the usual beginning lesion. *Nocardia aster-*

Table 17-7. CLASSIFICATION OF ATYPICAL MYCOBACTERIA

Group	Example	Principal lesion
I. Photochromogens.....	*Mycobacterium kansasii*	Pulmonary disease
II. Scotochromogens.....	*Mycobacterium scrofulaceum*	Cervical lymphadenitis
III. Nonchromogenic	*Mycobacterium intracellulare* (Battey bacillus)	Pulmonary disease
IV. Rapid growers........	*Mycobacterium marinum*	Swimming pool skin granuloma

oides may gain a foothold after prolonged steroid therapy for other conditions, or following vigorous chemotherapy for infections or neoplasms. Characteristically, the *Nocardia* produces a more acute infection than the *Actinomyces,* with necrosis and abscess formation. Hemoptysis occurs in a quarter of the patients, and metastatic involvement of the central nervous system is common. The patient can present with a mass in the chest wall from the progressive extension of the pulmonary lesion. Again, the chest x-ray is nonspecific and the infection may resemble either neoplasm or tuberculosis.

Surgical resection is rarely required, and when it has been performed the underlying reason has generally been that of providing a diagnosis for an individual at risk for lung cancer. Either sulfadiazine or sulfamerazine is the drug of choice, and the majority of lesions respond satisfactorily to a prolonged course of the drug.

FUNGOUS INFECTIONS

Pulmonary infections due to fungi are generally in the form of chronic granulomatous lesions that resemble tuberculosis. Their roentgenographic appearance often raises the possibility of a neoplasm and makes it necessary to follow an aggressive course for diagnosis. An increased use of steroid therapy and antibiotics has been blamed for a greater incidence of generalized fungous infections in recent years.

Histoplasmosis must be considered the most frequent pulmonary mycotic infection in this country because of the estimated millions of persons who are said to have a positive skin test. The disease has a high incidence of subclinical infection in the Mississippi and Ohio River Valleys, as reflected by the pulmonary and hilar lymph node calcifications that represent healed or arrested disease. Erosion of a calcified lymph node into a bronchus may occur rarely, with the production of hemoptysis. A *broncholith* produced by this mechanism can obstruct the bronchial lumen and result in segmental or lobar suppuration. The *Histoplasma capsulatum* may produce a rounded solitary granuloma with a necrotic center that grossly resembles a tuberculoma. Figure 17-62 shows a histoplasmoma that was resected from a forty-two-year-old construction engineer who moved to the Ohio Valley a year earlier. An attempt at diagnosis by percutaneous needle biopsy had failed. His skin test and the complement-fixation titer both were positive, but he was a heavy smoker with a family history of lung cancer. Drug therapy is generally not required for localized lesions, whether or not they are resected.

A rare patient develops a progressive granulomatous and cavitary form of histoplasmosis that resembles tuberculosis in many respects. The lesions are predominant in the upper lobes and frequently bilateral. Sputum smears may show the organisms, and the diagnosis is supported by a rising complement-fixation titer. Untreated, this form of the disease can progress to a fatal outcome. However, amphotericin B is effective in the great majority of cases, and slow healing may follow a prolonged course of therapy to maximum dosage. For the patient whose sputum remains positive, and for those who develop bronchiectasis or major hemoptysis, pulmonary resection is indicated.

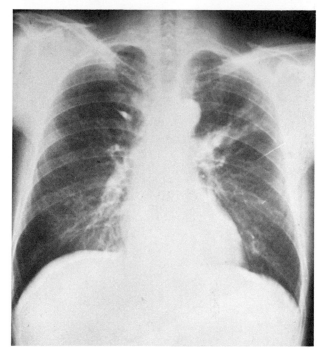

Fig. 17-61. The chest x-ray in this patient with proved pulmonary actinomycosis shows an infiltrate in the anterior segment of the left upper lobe.

North American blastomycosis is seen principally in the Central and Southeastern United States as a mycotic disease with pulmonary involvement alone, with cutaneous lesions, or with any combination of pulmonary, skin, and systemic disease. The *Blastomyces dermatitidis* can be demonstrated in the sputum and in pus or scrapings from skin lesions. Granulomatous lesions in the lungs may become confluent with cavitation. On the chest x-ray the findings may be an infiltrate, a perihilar consolidation, or a lesion with multiple cavities that can resemble tuberculosis. The pulmonary lesion may be mistaken for a bronchogenic neoplasm (Fig. 17-63), and it can extend into the mediastinal structures.

The diagnosis is often made because of modest respiratory symptoms and chest x-ray findings that prompt a complete work-up. A complement-fixation test is available that shows increasing titers with a pulmonary lesion. The blastomycin skin test is of limited value because patients with well-developed lesions often fail to react to the antigen. Chemotherapy with either 2-hydroxystilbamidine or amphotericin B is effective in almost all patients. Resection is occasionally indicated if there is a strong suspicion of malignancy or if there is no response to drug therapy.

Coccidioidomycosis is another fungal disease with principal pulmonary involvement and a strong geographical association. *Coccidioides immitis* is distributed in the Southwest, including California, and the fungus may produce a subclinical infection sufficient to convert the skin test to positive. An acute bronchopulmonary disease ("valley fever") and granulomatous lesions that have considerable resemblance to tuberculosis are additional forms of the disease. The diagnosis is suggested by residence or even

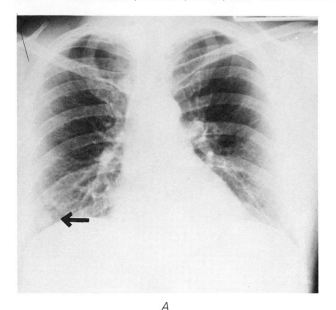

A

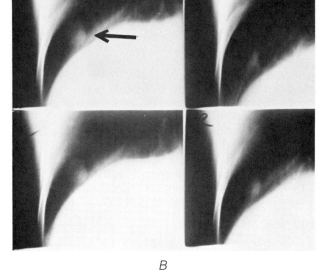

B

Fig. 17-62. Histoplasmosis. *A*. The posteroanterior chest x-ray shows a faint round lesion in the right lower lobe. *B*. Tomograms demonstrate the lesion clearly and show its sharp borders. *C*. The lesion was removed by wedge resection; the cut surface shows a histoplasmoma.

C

a brief visit in the endemic area coupled with a rising complement-fixation titer, a positive skin test, and the presence of the organisms in the sputum.

The mainstay of treatment for progressive coccidioidomycosis is amphotericin B. Pulmonary resection is required when the probability of neoplasm cannot be excluded, and for the management of recurrent hemoptysis, pneumothorax, or progressive cavitation.

The surgical significance of *aspergillosis* is related to the propensity of the *Aspergillus fumigatus* (and a few other species) to invade preexisting pulmonary cavities due to tuberculosis, histoplasmosis, chronic lung abscess, or even neoplasm. An accumulation of mycelia and exudate progressively fills the cavity to form a mycetoma, or "fungus ball," which can be recognized radiographically by a thin rim of air surrounding the mass (Fig. 17-64). Recurrent hemoptysis is often associated with this form of aspergillosis, and it may necessitate pulmonary resection. For those

patients with compromised pulmonary function the significance of the blood spitting must be carefully judged. If pulmonary resection seems formidable, a trial of amphotericin B may be warranted. An alternate or subsequent treatment is the performance of cavernostomy by which the cavity can be evacuated through the chest wall and a portal established for dressings and topical chemotherapy. While management of this type is time-consuming it may give excellent results.

Cryptococcosis is best known for the serious central nervous system infections that are its hallmark. The lungs are the usual route of infection with the *Cryptococcus neoformans,* and occasionally an infiltrative or solitary nodular lesion is removed because of a suspicion of malignancy. Other organisms, including *Candida albicans, Sporotrichum schenkii,* and *Geotrichum candidum,* are occasionally responsible for pulmonary infections that may proceed to cavitation or to other complications that require consideration for operative treatment. In a high percentage of cases factors such as prolonged steroid therapy, immunosuppression, or diabetes mellitus seem to have an effect on the initiation and course of the disease.

SOLITARY PULMONARY NODULES

A perplexing yet intriguing problem in pulmonary disease is presented by the patient with an asymptomatic solitary pulmonary nodule on the chest x-ray. Also referred to as a "coin lesion," the solitary pulmonary nodule (SPN) is an abnormal density up to 4 cm in diameter and rounded or ovoid in appearance (Fig. 17-65). The lesion may be located in any region of the lung, and to qualify as an SPN it should have delineated margins that need not be pencil sharp. Further, the density should be free of cavitation or associated lung infiltrates. Eccentric flecks of calcium may be present, but lesions that are largely calcified or that have concentric calcium rings are not considered.

The stimulus for a high interest in the patient with an SPN has come from the superior cure rate for bronchogenic carcinoma when pulmonary resection is performed at that stage of its growth. Therefore, when a chest x-ray shows a nodular density not present on previous films, a possibility of neoplasm must be given early consideration. Demonstrating that the lesion is of recent development depends upon the availability of previous chest x-rays, or the official report at the least. Occasionally, the review of an earlier film will show a faint, small lesion that was overlooked originally but now provides an indication of growth rate. When previous x-rays document radiologic stability of a solitary nodule for 2 years or more, this is a strong indication that the lesion is benign.

Unfortunately, the differential diagnosis of an SPN includes many entities, among which are pulmonary hamartoma, granuloma, pulmonary arteriovenous fistula, pulmonary infarct, and benign and malignant tumors. It would be desirable to have a correct diagnosis for every patient, but it is critical only for those with a malignant lesion. Extensive experience with this problem has allowed some basic information to be accumulated: (1) a significant percentage of the nodules will prove to be malignant tumors, either primary or metastatic. In the Veterans Administration–Armed Forces Cooperative Study, 51 percent of the resected lesions were primary bronchogenic carcinoma in patients older than fifty years. The subjects were all males,

and most of them were moderate to heavy cigarette smokers. (2) For patients under the age of thirty-five years the likelihood that a nodule is malignant is only 1 to 2 percent. (3) The great majority of benign nodules are granulomas, some of which prove to be histoplasmosis, tuberculosis, or fungal lesions. (4) Roentgenologic differentiation of benign from malignant lesions is usually not possible. (5) A 5-year cure rate greater than 50 percent can be expected for those peripheral bronchogenic carcinomas that are less than 2 cm in diameter when resected. (6) Resection of solitary metastatic neoplasms may be associated with a significant survival rate. Some difference of opinion exists about the approach to management of patients with an SPN that either was not present on previous x-rays or has increased in size during an interval of several months. With an enthusiasm to improve the cure rate of lung cancer some groups have advocated an early thoracotomy with resection of the lesion for all patients above thirty to thirty-five years of age. Because an aggressive surgical policy results in the removal of a high percentage of benign lesions, others have proposed a conservative approach with greater emphasis on diagnostic techniques and observation. Sputum cytology may yield a diagnosis in fewer than 50 percent of those patients with a primary malignant SPN if an aggressive program is followed. Failure to demonstrate malignant cells does not exclude a neoplasm, however, and bronchial brushing is a more productive technique if the method is available. The increasing skill with flexible fiberoptic bronchoscopy has allowed more widespread use of brush

Fig. 17-63. North American blastomycosis. *A*. The posteroanterior chest x-ray shows a mass in the right field adjacent to the heart border. *B*. The tomogram is consistent with a neoplasm, but pulmonary resection showed active blastomycosis in the middle lobe.

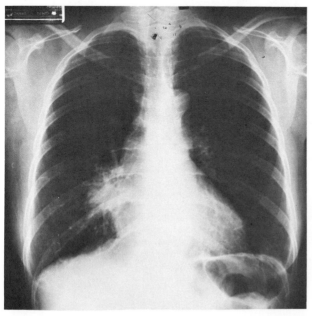

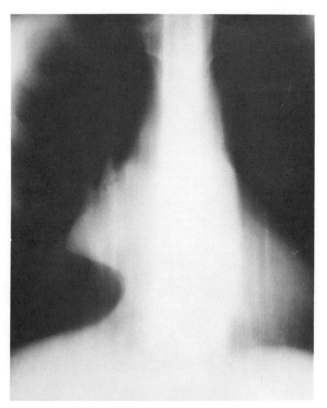

A

B

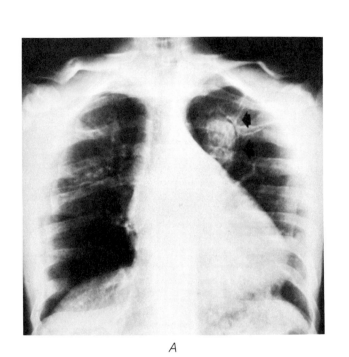

A

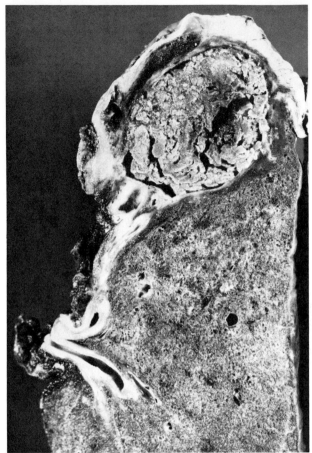

B

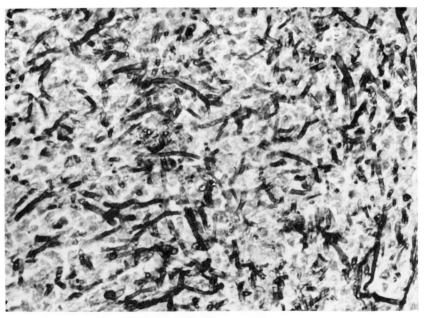

C

Fig. 17-64. A "fungus ball" due to *Aspergillus fumigatus. A.* The lordotic-view chest x-ray shows a probable fungus ball in a patient with recurrent hemoptysis. *B.* A cut section of the resected upper lobe confirms the presence of a fungus ball in an old fibrotic cavity. *C.* The microscopic section of the cavity wall stained for fungi shows the mycelia infiltrating the tissue. (×580).

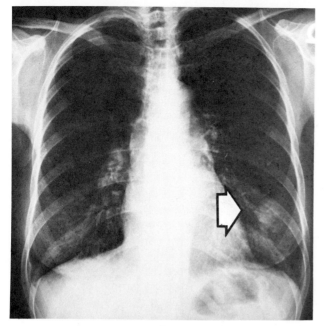

A

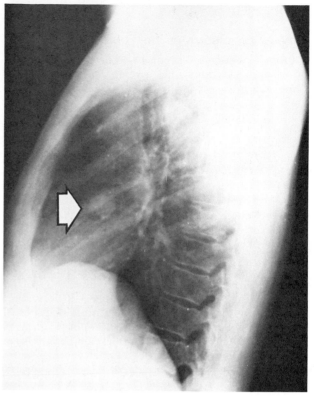

B

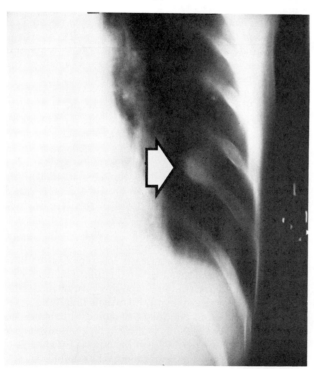

C

Fig. 17-65. A solitary pulmonary nodule. *A* and *B*. The postero-anterior and lateral chest x-rays show a round density in the lingula that had not been present on the patient's previous x-rays. *C*. The lesion is homogeneous, with smooth borders, on tomograms. A wedge resection showed the lesion to be a resolving pulmonary infarct.

biopsy, with a corresponding decrease in the need for diagnostic thoracotomy. Percutaneous needle-aspiration biopsy under fluoroscopic guidance is appropriate for lesions with a diameter of nearly 2 cm or more. If the biopsy material is suggestive, clearly shows a malignant lesion, or is nonspecific, resection is warranted. Only if the aspirated material shows a specific benign process is a plan of ob-

servation warranted in the older patient who smoked cigarettes.

Another approach to the patient with an undiagnosed coin lesion is based on observation of the growth rate of the lesion and calculation of the time necessary for doubling its volume. Serial roentgenograms provide the data for calculation of growth rate, and it is generally possible to detect that a lesion is growing within a few weeks. It has been demonstrated that the doubling time of a malignant nodule is usually between 37 and 465 days. Therefore, if the lesion under review is growing more slowly or more rapidly than this, the evidence is in favor of benignancy. Advocates of a conservative approach insist that present knowledge supports the concept that a pulmonary nodule can be watched safely for a period of time to determine whether it is growing. There has not been widespread acceptance of this method of watchful waiting.

Presently, a reasonable approach includes the concept that if there is a significant chance of malignancy (older patient, large lesion, long smoking history), early thoracotomy is appropriate. If the chance of malignancy is small, then needle biopsy and bronchial brush biopsy are appropriate, with watchful waiting and observation under limited circumstances.

Neoplasms

PRIMARY CARCINOMA OF THE LUNG

From a position of infrequent occurrence before 1900, bronchogenic carcinoma has become the leading cause of death due to cancer in this country. It is estimated that more than 85,000 persons died of lung cancer in 1976. Until the present decade, the disease was infrequent in women, but it now accounts for approximately 5 percent of all female cancer. In addition to the concern caused by its steady increase in frequency, bronchogenic carcinoma has also been disheartening because of its low cure rate. Only 5 to 8 percent of patients survive for 5 years after the diagnosis is confirmed. The remarkable aspect of lung cancer is its clear relationship to cigarette smoking, together with the fact that knowledge of this association has had so little effect on the frequency of tobacco use.

Though it seems certain that 90 percent or more of bronchogenic carcinomas are due to tobacco smoking, it is not so clear why a long period of exposure is generally required. The great majority of patients have smoked cigarettes for more than 20 years when the diagnosis of bronchogenic carcinoma is first made. Equally puzzling is the fact that most smokers do not develop clinical bronchogenic carcinoma, even if they have evidence of severe bronchitis or emphysema. Hundreds of separate organic compounds have been identified in cigarette smoke, and many have been shown to have carcinogenic potential. Since there has been little success in discouraging the smoking habit, considerable research is now directed at altering the composition of cigarette tobacco and the inhaled smoke.

Other studies have implicated chromium, nickel, asbestos, arsenic, radioactive minerals, and hydrocarbon distillates of coal and petroleum in the causation of bronchogenic carcinoma. Individuals working in the mining or processing of these materials may increase their hazard even further by heavy cigarette smoking. A cocarcinogen concept of respiratory viruses working in concert with tobacco smoke to produce bronchial neoplasia has been partly supported by experimental work in the recent past.

PATHOLOGY. Most primary lung carcinomas arise from the surface epithelium of the bronchial tree (bronchogenic). Table 17-8 shows a histopathologic classification of lung tumors developed as a working guide by a panel of the World Health Organization. Noteworthy is the fact that the term *bronchial adenoma,* which formerly referred to bronchial carcinoid, cylindroma, and mucoepidermoid tumors, has been eliminated. The latter two neoplasms are considered to be of bronchial-gland origin.

Several forms of atypical epithelial proliferation are thought to precede pulmonary neoplasms, and the identification of these processes in a patient may heighten the suspicion that a tumor is present. Carcinoma in situ is probably the fully developed expression of squamous metaplasia and dysplasia. These processes have been considered to be a frequent precursor of squamous bronchogenic carcinoma. A type of atypical epithelial proliferation of

Table 17-8. HISTOPATHOLOGIC CLASSIFICATION OF LUNG TUMORS (WHO CLASSIFICATION)

1. Epidermoid carcinoma
2. Small-cell anaplastic carcinoma
3. Adenocarcinoma
4. Large-cell carcinoma
    a. Solid tumors with mucinlike content
    b. Solid tumors without mucinlike content
    c. Giant-cell carcinoma
    d. "Clear"-cell carcinoma
5. Combined epidermoid and adenocarcinoma
6. Carcinoid tumor
7. Bronchial gland tumors
    a. Cylindroma
    b. Mucoepidermoid tumor
    c. Others
8. Papillary tumors of the surface epithelium
9. "Mixed" tumors and carcinosarcomas
10. Sarcoma
11. Unclassified
12. Mesotheliomas
    a. Localized
    b. Diffuse
13. Melanoma

cuboidal or columnar cells is referred to as acinar proliferation. Interstitial fibrosis and honeycombing of the lung are especially associated with this process, and the atypical proliferation develops as a regenerative process lining the remodeled air spaces. Finally, an atypical proliferation of Kultschitzsky cells is associated with development of the carcinoid tumors.

Bronchogenic carcinomas develop twice as frequently in the upper lobes as in the lower lobes, and the neoplasms may be present for several years before symptoms occur. In fact, it has been estimated that a tumor nodule must go through approximately 30 doublings to become 1 cm in diameter, a size that is large enough to be seen on the routine chest x-ray. If true, this could mean that many pulmonary tumors may have been present for as long as 8 years before discovery. Slow growth of this type is most often a characteristic of *epidermoid* (squamous) carcinoma. The epidermoid type of bronchial tumor resembles squamous epithelium and is therefore considered to arise after a preliminary squamous metaplasia has replaced the normal respiratory pseudostratified epithelium. The degree of differentiation in epidermoid neoplasms varies widely, and an occasional lesion is so highly anaplastic that its designation as an epidermoid tumor is speculative. Squamous cell carcinoma has been the most prevalent type of lung cancer in the United States, even though the criteria for classification used by individual pathologists has influenced its incidence at different institutions. Reports from several large medical centers, however, have documented a progressive increase in the incidence of adenocarcinoma, suggesting that it may replace the epidermoid tumor as the leading pulmonary neoplasm.

An epidermoid tumor has a tendency to present either as a central bulky neoplasm associated with bronchial obstruction or as an expanding peripheral lesion that develops cavitation. When centrally located, the tumor may involve the peribronchial and hilar lymph nodes by direct extension rather than by lymphatic permeation. Central necrosis and cavitation may also occur in the tumors that arise near the pulmonary hilum, and evidence of metastases may be absent even with tumors of very large size. When the tumor is located in the periphery, the slow growth rate and late metastasis characteristic of squamous cell carcinoma may allow selected patients to have operative removal for cure even with localized chest-wall invasion. The Pancoast syndrome represents a specific example of this circumstance wherein a tumor in the superior pulmonary sulcus may invade the brachial plexus, the upper two ribs or transverse processes, and the vascular structures at the thoracic apex.

Adenocarcinoma of the lung generally arises in the subsegmental bronchi away from the pulmonary hilum. These tumors are often acinar in structure, with or without mucin production. In the absence of a smoking history or occupational exposure to known bronchogenic carcinogens, a malignant bronchial neoplasm has a high likelihood of this classification. Pulmonary adenocarcinoma is especially prevalent in women, and the age distribution is purportedly greater than that of epidermoid tumors. Growth may be rapid, and early metastasis by the vascular route is common. Occasionally an adenocarcinoma may undergo symmetrical expansion in the lung periphery to reach a size and configuration that led to its designation as a "cannonball" tumor in earlier days. When an adenocarcinoma is anaplastic in appearance the pathologist may be hard-pressed to determine the classification with light microscopy alone. This is also true with other types of bronchogenic carcinoma, and multiple sections taken from separate areas of the same neoplasm may suggest a different classification for each area.

The pulmonary neoplasms that are designated as *bronchioloalveolar* tumors are considered by many to be variants of adenocarcinoma. For years, bronchioloalveolar cell carcinoma has been described as occurring in two forms, localized and diffuse, without a completely satisfactory explanation of the relationship between them. The localized tumor develops as a slowly growing peripheral neoplasm that is highly differentiated. Electron microscopy has been reported to show cellular features suggestive of alveolar origin in some instances, while other tumors have contained atypical Clara cells suggestive of an origin in bronchioles. Resection of the solitary or localized tumor has given a 5-year cure rate of approximately 50 percent. This contrasts remarkably with the diffuse form of bronchioloalveolar cell carcinoma, in which there is rapid dissemination of the neoplasm in one or both lungs, with no possible consideration of operative treatment. While the two forms of this neoplasm may be similar by microscopic appearance, the behavior necessarily raises the issue of whether they are two separate pulmonary tumors. Speculation that the diffuse form could represent uncontrolled metastases from an original single lesion developing after an unknown interval of time has not been corroborated to general satisfaction. Either multicentric origin or some other variant of biologic behavior that sets the diffuse neoplasm apart from the localized tumor seems more plausible.

The *small-cell anaplastic* carcinoma, sometimes referred to as "oat cell carcinoma," is a highly malignant, rapidly growing neoplasm that is most often central in location because of origin from a proximal bronchus. In addition to early spread by hilar and mediastinal lymph-node involvement, this tumor aggressively invades local structures and is disseminated by early vascular invasion. Because of its rapid growth and spread, many consider the oat cell carcinoma to have no place among the bronchogenic tumors that are treated by surgical resection.

Large-cell anaplastic bronchogenic carcinomas may have either a central or a peripheral location similar to epidermoid tumors. Mucin-producing cells are not uncommon, but this is not sufficient to classify these tumors as a variant of adenocarcinoma. Grouped with the large-cell neoplasms are the less common "giant-cell" bronchogenic tumors. The name for these highly malignant cancers is derived from the giant, multinucleated cells that characterize their microscopic appearance.

The term "scar carcinoma" has been used increasingly in recent years to refer to the concept that lung cancer occasionally arises at the site of previous pulmonary disease. This might be considered analogous to the circumstance of skin cancer arising in a burn scar. Therefore, when a patient with previous pulmonary tuberculosis develops a neoplasm in the same area that was scarred by the tuberculous process, there is generally a speculation about the cause-and-effect relationship. The majority of such lesions have been adenocarcinoma or bronchiolar cell carcinoma, but there is not yet convincing proof that the concept is valid.

CLINICAL MANIFESTATIONS. Bronchogenic carcinoma is seen predominantly in men of forty-five to sixty-five years of age with a peak incidence at fifty-five to sixty years. It is not rare in men less than forty-five years old, and the diagnosis is being made with increasing frequency in women who are in their fifth decade. The disease is discovered incidentally in a patient without symptoms in about 5 percent of cases. Such discovery is by means of chest x-ray for the greatest number of patients, but sputum cytology occasionally leads to the eventual identification of an otherwise occult tumor.

Because intermittent or chronic cough is so common among long-term smokers it may be difficult to establish an onset of symptoms. Nevertheless, about three-fourths of patients with bronchogenic carcinoma must be said to have coughing as a principal symptom. Hemoptysis in the form of blood streaking of sputum occurs in about half of all patients, but massive hemoptysis or spitting of blood clots is unusual. Chest pain of a dull, nonspecific type is described by some patients whose tumor is subsequently found to be free of chest-wall involvement. When there is invasion of the parietal pleura or chest wall the patient may have mild to severe pain that is either localized or radicular in form. Fever and purulent sputum may mark an increase of symptoms in the patient whose tumor is producing major bronchial obstruction, and wheezing or stridor may also be present.

Involvement of the left recurrent laryngeal nerve (rarely the right nerve), either by direct tumor invasion or by

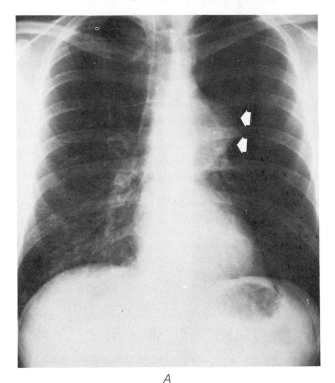

A

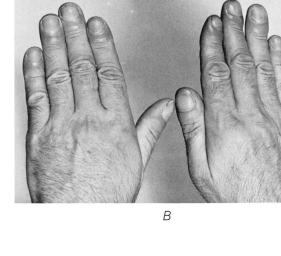

B

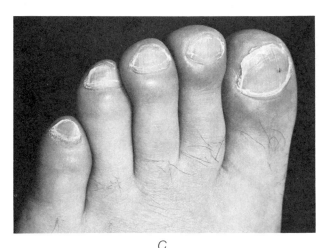

C

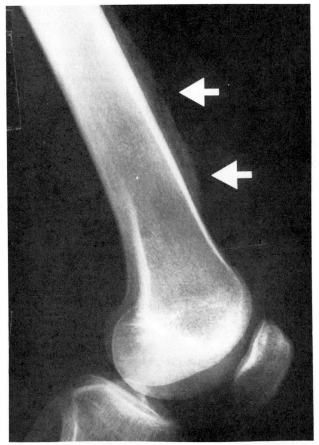

D

extension from a metastatic lymph node, may result in hoarseness that is often minimized by the patient. Direct tumor extension into the superior vena cava or its compression by the expanding neoplasm produces early symptoms of edema of the eyes and prominence or distension of the superficial veins over the upper part of the body. Dyspnea occurring as a symptom of bronchogenic carcinoma is usually associated with a large pleural effusion, paralysis of a hemidiaphragm due to phrenic nerve invasion, or major bronchial obstruction.

A loss of appetite accompanied by weight loss of more than a few pounds is an ominous sign in the patient with a bronchial neoplasm; such patients usually have either an unresectable tumor or systemic metastases. A deliberate

Fig. 17-66. Pulmonary hypertrophic osteoarthropathy associated with oat cell carcinoma. *A.* The chest x-ray in a thirty-nine-year-old man shows a left hilar mass that proved to be oat cell carcinoma on bronchial biopsy. *B.* Painful clubbing of the fingers and toes developed during an interval of approximately 3 months. *C.* A close-up of the patient's foot demonstrates clubbing of the toes. *D.* The arrow points to the new bone formation on the femur.

search should be made for evidence of spread by isotope scanning and computed tomography. Because the metastatic spectrum of these tumors is so wide, almost any imaginable symptom can be produced. A rare patient may develop pulmonary hypertrophic osteoarthropathy with clubbing of the digits (Fig. 17-66). Evidence of metastases may be absent, and the process may be partially reversed if the tumor is resected.

A small percentage of patients with bronchogenic carcinoma present with *extrapulmonary nonmetastatic* manifestations that are considered due to elaboration of hormone-like substances by the neoplastic cells (Fig. 17-67). The occurrence of these signs and symptoms does not imply systemic spread of the bronchogenic tumor, and resection of the lesion is generally associated with a regression of the symptoms. Ultrastructural studies have demonstrated the presence of neurosecretory-type granules in the cells of many anaplastic tumors, and the more striking clinical symptoms are associated with oat cell carcinomas. An example is a Cushing-like syndrome which differs from the classic Cushing's syndrome by an older age incidence, a greater frequency in males, and a more rapid clinical course. The ectopic adrenocorticotropic hormone that has been demonstrated in the oat cell tumors appears indistinguishable from the normal hormone. An inappropriate antidiuresis associated with the anaplastic small-cell carcinoma occasionally results in the symptoms of water intoxication with hyponatremia and increasing cerebral symptoms. The carcinoid syndrome has been reported in a few patients with oat cell carcinoma, and either 5-hydroxytryptamine or 5-hydroxytryptophan may be secreted.

Hypercalcemia caused by a parathormone-like polypeptide has most often been associated with squamous bronchogenic carcinoma. Tender gynecomastia and ectopic gonadotropin secretion have been identified with large-cell anaplastic carcinoma. Satisfactory resection of the squamous neoplasm reverses the hypercalcemia, but it may return if the tumor recurs. A group of carcinomatous neuromyopathies is included in the nonmetastatic manifestations of lung cancer, and their incidence is thought to be as high as 15 percent. The symptoms may be subtle or somewhat overshadowed by the pulmonary complaints. Thus, the patient with bronchogenic carcinoma who mentions weakness along with his cough and chest pain is usually not questioned in detail about the characteristics of the weakness. This is the principal symptom, however, of a myasthenia-like syndrome that is probably due to a defect in neuromuscular conduction. Peripheral and central neuropathies also occur, and their differentiation from the symptoms of metastatic lesions can be important. With the former, pulmonary resection may be possible and result in disappearance of the symptoms.

DIAGNOSIS. In recent years the trend has been toward a maximal effort at obtaining a cytologic or tissue diagnosis of lung carcinoma before subjecting the patient with a suspected tumor to thoracotomy. Even further, mediastinoscopy and mediastinotomy have found increasing use to determine the presence of hilar and mediastinal spread of tumor, with a corresponding decrease in frequency of fruitless exploratory thoracotomy. Unfortunately, bron-

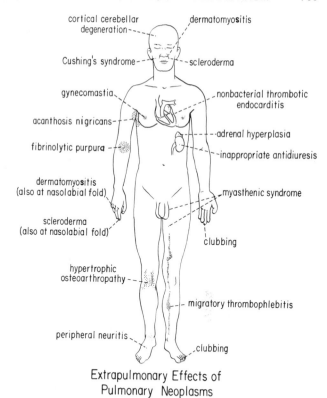

Extrapulmonary Effects of
Pulmonary Neoplasms

Fig. 17-67. Various extrathoracic nonmetastatic manifestations of bronchogenic carcinoma occur, but their frequency varies and they are often overlooked. (*From J. H. Kennedy, Extrapulmonary Effects of Cancer of the Lung and Pleura, J Thorac Cardiovasc Surg, 61:514, 1971, with permission of the author and publisher.*)

chogenic carcinoma has no characteristic or unique radiographic appearance. Therefore, thought must be given to the possibility of carcinoma with almost any type of pulmonary infiltrate, nodule, mass, or atelectasis. A pyogenic lung abscess secondary to aspiration may closely mimic the appearance of cavitated epidermoid carcinoma, even with tomography (Fig. 17-68). Some help with differentiation is obtained when the wall of the cavitated lesion is irregularly thickened with projections of tumor into the cavity. In those incidences when attempts to obtain cytologic evidence of neoplasm have failed, and factors such as young age or alcoholism increase the likelihood of a true abscess, it may be proper to treat the patient for a short interval with antibiotics. Some modest improvement in the appearance of the chest x-ray and the patient's condition does not exclude carcinoma. Close observation must be continued, along with serial studies of sputum cytology.

The cytologic examination of properly obtained and preserved sputum specimens may yield a high percentage of positive diagnoses in patients with bronchial carcinoma. By examining serial daily specimens, often combined with chest physiotherapy to increase the yield of sputum, a cytologic diagnosis may be made in as many as two-thirds of patients. Bronchoscopy is the fundamental diagnostic technique for patients with suspected carcinoma, and the development of the flexible fiberscope has increased the

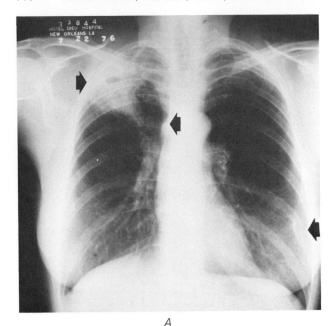

A

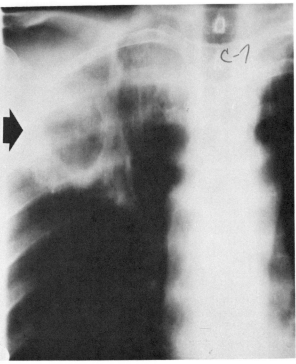

B

Fig. 17-68. Lung abscess masquerading as bronchogenic cancer. *A.* The posteroanterior chest x-ray shows a mass with a small cavity in the right apex, mediastinal lymph nodes (*arrow*). Several healed rib fractures are seen (*arrow*), and the patient was known to be a "social drinker." *B.* A tomogram confirms the presence of a cavity and suggests that the walls are thick. *C.* A chest x-ray 7 months later shows that the abscess has healed with antibiotic therapy. The decision to treat for abscess rather than for lung cancer hinged on the history of alcoholism.

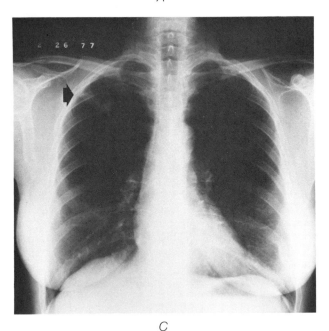

C

positive diagnosis yield to better than 70 percent in some hands. These results include bronchial brushing and cytologic studies of bronchial washings that may be obtained at the same time. The endoscopist must determine the proximal extent of a visualized neoplasm because the patient's operability may be governed by the closeness of the tumor to the tracheal carina.

Small peripheral lesions often present a problem in diagnosis; this was discussed in the preceding section on solitary pulmonary nodules. An infrequent dilemma occurs when a patient is found to have persistently positive sputum cytology without a visible lesion on the chest x-rays. Other sources of the malignant cells, such as the nasophar-

ynx or piriform sinuses, have to be eliminated, and careful flexible bronchoscopic examination may need to be performed at intervals of 4 to 8 weeks. Selective bronchial brushing or selective washing may localize the lesion, but exfoliated cells can become displaced into a bronchus other than the one of origin. This suggests caution in planning a major resection on the basis of these techniques alone.

Percutaneous transthoracic needle biopsy as a technique for obtaining a tissue diagnosis is increasingly accepted for patients who are not considered operable because of tumor extent, evidence of metastases, or general factors such as age. For patients who are considered to be candidates for resection there is widespread resistance to needle biopsy among surgeons. This is based on the possibility of tumor seeding in the pleural cavity or the needle track through the chest wall. Though this rarely happens, many thoracic surgeons are influenced by recollection of a single occurrence. Pneumothorax is the most frequent problem following needle biopsy, but less than half of the patients with this complication require treatment. In a series of 5,300 percutaneous biopsies performed in 2,726 patients, Sinner reported a definitive diagnosis in 90.7 percent, with pneumothorax occurring in 27.2 percent. Two percent of the patients had hemoptysis, and one subcutaneous tumor implant occurred in the more than 1,200 patients with malignant lesions.

A pleural effusion in the presence of a suspected or confirmed pulmonary cancer is generally an indication of extensive tumor that is producing pleural or mediastinal invasion. However, an effusion can occur as a consequence of bronchial obstruction with atelectasis or infection. The fluid should be examined for the presence of blood and malignant cells with a simultaneous pleural needle biopsy if feasible. A demonstration of malignant cells in the effusion occurs in approximately half the patients with visceral or parietal pleural invasion by the neoplasm.

It is unfortunate that approximately 50 percent of all patients with bronchogenic cancer are beyond consideration for operative treatment when the opportunity for definitive diagnosis is first presented. For this reason diagnosis includes a conscientious effort to determine whether localized or metastatic spread has occurred. This is based on a careful history, a meticulous examination for suggestive lymph nodes, and a consideration of how detailed the work-up should be. Some physicians recommend a routine roentgenographic bone survey for all patients who might be considered for operative treatment. This is based on the known incidence of 21 percent skeletal involvement in autopsy series and the frequency of bone metastases in patients who are followed after pulmonary resection. In the absence of skeletal symptoms this has not been sufficiently productive to justify the cost. The same principle applies to the routine use of brain and liver scans. Scanning with radioactive gallium has been disappointing for revealing unsuspected metastases, but some groups use gallium scans to help in the decision to perform mediastinoscopy or mediastinotomy. There should be no hesitancy to utilize any or all of these techniques to survey for metastatic spread in the presence of suggestive symptoms, or if the patient's general condition suggests systemic spread. With any question of a metastasis an attempt at biopsy should be considered before treatment for the primary neoplasm is planned.

TREATMENT. Bronchogenic carcinoma can be cured by pulmonary resection. Though the preceding statement is true, many qualifiers must be added. In general, the factors that determine the likelihood of cure are (1) the cell type, (2) tumor size, (3) lymph-node metastases, (4) direct extension of tumor to adjacent structures, and (5) distant metastases. These factors are the same for malignant neoplasms arising in any region of the body and are listed here to indicate that the approach to treatment depends on an assessment of individual factors as well as the constellation of factors. For example, if bronchoscopic biopsy of the neoplasm shows that it is a small-cell anaplastic carcinoma (oat cell), the majority of surgeons would consider the patient not a candidate for surgery.

Unfortunately, any consideration of operative treatment for cure is impossible in about half of all patients with bronchogenic carcinoma at the time of hospital admission. These patients have centrally located neoplasms with evidence of mediastinal extension, symptoms of distant metastases, or compromised cardiopulmonary function that precludes a major pulmonary resection. A primary goal of the patient's work-up is to confirm the suspected diagnosis of carcinoma by means other than exploratory thoracotomy. Mediastinotomy and mediastinoscopy are occasionally used to obtain a tissue diagnosis in the patient with a pulmonary lesion whose sputum cytology and bronchoscopic procedures have failed to give a positive yield. Thus, there is an overlap of the diagnostic procedures with the techniques for establishing the patient's suitability for operation. Despite a proper application of all reasonable diagnostic procedures, 10 to 20 percent of patients will undergo thoracotomy without a proved diagnosis before operation.

Factors such as the patient's age and tumor extension outside the lung vary in their influence on the decision of individual surgeons to attempt pulmonary resection. Though there is increasing risk of morbidity and mortality for those who undergo major pulmonary resection after sixty years of age, it has been demonstrated that patients of seventy years and beyond tolerate lobectomy with an acceptable mortality rate. Invasion of either the phrenic or the recurrent laryngeal nerve is considered a contraindication to thoracotomy by the majority of surgeons. This is not totally accepted, and because the phrenic nerve involvement is most often along its course over the pericardium, the latter can be resected en bloc with the lung in selected patients.

Direct extension of tumor into the chest wall may be considered a contraindication to attempted resection in the presence of other risk factors. When the tumor is a well-differentiated squamous carcinoma, however, cure is occasionally achieved by localized chest-wall resection, thus justifying an aggressive approach for selected patients.

Though total pneumonectomy would seem to be the ideal operation for bronchogenic carcinoma, it carries a significantly higher mortality rate than lobectomy (Fig. 17-69). For this reason, and because the survivors have a greater ventilatory handicap after the removal of an entire lung, most surgeons have come to accept lobectomy as the procedure of choice for bronchial cancer. This applies only to those patients whose tumor can be adequately removed by lobectomy. Brock has emphasized that a routine adherence to the concept of lobectomy can compromise the chance for cure of some patients. Lobectomy sharply limits the extent of en bloc lymph-node removal that can be performed, and it is clear that hilar and mediastinal nodal metastases have a marked effect on 5-year survival. Radical pneumonectomy, as described by Brock, provides for removal of anterior and posterior mediastinal lymph nodes along with excision of the ipsilateral tracheobronchial nodes. This represents an extensive resection of the lymphatic field, but there is no agreement among surgeons about the selection of patients for the radical procedure. Table 17-9 from a recent report by Lord Brock shows the results in an extensive personal series of patients who underwent lobectomy, simple pneumonectomy, or radical pneumonectomy. The 5-year survival rates are impressive, but the patients who underwent resection represented only a small fraction of all those seen with lung cancer during the study period.

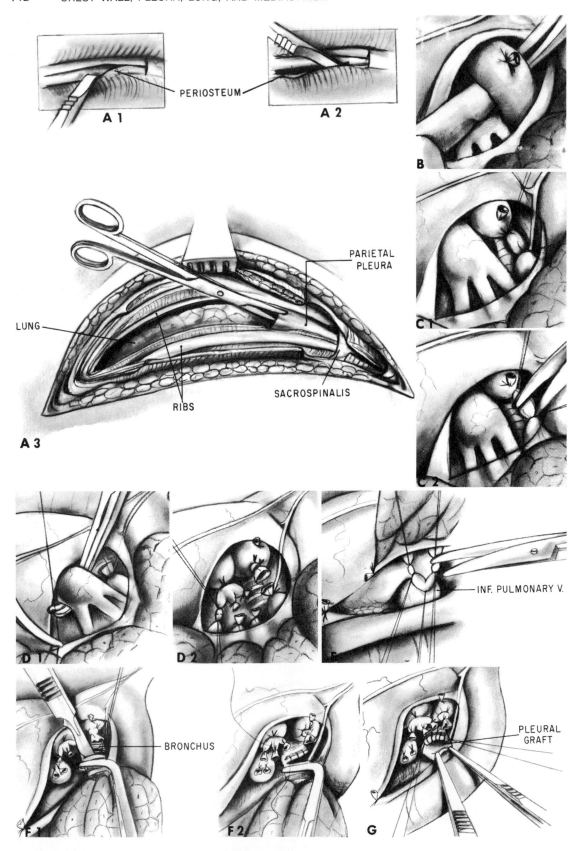

PERIOSTEUM

A 1

A 2

B

PARIETAL
PLEURA

LUNG

SACROSPINALIS

RIBS

A 3

C 1

C 2

D 1

D 2

E

INF. PULMONARY V.

F 1

BRONCHUS

F 2

G

PLEURAL
GRAFT

Table 17-9. COMPARATIVE RESULTS
IN 293 PATIENTS OPERATED ON
FOR BRONCHOGENIC CARCINOMA

Operation	*Total no. of patients*	*Mortality, %*	*5-year survival, %*	*Still alive*
Lobectomy...........	86	3.5	41	10
Simple pneumonectomy.	89	30.00	30	2
Radical pneumonectomy.	118	15.25	39	11
Total	293	13.00	32	23

SOURCE: Reproduced from Lord R. Brock, Long Survival after Operation for Cancer of the Lung, *Br J Surg,* **62**:1, 1975, by permission of the author and publisher.

Not infrequently, the surgeon is confronted with a circumstance in which the patient's neoplasm is relatively small but its growth has obviated the likelihood of cure with less than pneumonectomy. If the patient is young there is usually little hesitancy about removing the entire lung, especially if the pulmonary function studies are satisfactory. For an elderly patient, however, there is greater caution, and the decision may have to be supported by a combination of experience and objective data. Figure 17-70 shows the preoperative chest x-rays of a seventy-one-year-old obese man whose pulmonary function values were as follows:

	Predicted, L	*Observed, L*	*% Predicted*
Vital capacity	4.2	3.5	83
FEV$_1$ second	2.8	2.6	93
Maximal voluntary ventilation	123	149	121
Peak flow	510(L/min.)	560(L/min.)	110

Fig. 17-69. Resection of lung. *A.* Opening into pleural cavity: (1) periosteum incised over the rib; (2) subperiosteal resection being performed; (3) pleura opened through bed of resected rib. *B.* Freeing of pulmonary artery from adjacent structures. *C.* Ligation and division of pulmonary artery: (1) artery doubly ligated with an adequate distance between the two ligatures; (2) artery transected between two ligatures. *D.* Peripheral dissection of pulmonary artery to increase safety factor: (1) branches of pulmonary artery and main pulmonary artery identified; (2) branches individually double-ligated and transected. *E.* Division of pulmonary vein. Double ligatures are on inferior pulmonary vein which is to be transected. *F.* Transection of bronchus. This is performed after ligation of pulmonary arteries and veins. Diagram indicates bronchial transection during a left pneumonectomy. (1) Clamp is applied to bronchus distad, and as the bronchus is transected, the proximal end is closed with interrupted sutures in order to avoid a widely open bronchus with its associated ventilatory disturbance; alternately, the bronchus may be closed with an automatic stapler. (2) Progression of bronchial transection. *G.* Pleural flap placed over sutured bronchial stump.

At operation the upper-lobe tumor had extended across the major fissure to invade the lower lobe. Despite his age and obesity, his excellent pulmonary function and vigorous life-style suggested that he would tolerate pneumonectomy satisfactorily. More than 2 years following removal of his left lung with the epidermoid carcinoma he plays golf three times weekly and has shown no sign of recurrence.

For purposes of contrast, Fig. 17-71 shows the preoperative chest x-rays of a fifty-five-year-old man with a suspected carcinoma in the right pulmonary apex. He was smoking two packages of cigarettes daily and had clinical manifestations of significant chronic airways disease. After 2 weeks of sharply reduced smoking, chest physical therapy, and antibiotic treatment for his bronchitis, the following pulmonary function values were obtained:

	Predicted, L	*Observed, L*	*% Predicted*
Vital capacity.......	4.1	4.1	100
FEV$_1$ second........	3.1	2.0	65
Maximal voluntary ventilation.........	135	70	52

The marked reductions in his expiratory flow rates indicated that pneumonectomy would carry a prohibitive risk if the neoplasm had spread to the hilum. Therefore, a preliminary mediastinotomy was done, and no evidence of tumor was found in the pulmonary hilum or the right mediastinal lymph nodes. A subsequent right upper lobectomy was well tolerated, and the neoplasm was found to be a bronchioloalveolar cell carcinoma without lymph-node involvement.

Paulson has emphasized the great importance of selectivity in the surgical treatment of lung cancer. This requires a maximum use of preoperative evaluation through tomography, mediastinotomy, or mediastinoscopy, occasional pulmonary angiography, and acknowledgment of the differing biologic behavior of the different histologic types. The goal is to avoid exploratory thoracotomy in those patients whose tumor cannot be resected for cure. Figure 17-72 shows a comparison of survival for two 10-year time periods according to the stage of lymph-node involvement. For patients without lymph-node metastases (stage 0) the 5-year survival increased from 31 percent during the first period to 45 percent during the second 10-year era. For those with hilar node involvement (stage 1-2) the 5-year survival rate increased from 22 to 30 percent during the same time frames. Patients with mediastinal nodal involvement (stage 3) had very low survival rates in both decades.

Figure 17-73, also from Paulson's extensive experience, shows a survival comparison according to central or peripheral location of the patient's neoplasm, with relation to the extent of resection. The ability to perform lobectomy for a centrally located neoplasm generally implies a small tumor and a favorable cell type (epidermoid, most frequently). None of the 45 patients who underwent resection for small-cell undifferentiated carcinoma survived for 5 years. Interestingly, in a recent report by Shields, if oat cell

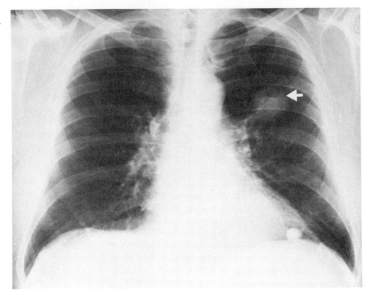

A

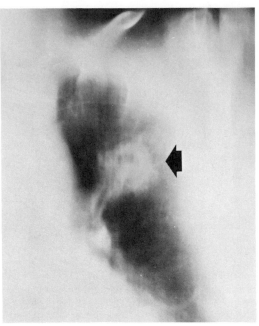

B

Fig. 17-70. *A.* The posteroanterior chest x-ray shows a mass in the left upper lobe that is compatible with pulmonary carcinoma. *B.* A tomogram indicates cavitation in the lesion compatible with epidermoid carcinoma. The diagnosis was confirmed by examination of the resected left lung.

cancer is discounted, the cell type per se had little or no significant influence on survival when curative resection was performed and lymph-node involvement was absent. A barely significant difference was noted in favor of squamous carcinoma when lymph nodes were involved.

A uniform method for staging lung cancer, based on the full definition of the extent of disease, is fundamental to the evaluation of treatment methods. Table 17-10 shows the definitions for tumor size and for lymph-node and distant metastases described by the American Joint Committee for Cancer Staging. From these definitions the extent of the neoplasm in any individual patient may be described as Stage I, II, or III as shown in Table 17-11. General adoption of this system should improve the meaning of reports on treatment results from differing medical centers. The place of radiation therapy in bronchogenic carcinoma is not easily defined. A hope for improved survival by combining preoperative radiation with resection has not been realized for the usual lung cancer patient. A generally recognized exception to this conclusion is the patient with Pancoast's syndrome, in whom preoperative radiation often relieves pain and allows a subsequent resection with a modest chance for long-term survival. Some surgeons also feel that preoperative radiotherapy is of benefit for the patient with chest-wall involvement in any location. Although firm data to prove its efficacy are still lacking, most surgeons request postoperative radiation therapy for those patients whose resection specimens show metastases to the hilar or mediastinal lymph nodes. The most extensive use of radiation therapy in lung cancer is for attempted palliation in those patients with extensive disease that precludes operation, or for those whose neoplasms are unresectable when thoracotomy is performed. In the occasional patient whose disease is still localized in the thorax, prolonged palliation may be achieved. Investigative work on therapy using particles with high linear energy transfer and interstitial implanta-

tion of radioactive ^{125}I is currently under assessment for local control of lung cancer.

Until very recently chemotherapy had little to offer for the patient with bronchogenic carcinoma. Now, the application of multiple-agent therapy has shown success in palliation of the condition of some patients with small-cell anaplastic carcinoma and disseminated epidermoid cancer. The successful chemotherapeutic programs have featured two characteristics: (1) a combination of agents that have shown some activity singly in at least one histologic type of lung carcinoma, but have different pharmacologic actions, and (2) the use of drugs that are active at different points within the cycle of cell division, and which are administered in a fashion to potentiate their cytotoxic activity. The combination of vincristine and bleomycin has proved to be effective for epidermoid carcinoma with use of a drug-scheduling technique that provides sequential administration of vincristine followed by the bleomycin. Other multiple-drug programs that include Adriamycin (doxorubicin HCL), bleomycin, nitrosureas, vincristine, and nitrogen mustard may show effective activity against epidermoid carcinoma as well as small-cell anaplastic cancer in at least 50 percent of patients. Significant palliation is often limited to 15 to 25 percent of patients, but chemotherapy is often used only in the far-advanced cases. At present, effective drug therapy for primary adenocarcinoma and large-cell undifferentiated carcinoma is lacking.

Concepts of adjuvant therapy are not new, and it is very disappointing that an effective systemic control of bronchogenic carcinoma is not available for routine use in those

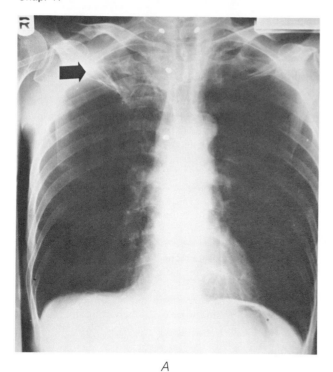

A

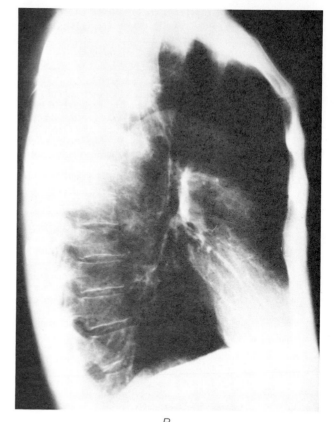

B

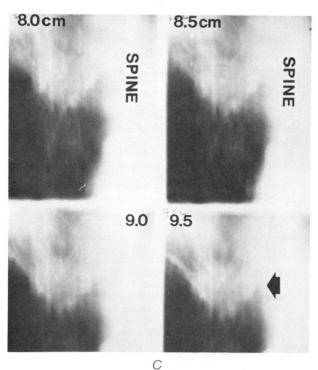

C

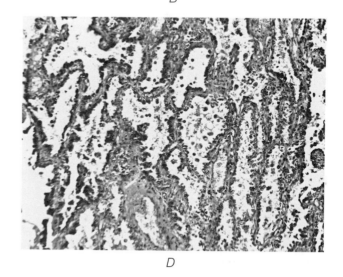

D

Fig. 17-71. *A.* The posteroanterior chest x-ray shows an indeterminate lesion in the right apex of this fifty-five-year-old man with compromised pulmonary function. *B.* A lateral chest x-ray suggests a posterior location of the lesion and radiographic features of chronic lung disease. *C.* A tomogram indicates that the lesion is a solid mass with features of malignancy. *D.* Microscopic examination of the tumor in the lobectomy specimen showed a bronchioloalveolar cell carcinoma. (×250.)

Table 17-10. DEFINITIONS OF T, N, AND M
CATEGORIES FOR CARCINOMA OF THE LUNG

Type	Definition
T—primary tumors:	
T0	No evidence of primary tumor
TX	Tumor proved by presence of malignant cells in bronchopulmonary secretions but not visualized roentgenographically or bronchoscopically, or any tumor that cannot be assessed
TIS	Carcinoma in situ
T1	A tumor 3 cm or less in diameter, surrounded by lung or visceral pleura and without invasion proximal to a lobar bronchus at bronchoscopy
T2	A tumor more than 3 cm in diameter, or any size with visceral pleural invasion or associated atelectasis or obstructive pneumonitis that extends to the hilar region but involves less than the entire lung; at bronchoscopy the proximal extent of tumor must be within a lobar bronchus or at least 2 cm distal to the carina
T3	A tumor of any size with extension into an adjacent structure such as the parietal pleura, chest wall, diaphragm, or mediastinum and its contents; or demonstrated bronchoscopically to involve a main bronchus less than 2 cm distal to the carina; any tumor associated with atelectasis or obstructive pneumonitis of an entire lung or with pleural effusion
N—regional lymph nodes:	
N0	No demonstrable metastasis to regional lymph nodes
N1	Metastasis to lymph nodes in the peribronchial or ipsilateral hilar region, or both, including direct extension
N2	Metastasis to mediastinal lymph nodes
M—distant metastasis:	
M0	No distant metastasis
M1	Distant metastasis such as supraclavicular, or contralateral hilar lymph nodes, lung, brain, etc.

patients who undergo pulmonary resection. Whether systemic therapy will take the form of antitumor agents or enhancement of the patient's innumocompetence is only speculated.

IMMUNOLOGY OF PULMONARY CARCINOMA. Recent studies have emphasized the important but not clearly defined role of immunodeficiency in the prognosis of patients with many forms of cancer. An impaired reaction to delayed cutaneous hypersensitivity testing with 2-4-dinitrochlorobenzene has been demonstrated in many lung cancer patients, and those who are unable to become sensitized to this antigen often have unresectable neoplasms. Impaired lymphocyte transformation with in vitro stimulation by several antigens and mitogens has also demonstrated a marked decrease in immunocompetence in patients with pulmonary carcinoma. One of the mechanisms of immune deficiency is thought to be the presence of circulating immunosuppressive factors in the serum of the lung cancer patient. Whether such factors might be produced by the neoplasm is only speculative. The observation some years ago of improved survival in patients who develop pleural empyema after pulmonary resection for bronchogenic cancer seems to coincide with current concepts. Presumably the mechanism that increased the cure rate in those patients with postoperative empyema was an immunostimulation.

On the basis of the observations just described, clinical trials are under way to evaluate the usefulness of immunostimulation as adjuvant therapy in patients who undergo pulmonary resection for carcinoma. McKneally has utilized intrapleural BCG and shown a significant improvement in the 1-year recurrence rate of tumor. Two other nonspecific immunopotentiators, formalized *Corynebacterium parvum*, and L-tetramisole (levamisole) are being used in clinical trials. The early results are encouraging, and it is possible that combinations of both immunotherapy and chemotherapy may be appropriate to supplement the surgical treatment of bronchial cancer.

BRONCHIAL CARCINOID TUMOR

Carcinoid neoplasms of the bronchus arise from Kultschitzsky-type cells and histologically resemble the carci-

Table 17-11. STAGE GROUPING IN CANCER
OF THE LUNG

Type	Definition
Occult carcinoma:	
TX N0 M0	An occult carcinoma with bronchopulmonary secretions containing malignant cells but without other evidence of the primary tumor or evidence of metastasis to the regional lymph nodes or distant metastis
Stage I:	
TIS N0 M0	Carcinoma in situ
T1 N0 M0	A tumor that can be classified T1
T1 N1 M0	without any metastasis or with
T2 N0 M0	metastasis to the lymph nodes in the ipsilateral hilar region only, or a tumor that can be classified T2 without any metastasis to nodes or distant metastasis
Stage II:	
T2 N1 M0	A tumor classified as T2 with metastasis to the lymph nodes in the ipsilateral hilar region only
Stage III:	
T3 with any N or M	Any tumor more extensive than T2,
N2 with any T or M	or any tumor with metastasis to
M1 with any T or N	the lymph nodes in the mediastinum, or with distant metastasis

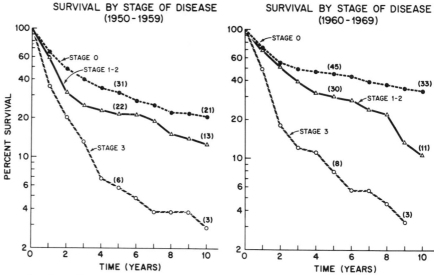

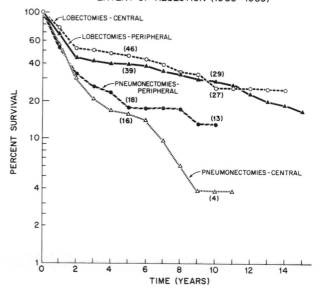

Fig. 17-72. A comparison of survival after operation for patients with lung cancer during two consecutive decades. The staging is based on lymph-node involvement, and for patients with positive hilar nodes the 5-year survival increased from 22 to 30 percent. (*From D. L. Paulson and J. S. Reisch: Long Term Survival after Resection for Bronchogenic Carcinoma, Ann Surg, 184:324, 1976, with permission of author and publisher.*)

noid tumors of the small intestine. Along with cylindroma and mucoepidermoid tumors, the bronchial carcinoid was formerly referred to as a bronchial adenoma. This designation was awkward because the term *adenoma* implied a fundamental quality of benignancy that was not in keeping with the high incidence of malignant behavior shown by cylindroma and mucoepidermoid tumors. Further, a small number of bronchial carcinoids has shown metastases to regional lymph nodes, with the result that reference was occasionally made to "metastasizing bronchial adenomas." The recent classification of lung tumors (Table 17-8) eliminates the designation of adenomas, but many years may be required to discard the term from common usage.

More than 80 percent of carcinoids arise in the major proximal bronchi, but peripheral origin beyond cartilage containing bronchi does occur. The tumors grow slowly and protrude into the bronchial lumen to a degree that makes symptoms and signs of bronchial obstruction the principal form of clinical presentation. Unusual vascularity often is associated with significant hemoptysis as a presenting complaint. In addition, the vascularity gives the tumor a deep pink or red color when visualized through a bronchoscope, and biopsy can result in substantial bleeding (Fig. 17-74).

The extent of bronchial-wall involvement is variable, but there is usually some invasion of the underlying cartilages by the neoplasm. Rarely, a direct extension of tumor through the bronchial wall can result in invasion of adjacent mediastinal structures. Regional lymph-node deposits are found in approximately 10 percent of patients, but liver metastases have been reported in only a few percent. Because bronchial carcinoids and oat cell cancer both are thought to arise from Kultschitzsky-type cells, there has

been speculation about their relationship. In their usual form these two neoplasms are widely separated in character. Nevertheless, a few carcinoids have been reported in which some part of the tumor had an anaplastic appearance. Further, a few patients with a bronchial carcinoid have had a Cushing-like syndrome that seemed attributable to the tumor.

Although the average age of patients with a carcinoid tumor is approximately forty years, the neoplasm does occur in children. Commonly, the clinical presentation is a result of bronchial obstruction with infection and pulmonary atelectasis. Sputum cytology is negative, but more

Fig. 17-73. A comparison of survival after operation for lung cancer based on location of the tumor. (*From D. L. Paulson and J. S. Reisch, Long Term Survival after Resection for Bronchogenic Carcinoma, Ann Surg, 184:324, 1976, with permission of author and publisher.*)

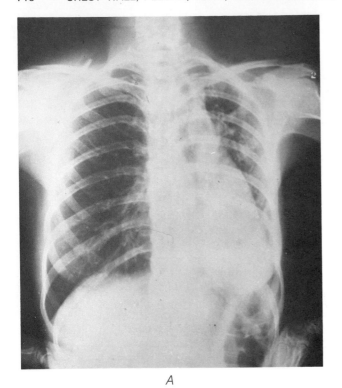

A

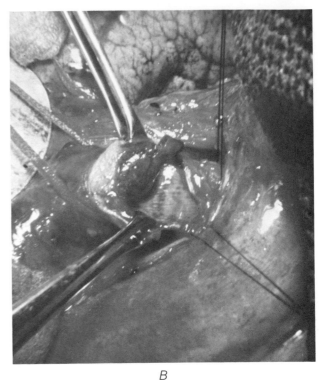

B

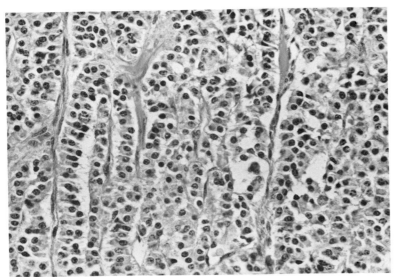

C

Fig. 17-74. A forty-two-year-old woman with a bronchial carcinoid tumor. *A.* The chest x-ray shows collapse of the left lower lobe and shift of the mediastinum to that side. *B.* Bronchotomy of the left stem bronchus confirmed an obstruction of the lower-lobe bronchus by the vascular tumor projecting from the bronchus between the Allis clamps. *C.* Histologic examination of the neoplasm showed it to be a benign carcinoid tumor. (×400.)

than 80 percent of the lesions can be visualized by bronchoscopy. The carcinoid syndrome is produced in a rare patient, but this can occur without extrathoracic metastases. It is wise to measure daily urinary 5-HIAA excretion and blood serotonin level, but these can be clearly elevated without corresponding symptoms.

The only treatment for bronchial carcinoid tumor is surgical resection. Neither the primary neoplasm nor lymph-node metastases are sensitive to radiation therapy. Lobectomy is an acceptable operation, but Jensik has correctly emphasized the low potential for malignancy of the carcinoid neoplasm. He has advocated the use of conservative procedures such as sleeve resection or local bronchial excision with bronchoplasty whenever feasible (Fig. 17-75). Occasionally, a critical location of the neoplasm makes pneumonectomy unavoidable. The mortality rate for operation is low, and the expected long-term survival rate is close to 90 percent.

TUMORS OF BRONCHIAL GLAND ORIGIN

Cylindroma, or adenocystic carcinoma, and mucoepidermoid tumors are the commonest neoplasms arising from the bronchial glands. Their location is predominantly central, and they are said to take origin only from bronchi containing cartilage. Both neoplasms may show a spectrum of behavior from benign to malignant, with regional and distant metastases. The treatment is surgical resection, including en bloc removal of regional lymph nodes when possible. Though the long-term cure rate is considerably higher than that of primary carcinoma of the lung, it does not equal the results in bronchial carcinoid.

Other rare tumors of bronchial gland origin are occasionally reported; the majority seem to be forms of adenocarcinoma.

CARCINOSARCOMA

An interesting but very infrequent group of pulmonary neoplasms are designated as carcinosarcomas because of their mixed components. Both epithelial and mesenchymal types of tissue comprise the neoplasms, and electron microscopy has confirmed that the sarcomatous elements are not simply transformed components of epithelial origin. The term *blastoma* has recently been used for some tumors

that show histologic evidence of association with embryonal tissue.

Carcinosarcomas may be located in the lung periphery or in proximal bronchi, and they have been reported in a wide age range, including children. The treatment is surgical resection, and a cure rate generally exceeding that for bronchogenic carcinoma can be expected.

SARCOMA

A variety of mesodermal sarcomas and tumors of reticuloendothelial origin may occur in the lungs. As a group these tumors represent approximately 1 percent of all primary neoplasms removed at operation. The age range of presentation is considerably wider than that for bronchogenic carcinoma, and the tumors may arise anywhere in the lung or bronchial tree. Difficulty with true histologic identification of the neoplasms is not rare, and they may be mistaken for highly undifferentiated carcinomas or metastatic neoplasms.

In general, the symptoms may be the same as those expected with primary carcinomas, but there is no distinct association with cigarette smoking. When the tumors develop as intrabronchial polypoid neoplasms, the symptoms of bronchial obstruction lead to earlier diagnosis and, therefore, a relatively higher cure rate after resection. Leiomyosarcomas, for example, had a 5-year cure rate of approximately 40 percent in McNamara's report.

Lymphosarcoma and *reticulum cell sarcoma* may rarely develop in the lung without evidence of tumor elsewhere.

Fig. 17-75. Operative procedures to conserve pulmonary tissue in patients with bronchial carcinoid. *A.* Sleeve resection of tumor from left main bronchus. *B.* Superior segmentectomy and middle lobectomy with bronchial anastomosis. (*From R. J. Jensik, L. P. Faber, C. M. Brown, and C. F. Kittle, Bronchoplastic and Conservative Resectional Procedures for Bronchial Adenoma, J Thorac Cardiovasc Surg, 68:556, 1974, with permission of the author and publisher.*)

LEFT BRONCHIAL TREE

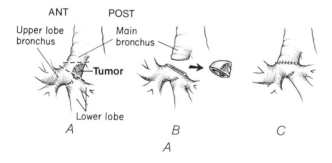

A

RIGHT BRONCHIAL TREE

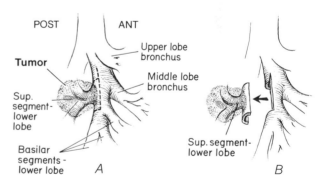

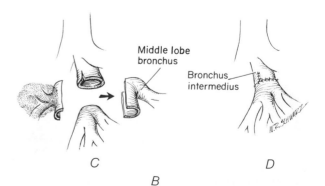

B

Routine chest x-rays discover an asymptomatic pulmonary lesion in a number of patients; other lesions become symptomatic because of pressure of the growing tumor or lymph nodes on adjacent structures. There is no characteristic roentgenographic appearance, and the diagnosis is rarely suspected from sputum cytology or bronchoscopy. Percutaneous needle biopsy may give the diagnosis with either neoplasm.

A sufficient number of lymphosarcomas are localized to make the prognosis good after pulmonary resection. A 5-year survival exceeding 50 percent may be anticipated, but the results with reticulum cell sarcoma are not as good because the neoplasm is less often resectable.

Hodgkin's disease frequently involves the lung, and a rare patient is seen in whom a solitary pulmonary lesion is unassociated with other evidence of tumor. If resection has been performed, the patient should have complete staging of the disease so that decisions regarding additional therapy can be made.

Fibrosarcoma, rhabdomyosarcoma, neurofibrosarcoma, and other tumors of mesodermal origin may occur rarely in the lung but without specific clinical presentation. The treatment is surgical resection, and the prognosis depends on the stage at which the neoplasm was discovered.

BENIGN TUMORS

The *hamartoma* (chondroadenoma), among the commonest benign pulmonary tumors, has a characteristic peripheral location (Fig. 17-76). Very slow growth and striking male preponderance are additional features. Although they have been reported in children, hamartomas have their greatest age incidence between forty and sixty years. An absence of symptoms is the rule, and the great

Fig. 17-76. This posteroanterior chest x-ray shows a smooth round density in the midlung field that proved to be a hamartoma when removed by wedge resection.

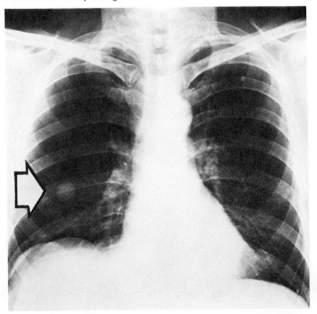

majority are discovered on chest x-rays taken for another purpose.

The major component of the hamartoma is cartilage, and it is often possible to shell the tumor out of the lung parenchyma. Epithelial elements are generally present, and there may be fat, muscular, or fibrous tissue interspersed. Removal by wedge resection is generally performed as the diagnostic procedure.

Neurofibromas may occur in the lung parenchyma, particularly in patients with neurofibromatosis. *Sclerosing hemangiomas, plasma cell granulomas, lipomas,* and rare examples of a few other neoplasms complete the list of benign tumors that may arise in the parenchyma. Many of the same neoplasms may develop in a major bronchus and present as a polypoid lesion. The *granular cell myoblastoma* is an example of this type of development in which the clinical presentation is that of bronchial obstruction. Lobar resection is often necessary because of the effects of chronic infection.

METASTATIC TUMORS

Metastases to the lungs are common during the clinical course of many uncontrolled primary neoplasms of extrathoracic origin. In some patients death occurs with pulmonary metastases in the absence of any other foci of recurrent tumor. Further, it has now been demonstrated that surgical resection of one or more pulmonary metastases can result in a significant 5-year survival rate for patients with several types of carcinomas or sarcomas. Unfortunately, in many communities there does not appear to be a general appreciation of the potential for cure that may result from an application of this knowledge.

The initial experience with surgical treatment of pulmonary metastases was based on the principle that resection was indicated only in those patients with a solitary metastasis, in whom a year or more had passed between control of the primary tumor and appearance of the metastasis. Occasionally, patients with an apparent solitary metastasis were observed for prolonged intervals so that any subclinical metastases could become apparent. Though a conservative approach of this type has most likely avoided fruitless thoracotomy for some patients who did have additional metastases, it also may have allowed additional metastases to develop from the lesion that was being observed. The occurrence of secondary metastases from a primary metastasis has been demonstrated to the satisfaction of most observers. Therefore, this phenomenon must now be considered in the decision about treatment for individual patients.

The original recommendation to consider for resection only those patients whose metastasis appeared approximately one year or more after control of the primary tumor has been challenged by more recent results. Five-year survivors have been reported who had their pulmonary metastasis resected within several months after resection of the primary neoplasm. It seems likely that the origin of the primary tumor and the biologic behavior of the individual neoplasm are the major factors in the prognosis for survival. Morton has shown that the measurement of the tumor doubling time (TDT) provides an accurate method for judging the biologic behavior of a neoplasm in the individual patient. From an experience with 60 patients who underwent resection for multiple pulmonary metastases, it was concluded that aggressive surgical resection is indicated when TDT is greater than 40 days. In that series, the estimated 5-year survival was approximately 60 percent for patients whose TDT exceeded 40 days.

Differing results in the literature have not allowed firm conclusions to be drawn regarding the tumors that offer the best change for cure with resection of metastases. In children the likelihood of 5-year survival after resection of single or multiple metastases from extremity sarcomas has seemingly been enhanced by effective chemotherapy. Breast carcinoma has not given favorable results in the experience of most surgeons, and the prognosis after resection of metastases from renal and colon neoplasms has varied widely.

The problem to be considered in a patient who presents with a solitary pulmonary nodule, either synchronous or metachronous with an extrathoracic cancer, is whether it is a metastasis, a primary pulmonary tumor, or a nonneoplastic lesion (Fig. 17-77). In a report on 54 colon cancer patients who had a solitary lung shadow at the Sloan-Kettering Cancer Center, 25 patients had colon cancer metastases and 29 had primary lung carcinoma. Resection of the metastases resulted in a 35 percent 5-year survival. In the absence of strong evidence to support a conclusion that the pulmonary lesion is nonneoplastic, an aggressive surgical approach is warranted under these circumstances.

In the evaluation of patients to be considered for resection of pulmonary metastases, the exclusion of metastases to other sites should be as thorough as possible. Besides the standard roentgenographic and radioisotopic surveys for metastatic disease, bone marrow biopsy, lymphangiography, and other special procedures may be indicated, depending on the known biologic behavior of the primary neoplasm. Metastatic neoplasms result in positive sputum cytology or positive bronchial washings much less frequently than primary lung cancers. If preoperative confirmation of the diagnosis is imperative, percutaneous needle biopsy may offer the greatest chance for success.

In all events it is important to assess the extent of the pulmonary lesions before operation. Standard x-ray tomography is rapidly being supplanted by computed tomography for this purpose. Although the survival rate for individuals who had bilateral metastases was not found to be significantly different (statistically) from those with unilateral metastases by Takita, other factors become operative (Fig. 17-78). Previously, the recommended approach for patients with bilateral lesions was that of staged thoracotomies and an interval of several weeks or months. The results achieved by Takita and his associates with a series of patients having simultaneous resection of bilateral metastases through a median sternotomy provides strong support for the single-stage operation.

McCormack has recently reported on 188 patients who underwent single or multiple thoracotomies for metastatic carcinoma from multiple sites of origin (Fig. 17-79). Only 26 patients had one or more metastases in each lung at the time of the first thoracotomy. The overall 5-year survival

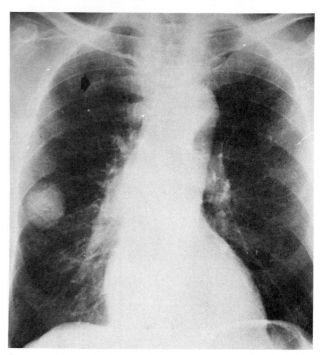

Fig. 17-77. This chest x-ray shows a large round density in the right lung of a patient who had undergone abdominoperineal resection for anal carcinoma 2 years earlier. The arrow points to a small density in the upper lobe area that was not detected before his right thoracotomy. Both lesions were removed by wedge resection and proved to be metastases from the anal neoplasm. There has been no further evidence of neoplasm in 18 months.

Fig. 17-78. Even though the survival rate after resection of unilateral metastases was not significantly different from that of patients with bilateral metastases, the data of Takita do show a trend that coincides with the experience of other surgeons. (*From H. Takita et al., The Surgical Management of Multiple Lung Metastases, Ann Thorac Surg, 24:359, 1977, with permission of the author and publisher.*)

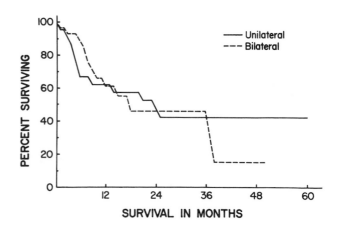

Multiple Lung Metastases: Survival by Unilateral vs. Bilateral Disease

Extent of Pulmonary Metastases at Initial Thoracotomy

Primary Site	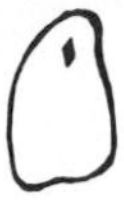	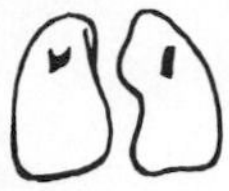	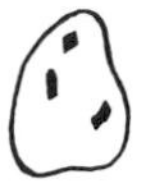	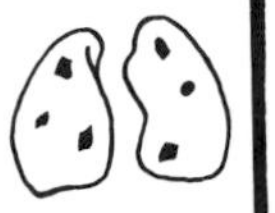	Number of Patients
Colon and Rectum	23	1	10	6	40
Melanoma	23	0	5	1	29
Breast	24	0	3	1	28
Testis	8	0	14	3	25
Head and Neck	10	0	12	1	23
Kidney	6	1	4	5	16
Bladder	2	0	4	2	8
Other	8	0	6	5	19
TOTAL	104	2	58	24	188

Fig. 17-79. The origin of the primary tumors and the unilateral or bilateral extent of pulmonary metastases at the time of the initial thoracotomy in 188 patients reported from the Sloan-Kettering Cancer Center. (*Reproduced from P. M. McCormack et al., Pulmonary Resection in Metastic Carcinoma, Chest, 73:163, 1978, with permission of the author and publisher.*)

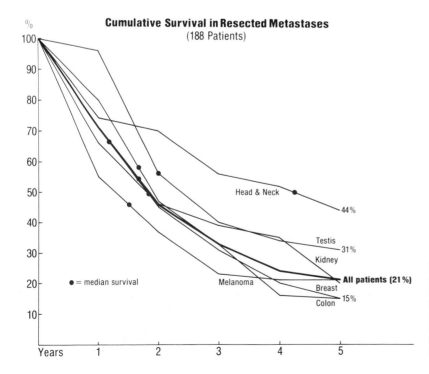

Cumulative Survival in Resected Metastases
(188 Patients)

Fig. 17-80. The overall 5-year survival in 188 patients who underwent resection of pulmonary metastases was 21 percent, but those who had primary tumors in the head and neck had a 44 percent survival. (*Reproduced from P. M. McCormack et al., Pulmonary Resection in Metastatic Carcinoma, Chest, 73:163, 1978, with permission of the author and publisher.*)

with resected solitary metastases was 21 percent, and that for multiple metastasis was 15 percent. As shown in Fig. 17-80, the overall rate of survival for all groups in her series was also 21 percent, but there was a significant difference between the groups according to tumor origin.

The extent of pulmonary resection for metastatic lesions is determined by the location of the lesions, the patient's pulmonary function, and the number of metastases. For a solitary lesion it may be necessary to do a lobectomy to distinguish between metastatic and primary carcinoma. Pneumonectomy is rarely indicated. For the majority of patients with multiple lesions, wedge resections must be done to conserve pulmonary tissue (Fig. 17-81).

Most recently a concept of "debulking" the lungs has developed in which the goal is to remove as much tumor volume as possible in the patient with extensive pulmonary metastases. Operation is then followed by intense chemotherapy with the hope of controlling tumor growth and prolonging survival. The preliminary results from this approach have been inconclusive to date except for isolated cases. Nevertheless, the concept seems valid and experience will lead to the proper selection of patients.

TRACHEA

Because of its singular importance to life and its relatively vulnerable position in the neck, the trachea must be considered among the few really vital structures in the body. Considering these facts one would have to say that it has been a relatively silent organ when compared to the attention demanded by the heart, the liver, etc. Research effort and money devoted to solution of the diseases or disorders affecting the trachea have been minuscule in comparison to that expended for other organs that are no more critical to human survival.

The adult trachea varies in length from approximately 10 to 13 cm, with an internal diameter of 2.3 cm laterally and 1.8 cm anteroposteriorly. There are generally 18 to 22 cartilaginous rings, but some degree of lateral fusion between adjacent rings, or lateral division of single rings is not infrequent. The flexible character of the trachea is complemented by its ability to maintain an adequate lumen during the extremes of neck motion and externally applied pressure. Loss of the cartilaginous support takes away the property of lumen integrity and is the principal threat to adequate tracheal function after injuries or benign disease.

The blood supply of the trachea is not generous, and this must be given major attention in operations involving repair or reconstruction. The cervical trachea receives its major blood supply from the inferior thyroid artery; the lower part of the trachea is supplied by bronchial arteries.

The most common significant congenital disorders of the trachea are the *tracheoesophageal fistulas* associated with esophageal atresia. Management of the tracheal part of these abnormalities consists essentially of interrupting the fistula and closing the posterior membranous wall of the trachea. It is the management of the esophagus that constitutes the long-term problem; that is discussed elsewhere.

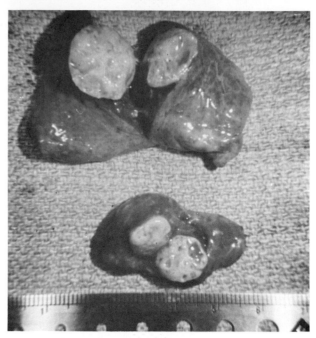

Fig. 17-81. Two small metastases that were wedged from the left lung in a thirty-four-year-old woman who previously had amputation of her left leg for an alveolar cell sarcoma.

Several forms of *congenital tracheal stenosis* may occur, often associated with other congenital anomalies. Congenital webs in the form of diaphragms may produce acute or chronic obstruction in newborns as well as older children. In addition, three types of stenosis involving the tracheal wall have been described: (1) funnel stenosis in which the distal trachea tapers to a very small lumen above the carina; (2) segmental stenosis, which may occur at any level; and (3) hypoplasia of the entire tracheal length. Obstruction of the trachea can occur in association with anomalous origin of the left pulmonary artery from the right pulmonary artery (pulmonary artery sling) and passage of the left artery behind the trachea. Several types of vascular ring malformations may produce partial tracheal obstruction.

Diagnosis of tracheal abnormalities depends on a suspicion of the anomalies and the use of air tracheograms, fluoroscopy, and careful bronchoscopy. Obviously there is a danger that the attempts at diagnosis can convert a partial obstruction to near-total obstruction and a critical emergency. Corrective operative procedures must be highly selective in infants, and reconstruction of the trachea is seldom attempted in small children. Tracheostomy or careful dilatations are the usual procedures done for intrinsic tracheal obstruction, and they must be done with the concept of subsequent reconstruction in mind.

Penetrating or blunt trauma to the neck or thorax may produce tracheal injuries that vary from localized contusion with submucosal hematoma to penetrating defects and complete interruption. An alertness to the significance of dyspnea, coughing, blood spitting, wheezing, or stridor should lead to emergency bronchoscopy or exploration of the trachea in patients with trauma. Simple penetrating injuries may require tracheostomy, or occasionally with small wounds of minor consequence, only the placement of a drain to the point of injury. Rarely, a complete division of the trachea allows the patient to survive for a period of hours to weeks before the diagnosis is made. Reanastomosis with appropriate tracheoplasty is the goal of management. A complementary tracheostomy may be required.

The complications of tracheostomy have constituted the principal need for tracheal reconstruction since the era of mechanical ventilation started. Table 17-12 lists the complications of tracheostomy according to the time period in which they are usually seen. Improved tracheostomy tubes and tracheostomy care have reduced the frequency of many of these complications. Unfortunately, acquired tracheoesophageal fistula, tracheo-innominate artery fistula, and tracheal stenosis have not been eliminated. The development of a tracheoesophageal fistula rarely occurs before the second or third week after tracheostomy has been performed. Pressure from an overinflated tracheostomy balloon cuff, trauma to the posterior tracheal wall from the tube and from suction catheters, and an indwelling nasogastric tube are factors in the development of the fistula. Repeated aspiration through the fistula produces severe pulmonary infection, while the positive-pressure ventilation forces excessive amounts of air into the gastrointestinal tract. Confirmation of the suspected diagnosis is usually accomplished with endoscopy, and treatment most often requires urgent division of the fistula with repair of both structures.

Massive hemorrhage resulting from a tracheo-innominate artery fistula may be preceded by one or more minor bleeding episodes. This is a highly lethal complication, but survivors with emergency operation are being reported with increasing frequency. A fistula is most likely to occur if tracheostomy is performed below the fourth tracheal ring. Direct erosion of the inner curve of the tube into the innominate artery is the usual mechanism of the fistula. Control of bleeding should be attempted by adjustment of the tube position and reinflation of the cuff. If this is unsuccessful, it is necessary to insert a finger into the pretracheal space and compress the artery against the

Table 17-12. COMPLICATIONS OF TRACHEOSTOMY

1. Complications of the operative procedure
   a. Cardiac arrhythmias and arrest
   b. Hemorrhage
   c. Injury to adjacent structures
   d. Incorrect tracheal incision
   e. Pneumothorax
2. Early postoperative complications
   a. Tube obstruction
   b. Displaced tube
   c. Aspiration
   d. Tracheobronchial infection
   e. Tracheoesophageal fistula
   f. Tracheo-innominate artery fistula
3. Late complications
   a. Persistent stoma
   b. Tracheal stenosis
   c. Tracheomalacia
   d. Granuloma

sternum while preparations are made for median sternotomy and direct operative control of the innominate artery.

Tracheal obstruction becomes apparent only after decannulation, and it may occur immediately or gradually over a period of days or weeks. While the development of large-volume, low-pressure balloon cuffs has sharply reduced the frequency of posttracheostomy obstruction, the complication has not been eliminated. The location of the site of obstruction in the majority of patients has changed from the area of balloon cuff–tracheal wall contact to the site of the tracheal stoma. Even so, examples of tracheal stenosis at the cuff site are still seen because of circumferential fibrous stricture or tracheomalacia resulting from overinflation of so-called "soft cuffs." The ready availability of pressure manometers to allow frequent monitoring of intracuff pressure has not completely prevented a misconception that the first approach to unsatisfactory ventilation in a respirator patient is the addition of air to the balloon cuff. Development of the foam-cuff tracheostomy tubes may help reduce even further the incidence of tracheal injury at the site of contact of the cuff with the tracheal wall.

Obstruction at the stomal site may be due to excessive granulation tissue, tracheomalacia, or fibrous stricture (Fig. 17-82). Factors that have been implicated in producing stomal stenosis are related to the type of incision made in the trachea, severity of infection at the tracheostomy site, possible protrusion of the balloon cuff through the stoma, and duration of the indwelling tube. There are no clear data to define the specific role of any of these factors, and different investigations support different types of tracheal incisions.

Recognition or suspicion of tracheal stenosis before a critical obstruction forces emergency tracheostomy can significantly reduce the complexity of tracheal resection and repair. Dilatation is usually not successful for management of severe stenosis, but recent experience with local steroid administration, dilatation, and intraluminal stenting has given encouraging results. Two other techniques currently being evaluated for treatment of localized strictures are endotracheal cryotherapy and endoscopic laser treatment. Both methods have shown promise for correctly selected patients. In addition, laser therapy may have application for management of benign and malignant tracheal tumors.

The usual management for acquired tracheal stenosis with a lumen diameter of 1.5 cm or less is resection of the stenotic area with end-to-end reanastomosis. This can generally be done through a cervical incision that incorporates the tracheostomy scar. Approximately 4.5 to 5 cm of trachea can be resected and still allow primary anastomosis, but a partial sternotomy may be required for adequate mobilization. In a rare patient the extent of tracheal stenosis, including its length, may block the attempt to do a reanastomosis. This has usually resulted in multiple operations utilizing several techniques for attempted tracheal reconstruction. The results have often been poor, and the patient was left with a permanent tracheostomy. A tracheal prosthesis of silicone rubber recently developed by Neville has shown promise for relief of this problem and for

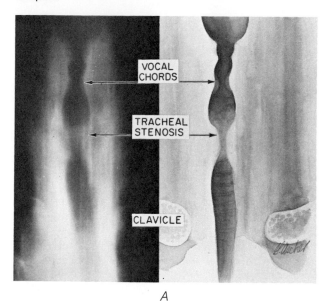

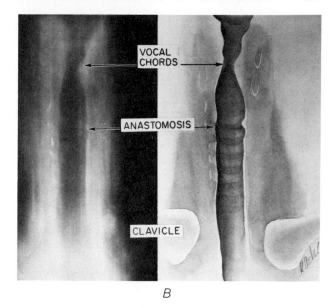

A

B

Fig. 17-82. Resection and the anastomosis of the trachea for tracheostomy stomal stenosis. *A.* A tomogram of the cervical trachea demonstrates the area of stenosis. *B.* A postoperative tomogram shows restoration of a normal tracheal lumen after resection and end-to-end anastomosis.

tracheal replacement in patients with carcinoma involving that structure (Fig. 17-83). Neville has been successful in achieving a "take" of the prosthesis in a modest group of patients; this represents significant progress in the area of tracheal surgery.

Fig. 17-83. *A.* An operative photograph furnished by Dr. William Neville shows a tracheal prosthesis that has been used to replace a length of the cervicomediastinal trachea. *B.* The drawing shows the relationship of the tracheal prosthesis to the aorta and innominate artery. *(From W. E. Neville et al., Prosthetic Reconstruction of the Trachea and Carina, J Thorac Cardiovasc Surg, 72:525, 1976, with permission of the author and publisher.)*

Tumors

Primary tracheal tumors are uncommon. The trachea is more frequently involved secondarily by direct extension of neoplasms arising in the bronchi, the esophagus, the larynx, or the thyroid gland. Of the primary tumors that do arise in the trachea more than 80 percent are malignant, with squamous cell carcinoma and cylindroma (adenocystic carcinoma) constituting the great majority. The commonest benign primary tumors are squamous papillomas and fibromas. Included among the other benign and malignant neoplasms are carcinoid tumor, chondroma, adenocarcinoma, mucoepidermoid tumor, giant-cell myoblastoma, chondrosarcoma, plasmacytoma, hemangioma, squamous papillomatosis, and fibrosarcoma.

The clinical manifestations of primary tracheal neo-

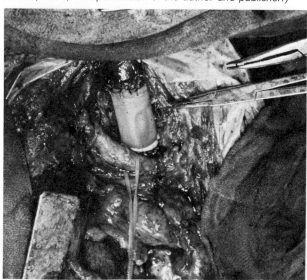

A

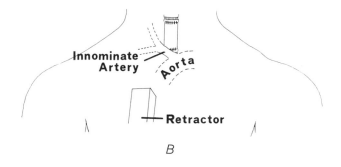

B

plasms are essentially the signs and symptoms of airway obstruction. Dyspnea on exertion may be the first evidence of developing obstruction, but cough, wheezing, and inspiratory stridor are frequently the complaints that cause the patient to seek help. Occasionally hemoptysis is the precipitating event, or it may be respiratory infection due to major obstruction of a mainstem bronchus. The chest x-rays are frequently of no help unless one requests laminagrams of the trachea because of the wheezing or stridor. Sputum cytology should be requested in the diagnostic work-up, but bronchoscopy should not be unduly delayed while numerous indirect techniques for diagnosis are performed. Because bronchoscopy can precipitate critical tracheal obstruction, however, the procedure should be carefully planned, with preparations made to proceed to definitive operation if indicated.

Pulmonary-function studies may have little meaning in the patient with high-grade tracheal obstruction, but they should be obtained if the patient's condition is satisfactory. With performance of flow-volume loops, significant obstruction will be indicated by plateaus of inspiration and expiration and flattening of the peak flow.

The goal of surgical treatment is complete resection of the neoplasm and restoration of tracheal continuity. From the bronchoscopic examination and biopsy the tumor should be identified sufficiently to plan the operative approach. Occasionally, tantalum bronchograms and tracheograms assist in the planning. Upper tracheal neoplasms are usually approached through a cervical incision, combined with median sternotomy as necessary. Lower tracheal tumors are generally operated upon through a right lateral thoracotomy. If possible a sleeve resection is done with end-to-end reanastomosis. When a more extensive resection is required, the technique of Moghissi for tracheal reconstruction with a Marlex mesh–pericardial graft may be employed (Fig. 17-84). The success reported by this author for reconstruction after major tracheal resection with both primary and secondary tumors is impressive. With a total experience of 27 patients, some of whom are alive and well from 3 to 7 years after resection for carcinoma, Moghissi suggests that an aggressive approach to tracheal resection is well justified.

For squamous carcinoma of the trachea, radiation may give temporary tumor control. At present, there is considerable hope that the chemotherapy programs that are showing improved results in bronchogenic carcinoma will also be helpful in tracheal neoplasms.

MEDIASTINUM

The mediastinum is the extrapleural space between the two pleural cavities, bordered on each side by parietal pleura and containing the heart and great vessels, trachea, esophagus, vagus nerves and sympathetic chains, the thymus gland, and a lymphatic network consisting of several groups of lymph nodes and the thoracic duct. In this complex area between the thoracic inlet and diaphragm, the heart and great vessels develop, the pulmonary diverticulum arises from the primitive foregut, and the caudal branchial arches develop. It is not surprising that many congenital anomalies are found within the mediastinum.

For purposes of classification, it is customary to divide the mediastinum into several areas. Traditional anatomists have considered the mediastinum to have superior, anterior, posterior, and middle segments. It has become obvious that this classification relies upon criteria that do not coincide with clinical behavior. For this reason, Burkell and his associates have suggested that the mediastinum be subdivided into the three major areas illustrated in Fig. 17-85. With this modification, the anterior part of the superior mediastinum is incorporated into the anterior mediastinum, and the boundary of the posterior mediastinum is extended cephalad. This is more in keeping with the actual distribution of the clinical lesions and allows the three regions to be described as follows:

1. The anterior mediastinum—bounded by the posterior surface of the sternum anteriorly, the anterior border of the upper dorsal vertebrae posteriorly, and an oblique line running along the

Fig. 17-84. Tracheal reconstruction after major resection for carcinoma. *A.* The drawings show the technique used by Moghissi for reconstruction of the trachea with a composite Marlex mesh–pericardial graft after resection of a primary tracheal neoplasm. *B.* Resection of the lateral tracheal wall en bloc with a right upper-lobe carcinoma may be repaired with the Marlex mesh–pericardial graft. (*From W. E. Neville et al., Prosthetic Reconstruction of the Trachea and Carina, J Thorac Cardiovasc Surg, 72:525, 1976, with permission of the author and publisher.*)

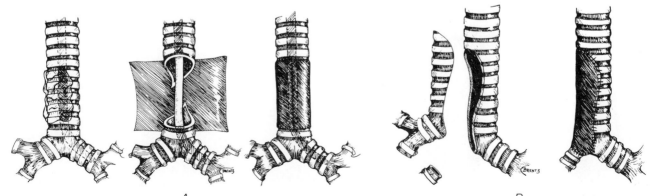

A   *B*

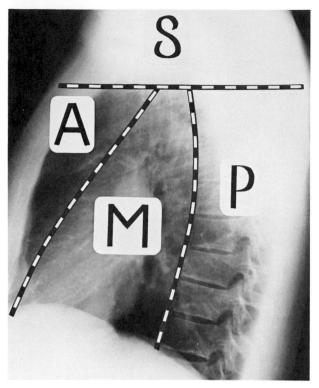

A

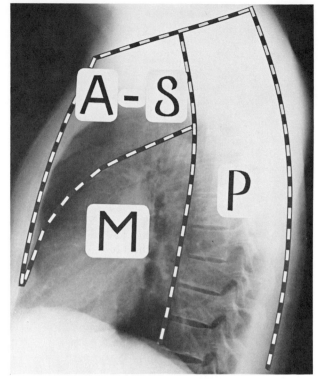

B

Fig. 17-85. The anatomic divisions of the mediastinum. *A.* The traditional consideration of the mediastinum provides for its division into superior (*S*), anterior (*A*), middle (*M*), and posterior (*P*) compartments. *B.* The anatomic divisions that Burkell and associates have suggested are shown as a cephalad extension of the posterior compartment, and a combination of the anterior and superior compartments (*A-S*). [*From C. C. Burkell, J. M. Cross, H. P. Kent, and E. N. Nanson, Mass Lesions of the Mediastinum, in M. M. Ravitch (ed.), "Current Problems in Surgery," Yearbook Medical Publishers, Inc., Chicago, June 1969, by permission of author and publisher.*]

anterior border of the heart with continuation upwards and posteriorly until it reaches the border of the dorsal vertebrae.

2. The posterior mediastinum—bounded posteriorly by the anterior surface of the curve of the ribs, anteriorly by a line drawn along the anterior border of the bodies of the dorsal vertebrae, and inferiorly by the diaphragm.

3. The middle mediastinum—a roughly triangular area with its base on the diaphragm and bounded front and back by the anterior and posterior compartments.

In addition to mass lesions, the principal concern for the surgeon, the mediastinum may be the site of acute and chronic infections, congenital malformations, and aneurysms.

Mass Lesions

The clinical presentation of primary mediastinal tumors and cysts varies from the asymptomatic and nonspecific systemic complaints to symptoms that are nearly pathognomonic for syndromes specifically associated with mediastinal lesions. Roughly 50 percent of mediastinal tumors and cysts are symptomatic in adults, with the figure being closer to two-thirds in children. Malignant tumors are more often symptomatic than benign ones, and the most common symptoms are related to compression of adjacent mediastinal structures. Chest pain is common, and many patients have respiratory symptoms caused by displacement or erosion of the tracheobronchial tree. In infants and children symptoms of cough, stridor, and dyspnea are prominent because even a small mass may readily encroach on their compressible airways. Other frequent manifestations include dysphagia, due to displacement of the esophagus, superior vena caval obstruction, recurrent nerve palsy, and Horner's syndrome. Less frequently a mediastinal neoplasm is discovered because of systemic symptoms such as hypertension due to a pheochromocytoma, hypoglycemia resulting from secretion of an insulin-like substance, or a Pel-Ebstein fever due to Hodgkin's disease.

In most cases, the definitive diagnosis of a mediastinal mass has to await histologic examination. However, every effort should be made to localize the lesion, assess its site of origin, and evaluate its relationship to surrounding structures. The diagnostic evaluation of a patient with a mediastinal mass lesion begins with a complete history and physical examination. Further investigation of these patients should follow a logical sequence proceeding from simpler to more complicated techniques.

The routine chest x-rays in anteroposterior and lateral projections are usually the most useful diagnostic procedures. The localization is of diagnostic value since certain tumors or cysts have a predilection for arising in specific regions of the mediastinum (Fig. 17-86). Not infrequently

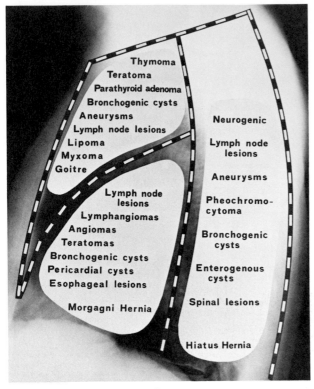

Thymoma
Teratoma
Parathyroid adenoma
Bronchogenic cysts
Aneurysms
Lymph node lesions
Lipoma
Myxoma
Goitre

Neurogenic

Lymph node lesions

Aneurysms

Pheochromo-cytoma

Lymph node lesions
Lymphangiomas
Angiomas
Teratomas
Bronchogenic cysts
Pericardial cysts
Esophageal lesions

Bronchogenic cysts

Enterogenous cysts

Morgagni Hernia

Spinal lesions

Hiatus Hernia

A

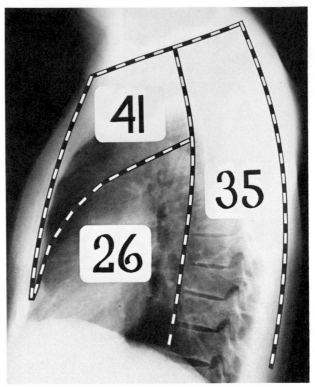

B

Fig. 17-86. *A*. Mediastinal lesions have a tendency to occur in specific areas; this figure indicates the expected location of the most frequently occurring lesions. *B*. The numbers shown in the mediastinal compartments indicate the distribution of lesions in 102 patients reported by Burkell and associates. [*From C. C. Burkell, J. M. Cross, H. P. Kent, and E. N. Nanson, Mass Lesions of the Mediastinum, in M. M. Ravitch (ed.), "Current Problems in Surgery," Yearbook Medical Publishers, Inc., Chicago, June 1969, by permission of author and publisher.*]

the precise localization is obscured because of overlying or adjacent structures, thus making it necessary to obtain further radiologic studies. Tomography may be useful in delineating middle mediastinal masses from normal hilar structures and in clarifying the presence of rib erosion or vertebral deformity in association with posterior neurogenic lesions. A barium swallow may show invasion, compression, or displacement of the esophagus resulting from either intrinsic or extrinsic lesions (Fig. 17-87). Fluoroscopy can be helpful for distinguishing mediastinal from pulmonary lesions in that a primary lung lesion will move with respiration in association with the adjoining lung parenchyma. Recently, computerized axial tomography has been helpful in certain cases because relative densities can be measured and vascular attachments can be assessed. Of further aid in assessing vascularity are angiocardiography and thoracic aortography. Pneumomediastinum has found application as a means of differentiating a true mediastinal mass from a normally enlarged thymus in infants. For patients with posterior mediastinal lesions, especially those with neurologic symptoms, myelography may be indicated in the diagnostic work-up.

Radioisotope scanning may be important in evaluating some patients, especially those with superior mediastinal lesions that may be substernal thyroid abnormalities. A recent development is the use of radioactive gallium to evaluate lymphadenopathy.

Ultrasonography is a noninvasive way to evaluate the density of a mediastinal lesion, such as differentiating a pericardial cyst from a primary tumor, but it has been shown that the technique is imperfect.

As noted previously, the above diagnostic procedures must be supplemented by tissue biopsy for precise diagnosis. Several techniques have been described for obtaining tissue, including needle biopsy, needle aspiration, anterior mediastinal exploration, and mediastinoscopy. Each method has specific advantages and disadvantages but the overall value of each probably depends most on the experience and expertise of the individual performing the procedure. The important role of exploratory thoracotomy as a diagnostic test should be emphasized, and the demonstration of a mediastinal mass may be sufficient indication for operative intervention. In modern practice there is no rationale for serial chest x-rays or the trial use of irradiation as a diagnostic technique.

ANTERIOR MEDIASTINAL LESIONS

Figure 17-86 shows those lesions which are most common in this area.

Thymoma

Thymomas are the most common neoplasms arising in the anterior mediastinum and comprise approximately 20 percent of all primary mediastinal tumors and cysts. There is an equal frequency of occurrence in males and females, with a peak incidence between ages forty and sixty years. These tumors do not have a characteristic radiologic appearance (Fig. 17-88), and the clinical presentations can be numerous and varied. Less than one-third are asympto-

Fig. 17-87. Mediastinal bronchogenic cyst. *A.* The anteroposterior view of this barium esophagogram shows lateral displacement of the distal esophagus in an eighteen-year-old man who had slowly progressive dysphagia. *B.* The lateral view demonstrates mild dilatation of the esophagus and a rapid tapering at the site of obstruction just above the diaphragm. *C.* A tomogram shows an egg-shaped mass overlying the vertebral column. *D.* The cystic lesion removed through a left thoracotomy was filled with mucoid material and was lined by typical pseudostratified respiratory epithelium.

matic at the time of diagnosis. Some patients present with compression effects such as chest pain, cough, dyspnea, or superior vena caval obstruction, but the majority have symptoms referable to one of the several systemic syndromes associated with thymoma. The most common of these is myasthenia gravis, the incidence being reported to vary from 10 to 50 percent. Conversely, the reported incidence of thymomas in patients with myasthenia gravis ranges from 8 to 15 percent. It is of interest that a thymoma can occur prior to, concomitant with, or subsequent to the onset of symptoms of myasthenia gravis. Unfortunately, myasthenic patients with thymoma derive less symptomatic benefit from thymectomy than patients without tumors.

The histologic classification of thymomas remains a

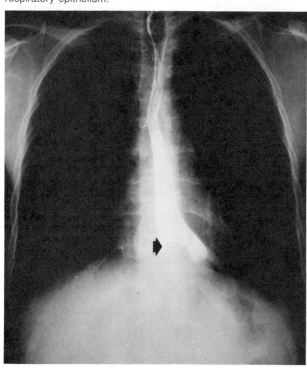

A

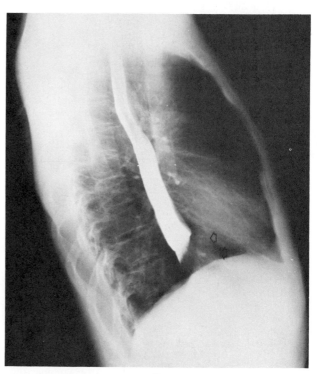

B

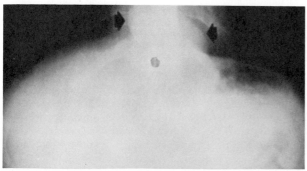

C

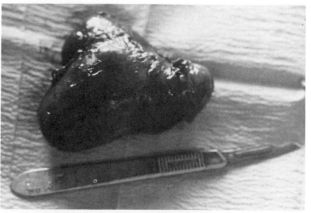

D

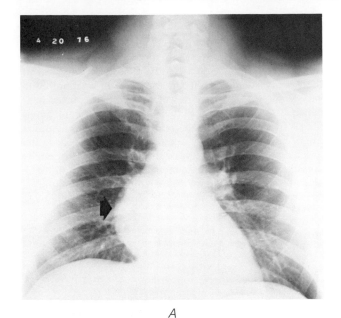

A

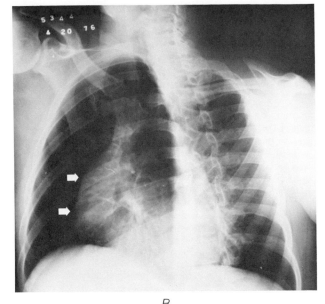

B

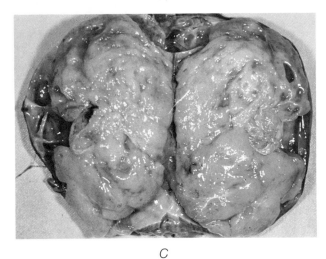

C

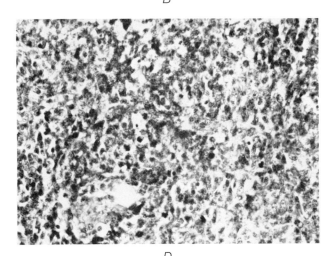

D

controversial problem. A categorization of thymomas into as many as 13 different types has been proposed; however, the prevalent opinion is to classify thymic neoplasms simply on the basis of the predominance of epithelial or lymphocytic cells. Thus, they may be typed as predominantly epithelial, lymphocytic, or mixed. Furthermore, there is no confirmed association between histologic appearance and biologic behavior. The important clinical classification of thymomas is that of benign or malignant, but the microscopic appearance is unreliable for this purpose. Benign tumors comprise 50 to 65 percent of all thymomas, they are well encapsulated, and they do not invade adjacent mediastinal structures. Tumors are designated as malignant when they locally infiltrate the pericardium, pleura, great vessels, heart, or chest wall.

The presence of a thymoma is sufficient indication for exploration regardless of whether or not the patient has an associated syndrome. A median sternotomy is the preferred approach because the extent of resection can be deter-

Fig. 17-88. A benign thymoma in a thirty-two-year-old man. *A.* The posteroanterior chest x-ray, taken because of persistent cough, showed a large smooth mass contiguous with the right heart border. *B.* An oblique projection again suggests that the mass is closely attached to the pericardium. *C.* The tumor was removed, along with the remnants of the thymus, through a high right thoracotomy. This photograph of the open neoplasm shows that it was a well-encapsulated fleshy neoplasm. *D.* Histologic examination of the tumor shows a predominance of lymphocytic elements that justifies its classification as a lymphocytic type of thymoma.

mined only at the time of operation. Encapsulated tumors should be completely resected, along with the entire thymus and the adjacent adipose tissue of the anterosuperior mediastinum. If the thymoma is invasive, complete resection should be attempted by excising all nonvital structures involved by contiguous spread. Radiation therapy in doses of 4,000 to 6,500 r is usually given postoperatively to patients with invasive tumors.

Lymphomas

Mediastinal lymph-node involvement is a frequent manifestation of disseminated lymphoma. In 50 percent of patients with Hodgkin's disease, there is evidence of mediastinal involvement; however, with the advent of accurate clinical staging, the mediastinum has been shown to be the sole site of involvement in only 5 percent of patients. Lymphomas are usually located in the anterior mediastinum but may present as hilar masses in the middle mediastinum, or even less frequently in the posterior compartment. Mediastinal lymphomas can occur at any age but most commonly are seen in the third or fourth decades of life with associated symptoms of cough, chest pain, fever, or weight loss. The diagnosis of mediastinal involvement by disseminated lymphoma is often inferred from the chest x-rays along with cervical lymph-node biopsy, bone marrow aspiration, or liver biopsy. When the tumor is confined to the mediastinum, thoracotomy or mediastinal exploration by anterior mediastinotomy or mediastinoscopy is required to obtain tissue for diagnosis.

Teratodermoid Tumors

A teratoma is a neoplasm composed of multiple tissues foreign to the area in which the teratoma is found. Mediastinal teratomas are believed to arise from cells originating from the branchial cleft and pouch in association with the thymus gland. The mediastinum is second to the gonads as the most frequent location of teratomas in adults, and to the sacrococcygeal area in children (Fig. 17-89). These tumors are most frequently found in the anterior mediastinum at the level of the pericardial reflection, but a rare teratoma is located intrapericardially in the posterior mediastinum. The term *dermoid cyst* is used to describe those lesions that are primarily cystic with a composition that varies in relative amounts of epidermis and dermal glands, hair, and sebaceous material. Careful histologic examination will often reveal that ectodermal elements predominate, but remnants of mesodermal and endodermal tissue are also present. Predominantly solid teratomas have a more complex structure and may contain well-differentiated elements of teeth, bone, cartilage, mucus or salivary glands, muscle, fibrous and lipoid tissue, nerve, thymus, pancreas, and lung.

Teratodermoid tumors occur most frequently in adolescents or young adults and with equal incidence in both sexes. Approximately 80 percent are benign. There is no correlation between the age of the patient or the size of the tumor and malignancy. Although not specific for teratocarcinomas, the most reliable diagnostic tests for suggesting malignancy preoperatively are the serum levels of alphafetoprotein and carcinoembryonic antigen. Elevated levels of these glycoproteins are due to their secretion by the malignant components of the tumor, most often adenocarcinoma.

Radiographically, the cystic lesions are well circumscribed, with a smooth outline that projects to either side of the sternum in the posteroanterior view. The solid lesions may be smooth and lobulated, or they may appear irregular.

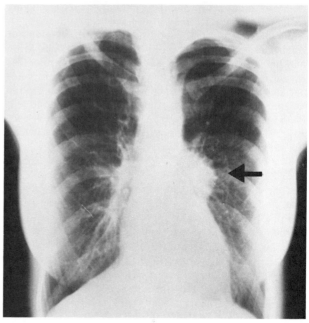

Fig. 17-89. A mediastinal teratoma in a twenty-five-year-old woman. Chest x-rays taken for nonspecific respiratory symptoms showed a smooth mass overlying the pulmonary artery. Pulmonary arteriography was normal, and the lesion was removed through a median sternotomy.

Operative resection is the definitive treatment for all teratodermoid tumors. Even if benign, the tumors often are attached to the pericardium or thymus, and portions of these structures must be removed with the specimen. Malignant teratomas often invade the pericardium, heart, or superior vena cava, making curative resection impossible. The prognosis for all malignant teratomas is poor because the tumors tend to recur locally and to metastasize early.

Germ Cell Tumors

The entire spectrum of germ cell tumors may arise in extragonadal sites, and when they occur in the thorax, they are located in the anterior mediastinum. Though the histogenesis of such extragonadal germ cell tumors is unknown, most authorities agree that the lesions do not represent metastases from a primary gonadal site.

Seminoma is the most common germinal tumor, usually affecting young men between the ages of twenty to thirty years. Most patients are symptomatic at the time of diagnosis, with retrosternal chest pain, weight loss, hoarseness, or evidence of superior vena caval obstruction. The chest x-ray may show a large anterior mediastinal mass, but there are no pathognomonic features. Clinically and roentgenographically these tumors must be differentiated from thymic neoplasms and lymphomas. They commonly metastasize to the pleura, chest wall, lymph nodes, liver, bone, and retroperitoneum. Most often, only partial excision can be accomplished because of regional and distant spread. Seminomas are highly radiosensitive, and even if complete excision is done postoperative radiation therapy is mandatory.

Choriocarcinoma and embryonal carcinoma are highly malignant neoplasms that also have a predilection for young males. Almost all patients present with symptoms of cough, chest pain, shortness of breath, or hemoptysis. More than half the male patients have gynecomastia and widespread metastases at the time of diagnosis. Choriocarcinomas always produce human chorionic gonadotropin, while the embryonal carcinomas often release alpha-fetoprotein or carcinoembryonic antigen. These tumors are rarely sensitive to irradiation or chemotherapy, and they usually lead to a rapidly fatal course.

Mesenchymal Tumors

A variety of mesenchymal tumors arise in the mediastinum, and as a group they comprise approximately 7 percent of all primary mediastinal tumors and cysts. Lipomas are the most frequently encountered, with three out of four occurring in the anterior mediastinum. Because of soft consistency and lack of fixation to adjacent structures, they may reach enormous size before causing symptoms. When symptoms do occur they are nonspecific in type, such as chest pain and dyspnea. Operative resection of these lesions is curative.

Other mesenchymal tumors which have been reported in the mediastinum include liposarcoma, fibroma, fibrosarcoma, mesothelioma, myxoma, xanthogranuloma, leiomyosarcoma, and rhabdomyosarcoma.

Tumors of blood-vascular and lymph-vascular origin are included among the mesenchymal neoplasms of the anterior mediastinum. The several types of hemangiomas—capillary, cavernous, and venous—are differentiated by the size of the vascular spaces and the presence or absence of smooth muscle cells in the vessel walls. Operative excision is the treatment of choice for both benign hemangiomas and the rare malignant hemangiopericytoma.

The tumors of lymph-vascular origin may be thin-walled, unilocular cysts or multilocular tumors intimately related to surrounding structures. They usually present as a rounded or lobulated mass of homogeneous density on the chest x-ray. The most common variety is the benign lymphangioma, also known as cystic hygroma.

Endocrine Tumors

The two types of endocrine tumors most frequently found in the anterior mediastinum are those of thyroid and parathyroid origin. Perhaps 10 percent of parathyroid adenomas are located in the mediastinum, although many of these may be approached by a cervical incision. They are usually in close association with the upper pole of the thymus gland, a result of their common embryologic origin from the third branchial cleft. It is rare for a parathyroid tumor to present as a mediastinal mass. Instead, a patient with signs and symptoms of hyperparathyroidism will be found to have an adenoma located in the mediastinum after a negative cervical exploration.

Thyroid tumors found in the mediastinum are usually substernal extensions of the cervical gland. True aberrant thyroid tissue is found in the mediastinum only infrequently, and the blood supply in this location is derived from the great vessels. Theoretically, the mediastinal thyroid could represent all of the thyroid tissue that a patient has, but this can easily be determined by means of a radionuclide scan. The latter test should be a routine part of the work-up in any patient who presents with an otherwise undiagnosed mass high in the anterior mediastinum.

MIDDLE MEDIASTINAL LESIONS

Some of the lesions that have been described as occurring in the anterior mediastinum may also develop in the middle mediastinum (Fig. 17-86). Pericardial cysts, esophageal lesions, and Morgagni hernias are unique to the middle compartment.

Cysts

Collectively, congenital cysts comprise approximately 20 percent of primary mediastinal mass lesions. Included in this group are cysts of pericardial, bronchogenic, enteric, and nonspecific origin. *Pericardial cysts* are the most common. Whatever the developmental defect may be, the result is usually a solitary cyst adjacent to the pericardium with a diameter of 3 to 6 cm. Such cysts usually contain a clear fluid and occasionally communicate with the pericardium. Histologically, the cyst wall is composed of a single layer of mesothelial cells. Pericardial cysts, despite their congenital origin, are usually first detected in adult life as an incidental finding on a routine chest x-ray. The most frequent location is at the right cardiophrenic angle. Operative removal is indicated primarily for diagnosis. Accumulated experience with more recent technologies for diagnosis, computed tomography, and ultrasound, for example, may allow confident observation in the future.

Bronchogenic cysts may arise in any location in the mediastinum or lung parenchyma, but they are usually located posterior or inferior to the carina. Rarely, there is communication with the tracheobronchial tree. Bronchogenic cysts are recognized most often in young adults, and symptoms are usually the result of compression by the cyst, with cough, wheezing, dyspnea, or even dysphagia. The cysts are uncommon in infancy, but lesions in a critical position may cause life-threatening respiratory embarrassment. Infection of the cyst may develop and make distinction from a lung abscess very difficult. All bronchogenic cysts should be removed. If the cyst has been infected, dense adhesions in the hilar area can make dissection difficult and require pulmonary resection.

Hernias through the foramen of Morgagni are most often discovered as incidental retrosternal masses on chest x-rays taken for other purposes. Alternately, a herniation of omentum or retroperitoneal fat may be found during a thoracotomy. Even less frequently the transverse colon becomes displaced into the right or left side of the chest through the foramen of Morgagni, and it may then appear as an anterior mediastinal mass on the plain films. Retrosternal pain is sometimes produced and requires operative treatment. When the diagnosis is made preoperatively, an abdominal approach is recommended.

Esophageal lesions and aneurysms are discussed in other chapters.

POSTERIOR MEDIASTINAL LESIONS

Neurogenic Tumors

The several types of neurogenic tumors are the most common neoplasms arising in the mediastinum, accounting for approximately 21 percent of all primary mediastinal tumors and cysts. Classically, neurogenic tumors arise from either the intercostal nerves or the sympathetic ganglia, and they are usually located in the paravertebral gutter (Fig. 17-90). Though the peak incidence is in adult life, the tumors may be seen in children and older persons. An incidence of malignancy between 10 and 20 percent can be estimated from analysis of several reports, with the greater likelihood of malignancy in children. In adults, it is more common for neurogenic tumors to be discovered as an incidental finding. When symptoms are present, the most common complaint is chest pain due to compression of an intercostal nerve or erosion of adjacent bone. Pleural effusion may be found with both benign and malignant lesions, but a bloody effusion is usually a sign of malignancy. The intraspinal component of a "dumbbell" tumor can compress the cord, causing paresthesias and weakness.

Neurogenic tumors may produce systemic syndromes secondary to the endocrine functions of the tumor; e.g., the production of catecholamine by a pheochromocytoma, vanillylmandelic acid by gangliosarcomas and neuroblastomas, and immunoreactive insulin by neurosarcomas.

Neurilemomas are the most common neurogenic tumors, occurring usually in the third to fifth decades of life. They arise from Schwann cells of the nerve sheath and are also called *schwannomas*. The neurilemomas are well encapsulated and are seen on chest films as dense, homogeneous, circumscribed masses in the posterior mediastinum.

Neurofibromas contain nerve elements as well as nerve-sheath cells. They are poorly encapsulated, but radiographically resemble neurilemomas. Neurofibromas of the mediastinum may be one manifestation of generalized neurofibromatosis; however, if a patient with known von Recklinghausen's disease is found to have a posterior mediastinal mass, this more likely represents a *meningocele*, not a neurofibroma. Because of the infiltrating growth of these tumors, complete operative excision is often difficult.

When a neurofibroma or neurilemoma undergoes malignant degeneration, it becomes a *neurosarcoma*. The frequency of malignant change varies from 25 to 30 percent. There is an increased incidence of neurosarcoma associated with generalized neurofibromatosis, and a malignant neoplasm is more often found in older patients. Patients with neurosarcoma have a poor survival rate because of rapid tumor growth and invasion of adjacent mediastinal structures.

Ganglioneuromas originate from a sympathetic ganglion and are composed of mature ganglion cells and nerve fibers. They occur in patients of a younger age group than tumors of nerve-sheath origin and may become very large before causing symptoms. Roentgenographically, a ganglioneuroma often has a triangular configuration, with the broad base toward the mediastinum. In the lateral projection, they are poorly defined because of the radiographic density of the vertebrae. There is no association between endocrine function and malignancy.

Neuroblastomas are the most poorly differentiated malignant tumors arising from the sympathetic nervous system, and approximately 10 percent occur as a primary

Fig. 17-90. A neurilemoma of the posterior mediastinum. *A.* The posteroanterior chest x-ray suggests a dense mass behind the heart. *B.* A tomogram shows the somewhat lobulated appearance of the tumor in the paravertebral gutter.

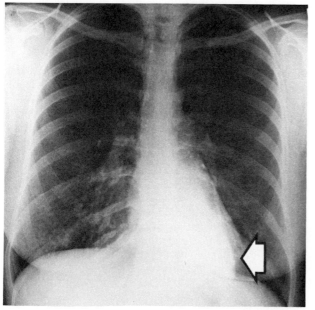

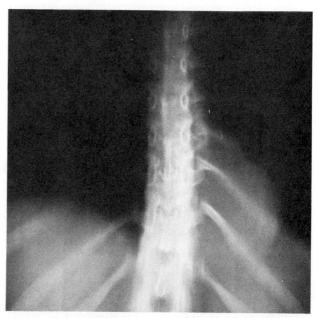

A

B

lesion in the mediastinum. More than 75 percent occur in children less than four years of age, often with symptoms of fever, vomiting, diarrhea, and cough. Metastases to bone, brain, liver, and regional lymph nodes may be present at the time of diagnosis, and direct invasion of the spinal cord with resultant neurologic deficit is not uncommon. Evidence of catecholamine excretion by the tumor is manifested by systemic hypertension.

Mediastinal neuroblastomas are often unresectable at the time of diagnosis, because of either local invasion or distant metastases. However, the tumors are usually radiosensitive, and long-term survival may follow postoperative radiation therapy. Interestingly, mediastinal neuroblastomas have a more favorable prognosis than neuroblastomas originating at other sites.

Less than 1 percent of all *pheochromocytomas* occur in the mediastinum, but the tumors are most often situated in the posterior region. Clinically, these tumors are no different from the intraabdominal lesions.

The therapy of benign neurogenic tumors is complete excision through a standard posterolateral thoracotomy. The preoperative evaluation should include careful radiographic visualization of the thoracic spine so that any enlargement of the interspinal foramina adjacent to the neoplasm may be detected. If there is an intraspinal component, this portion should be excised prior to thoracotomy, because manipulation of the intrathoracic tumor may cause swelling or bleeding in the spinal canal and precipitate cord compression.

Enteric Cysts

In addition to neurogenic lesions, the posterior mediastinum is the usual location of enteric cysts. These cysts can be located at any level of the posterior mediastinum adjacent to the esophagus, but only rarely is there a communication with that structure. Approximately 60 percent occur in infants less than one year of age, and symptoms of tracheal or esophageal obstruction are common. The cysts usually contain a clear, colorless mucoid fluid. Occasionally, a lining of aberrant gastric mucosa leads to peptic ulceration and perforation of the adjacent bronchial or esophageal lumen, with resulting hemoptysis or hematemesis. Erosion into adjacent lung parenchyma can result in a lung abscess.

Operative removal of the cysts is always indicated, and the surgical approach depends on the level of the lesion as well as its projection toward either hemithorax. Previous episodes of inflammation may result in fibrous tissue proliferation that interferes with dissection of the lesion away from adjacent structures.

Acute Mediastinitis

Acute suppurative mediastinitis is a serious and potentially fatal infection that is generally distributed in the superior or posterior mediastinum. The areolar tissues of the mediastinum have little ability to deal with infection, but the mediastinal pleura on each side serves as a temporary barrier to the spread of the infection into one or both pleural cavities. The mechanism of infection is usually from contamination of the mediastinum due to (1) perforation of the cervical or thoracic esophagus during instrumentation; (2) esophageal perforation by foreign body; (3) leakage of an esophageal suture line following operative procedures; (4) inferior extension of a cervical suppuration; (5) spread of infection into the soft tissues from an infection involving the ribs, sternum, or vertebra; (6) mediastinal extension of pleural or pulmonary infection; (7) external trauma; and (8) spontaneous esophageal rupture (Boerhaave's syndrome).

Chills and fever, shock, tachycardia, dull or severe chest pain, and soft tissue crepitus in the suprasternal notch may progress rapidly in the patient with continuing contamination from esophageal perforation. The chest x-ray will usually show widening of the superior mediastinum as well as air in the tissue planes. As the infection spreads, pleuritic pain often occurs, associated with effusion. Thoracentesis or tube thoracostomy may become necessary to relieve both the pleural sepsis and respiratory distress.

Acute infections which involve the lower mediastinum, as seen with perforation of the distal esophagus, produce less definite signs and symptoms. The pain may be subxiphoid or epigastric, and the tenderness and muscle rigidity of the upper part of the abdomen may suggest an acute intraabdominal process. Crepitus is often absent or late in appearance, and gastric contents escaping through the esophageal laceration may not penetrate the pleura for 24 hours or longer.

Acute infections of the mediastinum require immediate and vigorous management if prolonged and complicated convalescence or death is to be avoided. Without continued contamination, localized acute mediastinitis may resolve completely with massive broad-spectrum antibiotic coverage. Most surgeons, however, recommend immediate exploration for mediastinitis associated with esophageal injury. A more detailed discussion of the management of esophageal perforation is given in Chap. 25.

Chronic Mediastinitis

Chronic inflammation and fibrosis in the mediastinum is most often the result of a specific granulomatous infection such as tuberculosis, histoplasmosis, or other mycotic infections. *Sclerosing mediastinitis* and *fibrosing mediastinitis* are terms that have developed common usage with continuing mediastinal inflammation because of the clinical effects of the process. Analysis of cases suggests that the mediastinitis begins as an extension of infection from involved mediastinal, tracheobronchial, or hilar lymph nodes. Though histoplasmosis and tuberculosis are thought to be the most frequent initiators of the process, it has been unusual to prove the relationship in individual patients by demonstration of the organisms.

The more notable clinical presentations are usually the result of progressive fibrosis with obstruction of the superior vena cava, the esophagus, or the pulmonary veins. Symptoms of chest pain, fever, exercise intolerance, and dysphasia may occur to correlate with mediastinal widening on standard chest x-rays. A clinical picture of superior vena caval obstruction may occur, however, in the absence of significant changes on the x-rays. Angiography and tomography are usually helpful in demonstrating the underlying process, but operative exploration may be required to define the morphologic and etiologic diagnosis.

The treatment depends on the determination of the cause of the mediastinitis, its degree of activity, and the functional effects. Obstruction of the superior vena cava or esophagus may require operative relief, or rarely, pericardiectomy may be necessary to relieve constrictive pericarditis.

Superior Vena Caval Obstruction

In this country the great majority of patients who develop obstruction of their superior vena cava have bronchogenic cancer. It is estimated that 10 to 15 percent of those with lung cancer will develop caval obstruction before death. Primary neoplasms of the right upper lobe are the most frequent tumors that involve the vena cava, but metastatic tumor and lymphomas account for a larger number than do benign lesions. Thoracic aortic aneurysms, including dissecting aneurysms, occasionally compress the vena cava, and rarely a benign tumor is responsible for the obstruction. The mechanism of obstruction varies from simple compression to malignant invasion and thrombosis. Rarely, thrombosis may accompany a septic thrombophlebitis due to drug injections in an addict or a contaminated central venous catheter. Fibrosing mediastinitis may lead to thrombotic occlusion, and this complication can apparently occur in the presence of polycythemia without an associated obstruction.

Headache, confusion, discomfort on bending over, swelling of facial structures, and distended veins in the upper half of the body are common clinical presentations of superior caval obstruction. Sudden occlusion can lead to rapid development of cerebral edema, intracranial thrombosis, and death. A suspected diagnosis of caval obstruction should be confirmed by venography regardless of cause.

For patients with proved malignant neoplasms the aggressiveness of therapy for relief of caval obstruction depends on the stage of their disease. Most of those with bronchogenic carcinoma will receive only temporary relief from radiation therapy combined with nitrogen mustard or other adjuvants. A rare patient with a controlled or slowly growing malignancy can benefit from a combination of radiation therapy and a vascular graft that bypasses the superior vena cava. For patients with nonmalignant caval obstruction it is reasonable to consider treatment with diuretics, salt restriction, and a Fowler's position in bed while collateral venous channels have an opportunity to develop. Failing this, operative reconstruction of the superior vena cava or a bypass graft may be done.

References

Introduction

Meade, R. H.: "A History of Thoracic Surgery," Charles C Thomas, Publisher, Springfield, Ill., 1961.

Anatomy of the Thorax and Pleura

Blevins, C. E.: Anatomy of the Thorax and Pleura, in T. W. Shields, (ed.), "General Thoracic Surgery," Lea & Febiger, Philadelphia, 1972.

Grant, J. C. B. and Basmajian, J. V.: "Grant's Method of Anatomy," 7th ed., The Williams & Wilkins Company, Baltimore, 1965.

Thoracic Incisions

Thurer, R. J., Bognolo, D., Vargus, A., Isch, J. H. and Kaiser, G. A.: The Management of Mediastinal Infection following Cardiac Surgery, *J Thorac Cardiovasc Surg,* **68:**962, 1974.

Evaluation of the Thoracic Surgical Patient

Boren, H. G., Kory, R. C. and Syner, J. C.: The Veterans Administration–Army Cooperative Study of Pulmonary Function: II. The Lung Volume and Its Subdivisions in Normal Men, *Am J Med,* **41:**96, 1966.

Miller, R. N.: Evaluation of Pulmonary Impairment in the Surgical Candidate, *Med Clin North Am,* **46:**885, 1962.

Mittman, C.: Assessment of Operative Risk in Thoracic Surgery, *Am Rev Resp Dis,* **84:**197, 1961.

Olsen, G. N., Block, A. J., Swenson, E. W., Castle, J. R., and Wynne, J. W.: Pulmonary Function Evaluation of the Lung Resection Candidate: A Prospective Study, *Am Rev Resp Dis,* **111:**379, 1975.

Petty, T. L.: "Pulmonary Diagnostic Techniques," Lea & Febiger, Philadelphia, 1975.

Thoracic Injuries

Blaisdell, F. W., and Lewis, F. R., Jr.: "Respiratory Distress Syndrome of Shock and Trauma," W. B. Saunders Company, Philadelphia, 1977.

Bryant, L. R., Spencer, F. C., Boyd, A. D., and Daly, J. F.: Tracheostomy and Assisted Ventilation, in D. L. Sabiston, Jr. and F. C. Spencer (eds.), "Gibbon's Surgery of the Chest," W. B. Saunders Company, Philadelphia, 1976.

Grover, F. L., Richardson, J. D., Fervel, J. G., Arom, K. V., Webb, G. E., and Trinkle, J. K.: Prophylactic Antibiotics in the Treatment of Penetrating Chest Wounds, *J Thorac Cardiovasc Surg,* **74:**528, 1977.

Hankins, J. R., McAslan, T. C., Ayella, R., Cowley, R. A., and McLaughlin, J. S.: Extensive Pulmonary Laceration Caused by Blunt Trauma, *J Thorac Cardiovasc Surg,* **55:**16, 1968.

Naclerio, E. A.: "Chest Injuries," Grune & Stratton, Inc., New York, 1971.

Neugebauer, M. K., Fasburg, R. G., and Trummer, M. J.: Routine Antibiotic Therapy following Pleural Space Intubation, *J Thorac Cardiovasc Surg,* **61:**882, 1971.

Patterson, L. T., Schmitt, H. J., Jr., and Armstrong, R. G.: Intermediate Care of War Wounds of the Chest, *J Thorac Cardiovasc Surg,* **61:**882, 1971.

Ruckley, C. V., and McCormack, R. J. M.: The Management of Spontaneous Pneumothorax, *Thorax,* **21:**139, 1966.

Shackford, S. R., Smith, D. E., Zarins, C. K., Rice, C. L. and Virgilio, R. W.: The Management of Flail Chest: A Comparison of Ventilatory and Non-ventilatory Treatment, *Am J Surg,* **132:**759, 1976.

Sladen, A.: Methylprednisolone: Pharmacologic Doses in Shock Lung Syndrome, *J Thorac Cardiovasc Surg,* **71:**300, 1976.

Thomas, A. N., and Stephens, B. G.: Air Embolism: A Cause of Morbidity and Death after Penetrating Chest Trauma, *J Trauma,* **14:**633, 1974.

Waldo, W. J., Harlaftis, N. N. and Symbas, P. N.: Systemic Air Embolism: Does It Occur after Experimental Penetrating Lung Injury? *J Thorac Cardiovasc Surg,* **71:**96, 1976.

Wise, L., Connors, J., Hwang, Y. H., and Anderson, C.: Traumatic Injuries to the Diaphragm, *J Trauma,* **13:**946, 1973.

Chest Wall

Congenital Deformities of the Chest Wall

Beiser, G. C., Epstein, S. E., Stempter, M. D., Goldstern, R. E., Noland, S. P., and Levitsky, S.: Impairment of Cardiac Function with Pectus Excavatum with Improvement after Operative Correction, *N Engl J Med,* **287:**267, 1972.

Haller, J. A., Jr., Peters, G. N., Mazur, D., and White, J. J.: Pectus Excavatum, *J Thorac Cardiovasc Surg,* **60:**375, 1970.

Ravitch, M. M.: Disorders of the Sternum and the Thoracic Wall, in D. L. Sabiston, Jr., and F. C. Spencer (eds.), "Gibbon's Surgery of the Chest," 3d ed., W. B. Saunders Company, Philadelphia, 1976.

Stallworth, J. M., Quinn, G. J., and Aiken, A. F.: Is Rib Resection Necessary for Relief of Thoracic Outlet Syndrome? *Ann Surg,* **185:**581, 1977.

Urschel, H. C., Jr., Razzuk, M. A., Wood, R. E., Parekh, M., and Paulson, D. L.: Objective Diagnosis (Ulnar Nerve Conduction Velocity) and Current Therapy of the Thoracic Outlet Syndrome, *Ann Thorac Surg,* **12:**608, 1971.

Weg, J. G., Krumholz, R. A., and Harkleroad, L. E.: Pulmonary Dysfunction in Pectus Excavatum, *Am Rev Resp Dis,* **96:**936, 1967.

Chest-Wall Tumors

Adkins, P. C.: Tumors of the Chest Wall, in T. W. Shields (ed.), "General Thoracic Surgery," Lea & Febiger, Philadelphia 1972.

Burnard, R. J., Martini, N., and Beattie, E. J., Jr.: The Value of Resection in Tumors Involving the Chest Wall, *J Thorac Cardiovasc Surg,* **68:**530, 1974.

Martini, N., Huvos, A. G., Smith, J., and Beattie, E. J., Jr.: Primary Malignant Tumors of the Sternum, *Surg Gynecol Obstet,* **138:**391, 1974.

Pleura

Bryant, L. R., Chicklo, J. M., Crutcher, R. R., et al.: Management of Thoracic Empyema, *J Thorac Cardiovasc Surg,* **55:**850, 1968.

Craenen, J. M., Williams, T. E., Jr., and Kilman, J. W.: Simplified Management of Chylothorax in Neonates and Infants, *Ann Thorac Surg,* **24:**275, 1977.

Green, R. A., and Johnson, R. F.: Diseases of the Pleura, in G. L. Baum (ed.), "Textbook of Pulmonary Diseases," 2d ed., Little, Brown and Company, Boston, 1974.

Sahn, S. A.: Evaluation of Pleural Effusions and Pleural Biopsy, in T. L. Petty (ed.), "Pulmonary Diagnostic Techniques," Lea & Febiger, Philadelphia, 1975.

Shearin, J. C., Jr., and Jackson, D.: Malignant Pleural Mesothelioma: Report of 19 Cases, *J Thorac Cardiovasc Surg,* **71:**621, 1976.

Lungs and Trachea

Anatomy and Diagnostic Techniques

Arom, K. V., Franz, J. L., Grover, F. L., and Trinkle, J. K.: Subxiphoid Anterior Mediastinal Exploration, *Ann Thorac Surg,* **24:**289, 1977.

Bartlett, J. G., Rosenblatt, J. D., and Finegold, S. M.: Percutaneous Transtracheal Aspiration in the Diagnosis of Anaerobic Pulmonary Infection, *Ann Intern Med,* **79:**535, 1973.

Boyden, E. A., and Tomsett, D. H.: Congenital Absence of the Medial Basal Bronchus in a Child: With Preliminary Observations on Postnatal Growth of the Lungs, *J Thorac Cardiovasc Surg,* **43:**517, 1962.

Neff, T. A.: Needle Lung Biopsy, in T. L. Petty (ed.), "Pulmonary Diagnostic Techniques," Lea & Febiger, Philadelphia, 1975.

Nohl, H. C.: "The Spread of Carcinoma of the Bronchus," Lloyd Luke, London, 1962.

Nohl-Oser, H. C.: The Lymphatic Spread of Carcinoma of the Bronchus, in "International Symposium of Mediastinoscopy," Odense University Press, Odense, Denmark, 1970.

Sinner, W. N.: Wert und Bedeutung der perkutanen transthorakalen Nadelbiopsie, *Fortschr Geb Roentgenstr Nuklearmed,* **123:**197, 1975.

Stanford, W., Steele, S., Armstrong, R. G., and Larsen, G. L.: Mediastinoscopy: Its Application in Central versus Peripheral Thoracic Lesions, *Ann Thorac Surg,* **19:**121, 1975.

Congenital Disorders

Glenn, W. L., Liebow, A. A., and Lindskog, G. E.: "Thoracic and Cardiovascular Surgery with Related Pathology," 3d ed., Appleton-Century-Crofts, Inc., New York, 1975.

Michelson, E.: Clinical Spectrum of Infantile Lobar Emphysema, *Ann Thorac Surg,* **24:**182, 1977.

Pulmonary Infections

Baum, G. L.: "Textbook of Pulmonary Diseases," 2d ed., Little, Brown and Company, Boston, 1974.

Elkadi, A., Salas, R., and Almond, C. H.: Surgical Treatment of Atypical Pulmonary Tuberculosis, *J Thorac Cardiovasc Surg,* **72:**435, 1976.

Fosburg, R. G., Baisch, B. F., and Trumner, M. J.: Limited Pulmonary Resection for Coccidioidomycosis, *Ann Thorac Surg,* **7:**420, 1969.

Glenn, W. L., Liebow, A. A., and Lindskog, G. E.: "Thoracic and Cardiovascular Surgery with Related Pathology," 3d ed., Appleton-Century-Crofts, Inc., New York, 1975.

Groff, D. B., and Marquis, J.: Transtracheal Drainage of Lung Abscesses in Children, *J Pediatr Surg,* **12:**303, 1977.

Larsen, R. E., Bernatz, P. E., and Gerasi, J. E.: Results of Surgical and Nonoperative Treatment for Pulmonary North American Blastomycosis, *J Thorac Cardiovasc Surg,* **51:**714, 1966.

Prather, J. R., Eastridge, C. E., Hughes, F. H., Jr., et al.: Actinomycosis of the Thorax: Diagnosis and Treatment, *Ann Thorac Surg,* **9:**307, 1970.

Sealy, W. C., Bradham, R. R., and Young, W. G., Jr.: The Surgical Treatment of Multisegmental and Localized Bronchiectasis, *Surg Gynecol Obstet,* **123:**80, 1966.

Solit, R. W., McKeown, J., Jr., Smullens, S., et al.: The Surgical Implications of Intracavity Mycetoma (Fungus Balls), *J Thorac Cardiovasc Surg,* **62:**411, 1971.

Sutaria, M. K., Polk, J. W., Reddy, P., et al.: Surgical Aspects of

Pulmonary Histoplasmosis: A Series of 110 Cases, *Thorax,* **25:**31, 1970.

Takaro, T.: Mycotic Infections of Interest to Thoracic Surgeons: Collective Review, *Ann Thorac Surg,* **3:**71, 1967.

Tunell, W. P., Koh, Y. C., and Adkins, P. C.: The Dilemma of Coincident Active Pulmonary Tuberculosis and Carcinoma of the Lung, *J Thorac Cardiovasc Surg,* **62:**563, 1971.

Solitary Pulmonary Nodules

Higgins, G. A., Shields, T. W., and Keehn, R. J.: The Solitary Pulmonary Nodule: Ten-Year Follow-up of Veterans Administration–Armed Forces Cooperative Study, *Arch Surg,* **110:**570, 1975.

Lillington, G. A., and Stevens, G. M.: The Solitary Nodule: The Other Side of the Coin, *Chest,* **70:**322, 1976.

Nathan, M. H.: Management of Solitary Pulmonary Nodules: An Organized Approach Based on Growth Rate and Statistics, *JAMA,* **227:**1141, 1974.

Primary Carcinoma of the Lung

Armentrout, S. A.: Chemotherapy in Carcinoma of the Lung, *Chest,* **71:**638, 1977.

Bates, M.: Results of Surgery for Bronchial Carcinoma in Patients Aged 70 and Over, *Thorax,* **25:**77, 1970.

Bell, J. W.: Positive Sputum Cytology and Negative Chest Roentgenograms: A Surgeon's Dilemma, *Ann Thorac Surg,* **9:**149, 1970.

Brock, Lord: Long Survival after Operation for Cancer of the Lung, *Br J Surg,* **62:**1, 1975.

Holmes, E. C.: Immunology of Lung Cancer, *Chest,* **71:**643, 1977.

Kennedy, J. H.: Extrapulmonary Effects of Cancer of the Lung and Pleura, *J Thorac Surg,* **61:**514, 1971.

McKneally, M. F., Maver, C., and Kausal, H. W.: Regional Immunotherapy with Intrapleural BCG for Lung Cancer: Surgical Considerations, *J Thorac Cardiovasc Surg,* **72:**333, 1976.

Mountain, C. F.: Assessment of the Role of Surgery for Control of Lung Cancer, *Ann Thorac Surg,* **24:**365, 1977.

Paulson, D. L., and Reisch, J. S.: Long Term Survival after Resection for Bronchogenic Carcinoma, *Ann Surg,* **184:**324, 1976.

——— and Urschel, H. C., Jr.: Selectivity in the Surgical Treatment of Bronchogenic Carcinoma, *J Thorac Cardiovasc Surg,* **62:**554, 1971.

Pearson, F. G., Thompson, D. W., and Delarne, N. C.: Experience with the Cytologic Detection, Localization and Treatment of Radiographically Undemonstrable Bronchial Carcinoma, *J Thorac Cardiovasc Surg,* **54:**371, 1967.

Shields, T. W., Yee, J., Conn, J. H., and Robinette, C. D.: Relationship of Cell Type and Lymph Node Metastasis to Survival after Resection of Bronchial Carcinoma, *Ann Thorac Surg,* **20:**501, 1975.

Bronchial Carcinoid and Tumors of Bronchial-Gland Origin

Axelsson, C., Burcharth, F., and Johansen, A.: Mucoepidermoid Lung Tumors, *J Thorac Cardiovasc Surg,* **65:**902, 1973.

Heilbrunn, A., and Crosby, I. K.: Adenocystic Carcinoma and Mucoepidermoid Carcinoma of the Tracheobronchial Tree, *Chest,* **61:**145, 1972.

McConaghie, R. J.: The Malignant Carcinoid Syndrome Associated with a Metastasizing Bronchial Adenoma: Report of a Case, *J Thorac Cardiovasc Surg,* **43:**303, 1962.

Meffert, W. G., and Lindskog, G. E.: Bronchial Adenoma, *J Thorac Cardiovasc Surg,* **59:**588, 1970.

Turnbull, A. D., Huvos, A. G., Goodner, J. T., et al.: The Malignant Potential of Bronchial Adenoma, *Ann Thorac Surg,* **14:**453, 1972.

Miscellaneous Lung Tumors

Arrigoni, M. G., Woolner, L. B., Bernatz, P. E., et al.: Benign Tumors of the Lung: A Ten-Year Surgical Experience, *J Thorac Cardiovasc Surg,* **60:**589, 1970.

Davis, P. W., Briggs, J. C., Seal, R. M. E., et al.: Benign and Malignant Mixed Tumours of the Lung, *Thorax,* **27:**657, 1972.

Guccion, J. G., and Rosen, S. H.: Bronchopulmonary Leiomyosarcoma and Fibrosarcoma: A Study of 32 Cases and Review of the Literature, *Cancer,* **30:**836, 1972.

Iverson, R. E., and Straehley, C. J.: Pulmonary Blastoma: Long-term Survival of Juvenile Patient, *Chest,* **63:**436, 1973.

Kakos, G. S., Williams, T. E., Jr., Assor, D., et al.: Pulmonary Carcinosarcoma: Etiologic Therapeutic and Prognostic Considerations, *J Thorac Cardiovasc Surg,* **61:**777, 1971.

Koutras, P., Urschel, H. C., Jr., and Paulson, D. L.: Hamartoma of the Lung, *J Thorac Cardiovasc Surg,* **61:**768, 1971.

McNamara, J. J., Paulson, D. L., Kingsley, W. B., et al.: Primary Leiomyosarcoma of the Lung, *J Thorac Cardiovasc Surg,* **57:**635, 1969.

Martini, N., Hajdu, S. I., and Beattie, E. J., Jr.: Primary Sarcoma of the Lung, *J Thorac Cardiovasc Surg,* **61:**33, 1971.

Ostermiller, W. E., Comer, T. P., and Barker, W. L.: Endobronchial Granular Cell Myoblastoma: A Report of Three Cases and Review of the Literature, *Ann Thorac Surg,* **9:**143, 1970.

Metastatic Pulmonary Neoplasms

Beattie, E. J., Martini, N., and Rosen, G.: The Management of Pulmonary Metastases in Children with Osteogenic Sarcoma with Surgical Resection Combined with Chemotherapy, *Cancer,* **34:**618, 1975.

Cahan, W. G., Castro, E. B., and Hajdu, S. I.: The Significance of a Solitary Lung Shadow in Patients with Colon Carcinoma, *Cancer,* **33:**414, 1974.

McCormack, P. M., Bains, M. S., Beattie, E. J., and Martini, N.: Pulmonary Resection in Metastatic Carcinoma, *Chest,* **73:**163, 1978.

Morton, D. L., Joseph, W. L., Ketcham, A. S., Geelhoed, G. W., and Adkins, P. C.: Surgical Resection and Adjunctive Immunotherapy for Selected Patients with Multiple Pulmonary Metastasis, *Ann Surg,* **178:**360, 1973.

Ochsner, A., and DeBakey, M.: Significance of Metastasis in Primary Carcinoma of the Lungs, *J Thorac Surg,* **11:**357, 1942.

Roth, J. A., Silverstein, M. J., and Morton, D. L.: Metastatic Potential of Metastases, *Surgery,* **79:**669, 1976.

Takita, H., Merrin, C., Didalkar, M. S., Douglass, H. O., and Edgerton, F.: The Surgical Management of Multiple Lung Metastases, *Ann Thorac Surg,* **24:**359, 1977.

Trachea

Bryant, L. R., Trinkle, J. K., and Dubilier, L.: Reappraisal of Tracheal Injury from Cuffed Tracheostomy Tubes, *JAMA,* **215:**625, 1971.

Grillo, J. C.: Congenital Lesions, Neoplasms and Injuries of the Trachea, in Gibbon, J. H., Jr., Sabiston, D. C., Jr., and Spencer, F. C. (eds.), "Surgery of the Chest," 3d ed., W. B. Saunders Company, Philadelphia, 1976.

Hajdu, S. K., Huvos, A. G., Goodner, J. T., Foote, F. W., Jr., and

Beattie, E. J., Jr.: Carcinoma of the Trachea: Clinicopathologic Study of 41 Cases, *Cancer,* **25:**1448, 1970.

Moghissi, K.: Personal communication.

———: Tracheal Reconstruction with a Prosthesis of Marlex Mesh and Pericardium, *J Thorac Cardiovasc Surg,* **69:**499, 1975.

Neville, W. E., Bolanowski, P. J., and Soltanzadeh, H.: Prosthetic Reconstruction of the Trachea and Carina, *J Thorac Cardiovasc Surg,* **72:**525, 1976.

Pearson, F. G., Thompson, D. W., Weissbert, D., Simpson, W. J. K., and Kergin, F. G.: Adenoid Cystic Carcinoma of Trachea: Experience with 16 Patients Managed by Tracheal Resection, *Ann Thorac Surg,* **18:**16, 1974.

Rodgers, B. M., Rosenfeld, M., and Talbert, J. L.: Endobronchial Cryotherapy in the Treatment of Tracheal Strictures, *J Pediatr Surg,* **12:**443, 1977.

Webb, W. R., Ozdemir, I. A., Ikins, P. M., and Parker, F., Jr.: Surgical Management of Tracheal Stenosis, *Ann Surg,* **179:**819, 1974.

Mediastinum

Burkell, C. C., Cross, J. M., Kent, H. P., and Nanson, E. N.: Mass Lesions of the Mediastinum, in M. M. Ravitch (ed.), "Current Problems in Surgery," Yearbook Medical Publishers, Inc., Chicago, June 1969.

Effler, D. B., and Groves, L. K.: Superior Vena Caval Obstruction, *J Thorac Cardiovasc Surg,* **43:**574, 1962.

Filler, R. M., Troggis, D. G., Jaffe, W., and Vawter, G. F.: Favorable Outlook for Children with Mediastinal Neuroblastoma, *J Pediatr Surg,* **7:**136, 1972.

Gomes, M. N., and Hufnagel, C. A.: Superior Vena Cava Obstruction, *Ann Thorac Surg,* **20:**344, 1975.

Grimes, O. F.: Infections of the Mediastinum and the Superior Vena Caval Syndrome, in T. W. Shields (ed.), "General Thoracic Surgery," Lea & Febiger, Philadelphia, 1972.

Kirwan, W. O., Walbaum, P. R., and McCormack, R. J.: Cystic Intrathoracic Derivatives of the Foregut and Their Complications, *Thorax,* **28:**424, 1973.

Sakulsky, S. B., Harrison, E. G., Jr., Dinea, D. E., and Payne, W. S.: Mediastinal Granuloma, *J Thorac Cardiovasc Surg,* **54:**279, 1967.

Wychulis, A. R., Payne, W. S., Clagett, O. T., and Woolner, L. B.: Surgical Treatment of Mediastinal Tumors: A 40-Year Experience, *J Thorac Cardiovasc Surg,* **62:**379, 1971.

Chapter 18

Congenital Heart Disease

by **Frank C. Spencer**

INTRODUCTION

With the declining incidence of rheumatic fever, congenital heart disease has become the most common form of heart disease seen in children. In several studies the frequency has been found to be about 3 cases of congenital heart disease occurring in every 1,000 live births. The frequency is about ten times greater in members of the same family than in the normal population, and a convenient approximation of risk of occurrence in younger siblings of a child with congenital heart disease is about 2 percent. In most patients the etiologic factor is unknown.

Rubella occurring in the first trimester of pregnancy is one of the few infectious diseases known to cause congenital heart disease. It produces the well-recognized syndrome of mental deficiency, deafness, cataracts, and congenital heart disease, usually a patent ductus arteriosus. Mongolism is another congenital abnormality associated with a high incidence of congenital heart disease. Usually congenital heart disease occurs as an isolated malformation resulting from defective embryonic development without known cause.

The surprisingly short period of time during which cardiac development occurs in uterine life should be emphasized, for virtually all the fetal heart structures are formed between the third and eighth week of pregnancy, a time interval of only 5 weeks. Atrial or ventricular septal defects result from incomplete formation of the respective septa, while transposition and other anomalies of the aorta result from abnormalities in the spiral division of the primitive bulbus cordis. Although there are six branchial aortic arches, all atrophy with the exception of the fourth left arch, remaining as the aorta, and the sixth left arch, remaining as the ductus arteriosus. Malformations with vascular rings arise from different remnants of these embryonic branchial arches.

The fetal circulation has several distinctive features, which may persist in association with congenital heart disease in adults. In embryonic life the lungs are collapsed, with a high vascular resistance, and pulmonary blood flow is small. Most of the blood returning through the inferior vena cava to the right atrium goes through the foramen ovale into the left atrium and thence to the left ventricle. Also, most of the blood expelled from the right ventricle into the pulmonary artery is shunted through the ductus arteriosus into the descending thoracic aorta. At birth, with expansion of the lungs, there is a fall in pulmonary vascular resistance, although the vascular resistance does not decrease to that normally found in older individuals for the first 1 to 3 years of life. There is a corresponding persistence during this time of the fetal histologic-structure of the pulmonary arteries, characterized principally by an abundance of smooth muscle in the media of the arterial wall. Persistence of the fetal histologic structure of the pulmonary arterioles has been associated with pulmonary hypertension in small children.

With expansion of the lungs, the ductus arteriosus normally closes in the first few days after birth. It remains patent in only a small percentage of individuals, but this is one of the most common forms of congenital heart disease. The foramen ovale is a slitlike channel which is automatically sealed when left atrial pressure becomes higher than right atrial pressure and normally permits the flow of blood only from the right atrium to the left atrium, not in the reverse direction. Patency of the foramen ovale, usually an innocuous defect, remains throughout adult life in at least 10 to 20 percent of patients. With elevation of right atrial pressure above left atrial pressure from any cause, the foramen ovale may be stretched open and create a right-to-left shunt from the right atrium to the left atrium, resulting in cyanosis from shunting of unoxygenated blood. This characteristically occurs in patients with pulmonic valvular stenosis when right ventricular failure develops and right atrial pressure rises above left atrial pressure.

Although a large number of congenital heart defects have been recognized and classified, in a large pediatric cardiac clinic seven malformations will be found to comprise the majority of abnormalities seen. Ventricular septal defect, with or without pulmonic stenosis, is by far the most common, representing 20 percent or more of all patients. The other six malformations, each occurring in 10 to 15 percent of patients, are atrial septal defect, pulmonic valvular stenosis, aortic valvular stenosis, patent ductus arteriosus, coarctation of the aorta, and transposition of the great vessels. The frequency of different defects varies somewhat with the age of the patient studied; transposition of the great vessels is a much more common disease in the newborn, as many do not survive beyond six months of age.

Classification

Congenital heart disease may be conveniently classified by the type of anatomic abnormality present, which in turn produces a distinct physiologic disturbance, as follows: (1) obstructive lesions predominantly restrict the flow of blood, with corresponding increased work loads on the obstructed ventricular chamber; (2) left-to-right shunts occur through uncomplicated septal defects; (3) right-to-left shunts result from combination of a septal defect with obstruction to ventricular emptying; (4) complex malformations, as the name indicates, are more extensive disturbances of the structure of the heart from gross errors in development. These include abnormal origin or atresia of the aorta or pulmonary artery and hypoplasia or atresia of the right or left ventricle and the corresponding tricuspid and mitral valves.

Pathophysiology

Four stages in the severity of congenital heart disease often can be recognized. Initially, there may be only abnormal physical findings. In milder forms of congenital heart disease, such as trivial pulmonic valvular stenosis, there may never be any sign of heart disease except the characteristic systolic murmur. In the second stage of severity, physiologic disturbances can be measured by cardiac catheterization, such as pressure gradients across stenotic pulmonic or aortic valves, increased blood flow through shunts occurring through atrial or ventricular septal defects, or elevation in pulmonary artery pressure as pulmonary hypertension evolves. Sooner or later, these physiologic abnormalities produce corresponding anatomic changes (the third stage in severity) manifested principally by cardiac enlargement with hypertrophy of the right or left ventricle, best measured by the electrocardiogram and roentgenogram. With the development of pulmonary hypertension, histologic changes occur in the media and intima of the pulmonary arterioles. Only in the fourth stage do symptoms of cardiac failure appear.

This late appearance of symptoms is an important consideration in evaluating children with congenital heart disease, for parents are normally apprehensive about consenting to complex diagnostic studies or operative procedures on a child who seems, to the inexperienced eye, to have little disability. Postponing therapy until a child is disabled to a point that is clinically obvious may result in irreversible changes in ventricular muscle, for severe hypertrophy of the right or left ventricle does not always regress completely following surgical correction of the basic cause, such as pulmonic or aortic stenosis. Even more serious is an increase in pulmonary vascular resistance, which, with present therapy, is often irreversible.

The three main physiologic disturbances resulting from congenital heart disease are (1) obstruction to emptying of the ventricles, (2) left-to-right shunts with increase in pulmonary blood flow and corresponding decrease in systemic blood flow, and (3) right-to-left shunts producing oxygen unsaturation of the arterial blood. Each of these physiologic disturbances is considered in detail in subsequent sections. Also, with all forms of congenital heart disease there is an increased susceptibility to bacterial endocarditis, because the anatomic malformation creates a localized turbulent flow of blood predisposing to local deposition of bacteria during a transient bacteremia.

OBSTRUCTIVE LESIONS. The most common disorders are pulmonic valvular stenosis, aortic valvular stenosis, and coarctation of the aorta. These impede emptying of the involved ventricular chamber, resulting in what has been termed "systolic" overloading and corresponding concentric hypertrophy of the ventricle. As the ventricular response is predominantly concentric hypertrophy, cardiac enlargement cannot be detected by clinical means, and often the chest roentgenogram is only slightly abnormal. The electrocardiogram is a most useful guide, however, indicating the degree of ventricular hypertrophy which has occurred. With progressive left ventricular hypertrophy angina pectoris may occur, with susceptibility to arrhythmias and even sudden death. Cardiac failure is a late and often preterminal manifestation.

LEFT-TO-RIGHT SHUNTS. As pressures in the left atrium and left ventricle are normally greater than those in the right atrium and right ventricle, a defect in either the atrial or ventricular septum results in a shunt of oxygenated blood from the left side of the heart to the right side. This causes pulmonary congestion from an increase in pulmonary blood flow and often a corresponding decrease in systemic blood flow. Cyanosis, of course, does not occur. With the increase in pulmonary blood flow there is a tendency to develop pulmonary hypertension, varying both with the type of defect and with the individual patient. The most common defects producing left-to-right shunts are atrial septal defects, with or without anomalous pulmonary veins, ventricular septal defects, and patent ductus arteriosus.

Pulmonary Congestion. A shunt becomes physiologically significant when the pulmonary blood flow is 1.5 to 2.0 times as great as the systemic blood flow. Large shunts may produce a pulmonary blood flow three to four times greater than systemic blood flow, with a calculated pulmonary blood flow of even 10 to 15 liters/minute/square meter of body surface. The resulting pulmonary congestion produces a susceptibility to bacterial infection; recurrent bouts of pneumonia may occur in the first few years of life. Beyond early childhood, however, high pulmonary blood flows may be associated with surprisingly little disability for a period of time. With the increase in pulmonary blood flow there is a corresponding enlargement of the involved ventricle (right ventricle with atrial septal defect, left ventricle with patent ductus arteriosus, both ventricles with ventricular septal defect), resulting in so-called "diastolic" overloading of the ventricle, with cardiac dilatation rather than hypertrophy. The dilatation can be more easily recognized on clinical examination and on the chest roentgenogram than its counterpart, concentric hypertrophy. The changes in the electrocardiogram are often less prominent than those seen with concentric hypertrophy. Cardiac failure tends to occur somewhat earlier in the course of the disease than with concentric hypertrophy, and the prognosis with medical therapy is somewhat better than that for predominantly obstructive lesions.

Pulmonary Hypertension. With the increase in pulmonary blood flow there is a tendency to develop pulmonary hypertension. Although the mode of development has been a subject of intense study for over two decades, many factors remain unknown. An excellent analysis of the functional pathology of the pulmonary vascular bed was published by Edwards in 1957. Pulmonary hypertension may result from at least three factors: (1) an increase in pulmonary blood flow, (2) histologic changes in the pulmonary vascular bed with corresponding anatomic restriction of distensibility of the pulmonary vessels, or (3) pulmonary venous obstruction. It should be emphasized that the most important consideration in evaluating the pulmonary circulation is the pulmonary vascular resistance, not the systolic pulmonary arterial pressure per se. Pulmonary hypertension resulting from an increase in pulmonary blood flow subsides as soon as the cardiac defect producing the increase in

blood flow is corrected. Pulmonary hypertension due to increased pulmonary vascular resistance from a decrease in distensibility of the pulmonary vascular bed is often irreversible, however. When severe, surgical therapy may be of limited value or even contraindicated. Hence, in evaluating pulmonary hypertension, the significant physiologic measurement is the degree of change in the pulmonary vascular resistance, as calculated from the relation between flow and pressure, and not the absolute level of the pulmonary artery pressure per se.

Normally pulmonary arterioles are very distensible and can accommodate an increase in pulmonary blood flow up to three times normal values without any increase in pressure. Further distensibility is limited by the fibrous tissue in the adventitial sheath surrounding the arterioles. In infants and young children with pulmonary hypertension the prominent histologic change in the pulmonary arterioles is hypertrophy of the smooth muscle of the media of the arteriolar wall, which is similar to that normally found in embryonic life. Some feel that these histologic changes represent merely a failure of involution of the normal fetal pattern. In older children and adults, thickening of the intima occurs also, with associated fibrosis, and has a more serious prognosis, for such histologic changes are often irreversible and may not improve even after the underlying cause has been corrected.

More significant than the increase in pulmonary blood flow, however, is the pressure under which blood is expelled into the pulmonary artery, for pulmonary hypertension is much more frequent with ventricular septal defects than with atrial septal defects which produce a similar increase in pulmonary blood flow. In general, the incidence of hypertension with secundum atrial septal defects in children is about 5 percent, with atrioventricular canal defects about 10 percent, and with ventricular septal defects about 25 percent, as reported by Nadas.

In addition, there is an individual variation in susceptibility to development of pulmonary hypertension, for some children with a large ventricular septal defect and a large increase in pulmonary blood flow will not develop any change in pulmonary vascular resistance, while others with a smaller septal defect will develop significant pulmonary hypertension at an early age. Finally, there are unexplained variations in pulmonary hypertension for which no known cause can at present be discerned. In some children pulmonary hypertension is apparently present from birth and remains for several years without any change. In others pulmonary hypertension found at birth may be found to have regressed spontaneously when the patient is studied at repeat cardiac catheterization some years later. In most patients, however, pulmonary hypertension gradually but progressively increases in severity, eventually becoming incurable.

The earliest age at which pulmonary vascular changes become irreversible is both variable and uncertain, but certain defects such as truncus arteriosus or transposition apparently may produce permanent changes in some patients by the age of one year. With advances in surgical therapy, most lesions producing an increase in pulmonary vascular resistance, such as ventricular septal defect, patent ductus arteriosus, or aortopulmonary window, should be surgically corrected in the first two years of life. With simple atrial secundum defect, however, operation at such an early age is virtually never necessary, illustrating the unknown etiologic factors in the development of increase in pulmonary vascular resistance.

Restriction in Systemic Blood Flow. With large left-to-right shunts there is often a decrease in systemic blood flow, frequently associated with a retardation in normal growth and development. This is more prominently seen in children with a patent ductus arteriosus or an atrial septal defect. The appearance of frail, underweight children with atrial septal defect has been termed the *gracile* habitus. Although mental retardation is slightly more common in children with congenital heart disease, beyond this association there is no evidence that congenital heart disease retards mental development. Unfortunately, correction of the cardiac defect does not result in any improvement in mental function. There is, however, often a substantial increase in growth and weight once the cardiac defect has been corrected.

RIGHT-TO-LEFT SHUNTS. Right-to-left shunts of venous blood directly into the systemic circulation, producing arterial hypoxemia and cyanosis, result from the combination of an intracardiac septal defect with obstruction to normal flow of blood into the pulmonary artery. The classic example is the tetralogy of Fallot, a combination of ventricular septal defect and pulmonic stenosis. Other cyanotic disorders include the more complex malformations, such as transposition of the great vessels, tricuspid atresia, truncus arteriosus, and total anomalous drainage of the pulmonary veins. Right-to-left shunts produce a large number of physiologic disturbances because of the anoxia resulting from chronic hypoxemia in the arterial blood. These are considered in detail in the following paragraphs. It should be emphasized that all these disturbances result from deficient oxygen transport to tissues of the body. With right-to-left shunts there is no increase in cardiac output, and often the pulmonary blood flow is less than normal. Hence cardiac failure is rare with an uncomplicated right-to-left shunt, in contrast to its inevitable eventual occurrence with left-to-right shunts.

Cyanosis. This is the most prominent feature of a right-to-left shunt. The degree of cyanosis depends upon both the degree of anoxia and the blood hemoglobin concentration, for the visible intensity of cyanosis is determined by the number of grams of reduced hemoglobin in the circulation. It has been estimated that about 5 Gm of reduced hemoglobin is required to produce visible cyanosis. Normally in the capillaries about 2.25 Gm of reduced hemoglobin is present, so with an average hemoglobin concentration of 15 Gm/100 ml of blood, a decrease in arterial oxygen from the normal range of nearly 95% to 75% is needed to produce visible cyanosis. In the presence of anemia, however, a more severe degree of anoxia is required to produce visible cyanosis, while with polycythemia and hemoglobin concentrations of 20 Gm/100 ml of blood or more, severe cyanosis may represent less serious anoxia.

Cyanosis has been conveniently grouped into "central"

and "peripheral" types. *Peripheral* cyanosis results simply from a decrease in cardiac output with sluggish regional flow of blood through the capillary circulation, as a result of which more oxygen is extracted and a greater amount of reduced hemoglobin is present. This type of cyanosis occurs with conditions producing a low cardiac output, such as mitral stenosis, and varies with the condition of the patient. It is usually more prominent in certain regions of the body, such as the tips of the fingers, the lips, or the lobes of the ears.

Central cyanosis results either from a defect in oxygenation of blood in the lungs or from an intracardiac shunt. Cyanosis resulting from pulmonary insufficiency can usually be recognized from its prompt improvement when the patient breathes 100% oxygen, increasing the efficiency of pulmonary ventilation. In the catheterization laboratory it can be recognized from the finding that oxygen saturation of blood in the left atrium is less than 95%. Pulmonary insufficiency from cardiac disease occurs only with severe pulmonary congestion from cardiac failure or far advanced pulmonary vascular disease.

An intracardiac shunt, permitting direct entry of venous blood into the systemic circulation, is the cause of central cyanosis in most patients. The intensity of the cyanosis is related to the volume of pulmonary blood flow, for ultimately cyanosis depends upon the relative proportions of unoxygenated and oxygenated blood in the arterial circulation. Even though a large intracardiac shunt is present, an increase in pulmonary blood flow to produce a larger amount of oxygenated blood can substantially reduce cyanosis and improve oxygen transport. This was dramatically demonstrated by Blalock with the systemic-pulmonary artery anastomosis for tetralogy of Fallot.

Two distinctive changes which inevitably result with chronic cyanosis are clubbing of the digits and polycythemia. The triad of cyanosis, clubbing, and polycythemia is a familiar one in children with congenital heart disease. Clubbing of the digits, or hypertrophic osteoarthropathy, is an unusual change in the appearance and structure of the digits, consisting of a rounding of the tips of the fingers and toes, as well as a thickening of the ends, associated with deposition of fibrous tissue. In addition, there may be a pronounced convexity of the fingernails. Histologically, the fingers have increased numbers of capillaries, with a large number of tiny arteriovenous aneurysms. Clubbing is usually not prominent until a cyanotic child is one to two years of age, but in some instances of severe anoxia it may evolve within several weeks. It usually gradually subsides following correction of the intracardiac defect.

Polycythemia is a fortunate physiologic response of the bone marrow to chronic anoxia, as an increase in red cell and hemoglobin concentration increases the ability of the blood to transport oxygen. Hematocrit readings of 60 to 70 percent are frequent with chronic cyanosis, and readings exceeding 80 percent are found in extreme cases. There is a parallel rise in viscosity of the blood, with restriction to the flow of blood as the hematocrit reading increases. Once the hematocrit reading exceeds 75 to 80 percent, the increased viscosity constitutes a significant hazard, for transitory dehydration in an infant with a hematocrit reading above 80 percent may precipitate cerebral venous thrombosis and permanent neurologic injury, apparently from formation of thrombi in the viscous blood.

Limitation of Exercise Tolerance. A decrease in exercise tolerance, with dyspnea on exertion, is characteristic of cyanotic heart disease, for the circulation is unable to increase oxygen transport with exercise. The severity of the disability, or its progression, can be conveniently measured in terms of the patient's ability to walk a measured distance. Associated with exertional dyspnea is squatting, a phenomenon first emphasized by Taussig. The cyanotic child quickly learns that dyspnea on walking can be lessened by assuming a squatting position. Physiologic studies indicate that squatting produces an increase in peripheral vascular resistance, with a corresponding increase in pulmonary blood flow. Squatting is most commonly seen in tetralogy of Fallot, less frequently in other cyanotic conditions.

Neurologic Damage. Periodic episodes of unconsciousness, termed *cyanotic spells,* are grave signs of cerebral anoxia. They often appear in the third to fourth month of life in severely cyanotic children, even in the first few weeks of life with extreme anoxia, but are rare after the fifth to sixth year of life. They characteristically occur at different times, not always associated with exertion, and evolve as episodes of crying, deepening cyanosis, and coma, lasting a few minutes to a few hours. Such episodes are extremely grave, for although recovery may ensue promptly, the spells are recurrent, and any spell may either terminate fatally or result in permanent neurologic injury. Emergency surgical treatment to improve the oxygen content of the arterial blood is strongly indicated.

Another cause of neurologic injury in cyanotic children is brain abscess, for which there is increased susceptibility especially in children with tetralogy of Fallot. The increased susceptibility is partly related to direct access of bacteria in the venous circulation to the arterial circulation through the right-to-left shunt. This is probably not the entire explanation, however, for a similar increased frequency does not occur in other cyanotic conditions. A localized infarct with subsequent bacterial infection may explain the evolution in some patients.

Another rare cause of cerebral injury is paradoxic embolism through an intracardiac defect, in which a thrombus migrating in the venous circulation, which would normally produce a pulmonary embolus, traverses an intracardiac defect and lodges in the cerebral circulation. Hence permanent neurologic injury, most often seen as hemiplegia, is not uncommon in children with chronic severe cyanosis, constituting a strong indication for early surgical therapy when possible.

Other Changes. In older children with severe cyanosis there is a striking increase in bronchial circulation, apparently a compensatory response to the chronic decrease in pulmonary blood flow. The myriads of collateral vessels, often constituting a mass of varicosities in the mediastinum, are principally of surgical significance because of the risk of bleeding during operation. They may be associated with epistaxis in some children, but hemoptysis is rare because the pulmonary blood flow is usually less than normal, even though the bronchial circulation is greatly increased.

Finally, with chronic polycythemia in children older than ten to fifteen years of age, multiple defects in blood coagulation occur, with abnormalities in several aspects of the blood-clotting mechanism. Clinically this may result in mild gastrointestinal bleeding, but the major significance is the increased susceptibility to hemorrhage following surgical procedures.

Clinical Examination

HISTORY. In obtaining the history of a patient with congenital heart disease, the presence of abnormal factors during pregnancy, especially during the first trimester, should be noted. Rubella in the first trimester has been emphasized because of the high incidence of cardiac and other defects. In some disorders, notably hypertrophic muscular aortic stenosis, there is a definite familial history of the disorder. Also, with the majority of patients with congenital heart disease there is about a 2 percent associated occurrence of congenital heart disease in other members of the same family. In most patients, however, no etiologic factors can be found.

The age at which a cardiac murmur was detected for the first time should be carefully noted, and the reliability of this observation should be estimated. Similarly the time of appearance of cyanosis is of significance, whether at birth or subsequently during infancy. Variations in the appearance of cyanosis, as well as its location, are also important. In some patients cyanosis may be recognized at birth, then disappear for months or years, and finally appear again.

A decrease in exercise tolerance manifested by dyspnea on exertion, is a common symptom and a convenient indication of the severity of the disorder in patients with right-to-left shunts. Squatting can be readily identified by the parents. Symptoms of lesser degrees of restriction in physical capacity, such as undue fatigability or inability to participate in exercise, should be noted, although the ability of many children with large left-to-right shunts to participate vigorously in athletics is impressive. Feeding habits and the pattern of weight are also important features.

Previous neurologic episodes such as cyanotic spells, cerebral embolism, brain abscess, or other signs of cerebral injury should be noted.

Finally, episodes of infection occurring as pneumonia, bacterial endocarditis, or rheumatic fever should be ascertained.

PHYSICAL EXAMINATION. Abnormalities in growth and development should be particularly assessed, because these are among the most common signs of cardiac disease. Cyanosis, with clubbing or polycythemia, may be obvious or may require close scrutiny for detection. On examination of the heart, any deformity of the left costal cartilages, indicating long-standing cardiac enlargement, should be noted. Palpation for a thrill is particularly important, for its presence almost uniformly indicates significant underlying cardiac disease. Cardiac size should be estimated, although this is difficult in small children and infants and is best determined by the roentgenogram. Systolic murmurs are commonly found but often are of little diagnostic significance. Basal systolic murmurs occur with pulmonic stenosis, aortic stenosis, patent ductus in infants, and co-arctation of the aorta. A murmur along the left sternal border is particularly prominent with ventricular septal defect. With systolic murmurs the type of murmur, location, and transmission are of particular importance. Diastolic murmurs are infrequent in infants but when present are especially significant. They may occur from aortic insufficiency with prolapse of an aortic cusp, with pulmonic insufficiency from long-standing pulmonary hypertension, or in association with a systolic murmur as the continuous murmur of a patent ductus arteriosus. The cardiac sounds, especially the second sound at the base, may be of importance in certain conditions. The pulmonic second sound is increased with pulmonary hypertension, decreased or absent with pulmonic stenosis or atresia. Variation in splitting of the second sound may be recognized by experienced observers and is of diagnostic importance, especially with atrial septal defect. Disturbances of rhythm are infrequent. The gallop rhythm with its ominous prognosis is seen in terminal forms of cardiac disease.

Examination of the lungs may detect rales from cardiac failure in large left-to-right shunts, but characteristically no abnormalities are found in the lungs with right-to-left shunts producing cyanosis. The hallmark of congestive failure in children is hepatic enlargement, occurring with

Fig. 18-1. Chest roentgenogram of child with tetralogy of Fallot, showing typical cardiac silhouette (sabot-shaped heart). Features include heart of normal size with prominent apex from right ventricular hypertrophy. There is increased concavity at base of heart because pulmonic stenosis produces decrease in size or absence of shadow normally seen from pulmonary artery. Vascularity of lung fields may be normal or decreased. (*Courtesy of Dr. Raymond M. Abrams, Department of Radiology, New York University Medical Center.*)

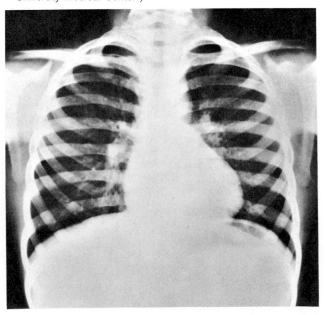

surprising rapidity and regressing rapidly as failure improves. Hence estimation of the presence and extent of hepatic enlargement is of particular importance. Often hepatic enlargement precedes the detection of audible rales, in contrast to adult forms of cardiac disease. Similarly, edema is usually less prominent clinically than hepatic enlargement.

In the extremities, the presence and quality of the radial, femoral, and pedal pulses should be noted. Faint pulses are characteristic of aortic stenosis. With coarctation, radial pulses are prominent while femoral pulses are weak or absent. Easily palpable, bounding pulses are characteristic of defects producing an abnormal exit of blood from the aorta during diastole, such as patent ductus arteriosus, aortic insufficiency, or a ruptured aneurysm of the sinus of Valsalva. These are associated with an increase in pulse pressure, usually due to a decrease in diastolic pressure. Normally the systolic blood pressure in infants is in the range of 70 to 90 mm Hg, rising to about 100 mm Hg in the first five years of life and subsequently to the normal adult level of 120 mm Hg in the next few years. Diastolic pressures are usually in the range of 55 to 60 mm Hg.

Examination of the digits is particularly useful with cyanosis, because clubbing is inevitable with chronic severe cyanosis.

LABORATORY STUDIES. A noninvasive diagnostic tripod for congenital heart disease consists of the clinical examination, the chest roentgenogram, and the electrocardiogram. These three modalities are all important in arriving at the correct diagnosis. In the roentgenogram, contour of the heart, cardiac size, and vascularity should be particularly noted. Infrequent abnormalities include pleural effusion and notching of the ribs in coarctation of the aorta. Cardiac size is best estimated from the cardiothoracic ratio; a ratio greater than 0.5 indicates cardiac enlargement. In infants a cardiac shadow with a transverse diameter greater than 5.5 cm indicates cardiac enlargement. In oblique views with fluoroscopy, cardiac enlargement involving the atria, right ventricle, left ventricle, or both ventricles may be estimated. Enlargement of the left atrium occurs with mitral insufficiency, ventricular septal defect, patent ductus arteriosus, or any form of left ventricular failure. Left ventricular enlargement is characteristic of aortic disease, mitral insufficiency, coarctation of the aorta, patent ductus arteriosus, ventricular septal defect, or tricuspid atresia. Right atrial enlargement is especially prominent in Ebstein's malformation and also occurs in tricuspid atresia, atrial septal defect, and pulmonic stenosis. Selective enlargement of the right ventricle is frequent with pulmonic stenosis, pulmonary hypertension from any cause, atrial septal defect, and ventricular septal defect.

Changes in cardiac contour may be characteristic in certain conditions. The sabot-shaped heart of tetralogy of Fallot results from hypertrophy of the right ventricle in association with a small pulmonary conus (Fig. 18-1). The egg-shaped heart of transposition of the great vessels (Fig. 18-2) is caused by enlargement of the right ventricle and right atrium, with a narrow shadow at the base from the anteroposterior relation between the aorta and the pulmonary arteries. With total anomalous drainage of the pulmonary venous return, a figure-of-eight abnormality (Fig. 18-3), composed of a large left superior vena cava in the upper mediastinum separate from the cardiac shadow, is characteristic.

The size of the pulmonary vessels and the pulmonary vascularity are also important. This can be estimated by fluoroscopy, where the vigor of the pulsations can be observed. Defects with an increased pulmonary blood flow and pulmonary hypertension can be easily differentiated from conditions associated with a normal or a decreased pulmonary blood flow.

The electrocardiogram is the best guide to the presence of ventricular hypertrophy. Selective hypertrophy of the left ventricle, as in aortic valvular stenosis, or selective hypertrophy of the right ventricle, as in pulmonic valvular stenosis, can be recognized and also correlated with the degree of stenosis. Bundle branch block, typically seen as a right bundle branch block with an atrial septal defect, also occurs in certain conditions.

Cardiac catheterization with cineangiography is essential for a complete evaluation. With cardiac catheterization, intracardiac pressures can be determined; abnormal shunts of blood can be recognized, and the ratio between pulmonary and systemic blood flow determined. Direct passage of the catheter into an abnormal chamber, such as a patent ductus arteriosus, may provide visual confirmation of the diagnosis. Mitral or aortic insufficiency are best evaluated

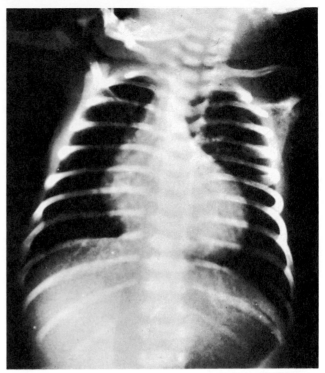

Fig. 18-2. Chest roentgenogram of child with transposition of great vessels, showing egg-shaped heart with large ventricular silhouette and small "waist," which results from abnormal location of aorta directly anterior to pulmonary artery. (*Courtesy of Dr. Raymond M. Abrams, Department of Radiology, New York University Medical Center.*)

by cineangiography. Dye-dilution curves, once widely used, are now seldom done, as simpler and more precise diagnostic methods have evolved.

In the normal heart the right atrial systolic pressure does not exceed 5 mm Hg, while left atrial pressure is in the

Fig. 18-3. *A.* Chest roentgenogram of child with total anomalous drainage of pulmonary veins through left superior vena cava. Shadow in left upper mediastinum is due to dilated left superior vena cava. *B.* Angiogram demonstrates left superior vena cava emptying into greatly dilated left innominate vein. This x-ray appearance is pathognomonic of total anomalous drainage of pulmonary veins into left superior vena cava. (*Courtesy of Dr. Raymond M. Abrams, Department of Radiology, New York University Medical Center.*)

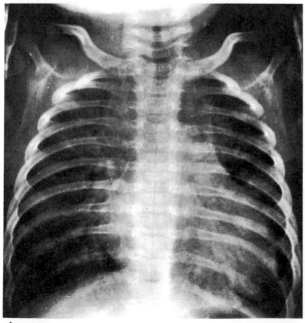

A

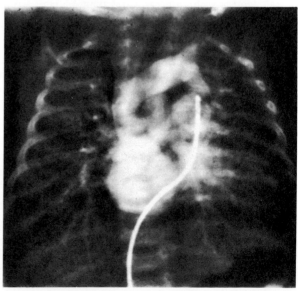

B

range of 5 to 10 mm Hg. In the normal right ventricle systolic pressure ranges from 15 to 30 mm Hg, while in the left ventricle pressures average 80 to 130 mm Hg systolic and 5 to 10 mm Hg diastolic. Continuous pressure recordings as a catheter is withdrawn from one cardiac chamber to another can readily detect the presence of stenosis; pulmonic stenosis can be measured as a catheter is withdrawn from the pulmonary artery to the right ventricle, and aortic stenosis as a catheter is withdrawn from the left ventricle into the aorta. Combined right- and left-heart catheterization is usually done with the introduction of a catheter through a systemic vein into the right side of the heart, combined with introduction of another catheter from a peripheral artery into the aorta and across the aortic valve into the left ventricle to obtain information from both the right and left sides of the heart simultaneously.

All variations from the normal pulmonary and systemic flow of 3 liters/minute/square meter of body surface may occur with intracardiac shunts. A rise in oxygen saturation of 1 vol % between cardiac chambers is usually sufficient evidence to diagnose an intracardiac left-to-right shunt. Smaller shunts may be detected with a hydrogen electrode. A pulmonary blood flow one and one-half to two times greater than systemic blood flow is associated with mild physiologic disturbances and is on the borderline of indications for surgical correction. Defects producing greater pulmonary blood flows are uniformly recommended for operation. From the combination of pulmonary blood flow and pulmonary pressure, pulmonary vascular resistance can be calculated, which with pulmonary hypertension is one of the most significant physiologic measurements influencing prognosis.

The most precise physiologic evaluation of the degree of valvular stenosis is obtained by calculation of the functional cross-sectional area of the stenotic valve orifice, as elucidated by Gorlin and Gorlin in 1951. A normal mitral valve has a functional cross-sectional area of about 5 cm²; mitral stenosis with an area of less than 1.5 cm² is functionally significant. In the aortic valve, normally with a cross-sectional area of 3 to 4 cm², a stenosis producing an opening of less than 0.8 cm² is functionally significant. Similarly, in the pulmonic valve, with a normal cross-sectional area of 2 to 4 cm², a stenosis producing an opening of less than 0.8 cm² is functionally significant.

Principles of Operative and Postoperative Care of Infants

Certain principles of management specifically pertain to infants undergoing cardiovascular surgery. For general principles of operative monitoring, extracorporeal circulation, cardiac massage, and defibrillation, Chap. 19 on acquired heart disease should be consulted.

OPERATIVE MANAGEMENT. Four important aspects of operative care are temperature control, fluid administration, prevention of air emboli, and serial blood-gas monitoring. Temperature control is essential in infants, especially in air-conditioned operating rooms, because body temperature will quickly decrease to 32 to 34°C when the

infant is anesthetized and shivering mechanisms abolished. Constant recording of the temperature with an electric esophageal or rectal probe is mandatory, and some method of warming the infant, preferably a water mattress, should routinely be employed.

Fluids must be administered with unusual precision; a 3-kg infant in cardiac failure should have no more than 20 to 40 ml of fluid in excess of measured losses during an operative procedure.

The danger of air embolism is frequently overlooked in cyanotic infants with right-to-left shunts, in whom air emboli can bypass the heart and lungs to enter the cerebral or the coronary circulation. With intravenous therapy, much care is required to prevent small air emboli, which almost routinely occur with the usual intravenous therapy during an operation. Only a few small bubbles, if lodged in a coronary artery, can precipitate ventricular fibrillation.

Serial measurement of the pH and the oxygen and carbon dioxide tensions of central venous blood, usually at 20- to 30-minute intervals during an operation, is perhaps the most essential part of monitoring. Metabolic and respiratory acidosis are extremely frequent in seriously ill infants and may quickly become intensified with compression of the lung, ineffective cardiac contraction, or hypovolemia. A pH of central venous blood below 7.30 should be promptly corrected by appropriate ventilation, bicarbonate infusion, cessation of anesthesia, or other measures to increase cardiac output. In the author's experience, changes in pH always well antedate cardiac arrest or ventricular fibrillation. With serial monitoring of blood-gas tensions during operation, desperately ill anoxic children may tolerate procedures which ordinarily would terminate in cardiac arrest or fibrillation.

POSTOPERATIVE CARE. Four important principles are constant observation, monitoring of the electrocardiogram, routine measurement of blood-gas tensions, and respiratory therapy.

Constant observation of the seriously ill infant by experienced staff on a 24-hour basis is mandatory. This includes observation of adequacy of ventilation, blood-gas tensions, fluid therapy, and arrhythmias appearing on the electrocardiogram. Ventricular fibrillation can appear virtually without warning but can be corrected, usually with electric cardioversion, if therapy can be started within 1 to 3 minutes. With a policy of constant observation, fibrillation has often been corrected with subsequent recovery in infants who otherwise would surely have succumbed to transitory ventricular arrhythmias following operation.

Serial measurement of blood-gas tensions by analysis of blood samples withdrawn through a central venous catheter, usually introduced through the saphenous vein and the inferior vena cava, is the best measurement of adequacy of ventilation and circulation. Venous carbon dioxide tensions above 45 mm Hg promptly develop with inefficient ventilation, and pH values below 7.30 quickly occur with either metabolic or respiratory acidosis. These changes far antedate any obvious clinical alteration in pulse or blood pressure and accordingly permit more effective therapy. Whether changes in pH and gas tensions are due to metabolic or respiratory causes can be determined by clinical evaluation and by gas analysis of peripheral arterial blood.

Proper ventilation is perhaps the most difficult postoperative problem in the infant following a thoracotomy. Secretions are difficult to remove, the tracheobronchial passages are so small that instrumental manipulation is difficult and can precipitate occlusive edema, and infants quickly develop cardiac arrest with transient anoxia or respiratory acidosis. Many advances in respiratory therapy of infants have been made in the past 5 to 7 years. These include mechanical respirators specifically designed for infants, the continuous positive-pressure breathing system developed by Gregory, and intermittent mandatory ventilation.

The following methods of management have been found useful, but the mode of application varies widely with individual patients. Adequate humidity, with the infant kept in a dense mist right from the time of operation, is essential. An endotracheal tube may be left in place for an indeterminate length of time following operation to assist ventilation and removal of secretions. Some have left endotracheal tubes in position for days or weeks, but the author prefers a much shorter period, usually less than 24 to 48 hours. When an endotracheal tube is left in position, it may require changing every 6 to 12 hours if inspissated secretions occlude the tip of the tube.

Translaryngeal aspiration of the trachea, accomplished with a laryngoscope to permit direct introduction of a soft catheter between the vocal cords into the trachea, is a valuable technique. It must be done by experienced personnel; otherwise trauma and edema of the vocal cords will quickly develop. It is simpler than bronchoscopy, less traumatic, and can be repeated frequently.

Tracheostomy should be avoided if possible but should be done if secretion cannot be adequately removed otherwise. With a precise technique avoiding excision of any tracheal cartilage, complications are far less frequent than in the past. At the University of South Africa in Cape Town, an extensive experience with tracheostomy and mechanical ventilation for several weeks in the treatment of neonatal tetanus has clearly demonstrated the safety of a properly performed tracheostomy.

OBSTRUCTIVE LESIONS

Pulmonic Stenosis

HISTORICAL DATA. In 1948 Brock and Sellors independently performed the first successful valvulotomies for pulmonic valvular stenosis, using a valvulotome through a transventricular approach. In 1954 Swan and Zeavin used hypothermia and venous inflow occlusion. These facts are of historical interest only, for operation with extracorporeal circulation is almost always the best approach. Rarely, a moribund infant may be best treated with one of the simpler methods.

INCIDENCE AND ETIOLOGY. Pulmonic stenosis is a common disease, representing about 10 percent of all patients with congenital heart disease. However, it was once considered a very rare disease. Taussig, in her monograph in

1947, wrote that she had not had an opportunity to study a proved case herself. The now well-established frequency of the disease indicates how interest in and recognition of a disorder is influenced by the diagnostic methods available.

There are no known significant etiologic factors.

PATHOLOGIC ANATOMY. Pulmonic stenosis was once considered to be a simple pathologic disorder due to stenosis of the pulmonary valve in most patients. From clinical experience, combined with the development of excellent angiography in recent years, it is now apparent that this simplistic concept was often erroneous and that pulmonic stenosis is a wide spectrum of disorders involving the pulmonary artery, pulmonary valve complex, and right ventricular muscle. For effective therapy these areas must be evaluated both with angiography and also at operation.

The most common variety is stenosis from fusion of the pulmonary valve cusp (Fig. 18-4). Frequently there is some hypoplasia of the main pulmonary artery, which normally should be larger than the aorta. Stenosis of the distal pulmonary artery is fortunately uncommon and is described subsequently.

Hypoplasia of a pulmonic annulus, in addition to stenosis of the valve leaflets, is important to recognize, and Kirklin and associates have recently reported a mathematical guideline of normal and abnormal cross-sectional areas of the pulmonic valve for different body weights. In the ventricle there may be a discrete infundibular stenosis (Fig. 18-5), obstruction from severe hypertrophy of ventricular muscle or combined with fibrosis, or, rarely, an anomalous papillary muscle. Hence at operation, all potential areas of stenosis should be carefully examined.

Pulmonary valvular stenosis results from fusion of the three semilunar cusps of the pulmonic valve to form a

Fig. 18-4. Pulmonic valvular stenosis with fused valve cusps creating central stenotic opening. Annulus of pulmonic valve ring is normal. (*Adapted from W. H. Cole and R. M. Zollinger, "Textbook of Surgery," Appleton-Century-Crofts, Inc., New York, 1963, 8th ed., p. 935.*)

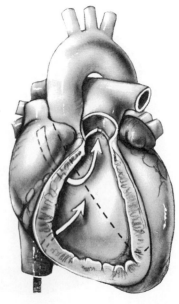

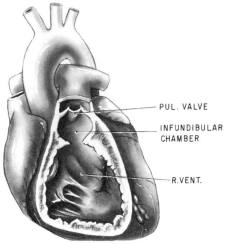

Fig. 18-5. Types of subvalvular or infundibular pulmonic stenosis. Infundibular stenosis may result in a discrete chamber between stenotic area and pulmonic valve. (*Adapted from W. H. Cole and R. M. Zollinger, "Textbook of Surgery," Appleton-Century-Crofts, Inc., New York, 1963, 8th ed., p. 936.*)

dome with a central opening usually 1 to 3 mm in diameter. In infants with severe obstruction only a pinpoint orifice may be present, while in milder forms the orifice may be 7 to 10 mm in diameter (Fig. 18-6). It has been estimated that the pulmonary valve orifice must be reduced to about one-third of normal size before significant physiologic obstruction results. Normally the three valve cusps are well formed, although variation in size is frequent. Variants include a bicuspid valve or, rarely, a fused dome-like structure with a central opening and only vestigial

Fig. 18-6. Pulmonic valvular stenosis exposed at operation following incision of pulmonary artery. Dome-shaped structure produced by fusion of valve cusps, with small central opening, is clearly shown. Suction tip has been placed in distal pulmonary artery.

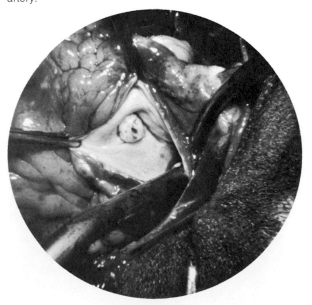

commissures. Some patients develop varying degrees of poststenotic dilatation of the main pulmonary artery. The mechanism of poststenotic dilatation was well elucidated by Holman in 1954, being related to increased lateral pressure resulting from deceleration of high velocity of flow through a small orifice. Other factors, however, must be present, for the degree of dilatation does not correspond to the severity of stenosis. Occasionally an asymptomatic patient in the fourth or fifth decade is seen following the detection of a mediastinal mass on a chest roentgenogram, who on later study will be found to have mild pulmonic stenosis with extensive poststenotic dilatation.

Compensatory hypertrophy of the right ventricle to eject blood through the stenotic orifice occurs regularly. In severe, chronic stenosis the massive ventricular hypertrophy (1 to 2 cm), may significantly reduce the lumen of the right ventricular cavity, constituting an additional element of obstruction to the flow of blood.

Isolated infundibular stenosis occurs in 5 to 10 percent of patients with pulmonic stenosis. It consists of a discrete fibrous diaphragm with a 3- to 6-mm central opening in the outflow tract of the right ventricle located 2 to 5 cm proximal to the pulmonic valve. The most frequent location is at the site of the crista supraventricularis. With infundibular stenosis, an "infundibular chamber" exists in the right ventricle between the site of stenosis and the pulmonic valve (Fig. 18-7). Detection of this chamber on cardiac catheterization or angiography readily confirms the diagnosis.

A patent foramen ovale is present in at least 50 percent of patients. This often is a slitlike opening apparently stretched open from the increased right ventricular pressure and dilatation of the right atrium. Rarely, a larger typical atrial septal defect, 1 to 3 cm in diameter, is present, Other associated abnormalities such as patent ductus arteriosus are rare.

PATHOPHYSIOLOGY. The physiologic disturbance is obstruction to flow of blood from the right ventricle with resulting hypertrophy of the right ventricle. Initially the severity of the obstruction is related to the diameter of the stenotic orifice. Right ventricular pressures of 75 to 100 mm Hg are found with moderate pulmonic stenosis, while severe obstruction results in right ventricular pressures of 100 to 200 mm Hg, and levels as high as 270 mm Hg have been recorded. With growth of the patient, two additional elements of obstruction occur. One of these is progressive hypertrophy of the right ventricle, until subsequently the contraction of the hypertrophied muscle of the right ventricular outflow tract also constitutes an obstruction to the flow of blood. The other factor is a relative one related to the growth of the child with corresponding increase in the flow of blood. Hence a 3- to 4-mm opening tolerated by an infant may produce serious symptoms in a child of twelve to fourteen years.

With the obstruction to the flow of blood, over one-half the patients have a patent foramen ovale with a right-to-left shunt producing unsaturation of the arterial blood. When the shunt through the foramen ovale is large, visible cyanosis develops, followed by polycythemia and clubbing. The usual clinical story is a progressive increase in cyanosis over a period of years, insidiously appearing in early child-hood and gradually increasing in severity.

Overt cardiac failure seldom occurs in children except in infancy. In infants with a pinpoint opening in the pul-monary valve, severe failure may constitute an emergency indication for pulmonic valvulotomy to prevent immediate death. Cardiac failure gradually becomes more common in older children and young adults, as cardiac reserve is progressively decreased.

CLINICAL MANIFESTATIONS. Symptoms. Dyspnea on exertion is the dominant symptom, increasing in severity as the cardiac reserve fails. Easy fatigability is common but less precise. Dizziness and/or syncope are occasionally seen; chest pain is infrequent. The history of the develop-ment of cyanosis may be characteristic. Cyanosis may have been noted in infancy, due to a right-to-left shunt through a foramen ovale, which subsequently disappeared as the foramen ovale closed. In later years, as right ventricular pressure increases and atrial dilatation occurs, the foramen ovale is gradually stretched open, resulting in the insidious appearance and progression of cyanosis as the right-to-left shunt progressively increases in magnitude. With chronic cyanosis, clubbing and polycythemia appear.

Sudden death in childhood has been reported but fortu-nately is rare. Symptoms of overt cardiac failure are rarely seen in children except in infancy but may be present in adults with severe stenosis.

Physical Examination. The characteristic finding is a harsh, loud systolic murmur heard best in the second left intercostal space and widely transmitted to the neck and adjacent areas. The murmur is of the ejection type, the peak intensity varying with the severity of the stenosis. Usually in infancy it can be clearly detected, although in advanced failure it may be faint. The pulmonic second sound is characteristically weak or absent. Diastolic mur-murs are almost never heard. With increasing cardiac hypertrophy, the forceful contractions of the right ventricle can be palpated along the left sternal border. Cyanosis is present in varying degrees in patients with a patent fora-men ovale and in the neglected chronic case is associated with polycythemia and clubbing.

Signs of cardiac failure, with hepatomegaly and edema, are usually found only in adults with severe obstruction.

LABORATORY FINDINGS. The chest roentgenogram characteristically shows cardiac enlargement confined to the right ventricle, although this is not marked until cardiac reserve fails. In older patients the poststenotic dilatation of the pulmonary artery, often unusually prominent in the left pulmonary artery, may be seen in association with normal or decreased vascularity of the peripheral lung fields. Changes in cardiac size are of particular importance, because cardiac enlargement precedes the onset of symp-toms. In infants, marked cardiac enlargement may occur within only a few months.

The electrocardiogram is of great value in assessing the severity of the obstruction, for signs of right ventricular hypertrophy are regularly present. With severe disease a right ventricular strain pattern with changes in the ST segment and T waves becomes apparent.

Cardiac catheterization and angiography are, of course,

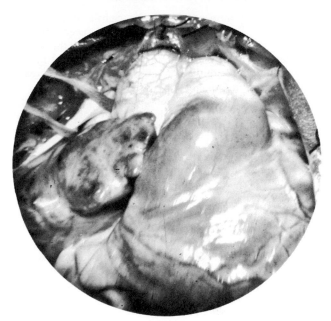

Fig. 18-7. Heart with infundibular stenosis. Site of infundibular stenosis is visible as area of constriction in outflow tract of right ventricle. Infundibular chamber, consisting of dilated right ven-tricular muscle, is located between infundibular stenosis proxi-mally and pulmonary vein distad.

necessary to define precisely the severity of the condition and the associated abnormalities. With moderate disease, a right ventricular systolic pressure of 100 mm Hg or more, associated with a systolic gradient across the stenotic pul-monary valve of 80 to 90 mm Hg, is frequent. With severe disease, systolic ventricular pressures may even exceed 200 mm Hg. The presence of a foramen ovale can be detected by noting oxygen unsaturation in the arterial blood. A right ventricular pressure exceeding systemic pressure almost always indicates an intact ventricular sep-tum, although unusual exceptions have been recorded.

On angiography, as mentioned earlier, several structures should be carefully noted. These include the degree of stenosis of the right ventricular outflow tract by the hyper-trophied muscle, especially noting any signs of a focal infundibular stenosis. The size of the pulmonary valve ring, the main pulmonary artery, and the distal pulmonary artery should also be carefully analyzed. The recognition of the frequency of multiple sites of obstruction constitutes a significant advance in effective therapy in recent years.

DIAGNOSIS. The diagnosis can usually be made with certainty in the presence of a loud systolic murmur with a weak pulmonic second sound, combined with roentgeno-graphic evidence of enlargement of the right ventricle and electrocardiographic signs of right ventricular hypertrophy. An atrial septal defect or pulmonary hypertension may be confused with pulmonic stenosis, but the quality of the pulmonic second sound is a helpful guide. Ebstein's anom-aly of the tricuspid valve is a rare malformation which can simulate pulmonic stenosis; catheterization and angi-ography are required to establish the correct diagnosis.

Differentiating pulmonic stenosis from tetralogy of

Fallot is a common problem when right-to-left shunting of blood through a foramen ovale has produced cyanosis. Cyanosis is usually a more prominent feature of the history with tetralogy of Fallot; cardiac enlargement and failure also are unusual with the latter. Cardiac angiography readily establishes the diagnosis.

TREATMENT. Indications for Operation. With mild pulmonic stenosis associated with a heart of normal size and no signs of hypertrophy of the right ventricle on the electrocardiogram, no treatment has been found necessary. Johnson and associates described the benign course of trivial pulmonic stenosis in a significant group of patients followed over many years. If there are electrocardiographic signs of significant right ventricular hypertrophy, cardiac catheterization should be done. Operation is usually recommended if the systolic pressure gradient across the stenotic pulmonary valve is greater than 50 mm Hg. It should be emphasized that the severity of the obstruction often increases with growth of the child, so a physiologically insignificant stenosis in a young child may become more significant in later childhood.

Operative Technique. Except for the rare emergency operation in an infant, all operations are done with extracorporeal circulation through a median sternotomy. The closed technique with the valvulotome developed by Potts (Fig. 18-8) is rarely used.

Our operative approach at New York University has undergone considerable modifications in the last few years following unsatisfactory results in unusual patients with severe obstruction in whom, although angiography indicated an isolated stenosis, multiple points of obstruction were found at operation. The approach currently used is briefly described in the following paragraphs.

With cardiopulmonary bypass established and body temperature lowered to 30°C, a small left ventricular vent is inserted to facilitate both decompression of the left ventricle and removal of any intracardiac air which might lodge in the left ventricle if a small unrecognized septal defect is present.

Initially, the atrial septum is palpated through a small stab wound in the right atrium to detect a foramen ovale. If present, this is sutured.

The size of the pulmonary artery in comparison to the aorta is carefully noted. If it is smaller than normal, a longitudinal arteriotomy is made and subsequently closed with a patch of pericardium or Dacron to produce a pulmonary artery of normal diameter. The size of the distal pulmonary artery is carefully measured with graduated Hegar dilators, and any stenoses found are corrected.

The external appearance of the pulmonary valve ring is carefully noted, as a hypoplastic annulus will require division of the ring and insertion of a patch. This is especially emphasized because occasionally excellent angiograms have been found to be misleading in this regard.

Contrary to our previous technique of either avoiding a ventriculotomy or using a transverse ventriculotomy, our preferred approach now is to make a short longitudinal ventriculotomy, beginning near the pulmonic annulus and extending proximally to the right ventricle for no more than 4 to 5 cm. Division of any significant coronary arteries is carefully avoided. Limiting the ventriculotomy to a short one in the outflow tract results in less impairment of ventricular function. Its use, however, usually requires closure of the ventriculotomy with a small woven Dacron patch. Through the vertical ventriculotomy, the pulmonic valve can often be adequately visualized and the commissures incised without opening the pulmonary artery. In addition, any areas of subcommissural fusion can be divided. If the valve ring is found to be hypoplastic according to the diameter guidelines recently published by Pacifico, Kirklin, and Blackstone, the ventriculotomy can be extended across the pulmonic annulus.

The short vertical ventriculotomy not only maintains ventricular function better but also, when combined with a patch, permits relief of the stenosis without radical excision of right ventricular muscle.

During the procedure, the aorta is intermittently occluded for periods of 10 to 15 minutes, venting the aorta through a small stab wound with a catheter when the aortic clamp is released, while compressing the coronary arteries to avoid air embolism and then defibrillating the heart and allowing it to beat for a few minutes before proceeding. Defibrillating the heart and allowing it to beat at 15- to 20-minute intervals for a few minutes seemingly has resulted in far less right ventricular failure than seen in the past, for subendocardial coronary blood flow is probably significantly impaired in a severely hypertrophied right ventricle with prolonged fibrillation. Care is taken to be certain that no air is present in the left ventricle before the heart is defibrillated.

With this approach, making certain that obstruction has been appropriately corrected in all areas, i.e., the right ventricle, the pulmonic annulus, the pulmonic valve, the main pulmonary artery, and its branches, even the most severe forms of pulmonic stenosis with right ventricular pressures exceeding 200 mm Hg can be promptly corrected with little cardiac failure afterward. Pressures are routinely checked, with the goal of obtaining a residual gradient between the right ventricle and pulmonary artery of less than 40 mm Hg.

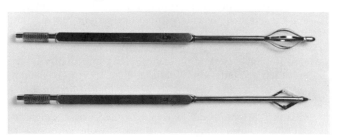

Fig. 18-8. Dilator and valvulotome developed by Potts for pulmonic valvulotomy. Calibrated swivel mechanism permits precise opening or closing of instruments.

Postoperative Course. With the exception of emergency operations in infants, the operative risk is very low, approaching 1 to 2 percent, and most patients have an uneventful convalescence.

After recovery from operation, symptomatic improvement is usually prompt. A systolic murmur almost always remains audible, and a faint diastolic murmur of no known physiologic significance frequently can be heard. The electrocardiogram will show signs of gradual regression of right ventricular hypertrophy, although such changes may require 1 to 3 years to evolve completely. Often there is little change in the heart size as seen on the chest roentgenogram, unless cardiac dilatation from failure was present before operation. If significant right ventricular hypertension remains after valvulotomy, cardiac catheterization should be performed after 6 months to 1 year to evaluate the degree of residual hypertension. In the majority of patients the systolic pressure in the right ventricle will subsequently be found to be less than 50 mm Hg.

A study of a group of 108 patients reported by Tandon and associates included only 10 percent with significant residual abnormalities on the electrocardiogram or roentgenogram. Postoperative catheterization studies performed upon 22 patients demonstrated only 1 with significant hypertension in the right ventricle.

STENOSIS OF THE PULMONARY ARTERY

Focal stenosis of the pulmonary artery or its peripheral branches, either single or multiple, has been recognized as an unusual condition since the development of selective angiocardiography. An early review by Franch and Gay in 1963 reported experiences with 11 patients and found 90 previously reported cases.

The physiologic disability depends upon the severity of the stenosis and the artery involved. Usually no limitation is present unless multiple stenoses involving both pulmonary arteries are present.

Although plastic reconstruction of multiple stenoses can be done, long-term results are yet uncertain. The operative technique is not complicated, and one of the first such operations was reported by McGoon and Kincaid in 1964. However, recurrence of the stenosis at the site of patch grafting has been described in several reports, so the indications and the best method of patch grafting remain uncertain at this time.

Congenital Aortic Stenosis

HISTORICAL DATA. Adequate surgical treatment of congenital aortic stenosis was not possible until the development of extracorporeal circulation. In 1955 Swan and associates and Lewis independently performed valvulotomy under hypothermia, but this approach was quickly discarded in favor of the more precise approach possible with cardiopulmonary bypass. By 1958, Spencer et al. had reported successful operation upon 12 children without any mortality.

INCIDENCE AND ETIOLOGY. Congenital aortic stenosis is a common congenital cardiac anomaly, representing 8 to 10 percent of all patients with congenital heart disease. For unknown reasons it is three to four times more frequent in males than in females. By contrast, congenital aortic regurgitation is an extremely rare lesion. The four patients with isolated congenital aortic regurgitation reported by Frahm and associates in 1961 were the first reported in whom the diagnosis was firmly established during life.

There are no known causative factors associated with valvular or subvalvular aortic stenosis. Only in the unusual forms of supravalvular or diffuse muscular stenosis are there associated factors suggesting a genetic basis for the disease. Rheumatic fever is rarely a cause of isolated aortic stenosis; it usually causes associated disease of the mitral valve.

PATHOLOGIC ANATOMY. In valvular stenosis the valve cusps are often well formed but are fused along the commissures to produce an opening varying from 2 to 6 mm in diameter. The pattern of fusion of the commissures is similar in many patients. The commissure between the right and left coronary cusps is often the least developed, the valve functioning as a bicuspid valve. Commissural fusion between the right and noncoronary cusps is usually moderate, and fusion between the left and noncoronary cusps is usually the least extensive. The valve cusps are usually thicker than normal cusps but have adequate mobility. Calcification is common in adults but is almost never seen before seventeen to eighteen years of age. In most patients the aortic annulus is of normal diameter, but mild poststenotic dilatation of the ascending aorta is common (42 percent of 100 patients reported by Braunwald et al.). Fortunately, only in a minority of patients are the more bizarre, extreme forms of valvular stenosis seen, with a hypoplastic annulus, unusual valve cusps with absence of commissures, and associated hypoplasia of the left ventricle.

Subvalvular stenosis usually occurs as a narrow ring of fibrous tissue, varying in length from a "ring" to a short "tunnel," 1 to 2 cm proximal to the aortic valve cusps. The orifice varies from 4 to 8 mm. The aortic outflow tract is usually of normal diameter proximal and distal to the stenotic ring, although muscular hypertrophy may be prominent in older patients. In some patients the base of the aortic cusps is immediately adjacent to the stenotic ring and must be protected from injury during surgical excision of the stenosis. Two other anatomic relations are of particular importance during surgical excision. Beneath the noncoronary cusp where the stenotic ring is attached to the ventricular septum, the conduction bundle is present and may easily be injured. Beneath the left coronary cusp the ring is attached to the base of the aortic leaflet of the mitral valve, which is also susceptible to injury.

Associated cardiac malformations are found in 15 to 20 percent of patients, being more frequent with valvular stenosis than with subvalvular stenosis. The most frequent associated conditions are patent ductus, coarctation, ventricular septal defect, and pulmonic stenosis.

PATHOPHYSIOLOGY. The physiologic limitations from aortic stenosis are directly related to the severity of obstruction. Mild stenosis of little physiologic significance can occur with "typical" findings on examination. At the other extreme, severe obstruction can cause death from congestive heart failure in infants or sudden death in older children. The severity of the stenosis can be quantitated only by left heart catheterization; it is usually expressed in terms of the peak systolic gradient between the left ventricle and the ascending aorta. A gradient of less than 40 mm Hg is usually associated with such mild disability that operation is not recommended. In such patients cardiac output should be measured as well as the pressure gradient in order to calculate the functional cross-sectional area of the aortic valve. A functional cross-sectional area less than $0.5 \text{ cm}^2/\text{m}^2$ of body surface should usually be surgically corrected. Systolic pressure gradients of 50 to 75 mm Hg are usual with aortic stenosis of moderate severity, while gradients exceeding 100 mm Hg may be found with severe stenosis.

Depending upon the degree of stenosis, there is resulting hypertrophy of the left ventricle. Cardiac failure may occur in infants and is often fatal: 19 of 25 infants with cardiac failure reported by Peckham et al. died from their illness. Operation is urgently indicated in these severely ill infants. The stenosis in infants is almost always valvular, not subvalvular, and is often associated with additional cardiac malformations.

Between the ages of two and ten there are usually few or no signs of impairment of function of the left ventricle. In older children symptoms representing limited cardiac reserve and a restriction in coronary or cerebral blood flow become increasingly common, although overt congestive heart failure is rare. Sudden death may occur in children, apparently from ventricular fibrillation. The frequency of sudden death varies with different reports. Braverman and Gibson reported 6 deaths in 73 patients, an 8.2 percent mortality rate. Nadas estimated the incidence of sudden death in his group of 250 patients as 7.5 percent. The lowest incidence of sudden death was reported by Peckham et al., who observed only 4 deaths in a group of 300 patients, approximately 1 percent. The occurrence of sudden death has not always correlated with clinical signs of severity of obstruction, so the risk of this tragedy cannot be predicted with certainty.

In young adults calcification of the fused valve cusps occurs with increasing frequency and probably approaches 100 percent in the third and fourth decades. Calcification adds the element of rigidity to the obstruction formerly originating only from the small size of the orifice. Consequently patients in the third or fourth decades may be seen with severe symptoms who have a history of a cardiac murmur during childhood without symptoms. It is now recognized that with the declining frequency of rheumatic fever, most adults with isolated calcific aortic stenosis represent calcification of a congenitally deformed valve. In the past year, the author has operated upon one patient over seventy-five years of age who had calcific aortic stenosis with the classic commissural abnormalities of a congenital deformity, well illustrating the long period of time that may elapse before rigidity from progressive calcification produces significant stenosis.

CLINICAL MANIFESTATIONS. Symptoms. Many young children with significant aortic stenosis are asymptomatic.

The most common symptoms are fatigue, dyspnea, angina pectoris, and syncope. These were found in 30 to 50 percent of a group of 100 patients studied by Braunwald et al. In most of these patients the systolic gradient was greater than 50 to 70 mm Hg.

Physical Examination. The four principal physical findings are a basal systolic murmur, palpable thrill, forceful left ventricular impulse, and narrow pulse pressure. The systolic murmur is a harsh, ejection-type murmur usually heard best in the second right interspace and is widely transmitted to the neck and arms. In infants and young children it may be loudest to the left of the sternum. A thrill can be felt in over 80 percent of patients. The left ventricular impulse is usually forceful and heaving. The pulse pressure was found to be decreased from the normal value of 30 mm Hg in 38 percent of 300 patients studied by Peckham and associates but was considered normal in 54 of 67 patients studied by Nadas.

An early diastolic murmur can be heard in about 20 percent of patients but is usually of no physiologic significance. For unknown reasons, it is considerably more frequent with subvalvular stenosis than with valvular stenosis.

LABORATORY FINDINGS. The electrocardiogram is the most sensitive guide to the severity of aortic stenosis but has distinct limitations. The usual abnormalities are signs of left ventricular hypertrophy, subsequently followed by depression of the ST segment and inversion of T waves. In about 75 percent of patients in whom the gradient exceeded 50 mm Hg, a left ventricular strain pattern was present. The limitations of electrocardiography have been emphasized by Braunwald and associates, for in some patients with severe obstruction the electrocardiogram may show few abnormalities.

The chest roentgenogram is frequently normal. In about one-half the patients slight enlargement of the left ventricle can be recognized, with a cardiothoracic ratio greater than 50 percent. Mild dilatation of the ascending aorta may be detected in 30 to 40 percent of patients. Calcification of the stenotic valve is rarely found except in adults.

Cardiac catheterization is necessary to determine whether operation is indicated. The critical determination is measurement of the systolic gradient between the left ventricle and the ascending aorta. With gradients of less than 50 mm Hg, cardiac output should be determined to permit calculation of the functional cross-sectional area of the aortic valve. It may be possible to differentiate valvular from subvalvular stenosis by noting changes in pressure as a catheter is withdrawn from the apex of the left ventricle into the aorta, but this information is of little value to the surgeon, as the two areas are immediately adjacent to each other and can be easily identified at operation. Usually on catheterization the pulmonary artery pressure, left atrial pressure, and cardiac output are normal. The left ventricular pressure is elevated when severe stenosis with early cardiac failure is present.

DIAGNOSIS. The diagnosis can be made with confidence in the presence of the characteristic murmur, thrill, left ventricular impulse, and narrow pulse pressure. Confirmation can be obtained from the chest roentgenogram and electrocardiogram, reserving cardiac catheterization to assess the severity of the obstruction. In infants, when the murmur is loudest to the left of the sternum, catheterization may be required to differentiate from ventricular septal defect or pulmonic valvular stenosis.

TREATMENT. Infants in congestive heart failure should usually be operated upon with a pump-oxygenator once the diagnosis has been established. The mortality from nonoperative therapy is extremely high, 19 of 25 patients having died in a series reported by Peckham et al. Before operation, catheterization is required to differentiate the condition from coarctation of the aorta or the hypoplastic left heart syndrome.

In most children operation is considered because of mild symptoms or the presence of changes in the electrocardiogram. A final decision can be made after left heart catheterization; operation is usually performed if the peak systolic gradients are greater than 40 to 50 mm Hg.

Operative Technique. Operation is performed with cardiopulmonary bypass, using a median sternotomy incision. After bypass is established, the temperature is lowered to about 25°C and a vent is inserted into the apex of the left ventricle to aspirate blood from the operative field. Subsequently the ascending aorta is clamped and opened with a curved incision, which is extended down into the noncoronary sinus but does not go to the base of the sinus. Extending the incision into the depth of the noncoronary sinus may increase exposure but theoretically may result in prolapse of the noncoronary cusp when the aortic circumference is narrowed by suture of the aortotomy.

Coronary perfusion was occasionally used in the past but has now been abandoned in favor of the potassium cardioplegia technique, injecting the cold (4°C) potassium cardioplegic mixture into the coronary ostia to stop the heart and lower the myocardial temperature below 20°C. With this technique, periods of ischemia for as long as 45 to 60 minutes seem completely safe.

Calibrated Hegar dilators are useful for measuring the diameter of the stenotic orifice both before and after commissurotomy. If an orifice admitting a #16 or #18 Hegar dilator can be obtained by commissurotomy, corresponding to a cross-sectional area nearly 2 cm², the obstruction will have been adequately relieved. (This, of course, varies with body size.) Even a larger opening is preferable, of course, if this can be obtained without risking the production of aortic insufficiency. Measuring the stenotic orifice before commissurotomy provides a good guide to the length of commissural incision necessary to obtain the desired opening.

With valvular stenosis, the fused commissures are gradually incised with a small (#15) knife blade, the fused commissure being incised exactly along the center of the fibrous raphe in order to have a thick margin on each of the two cusps which are thus separated (Fig. 18-9). Attempted division of the fused commissures with scissors will often result in division of the area to one side of the area of fusion and increase the likelihood of insufficiency. As far as possible, the incision of the commissures should be limited to areas where the commissures are well formed. When necessary, the commissural incisions may be carried

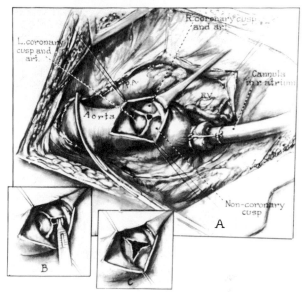

Fig. 18-9. *A.* Operative exposure of congenital aortic stenosis. Stenotic aortic valve has been exposed through longitudinal aortotomy. Fused commissures between three aortic cusps are clearly seen, with small central opening. *B* and *C.* Commissurotomy performed with knife, with center of fused commissures carefully incised and incision avoided in areas where commissures are not well developed. (*Reprinted by permission of The C. V. Mosby Company, St. Louis, from F. C. Spencer, C. A. Neill, and H. T. Bahnson, The Treatment of Congenital Aortic Stenosis with Valvulotomy during Cardiopulmonary Bypass, Surgery, 44:116, 1958.*)

completely to the aortic wall or, if not necessary, can be stopped 1 to 3 mm away. With the classic bicuspid valve, the commissure between the right and left coronary cusps is not well developed, and only a 2- to 4-mm incision, or no incision at all, may be made in this area, leaving the valve as a bicuspid valve. It is better to relieve the stenosis incompletely than to produce severe aortic insufficiency. Starr and associates have reported disappointing long-term results if significant insufficiency is produced at operation, with patients often requiring aortic valve replacement within a few years because of progressive cardiac enlargement and failure. In most patients, however, a stenosis can be adequately relieved by selective incision of the fused commissures without producing significant insufficiency. In one group of 23 patients studied, limited incision of the commissures was performed in 15 and obtained a satisfactory reduction in pressure gradient. The technique of commissurotomy is emphasized in some detail, for most difficulties with aortic insufficiency following aortic valvulotomy have resulted from inept valvulotomies rather than from the pathologic anatomy.

With subvalvular stenosis the valve cusps can be carefully retracted and the fibrotic ring excised. The tissue between the base of the valve cusps and the fibrotic ring must be clearly visualized to avoid injury of the base of the aortic valve cusps. The ring may consist of thin fibrous tissue, easily removed, or it may be a thick fibrotic structure requiring excision with a knife and rongeur. The surgical anatomy is of crucial importance in this area, for

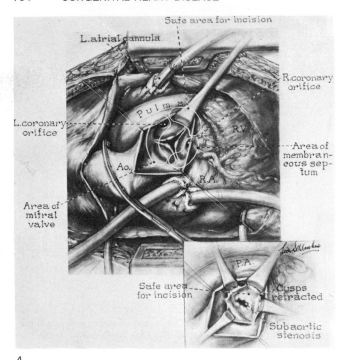

A

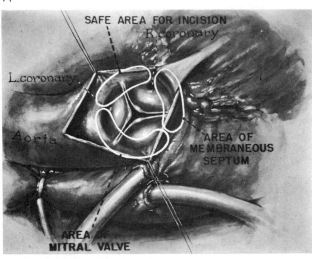

B

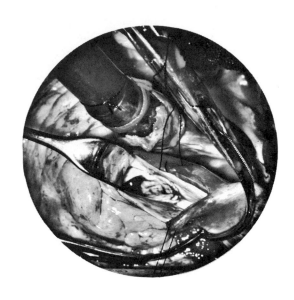

C

Fig. 18-10. *A.* Operative exposure of congenital subaortic stenosis. Valve cusps are normal. Insert shows membranelike subaortic stenosis exposed by retraction of valve cusps. (*From Am Surg, 26:210, 1960.*) *B.* Diagram of pertinent surgical anatomy with subaortic stenosis. Beneath noncoronary cusps and part of left coronary cusp is aortic leaflet of mitral valve. Beneath part of right coronary cusp is membranous septum. Only in area beneath commissure between right and left coronary cusps is limited zone where underlying ventricular muscle can be safely excised. Failure to observe these landmarks can result in injury to mitral valve or to membranous septum with conduction bundle. *C.* Subaortic stenosis exposed at operation. Aorta has been opened with longitudinal aortotomy and retractor inserted to retract normal aortic cusps. Diaphragmlike subaortic stenosis can be clearly seen with small pinpoint central opening. (*Reprinted by permission of C. V. Mosby Co. from F. C. Spencer, C. A. Neill, and H. T. Bahnson, The Treatment of Congenital Aortic Stenosis with Valvulotomy during Cardiopulmonary Bypass, Surgery, 44: 117, 1958.*)

only in a narrow zone constituting less than 20 percent of the circumference of the stenotic ring can excision be safely carried into the underlying ventricular wall. This corresponds to the area beneath the commissure between the right and left coronary cusps (Fig. 18-10). Radical excision of the fibrotic ring beneath the left coronary cusp will perforate the aortic leaflet of the mitral valve, producing severe or fatal mitral insufficiency. Radical excision beneath the noncoronary cusp and part of the right coronary cusp will injure the ventricular septum, creating either a complete heart block or ventricular septal defect. The most useful instrument for excising the stenotic ring is a right-angled rongeur with a swivel for rotating the instrument to an appropriate angle (Fig. 18-11). With good exposure, an unhurried approach, and appropriate instru-

ments, a stenotic area can be regularly excised satisfactorily. Optical magnification and focal illumination with a headlight are excellent adjuncts in small children.

The aortotomy is sutured with a continuous Prolene suture. A small opening is left for removal of air. Following closure of the aortotomy, induced electrical ventricular fibrillation is carefully maintained with electrodes on the heart. The heart is then allowed to fill with blood by stopping the suction on the left ventricular vent, after which it is gently massaged to expel air from the ventricle and the aorta through the small opening remaining in the aortotomy. While compressing the right coronary artery digitally, the aortic clamp is cautiously removed and any remaining air expelled through the aortic vent site, which can later be sutured.

Following removal of the aortic clamp and meticulous removal of air from the heart, the heart can be defibrillated. Subsequently the left ventricular vent is removed and bypass slowed and stopped.

Following bypass, with a systemic pressure over 100 mm Hg, the residual gradient across the aortic valve can be measured by needle puncture of the left ventricle and the aorta. The residual gradient should be less than 40 mm Hg, and is often very small.

Postoperative care is little different from that for thoracotomy for other conditions. Arrhythmias or mild congestive failure may occur, but are infrequent.

The risks of operation are small and the results good. Nadas reported that only 2 of 54 patients with uncomplicated aortic stenosis died following operation. Some have expressed pessimism and dissatisfaction with operations for aortic stenosis, but the experience of the author has been most favorable. In a series exceeding 75 patients over the past several years, there have been no deaths among those with valvular stenosis, a satisfactory reduction in systolic gradient was achieved in almost all, and only a few have some aortic insufficiency. With subvalvular stenosis, there have been no operative deaths in several years. Earlier, deaths occurred in isolated patients from injury to adjacent anatomic structures, such as the mitral valve or attached aortic cusp, but with the present technique such injuries can be avoided.

Postoperative Course. Electrocardiographic changes may show improvement in some patients after recovery from operation, but in others little change may occur. The failure to show electrocardiographic improvement may indicate that operation should have been performed earlier than is customary. Changes in heart size on the chest roentgenogram are usually negligible. Usually a systolic murmur is audible, and a faint diastolic murmur without any signs of significant aortic insufficiency may be heard.

The long-term prognosis for these patients is yet unknown, although some patients have now survived for over 15 years after operation and recurrence of the stenosis has not been observed. A more probable complication is the eventual development of progressive aortic insufficiency from fibrosis and contraction of the thickened aortic cusp, ultimately requiring valvular replacement. To date, this has not occurred in a significant number of patients. Similarly, the persistence of abnormal changes in the electrocardiogram following operation has not been associated with any serious long-term complications.

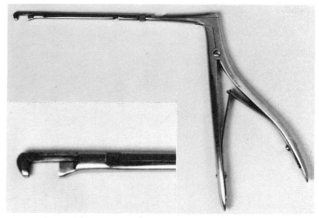

Fig. 18-11. Right-angled sharp rongeur used for excision of subaortic stenosis. Swivel mechanism permits rotation of instrument to obtain proper exposure.

SUPRAVALVULAR AORTIC STENOSIS

Supravalvular aortic stenosis is the rarest form of aortic stenosis, although it has been recognized with increasing frequency in recent years. The first successfully treated patient was reported by McGoon and Kirklin in 1956, and 10 years later Rastelli et al. reported surgical experience with 16 patients. At that time a total of 88 cases were found in the medical literature, 51 of which had been treated surgically. In most patients there are no known etiologic factors. Both sexes are equally involved. In about 20 percent of patients there is a peculiar facies consisting of a broad forehead, heavy cheeks, protuberant lips, and pointed chin. This facies is similar to that found with idiopathic hypercalcemia of infancy, and experimental induction of hypercalcemia in rats may produce a vascular lesion resembling supravalvular aortic stenosis. Most but not all patients with the characteristic facies are mentally deficient.

There is considerable variation in the type of aortic obstruction in different patients. In a review of 68 cases, Peterson et al. found three types: membranous, 9 cases; diffuse hypoplastic, 14 cases; hourglass, 45 cases (Fig. 18-12). Surgical results with the diffuse hypoplastic type to date have not been very good. The left ventricular-aortic valve conduit has been used for some forms of severe

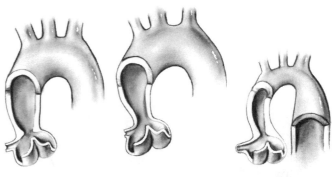

Fig. 18-12. Different types of supravalvular aortic stenosis, obstruction varying from localized constriction near aortic valve to diffuse hypoplasia of ascending aorta. (*Adapted from G. C. Rastelli et al., J Thorac Cardiovasc Surg, 51:878, 1966.*)

LOCALIZED   DIFFUSE

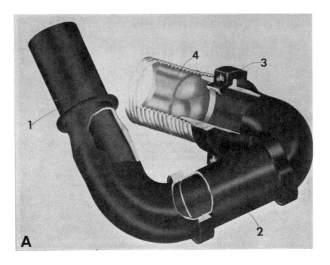

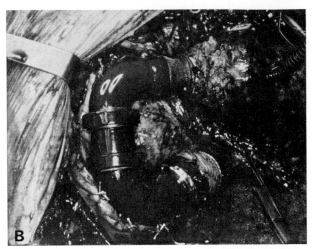

Fig. 18-13. *A.* Drawing of left ventricular aortic prosthesis coupled to valved Dacron conduit. (1) Inflow tube to be inserted through left ventricular apex to body of ventricle. (2) Curved part of prosthesis with movable outflow connection. (3) Clamp used to fix Dacron graft in place. (4) Dacron graft containing xenograft valve. *B.* Operative photograph showing left ventricular aortic prosthesis in place during cardiopulmonary bypass. Catheter used to decompress left ventricle can be seen entering lateral wall (on right). Vascular clamp placed beneath aortic anastomosis is visible at bottom of photograph. (*From W. F. Bernhard et al., J Thorac Cardiovasc Surg, 69:223, 1975.*)

obstruction to left ventricular outflow in the past two or three years by several investigators, including Weldon and Cooley and Bernhard and associates, and may be used for such patients in the future (Figs. 18-13, 18-14).

A new technique for insertion of a prosthetic aortic valve in patients with a hypoplastic aortic valve ring was reported by Konno in 1975. He described an ingenious method of extending the aortotomy down into the upper ventricular septum by a complex approach in which the anterior wall of the right ventricular outflow tract is also incised (Fig. 18-15). Favorable experiences have also been described by others, so initial experience with this technique seems sound. Most successful operations have been with the hourglass type, in which constriction of the aorta is found as a shelflike thickening and hypertrophy of the plica at the upper margin of the sinuses of Valsalva. The

Fig. 18-14. Technique for modifying a commercially available valve-bearing arterial prosthesis for use as an apical-aortic shunt. (1) A metal cylinder is drawn over a cloth cylinder. (2) The cloth is doubled over the metal cylinder in porous polyester cloth. (3) The cloth-covered cylinder is sewn to the prosthesis and a ring of felt is used to cover the junction. (*From W. P. Dembitsky et al., Ann Surg, 184:317, 1976.*)

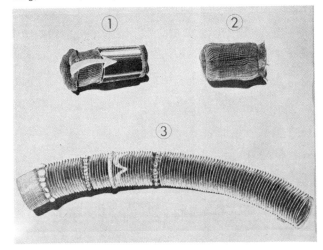

outer diameter of the aorta may be normal or reduced. The stenotic ridge has thickened intima and hypertrophy of the media, with an increase in fibrous and elastic tissue.

Associated abnormalities are frequent. In about one-third of the patients abnormalities of the aortic valve cusps are present, frequently consisting of adherence of part of one of the free margins of the cusps to the aortic wall, which, when extensive, can result in aortic regurgitation. The coronary arteries are abnormal in over one-half the patients. Often the right coronary artery is markedly dilated and tortuous, with hypertrophy of the media and intima which produce narrowing of the lumen. Focal stenotic lesions of the branches of the aortic arch and of the peripheral branches of the pulmonary arteries have also been found.

The usual symptoms are either angina or syncope, as with other forms of aortic stenosis. Death usually either has been sudden, suggesting an arrhythmia, or has resulted from congestive heart failure. Physical examination provides no clues to the diagnosis except when the typical facies, first described by Williams and associates in 1961, is present. A precise diagnosis can be established only by aortography.

A satisfactory operation can be accomplished in the localized type of stenosis by widening the stenotic area by the insertion of a patch of Dacron or pericardium. Complete excision of the stenotic ridge is not possible because of the attachment of the aortic valve cusps (Fig. 18-16). Although some have reported sudden death of patients after such an operation, a report by Rastelli et al. in 1966 stated that 15 of 16 patients survived operation, and in subsequent follow-up evaluation 13 of the 15 were consid-

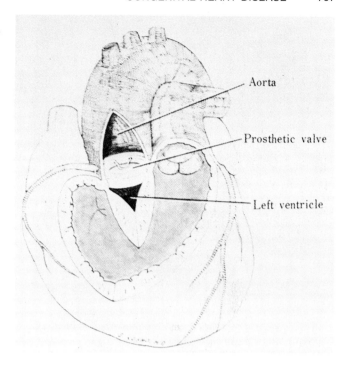

Fig. 18-15. Prosthetic valve is placed in subcoronary position. (*From S. Konno et al., J Thorac Cardiovasc Surg, 70:909, 1975.*)

ered to have had a good result (Fig. 18-17). In 1977 Doty described a more complex form of reconstruction of the aorta for severe supravalvular stenosis. This may be applicable for some of the more complex forms of obstruction.

IDIOPATHIC HYPERTROPHIC SUBAORTIC STENOSIS

This disease is basically a myopathy involving the left ventricle, with secondary obstruction of the left ventricular outflow tract. The hypertrophy is not uniform but may be most extensive in the septum, in some patients producing obstruction of the right ventricular outflow tract as well.

There is a familial history, in 30 to 40 percent of patients, of puzzling forms of heart disease in other members of the family, often terminated by sudden death at an early age. In one group of 27 patients reported by Braunwald et al., a positive familial history was found in 10. Often there is no sign of heart disease in childhood, with symptoms and physical findings appearing in later years, apparently as the hypertrophy of the left ventricle progresses. Pathologically, the heart shows massive ventricular hypertrophy with virtual obliteration of the lumen. The histologic structure of the hypertrophied muscle fibers is not distinctive. Although little is known of the natural history of the disease, the

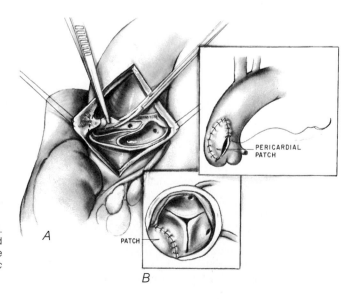

Fig. 18-16. Operation for localized supravalvular aortic stenosis. Stenotic area is widened by making longitudinal aortotomy and inserting pericardial patch. Partial excision of stenotic membrane is also shown. (*Adapted from G. C. Rastelli et al., J Thorac Cardiovasc Surg, 51:875, 1966.*)

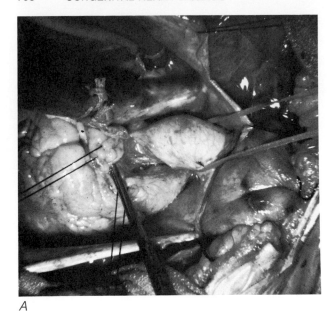

A

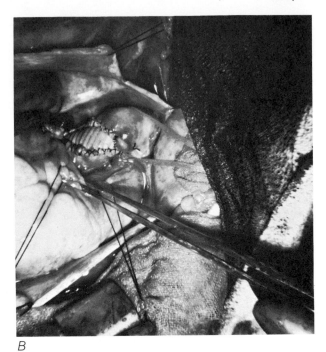

B

Fig. 18-17. *A.* Operative photograph of the unusual lesion of supravalvular aortic stenosis. The waistlike narrowing of the ascending aorta just above the aortic valve can be clearly seen. *B.* Operative photograph of correction of supravalvular aortic stenosis by insertion of a Dacron patch to widen the area. The aortic valve gradient was reduced from 80 to near 30 mm Hg.

usual course has not been a favorable one, with death occurring at an early age.

The symptoms differ little from those of patients with the usual form of aortic stenosis, including syncope, angina, and dyspnea. On physical examination a systolic murmur, of medium intensity near the apex but not prominent at the base of the heart in the aortic area, may first arouse suspicion that a valvular stenosis is present. The chest roentgenogram will usually show some enlargement of the left ventricle, while the electrocardiogram shows left ventricular hypertrophy with depression of the ST segment and inversion of the T waves.

Diagnosis is best established by cardiac catheterization and angiography. On catheterization a gradient can usually be demonstrated over an area in the proximal outflow tract of the left ventricle. The systolic gradient may vary from 50 to 150 mm Hg, the average value being 80 to 90 mm Hg. An increase in the pressure gradient can characteristically be produced by the infusion of isoproterenol, apparently resulting from a more forceful contraction of the left ventricle. Cardiac angiography will show striking hypertrophy of the left ventricle, with a small lumen.

Operation is indicated in the presence of symptoms when there is a systolic gradient of more than 50 mm Hg. Although operation can relieve the left ventricular obstruction, it of course does not alter the basic disease of diffuse progressive ventricular hypertrophy.

The best operative results have been obtained with the technique developed by Morrow and associates. Their experience has been extensive, and catheterization studies 2 to 3 years after operation have demonstrated that recurrence of the obstruction is rare. At operation a trough of ventricular muscle is excised, going from the base of the aortic cusp into the ventricular cavity (Fig. 18-18). This procedure has been found to be superior to a variety of others attempted, including simple myotomy through the aorta, myotomy performed through a radical ventriculotomy, and even mitral valve replacement.

Coarctation of the Aorta

HISTORICAL DATA. In 1928 the characteristic features of coarctation of the aorta were outlined by Abbott in her classic analysis of 200 cases, including postmortem examinations. In 1944 and 1945 Blalock and Park, Gross, and Crafoord and Nylin all independently contributed to the first successful surgical treatment of coarctation by excision and direct anastomosis. Subsequently Gross provided a strong impetus to the study of vascular grafts by successfully using aortic homografts for patients with coarctation in whom direct anastomosis could not be performed.

INCIDENCE AND ETIOLOGY. Coarctation is one of the most common congenital abnormalities, occurring in 10 to 15 percent of patients with congenital heart disease. It is approximately twice as frequent in males as in females.

The exact cause of coarctation is unknown, but proximity of the coarctation to the ligamentum arteriosum has supported the most popular theory, that coarctation is an aberrant extension of the same fibrotic process that converts a patent ductus into a ligamentum arteriosum. Some observations indicate that a coarctation may increase in severity with time as a result of progressive thickening of the intima.

PATHOLOGIC ANATOMY. In most patients the coarctation is located as a diaphragmlike constriction in the first 2 to 4 cm of thoracic aorta distal to the left subclavian artery. Usually there is a 1- to 3-mm lumen, although complete occlusion may be present. On histologic examination the intima and media are both found to be markedly thickened. In older patients fibrosis and calcification may be found in the adjacent aortic wall. Usually the ligamentum arteriosum is attached to the medial surface of the aorta at the site of coarctation, although it may be inserted slightly above or below. The ligamentum clearly anchors the coarctation in this area, for when surgically divided, the two ends retract sharply, indicating the degree of tension previously exerted.

The aorta distal to the coarctation is usually dilated, more so in older patients; rarely it develops into an aneurysm. A striking feature of coarctation, becoming more prominent in older patients, is the large, dilated intercostal arteries which enter the distal aorta. As these vessels dilate, there is progressive thinning of the arterial wall, frequently resulting in the development of small aneurysms in adult patients.

The proximal aorta between the coarctation and the left subclavian artery is usually smaller than the distal aorta and may be hypoplastic, requiring excision along with the coarctation to relieve the obstruction completely.

The striking clinical characteristics of coarctation of the aorta are related to the growth of collateral circulation around the site of obstruction. These tributaries predominantly arise from the subclavian arteries and anastomose with the intercostal and epigastric vessels to enter the distal aorta. The development of collateral circulation through the intercostal arteries results in the characteristic "notching" of the ribs seen on the chest roentgenogram in patients over eight to ten years of age, virtually pathognomonic of coarctation.

A variety of unusual forms of coarctation are occasionally seen. A coarctation may extend proximally to involve the left subclavian artery or even left carotid and innominate artery, constituting an *interruption of the aortic arch*. In 1976 the different forms of this severe type of obstruction were well classified in the report by Fishman and associates.

A separate severe anomaly, often fatal in the first few months of life unless recognized and treated, is the so-called "preductal" coarctation, in which a number of severe anomalies are present. A large patent ductus supplies the distal aorta, with the coarctation proximal to this. Often additional severe cardiac defects are present. The syndrome, though rare, is well described in the textbook by Taussig. In the few patients surviving infancy, cyanosis may be recognized as localized in the lower half of the body.

PATHOPHYSIOLOGY. In infants, left ventricular failure may result from the obstruction to emptying of the left ventricle created by the coarctation. This is often fatal if untreated. Subsequently, enlarging collateral circulation partly relieves the obstruction; thus congestive failure is rare after the first year of life until late childhood or early adult life.

In infants with a preductal coarctation, severe symptoms are present, with pulmonary congestion, cardiac failure, and cyanosis. These disabilities cause death in the majority of infants unless effective surgical therapy can be performed. The disabilities result from the coarctation, the large patent ductus entering the distal aorta, and the other

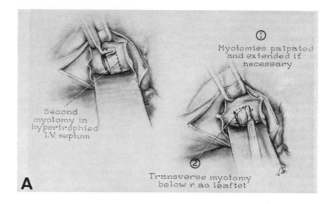

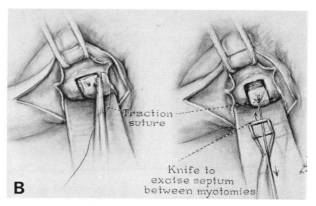

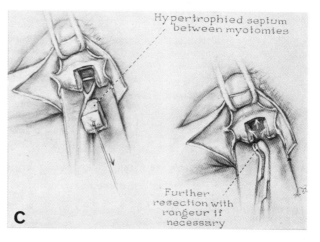

Fig. 18-18. *A.* Second myotomy is made about 1 cm to right (clockwise) of first. Incisions are then deepened if necessary by digital splitting of muscle fibers. Myotomies are usually 12 to 15 mm in depth at most prominent aspect of septum. Transverse incision is then made at base of valve leaflet connecting proximal portions of the two myotomies. *B.* Bar of muscle isolated between incisions is held by traction suture as shown or by suitable clamp. Muscle is freed with rectangular knife (devised by Stinson) or with special angled rongeur. *C.* As traction is made on muscle bar, rectangular knife is pushed toward apex, freeing muscle bar from its anterior attachments to septum. Apical portion of resection is often more easily accomplished with rongeur, which may be introduced via aorta or via apical stab wound. In latter case, rongeur is positioned and directed by left index finger passed through valve ring. (*From A. G. Morrow et al., Circulation, 52:88, 1975.*)

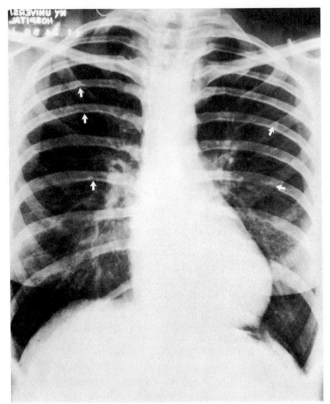

Fig. 18-19. Chest roentgenogram in patient with coarctation of aorta, demonstrating classic notching of ribs from enlarged intercostal arteries. This roentgen appearance is virtually pathognomonic of coarctation of aorta, as it is rarely produced by any other condition. (*Courtesy of Dr. Raymond M. Abrams, Department of Radiology, New York University Medical Center.*)

associated cardiac malformations so frequently present, such as ventricular septal defect, fibroelastosis, or even transposition of the great vessels.

The hypertension from the coarctation causes rapid degenerative changes in the proximal aorta at such a rate that children in their early teens may have severe fibrosis that complicates surgical repair. Although some patients may live until the fifth or sixth decade, the average life expectancy is between 30 or 40 years. Before surgical therapy was possible, approximately 25 percent of untreated patients died from rupture of the aorta, 25 percent from cardiac failure, 25 percent from rupture of intracranial aneurysms, and 25 percent from superimposed bacterial endocarditis.

CLINICAL MANIFESTATIONS. Symptoms. Many children are asymptomatic for long periods of time despite severe hypertension and the progressive degenerative changes occurring in the aorta. When symptoms are present, headache, dizziness, and epistaxis are the most common. Dyspnea on exertion or occasionally chest pain may be mentioned. Claudication in the lower extremities is infrequent despite the restriction of peripheral blood flow.

Physical Findings. The combination of hypertension in the upper extremities and absence or decrease of pulses in the lower extremities in a child immediately suggest the

diagnosis of coarctation. In less severe forms measurements of the blood pressure in the upper and lower extremities may be required to confirm the diagnosis. Normally the blood pressure in the lower extremities is slightly higher than in the upper. Prominent pulsations are usually visible in the neck, and examination of the muscles of the shoulder girdle, especially the latissimus dorsi and suprascapular muscles, will often reveal visible and palpable pulsations. Auscultation over these sites may detect a bruit. A systolic murmur, the origin of which is often obscure, is usually widely audible over the left hemithorax. It may result from the coarctation, an associated abnormality of the aortic valve, or dilated, tortuous arteries.

LABORATORY STUDIES. The chest roentgenogram in older patients may automatically establish the diagnosis by demonstrating bilateral notching of the ribs (Fig. 18-19). Notching of the ribs from other causes is extremely rare. Left ventricular hypertrophy also may be evident. The electrocardiogram shows signs of left ventricular hypertrophy or strain.

In most patients the diagnosis can be made from the clinical findings in combination with the roentgenogram and the electrocardiogram. Cardiac catheterization and aortography should be done routinely to detect additional anomalies and to outline the location and extent of the obstruction.

TREATMENT. The ideal age for operation is between five and seven years, preferably before the child begins to attend school. There is little reason and some risk in postponing operation beyond this time.

In adults, operation is complicated by the extensive degenerative changes of calcification and fibrosis. If these are so extensive that direct anastomosis is not feasible, a bypass graft with Dacron is preferable to attempting excision of the coarctation and insertion of a direct graft.

In the majority of infants with congestive failure, operation should be performed unless response to medical therapy is prompt. This may require operation within the first few weeks of life. Often there is an associated ventricular septal defect with a large increase in pulmonary blood flow; so banding of the pulmonary artery may be necessary at the time the coarctation is resected. When operation is performed in infants, there may be a recurrence as the child grows older, even though interrupted sutures are used to perform the anastomosis.

Operative Technique. A left posterolateral thoracotomy in the fourth intercostal space is used, usually dividing the fourth rib posteriorly in older patients (Fig. 18-20). After the lung is retracted inferiorly, the coarctation is usually obvious, with the indentation mediad at the site of insertion of the ligamentum arteriosum, and large, tortuous intercostal arteries entering the distal aorta (Fig. 18-21). After incision of the mediastinal pleura, the vagus nerve is retracted mediad; the aorta proximal to the left subclavian artery, the left subclavian artery, the ligamentum arteriosum, and the distal aorta are serially mobilized and encircled with tapes. The recurrent nerve coursing around the ligamentum arteriosum is usually not seen if dissection is kept close to the aorta but should be identified and protected if more extensive dissection is performed. Injury of

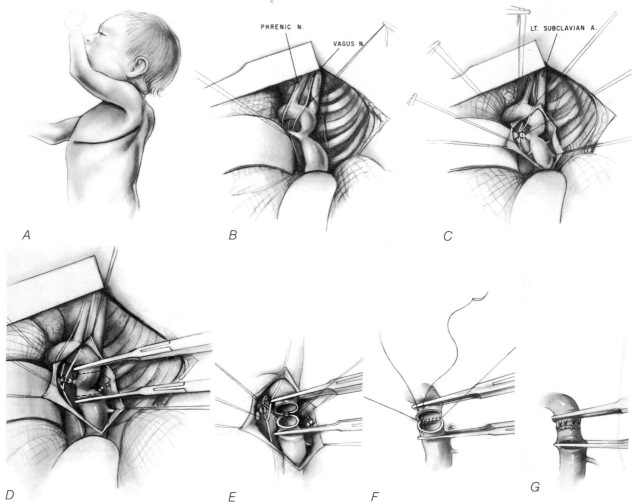

Fig. 18-20. Excision of coarction of aorta. *A.* Chest is opened with posterolateral incision in fourth intercostal space. *B.* Once chest has been opened and lung retracted, site of coarctation is often visible where aorta is angulated inward toward mediastinum just distal to left subclavian artery. This is site where ligamentum arteriosum is inserted. *C.* After incision of mediastinal pleura overlying coarctation, vessels are isolated proximal and distal to coarctation and ligamentum arteriosum is mobilized and divided. Recurrent laryngeal nerve, often not seen during operative procedure, is displaced mediad with vagus nerve. *D.* After division of ligamentum arteriosum, vascular occlusion clamps are applied to aorta proximal and distal to site of coarctation. Often it is necessary to apply proximal clamp to aorta between left carotid and left subclavian arteries, separately occluding left subclavian artery, in order to excise widely the narrowed segment of aorta. *E.* End-to-end anastomosis is constructed with continuous or interrupted sutures of silk. *F.* After completion of posterior row of anastomosis, interrupted sutures are often used in anterior row in young children to permit growth of anastomosis. *G.* Final view of completed anastomosis.

the thoracic duct may also occur if dissection is not kept next to the aorta. The proper plane for dissection of the aorta is between the adventitia and the media. This will avoid injury to the thoracic duct in the majority of patients. If the aorta is sharply angulated, division of the ligamentum will provide sufficient mobility. This may be done

before the aorta is occluded; otherwise the ligamentum may be divided at the same time that the coarctation is excised. Dissection of the distal aorta is the greatest hazard in the operation because of friable intercostal arteries. In older patients, intercostal aneurysms occur. Such aneurysms were found in 45 of 487 patients operated upon by Gross and associates. Usually the aorta can be mobilized sufficiently beyond the intercostal arteries. The intercostals are then individually isolated and can be separately occluded during performance of the anastomosis. Division of the intercostal arteries can be done but is seldom necessary.

One of the most feared hazards with operation for coarctation is paraplegia, fortunately rare. In a survey of published reports by Brewer et al., paraplegia has been reported to occur in approximately 0.5 percent of patients following operation (1 patient in 200). Although the author has personally never had a postoperative neurologic complication, for several years the pressure in the aorta has been routinely monitored during excision of the coarctation by inserting a small catheter in the distal aorta before it is occluded. Though significant data are not available, it seems probable that there is little risk of neurologic injury if the distal aortic pressure remains above 60 mm, although

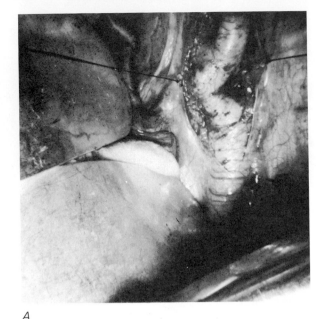

A

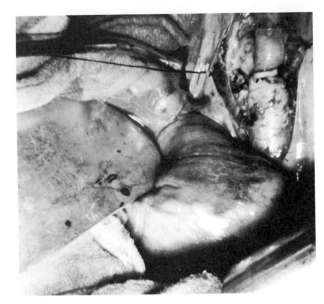

B

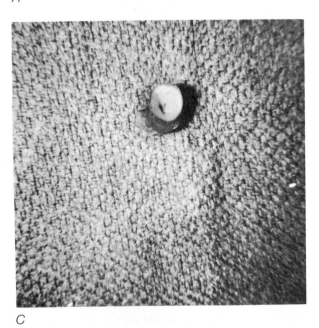

C

Fig. 18-21. *A.* Typical coarctation of aorta in child. Dilated sub-clavian artery is visible at top of field. At area of coarctation, aorta is angulated into mediastinum, where ligamentum arteriosum is inserted. *B.* Aortic anastomosis performed after excision of co-arctation. Anastomosis is made at point of origin of left subclavian artery. *C.* Resected coarctation of aorta, showing narrow lumen which was present.

the pressure has been found to vary widely, from as low as 30 mm to levels greater than 60 mm. Another safeguard is the fact that neurologic injury is virtually unknown if the aorta is occluded for less than 20 minutes. Hence it would seem wise to limit periods of aortic occlusion to less than 20 minutes if the distal pressure is less than 50 to 60 mm, or otherwise to employ a temporary shunt, as recommended by Hughes and Reemtsma.

With these precautions regarding paraplegia, once the vessels have been adequately mobilized, occluding vascular clamps are applied to the left subclavian artery, the proxi-mal aorta, and the distal aorta, after which the coarctation is excised. The objective with excision, of course, is to obtain an anastomotic lumen as large as the proximal

aorta. Often this can be done in children by excising as much as 5 cm of the proximal aorta up to the level of the left subclavian artery and performing a primary anasto-mosis (Fig. 18-22). In older children, with fibrosis and decreased elasticity of the aorta, only 2.5 to 3.0 cm of aorta may be excised.

An end-to-end anastomosis is usually done with contin-uous and interrupted sutures of polypropylene (Prolene), using interrupted sutures especially in small children to provide the best opportunity for subsequent growth of the anastomosis.

Following completion of the anastomosis and removal of vascular clamps, the blood pressure is measured proxi-mal and distal to the anastomosis to confirm that no significant gradient remains. In addition, the circumference of the anastomosis is measured and compared to that of the proximal aorta. If a gradient of more than 5 to 10 mm Hg is present and the circumference is smaller than the proximal aorta, clamps are reapplied after a short period of time, one or two sutures are removed from the anterior suture line, and a short anterior arteriotomy is made. This permits insertion of an appropriate patch of Dacron, widening the lumen sufficiently to construct an anastomosis equal to the proximal aorta. The combination of anastomosis and selective patch grafting is a valuable technique that permits complete correction of the obstruction without the insertion of a vascular graft. Less than 10 percent of children have an obstruction so diffuse that primary insertion of a graft is necessary. Schuster and Gross inserted grafts in 70 patients, 14 percent of their series, with excellent results over periods of observation as long as 12 years. Crafoord and Nylin employed grafts in only 1.0 percent of patients, while Brom reported the use of grafts in 5.0 percent.

A useful guideline for criteria of inadequate anastomosis in children was reported in 1965 by Brom, who observed from experience with over 1,000 operations for coarctation that recurrence was unlikely if the anastomosis had a circumference greater than 40 mm.

Postoperative Course. Antibiotics are given routinely during operation and for 3 to 4 days afterward. Patients usually recover rapidly and are discharged from the hospital in 10 to 12 days.

Fig. 18-22. *A.* Preductal coarctation exposed at emergency operation on thirteen-day-old infant. Large patent ductus equal in diameter to descending aorta is present. Proximal to patent ductus is coarctation of aorta with narrow proximal aortic segment and narrow subclavian artery. *B.* Appearance after excision of coarctation and suture of patent ductus arteriosus. Anastomosis was constructed proximally at point of origin of left subclavian artery from aorta.

Often there is a "paradoxical" hypertension to some extent in the first 48 to 72 hours after operation. This was first recognized by Sealy. Apparently it is related to a sudden perfusion of visceral arteries, previously functioning with a lower perfusion pressure. If this is untreated, a number of complications can occur, including intermittent abdominal pain or even intestinal necrosis in its extreme form, probably due to a mesenteric arteritis. With recognition of the syndrome and prompt treatment with appropriate antihypertensive medications, usually reserpine, serious complications are virtually unknown. Brom reported the abdominal pain syndrome in 16 of 548 patients, none of whom required laparotomy. With the liberal use of antihypertensive medications, the author has not seen any significant abdominal problems in the past 10 years.

With present techniques, the risk of operation is small and long-term results are excellent. In the series of 487 resections reported by Schuster and Gross, operative mortality was 4 percent. On long-term follow-up, 4 percent of the patients had systolic pressures above 150 mm Hg, 36 percent had values between 130 and 150 mm Hg, and 60 percent had pressures below 130 mm Hg. Crafoord and Nylin reported experiences with 249 patients, with a 4.5 percent mortality, and Brom reported experiences with 530 patients and a mortality of slightly greater than 3 percent. In a long-term evaluation of 350 patients, Brom found only 42 with some residual hypertension. At New York University, of patients operated upon beyond the first year of life, there has been no mortality and no significant complications since 1963.

Vascular Rings

HISTORICAL DATA. Although the clinical significance of vascular rings was recognized by Abbott in her classic survey of congenital heart disease in 1932, surgical therapy

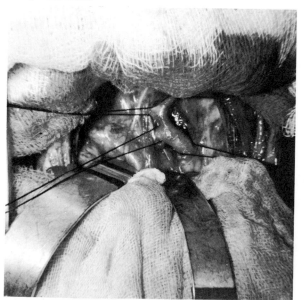

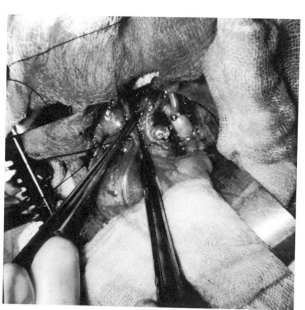

A   *B*

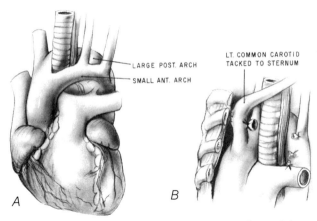

Fig. 18-23. Double aortic arch with small anterior and large posterior limb. *A.* Anterior view of double aortic arch with small anterior limb. *B.* Exposure after division of small anterior arch between left carotid and left subclavian artery, followed by displacement of carotid artery anteriorly toward sternum. (*Adapted from R. E. Gross, "The Surgery of Infancy and Childhood," W. B. Saunders Company, Philadelphia, 1953, p. 917.*)

was first successfully used with the division of a double aortic arch by Gross in 1945. Gross subsequently made many contributions to diagnosis and therapy of vascular rings, classifying and illustrating with clarity and precision the various anomalies found.

INCIDENCE AND ETIOLOGY. Vascular rings are fairly common among patients with congenital heart disease. Nadas reported seeing over 50 such patients during a

period of 10 years. Embryologically, the vascular rings result from variation in the formation of the aorta and pulmonary artery from the six embryonic aortic arches. In view of the fact that six aortic arches exist in the embryo, it is surprising that such abnormalities are not even more frequent. In embryonic life six pairs of aortic arches appear and disappear as the heart migrates caudad. The first two arches disappear before the fifth and sixth have developed, and the fifth never fully develops. Only the third, fourth, and sixth are significant in normal development. Ultimately the right common carotid artery arises from the third arch and the innominate from the right fourth. The left fourth contributes to the transverse aortic arch, while the ductus arteriosus originates from the sixth aortic arch.

PATHOLOGIC ANATOMY. Five types of vascular anomalies of clinical significance have been recognized: (1) double aortic arch; (2) right aortic arch with left ligamentum arteriosum; (3) retroesophageal subclavian artery; (4) anomalous origin of innominate artery; and (5) anomalous origin of left common carotid artery. The last two conditions, anomalous origin of the innominate or of the left common carotid artery, are rare malformations in which the origin of the artery from the aortic arch is such that the trachea is compressed. Briefly, surgical correction can be achieved by mobilizing the vessel and suturing it in

Fig. 18-24. *A.* Double aortic arch with large anterior arch. *B.* Small posterior arch, compressing esophagus. *C.* Appearance after division of small posterior arch. (*Adapted from R. E. Gross, "The Surgery of Infancy and Childhood," W. B. Saunders Company, Philadelphia, 1953, p. 918.*)

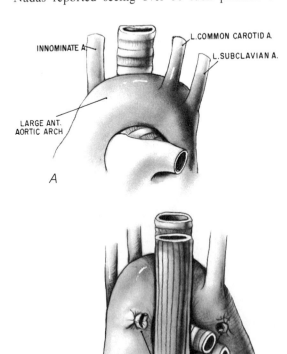

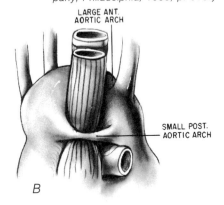

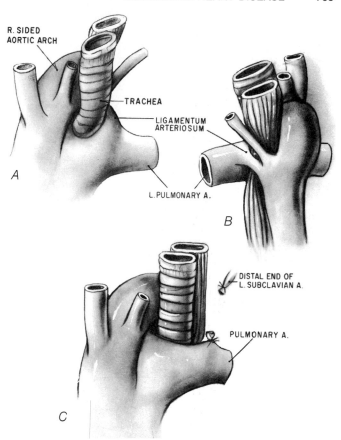

Fig. 18-25. *A.* Right aortic arch with left posterior ligamentum arteriosum. *B.* Posterior view of ligamentum arteriosum extending from right aortic arch to left pulmonary artery, compressing esophagus. Small left subclavian artery arising close to ligamentum arteriosum is also present. *C.* Appearance after division of ligamentum arteriosum and subclavian artery. (*Adapted from R. E. Gross, "The Surgery of Infancy and Childhood," W. B. Saunders Company, Philadelphia, 1953, p. 923.*)

a more normal position. The other three conditions are considered here in more detail.

A double aortic arch, with one limb anterior to the trachea and the other limb posterior to the esophagus (Figs. 18-23 and 18-24), is usually the most severe malformation, producing symptoms in early infancy. Usually one limb is smaller than the other. Often the thoracic aorta descends on the right rather than on the left.

A right aortic arch with a retroesophageal ligamentum arteriosum is an important anomaly, often producing symptoms in later childhood (Fig. 18-25). A retroesopha-

geal subclavian artery, usually consisting of a right subclavian artery originating beyond the left subclavian artery and coursing posterior to the esophagus to the right arm, is a common anomaly but usually does not cause symptoms (Fig. 18-26).

CLINICAL MANIFESTATIONS. Symptoms from vascular rings are usually due to respiratory obstruction from compression of the trachea. Less frequently, there is difficulty in swallowing from compression of the esophagus.

Symptoms. Infants with a double aortic arch often develop respiratory difficulty in the first few months of life

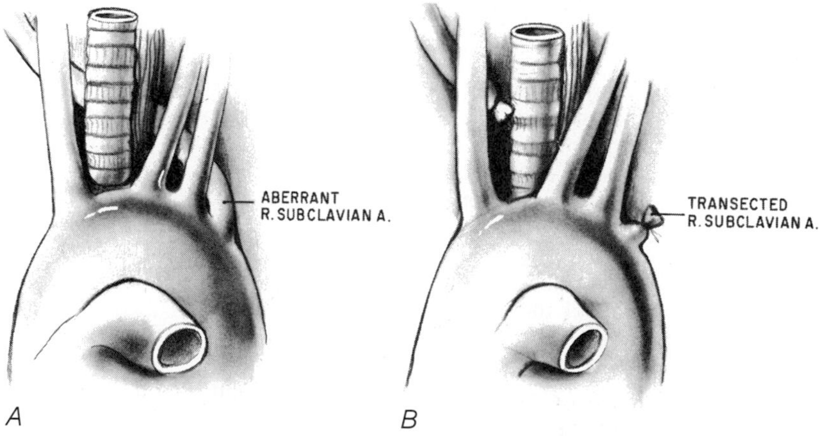

Fig. 18-26. *A.* Retroesophageal right subclavian artery, anomalous vessel arising from aortic arch distal to left subclavian artery. *B.* Appearance after division of anomalous vessel with retraction of distal stump to right of trachea. (*Adapted from R. E. Gross, "The Surgery of Infancy and Childhood," W. B. Saunders Company, Philadelphia, 1953, p. 932.*)

and become seriously ill. Episodes of serious respiratory distress, with "crowing" respirations, are common. During these attacks the infant prefers to lie in hyperextension, and there is visible retraction of the intercostal and supra-clavicular spaces with inspiration. Feeding may precipitate such episodes, perhaps from flexing of the neck, and attempts at feeding may be interrupted by vomiting, and cyanosis, probably from aspiration. Because of the feeding difficulties, infants soon become underweight and malnourished.

Symptoms developing after infancy are more gradual in onset, with intermittent episodes of respiratory compression, at times precipitated by a respiratory infection. Mild difficulty in swallowing may be present, but this is seldom prominent. Recurrent pneumonic infections occur, perhaps from aspiration. The mildest clinical picture is seen with the retroesophageal subclavian artery, which may cause only mild or intermittent dysphagia for long periods of time. Some patients may be symptomatic in infancy and spontaneously recover with growth.

Physical Examination. The physical examination is within normal limits unless respiratory distress is present. During such episodes, the infant remains with the back arched and the neck extended. Attempts to flex the neck may precipitate severe dyspnea and cyanosis. Stridor is usually obvious. There are no abnormalities in the heart or peripheral circulation.

LABORATORY STUDIES. The chest roentgenogram is normal unless aspiration pneumonia is present, and the electrocardiogram is normal. Examination of the esophagus with a barium swallow usually establishes the diagnosis by demonstrating a typical area of compression from the retroesophageal vessel, usually at the level of the third or fourth thoracic vertebra. Such a finding is virtually all that is needed to establish the diagnosis of a vascular ring. To determine whether the ring is responsible for the symptoms may require further study. Tracheal compression may be defined with a tracheogram. In the anterior view, compression may be noted laterally, but the lateral tracheogram provides the best evidence for the vascular ring, demonstrating anterior compression of the trachea a short distance above the carina. The demonstration of anterior compression of the trachea combined with posterior compression of the esophagus firmly establishes the diagnosis of a vascular ring. Aortography can then precisely delineate the abnormal vessels.

TREATMENT. Since a vascular ring has no physiologic significance, no treatment is needed in the absence of symptoms. If symptoms are mild, their origin may be uncertain, and an observation period is required to be sure that other difficulties are not responsible. If obvious respiratory compression is present, operation should be performed promptly, however, because death from aspiration can occur.

Operative Technique. The preferred operative approach is through a left lateral thoracotomy, usually the fourth intercostal space. An important feature of the operation is to dissect the aortic arch completely and identify the innominate artery, the left common carotid artery, and both subclavian arteries. Opening the pericardium will facilitate identification of these vessels. The vagus nerve should be traced to the recurrent laryngeal nerve and, usually, the ligamentum arteriosum divided. Removal of part of the thymus gland will facilitate exposure. It should be emphasized that operative correction is more than simple division of an abnormal ring, because fibrosis surrounding the adventitia of the abnormal vessel may cause continued compression unless the vessels are widely mobilized and all possible compression relieved.

With a double aortic arch, the smaller of the two arches should be divided. Usually, with a left descending aorta, the anterior arch is smaller and should be divided between the left common carotid and left subclavian artery, after which the mobilized anterior arch can be sutured to the posterior surface of the anterior chest wall to prevent compression of the trachea. If the posterior arch is smaller, it can be divided behind the esophagus. With a right descending thoracic aorta, almost always the posterior arch is the smaller of the two.

With a right aortic arch and a retroesophageal ligamentum arteriosum, division of the ligamentum arteriosum, combined with mobilization of the abnormal vessels, may be all that is necessary. In some patients the left subclavian artery may be in a retroesophageal location and should also be divided. A nubbin of aorta, constituting an aortic diverticulum, has been found in a retroesophageal location in some patients and may require amputation to relieve compression.

With a retroesophageal subclavian artery as an isolated anomaly, simple division of the artery is all that is necessary. Division of this artery through a cervical incision, followed by reimplantation into the right carotid artery, has been reported.

Postoperative Course. Postoperative care consists primarily of careful attention to respiration, with the infant kept in a highly humidified atmosphere and tracheal secretions aspirated. Tracheostomy should be avoided if at all possible. If serious tracheal compression was present before operation, serious difficulties may develop after operation if extensive dissection around the trachea was necessary, creating postoperative edema. In such cases the patient may require unusually vigilant care for 24 to 72 hours because of edema of the trachea. After recovery from operation, symptoms promptly disappear without further disability. The risk of operation is primarily related to the age of the patient and the severity of compression of the trachea. Excellent results in a group of 70 patients have been reported by Gross, who had only 5 postoperative deaths, all of which occurred in a group of 26 infants with double aortic arches.

LEFT-TO-RIGHT SHUNTS (ACYANOTIC GROUP)

Atrial Septal Defects

A variety of malformations involve the atrial septum or the pulmonary veins and result in a left-to-right shunt of blood from the systemic to the pulmonary circulation.

These include atrial septal defects of the secundum type, anomalous drainage of the pulmonary veins, ostium primum defects, and atrioventricular canal malformations. These defects are serially considered below. The physiologic disturbance is identical with secundum-type atrial defects and with anomalous pulmonary veins, consisting simply in a left-to-right shunt. With ostium primum defects and atrioventricular canals, mitral and tricuspid insufficiency are present in addition to the left-to-right shunt.

SECUNDUM DEFECTS

HISTORICAL DATA. Several ingenious attempts were made to close atrial septal defects by closed techniques from 1947 to 1953, but only following the successful closure of an atrial septal defect by Lewis in 1953 under direct vision with inflow occlusion and hypothermia did a method of surgical closure become firmly established. In the same year Gibbon employed the pump-oxygenator successfully for the first time in man to suture an atrial septal defect. In subsequent years a large number of patients were successfully operated upon by using hypothermia to permit interruption of the circulation for 5 to 10 minutes, but extracorporeal circulation quickly became the preferred technique because of the additional time available to close the septal defect and also to correct any additional malformations which may be encountered.

INCIDENCE AND ETIOLOGY. Atrial septal defects are among the most common cardiac malformations, representing 10 to 15 percent of all cases of congenital heart disease. They are approximately twice as frequent in females as in males. Embryologically, the secundum defects result from failure of the septum secundum to develop completely.

PATHOLOGIC ANATOMY. Atrial septal defects vary widely in size and location. A "high" defect near the entrance of the superior vena cava is commonly referred to as a sinus venosus type of defect and is usually associated with anomalous entry of the superior pulmonary veins into the vena cava. The majority of secundum defects are located in the midportion of the atrial septum. "Low" defects are near the point of entry of the inferior vena cava, and caution must be taken in closing such defects to avoid compromising the entry of the inferior vena cava into the right atrium. Defects vary from as small as 1 cm in diameter to virtual absence of the atrial septum, but most are 2 to 3 cm. A foramen ovale should not be considered an atrial septal defect, for it is a normal opening in 15 to 25 percent of adult hearts. Because of its slitlike construction, a normal foramen ovale allows shunting of blood only from right to left. In some patients the atrial septum is fenestrated with multiple defects.

Anomalous pulmonary veins entering the right atrium are frequent, occurring in 10 to 15 percent of patients with atrial septal defects. An unusual variant of atrial septal defect is seen when a secundum defect occurs in association with mitral stenosis, the so-called Lutembacher's syndrome. The mitral stenosis retards flow of blood from the left atrium to the left ventricle and results in an enormous shunt of blood through the septal defect, with massive dilatation of the pulmonary arteries. With present diagnostic techniques, this syndrome has become rare.

PATHOPHYSIOLOGY. An atrial septal defect results in a left-to-right shunt of blood from the left atrium to the right atrium because of the pressure-volume characteristics of the left and right ventricles. The thick-walled left ventricle is less distensible than the right ventricle; with a closed atrial septum, left atrial pressure is normally 8 to 10 mm Hg, while right atrial pressure is 4 to 5 mm Hg. This difference in distensibility of the two ventricles results in a left-to-right shunt when an atrial septal defect is present. However, during infancy and the first few years of life the structure of the right ventricle more closely resembles the left ventricle, and usually only a small shunt is present. For this reason atrial septal defects are commonly not recognized during the first few years of life.

Depending upon the size of the atrial defect, as well as the difference in distensibility of the two ventricles, the size of the left-to-right shunt may vary from as little as 1 liter to as high as 20 liters/minute. Most septal defects have a pulmonary blood flow two to four times greater than the systemic blood flow. The great reduction in systemic blood flow may result in retardation of normal growth and development, with the so-called gracile habitus seen in some children with a large atrial septal defect. The increase in pulmonary blood flow increases susceptibility to pneumonia and also causes dyspnea on exertion. For unknown reasons patients are susceptible to rheumatic fever, but fortunately bacterial endocarditis is rare. Arrhythmias of different types are also frequently seen.

With the increased pulmonary blood flow, pulmonary vascular resistance in children is usually less than normal, but it gradually increases. Pulmonary hypertension is found in less than 5 percent of children with this condition but occurs in 20 to 25 percent of adult patients as fibrotic changes develop in the pulmonary vessels. Cardiac failure is similarly unusual in children but becomes more frequent in the second and third decades. It has been estimated that the average life span of an untreated patient with an atrial septal defect is about 40 years.

Some patients are seen in the fourth, fifth, or sixth decades for the first time with a previously unrecognized atrial septal defect. In these older patients, arrhythmias are especially common, a result of long-standing hypertrophy of the right atrium. Even in patients in the sixth decade a good result may be obtained following operation if increase in pulmonary vascular resistance has not occurred. However, arrhythmias may continue.

CLINICAL MANIFESTATIONS. Symptoms. Symptoms are uncommon in the first few years of life because the shunt may be small until the right ventricular hypertrophy of embryonic life has subsided. Frequently children with large shunts are physically active and completely free of symptoms. In a report of 275 surgically treated patients with hemodynamically significant atrial defects, Sellers et al. found 113 asymptomatic. The most frequent symptoms are fatigue, palpitations, and exertional dyspnea. Slow growth and development may also be noted by the parents. In adults overt signs of congestive heart failure gradually appear, often with the first pregnancy.

Physical Examination. A soft systolic murmur is usually audible in the second or third left intercostal space. In the first few years of life this murmur may be scarcely detectable or may be diagnosed as a functional murmur. The murmur arises at the pulmonary valve from the increased flow of blood through the valve. The second pulmonic sound is characteristically widely split, and "fixed" splitting (not varying with respiration) is characteristic of the disorder. Slight to moderate cardiac enlargement is present with large defects. With large defects the cardiac enlargement may produce a distinct prominence of the left costal cartilages. The physical habitus of such patients is often thin, with long, narrow bones and limited muscular development—the gracile habitus.

LABORATORY FINDINGS. The chest roentgenogram shows mild to moderate cardiac enlargement limited to the right ventricle. The pulmonary artery is prominent, with increased vascularity in the lung fields. The electrocardiogram typically shows a right axis deviation with a right bundle branch block. Mild but not severe right ventricular hypertrophy is usually evident.

On cardiac catheterization the diagnosis can be confirmed by finding a rise in oxygen saturation of 1.5 to 2.0 vol % between the superior vena cava and right atrium. During catheterization the presence of anomalous veins should be noted, although the diagnosis cannot always be established with certainty. The right ventricular systolic pressure in children is usually 30 to 40 mm Hg. With large shunts there may be a 20 to 40 mm Hg gradient across a normal pulmonary valve as a result of the large flow of blood. Selective angiography with injection of dye into the pulmonary artery may disclose opacification of the right atrium as dye flows from the left atrium through the defect.

DIAGNOSIS. Diagnosis in infancy is virtually impossible on clinical grounds, because the systolic murmur is not distinctive. In older children the diagnosis can be made with reasonable certainty from the combination of a soft systolic murmur with fixed splitting of the pulmonic second

sound. These physical findings, combined with the chest roentgenogram and electrocardiogram, provide firm support for the diagnosis. A left axis deviation on the electrocardiogram immediately suggests that an ostium primum malformation is present.

TREATMENT. Indications. Since many children are asymptomatic, operation is frequently recommended on the basis of clinical findings and laboratory determination of the size of shunt present. Operation is usually performed if the pulmonary blood flow is one and one-half to two times greater than the systemic blood flow. The only contraindication to operation is the presence of severe pulmonary hypertension with an elevated pulmonary vascular resistance, fortunately almost unknown in children. In adults, if the pulmonary vascular resistance has increased to where pulmonary blood flow is only slightly greater than systemic flow, operation is hazardous, and patients who survive often show little benefit. However, if pulmonary blood flow is still significantly increased despite the presence of pulmonary hypertension, operation may be beneficial, although the operative risk is considerably greater than with uncomplicated atrial septal defect and improvement does not occur to an equal degree in all patients.

Operative Technique. All patients are operated on with extracorporeal circulation. A sternotomy or a right thoracotomy in the fourth intercostal space is used. Once bypass has been established, a finger is introduced into the right atrium through a stab wound to identify the pathologic anatomy, noting the atrial septal defect, the coronary sinus, the location of the pulmonary veins, the mitral and tricuspid valves, and the ventricular septum. Palpation beforehand minimizes the need for exploration of the heart once it has been opened and similarly lessens the hazards of air embolism.

At a perfusion temperature of 30°C, the heart is fibrillated, the aorta clamped, and the atrium opened widely to identify the margins of the defect (Fig. 18-27). In at least 90 percent of patients, closure can be done with a simple continuous suture, preferably polypropylene (Prolene). If

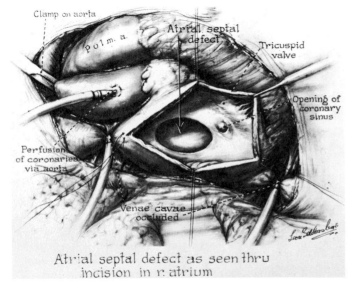

Fig. 18-27. Atrial septal defect of secundum type exposed at operation. Operation illustrated was performed under hypothermia several years ago with perfusion of aorta with oxygenated blood. Such operations are now performed with cardiopulmonary bypass. Large oval opening in atrial septum superior to coronary sinus is type usually found with secundum-type defects.

direct suture is not possible, a prosthetic patch of knitted Dacron or pericardium can be inserted.

Care is taken during operation to avoid aspiration of blood from the left atrium. As the suture line is completed, the lungs are ventilated and the aorta unclamped to expel blood from the left atrium into the right atrium and provide an additional protection against trapping air in the left atrium. With these safeguards, no problems with air embolism have occurred in several years.

Subsequently, after bypass has been stopped, correction of the left-to-right shunt can be confirmed by aspirating blood from the superior vena cava and pulmonary artery and demonstrating similar oxygen concentration in the two samples. Left atrial pressure should be measured afterward and serially monitored if elevated.

Postoperative Course. Postoperative convalescence is uncomplicated and recovery from any signs of cardiac disability is prompt in the usual patient with uncomplicated atrial septal defect.

The risk of operation with extracorporeal circulation is surprisingly small. Several groups have reported series of more than 100 patients operated upon with a mortality of 1 to 3 percent. Gerbode et al. reported one death in 77 patients, and Sellers et al. a 1.8 percent mortality in uncomplicated atrial defects in a group of 275 patients. In the author's experience with more than 100 secundum defects, no deaths have occurred in the past decade.

ANOMALOUS DRAINAGE OF PULMONARY VEINS

Partial and total anomalous drainage of the pulmonary veins are distinct clinical entities and are presented separately in the following sections. The physiologic handicap from partial drainage of the pulmonary veins resembles atrial septal defect, while total anomalous drainage is a much more serious physiologic derangement, often fatal in the first few months of life.

Partial anomalous drainage is frequent, occurring in 10 to 15 percent of patients with atrial septal defect. Total anomalous drainage, however, is much less common.

HISTORICAL DATA. Although anomalous pulmonary veins have been recognized at postmortem examinations for decades, emphasis was focused on clinical features by the analysis by Brody of 106 cases in 1942. Before open cardiac surgery was possible, only a few cases of successful surgical correction were reported. One of the first of these was reported in 1951 by Muller, who successfully implanted an anomalous left pulmonary vein into the left atrium. Subsequently, with operations performed under hypothermia, partial anomalous drainage of pulmonary veins, usually into the right atrium or superior vena cava, could be corrected by changing the position of the atrial septum. Successful correction of total anomalous pulmonary venous drainage, however, was accomplished only with extracorporeal circulation. A modification of the technique reported by Cooley and Ochsner in 1957 has subsequently proved to be the most useful.

PARTIAL ANOMALOUS DRAINAGE OF PULMONARY VEINS. Pathologic Anatomy. Anomalous drainage of the right pulmonary veins occurs approximately twice as frequently as that involving the left. Anomalous right pulmo-

nary veins usually enter the superior vena cava inferior to the point of entry of the azygos vein, the right atrium, or the inferior vena cava. Anomalous left pulmonary veins commonly enter a persistent left superior vena cava or innominate vein or, more rarely, the coronary sinus. Partial anomalous drainage usually involves only the veins from one lung, but a few unusual examples of partial drainage of pulmonary veins from both lungs have been described. One of the most detailed reports of the pathologic anatomy of anomalous pulmonary veins was published by Blake et al. in an analysis of data from the Armed Forces Institute of Pathology. In a group of 113 patients with anomalous pulmonary venous return, a total of 27 different variations were found, emphasizing the wide variation in physiologic derangement which occur.

Anomalous right pulmonary veins entering the superior vena cava are almost always associated with a characteristic high atrial septal defect at the point of entry of the superior vena cava, which has been termed a sinus venosus defect because of its embryologic origin. Pulmonary veins entering the right atrium are also usually associated with an atrial septal defect of the secundum type. Only rarely are anomalous pulmonary veins found with an intact atrial septum. Pulmonary veins entering the inferior vena cava usually communicate through a single channel with the inferior vena cava near the diaphragm.

An unusual variant of anomalous right pulmonary veins entering the inferior vena cava, in association with other anomalies, has been described as a "scimitar" syndrome, a term emphasizing a characteristic radiologic appearance resulting from the shadow of the anomalous vein parallel to the right border of the heart. Although this roentgenographic appearance is suggestive, other abnormalities may have a similar appearance. The malformation is often associated with defective development of the right lung and anomalous origin of the pulmonary arteries from the aorta. The physiologic disturbance is not severe, because the amount of blood shunted through the hypoplastic lung is small.

Pathophysiology. With partial anomalous drainage of the pulmonary veins, the volume of blood shunted is usually less than 50 percent of normal pulmonary blood flow, because less than one-half the pulmonary veins are involved. Hence the abnormal physiology is a left-to-right shunt identical to that of an atrial septal defect.

Clinical Manifestations. The symptoms and signs are identical to those of an atrial septal defect, and clinical separation of the two entities is not possible. Cardiac catheterization is the only method for establishing a precise diagnosis. Direct entry of an anomalous vein by the cardiac catheter may be diagnostic, especially if the vein is entered from the superior vena cava. In the right atrium, one often cannot be certain whether or not the catheter has traversed an atrial septal defect before entering the pulmonary vein. Selective angiography may confirm the diagnosis in some patients.

Treatment. A single anomalous pulmonary vein, usually from the right upper lobe entering the superior vena cava, is physiologically harmless and does not require treatment. More extensive malformations are usually operated upon in conjunction with closure of an atrial septal defect. Anomalous veins entering the right atrium can be corrected by insertion of a prosthetic patch so that the defect is closed and the pulmonary veins enter the left atrium. Pulmonary veins entering the superior vena cava in association with a sinus venosus defect can be corrected by the application of a prosthetic patch, preferably of pericardium, to shunt blood into the left atrium (Fig. 18-28). Anomalous veins entering the inferior vena cava are usually treated by division of the aberrant channel and direct implantation into the left atrium.

TOTAL ANOMALOUS DRAINAGE OF PULMONARY VEINS. Pathologic Anatomy. Darling et al. have classified anatomically the types of total anomalous drainage of pulmonary veins according to location. Supracardiac drainage occurs in 55 percent of cases, paracardiac in 30 percent, and infracardiac in 12 percent. Multiple sites of entry are found in 3 percent.

With the supracardiac type of drainage, the most common point of entry of the anomalous veins is into a left vertical vein which in turn enters the left innominate vein. Rarely, the common anomalous venous trunk may drain directly into the posterior aspect of a right superior vena cava. With paracardiac drainage, the anomalous veins may enter the right atrium directly or, more rarely, may drain into the coronary sinus. With infracardiac drainage the pulmonary venous blood usually enters the inferior vena cava through a common channel traversing the diaphragm to connect with a hepatic vein or the portal vein.

Pathophysiology. Life is possible with total anomalous pulmonary venous drainage only as long as an atrial septal defect, often only a foramen ovale, is present. In addition, pulmonary venous hypertension often exists because of constriction of the point of entry of the anomalous pulmonary veins into the systemic venous system, which in turn results in pulmonary hypertension. With adequate communication between the anomalous pulmonary veins and the systemic venous circulation and a large atrial septal defect, patients may do surprisingly well for a period of time, the disability resembling that from a large atrial septal defect. This fortunate situation occurs in about 20

percent of patients. In the majority (80 percent) severe pulmonary hypertension is present; half these patients die in the first 3 months of life, and most within the first year. Cardiac failure develops with great rapidity, and cyanosis, varying with the degree of pulmonary blood flow, is frequent.

Clinical Manifestations. The dominant findings are a seriously ill infant with congestive failure, cyanosis, and rapidly progressive cardiac enlargement. In infants a murmur may not be audible. Hepatic enlargement is frequent.

The chest roentgenogram may be diagnostic when there is significant dilatation of the left vertebral and left innominate veins, creating a characteristic double contour on the x-ray termed a "snowman" appearance (Fig. 18-3).

Occasionally, with severe pulmonary venous obstruction, pulmonary congestion may be so severe in the infant as to suggest miliary tuberculosis. Diagnosis can be confirmed by cardiac catheterization. The hallmark of the physiologic disturbance in total anomalous pulmonary venous drainage is an almost identical oxygen content of the right atrium, pulmonary artery, and femoral artery because of complete mixing of oxygenated and unoxygenated blood in the right atrium before entering the left atrium through an atrial septal defect. Pulmonary hypertension is common. Also, the right atrial pressure is usually greater than the left atrial pressure.

Treatment. Infants with total anomalous pulmonary venous drainage may not survive more than the first few days or weeks of life without operation, so operation is often performed under emergency or desperate circumstances. Enlarging the atrial septal defect by the balloon septos-

Fig. 18-28. *A.* Sinus venosus type of atrial septal defect located near junction of superior vena cava with right atrium. Defect is partly obscured by crescentic lower margin. Anomalous pulmonary veins from right upper lobe enter superior vena cava near its juncture with right atrium. *B.* Prosthetic patch can be applied to encompass both atrial septal defect and ostia of anomalous pulmonary veins, avoiding undue constriction of point of entry of superior vena cava into right atrium. *C.* Final view of prosthetic patch which excludes anomalous veins and atrial septal defect from right atrium. (*Adapted from C. D. Benson et al., "Pediatric Surgery," vol. I, Year Book Medical Publishers, Inc., Chicago, 1962, p. 439.*)

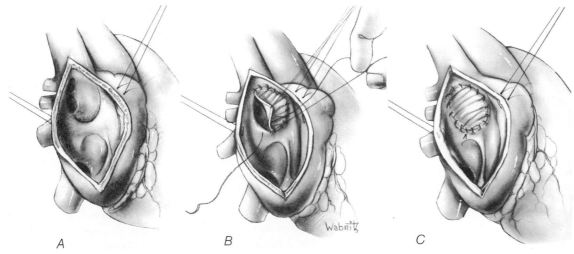

A   *B*   *C*

tomy technique of Rashkind may provide valuable palliation but unfortunately is not always successful. When
surgical correction is done in infants, the deep hypothermia–circulatory arrest technique, well developed by
Barratt-Boyes and his colleagues, is the preferred approach, for extracorporeal circulation is often not well
tolerated in infants.

When the pulmonary veins drain into a left vertical vein,
surgical correction includes creation of a long (2.5 to
3.0 cm) side-to-side anastomosis between the anomalous
pulmonary veins and the left atrium (Fig. 18-29), followed
by closure of the atrial septal defect and ligation of the left
vertical vein. A similar procedure is followed with the
unusual condition of drainage of the pulmonary veins into
a single vein that courses beneath the diaphragm to join
the portal venous system. If anomalous veins enter the
right atrium or the coronary sinus, surgical reconstruction
can be more simply performed (Fig. 18-30).

In infants, operative mortality has remained high, in the
range of 30 to 50 percent. Most deaths are associated with
pulmonary congestion and insufficiency. Beyond the first
year of life, operative risk is small, approaching that of
atrial septal defect if there is not a great increase in pulmonary vascular resistance. In 1975 Wukasch, Cooley, and
associates reported experiences with 125 patients with an
operative mortality in the first year of life remaining near
50 percent. By contrast, several groups have reported reasonable mortality rates in infants requiring operation before the age of 6 months, often employing the technique of
deep hypothermia and circulatory arrest. Kirklin stated in
1976 that he and his associates had not had a death in
patients over 6 months of age since 1967.

OSTIUM PRIMUM DEFECT

Primum defects are relatively infrequent, occurring in 4
to 5 percent of patients with defects in the atrial septum.
One of the first papers to emphasize clinical differentiation
of ostium primum from secundum defects was published
in 1956 by Blount and associates.

Ostium primum defects are often found in children with
mongolism, occurring in 20 to 30 percent. Except for this
unusual association, no etiologic factors are known.

A primum defect results from incomplete formation of
the mitral and tricuspid valves and the atrial and ventricular septa from the embryonic endocardial cushions. In
embryonic life the endocardial cushions develop as dorsal
and ventral partitions to separate the single atrium and
ventricle of the embryo and join with the ventricular and
atrial septa to form the normal four cardiac chambers. A
synonym for ostium primum defects and the more severe
associated malformation, atrioventricular canal, is *endocardial cushion defect,* partial (ostium primum) or complete
(atrioventricular canal).

PATHOLOGIC ANATOMY. The two significant defects are
a cleft in the anterior leaflet of the mitral valve and a low,
crescent-shaped defect in the atrial septum (Fig. 18-31*A*).
The sicklelike superior border of an ostium primum defect
can be easily recognized on palpation at the time of surgical correction. The cleft in the anterior leaflet of the mitral
valve may be partial, extending for a short distance from

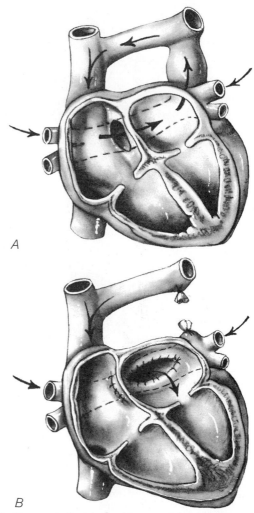

A

B

Fig. 18-29. *A.* Abnormal physiology with anomalous drainage of
pulmonary veins into left superior vena cava. All pulmonary venous blood flows through left innominate vein into large right
superior vena cava and can enter systemic circulation only
through atrial septal defect, usually foramen ovale. *B.* At operation, wide opening is made between posteriorly located common
pulmonary venous trunk and left atrium, after which opening in
atrial septum is closed and left superior vena cava divided.
(*Adapted from C. D. Benson et al., "Pediatric Surgery," vol. I,
Year Book Medical Publishers, Inc., Chicago, 1962, p. 446.*)

the ventricular septum, or complete, separating the mitral
valve leaflet into anterior and posterior halves.

Chordae tendineae are usually attached to the margins
of the cleft and in some fortunate patients may prevent
significant mitral insufficiency. In other patients, usually
those with more severe malformations, abnormal chordae
tendineae are present.

An associated partial or complete cleft in the tricuspid
valve is also frequently seen. Conduction abnormalities
from fibrosis or distortion of the conduction bundle, characteristically located along the posterior rim of the septal
defect, are common.

Primum defects are anatomically distinguished from the
more severe atrioventricular canal malformation by the

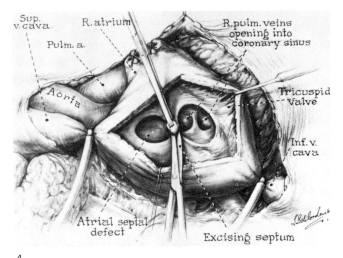

A

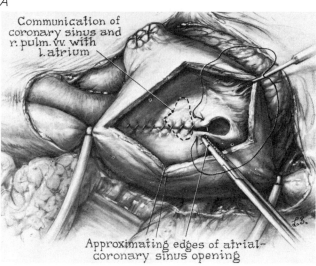

B

Fig. 18-30. *A.* Total anomalous drainage of pulmonary veins into coronary sinus. With this anomaly, atrial septal defect, usually foramen ovale, must be present to maintain life. It is possible to correct anomaly by excision of septum between foramen ovale and dilated coronary sinus. *B.* After excision of septum between foramen ovale and coronary sinus, resulting opening can be closed by suture of atrial septum, thus diverting all pulmonary venous blood, as well as blood draining from coronary sinus, into left atrium.

presence of distinct, separate mitral and tricuspid valve rings and an intact ventricular septum. With an atrioventricular canal malformation there is an additional defect in the ventricular septum, as well as extensive abnormalities of the mitral and tricuspid valve leaflets.

PATHOPHYSIOLOGY. The physiologic abnormalities are a left-to-right shunt combined with mitral insufficiency. When mitral insufficiency is minimal, the malformation is identical with that of atrial septal defect of the secundum type. When mitral insufficiency is severe, left ventricular failure and pulmonary hypertension appear early in life and produce a much more severe impairment of cardiac function than is seen in secundum-type septal defects. Increase in pulmonary vascular resistance with pulmonary hypertension may develop but is more frequent with atrioventricular canals.

CLINICAL MANIFESTATIONS. Symptoms. A variety of clinical profiles occur, varying with the degree of mitral insufficiency. When mitral insufficiency is minimal, the clinical picture is similar to that of atrial septal defect of the secundum type. Before the advent of precise diagnostic techniques, ostium primum defects were often first recognized at operation. With significant mitral insufficiency, cardiac failure with pulmonary congestion, dyspnea, recurrent bouts of pneumonia, and retardation of growth may be prominent in the first years of life.

Physical Examination. On physical examination moderate cardiac enlargement is often found, with a thrill near the apex. A harsh apical systolic murmur from mitral insufficiency is usually present and should arouse suspicion of an ostium primum defect. An additional systolic murmur may be heard along the left sternal border. The intensity of the pulmonic second sound is often increased. With cardiac failure, signs of pulmonary congestion and hepatic enlargement are found. Growth is frequently retarded.

LABORATORY FINDINGS. The chest roentgenogram usually shows moderate cardiac enlargement, involving both the right and the left ventricle. Increased pulmonary vascularity is also common. The most useful diagnostic guide is provided by the electrocardiogram, which shows both right and left ventricular hypertrophy, with a left axis deviation. In the vectorcardiogram the inscription in the

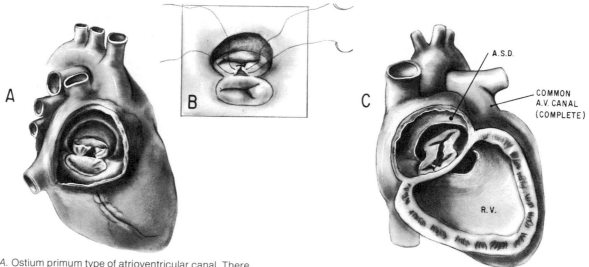

Fig. 18-31. *A.* Ostium primum type of atrioventricular canal. There is a cleft in anterior mitral leaflet, but ventricular septum is intact. *B.* Method of repair of cleft valve with interrupted sutures to produce competent mitral valve. Classic crescent-shaped atrial septal defect superior to valve ring is shown. *C.* Appearance of complete atrioventricular canal, showing complete division of mitral and tricuspid valves in association with atrial septal defect and ventricular septal defect. (*Adapted from D. C. McGoon et al., Am J Cardiol, 6:598, 1960.*)

frontal plane is in a counterclockwise loop, a finding almost pathognomonic of ostium primum defect. Conduction defects with prolongation of the P-R interval are frequent. These electrocardiographic abnormalities are due primarily to the conduction defect and not to the associated left ventricular hypertrophy.

On cardiac catheterization a left-to-right shunt is found at the atrial level; frequently the catheter will enter the left atrium or left ventricle. The pulmonary blood flow is frequently two to three times greater than systemic flow. Mitral insufficiency, suggested by prominent V waves in the left atrial pressure tracing, is best confirmed by injection of contrast media into the left ventricle.

DIAGNOSIS. The diagnosis usually can be made with reasonable certainty from the clinical picture of a child with cardiac enlargement, a left-to-right shunt with an apical systolic murmur, and an electrocardiogram showing left axis deviation with a frontal-plane counterclockwise loop in the vectorcardiogram. Differential diagnosis should exclude ventricular septal defect and atrial septal defect of the secundum type.

TREATMENT. In most patients operative correction of the defect should be performed between the ages of four and six years. Rarely, an adult is seen in the third or fourth decade with a history of little disability from a primum defect, but such patients are those in whom mitral insufficiency has been minimal and the clinical course has been more similar to the benign secundum-type defect. In most patients the combination of a left-to-right shunt with mitral insufficiency results in progressive cardiac enlargement and failure in childhood.

Operative Technique. Operation is performed with extra-

corporeal circulation, using a median sternotomy incision. The three principal objectives are correction of the mitral insufficiency, closure of the septal defect, and avoidance of the production of heart block from injury to the conduction bundle along the posterior margin of the septal defect. Incomplete correction of the mitral insufficiency can be disastrous. Closure of the septal defect with residual severe mitral insufficiency may produce severe or fatal pulmonary edema, because decompression of the left atrium into the right atrium has been abolished by closure of the defect.

Usually, operation is performed with intermittent aortic occlusion for 10 to 15 minutes at 30°C, alternating with periods of aortic unclamping and cardiac contraction. Appropriate measures are taken to avoid an air embolism. The right atrium is widely opened, and the septal defect, cleft in the mitral valve, associated cleft in the tricuspid valve, and ventricular septum are carefully examined. Initially the cleft in the mitral valve is closed with interrupted sutures placed from the ventricular septum out to the free margin of the mitral orifice (Fig. 18-31*B*), the points of insertion of the chordae tendineae being carefully noted. Usually a left ventricular vent is inserted through the apex of the left ventricle to avoid production of air embolism once the mitral valve has been rendered competent by closure of the cleft. After repair of the cleft mitral valve, the septal defect is repaired with a patch of pericardium inserted with interrupted sutures. Along the posterior rim near the conduction bundle the sutures are inserted superficially to the left of the rim of the defect along the annulus of the mitral valve, the electrocardiogram being checked after the sutures are inserted to avoid producing a conduction injury. A defect in the tricuspid valve is frequent but usually is not amenable to repair by direct suture. Air should be completely evacuated from the left atrium as closure of the septal defect is completed.

Postoperative Course. If adequate correction of the mitral insufficiency is accomplished and production of heart block avoided, postoperative recovery is usually uneventful and similar to that for closure of other septal defects. A conduction injury is a grave complication, but rare. It should be treated at operation by the temporary insertion of a pacemaker. If a complete heart block should persist, a permanent pacemaker should be inserted. Some patients have a residual systolic murmur, and some of these will be found on subsequent study to have significant mitral regurgitation. A small percentage of such patients require mitral valve replacement in the next 5 to 10 years. The functional results in the majority of patients, however, are satisfactory. At the Mayo Clinic, McGoon and associates in 1973 reported long-term results in 232 patients, the majority of whom had maintained an excellent result following operation. The operative mortality is less than 5 percent. At New York University since 1963, there have been no deaths or complete heart blocks following operation.

In early experiences with surgical repair, an unusual syndrome of severe hemolytic anemia was recognized in a small percentage of patients following repair of an ostium primum defect. This striking clinical picture resulted from residual mitral insufficiency accidentally oriented so that the regurgitant jet of blood struck the prosthetic patch closing the septal defect and intermittently dislodged fibrin from the surface of the patch with each systolic jet. Although rare, such a syndrome should be recognized, for reoperation and closure of the residual insufficiency is curative.

PERSISTENT ATRIOVENTRICULAR CANAL

This malformation is a more extensive error in development of the endocardial cushions, consisting of a large common defect involving both the atrial and ventricular septa, and extensive defects in the mitral and tricuspid valves (Fig. 18-31C). These are often connected across the incomplete septa to form large common valve leaflets in the anterior and posterior portions of the heart. The great variation in valve deformities in these patients was well described by Rastelli et al. in an analysis of 30 postmortem specimens. The physiologic defect is a left-to-right shunt at both the atrial and ventricular levels, resulting in cardiac failure in early life as well as pulmonary vascular obstruction and pulmonary hypertension. The severity of the malformation depends upon the extent of the mitral insufficiency and the size of the ventricular septal defect. In infants with severe deformities the course is a severe one, with death in the first few months of life, while patients with less severe lesions do reasonably well for the first few years of life.

An atrioventricular canal, rather than an ostium primum defect, may be suspected from the malignant clinical course of severe cardiac failure and cardiac enlargement in the first one or two years of life. Diagnosis is established principally by cardiac catheterization and angiography, demonstrating both a ventricular septal defect and mitral insufficiency.

Several years ago results of operative correction were very poor, the mortality exceeding 75 percent in infants. Prosthetic valves were employed in a few infants but with similarly unimpressive results. Great advances have been made in surgical therapy in recent years, due principally to the techniques of surgical correction developed by Rastelli et al. and McGoon, which have reduced mortality to a range of 10 to 15 percent in patients over 2 years of age.

Similar results have been reported by Mills in a smaller series. The original publication should be consulted for details of operative techniques. The essential steps include insertion of a large prosthetic patch, which is attached to the underlying ventricular septum, following which the valve is reconstructed and attached to the patch at an appropriate level, with subsequent closure of the atrial septal defect.

In 1976 Kirklin stated that the policy of his department for a long time had been that of primary repair of the complete atrioventricular canal at whatever age operation was required and elective repair in all patients by age 2. Results in a small series of infants have been quite good since 1974, in striking contrast to experiences before that time.

Ventricular Septal Defect

HISTORICAL DATA. A description by Roger in 1879 of two patients with ventricular septal defect led to the eponymic designation *Roger's disease* and emphasized the asymptomatic nature of the disease when the ventricular septal defect is small. Further contributions to clinical characterization of the syndrome were made by Abbott in 1932, by Taussig in 1947, and later by Selzer and by Wood. Surgical closure became possible with the development of the pump-oxygenator in 1955. In recent years the frequency of spontaneous closure of ventricular septal defects has been well delineated. It is now clear that spontaneous closure of septal defects, once thought to be a rare phenomenon, may occur in the first few years of life in a significant percentage of patients, so patients with few symptoms and without pulmonary hypertension may be safely observed for 3 to 4 years for signs of spontaneous closure.

INCIDENCE AND ETIOLOGY. There are no known significant etiologic factors, although ventricular septal defect is a common form of congenital heart disease, constituting 20 to 30 percent of all cases in various cardiac clinics.

PATHOLOGIC ANATOMY. Five types of ventricular septal defect have been recognized, depending upon the location in the ventricular septum: membranous septum defect; defect anterior to the crista supraventricularis near the pulmonic valve; posterior ventricular septum defect; low muscular defect; and left ventricular–right atrial defect. Defects in the membranous septum are by far the most frequent (85 to 90 percent of patients), the other types being seen only infrequently.

Defects in the membranous septum (Fig. 18-32, type B) are located posterior to the crista supraventricularis. With small defects a rim exists superiorly, while large defects are extremely close to the base of the septal leaflet of the tricuspid valve on the right and the mitral valve on the left. The bundle of His, of critical importance to the surgeon, is located at the posterior and superior rim of the defect, where it bifurcates into the right and left conduction bundles. The septal defects are located beneath the right aortic cusp or beneath the junction of the right aortic and septal cusps. Often these cusps are easily visible through the defect and must be protected from injury during surgical repair. The degree of dextroposition of the aorta varies widely. With some defects the aortic valve is not visible at all. At the other extreme are those defects in which the aorta partly arises from the right ventricle. This type is common with tetralogy of Fallot.

Anterior ventricular septal defects (Fig. 18-32, type A) occur anterior to the crista supraventricularis near the pulmonic valve. Surgical closure is simple because the defect is a safe distance from the conduction bundle. Posterior ventricular septal defects (Fig. 18-32, type C) are posterior to the papillary muscle of the conus and beneath the tricuspid valve. Often the rim is partly or completely muscular. Exposure is awkward but can be accomplished with appropriate retraction. Muscular ventricular septal defects (Fig. 18-32, type D) are located inferiorly in the ventricular septum and are often multiple. In the most extreme form, the "Swiss cheese" type of septum, there are multiple tiny serpentine communications which make complete surgical closure difficult or perhaps impossible. Left ventricular–right atrial defects are the rarest of all, consisting of a communication between the left ventricle and the right atrium through the membranous septum superior to the annulus of the tricuspid valve. Such defects are small but are associated with a large shunt because of the great difference in pressure between the left ventricle and right atrium. Once these defects are recognized, closure by direct suture is simple.

The size of ventricular septal defects varies from as small as 0.3 cm to greater than 3 cm. A diameter of 0.8 to 1 cm is a convenient one for separating "small" and "large" septal defects, for those smaller than 1 cm are often associated with a pulmonary blood flow less than twice systemic blood flow and few cardiac abnormalities. "Small" defects are seen in about 25 percent of patients. Defects larger than 1 cm, corresponding to about one-half the diameter of the aortic valve orifice, are regularly associated with more severe physiologic disturbances.

Histologic changes in the pulmonary vasculature are an important part of the pathologic anatomy, for these are related to the evolution of pulmonary hypertension. Young children with pulmonary hypertension have prominent smooth muscle in the media of the pulmonary arterioles, resembling that found in the pulmonary vasculature during fetal life. In subsequent years, with continued pulmonary hypertension, proliferative changes appear in the intima, becoming more prominent in late childhood and early adult life. The intimal proliferative changes apparently represent a permanent increase in pulmonary vascular resistance, with irreversible pulmonary hypertension. Though the pathogenesis of pulmonary hypertension has been studied intensely, the sporadic appearance and erratic course among different patients with similar defects remains a mystery.

Associated anomalies with ventricular defects are common. These include patent ductus arteriosus, coarctation of the aorta, atrial septal defect, mild infundibular stenosis of the right ventricle, and aortic insufficiency from prolapse

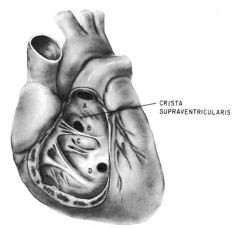

Fig. 18-32. Common types of ventricular septal defect. Most common is type B, with defect lying just proximal to crista supraventricularis. Type A defects are located immediately proximal to pulmonic valve. Type C defects are located beneath septal leaflet of tricuspid valve. Type D defects are in muscular part of ventricular septum and are often multiple. (*Adapted from J. W. Kirklin et al., J Thorac Surg, 33:45, 1957.*)

of an aortic valve cusp into the ventricular septal defect. Recognition of the additional anomalies is an obviously important part of preoperative diagnosis and planning prior to surgical correction.

PATHOPHYSIOLOGY. Since normally the systolic left ventricular pressure is about four times greater than the systolic right ventricular pressure, a ventricular septal defect results in a left-to-right shunt of blood from the left ventricle into the pulmonary circulation, producing a pulmonary blood flow greater than systemic blood flow. The size of the left-to-right shunt varies with both the size of the defect and the pulmonary vascular resistance. With a septal defect less than 1 cm in diameter, the pulmonary blood flow may be only about $1\frac{1}{2}$ times systemic blood flow, and few physiologic changes result. With septal defects greater than 1 cm in diameter and a pulmonary blood flow more than twice systemic flow, a strain on cardiac function becomes obvious. With huge septal defects, pulmonary blood flow may be four to five times greater than systemic flow, producing severe pulmonary congestion and heart failure.

The two major changes from a ventricular septal defect are cardiac failure and pulmonary hypertension. In infancy severe cardiac failure develops if a large defect is present. This may be fatal in some unless surgical therapy, either closure of the defect or banding of the pulmonary artery, is performed. Surgical closure of ventricular septal defects in severely symptomatic infants has been safely accomplished in recent years, using the technique of deep hypothermia and partial or complete circulatory arrest. A considerable experience with this technique has been reported by Barratt-Boyes and also by Kirklin, clearly indicating that in the majority of patients such defects may be safely closed in the first 1 to 2 years of life, rather than banding the pulmonary artery. After the first year of life, chronic pulmonary congestion may persist with large defects, resulting in recurrent pulmonary infections and limitation of growth and development. Death from congestive heart failure is unusual in children after the first year of life. In adults, however, congestive heart failure is frequent.

Pulmonary hypertension from progressive sclerosis of the pulmonary vascular bed is the other major pathologic change. As mentioned earlier, the principal histologic changes are in the pulmonary arterioles, with hypertrophy of the smooth muscle of the media and proliferation of the intima. These evolve slowly during childhood, becoming more prominent in the late teens and early adult life. Rarely, such changes may progress to an "irreversible" degree in the first few years of life. The cause of this great variability is unknown.

As pulmonary vascular resistance increases to approach systemic vascular resistance, definite changes in blood flow result, for right-to-left shunting through the defect appears in association with the predominant left-to-right shunt. This right-to-left shunt produces unsaturation of the peripheral arterial blood. When the pulmonary vascular resistance and the systemic vascular resistance are nearly equal, a *balanced shunt* results. Ultimately, when pulmonary vascular resistance has risen to exceed systemic vascular resistance, the right-to-left shunt is predominant, resulting in cyanosis, clubbing, and polycythemia. This advanced inoperable disease, formerly termed the Eisenmenger syndrome, is now recognized as simply the end stage of progressive pulmonary hypertension from a large left-to-right shunt. It usually results from a ventricular septal defect but can also occur from a neglected patent ductus arteriosus, atrial septal defect, or other malformations. With severe pulmonary hypertension, death usually occurs at about forty years of age from cardiac failure, respiratory infection, or hemoptysis. The natural course of disease in these patients has been well documented by Wood.

An increased susceptibility to bacterial endocarditis has been long recognized with ventricular defects and is the only known physiologic handicap from a small one. The susceptibility results from the jet of blood through the defect striking the right ventricular wall; bacterial fungations form here. The estimated frequency of the disease varies widely, from 15 to 30 percent, but the risk emphasizes the importance of prophylactic chemotherapy.

Patients with mild infundibular stenosis and a ventricular septal defect are in the midportion of the spectrum of malformations extending from ventricular septal defect at one end to tetralogy of Fallot at the other. The clinical picture varies with severity of the infundibular stenosis. As long as the infundibular stenosis is mild, pulmonary blood flow exceeds systemic blood flow, and the patient is acyanotic. However, if infundibular stenosis is more severe, with a systemic blood flow greater than pulmonary blood flow, cyanosis develops. Cases in this intermediate zone are often termed *acyanotic* tetralogies of Fallot.

The ultimate life expectancy of patients with a ventricular septal defect is unknown, but it appears that average life expectancy of patients with a pulmonary blood flow more than twice the systemic blood flow is near forty years of age. Death is from pulmonary hypertension, cardiac failure, or endocarditis.

CLINICAL MANIFESTATIONS. Symptoms. Patients with a small ventricular septal defect (0.3 to 0.8 cm in diameter) are often asymptomatic and enjoy unrestricted physical activity. Those with larger defects are usually symptomatic. Dyspnea on exertion with easy fatigability is most common, often accompanied by frequent pulmonary infections. Severe cardiac failure is usually seen only in infants or in adults, although chronic pulmonary congestion may occur throughout early childhood. Hemoptysis occurs only in older children or adults with severe pulmonary hypertension. In these unfortunate patients it is a frequent cause of death in the third and fourth decades.

Physical Findings. A loud, harsh, pansystolic murmur is typically present along the left sternal border in the third and fourth intercostal spaces. Frequently a thrill is palpable. The pulmonic second sound varies with pulmonary vascular resistance and may even be palpable when pulmonary vascular resistance is markedly elevated. Intensity of the systolic murmur also varies with the pulmonary vascular resistance, diminishing in many patients as the pulmonary vascular resistance increases. In some patients there is a paradoxic variation between signs and symptoms: pronounced physical findings with a loud murmur and thrill in an asymptomatic child, but a murmur of less intensity without a thrill with severe pulmonary hypertension.

Retardation of growth may be obvious, accompanied by rales from chronic pulmonary congestion and hepatic enlargement. Some cardiac enlargement is regularly present. When severe, it may produce a visible deformity of the left costal cartilages. Basal diastolic murmurs are infrequent but can originate from two sources: A murmur of aortic insufficiency can develop from prolapse of an aortic cusp into the underlying ventricular septal defect. Alternately, a murmur resulting from pulmonic insufficiency may appear with far advanced pulmonary hypertension.

LABORATORY FINDINGS. The chest roentgenogram with a small ventricular septal defect is usually normal. With larger defects, enlargement of both ventricles becomes visible, especially as pulmonary vascular resistance increases. When the pulmonary blood flow is significantly increased, there is visible enlargement of the pulmonary artery and its tributaries, pulmonary congestion, and enlargement of the left atrium.

The electrocardiogram varies with both the pulmonary blood flow and the pulmonary vascular resistance. With a small defect it is normal. A large pulmonary blood flow produces left ventricular hypertrophy, while an increase in pulmonary vascular resistance induces right ventricular hypertrophy. Often hypertrophy of both ventricles is evident, and the axis of the electrocardiogram varies with the relative degree of ventricular hypertrophy. Predominant right ventricular hypertrophy and a right axis deviation appear with severe pulmonary hypertension.

Cardiac catheterization confirms the diagnosis and assesses the extent of the left-to-right shunt and the pulmonary vascular resistance. A rise in oxygen saturation of more than 1 vol % between the right atrium and the right ventricle establishes the diagnosis, and calculation of the ratio between the pulmonary blood flow and the systemic blood flow will indicate both the size of the shunt and the pulmonary vascular resistance. At times the catheter may actually traverse the septal defect. Selective angiography, usually by injection of dye directly into the left ventricle from a catheter advanced from the aorta across the aortic valve, can opacify the defect.

DIAGNOSIS. The diagnosis is suggested by the loud systolic murmur along the left sternal border, often with a thrill. Similar physical findings may be present with aortic stenosis in infancy, infundibular pulmonic stenosis, or an ostium primum defect. An atrial septal defect usually has a softer systolic murmur near the base of the heart. Confirmation of the diagnosis requires cardiac catheterization, although the changes in the chest roentgenogram and electrocardiogram are helpful.

TREATMENT. Indications for Operation. Operation should be performed in the first 1 to 2 years of life for infants with either severe congestive failure or an increase in pulmonary vascular resistance. There are good data to indicate that an increase in pulmonary vascular resistance will regress if surgical correction is performed before 2 years of age, but there may be irreversible injury to the pulmonary vascular bed if operation is postponed beyond 2 years.

If symptoms are not disabling and pulmonary vascular resistance is not increased, the preferred time for operation is between 4 and 6 years of age. Often a period of observation is indicated to determine whether the defect will close spontaneously. Once observation has demonstrated that the defect is a persistent one, operation is usually done if the pulmonary blood flow is more than one and one-half to two times greater than normal. With smaller defects, operation is usually not recommended unless there is a demonstrated susceptibility to endocarditis, the only known hazard of a small ventricular septal defect.

In the unfortunate patients with marked elevation of pulmonary vascular resistance, the hazard of operation is increased and the benefit decreased. Criteria of inoperability vary among different institutions, but generally patients with a pulmonary vascular resistance greater than one-half the systemic resistance have a high operative mortality and little benefit from operation. With the increasing awareness of the problem and the ready availability of excellent diagnostic facilities, such unfortunate children are becoming increasingly rare, as most cases are detected and the patients successfully operated on within the first few years of life.

Technique of Operation. The operation is performed through a median sternotomy with extracorporeal circulation. If a patent ductus arteriosus, a commonly associated defect in infants, has been found by preoperative catheterization and angiography, this must be closed at the start of bypass before the ventricle is opened.

In selecting the site of ventriculotomy, the most important consideration is to avoid division of any underlying significant coronary arteries, for anomalous coronary arteries are frequent. The most common anomaly is the origin of the left anterior descending from the right coronary artery, division of which is often fatal. With these considerations, a transverse, longitudinal, or oblique ventriculotomy can be made. If the coronary anatomy is satis-

factory, the author prefers a short transverse incision. If a longitudinal ventriculotomy is performed, it should be in the infundibular part of the right ventricle and near the anterior descending coronary.

An alternate approach is closure of the ventricular septal defect through the right atrium. This is strongly indicated when pulmonary vascular resistance is significantly increased, to avoid any transitory injury to the right ventricle. In some institutions this technique is almost routinely employed, although it is more awkward than operation through a ventriculotomy.

A left ventricular vent is routinely used to aspirate blood from the operative field and facilitate removal of intracardiac air. A variety of surgical techniques have been employed successfully. The author's preference is for intermittent cardiac ischemia, intermittently occluding the aorta 10 to 15 minutes at a temperature of 30°C. This has the advantage of having the heart intermittently contract, with monitoring of the electrocardiogram to protect against heart block. Excellent results have been obtained by several groups with techniques of hypothermia and prolonged cardiac arrest, carefully placing the sutures to the right of the ventricular septum posteriorly to avoid heart block. In the author's personal experience there have been no complete heart blocks in the past decade.

Once the septal defect, usually located in the membranous septum posterior to the crista supraventricularis, has been identified, an oval patch of knitted Dacron is inserted with mattress sutures posteriorly and a continuous suture anteriorly, preferably polypropylene (Prolene) (Fig. 18-33).

Posteriorly, the sutures are inserted through the base of the septal leaflet of the tricuspid valve to the right of the posterior margin of the defect, avoiding the posterior superior angle where the conduction bundle is located. A useful surgical guide for avoiding the conduction bundle, described by Barratt-Boyes, is to identify the fibrous trigone located at the bottom of the noncoronary aortic sinus, inspecting this area through the ventricular septal defect with a dry, still operative field. The conduction bundle passes through this fibrous trigone and then along the area where the membranous ventricular septum joins the muscular septum posteriorly. Projecting an imaginary line between the fibrous trigone and the papillary muscle of the conus and subsequently inserting sutures to the right of this imaginary line avoids injury to the conduction bundle. This can be confirmed by observing the electrocardiogram after the posterior sutures are inserted but before the prosthetic patch is tied in position. The anterior portion of the closure can be simply done with a continuous suture. After the patch is inserted, adequacy of closure, as well as the presence of additional defects, can be checked by temporarily occluding the aorta, aspirating air through the left ventricular vent, and then forcefully injecting saline solution retrograde through the left ventricular vent into the left ventricle to distend the ventricular septum. This technique, used for several years, has been a valuable adjunct and has identified additional defects in several patients.

Subsequently, after closing the ventriculotomy and stopping the bypass, adequacy of closure can be confirmed by

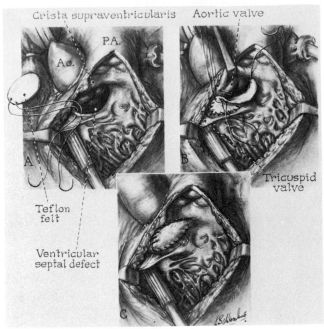

Fig. 18-33. *A.* Ventricular septal defect exposed through longitudinal ventriculotomy. Cusps of aortic valve are clearly visible through large defect. Closure is carried out with prosthetic patch of Teflon felt. First sutures are inserted in posterosuperior margin where conduction bundle is located. Often sutures are placed to right of margin of defect, through base of septal leaflet of tricuspid valve. Heart is beating while sutures are inserted, in order to observe conduction disturbances on electrocardiogram. *B.* Subsequent sutures around margins of defect may be interrupted or continuous sutures. In aortic valve area, care is taken to insert sutures directly into aortic annulus, avoiding injury to valve cusps. *C.* Final position of prosthetic patch.

demonstrating a similar oxygen content of blood samples withdrawn simultaneously from the right atrium and the pulmonary artery.

The combination of ventricular septal defect with aortic insufficiency from prolapse of an aortic valve cusp is fortunately rare. The lesion is often a progressive one due to continued herniation of an aortic valve cusp, usually the right coronary cusp, into the underlying ventricular septal defect. Surgical correction can usually be done without insertion of a prosthetic aortic valve, even though some aortic insufficiency remains. A detailed report of the experience of the author, Bahnson, and Weldon with this condition was published in 1973 (Fig. 18-34). In the subsequent years, continued experience has been satisfactory.

Postoperative Course. A temporary pacemaker wire is routinely left in the ventricle before the thoracotomy incision is closed. If bradycardia appears, with a rate lower than 70 to 80 per minute, pacing is done for 1 to 2 days, as necessary. Transitory conduction disturbances often subside within 24 to 48 hours. A report years ago by Lillehei et al. indicated the grim prognosis with complete heart block. If a complete heart block persists for as long as 3 weeks after operation, a permanent pacemaker should be inserted before the patient is discharged from the hospital,

for the risk of sudden death is great even though the patient is asymptomatic.

Digitalis is usually given after operation, as some degree of right ventricular failure is common, especially if significant pulmonary hypertension was present. In most patients convalescence is uneventful.

The risk of operation increases if pulmonary vascular resistance is increased, but with earlier diagnosis and treatment such complicated problems are fortunately becoming rare. With normal pulmonary vascular resistance, postoperative mortalities as low as 1 to 2 percent have been reported. Similar results have been obtained at New York University. However, when the pulmonary vascular resistance is significantly elevated, the risk of operation rises, approaching 15 to 30 percent if pulmonary vascular resistance is as much as one-half systemic resistance.

Following recovery from operation, patients without an increase in pulmonary vascular resistance have a dramatic regression of all signs of cardiac disease. Heart size and the vascularity of the lung fields both return to normal. A right bundle branch block usually persists on the electrocardiogram as a consequence of insertion of sutures to the right of the margin of the septal defect. Life expectancy is probably that of a normal person. In patients with increased pulmonary vascular resistance, there may be regression in some. In general, the pulmonary vascular resistance decreases in about one-third of the patients, remains stationary in about one-third, and actually increases in the remainder, probably representing an inherent disease in the pulmonary vasculature separate from that due to the previous left-to-right shunt.

Patent Ductus Arteriosus

HISTORICAL DATA. Gibson, in Edinburgh, first reported in 1900 the classic clinical findings of a patent ductus arteriosus, but it was not until 1937 that Strieder first attempted ligation of the ductus in a patient with bacterial endocarditis. This patient died on the fourth postoperative day, but the following year Gross successfully ligated the patent ductus of a seven-year-old girl.

INCIDENCE AND ETIOLOGY. Patent ductus arteriosus is one of the most common forms of congenital heart disease, occurring once in about every 4,000 births and constituting about 15 percent of all cases of congenital heart disease. For unknown reasons it is two to three times more frequent in females than in males.

The patent ductus arteriosus, which develops as an embryologic remnant of the sixth left aortic arch, is an important normal fetal pathway connecting the pulmonary artery at its bifurcation to the aorta just beyond the origin of the left subclavian artery. Through this channel in embryonic life blood bypasses the collapsed lungs, flowing directly from the pulmonary artery into the aorta. With the expansion of the lungs at birth, the ductus normally closes within a few days, becoming fibrotic ligamentum arteriosum. The physiologic stimuli responsible for closure of the ductus have been studied in detail. Apparently changes in oxygen tension of the arterial blood exert a

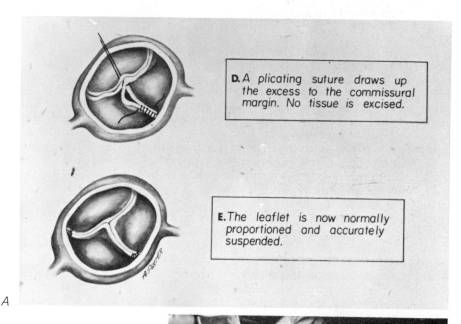

D. A plicating suture draws up the excess to the commissural margin. No tissue is excised.

E. The leaflet is now normally proportioned and accurately suspended.

A

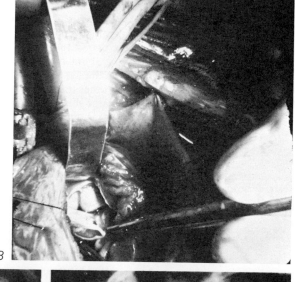

B

Fig. 18-34. *A.* Diagram of concept of one method of repair of the prolapsed valve cusp, developed by Weldon at Washington University in St. Louis. *B.* Operative view of the prolapsed aortic cusp through a right ventriculotomy, showing the cusp prolapsing into the ventricular septal defect. Partial occlusion of the ventricular septal defect by the prolapsing cusp is one reason that the left-to-right shunt is not large. *C.* Pre- and postoperative aortograms showing massive aortic insufficiency before operation and no insufficiency whatever several months later.

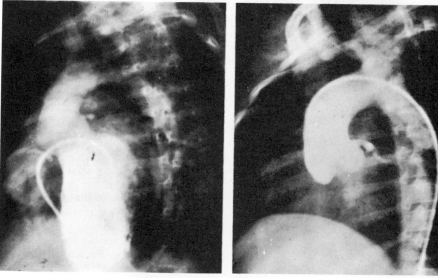

C

profound stimulus on the closure. The most important cause of closure, however, is probably related to the distinctive histologic structure of the wall of the ductus, which is different from that of either the pulmonary artery or the aorta. As the ductus closes, the wall of the ductus contracts, the internal elastic membrane fragments, and smooth muscle projects into the lumen as progressive fibrosis obliterates the patent channel.

If rubella occurs during the first trimester of pregnancy, a well-recognized syndrome of congenital defects can occur, including mental retardation, cataracts, and a patent ductus. For the majority of patients, however, the cause of persistent patency is unknown.

PATHOLOGIC ANATOMY. The diameter of a ductus ranges from as small as 2 to 3 mm to greater than 1 cm. Usually it is 5 to 7 mm. The length is usually slightly greater than the width, although in some cases the ductus is unusually short, creating some technical hazard at the time of surgical correction (Fig. 18-35).

Associated anomalies occur in approximately 15 percent of cases; the most common are ventricular septal defect and coarctation of the aorta.

PATHOPHYSIOLOGY. Depending upon the diameter of the ductus, a varying amount of blood is shunted from the aorta to the pulmonary artery, constituting a left-to-right shunt. In a large ductus, the shunt may constitute 50 to 70 percent of the output from the left ventricle, with resulting decrease of blood flow to other tissues and retardation of development. With such large shunts, the pulmonary blood flow may reach levels as high as 10 to 15

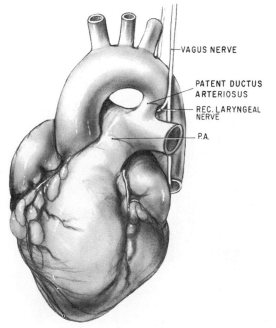

Fig. 18-35. Patent ductus arteriosus as regularly found just distal to left subclavian artery between aorta and pulmonary artery. It is encircled by recurrent laryngeal nerve, a useful surgical landmark in isolating patent ductus in mediastinal tissues. (*Adapted from R. E. Gross, "The Surgery of Infancy and Childhood," W. B. Saunders Company, Philadelphia, 1953, p. 807.*)

VAGUS NERVE
PATENT DUCTUS ARTERIOSUS
REC. LARYNGEAL NERVE
P.A.

liters/minute. The symptomatology is directly proportional to the size of the shunt.

A large patent ductus in infants may result in serious or even lethal heart failure. However, after the age of two years heart failure is rare until adult life, although symptoms of limited cardiac reserve may occur.

In infancy the high pulmonary vascular resistance of fetal life subsides gradually in the first 1 to 2 years after birth. During this time only a systolic murmur may be audible. In some infants the increased pulmonary blood flow from the ductus causes the pulmonary vascular resistance to remain elevated and even increase, with resulting pulmonary hypertension. Usually the pulmonary vascular resistance will decrease to normal levels following surgical division of the ductus, but in older patients only a partial regression toward normal levels may occur. With a long-neglected patent ductus pulmonary resistance may, rarely, increase to exceed systemic vascular resistance, resulting in a "reversed" ductus, with blood flowing from the pulmonary artery to the descending thoracic aorta to produce cyanosis in the lower half of the body. Fortunately this is now almost unknown, for diagnosis and treatment are carried out at an early age.

An unusual feature of a patent ductus is susceptibility to development of bacterial endocarditis from viridans streptococci. Although this is most common in the second or third decade, it may occur rarely in children. It has been estimated that in untreated cases such an infection would ultimately develop in 20 to 25 percent of patients. The localization of the infection apparently is related to turbulent blood flow where blood forcefully ejected from the aorta through the ductus strikes the wall of the pulmonary artery. The fungations of bacterial endocarditis usually begin in this location, with septicemia initially limited to the lungs until systemic spread occurs. Fortunately such infections can usually be promptly controlled with antibiotic therapy.

With the dual tendency to develop either heart failure or bacterial endocarditis, it has been estimated that the life expectancy of a seventeen-year-old patient with a patent ductus is approximately one-half that of a normal individual.

CLINICAL MANIFESTATIONS. Symptoms. In infants a large patent ductus may cause serious heart failure, but many older children are asymptomatic. When symptoms are present, the most common are palpitations, fatigue, and dyspnea. More definite symptoms of congestive heart failure are usually seen only in adult patients. In the female these often appear during the first pregnancy. The author has successfully operated on one patient over sixty years of age who first developed signs of congestive failure after age sixty. Fortunately, though advanced cardiac failure was present, full recovery ensued after closure of the ductus.

Physical Examination. The hallmark of a patent ductus is the continuous murmur. This murmur is one of the most distinctive signs in clinical medicine, and usually a patent ductus can be diagnosed with confidence simply on this basis. Because of the continuous quality of the murmur it is often described as a "machinery" murmur. It is a harsh, rasping sound, accentuated in systole and diminishing in diastole. It is best heard in the second left intercostal space but is normally widely transmitted over the chest and into the neck. In many patients the murmur is so loud that it is associated with a palpable thrill. Often in infants either no murmur or only a systolic murmur can be heard until the age of one or two years, after which a continuous murmur may be detected for the first time. The absence of the diastolic component of the murmur during infancy is due to persistent elevation of the pulmonary vascular resistance, which limits flow of blood through the ductus during diastole.

A wide pulse pressure is usually found with a large ductus, resulting from a decrease in diastolic pressure. In the extremely large ductus the diastolic pressure may approach very low levels and be associated with peripheral vascular findings similar to those of severe aortic insufficiency.

Cyanosis is never present with an uncomplicated patent ductus. The presence of cyanosis indicates either an associated cardiac anomaly, such as tetralogy of Fallot, or a marked increase in pulmonary vascular resistance, either from progressive sclerosis of the pulmonary arteriolar bed or from congestive heart failure. The severity of the arterial hypoxia which can result from heart failure in infants often has not been recognized. Arterial oxygen saturations as low as 75% may occur with the severe pulmonary congestion of heart failure.

LABORATORY FINDINGS. With a small patent ductus the chest roentgenogram may be normal. With a larger ductus the pulmonary conus is prominent, the left ventricle is enlarged, and the pulmonary vascular markings are increased, all indicating a large left-to-right shunt. On fluoroscopy a "hilar dance" may be observed. The electrocardiogram is often normal with a small ductus but will show left ventricular hypertrophy with a larger one. Cardiac catheterization can readily localize the left-to-right shunt to the pulmonary artery and differentiate the condition from a ventricular septal defect or an atrial septal defect. Often with appropriate manipulation the cardiac catheter can be passed through the patent ductus, visually confirming the diagnosis. Aortography is the most definitive diagnostic measure, visually demonstrating the flow of dye from the aorta through the ductus into the pulmonary arteries (Fig. 18-36). It is of particular value with severe pulmonary hypertension, when only a systolic murmur may be audible.

DIAGNOSIS. In most patients the diagnosis can be made with confidence from the clinical findings combined with the chest roentgenogram and the electrocardiogram. Cardiac catheterization with aortography should then be done both for confirmation and for detection of additional anomalies.

There are several rare conditions which may produce a continuous murmur simulating a patent ductus arteriosus and requiring cardiac catheterization and angiography for differentiation from a patent ductus. These include an aortic-pulmonary window, a ventricular septal defect with a prolapsed cusp causing aortic insufficiency, a ruptured aneurysm of the sinus of Valsalva, and a coronary arterio-

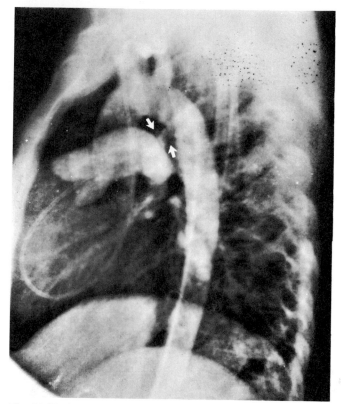

Fig. 18-36. Aortogram performed by injection of dye into aorta demonstrates patent ductus arteriosus, as indicated by arrows, with opacification of pulmonary artery. (*Courtesy of Dr. Raymond M. Abrams, Department of Radiology, New York University Medical Center.*)

venous fistula. Most of these conditions create a physiologic left-to-right shunt and hence a continuous murmur simulating a patent ductus.

TREATMENT. In most patients over two to three years of age, a patent ductus should be surgically corrected as soon as convenient after the diagnosis has been made. The operative risk is low and the results are excellent. In infants, operation should be performed if serious heart failure is present.

The only contraindication to operation, rarely seen, is cyanosis. Cyanosis may be due to an associated cardiac anomaly such as tetralogy of Fallot, in which case the patent ductus is an important ancillary source of blood flow to the lungs. Cyanosis can also develop with a reversed ductus when pulmonary vascular resistance has increased to exceed systemic vascular resistance, as a result of which blood flows from the pulmonary artery to the aorta and creates cyanosis in the lower half of the body. A reversed ductus cannot be safely closed, for the patent ductus partly decreases the pulmonary hypertension, shunting blood from the pulmonary artery to the aorta. Attempted surgical closure usually results in immediate death. Fortunately, with early operations for patent ductus, such advanced pulmonary vascular disease is almost unknown. The author has not seen such a patient in the past 15 years.

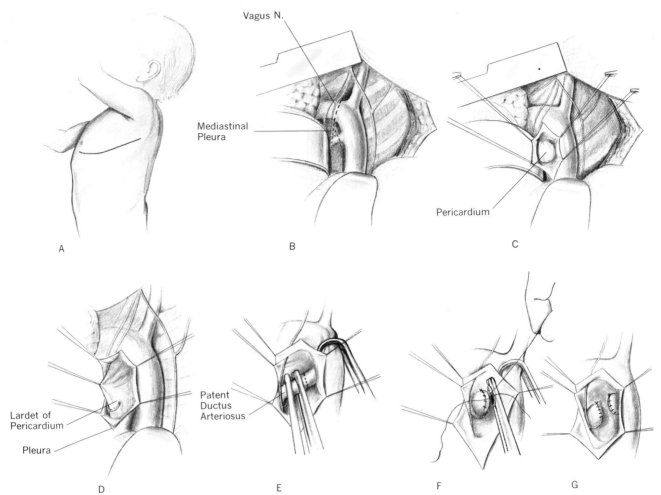

Fig. 18-37. Division of patent ductus arteriosus. *A.* Chest is opened with left posterolateral incision in fourth intercostal space. *B.* Once lung has been retracted, mediastinal pleura is incised longitudinally parallel to vagus nerve. *C.* Initial dissection is along vagus nerve to expose widely the recurrent laryngeal nerve originating from vagus and passing beneath ductus. Wide exposure of recurrent laryngeal nerve is essential part of operative procedure. *D.* After dissection of recurrent laryngeal nerve, lappet of pericardium overlying ductus is freed by sharp dissection proximally to expose pulmonary artery. *E.* Subsequently ductus is encircled, and vascular occlusion clamps are applied. *F.* Ductus is gradually divided and sutured, employing two rows of sutures. *G.* Final view of divided ends of ductus with recurrent laryngeal nerve well exposed.

With bacterial endocarditis, intensive antibiotic therapy will effect cure in most patients; operation can then be more safely performed several weeks later. If the endocarditis cannot be controlled with antibiotic therapy, operation should be undertaken as a last resort, although operations upon a friable, infected ductus have a high mortality rate from hemorrhage or subsequent infection.

Operative Technique. The operation is preferably done through a posterolateral thoracotomy in the fourth intercostal space, although a left anteriolateral thoracotomy in the third intercostal space has been satisfactorily used in previous years. The author's preferred operative technique is shown in detail in Fig. 18-37.

Patients in the third and fourth decade with pulmonary hypertension and sclerosis or calcification of the ductus constitute a difficult and dangerous technical problem because of friability of the ductus, especially at its junction with the pulmonary artery. Lacerations in this artery may quickly result in fatal hemorrhage. A temporary aortic shunt, either a left atrial–femoral artery bypass or the Gott aortic shunt, can be employed to permit temporary occlusion of the aorta above and below the ductus, which can be safely occluded with a single clamp placed near its junction with the aorta. The ductus can then be divided at its point of origin from the aorta, or alternately, the aorta can be incised and the orifice of the ductus obliterated with a patch applied from within the aorta.

Ligation of a patent ductus with multiple ligatures, well developed by Blalock, is now rarely used but is an effective technique in most patients. The original technique included four separate ligatures, with two purse-string sutures at the aortic and pulmonary artery ends of the ductus, followed by two transfixion ligatures on the remaining portions of the ductus.

In 1971 the author treated a sixty-five-year-old patient with congestive failure and extensive calcification of both the aorta and a large patent ductus. Even simple application of vascular clamps to the calcified vessels seemed unusually hazardous. Accordingly, the ductus was effectively obliterated with multiple mattress sutures placed through Teflon felt surrounding the ductus. The patient has subsequently remained well.

As illustrated in Fig. 18-37, a valuable technical point for safe division of any patent ductus is the application of a vascular clamp tangentially onto the aorta a few millimeters from the ductus, rather than on the ductus itself. This method of application of the clamp avoids the problem of a short ductus.

Postoperative Course. With an uncomplicated ductus, the operative risk is surprisingly small. As early as 1953 Gross reported experience with 611 patients, with a mortality rate of less than 0.5 percent in those with neither cardiac failure nor infection before operation. Similar figures were described by Jones in a total series of 909 patients. When patent ductus is associated with other abnormalities, a condition encountered in infants with cardiac failure, operative mortality is higher. At New York University there has been no mortality or serious complications following division of an uncomplicated patent ductus in several years.

Convalescence following operation is usually uneventful, most patients leaving the hospital within 7 to 10 days. A functional systolic murmur may remain audible in a few patients. This may be related to a localized irregularity in the wall of the pulmonary artery where the ductus was present. The electrocardiogram usually returns to normal within a few months. From data now available from over 30 years' experience, it appears that cardiac function becomes normal once the ductus has been surgically obliterated.

RIGHT-TO-LEFT SHUNTS (CYANOTIC GROUP)

Tetralogy of Fallot

HISTORICAL DATA. Tetralogy of Fallot was described as long ago as 1671 by Stensen, but it was not until 1888 that the combination of abnormalities regularly present was emphasized by Fallot. Effective therapy first became possible in 1944, when Blalock dramatically demonstrated that much benefit could be obtained by anastomosis of the subclavian artery and pulmonary artery to create an artificial ductus arteriosus. This operation was developed following the suggestion of Taussig, who had noted an increase in symptoms in infants when a patent ductus arteriosus spontaneously closed. Thereafter the operation was referred to as the *Blalock-Taussig procedure.* It constitutes one of the milestones in cardiac surgery. Subsequently over 1,500 such procedures were performed at the Johns Hopkins Hospital, and experience with these operations led to the development of many other aspects of cardiac surgery. Subsequent contributions were made by Potts et al., who developed an aortic-pulmonary side-to-side anastomosis, especially applicable to infants, and by Brock, who introduced partial excision of the infundibular obstruction. With the development of extracorporeal circulation, correction of the tetralogy first became possible in 1954–1955 and is now the preferred operation.

INCIDENCE AND ETIOLOGY. Tetralogy of Fallot is one of the most common cyanotic malformations, constituting over 50 percent of all cases of cyanotic heart disease. In cyanotic children who survive beyond the first 2 years of life, a tetralogy of Fallot is present in 70 to 75 percent. There are no known etiologic factors.

PATHOLOGIC ANATOMY. The four features of the tetralogy from which the name originates are obstruction of the outflow tract of the right ventricle, a ventricular septal defect, dextroposition of the aorta, and hypertrophy of the right ventricle. The right ventricular obstruction is severe enough to increase right ventricular systolic pressure to equal left ventricular systolic pressure. The ventricular septal defect is large (2 to 3 cm), approximately equaling the diameter of the orifice of the aortic valve. Right ventricular hypertrophy is the natural consequence of the severe obstruction to emptying of the right ventricle; dextroposition of the aorta is an anatomic variant of probably little physiologic significance.

The right ventricular obstruction may be an infundibular stenosis, a valvular stenosis, or a combined lesion (Fig. 18-38). Often it is a localized obstruction, although less frequently a diffuse stenosis of the entire right ventricular outflow tract is present. In one series of patients, Brock found a localized infundibular stenosis in slightly less than 50 percent of patients, a valvular stenosis in 35 percent, and a combined lesion in 22 percent. The pulmonary artery is often smaller than normal, while the diameter of the aorta is larger than normal. When a localized infundibular stenosis is present, an "infundibular chamber" exists between the right ventricle proximal to the stenosis and the pulmonary valve distad.

The ventricular septal defect is almost always located proximal to the crista supraventricularis and is usually 2 to 3 cm in diameter. The aortic cusps are readily seen through the defect, varying with the degree of dextroposition which is present.

With the decrease in pulmonary blood flow, there is striking enlargement of the bronchial arteries and other routes of collateral circulation to the lungs, creating extensive varicosities throughout the mediastinum and chest wall. In some older children with severe cyanosis, a progressive occlusive disease also develops in the peripheral pulmonary arteries. Absence of the left pulmonary artery has been found in a small number of patients, and in others one or more focal stenoses may be found in either one or both the pulmonary arteries.

Anomalous coronary arteries are also frequent, especially in the outflow tract of the right ventricle, where they are of particular surgical significance. A right aortic arch, for unknown reasons, occurs in about 25 percent of patients. An atrial septal defect is also frequent, at times referred to as part of a pentalogy of Fallot, although the malformation differs little physiologically from the tetralogy. It is noteworthy that although a patent ductus arteriosus may be essential to life, it gradually closes in almost all patients during the first few months of life, often with a disastrous increase in the severity of anoxia.

PATHOPHYSIOLOGY. Physiologically, a tetralogy of Fallot is a combination of a large ventricular septal defect

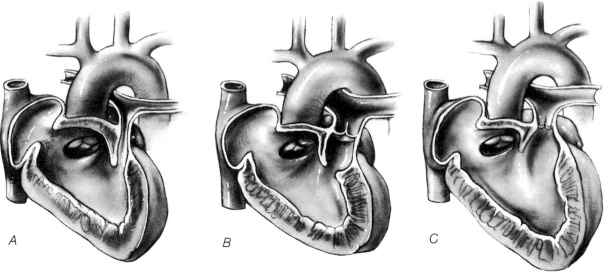

A   *B*   *C*

with an obstruction in the right ventricular outflow tract of sufficient severity to elevate right ventricular systolic pressure to equal left ventricular systolic pressure. Venous blood entering the right ventricle then is shunted directly into the aorta to produce cyanosis. In addition to cyanosis, the malformation decreases pulmonary blood flow and hence limits the ability of the lungs to absorb oxygen. The inability to increase pulmonary blood flow constitutes the basis for the severe intolerance of exercise. The large ventricular septal defect has a separate influence, in that right ventricular pressure almost never exceeds left ventricular pressure, in contrast to isolated pulmonic valvular stenosis. Hence cardiac enlargement and cardiac failure are rare. Only a few unusual patients have been reported in whom the malformation was such that right ventricular pressure exceeded left ventricular pressure.

The severity of the anoxia varies with the degree of reduction in pulmonary blood flow. Arterial oxygen saturations of 70 to 85% are seen in older children, but in younger children, who may not survive through infancy without operation, astonishingly low arterial oxygen saturations are encountered. Saturations of 30 to 35% may be seen in patients who can walk only a short distance, and levels of 20 to 25% are found in some infants who are unable to walk. Saturations as low as 10% have been recorded, usually associated with loss of consciousness from cerebral anoxia. With exercise, there is often a precipitous fall in arterial oxygen saturation, decreasing from a resting level of 70% to 20 to 25%, which clearly indicates the physiologic basis for exertional dyspnea.

Chronic anoxia produces compensatory polycythemia and, subsequently, clubbing of the extremities. Polycythemia is seldom apparent until after two years of age, but later hematocrit readings varying from 60 to 75 percent are common. Wide variations in hematocrit readings are found, ranging from normal with mild tetralogies to readings as high as 85 to 90 percent in the most severe forms.

The degree of cyanosis increases significantly in the first few years of life, for visible cyanosis is proportional to the number of grams of unsaturated hemoglobin in the pe-

Fig. 18-38. Different types of right ventricular obstruction in tetralogy of Fallot. *A.* Combined obstruction from hypoplasia of pulmonic annulus in association with diffuse stenosis of outflow tract of right ventricle. This type of diffuse stenosis is commonly found and often requires insertion of prosthetic patch to widen annulus. *B.* Localized stenosis of infundibulum of right ventricle, with "infundibular chamber" distal to this which is proximal to normal pulmonic valve. *C.* Pulmonic stenosis of valvular type in association with normal right ventricular outflow tract. (*Adapted from C. D. Benson et al., "Pediatric Surgery," vol I, Year Book Medical Publishers, Inc., Chicago, 1962, p. 463.*)

ripheral circulation and not to the actual oxygen concentration. Hence severe cyanosis is visible only after polycythemia has developed. The time of appearance has been used by Nadas for a convenient grouping of the clinical course of the disease. About one-third of patients are cyanotic at birth, another one-third become cyanotic in the first year of life, and one-third develop cyanosis only subsequently in childhood. Patients who are cyanotic at birth have severe anoxia and often do not survive infancy unless operation is performed. Patients who become cyanotic in the first year of life have a milder course but are seriously disabled, while those who develop cyanosis in later years may have little incapacity and little polycythemia—a so-called "pink" tetralogy. These patients, of course, have only moderate reduction in pulmonary blood flow.

The main threat to life in the first years of life is a cerebral vascular accident, either from cerebral thrombosis or from a localized infarct from anoxia. In severe cases, cyanotic "spells" are seen in which the infant becomes deeply cyanotic and comatose. Spontaneous recovery usually occurs, but death or hemiplegia may ensue.

Brain abscess is another serious, often lethal, complication to which patients are peculiarly susceptible. The right-to-left shunt, bypassing the lungs and providing direct access for bacteria into the venous blood to the arterial circulation, is the most convenient explanation of the high incidence of brain abscess, although localized cerebral infarcts may also play a role in etiology.

Cardiac failure is extremely rare with tetralogy, and

its presence always brings into question the accuracy of the diagnosis. It is seen in a few adults in the second or third decade but is virtually unknown in children. There is also a susceptibility to bacterial endocarditis, as with other cardiac malformations.

Life expectancy without treatment is relatively short. Infants cyanotic at birth formerly seldom lived beyond the first decade. Those becoming cyanotic in the first year of life might survive to early adult life, while those becoming cyanotic in later years would occasionally survive into the third or fourth decade or, rarely, beyond. In older, chronically cyanotic patients, other physiologic signs of chronic anoxia appear, with disturbances in the blood-clotting mechanism and secondary hemorrhage in the gastrointestinal tract.

CLINICAL MANIFESTATIONS. Symptoms. Almost all patients are symptomatic. Dyspnea and cyanosis, markedly aggravated by exertion, are the outstanding features. Two additional characteristics are cyanotic spells and squatting. Cyanotic spells are episodes of sudden increase in intensity of cyanosis, followed by unconsciousness, usually with spontaneous recovery within a few minutes or hours. Such episodes, representing acute cerebral anoxia, may be fatal or may result in hemiplegia. They are frequent in infants but seldom occur in older children, probably because symptomatic infants seldom survive without treatment. Squatting is an impressive characteristic, for children learn quickly to relieve dyspnea by assuming a squatting position. The physiologic benefit from squatting, apparently a redistribution of blood flow, is not clear. Walking for short distances, interrupted by squatting, is a well-recognized hallmark of the tetralogy. Hemoptysis is a rare symptom, occurring usually in older children with marked varicosities of the bronchial circulation.

Physical Examination. On physical examination the obvious features are cyanosis of varying severity and clubbing of the digits. The heart usually has a normal size, rate, and rhythm. A systolic murmur of grade II to III intensity is commonly present along the left sternal border at the third or fourth intercostal spaces, and a thrill is present in about one-half the patients. With severe pulmonic stenosis or pulmonary atresia, the murmur may be faint or even absent because of absence of flow through the pulmonic orifice. The second pulmonic sound is weak or absent, while the aortic second sound is increased above normal intensity.

LABORATORY FINDINGS. The chest roentgenogram shows a heart of normal size with an unusual contour, termed the *coeur en sabot,* or sabot-shaped heart (Fig. 18-1). This indicates the characteristic enlargement due to selective hypertrophy of the right ventricle, combined with a concavity in the area where the pulmonary artery is normally located. The lung fields often show decreased vascularity.

The electrocardiogram is always abnormal, showing right ventricular hypertrophy of varying severity with right axis deviation.

Cardiac catheterization demonstrates several characteristic features. A slight left-to-right shunt may be detected at the ventricular level in mild cases, but often no left-to-right intracardiac shunt is present. A large right-to-left shunt is indicated by arterial unsaturation. The right ventricular systolic pressure is usually identical with the left ventricular systolic pressure, while pulmonary artery pressure is decreased below normal levels, resulting in a large systolic pressure gradient between the right ventricle and pulmonary artery. The pulmonary blood flow is decreased, varying with the severity of the disorder. The degree of decrease in pulmonary blood flow will be found to parallel the severity of the arterial oxygen saturation. The hematocrit is usually between 60 and 75 percent, with a range from 45 to 90 percent.

Selective angiocardiography is of great importance in planning surgical correction, for the location of the right ventricular obstruction, either infundibular, valvular, or diffuse, can be outlined. The presence of associated abnormalities in the pulmonary arteries should be particularly noted. Simultaneous opacification of the aorta and pulmonary arteries when dye is injected into the right ventricle is typical of tetralogy of Fallot (Fig. 18-39).

DIAGNOSIS. The diagnosis can usually be made with certainty from clinical examination combined with roentgenogram and electrocardiogram. The important clinical features are cyanosis with severe exertional dyspnea and squatting. The important physical findings are a heart of normal size with a systolic murmur. Roentgenographic

Fig. 18-39. Cardiac angiogram in patient with tetralogy of Fallot, demonstrating large ventricular septal defect. Dye has been injected through catheter in right ventricle. Dye flows through large ventricular septal defect into left ventricle. Pulmonic stenosis which was present is not visible on this angiogram. (*Courtesy of Dr. Raymond M. Abrams, Department of Radiology, New York University Medical Center.*)

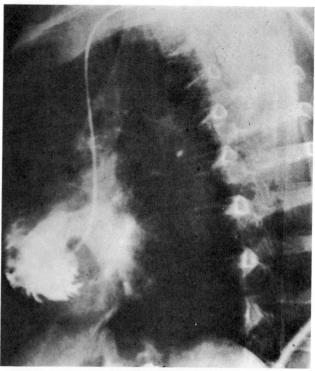

findings demonstrate a heart of normal size with decreased vascularity of the lung fields, while the electrocardiogram shows right ventricular hypertrophy. Cardiac catheterization and angiography should be done routinely to confirm the diagnosis and precisely define the pathologic anatomy.

Other cyanotic conditions to be distinguished from the tetralogy include tricuspid atresia, transposition of the great vessels, and pulmonic valvular stenosis with a patent foramen ovale. Tricuspid atresia can be suspected from the electrocardiogram, which characteristically shows a left axis deviation. Transposition often has cardiac enlargement and vascular lung fields, although cardiac catheterization is required for precise evaluation. Pulmonic valvular stenosis with a patent foramen ovale is suggested by the presence of cardiac enlargement with signs of cardiac failure. The most important feature in differentiating the tetralogy from other cyanotic malformations is the fact that the heart with a tetralogy is of normal size.

TREATMENT. Indications for Operation. Infants with cyanotic spells from anoxia require emergency operation to prevent death or hemiplegia. At present some type of shunt procedure is preferable, although a few groups have explored corrective operations even in the first few months of life. The best type of shunt in these critically ill infants, usually under four months of age, remains uncertain. The side-to-side anastomosis between the ascending aorta and the right pulmonary artery, developed by Waterston, is almost always possible but fraught with serious complications because the margin of safety between an adequate shunt and an excessively large shunt, producing serious or

lethal cardiac failure, is small (Fig. 18-40). Despite a number of variations, almost all groups report a mortality above 20 percent with the Waterston procedure in the first few months of life, so this has been virtually abandoned at New York University.

The Potts operation of aortic–pulmonary side-to-side anastomosis is also rarely used because of both the technical difficulties of construction and subsequent problems of dismantling such a shunt at the time of corrective surgery (Fig. 18-41).

The subclavian–pulmonary anastomosis of Blalock has been used more and more in infants (Fig. 18-42) but is not always technically feasible with small subclavian arteries.

At New York University for the past few years a homograft vein has been successfully used in several patients to establish a shunt between the ascending aorta and the pulmonary artery. This approach has several attractive features and may well become the procedure of choice.

Beyond six months of age, the increasing tendency is for primary corrective operation rather than performance of a shunt. Excellent data have been reported from several centers supporting this approach.

At New York University, the Blalock shunt is still employed in some children between six and twenty-four months of age with complex tetralogies, although the tendency is increasingly in favor of primary correction. Certainly beyond two years of age primary correction is considered the procedure of choice by most groups, although Chiariello in 1975, reviewing a 5-year experience with 403 patients operated on in Houston, Tex., still considered the

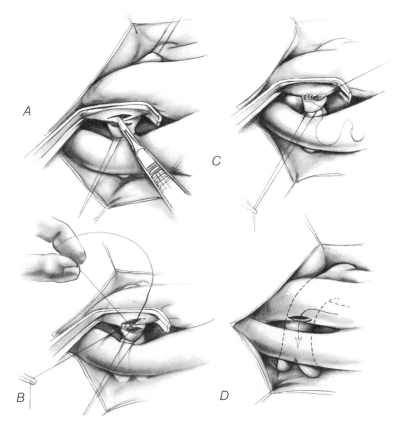

Fig. 18-40. Side-to-side anastomosis between ascending aorta and right pulmonary artery. *A.* Tangential clamp has been applied to ascending aorta, which is then incised for 4 to 5 mm. Corresponding incision is then made in right pulmonary artery, which has been occluded with proximal and distal ligatures. *B.* Posterior row of anastomosis is constructed with continuous suture of 5-0 silk. *C.* Anterior anastomosis may be done with interrupted or continuous sutures. *D.* Diagram of final anastomosis, depicting flow of blood from aorta into pulmonary artery. (*Adapted from D. A. Cooley and G. L. Hallman, "Surgical Treatment of Congenital Heart Disease," Lea & Febiger, Philadelphia, 1966, p. 128.*)

optimal age for elective correction to be between six and ten years.

Technique of Corrective Operation. A median sternotomy incision is preferred. If a previous shunt operation has been performed, the anastomosis is isolated before extracorporeal circulation is begun and subsequently occluded during bypass before the heart is opened. Once the pericardium has been opened, the outflow tract of the right ventricle is carefully examined for anomalous coronary arteries, selecting an incision in the right ventricle to avoid dividing any such arteries. Only rarely is the anatomy of the coronary circulation such that a ventriculotomy cannot be safely performed. In such instances the approach may be through the right atrium. Edmunds reported, in 1976, successful experiences with 15 patients using the transatrial approach.

Five potential zones of obstruction to flow of blood to the lungs should be considered for surgical correction, the location, the severity, and number varying with each patient. These include fusion of the pulmonary valve leaflets; a hypoplastic pulmonic annulus; varying degrees of infundibular stenosis in the right ventricle, either fibrous or muscular; hypoplastic main pulmonary artery; or hypoplastic distal pulmonary arteries. Precise selective angiocardiograms are of great value before operation in identifying these zones of obstruction.

For several years a high transverse ventriculotomy was employed but has been abandoned in favor of a short (4 to 5 cm) high vertical ventriculotomy stopping near the pulmonic annulus and being limited almost to the infundibular portion of the right ventricle. This incision is routinely closed with an appropriate Dacron patch. This approach of a short high vertical ventriculotomy combined with insertion of a prosthetic patch requires a less radical excision of the hypertrophied right ventricular musculature and better preserves ventricular function. Large muscle bundles of the hypertrophied crista supraventricularis are excised, but the infundibulectomy is considerably less radical than working through a transverse ventriculotomy.

If the pulmonic valve ring is of adequate size, the fused commissures of the pulmonic valve may be divided through the ventriculotomy without opening the pulmonary artery. Otherwise a separate incision is made in the pulmonary artery to facilitate appropriate commissurotomies.

A crucial part of the operation is deciding whether the diameter of the pulmonic valve ring is adequate. Sizing of the diameter of the pulmonic ring with graduated Hegar dilators has been used by our group for several years and has been similarly endorsed by several others. Kirklin and associates in 1976 precisely described the relationships between body weight and a pulmonic annulus of adequate size. These measurements are particularly useful for smaller children. In larger children, a pulmonic valve ring that will accommodate a No. 16 Hegar dilator, representing a cross-sectional area of slightly less than 2 cm², is satisfactory.

If the pulmonic annulus is hypoplastic, the ventriculotomy is extended accordingly across the annulus into the pulmonary artery and an appropriate patch applied.

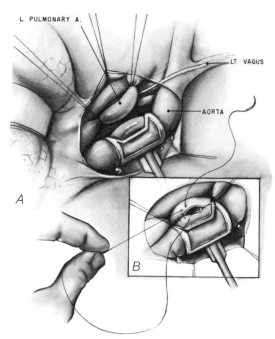

Fig. 18-41. Potts type of aortic-pulmonary anastomosis. *A.* Partial-occlusion clamp has been applied to aorta, and segment of pulmonary artery has been occluded by traction on ligatures. *B.* After approximation of two vessels, side-to-side anastomosis is constructed. Size of anastomosis is critical, an aortic incision 4 mm long being used in infants and one 6 mm in older children. This type of anastomosis is avoided whenever possible because of difficulties in dividing it during subsequent corrective surgery with cardiopulmonary bypass.

Following correction of the infundibular obstruction, the ventricular septal defect is closed in a manner identical to that described previously for ventricular septal defect. Adequacy of closure is confirmed by retrograde injection of saline solution through a left ventricular vent while the aorta is temporarily clamped. With the technique of closure of the septal defect as described, there has been no permanent heart block in any patient in the author's experience in the past decade.

If the diameter of the main pulmonary artery is less than 2 cm, it is also widened to an appropriate degree with a patch which may be extended when necessary beyond the bifurcation of the artery onto the left pulmonary artery.

Our preference for the prosthetic patch is a section of woven tubular Dacron graft, popularized by Kirklin. Pericardium is also a satisfactory material in most patients but has been associated with the subsequent formation of aneurysms in a small number of patients, usually with residual pulmonary hypertension.

Following closure of the ventriculotomy and removal of air from all cardiac chambers, extracorporeal circulation is stopped and intracardiac pressure is measured to confirm that right ventricular obstruction has been corrected. The right ventricular systolic pressure should be reduced to less than 60 to 70 percent of left ventricular systolic pressure. If right ventricular pressure is still elevated above this level, more adequate correction of the ventricular obstruction is

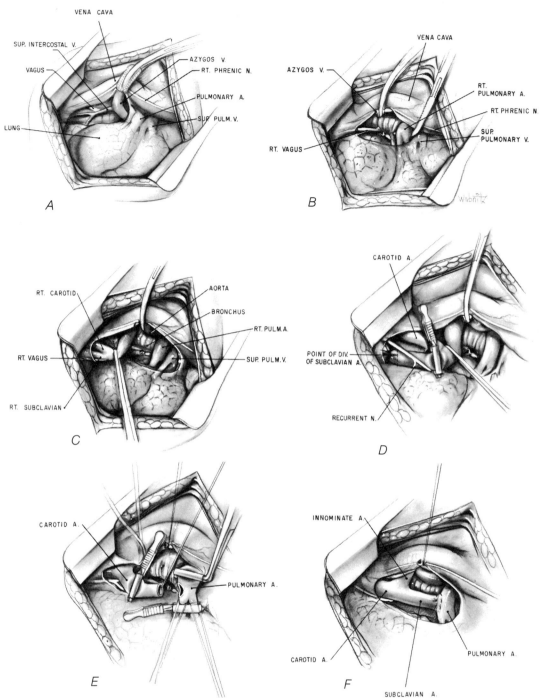

Fig. 18-42. Blalock procedure. *A.* Dissection is begun by isolation of azygos vein, followed by incision of mediastinal pleura in front of pulmonary artery. *B.* Pulmonary artery is isolated in hilum, dissecting artery distally to beyond point of origin of upper lobe branch. Medially, artery is freed well into mediastinum in order to permit displacement of artery superiorly during construction of anastomosis. Traction on stump of divided azygos vein retracts superior vena cava to expose pulmonary artery in mediastinum. *C.* Subclavian artery is mobilized at apex of thorax, mobilizing carotid artery and subclavian artery down into mediastinum. Wide mobilization of carotid artery greatly facilitates subsequent performance of anastomosis. Vagus and recurrent nerves are protected during this dissection. *D.* After mobilization of carotid and subclavian arteries, tributaries of subclavian arteries are ligated, vertebral artery being ligated separately to avoid retrograde flow of blood from vertebral artery distad into arm, producing subclavian "steal" abnormality. *E.* After division of subclavian artery, longitudinal arteriotomy is made in pulmonary artery. Adventitia is carefully cleared from subclavian artery before performance of anastomosis. *F.* Appearance of completed anastomosis. Anterior row of anastomosis is usually made with interrupted sutures of 5-0 silk to permit growth of anastomosis. With wide mobilization of carotid artery superiorly and pulmonary artery inferiorly, satisfactory anastomosis can be accomplished with sublcavian artery as short as 1 to 1.5 cm in length. Vein graft is rarely necessary.

necessary. Otherwise fatal depression of cardiac output from right ventricular failure may occur in the early postoperative course. In most patients following bypass a satisfactory result is obtained, with a systolic pressure near 100 mm, a right ventricular systolic pressure between 35 and 50 mm, and a pulmonary artery systolic pressure of 20 to 25 mm.

Postoperative Course. Following operation, particular attention is required in the first 24 hours to intrathoracic bleeding, because older cyanotic patients have an increased hemorrhagic tendency from the long-standing polycythemia. Transfusion of fresh frozen plasma, often combined with platelet transfusions, is the best therapy. Close observation is necessary to avoid intrathoracic accumulation of blood with cardiac tamponade.

Adequacy of cardiac output is monitored by observing blood pressure, blood-gas concentrations in mixed venous blood, and urine output. Blood is transfused in sufficient amounts to keep central venous pressure near 12 to 15 mm Hg if necessary, possibly at higher levels. If cardiac output is inadequate despite these measures, small amounts of isoproterenol or epinephrine are infused (1 to 2 μg/minute). Acidosis is not a significant problem if cardiac output remains adequate. Assisted ventilation may be required for a few hours but seldom for longer.

Some degree of right ventricular failure is commonly encountered. Hence, digitalis is routinely given, combined with bedrest and restriction of sodium intake.

The risk of operation varies with the age of the patient and the degree of cyanosis, reflecting the severity of the right ventricular obstruction. The risk is only 3 to 5 percent in older children but larger in smaller ones with severe cyanosis. The excellent monograph by Kirklin et al. contains much data regarding experiences with tetralogy of Fallot. Large clinical series showing low operative mortality have also been published by Kirklin et al., Malm et al., Shumway et al., and McGoon et al.

Following recovery from operation, dramatic improvement is obvious. Cyanosis is, of course, absent, and exercise tolerance within a few months approaches that of a normal individual. If cardiac failure is significant following operation, convalescence may be slow for several weeks. Some cardiac enlargement may remain, but long-term studies show that most patients have excellent cardiac function. The tolerance for pulmonic insufficiency which results if the pulmonic annulus is incised and a prosthetic patch inserted is surprisingly good. Ultimate prognosis in such patients is uncertain, though some have now survived for over 20 years with continuing good results. Some groups have inserted homograft valves at the time of operation to avoid pulmonic insufficiency, but there is not sufficient evidence to warrant this as a routine procedure.

COMPLEX MALFORMATIONS

Transposition of the Great Vessels

HISTORICAL DATA. The clinical syndrome of transposition of the great vessels was clearly described by Taussig in 1938. The first surgical procedure to achieve significant benefit, creation of an atrial septal defect, was reported by Blalock and Hanlon. Another palliative surgical procedure, no longer used, was developed by Baffes, who transposed the inferior vena cava and the right pulmonary veins. Senning, in 1957, first completely corrected transposition of the great vessels by repositioning the atrial septum, but mortality was prohibitively high. Further experience with a modification of the technique was reported by Senning in 1975. Mustard, in 1964, developed a method of reconstructing the atrial cavity which has produced the best clinical results to date.

INCIDENCE AND ETIOLOGY. Transposition of the great vessels is one of the most frequent causes of cyanotic heart disease in the newborn, constituting 30 to 40 percent of all cases. It is the most common cause of cardiac failure in the newborn. As many patients die in infancy, it is much less common after the first two years of life.

Transposition of the aorta and pulmonary arteries results from abnormal division of the bulbar trunk in embryologic development, occurring between the fifth and seventh uterine week. Etiologic factors are unknown. It is about four times more frequent in males than in females.

PATHOLOGIC ANATOMY. With transposition of the arteries, the aorta originates from the right ventricle and the pulmonary artery from the left ventricle (Fig. 18-43). As a result of these abnormal locations, venous blood returning through the venae cavae to the right atrium enters the right ventricle and is then propelled directly into the aorta. Oxygenated blood returning from the lungs through the pulmonary veins to the left atrium enters the left ventricle and is then expelled through the pulmonary artery again to the lungs. This dual, parallel circulatory arrangement is obviously incompatible with life without communication between the pulmonary and systemic circulations. Three possible communications exist, a patent ductus arteriosus, an atrial septal defect or foramen ovale, or a ventricular septal defect. One or more of these, of course, must exist for the infant to survive even a few hours after birth. Normally a patent ductus is present for a few weeks after birth in over one-half the patients. A foramen ovale is frequently found, and a ventricular septal defect occurs in 50 to 70 percent of patients, varying with the group of patients studied.

Associated anomalies are common. One of the most frequent of these, pulmonic stenosis, occurs so commonly as to constitute a well-defined variant of the syndrome, because the prognosis is unusually favorable in such patients. A wide variety of other anomalies may occur, including coarctation of the aorta, pulmonary atresia, and dextrocardia.

PATHOPHYSIOLOGY. The two basic physiologic handicaps with transposition are severe anoxia from inability to transport oxygen from the lungs to the tissues of the body and progressive cardiac failure. The severe and rapidly progressive cardiac failure results partly from a high cardiac output and partly from the fact that the coronary arteries are filled with unoxygenated blood with resulting myocardial anoxia. The relative severity of the anoxia and the cardiac failure varies with the nature of the intracardiac

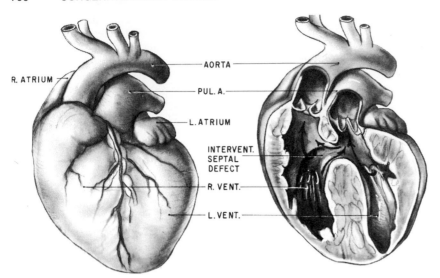

Fig. 18-43. Transposition of great vessels, with aorta arising from right ventricle and pulmonary artery from left ventricle. Ventricular septal defect permits communication between pulmonic and systemic circulations; otherwise condition would be incompatible with life after birth. (*Adapted from H. B. Taussig, "Congenital Malformations of the Heart," 3d ed., Harvard University Press, Cambridge, 1960, p. 149.*)

communications and valvular stenoses. Nadas has found in his group of patients that cardiac failure was present at birth in 80 percent. Because of the severe cardiac failure and anoxia, physical development is severely retarded.

Transposition is a lethal condition, and a high percentage of patients die within the first 1 to 3 months of life. Mustard et al. estimated that 90 percent of their patients died within 7 months. A survey by Hanlon and Blalock in 1948 found only six patients reported in the literature at that time who had lived beyond ten years of age.

Nadas has conveniently grouped patients into four clinical categories related to prognosis. Those with an intact ventricular septum do poorly because of inadequate mixing of the pulmonary and systemic circulations. Similarly, those with a large ventricular septal defect do badly because of excessive pulmonary blood flow. Pulmonary hypertension in this group of patients is also associated with a poor prognosis. The most favorable prognosis is associated with a ventricular septal defect combined with pulmonic stenosis. This combination permits mixing of the pulmonary and systemic circulations through the ventricular septal defect, while the pulmonic stenosis prevents excessive pulmonary blood flow with pulmonary congestion and secondary pulmonary hypertension.

CLINICAL MANIFESTATIONS. Symptoms. A high percentage of infants are cyanotic at birth (80 percent in Nadas' series), and cardiac failure is similarly frequent. Cyanosis appears in most other patients in the first year of life. There is a corresponding severe retardation of growth and development, and anoxic spells of unconsciousness are frequent. Mental development, however, is not impaired. The most prominent symptoms are cyanosis and dyspnea. In children who survive beyond the first two years of life, clubbing and polycythemia appear.

Physical Findings. Cyanosis is frequently obvious on inspection and is often severe. In older children clubbing and polycythemia are similarly evident. Signs of congestive failure are almost always found, with cardiac enlargement, hepatomegaly, and pulmonary congestion. A systolic murmur is usually present but is variable and not diagnostic.

It can result from any of the different intracardiac communications which may be present. Severe retardation of physical development is obvious in older infants.

Absence of a murmur, often indicating absence of an intracardiac communication, indicates a particularly unfavorable prognosis because of inadequate communication between the pulmonary and systemic circulations.

LABORATORY FINDINGS. The chest roentgenogram shows cardiac enlargement, often with a distinctive silhouette, and pulmonary congestion. The contour of the heart has been described as "egg-shaped" and results from the prominent right ventricle projecting into the left side of the chest and the dilated right atrium bulging into the right side. The base of the cardiac shadow, termed the "waist," may be unusually narrow because of the location of the aorta directly in front of the pulmonary artery, rather than the conventional side-to-side relationship seen in the normal cardiac shadow (Fig. 18-2).

The electrocardiogram consistently shows severe right ventricular hypertrophy. Left ventricular hypertrophy varies with the pulmonary blood flow or with the presence of pulmonary valvular stenosis.

Cardiac catheterization reveals several distinctive features. It may not be possible to enter all four cardiac chambers because of the malformations. The systolic pressure in the right ventricle is the same as in the aorta, while that in the left ventricle varies with the size of the ventricular septal defect and the presence of pulmonic stenosis. The oxygen saturation in the pulmonary artery is increased, and a hallmark of the condition is the fact that oxygen saturation in the pulmonary artery is greater than that in the femoral artery. Varying degrees of arterial oxygen unsaturation are regularly found, ranging from as low as 12% to as high as 85%. Angiocardiography provides the best means for confirming the diagnosis, for it classically demonstrates the anterior origin of the aorta from the right ventricle, with the more faintly visualized pulmonary artery lying posterior to the aorta.

DIAGNOSIS. The diagnosis of transposition can be immediately considered in a seriously ill, cyanotic infant with cardiac enlargement and congestive heart failure. In older children the retardation of physical development is striking. It must be differentiated from tetralogy of Fallot, tricuspid atresia, and total anomaly of venous return. Tetralogy of Fallot is readily identified in many patients by the normal cardiac size and the absence of cardiac failure. Tricuspid atresia is easily recognized by the characteristic left axis deviation on the electrocardiogram. Total anomalous drainage of the pulmonary veins may require cardiac catheterization to establish the diagnosis with certainty.

TREATMENT. Indications for Operation. For several reasons transposition may be classified into four broad groups, as follows: (1) Intact ventricular septum, patent foramen ovale; (2) ventricular septal defect; (3) ventricular septal defect and pulmonic stenosis; and (4) complex transposition, one of the previous three forms in association with other severe defects such as coarctation of the aorta.

The most urgent problems are seen with an intact ventricular septum, for the only communication between the pulmonary and systemic circulations is through the foramen ovale. In these patients, balloon septostomy provides dramatic, though not permanent, improvement. In the other groups, balloon septostomy is of considerably less value.

Because of the high fatality rate in the first month of life, some type of surgical procedure must be done to increase communication between the pulmonary and systemic circulations at the time the diagnosis is established in the catheterization laboratory. The simplest procedure is the balloon septostomy, enlarging the foramen ovale or atrial septal defect present by passing a deflated balloon catheter through the defect into the left atrium, inflating the balloon, and forcefully pulling the inflated balloon across the septum to enlarge the opening. This ingenious technique was developed by Rashkind and has greatly helped in the initial treatment of these seriously ill infants. In most instances, balloon septostomy probably should be routinely done at the time of cardiac catheterization to establish the diagnosis.

When balloon septostomy is ineffective, an atrial septal defect may be created by the Blalock-Hanlon technique. With the attractive simplicity of balloon septostomy, this procedure is now performed much less frequently than in the past. The operative procedure is illustrated in Fig. 18-44. A right thoracotomy is performed, after which the pericardium is opened and the superior and inferior pulmonary veins are isolated. The atrial septum is identified at the point of entry of the right pulmonary veins and a vascular clamp applied to isolate a segment of both the right and left atria at this point. Parallel incisions are then made in the right atrium and pulmonary vein through the septum, after which the two incisions are connected and a portion of the septum is incised, creating a defect 1 to 2 cm in diameter. Although this procedure has provided dramatic palliation in many patients for 6 to 12 months, results are often not sustained. Hence the present trend is to consider total surgical correction if balloon septostomy is inadequate.

In patients with a large ventricular septal defect resulting

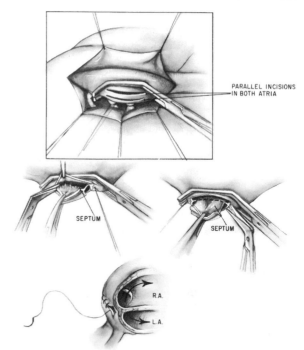

Fig. 18-44. Creation of atrial septal defect (Blalock-Hanlon Technique). Right pulmonary veins are mobilized and occluded by traction on ligatures. Pulmonary artery and right main bronchus are also occluded to avoid congestion of lungs during occlusion of pulmonary veins. Tangential occlusion clamp is applied to right and left atria, enclosing atrial septum. Separate incisions are then made in right atrium and left atrium. Exposed atrial septum is then removed, temporarily releasing clamp in order to withdraw more septum from between its jaws and create larger defect. After excision of this septum, incision is sutured, creating large atrial septal defect. (*Adapted from D. A. Cooley et al., Arch Surg, 93:704, 1966.*)

in flooding of the lung fields from excessive pulmonary blood flow, total correction may be considered or banding of the pulmonary artery may be done as a palliative procedure. Conversely, if pulmonic stenosis is present with severe reduction in pulmonary blood flow, a palliative subclavian-pulmonary anastomosis may be done.

Corrective Operations. All the previously described procedures are palliative only. If the ventricular septum is intact, many patients do reasonably well with a large atrial septal defect up to two to three years of age, and then total correction may be undertaken. In patients with ventricular septal defects, however, operation must be employed at an earlier age unless banding of the pulmonary artery is performed. Otherwise irreversible changes in the pulmonary vascular bed may develop before two years of age.

Dramatic advances have been made in recent years with the total correction of transposition in the first 1 to 2 years of life. In some instances operation has been successfully performed in the first 2 to 3 months of life, although operative mortality is higher. Performance of these complex procedures in small infants has been greatly facilitated by the deep hypothermia–circulatory arrest technique, developed extensively by Barratt-Boyes and his colleagues.

Data from several sources, including Barratt-Boyes, Kirklin, and Stark, now indicate that excellent results can be obtained by operation in the first 2 years of life. A more conservative approach is to perform palliative procedures described in earlier paragraphs, delaying the corrective procedure until the child is older. The strongest factor in support of early operation is the development of irreversible changes in the pulmonary vascular bed within the first 1 to 2 years of life in some patients. At New York University we have increasingly favored total surgical correction performed within the first 2 years of life.

A second important concept is that the durability of the Mustard baffle procedure, first reported in 1964, seems well established. In 1976 Mustard reported catheterization studies on 14 patients 4 to 10 years after the baffle operation, with continuing good results. Several technical modifications of the method of insertion of the baffle for the Mustard procedure are beyond the scope of this report, but complications from obstruction of either the pulmonary veins or the vena cavae have been described by several groups.

In 1975 Jatene, in South America, reported a successful surgical correction in an infant by switching the aorta and pulmonary arteries, with transposition of the abnormal coronary arteries. To date, attempts by others with this technique have had a prohibitive mortality; however, this method of total correction remains an attractive goal for the future.

Tricuspid Atresia

PATHOLOGIC ANATOMY. Tricuspid atresia is a rare form of congenital heart disease (Fig. 18-45) affecting 3 to 8 percent of children with cyanotic heart disease. However, series of 100 to 150 cases have been analyzed and reported from different cardiac centers. The basic abnormality is atresia of the tricuspid valve. Often only a dimple is found in the right atrial cavity where the tricuspid valve orifice is normally located. Several other cardiac malformations are associated with tricuspid atresia, and the severity of the disease varies with the associated malformations. The right ventricle is always underdeveloped, even absent, its place being taken by a solid mass of hypoplastic muscle. In other patients it exists as a small chamber, either a blind sac or one communicating with the left ventricle through a ventricular septal defect. The pulmonary artery and pulmonary valve are atretic with severe right ventricular hypoplasia, the pulmonary circulation being maintained through the ductus arteriosus. When a small right ventricular cavity is present, a normal pulmonary valve may be found. The ventricular septum is intact with right ventricular hypoplasia, but with a rudimentary ventricular chamber a septal defect is usually present. There is often an associated transposition of the great vessels. Edwards and Bargeron have described four anatomic variants of tricuspid atresia, differing in the presence of a ventricular septal defect, pulmonic stenosis, or transposition of the great vessels. An atrial septal defect must, of necessity, be present to maintain life. This may consist of a foramen ovale stretched open by a high right atrial pressure, a small atrial septal defect, or virtual absence of the atrial septum.

PATHOPHYSIOLOGY. The basic physiologic disturbance results from complete mixing of systemic venous blood and pulmonary venous blood in the left atrium, as blood returning to the right atrium is diverted by the hypoplastic tricuspid orifice through the atrial septal defect into the left atrium. The severity of the resulting cyanosis varies with the pulmonary blood flow. Cyanosis and anoxia are severe with pulmonary atresia, while they may be minimal with an adequate pulmonary blood flow. The hypoplastic right ventricle which is uniformly present is the most valuable clue to the diagnosis. An additional significant physiologic disturbance is the elevated right atrial pressure resulting from flow of systemic venous blood through the atrial septal defect and into the left ventricle. The right atrial pressure may be elevated 5 to 10 mm Hg if only a foramen ovale is present, resulting in hepatic enlargement and other signs of right-sided heart failure.

CLINICAL MANIFESTATIONS. Symptoms. The disease is a severe one, and most infants die in the first few months of life as the patent ductus arteriosus closes, unless an operation is performed. The severity of the malformation varies with the degree of reduction in pulmonary blood flow, which in turn is related to the degree of hypoplasia of the right ventricle. The patients are usually cyanotic at birth and have exercise intolerance, retarded development, and frequent anoxic spells of unconsciousness. Hemiplegia may develop after a severe anoxic spell. Death occurs during an anoxic episode or results from congestive heart failure. In older children endocarditis may occur.

The prominent symptoms are cyanosis and dyspnea with intolerance to exercise, squatting, and limited growth and development.

Physical Examination. On physical examination there is slight to moderate cardiac enlargement. A moderate systolic murmur along the left sternal border is present in about one-half the patients but is of no diagnostic significance. It presumably arises either from flow through the atrial septal defect or possibly from flow through a stenotic pulmonic valve. Absence of a murmur often indicates an unusually poor prognosis. The second heart sound is unusually "pure" because the pulmonic second sound is weak or absent. A particularly significant diagnostic finding is hepatic enlargement and other signs of right-sided failure, especially in association with absence of any signs of pulmonary congestion or left-sided failure.

LABORATORY FINDINGS. The chest roentgenogram regularly shows cardiac enlargement, and on fluoroscopy it may be possible to detect that the enlargement is predominantly in the left ventricle. There is decreased vascularity in the lung fields. The electrocardiogram is the most important diagnostic tool, for left ventricular hypertrophy and left axis deviation are uniformly present, in contrast to the classic right ventricular hypertrophy of most forms of cyanotic heart disease. There are often unusually tall, peaked P waves, indicating right atrial hypertrophy in association with a small atrial septal defect or foramen ovale. On cardiac catheterization there is a right-to-left

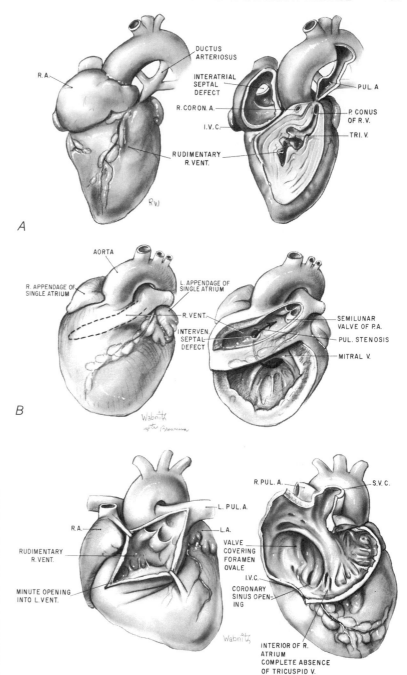

Fig. 18-45. *A.* Tricuspid atresia with rudimentary right ventricle, pulmonary atresia, and vestigial pulmonary artery which does not communicate with hypoplastic right ventricular cavity. *B.* Tricuspid atresia in which pulmonary artery is normally formed and arises from rudimentary right ventricular cavity. Small ventricular septal defect is present, permitting flow of blood from normal left ventricular cavity through rudimentary right ventricular cavity into pulmonary artery. *C.* Tricuspid atresia with rudimentary right ventricle in which normal pulmonary artery with normal pulmonic valves arises from rudimentary right ventricle. Right atrial cavity is dilated, with absence of tricuspid valve. (*Adapted from H. B. Taussig, "Congenital Malformations of the Heart," 2d ed., Harvard University Press, Cambridge, 1960, pp. 77–79.*)

shunt at the atrial level, with some elevation of the right atrial pressure. The right atrial pressure is higher than the left atrial pressure if only a foramen ovale is present. Characteristically it is impossible to advance the catheter into the right ventricle because of the tricuspid atresia. Selective angiocardiography establishes the diagnosis by demonstrating flow of blood from the right atrium to the left atrium and into the left ventricle.

DIAGNOSIS. Diagnosis can be reasonably well estab-

lished from the combination of clinical cyanosis with left ventricular hypertrophy shown on the electrocardiogram. The usual differential diagnosis is from tetralogy of Fallot or from transposition of the great vessels, with the electrocardiogram and other clinical features providing the best diagnostic clues. Confirmation can be obtained by catheterization and angiography.

TREATMENT. As the malformation is often incompatible with life once the ductus arteriosus closes, emergency operations in infants undergoing cyanotic spells are often necessary. In the rare patient who survives the first year of life without operation, the presence of cyanosis and severe retardation of growth are the usual indications for operation.

Operative Procedures. With this severe malformation, most operative efforts have been to provide effective palliation for a few years. The long-term results have been uncertain. Some encouragement, however, came from the initial report by Fontan in 1971 of a more effective corrective procedure, inserting a valve conduit between the right atrium and pulmonary artery in older children. The importance of palliative procedures has been enhanced, as, if successful, these procedures may support the patient for several years until the child is large enough for a Fontan-type operation or some other more effective corrective procedure.

In infants and small children, the Potts type of aortopulmonary shunt seems to provide the best results over several years, probably because of the gradual enlargement in size of the Potts anastomosis. These data were well demonstrated in an analysis of Williams et al., in 1975, of experiences with 104 patients in Toronto with different types of shunts. The results seem superior to those obtained from either the subclavian–pulmonary anastomosis or the aortopulmonary anastomosis. A similar preference for the Potts anastomosis was reported by Kyger and associates in 1975 in a series of 105 patients operated on.

The cable-pulmonary shunt developed by Glenn provides excellent palliation for 5 to 7 years and is most effective in older children (Fig. 18-46). Its future after this time, as collateral circulation enlarges, is uncertain. It has the distinct advantage of not increasing cardiac work. Hence, if there are signs of cardiac failure, this should be considered the procedure of choice.

Postoperative Course. The risk of operation in infants is significant because of the severity of the malformation; an operative mortality of 10 to 20 percent is common. Long-term evaluation of patients surviving operation has shown substantial improvement in 60 to 70 percent. In the next

few years more effective and sustained results may be obtained with valve-conduit procedures of the Fontan type.

RARE MALFORMATIONS

Cor Triatriatum

Cor triatriatum is a rare malformation. In 1960 a review by Niwayama found only 36 cases, and in 1965 McGuire et al. stated that only about 10 cases had been recognized in adult patients.

PATHOLOGIC ANATOMY. The anomaly results from incomplete absorption of the embryonic common pulmonary vein into the left atrium, so that it remains as an additional cardiac chamber superior and posterior to the normal left atrium. The pulmonary veins enter this accessory chamber, which communicates with the left atrium through a tiny opening, often only 3 to 4 mm in diameter. The mitral valve and atrial appendage are normal. The foramen ovale almost always opens into the left atrium and not into the accessory chamber.

CLINICAL MANIFESTATIONS. The disease is a severe one, with rapid progression of pulmonary congestion, pulmonary hypertension, and heart failure. Over 50 percent of affected infants do not survive the first year of life. Symptoms are identical to those of mitral stenosis, although in the few older patients who have been studied, hemoptysis has been an unusually prominent feature. On physical

Fig. 18-46. Anastomosis between superior vena cava and right pulmonary artery. *A.* Tangential clamp has been applied to superior vena cava to include origin of azygos vein. Right pulmonary artery has been divided, and end-to-end anastomosis will be constructed. *B.* Posterior row of anastomosis is constructed with continuous 5-0 silk suture. *C.* Completed posterior row of anastomosis. *D.* Anterior row of anastomosis is constructed with interrupted sutures to permit growth of anastomosis. After removal of occluding clamps, superior vena cava is doubly ligated at point of juncture with right atrium. (*Adapted from W. W. L. Glenn, N Engl J Med, 259:117, 1958.*)

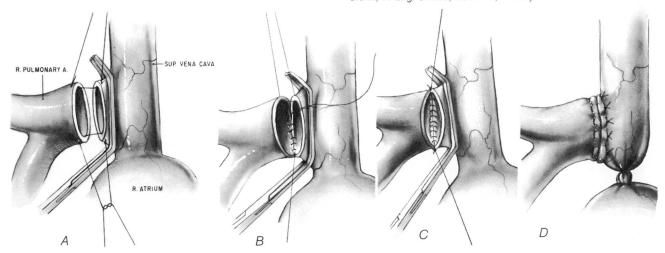

R. PULMONARY A. —SUP. VENA CAVA

R. ATRIUM

A   *B*   *C*   *D*

examination a typical diastolic rumbling murmur of mitral stenosis is usually not present, although a systolic murmur is audible. The absence of a typical murmur, combined with the presence of a sinus rhythm, should raise the suspicion that something other than mitral stenosis is present. A forceful impulse may be palpable in the left parasternal area because of marked right ventricular hypertrophy.

LABORATORY FINDINGS. The roentgenogram shows pulmonary congestion with enlargement of the right ventricle, and the electrocardiogram shows right ventricular hypertrophy. The diagnosis can be established at catheterization by the finding of elevated pulmonary artery pressure as well as an increased wedge pressure (often 25 to 30 mm Hg), *combined with a normal pressure in the left atrium.* Selective angiocardiography will disclose the accessory chamber superior and posterior to the normal left atrium.

DIAGNOSTIC CONSIDERATIONS. By far the most common condition that obstructs flow of blood from the pulmonary veins into the left ventricle is mitral stenosis. In the differential diagnosis, however, three rare conditions should be considered: stenosis of the pulmonary veins, cor triatriatum and supravalvular stenosing ring of the left atrium. Although all these are rare, if they are recognized, surgical treatment is relatively simple. With the precise diagnostic catheterization and angiographic methods now available, it may be hoped that earlier diagnosis and successful treatment will be reported more frequently in the next few years than it has in the past.

TREATMENT. Operation should be performed as soon as the diagnosis is established, because most patients succumb to cardiac failure at an early age. Although a successful operation was performed by Lewis and one by Vineberg in 1956, the collective review published in 1960 by Niwayama found a total of only five successful operations at that time. In 1964 Grondin et al. reported experiences with six cases, four of whom had been operated upon, with three survivors.

The operative procedure is theoretically a simple one, consisting of enlarging the small opening between the accessory atrium and the normal left atrium. It should ideally be performed with cardiopulmonary bypass, to permit extensive excision of the obstructing membrane. The few reported survivors have been asymptomatic.

Congenital Mitral Stenosis

Congenital mitral stenosis is a rare lesion which frequently results in congestive heart failure and death in the first year of life. Ferencz et al., in 1954, found 34 patients previously reported and described nine additional cases. Nadas has studied five cases, and Daoud and associates in 1963 described experiences with seven. In 1967 Tsuji et al. stated that 131 cases had been reported. Two additional patients who had been successfully operated upon were described, making a total of 41 patients operated upon with 21 known survivors.

In 1975 Khalil reported operative experiences with nine patients at the Ohio State University Hospital, with five

survivors, and in 1976, Carpentier reported an extensive experience with 47 children with congenital mitral lesions, in 14 of whom mitral stenosis was the dominant finding.

PATHOLOGIC ANATOMY. The wide spectrum of abnormalities which may be found is well described in the excellent report by Carpentier, probably the most extensive experience in the world with congenital mitral valve abnormalities. The abnormalities present include commissural fusion, abnormalities in the development of the leaflets (such as a parachute valve), and defects in the chordae tendinae and papillary muscles.

If the leaflets are well developed, commissurotomy and a reconstructive procedure may be feasible. With severe abnormalities, valve replacement may be necessary. In the extensive experience reported by Carpentier, valve reconstruction was possible in 38 patients, while valve replacement was necessary in 9. In most reports, valve replacement has been required much more frequently.

CLINICAL MANIFESTATIONS. Symptoms often appear in infancy, with dyspnea, pulmonary congestion, and repeated pneumonic infections. In milder forms of stenosis, symptoms may appear only in later childhood. On physical examination an apical diastolic rumbling murmur is almost always found and provides the best clue to the diagnosis. A thrill is also frequent. An associated systolic murmur, probably from concomitant mitral insufficiency, is common. Sinus rhythm is usually present.

LABORATORY FINDINGS. The main abnormality on the chest roentgenogram is enlargement of the left atrium, with some associated enlargement of the right ventricle. The electrocardiogram will demonstrate right ventricular hypertrophy and right axis deviation. On cardiac catheterization the diagnosis can be confirmed by the finding of an elevated pulmonary artery pressure and pulmonary capillary pressure. Selective angiography may outline the dilated left atrium.

TREATMENT. Operation should be avoided in infancy or early childhood because of the complexity of prosthetic valve replacement, which may be required in the young child. However, severe symptoms may necessitate operation at an early age. The excellent article by Carpentier should be consulted for the techniques of mitral valve reconstruction which he has employed. If a prosthetic valve is inserted, replacement with a larger prosthesis will almost certainly be necessary within a few years.

Aortic-Pulmonary Window

Several terms have been applied to this rare anomaly, including *aortopulmonary fenestration, aorticopulmonary fistula*, and *aortic septal defect.* It is an unusual lesion and has been recognized only with the development of diagnostic and surgical techniques for patent ductus arteriosus. In a group of 100 patients with a diagnosis of patent ductus arteriosus, 1 will usually be found to have an aortic-pulmonary window. A comprehensive report by Skall-Jensen in 1958 found 62 cases in the medical literature. One case was successfully treated by ligation by Gross in 1948, and another was treated by division and suture by Scott and

Sabiston in 1951 (Fig. 18-47), but correction with extracorporeal circulation is now the preferred procedure. Three such patients were reported by Cooley et al. in 1957. In 1962, Morrow and associates found 71 reported cases, 27 of whom had been operated upon. In 1976 Clark reported experiences with seven patients, all surviving operation. In five, the defect was closed with a Dacron patch through a transaortic approach, which was considered to be the best surgical technique.

PATHOLOGIC ANATOMY. Embryologically, the defect results from incomplete development of the spiral septum dividing the primitive truncus arteriosus into the aorta and the pulmonary artery. Persistent truncus arteriosus is a more severe malformation of similar cause but represents incomplete development of both the spiral septum in the truncus arteriosus and the bulbar septum in the bulbus cordis. In persistent truncus arteriosus there is both a ventricular septal defect and a failure of formation of the separate aortic and pulmonic valves, while in aortic-pulmonary window the aortic and pulmonic valves are normally formed, although a separate ventricular septal defect has been found in some patients.

The opening, or "window," between the aorta and the pulmonary artery may vary in diameter from 5 to 30 mm. It may be located proximally near the ostia of the coronary arteries and the pulmonic valve, or it may be as much as 2 cm distal to these structures.

PATHOPHYSIOLOGY. The defect produces a large left-to-right shunt similar to that of a patent ductus arteriosus. The course is a more malignant one, however, because the shunt is usually larger than that seen in the usual patent ductus, resulting in the rapid development of pulmonary hypertension, increase in pulmonary vascular resistance, and cardiac failure.

CLINICAL MANIFESTATIONS. The clinical findings may be identical to those found in patent ductus arteriosus, with a continuous murmur, wide pulse pressure, left ventricular enlargement, and pulmonary congestion. Often only a systolic murmur is present, however, because of severe pulmonary hypertension. Usually the condition is diag-

nosed as patent ductus arteriosus until cardiac catheterization, angiography, or surgical exploration discloses the correct diagnosis.

LABORATORY FINDINGS. At catheterization the findings are identical to those with a patent ductus arteriosus unless the cardiac catheter can be manipulated through the defect into the aorta, in which case the catheter takes a characteristic course to enter either the ascending aorta or the innominate artery; in patent ductus arteriosus, the catheter enters the aorta distal to the left subclavian artery and usually goes into the descending thoracic aorta. This observation of the course of the catheter can visually establish the diagnosis.

Angiography can also confirm the diagnosis, demonstrating dye flowing from the aorta into the pulmonary artery near the aortic valve rather than in the usual location distal to the left subclavian artery.

DIAGNOSIS. Differential diagnosis must exclude persistent truncus arteriosus, ventricular septal defect with a prolapsed aortic cusp, and patent ductus arteriosus. The exact diagnosis can be made only upon cardiac catheterization and angiography.

TREATMENT. Usually operation should be performed as soon as the diagnosis has been established, because irreversible changes in pulmonary vascular resistance develop rapidly. There is a paucity of data about the natural history of the disease because of its rarity and recent recognition, but irreversible changes in the pulmonary arterioles have been seen as early as three or four years of age. The author has had one three-year-old patient who died within a few hours from elevated pulmonary vascular resistance following an uncomplicated division and suture of a large aortic-pulmonary window with extracorporeal circulation, and Gross has reported similar experiences with two patients.

Operation should be performed with extracorporeal circulation because of the unpredictable variation in friability of the vascular structures. Once cardiopulmonary

Fig. 18-47. Aortic-pulmonary fistula, showing large communication between aorta and pulmonary artery near base of heart. (*Adapted from H. W. Scott and D. C. Sabiston, J Thorac Surg, 25:26, 1953.*)

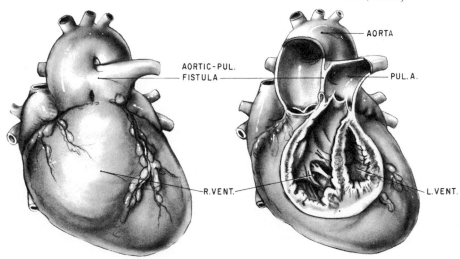

AORTA

AORTIC-PUL. FISTULA — — PUL. A.

R.VENT. — — L.VENT.

bypass has been established, the aorta can be occluded distal to the window, lowering the pressure in the pulmonary artery.

The window may then be divided and the aortic and pulmonary openings sutured. If possible, tangential vascular clamps may be applied to the aorta and pulmonary artery at the site of the window before it is divided, but simple division is usually preferable. The main precaution is evacuation of air from the aorta before circulation is reestablished. Shumway has reported an alternate technique of opening the pulmonary artery and suturing the opening without dividing it. The alternate approach of opening the aorta and applying a patch to the opening, suggested by Wright in 1968 and endorsed by Clark, as mentioned earlier, seems to be reasonable.

The risk of operation is proportional to the increase in pulmonary vascular resistance and is probably in the range of 15 to 20 percent. Gross has operated upon seven patients with two fatalities, both in patients who had an elevated pulmonary vascular resistance. Following recovery from operation, prognosis is apparently as favorable as that found with patent ductus arteriosus.

Ruptured Aneurysm of Sinus of Valsalva

This unusual entity produces a distinct syndrome which can be readily diagnosed and effectively treated. Before the advent of extracorporeal circulation it usually caused death from cardiac failure within 1 to 2 years after onset. An aneurysm of the sinus of Valsalva can result from syphilis or other infections; at present most are congenital in origin.

A detailed review by Sawyer et al. in 1957 found 47 patients with congenital aneurysms, but the natural increased interest in diagnosis and therapy which followed the first successful surgical closure in 1956 has led to more widespread recognition. Paton and associates stated in 1965 that since the first operation performed, there had been reports of 91 additional patients operated upon and at least 60 other cases had been described.

PATHOLOGIC ANATOMY. The normal sinus of Valsalva is composed of an aortic valve cusp medially and the aortic wall laterally, which joins the annulus fibrosus of the aortic valve ring inferiorly. In embryonic development the developing ventricular septum inferiorly meets the spiral septum superiorly which separates the aorta and the pulmonary arteries. Incomplete merger of these two structures results in a ventricular septal defect in the membranous septum. An aneurysm of the sinus of Valsalva results from a less severe malformation of the same type, for the media of the aortic wall does not extend down to the annulus of the aortic valve ring. As might be expected, however, an associated ventricular septal defect is often found.

The right coronary sinus is involved in about 70 percent of patients, and rupture occurs into the right ventricle. The noncoronary sinus is involved in about 20 percent of patients, with rupture occurring into the right atrium. Involvement of the left coronary sinus is rare, and rupture into the left atrium or left ventricle is very unusual.

CLINICAL MANIFESTATIONS. Until rupture occurs, an aneurysm of the sinus of Valsalva does not cause any disability, and diagnosis can be made only accidentally during aortography performed for other reasons. The average age at rupture is thirty-one years, although a few such instances have been reported in childhood. Rupture usually occurs without known cause and is soon followed by cardiac failure. Once cardiac failure develops, life expectancy without surgical correction is about 1 year.

At the time of rupture there may be transitory pain in the chest, subsequently followed by dyspnea and palpitation, although in some patients the first symptom is dyspnea. Subsequently other symptoms of congestive heart failure appear. On physical examination, the important abnormality is the characteristic parasternal murmur, often accompanied by a palpable thrill. The murmur may be continuous or may be a to-and-fro murmur with a somewhat louder component in diastole. It is often located somewhat lower than the usual murmur of a ductus arteriosus, being heard in the third, fourth, or fifth parasternal spaces to the right or left of the sternum, depending upon the point of rupture of the aneurysm. The murmur is unusually superficial in location and is widely transmitted. These unusual qualities may lead to the suspicion that it is not arising from the usual patent ductus arteriosus. Other physical findings, including a wide pulse pressure, cardiac enlargement, and pulmonary congestion, resemble those of a patent ductus arteriosus.

LABORATORY FINDINGS. Cardiac enlargement and pulmonary congestion are noted on the roentgenogram, and cardiac hypertrophy on the electrocardiogram. On cardiac catheterization, a left-to-right shunt can be identified at the atrial or ventricular level. Diagnosis is best established by selective aortography, demonstrating the leakage of dye from the aorta into the involved cardiac chamber (Fig. 18-48). The differential diagnosis must exclude patent ductus arteriosus and aortic-pulmonary window.

Fig. 18-48. Aortogram confirms diagnosis of ruptured aneurysm of sinus of Valsalva by demonstrating flow of dye from region of aortic sinuses to right atrium. (*Courtesy of Dr. Raymond M. Abrams, Department of Radiology, New York University Medical Center.*)

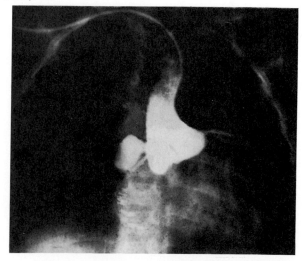

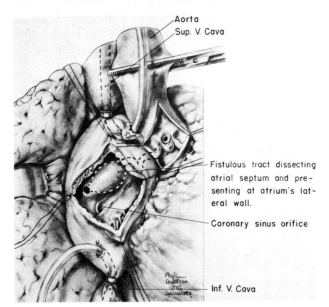

Fig. 18-49. Diagram of unusual type of ruptured aneurysm of sinus of Valsalva. Aneurysm arose from left coronary cusp and developed fistulous tract before rupture into right atrium. Operative closure was performed by opening aorta and closing opening directly. (*From Ann Surg, 152:965, 1960.*)

TREATMENT. Operative correction should be performed as soon as the diagnosis has been established. This is done with extracorporeal circulation through a median sternotomy incision. The basic objective at operation is to close the defect in the aortic wall at the mouth of the aneurysm by attaching the aortic media superiorly to the aortic ring

Fig. 18-50. Four anatomic types of truncus arteriosus. (*From R. A. Poirier et al., J Thorac Cardiovasc Surg, 69:169, 1975.*)

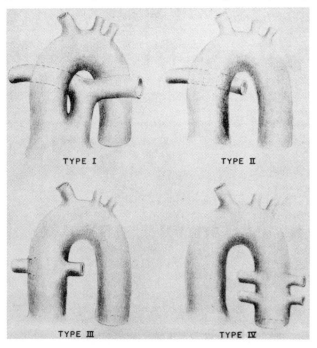

below (Fig. 18-49). Although initially operations were usually performed by approaching the lesion through the right atrium or right ventricle, excising the fistulous sac and suturing the opening, a transaortic approach, as suggested by Shumacker et al., permits a more precise closure, assuring adequate repair of the aortic wall without any risk of injury to the aortic valve cusps. The author has seen recurrence of the lesion in one young woman, occurring a few months after the aortic opening was closed by direct suture. With a large opening, transaortic closure with a Dacron patch may be preferable to direct suture. A concomitant ventricular septal defect may frequently be found and repaired at the same operation. The operative risk is small and the results have been excellent.

Truncus Arteriosus

Truncus arteriosus is a rare malformation resulting from failure of division of the fetal arterial channel into the aorta and pulmonary arteries and the left and right ventricles. Therapy of this condition is a good example of the rapid changes in cardiac surgery. When the first edition of this book was written in 1969, only palliative therapy was possible. Since that time McGoon and associates have developed a technique of surgical correction with an aortic homograft which has been successfully applied to a significant number of patients.

PATHOLOGIC ANATOMY. In this condition the entire circulation, including the coronary arteries, the pulmonary arteries, and the systemic arteries, arises from a common arterial trunk. There is always a ventricular septal defect, and a single ventricle occurs in 15 to 20 percent of patients. Only one semilunar valve is present, usually with four cusps, although the number may vary from two to six. Four anatomic types of truncus have been described, according to how the pulmonary arteries arise from the aorta. These are well illustrated in the publication by Poirier in 1975 (Fig. 18-50).

"Pseudotruncus" has been used by some to describe a condition in which a single large artery originates from the base of the heart, but the pulmonary arteries are absent and pulmonary blood flows through enlarged bronchial vessels. Others consider the condition as pulmonary atresia or a variant of severe tetralogy of Fallot.

PATHOPHYSIOLOGY. The disability with this condition is a severe one, with 70 to 80 percent of infants dying within the first year of life, usually from congestive heart failure. Incompetence of the truncal valve contributes to death in many of this group.

As blood entering the aorta is a mixture of blood from the systemic circulation and the pulmonary circulation, arterial oxygen unsaturation is always present, the degree varying with the volume of pulmonary blood flow. If large pulmonary arteries originate from the aorta, initially there is a large pulmonary blood flow with minimal cyanosis. Subsequently there is a progressive rise in pulmonary vascular resistance with diminution of pulmonary blood flow and increase in cyanosis. Hence the degree of cyanosis is directly related to the volume of pulmonary blood flow.

Severe pulmonary vascular disease develops rapidly in

many patients, some of whom probably become inoperable before 2 to 3 years of age.

CLINICAL MANIFESTATIONS. Disability is evident in infancy, with cyanosis and dyspnea on exertion and retardation of growth and development. On physical examination, loud systolic and diastolic murmurs are audible over the base of the heart, often as a to-and-fro murmur rather than a true continuous murmur. In older children, continuous murmurs may be best heard over one or both lungs, originating from collateral circulation to the lungs; as emphasized by Taussig, this is virtually diagnostic of the malformation. The second heart sound is "pure" and increased in intensity.

LABORATORY FINDINGS. The chest roentgenogram and electrocardiogram show both right and left ventricular enlargement. Cardiac catheterization will demonstrate a left-to-right shunt in the ventricle with a systolic pulmonary artery pressure equal to aortic systolic pressure. The abnormal vessels can be outlined with selective angiography, but precise studies are required to demonstrate with certainty the exact point of origin of the pulmonary arteries.

In acyanotic children the condition must be differentiated from patent ductus arteriosus or an aortic-pulmonary window. With severe cyanosis, pulmonary atresia, tricuspid atresia, and transposition of the great vessels must be considered.

TREATMENT. The operation developed by McGoon et al. consists of construction of a new pulmonary artery with a valved conduit, preferably a Dacron tube with a glutaraldehyde preserved porcine heterograft (Hancock prosthesis). Employing extracorporeal circulation, the pulmonary arteries are detached from the aorta. The right ventricle is then opened in the outflow tract. The ventricular septal defect is then closed so that the aorta originates only from the left ventricle. The homograft with the aortic valve is then attached to the opening in the right ventricle, and distally is connected to the right and left pulmonary arteries, creating a new pulmonary artery.

Operative mortality has been low in the selective group of patients operated upon between five and ten years of age, in whom the pulmonary vascular resistance is less than 0.6 percent of systemic vascular resistance. However, this is a selective group of patients because, as indicated earlier, there is both a high mortality in infancy and also rapid development of irreversible pulmonary vascular disease in many. These considerations were well reviewed in the reports by Poirier in 1975 and by Applebaum in 1976.

Banding of the pulmonary arteries in infancy to protect the pulmonary vascular bed has a surprisingly high mortality, nearly 50 percent from different reports according to Applebaum, and also a significant mortality at the time of attempted correction at a later date. Hence the increasing tendency is to perform corrective surgery with a valve conduit at an earlier age, probably between two and three years, or in the first years of life if symptoms are severe. This has been accomplished in several patients described by Ebert in 1976.

When a conduit is inserted in such small children, it will have to be replaced as the child grows older; however,

Marcelletti and McGoon reported in 1976 that 22 aortic homograft conduits had been successfully replaced with a Dacron conduit.

Single Ventricle

A single ventricle is a rare, severe malformation for which corrective surgery has only recently become possible with the construction of a new ventricular septum [Malm]. Nadas found only 10 cases in a group of 577 patients.

PATHOLOGIC ANATOMY. The anomaly consists of a single functioning ventricular chamber into which both atrioventricular valves enter. Connected to the functioning ventricle is a rudimentary outlet chamber located in the position normally occupied by the outflow tract of the right ventricle. From this rudimentary chamber one or both of the great vessels may arise. Transposition of the aorta and pulmonary artery occurs in over one-half the patients. The clinical profile varies widely, depending upon whether or not the arteries are transposed and whether the artery arising from the rudimentary outlet chamber is of normal diameter or hypoplastic.

PATHOPHYSIOLOGY. The two physiologic characteristics are admixture of oxygenated and unoxygenated blood in the common ventricle before entering the aorta, and pulmonary hypertension resulting from origin of the pulmonary artery and the aorta from the same ventricle. The degree of cyanosis depends upon the pulmonary blood flow.

CLINICAL MANIFESTATIONS. Infants with an increased pulmonary blood flow, occurring when the aorta arises from the rudimentary outlet chamber and the pulmonary artery from the functioning ventricle, may be acyanotic but disabled from pulmonary congestion and cardiac failure. Conversely, with a decreased pulmonary blood flow from a hypoplastic pulmonary artery, cyanosis may be severe and the clinical picture dominated by signs of anoxia. Much variation between these two extremes is seen because of other anomalies frequently present. A single ventricle per se is most unusual, for concomitant cardiac malformations are frequent.

The disability is severe and associated with cardiac failure or cyanosis. In a group of 85 patients reviewed by Campbell and associates, over one-half died in the first year of life, although 18 lived to be twenty years of age. On physical examination variable systolic murmurs and cardiac enlargement are found, but variation in the murmurs precludes any diagnostic significance.

LABORATORY FINDINGS. The roentgenogram demonstrates cardiac enlargement, and the electrocardiogram shows left or right ventricular hypertrophy. Great variation is present, depending upon the relation of the aorta and pulmonary artery to the common ventricle and the rudimentary outlet chamber. The best diagnostic information is obtained on cardiac catheterization, with a rise in oxygen concentration of 4 to 5 vol % noted when a catheter is advanced from the atrium into the common ventricle. Similar pressures may be found in the aorta and pulmonary artery. Selective angiography may demonstrate the rudimentary outlet chamber.

TREATMENT. In the past few years, single ventricle has been successfully corrected in a few selected cases by construction of a new ventricular septum. To avoid complete heart block, the course of the conduction bundle should be electrically mapped at the time of operation as noted by Malm. Though experience thus far is limited, it indicates the ever-widening horizon of possibilities of correction of anomalies which in the past could only be treated by palliative methods.

Ebstein's Anomaly

This peculiar and unusual anomaly was described by Wilhelm Ebstein in 1866 following postmortem examination of a nineteen-year-old cyanotic youth who had died with signs of tricuspid insufficiency. Although the anomaly is uncommon, with improvement in cardiac diagnostic techniques it has been recognized with increased frequency. Vacca and associates in 1958 found the total number of cases reported to be 108. The cause is unknown.

PATHOLOGIC ANATOMY. The anomaly consists of a downward displacement of part of the tricuspid valve, creating a third chamber in the right side of the heart. Usually the anterior leaflet of the tricuspid valve arises normally from the tricuspid annulus and may be abnormally large and prominent. It has been described as sail-like. The septal and posterior leaflets, however, are not attached to the normal tricuspid annulus but arise from the wall of the right ventricle at a varying distance from the true annulus. These two cusps may be small and adherent to the wall of the ventricle, with little functional ability (Fig. 18-51). The segment of right ventricular wall between the true annulus of the tricuspid valve and the origin of the displaced leaflets is then functionally a part of the right atrium and has been termed the *atrialized* ventricle. The wall of this part of the ventricle may be unusually thin. The foramen ovale is usually patent, and often an atrial septal defect is also present.

The malformation varies widely in severity, depending upon the relative size of the atrialized ventricle above the tricuspid valve and the functioning right ventricle below the abnormal valve. The anatomic spectrum of malforma-

tions which may be seen has been well illustrated by Taussig.

PATHOPHYSIOLOGY. The main physiologic disturbance is inadequate cardiac output from the right ventricle. This is probably due to both the tricuspid insufficiency and the paradoxic contraction of the atrialized segment of the right ventricle. Less significant causes are the small size of the functioning right ventricle and the frequent arrhythmias. With the low cardiac output and tricuspid insufficiency, the right atrium becomes massively dilated, and cyanosis of moderate degree is usually present because of a right-to-left shunt through the foramen ovale. The cyanosis tends to become more severe in later years of life, probably because of progressive right ventricular failure.

CLINICAL MANIFESTATIONS. The clinical course is often a severe one, although some adults survive for many years. Analysis of reported cases has found that about 40 percent of patients die in the first decade and 30 percent in the next. Death occurs from congestive failure in about one-third of patients, and at least another third may die suddenly from an arrhythmia.

The predominant symptoms are fatigue, with gradual increase in exertional dyspnea and cyanosis over the years. Symptoms may be present in some patients during early childhood, while in others they appear only after the first decade. Signs of right-sided failure gradually become more evident. Physical examination discloses soft, blurred systolic and diastolic murmurs along the left sternal border,

Fig. 18-51. *A.* Normal heart showing septal and posterior leaflets of tricuspid valve. *B.* Pathologic anatomy in Ebstein's malformation, with displacement of diminutive septal and posterior leaflets down into normal right ventricular cavity. Large anterior leaflet is not shown. *C.* Abnormal pathologic anatomy in Ebstein's malformation. There is large "saillike" anterior leaflet with hypoplastic septal and posterior leaflets, which are often displaced downward into ventricle, creating third cardiac chamber interposed between right atrium and functioning right ventricle. (*Adapted from K. L. Hardy et al., J Thorac Cardiovasc Surg, 48:931, 1964.*)

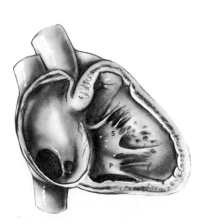

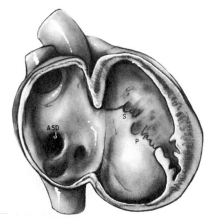

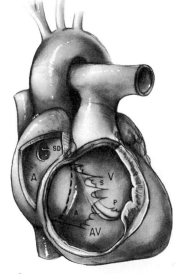

A   *B*   *C*

with muffled heart sounds and signs of feeble, ineffective cardiac contractions. The cardiac size is usually increased. The findings have been appropriately compared to those with a large pericardial effusion. Cyanosis and clubbing may be found but are usually not severe.

Nadas has stated that the auscultatory findings are pathognomonic of the condition. He emphasizes three findings: a slow cardiac rate with a triple or quadruple rhythm, a systolic murmur of tricuspid regurgitation, and frequently a low-pitched diastolic murmur.

LABORATORY FINDINGS. The roentgenogram may be remarkable for the great enlargement of the right side of the heart, including a huge right atrium and the atrialized part of the right ventricle. The pulmonary artery segment is often small, and the vascularity in the lung fields is less than normal. On fluoroscopy, feeble cardiac contractions are frequently seen. The electrocardiographic findings are also considered to be typical. Conduction disturbances with prolonged P-R interval and partial right bundle branch block are common. Right ventricular hypertrophy is absent after infancy, but the left chest leads show average potentials.

Cardiac catheterization may be hazardous; deaths from arrhythmias have occurred in several laboratories. Alertness to the possibility, however, in combination with use of electric defibrillators, has greatly decreased the risk of catheterization. With catheterization, a right-to-left shunt at the atrial level, with resulting arterial hypoxemia, is found in 25 to 50 percent of patients. Interestingly enough, the contour of the right atrial pressure wave may not be strikingly abnormal, perhaps because of the damping effect of the large cavity of the right atrium on the blood regurgitating through the incompetent tricuspid orifice. The abnormal course of the cardiac catheter in the atrialized part of the right ventricle can be of diagnostic significance, and with selective angiography, the huge right atrium can be outlined. Diagnosis can usually be made with certainty on the basis of the typical physical findings, combined with the abnormalities observed on the roentgenogram and electrocardiogram and those found at cardiac catheterization.

TREATMENT. A suggestion made by Hunter and Lillihei in 1958 to exclude the atrialized ventricle from the circulation seemingly remains sound, but there is a disappointing lack of data demonstrating good surgical results. Hardy and associates reported one successful operation in 1964 and Bahnson and associates two additional operations in 1965. Hardy subsequently operated on a few additional patients. Replacement of the abnormal valve with a prosthetic valve was performed by Barnard, and Timmis and associates combined prosthetic replacement with elimination of the atrialized ventricle in one patient.

Surprisingly little progress has been made in the surgical treatment of Ebstein's disease since the previous edition of this textbook. The report by MacFaul from the Mayo Clinic in 1976, summarizing experiences with 16 patients, expresses the continuing uncertainty about indications for operation as well as the best method of approach. Five patients had valve replacement performed, but only one survived, while much better results were obtained with

tricuspid annuloplasty and plication of the atrialized segment. However, two of seven patients who survived operation died suddenly with arrhythmias at a later date.

The four basic problems with Ebstein's anomaly are the insufficiency of the right ventricle from the atrialized segment, tricuspid insufficiency, arrhythmias, and the atrial septal defect. The atrial septal defect is surely the least important, except for the occasional instance of paradoxical embolization, although this is the mechanism of cyanosis in these patients, permitting right-to-left shunting if the right ventricle fails.

It seems clear that there is wide variation in the pathologic anatomy, making individualization of different patients necessary, as emphasized by Bahnson. A second therapeutic point is that the atrialized segment of the right ventricle must be appropriately treated if it is enwalled and moves paradoxically, treating this either by excision or by plication. On the other hand, if the segment is thick-walled with little paradoxical motion, treatment may not be necessary. This variation in the severity of the atrialized segment may explain the finding in some patients that valve replacement alone is sufficient, while in others it has promptly resulted in a fatality, perhaps because the incompetent right ventricle could no longer decompress through the insufficient tricuspid valve.

An additional therapeutic point is the malignant nature of the arrhythmias of some patients. Possibly earlier operation before right atrial hypertrophy becomes severe might be helpful, but this is only a hypothesis. Helpful advances in electrical mapping of the abnormal pathways are another possibility. A third possibility is that prostheses used in the past may have contributed to subsequent arrhythmias as the right ventricle decreases in size, as has been seen with other complications with ball-valve prostheses in the tricuspid position. Hence the tricuspid prosthesis of choice at present would seem to be a heterograft. An alternative approach is a form of annuloplasty, perhaps employing the Carpentier ring in severe cases.

Anomalies of the Coronary Arteries

ANOMALOUS ORIGIN OF LEFT CORONARY ARTERY FROM PULMONARY ARTERY

The first case of this unusual malformation was described by Abrikosov in 1911, but little clinical interest evolved until Bland et al. in 1933 described the clinical features of the syndrome and emphasized its similarity to myocardial infarction in adults. Over 50 cases were reviewed by Keith in 1959. A significant advance was made by Sabiston et al. in 1959 when they conclusively demonstrated retrograde flow of blood from the anomalous left coronary artery into the pulmonary artery, a theoretical possibility previously mentioned by several investigators. Subsequently, in two older children, four and five years of age, the ideal operation was accomplished by Cooley and associates, who detached the coronary artery from the pulmonary artery and connected it to the aorta by means of an interposed graft (Fig. 18-52).

PATHOLOGIC ANATOMY AND PHYSIOLOGY. The disease

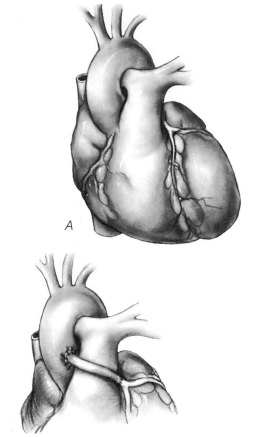

Fig. 18-52. *A.* Anomalous left coronary artery arising from pulmonary artery. *B.* Vein graft is used to anastomose coronary artery to aorta. This theoretically ideal operation has rarely been accomplished as yet. (*Adapted from D. A. Cooley et al., J Thorac Cardiovasc Surg, 52:805, 1966.*)

is a severe one, and the majority of affected children die in the first year of life. The left ventricle is usually grossly dilated, with a thin fibrotic wall showing multiple areas of infarction. Other abnormalities are secondary to chronic congestive failure. Apparently the serious physiologic handicap from origin of the left coronary artery from the pulmonary artery is the low perfusion pressure and not the low oxygen content of blood in the coronary artery, because even more severe degrees of oxygen unsaturation in severely cyanotic children do not produce gross injury to the muscle of the left ventricle. The demonstration that the flow of blood may be retrograde through the coronary artery into the pulmonary artery indicates that the anomaly actually siphons oxygenated blood away from the ischemic myocardium. Retrograde flow is proved by finding a higher oxygen content in blood in the coronary artery than in the pulmonary artery, and also by demonstrating a *rise* in pressure in the coronary artery when its origin from the pulmonary artery is occluded. Survival of a few patients beyond infancy apparently results from an abundant collateral circulation with the right coronary artery, so that the left ventricle is supplied with blood first entering the right coronary artery and then flowing through collateral

channels into tributaries of the left coronary artery. Anomalous origin of the *right* coronary artery from the pulmonary artery is apparently an innocuous condition and compatible with normal longevity.

CLINICAL MANIFESTATIONS. Dyspnea and other symptoms often appear in the first 3 months of life. Characteristically, acute episodes may occur with feeding, between which the infant is completely normal. During these episodes there may be colicky pain, tachypnea, cyanosis, pallor, and sweating, apparently a syndrome resembling angina pectoris. Subsequently, with chronic congestive failure, tachypnea becomes a chronic symptom. On examination, obvious cardiac enlargement is found, with muffled heart sounds. Frequently no murmurs are audible.

LABORATORY FINDINGS. The chest roentgenogram will confirm the extensive enlargement of the ventricle. The electrocardiogram may be diagnostic, demonstrating inversion of the T waves and prominent Q waves in certain precordial leads. The diagnosis can be confirmed by catheterization and coronary arteriography, demonstrating the abnormal origin of the left coronary artery, a small left-to-right shunt at the level of the pulmonary artery, and dilatation of the left ventricle, often with a thin wall from multiple infarctions. On angiography the right coronary artery in older children will be dilated and tortuous, with dye filling the right coronary artery and subsequently opacifying the left coronary artery.

TREATMENT. Patients should obviously be operated on as soon as the condition is recognized, for it is frequently lethal in the first year of life. Ligation of the anomalous coronary artery can be done if reconstruction is not feasible. One study by Likar and associates of 27 patients who underwent ligation of anomalous artery included 20 infants, 11 of whom died after operation; but this report, published in 1966, is surely not representative of what might be achieved with present techniques.

With present techniques of microsurgery it would seem that reconstruction should be possible in the majority of infants, using the "button" concept of detaching the anomalous left coronary artery from the pulmonary artery with a button of wall of the pulmonary artery to facilitate reconstruction. This is well discussed in the 1976 report by Doty of reconstruction in a ten-month-old child.

Cooley first demonstrated possibilities with vein-graft reconstruction of the coronary artery and in 1975 summarized his experiences with 15 patients. Though initial results have been good, long-term results with the saphenous vein graft are disappointing, probably because of the disproportion in size.

The subclavian artery would seem far preferable and at present would seem to be the ideal graft. As discussed in the report by Doty, this has been used in a variety of methods, mobilizing either the left subclavian or the right subclavian artery as in the classic subclavian–pulmonary anastomosis.

The author has successfully used a free graft of subclavian artery in one patient, placing the free arterial graft *behind* the pulmonary artery, rather than in front, which makes it possible to use a much smaller graft. A similar technique has been reported by Bahnson. Hence, at present, although few data are available, the ideal form of reconstruction would seem to be detachment of the anomalous coronary with a button of arterial wall, followed by anastomosis to the subclavian artery, either directly to the mobilized subclavian artery or as a free graft of subclavian artery, placing the subclavian graft behind the pulmonary artery, if the graft is too short to reach the aorta otherwise.

CORONARY ARTERIOVENOUS FISTULA

Information concerning this unusual anomaly was crystallized in 1960 by Gasul and associates in their collective review of 52 cases.

PATHOLOGIC ANATOMY AND PHYSIOLOGY. The abnormality consists of a direct communication between a coronary artery and a cardiac chamber through one or more abnormal openings. Usually the coronary fistula opens into the right atrium or right ventricle, constituting a left-to-right shunt. Rarely it enters the left atrium or left ventricle, causing signs of mild aortic insufficiency. With the increased blood flow through the arteriovenous fistula there is dilatation of the coronary arteries, which become progressively elongated and tortuous (Fig. 18-53). Astonishing degrees of dilatation, with vessels 1 to 2 cm in diameter, have been reported.

When the fistula opens into the right side of the heart, the resulting left-to-right shunt is small, but with subsequent dilatation of the parent artery the shunt may eventually become large enough to cause significant cardiac enlargement.

CLINICAL MANIFESTATIONS. Although the arteriovenous fistula may cause myocardial ischemia from blood preferentially flowing through the fistula rather than through the myocardial capillaries, this is uncommon. Several patients with minor hemodynamic disability have been reported living normal lives without symptoms. When the fistula is large, however, significant cardiac symptoms appear, both from the left-to-right shunt and from the myocardial ischemia.

The most common symptoms are fatigue and dyspnea. On physical examination the significant finding is a continuous murmur that seems unusually loud and superficial, especially in combination with absence of symptoms and minimal signs of cardiac disability. The location of maximal intensity of the murmur varies with the site of the fistula; it usually is at a lower level than that of the typical patent ductus arteriosus.

LABORATORY FINDINGS. The chest roentgenogram may be normal or may show only slight cardiac enlargement. Similarly, the electrocardiogram may be normal or may show minimal signs of ventricular hypertrophy. Cardiac catheterization can detect the site of the left-to-right shunt and thereby identify the chamber into which the fistula empties. The most definitive study is coronary arteriography, outlining both the site of the fistula and the course of the abnormal vessels. The degree of dilatation and tortuosity in some patients is most impressive.

TREATMENT. If a patient is asymptomatic with no signs of cardiac disability, operation is not urgent. Some have been managed simply by continued observation. However, as the usual course is continued enlargement of the fistula,

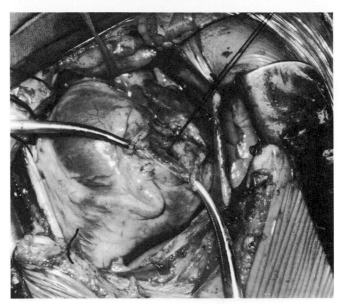

Fig. 18-53. Arteriovenous fistula of right coronary artery. Enlarged, tortuous right coronary artery is clearly visible over surface of right ventricle. Fistulous communication directly into right ventricle was found, as illustrated by ligatures, and ligated.

with progressive hemodynamic disability, elective repair is preferable in most instances (Fig. 18-54).

A 1971 review by Oldham et al. well summarized clinical experiences. In a review of over 200 reported cases, including their own personal experiences with 12 cases, 183 of the fistulas entered the right side of the heart, and only 17 entered one of the chambers of the left side. A significant point facilitating surgical treatment is the fact that almost all fistulas had a single, rather than multiple, point of entry into the heart. The shunt was seldom large, with the pulmonary blood flow usually increased to about twice normal. Congestive heart failure appeared in two age groups, either in infancy or after forty years of age. The latter group probably resulted from progressive enlargement of the fistula. However, in the overall series there was a history of congestive heart failure in only 14 percent of the patients, and angina in 7 percent.

Precise coronary angiography has greatly facilitated treatment. The single point of entry of the fistula can be identified by angiography. Surgical dissection in this area can often locate the abnormal vessel and occlude it but preserve continuity of the involved coronary artery. Of 116 reported cases undergoing operation, only four deaths have occurred.

Little change in the status of the treatment of coronary arteriovenous fistula has occurred since 1974. The author has treated one patient over fifty years of age with congestive heart failure who has subsequently remained asymptomatic in the three years since occlusion of the fistula. A few other patients have been treated at New York University with an uneventful course. In all instances it has been possible to isolate the fistula and occlude it by the combination of precise angiography and appropriate dissection at operation, maintaining continuity of the involved coronary

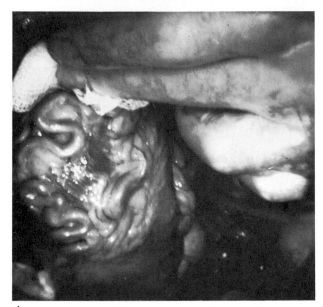

A

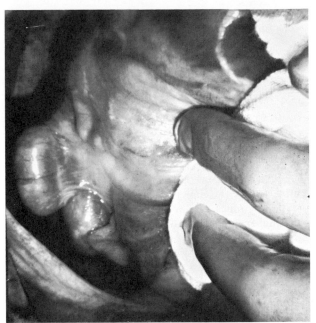

B

Fig. 18-54. *A.* Operative photograph of the tortuous coronary vessels with a coronary arteriovenous fistula in a woman in the fifth decade who was virtually asymptomatic. *B.* Operative photograph of the site of entry of the fistula into the right ventricle near the apex of the heart. This was eliminated by simple ligature.

artery. Sudden death has been reported months following closure of a fistula in a patient with large dilated coronary arteries, presumably a case of arrhythmia. This may constitute an additional indication for early operation in these patients, once the diagnosis has been made, as the risk of operation is small and the results excellent.

Corrected Transposition

This unusual anomaly has been studied in detail in recent years, principally because of the influence of its unusual anatomic features on the surgical treatment of associated cardiovascular malformations. The clinical features of the syndrome were well summarized by Anderson et al. in their report of 14 patients in 1957. An additional group of 33 cases was reported by Schiebler and associates in 1961.

PATHOLOGIC ANATOMY AND PHYSIOLOGY. In this malformation the aorta and pulmonary artery are transposed to lie in a relation exactly the opposite of that normally occurring. The aorta arises from the anterior left border of the heart and the pulmonary artery from the right and posterior area of the heart (Fig. 18-55). The ventricle from which the aorta arises has the anatomic characteristics of a normal trabeculated right ventricle, and that from which the pulmonary artery arises resembles a left ventricle. The atrioventricular valves are similarly reversed, with the tricuspid valve opening into the aortic ventricle and the mitral valve opening into the pulmonary ventricle. Venous drainage into the atria, however, is normal; so despite the abnormal anatomic relations, the circulation is normal. Venous blood returns to the right atrium, flows through the mitral valve into an anatomic "left" ventricle, and is expelled into the pulmonary artery. From the lungs blood returns through the pulmonary veins to the left atrium, flows across a tricuspid valve into an anatomic "right" ventricle, and is expelled into the aorta. The anatomic

relations of the coronary arteries are also reversed, the right coronary artery arising anteriorly and the left coronary artery posteriorly and the noncoronary sinus being located at the anterior left border of the heart.

The significance of the malformation is primarily in the high incidence of associated abnormalities, for some additional malformation is almost always present. Nadas has stated that at least 50 percent of patients with this condition have mitral insufficiency, perhaps as a result of the tricuspid valve being poorly designed to withstand systemic ventricular pressures. A ventricular septal defect is common, and a wide variety of other malformations may be seen. Conduction defects are frequent. Approximately one-third of the patients have a first- to third-degree heart block, and another third have different types of arrhythmias, such as paroxysmal atrial tachycardia.

CLINICAL MANIFESTATIONS. The symptoms are principally determined by the associated malformations. In the unusual case of "pure" corrected transposition, there are no symptoms except for those resulting from the cardiac arrhythmias. Physical examination similarly discloses no abnormalities, except that the cardiac second sound to the left of the sternum is unusually loud because it originates from closure of the aortic valve.

LABORATORY FINDINGS. On the roentgenogram there is an unusual contour at the base of the heart from the unusual relation of the great vessels, but often this is not distinctive enough to be diagnostic. The electrocardiogram is almost always abnormal and is one of the best diagnostic guides. Conduction disturbances, arrhythmias, and unusual

NORMAL

CORRECTED TRANSPOSITION

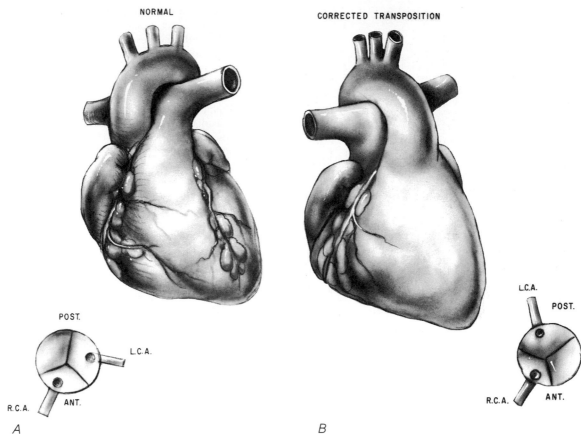

POST.

L.C.A.

R.C.A.   ANT.

A

L.C.A.

POST.

R.C.A.   ANT.

B

Fig. 18-55. *A.* Normal cardiac anatomy with pulmonary artery arising from right ventricle and aorta from left ventricle. Comparison with *B* shows that in corrected transposition, relative positions of aorta and pulmonary artery are reversed. *B.* In corrected transposition of great vessels, aorta arises anteriorly from ventricle that has anatomic characteristics of right ventricle. Pulmonary artery arises posteriorly and to right of aorta—reverse of normal anatomic arrangement. Insert depicts origin of coronary arteries in corrected transposition. (*Adapted from A. S. Nadas, "Pediatric Cardiology," W. B. Saunders Company, Philadelphia, 1964, p. 714.*)

patterns of ventricular hypertrophy in the precordial leads may all suggest the diagnosis. Diagnosis can be firmly established by angiography, which will demonstrate the aorta to the left of the pulmonary artery.

TREATMENT. The importance of this condition is predominantly related to the other anatomic defects often present. With ventricular septal defect, there is a high frequency of complete heart block, which occurs spontaneously during the course of the disease in some patients but is especially hazardous surgically because of the abnormal location of the conduction bundle. A significant contribution was reported by Waldo et al. in 1975, using electrophysiologic studies to map the course of the conduction bundle and finding the conduction system in the anterior rim of the defect. Clearly, mapping of the conduction bundle should be an important part of surgical operations performed for closure of a septal defect in patients with corrected transposition.

Kirklin and associates have had one of the most exten-

Fig. 18-56. Diagram of anomalous origin of left pulmonary artery from right pulmonary artery. Anatomic relationship of left pulmonary artery to trachea and esophagus is also shown. (*From F. L. Grover et al., J Thorac Cardiovasc Surg, 69:295, 1975.*)

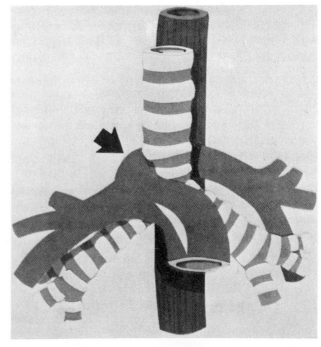

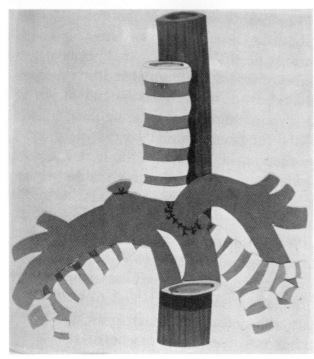

Fig. 18-57. Diagram of anatomy at completion of operation. Note that proximal stump of left pulmonary artery is to right of trachea after having been dissected free. Distal left pulmonary artery has been anastomosed to side of main pulmonary artery. (*From F. L. Grover et al., J Thorac Cardiovasc Surg, 69:295, 1975.*)

sive experiences with operations with corrected transposition, reporting 17 patients in 1976. With tetralogy of Fallot in the presence of corrected transposition, the location of the coronary vessels may preclude use of the usual operative approach, but the insertion of a valve conduit may make surgical correction possible.

In the absence of other anatomic defects, many patients with corrected transposition do well for some decades but subsequently develop mitral insufficiency and may require prosthetic valve replacement at that time.

Double Outlet Right Ventricle

Double outlet right ventricle was not included in the previous edition of this book, but significant advances have been made in the recognition of this anomaly. The classification developed by Van Praagh has been especially useful in recognizing the different variants of this syndrome, with appropriate modifications for effective surgical treatment. The reader is referred to the excellent recent article by Stewart in 1976, a collective review with 68 references, which provides an up-to-date summary of the present status of knowledge of this unusual but surgically significant lesion.

Pulmonary Artery Sling

This unusual anomaly, not included in the previous edition, is briefly mentioned here because of the facility of its recognition with modern angiography and the simplicity of surgical correction.

The condition is essentially an aberrant origin of the left pulmonary artery, arising from the right pulmonary artery and passing between the trachea and esophagus to the left lung, forming a "sling" around the distal trachea and producing respiratory distress. The anomaly is usually fatal in the first year of life if not corrected then. In 1975, Grover and associates reported data on the eighteenth survivor of correction of this anomaly (Figs. 18-56 and 18-57). In their report they mention that 63 patients with the anomaly have been reported, one-half of whom had additional anomalies. Twenty of twenty-three unoperated patients died. Twenty-six had definite anatomic correction, with eight hospital deaths and one late death.

References

General

Abbott, M. E.: "Atlas of Congenital Cardiac Disease," The American Heart Association, New York, 1936.

Benson, C. D., Mustard, W. T., Ravitch, M. M., Snyder, W. H., and Welch, K. J. (eds.): "Pediatric Surgery," 2d ed., Year Book Medical Publishers, Inc., Chicago, 1971.

Breckenridge, I. M., Oelert, H., Graham, G. R., Stark, J., Waterston, D. J., and Bonham-Carter, R. E.: Open Heart Surgery in the First Year of Life, *J Thorac Cardiovasc Surg*, **65**:58, 1973.

Cooley, D. A., and Hallman, G. L.: "Surgical Treatment of Congenital Heart Disease," Lea & Febiger, Philadelphia, 1966.

Dammann, J. F., Jr.: Pulmonary Hypertension in C. D. Benson et al. (eds.), "Pediatric Surgery," 2d ed., vol. 1, Year Book Medical Publishers, Inc., Chicago, 1971.

Edwards, J. E.: Functional Pathology of the Pulmonary Vascular Tree in Congenital Cardiac Disease, *Circulation*, **15**:164, 1957.

Gorlin, R., and Gorlin, S. G.: Hydraulic Formula for Calculation of the Area of the Stenotic Mitral Valve, Other Cardiac Valves, and Central Circulatory Shunts: I, *Am Heart J*, **41**:1, 1951.

Gross, R. E.: "The Surgery of Infancy and Childhood," W. B. Saunders Company, Philadelphia, 1953.

Keith, J. D., Rowe, R. D., and Vlad, P.: "Heart Disease in Infancy and Childhood," 2d ed., The Macmillan Company, New York, 1967.

Nadas, A. S.: "Pediatric Cardiology," 2d ed., W. B. Saunders Company, Philadelphia, 1963.

Stewart, S., III, Edmunds, L. H., Jr., Kirklin, J. W., and Allarde, R. R.: Spontaneous Breathing with Continuous Positive Airway Pressure after Open Intracardiac Operations in Infants, *J Thorac Cardiovasc Surg*, **65**:37, 1973.

Taussig, H. B.: "Congenital Malformations of the Heart," 2d ed., Harvard University Press, Cambridge, Mass., 1960.

Pulmonic Stenosis

Brock, R. C.: Pulmonary Valvulotomy for the Relief of Congenital Stenosis: Report of Three Cases, *Br Med J*, **1**:112, 1948.

Engle, M. A., Holswade, G. R., Goldberg, H. P., Lukas, D. S., and Glenn, F.: Regression after Open Valvotomy of Infundibular Stenosis Accompanying Severe Valvular Pulmonic Stenosis, *Circulation,* **17:**862, 1958.

Gilbert, J. W., Morrow, A. G., and Talbert, J. L.: The Surgical Significance of Hypertrophic Infundibular Obstruction Accompanying Valvular Pulmonic Stenosis, *J Thorac Cardiovasc Surg,* **46:**457, 1963.

Holman, E.: On Circumscribed Dilation of an Artery Immediately Distal to a Partially Occluding Band: Poststenotic Dilatation, *Surgery,* **36:**3, 1954.

Johnson, L. W., Grossman, W., Dalen, J. E., and Dexter, L.: Pulmonic Stenosis in the Adult: Longterm Followup Results, *N Engl J Med,* **287:**1159, 1972.

Nadas, A. S.: Pulmonic Stenosis: Indications for Surgery in Children and Adults, *N Engl J Med,* **287:**1196, 1972.

Pacifico, A. D., Kirklin, J. W., and Blackstone, E. H.: Primary Patch Enlargement of the Pulmonary Valve Ring in the Repair of the Tetralogy of Fallot. Paper presented at the American Association for Thoracic Surgery, Ontario, Canada, April 1977.

Sellors, T. H.: Surgery of Pulmonic Stenosis, *Lancet,* **1:**988, 1948.

Spencer, F. C., and Bahnson, H. T.: Intracardiac Surgery Employing Hypothermia and Coronary Perfusion Performed on 100 Patients, *Surgery,* **46:**987, 1959.

Swan, H., and Zeavin, I.: Cessation of Circulation in General Hypothermia, *Ann Surg,* **139:**385, 1954.

Tandon, R., Nadas, A. S., and Gross, R. E.: Results of Open Heart Surgery in Patients with Pulmonic Stenosis and Intact Ventricular Septum: A Report of 108 Cases, *Circulation,* **31:**190, 1965.

Stenosis of the Pulmonary Artery

Franch, R. H., and Gay, B. B.: Congenital Stenosis of the Pulmonary Artery Branches, *Am J Med,* **35:**512, 1963.

McGoon, D. C., and Kincaid, O. W.: Stenosis of Branches of the Pulmonary Artery: Surgical Repair, *Med Clin North Am,* **48:**1083, 1964.

Wallsh, E., Reppert, E. H., Doyle, E. F., and Spencer, F. C.: "Absent" Left Pulmonary Artery with Tetralogy of Fallot, *J Thorac Cardiovasc Surg,* **55:**333, 1968.

Congenital Aortic Stenosis

Braunwald, E., Goldblatt, A., Aygen, M. M., Rockoff, S. D., and Morrow, A. G.: Congenital Aortic Stenosis: Clinical and Hemodynamic Findings in 100 patients, *Circulation,* **27:**426, 1963.

Braverman, I. B., and Gibson, S.: The Outlook for Children with Congenital Aortic Stenosis, *Am Heart J,* **53:**487, 1957.

Frahm, C. J., Braunwald, E., and Morrow, A. G.: Congenital Aortic Regurgitation: Findings in Four Patients, *Am J Med,* **31:**63, 1961.

Lawson, R. M., Bonchek, L. I., Menashe, V., and Starr, A.: Late Results of Surgery for Left Ventricular Outflow Tract Obstruction in Children, *J Thorac Cardiovasc Surg,* **71:**334, 1976.

Peckham, G. B., Keith, J. D., and Evans, J. R.: Congenital Aortic Stenosis: Some Observations on the Natural History and Clinical Assessment, *J Can Med Assoc,* **90:**639, 1964.

Spencer, F. C., Neill, C. A., and Bahnson, H. T.: The Treatment of Congenital Aortic Stenosis with Valvulotomy during Cardiopulmonary Bypass, *Surgery,* **44:**109, 1958.

———, ———, Sank, L., and Bahnson, H. T.: Anatomical Varia-

tions in 46 Patients with Congenital Aortic Stenosis, *Am Surg,* **26:**204, 1960.

Supravalvular Aortic Stenosis

Bernhard W. F., Poirier, V., and LaFarge, C. G.: Relief of Congenital Obstruction to Left Ventricular Outflow with Ventricular-Aortic Prosthesis, *J Thorac Cardiovasc Surg,* **20:**136, 1975.

Dembitsky, W. P., and Weldon, C. S.: Clinical Experience with the Use of a Valve-bearing Conduit to Construct a Second Left Ventricular Outflow Tract in Cases of Unresectable Intraventricular Obstruction, *Ann Surg,* **184:**317, 1976.

Doty, D. B., Polansky, D. B., and Jensen, C. B.: Supravalvular Aortic Stenosis: Repair by Extended Aortoplasty. Paper presented at the American Association for Thoracic Surgery, Ontario, Canada, April 1977.

Keane, J. F., Fellows, K. E., LaFarge, C. G., Nadas, A. S., and Bernhard, W. F.: The Surgical Management of Discrete and Diffuse Supravalvar Aortic Stenosis, *Circulation,* **54:**112, 1976.

Morrow, A. G., Waldhausen, J. A., Peters, R. L., Bloodwell, R. D., and Braunwald, E.: Supravalvular Aortic Stenosis, *Circulation,* **20:**1003, 1959.

Peterson, T. A., Todd, D. C., and Edwards, J. E.: Supravalvular Aortic Stenosis, *J Thorac Cardiovasc Surg,* **50:**734, 1965.

Rastelli, G. C., McGoon, D. C., Ongley, P. A., Mankin, H. T., and Kirklin, J. W.: Surgical Treatment of Supravalvular Aortic Stenosis: Report of 16 Cases and Review of Literature, *J Thorac Cardiovasc Surg,* **51:**873, 1966.

Williams, J. C. P., Barratt-Boyes, B. G., and Lowe, J. B.: Supravalvular Aortic Stenosis, *Circulation,* **24:**1311, 1961.

Idiopathic Hypertrophic Subaortic Stenosis

Barratt-Boyes, B. G., Neutze, J. M., and Harris, E. A. (eds.): "Heart Disease in Infancy," The Williams and Wilkins Company, Baltimore, 1973.

Bigelow, W. G., Trimble, A. S., Auger, P., Marquis, Y., and Wigle, E. D.: The Ventriculomyotomy Operation for Muscular Subaortic Stenosis: A Reappraisal, *J Thorac Cardiovasc Surg,* **52:**514, 1966.

Braunwald, E., Brockenbrough, E. C., and Morrow, A. G.: Hypertrophic Subaortic Stenosis: A Broadened Concept, *Circulation,* **26:**161, 1962. (Editorial.)

Frye, R. L., Kincaid, O. W., Swan, H. J. C., and Kirklin, J. W.: Results of Surgical Treatment of Patients with Diffuse Subvalvular Aortic Stenosis, *Circulation,* **32:**52, 1965.

Kelly, D. T., Barratt-Boyes, B. G., and Lowe, J. B.: Results of Surgery and Hemodynamic Observations in Muscular Subaortic Stenosis, *J Thorac Cardiovasc Surg,* **51:**353, 1966.

Kirklin, J. W., in B. G. Barratt-Boyes, J. M. Neutze, and E. A. Harris (eds.): "Heart Disease in Infancy," The Williams and Wilkins Company, Baltimore, 1973.

Konno, S., Imai, Y., Iada, Y., Nakajima, M., and Tatsuno, K.: New Method for Prosthetic Valve Replacement in Congenital Aortic Stenosis Associated with Hypoplasia of the Aortic Valve Ring, *J Thorac Cardiovasc Surg,* **70:**909, 1975.

Morrow, A. G., Reitz, B. A., Epstein, S. E., Henry, W. L., Conkle, D. M., Itscoitz, S. B., and Redwood, D. R.: Operative Treatment in Hypertrophic Subaortic Stenosis: Technics and Results of Pre- and Postoperative Assessments in 83 Patients, *Circulation,* **52:**88, 1975.

Coarctation of the Aorta

Abbott, M. E.: Coarctation of the Aorta of the Adult Type: II. A Statistical Study and Historical Retrospect of 200 Recorded Cases, with Autopsy, of Stenosis or Obliteration of the Descending Arch in Subjects above the Age of Two Years, *Am Heart J,* **3**:392, 1928.

Allard, J. R., Williams, R. L., and Dobell, A. R. C.: Interrupted Aortic Arch: Factors Influencing Prognosis, *Ann Thorac Surg,* **21**:243, 1976.

Blalock, A., and Park, E. A.: The Surgical Treatment of Experimental Coarctation (Atresia) of the Aorta, *Ann Surg,* **119**:445, 1944.

Brewer, L. A., III, Fosburg, R. G., Mulder, A. G., and Verska, J. J.: Spinal Cord Complications following Surgery for Coarctation of the Aorta: A Study of 66 Cases, *J Thorac Cardiovasc Surg,* **64**:368, 1972.

Brom, A. G.: Narrowing of the Aortic Isthmus and Enlargement of the Mind, *J Thorac Cardiovasc Surg,* **50**:166, 1965.

Crafoord, C., and Nylin, G.: Congenital Coarctation of the Aorta and Its Surgical Treatment, *J Thorac Surg,* **14**:347, 1945.

DeBakey, M. E., Garrett, H. E., Howell, J. F., and Morris, G. C.: Coarctation of the Abdominal Aorta with Renal Arterial Stenosis: Surgical Considerations, *Ann Surg,* **165**:830, 1967.

Fishman, N. H., Bronstein, M. H., Berman, W., Roe, B. B., et al.: Surgical Management of Severe Aortic Coarctation and Interrupted Aortic Arch in Neonates, *J Thorac Cardiovasc Surg,* **71**:35, 1976.

Gross, R. E.: Coarctation of the Aorta: Surgical Treatment of One Hundred Cases, *Circulation,* **1**:41, 1950.

Hughes, R. K., and Reemtsma, K.: Correction of Coarctation of the Aorta: Manometric Determination of Safety during Test Occlusion, *J Thorac Cardiovasc Surg,* **62**:31, 1971.

Schuster, S. R., and Gross, R. E.: Surgery for Coarctation of the Aorta: A Review of 500 Cases, *J Thor Cardiovasc Surg,* **43**:54, 1962.

Sealy, W. C., Harris, J. S., Young, W. G., and Callaway, H. A.: Paradoxical Hypertension following Resection of Coarctation of the Aorta, *Surgery,* **42**:135, 1957.

Vascular Rings

Gross, R. E.: Arterial Malformations Which Cause Compression of the Trachea or Esophagus, *Circulation,* **11**:124, 1955.

Mahoney, E. B., and Manning, J. A.: Congenital Abnormalities of the Aortic Arch, *Surgery,* **55**:1, 1964.

Shumacker, H. B., Jr., and Burford, T. H.: Unusual Sequel to Operative Intervention for Vascular Ring, *J Thorac Cardiovasc Surg,* **65**:124, 1973.

Atrial Septal Defects: Secundum Defects

Gerbode, F., Harkins, G. A., Ross, J. K., and Osborn, J. J.: Experience with Atrial Septal Defects Repaired with the Aid of Cardiopulmonary Bypass, *Arch Surg,* **80**:846, 1960.

Gibbon, J. H., Jr.: Application of a Mechanical Heart and Lung Apparatus to Cardiac Surgery, *Minn Med,* **37**:171, 1954.

Sellers, R. D., Ferlic, R. M., Sterns, L. P., and Lillehei, C. W.: Secundum Type Atrial Septal Defects: Results with 275 Patients, *Surgery,* **59**:155, 1966.

Spencer, F. C., and Bahnson, H. T.: Intracardiac Surgery Employing Hypothermia and Coronary Perfusion Performed on 100 Patients, *Surgery,* **46**:987, 1959.

Anomalous Drainage of Pulmonary Veins

Bahnson, H. T., Spencer, F. C., and Neill, C. A.: Surgical Treatment of 35 Cases of Drainage of Pulmonary Veins to the Right Side of the Heart, *J Thorac Cardiovasc Surg,* **36**:777, 1958.

Blake, H. A., Hall, R. C., and Manion, W. C.: Anomalous Pulmonary Venous Return, *Circulation,* **32**:406, 1965.

Brody, H.: Drainage of the Pulmonary Veins into the Right Side of the Heart, *Arch Pathol,* **33**:221, 1942.

Cooley, D. A., Hallman, G. L., and Leachman, R. D.: Total Anomalous Pulmonary Venous Drainage, *J Thorac Cardiovasc Surg,* **51**:88, 1966.

——, and Ochsner, A., Jr.: Correction of Total Anomalous Pulmonary Venous Drainage: Technical Considerations, *Surgery,* **42**:1014, 1957.

Darling, R. C., Rothney, W. B., and Craig, J. M.: Total Pulmonary Venous Drainage into the Right Side of the Heart: Report of 17 Autopsied Cases Not Associated with Other Major Cardiovascular Anomalies, *Lab Invest,* **6**:44, 1957.

El-Said, G., Mullins, C. E., and McNamara, J. J.: Management of Total Anomalous Pulmonary Venous Return, *Circulation,* **45**:1240, 1972.

Gott, V. L., Lester, R. G., Lillehei, C. W., and Varco, R. L.: Total Anomalous Pulmonary Venous Return: An Analysis of 30 Cases, *Circulation,* **13**:543, 1956.

Muller, W. H.: Surgical Treatment of Transposition of Pulmonary Veins, *Ann Surg,* **134**:683, 1951.

Wukasch, D. C., Deutsch, M., Reul, G. J., Hallman, G. L., and Cooley, D. A.: Total Anomalous Pulmonary Venous Return, *Ann Thorac Surg,* **19**:622, 1975.

Ostium Primum Defect and Persistent Atrioventricular Canal

Alfieri, O., and Subramanian, S.: Successful Repair of Complete Atrioventricular Canal with Undivided Anterior Common Leaflet in a Six-month-old Infant, *Ann Thorac Surg,* **19**:92, 1975.

Blount, S. G., Jr., Balchum, O. J., and Gensini, G.: Persistent Ostium Primum Atrial Septal Defect, *Circulation,* **13**:499, 1956.

Braunwald, N. S., and Morrow, A. G.: Incomplete Persistent Atrioventricular Canal, *J Thorac Cardiovasc Surg,* **51**:71, 1966.

Castaneda, A. R., Nicoloff, D. M., Moller, J. H., and Lucas, R. V., Jr.: Surgical Correction of Complete Atrioventricular Canal Utilizing Ball-Valve Replacement of the Mitral Valve: Technical Considerations, *J Thorac Cardiovasc Surg,* **62**:926, 1971.

Cooley, D. A., and Hallman, G. L.: "Surgical Treatment of Congenital Heart Disease," Lea & Febiger, Philadelphia, 1966.

Gerbode, F., Sanchez, P. A., Arguero, R., Kerth, W. J., Hill, J. D., and deVries, P. A.: Endocardial Cushion Defects, *Ann Surg,* **167**:486, 1967.

Levy, M. J., Cuello, L., Tuna, N., and Lillehei, C. W.: Atrioventricularis Communis, *Am J Cardiol,* **14**:587, 1964.

McGoon, D. C.: Atrioventricular Canal, in D. C. Sabiston and F. C. Spencer (eds.), "Gibbon's Surgery of the Chest," W. B. Saunders Company, Philadelphia, 1976.

McMullan, M. H., McGoon, D. C., Wallace, R. B., Danielson, G. K., and Weidman, W. H.: Surgical Treatment of Partial Atrioventricular Canal, *Arch Surg,* **107**:705, 1973.

Mills, N. L., Ochsner, J. L., and King, K. D.: Correction of Type C Complete Atrioventricular Canal: Surgical Considerations, *J Thorac Cardiovasc Surg,* **71:**20, 1976.

Neill, C. A.: Postoperative Hemolytic Anemia in Endocardial Cushion Defects, *Circulation,* **30:**801, 1964.

Rastelli, G. C., Kirklin, J. W., and Titus, J. L.: Anatomic Observations on Complete Form of Persistent Common Atrioventricular Canal with Special Reference to Atrioventricular Valves, *Mayo Clin Proc,* **41:**296, 1966.

———, Weidman, W. H., and Kirklin, J. W.: Surgical Repair of the Partial Form of Persistent Common Atrioventricular Canal, with Special Reference to the Problem of Mitral Valve Incompetence, *Circulation,* **31:**31, 1965.

Ventricular Septal Defect

Barratt-Boyes, B. G., Neutze, J. M., Clarkson, P. M., Shardey, G. C., and Brandt, P. W. T.: Repair of Ventricular Septal Defect in the First Two Years of Life Using Profound Hypothermia–Circulatory Arrest Technics, *Ann Surg,* **184:**376, 1976.

Bloomfield, D. K.: The Natural History of Ventricular Septal Defect in Patients Surviving Infancy, *Circulation,* **29:**914, 1964.

Cartmill, T. B., DuShane, J. W., McGoon, D. C., and Kirklin, J. W.: Results of Repair of Ventricular Septal Defect, *J Thorac Cardiovasc Surg,* **52:**486, 1966.

Cooley, D. A., and Hallman, G. L.: "Surgical Treatment of Congenital Heart Disease," Lea & Febiger, Philadelphia, 1966.

Hallman, G. L., Cooley, D. A., and Bloodwell, R. D.: Two-stage Surgical Treatment of Ventricular Septal Defect: Results of Pulmonary Artery Banding in Infants and Subsequent Open-Heart Repair, *J Thorac Cardiovasc Surg,* **52:**476, 1966.

———, ———, Wolff, R. R., and McNamara, D. G.: Surgical Treatment of Ventricular Septal Defect Associated with Pulmonary Hypertension, *J Thorac Cardiovasc Surg,* **48:**588, 1964.

Lillehei, C. W., Anderson, R. C., Eliot, R. S., Wang, Y., and Ferlic, R. M.: Pre- and Postoperative Cardiac Catheterization in 200 Patients Undergoing Closure of Ventricular Septal Defects, *Surgery,* **63:**69, 1968.

———, Sellers, R. D., Bonnabeau, R. C., Jr., and Eliot, R. S.: Chronic Postsurgical Complete Heart Block: With Particular Reference to Prognosis, Management, and a New P-Wave Pacemaker, *J Thorac Cardiovasc Surg,* **46:**436, 1963.

McGoon, D. C.: Closure of Patent Ductus during Open-Heart Surgery, *J Thorac Cardiovasc Surg,* **48:**456, 1964.

Spencer, F. C., Doyle, E. F., Danilowicz, D. A., Bahnson, H. T., and Weldon, C. S.: Longterm Evaluation of Aortic Valvuloplasty for Aortic Insufficiency and Ventricular Septal Defect, *J Thorac Cardiovasc Surg,* **65:**15, 1973.

Walker, W. J., Garcia-Gonzalez, E., Hall, R. J., Czarnecki, S. W., Franklin, R. B., Das, S. K., and Cheitlin, M. D.: Interventricular Septal Defect: Analysis of 415 Catheterized Cases, *Circulation,* **31:**54, 1965.

Wood, P.: The Eisenmenger Syndrome, *Br Med J,* **2:**701, 1958.

Patent Ductus Arteriosus

Blalock, A.: Operative Closure of the Patent Ductus Arteriosus, *Surg Gynecol Obstet,* **82:**113, 1946.

Dammann, J. F., Jr.: Berthrong, M., and Bing, R. J.: Reverse Ductus, *Bull Johns Hopkins Hosp,* **92:**128, 1953.

Gross, R. E.: "The Surgery of Infancy and Childhood: Its Principles and Techniques," W. B. Saunders Company, Philadelphia, 1953.

——— and Hubbard, J. P.: Surgical Ligation of a Patent Ductus Arteriosus: Report of First Successful Case, *JAMA,* **112:**729, 1939.

Jones, J. C.: Twenty-five Years Experience with the Surgery of Patent Ductus Arteriosus, *J Thorac Cardiovasc Surg,* **50:**149, 1965.

Touroff, A. S. W., and Vesell, H.: Subacute Streptococcus Viridans Endarteritis Complicating Patent Ductus Arteriosus: Recovery following Surgical Treatment, *JAMA,* **115:**1270, 1940.

Tetralogy of Fallot

Bahnson, H. T., Spencer, F. C., and Neill, C. A.: Surgical Treatment and Follow-up of 147 Cases of Tetralogy of Fallot Treated by Correction, *J Thorac Cardiovasc Surg,* **44:**419, 1962.

Blalock, A.: Surgical Procedures Employed and Anatomical Variations Encountered in the Treatment of Congenital Pulmonic Stenosis, *Surg Gynecol Obstet,* **87:**385, 1948.

——— and Taussig, H. B.: The Surgical Treatment of Malformations of the Heart in Which There Is Pulmonary Stenosis or Pulmonary Atresia, *JAMA,* **128:**189, 1945.

Brock, R. C.: Pulmonary Valvulotomy for the Relief of Congenital Pulmonary Stenosis: Report of Three Cases, *Br Med J,* **1:**1121, 1948.

Chiariello, L., Meyer, J., Wukasch, D. C., Hallman, G. L., and Cooley, D. A.: Intracardiac Repair of Tetralogy of Fallot, *J Thorac Cardiovasc Surg,* **70:**529, 1975.

Cooley, D. A., and Hallman, G. L.: "Surgical Treatment of Congenital Heart Disease," Lea & Febiger, Philadelphia, 1966.

Ebert, P. A., and Sabiston, D. C.: Surgical Management of the Tetralogy of Fallot: Influence of a Previous Systemic-Pulmonary Anastomosis on the Results of Open Correction, *Ann Surg,* **165:**806, 1967.

Edmunds, L. H., Saxena, N. C., Friedman, S., Rashkind, W. J., and Dodd, P. F.: Transatrial Resection of the Obstructed Right Ventricular Infundibulum, *Circulation,* **54:**117, 1976.

Kirklin, J. W.: "Tetralogy of Fallot," W. B. Saunders Company, Philadelphia, 1971.

———, Wallace, R. B., McGoon, D. C., and DuShane, J. W.: Early and Late Results after Intracardiac Repair of Tetralogy of Fallot, *Ann Surg,* **162:**578, 1965.

Lillehei, C. W., Levy, M. J., Adams, P., and Anderson, R. C.: Corrective Surgery of Tetralogy of Fallot: Longterm Follow-up by Postoperative Recatheterization in 69 Cases and Certain Surgical Considerations, *J Thorac Cardiovasc Surg,* **48:**556, 1964.

Malm, J. R., Blumenthal, S., Bowman, F. O., Jr., Ellis, K., Jameson, A. G., Jesse, M. J., and Yeoh, C. B.: Factors That Modify Hemodynamic Results in Total Correction of Tetralogy of Fallot, *J Thorac Cardiovasc Surg,* **52:**502, 1966.

Potts, W. J., Smith, S., and Gibson, S.: Anastomosis of the Aorta to a Pulmonary Artery: Certain Types in Congenital Heart Disease, *JAMA,* **132:**627, 1946.

Shumway, N. E., Lower, R. R., Hurley, E. J., and Pillsbury, R. C.: Results of Total Surgical Correction of Fallot's Tetralogy, *Circulation,* **31:**I-57, 1965.

Wolf, M. D., Landtman, B., Neill, C. A., and Taussig, H. B.: Total

Correction of Tetralogy of Fallot: Follow-up Study of 104 Cases, *Circulation,* **31:**385, 1965.

Transposition of the Great Vessels

Baffes, T. G., Riker, W. L., Boer, A. D., and Potts, W. J.: Surgical Correction of Transposition of the Aorta and the Pulmonary Artery, *J Thorac Cardiovasc Surg,* **34:**469, 1957.

Barratt-Boyes, B. G., Neutze, J. M., and Harris, E. A.: "Heart Disease in Infancy," The Williams and Wilkins Company, Baltimore, 1973.

Blalock, A., and Hanlon, C. R.: The Surgical Treatment of Complete Transposition of the Aorta and the Pulmonary Artery, *Surg Gynecol Obstet,* **90:**1, 1950.

Cooley, D. A., Hallman, G. L., Bloodwell, R. D., and Leachman, R. D.: Two Stage Surgical Treatment of Complete Transposition of the Great Vessels, *Arch Surg,* **93:**704, 1966.

Cornell, W. P., Maxwell, R. E., Haller, J. A., and Sabiston, D. C.: Results of the Blalock-Hanlon Operation in 90 Patients with Transposition of the Great Vessels, *J Thor Cardiovasc Surg,* **52:**525, 1966.

Edwards, W. S., Bargeron, L. M., and Lyons, C.: Reposition of Right Pulmonary Veins in Transposition of Great Vessels, *JAMA,* **188:**522, 1964,

Glenn, W. W. L., Ordway, N. K., Talner, N. S., and Call, E. P.: Circulatory Bypass of the Right Side of the Heart, *Circulation,* **31:**172, 1965.

Godman, M. J., Friedli, B., Pasternac, A., Kidd, B. S. L., Trusler, G. A., and Mustard, W. T.: Hemodynamic Studies in Children Four to Ten Years after the Mustard Operation for Transposition of the Great Arteries, *Circulation,* **53:**532, 1976.

Hanlon, C. R., and Blalock, A.: Complete Transposition of Aorta and Pulmonary Artery: Experimental Observations on Venous Shunts as Corrective Procedures, *Ann Surg,* **127:**385, 1948.

Hermann, V., Laks, H., Kaiser, G. C., Barner, H. B., and Willman, V. L.: The Blalock-Hanlon Procedure: Simple Transposition of the Great Arteries, *Arch Surg,* **110:**1387, 1975.

Jatene, A. D., Fontes, V. F., Paulista, P. P., et al.: Successful Anatomic Correction of Transposition of the Great Vessels: A Preliminary Report, *Arq Bras Cardiol,* **28:**461, 1975.

McGoon, D. C.: Intraventricular Repair of Transposition of the Great Arteries, *J Thorac Cardiovasc Surg,* **64:**430, 1972.

Merendino, K. H., Jesseph, J. E., Herron, P. W., Thomas, G. I., and Vetto, R. R.: Interatrial Venous Transposition, *Surgery,* **42:**898, 1957.

Moss, A. J., Maloney, J. V., Jr., and Adams, F. H.: Transposition of the Great Vessels, *Ann Surg,* **153:**183, 1961.

Mustard, W. T.: Progress in the Total Correction of Complete Transposition of the Great Vessels, *Vasc Dis,* **3:**177, 1966.

———, Keith, J. D., Trusler, G. A., Fowler, R., and Kidd, L.: The Surgical Management of Transposition of the Great Vessels, *J Thorac Cardiovasc Surg,* **48:**953, 1964.

Senning, A.: Surgical Correction of Transposition of the Great Vessels, *Surgery,* **45:**966, 1959.

———: Surgical Correction of Transposition of the Great Vessels, *Surgery,* **59:**334, 1966.

Stark, J., de Leval, M. R., Waterston, D. J., Graham, G. R., and Bonham-Carter, R. E.: Corrective Surgery of Transposition of the Great Arteries in the First Year of Life, *J Thorac Cardiovasc Surg,* **67:**673, 1974.

Tricuspid Atresia

Fontan, F., and Baudet, E.: Surgical Repair of Tricuspid Atresia, *Thorax,* **26:**240, 1971.

Glenn, W. W. L., Ordway, N. K., Talner, N. S., and Capp, E. P.: Circulatory Bypass of the Right Side of the Heart: Shunt between Superior Vena Cava and Distal Right Pulmonary Artery; Report of Clinical Application in 38 Cases, *Circulation,* **31:**172, 1965.

Kyger, E. R., Reul, G. J., Sandiford, F. M., Wukasch, D. C., Hallman, G. L., and Cooley, D. A.: Surgical Palliation of Tricuspid Atresia, *Circulation,* **52:**685, 1975.

Williams, W. G., Rubis, L., Trusler, G. A., and Mustard, W. T.: Palliation of Tricuspid Atresia, *Arch Surg,* **110:**1383, 1975.

Cor Triatriatum

Grondin, C., Leonard, A. S., Anderson, R. C., Amplatz, K. A., Edwards, J. E., and Varco, R. L.: Cor Triatriatum: A Diagnostic Surgical Enigma, *J Thorac Cardiovasc Surg,* **48:**527, 1964.

McGuire, L. B., Nolan, T. B., Reede, R., and Dammann, J. F.: Cor Triatriatum as a Problem of Adult Heart Disease, *Circulation,* **31:**263, 1965.

Niwayama, G.: Cor Triatriatum, *Am Heart J,* **59:**291, 1960.

Oglietti, J., Reul, G. J., Leachman, R. D., and Cooley, D. A.: Supravalvular Stenosing Ring of the Left Atrium, *Am Thorac Surg,* **21:**421, 1976.

Congenital Mitral Stenosis

Carpentier, A., Branchini, B., Cour, J. C., Asfaou, E., et al.: Congenital Malformations of the Miral Valve in Children, *J Thorac Cardiovasc Surg,* **72:**854, 1976.

Daoud, G., Kaplan, S., Perrin, E. V., Dorst, J. P., and Edwards, F. K.: Congenital Mitral Stenosis, *Circulation,* **27:**185, 1963.

Ferencz, C., Johnson, A. L., and Wiglesworth, F. W.: Congenital Mitral Stenosis, *Circulation,* **9:**161, 1954.

Khalil, K. G., Shapiro, I., and Kilman, J. W.: Congenital Mitral Stenosis, *J Thorac Cardiovasc Surg,* **70:**40, 1975.

Tsuji, H. K., Shapiro, M., Redington, J. V., and Kay, J. H.: Congenital Mitral Stenosis: Report of Two Cases and Review of the Literature, *J Thorac Cardiovasc Surg,* **53:**850, 1967.

Aortic-Pulmonary Window

Clarke, C. P., and Richardson, J. P.: The Management of Aortopulmonary Window, *J Thorac Cardiovasc Surg,* **72:**48, 1976.

Cooley, D. A., McNamara, D. G., and Latson, J. R.: Aorticopulmonary Septal Defect, *Surgery,* **42:**101, 1957.

Gross, R. E.: Surgical Closure of an Aortic Septal Defect, *Circulation,* **5:**858, 1952.

Morrow, A. G., Greenfield, L. J., and Braunwald, E.: Congenital Aortopulmonary Septal Defect: Clinical and Hemodynamic Findings, Surgical Technique, and Results of Operative Correction, *Circulation,* **25:**463, 1962.

Putnam, T. C., and Gross, R. E.: Surgical Management of Aortopulmonary Fenestration, *Surgery,* **59:**727, 1966.

Scott, H. W., and Sabiston, D. C.: Surgical Treatment for Congenital Aortico-pulmonary Fistula, *J Thorac Cardiovasc Surg,* **25:**26, 1953.

Skall-Jensen, J.: Congenital Aortico-pulmonary Fistula: A Review of the Literature and Report of Two Cases, *Acta Med Scand,* **160:**221, 1958.

Ruptured Aneurysm of Sinus of Valsalva

Gerbode, F., Osborn, J. J., Johnston, J. B., and Kerth, W. J.: Transaortic Approach for the Repair of Ruptured Aneurysms of the Sinus of Valsalva, *Ann Surg,* **161**:946, 1965.

Lillehei, C. W., Stanley, P., and Varco, R. L.: Surgical Treatment of Ruptured Aneurysms of the Sinus of Valsalva, *Ann Surg,* **146**:459, 1957.

Paton, B. C., MacMahon, R. A., Swan, H., and Blount, S. G.: Ruptured Sinus of Valsalva, *Arch Surg,* **90**:209, 1965.

Sawyer, J. L., Adams, J. E., and Scott, H. W.: Surgical Treatment for Aneurysms of Aortic Sinuses with Aorticoatrial Fistula, *Surgery,* **41**:126, 1957.

Shumacker, H. B., King, H., and Waldhausen, J. A.: Transaortic Approach for the Repair of Ruptured Aneurysms of the Sinus of Valsalva, *Ann Surg,* **161**:946, 1965.

Spencer, F. C.,Blake, H. A., and Bahnson, H. T.: Surgical Repair of Ruptured Aneurysm of Sinus of Valsalva in Two Patients, *Ann Surg,* **162**:963, 1960.

Truncus Arteriosus

Applebaum, A., Bargeron, L. M., Pacifico, A. D., and Kirklin, J. W.: Surgical Treatment of Truncus Arteriosus with Emphasis on Infants and Small Children, *J Thorac Cardiovasc Surg,* **71**:436, 1976.

Ebert, P. A., Robinson, S. J., Stanger, P., and Engle, M. A.: Pulmonary Artery Conduits in Infants Younger than Six Months of Age, *J Thorac Cardiovasc Surg,* **72**:351, 1976.

Marcelletti, C., McGoon, D. C., and Mair, D. D.: The Natural History of Truncus Arteriosus, *Circulation,* **54**:108, 1976.

McGoon, D. C., Wallace, R. B., and Danielson, G. K.: The Rastelli Operation: Its Indications and Results, *J Thorac Cardiovasc Surg,* **65**:65, 1973.

Poirier, R. A., Berman, M. A., and Stansel, H. C.: Current Status of the Surgical Treatment of Truncus Arteriosus, *J Thorac Cardiovasc Surg,* **69**:169, 1975.

Single Ventricle

Campbell, M. G., Reynolds, G., and Trounce, J. R.: Six Cases of Single Ventricle with Pulmonary Stenosis, *Guys Hosp Rep,* **102**:99, 1953.

Edie, R. N., and Malm, J. R.: Surgical Repair of Single Ventricle, *J Thorac Cardiovasc Surg,* **66**:350, 1973.

———— and ————: Surgical Repair of Single Ventricle, in B. S. L. Kidd and R. D. Rowe (eds.): "The Child with Congenital Heart Disease after Surgery," Futura Publishing Co., Mount Kisco, N.Y., 1976.

McGoon, D. C., Danielson, G. K., Ritter, D. G., Wallace, R. B., Maloney, J. D., and Marcelletti, C.: Correction of the Univentricular Heart Having Two Atrioventricular Valves, *J Thorac Cardiovasc Surg,* **74**:218, 1977.

Ebstein's Anomaly

Bahnson, H. T., Bauersfeld, S. R., and Smith, J. W.: Pathological Anatomy and Surgical Correction of Ebstein's Anomaly, *Circulation,* **31**(*Suppl 1*):3, 1965.

Barnard, C. N., and Schrire, V.: Surgical Correction of Ebstein's Malformation with Prosthetic Tricuspid Valve, *Surgery,* **54**:302, 1963.

Hardy, K. L., May, I. A., Webster, C. A., and Kimball, K. G.: Ebstein's Anomaly: A Functional Concept and Successful Definitive Repair, *J Thorac Cardiovasc Surg,* **48**:927, 1964.

Hunter, S. W., and Lillehei, C. W.: Ebstein's Malformation of the Tricuspid Valve, *Dis Chest,* **33**:297, 1958.

Timmis, H. H., Hardy, J. D., and Watson, D. G.: The Surgical Management of Ebstein's Anomaly, *J Thorac Cardiovasc Surg,* **53**:385, 1967.

Vacca, J. B., Bussmann, D. W., and Mudd, J. G.: Ebstein's Anomaly: Complete Review of 108 Cases, *Am J Cardiol,* **2**:210, 1958.

Anomalous Origin of Left Coronary Artery from Pulmonary Artery

Bland, E. F., White, P. D., and Garland, J.: Congenital Anomalies of Coronary Arteries: Report of an Unusual Case Associated with Cardiac Hypertrophy, *Am Heart J,* **8**:787, 1933.

Chiarello, L., Meyer, J., Reul, G. J., Hallman, G. L., and Cooley, D. A.: Surgical Treatment for Anomalous Origin of Left Coronary Artery from Pulmonary Artery, *Am Thorac Surg,* **19**:443, 1975.

Cooley, D. A., Hallman, G. L., and Bloodwell, R. D.: Definitive Surgical Treatment of Anomalous Origin of Left Coronary Artery from Pulmonary Artery, *J Thorac Cardiovasc Surg,* **52**:798, 1966.

Doty, D. B., Chandramouli, B., Schieken, Lauer, R. M., and Ehrenhaft, J. L.: Anomalous Origin of the Left Coronary Artery from the Right Pulmonary Artery, *J Thorac Cardiovasc Surg,* **71**:787, 1976.

Likar, I., Criley, J. M., and Lewis, K. B.: Anomalous Left Coronary Artery Arising from the Pulmonary Artery in Adults: A Review of the Therapeutic Problems, *Circulation,* **33**:727, 1966.

Neches, W. H., Matthews, R. A., Park, S. C., Lenox, C. C. et al.: Anomalous Origin of the Left Coronary Artery from the Pulmonary Artery: A New Method of Surgical Repair, *Circulation,* **50**:582, 1974.

Sabiston, D. C., Neill, C. A., and Taussig, H. B.: The Direction of Blood Flow in Anomalous Left Coronary Artery Arising from the Pulmonary Artery, *Circulation,* **22**:591, 1960.

Coronary Arteriovenous Fistula

Effler, D. B., Sheldon, W. C., Turner, J. J., and Groves, L. K.: Coronary Arteriovenous Fistulas: Diagnosis and Surgical Management; Report of Fifteen Cases, *Surgery,* **61**:41, 1967.

Gasul, B. M., Arcilla, R. A., Fell, E. H., Lynfield, J., Bicoff, J. P., and Luan, L. L.: Congenital Coronary Arteriovenous Fistula: Clinical, Phonocardiographic, Angiocardiographic, and Hemodynamic Studies in Five Patients, *Pediatrics,* **25**:531, 1960.

Hallman, G. L., Cooley, D. A., and Singer, D. B.: Congenital Anomalies of the Coronary Arteries: Anatomy, Pathology, and Surgical Treatment, *Surgery,* **59**:133, 1966.

Oldham, H. N., Jr., Ebert, P. A., Young, W. G., and Sabiston, D. C., Jr.: Surgical Management of Congenital Coronary Arteriovenous Fistula, *Ann Thorac Surg,* **12**:503, 1971.

Corrected Transposition

Anderson, R. C., Lillehei, C. W., and Lester, R. G.: Corrected Transposition of the Great Vessels of the Heart: A Review of 17 Cases, *Pediatrics,* **20**:626, 1957.

Fox, L. S., Kirklin, J. W., Pacifico, A. D., Waldo, A. L., and Bargeron, L. M.: Intracardiac Repair of Cardiac Malformations with Atrioventricular Discordance, *Circulation,* **54:**123, 1976.

Schiebler, G. L., Edwards, J. E., Burchell, H. B., DuShane, J. W., Ongley, P. A., and Wood, E. H.: Congenital Corrected Transposition of the Great Vessels: A Study of 33 Cases, *Pediatrics,* **27:**851, 1961.

Waldo, A. L., Pacifico, A. D., Bargeron, L. M., James, T. N., and Kirklin, J. W.: Electrophysiological Delineation of the Specialized A-V Conduction System in Patients with Corrected Transposition of the Great Vessels and Ventricular Septal Defect, *Circulation,* **52:**435, 1975.

Double Outlet Right Ventricle

Stewart, S.: Double Outlet Right Ventricle, *J Thorac Cardiovasc Surg,* **71:**355, 1976.

Van Praagh, R., Perez-Trevino, C., Reynolds, J. L., et al.: Double Outlet Right Ventricle with Subaortic Ventricular Septal Defect and Pulmonary Stenosis, *Am J Cardiol,* **35:**42, 1975.

Pulmonary Artery Sling

Grover, F. L., Norton, J. B., Webb, G. E., and Trinkle, J. K.: Pulmonary Sling: Case Report and Collective Review, *J Thorac Cardiovasc Surg,* **69:**295, 1975.

Chapter 19

Acquired Heart Disease

by **Frank C. Spencer**

INTRODUCTION: CLINICAL MANIFESTATIONS

With the development of prosthetic cardiac valves, the scope of surgical therapy for heart disease was greatly enlarged. An additional major advance was the development of bypass grafting for coronary artery disease, starting in the year 1967–1968 and now widely employed.

Present frontiers include corrective operations for severe cardiac malformations in infancy, cardiac transplantation, and the development of an artificial heart. This steadily expanding scope of cardiac surgery requires that the surgeon become familiar with features of cardiac disease that have traditionally been the province of the cardiologist. Accordingly, basic clinical features of cardiac disease, which classically are found only in a textbook of cardiology, are briefly presented in this section. The objective is not to train a surgeon as an amateur cardiologist but to enable the surgeon to be familiar enough with the clinical manifestations of cardiac disease to recognize gross abnormalities and to appreciate further the great importance of having a cardiologist as an integral part of a cardiac surgical team. Unless a cardiologist works closely with a cardiac surgeon, many surgical mishaps can occur which otherwise might be prevented or promptly treated, such as arrhythmias or myocardial infarction.

The five major methods of evaluating a patient with heart disease can be conveniently grouped as history, physical examination, electrocardiogram, radiologic studies, and special diagnostic tests, especially cardiac catheterization and cineangiography. In this introductory section the major characteristics of cardiac disease, as elicited by the history, physical examination, and laboratory studies, will be briefly described. For additional details, a textbook of cardiology should be consulted.

HISTORY. It is particularly important to determine the degree of disability present and its rate of progression. These considerations are especially pertinent to a decision as to the advisability of surgical intervention, especially if the contemplated operative procedure would require insertion of a prosthetic mitral or aortic valve. The hazard of thromboembolism with prosthetic valves, though decreased to the range of 2 to 4 percent since about 1970, still limits their use to patients seriously disabled or to those developing marked cardiac enlargement. The relative freedom from thromboembolism of the glutaldehyde-preserved porcine heterograft prosthesis, used with increasing frequency in the past 5 years, has further expanded the indications for valve replacement.

Dyspnea, fatigue, edema, and *cyanosis* are all usually manifestations of decreased cardiac output and congestive heart failure. *Pain* is an especially prominent feature with coronary artery disease. *Palpitation* and *syncope* occur with many forms of heart disease, especially with disturbances of rhythm. *Hemoptysis* can result from either cardiac or pulmonary causes. Each of these disorders will be briefly discussed.

Dyspnea on exertion is an extremely common symptom with heart disease, resulting from pulmonary congestion from elevation of left atrial pressure with increased physical activity. The degree of exertion required to cause dyspnea, especially with any changes in recent months, should be carefully noted. Other clinical manifestations of pulmonary congestion include cough, orthopnea, paroxysmal nocturnal dyspnea, or frank pulmonary edema. In considering the possible causes of dyspnea, it should be remembered that probably the most common cause is an anxiety syndrome, not heart disease. This can usually be determined by careful examination. *Fatigue,* probably a reflection of decrease in cardiac output, is a more subtle sign of limited cardiac function than dyspnea and may be the only complaint when the patient has subtly restricted his physical activities to avoid dyspnea. Patients following a sedentary existence can tolerate serious cardiac disease for long periods of time without having any other symptoms from a significant underlying hemodynamic disturbance.

Cyanosis may appear with acute pulmonary congestion but is usually variable and not a reliable guide to the type or severity of cardiac disease. It is a more reliable and significant finding in patients with congenital heart disease. *Edema* is a late symptom of congestive heart failure, for it can be detected clinically only after 10 lb or more of extracellular fluid have accumulated. Few symptoms may result from the presence of edema except for generalized aching and discomfort from the increased weight of the legs.

Chest pain is a particularly significant symptom which must be closely analyzed. Angina pectoris is one of the most frequent causes and, in perhaps 75 percent of patients, can be readily diagnosed from the characteristic symptoms. It usually occurs as a substernal pain or constriction provoked by exercise, eating, emotion, or exposure to cold. The discomfort commonly lasts 1 to 4 minutes and may be immediately relieved by sublingual administration of nitroglycerin. In perhaps 20 to 25 percent of patients a bizarre discomfort develops with radiation of pain to numerous unusual locations, such as the ear, the right hand, or the epigastrium. In such patients establishing the correct diagnosis may challenge the most experienced cardiologist and require laboratory evaluation with exercise electrocardiography or coronary arteriography.

Other frequent causes of chest pain include myocardial infarction, dissecting aneurysm, pericarditis, or pulmonary infarction. As with dyspnea, anxiety is a frequent cause for a precordial discomfort described as pain or "tightness," and its frequency must be appreciated in considering the differential diagnosis. Other noncardiac conditions which may be easily confused with angina pectoris are diseases of the esophagus or, less frequently, biliary disease.

Palpitation is a generalized term for the patient's becoming aware of cardiac contractions. Rarely this occurs in a thin-chested individual without cardiac disease. Usually it results from increased force of left ventricular contraction as a result of underlying heart disease or from a cardiac arrhythmia, such as an extrasystole. Its significance is re-lated to the underlying disease or disturbance which produces the discomfort. *Syncope* may result from several cardiac diseases, the most important of which are aortic stenosis, heart block, mitral stenosis, tetralogy of Fallot, or rarely pulmonary hypertension. It is a particularly ominous symptom in patients with aortic stenosis, for the life expectancy of such patients is brief unless surgical therapy is performed. In evaluating the significance of syncope, the possibility of epilepsy or cerebrovascular disease must be considered.

Hemoptysis, an alarming symptom, often results from pulmonary disease. The four most frequent disorders are tuberculosis, bronchogenic carcinoma, bronchiectasis, and pneumonia. The two cardiac conditions most commonly associated with hemoptysis are mitral stenosis and pulmonary infarction. Patients with fulminating pulmonary edema may expectorate a pink, frothy sputum as a result of rupture of pulmonary capillaries into the alveoli, but the frothy sputum of pulmonary edema can be easily distinguished from the blood clots expectorated with frank hemoptysis.

PHYSICAL EXAMINATION. The general body habitus of the patient should be carefully noted. A number of unusual genetic syndromes are associated with cardiac disease. Most of these are described in recent textbooks of cardiology. The Marfan syndrome is a familiar example of a disorder of connective tissue which may cause either a dissecting aneurysm or aortic insufficiency.

The prominence of the neck veins is a guide to venous pressure. With a normal venous pressure of 2 to 10 mm Hg, the internal jugular vein is visible for only 2 to 3 cm above the level of the clavicle. With obviously distended veins, measurement of central venous pressure should be considered. In patients with tricuspid valvular disease, the experienced cardiologist can detect prominent *a* waves in the jugular pulse generated from forceful contractions of the right atrium. Peripheral edema can be best noted in the legs, but in patients confined to bed edema may be more prominent in the flanks or buttocks.

Much information can be obtained from a careful examination of the peripheral pulse and the blood pressure. A disturbance of cardiac rhythm, such as atrial fibrillation, can be recognized from the pulse and then investigated more thoroughly by auscultation of the heart and study of the electrocardiogram. Pulsus alternans, a rhythmic alternation between a forceful pulse and a weak one, is a significant sign of serious left ventricular failure. A small, weak pulse is found with cardiac disease associated with a low cardiac output, increased peripheral vascular resistance, and a narrow pulse pressure. This may occur with myocardial failure, aortic stenosis, mitral stenosis, or cardiac tamponade. A forceful, bounding pulse results when there is an increased cardiac output with a wide pulse pressure and decreased peripheral vascular resistance. This is classically seen with aortic insufficiency but is also a prominent feature in any disease associated with a decreased peripheral vascular resistance, such as patent ductus arteriosus, peripheral arteriovenous fistula, hyperthyroidism, or pregnancy.

Inspection and palpation of the precordium is another

important part of the cardiac examination. Some cardiologists have almost discarded percussion of the cardiac shadow because of the wide range of normal findings among persons of different habitus and have found more significant information by careful inspection and palpation. Cardiac pulsations should be observed for their location, timing, amplitude, and distribution. Normally, the apical impulse is near the midclavicular line and can be detected as a moderately forceful tapping sensation in early systole over an area 2 to 3 cm in diameter. With left ventricular hypertrophy, as with aortic stenosis or insufficiency, both the size and vigor of the left ventricular impulse are increased. With right ventricular hypertrophy, a prominent parasternal impulse, which some cardiologists consider a better index of right ventricular hypertrophy than the electrocardiogram, can be felt. In the presence of marked dilatation of the heart from congestive heart failure, palpation becomes less reliable because of the diffuse nature of the cardiac impulse.

Characteristic thrills develop with certain types of valvular disease. The more common of these are the thrill in the aortic area from aortic stenosis, a similar one in the pulmonic area with pulmonic stenosis, and less frequently a diastolic thrill at the apex with mitral stenosis.

Auscultation is a very important part of the cardiac examination, because some serious disorders, such as mitral stenosis or aortic insufficiency, can be firmly diagnosed best by detection of the characteristic murmur. In auscultation the cardiac sounds should be carefully analyzed and any murmurs identified. A convenient method for beginning the examination is to identify the first and second sounds by auscultation at the base of the heart. Normally the second sound, produced by closure of the aortic and pulmonic valves, is of a higher pitch and shorter duration than the first sound, produced by seating of the mitral and tricuspid valves. If uncertainty exists, simultaneous palpation of the carotid pulse will identify the two sounds. Splitting of the pulmonic second sound is a familiar characteristic of conditions which increase pulmonary blood flow, especially atrial septal defect.

In defining the characteristics of a murmur, the timing, duration, intensity, and location are of particular significance. Aortic and pulmonic stenosis each produce so-called "diamond-shaped" murmurs, representing an early rise and late decline in intensity. Mitral insufficiency, by contrast, produces a loud apical systolic murmur without the characteristic sharp decrease heard in aortic stenosis. The diastolic murmur of aortic insufficiency is usually best heard along the left sternal border, while the typical diastolic murmur of mitral stenosis may be sharply localized at the cardiac apex. Murmurs of tricuspid stenosis and insufficiency often are similar to the more frequently encountered murmurs of mitral stenosis or insufficiency, except that they also may be audible near the lower end of the sternum and can be accentuated during inspiration. Confirmation of the diagnosis usually requires cardiac catherization. A murmur of ventricular septal defect is usually a harsh holosystolic murmur near the lower border of the sternum, while the murmur of an atrial septal defect creased pulmonary blood flow. The classic murmur of patent ductus arteriosus is a continuous murmur best heard in the left second or third intercostal space.

Functional murmurs are especially common in conditions with an increase in cardiac output, such as hyperthyroidism, anemia, or pregnancy. In general these are short systolic murmurs which may be audible at the apex or in the pulmonic area. Their differential diagnosis, which may necessitate cardiac catheterization, is beyond the scope of this presentation.

Two infrequent findings on auscultation are a pericardial friction rub or a gallop rhythm. A friction rub is particularly common after cardiac operations and may be unassociated with any other clinical signs, originating from resorption of fluid in the pericardium. In other patients it may indicate the so-called "pericardiotomy syndrome," which frequently occurs following cardiac surgical procedures. A gallop rhythm is of particular importance, because its presence usually indicates serious disease of the myocardium, such as myocardial infarction or impending cardiac failure.

ELECTROCARDIOGRAPHY. The electrocardiogram will be mentioned only briefly, for its proper interpretation requires the careful analysis of an experienced cardiologist. Disorders of cardiac rhythm are extremely common following cardiac surgical procedures, and a wide variety of rhythms can occur in a patient over a period of several hours. In analysis of the electrocardiogram, the cardiac rate, rhythm, and electrical axis should be noted. It is particularly useful for detection of hypertrophy of either the right or left ventricle. Conduction defects, such as right or left bundle branch block, can be diagnosed only by electrocardiography. With serious coronary artery disease, either as chronic coronary artery disease or with acute myocardial infarction, the electrocardiogram may provide the only positive laboratory findings.

RADIOLOGY. The chest roentgenogram provides many valuable guides in evaluation of cardiac disease. Determination of heart size is of basic importance, for cardiac enlargement immediately establishes the presence of cardiac disease. Alterations in cardiac contour occur with different diseases. Normally the right border of the heart is formed by the superior vena cava and the right atrium, and the left border by the aorta, pulmonary artery, and left ventricle. Selective enlargement of any of the four cardiac chambers is best recognized by oblique or lateral views. In the left anterior oblique position, enlargement of the left ventricle can be recognized as a posterior shadow against the spine, while an enlarged right ventricle can be seen bulging anteriorly into the retrosternal space. Enlargement of the left atrium is best recognized in the lateral view, by simultaneous opacification of the esophagus with barium, as it produces a characteristic concave indentation of the esophagus. Enlargement of the right atrium, bulging into the right hemithorax, can be easily seen in the usual posteroanterior view.

In analysis of the cardiac shadow, detection of calcification is of particular importance. Calcification of the aortic or mitral valves is very common with long-standing rheumatic disease. With constrictive pericarditis most patients will have visible areas of calcification.

Analysis of the pulmonary circulation provides many valuable guides to the status of the circulation. Pulmonary venous congestion develops when left atrial pressure is chronically elevated above the upper limit of normal of 12 mm Hg. With severe mitral stenosis, a typical picture of engorged pulmonary veins may be readily recognized. When severe left atrial hypertension is present, edema forms in the lungs in both the alveoli and the interstitial tissues. Edema accumulating in the interlobar planes forms transverse linear opacities on the chest roentgenogram which are perpendicular to the surface of the pleura, the so-called "Kerley lines." Their presence usually indicates a left atrial pressure exceeding 20 mm Hg.

The prominenence of the pulmonary arteries is also of particular significance. Marked enlargement of the pulmonary arteries may occur with either an increase in pulmonary blood flow or an increase in pulmonary vascular resistance with pulmonary hypertension. Normally, the central pulmonary arteries are three to five times larger than the peripheral arteries. With an increase in pulmonary blood flow, as with an atrial septal defect, both the central and peripheral pulmonary arteries are symmetrically enlarged. With an increase in pulmonary vascular resistance and pulmonary hypertension, the central pulmonary arteries may become strikingly enlarged, while the peripheral pulmonary arteries do not distend, producing a striking disproportion in the size of the two vessels. An estimation of the pulmonary blood flow by fluoroscopy is of particular importance in the presence of congenital heart disease. Wide variations are seen, ranging from the avascular lung fields with tetralogy of Fallot to the plethoric lung fields of ventricular or atrial septal defect.

CARDIAC CATHETERIZATION AND CINEANGIOGRAPHY. These two techniques have greatly advanced the precision of diagnosis of cardiac disease. Only by these studies can many cardiac disorders be properly diagnosed and quantitatively analyzed. It is our practice to perform cardiac catheterization and angiography upon virtually every patient undergoing cardiac surgical treatment to assess the hemodynamic disturbance, confirm the diagnosis, and detect any associated cardiac disease. This liberal policy has provided numerous dividends in the care of patients both during and following operation.

Cardiac catheterization, by obtaining oxygen concentration and pressure in different cardiac chambers, can establish the diagnosis of an intracardiac shunt, such as an atrial or ventricular septal defect, or the presence of a valvular stenosis, such as pulmonic stenosis, mitral stenosis, or aortic stenosis. The presence of cardiac failure, as indicated by an elevation of left atrial pressure, or pulmonary hypertension can also be measured. It is not of great value for analysis of aortic or mitral insufficiency, except to detect the development of cardiac failure.

Cineangiography, however, provides the best method for analysis of aortic or mitral insufficiency, visually demonstrating the amount of dye refluxing through the incompetent valve. In patients over forty years of age, simultaneous coronary arteriography is routinely done to evaluate the presence of associated coronary atherosclerosis.

The combination of cardiac catheterization and cineangiography in a well-equipped cardiac catheterization laboratory is an essential component of any cardiac surgical unit.

PATHOPHYSIOLOGY

A detailed analysis of the pathophysiology of mitral and aortic disease is presented in those respective sections. Accordingly, only a brief discussion of certain broad principles of pathophysiology of acquired heart disease is presented here.

As stated earlier, the degree of incapacity of a patient with cardiac disease should be carefully evaluated in deciding that an operation should be performed. Many patients with aortic or mitral disease can function well for years and should be treated by nonoperative methods until the disease has progressed to an incapacitating stage. The reason for this conservatism, which may change in the future, is the significant frequency of thromboemboli with prosthetic cardiac valves. Hence, an operation which entails insertion of a prosthetic cardiac valve should be postponed as long as a patient can carry out his normal activities with appropriate medical therapy. One exception to this policy is the presence of progressive cardiac enlargement. As very large hearts of 750 to 1,000 Gm may not decrease after operation, surgery is being performed earlier in some patients with only moderate symptoms but with progressive cardiac enlargement.

Conversely, it is important to realize that with present surgical techniques an operation almost always can be performed, even though advanced, severe cardiac failure is present. The immediate risk of operation is increased, but possibilities for rehabilitating a patient are fairly good, even though he is bedridden with severe edema from far advanced congestive failure. Our most extreme example of this is a patient who lost 80 pounds of edema fluid during prolonged preoperative treatment before undergoing an uneventful mitral valve replacement. The most important principle in operating upon such patients is to be certain that all existing valvular pathologic conditions are corrected, for multivalvular disease is common with intractable congestive failure. In some patients replacement of three cardiac valves, the mitral, aortic, and tricuspid, is necessary.

With mitral stenosis, different considerations apply, because many such patients can be effectively treated by commissurotomy. Accordingly, operation should be planned whenever the diagnosis is made if any symptoms are present. Surgical therapy should be especially considered once atrial fibrillation has occurred because of the risk of thromboembolism. Before either anticoagulant or surgical therapy was available, approximately 25 percent of patients with mitral stenosis ultimately died from cerebral embolism.

With aortic stenosis or insufficiency, once symptoms such as dyspnea, syncope, or chest pain have appeared, operation should be performed quickly, because sudden death is a real possibility. This is particularly true with aortic stenosis. Sudden death of patients with aortic stenosis either contemplating or scheduled for operation still occurs with distressing frequency.

Pulmonary hypertension is of considerably different significance with acquired heart disease than with congenital heart disease. With ventricular septal defect an elevated pulmonary vascular resistance may or may not decrease following closure of the defect. With pulmonary hypertension from mitral stenosis, however, even in its more severe forms with a pulmonary artery systolic pressure exceeding 100 mm Hg, improvement almost invariably occurs following adequate correction of the stenosis.

The heart size and presence of congestive failure are important indices of long-term rehabilitation following successful cardiac valvular surgical treatment. Unfortunately in most patients disabled by the disease significant cardiac enlargement has developed. A small percentage of patients with mitral disease following valvular replacement will have permanent cardiac disability, requiring careful limitation of physical activities and administration of diuretics. Whether this permanent disability reflects a rheumatic myocarditis or a permanent injury to the myocardium from long-standing valvular disease is unknown. Similarly, with aortic valvular disease and severe cardiac enlargement, sometimes to weights of 700 to 900 Gm, sudden death remains an ominous possibility following operation, especially in the first year. Death is probably due to a disturbance of rhythm from the severely hypertrophied left ventricle. As mentioned earlier, the probable solution for this group of patients is performance of operation at an earlier date, which will surely be done when cardiac valvular prostheses are completely free from the risk of thromboembolism.

PHYSIOLOGY OF EXTRACORPOREAL CIRCULATION

HISTORICAL DATA. The pioneering imagination and efforts of Gibbon were largely responsible for the development of extracorporeal circulation. In 1932, Gibbon initiated laboratory investigations which continued for over 20 years until the first successful open heart operation in man was performed by him in 1953. Subsequent developments were rapid, with the brief use of cross circulation by Lillehei and associates at the University of Minnesota in 1954, followed a short time later by the development of the bubble oxygenator by DeWall, who was working in the group with Lillehei. Kirklin and associates at the Mayo Clinic first began routine, successful use of the Gibbon oxygenator in 1955. The disc oxygenator was developed in Sweden by Bjork and Crafoord and introduced to the United States by Kay and Cross. Since 1970, disposable bubble oxygenators have been adopted almost universally.

PUMPS. The majority of heart-lung machines utilize a simple roller pump, originally developed by DeBakey. The resulting flow is almost nonpulsatile, with a pulse pressure of about 15 mm Hg. A variety of other pumps have been employed, with no clear demonstration of any advantages over the simple roller pump. A recurrent physiologic question has been the importance of a pulsatile flow in the normal circulation. Available experimental data indicate that over long periods of time a pulsatile flow may be of importance, but for periods of 1 to 4 hours a nonpulsatile flow seems adequate. The gradual increase in vasomotor tone which occurs during extracorporeal circulation may be a physiologic response to nonpulsatile perfusion.

OXYGENATORS. Since 1970 the disposable bubble oxygenator has become the most widely used type (Fig. 19-1). Technical improvements in the removal of bubbles from blood following oxygenation have made it possible to perfuse with surprisingly little difficulty for as long as 4 to 6 hours. Disposable membrane oxygenators have also been developed and are used frequently in some centers, particularly for infants, but are somewhat more cumbersome than disposable oxygenators.

PRIMING SOLUTIONS. Originally heart-lung machines were primed with heparinized blood collected within 24 hours before the time of operation, adding 20 mg heparin for each 500 ml blood used. Citrated blood (first demonstrated by Maloney and associates) is now used almost routinely, except in small infants. Some degree of hemodilution is now used routinely during perfusion by most groups. A variety of substances, such as dextrose-water, Ringer's lactate, and other solutions have been used. Our preference is for modified Ringer's lactate solution (Plasmalyte), which closely approximates the electrolyte composition of blood. Serum albumin is also added; so the priming mixture closely resembles plasma. Our preferred technique is to prime the pump-oxygenator with the electrolyte solution up to 40 ml/kg, which is adequate for adult patients but not adequate to fill the oxygenator in smaller children. Once bypass has started, blood is added as needed, but blood is not placed in the oxygenator until the time for initiation of bypass, to avoid prolonged contact of blood with the plastic surfaces of the oxygenator. Blood or packed red cells are added as necessary to keep the hematocrit reading between 20 and 25 percent. If there is significant hypotension, blood or albumin may be added to increase the oncotic pressure of the perfusate.

TECHNIQUE OF PERFUSION. Heparin, 3 mg/kg body weight, is given before the venous and arterial cannulae are inserted. Venous blood is aspirated by gravity or pump drainage through large cannulae inserted into the right atrium, except in some children and young adults, and advanced into the venae cavae. Oxygenated blood is returned to the arterial circulation, usually through a cannula directly inserted into the ascending aorta. Once widely popular, femoral artery cannulation has been almost abandoned to avoid the rare but dangerous complication of retrograde dissection of the aorta. Perfusion is done at a flow rate of about 2.500 ml/m^2/minute, providing a flow rate between 4 and 5 liters/minute for adults of normal size. Oxygen flow rates through the oxygenator are adjusted to produce an arterial oxygen tension near 100 mm Hg. Temperature is controlled with a heat exchanger in the circuit and is often lowered to 30 to 32°C. This moderate

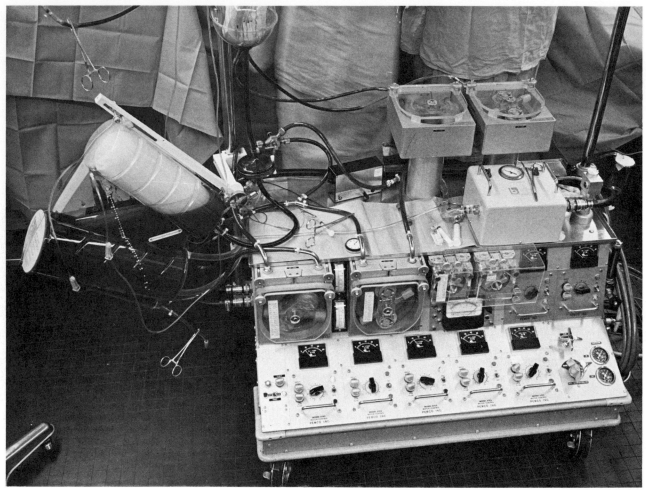

Fig. 19-1. Photograph of heart-lung machine, showing the Bentley bubble oxygenator with DeBakey roller pumps. The filters in the coronary suction return are also visible.

hypothermia increases the tolerance of the heart to ischemia produced by temporary occlusion of the ascending aorta in order to permit better visualization of intracardiac structures. Intracardiac blood is aspirated with a suction apparatus, filtered, and returned to the oxygenator.

During perfusion a number of modalities are monitored. Arterial pressure is monitored with a catheter previously inserted into a peripheral artery. Venous pressure in the superior vena cava is carefully observed to be certain that there is no obstruction to return of blood from the brain. The electrocardiogram and electroencephalogram are also monitored. Mean arterial pressure usually decreases sharply with the onset of perfusion, apparently from vasodilatation, and then subsequently rises to levels varying between 50 and 80 mm Hg. The importance of the actual level of mean arterial pressure, as long as flow rate is adequate, is debated. For several years we have preferred to maintain a mean perfusion pressure near that existing before bypass, achieving this by increasing the flow rate, increasing the volume of fluid in the patient, or infusing small amounts of vasopressor agents. This seems especially important in older patients with a history of hypertension or stroke and is of less importance in younger patients and children. There is a wide variability in the blood pressure

response to perfusion. Within a short period of time the blood pressure may stabilize. Some patients develop signs of progressive vasoconstriction after 1 to 2 hours. An occasional patient has a puzzling hypotension which requires rigorous therapy.

Oxygen and carbon dioxide tensions are periodically measured in the venous blood returned to the oxygenator and the oxygenated blood returned to the patient. Preferably the arterial oxygen tension should be near 100 mm Hg and the carbon dioxide tension 30 to 35 mm Hg. Venous blood returning to the heart-lung machine with the described flow rate will usually have an oxygen saturation greater than 50 percent. With flow rates and oxygen saturations in this range, metabolic acidosis of significant degree does not occur.

Heparin is gradually metabolized by the body; so, additional heparin is given each hour of perfusion in a dose of 1 mg/kg body weight. During perfusion the lungs are kept stationary in a partially inflated position with intermittent periods of inflation.

Termination of Perfusion. As perfusion is stopped, left atrial pressure is measured and blood transfused from the heart-lung machine until a left atrial pressure adequate to maintain cardiac output is obtained. The left atrial pressure needed will vary according to that existing before bypass. This technique has been found a better guide to adjustment of blood volume than either blood volume measurement or careful, balanced measurements of blood withdrawn versus blood transfused. Heparin is then neutralized with protamine. Initially 3 mg of protamine/kg is given, regardless of the total amount of heparin administered, assuming that the rate of heparin metabolism approximately equals the rate at which additional heparin is given. A protamine titration is then carried out and additional small amounts of protamine given as indicated. Several reports have emphasized the wide variations in response of patients to both heparin and protamine; so flexibility in management of the individual patient is necessary.

TRAUMA FROM PERFUSION. Extracorporeal circulation produces trauma to the blood, primarily from the exposure of blood to gas in the oxygenator and from the use of suction to aspirate intracardiac blood. At present tolerance for extracorporeal circulation is in the range of 6 to 8 hours; some patients undergo a very long perfusion with surprisingly few metabolic defects, but others show definite signs of physiologic injury after 6 hours of perfusion. Experimental studies of the capillary microcirculation during perfusion have found a progressive sludging of the blood elements, producing stasis and obstruction to capillary blood flow. The concentration of hemoglobin in the plasma is an index of hemolysis occurring during perfusion and may rise 40 to 50 mg/hour perfusion, the amount varying with the volume of urine secreted during perfusion. Some derangement of the clotting mechanisms invariably occurs and is reflected by an increased bleeding tendency afterward even though heparin activity has been neutralized. The coagulation defects, usually from multiple sources, subside within 6 to 12 hours. Bleeding problems are far less frequent than in previous years because of an appreciation of the vulnerability of platelets to injury from a wide variety of medications, especially aspirin, combined with availability of platelets and frozen plasma for correction of coagulation disorders. Fat embolism also has been demonstrated, although the significance is uncertain. Denaturation of plasma proteins occurs from the trauma at the gas-blood interphase and is probably responsible for some of the subtle physiologic changes with long perfusions.

In the past few years several studies have demonstrated microaggregates in the blood in the oxygenator, which can be partly removed with special filters in the pump circuit. Filters of different porosity are now widely used clinically, but their importance is yet uncertain. Our preference is for the Dacron wool (Swank) filter in the coronary suction line, but filters are not used in the venous or arterial lines.

The clinical counterparts of trauma with long perfusions have manifestations in different organs. A bleeding tendency develops, the degree varying with the duration of perfusion and the degree of trauma. This subsides within 12 to 18 hours. A mild degree of renal insufficiency is common after long perfusions, varying with flow rate during perfusion, blood trauma, and acidosis. Fortunately this is usually reversible. Varying degrees of respiratory insufficiency can develop with long perfusions. The cause is not completely clear and is probably related to multiple factors. Postoperatively, some patients require mechanical ventilation for a few hours but seldom for more than 8 to 12 hours. The central nervous system also becomes injured with long perfusions, as a result of which a variety of generalized neurolgic signs may appear. One of the most interesting of these is a psychosis, appearing unpredictably in a few patients, with all the symptoms of a severe toxic psychosis; fortunately this subsides within 2 weeks after operation.

RISK OF PERFUSION. At present the risk from extracorporeal circulation for 1 to 2 hours is extremely small, in the range of less than 1 percent. This low risk represents an astonishing achievement, especially when compared with the fact that as late as 1950 to 1952 the entire concept of extracorporeal circulation was purely hypothetic. Perhaps the most common complication is the development of serum hepatitis, related to the amount of blood used to prime the oxygenator and perform the operation. With longer periods of perfusion, the risk of perfusion per se gradually increases, though perfusion for as long as 6 hours is well tolerated in some patients. In some patients with severe respiratory insufficiency, partial perfusion with extrathoracic cannulation and a membrane oxygenator has been performed for as long as 7 to 8 days.

POSTOPERATIVE CARE AND COMPLICATIONS FOLLOWING EXTRACORPOREAL CIRCULATION

Postoperative care following extracorporeal circulation involves problems which are not encountered following other surgical procedures. Part of the complications arise from the use of extracorporeal circulation, involving several units of blood and moderate trauma to the blood, the degree varying with the duration of extracorporeal circulation as well as with the type of oxygenator. In general, extracorporeal circulation for 2 to 4 hours is well tolerated; periods of 4 to 6 hours may have moderate but reversible complications, while periods for 6 to 9 hours approach the physiologic limits compatible with survival with present pump-oxygenators. The complications are also related to the type of disease which is treated by open cardiotomy and often occur in patients with chronic congestive failure with the attendant impaired function of many organ systems.

GENERAL PROCEDURES. Following these operations, as with most major surgical procedures, temperature, pulse, blood pressure, and respirations are frequently measured. Intraarterial pressure recording is often used for 24 to 48 hours, because residual vasoconstriction following extracorporeal circulation may make auscultatory methods for blood pressure measurement difficult and unreliable. Central venous pressure is routinely measured. In addition, since 1958 or 1960, small polyvinyl catheters frequently have been left in the left atrium and pulmonary artery for 24 to 48 hours to measure oxygen and carbon dioxide tensions in left atrial and mixed venous blood, as well as to measure pulmonary artery and left atrial pressures. The oxygen saturation of mixed venous blood, representing the ability of the respiratory and circulatory systems to supply oxygen requirements, is a particularly useful guide, especially in seriously ill patients. Left atrial pressure is of more value than central venous pressure, especially with isolated left ventricular failure. Pulmonary artery diastolic pressure in most patients parallels left atrial pressure and may be substituted for direct measurement of left atrial pressure in many patients, but this relationship should be checked while the heart is exposed.

Chest roentgenograms are frequently made to evaluate hemothorax, pleural effusion, or atelectasis. The electrocardiogram is regularly monitored on an oscilloscope for varying periods of time because of the frequency of cardiac arrhythmias. Hematocrit, serum electrolyte concentrations (sodium, potassium, carbon dioxide, and chloride), and blood urea nitrogen (BUN) levels are serially measured.

Antibiotics are regularly given in large amounts during the operative procedure and for different lengths of time after operation. Although routines for antibiotic therapy vary widely among different institutions, we have preferred to administer oxacillin, 4 to 8 Gm daily, and more recently cephalothin, 2 Gm daily, for approximately 2 to 4 days following insertion of valvular prostheses. Digitalis is given routinely to patients who previously have been in congestive failure. Anticoagulant therapy is regularly used with valvular prostheses and continued for varying periods of time. It is usually begun 2 to 4 days after operation.

SPECIFIC COMPLICATIONS. Bleeding Syndromes. Although heparin is routinely neutralized with protamine following extracorporeal circulation, it is important to realize that blood-clotting mechanisms are abnormal for 8 to 12 hours following bypass. Unusually diligent care is required following extracorporeal circulation to obtain hemostasis before incisions are sutured, necessitating much more attention than after usual operations. The exact basis for the deficient clotting mechanisms is not certain, since detailed studies of the different components of the blood responsible for normal clotting show some derangement of several components, without any specific correctible factor. Residual heparin activity, the so-called "heparin rebound phenomenon," probably occurs in some patients. When serious defects of blood coagulation persist after operation, transfusion with fresh frozen plasma or platelets is the most effective therapy. Fortunately, the clotting derangements are transitory and will disappear in the majority of patients within a few hours.

Because of the bleeding tendency, unusual care is required to measure blood loss serially and transfuse appropriate amounts of blood. Soft plastic sump tubes are now used regularly in the mediastinum and pericardium after operation and seem superior to previous drainage techniques.

With the extensive bleeding, the possibility of cardiac tamponade from blood clots accumulating in the pericardium should be considered. The usual findings with cardiac tamponade include hypotension, elevated venous pressure, and a wide mediastinal shadow on the chest roentgenogram. In doubtful cases reoperation may be required to confirm or exclude the diagnosis. In most patients the right or left pleural cavity is opened at operation to lessen the subsequent risk of cardiac tamponade. Closure of the pericardium may be accomplished in many patients without undue constriction of the heart and has been found by Cunningham and others to lessen the frequency of tamponade.

The usual blood loss following operation is in the range of 400 to 800 ml, although this varies widely among individual patients. A blood loss exceeding 1 liter usually indicates active intrathoracic hemorrhage requiring reoperation. With improvements in pump-oxygenators and surgical technique, the frequency of reoperation for postoperative hemorrhage has greatly decreased.

Cardiac Failure. *Low-Cardiac-Output Syndrome.* In the early period of open heart surgery, a low-cardiac-output syndrome frequently developed. With increasing experience, however, the syndrome has progressively decreased in frequency and is now rarely encountered except in association with specific causes, most of which can be prevented. The normal cardiac output is near 3 liters/m^2/minute. Following cardiac surgical procedures, there may be a decrease to 2 liters/m^2/minute with moderate cardiac failure or to as low as 1 to 1.5 liters/m^2/minute with severe depression of cardiac function. With low cardiac output and deficient perfusion of different organs, a number of metabolic disturbances appear. There is hypotension, vasoconstriction, oliguria, and metabolic acidosis. After varying periods of time, ranging from a few hours to 1 to 2 days, death may result from either progressive hypotension or cardiac arrest.

Although a number of complex hypotheses were developed to explain the low-output syndrome, it is now realized that most of the causative factors are preventable. In the past 2 or 3 years, significant advances in myocardial preservation have been made. Undoubtedly, the most frequent cause of the low-output syndrome is some form of myocardial injury occurring insidiously at operation. Even with advanced cardiac failure, the majority of patients will maintain an adequate cardiac output following operation if the entire underlying valvular pathologic condition is corrected and significant injury to the heart does not occur during operation. Failure to correct the valvular pathologic condition completely, especially before the advent of satisfactory prosthetic cardiac valves, was a frequent cause of cardiac failure. Another frequent cause was hypovolemia.

Although a number of methods to adjust blood volume have been used following extracorporeal circulation, including blood volume determinations and careful fluid balance measurements, the most reliable technique has been transfusion of fluid to elevate the central venous pressure or left atrial pressure to normal or moderately high levels. Preoperatively, many patients with aortic or mitral valvular disease may have a mean left atrial pressure of 15 to 20 mm Hg, and at times even higher levels (20 to 40 mm Hg). As this pressure represents the pressure distending the left ventricle in diastole and hence determining stroke volume and cardiac output, transfusion to similar levels may be required following operation to maintain a satisfactory cardiac output. In retrospect, failure to transfuse adequate fluid was a frequent unrecognized cause of the low-output syndrome.

Coronary air emboli, transection of coronary arteries during a ventriculotomy, or prolonged cardiac ischemia from temporary aortic occlusion are all insults which can depress cardiac function but can be avoided in carefully executed operative procedures. With congenital heart disease, a greatly increased pulmonary vascular resistance, as with a ventricular septal defect and pulmonary hypertension, can severely impair cardiac function after operation and in some patients can result in death. Fortunately, with acquired valvular disease an irreversible increase in pulmonary vascular resistance almost never occurs.

An inadequate cardiac output can be suspected if hypotension, oliguria, or acidosis develops. Acidosis following operation is virtually unknown in the presence of an adequate cardiac ouput, for the acidosis results from production of lactate, pyruvate, and similar anions by anaerobic metabolism. A more precise method for evaluating the low-cardiac-output syndrome is either by direct measurement of cardiac output or by measurement of oxygen saturation of mixed venous blood obtained from the pulmonary artery through an indwelling catheter implanted at operation. The oxygen saturation of mixed venous blood, normally greater than 60 percent, is only an approximation of cardiac output, for it varies with the adequacy of ventilation, the blood volume, the hematocrit, and temperature. However, the oxygen saturation is an extremely useful guide, because it reflects how well the circulation is supplying the oxygen requirements of the body tissues. An oxygen saturation in the range of 50 to 80 percent (P_{O_2} 25 to 30 mm) indicates a moderate deficiency in oxygen transport, while a saturation in the range of 40 to 50 percent (P_{O_2} less than 25 mm) represents a serious deficiency and may be associated with a fatal outcome unless corrected.

Therapy of the low-cardiac-output syndrome includes transfusion of fluid to elevate the central venous pressure to an appropriate level, usually 10 to 12 mm Hg, or the left atrial pressure to 15 to 20 mm Hg. Acidosis which has developed can be corrected by infusion of sodium bicarbonate (50 to 200 mEq). If a low cardiac output remains despite transfusion of appropriate fluid, cardiac inotropic drugs, such as epinephrine or isoproterenol, may be cautiously administered, usually in the range of 1 to 3 μg/minute in adult patients. Premature use of inotropic drugs and vasopressors, such as norepinephrine or metaraminol, in the past perhaps accentuated the severity of the low-cardiac-output syndrome because hypovolemia was not recognized and was further masked by elevation of the blood pressure.

If respiratory insufficiency is present, as manifested by dyspnea or abnormalities in the oxygen and carbon dioxide tensions of arterial blood, artificial ventilation may be required. This is usually done initially by insertion of an endotracheal tube following appropriate sedation of the patient. Tracheostomy is rarely necessary. Digitalis, usually digoxin, should be administered to full therapeutic doses, although the immediate effect on cardiac output is often not significant.

The intraaortic balloon pump has been adopted widely in the last 3 or 4 years to provide an effective method of circulatory support by increasing cardiac index 0.5 to 0.7 liters/minute. Such support may be used for several days or longer and is undoubtedly lifesaving in certain critically ill patients.

Cardiac Arrhythmias. Minor arrhythmias, such as atrial fibrillation or a nodal rhythm, are very common after open heart surgical procedures. An important feature of postoperative care is constant, 24-hour-a-day, visual monitoring of the cardiac rhythm on an oscilloscope for 2 to 3 days following operation. Only by constant visual observation can serious arrhythmias be promptly detected, because such arrhythmias may develop in the presence of a normal cardiac output and without any other signs of circulatory failure.

Tachycardia, either as a sinus rhythm or rapid atrial fibrillation, may result from inadequate amounts of digitalis. Ventricular extrasystoles are the most common serious arrhythmias, because their appearance may herald the developing of more serious arrhythmias, such as bigeminy, ventricular tachycardia, or ventricular fibrillation. Digitalis toxicity is probably the most frequent cause of ventricular arrhythmias, resulting from varying sensitivity to digitalis after operation in relation to changes in plasma potassium concentration. Hypokalemia is particularly frequent, because patients in cardiac failure preoperatively may have significant depletion of body stores of potassium from chronic diuretic therapy.

Mild disturbance of cardiac rhythm from digitalis toxicity will subside following restriction of digitalis and administration of supplemental potassium. Intravenous lidocaine, 1 to 3 mg/minute, is a valuable form of therapy for temporary control of arrhythmias, although the drug is quickly metabolized. In selected arrhythmias the beta-blocking drug propranolol is of great value. Procainamide, in doses varying from 2 to 6 Gm/day, is also useful for more lasting control. In serious circumstances with ventricular tachycardia or other rhythms refractory to other forms of therapy, electrical cardioversion is invaluable.

Chronic Cardiac Failure. When the patient becomes ambulatory a few days after operation, fluid retention commonly becomes evident, especially if sodium intake is not carefully restricted. This can be easily detected by noting the appearance of edema in the flanks, hips, and legs. Weighing the patient daily is an important part of routine postoperative care. The edema usually responds promptly to diuretic therapy and restriction of sodium, but some patients with severe chronic cardiac failure before operation may require long periods of care before edema no longer develops.

Respiratory Insufficiency. Some disturbance of pulmonary function is very common following extracorporeal circulation. The frequency varies widely with different groups and also at different periods of time. The simplest numerical expression of the pulmonary dysfunction is indicated by the alveolar-arterial oxygen gradient, representing impaired diffusion of oxygen from the alveoli into the pulmonary venous blood. There are undoubtedly many causes of the pulmonary dysfunction, some of which are not well understood. Overtransfusion with resulting elevation of left atrial pressure and pulmonary congestion is one of the most frequent causes. Inadequate removal of pulmonary secretions, with resulting atelectasis and infection, is another. Microemboli or fat emboli are less well understood possible causative factors.

Ventilation through an indwelling endotracheal tube for 24 to 48 hours has much decreased the need for tracheostomy. The most effective measures for avoiding pulmonary congestion following operation are the familiar ones of humidification of inspired gas, usually with an oxygen mask, and diligent removal of tracheobronchial secretions, including frequent turning of the patient with coughing and deep breathing. Nasotracheal aspiration with a catheter may be done if necessary. Bronchoscopy is rarely necessary.

Postoperative Fluids. Fluids are restricted moderately during the first 48 hours following operation, though less stringently than in the past. An average intake would be about 30 to 35 ml/kg/24 hours, although wide variation exists. Oral intake is minimized for the first 24 hours after operation because of the risk of gastric dilatation with vomiting and aspiration.

Renal Function. Hourly urine output is carefully measured for 1 to 2 days after operation, preferably keeping the average urine output greater than 30 ml/hour. A transitory elevation of BUN level to 25 to 35 mg/100 ml is commonly seen after complex operative procedures, although the frequency has much decreased with the use of hemodilution priming of the pump-oxygenator. The renal injury may be produced by deficient perfusion, excessive hemolysis, or a transfusion incompatibility. Significant renal failure often presents a high-output renal failure, with daily secretion of 1 to 2 liters of dilute urine, associated with progressive elevation in BUN level. The degree of renal insufficiency in such circumstances can be most simply evaluated by performance of a simple urea clearance test, comparing the simultaneous urea concentration in the blood and the urine. Normally, urea concentration should be at least fifteen to twenty times greater in the urine than in the blood; a urea concentration less than ten times greater in the urine than in the blood usually represents a severe degree of renal insufficiency.

If serious renal insufficiency evolves, peritoneal dialysis is employed at an early stage, often within 2 to 3 days after operation with BUN levels of 75 to 90 mg/100 ml. Postponement of peritoneal dialysis, with progressive increase of BUN concentration above 100 mg/100 ml, may be associated with serious or even fatal cardiac arrhythmias. As the risk of arrhythmias cannot be predicted for an individual patient, the routine use of early dialysis has been of significant benefit. With frequent dialysis, recovery from the renal injury almost always takes place.

Oliguric renal failure of severe degree has a much more ominous prognosis, with a mortality rate exceeding 50 to 70

percent. Fortunately, this is rare. In some instances the etiology remains uncertain.

Fever. There is almost always some fever following extracorporeal circulation, temperatures of 38 to 39°C being very common in the first 1 to 3 days after operation. In some patients, unexplained fevers of 39 to 40°C may develop, probably as a result of minute areas of atelectasis. Contamination of the heart-lung machine with pyrogens was a frequent cause of fever in the early experiences with open heart operations but with disposable oxygenators now occurs rarely. Significant fever, with its detrimental effects on metabolic requirements, can be most simply controlled by the use of a hypothermia mattress beneath the patient through which cold fluid can be circulated at appropriate intervals.

Fever persisting beyond a few days after operation is commonly found to be due to atelectasis or a pleural effusion. Another frequent cause of fever is the so-called "pericardiotomy syndrome," which may develop in any patient in whom the pericardium has been opened at operation, even if extracorporeal circulation has not been employed. This puzzling syndrome, the cause of which still remains unknown despite numerous investigations, may be associated with sustained fever, a pericardial friction rub, and pericardial and pleural effusions. The white blood cell count may be increased in some patients, while in others it is normal or decreased to 5,000 to 7,000 white blood cells per cubic millimeter. In a minority of patients abnormal lymphocytes appear, the recognition of which greatly facilitates the diagnosis. Most patients respond promptly to administration of 50 to 60 mg prednisone daily, which is frequently employed for both a diagnostic and therapeutic test. Prednisone is given for 3 to 4 days and then stopped to see if fever recurs. Recurrences are not uncommon and may require administration of smaller amounts of prednisone, 10 to 20 mg daily, for several days.

Urinary tract infection is another frequent cause of postoperative fever and can be easily recognized by microscopic examination of the urine and appropriate bacterial cultures. With fever continuing more than a few days after operation, the dread question of bacterial endocarditis must always be considered. The diagnosis can be established or excluded only by serial blood cultures, which should routinely be done with persistent unexplained fever. Fortunately in recent years bacterial endocarditis has become extremely rare. With routine use of large amounts of antibiotics both during and following cardiac operations, staphylococcal endocarditis has almost disappeared. Rarely a fungal endocarditis, usually organisms of the *Candida* group, appears and is often lethal. Since our unit adopted the practice of stopping prophylactic antibiotics within 3 to 4 days after operation, as opposed to 7 to 14 days, fungal endocarditis has virtually disappeared.

Central Nervous System. Probably the most common cause of injury to the central nervous system following extracorporeal circulation is air embolism associated with incomplete evacuation of air from the cardiac chambers. It is extraordinarily difficult to remove all intracardiac air, because air pockets may be loculated in pulmonary veins, the left atrium, or the left ventricle. Rarely air accumulating in the right side of the heart with a functioning right ventricle may be propelled through the pulmonary vascular bed into the left side of the heart. Prevention of air embolism is more difficult when previous operations have been performed, producing adhesions which fix the heart in the pericardial cavity and limit manipulation and massage of the heart at the end of perfusion to displace air pockets. Use of both a left ventricular vent and an aortic vent, which function while the heart is beating, is a valuable method of protection from air emboli, since in some patients all air is not completely removed until the heart begins to beat.

Another cause of focal neurologic injury is calcium emboli, especially in patients with calcific aortic stenosis in whom extensive fragmentation of the calcific valve may occur as it is removed, often piecemeal, with rongeurs. Thrombi in the left atrium, usually in patients with chronic mitral stenosis, are another cause of emboli unless they are carefully removed. Fortunately, all these forms of cerebral injury are avoidable with a carefully planned and executed procedure.

With extracorporeal circulation for 5 to 6 hours or longer, especially when associated with significant trauma to the blood from extensive use of intracardiac suction, a diffuse depression of cerebral function may occur, almost always subsiding without residual neurologic injury in a few days. The exact cause of this difficulty is unknown but is probably sludging of blood elements in cerebral capillaries with focal areas of circulatory stasis. Fat emboli have been long considered as a possible cause, but their significance remains uncertain.

A curious postperfusion psychosis may develop in some patients, with all the emotional symptoms of a psychotic syndrome. Intensive therapy with appropriate sedation and physical restraints to avoid bodily harm is necessary. Fortunately such emotional disturbances almost always subside within 2 weeks after operation. They probably also result from diffuse disturbances in cerebral microcirculation.

With focal injuries to the central nervous system, convulsions are frequent and should be anticipated in therapy. With severe injuries, a tracheostomy is usually performed to facilitate removal of bronchial secretions and assist ventilation. In a seriously ill, comatose patient, a sustained convulsion with anoxia can precipitate a serious or fatal cardiac arrhythmia. This can be avoided if a tracheostomy with mechanical ventilation is performed prophylactically. Convulsions usually can be controlled satisfactorily with appropriate amounts of diphenylhydantoin (Dilantin) or phenobarbital. With neurologic injuries fever of 39 to 40°C is common but can be controlled simply by the use of a hypothermia mattress. A massive neurologic injury may be fatal, but less severe ones are seldom permanent. Although intensive care may be necessary for 3 to 4 weeks, virtually complete recovery usually results. If a neurologic deficit persists more than a month after operation, full recovery seldom occurs.

Gastrointestinal Disturbances. A mild paralytic ileus is frequent for the first 24 hours after operation, and for this reason patients are usually not allowed fluids by mouth for this period of time. Otherwise, gastric dilatation with the risk of vomiting and aspiration can occur. After this period of time, gastrointestinal disturbances are infrequent. Rarely, in seriously ill patients, a stress ulcer with serious gastrointestinal hemorrhage can develop. However, the routine use of a bland (antiulcer) diet, combined with antacid medications for the first few days after operation, has greatly decreased the frequency of this ulcer. Perforation of a stress ulcer, a rare and often fatal complication, has not been seen in our unit for several years.

Anemia. Often following operation there is a daily decrease in hematocrit to levels of 28 to 32 percent. Blood transfusion in appropriate amounts is usually given for severe anemia, while oral therapy with iron is sufficient for most patients. Although anemia can result from many causes, it is usually due to an accelerated rate of blood cell destruction, probably from trauma to the red blood cells during extracorporeal circulation.

Anticoagulant Therapy. Although policies vary at different cardiac centers, most patients with prosthetic valves are routinely started on anticoagulants in the 2 to 4 days following operation. Since 1971, with the use of cloth-covered valves, anticoagulant programs have varied widely among different centers, and the overall frequency of major thromboembolism is only 1 to 3 percent. At New York University, sodium warfarin is continued permanently for patients with prosthetic valves; when porcine heterografts are employed, the drug is prescribed for about 3 months following operation. Dosage levels are adjusted to maintain the prothrombin time at about two to two-and-a-half times normal. Once the dosage requirement for warfarin has stabilized, usually within 4 to 6 weeks after operation, aspirin, 0.6 Gm twice daily, is begun and continued daily for 2 years to minimize the hazard of platelet emboli.

CARDIAC ARREST AND VENTRICULAR FIBRILLATION

Cardiac arrest and ventricular fibrillation are considered together in this section because either of these catastrophes produces immediate cessation of the circulation. An injury causing generalized cardiac depression, such as anoxia, is more likely to lead to cardiac arrest, while agents increasing myocardial irritability, such as digitalis intoxication, are more likely to produce ventricular fibrillation. Diagnosis and treatment for the two conditions are, however, very similar.

HISTORICAL DATA. The first successful cardiac resuscitation was performed in 1901 by Igelsrud in Norway, but for many years this remained an isolated therapeutic triumph. The first successful case of electrical defibrillation was reported by Beck in 1947. In 1960 a dramatic advance in cardiac resuscitation occurred when Kouwenhoven, Jude, and Knickerbocker, working as a group at the Johns Hopkins Hospital, first introduced the concept of closed-chest massage. The same group also contributed greatly to the simultaneous development of methods of closed-chest defibrillation. The applicability of closed-chest cardiac massage and defibrillation has greatly enlarged the feasibility of cardiac resuscitation and has made it a responsibility of every physician to become familiar with these techniques. Resuscitative techniques have been successfully taught to large numbers of nonmedical personnel and have been applied effectively in many instances.

PATHOGENESIS. Etiology. A great many agents may cause cardiac arrest. The more frequent of these will be briefly mentioned.

Coronary Thrombosis. Coronary thrombosis, with or without myocardial infarction, may induce either cardiac arrest or ventricular fibrillation and is a frequent cause of cardiac arrest refractory to all forms of therapy.

Anoxia. The depressant effect of anoxia on the myocardium is a frequent major underlying factor in producing cardiac arrest. This can occur from many causes, including depression of respiration, airway obstruction, and aspiration of gastric contents.

Drugs. Several drugs may produce either ventricular fibrillation or cardiac arrest when excessive amounts are used or when an abnormal sensitivity to the drug is present. Digitalis is one of the most prominent of this group, for the sensitivity of the myocardium to digitalis varies with the serum electrolyte concentrations, especially potassium.

Serum Electrolyte Abnormalities. Either deficiency or excess of potassium can cause cardiac arrest. The effects of the abnormal potassium concentration are significantly influenced by the existing concentration of calcium ions, and also by the presence of acidosis or alkalosis.

Anesthesia. Almost any anesthetic agent in excessive amounts will depress the myocardium and precipitate cardiac arrest. Statistical surveys have disclosed that cardiac arrest occurs in approximately 1 in every 1,500 operations.

Bradycardia. A profound bradycardia, with a heart rate below 60 beats per minute, may result in ventricular extrasystoles, subsequently followed by ventricular tachycardia or fibrillation. This is frequently seen in patients with a complete heart block unless the heart rate is increased by electrical or chemical stimulation.

Cardiac Catheterization. Ventricular fibrillation is an infrequent but well-recognized complication of cardiac catheterization or angiocardiography, usually developing during manipulation of the cardiac catheter into different cardiac chambers.

Reflex Mechanisms. On many occasions cardiac arrest has developed in association with some event which stimulated the vagus nerve. Such episodes include endotracheal suctioning, insertion of a gastric tube, or vomiting. It is doubtful that a vagal reflex per se can ever arrest a normal heart. In the laboratory, normal hearts can be arrested for only a few seconds even with continuous electrical stimulation of the vagus nerve. It is probable in clinical circumstances that only a myocardium seriously injured from other causes will be arrested or fibrillated during some event which stimulates the vagus nerve.

Aberrant Electric Currents. When implanted pacemaker wires traverse the chest wall, faulty electrical mechanisms associated with monitoring, electrocardiography, or electrocautery can be responsible for fibrillating the heart. Malfunction of an implanted pacemaker is yet another cause.

Pathophysiology. The cerebral anoxia resulting from cessation of circulation produces significant brain injury within 3 to 4 minutes, depending upon the temperature. Periods of anoxia for 6 to 8 minutes may produce extensive but reversible brain damage, whereas longer periods regularly cause irreversible brain injury. Myocardial anoxia is, of course, also present but is of little clinical significance as compared to the central nervous system injury.

DIAGNOSIS. Since brain injury will develop following 3 to 4 minutes of cardiac arrest, it is imperative that a diagnosis be made rapidly and therapy begun. The physician considering a diagnosis of cardiac arrest should either confirm or exclude it within 30 to 60 seconds and act accordingly. In most patients the diagnosis can be simply made. There is an abrupt disappearance of peripheral pulses, most easily confirmed by palpation of the femoral or carotid arteries. Loss of consciousness quickly occurs, as well as absence of respiratory activity except for a few agonal gasps. Auscultation of the chest readily demonstrates that no cardiac sounds are audible. Complex diagnostic maneuvers which require larger amounts of time should be avoided. It should be emphasized that the *electrocardiogram is of little value for the diagnosis of cardiac arrest,* for electrical activity can continue on the electrocardiogram for some minutes after effective cardiac contractions have ceased. The main value of the electrocardiogram is to demonstrate the presence of ventricular fibrillation, because cardiac arrest can be differentiated from ventricular fibrillation only by the electrocardiogram or by direct inspection of the myocardium.

The most common differential diagnosis from cardiac arrest is the presence of extreme bradycardia with hypotension, as in someone who has fainted or developed anaphylactic shock from a hypersensitivity syndrome. Usually differentiation is not difficult, for although profound peripheral vascular collapse is present, there is some respiratory activity and not a total loss of consciousness.

TREATMENT. Ventilation. The most urgent first step in treatment of cardiac arrest is to provide adequate oxygenation (Fig. 19-2). It is futile to begin cardiac massage without ventilation of the lungs, although under the pressures of extreme circumstances, this obvious fact is often overlooked. Ventilation is most readily accomplished by mouth-to-mouth insufflation of the lungs. This can be begun immediately and continued until less laborious methods can be arranged. Most cardiac resuscitation kits include a laryngoscope and an endotracheal tube which can be inserted by any physician with moderate experience. Until an endotracheal tube can be inserted, however, mouth-to-mouth ventilation should be continued. Attempts to perform a hurried tracheostomy should not be made unless there is an obstruction at the larynx. Tracheostomy under emergency circumstances can be surprisingly difficult and quickly waste the precious few minutes available for preserving cerebral function. If an endotracheal tube cannot be inserted, a cricothyroidotomy, rather than an emergency tracheostomy, is probably preferable, as evidenced by the report of Brantigan and Grow.

Cardiac Massage. Closed-chest massage should be used in the majority of patients. Its efficacy depends upon intermittent compression of the heart between the sternum and the vertebral column, with lateral motion of the heart limited by the pericardium. For performing cardiac massage, the patient must be on a firm surface, such as the floor or a board under his shoulders. Certain points of technique are essential. The heel of the hand should be applied over the lower third of the sternum with the other hand above it to depress the sternum intermittently for 3 to 4 cm (Fig. 19-3). Sternal compression should be brisk, depressing the sternum sharply and then releasing it to permit cardiac filling. Compression of the sternum at a lower level near the xyphoid process may injure the liver, while compression more superiorly or laterally over the chest will result in multiple fractures of the ribs. Massage should be at a rate of about 60 per minute; more than one person is usually required, since the person performing massage will fatigue quickly. The amount of force applied should be gauged by palpation of a peripheral pulse, usually the femoral. Some caution is required to be certain that a regurgitant pulse in the femoral vein is not confused with a pulse in the femoral artery, because a strong retrograde pulse wave can be propagated down the vena cava during massage. Massage should be continued for as long as cardiac resuscitation remains feasible, especially if cerebral function is intact. A definite time limit cannot be given beyond which cardiac massage should be abandoned, although most successful cardiac resuscitations are accomplished within a few minutes. On one occasion we partici-

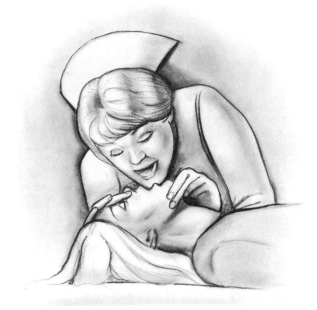

Fig. 19-2. Technique of mouth-to-mouth ventilation. The chin of the patient must be held forward with one hand to prevent obstruction of the nasopharynx by backward displacement of the tongue. The nostrils need to be occluded with the other hand. The head should be extended on the cervical spine to avoid obstruction in the nasopharynx.

pated in a successful cardiac resuscitation which required 2 hours and 20 minutes of direct massage before a fibrillating heart could be successfully defibrillated. The patient was still well 20 years later.

Open cardiac massage, performed through a lateral thoracotomy in the left fourth or fifth intercostal space, is seldom needed. It should, however, be used if there is an open pericardium, cardiac tamponade, or massive intrathoracic hemorrhage.

Drugs and Fluids. Epinephrine, sodium bicarbonate, and calcium are the most useful agents. Epinephrine, 1 to 2 ml of 1:10,000 dilution, may be injected directly into the heart or into a peripheral vein. Calcium, 3 to 4 ml of a 10% solution, is a similarly powerful stimulant of myocardial contraction. Acidosis is especially common with

Fig. 19-3. *A.* Closed-chest massage. The heel of the hand should be used to compress intermittently the lower portion of the sternum toward the vertebral column. The effectiveness of the compression should be monitored by palpation of a peripheral pulse by another member of the team. Artificial ventilation must be performed at the same time. *B.* Cross section of chest showing the anatomic basis for closed-chest massage. The heart is seen suspended in the midthorax between the sternum anteriorly and the vertebral column posteriorly. The pericardium must be intact for closed-chest massage to be effective. *C.* Compression of the heart as the sternum is depressed downward toward the vertebral column.

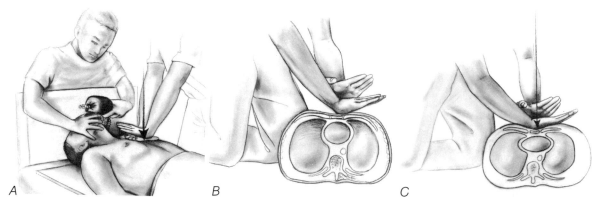

A   B   C

cardiac arrest and may require vigorous therapy to restore a normal pH before effective cardiac contractions can be obtained. Sodium bicarbonate, in amounts as large as 200 to 300 mEq, may be required if severe acidosis is present. Rapid intravenous infusion of fluids, up to 1 liter or more, is usually of value, especially if hypovolemia was present before cardiac arrest occurred. An intravenous infusion of vasopressors, usually 1 to 4 μg/minute of norepinephrine or epinephrine, is frequently of value. Other drugs, such as atropine or digitalis, are usually of little benefit.

Defibrillation. In the presence of ventricular fibrillation, which can be confirmed only by the electrocardiogram or by direct inspection of the myocardium, electrical defibrillation is required. This can be accomplished in the closed chest by applying electrodes over the base and apex of the heart or by applying one large electrode posteriorly near the vertebral column and a smaller electrode anteriorly near the cardiac apex (Fig. 19-4). Defibrillation can be done with either alternating or direct current, although studies in recent years have indicated that direct current defibrillation is preferable (approximately 400 joules). With an open chest, direct defibrillation can be easily accomplished by application of electrodes to the heart and administration of an appropriate electric impulse, usually 110 to 120 volts for 0.1 second. The usual cause of failure to defibrillate is either an anoxic or an acidotic myocardium. Vigorous massage before application of the electric shock may be required to oxgenate the myocardium sufficiently. Acidosis can be corrected with bicarbonate. Injection of epinephrine may also stimulate myocardial tone and enhance subsequent defibrillation. Unless a coronary thrombosis has occurred, it should be possible to defibrillate almost all fibrillating hearts, although the ensuing

Fig. 19-4. Technique of closed-chest defibrillation. One electrode paddle is applied at the apex of the heart and the other at the base. The most common errors are inadequate electrical contact between the electrodes and the skin or inadequate amounts of current.

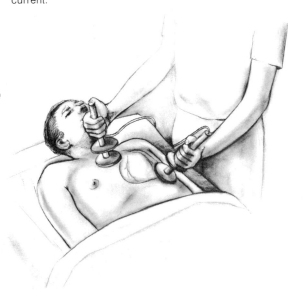

cardiac arrest may be refractory to therapy. Inability to defibrillate is usually due to one or more correctible causes, such as inadequate electric stimulus, inadequate application of electrodes, anoxic myocardium, or acidosis. The heart should be observed closely when the electric shock is applied. If adequate current is transmitted through the myocardium, the fibrillations will cease almost immediately, though they may recur. If the fibrillations are not stopped completely for a short period, enough current has not been transmitted, and the stimulus should be adjusted accordingly. Causes of inadequate current include the voltage applied, the electrodes, and the manner in which the electrodes are applied to the heart.

Therapy following Cardiac Resuscitation. Following restoration of an adequate heartbeat, careful note should be made of the presence of injury to the central nervous system. This is usually indicated by continuing coma. Patients with significant brain injury are best treated by mild hypothermia, lowering the body temperature to 33 to 34°C and maintaining this temperature for 3 to 4 days. There are abundant experimental data indicating that this mild degree of hypothermia will significantly enhance recovery from cerebral injury. Hypothermia should be begun soon, because hyperthermia to 39 to 40°C often develops within 2 to 4 hours. Massive doses of a steroid, e.g., 2 to 3 Gm of prednisone, should be given every 6 to 8 hours for 24 to 48 hours to minimize cerebral edema. The efficacy is difficult to measure, although steroids have been shown to be beneficial in experimental cerebral edema.

Continuous visual monitoring of the cardiac rhythm with an oscilloscope is essential, because arrhythmias are frequent and some can progress to ventricular fibrillation unless promptly treated. Intravenously administered lidocaine, 1 mg/minute, and procainamide are both very useful drugs for suppressing cardiac arrhythmias. Adequacy of cardiac output and ventilation can be monitored by periodic measurment of arterial and central venous blood-gas concentrations (P_{O_2}, P_{CO_2}, and pH).

Fluid therapy should be carefully regulated, depending upon the blood volume and the renal function. Excessive fluids may intensify cerebral edema. Adequacy of ventilation should be carefully assessed, because anoxia can readily precipitate another episode of cardiac arrest. In comatose patients, a tracheostomy is usually performed, and frequent assisted ventilation with a mechanical respirator is performed for 2 to 3 days.

PROGNOSIS. Unless a myocardial thrombosis or some other irreversible injury is present, the majority of patients in whom cardiac arrest has developed may be effectively treated if the correct diagnosis is made promptly.

When a reversible cardiac injury is present, as with overdose of an anesthetic agent, cardiac resuscitation is almost uniformly possible if begun quickly. Similarly, ventricular fibrillation from a variety of mechanisms can be promptly and effectively treated by external defibrillation if defibrillation is done before severe myocardial anoxia has developed. The usual cause of failure of defibrillation is the presence of an underlying myocardial thrombosis.

MITRAL STENOSIS

HISTORICAL DATA. A valiant effort to treat mitral stenosis by excising a portion of the valve with a valvulotome was made by Cutler and Levine in 1923, but the resulting mitral insufficiency caused a prohibitive operative mortality. Souttar, in 1925, performed a digital commissurotomy in one patient. Thereafter surgical efforts virtually ceased for over 20 years until 1948–1949 when Harken et al. and Bailey independently demonstrated the value of digital commissurotomy. These early commissurotomies, often limited in extent, frequently produced striking clinical improvement, even though mitral stenosis frequently recurred within 5 years. A transventricular mitral dilator developed around 1957 produced a more extensive commissurotomy and was widely adopted. Subsequently the increasing safety of cardiopulmonary bypass made commissurotomy under direct vision the procedure of choice in most centers, though some groups still obtain excellent results with a closed commissurotomy. When a closed commissurotomy is undertaken, the heart-lung machine is usually kept on a standby basis to permit use of cardiopulmonary bypass if closed commissurotomy becomes hazardous or is unsuccessful. When the mitral valve has been virtually destroyed by fibrosis and calcification, effective commissurotomy is not possible, and replacement with a prosthetic valve is necessary.

ETIOLOGY. All evidence indicates that mitral stenosis is almost always due to rheumatic fever, even though a definite history of rheumatic fever can be obtained in only about 50 percent of patients. Congenital mitral stenosis is very rare, less than 300 cases having been reported. After the initial episode of rheumatic fever, symptoms of mitral stenosis may not appear for 10 or more years but may develop as soon as 3 years in some patients and as late as 25 years in others. Selzer and Cohn, in an excellent review of clinical characteristics of mitral stenosis, have suggested that scarring of the mitral valve from rheumatic fever may cause turbulent flow of blood which in turn causes progressive scarring and contraction over many years; this would explain the appearance of severe mitral stenosis 20 to 30 years after the last known bout of rheumatic fever.

PATHOLOGY. Although rheumatic fever produces a pancarditis, involving pericardium, myocardium, and endocardium, the most serious permanent injury results from the endocarditis. Permanent myocardial injury following recovery from acute myocarditis is ill defined and apparently seldom of clinical significance. Endocarditis produces ulceration of the endocardium along the edges of the valve leaflets where they normally appose in systole. Tiny, 1- to 2-mm nodules of fibrin and platelets accumulate and may progress to fusion of the leaflets at the commissures. A more serious injury evolves from extensive valvulitis with fibrosis and contraction of the body of the leaflets, compounded in subsequent years with calcification and decreasing leaflet mobility. Inflammation of the chordae tendineae similarly leads to fibrosis with contraction, thickening, and fusion. With severe disease the chordae contract to such an extent that the valve leaflets are pulled down to appose the tips of the underlying papillary muscles.

In many patients mitral stenosis gradually increases in severity over many years, at times more than 20. Previously these progressive changes were considered due to clinically silent episodes of rheumatic fever. A more plausible current hypothesis is that the changes are hemodynamic in origin, resulting from turbulent flow of blood originally produced by the initial inflammation and scarring.

The possibilities of surgical correction of mitral stenosis vary greatly with the nature of the valve injury. When simple fusion of the commissures is the only lesion, mitral commissurotomy is highly successful. With concomitant fibrosis and rigidity of the leaflets, commissurotomy is less effective. If the chordae tendineae have contracted and fused to make the leaflets immobile, commissurotomy may be impossible. With such advanced pathology replacement of the diseases valve with a prosthesis is necessary. How often this is required varies with the type of patient operated on. When operation is performed fairly "early" in the course of the disease, valvular reconstruction, rather than replacement, should be possible in the majority of patients, i.e., 85 to 90 percent.

PATHOPHYSIOLOGY. A normal mitral valve has a cross-sectional area between 4 and 6 cm^2. Reduction of the cross-sectional area to 2 to 2.5 cm^2 constitutes the mildest form of mitral stenosis. Typical auscultatory findings are present, but the patient is often asymptomatic (Class I). Further reduction to the range of 1.5 to 2.0 cm^2 produces some symptoms (Class II disability); these are more severe with a cross-sectional area in the range of 1 to 1.5 cm^2. Patients with a cross-sectional area of less than 1 cm^2 are usually seriously disabled (Class IV). A valve area near 0.6 cm^2 is said to be the minimal size compatible with life.

Three significant physiologic events result from mitral stenosis—increase in left atrial pressure, decrease in cardiac output, and increase in pulmonary vascular resistance. Increase in left atrial pressure (normally less than 10 to 12 mm Hg) is the immediate consequence of mitral stenosis. The degree of elevation of left atrial pressure varies with three factors: (1) the cross-sectional area of the mitral orifice, (2) cardiac output, and (3) cardiac rate. These three factors represent physical laws determining pressure-flow relations through a stenotic orifice, namely, cross-sectional area of orifice, total volume of flow, and duration of time during which flow occurs. When left atrial pressure rises to exceed oncotic pressure of plasma (25 to 30 mm Hg), transudation of fluid across the pulmonary capillaries will occur. The result of this transudation depends upon the capacity of the pulmonary lymphatics to transport the additional fluid. When the fluid load exceeds the capacity of the lymphatic circulation, pulmonary edema results. Clinically, therefore, left atrial pressure and concomitant pulmonary symptoms vary with the degree of mitral stenosis, the cardiac output as influenced by exercise or emotion, and the length of diastole determined by cardiac rate.

As the oncotic pressure of plasma is 25 to 30 mm Hg,

about that of a column of blood 12 to 14 in. high, pulmonary congestion in the upright position may be much greater in the lower lobes of the lung than in the upper, for the average thorax is about 20 in. high. A patient with only basilar rales in the upright position may develop extensive pulmonary congestion when supine, with cough, dyspnea, or frank pulmonary edema. Hence, the pathogenesis of paroxysmal nocturnal dyspnea.

The cardiac output is fixed at a low level by the rigid stenotic orifice. With exercise, cardiac output cannot be increased significantly, and dyspnea results. The general fatigue and limitation of physical activity with mitral stenosis is a clinical reflection of this physiologic inability to increase cardiac output.

The degree to which pulmonary vascular resistance increases with mitral stenosis varies greatly among different patients. The cause for the variation is unknown. Some, with severe mitral stenosis, have little change, while in others vascular resistance increases to levels fifteen to twenty times greater than normal. This increased resistance is primarily a result of vasoconstriction in the pulmonary arterioles, ultimately intensified by hypertrophy of the media and intima. In far advanced cases recurrent pulmonary emboli may create additional obstruction, but this is uncommon. Fortunately, in the vast majority of patients, the increased vascular resistance either decreases greatly or disappears following surgical correction.

Two other serious disabilities which appear with chronic mitral stenosis are atrial fibrillation and systemic embolization. Atrial fibrillation is the usual ultimate consequence of the atrial hypertrophy produced by chronic left atrial hypertension. Fibrillation produces some decrease in cardiac output and also is often a prelude to more serious arrhythmias. The most serious consequence, however, is the development of thrombi, usually in the ineffectively contracting left atrial appendage. The frequency of thrombi varies both with the duration of mitral stenosis and the presence of atrial fibrillation. Utlimately thrombi develop in 15 to 20 percent of patients, after which episodes of arterial embolism appear with increasing frequency. Before either anticoagulant therapy or operation was possible, cerebral embolism caused death in 20 to 25 percent of patients dying from mitral stenosis.

CLINICAL MANIFESTATIONS. Symptoms. The most important symptom is *dyspnea.* This appears whenever mean left atrial pressure exceeds 30 mm Hg long enough to produce significant transudation of fluid into the pulmonary capillaries. Characteristically, it first appears with extreme exertion and subsequently, with more severe stenosis, occurs with lesser degrees of exertion. It may also appear with emotion or other circumstances which increase cardiac output.

Several other symptoms subsequently appear, all developing as a result of recurrent pulmonary congestion. A chronic *cough,* worse in the evenings in the recumbent position, is frequent, reflecting basilar congestion. *Orthopnea* and *paroxysmal nocturnal dyspnea* similarly reflect the influence of the upright position on the localization of pulmonary congestion. In the upright position, congestion may be limited to the lower lobes but becomes more diffuse in the supine position. Mobilization of peripheral edema from the lower extremities when the patient is supine intensifies the degree of pulmonary congestion. *Hemoptysis* is a frequent symptom, varying from expectoration of blood-tinged sputum to massive amounts of bright red blood, in unusual circumstances exceeding 1 liter. Fortunately such severe hemoptysis, although an alarming symptom, usually subsides spontaneously. Rarely, an emergency mitral valvotomy is required. Episodes of *pulmonary edema* occur when pulmonary congestion greatly exceeds the capacity of the pulmonary lymphatics. In contrast to hemoptysis, pulmonary edema may be fatal unless quickly and effectively treated.

When pulmonary vascular resistance rises to produce pulmonary hypertension, failure of the right side of the heart appears, manifested by venous distension, hepatic enlargement, and peripheral edema.

As mentioned earlier, atrial fibrillation develops eventually in most patients. Initially it may be transient, but ultimately in most patients chronic atrial fibrillation is the most common rhythm.

Arterial embolism is a constant threat, especially with atrial fibrillation, although emboli can occur with a sinus rhythm. Emboli evolve from stasis in the dilated left atrium, especially in the atrial appendage. Rarely, huge thrombi 5 to 10 cm in diameter may fill much of the left atrium and partly obstruct the ostia of the pulmonary veins.

Angina pectoris develops in about 10 percent of patients. The basic cause is unclear, for it is usually not due to associated coronary atherosclerosis. Possible mechanisms include a low cardiac output, impaired blood flow during diastole because of tachycardia, and recurrent small emboli to the coronary arteries.

Physical Examination. A patient with chronic, severe mitral stenosis may be thin and frail, with the muscular wasting characteristic of a chronic illness. Dilated neck veins are visible if congestive failure is present. Rubor and/or cyanosis are often seen over the fingers or lips. These signs reflect a chronic severe restriction in cardiac output, resulting in blood flowing slowly through peripheral capillary beds. Rales are frequently audible over the lung bases.

On examination of the heart, the cardiac size and the quality of the apical impulse are of particular importance. Often with pure mitral stenosis, the cardiac size is normal, and the apical impulse is normal or decreased in intensity. A forceful, heaving left ventricular impulse immediately suggests that associated disease, such as mitral insufficiency or aortic valvular disease with resulting ventricular hypertrophy, is present. With increased pulmonary vascular resistance, palpation of the left parasternal area may find a "lift," resulting from contraction of a hypertrophied right ventricle. The pulse rhythm may be regular but is usually atrial fibrillation.

The three significant auscultatory findings with mitral stenosis are the diastolic rumble, an opening snap, and an increased first sound. The apical diastolic rumble, at times sharply localized to an area at the apex only 2 to 3 cm in diameter, is the hallmark of mitral stenosis. It may be of grade I or II intensity in some patients, while in others it is unusually loud with a palpable thrill. The intensity of the murmur, however, does not correlate with the severity of the stenosis. Rarely "silent" mitral stenosis is present without an audible murmur. This results from a calcified, fibrosed valve with little mobility. The increased first sound, the origin of which is not certain, is another distinctive feature and is often the first auscultatory abnormality detected. The opening snap, closely following the second sound, is the third distinctive feature. In many patients careful auscultation can immediately establish the diagnosis of mitral stenosis by finding the triad of an opening snap, followed by a diastolic rumble, and an accentuated first sound.

A short apical systolic murmur may be heard in patients with pure mitral stenosis without any associated mitral insufficiency. Loud pansystolic murmurs, however, which are transmitted to the axilla usually indicate associated mitral insufficiency. A systolic murmur from tricuspid insufficiency may be confused with one arising from mitral insufficiency. The systolic murmur of tricuspid insufficiency, although audible at the apex with hypertrophy of the right ventricle, is usually heard equally well near the sternum and may be accentuated with deep inspiration.

Laboratory Studies. The initial change in mitral stenosis is dilatation of the left atrium (Fig. 19-5). Hence, detection of slight degrees of enlargement of the left atrium is of particular importance in establishing the diagnosis. Once it has been determined that the left atrium is enlarged, however, there is little correlation between the actual size of the left atrium and the severity of the mitral stenosis. Left atrial enlargement is best detected with a lateral chest roentgenogram exposed during oral administration of barium to outline the esophagus. Characteristically, the middle third of the esophagus is displaced backward to form a slight concave curve. With additional degrees of enlargement, the dilated left atrium may be visible as a double shadow in the posteroanterior roentgenogram, forming a separate dense shadow behind the normal shadow of the right atrium. The left border of the cardiac shadow also shows characteristic changes with mitral stenosis, for the normal concavity between the shadow of the aortic knob and the left ventricle becomes obliterated as both the left atrium and the pulmonary artery enlarge to produce a "straight" left heart border. The overall cardiac size may be normal, but lateral views can demonstrate enlargement of the right ventricle when pulmonary vascular resistance has increased. Calcification of the mitral valve is visible with chronic disease in older patients.

Careful roentgenographic scrutiny of the lung fields is of particular importance, for several abnormalities occur. Engorged pulmonary veins can be unusually prominent, often with a greater degree of dilatation in the veins to the upper lobes. With pulmonary hypertension the pulmonary arteries are also enlarged. With chronic, severe left atrial hypertension, dilated pulmonary lymphatics become visible as transverse lines across the lower lung fields, "Kerley lines," indicating significant left atrial hypertension.

The electrocardiogram is normal in some patients. The earliest change is an increased P wave from hypertrophy of the left atrium. Unfortunately, this is not consistent, and different studies have reported variation in the frequency of P-wave abnormalities from as low as 20 to 30 percent to as high as 70 to 80 percent. Only with increase in pulmonary vascular resistance does right ventricular hypertrophy produce distinct electrocardiographic changes, with the development of a right axis deviation. Hence, the electrocardiogram often is an inaccurate guide to the severity of the mitral stenosis. It is of particular value, however, in differential diagnosis, for signs of left ventricular hypertrophy immediately suggest some disease in addition to mitral stenosis, usually mitral insufficiency or aortic valvular disease.

Cardiac catheterization is required to evaluate mitral stenosis precisely, as well as for detecting the presence of additional valvular disease, such as mitral insufficiency or aortic valvular disease. Left atrial pressure is usually estimated from the pulmonary capillary "wedge" pressure, although alternatively the left atrium can be entered directly with a catheter, usually by puncture of the atrial septum. The left atrial pressure in isolated mitral stenosis is increased from the normal range of 5 to 10 mm Hg to levels of 20 to 30 mm Hg with severe stenosis, producing a diastolic pressure gradient between the left atrium and left ventricle of 10 to 20 mm Hg. It is important to realize that the left atrial pressure varies not only with the severity of the stenosis, but also with the cardiac output and the cardiac rate. Hence, evaluation of an isolated determination must include assessment of these additional factors. The most precise measurement is mathematical calculation of the cross-sectional area of the mitral valve, determined by the pressure gradient and the cardiac output. Angiography may demonstrate rigidity and limited mobility of the valve leaflets but is not of great diagnostic value. It is of particular value, however, in determining the presence of mitral insufficiency by noting the reflux of dye after injection into the left ventricle. Coronary arteriography is an important part of the evaluation of cardiac catheterization, especially in patients over forty years of age in whom coronary atherosclerosis may be present.

DIAGNOSIS. A diagnosis of mitral stenosis can usually be made with certainty on physical examination, with the finding of the triad of an opening snap, an apical diastolic rumble, and an increased first sound. These abnormalities often occur in association with a normal left ventricle, an enlarged left atrium, signs of pulmonary congestion, pulmonary hypertension, and right ventricular hypertrophy. The differential diagnosis should include associated mitral insufficiency, tricuspid insufficiency, or aortic valvular disease.

TREATMENT. Indications for Operation. Operation is usually recommended for any patient with symptoms, because the risk is small (1 to 3 percent) and the slight but definite hazard of cerebral embolism is always present. If peripheral embolism has occurred, operation should be performed as soon as the patient has recovered from the embolic episode, for sooner or later emboli almost always recur. Until operation is performed, continuous anticoagulant therapy should be employed.

Fortunately, mitral stenosis almost always can be successfully operated upon, no matter how far advanced the disease or how severe the pulmonary hypertension. The immediate risk of operation is increased with far advanced disease, but surviving patients nearly always show remarkable improvement, with a significant decrease in, or complete disappearance of, pulmonary hypertension.

General Considerations. Since 1971 at New York University almost all mitral valve operations have been performed with cardiopulmonary bypass. The "closed" commissurotomy, performed blindly with the index finger introduced through the left atrial appendage, has been virtually abandoned. For some years mitral operations were performed with the heart-lung machine on a "standby" basis: a closed commissurotomy was attempted first, but if it was unsatisfactory, cardiopulmonary bypass was employed. For several reasons, an open operation with cardiopulmonary bypass is now preferred. The risk of bypass is very small, approaching less than 1 percent. The hazard of emboli from thrombi in the atrium or calcium in the mitral valve is much less than with blind, digital commissurotomy. Of even greater importance, perhaps, is that a more effective commissurotomy can be performed as the commissures can be clearly separated, underlying fused

chordae separated, and a wide mitral orifice obtained without producing mitral insufficiency. Not all cardiac centers agree with this policy, however, and some continue to report excellent short-term results with the classic digital commissurotomy.

Technique of Open Mitral Commissurotomy. A median sternotomy incision is employed in almost all cases unless a previous sternotomy incision has been made, in which case a left thoracotomy is used. A sternotomy is preferred because of ready access to the heart, including palpation of the mitral and tricuspid valves, cannulation of the aorta and venae cavae, as well as access to the aortic valve if needed. Once cardiopulmonary bypass is established, body temperature is lowered to 30°C and the heart fibrillated. The left atrium is opened with a longitudinal incision in the interatrial groove, anterior to the point of entry of the right pulmonary veins. By extending the atriotomy beneath the superior vena cava above and the inferior vena cava below, adequate exposure of the mitral valve can be obtained. Usually the aorta is intermittently occluded for periods of 10 to 15 minutes to attain a dry, quiet heart. Before the aortic occlusion clamp is intermittently released, a small catheter vent is placed in the ascending aorta through a stab wound to remove accumulated air.

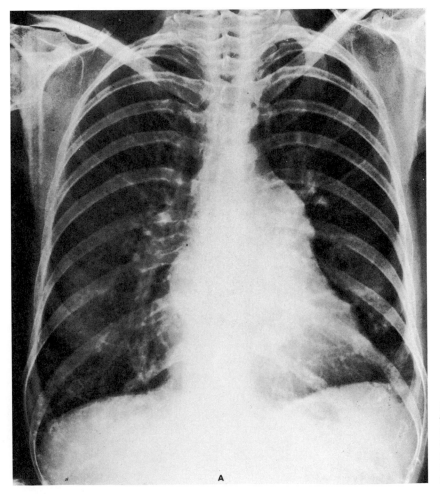

Fig. 19-5. *A.* Chest roentgenogram of a patient with mitral stenosis showing a heart of normal size. The prominent pulmonary artery along the left cardiac border is characteristic of this condition. The enlarged left atrium can be seen as a double density behind the shadow normally formed by the right atrium.

Periodically the heart is defibrillated and allowed to beat for 3 to 4 minutes, to permit adequate distribution of coronary blood flow.

Any thrombi in the atrium or atrial appendage are carefully removed before the mitral valve is approached. The atrial appendage, a potential source of postoperative emboli, is routinely excluded from the atrial cavity, either by closure of the orifice from within the atrium or by amputating the appendage outside the heart (Fig. 19-6).

The fused commissures of the mitral valve are best exposed by inserting sutures into both the aortic and mural leaflets for traction. By applying *horizontal,* not vertical, traction on the two leaflets, the fused commissures can be clearly visualized. The commissure is then carefully separated with a knife, often with a right-angled clamp held open below the commissure to identify chordae arising from the underlying papillary muscle and inserting on the adjacent leaflets. Division of any chordae is scrupulously avoided. A technical problem encountered in 25 to 30 percent of patients is fusion and contraction of the chordae beneath the commissures, often with the fused commissures virtually attached to the papillary muscle. In such instances the papillary muscle is carefully split with a knife for as much as 1 cm, carefully preserving the chordae to each leaflet. This, of course, greatly increases the efficacy of

the commissurotomy and is one of the attractive features of routine open operation.

The question of having produced mitral insufficiency following commissurotomy can be assessed by selective induction of aortic insufficiency, using a small plastic catheter (#10 French) with multiple side perforations over a length of 6 to 7 cm. The catheter is introduced into the ascending aorta through a stab wound and manipulated across the aortic valve into the left ventricle, occluding the aorta momentarily to permit collapse of the valve leaflets. With the catheter in its proper position, some perforations are in the aorta while the remainder are in the ventricle (Figs. 19-7 to 19-9). Then, when the aortic clamp is released, removing intraaortic air, blood refluxes through the catheter into the ventricle, ballooning the aortic leaflets of the mitral valve and seating it firmly against the mural leaflet. Areas of regurgitation can be readily identified and corrected, usually with direct sutures, although a few patients may require an annuloplasty.

As originally reported by Mullin in 1974, this method has been used for about 5 years and has greatly simplified valvuloplasty, permitting a bolder approach. Hence a wider opening can be safely produced. This, in turn, should minimize the likelihood of turbulent flow and recurrence in the future. For a long time the reliability of the method

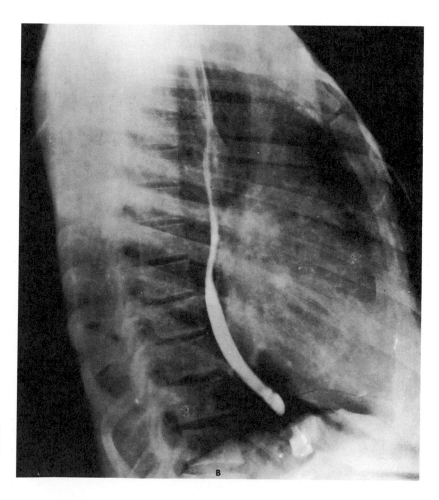

Fig. 19-5. *B.* Lateral roentgenogram of the same patient shows enlargement of the left atrium, producing a concave displacement of the esophagus, which has been filled with barium.

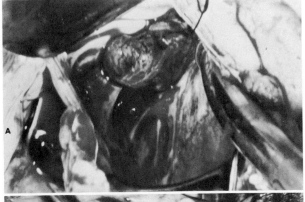

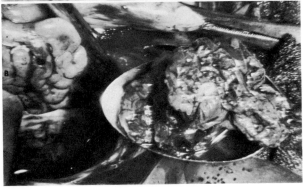

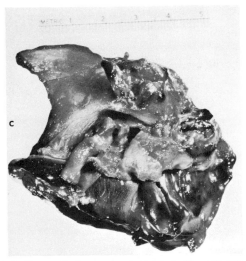

Fig. 19-6. Open mitral commissurotomy. *A.* The left atrium has been incised and the edges retracted. A small thrombus is present in the midportion of the field, demonstrating the pathologic condition which frequently causes cerebral embolism with mitral stenosis. *B.* Large clot found within the left atrium. With cardiopulmonary bypass functioning, the left atrium has been opened widely. The laminated clot is being removed with a large spoon. A clamp occluding the ascending aorta to avoid embolization of clot is visible at the top of the illustration. *C.* Large laminated clot removed at operation from a patient with mitral stenosis. The inability to detect the presence of such a clot before operation is the most cogent reason that all mitral commissurotomies should be performed with a pump-oxygenator as a "standby," to be employed if such a clot is found.

was routinely checked by subsequent digital palpation of the mitral valve with the heart beating and the systolic pressure near the preoperative level, but this now seems superfluous.

After discontinuing bypass, adequate correction of the mitral stenosis is confirmed by measuring left atrial and ventricular pressure by needle puncture and demonstrating elimination of the end-diastolic pressure gradient. This is an important check, surprisingly neglected in many reports, because with fibrosis and stiff mitral leaflets an opening that seems adequate may be restrictive because of the impaired mobility of the leaflets.

Following operation convalescence is usually benign, and the patient is discharged in 10 to 12 days. If atrial fibrillation is present, an attempt is made to convert it to a sinus rhythm. This is usually successful if chronic atrial fibrillation, with hypertrophy of left atrial musculature, has not been present.

Technique of Mitral Valve Replacement. An approach with a sternotomy incision similar to that for open commissurotomy is used. Mitral replacement, rather than commissurotomy, is almost always necessary if both insufficiency and stenosis are present. It is frequently needed for mitral stenosis with extensive calcification in the valve if the calcification is in the commissures, while calcification in the leaflets does not preclude effective commissurotomy. When replacement is done, the valve is excised by incising it a few millimeters from the annulus with a circumferential incision, which often removes the entire valve intact (Fig. 19-10). Underlying papillary muscles are divided near their apexes. A ball-valve prosthesis is used almost routinely, though excellent results also have been reported with a disc prosthesis. The ball-valve prosthesis has the advantages of longer experience in its use and less likelihood of prosthetic failure, which has been more frequent with a disc prosthesis. The problem of a small left ventricle with mitral stenosis has been avoided by careful selection of a valve of appropriate size. Rarely an obstructing collar of muscle in the wall of the left ventricle has been excised to avoid possible protrusion of muscle into the cage of the prosthesis. With these precautions a ball-valve prosthesis has functioned well. Some have proposed that ventricular function is better with a disc than with a ball-valve prosthesis, but data demonstrating a significant difference are meager (Figs. 19-11 and 19-12).

The prosthesis is inserted with a series of 12 to 18 mattress sutures of Dacron, with a pledget in each mattress suture to avoid the suture's cutting through a friable annulus (Fig. 19-13). Before pledgeted mattress sutures were routinely employed, significant postoperative insufficiency from suture leaks continued to occur, but the routine use of pledgets has virtually eliminated this complication. An alternative technique, widely and effectively used by others, is to insert 25 to 30 simple interrupted sutures. Care is taken to insert the sutures in the annulus, but no deeper, to avoid injury to the coronary sinus, the circumflex coronary artery, or the conduction bundle. Once the prosthesis has been tied in position, the motion of the ball in the cage is carefully checked to be certain that no muscle bundles in the ventricular cavity protrude into the cage

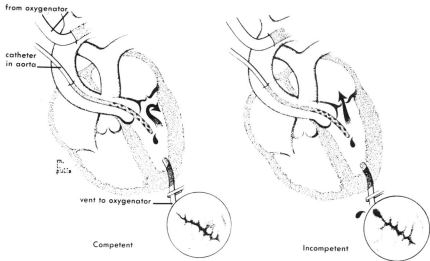

Fig. 19-7. Assessment of mitral regurgitation utilizing controlled aortic insufficiency to close mitral valve.

and restrict motion of the ball. With this important precaution, so-called postoperative thrombosis of a prosthetic valve has not been seen.

As the atriotomy is closed, air is removed from the heart with the conventional Foley catheter left across the mitral valve, but in addition the apexes of both the left ventricle and the ascending aorta are vented to remove air, as the simple use of the Foley catheter is not completely effective in removing air emboli. A catheter vent in the ascending aorta, rather than the needle vent previously used, has been found far more effective for prevention of air embolism.

Fig. 19-8. A. Closure of left atrial appendage. B. Exposure of mitral valve with horizontal traction on sutures. C. Right-angle clamp guides incision.

Convalescence is usually benign except in patients with long-standing congestive failure where the cardiac output may be low for 1 to 2 days and require careful supportive care. Antibiotics are given for 3 to 5 days. Anticoagulation with sodium warfarin is begun about 4 days after operation and maintained with a prothrombin time near 20 seconds, a significantly lesser degree of anticoagulation than the former prothrombin levels near 30 seconds. This more conservative approach has less risk of anticoagulant hemorrhage but has not been associated with an increase in frequency of thromboembolism. Anticoagulation is continued permanently. Acetylsalicylic acid, 0.6 Gm twice daily, is also given for 1 to 2 years for possible inhibition of platelet aggregation. The frequency of thromboembolism has been small, in a range of 2 to 4 percent.

Most patients improve promptly after operation, obtaining the full therapeutic benefit within 3 to 6 months. Dur-

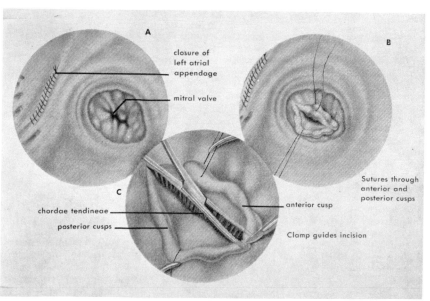

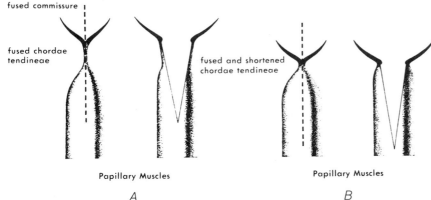

fused commissure

fused chordae
tendineae

fused and shortened
chordae tendineae

Papillary Muscles

Papillary Muscles

A

B

Fig. 19-9. *A.* Separation of fused chordae tendinae with incision into papillary muscle. *B.* Deeper incision into papillary muscle when valve leaflets are fused to underlying papillary muscle.

ing this time careful attention to salt intake and body weight is necessary, for renal excretion of sodium remains impaired for several weeks.

Within 6 months after operation most patients have little physical restriction of activity. However, a few, with chronic congestive failure and cardiac enlargement beforehand, continue to have some permanent limitation, apparently from irreversible myocardial injury before operation.

Different types of tissue valve have been used, including aortic homografts, fascia lata, dura mater, and most recently gluteraldehyde-preserved porcine heterografts.

Fig. 19-10. *A.* Excised mitral valve with severe calcification. When such calcification is present, satisfactory function can rarely be restored to the valve. *B.* Calcified mitral valve removed from another patient in whom prosthetic replacement of the mitral valve was necessary.

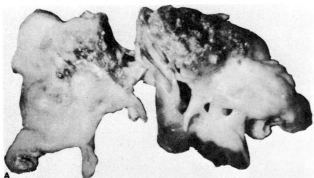

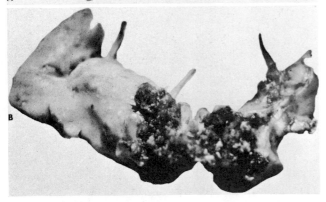

These are discussed in more detail in the following section on mitral insufficiency.

PROGNOSIS. Following an adequate mitral commissurotomy that does not produce insufficiency, long-term prognosis is very good. As the valve is not normal, long-term function will probably be determined by the degree of fibrosis in the leaflets and the chordae. If these fibrotic changes are extensive enough to produce significant turbulent flow of blood, eventual stiffening and calcification of the leaflets are likely. However, if disease is predominantly in the commissures, excellent long-term function may be expected. Formerly a recurrence rate of mitral stenosis as high as 30 to 40 percent within 5 years after operation was reported, but this group included a significant percentage of patients in whom commissurotomy was initially ineffective, either because of technique or because calcification and fibrosis prevented effective reconstruction, for which prosthetic replacement is now done.

With commissurotomy as now performed, recurrence at 5 years is probably near 10 percent, far less than that estimated in the past. In a group of patients operated upon by the author at the University of Kentucky between 1961 and 1966, reported in a larger series by Bryant and Trinkle in 1971, the recurrence rate was well under 10 percent. Similarly, Higgs and associates in 1970 and Morrow and Braunwald in a careful study of 45 patients from a series of 226 undergoing mitral commissurotomy found that true restenosis occurred in only 5 patients. As stated earlier, the frequent "restenosis" reported previously was often simply an ineffective commissurotomy. Valve complications which do occur at a later date, either restenosis or insufficiency, are probably due to fibrosis of the valve leaflets from turbulent flow of blood, much like that seen in a congenitally bicuspid aortic valve, and are not a result of recurrent rheumatic fever. Since 1966, the author has not had a single patient who developed recurrent stenosis of the mitral valve due to an inadequate commissurotomy.

Following prosthetic replacement of the mitral valve, the risk of endocarditis is small but permanent. Hence, prophylactic antibiotics should be routinely employed when episodes of transient bacteremia can be anticipated, as with

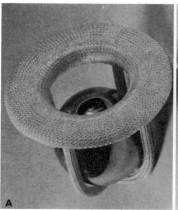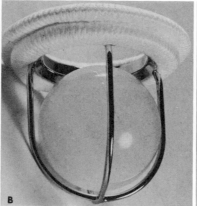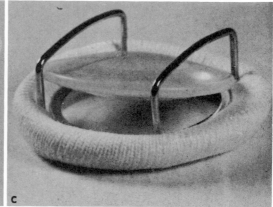

Fig. 19-11. *A.* Starr-Edwards mitral prosthesis. This prosthesis is completely covered with cloth and uses a steel ball. It is hoped that the complete covering of the prosthesis with cloth will decrease the incidence of thromboembolism. *B.* Mitral valve prosthesis with a Silastic ball used prior to 1967. In contrast to the prosthesis in *A*, the Teflon cloth does not cover the metallic ring and struts. *C.* Disc prosthesis. The disc prosthesis has a wider opening than a ball-valve prosthesis, and the cage does not protrude as far into the ventricle.

dental extraction or cystoscopy. Thromboembolism remains a small but definite hazard. For this reason anticoagulants are used permanently, as described in the earlier paragraphs. A detailed report by Starr in 1971 of all experiences with mitral valve replacement, beginning with the first model prosthetic valve in 1961, confirms the durability of prosthetic mitral replacement (Figs. 19-14 and 19-15).

In 1977, Isom et al. reported the long-term follow-up of 1,375 cloth-covered ball-valve replacements. The 5-year survival following mitral valve replacement was 71 percent.

MITRAL INSUFFICIENCY

HISTORICAL DATA. A number of ingenious attempts to treat mitral insufficiency surgically by a closed approach were made before cardiopulmonary bypass became clinically feasible in 1955. Since that time an open approach with cardiopulmonary bypass has been uniformly used. Prosthetic replacement of the insufficient valve is usually necessary, especially if calcification of the valve has occurred. In some patients with mobile valve leaflets it may be possible to correct the insufficiency with an annuloplasty. Long-term results following annuloplasty in selected cases have been reported by Merendino and by Reed et al. The Carpentier annuloplasty has provided another method of reconstruction rather than replacement.

ETIOLOGY. Mitral insufficiency is usually rheumatic in origin, although a definite history of rheumatic fever can be obtained in only somewhat over one-half of the patients. Other causes of mitral insufficiency include prolapse of the mitral valve, bacterial endocarditis, rupture of chordae tendineae, and papillary muscle dysfunction from extensive occlusive disease of the coronary arteries. Bacterial endocarditis can be suspected when protracted fever is associated with the development and persistence of the systolic murmur of mitral insufficiency, but the diagnosis can be proved only by identification of the bacterial organism in serial blood cultures. Rupture of chordae tendineae is an unusual but important cause of mitral insufficiency in older patients. Clinically it simulates rheumatic mitral insufficiency closely, but the acute onset in an older patient without previous signs of cardiac disease should suggest the diagnosis. Papillary muscle dysfunction is usually associated with obvious extensive disease of the coronary arteries, causing either cardiac dilatation and failure or myocardial infarction.

In the past decade the surprising frequency of some degree of prolapse of the mitral valve has become widely recognized. It occurs to a slight degree in as many as 5 to 10 percent of the normal population. Fortunately, in the majority of patients the hemodynamic disturbance is minimal. In older patients, however, it has become an increasingly common cause of severe insufficiency requiring valve replacement.

PATHOLOGIC ANATOMY. The basic changes with rheumatic fever have been described under Pathology in the preceding section, Mitral Stenosis. Several alterations in the normal mitral valve, either singly or in combination, may produce mitral insufficiency. These include fibrosis and retraction of the valve leaflets, extensive calcification limiting mobility of the valve leaflets, fibrosis and contraction of the chordae tendineae, rupture of the chordae tendineae, or dysfunction of the papillary muscles. Although seldom a primary cause, dilatation of the mitral annulus develops with mitral insufficiency and accordingly intensifies the insufficiency over a period of time as progressive dilatation of the annulus occurs. The reason that rheumatic endocarditis produces mitral stenosis in one patient and mitral insufficiency in another is unknown and is probably fortuitous.

PATHOPHYSIOLOGY. The basic physiologic change is systolic elevation of left atrial pressure as blood regurgitates through the incompetent mitral valve during ventricular systole. The ventricular pressure spike is commonly to levels of 30 to 40 mm Hg, but levels as high as 80 to 90 mm Hg have been recorded. In diastole the left atrial pressure drops sharply to approach the left ventricular

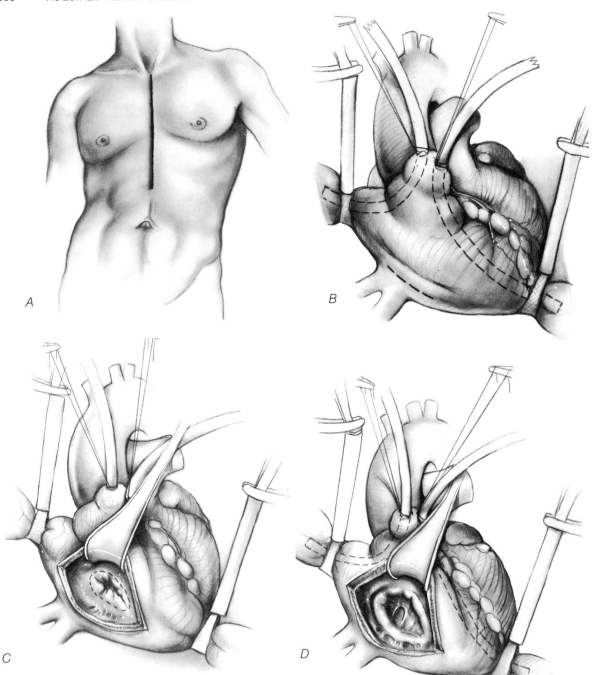

Fig. 19-12. Insertion of mitral valve prosthesis. *A*. A median sternotomy is the preferred incision, providing ready access to all
areas of the heart. *B*. Cannulae are introduced through the atrial
wall into the venae cavae. Normally these are not snared with
encircling tapes unless a patent foramen ovale is encountered
which causes aspiration of air from the opened left atrium into
the right atrium. *C*. The mitral valve is exposed with an incision
in the left atrium anterior to the point of entry of the right pulmonary veins. Exposure is facilitated by intermittent occlusion of the
aorta, which will arrest and stop the heart, and also decrease
the amount of blood in the operative field. *D*. The mitral valve
with the papillary muscles is completely excised, leaving a small
rim of annulus. The cavity of the left ventricle is carefully inspected and a prosthesis of appropriate size chosen, making
certain that the cage of the prosthesis can be readily accommodated in the ventricular cavity. *E*. A Starr-Edwards ball-valve
prosthesis, cloth-covered and with a steel ball, is preferred. It is
inserted with 12 to 15 mattress sutures of #0 Dacron. Often
the mattress sutures are buttressed with Teflon felt on the ventricular surface (not shown). *F*. Following insertion of the valve,
a Foley catheter is placed across the valve to keep the valve
incompetent and avoid air embolism. *G*. Final view of the valve
in position before closure of the atriotomy. *H*. The atriotomy
incision is closed around the Foley catheter, after which the heart
is allowed to fill with blood and displace air. Subsequently the
Foley catheter is removed, which permits the left ventricle to
contract normally. (Figure continued on next page.)

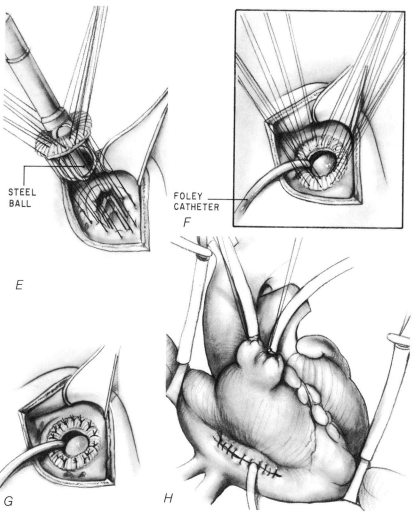

STEEL
BALL

FOLEY
CATHETER

E

F

G

H

Fig. 19-12. Continued.

diastolic pressure, although a small gradient usually remains because of the large blood flow through the mitral valve during diastole. Mean left atrial pressure is usually 15 to 25 mm Hg. The mitral regurgitation produces enlargement of the left atrium, although for unknown reasons the degree of left atrial enlargement varies greatly among different patients and is not proportional to the degree of regurgitation. In some patients with significant regurgitation only slight left atrial enlargement is present, while in others giant left atria evolve, enlarging to contact the right chest wall. In contrast to mitral stenosis, pulmonary vascular changes appear rather late in the course of the disease, perhaps as a result of a large left atrium absorbing much of the kinetic energy of the regurgitating blood without sustained elevation of left atrial pressure. Fortunately, the dilated left ventricle with mitral insufficiency may function adequately for surprisingly long periods of time, maintaining the left ventricular diastolic pressure near the normal range of 8 to 12 mm Hg until eventually left ventricular failure appears.

As there is little stasis of blood in the left atrium, in contrast to mitral stenosis, left atrial thrombosis and arterial embolism are much less frequent than with mitral stenosis.

CLINICAL MANIFESTATIONS. Symptoms. In some patients mild mitral insufficiency may be present without significant disability. This results from minimal rheumatic injury to the mitral leaflets, producing a systolic murmur but few other hemodynamic alterations. In a number of patients, mitral valve prolapse may have been misdiagnosed as rheumatic in origin. With developments in echocardiography, the differential diagnosis can be made readily. Such patients have an increased susceptibility to bacterial endocarditis, but in the absence of symptoms or cardiac enlargement additional therapy is not needed. With more significant mitral insufficiency, the most common symptoms are fatigue, dyspnea on exertion, and palpitation. Often these symptoms remain mild for long periods of time, despite impressive physical signs of mitral insufficiency and cardiac enlargement. Eventually left ventricular failure and increase in pulmonary vascular resistance both develop and intensify the cardiac disability. Respiratory symptoms then become prominent, with increasing dyspnea, cough, and paroxysmal nocturnal dysp-

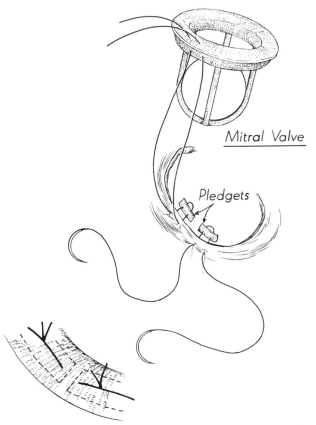

Fig. 19-13. Technique for suturing a mitral valve prosthesis with Dacron pledgets seated below the mitral annulus.

nea, all of which are essentially similar to those occurring with mitral stenosis and are described in more detail in that section.

Physical Examination. The two characteristic features of mitral insufficiency are the apical systolic murmur and the increased force of the apical impulse. The systolic murmur is heard best at the apex, which is often displaced downward and to the left from enlargement of the left ventricle. It is well transmitted to the axilla. The quality is of a harsh, blowing type. With severe insufficiency, the murmur is pansystolic, appearing immediately after the first sound and continuing until the second sound. The intensity of the murmur does not correlate with the severity of the regurgitation, but the pansystolic characteristic does. Murmurs not extending completely through systole are seen with less serious degrees of regurgitation. The systolic murmur is a highly characteristic feature of mitral insufficiency and is absent only in most unusual circumstances. A diastolic murmur is usually present in addition, resulting from increased flow across the mitral valve as a result of blood regurgitated into the atrium during systole. The absence of an opening snap and the normal quality of the first heart sound both suggest that the diastolic murmur is due to increased flow of blood rather than anatomic mitral stenosis.

The apical impulse is typically forceful, prolonged, and

Fig. 19-14. *A.* Autopsy photograph of a Starr-Edwards valve prosthesis inserted before 1966, showing the tendency for original model of the prosthetic valve to develop extensive thromboembolism. Surprisingly enough the patient had had no clinical signs of emboli although myriads of scars were found in the kidneys at autopsy. Death occurred 7 years after operation, following a pulmonary infection. Thrombi extending from the ring of the prosthesis down the struts to the apex are clearly seen. *B.* Atrial view of valve, showing thrombi over approximately two-thirds of the metallic ring. Development of such thrombi was the principle reason for the development of cloth-covered prosthetic valves.

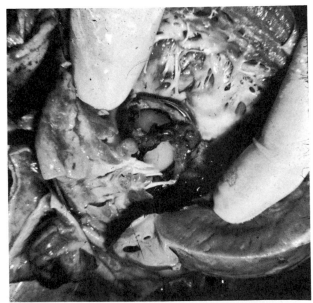

A

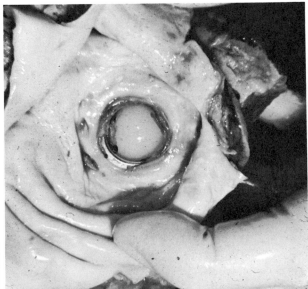

B

diffuse, occupying an area 3 to 4 cm². The first heart sound is usually normal, although it has been reported as decreased or absent, usually from confusion with the early onset of the systolic murmur. Atrial fibrillation is frequent with chronic disease.

Laboratory Examinations. The chest roentgenogram will show enlargement of both the left ventricle and the left atrium (Fig. 19-16). As mentioned earlier, in some patients for unknown reasons a giant enlargement of the left atrium occurs, with an atrial chamber extending to the right chest wall and producing a grotesque deformity of the cardiac shadow. Calcification of the regurgitant valve is infrequent, although with combined lesions of stenosis and insufficiency, calcification is common. Visible changes in the pulmonary vasculature are often minimal except with advanced disease.

The electrocardiogram is unfortunately variable and may not contribute greatly to assessment of the severity of the disease. In about 50 percent of patients there is definite left ventricular hypertrophy. Significant insufficiency may be present, however, with a normal electrocardiogram, or in some patients a right axis may develop as a result of pulmonary vascular changes. Atrial fibrillation is frequent.

Mitral insufficiency is best quantified by cardiac catheterization with cineangiography. Only by injection of dye into the left ventricle, with evaluation of the degree of reflux into the atrium, can the degree of insufficiency be best estimated. This is far superior to complex studies with indicator dilution dye curves. The left atrial pressure tracing with mitral insufficiency is greatly altered, usually with a prominent V wave developing from regurgitation of blood during systole. During diastole the left atrial pressure decreases sharply to approach left ventricular diastolic pressure, but usually some gradient remains throughout diastole because of increased flow of blood across the mitral valve.

DIAGNOSIS. The diagnosis of mitral insufficiency can be made with reasonable certainty from the characteristic systolic murmur radiating to the axilla in association with evidence of left ventricular hypertrophy obtained by palpation, the chest roentgenogram, or the electrocardiogram. The degree of severity of the insufficiency is best quantitated with cineangiography. When multivalvular disease is present, cardiac catheterization and angiography are needed to delineate the relative severity of the different valvular lesions.

TREATMENT. Indications for Operation. An acceptable operation for mitral insufficiency was not routinely available until the pioneering work of Starr and Edwards first developed a mitral valve prosthesis in 1961. With the mitral prostheses available between 1961 and 1966, the 5-year survival was only about 50 percent.

Over the past 5 to 7 years, the cloth-covered valve has been modified several times, the most recent modification being a "track" valve (Fig. 19-17). A tilting disc valve, the Bjork-Shiley, which is the most popular, is an excellent prosthesis and provides a wider orifice than is available with most ball valves (Fig. 19-18). The gluteraldehyde-preserved porcine heterograft has become increasingly

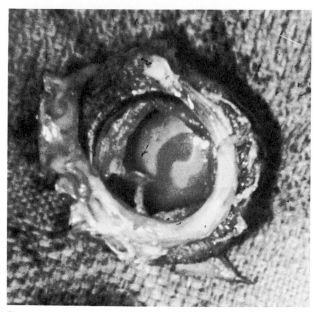

Fig. 19-15. Operative photograph of a Kay-Shiley disc prosthesis removed over 2 years after insertion because of recurrent emboli. Extensive thrombi, easily detached from the metallic surface of the prosthesis, are present. Development of these thrombi, intermittently dislodging into the circulation, is the principal reason for the development of cloth-covered prostheses.

Fig. 19-16. Chest roentgenogram of a patient with mitral insufficiency. The distinctive features include an enlarged cardiac shadow with a prominent pulmonary artery. The shadow of the left atrium is visible in the right border of the cardiac shadow behind the shadow of the right atrium. The pulmonary vascular markings are prominent.

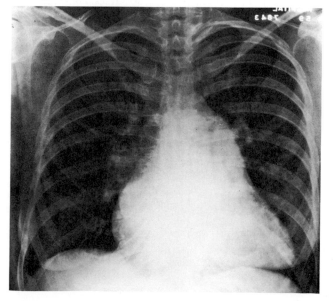

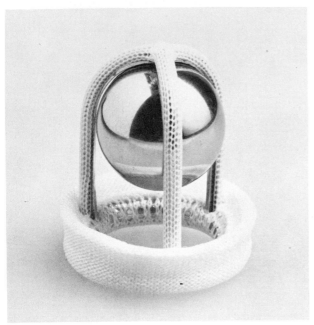

Fig. 19-17. Starr-Edwards composite track valve available since 1972. Cloth covers the exterior portion of the valve cage and a metallic track is provided on the inner surface of each cage strut.

popular in the last 5 years and is now used at many centers as the valve of choice, because all other types of prosthetic valve require anticoagulation (Fig. 19-19).

Most patients at New York University have received cloth-covered steel ball valves (Fig. 19-20). The cloth usually becomes covered with a translucent layer of compacted fibrin less than 1 mm thick. This surface is very resistant to thromboembolism. Problems with cloth wear, hemolysis, and endocarditis have occurred in a minority of patients and there is limited enthusiasm for the prosthesis. Because of the limitations of all prostheses and the limited data about their 5- to 10-year durability, operation is usually recommended only for progressive disability resistant to customary medical therapy.

Fig. 19-18. Bjork-Shiley tilting disc valve.

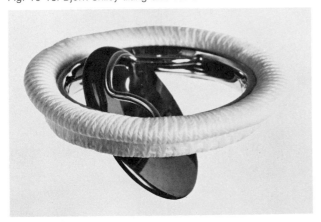

Medical therapy includes appropriate use of digitalis, diuretics, and restriction of sodium intake in the presence of heart failure. Arrhythmias, usually atrial fibrillation, require frequent therapy, both to control tachycardia and to attempt conversion of the arrhythmia to a sinus mechanism.

Technique of Operation. The technique for mitral valve replacement was described under Mitral Stenosis and will not be repeated in detail here. In general, operation is performed through a median sternotomy, occasionally a right thoracotomy. The main precautions during mitral replacement are to anchor the prosthetic valve adequately in position to prevent subsequent partial dislodgment with recurrent mitral insufficiency and to avoid air embolism. Until recent years the prevalence of the two complications cited resulted in an operative mortality of 15 to 20 percent; now it is near 5 percent. Following operation anticoagulant therapy is begun on the fourth or fifth postoperative day and continued indefinitely.

In 10 to 15 percent of patients a mitral annuloplasty may be employed, rather than prosthetic replacement of the valve. Such patients are usually younger, with a dilated mitral annulus and mobile valve leaflets with little or no calcification. Several techniques of annuloplasty have been described, with the objective of producing a small, competent mitral orifice. In general, heavy sutures are used, often including more of the annulus of the mural leaflet rather than the aortic leaflet, because the aortic leaflet often has more mobility than the smaller mural leaflet. When annuloplasty can be satisfactorily performed, excellent long-term results may be obtained. Unfortunately, in many patients the insufficiency cannot be completely corrected at the first operation; also, it may recur at a later date. The Carpentier ring annuloplasty, developed in France, has not to date been widely used in this country.

Ruptured chordae tendineae causing mitral insufficiency create a special surgical problem, varying with the number and location of the chordae ruptured (Fig. 19-21). McGoon has described a technique of plication of the flail mitral leaflet which is applicable in some patients. Kay and Egerton have described other methods of repair, including suture of the flail leaflet directly to the underlying papillary muscle. In some patients excision of the valve with prosthetic replacement is necessary. Long-term results are usually excellent.

PROGNOSIS. Recovery from operation is usually followed by excellent rehabilitation. There is subsidence of pulmonary vascular changes and of signs of cardiac failure. For unknown reasons, however, cardiac function does not return to completely normal values, perhaps because of the rigid ring of the prosthesis in the mitral annulus or because of irreversible myocardial injury from longstanding mitral insufficiency. Most patients have few, if any, restrictions on physical activity. (For specific data following prosthetic valve replacement, see Prognosis, under Mitral Stenosis.)

Careful long-term management is required to supervise anticoagulant therapy, to detect any signs of malfunction of the prosthesis, and to protect from endocarditis during episodes of transient bacteremia by using prophylactic antibiotics.

Five-year survival following mitral valve replacement varies widely with the stage of the disease at which operation is performed. With Class II patients it is about 90 percent; with Class III, nearly 70 percent; and with Class IV, only about 50 percent.

AORTIC STENOSIS

HISTORICAL DATA. Effective treatment of aortic valve disease first became acceptable in 1961 with the development of satisfactory prosthetic valves by Starr and Edwards and by Harken and associates. Earlier attempts to correct aortic valvular disease by cusp replacement with prosthetic cusps of Teflon cloth or by extensive debridement of calcific material from calcified valve cusps initially gave satisfactory results in many patients, but a high failure rate within 1 to 2 years following operation led to abandonment of these techniques as soon as a satisfactory prosthetic valve became available.

With all prosthetic valves, the major limitation is thromboembolism. With the improvements in prosthetic valves in the past few years, especially with the use of cloth covering, thromboembolism has decreased to a range of 1 to 3 percent. Endocarditis following transient bacteremia remains a small but definite risk.

The most exciting data in recent years are those on the continuing excellent results obtained with the gluteraldehyde-preserved porcine heterograft, developed especially by the Hancock Laboratories. Aortic homograft valves have been discarded by many groups but are still preferred by Barratt-Boyes.

ETIOLOGY. A definite history of rheumatic fever can be obtained in only 30 to 50 percent of all patients, but the fact that associated mitral valve disease also is found in 30 to 50 percent of patients with aortic disease supports the relative frequency of rheumatic infection.

In the majority of other patients, calcification superimposed on a mild congenital aortic stenosis is probably the most frequent cause, rather than unrecognized rheumatic fever. In almost all untreated patients with congenital aortic stenosis, calcification in the aortic leaflets develops after thirty years of age. This adds an element of valve cusp rigidity to the obstruction already present because of congenital fusion. It is now clear that this calcification may gradually increase over several decades. Several patients in the sixth and seventh decades of life have been followed with a heart murmur since childhood but without symptoms until 2 or 3 years before operation, at which time a calcified bicuspid valve was found.

In patients in the seventh and eighth decades, an aortic systolic murmur, resulting from mild fibrosis and calcification of the valve leaflets, is extremely common. Only rarely, however, does this form of atherosclerosis in the elderly produce significant obstruction.

PATHOLOGY. The basic pathology of rheumatic fever has been detailed under Mitral Stenosis. The pathologic process with aortic valvulitis is similar, with ulceration of the endocardium developing over the valve leaflets where the margins normally appose in diastole. Tiny, beadlike

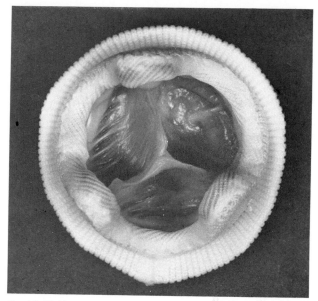

Fig. 19-19. Hancock gluteraldehyde-preserved porcine xenograft, now the valve of choice in many centers.

vegetations form and produce fusion of the commissures as healing takes place. Fibrosis and stiffening of the leaflets may develop as well as fusion of the commissures, both features producing obstruction to the flow of blood. In subsequent years superimposed calcification of the diseased leaflets, probably from turbulent flow of blood, regularly occurs and creates further rigidity of the valve cusps.

Mitral valve disease, either stenosis or insufficiency, is found in a high percentage of patients with aortic disease, indicating the underlying rheumatic cause. In older patients coronary atherosclerosis may be present, although the incidence is no greater than that in the normal population. When extensive coronary atherosclerosis is present in association with aortic stenosis of only moderate severity,

Fig. 19-20. Starr-Edwards cloth-covered steel ball aortic prostheses. *A.* The Starr-Edwards aortic ball-valve prosthesis developed in the latter part of 1967. The prosthesis is completely covered with Teflon cloth. A metal ball is used. *B.* The Starr-Edwards ball-valve prosthesis used prior to 1967. The ball is composed of silastic. The Teflon cloth, in contrast to the valve shown in *A*, only partially covers the metal surfaces of the prosthesis.

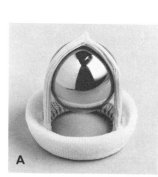

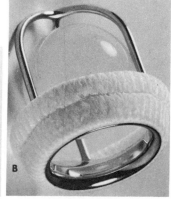

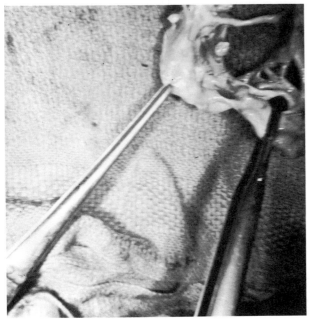

Fig. 19-21. Operative photograph of mitral valve showing rupture of a major chordae, creating severe mitral insufficiency. In some such patients, plication of the mitral leaflet will obviate mitral replacement.

it may be difficult to determine which of the two lesions is responsible for the symptoms.

PATHOPHYSIOLOGY. The normal aortic valve has a cross-sectional area of 2.5 to 3.5 cm². Moderately severe aortic stenosis is present when the valve orifice has been narrowed to a cross-sectional area of 0.8 to 1 cm², which is associated with a systolic gradient of about 50 mm Hg at a moderate cardiac output. Severe aortic stenosis exists if the cross-sectional area has been reduced to 0.5 to 0.7 cm², which requires a systolic pressure gradient near 150 mm Hg to produce a moderate cardiac output. When stenosis of such severity is present, increases in ventricular systolic pressure are very ineffective in producing further increases in cardiac output. A left ventricular systolic pressure of 250 mm Hg is near the maximum that a left ventricle can sustain for any period of time.

With the increased cardiac work imposed by the stenosis, there is progressive concentric ventricular hypertrophy but little cardiac dilatation, as a result of which the heart size may be near normal on the conventional chest roentgenogram. The cardiac output is often normal, though the left ventricular diastolic pressure is frequently elevated above the normal of 12 mm Hg, especially during exercise, because of the extensive muscular hypertrophy. Left atrial pressure may be temporarily elevated, but sustained elevation of left atrial pressure with production of pulmonary edema is a late and often a preterminal manifestation. Similarly, pulmonary vascular disease is infrequent. In contrast to mitral stenosis, a patient with aortic stenosis may have relatively few symptoms for a long period of time, but when cardiac decompensation with pulmonary congestion appears, a fatal outcome often ensues within a few months.

The quality of the pulse is frequently altered with aortic stenosis because of the restriction to ventricular ejection. The typical changes include a pulse wave of low amplitude, a slow rate of rise, and a rounded peak.

Myocardial ischemia, manifested as angina pectoris, is frequent in aortic stenosis from a combination of factors. These include increase in left ventricular work, myocardial hypertrophy with resulting fewer capillaries per gram of myocardium, decreased aortic pressure in diastole, during which the majority of coronary blood flow usually occurs, and in some patients superimposed atherosclerosis. Because of the myocardial ischemia, aortic stenosis is a most treacherous lesion, for sudden death is *always* a possibility. The risk varies with the severity of the disease but is always present, even with mild aortic stenosis. It is much more frequent with aortic stenosis than with any other form of acquired valvular heart disease.

CLINICAL MANIFESTATIONS. Symptoms. Characteristically there is a prolonged latent period in the development of aortic stenosis. For perhaps 10 to 20 years classic physical findings may be present with slight dyspnea on exertion as the only symptom. The turning point in the illness is heralded by the appearance of one or more of three symptoms: angina pectoris, syncope, or left ventricular failure. Sudden death, which accounts for about 20 percent of fatalities from aortic stenosis, becomes much more of a threat once these symptoms are present, although sudden death is an ever-present hazard in any patient with aortic stenosis. Once angina or syncope appears, the average life expectancy for the untreated patient is 3 to 4 years. Left ventricular failure is an even more serious symptom, death usually occurring within 1 to 2 years, although great variations are seen among different patients, ranging from periods as short as 1 week to as long as 10 years.

Syncope develops in about one-third of the patients. In a minority of patients syncope may result from a conduction abnormality, arising from involvement of the atrioventricular node by calcium spicules deposited on the stenotic valve. Usually syncope develops with effort, and it is commonly associated with angina pectoris. Once left ventricular failure has developed, syncopal attacks may be precipitated by very little effort and are of the gravest significance.

Angina pectoris develops in about two-thirds of the patients, representing myocardial ischemia from an inadequate cardiac output. With protracted angina, small areas of muscle necrosis may evolve, ultimately represented as myocardial fibrosis; infrequently large areas of silent infarction occur.

Left ventricular failure is a grave development and demands immediate therapy. Many patients do not survive long enough to develop associated right ventricular failure. Atrial fibrillation, developing as a consequence of prolonged elevation of left atrial pressure, is similarly a grave event, as it indicates an advanced stage of left ventricular failure.

Physical Examination. The classic physical finding with aortic stenosis is the systolic diamond-shaped ejection murmur produced by blood forced through the stenotic orifice. The murmur is usually heard best in the aortic area to the right of the sternum but in some patients is loudest at the cardiac apex. The intensity of the murmur varies from grade II to grade IV but has no correlation with the severity of the stenosis. Loud murmurs are associated with a palpable thrill and are readily transmitted to the carotid arteries. The aortic second sound is soft but can be detected in 70 to 80 percent of patients. A grade I to II diastolic murmur of aortic insufficiency can often be heard along the left sternal border.

The apical impulse has distinctive features. It is usually in a normal position, for cardiac size is not increased. Palpation of the apical contraction detects a prolonged heave but not a forceful thrust such as is found with ventricular dilatation from aortic or mitral insufficiency. In many patients the blood pressure is normal. Only with advanced stenosis is the pulse pressure significantly narrowed to less than 30 mm Hg.

Laboratory Studies. The chest roentgenogram often demonstrates a heart of normal size. Gross cardiac enlargement, resulting from ventricular dilatation and failure, is associated with an ominous prognosis. Mild degrees of left atrial enlargement are often found. Calcification of the aortic valve should be almost routinely visible in patients over thirty-five years of age. If calcification is not found, the validity of the diagnosis should be seriously questioned.

With advanced disease the electrocardiogram will show signs of left ventricular hypertrophy, including increased voltage of the QRS complex, in association with ST-segment and T-wave abnormalities. With less advanced stenosis, however, the changes may be much less specific, and in some dangerously ill patients the electrocardiogram is virtually normal. In older patients the prevalence of ST-segment and T-wave abnormalities from coronary artery disease makes correlation of the electrocardiogram with the severity of the aortic stenosis difficult. A left bundle branch block is occasionally seen in some patients with advanced stenosis.

Cardiac catheterization to determine the pressure gradient between the left ventricle and the aorta is required to estimate the severity of the stenosis. With mild aortic stenosis, a systolic pressure gradient of only 30 to 40 mm Hg is found, while severe stenosis may have a pressure gradient exceeding 100 mm Hg. Actually, the severity is best correlated with the cross-sectional area of the valve, calculated from simultaneous measurement of pressure gradient and cardiac output. In most patients simple determination of the gradient is sufficient if the patient is in a resting, basal state. At the time of catheterization the presence of mitral disease can also be determined, as well as associated aortic insufficiency. When feasible, coronary arteriography should be done in association with aortogra-phy to detect associated coronary vascular disease.

DIAGNOSIS. A diagnosis of aortic stenosis can usually be made with certainty from detection of the characteristic ejection-type systolic murmur in the aortic area, associated with findings of left ventricular hypertrophy. Supportive evidence can be obtained from the chest roentgenogram, demonstrating calcification of the aortic valve and often a heart of normal size. The electrocardiogram will usually show variable degrees of left ventricular hypertrophy.

The diagnosis can be confirmed by cardiac catheterization, which also provides the only precise method of measuring the severity of the stenosis. In some patients with aortic systolic murmurs, especially those in the seventh and eighth decades, catheterization will demonstrate that significant obstruction is not present.

TREATMENT. Indications for Operation. Once a clinical diagnosis of aortic stenosis has been made, usually cardiac catheterization should be performed to measure the severity of the obstruction. Subsequent management of the patient depends upon the symptoms, the severity of the obstruction, and the degree of cardiac hypertrophy. Operation is recommended with a gradient exceeding 50 mm Hg, though some such patients are virtually asymptomatic.

Once syncope, angina, or congestive heart failure has appeared, operation should be performed promptly because of the high incidence of sudden death.

Technique of Operation. Detailed preoperative care is not often necessary. If diuretic therapy has been employed, supplemental potassium is usually given before operation to avoid postoperative hypokalemia and arrhythmias. Patients are usually hospitalized 2 to 3 days in advance of the scheduled operation.

A median sternotomy incision is usually employed, with cannulation of the venae cavae for withdrawal of venous blood from the patient to the pump-oxygenator and cannulation of the ascending aorta for return of arterial blood from the pump-oxygenator to the patient (Fig. 19-22). Before bypass is instituted, left atrial pressure is measured to indicate the degree of left ventricular failure. The preoperative left atrial pressure is a convenient guide to postoperative infusion of fluids, because left atrial pressure reflects the diastolic filling pressure of the left ventricle. With severe cardiac failure a mean left atrial pressure of 20 to 30 mm Hg may be present, and following operation elevation of left atrial pressure to similar levels by infusion of fluids may be required for a short time to maintain an adequate cardiac output.

Once cardiopulmonary bypass has been instituted, a vent is placed in the apex of the left ventricle to aspirate blood. The ascending aorta is then occluded distad and incised with an oblique incision which extends proximally into the noncoronary sinus. Perfusion of the left and right coronary arteries is then instituted following cannulation with Silastic coronary cannulae of appropriate size. Perfusions at 100 to 150 ml/minute are used in each artery, depending upon the size of the left ventricle (Fig. 19-23).

In recent years the technique of topical hypothermia, long used by Shumway and associates, has become in-

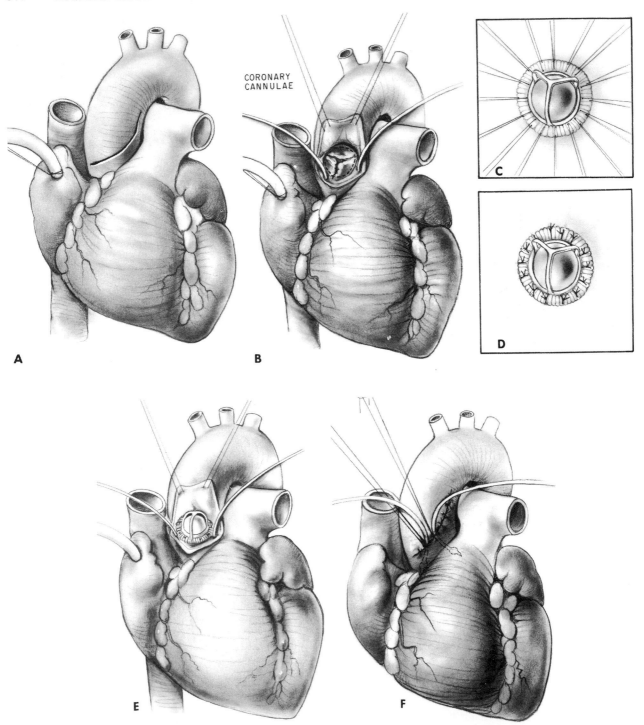

Fig. 19-22. Insertion of aortic valve prosthesis. *A.* Cardiopulmonary bypass is instituted following cannulation of the right atrium with a single large cannula. Usually the ascending aorta is cannulated for arterial return (not shown). The aorta is opened with an oblique incision, initially begun about a centimeter above the right coronary artery. *B.* The right and left coronary arteries are cannulated with Silastic coronary cannulae, held in position with purse-string sutures about the coronary ostia. Coronary perfusion is then begun at a rate of 200 to 250 ml/minute in each coronary artery. The aortic valve is then excised, with care to avoid the loss of any calcific fragments into the ventricle which might subsequently embolize. *C.* The Starr-Edwards ball valve which is normally used. *D.* Valve sutured in position. *E.* Final position of the valve. Care is taken, as the valve is tied in position, to seat the valve well below the coronary ostia, actually farther below than is shown here. *F.* The aortotomy is closed around the coronary cannulae, encircling each one with a mattress suture. Subsequently the contracting heart is allowed to fill with blood and expel air from the heart before the cannulae are removed.

creasingly popular. Hypothermic cardiac arrest, often combined with potassium cardioplegia, has become the most popular method of myocardial preservation, though the author and McGoon, among others, prefer coronary perfusion in routine cases unless significant coronary disease or coronary anomalies are present. There are seemingly valid data from several sources to indicate that myocardial ischemia for 1 hour is well tolerated if the myocardial temperature, as measured by an indwelling thermistor, is kept below 20 to 25°C.

The stenotic aortic valve is then completely removed (Fig. 19-24). Only in a small percentage of cases is simple fusion of the valve commissures found which can be treated by commissurotomy. In most patients there is extensive destruction of the valve cusps with superimposed calcification; complete removal has been found the only satisfactory therapy (Fig. 19-25). Removal of the calcified valve requires great care to avoid losing fragments of calcium into the left ventricle which could subsequently be embolized into the peripheral circulation. A gauze pack is routinely placed in the ventricle before removal of the valve is begun. Subsequent removal of the pack often reveals several fragments of calcium which have been dislodged during removal of the valve and would otherwise have been lost in the left ventricle.

Following removal of the diseased valve, a prosthetic ball valve of appropriate size is selected. It is important that the valve fit easily into the aortic lumen, choosing one that is neither too large nor too small. Once the appropriate valve has been chosen, 12 to 15 mattress sutures of 2-0 Dacron are placed in the valve annulus and inserted into the prosthetic valve. Each mattress suture is buttressed with a small pledget of Dacron cloth to avoid tearing of the

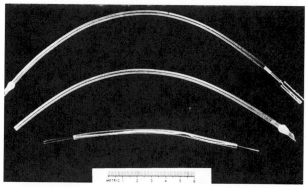

Fig. 19-23. Silastic coronary cannulae used to cannulate the coronary arteries at operation for coronary perfusion. Once the cannulae are inserted, slight tension is applied through the snare shown here to a purse-string suture of 4-0 silk which has been sutured about the coronary ostium. If a short left coronary artery is present, the tip of the cannula is amputated back to the ball to avoid inadvertent perfusion of only one tributary of the left coronary artery.

sutures through the annulus (Fig. 19-26). During seating of the valve, care is taken to seat the valve well below the coronary ostia and to avoid any tilting of the valve in its final position. Following closure of the aortotomy, air is displaced from the left ventricle, the coronary cannulae are removed, effective cardiac contraction is restored, and bypass gradually is slowed and stopped (Fig. 19-27).

Coronary perfusion is maintained throughout operation at a flow rate of 250 to 300 ml/minute and a temperature of 32 to 34°C, interrupting perfusion for 5 to 10 minutes when necessary for adequate exposure. In the past three to four years, abundant data have demonstrated that subendocardial coronary blood flow is seriously impaired in fibrillating hypertrophied hearts. Accordingly, the author and many others have abandoned the use of ventricular fibrillation and keep the heart beating throughout the

Fig. 19-24. A. Stenotic aortic valve exposed during cardiopulmonary bypass through a transverse aortotomy. The valve orifice has been almost obliterated by calcification and apposition of the cusps. B. Calcified aortic valve in another patient exposed through a transverse aortotomy. Fusion has produced a small eccentric rigid ostium which is both stenotic and insufficient.

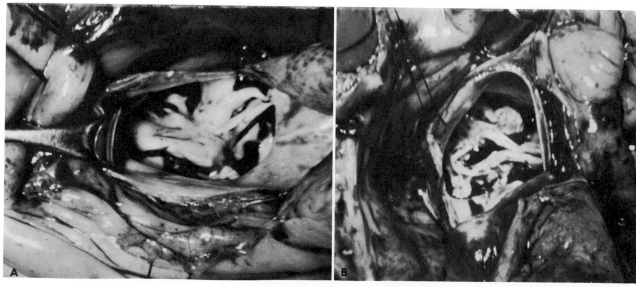

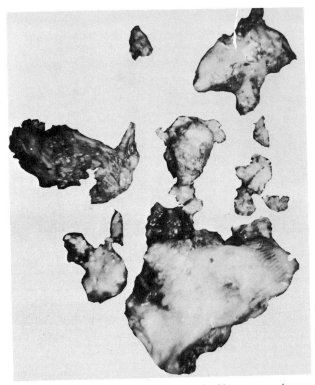

Fig. 19-25. Calcified fragments removed with rongeurs from a patient with severe aortic stenosis. The multiplicity of such fragments emphasizes the grave risk of embolization of calcified material during aortic valve replacement with reduction of severe or fatal neurologic injury. Careful packing of the ventricle with gauze before removal of the calcified valve is essential.

entire procedure. In the rare instance when this cannot be done, coronary perfusion is abandoned and the potassium cardioplegia technique substituted.

Following bypass, blood is transfused to elevate left atrial pressure to a level adequate to maintain a satisfactory cardiac output. The actual mean left atrial pressure required varies with that existing before bypass but is usually between 10 and 20 mm Hg. The left atrial pressure has been found a more valuable guide for postoperative fluid infusion than measurement of blood volume or blood loss.

Postoperative Care. After initial adjustment of blood volume following operation, convalescence may be uneventful. Arrhythmias are among the more frequent complications. Because they are serious and can be fatal if untreated, early detection by 24-hour monitoring of the cardiac rhythm with an oscilloscope in a cardiac intensive care unit is necessary. Arrhythmias are often related to changes in electrolyte concentration, such as decreased potassium concentration and varying sensitivities to digitalis. The most frequently employed therapeutic measures include supplemental potassium, intravenously administered lidocaine for short-term therapy, procainamide, or propranolol.

Anticoagulant therapy is begun with sodium warfarin 4 days after operation, keeping the prothrombin time in the conservative range of 20 to 25 seconds, and continued permanently. Elevation of the prothrombin time to 25 to 30 seconds has resulted in serious hemorrhage in a few patients, especially in the early postoperative course. Acetylsalicylic acid, 0.6 Gm twice a day, is given for 1 to 2 years to inhibit platelet aggregation, for such aggregates

Fig. 19-26. Schematic representation of technique for suturing the aortic valve with Dacron pledgets seated below the aortic annulus.

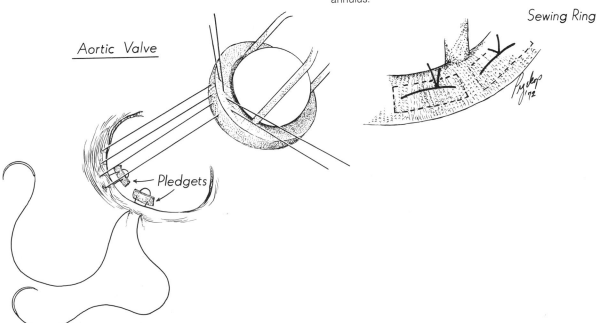

rather than fibrin appear to be the most frequent cause of thromboembolism with cloth-covered prostheses.

Within 3 to 4 months after operation the majority of patients are asymptomatic, with a normal range of physical activities. Careful long-term medical supervision is essential, however, especially in patients with marked cardiac hypertrophy. Actually there is a greater risk of death during the first year after leaving the hospital than from the operation itself. With severely hypertrophied hearts, arrhythmias remain a constant problem for months or longer and may be fatal if not treated. A mild degree of salt restriction and diuretic therapy may also be required if cardiac enlargement was severe beforehand. The rate of increase of physical activity should be determined from the patient's symptoms, heart size, and signs of left ventricular hypertrophy on the electrocardiogram.

PROGNOSIS. The average operative mortality for aortic valve replacement is in the range of 5 to 8 percent. It may be much higher in patients with far advanced disease from cardiac failure or less than 5 percent in good-risk patients. Probably the major factor influencing operative mortality is the ability to avoid serious myocardial ischemia. In 1965, McGoon et al. reported an impressive series of 100 consecutive aortic replacements without *any* operative mortality.

Most patients show a surprising degree of recovery following operation, and many subsequently have virtually no limitation of physical activity. With severe cardiac enlargement, however, there remains a risk of sudden death, even beyond 1 year after operation. This is probably due to arrhythmias, for the cause is often not found at postmortem examination.

AORTIC INSUFFICIENCY

ETIOLOGY. The most common cause of aortic insufficiency is rheumatic fever. A definite history of this illness can be obtained from 60 to 70 percent of patients. In the past, syphilis was a frequent cause, but it is now rare. Bacterial endocarditis produces insufficiency from destruction and perforation of valve cusps. Though formerly operation was strenuously avoided until the bacterial infection had been controlled, operation is now being performed much earlier, at times within the first 7 to 10 days of the illness in patients with life-threatening insufficiency. This is only possible, of course, if effective antibiotic therapy is used.

A dissecting aneurysm produces insufficiency by dissection of the aortic wall with detachment and prolapse of the valve cusps. Usually the noncoronary cusp is involved most. Diseases producing dilatation of the aortic annulus create insufficiency by preventing effective coaptation of the valve cusps in diastole. This is typically seen in the Marfan syndrome and also in less well defined diseases in which there is an isolated unexplained dilatation of the aortic annulus and ascending aorta. A similar pathologic process develops in a small percentage of patients with rheumatoid arthritis. Not infrequently a patient is seen with a "floppy valve," a connective tissue degeneration of the valve cusps resulting in elongation and prolapse with-

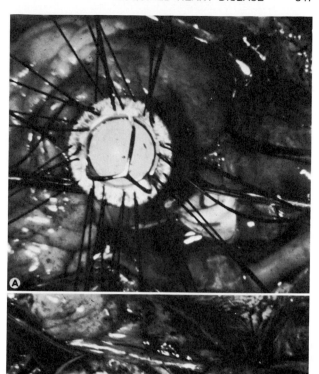

Fig. 19-27. *A.* A Starr-Edwards ball valve being inserted in the operation shown in Fig. 18-17*B* following excision of the calcified valve. The operation was performed in 1963. The patient has done well since that time. *B.* The aortic ball valve in position.

out any signs of infection or fibrosis. Congenital aortic insufficiency is very rare.

PATHOLOGY. Normal function of the aortic valve depends upon sufficient mobility and length of the cusps so that the centers of the three cusps appose in diastole. With fibrosis and retraction of the cusps, varying degrees of distortion produce an incompetent valve (Fig. 19-28). It is probable that the turbulent blood flow produced by the initial distortion of the cusps results in progressive fibrosis, stiffening, and eventual calcification, all of which result in a gradual increase in the degree of insufficiency. In the Marfan syndrome and other diseases associated with dilatation of the aortic annulus, the basic disturbance is stretching of the aortic valve ring, as a result of which the valve cusps can no longer meet centrally (Fig. 19-29).

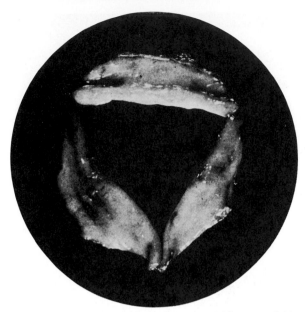

Fig. 19-28. Three aortic valve cusps removed from an eighteen-year-old boy with rheumatic aortic insufficiency. The contracted free margins of each cusp are clearly shown, illustrating the mechanism of production of aortic insufficiency from contracture and retraction of the free margins of the aortic valve cusps.

The cardiac response to blood regurgitating into the left ventricle in diastole is an increase in left ventricular stroke volume, accomplished by dilatation of the heart. Progressive dilatation of the left ventricle gradually evolves. This response is quite different from that occurring with aortic stenosis, where there is concentric muscular hypertrophy but little increase in ventricular diastolic volume.

PATHOPHYSIOLOGY. Surprisingly large volumes of blood can regurgitate through an incompetent orifice of less than 1 cm² because of the large differential in diastolic pressure between the aorta and the left ventricle. The actual amount of blood regurgitating with each cardiac cycle can be only approximated by existing techniques, such as dye-dilution measurements, or experimentally with flow meters. The initial adjustment of the heart is an increase in diastolic fiber length and a corresponding increase in stroke volume. There is little elevation in left ventricular diastolic pressure until cardiac failure begins to develop. In the absence of elevation of left ventricular diastolic pressure, there is accordingly no increase in left atrial pressure or pulmonary congestion. Hence, in contrast to mitral disease, symptoms of pulmonary congestion appear only in the terminal stages, once left ventricular failure has occurred.

The amount of blood regurgitating during diastole varies not only with the size of the incompetent orifice but also with the degree of peripheral vasodilatation and the heart rate. Tachycardia has a somewhat beneficial effect, for diastole is shortened and less time is available for blood to regurgitate into the ventricle. Peripheral vasodilation apparently is a compensatory mechanism by which peripheral resistance and the amount of blood regurgitating into the ventricle are decreased. It is often a prominent clinical finding.

With advanced aortic insufficiency and marked dilatation of the left ventricle, some mitral insufficiency may develop from dilation of the annulus of the mitral valve. When severe cardiac failure is present, with elevation of left ventricular end-diastolic pressure above 20 mm Hg, clinical findings of aortic insufficiency may actually decrease, for the total volume of blood regurgitating during diastole decreases as the left ventricular diastolic pressure rises.

CLINICAL MANIFESTATIONS. Symptoms. Although there is considerable variability among different patients, in general the symptom-free period after the appearance of aortic insufficiency averages about 10 years. With the onset of symptoms, death occurs in about 5 years, but the variability is great. Although in a large group, about 40 percent of patients will be dead within 10 years and over 50 percent within 20 years, another 25 percent may live for 20 years with very few symptoms. The terminal illness is usually a progressive downhill course from increasing cardiac failure, but sudden death occurs in about 5 percent.

The earliest symptom is palpitations because of the forceful contractions of the dilated left ventricle. Dyspnea on exertion is another early symptom, gradually increasing as the disease progresses. Angina pectoris is common in the later stages from myocardial ischemia, developing from the decreased coronary blood flow during diastole as well as the large size of the left ventricle. Peripheral vasomotor phenomena, including episodes of severe sweating and intolerance to heat, are common.

Physical Examination. The cardiac rhythm is usually normal. With significant aortic insufficiency palpation readily discloses a prominent cardiac impulse, located downward and to the left of the normal location because of dilatation of the left ventricle. The hallmark of aortic insufficiency is the high-pitched, decrescendo diastolic murmur along the left sternal border. The murmur starts immediately after the second sound and may be confused with it. The length of the murmur correlates approximately with the severity of the insufficiency; those lasting only through early diastole represent less severe degrees of regurgitation. Having the patient lean forward while listening along the left sternal border makes the murmur more audible. With faint high-pitched murmurs, having the patient stop breathing momentarily is helpful. If the murmur is loudest to the right of the sternum, dilatation of the aortic ring, as in the Marfan syndrome, is likely. As mentioned earlier, with advanced cardiac failure and increase in the left ventricular diastolic pressure, the intensity of the diastolic murmur may decrease to actually become inaudible in terminal stages. A systolic murmur of the ejection type, moderate in intensity, is frequently heard, arising from increased volume of blood expelled from the left ventricle, not from anatomic aortic stenosis.

Examination of the peripheral arterial circulation reveals many positive findings. The pulse pressure is increased, partly from an increase in systolic pressure, but principally from a decrease in diastolic pressure from the normal range near 80 mm Hg. The diastolic pressure may

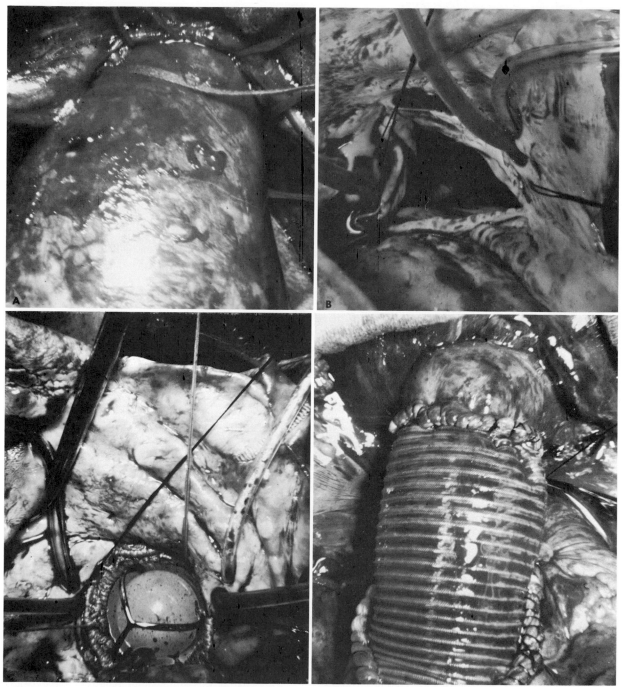

Fig. 19-29. *A.* Aneurysm in the ascending aorta in a patient with the Marfan syndrome. Marked dilatation of the proximal ascending aorta has developed, stretching the aortic annulus and producing aortic insufficiency. The distal ascending aorta, proximal to the innominate artery, is nearly normal in diameter and has been encircled with an umbilical tape. The left innominate vein is retracted at the top of the field. *B.* With the patient on cardiopulmonary bypass, the aorta has been clamped and the aneurysm opened. The aortic annulus is shown with the stretched leaflets producing total insufficiency. Silastic coronary cannulae have been inserted into each coronary ostium for coronary perfusion while reconstruction is performed. *C.* A Starr-Edwards ball valve in position which has been inserted following excision of the insufficient valve leaflets. The coronary perfusion cannulae are still in position. *D.* Following insertion of the aortic valve, the ascending aorta was reconstructed with a short prosthesis of Dacron cloth. The distal suture line is just proximal to the origin of the innominate artery.

be as low as 40 mm Hg, but true diastolic pressure is never less than 30 to 35 mm Hg, as measured by direct arterial puncture. Auscultatory findings of a diastolic pressure of zero results from dilatation of peripheral arteries. The exact level of diastolic pressure does not correlate closely with the severity of the aortic insufficiency. For example, a blood pressure of 130/65 mm Hg may be present with either moderate or severe insufficiency. This lack of correlation is due to the influence of peripheral resistance. With vasodilatation, diastolic pressure may be low without marked regurgitation, while with severe vasoconstriction diastolic pressure may be higher but with severe regurgitation.

With significant insufficiency, peripheral pulses are easily visible, forceful, and bounding. "Pistol shot" sounds are readily heard with the bell of the stethoscope over peripheral arteries. A wide variety of other auscultatory phenomena have been described, all of which indicate vasodilatation and a hyperactive peripheral circulation.

Laboratory Studies. The chest roentgenogram usually shows enlargement of the left ventricle, with the apex displaced downward and to the left. Serial chest roentgenograms over months or years is the best method for evaluating progression of the disease. Lateral views are required to appreciate fully the degree of enlargement of the left ventricle because of its posterior location. The electrocardiogram may be normal with early aortic insufficiency, but with more advanced disease and the appearance of symptoms there are signs of left ventricular hypertrophy with abnormalities in the ST-T segments. The cardiac rhythm is usually sinus. Atrial fibrillation is rare. Its presence suggests either terminal aortic insufficiency or concomitant mitral valve disease.

Cardiac catheterization may show no abnormalities in

Fig. 19-30. Operative photograph of a Silastic ball removed from an aortic valve prosthesis, inserted before 1966. Development of a diastolic murmur fortunately led to reoperation before fatal embolization of the fragmented Silastic ball occurred. With improvement in Silastic ball prostheses this complication has been virtually unknown since 1966.

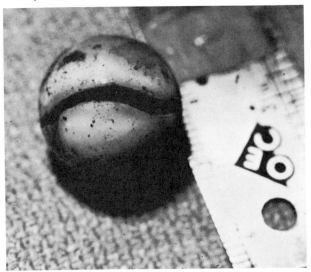

the early stages of the disease when left ventricular diastolic pressure is normal. With cardiac failure and elevation of the left ventricular diastolic pressure to 15 to 20 mm Hg, there is corresponding elevation of left atrial pressure. The best method for quantitating the degree of insufficiency is aortography, injecting dye into the ascending aorta and visually estimating the degree of reflux into the ventricle. Though subjective, this method is quite satisfactory for most clinical decisions.

DIAGNOSIS. A diagnosis can be readily made when the characteristic diastolic murmur is heard along the left sternal border. Quantitation of the degree of insufficiency, however, is more difficult. Mild insufficiency exists when only a murmur is audible without any changes in pulse pressure. Such patients may be treated optimistically, as their only serious risk is that of developing bacterial endocarditis. With more significant insufficiency, a diastolic murmur extending throughout diastole is audible in association with a decrease in diastolic blood pressure and prominent peripheral pulses. Cardiac enlargement as well as changes in the electrocardiogram of left ventricular hypertrophy are usually present. The degree of enlargement of the left ventricle is probably the most reliable indicator of the severity of the disease.

A significant surgical problem exists regarding the degree of aortic insufficiency when concomitant mitral valve disease requires operation. In such patients a decision needs to be made whether or not to replace the diseased aortic valve as well as the diseased mitral valve. Aortography is the best method for estimating the degree of insufficiency but is not totally accurate. A final decision must be made at operation, approaching the heart through a median sternotomy incision and noting the amount of blood regurgitating through the aortic valve after the mitral valve has been removed.

TREATMENT. Surgical treatment is recommended ordinarily only when symptoms become significant. In some patients progressive enlargement of the left ventricle develops with surprisingly few symptoms. Probably these patients should be operated upon to avoid extreme degrees of left ventricular hypertrophy, with heart weights approaching 900 to 1,000 Gm. Once symptoms become significant, surgical therapy should be prompt because of the rapid downhill course of the disease in most symptomatic patients.

When operation is performed, we prefer prosthetic replacement with a cloth-covered ball valve of the Starr-Edwards variety (Fig. 19-30). With small aortic roots, the disc valve of the Bjork-Shiley type is useful. Tissue prostheses, such as homografts and porcine heterografts, are described in the preceding section, Aortic Stenosis. They have been widely and effectively used by several groups.

TRICUSPID STENOSIS AND INSUFFICIENCY

ETIOLOGY. Organic disease of the tricuspid valve is almost always due to rheumatic fever. With the exception of septic endocarditis, usually in drug addicts, it virtually never occurs as an isolated lesion, but only in association with extensive disease of the mitral valve. With mitral disease the frequency of associated tricuspid disease is near 10 to 15 percent, although an incidence as high as 30 percent has been reported.

Tricuspid insufficiency is the more common lesion encountered, while pure stenosis is infrequent. Rarely, both stenosis and insufficiency are present.

Functional tricuspid insufficiency is actually more common than insufficiency from organic disease. It develops from dilatation of the tricuspid annulus and right ventricle as a result of pulmonary hypertension and right ventricular failure. The hypertension is usually a consequence of mitral valve disease with elevated left atrial pressure.

A more recent etiologic factor in isolated tricuspid disease is bacterial endocarditis among heroin addicts. This presents many very special problems because of the repeated infections which such patients tend to sustain.

PATHOLOGY. With tricuspid stenosis the pathologic changes are similar to those found with the more familiar mitral stenosis. There is fusion of the commissures to form a small central opening 1 to 1.5 cm in diameter. As right atrial pressure is normally only 4 to 5 mm Hg, significant tricuspid stenosis may be present with a valve orifice considerably larger than that seen with mitral stenosis.

Tricuspid insufficiency results from fibrosis and contraction of the valve leaflets, often in association with shortening and fusion of chordae tendineae. Calcification is rare. With dilation of the tricuspid annulus the valve leaflets appear stretched, but otherwise are pliable and seemingly normal even though serious regurgitation is present. An unexplained fact, however, is that such valves may not regain competence after correction of mitral valve disease and restoration of pulmonary artery systolic pressure to normal.

PATHOPHYSIOLOGY. With tricuspid stenosis the mean right atrial pressure is elevated to 10 to 20 mm Hg. The higher pressures are found with a tricuspid valve orifice smaller than 1.5 cm^2 and a mean diastolic gradient between the atrium and ventricle of 5 to 15 mm Hg. When mean right atrial pressure remains above 10 mm Hg, edema and ascites usually appear.

Moderate degrees of tricuspid insufficiency may be tolerated surprisingly well because the regurgitant blood is dissipated into the systemic veins with little adverse influence on circulation except for a decrease in cardiac output. This is in striking contrast to mitral insufficiency, where the regurgitating blood produces pulmonary congestion. The significance of tricuspid insufficiency alone is difficult to evaluate because it is almost always seen in association with the more serious mitral valve disease. However, rarely tricuspid insufficiency results from an isolated traumatic injury. Such patients may tolerate the disease well for many years, the only physiologic disturbance being elevation of venous pressure and a decrease in cardiac output.

CLINICAL MANIFESTATIONS. Symptoms. The symptoms of tricuspid valve disease are similar to those of failure of the right side of the heart resulting from the associated mitral valve disease. Prominent features include elevation of venous pressure with edema, ascites, and hepatomegaly.

As similar findings occur from failure of the right side of the heart without disease of the tricuspid valve, the concomitant presence of tricuspid disease may be easily overlooked. The general effects of tricuspid disease are to increase the severity of failure of the right side of the heart. Otherwise the clinical course is similar to that seen with isolated mitral stenosis or insufficiency.

Physical Examination. The characteristic murmur of tricuspid stenosis is best heard as a diastolic murmur at the lower end of the sternum. It is a low-pitched murmur of medium intensity and can easily be overlooked as it is well localized at the lower end of the sternum. During inspiration the intensity of the murmur increases as the volume of blood returning to the heart is temporarily increased by an increase in intrathoracic negative pressure. Tricuspid insufficiency produces a prominent systolic murmur at the lower end of the sternum and also at the cardiac apex, where it may be confused with the systolic murmur of mitral insufficiency. The murmur is often seen in association with an enlarged pulsating liver and prominent engorged peripheral veins. A prominent jugular pulse, especially when the cardiac rhythm is sinus, may be the best clue to unsuspected tricuspid disease.

Laboratory Studies. The chest roentgenogram and electrocardiogram may show enlargement of the right side of the heart, but this does not differentiate tricuspid disease from cardiac enlargement caused by pulmonary hypertension secondary to mitral disease. Cardiac catheterization and cineangiography are the most precise ways of establishing the diagnosis. At catheterization the presence of tricuspid stenosis can be established by measuring the diastolic gradient between the atrium and the ventricle. As the gradient may be quite small (5 to 7 mm Hg), careful measurements are necessary.

With serious tricuspid insufficiency, the contour of the right atrial pressure tracing is altered by the regurgitating of blood during systole. If the right atrium is large, however, significant regurgitation may be present with little alteration in contour of the right atrial pressure tracing; so a normal pressure tracing does not exclude significant insufficiency. Cineangiography is the best method for detecting insufficiency, noting the degree of reflux of dye into the atrium when dye is injected into the ventricle.

DIAGNOSIS. The diagnosis can be made with reasonable certainty if the characteristic systolic or diastolic murmurs are audible at the lower end of the sternum, especially in association with an enlarged, pulsating liver. Confirmatory studies are best obtained by catheterization and angiography. A good surgical routine at the time of mitral valve operation is to palpate the tricuspid valve through the right atrium before bypass is started to confirm or exclude the presence of tricuspid disease.

TREATMENT. Tricuspid disease is surgically treated at the time of correction of more serious mitral disease. Rarely the aortic valve is also involved; so replacement of three cardiac valves is necessary. There is not a uniform opinion about the necessity for treating minor to moderate degrees of tricuspid insufficiency secondary to pulmonary hypertension from mitral disease. Some have felt that correction of mitral valve disease, followed by regression of the pulmonary hypertension, would decrease the degree of tricuspid insufficiency to clinically unimportant levels. Braunwald and associates reported results with operation upon 23 patients with tricuspid disease, 4 of whom had an annuloplasty while 19 had no therapy other than correction of the mitral disease. Fairly good clinical results were obtained. With extensive tricuspid insufficiency, however, almost all surgeons have concluded that tricuspid replacement or annuloplasty, should be performed at operation because a significant impairment of cardiac output from untreated tricuspid insufficiency jeopardizes the patient's opportunity for recovery following mitral replacement.

Tricuspid stenosis may be treated by simple commissurotomy, usually opening the commissure between the anterior and septal leaflets and the commissure between the posterior and septal leaflets, but leaving the fused commissure between the anterior and posterior leaflets. Opening of this commissure usually produces insufficiency. Hence, following commissurotomy the valve functions as a bicuspid one.

With organic disease of the tricuspid valve producing tricuspid insufficiency, surgical correction has usually been ineffective except with prosthetic replacement. For a long time the ball-valve prosthesis seemed satisfactory in the tricuspid position, much as in the mitral position. However, late thrombosis of the tricuspid ball-valve prosthesis months or years after operation has been reported by several groups. This is presumably caused by decrease in size of the right ventricle with resulting impairment of motion of the ball within the cage of the prosthesis (Fig. 19-31). For this reason most groups have abandoned the use of the ball-valve prosthesis.

A disc prosthesis may be used but carries an increased risk of thrombosis because of the low pressures in the right side of the heart. For this reason, the prosthesis of choice at present is the gluteraldehyde-preserved porcine heterograft. This does not require anticoagulants, and a durability of up to 5 or 6 years is well established.

During insertion of the prosthetic valve, along the septal leaflet where the conduction bundle is located between the coronary sinus and the ventricular septum, sutures are placed through the base of the septal leaflet rather than through the annulus to avoid injury of the conduction bundle and production of heart block (Fig. 19-32). As arrhythmias are frequent after operation, two pacemaker wires are routinely left in the ventricle.

When moderate tricuspid insufficiency with pulmonary hypertension is present and the leaflets of the tricuspid valve appear normal but the annulus is dilated, an annuloplasty is preferable. Our results with posterior leaflet annuloplasty, as reported by Boyd et al., have been consistently good. Others have preferred the more complex annuloplasty techniques, using either the Carpentier ring or the method of annuloplasty developed by DeVega. Considerable pessimism had been expressed about the durability of annuloplasty, but enough long-term data are now available to indicate that annuloplasty is a sound procedure of permanent benefit.

An astonishing observation of some physiologic importance concerning tricuspid function is the finding reported by Arbulu and associates that total excision of the tricuspid

Fig. 19-31. *A.* Chest roentgenogram of a patient following prosthetic replacement of the mitral and tricuspid valves. The mitral valve has been replaced with a Starr-Edwards ball-valve prosthesis. A Kay-Shiley disc prosthesis was used for the tricuspid valve. *B.* Lateral-roentgenogram showing the mitral and tricuspid valves in position.

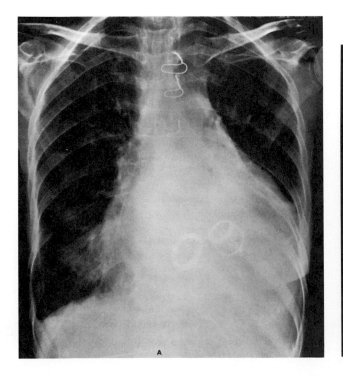

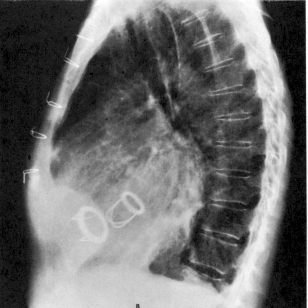

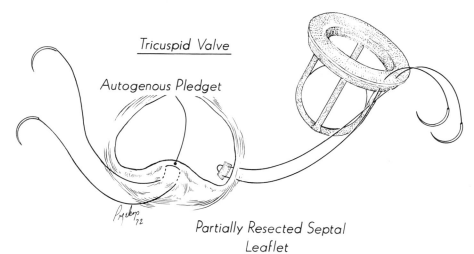

Fig. 19-32. Technique for suturing the tricuspid valve prosthesis with Dacron pledgets seated below the tricuspid annulus. The pledgets are used in all areas except the area of the partially resected septal leaflet, which is used as an autogenous pledget to avoid the conduction bundle and the production of heart block.

valve *without replacement* could be tolerated for at least short periods of time. These observations were made in treating the difficult problem of tricuspid valve endocarditis in heroin addicts, where repeated septic injections had resulted in endocarditis of the tricuspid valve. Chemotherapy in such instances has often been futile, and prosthetic replacement frequently resulted in reinfection. These writers made the significant observation that the value could simply be excised with fair cardiac function for at least several months. They reported one survivor who was without a tricuspid valve for 10 months. However, there is definite disability, therefore a two-stage procedure for the treatment of endocarditis seems to be the method of choice. Initially, all diseased valvular tissue is excised to eradicate the endocarditis, and an elective prosthetic replacement is done a few weeks later.

MULTIVALVULAR HEART DISEASE

With rheumatic heart disease, more than one cardiac valve is frequently involved. The physician must remain alert to this possibility, for prominent signs of disease of one valve can readily mask disease of additional valves. For this reason, cardiac catheterization and cineangiography are used to evaluate the function of all four cardiac valves to determine stenosis or insufficiency. In addition, at the time of operation other valves can be inspected or palpated. This is one of the great advantages of the sternotomy incision, which provides ready access to all cardiac chambers. The precise recognition of multivalvular disease is of considerable therapeutic importance, for widespread clinical experience has demonstrated that failure to correct all significant valvular disease at the time of operation significantly increases the surgical mortality.

A variety of clinical syndromes can be produced by

different combinations of valvular disease. Often the clinical diagnosis can be only suspected and must be decided either by cardiac catheterization and angiography or operative exploration. The more common types of multivalvular disease will be briefly mentioned.

AORTIC DISEASE WITH FUNCTIONAL MITRAL INSUFFICIENCY. With dilatation of the left ventricle from cardiac failure due to aortic insufficiency, rarely from aortic stenosis, dilatation of the mitral annulus can produce a functional mitral insufficiency without intrinsic disease of the mitral valve. Such insufficiency may regress following repair of the aortic lesion, or it may be corrected by annuloplasty at operation, narrowing the annulus to normal dimensions by placing sutures at the stretched commissures. Replacement of the stretched but normal mitral valve is not often necessary. Usually the procedure can be decided by palpation of the mitral valve in the functioning, beating heart by introducing a finger into the left atrium through a stab wound in the intraatrial groove, just before cardiopulmonary bypass is started.

A convenient approach for assessing the magnitude of functional mitral insufficiency is to palpate the mitral valve in the beating heart by introducing a finger into the left atrium through a stab wound in the intraatrial groove just before bypass is started. There is some danger of hemorrhage with this maneuver, and preparations for initiating bypass should be complete before the finger is introduced. If uncertainty remains, the mitral valve can be palpated in a similar manner after the aortic valve has been replaced and bypass stopped. In recent years we have found that annuloplasty is seldom necessary in the absence of organic disease of the mitral valve.

AORTIC STENOSIS AND MITRAL STENOSIS. When these two stenotic lesions coexist, the clinical signs of mitral stenosis often overshadow those of aortic stenosis, for the volume of blood entering the left ventricle is restricted by the stenotic mitral valve. Hence, functionally severe aortic stenosis may be present with minimal physical findings and a systolic pressure gradient between the left ventricle and aorta or only 20 to 40 mm Hg. Calculation of the cross-sectional area of the aortic valve by simultaneous measurement of cardiac output will quantitate the degree of aortic stenosis present. In uncertain instances, at the end of operative correction of the mitral stenosis, the aortic valve should be examined, either by pressure measurements or by inspection. Overlooking significant aortic stenosis at the time of correction of mitral stenosis can easily result in death early in the postoperative period.

AORTIC INSUFFICIENCY AND MITRAL STENOSIS. With prominent aortic disease, an underlying mitral stenosis can easily be masked because the classic diastolic rumble of mitral stenosis is overshadowed by the prominent aortic murmurs. Cardiac catheterization will usually detect significant mitral stenosis beforehand. If uncertainty remains, however, the mitral valve may be readily palpated or inspected through a short incision in the left atrium at the time of surgical correction of aortic valve disease.

MITRAL STENOSIS WITH TRICUSPID DISEASE. When signs of mitral disease are prominent, tricuspid disease can be easily overlooked. As mentioned earlier, the most significant clinical signs of tricuspid disease are a systolic or diastolic murmur at the lower end of the sternum, especially one accentuated during inspiration. Often the jugular veins are prominent with systolic pulsations, in combination with an enlarged, pulsating liver. These clinical signs, however, are not precise. Catheterization and angiography may establish the diagnosis, but again the technique is not totally reliable. The pressure gradient with significant tricuspid stenosis may be small, and tricuspid insufficiency can be assessed by angiography only by introducing a catheter across the triscupid valve to inject dye into the

right ventricle, a procedure which in itself may produce some tricuspid insufficiency. For these reasons, routine palpation of the tricuspid valve at the time of operation on the mitral valve is preferred. This is technically simple and quickly confirms or excludes the presence of tricuspid disease.

TRIVALVULAR DISEASE. In some unfortunate patients, significant disease of the mitral, aortic, and tricuspid valves is present. Such patients are usually in far advanced cardiac failure with generalized cardiomegaly. Hence, detection and surgical correction of all three valvular lesions is of critical importance if the patient is to survive operation. Attempting to shorten and simplify the operative procedure by not correcting all three diseased valves is usually unsatisfactory. Triple valve replacement, however, is an operative procedure of significant complexity and magnitude and has a mortality in the range of 15 to 20 percent, primarily because patients requiring triple valve replacement are usually critically ill with far advanced chronic congestive failure and extensive cardiomegaly. In such patients cardiac function often improves slowly over weeks or even months after operation (Fig. 19-33).

CARDIAC TRAUMA

HISTORICAL DATA. In 1896 Rehn first successfully sutured a stab wound of the heart, but for over 20 years this remained principally an isolated historic achievement until developments in anesthesia, blood transfusion, and

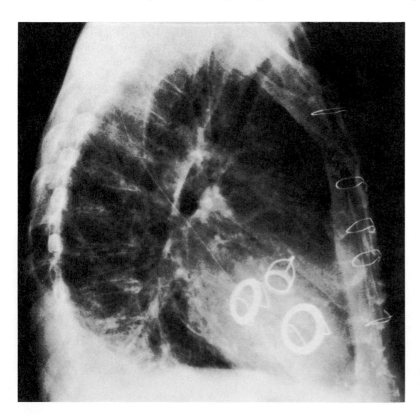

Fig. 19-33. Lateral roentgenogram in a patient with prosthetic replacement of the mitral, tricuspid, and aortic valves. The mitral and tricuspid valves were replaced with Kay-Shiley disc prostheses, while the aortic valve was replaced with a Starr-Edwards ball-valve prosthesis.

other surgical advances made thoracotomy progressively safer, especially after 1940. In 1943 Blalock and Ravitch recognized that many patients survived a penetrating injury of the heart because pericardial tamponade developed and prevented exsanguination. Their introduction of pericardial aspiration as a form of definitive treatment greatly lowered mortality from penetrating cardiac injuries. Asfaw et al., in 1975, reported experiences with 12 cases of traumatic intraventricular defects and reviewed previous published reports. Improvements in diagnosis, resuscitative therapy for shock, anesthesia, and operative technique have all contributed to lower mortality from cardiac injuries in recent years. At present, pericardial aspiration is used primarily in resuscitation before operating on the patient. It is used much less frequently as definitive therapy. The risks from a negative exploratory thoracotomy are small and outweigh the hazards of recurrent tamponade or of overlooking multiple injuries if nonoperative therapy is employed.

ETIOLOGY. Patients with penetrating cardiac injuries who are still alive when first seen by a physician usually have stab wounds from a small instrument such as an ice pick or small knife. Less common are similar injuries from low-velocity bullets, but injuries from high-velocity bullets or large knives often cause immediate death from exsanguination. Nonpenetrating cardiac injuries result from blunt trauma to the chest wall, the most frequent of which is the "steering wheel" injury from contusion of the chest wall by impact against the steering wheel in an automobile accident.

PATHOLOGY. Because of its anterior position, the right ventricle is the cardiac chamber most frequently injured with penetrating wounds. In surviving patients most wounds are penetrating rather than perforating wounds. Nonpenetrating crushing injuries usually cause diffuse contusion of the myocardium. With nonpenetrating injuries of severe force, however, actual cardiac lacerations occur, usually fatal. Rarely, a surviving patient is seen with a laceration of the tricuspid valve, the right atrium, or even the ventricular septum.

PATHOPHYSIOLOGY. The three principal physiologic disturbances following a cardiac injury are intrathoracic hemorrhage, pericardial tamponade, and cardiac failure. Hemorrhage of varying degree, of course, is present with every cardiac injury. The clinical signs are usually obvious with profound shock; death often occurs before definitive treatment can be started. Cardiac tamponade is frequently the dominant physiologic injury in surviving patients because patients surviving long enough for therapy often do so because tamponade has delayed or stopped the bleeding from the cardiac laceration. Tamponade quickly occurs because the normal pericardium can accommodate only 100 to 250 ml of blood. As the intrapericardial pressure rises with continuing tamponade, there is a progressive fall in cardiac output. Careful experimental studies by Isaacs found that elevation of intrapericardial pressure to 17 cm saline solution virtually stopped cardiac output unless venous pressure was elevated by infusion of fluid. This restriction of cardiac output results from prevention of diastolic filling of the ventricles, not from impaired venous flow into atria from the venae cavae.

Impaired cardiac function from the penetrating injury per se is unusual. It is seen only with the rare instance of injury of specific structures, such as a major coronary artery, a heart valve, or the cardiac conduction bundle.

CLINICAL MANIFESTATIONS. Symptoms. Patients with a cardiac injury may collapse immediately in profound shock or develop shock more gradually over a period of 1 to 2 hours. The clinical appearance of some patients with tamponade is initially deceptive, for they may appear only moderately ill and then collapse suddenly with an imperceptible blood pressure. This rapid change is due to the fact that once the pericardial cavity becomes distended, only 5 to 10 ml additional fluid is sufficient to raise the intrapericardial pressure to the critical zone of 17 to 18 cm saline solution, where cardiac output falls to very low levels.

The most frequent symptoms are the familiar ones of shock, including weakness, thirst, and restlessness. Chest pain is seldom severe. An unusual degree of restlessness, at times with the patient wildly rolling about, in contrast to the usual quiet, apathetic state of patients in hemorrhagic shock, perhaps results from cerebral anoxia produced by both arterial hypotension and venous hypertension.

Physical Examination. If tamponade is not present, the findings are those of hemorrhagic shock, hypotension with collapsed peripheral veins, and intense vasoconstriction. Tamponade is immediately suggested by finding hypotension combined with venous hypertension, indicated by visible, dilated neck and arm veins. The chest roentgenogram often shows little cardiac enlargement with tamponade, because the pericardium does not distend easily. A hemothorax is common, especially if there is concomitant injury of the lung or if the laceration is large enough for blood to drain from the pericardium into the pleural space. Particular care should be taken in examining the film for the presence of a small foreign body. The electrocardiogram is often normal, except for the rare patient with injury of a coronary artery or the conduction bundle. Fluoroscopy, once a popular technique for evaluating tamponade, has been virtually abandoned because of the time required and the lack of precision. Accurate measurement of central venous pressure, an important early measurement in the treatment of any patient with hemorrhagic shock, may quickly establish or exclude tamponade. A venous pressure above 10 cm saline solution suggests the diagnosis, while one above 15 cm is virtually diagnostic.

DIAGNOSIS. With the combination of arterial hypotension and venous hypertension, combined with other clinical findings, cardiac tamponade can be diagnosed with considerable accuracy. The differential diagnosis includes venous hypertension from overtransfusion, cardiac failure, or pulmonary embolism. If tamponade is a possibility, the pericardium should be aspirated promptly, at times within 5 to 10 minutes after the patient is first seen in the emergency department. Aspiration both confirms the diagnosis and partially relieves the tamponade.

In urgent instances where death is imminent and the presence of tamponade uncertain, a subxiphoid incision can be made in the linea alba and the pericardial cavity entered by making a small opening in the diaphragm immediately behind the xiphoid process. This can be quickly done and the pericardial cavity digitally explored. This is particularly helpful when large clots in the pericardium make needle aspiration ineffective.

The diagnosis of chronic or subacute cardiac tamponade is difficult. The question may arise several days after a penetrating thoracic injury which initially was not thought to have entered the pericardium. It more commonly arises after cardiac surgery, usually several days after operation when the question of intrathoracic bleeding no longer exists. As with acute tamponade, the clinical findings are a decreased cardiac output with hypotension and elevation of venous pressure. The usual condition to be differentiated from chronic tamponade is cardiac failure, more rarely pulmonary embolism. Several years of experience have indicated the great variation in clinical signs with chronic tamponade and the unreliability of such findings as a paradoxic pulse, changes in intensity of cardiac sounds, or size of the cardiac silhouette on the chest roentgenogram. The safest approach seems to be the realization that in the presence of decreased cardiac output and elevated venous pressure tamponade cannot be excluded with 100 percent certainty except by thoracotomy. Simply being aware of these diagnostic limitations is particularly important in treating a patient for supposedly congestive failure who does not respond to the usual therapy of digitalis and diuretics. In uncertain instances the pericardial cavity must be explored, either by needle aspiration, subxiphoid digital aspiration, or formal thoracotomy.

TREATMENT. With shock from penetrating cardiac injuries, therapy includes intravenous infusion of fluids, administration of catecholamines to stimulate myocardial contractility, pericardial aspiration, and thoracotomy. Appropriate amounts of fluid, 1 to 3 liters of electrolyte or blood, should be infused rapidly to elevate venous pressure and thus enhance cardiac filling, despite the elevated intrapericardial pressure. Cardiac filling results from the difference between venous pressure and intrapericardial pressure; hence, elevation of venous pressure by intravenously infused fluids will partly correct the impaired myocardial filling from the elevated pericardial pressures. For patients in extremis with bradycardia and impending cardiac arrest, probably from impaired coronary blood flow, catecholamines such as epinephrine or isoproterenol may be useful for short periods of time.

When a moribund patient with possible tamponade is first seen, pericardial aspiration should be done immediately. One of the most dramatic experiences in surgery is to aspirate as little as 10 to 15 ml blood from the pericardium of a moribund patient with an imperceptible blood pressure and see a prompt rise in blood pressure to 70 to 80 mm Hg and a return of consciousness. Aspiration is best done through a subxiphoid approach, inserting a 16- or 18-gauge needle slowly upward in the angle between the xiphoid process and the left costal margin. Ideally, the electrocardiogram should be monitored for an arrhythmia during the procedure. As the needle is angled upward, a sense of resistance can be noted as the diaphragm and pericardium are traversed. Varying amounts of blood may be obtained, ranging from as little as 10 ml to as much as 300 to 400 ml. The blood obtained from the pericardium may not clot, while blood obtained from inadvertent puncture of the heart, usually the right ventricle, does.

As mentioned earlier, when tamponade is likely but aspiration is ineffective, a prompt subxiphoid digital exploration should be done, making a short incision in the linea alba, separating the diaphragm behind the xiphoid process, and digitally entering the pericardium. The technique is well described by Berger et al.

Immediate thoracotomy should be considered and the operating room notified as soon as a patient is seen with a penetrating cardiac injury, because of the unpredictability of either continued hemorrhage or tamponade. Final decision about thoracotomy can be made after initial response to intravenously administered fluids.

Some patients with massive hemorrhage from cardiac wounds are near death on arrival in an emergency department and are often seen alive only because they were injured not far from the hospital. In such patients immediate thoracotomy in the emergency room, often with minimal aseptic technique, may be lifesaving. Once hemorrhage has been controlled by digital pressure or temporary suture, resuscitation can proceed in a more orderly fashion, usually followed by closure of the incision in the operating room. Since 1970, at Bellevue Hospital, several such patients have recovered uneventfully after immediate thoracotomy who clearly would not have survived otherwise.

Separate from the necessity of immediate thoracotomy for massive hemorrhage is the question of elective thoracotomy for penetrating cardiac injuries with tamponade. Data clearly indicate that 60 to 70 percent of the patients with tamponade can be safely treated by serial aspiration. In 1959 Isaacs reported that in a group of 60 patients with cardiac injuries treated at The Johns Hopkins Hospital, 40 had symptoms of tamponade for which aspiration was successful treatment in 75 percent; there was only one death in this group. However, there has been a gradual trend in recent years to perform thoracotomy upon virtually all patients with penetrating injuries and tamponade. The risk of thoracotomy is very small, probably no more than 1 to 2 percent, and the likelihood of delayed bleeding and recurrent tamponade small.

Sugg et al. in 1968 presented convincing data that routine thoracotomy gave overall better results in most institutions than selective thoracotomy for patients judged to have continuing hemorrhage or recurrent tamponade. In 1971 Beall et al. described a similar trend at Baylor University, where thoracotomy is now done almost routinely, rather than repeated pericardiocentesis.

Myocardial contusion from blunt thoracic trauma should be treated much as an acute myocardial infarction, with bed rest and serial observations with blood-enzyme measurements and the electrocardiogram. Complete recovery after a period of weeks can be expected in most patients. Rarely blunt injury may be associated with signs of intrapericardial bleeding from a laceration. Such instances are unusual, but because of the unpredictable nature of the laceration a pump-oxygenator should be available, and attachment of the pump-oxygenator to the femoral vessels in the thigh before the chest is opened should be considered. Without the pump-oxygenator, fatal hemorrhage may occur when the pericardium is opened if the laceration is too extensive to be promptly controlled by digital pressure. A recent report by Drapanas dramatically illustrates the utility of the pump-oxygenator in such injuries.

COMPLICATIONS. In the absence of injury of a discrete cardiac structure, recovery in most patients following suture of a cardiac laceration is uneventful. Formerly in those treated by serial aspiration alone, 15 to 20 percent developed a pericardiotomy syndrome with fever and effusion, lasting for several days to a few weeks but eventually resulting in complete recovery. Septic pericarditis from bacterial infection is very rare, and constrictive pericarditis has occurred as a late complication in only a few patients.

Foreign Bodies

Foreign bodies remaining in the heart after injury have naturally attracted much interest because of the unusual circumstances and the profound psychologic influences of having a missile embedded in the heart. Following World War II, Harken published a careful analysis of extensive experiences with foreign bodies, defining the complications and the indications for removal at that time. A reevaluation of the problem was published by Holdeger et al. in 1966. Data clearly indicate that symptomatic foreign bodies smaller than 1 cm are innocuous and can be safely left alone. Larger foreign bodies or those associated with a pericardial effusion or signs of pericarditis are best removed. Occasionally foreign bodies migrate in the circulation, moving from a large vein to the right ventricle or to a pulmonary artery.

In 1966 Bland and Beebe published a significant report of the 20-year course of 40 patients with foreign bodies remaining in the heart after World War II. All patients survived. A major complication occurred in only 1 patient, in whom a shell fragment in the left pulmonary artery moved to the right pulmonary artery and eroded the bronchus. The electrocardiogram became normal in all but 2 patients. Only 1 patient, who had a distinct injury of the aortic valve, had persistent cardiac enlargement. However, the emotional disability was impressive, apparently related to the strain of living with a condition of uncertain prognosis. Almost all patients were seriously concerned, and 5 were incapacitated with anxiety neuroses. Because of this significant emotional disability and the safety of current cardiac surgical procedures, most foreign bodies of significant size should be electively removed.

CARDIAC TUMORS

Metastatic neoplasms are the most common cardiac neoplasms, occurring in 4 to 12 percent of the autopsies performed on patients with neoplastic disease. The most frequent primary cardiac tumor is *myxoma,* comprising 50 to 60 percent of all primary cardiac neoplasms. *Sarcomas* are found in 20 to 25 percent of cases, and *rhabdomyomas* in 10 to 15 percent. Benign but extremely rare neoplasms include fibromas, angiomas, lipomas, teratomas, and cysts.

The clinical significance of cardiac tumors is similar to that of many other cardiac lesions in that accurate diagnosis and successful treatment first became possible with the development of extracorporeal circulation. Before 1950 cardiac tumors were usually first diagnosed at autopsy. Several excellent reviews have previously summarized the pathologic findings and clinical features. A classic analysis was published by Yater in 1931, and a detailed French monograph was published by Mahaim in 1945. In 1949 Whorton described the clinical findings in 100 sarcomas of the heart, and in 1951 Prichard reviewed 150 lesions, most of which were metastatic in origin.

In 1953 Steinberg et al. reported the diagnosis of an atrial myxoma in three patients by angiocardiography. An unsuccessful attempt was made to remove the myxoma in one of the patients studied by Steinberg et al., and in 1952 another unsuccessful attempt was made by Bahnson. Both these efforts preceded the development of open heart surgery. The first successful removal of an atrial myxoma was performed by Crafoord in 1954, using extracorporeal circulation. Other successful reports quickly followed, and in 1967 Thomas et al. stated that there had been 126 attempted excisions of atrial myxomas, either planned or inadvertent, 85 of which had been successful.

With the safety of extracorporeal circulation and the refinement of diagnostic techniques, including selective angiocardiography and more recently echocardiography, diagnosis and surgical excision have been greatly simplified. Typical of several reports is one by Symbas et al. in 1976, describing experiences with 13 patients.

Myxoma

Sixty to seventy-five percent of cardiac myxomas develop in the left atrium, almost always from the atrial septum near the fossa ovalis. Most other myxomas develop in the right atrium. Less than 20 have been found in either the right or left ventricle. The curious predilection for a myxoma to develop from the rim of the fossa ovalis in the left atrium has been studied by several observers, but a satisfactory explanation has not been found.

Myxomas are apparently true neoplasms, although their similarity to an organized atrial thrombus led to considerable debate at one time about whether they represented a true neoplasm or not. Their occurrence in the absence of other organic heart disease, histochemical studies demonstrating mucopolysaccharide and glycoprotein, and a distinct histologic appearance all indicate that myxomas are true neoplasms. In 1976 Dang and Hurley reported 19 recurrences of a myxoma following surgical excision in 16 patients, conclusively establishing the low-grade malignant potential of the tumor.

PATHOLOGY. The tumors are usually polypoid, projecting into the atrial cavity from a 1- to 2-cm stalk attached to the atrial septum. The maximal diameter varies from 0.5 to 10 cm. Careful histologic study of the point of origin of the myxoma from the atrial septum has demonstrated that only the superficial layer of the septum is involved, and invasion of the septum does not occur. Frequently myxomas grow slowly, some patients having symptoms for 10 to 20 years. There is no tendency to invade other areas of the heart, and metastases have not occurred. The consistency of a myxoma is of surgical significance, for extreme friability has been found in some tumors, resulting in fatal embolization when the tumor was digitally manipulated.

Histologically, a myxoma is covered with endothelium and composed of a myxomatous stroma with large stellate cells mixed with fusiform or multinucleated cells. Mitoses are infrequent. Lymphocytes and plasmacytes are regularly found. Hemosiderin, a result of hemorrhage into the tumor, is also common.

PATHOPHYSIOLOGY. A myxoma may cause no difficulty until it grows large enough to obstruct the flow of blood through either the mitral or tricuspid valve, or fragments to produce peripheral emboli. The rarity of embolization is surprising, for an astonishing degree of to-and-fro motion of a myxoma swinging on a small pedicle with each cardiac contraction may occur. This has been vividly demonstrated by angiographic and fluoroscopic studies.

Because of its rarity, myxoma is almost always confused with a more frequent cardiac condition. Left atrial myxomas simulate mitral stenosis or insufficiency or idiopathic pulmonary hypertension. Right atrial myxomas are confused with tricuspid valvular disease or constrictive pericarditis. Because of the polypoid nature of the myxoma, intermittent obstruction of the mitral or tricuspid valve may occur, with resulting variation in symptoms, but this has not been observed frequently enough to be of much diagnostic significance.

CLINICAL MANIFESTATIONS. The clinical course of the patient with a myxoma may be protracted, with a variety of erroneous clinical diagnoses. The rate of development and variation in symptoms depend upon the growth of the tumor with the associated obstruction to cardiac filling and obstruction at the valve orifice. There are no characteristic symptoms or signs from which a precise diagnosis can be made. The usual findings are those of mitral valvular disease, with progressive dyspnea, cough, and subsequent cardiac failure with hepatic enlargement and edema.

In a few patients unusual signs of a generalized systemic disease have developed, with recurrent fever, weight loss, malaise, and abnormalities in serum proteins gradually evolving over 1 to 3 years. Why these symptoms should occur with a myxoma is not known.

Peripheral emboli occur in a minority of patients and in some are the first sign of a myxoma. A few instances have been described in which the diagnosis was first made as a result of histologic examination of a surgically removed embolus recognizing the characteristic myxomatous structure. Such a patient was recently treated in our unit.

On physical examination patients with a left atrial myxoma may have either a diastolic murmur suggesting mitral stenosis or a systolic murmur simulating mitral insufficiency. With a right atrial myxoma, hepatic enlargement and edema characteristic of constrictive pericarditis are frequent.

The electrocardiogram is often normal unless pulmonary hypertension from long-standing mitral valve obstruction has produced right ventricular hypertrophy. The chest roentgenogram may show enlargement of the left atrium with pulmonary congestion. Rarely on fluoroscopy calcification is visible. Echocardiography has been a significant advance in diagnosis, since most myxomas can be readily identified by this simple, noninvasive technique. Selective angiography may graphically confirm the diagnosis if the left atrium can be opacified satisfactorily, but unfortunately this cannot always be accomplished.

Differential diagnosis includes more frequent cardiac lesions, such as mitral stenosis or insufficiency, pulmonary hypertension, constrictive pericarditis, rheumatic fever, and bacterial endocarditis.

TREATMENT. Operation should be performed upon all patients once the diagnosis has been established. Extracorporeal circulation is routinely employed because of the grave risk of dislodging emboli into the arterial circulation.

A sternotomy or a right lateral thoracotomy is preferred. Once extracorporeal circulation has been established, ventricular fibrillation may be induced and the aorta clamped to avoid the risk of embolism of tumor fragments. Palpation of the lesion is avoided. In recent years we have adopted the operative approach described by Cooley in 1973. With bypass functioning, the right atrium is opened and the fossa ovalis incised to expose the stalk of the myxoma. The left atrium is opened in the interatrial groove. With the myxoma visualized, the segment of fossa ovalis from which the tumor arises is excised, after which the myxoma is removed through the incision in the left atrium. The defect in the atrial septum is closed with a small patch. This technique is simple, avoids manipulation of the tumor, and should prevent the rare recurrences which have been described.

Following operation the prognosis is excellent for complete recovery. Complete regression of severe pulmonary hypertension has been reported in several patients. One of the earliest cases, a fifty-seven-year-old patient operated upon in 1956, was well and asymptomatic 8 years later (Fig. 19-34).

Metastatic Neoplasms

Cardiac metastases have been found in 4 to 12 percent of autopsies performed for neoplastic disease. Although they have occurred from primary neoplasms developing in almost every known site of the body, the most frequent have been carcinoma of the lung or breast, melanoma, and lymphoma. Cardiac metastases involving only the heart are very unusual. Similarly, a solitary cardiac metastasis is infrequent; usually there are multiple areas of involvement. Cardiac involvement is particularly common with leukemia or lymphoma, developing in 25 to 40 percent of patients. All areas of the heart are involved with equal frequency except the cardiac valves, perhaps as a result of the absence of lymphatics in the valves.

Most patients have no symptoms of heart disease, even though large areas of myocardium are involved by an infiltrating neoplasm. A pericardial effusion, which is hemorrhagic in about 15 percent of patients, is the most frequent abnormality. This was found in 45 of 217 patients studied by Gassman and associates, but only 3 of these had cardiac tamponade. Symptoms from cardiac failure are the most common disability, but these developed in only 17 of the 217 patients in Gassman's series. Recurrent arrhythmias are infrequent. The electrocardiogram is similarly nonspecific, usually showing T-wave changes, although a wide variety of conduction abnormalities have been reported.

The diagnosis can be suspected in a patient with malignant disease in whom a hemorrhagic pericardial effusion develops. Identification of malignant cells in fluid aspirated from the pericardium can establish the diagnosis. Thoracotomy should be avoided if possible, because no effective treatment is available and death usually occurs from generalized metastatic disease within a few months. The cardiac involvement per se is seldom a significant factor in the terminal illness.

Sarcoma

Sarcomas of the heart constitute about 25 percent of all primary cardiac neoplasms. In 1962 Dong et al. reported that 178 cases had been described. Spindle cell and round cell sarcomas are the most frequent, but the entire range of mesenchymal tumors has been reported, including leiomyosarcoma and fibrosarcoma. The right atrium and right ventricle are the most frequent sites of involvement, usually with a diffuse infiltrating tumor that does not involve the cardiac valves. Valvular obstruction or embolization, in contrast to atrial myxoma, is infrequent. Metastatic spread to the mediastinum is frequent, with death occurring 1 month to 3 years after onset of symptoms. Symptoms usually evolve from obstruction of the venae cavae, pericardial effusion, or arrhythmias from invasion of the conduction system.

Sarcomas developing in the pericardium, usually mesotheliomas, are rare lesions that grow rapidly and cause symptoms from obstruction of the venae cavae. Invasion of the myocardium develops in the late stages of the tumor.

The diagnosis of a primary cardiac malignant tumor can be suspected in a patient in whom an unexplained hemorrhagic pericardial effusion develops, especially in association with a bizarre cardiac shadow on the roentgenogram. Thoracotomy is usually required to establish the diagnosis. Only rarely is effective therapy possible. Scannell and Grillo, in 1958, reported one fortunate experience in a child in whom exploration for pericardial effusion found a localized fibrosarcoma in the right atrial wall which was successfully excised. In 1966, we removed an angiosarcoma of the right side of the heart, invading the tricuspid valve, along with a large segment of right atrial wall. Reconstruc-

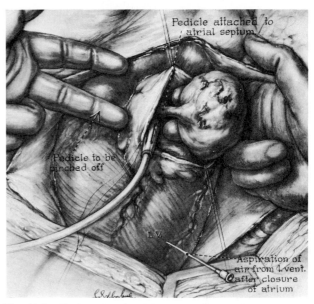

Fig. 19-34. Pedunculated atrial myxoma removed at operation in 1957. The patient has remained free of cardiac symptoms since that time. (*Reprinted from H. T. Bahnson, F. C. Spencer, and E. C. Andrus, Diagnosis and Treatment of Intracavitary Myxomas of the Heart, Ann Surg, 145:915, 1957, by permission of J. B. Lippincott Company, Philadelphia.*)

tion was with a pericardial patch graft, reattaching the tricuspid valve to the reconstructed annulus. Postoperative radiotherapy was given, following which the patient lived for 18 months before dying of widespread metastatic disease.

Rhabdomyoma

A cardiac rhabdomyoma is a rare lesion which is not a true tumor but is probably a focal arrest in maturation of cardiac muscle. Seventy such patients were reviewed by Prichard in 1951. The nodules have been termed *nodular glycogenic degeneration,* being interpreted as an example of localized glycogen storage disease. It is uncertain whether they are hamartomas or merely localized manifestations of glycogen storage disease.

The cardiac lesions may be solitary or multiple nodules, or may present as diffuse infiltration of the cardiac muscle. The nodules are not encapsulated but merge imperceptibly with the surrounding healthy myocardium. The lesions do not grow, and metastases do not occur.

On histologic examination, the nodules are composed of tubular muscle cells with large vacuoles in which the nuclei appear suspended by threads of cytoplasm, like spiders in a web, giving origin to the term "spider cell." About one-half of the patients have tuberous sclerosis of the brain. The clinical significance of the cardiac lesions is uncertain, for disability is usually due to the associated tuberous sclerosis. Sudden death has been reported in some patients who, at postmortem examination, were found to have a rhabdomyoma. Isolated instances of obstruction of the outflow tract of the right ventricle from a large rhabdomyoma requiring surgical excision have been reported.

Miscellaneous Tumors

Unusual benign lesions of the heart include fibromas, lipomas, angiomas, teratomas, and cysts. Fewer than 50 examples of each of these types of lesions have been reported. Fibromas have been found most frequently in the left ventricle, often as 2- to 5-cm nodules within the muscle. Sudden death, probably from a cardiac arrhythmia, has been reported with such tumors and may be the reason that only 18 percent of the reported tumors have been found in adults.

Lipomas are usually asymptomatic tumors found projecting from the epicardial or endocardial surface of the heart in older patients. Only about 30 such cases have been reported. Angiomas are commonly small, focal vascular malformations of no clinical significance, except four that have been found associated with a heart block. Pericardial teratomas and bronchogenic cysts are rare lesions that may cause symptoms from compression of the right atrium and obstruction of venous return. About 30 such patients have been reported in the surgical literature, most of them children. Some of the larger cysts, up to 10 cm in diameter, may produce grotesque deformities from extensive invagination of the right atrial wall.

CORONARY ARTERY DISEASE

HISTORICAL DATA. Since the late 1930s, different investigators have attempted to increase the blood supply of a heart ischemic from coronary atherosclerosis. Beck pioneered these efforts by attempting to develop vascular adhesions around the heart to introduce additional blood supply and to redistribute blood flowing through patent coronary vessels. Many unusual, imaginative, and sometimes bizarre procedures were tried. These included abrasion of the epicardium, painting the epicardium with phenol, insertion of talc or asbestos into the pericardial cavity, and wrapping omentum around the heart. Unfortunately, consistent benefit could not be demonstrated from any of these procedures, and virtually all have been abandoned. Perhaps the fundamental biologic reason for failure is the natural tendency for vascular adhesions to progressively fibrose and become more avascular with time.

In 1946, Vineberg developed a new concept for revascularizing the heart when he found that an internal mammary artery implanted in a tunnel in the myocardium of a dog would remain patent in a high percentage of cases. The operation of implantation of the internal mammary artery into the wall of the left ventricle in man was begun by Vineberg in 1950 and has been consistently employed by him since that time. Objective analysis of the results of arterial implantation was not possible until the development of coronary arteriography by Sones in the year 1958–1959. Demonstration by Sones that the implanted artery remained patent in the majority of patients and in

some patients connected with regional coronary arteries provided a stimulus to further investigation of methods of arterial implantation. Subsequently between 1960 and 1967 different arterial implants were extensively tried in several centers, but with the introduction of the bypass operation the procedure has greatly decreased in popularity and has been virtually abandoned in most institutions, including ours. The limited, often negligible, physiologic improvement in most patients is related to the fact that even though the artery remains patent in over 90 percent of patients, it often carries only a small amount of blood, as little as 5 to 10 ml/minute, to the myocardium. An occasional patient develops significant collateral circulation following implantation, and isolated instances have been reported in which the implanted artery clearly was of substantial benefit, carrying as much as 50 ml of blood per minute and causing obvious severe myocardial ischemia when temporarily interrupted. The reason for the wide variation in the development of collateral circulation after implantation has never been satisfactorily determined.

From 1956 to 1959 initial attempts were made with coronary endarterectomy to remove directly localized areas of obstruction caused by atherosclerotic plaques. Longmire and Cannon, Bailey, and others attempted such procedures, but results were discouraging because of a high operative mortality and a high rate of subsequent occlusion. Subsequent performance of such procedures with cardiopulmonary bypass, often combined with a pericardial roof patch, was satisfactory in a small percentage of patients but disappointing in many.

The development of the bypass operation for coronary occlusive disease from 1967 to 1968 was a dramatic achievement, for this represented the first such operation in which it was possible to immediately increase the blood flow to the myocardium. Most of the basic clinical investigations of the technique of bypass grafting evolved from studies in three centers in the United States during this period. Favaloro, discouraged with the limited application of endarterectomy and pericardial patch grafting, began using longer and longer segments of saphenous vein to bypass occlusive disease in the right coronary artery, eventually demonstrating that grafts could be effectively interposed between the aorta proximally and the termination of the right coronary artery at the posterior descending coronary artery distad. Johnson first showed that similar grafts could be effectively used for the left coronary artery, a most significant achievement, for previously all direct operative procedures upon the left coronary artery had had a prohibitive operative mortality well over 50 percent. At New York University, Green et al., following extensive experimental studies, first began direct anastomoses between the left internal mammary artery and the anterior descending coronary artery, using an end-to-side anastomosis. This procedure was not widely used by others for 2 to 3 years but subsequently greatly increased in popularity. The dramatic, virtually instantaneous relief of angina with bypass techniques led to performance of the procedure in thousands of patients in the past several years.

However, despite this widespread popularity, much remains unknown about the long-term results. For this reason considerable debate continues about indications and contraindications for bypass grafting, a question that will require several years' accumulation of data to answer.

ETIOLOGY AND PATHOGENESIS. Atherosclerosis is the cause of coronary occlusive disease in almost all patients. It is extremely common in the American male; autopsy studies of men killed in the Korean conflict who were between twenty and thirty years of age found some coronary atherosclerosis in 30 to 40 percent. The frequency gradually rises in men to approach 70 to 80 percent by seventy years of age. For a detailed analysis of the different theories concerning the cause of coronary disease, as well as its widely varying incidence according to race, sex, and other factors, recent monographs on epidemiology of atherosclerosis should be consulted.

The basic lesion is a segmental atherosclerotic plaque, often localized within the first 5 cm of the origin of the coronary arteries from the aorta. Involvement of the tributaries of the major coronary arteries, as well as the arterioles, is often minimal. This segmental localization makes bypass procedures possible. The atherosclerotic plaque is composed of focal deposits of lipid alternating with areas of fibrosis, perhaps a histologic reaction to the deposition of lipids. In older lesions spotty areas of calcification develop. Areas of intramural hemorrhage are visible in some lesions and often seem to precipitate thrombosis of the stenosed vessel.

The myocardial ischemia produced by coronary atherosclerosis results in a number of grave complications: sudden death, angina pectoris, myocardial infarction (with or without coronary thrombosis), and congestive heart failure. Any one or all of these events may occur unpredictably in a patient with coronary atherosclerosis.

Of these four, angina pectoris occurs most frequently. Patients experience a periodic discomfort, usually substernal, appearing typically with exertion, after eating, or with extreme emotion. Characteristically these symptoms subside within 3 to 5 minutes or may be dramatically relieved by sublingual nitroglycerin. In about 25 percent of patients, the symptoms are less typical and may have unusual areas of radiation to such remote areas as the teeth, the shoulder, the hand, or the epigastrium. Establishing a diagnosis of angina in such patients is difficult, perhaps impossible, without angiography, for results of the physical examination are usually normal. Differential diagnosis includes anxiety states, musculoskeletal disorders, and reflux esophagitis.

There is a constant risk of sudden death with angina pectoris: the risk varies both with the extent of disease and the degree of impairment of ventricular function, ranging from 2 percent to 10 to 15 percent per year. Often postmortem examination does not show any acute cause of death, such as myocardial infarction or coronary thrombosis. In such instances death is probably due to an acute disturbance of rhythm with terminal ventricular fibrillation.

Myocardial infarction, with or without thrombosis of a diseased coronary artery, is another frequent and often fatal complication. For a detailed discussion of myocardial infarction, a textbook of cardiology should be consulted.

Surgical procedures for acute myocardial infarction have been tried in a few instances, but thus far the procedures remain experimental. Results with bypass grafting seem best if it is performed within 6 hours after onset of infarction. Berg in 1976 reported operating on almost 100 such patients.

In some patients congestive heart failure develops and may become the principle disability, eventually causing death. Congestive failure may or may not be preceded by angina or a myocardial infarction. Probably congestive failure is a result of myriads of tiny myocardial infarctions, eventually destroying over one-third of left ventricular muscle mass. What determines angina as the dominant symptom in one patient and congestive failure in another is unknown. Repeated tiny emboli from an ulcerated atherosclerotic plaque have been suggested as one possible mechanism. Once congestive failure has developed, revascularization of the heart with bypass operations has been disappointing, for objective signs of improved cardiac function have been small in a few and negligible in most. Probably this unfortunate group of patients may be best treated by cardiac transplantation when advances in immunology make organ transplantation more feasible. At present congestive failure is significantly helped by operation only in patients with large left ventricular aneurysms.

DIAGNOSIS OF ANGINA PECTORIS. The history is the most important method for making the diagnosis, for usually there are no abnormal physical findings. With unusual symptoms, especially the absence of pain induced by exertion and relieved by nitroglycerin, laboratory studies are needed.

The electrocardiogram is normal at rest in about 70 percent of patients. Evaluation of changes in the electrocardiogram with graded exercise is a useful and widely used test, noting signs of ischemia in the cardiogram with increasing exercise, but the changes are difficult to quantitate. By far the most exact method for determining the presence and severity of coronary artery disease is selective coronary arteriography (Fig. 19-35). Coronary arteriography provided the first method for accurately determining the extent and severity of coronary disease in individual patients. Not only the presence of disease but progression and response to therapy over months or years can be evaluated by serial arteriograms. Since the introduction of arteriography, around 1958 or 1959, thousands of such procedures have been performed.

OPERATIVE PROCEDURES FOR CORONARY ARTERY DISEASE. Coronary Bypass Operations. *Indications and Contraindications.* There is some disagreement at present about indications for bypass grafting for angina. It is well established that operation can be performed in good-risk patients with a mortality of less than 3 percent and is followed by almost immediate and complete relief of angina in the majority of patients. Fifteen to twenty percent of vein grafts may occlude in the first year after operation, but thereafter the rate of occlusion is reduced. Although the 5-year patency data are meager, it appears that the patency rate approximates 60 percent.

Bypass grafting is widely used for patients with disabling angina unresponsive to conventional medical therapy, and

A

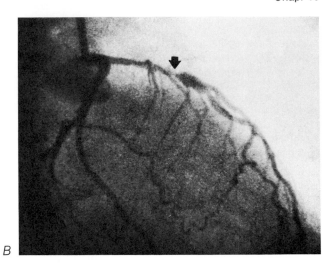

B

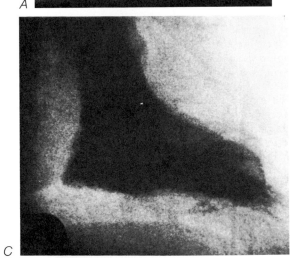

C

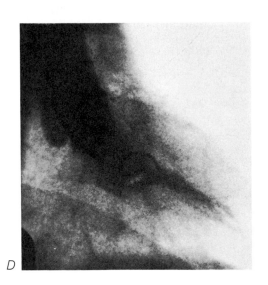

D

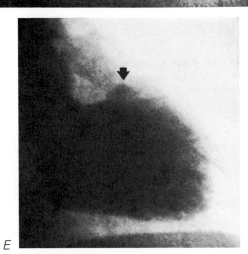

E

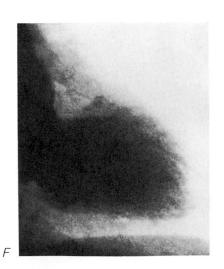

F

also for angina of increasing intensity, so-called preinfarction angina, for this is often a forerunner of acute myocardial infarction. At New York University most operations have been performed for patients in these two categories.

More uncertain is the use of bypass grafts for patients with mild, nonincapacitating angina or on a prophylactic basis in patients with few or no symptoms but with previous myocardial infarction and extensive occlusive disease seen on subsequent coronary arteriography. Some experienced groups routinely recommend operation for triple occlusive disease with few or no symptoms, while others, equally experienced, do not. In such patients the operation would provide protection from future myocardial infarctions, a very plausible hypothesis if the grafts remain patent for several years but one that has not yet been proved.

Severe congestive failure is a definite contraindication to operation, for the mortality is high and improvement small in surviving patients.

When a patient is considered for operation, coronary arteriography must be performed to determine the areas of obstruction, the size and patency of vessels beyond the area of obstruction, and the function of the left ventricle. Atherosclerotic obstruction is physiologically significant if the diameter of the vessel is narrowed more than 50 percent, corresponding to a reduction in cross-sectional area greater than 75 percent. The size and patency of vessels beyond the area of obstruction is also of importance, for patency rates after bypass grafting have been better with larger arteries in the range of 2 to 3 mm, as compared to 1 to 2 mm. However, ability to visualize vessels beyond an area of obstruction is a function of collateral circulation; so the angiographic evaluation is not precise. In some patients dissection at operation will find an adequate vessel beyond an area of obstruction not visualized by angiography because the flow of the injected dye was limited by sparse collateral circulation.

Multiple areas of obstruction are common. Nearly 50 percent of patients with severe angina have involvement of all three major coronary arteries, the anterior descending, the circumflex, and the right coronary.

Ventricular function, judged by contractility of the left ventricle during ventriculography, is a crucial part of preoperative evaluation, as it indicates the degree of previous muscle injury. In patients with normal ventricular function,

operative risk is less than 3 percent and the likelihood of improvement great. At the other extreme, severe impairment of ventricular function with congestive failure, representing infarction of areas of myocardium and replacement by scar, indicates an operative risk as high as 20 to 25 percent and far less likelihood of improvement.

Attempts have been made to quantitate the degree of impairment of ventricular function by measurement of ejection fractions, angiographically estimating the percentage of blood in the ventricle which is ejected during systole. Although this is an imprecise measurement, reduction of ventricular function to a point at which the ejection fraction is less than 0.15 to 0.20 indicates a serious operative risk. The degree of angina as compared with the degree of congestive failure is significant in deciding on operation.

Left ventricular end-diastolic pressure in patients with normal ventricular function is normal, less than 10 to 12 mm Hg. Some increase occurs with moderate failure, but the level of elevation varies so much with the medical management of congestive failure preceding catheterization that the actual value found at catheterization is not of precise prognostic value. Elevation beyond 20 to 25 mm Hg, however, indicates a poor prognosis. Nevertheless, over 100 such patients have been operated on at NYU with an operative risk near 10 percent and a 5-year survival of 83 percent.

Operative Technique. Coronary bypass operations are usually performed during extracorporeal circulation with the heart stilled either by inducing ventricular fibrillation or by ischemic arrest produced by temporary occlusion of the ascending aorta. Before bypass is started, a long segment of saphenous vein is removed from the thigh or leg, taking 15 to 20 cm of vein for each graft to be performed. It is reversed before insertion because of venous valves, attaching the distal end to the aorta. During bypass with the heart fibrillating, the left ventricle is decompressed with a vent to avoid overdistension. Either the aortic or the coronary anastomosis may be done first; our preference is to do the aortic first. The patent coronary artery beyond the area of obstruction is then dissected, and an arteriotomy about 1 cm long made. Care is taken to avoid dissecting the coronary artery from its bed, for inclusion of the surrounding soft tissue in the subsequent anastomotic suture line greatly aids hemostasis. The vein-coronary artery anastomoses are performed end-to-side with interrupted and continuous sutures of 6-0 or 7-0 synthetic suture material, usually Prolene. Three- to four-power optical magnification is routinely employed and greatly facilitates the performance of these small anastomoses. Following completion of the distal anastomosis, the vein graft is attached in gentle curves to the epicardium over the surface of the heart.

One theoretic objection to the use of vein grafts is the discrepancy in size between the vein and the artery, which results in turbulent flow. For example, if a 6-mm vein is anastomosed to a 2-mm artery, the rate of blood flow in the vein will be only one-ninth of that in the artery because of the difference in cross-sectional area. For this reason there has been an increased tendency to use veins from

Fig. 19-35. *A.* Right coronary artery, left anterior oblique projection. There is total obstruction of the vessel immediately distal to its aortic origin (arrow). A network of collateral vessels on the anterior surface of the right atrium and the right ventricle is apparent. *B.* Left coronary artery, right anterior oblique projection. There is severe narrowing of the left anterior descending coronary artery (arrow) distal to the origin of the second septal branch. *C.* Left ventricle in right anterior oblique projection in diastole. There is a normal contour of the chamber. *D.* Same ventricle in systole showing excellent contraction of all areas of the ventricle. *E.* Left ventricle in diastole, right anterior oblique projection. There is increased rounding of the ventricle and bulging of the anterolateral wall. A localized bulge on the superior portion of the anterolateral wall is evident (arrow). *F.* The same ventricle in systole. The degree of left ventricular contraction is generally markedly impaired.

the leg, with a diameter near 4 mm, rather than larger veins from the thigh. However, significant data regarding influence of the size of veins on long-term patency rates are not available.

Because of the frequency of multiple areas of occlusion, double or triple bypass grafts are used in most patients, usually attaching each graft separately to the aorta. At New York University in the past 5 years, during the performance of over 1,000 bypass procedures, nearly 50 percent of patients have had a triple bypass. With the techniques described, a graft can be attached to a vessel on almost any surface of the heart, the most difficult being the posterior wall of the left ventricle near the termination of the circumflex coronary artery. With optical magnification, grafts can be attached to vessels as small as 1 mm internal diameter. This fact, combined with the ability to attach grafts to any area of the heart, makes it possible to perform bypass grafts in the majority of patients with angina, over 95 percent of patients seen. The artery is technically inoperable when there are multiple areas of occlusion throughout the length of the artery, fortunately an unusual pattern of involvement.

Once the bypass grafts have been constructed, rate of blood flow is measured with a flowmeter. Though accuracy in the operating room is sometimes questionable, these measurements are of particular prognostic value, for there is good correlation between rate of flow and long-term patency. A mean flow rate of less than 20 ml/minute is associated with a high rate of subsequent occlusion, while high mean flow rates, greater than 70 to 80 ml/minute, have a much better prognosis. The flow rate, of course, varies with the size of the distal artery and the patency of the distal vascular bed. Patency rates have not been good with grafts attached to vessels as small as 1 mm in diameter, probably because of the small rate of flow.

Following operation careful observation in a cardiac intensive care unit is necessary to maintain adequate ventilation and cardiac output and to detect arrhythmias. Arrhythmias are quite frequent following operation but can

Fig. 19-36. Angiogram performed several months after left internal mammary–left anterior descending coronary bypass, showing a good flow from the internal mammary artery into the anterior descending coronary and its branches.

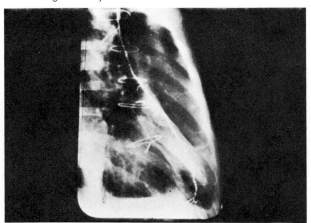

be controlled by appropriate measures. These include infusion of lidocaine, procainamide, digitalis, propranolol, and electrical cardioversion. In most patients convalescence is comparatively uneventful, with the patient leaving the hospital in 10 to 14 days. A pericardiotomy syndrome, with fever, pleural effusion, and pleural or pericardial friction rubs, occurs in a small percentage of patients but responds well to administration of prednisone in small amounts for several days.

Angiographic studies performed within 1 to 2 weeks after operation have found a patency rate well above 90 percent. However, angiograms performed 6 to 12 months later have found occlusion of 20 to 25 percent of vein grafts. Though extensive data are not yet available, with periods of observation now between 4 and 5 years in small numbers of patients, the rate of occlusion beyond the first year after operation apparently is small. Several factors may cause early or late thrombosis in a vein graft. These include technical factors at the time of operation in the construction of the anastomoses and ischemic injury to the vein during removal from its bed, such as excessive removal of adventitia or other mechanical trauma. As mentioned earlier, the size of the coronary artery grafted and the rate of flow through the vein graft both correlate reasonably well with late patency. A progressive fibrosis has been seen in some vein grafts, usually segmental in location, which progresses to complete obliteration within a few months. This curious histologic response at times is observed in one vein graft but not in others in the same patient. It probably represents segmental ischemic or mechanical injury to the vein at the time of operation. With appropriate care in removal of the vein graft, dissecting the vein gently and gradually distending it with cold heparinized blood, segmental stenosis has virtually disappeared in our unit over the past 3 to 4 years. Other factors influencing thrombosis of vein grafts include turbulent blood flow producing intimal proliferation at the anastomotic sites, pericardial adhesions, and theoretically progressive coronary atherosclerosis. The last factor, to date, has been rare.

With the natural concern about the significant rate of thrombosis of vein grafts, arterial grafts have been used with increasing frequency. The left internal mammary–anterior descending coronary anastomosis was first developed at New York University by Green and Tice and has been used consistently by Green since (Fig. 19-36). Since 1970 there has been increasing use of the internal mammary artery by several groups because of the long-term patency rates above 90 percent, a much more favorable finding than that with vein grafts. Unfortunately the internal mammary artery is small, and the rate of flow of blood is not as great as with vein grafts. However, the size of the internal mammary closely approximates that of the coronary artery in many patients. Another objection is the fact that use of the internal mammary is much more restrictive than that with free vein grafts. It is possible to attach the right internal mammary artery to the anterior descending, and the left internal mammary artery to the circumflex, but the right internal mammary will not reach to the termination of the right coronary on the posterior surface of the heart. For this reason, pedicled splenic arterial grafts have been tried, but the rate of occlusion within one year was prohibitive (40 to 50 percent). A search for other arterial grafts continues, and at this time a few experiences with the radial artery have been verbally reported but not published. At present the feasibility of bypass grafting has been thoroughly established, but undoubtedly the best technique for grafting will require long periods of comparison of data with different methods.

The critical question with coronary bypass grafting is, of course, the long-term protection from myocardial infarction and death. This will require several years of careful study. A cooperative study among several universities is currently being coordinated by the National Institutes of Health.

The total experience with elective coronary bypass at New York University between February 1968 and December 1975 included 1,172 patients; 98 percent of the cases were reassessed in 1976. Overall operative mortality over this $7\frac{1}{2}$-year period was 5 percent, decreasing to about 2 percent for the last few years. Hence a total of 1,111 patients left the hospital. Only 48 cardiac-related deaths subsequently occurred. Thus the long-term survival, calculated by the actuarial method and including operative deaths, was 88 percent at 5 years and 80 percent at 7 years. To further emphasize the surprisingly low late mortality, of each 95 patients discharged from the hospital, only 7 died from cardiac causes in the next 5 years, an annual mortality of 1.5 percent, closely paralleling the normal population. Although the study was not randomized, most patients were operated on for angina refractory to available medical therapy, and multiple coronary grafts were performed in over 80 percent of the group, indicating the extent and severity of disease. These data strongly indicate that coronary bypass does indeed prolong life. Similar data were recently reported by Jones et al. and by Mills and Ochsner.

When significant obstruction of the left main coronary artery is present, which fortunately occurs in only 5 to 10 percent of patients, virtually all published data agree that a bypass procedure should be done promptly, regardless of symptoms, because complete occlusion of the left main coronary is almost always fatal.

Other Operative Procedures. It is significant that when the previous edition of this textbook was published, most of the discussion of surgical procedures concerned implantation of a systemic artery into the myocardium, the Vineberg procedure. In the intervening years, with the dramatic results obtained with the bypass operation, the popularity of arterial implants has waned sharply. Almost none have been performed at New York University since 1970, primarily because bypass grafts can be used in the majority of patients. The implanted artery remains patent in the majority of patients, a range of 80 to 90 percent, but the amount of blood flowing through the implanted artery seems to be small in most. Hence, the degree of improvement in myocardial ischemia is disappointingly small. A few unusual exceptions have been cited where at repeat operation months or years later when disease developed in other areas, direct flow measurements of an implanted artery found blood flow as high as 50 ml/minute.

Endarterectomy, either with carbon dioxide gas or with mechanical strippers, is employed particularly on the right coronary artery but in selected instances on the left. The procedure now is done almost always in conjunction with bypass grafting to improve flow rates through the graft.

Operative procedures for acute myocardial infarction, performing bypass grafting within hours after the vessel has become occluded, are under evaluation. Experimentally, total ischemia to an area of myocardium produces irreversible necrosis within less than 1 hour; so the potential value of bypass grafting is to improve blood flow to critically ischemic areas which have not yet undergone necrosis. Excision of myocardial infarcts has been studied experimentally and in a few instances clinically, but results have usually been poor.

Intestinal bypass procedures to decrease absorption of cholesterol and to stop or even reverse the coronary atherosclerotic process have been cautiously but hopefully evaluated primarily by Buchwald and Varco and by others. Results are somewhat encouraging, but significant data are not yet available. Such observations require several years.

VENTRICULAR ANEURYSM

HISTORICAL DATA. A few early attempts to excise ventricular aneurysms by a closed technique were made before the development of pump-oxygenators, but a precise, safe surgical technique with a pump-oxygenator was first employed by Cooley et al. in 1958. Initially the operation was rarely done; by 1962 a total of only 28 cases operated upon had been reported. By 1965 Effler et al. reported that 61 patients with such aneurysms had been operated upon at the Cleveland Clinic. With coronary bypass, excision of such aneurysms has become commonplace, usually combined with bypass grafting. By 1971 the Cleveland Clinic group alone had performed over 300 such procedures.

ETIOLOGY. Almost all aneurysms develop as a complication of myocardial infarction (Fig. 19-37). The reported frequency with which an aneurysm develops after an infarction varies from 10 to 15 percent.

PATHOLOGY AND PATHOPHYSIOLOGY. Most of the aneurysms which have been surgically treated have been located in the anterior portion of the left ventricle in the area supplied by the anterior descending coronary artery. Aneurysms of the posterior portion of the ventricle, an area supplied by the circumflex artery, are much less frequent. It has been suggested that large aneurysms seldom arise in the posterior part of the left ventricle because of the attachments of the papillary muscles in this area, for a large infarction involving the attachments of the papillary muscles is usually fatal. Calcification may develop in the wall of a chronic aneurysm, but is not common. Lower recently described several uncommon types of ventricular aneurysms.

An aneurysm with an expansile wall can impair function of the left ventricle, since energy developed during contraction of the left ventricle is dissipated into expanding the wall of the aneurysm. This may be recognized by fluoroscopy. The resulting decrease in cardiac function can increase the severity of congestive heart failure. Mural

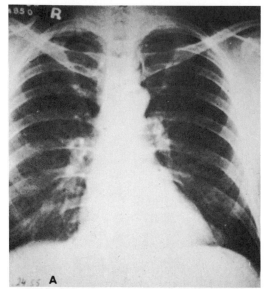

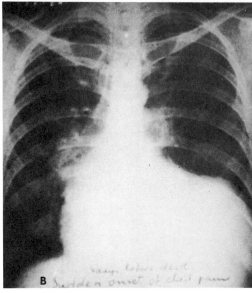

Fig. 19-37. Ventricular aneurysm. *A.* Chest roentgenogram showing a heart of normal size 2 days following an acute myocardial infarction. *B.* Chest roentgenogram showing cardiac enlargement from a large left ventricular aneurysm which progressively enlarged before a fatal episode of cardiac arrhythmia.

thrombi often develop in the aneurysm and may be a source of systemic embolization, although this is not frequent. Also, the aneurysm may enlarge and rupture, fortunately an uncommon complication. Rupture occurred in only 2 of 65 cases studied at autopsy by Abrams et al. Death in most patients with a left ventricular aneurysm is from further complications of the underlying coronary atherosclerosis, usually a subsequent myocardial infarction.

Prognosis of patients with an untreated left ventricular aneurysm was found by Schlichter et al. to be grim; 75 percent of the patients died within 3 years after the myocardial infarction. In contrast, a study of 65 patients by

Abrams et al. found a much more favorable prognosis; the 5-year survival rate following myocardial infarction was 69 percent, and in only 14 percent of the patients was death considered to be a complication of the aneurysm. The patients studied by Abrams et al., however, had small aneurysms in the posterior portion of the left ventricle, with an average diameter of 4 cm, which may explain the discrepancy in the two reports.

CLINICAL MANIFESTATIONS. Clinical findings are meager, often absent. A diffuse forceful apical impulse is seen in some. The chest roentgenogram may show a suspicious bulge in the area of the left ventricle, but with small aneurysms the roentgenogram may appear normal. The electrocardiogram shows only the changes of coronary artery disease with a previous myocardial infarction. Small aneurysms are probably often not recognized, and in only 4 of the 65 cases studied by Abrams et al. was the diagnosis made before autopsy. The size of the aneurysm ranged up to 8 cm, with an average diameter of 4 cm, and all were located in the posterior portion of the ventricle.

Diagnosis can be made principally by cineangiography, outlining the size, location, and expansile nature of the aneurysm. Simultaneous coronary arteriography is of significant value, indicating the extent of the coronary artery disease and the consequent risk of operation. Preferably the cardiac output should be measured at the time of cardiac catheterization, in order to evaluate subsequent improvement of the patient following operation. In equivocal cases evaluation by cineangiography and catheterization should form the basis for a decision to excise the aneurysm. It seems probable that small left ventricular aneurysms are of negligible physiologic significance, while larger ones significantly impair cardiac function. Operation should usually be postponed for a minimum of 3 months after the preceding myocardial infarction because of the friability of the ventricular muscle.

TREATMENT. Technique of Operation. A sternotomy incision is preferred. Dissection of adherent pericardium over the aneurysm, usually obliterating the major portion of the pericardial cavity overlying the left ventricle, is postponed until cardiopulmonary bypass is started. Once bypass is established, the heart is fibrillated and the left atrium opened to decompress the left heart (Fig. 19-38). Adhesions over the ventricle and aneurysm are divided to mobilize the heart. The aneurysm is then incised in its central portion and widely opened, carefully removing any laminated clot. If pericardial adhesions are extensive, the wall of the aneurysm is simply divided a short distance from the pericardial adhesions, leaving this part of the aneurysmal wall in situ and thus avoiding troublesome bleeding. Similarly, the wall of the aneurysm is divided about 2 cm from its junction with left ventricular muscle. When the opening of the aneurysm is sutured, most of the suture line includes the scar at the point of junction, and there is little compromise of the adjacent left ventricular muscle and no reduction in size of the left ventricular cavity (Fig. 19-39).

At New York University the frequency with which the wall of the aneurysm includes the area of the anterior descending coronary artery has been significant, for the scar may extend over into the ventricular septum. Preservation of the anterior descending coronary artery, often occluded proximally, may not be significant in some patients because the ventricular muscle supplied by the anterior descending coronary artery has been previously infarcted, but in other patients significant tributaries arise from this artery, especially to the ventricular septum. For this reason, before the aneurysm is excised, the anterior descending coronary artery is identified to avoid injury during excision of the aneurysm. Later, a bypass graft is attached if the artery is of adequate size. Following excision, the wall of the aneurysm is closed with two or three rows of continuous sutures, placing these through Teflon felt to reinforce the closure. Air is removed subsequently from the heart and the ventricle defibrillated.

This technique avoids several hazards associated with excision of an aneurysm. Extensive bleeding is avoided by cautiously dissecting adhesions without tearing the epicardium. There is no danger of reduction in size of the ventricular cavity or loss of functioning ventricular muscle from incorporation in the suture line to close the aneurysm, and the anterior descending coronary artery is revascularized. With these guidelines and precautions, operative excision has a very low mortality, and convalescence is usually uneventful. If the other coronary vessels, the right and the circumflex, are involved, bypass grafts are also inserted to these vessels.

The impressive advances made in the therapy of complications of myocardial infarction and ventricular aneurysms were well illustrated with a recent patient at New York University. The patient, seventy-seven years of age but previously in good health, sustained a massive myocardial infarction complicated by refractory congestive failure, a large ventricular aneurysm, multiple interventricular septal defects, left ventricular end-diastolic pressure of 30, cardiac index 1.2 liters/minute, and a pulmonary blood flow three times normal. At operation the aneurysm was excised, the ventricular septal defects closed with application of a large patch, and two bypass grafts done. Recovery was strikingly uneventful, and the patient remains in excellent health 4 months later.

PROGNOSIS. Substantial improvement has been reported following excision of large ventricular aneurysms. Actually this is the only cardiac operation in which preoperative congestive failure has been greatly improved by the surgical procedure. Disruption of the suture line with recurrence of the aneurysm has not been reported. In 1964 Cooley et al. reported experiences with 37 patients, with eight hospital deaths and five subsequent deaths. Thirteen patients at that time were living more than 3 years after operation, and substantial improvement had occurred in most of these. Catheterization studies before and after operation in seven patients showed an increase in cardiac output and regression of pulmonary hypertension, confirming the physiologic benefit following excision of large aneurysms.

In the past few years excision of aneurysms has become commonplace. Most patients undergoing excision of a left ventricular aneurysm now often have concomitant bypass grafting; so the benefit from excision of the aneurysm per se cannot be easily determined.

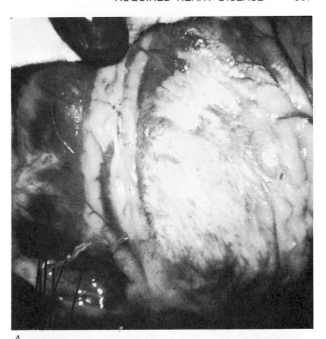

A

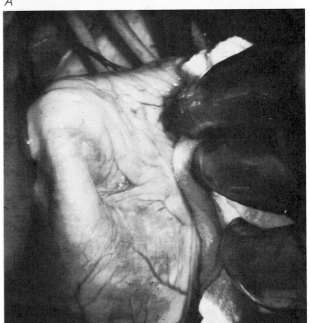

B

Fig. 19-38. *A.* Operative photograph of left ventricle, showing advanced destruction of the left ventricle from multiple myocardial infarcts. The heart has been turned upward so that the posterior surface of the left ventricle is exposed. *B.* During cardiopulmonary bypass, when suction was applied to the left ventricle, the ventricle collapsed readily, demonstrating that most of the ventricular muscle had been replaced by scar. The patient did not survive operation, and in retrospect it appears that the condition was probably inoperable because of extensive destruction of left ventricular muscle.

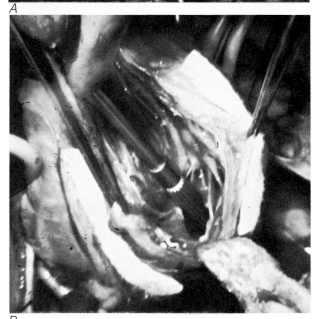

A

B

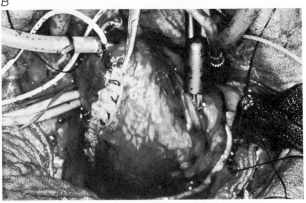

C

PERICARDITIS

Acute Pyogenic Pericarditis

A purulent infection of the pericardium has been reported for many centuries, and some of the earliest operations in thoracic surgery involved resection of costal cartilages to drain a purulent pericarditis. In recent years, with the widespread availability of antibiotics, purulent pericarditis has become a rare disease, and few institutions have experiences with more than a few cases. In 1961 Boyle and associates reviewed 414 cases reported in the literature and added 11 of their own. At that time their group of 11 patients constituted one of the largest single series ever reported.

Formerly pneumococcal pericarditis was one of the most common types and developed in association with a pneumonic infection in the lungs. Such infections are now infrequent. Staphylococcal infection, by contrast, usually occurs as a complication of generalized septicemia from a septic focus in another area of the body. Less frequent forms of pericarditis include a streptococcal pericarditis, now rarely seen, and infection with such unusual organisms as *Hemophilus influenzae* or *Salmonella.*

An unrecognized, untreated purulent pericarditis usually terminates fatally. The clinical picture is that of an acute septic course, which soon includes signs of a pericardial effusion and may progress to cardiac tamponade. Simply considering the possibility of the disease is probably the main factor in making a correct diagnosis. Once the diagnosis has been considered, needle aspiration of the pericardial cavity can confirm or exclude it. If uncertainty remains, a subxyphoid exploration can easily be done.

Both the rarity and the lethal nature of purulent pericarditis are well illustrated in the report by Rubin et al. of 18 cases, with only six patients surviving. The rarity was clearly indicated by the fact that only 14 patients were seen over a 14-year period. In eight of the patients the pericarditis developed as a complication after thoracic surgery; in others it developed from primary pleural mediastinal or pulmonary foci; in six it was a result of systemic bacteremia, probably the most difficult diagnosis of all. In these patients, resistance to infection was decreased because of other diseases, such as extensive burns or immunosuppressive therapy.

Treatment is with parenteral administration of appropriate antibiotics, combined with serial pericardial aspiration and instillation of antibiotics directly into the peri-

Fig. 19-39. *A.* Photograph of left ventricular aneurysm involving the posterior part of the left ventricle, an unusual location. *B.* The aneurysm has been excised, and the interior of the left ventricle is being inspected. The suction tip is within the ostium of the mitral valve, showing the proximity of the aneurysm to the mitral valve. The unusual occurrence of these aneurysms may be related to the fact that myocardial infarction in this area is often fatal because of concomitant mitral insufficiency. *C.* Completed repair of the aneurysm with a long suture line buttressed with Teflon felt. A coronary bypass graft is visible at the top of the field which was inserted into a branch of the circumflex coronary artery.

cardial cavity. In patients not responding to therapy, surgical drainage may be required, but this has not always been necessary.

Chronic Constrictive Pericarditis

HISTORICAL DATA. The first successful pericardiectomy was performed by Rehn in 1913, although the theoretical basis for the operation had been suggested some years before. Subsequently, the first pericardiectomy in the United States was performed by Churchill in 1929. Initial operations were limited in scope, partly because of differences in philosophy as to what part and how much of the constricted pericardium should be removed. In the 1960s routine performance of a radical pericardiectomy became widely accepted with considerable improvement in results.

ETIOLOGY. In most patients the cause is unknown. Possibly the disease represents the end stages of an undiagnosed viral pericarditis. Tuberculosis was formerly thought to be the most frequent cause, but in recent years it has been responsible for less than 20 percent of cases in most series. The author has personally never seen a proved case. Rarely, a traumatic hemopericardium can evolve to a constrictive pericarditis.

PATHOLOGY AND PATHOPHYSIOLOGY. The pericardial cavity is obliterated by dense scar tissue which encases and constricts the heart. In chronic cases areas of calcification develop in the fibrous tissue, resulting in an additional element of constriction.

The physiologic handicap from pericardial constriction is limitation of diastolic filling of the ventricles. Several sequelae result: Stroke volume is decreased with a resulting decrease in cardiac output, despite a compensatory tachycardia. Right ventricular diastolic pressure increases, with a corresponding increase in right atrial and central venous pressure, ranging from 15 to 40 cm water, the average elevation being 25 to 30 cm water. The venous hypertension produces hepatic enlargement, ascites, peripheral edema, and venous distension, accompanied by a gradual increase in blood volume.

CLINICAL MANIFESTATIONS. Symptoms. The disease is most common in patients in their second or third decade, but patients ranging from two to seventy-eight years have been reported. The youngest patient in our personal series of cases was three years old. The disease is a slowly progressive one with increasing ascites and edema. Fatigability and dyspnea on exertion are common complaints, but dyspnea is rare at rest. Ascites may be unusually severe. The diagnosis is easily confused with cirrhosis.

Physical Findings. Several unusual physical findings are commonly present. There may be striking enlargement of the liver with ascites, often in association with only moderate peripheral edema. Dilatation of peripheral veins is also prominent. Although these findings are the familiar ones of advanced congestive failure from heart disease, with constrictive pericarditis the usual cardiac findings are a heart of normal size without murmurs or abnormal sounds. Atrial fibrillation is present in about one-third of patients, and a pleural effusion in about one-half. The pulse pressure is normally decreased to a variable degree, and a paradoxic pulse, with obliteration of the pulse during deep inspiration, is found in a small percentage of patients.

Laboratory Findings. The venous pressure is regularly elevated to levels between 20 and 40 cm water. The electrocardiogram is not diagnostic but is almost always abnormal, with a low voltage and inversion of T waves. A chest roentgenogram often shows a heart of normal size, but calcification in the pericardium can be seen, often as a linear sheet, in about 50 percent of patients. Fluoroscopy may demonstrate decreased cardiac pulsations.

On cardiac catheterization several characteristic abnormalities are usually detected, although rarely these can also result from diffuse myocardial fibrosis from other causes. There is elevation of the right ventricular diastolic pressure to levels greater than one-third of right ventricular systolic pressure, and a corresponding increase in right atrial pressure. The contour of the right ventricular pressure pulse is characteristically altered, showing an early "dip" in diastole. A similarity of pressures in different cardiac chambers is frequently found, the right atrial pressure, the right ventricular diastolic pressure, the pulmonary artery diastolic pressure, and the pulmonary wedge pressure often being almost identical.

DIAGNOSIS. Once the diagnosis has been suspected from the clinical picture, it can usually be confirmed with findings from the electrocardiogram, chest roentgenogram, and catheterization data. Most diagnostic errors arise from failure to consider constrictive pericarditis, for it is a comparatively rare disease. The most frequent erroneous diagnoses are cirrhosis of the liver and congestive heart failure from other causes.

TREATMENT. Once the diagnosis has been established in a symptomatic patient, pericardiectomy should be performed. The incision may be a sternotomy or a bilateral thoracotomy in the left fifth and right fourth intercostal spaces with oblique division of the sternum. Bilateral thoracotomy provides ready exposure to all areas of the heart, but in recent years we have found sternotomy simpler and adequate. The objective is extensive removal of the constricting pericardium from both ventricles, extending from the right to the left pulmonary veins. Recently the adherent pericardium over the posterior (diaphragmatic) part of the ventricle also has been excised, thus removing the pericardium from the entire surface of both ventricles. Removal of the pericardium from the atria and the venae cavae is physiologically less important, although we remove most of this pericardium as well. Dissection over the thin-walled atria involves some hazard of perforation and hemorrhage and must be done with caution. Particular care is required over the coronary vessels, leaving a small segment of thickened pericardium if it cannot be satisfactorily mobilized from the underlying coronary arteries.

In performing pericardiectomy, where possible the plane of dissection should be *external* to the epicardium, which greatly decreases operative hemorrhage.

It is helpful to measure intracardiac pressures by direct needle puncture before and following pericardiectomy. With an extensive pericardiectomy, the characteristic pressure changes present before operation are either eliminated or greatly improved.

Following operation many patients improve immediately with a massive diuresis of edema fluid, but others recover more slowly and require careful restriction of sodium intake with appropriate diuretic therapy for several months before recovery. Atrophy of myocardial muscle fibers compressed by scar tissue has been considered a probable cause of the prolonged convalescence. In the past, inadequate removal of the scarred pericardium was undoubtedly the most frequent cause of a poor result. Some groups have used bypass to facilitate pericardiectomy, but to date we have not found this necessary. Copeland et al., reporting experiences in 1975, described the use of bypass to perform pericardiectomy in 11 patients with an excellent short-term result in all.

PROGNOSIS. The risk of operation varies with the age of the patient and the severity of the disease, but it is in the range of 10 to 12 percent. A good result can be anticipated in 80 to 85 percent of patients, although there is considerable discrepancy in the reports in the literature. In a series of 26 patients reported by Effler, 15 of the 26 obtained substantial improvement from operation while there was a total of nine early and late deaths. Schumacker and Roshe, however, have reported a total of 19 patients with 18 good results. In a long-term follow-up of 78 cases reported by Dalton et al., sustained improvement continuing over many years was found in patients initially obtaining a good result. A group of 40 cases has been reported from Vanderbilt University by Collins et al., including patients originally studied by Blalock and Burwell in 1941. Only 53 percent of 32 patients subjected to operation obtained an excellent result, but this series includes the early operations which are now considered inadequate. At New York University an excellent short-term result has been obtained in most patients, but detailed long-term data are not available.

HEART BLOCK AND PACEMAKERS

by Joseph N. Cunningham

HISTORICAL DATA. Surgical therapy of complete heart block with an electric pacemaker has evolved with astonishing rapidity in the past 20 years. In 1951 Callaghan and Bigelow developed a transvenous pacemaker which could be used to stimulate the sinoatrial node, and the following year Zoll first described successful treatment of ventricular standstill by external electrical stimulation of the heart through the intact chest wall. In 1958 Lillehei and associates demonstrated that direct cardiac pacing could be performed with an electrode implanted in the left ventricle, but long-term electrical stimulation with such electrodes traversing the chest wall ultimately resulted in infection. Between 1958 and the present, many investigators contributed to the development of implantable, battery-powered pacemakers, including Chardack, Zoll, Frank, Senning, Kantrowitz, Furman, Escher, and Parsonnet. Glenn has intensively studied radiofrequency stimulation of the heart with a transmitter through the intact chest wall, while Nathan and Center have evaluated pacemakers activated

from impulses arising in the atrium, which are subsequently transmitted to the ventricle. Furman and Schwedel, in 1959, described permanent pacing of the heart with a transvenous catheter wedged into the endocardial surface of the right ventricle. Since 1962 modifications of this technique have made it the procedure of choice, with the catheter implanted under local anesthesia and subsequently connected to an implanted pacemaker in a subcutaneous pocket.

In 1957 the first implantable pacemakers were being used. As of 1972, 120,000 implantations had been made in the United States alone, with a 15-year survival rate for that population of about 75 percent and an average age of approximately 70 years. Since 1972 an astronomical number of implantations have been performed. This appears to be a function not only of increased awareness on the part of the physician but also of new developments in pacemaker hardware, with increased battery longevity and improved electrode design the major factors in the increasing success and popularity of these procedures.

ETIOLOGY. Congenital heart block is extremely rare, less than 200 patients having been reported in the literature. Heart block from surgical trauma during repair of intracardiac defects has decreased in frequency but still remains a serious postoperative complication, usually resulting from direct injury to the bundle of His associated with repair of ventricular septal defects and occasionally with aortic valve replacement in the severely calcified aortic annulus. Heart block following myocardial infarction is usually transitory in surviving patients and requires no permanent pacing. Temporary pacing through a transvenous route is often indicated and can be performed with low morbidity. Infection or tumors have been reported in rare cases to cause heart block.

The most common cause of complete heart block in the elderly patient is degenerative fibrosis of the conduction system (75 to 80 percent of cases). The most common indication for implantation of pacemakers continues to be the occurrence of Stokes-Adams attacks; these have been the indication in 80 to 90 percent of patients requiring pacemakers.

PATHOLOGY AND PATHOPHYSIOLOGY. In normal cardiac conduction the cardiac impulse arises in the sinoatrial node located near the junction of the superior vena cava with the wall of the right atrium. The impulse is propagated through the wall of the right atrium to the atrioventricular (AV) node, lying medial to the ostium of the coronary sinus. From this node it travels along the bundle of His near the annulus of the tricuspid valve to pass through the central fibrous body of the ventricular septum near the junction of the muscular and membranous components. In this area the conduction bundle divides into the right and left bundles, which in turn travel to different areas of the respective ventricles. The most common surgical trauma producing complete heart block occurs during repair of a ventricular septal defect or an ostium primum defect. More rarely it occurs during prosthetic replacement of the aortic valve, mitral valve, or tricuspid valve, as there are areas along the annulus of each of these three valves where the bundle of His can be injured. Surgical injuries of either the right or the left conduction bundle are usually not of clinical significance.

Heart block, of whatever degree, may seriously impair cardiac output by any of a number of mechanisms. With complete heart block the resulting bradycardia, varying from 25 to as high as 60 beats per minute, depending on the idioventricular response, may decrease coronary and cerebral circulation. There may be progressive refractory congestive heart failure even with rates as high as 45, marked intolerance to exercise, and even symptoms of cerebrovascular insufficiency with syncope and convulsions. With complete AV dissociation there may be periods of transient ventricular asystole with cessation of cardiac output, syncope, convulsions, and death. In some patients, rather than standstill, there may be equally disastrous bouts of ventricular tachycardia or ventricular fibrillation, as ventricular "escape" mechanisms result from absence of normal AV conduction. In others there may be only periodic marked accentuation of the bradycardia. With lesser degrees of heart block, although the cardiac rate is usually normal, abrupt transition to complete AV dissociation with any of its complications can occur. Any one episode may be followed by complete recovery with resumption of the preattack rhythm or may result in death.

Attacks of syncope and convulsions due to sudden alterations of cardiac output from heart block have long been designated the *Stokes-Adams syndrome.* Some patients with low cardiac output from severe bradycardia become disabled with progressive cardiac failure but never develop Stokes-Adams syndrome.

It is a curious and as yet unexplained phenomenon that with ventricular standstill from heart block, mechanical or electrical energy delivered to the heart will result in intermittent ventricular contractions. Thus, even rhythmic thumping of the chest wall may result in 1:1 ventricular responses until the ventricles resume their intrinsic rhythmic contractions.

CLINICAL MANIFESTATIONS. Although some patients may be asymptomatic with a rate as low as 30 to 35 beats per minute, most patients have symptoms with a rate less than 45 per minute. Episodic Stokes-Adams attacks are the most frequent disability; between attacks the patient feels entirely well. During such episodes there is the sudden onset of syncope, often followed by convulsions. Examination reveals severe bradycardia or cardiac standstill. Recovery depends on the spontaneous return of cardiac contractions. In milder forms, recurrent syncope for a short period may be the only symptom. Then the differential diagnosis must consider heart block, aortic stenosis, simple syncope, carotid sinus syndrome, epilepsy, and occlusive arterial disease of the cerebral circulation. When complete heart block is present, the diagnosis can be quickly established by the electrocardiogram. When intermittent heart block or the presence of a "sick-sinus syndrome" (tachy-brady arrhythmia) is etiologic in the production of symptomatology, a 24-hour recording by Holter monitor may be necessary to determine the diagnosis. This test is performed by having the patient carry a portable ECG which produces a 24-hour recording of the intrinsic cardiac rhythm. The tape recording of the patient's rhythm can be quickly analyzed with a computer to determine what arrhythmia is present.

With intermittent heart block there may be no definite findings between syncopal attacks. However, certain electrocardiographic findings are suggestive. Trifascicular block, degrees of block less than complete AV dissociation, and the Mobius II type usually signify impending or intermittent AV dissociation. Attempts have been made to induce heart block under controlled conditions to confirm the diagnosis. One method reported by the author involved atrial pacing to rates of 120 or less, which ordinarily does not affect normal conduction.

Some patients become disabled from progressive heart failure simply as a result of inadequate cardiac output, while other patients tolerate rates of 40 to 50 beats per minute with no apparent symptoms. Dramatic improvement, with prompt diuresis of many liters of fluid, may follow insertion of a pacemaker.

TREATMENT. Physiology of Cardiac Pacemakers. The electrical resistance of the normal heart is 300 to 350 ohms, and the fibrillating threshold to electrical stimulation is at least ten times greater. The efficacy of cardiac pacemakers depends on the ability of the heart in ventricular standstill to respond to short bursts (2 milliseconds) of electric current, ideally less than $1\frac{1}{2}$ to 2 milliamperes. This amount of current is effective if delivered directly to the heart, but much larger currents are necessary to pace the ventricle directly through the chest wall, a method of pacing generally not employed at present.

Ventricular pacing may be accomplished by one of two methods, bipolar or unipolar. In the bipolar system both the positive and the negative pole of the electrode are in contact with the endocardium of the heart. In epicardial implantation, two separate electrodes (positive and negative) must be implanted. If unipolar pacing is desired, the tip of the endo- or epicardial electrode acts as the stimulating pole, while the cathode or indifferent pole is usually the ground plate on the generator implanted in the subcutaneous tissue. The choice of unipolar or bipolar pacing modes is purely a personal preference. Most cardiologists feel that use of a bipolar system allows more accurate reading of the patient's intrinsic underlying electrocardiogram, since the stimulus artifact when this system is used is much less than when a unipolar system is employed. Bipolar electrodes can be converted to unipolar systems at any point where indicated by simply capping off the lead which has the highest threshold and connecting the remaining lead to a unipolar generator, which is then implanted in the subcutaneous tissue.

Ventricular stimulation by current generator and electrode systems generally results in ventricular rates of 72 beats per minute. Such rates not only effectively override and suppress spontaneous ventricular activity of hearts in complete AV dissociation with rates of 45 or less but also prevent Stokes-Adams attacks due to complete ventricular standstill. Resultant improvement in cardiac output on the basis of rate increase alone may be as much as 50 to 80 percent. Frequently an impressive improvement in exercise tolerance, with regression of any overt signs of cardiac failure and even with diuresis, occurs. Despite the fixed rates of stimulation, variations in cardiac output are usually effectively achieved by variations in cardiac stroke volume in most patients. In some instances, however, variations in pacemaker rate and amplitude are necessary. The present availability of pacemakers with variable rate and amplitude settings now allows effective control of such syndromes as the tachy-brady arrhythmia type and syndromes characterized by refractory ventricular arrhythmias. In such patients, not only the rate but also the amplitude of the pacemaker generator may be increased to permit chronic "overdriving" of the arrhythmia. In the "sick-sinus syndrome," where the patient's rate often varies from 40 to 120 beats per minute, it is possible to control the bradycardia by use of a pacemaker which has been surgically implanted, while Inderal is given to control the intermittent bouts of tachycardia which these patients experience. An occasional patient with angina who is not a surgical candidate may be extremely sensitive to digitalis or propranolol. Such patients may require instillation of pacemakers with variable rate settings so that rates as low as 60 can be achieved by the pacemaker while the patient receives adequate doses of digitalis and propranolol for heart failure and/or angina.

Variations of the fixed-rate mode of delivery of the stimulus were sought to correct certain problems which became evident during early pacemaker experience. The most significant of these was a markedly decreased fibrillatory threshold to electric currents under certain conditions such as hypokalemia and acute myocardial infarction. In patients who either did not have complete AV dissociation at the time of pacemaker implant or had return of intermittent AV conduction after periods of electrical pacing, the coincidence of the fixed-rate stimulus with the "supernormal phase" of the cardiac cycle could precipitate ventricular fibrillation if the patient sustained an acute myocardial infarct or became hypokalemic. This led to the so-called "demand" pacemaker, which may be of the R-wave-suppressed or R-wave-triggered type. In both, the electrode acts as an element which senses beginning ventricular depolarization. In one, the pacemaker output is suppressed and no artifact appears on the electrocardiogram, while in the other the pacemaker discharge occurs during the refractory period of the heart and the artifact is seen on the electrocardiogram within the QR segment. This seems to have effectively eliminated the problem of pacemaker-induced arrhythmias in postinfarction patients or those with severe electrolyte abnormalities. Suppressing pacemaker discharge does not appear to significantly increase the life expectancy of the pacemaker generator.

Many currently used pacemaker generators are programmed to produce a fixed output and impulse at 72 beats per minute irrespective of ventricular response or activity. The generated impulse is either received or suppressed by the cardiac muscle in relation to the refractory period of the QRS complex. Fixed-rate pacemakers should only be used in patients who have not had documented evidence of competitive rhythms. This should be established by exercise testing, which will often reveal the presence of competitive arrhythmias in patients who had been presumed to have complete heart block. When using fixed-rate units,

efforts should be made to use low-output pacemakers to prolong the life of the generator. Demand pacemakers, on the other hand, are always indicated for patients with intermittent AV dissociation or block and for those who occasionally have competitive intrinsic rhythms of their own.

Asynchrony between atrial and ventricular contractions, which impairs cardiac output and limits the rate imposed by ventricular pacemakers, led to the development by Nathan and associates of the P-wave-activated pacemaker. This pacemaker senses atrial depolarization and delivers a subsequent synchronized stimulus to the ventricle which follows atrial activity in a timely electrical fashion, thereby resulting in optimal cardiac output. This system is more "physiologic." However, it requires more complex circuitry and implantation of electrodes in the atrium as well as the ventricle. Previously such implantation was possible only via thoracotomy. More recently, advances in technology have resulted in production of generator and electrode systems which may be adapted to either transthoracic or pervenous implantation. By either modality, a pair of electrodes (one in the atrium and one in the ventricle) is utilized to sense and stimulate in a synchronous fashion both atrial and ventricular contractions. This clever and extremely physiologic pacemaker system is most indicated in the patient whose cardiac output would otherwise be inadequate without the "atrial kick" prior to ventricular systole, most commonly the patient with severe chronic failure and heart block, or the younger person with heart block who is athletic. In the latter instance, exercise-induced increase in atrial activity is sensed by one electrode and transmitted in a similar fashion to the ventricular electrode. This allows for atrioventricular rates of 100 to 120 beats per minute with exercise.

Selection of Patients for Operation. Medical therapy of symptomatic complete heart block with myocardial stimulants such as isoproterenol has been associated with a high mortality. In one group of 100 patients treated before pacemakers were developed, 30 percent were dead in 6 months and 75 percent within 5 years. Heart block resulting from acute myocardial infarction usually can be treated by temporarily pacing the heart with an electrode catheter introduced through a peripheral vein and advanced into the right ventricle. The block usually disappears as the patient recovers from the infarction, and implantation of a permanent pacemaker is rarely indicated.

Heart block following intracardiac operations is a grave complication, requiring a pacemaker if the block is permanent. Most such problems develop at operation and can be prophylactically treated by leaving a temporary electrode wire in the ventricle before the thoracotomy or sternotomy incision is sutured. Stimulation can be given through the wire for several days, but prolonged use of the unit is inadvisable because of the risk of infection. It was found by Lillehei and associates, reporting experiences with 40 patients with complete heart block in 1963, that heart block lasting more than 1 month after operation is almost always permanent; until 1 month, some hope remains that complete block is temporary and may subside with healing of the intracardiac wound. Low-dose steroids (Dexamethasone 1 mg/hour) may be useful for reduction of edema of the conduction system and improvement in AV conduction during the first 24 hours postoperatively.

In some unfortunate patients complete block may develop several months after a cardiac operation, probably from progressive fibrosis near the conduction bundle. With a cardiac rate less than 50 beats per minute, it is probably wise to implant a permanent pacemaker before the patient leaves the hospital, especially if the block has persisted longer than 1 month after operation. A study of 20 patients discharged without pacemakers found an appalling mortality of 80 percent in subsequent years. Because of the complications of pacemaker use in a small child, some investigators have cautiously managed a few asymptomatic children without pacemaker implantation with better long-term results than those reported earlier by Lillehei and associates. However, ultrasmall units weighing 40 to 100 Gm are now available for implantation into small children. It is imperative to use epicardial electrodes with sufficient length to ensure that growth patterns do not result in need for electrode replacement. While pacemaker implantation in the small infant generally requires a minithoracotomy, the long-term results can be gratifying if sufficient electrode length is left to accommodate the child's growth. This, coupled with use of the previously mentioned small pacemaker generators, makes management of heart block in the infant or young child more promising than it was 5 years ago.

Technique of Endocardiac Catheter Pacing. Fluoroscopic placement of a transvenous endocardial electrode in the anterior wall of the right ventricle is the preferred method of pacemaker implantation at this time. The procedure can be performed with minimal risk (0.5 percent in large series). It is generally done under local anesthesia and, for reasons of sterility, should generally be done in the operating room or cardiac catheterization laboratory under totally aseptic techniques. Most large centers currently employ a C-arm fluoroscopic unit which enables a surgeon to place the electrode in proper position in the operating room or cardiac catheterization laboratory. Numerous reports by Lagergren, Furman, Parsonnet, Escher, and others have described experiences with large numbers of patients who underwent successful transvenous electrode placement with low mortality and morbidity rates.

The operative approach involves a semilunar incision, preferably made on the right side below the clavicle in the deltopectoral groove. A single incision is utilized to expose the right cephalic vein and at the same time fashion a subcutaneous tissue pocket inferiorly to implant the generator. If the cephalic vein is inadequate for electrode advancement, a separate incision can be made in the neck in the area of the external jugular vein to permit introduction of the pacemaker electrode and proper placement in the right anterior ventricular wall under fluoroscopy. Once the electrode is introduced into the right side of the heart through a pervenous route, it is necessary to position the tip of the electrode properly in the anterior and apical portion of the right ventricle. Care must be taken to ensure that the tip of the electrode is properly wedged into the right ventricle and does not move significantly with cardiac

pulsations or when the patient coughs or breathes deeply. Diaphragmatic contractions at the rate of 72 per minute, observed under fluoroscopy, should alert the surgeon to the possibility of perforation of the right ventricle. In this case the electrode should be withdrawn and replaced, as perforation generally does not occur. Once the electrode is wedged properly into a motionless area of the right ventricle, thresholds should be checked. With current equipment, thresholds for complete and consistent capture of less than 2 milliamperes should be obtained if electrode positioning and placement are correct. Care should be taken to ensure that the electrode not only paces but also adequately senses the intrinsic rhythm of the ventricle.

Once the electrode is properly placed, it is securely tied to the cephalic vein by suture ligature and then connected to the appropriate generator. The generator, in turn, is implanted in the subcutaneous pocket previously fashioned from the original semilunar incision in the deltopectoral area. It is generally advisable to seal the connections between the electrode and generator with silastic adhesive. Antibiotic lavage of the incisions and the subcutaneous pocket is carried out, and a simple mound closure follows. All patients should be placed on preoperative antibiotics for 12 to 24 hours and kept on antistaphylococcal drugs for at least 2 to 3 days following implantation. A closed, airtight occlusive dressing should be applied to the deltopectoral incision and not removed for 72 hours, since retrograde contamination by bacteria through the skin is a possibility. Many pacemaker-generator pockets collect serous fluid. Despite the appearance of fluid or hemotomas in the area, the cardinal rule is "never aspirate a pacemaker generator pocket." The hazards of introducing bacteria by aspiration of fluid from a pacemaker-generator pocket are obvious, and infection often ensues.

Technique of Direct Myocardial Implantation. In certain instances, endocardial electrode placement is not possible. Patients with pulmonary hypertension, extremely dilated right ventricles and right atria, or tricuspid regurgitation are usually poor candidates for endocardial electrode placement in the right ventricle, for there is a high frequency of electrode displacement in the first few days following operation. Also, a rare patient with endocardial fibrosis will prove to be an unsatisfactory candidate for endocardial pacing. In these instances, direct approach to ventricular pacing by implantation of epicardial electrodes is indicated. Small, coiled platinum-iridium electrodes of a fragile nature, often used in the past, have proved unsatisfactory after lengthy analysis; fracture of the electrode coils resulted at varying lengths of time after implantation. More recently, sutureless myocardial electrodes of the screw-in variety have been perfected (Medtronics), which allow for extremely fast implantation of epicardial electrodes through a minimal surgical approach. Generally, a subxiphoid approach through the "space of Lare," where the rectus abdominus muscles attach to the underside of the rib cage, is utilized. A transverse or diagonal incision in the left upper quadrant anterior to the left side of the rectus muscle is made just below the left costal arch. The rectus sheath is entered and the muscle retracted. With blunt dissection in a cephalad fashion, the free space anterior to the pericardium can be reached through the insertion of the rectus sheath and muscles on the costal arch. The pericardium can be opened in a T-shaped incision and the inferior wall of the right or left ventricle visualized. The screw-in electrode is mounted on a 12- to 15-inch applicator which allows placement of the electrode in the inferior wall of the ventricular muscle. Generally, three turns of the electrode are necessary to implant the corkscrew apparatus deeply into the ventricular muscle. Placement of the electrode in the left ventricle is preferable, as perforation of the corkscrew apparatus into the right ventricle may result in increased pacemaker thresholds. Three- to five-year follow-up on this type of epicardial electrode implantation would suggest that it is superior to the previously employed small coil electrodes implanted through a thoracotomy incision. There is no evidence of late electrode breakage, and the only negative aspect of such implantation is that late threshold rise after implantation may occur.

Implantation of epicardial electrodes by direct approach should be reserved for patients in whom endocardial electrode placement is inadvisable, as mentioned above. It is also ill-advised to use such an approach in the elderly patient, in whom chronic lung disease or other cardiac problems may exist. Implantation of electrodes by this approach usually requires general anesthesia for a brief period of 15 to 20 minutes and is best employed in the young, healthy patient who cannot tolerate endocardial pacing.

Temporary Cardiac Pacing. After an acute myocardial infarction associated with heart block, temporary cardiac pacing is preferably done by insertion of a transvenous electrode catheter under fluoroscopy through an internal jugular or subclavian vein approach. If transvenous catheter placement cannot be quickly achieved, direct insertion of an electrode via a transthoracic route through the third or fourth left intercostal space into the left ventricle is now routinely carried out. As a last resort, the heart can be stimulated directly through needles implanted subcutaneously over the anterior chest wall; this requires generators which produce considerable milliamperage output for pacing.

Postoperative Care. Following operation, electrocardiograms should be obtained promptly to determine that the pacemaker is functioning properly, and a chest x-ray should be obtained to confirm that the pacemaker electrode is correctly placed in the anterior portion of the right ventricle.

To protect from infection, antibiotics should be started before operation and continued for 3 or 4 days after operation, using the antistaphylococcal antibiotics. Dressings over the generator should be carefully sealed for about 72 hours because of the hazard of infection.

Subsequently, after recovery and discharge from the hospital, the patient should enroll in a pacemaker clinic for long-term follow-up. An alternate approach is for the patient to enroll in a telephonic pacemaker program, now being routinely offered by Intermedics, Medtronics, and others.

Complications of Pacemaker Implantation. Mortality rates for transvenous pacemaker implantation in most institutions are about 0.5 percent and for epicardial implantation between 1 and 2 percent. Morbidity likewise is quite low, ranging from 10 to 30 percent, depending on the series involved. The most common pacemaker complication is early electrode displacement when the transvenous approach is used, generally within the first 24 hours and infrequently at a later time. Electrode perforation may occur after transvenous implantation and often is indicated by diaphragmatic twitching or pacing and, more ominously, by signs of cardiac tamponade. Immediate electrode removal, with preparations if necessary for emergency thoracotomy, is indicated.

Rise in thresholds for endocardial electrodes usually occurs 1 to 2 months after implantation, with subsequent return of thresholds to preoperative levels. Since most generators put out 9 to 10 milliamperes of current, the early rise in threshold appears to be no problem. Late rise in thresholds of epicardial screw-in electrodes has been reported but does not appear to be a serious problem.

Erosion of the pacemaker generator or electrode in a thin person with sparse subcutaneous tissue has occurred, and implantation of the unit below the pectoralis muscle may be indicated in such persons. Infection is an inevitable consequence of erosion, and removal or replacement of the generator and electrode generally follows. Subclavian vein thombosis due to electrode implantation through the pervenous route has been reported and generally is of no consequence. Infectious complications of transvenous pacemaker insertion have been reported in about 5 percent of patients, usually involving the generator pocket. Occasionally bacteremia exists without subsequent evidence of clinical infection. Most cases can be treated effectively with adequate antibiotics. Pericarditis following implantation of epicardial pacemakers is frequent and probably occurs in 10 to 15 percent of the patients in the form of a postcardiotomy syndrome secondary to incision of the pericardium for electrode implantation.

Equipment malfunction continues to be the commonest cause of pacemaker failure. Fortunately, federal regulations (FDA) now require all companies to register their pacemakers, and failures of the generators are reported with regularity. All companies are about equal in terms of their failure or success rate.

Finally, an unusual cause of electrode displacement should be mentioned, the "pacemaker twiddler's syndrome." This occurs when the patient inadvertently turns the pulse generator over and over in its subcutaneous pocket in a manner that dislodges the endocardial or epicardial electrode.

PROGNOSIS. The long-term outlook following pacemaker implantation has progressively improved and now approaches that of patients with cardiac disease without conduction problems. There has been progressive improvement in the durability of pacemaker generators worn with the standard nickel-mercury-cadmium batteries, with a life span approaching 5 to 6 years. Recently lithium-powered units have been developed by most pacemaker companies which are guaranteed to last 6 years and will probably last 8 to 10 years. These units are more expensive, costing approximately $2,000, but are not only longer-lasting but also much smaller than other units, weighing 100 to 200 Gm. An additional significant development, principally at the research level at the present time, is the atomic energy–powered pacemaker, using plutonium 238 or promethium 137, which will last for 20 years or more. The units cost about $10,000 and are under careful federal regulation at present. They are tiny, weighing less than 100 Gm, and are particularly applicable for young patients who may require a generator for decades.

Two other recent developments in this rapidly changing field are also of significance. Programmable pacemakers have been developed which permit the physician to change the rate and amplitude of the pacemaker's generator externally by a radiofrequency beam. Hence the patient may use a rate of 65 to 70 beats per minute while sleeping and increase it to 80 to 90 beats per minute while playing tennis. Rechargeable generators are also now available in which a unit can be recharged once a month by a radiofrequency console, which can be kept at the patient's bedside at home. It is predicted that such rechargeable pacemakers will last for 8 to 10 years.

It is obvious that the entire field has not only developed rapidly but is making progress in several areas and will certainly constitute an important segment of cardiac surgery in the future.

ASSISTED CIRCULATION, AND ARTIFICIAL HEARTS

For certain forms of advanced heart disease, cure seems possible only with cardiac transplantation or the implantation of an artificial heart. This is true in some complex congenital anomalies, but most commonly in advanced coronary artery disease in which more than 40 percent of the left ventricular muscle mass has been destroyed. Significant experimental progress has been made with both forms of treatment, but ultimate solution remains unclear at this time. Both are active fields of laboratory investigation. Subsequent paragraphs briefly describe the status of these areas as of mid-1977.

THEORETIC CONSIDERATIONS. The concept of assisting the failing heart by pumping part or all of the circulation through a heart-lung machine as a parallel circuit is, on first glance, a simple and attractive one. One of the first observations of the possible beneficial effects of assisted circulation was made by Senning, who noted that an injured left ventricle incapable of supporting the circulation after an intracardiac operation might recover if extracorporeal circulation was continued for 30 to 60 minutes. Apparently the injury of the left ventricle was reversible.

Subsequent investigation of this seemingly simple hypothesis encountered many problems: First, attempting to "rest" a contracting left ventricle is a complex undertaking. Unless the left ventricle is decompressed during cardiopulmonary bypass, which requires the insertion of a can-

nula into the left atrium and left ventricle, blood will continue to accumulate in the left ventricle, which in turn will contract as a closed chamber against closed mitral and aortic valves. Left ventricular systolic pressure must then exceed that produced in the aorta by the extracorporeal pump, as a result of which oxygen requirements of the contracting left ventricle remain near those levels existing before the extracorporeal pump was used. Hence, although most of the circulation may be supplied from an extracorporeal pump, a contracting left ventricle intermittently ejecting a small amount of blood may metabolize a large amount of oxygen, and thus not be significantly "rested."

If a peripheral circulatory bypass is employed, as with a venoarterial circuit, the left ventricle can actually be harmed. Blood pumped into a peripheral artery from the extracorporeal pump may increase work requirements of the ventricle as it contracts and attempts to propel blood through the aortic valve, which is being maintained in a closed position by the pressure generated from the "assist" circulatory device. Electronic synchronization of the natural heart and the artificial heart so that the artificial heart infuses blood during diastole is physiologically of greater benefit.

A second hypothesis—that recovery of a failing heart would be aided by "resting" the heart with assisted circulation—has also been difficult to demonstrate. The most encouraging data are from experiments in which an acute, reversible injury has occurred, such as transient anoxia, where extracorporeal circulation for 30 minutes to 1 hour may permit recovery. With an extensive injury, such as a myocardial infarction, how long extracorporeal circulation would be required is unknown. It seems likely that bypass for several days may be necessary, during which time collateral circulation could develop around the acutely occluded coronary artery.

TECHNIQUES OF ASSISTED CIRCULATION. Intraaortic Balloon Pumping. In the past 5 or 6 years the most effective technique for assisted circulation has been intraaortic balloon pumping. A balloon catheter is inserted into a peripheral artery, usually the femoral, and advanced into the thoracic aorta. With electronic synchronization, the balloon is alternately inflated during diastole and deflated during systole. This intermittent inflation is of significant benefit to the peripheral circulation, but careful synchronization is essential. Inflation of the balloon during systole actually may harm the left ventricle as it attempts to open the aortic valve against the pressure generated by the inflating balloon. Early experimental and clinical studies with balloon pumping were reported by several investigators. In the past few years balloon pumping has been widely employed, as morbidity is small and the benefit, though limited, is critical to some patients. It seems to increase cardiac index about 0.5 to 0.7 liters and can be used for several days. We use the balloon pump often in our unit and firmly believe several patients would not have survived without it.

Left Heart Bypass. A decade ago Dennis demonstrated the benefits of assisted circulation with left heart bypass, withdrawing blood from the atrium and infusing it into a peripheral artery. Difficulties with closed chest cannulation of the left atrium, however, have thus far greatly limited application of the procedure. Several years ago the author and associates applied left heart bypass in a small group of patients by direct cannulation of the left atrium through a thoracotomy incision and employing perfusion for periods of 3 to 4 hours, but longer periods of perfusion were impractical because of the necessity for thoracotomy. At New York University, a special transvenous cannula has been developed by Glassman and associates which permits closed-chest cannulation of the left atrium through a modification of the transseptal puncture technique. First a standard transseptal left atrial puncture is done, introducing the needle and catheter through the femoral vein. A guide wire is subsequently introduced, after which the special large bore (28 F) catheter is advanced over the guide wire into the left atrium. With this large catheter bypass flow rates as great as 4 liters/minute have been obtained. This technical advance may increase the applicability of left heart bypass, especially as the circulatory support feasible is far greater than that attainable with intraaortic balloon pumping. At this time, it has had limited clinical application.

Litwak and associates in 1976 reported a new type of left heart bypass, used in patients who could not be weaned from the heart-lung machine at the time of operation. Especially designed silastic cannulae were left in the left atrium and femoral artery and brought through the chest wall, which was then closed. Pumping was done with a roller pump with silastic tubing, infusing enough heparin to keep the activated clotting time near 150 seconds and to prevent clotting in the pump, but not enough to cause serious bleeding. There is significant platelet destruction, however, requiring serial infusion of platelets. In their report they describe using the device in 14 patients, in some for 1 week or longer. Of the 14, nine could be weaned from the device, six left the hospital, and four remained alive at the time of the report, one 22 months after operation. We have unsuccessfully used the technique at New York University in three or four moribund patients and believe that, with some modification to lessen the destruction of platelets, it may have significant possibilities.

Peripheral Bypass. A peripheral bypass may be a venoarterial bypass in which venous blood is withdrawn, oxygenated, and returned into a peripheral artery. As indicated earlier, such perfusion should be synchronized to return blood during diastole. Alternatively, a venovenous bypass can be used, returning the blood from the oxygenator into a peripheral vein. Hill and associates have reported on extensive use of this technique for the treatment of acute pulmonary insufficiency, employing a membrane oxygenator and continuing perfusion for several days. In 1977 Hill and associates were still employing the technique, but to date ultimate survival has been poor, primarily because of lack of reversibility of the primary disease causing the acute respiratory insufficiency.

A number of other techniques have been attempted for assisted circulation, such as counterpulsation or synchronized application of external pressure to the extremities, but none have found widespread clinical use. The main limitation of all techniques is that short periods of assisted circulation seem of little value unless the underlying cardiac injury can be corrected.

ARTIFICIAL HEARTS. The ideal solution of many difficult cardiac problems would be a satisfactory mechanical heart, but this seems to be far on the horizon. The National Heart and Lung Institute for several years coordinated a large interdisciplinary program, studying many of the engineering, physical, chemical, and hematologic problems involved. Results were meager, however, primarily because of lack of basic knowledge that would make an artificial heart feasible at this time. One major obstacle, among many, is the inability to pump blood without the use of heparin. Continuous heparinization results in intractable bleeding, while pumping without heparin results in thromboembolism.

Experiences in an attempt to develop a nuclear-fuel support system were summarized by Norman and Huffman in 1972. Bernhard has precisely studied left ventricular bypass pumps in calves for several years and summarized his experience in 1975. The pump functioned successfully in 20 consecutive calves for at least 2 weeks, with an average flow rate of 5 liters/minute. One calf was maintained for over a year. The technique has subsequently been applied successfully to two or three patients.

Weldon and Cooley, as well as others, have successfully implanted conduits between the left ventricle and the aorta for severe forms of obstruction to left ventricular outflow, usually a hypoplastic aortic annulus. The conduit consists of a Dacron tube with a porcine heterograft. Long-term results are not yet available.

Studies of total replacement of the heart, rather than simple left heart bypass, have continued. Kolff and associates have periodically reported the status of their investigations, obtaining survivals for a few weeks, with death ultimately occurring either from thromboembolism or from infection. Excellent work has been done by Pierce and associates with left heart bypass pumps functioning in calves for several weeks, and significant progress is being made toward total heart replacement.

At present the most realistic immediate goal for artificial hearts is their use for bypassing the left heart for a few days or 1 or 2 weeks until the heart recovers from either operative injury or an acute infarction. If recovery is not possible, such a device would simply postpone inevitable death, so its use would require considerable judgment and caution.

References

Introduction; Clinical Manifestations

Gibbon, J. H., Jr., Sabiston, D. C., Jr., and Spencer, F. C.: "Surgery of the Chest," 2d ed., W. B. Saunders Company, Philadelphia, 1969.
Hurst, J. W., and Logue, R. B.: "The Heart, Arteries, and Veins," 2d ed., McGraw-Hill Book Company, New York, 1970.

Extracorporeal Circulation

Allen, J. G. (ed.): "Extracorporeal Circulation," Charles C Thomas, Publisher, Springfield, Ill., 1958.

Bahnson, H. T., and Spencer, F. C.: Extracorporeal Circulation, in C. D. Benson et al. (eds.), "Pediatric Surgery," vol. I, Year Book Medical Publishers, Inc., Chicago, 1962.

Boyd, A. D., Tremblay, R. E., Spencer, F. C., and Bahnson, H. T.: Estimation of Cardiac Output Soon after Intracardiac Surgery with Cardiopulmonary Bypass, *Ann Surg,* **150:**613, 1959.

Brantigan, C. O., and Grow, J. B.: Cricothyroidotomy: Elective Use in Respiratory Problems Requiring Tracheostomy, *J Thorac Cardiovasc Surg,* **71:**72, 1976.

Clowes, G. H. A., Jr.: Extracorporeal Maintenance of Circulation and Respiration, *Physiol Rev,* **40:**826, 1960.

DeWall, R. A., Warden, H. E., Varco, R. L., and Lillehei, C. W.: The Helix Reservoir Pump-Oxygenator, *Surg Gynecol Obstet,* **104:**699, 1957.

Ellison, L. T., Duke, J. F., III, and Ellison, R. G.: Pulmonary Compliance following Open-Heart Surgery and Its Relationship to Ventilation and Gas Exchange, *Circulation,* **35**(*Suppl 1*):217, 1967.

Gibbon, J. H., Jr.: Application of a Mechanical Heart and Lung Apparatus to Cardiac Surgery, *Minn Med,* **37:**171, 1954.

Jones, R. E., Donald, D. E., Swan, H. J. C., Harshbarger, H. G., Kirklin, J. W., and Wood, E. H.: Apparatus of the Gibbon Type for Mechanical Bypass of the Heart and Lungs: Preliminary Report, *Proc Staff Meetings Mayo Clin,* **30:**105, 1955.

McGoon, D. C., Moffitt, E. A., Theye, R. A., and Kirklin, J. W.: Physiologic Studies during High Flow, Normothermic, Whole Body Perfusion, *J Thorac Cardiovasc Surg,* **39:**275, 1960.

Porter, G. A., Kloster, F. E., Herr, R. H., Starr, A., Griswold, H. E., and Kimsey, J. A.: Renal Complications Associated with Valve Replacement Surgery, *J Thorac Cardiovasc Surg,* **53:**145, 1967.

———, Starr, A., Kimsey, J., and Lenertz, H.: Mannitol Hemodilution-Perfusion: The Kinetics of Mannitol Distribution and Excretion during Cardiopulmonary Bypass, *J Surg Res,* **10:**447, 1967.

Sachdev, N. S., Carter, C. C., Swank, R. L., and Blachly, P. H.: Relationship between Post-Cardiotomy Delirium, Clinical Neurological Changes, and EEG Abnormalities, *J Thorac Cardiovasc Surg,* **54:**557, 1967.

Spencer, F. C., Benson, D. W., Liu, W. C., and Bahnson, H. T.: Use of a Mechanical Respirator in the Management of Respiratory Insufficiency following Trauma or Operation for Cardiac or Pulmonary Disease, *J Thorac Cardiovasc Surg,* **38:**758, 1959.

Cardiac Arrest and Ventricular Fibrillation

Cunningham, J. N., Spencer, F. C., Zeff, R., Williams, C. D., Cukingnam, R., and Mullin, M.: Influence of Primary Closure of Pericardium after Open Heart Surgery on Frequency of Tamponade, Postcardiotomy Syndrome and Pulmonary Complications, *J Thorac Cardiovasc Surg,* **70:**119, 1975.

Joseph, W. L., and Maloney, J. V., Jr.: Extracorporeal Circulation as an Adjunct to Resuscitation of the Heart, *JAMA,* **193:**683, 1965.

Jude, J. R., and Elam, J. O.: "Fundamentals of Cardiopulmonary Resuscitation," F. A. Davis Company, Philadelphia, 1965.

Kouwenhoven, W. B., Jude, J. R., and Knickerbocker, G. G.: Closed Chest Cardiac Massage, *JAMA,* **137:**1064, 1960.

———, Milnor, W. R., Knickerbocker, G. G., and Chestnut, W. R.: Closed Chest Defibrillation of the Heart, *Surgery,* **42:**550, 1957.

Spencer, F. C., and Bahnson, H. T.: Treatment of Cardiac Arrest, in C. D. Benson et al. (eds.), "Pediatric Surgery," vol. I, p. 522, Year Book Medical Publishers, Inc., Chicago, 1962.

Williams, G. R., and Spencer, F. C.: The Clinical Use of Hypothermia following Cardiac Arrest, *Ann Surg,* **148:**462, 1958.

Zimmerman, J. M., and Spencer, F. C.: The Influence of Hypothermia on Cerebral Injury Resulting from Circulatory Occlusion, *Surg Forum,* **9:**216, 1958.

Mitral Stenosis

Bailey, C. P.: The Surgical Treatment of Mitral Stenosis (Mitral Commissurotomy), *Dis Chest,* **15:**377, 1949.

Bryant, L. R., and Trinkle, J. K.: Mitral Valvotomy in the Valve Replacement Era, *Ann Surg,* **173:**1024, 1971.

Cutler, E. C., and Levine, S. A.: Cardiotomy and Valvulotomy for Mitral Stenosis, *N Engl J Med,* **188:**1023, 1923.

Ellis, L. B., Harken, D. E., and Black, H.: A Clinical Study of 1000 Consecutive Cases of Mitral Stenosis Two to Nine Years after Mitral Valvuloplasty, *Circulation,* **19:**803, 1959.

Gerbode, F.: Transventricular Mitral Valvulotomy, *Circulation,* **21:**563, 1960.

Higgs, L. M., Glancy, D. L., O'Brien, K. P., Epstein, S. E., and Morrow, A. G.: Mitral Restenosis: An Uncommon Cause of Recurrent Symptoms following Mitral Commissurotomy, *Am J Cardiol,* **26:**34, 1970.

Kiser, I. O., Hoeksema, T. D., Connolly, D. C., and Ellis, F. H., Jr.: Long-Term Results of Closed Mitral Commissurotomy, *J Cardiovasc Surg,* **8:**263, 1967.

Logan, A., and Turner, R.: Surgical Treatment of Mitral Stenosis with Particular Reference to the Transventricular Approach with a Mechanical Dilator, *Lancet,* **2:**874, 1959.

Mullin, M. J., Engelman, R. M., Isom, O. W., Boyd, A. D., Glassman, E., and Spencer, F. C.: Experience with Open Mitral Commissurotomy in 100 Consecutive Patients, *Surgery,* **76:**974, 1974.

Nathaniels, E. K., Moncure, A. C., and Scannell, J. G.: A Fifteen-Year Follow-up Study of Closed Mitral Valvuloplasty, *Ann Thorac Surg,* **10:**27, 1970.

Nichols, H. T., Blanco, G., Morse, D. P., Adam, A., and Baltazar, N.: Open Mitral Commissurotomy: Experience with 200 Consecutive Cases, *JAMA,* **182:**268, 1962.

Olinger, G. N., Rio, F. W., and Maloney, J. V., Jr.: Closed Valvulotomy for Calcific Mitral Stenosis, *J Thorac Cardiovasc Surg,* **62:**357, 1971.

Roe, B. B., Edmunds, L. H., Jr., Fishman, N. H., and Hutchinson, J. C.: Open Mitral Valvulotomy, *Ann Thorac Surg,* **12:**483, 1971.

Selzer, A., and Cohn, K. E.: Natural History of Mitral Stenosis: A Review, *Circulation,* **45:**878, 1972.

Souttar, P. W.: The Surgical Treatment of Mitral Stenosis, *Br Med J,* **2:**603, 1925.

Spencer, F. C., Cortes, L., Marcarenhas, G., Ifuku, M., and Koepke, J.: The Mechanism of Thrombus Formation upon the Starr-Edwards Prosthetic Mitral Valve, *Ann Surg,* **165:**814, 1967.

Starr, A.: Mitral Valve Replacement with Ball Valve Prostheses, *J Thorac Cardiovasc Surg,* **64:**354, 1972.

——— and Edwards, M. L.: Mitral Replacement: Clinical Experience with a Ball Valve Prosthesis, *Ann Surg,* **154:**726, 1961.

————, Herr, R. H., and Wood, J. A.: Mitral Replacement: Review of Six Years' Experience, *J Thorac Cardiovasc Surg*, **54**:333, 1967.

Mitral Insufficiency

Anderson, A. M., Cobb, L. A., Bruce, R. A., and Merendino, K. A.: Evaluation of Mitral Annuloplasty for Mitral Regurgitation: Clinical and Hemodynamic Status Four to 41 Months after Surgery, *Circulation,* **26**:26, 1962.

Barnhorst, D. A., Oxman, H. A., Connolly, D. C., Pluth, J. R., Danielson, G. K., Wallace, R. B., and McGoon, D. W.: Long-term Follow-up of Isolated Replacement of Aortic or Mitral Valve with the Starr-Edwards Prosthesis, *Am J Cardiol,* **35**:228, 1975.

Bjork, V. O., Book, K., And Holmgren, A.: The Bjork-Shiley Mitral Valve Prosthesis, *Ann Thorac Surg,* **18**:379, 1974.

Bonchek, L. I., Anderson, K. P., and Starr, A.: Mitral Valve Replacement with Cloth-Covered Composite-Seat Prostheses, *J Thorac Cardiovasc Surg,* **67**:93, 1974.

Braunwald, N. S., and Bonchek, L. I.: Prevention of Thrombus Formation on Rigid Prosthetic Heart Valves by the Ingrowth of Autogenous Tissue, *J Thorac Cardiovasc Surg,* **54**:630, 1967.

Isom, O. W., Williams, C. D., Falk, E. A., Glassman, E., and Spencer, F. C.: Long-Term Evaluation of Cloth-covered Metallic Ball Prostheses, *J Thorac Cardiovasc Surg,* **64**:354, 1972.

————, Spencer, F. C., Glassman, E., Teiko, P., Boyd, A. D., Cunningham, J. N., and Reed, G. E.: Long-Term Results in 1375 Patients Undergoing Valve Replacement with the Starr-Edwards Cloth-Covered Steel Ball Valve Prosthesis, *Ann Surg,* **186**:310, 1977.

Kay, J. H., and Egerton, W. S.: The Repair of Mitral Insufficiency Associated with Ruptured Chordae Tendineae, *Ann Surg,* **157**:351, 1963.

McGoon, D. C.: Repair of Mitral Insufficiency Due to Ruptured Chordae Tendineae, *J Thorac Cardiovasc Surg,* **39**:357, 1960.

Pakrashi, B. C., Mary, D. A., Elmufti, M. E., Wooler, G. H., and Ionescu, M. I.: Clinical and Hemodynamic Results of Mitral Annuloplasty, *Br Heart J,* **36**:768, 1974.

Reed, G. E.: Repair of Mitral Regurgitation, *Am J Cardiol,* **31**:494, 1973.

————, Tice, D. A., and Clauss, R. H.: Asymmetric Exaggerated Mitral Annuloplasty: Repair of Mitral Insufficiency with Hemodynamic Predictability, *J Thorac Cardiovasc Surg,* **49**:752, 1965.

Starr, A.: Mitral Valve Replacement with Ball Valve Prostheses, *Br Heart J Suppl,* **33**:47, 1971.

—————— and Edwards, M. L.: Mitral Replacement: Clinical Experience with a Ball Valve Prosthesis, *Ann Surg,* **154**:726, 1961.

Stinson, E. B., Griepp, R. B., and Shumway, N. E.: Clinical Experience with a Porcine Aortic Valve Xenograft for Mitral Valve Replacement, *Ann Thorac Surg,* (In press.)

Zerbini, E. J.: Results of Replacement of Cardiac Valves by Homologous Dura Mater Valves, *Chest,* **67**:706, 1975.

Aortic Stenosis

Angell, W. W., Shumway, N. E., and Kosek, J. C.: A Five Year Study of Viable Aortic Valve Homografts, *J Thorac Cardiovasc Surg,* **64**:329, 1972.

Bahnson, H. T., Spencer, F. C., Busse, E. F. G., and Davis, F. W., Jr.: Cusp Replacement and Coronary Artery Perfusion in Open Operations on the Aortic Valve, *Ann Surg,* **152**:494, 1960.

Barnhorst, D. A., Oxman, H. A., Connolly, D. C., Pluth, J. R., Danielson, G. K., Wallace, R. B., and McGoon, D. W.: Long-Term Follow-up of Isolated Replacement of Aortic or Mitral Valve with the Starr-Edwards Prosthesis, *Am J Cardiol,* **35**:228, 1975.

Isom, O. W., Spencer, F. C., Glassman, E., Teiko, P., Boyd, A. D., Cunningham, J. N., and Reed, G. E.: Long-Term Results in 1375 Patients Undergoing Valve Replacement with the Starr-Edwards Cloth-Covered Steel Ball Valve Prosthesis, *Ann Surg,* **186**:310, 1977.

Magovern, G. J., Kent, E. J., Cromie, H. W., Cushing, W. B., and Scott, S.: Sutureless Aortic and Mitral Prosthetic Valves: Clinical Results and Operative Technique on 60 Patients, *J Thorac Cardiovasc Surg,* **48**:346, 1964.

McGoon, D. C., Ellis, F. H., and Kirklin, J. W.: Late Results of Operations for Acquired Aortic Valvular Disease, *Circulation,* **31**:108, 1965.

————, Pestana, C., and Moffitt, E. A.: Decreased Risk of Aortic Valve Surgery, *Arch Surg,* **91**:779, 1965.

Pacifico, A. D., Karp, R. B., and Kirklin, J. W.: Homografts for Replacement of the Aortic Valve, *Circulation,* **45**:I-36, 1972.

Senning, A.: Fascia Lata Replacement of Aortic Valves, *J Thorac Cardiovasc Surg,* **54**:465, 1967.

Starr, A., Edwards, M. L., McCord, C. W., and Griswold, H. E.: Aortic Replacement: Clinical Experience with a Semi-rigid Ball-Valve Prosthesis, *Circulation,* **27**:779, 1963.

————, Bonchek, L. I., Anderson, R. P., Wood, J. A., and Chapman, R. D.: Late Complications of Aortic Valve Replacement with Cloth-Covered, Composite-Seat Prostheses, *Ann Thorac Surg,* **19**:289, 1975.

Stinson, E. B., Griepp, R. B., Oyer, P. E., and Shumway, N. E.: Long-Term Experience with Porcine Aortic Valve Xenografts, *J Thorac Cardiovasc Surg,* **73**:54, 1977.

Zerbini, E. J.: Results of Replacement of Cardiac Valves by Homologous Dura Mater Valves, *Chest,* **67**:706, 1975.

Tricuspid Stenosis and Insufficiency

Arbulu, A., Thoms, N. W., and Wilson, R. F.: Valvulectomy without Prosthetic Replacement: A Lifesaving Operation for Tricuspid *Pseudomonas* Endocarditis, *J Thorac Cardiovasc Surg,* **64**:103, 1972.

Boyd, A. D., Engelman, R. H., Isom, O. W., Reed, G. E., and Spencer, F. C.: Tricuspid Annuloplasty, *J Thorac Cardiovasc Surg,* **68**:344, 1974.

Breyer, R. H., McClenathan, J. H., Michaelis, L. L., McIntosh, C. L., and Morrow, A. G.: Tricuspid Regurgitation, *J Thorac Cardiovasc Surg,* **72**:867, 1976.

Grondin, P., Lepage, G., Castonguay, Y., and Meere, C.: The Tricuspid Valve: A Surgical Challenge, *J Thorac Cardiovasc Surg* **53**:7, 1967.

————, Meere, C., Limet, R., Lopez-Bescos, L., Delcan, J. L., and Rivera, R.: Carpentier's Annulus and DeVega's Annuloplasty: End of the Tricuspid Challenge, *J Thorac Cardiovasc Surg,* **70**:852, 1975.

Isom, O. W., Spencer, F. C., Glassman, E., Teiko, P., Boyd, A. D.,

Cunningham, J. N., and Reed, G. E.: Long-Term Results in 1375 Patients Undergoing Valve Replacement with the Starr-Edwards Cloth-Covered Steel Ball Valve Prosthesis, *Ann Surg,* **186:**310, 1977.

Kay, J. H., Maselli-Campagna, G., and Tsuji, H. K.: Surgical Treatment of Tricuspid Insufficiency, *Ann Surg,* **162:**53, 1965.

Spencer, F., C., Shabetai, R., and Adolph, R.: Successful Replacement of the Tricuspid Valve 10 Years after Traumatic Incompetence, *Am J Cardiol,* **18:**916, 1966.

Starr, A., Herr, R., and Wood, J.: Tricuspid Replacement for Acquired Valve Disease, *Surg Gynecol Obstet,* **122:**1295, 1966.

Multivalvular Heart Disease

Bonchek, L. I., and Starr, A.: Ball Valve Prostheses: Current Appraisal of Late Results, *Am J Cardiol,* **35:**843, 1975.

Starr, A., McCord, C. W., Wood, J., Herr, R., and Edwards, M. L.: Surgery for Multiple Valve Disease, *Ann Surg.* **160:** 596, 1964.

Cardiac Trauma

Asfaw, I., Thoms, N. W., and Arbulu, A.: Interventricular Septal Defects from Penetrating Injuries of the Heart, *J Thorac Cardiovasc Surg,* **69:**450, 1975.

Bahnson, H. T., and Spencer, F. C.: Pericardial Aspiration and the Treatment of Acute Cardiac Tamponade from Penetrating Wounds in the Heart, in J. H. Mulholland, E. H. Ellison, and S. R. Freisen (eds.), "Current Surgical Management," W. B. Saunders Company, Philadelphia, 1957.

Beall, A. C., Jr., Gasior, R. M., and Bricker, D. L.: Gunshot Wounds of the Heart: Changing Patterns of Surgical Management, *Ann Thorac Surg,* **11:**523, 1971.

———, Ochsner, J. L., Morris, G. C., Jr., Cooley, D. A., and DeBakey, M. E.: Penetrating Wounds to the Heart, *J Trauma,* **1:**195, 1961.

Berger, R. L., Loveless, G., and Warner, O.: Delayed and Latent Postcardiotomy Tamponade: Recognition and Nonoperative Treatment, *Ann Thorac Surg,* **12:**22, 1971.

Blalock, A., and Ravitch, M. M.: A Consideration of the Nonoperative Treatment of Cardiac Tamponade Resulting from Wounds to the Heart, *Surgery,* **14:**157, 1943.

Bland, E. F., and Beebe, G. W.: Missiles in the Heart: A 20-Year Follow-up Report of World War II Cases, *N Engl J Med,* **274:**1039, 1966.

Boyd, T. F., and Strieder, J. W.: Immediate Surgery for Traumatic Heart Disease, *J Thorac Cardiovasc Surg,* **50:**305, 1965.

Harken, D. E.: Foreign Bodies in and in Relation to the Heart and Thoracic Vessels, *Surg Gynecol Obstet,* **83:**117, 1946.

Holdeger, W. F., Lyons, C., and Edwards, W. S.: Indications for Removal of Intracardiac Foreign Bodies, *Ann Surg,* **163:**249, 1966.

Isaacs, J. P.: Sixty Penetrating Wounds to the Heart: Clinical and Experimental Observations, *Surgery,* **45:**696, 1959.

Spencer, F. C.: Treatment of Chest Injuries, *Curr Probl Surg,* January, 1964.

——— and Kennedy, J. H.: War Wounds of the Heart, *J Thorac Cardiovasc Surg,* **33:**361, 1957.

Sugg, W. L., Ecker, R. R., Webb, W. R., Rose, E. F., and Shaw, R. R.: Penetrating Wounds of the Heart: An Analysis of 459 Cases, *J Thorac Cardiovasc Surg,* **56:**531, 1968.

Symbas, P. N., Harlaftis, N., and Waldo, W. J.: Penetrating Cardiac Wounds: A Comparison of Different Therapeutic Methods, *Ann Surg,* **183:**377, 1976.

Tabatznik, B., and Isaacs, J. P.: Post-Pericardiotomy Syndrome following Traumatic Hemopericardium, *Am J Cardiol,* **7:**83, 1961.

Cardiac Tumors

Bahnson, H. T., Spencer, F. C., and Andrus, E. C.: Diagnosis and Treatment of Intracavitary Myxomas of the Heart, *Ann Surg,* **145:**915, 1957.

Crafoord, C.: Case Report, *Int Symp Cardiovasc Surg Henry Ford Hosp,* p. 202, 1955.

Dang, C. R., and Hurley, E. J.: Contralateral Recurrent Myxoma of the Heart, *Ann Thorac Surg,* **21:**59, 1976.

Gassman, H. S., Meadows, R., and Baker, L. A.: Metastatic Tumors of the Heart, *Am J Med,* **19:**357, 1955.

Geha, A. S., Weidman, W. H., Soule, E. H., and McGoon, D. C.: Intramural Ventricular Cardiac Fibroma: Successful Removal in Two Cases and Review of the Literature, *Circulation,* **36:**427, 1967.

Gerbode, F., Keith, J. W., and Hill, J. D.: Surgical Management of Tumors of the Heart, *Surgery,* **61:**94, 1967.

Hanfling, S.: Metastatic Cancer to the Heart, *Circulation,* **22:**474, 1960.

Mahaim, I.: "Les Tumors et les polypes du coeur: Étude anatomo-clinique," Masson et Cie, Paris, 1945.

Prichard, R. W.: Tumors of the Heart, *Arch Pathol,* **21:**98, 1951.

Scannell, J. G., and Grillo, H. E.: Primary Tumors of the Heart, *J Thorac Cardiovasc Surg,* **35:**23, 1958.

Spencer, F. C.: The Heart, in T. F. Nealon (ed.), "Management of the Patient with Cancer," p. 537, W. B. Saunders Company, Philadelphia, 1965.

Steinberg, I., Dotter, C. T., and Glenn, F.: Myxoma of the Heart: Roentgen Diagnosis during Life in Three Cases, *Dis Chest,* **24:**509, 1953.

Symbas, P. N., Hatcher, C. R., Jr., and Gravanis, M. B.: Myxoma of the Heart: Clinical and Experimental Observations, *Ann Surg,* **183:**470, 1976.

Thomas, K. E., Winchell, C. P., and Varco, R. L.: Diagnostic and Surgical Aspects of Left Atrial Tumors, *J Thorac Cardiovasc Surg,* **53:**535, 1967.

Whorton, C. M.: Primary Malignant Tumors of the Heart, *Cancer,* **2:**245, 1949.

Yater, W. M.: Tumors of the Heart and Pericardium, *Arch Intern Med,* **48:**627, 1931.

Coronary Artery Disease

Berg, R., Kendall, R. W., Duvoisin, G. E., Ganji, J. H., Rudy, L. W., and Everhart, F. J.: Acute Myocardial Infarction: Surgical Emergency, *J Thorac Cardiovasc Surg,* **70:**432, 1975.

Buchwald, H., and Varco, R. L.: A Bypass Operation for Obese Hyperlipedemic Patients, *Surgery,* **70:**62, 1971.

Cheanvechai, C., Groves, L. K., Reyes, E. A., Shirey, E. K., and Sones, F. M., Jr.: Manual Coronary Endarterectomy: Clinical Experience in 315 Patients, *J Thorac Cardiovasc Surg,* **70:**524, 1975.

Dilley, R. B., Cannon, J. A., Kattus, A. A., MacAlpin, R. N., and Longmire, W. P.: The Treatment of Coronary Occlusive Disease by Endarterectomy, *J Thorac Cardiovasc Surg,* **50:**511, 1965.

Favaloro, R., Effler, D. B., Groves, L. K., Sones, F. M., Jr., and Fergusson, B. J. G.: Myocardial Revascularization by Internal Mammary Artery Implant Procedures, *J Thorac Cardiovasc Surg,* **54:**359, 1967.

Green, G. E., Stertzer, S. H., and Reppert, E. H.: Coronary Arterial Bypass Grafts, *Ann Thorac Surg,* **5:**443, 1968.

Grondin, C. M., Lesperance, J., Bourassa, M. G., and Campeau, L.: Coronary Artery Grafting with the Saphenous Vein or Internal Mammary Artery, *Ann Thorac Surg,* **20:**605, 1975.

Isom, O. W., Spencer, F. C., Glassman, E., Cunningham, J. N., Teiko, P., Reed, G. E., and Boyd, A. D.: Does Coronary Bypass Increase Longevity? *J Thorac Cardiovasc Surg,* **75**(1):28, 1978.

————, ————, ————, Dembrow, J. M., and Pasternack, B. S.: Long-Term Survival Following Coronary Bypass Surgery in Patients with Significant Impairment of Left Ventricular Function, *Circulation,* **51–52**(*Suppl 1*):141, 1975.

Jones, J. W., Ochsner, J. L., Mills, N. L., and Hughes, L.: Impact of Multiple Variables on Operative and Extended Survival Following Coronary Artery Surgery, *Surgery,* **83**(1):20, 1978.

Kouchoukos, N. T., and Kirklin, J. W.: Coronary Bypass Operations for Ischemic Heart Disease, *Mod Concepts Cardiovasc Dis,* **41:**47, 1972.

McNeer, J. F., Starmer, C. F., Bartel, A. G., Behar, V. S., Kong, Y., Peter, R. H., and Rosati, R. A.: The Nature of Treatment Selection in Coronary Artery Disease, *Circulation,* **49:**606, 1974.

Mills, N. L., and Ochsner, J. L.: Coronary Artery Bypass Surgery: 322 Consecutive Patients with No Hospital Mortality, *J La State Med Soc,* **128:**1, 1976.

Mundth, E. D., and Austen, W. G.: Surgical Measures for Coronary Heart Disease: Part I, *N Engl J Med,* **293:**13, 1975.

————, and Austen, W. G.: Surgical Measures for Coronary Heart Disease: Part II, *N Engl J Med,* **293:**75, 1975.

————, and Austen, W. G.: Surgical Measures for Coronary Heart Disease: Part III, *N Engl J Med,* **293:**124, 1975.

Oglietti, J., Angelini, P., Leachman, R. D., and Cooley, D. A.: Myocardial Revascularization, *J Thorac Cardiovasc Surg,* **71:**736, 1976.

Olinger, G. N., Po, J., Maloney, J. V., Jr., Mulder, D. G., and Buckberg, G. D.: Coronary Revascularization in "High-" versus "Low-Risk" Patients: Role of Myocardial Protection, *Ann Surg,* **182:**293, 1975.

Reul, G. J., Cooley, D. A., Sandiford, F. M., Kyger, E. R., III, Wukasch, D. C., and Hallman, G. L.: Aortocoronary Artery Bypass, *Arch Surg,* **111:**414, 1976.

Schimert, G., Vidne, B. A. and Lee, A. B., Jr.: Free Internal Mammary Artery Graft: Improved Surgical Technic, *Ann Thorac Surg,* **19:**474, 1975.

Slater, S. D., Sallam, A., Bain, W. H., Turner, M. A., and Lawrie, T. D. V.: Hemolysis with Bjork-Shiley and Starr-Edwards Prosthetic Heart Valves: Comparative Study, *Thorax,* **29:**624, 1974.

Spencer, F. C.: Bypass Grafting for Preinfarction Angina, *Circulation,* **40:**274, 1972.

————: Surgical Procedures for Coronary Atherosclerosis, *Prog Cardiovasc Dis,* **14:**399, 1972.

————, Green, G. E., Tice, D. A., and Glassman, E.: Surgical Therapy for Coronary Artery Disease, *Curr Probl Surg,* September, 1970.

————, ————, ————, Wallsh, E., Mills, N. L., and Glassman, E.: Coronary Artery Bypass Grafts for Congestive Heart Failure, *J Thorac Cardiovasc Surg,* **62:**529, 1971.

————, Isom, O. W., Glassman, E., Boyd, A. D., et al.: The Long-Term Influence of Coronary Bypass Grafts on Myocardial Infarction and Survival, *Ann Surg,* **180:**439, 1974.

Stiles, Q. R., Lindesmith, G. G., Tucker, B. L., Hughes, R. K., and Meyer, B. W.: Long-Term Follow-Up of Patients with Coronary Bypass Grafts, *Circulation,* **54**(*Suppl 3*):32, 1976.

Tecklenberg, P. L., Alderman, E. L., Miller, D. C., Shumway, N. E., and Harrison, D. C.: Changes in Survival and Symptom Relief in a Longitudinal Study of Patients after Bypass Surgery, *Circulation,* **51–52**(*Suppl. 1*):98, 1975.

Vineberg, A. M.: Technical Considerations for the Combined Operation of Left Internal Mammary Artery or Right and Left Internal Mammary Implantations with Epicardiectomy and Free Omental Graft, *J Thorac Cardiovasc Surg,* **53:**837, 1967.

Ventricular Aneurysm

Abrams, D. L., Edelist, A., Leuria, M. H., and Miller, A. J.: Ventricular Aneurysm: A Re-appraisal Based on a Study of 65 Consecutive Autopsy Cases, *Circulation,* **27:**164, 1963.

Cooley, D. A., Hallman, G. L., and Henly, W. S.: Left Ventricular Aneurysm Due to Myocardial Infarction: Experience with 37 Patients, *Arch Surg,* **88:**114, 1964.

Effler, D. B., Groves, L. K., and Favaloro, R.: Surgical Repair of Ventricular Aneurysm, *Dis Chest,* **48:**37, 1965.

Schlichter, J., Hellerstein, H. K., and Katz, L. N.: Aneurysm of the Heart: A Correlative Study of 102 Proved Cases, *Medicine,* **33:**43, 1954.

Pericarditis

Berger, R. L., Loveless, G., and Warner, O.: Delayed and Latent Postcardiotomy Tamponade: Recognition and Nonoperative Treatment, *Ann Thorac Surg,* **12:**22, 1971.

Boyle, J. D., Pearce, M. L., and Guze, L. B.: Purulent Pericarditis: Review of Literature and Report of 11 Cases, *Medicine,* **40:**119, 1961.

Collins, H. A., Woods, L. P., and Daniel, R. A.: Late Results of Pericardectomy, *Arch Surg,* **89:**921, 1964.

Copeland, J. G., Stinson, E. B., Griepp, R. B., and Shumway, N. E.: Surgical Treatment of Chronic Constrictive Pericarditis Using Cardiopulmonary Bypass, *J Thorac Cardiovasc Surg,* **69:**236, 1975.

Dalton, J. C., Pearson, R. J., and White, P. D.: Constrictive Pericarditis: A Review and Long-Term Follow-up of 78 Cases, *Ann Intern Med,* **45:**445, 1956.

Effler, D. B.: Chronic Constrictive Pericarditis Treated with Pericardectomy, *Am J Cardiol,* **7:**62, 1961.

Holman, E.: The Pericardium, in J. H. Gibbon (ed.), "Surgery of the Chest," chap. 24, 1st ed., W. B. Saunders Company, Philadelphia, 1962.

Rubin, R. H., and Moellering, R. C., Jr.: Clinical Microbiologic and Therapeutic Aspects of Purulent Pericarditis, *Am J Med,* **59:**68, 1975.

Heart Block and Pacemakers

Chardack, W. M., Gage, A. A., Federico, A. J., Schimert, G., and Greatbatch, W.: The Long-Term Treatment of Heart Block, *Prog Cardiovasc Dis,* **9**:105, 1966.

Corman, L. C., and Levison, M. E.: Sustained Bacteremia in Transvenous Cardiac Pacemakers, *JAMA,* **233**:264, 1975.

Furman, S., Escher, D. J., Solomon, S., and Schwedel, J. B.: Implanted Transvenous Pacemakers: Equipment, Technic and Clinical Experience, *Ann Surg,* **164**:465, 1966.

Glenn, W. W. L.: Cardiac Pacemakers and Heart Block, in J. H. Gibbon (ed.), "Surgery of the Chest," 1st ed., W. B. Saunders Company, Philadelphia, 1962.

Imparato, A. M. and Kim., G. E.: Electrode Complications in Patients with Permanent Cardiac Pacemakers, *Arch Surg,* **105**:705, 1972.

————, Reppert, E., and Spencer, F. S.: Rapid Atrial Pacing to Produce Heart Block, *Surgery,* **63(1)**:198, 1968.

Johnson, R. A., Hutter, A. M., Desanctis, R. W., Yurchak, P. M., Leinbach, R. C., and Hartone, J. W.: Chronic Overdrive Pacing and Control of Refractory Ventricular Arrhythmias, *Ann Intern Med,* **80**:380, 1974.

Lagergren, H., et al.: Three-hundred-five Cases of Permanent Intravenous Pacemaker Treatment for Adams-Stokes Syndrome, *Surgery,* **59**:494, 1966.

Lillehei, C. W., Sellers, R. D., Bonnabeau, R. C. and Eliot, R. S.: Chronic Postsurgical Complete Heart Block: With Particular Reference to Prognosis, Management, and a New P-wave Pacemaker, *J Thorac Cardiovasc Surg,* **46**:436, 1963.

Nathan, D. A., Center, S., Wu, C., and Keller, W.: An Implantable Synchronous Pacemaker for the Long Term Correction of Complete Heart Block, *Am J Cardiol,* **11**:362, 1963.

Parsonnet, J.: Power Sources for Implantable Cardiac Pacemakers, *Chest,* **61**:165, 1972.

Parsonnet, V., Feldman, S., Parsonnet, J., and Rothfeld, E.: Arrhythmias Induced by Exercise in Paced Patients, *Am Heart J,* **86**:76, 1974.

————, Furman, S., and Smyth, N.: Implantable Cardiac Pacemakers: Status Report and Resource Guideline, *Circulation,* **50**:A21, 1974.

Sowton, E., Hendrix, G., and Row, P.: Treatment with Implantable Cardiac Pacemakers, *Br Med J,* **3**:155, 1974.

Zoll, P. M.: Historical Development of Cardiac Pacemakers, *Prog Cardiovasc Dis,* **14**:421, 1972.

————, Frank, H. A., and Linenthal, A. J.: Four Year Experience with an Implanted Cardiac Pacemaker, *Ann Surg,* **160**:351, 1964.

Assisted Circulation and Artificial Hearts

Bergman, D., and Goetz, R. H.: Clinical Experience with a New Cardiac Assist Device: The Dual-Chambered Intra-aortic Balloon Assist, *J Thorac Cardiovasc Surg,* **62**:577, 1971.

Bernhard, W. F., Poirier, V., LaFarge, C. C., et al.: A New Method for Temporary Left Ventricle Bypass: Preclinical Appraisal, *J Thorac Cardiovasc Surg,* **70**:880, 1975.

————, Griepp, R. B., Stinson, E. B., and Shumway, N. E.: Clinical Transplantation of the Heart, *Ann Surg,* **176**:503, 1972.

Dembitsky, W. P., and Weldon, C. S.: Clinical Experience with the Use of a Valve-Bearing Conduit To Construct a Second Left Ventricular Outflow Tract in Cases of Unresectable Intraventricular Obstruction, *Ann Surg,* **184**:317, 1976.

Glassman, E., Engelman, R. M., Boyd, A. D., Lipson, D., Ackerman, B., and Spencer, F. C.: Method of Closed-Chest Cannulation of Left Atrium for Left Atrial-Femoral Artery Bypass, *J Thorac Cardiovasc Surg,* **69**:283, 1975.

Gold, H. K., Leinbach, R. C., Mundth, E. D., Sanders, C. A., and Buckley, M. J.: Reversal of Myocardial Ischemia Complicating Acute Infarction by Intra-aortic Balloon Pumping (IABP), *Circulation,* 1973.

Griepp, R. B., Stinson, E. B., Biever, C. P., Reitz, B. A., Copeland, J. G., Oyer, P. E., and Shumway, N. E.: Human Heart Transplant, *Ann Thorac Surg,* **22**:171, 1976.

Hall, D. P., Moreno, J. R., Dennis, C., and Senning, A.: An Experimental Study of Prolonged Left Heart Bypass without Thoracotomy, *Ann Surg,* **156**:190, 1962.

Hill, J. D., deLeval, M. R., Fallat, R. J., Bramson, M. L., Eberhart, R. C., Schulte, H. D., Osborn, J. J., Barber, R., and Gerbode, F.: Acute Respiratory Insufficiency: Treatment with Prolonged Extracorporeal Oxygenation, *J Thorac Cardiovasc Surg,* **64**:551, 1972.

Kaiser, G. C., Marco, J. D., Barner, H. B., Codd, J. E., Laks, H., and Willman, V. L.: Intraaortic Balloon Assistance, *Ann Thorac Surg,* **21**:487, 1976.

Liotta, D., Maness, J., Bourland, H., Rodwell, D., Hall, W. C., and DeBakey, M. E.: Recent Modifications in the Implantable Left Ventricle By-pass, *Trans Am Soc Artif Intern Organs,* **11**:284, 1965.

Litwak, R. S., Koffsky, R. M., Jurado, R. A., Lukban, S. B., et al.: Use of a Left Heart Assist Device after Intracardiac Surgery: Technique and Clinical Experience, *Ann Thorac Surg,* **21**:191, 1976.

Norman, J. C., Molokhia, F. A., Harmison, L. T., Whalen, R. L., and Huffman, F.: An Implantable Nuclear-fueled Circulatory Support System: I. Systems Analysis of Conception, Design, Fabrication, and Initial *In Vivo* Testing, *Ann Surg,* **176**:492, 1972.

Okura, T., Tjonneland, S., Fred, P. S., and Kantrowtiz, A.: U-shaped Mechanical Auxiliary Ventricle, *Arch Surg,* **95**:821, 1967.

Skinner, D. B., Anstadt, G. L., and Camp, T. F., Jr.: Applications of Mechanical Ventricular Assistance, *Ann Surg,* **166**:500, 1967.

Spencer, F. C., Eiseman, B., Trinkle, J. K., and Rossi, N. P.: Assisted Circulation for Cardiac Failure following Intracardiac Surgery with Cardiopulmonary Bypass, *J Thorac Cardiovasc Surg,* **49**:56, 1964.

Chapter 20

Diseases of Great Vessels

by Frank C. Spencer

ANEURYSMS OF THE THORACIC AORTA

Aneurysms of the thoracic aorta may be classified in five groups, varying with the anatomic location: (1) ascending aorta; (2) transverse aortic arch; (3) traumatic thoracic aorta, uniformly occurring distal to the left subclavian artery; (4) descending thoracic aorta; and (5) thoracoabdominal. The etiology, disability, and surgical approach all vary with these different types. Hence, each one is discussed separately.

Aneurysms of the Ascending Aorta

Aneurysms localized to the ascending aorta are often due to a degenerative connective tissue disease of the aortic media. This is seen typically as cystic medial necrosis, one manifestation of a generalized disorder in the Marfan syndrome, or as an isolated disease in Erdheim's cystic medial necrosis. Syphilitic destruction of the media of the aorta was formerly a frequent cause of such aneurysms but is now uncommon. Atherosclerotic aneurysms are seldom limited to the ascending aorta, usually evolving as diffuse fusiform lesions involving both the ascending aorta and the transverse arch.

PATHOLOGY. As an aneurysm develops in the proximal ascending aorta, dilatation of the annulus of the aortic valve often develops, stretching the cusps of the aortic valve apart and producing aortic insufficiency (Fig. 20-1). Often cardiac failure from aortic insufficiency is the significant disability, rather than enlargement of the aneurysm with rupture or compression of adjacent structures. Large saccular syphilitic aneurysms can enlarge and erode through the sternum (Fig. 20-2), but these are now rare.

Once aortic insufficiency has resulted from an aneurysm, progression of disability is fairly rapid with death from cardiac failure in 1 to 2 years in many patients unless operation is performed. In the Marfan syndrome, the degenerated wall of the aorta may also rupture and form a dissecting aneurysm. Before surgical therapy was available, most patients with the Marfan syndrome died from one of two complications—either dissecting aneurysm or aortic insufficiency.

CLINICAL MANIFESTATIONS. Patients are often asymptomatic when the diagnosis is made following detection of a mass on a chest roentgenogram performed for other purposes. Expanding saccular aneurysms may cause symptoms from compression of the superior vena cava or the trachea, but compression rarely occurs from fusiform aneurysms. Frequently, the first symptom is due to congestive heart failure from aortic insufficiency. Physical examination usually demonstrates no abnormalities except the aortic diastolic murmur and wide pulse pressure of aortic insufficiency.

DIAGNOSTIC FINDINGS. The diagnosis can be suspected from the chest roentgenogram, disclosing enlargement of the ascending aorta, but aortography is required to establish the exact diagnosis. The aortographic finding of a fusiform aneurysm in the proximal ascending aorta, tapering to an aorta of near-normal diameter at the level of the innominate artery, is virtually diagnostic of cystic medial necrosis (Fig. 20-3).

TREATMENT. Because of the progressive nature of the aortic insufficiency, operation should be performed as soon as possible after the diagnosis is made. The operative procedure must include both correction of the aortic insufficiency and excision of the aneurysm. This, of necessity, involves the use of extracorporeal circulation. If aortic insufficiency is minimal, simple excision of the aneurysm may be adequate.

At operation, once cardiopulmonary bypass has been started, the aorta can be occluded and the aneurysm excised. A critical point is whether the aorta proximally can be divided distal to the coronary ostia or whether excision should extend proximal to the ostia. Usually this decision can be made based on preoperative angiography.

If excision distal to the coronary ostia, which is preferable, can be done, the aorta is divided at this level. The author's preference is for cannulation of both coronary arteries and perfusion during the operative procedure. Others prefer a hypothermic cardioplegic technique, often with potassium.

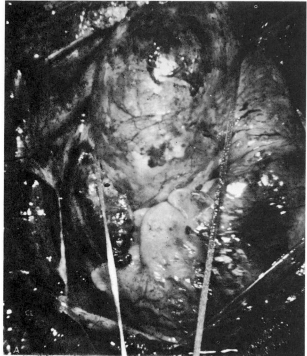

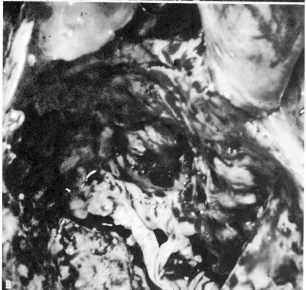

Fig. 20-1. Operative photograph of a patient with a large aneurysm of the ascending aorta. *A.* The aneurysm in the proximal aorta has been isolated and the aorta elevated by encircling umbilical tapes. *B.* Once the aorta has been incised, the incompetent aortic valve is exposed. The aortic insufficiency was produced by dilatation of the aortic annulus.

If aortic valve replacement is required, this is done initially, inserting the prosthetic valve of choice. Our preference is for the Starr-Edwards cloth-covered steel ball prosthesis. With a narrow aortic root, the tilting disc prosthesis of the Björk-Shiley type is preferred.

Subsequently, a preclotted, short, woven Dacron graft, usually about 10 cm long, is inserted to reestablish aortic continuity. Because the aortic wall is thinned by the disease in the media, care must be taken in performing the anastomosis to avoid serious or even fatal hemorrhage. Buttressing the suture lines with pledgets of Teflon felt (Fig. 20-4) is valuable. Other techniques are either preserving the wall of the aneurysm and wrapping it about the graft afterward or constructing a tube of pericardium and sewing this about the graft if there is serious hemorrhage.

Liddicott et al., in 1975, described excision of 100 ascending aortic aneurysms (including 45 dissecting aneurysms) over a period of 10 years. Concomitant replacement of the aortic valve was necessary in 63 patients. Of the 100 aneurysms, 69 were considered to be due to atherosclerosis, 22 to cystic medial necrosis, and 9 to syphilitic aortitis. The average follow-up of 82 surviving patients was 4.7 years, with an actuarial survival rate of 83 percent at 2 years and 70 percent at 8 years.

If the aneurysm extends proximal to the ostia of the coronary arteries, the complex composite operation developed by Dentall in 1968 and later described by Edwards in 1970 seems to be quite satisfactory. In this procedure an aortic prosthetic valve is placed inside a Dacron tube and the composite graft sutured to the aortic annulus. The distal anastomosis is to the distal aorta, and the ostia of the coronary artery are reimplanted into windows made in the side of the graft. The wall of the aneurysm is then closed around the graft. Zubiate and Kay, in 1976, reported experiences with six patients, and recently Kouchoukos et al. described operations on 25 patients with no operative

Fig. 20-2. Patient with a large syphilitic aneurysm eroding through the sternum and projecting beneath the skin. Fortunately such lesions are now rare. An attempt at operative extirpation of the lesion was unsuccessful because of hemorrhage.

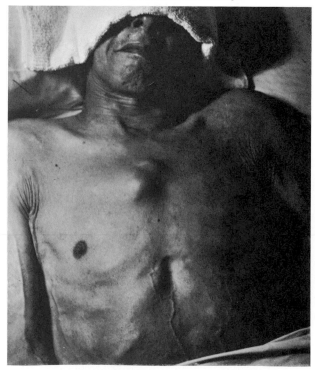

mortality. We have used the procedure several times and have found it quite satisfactory.

In 1975 Griepp et al. reported the use of deep hypothermia and circulatory arrest for simplifying the procedure in four patients, three of whom survived. His technique is shown in Fig. 20-5. Further experience with this method, which could simplify the operative approach, will be significant.

Aneurysms of the Transverse Aortic Arch

Aneurysms of the transverse aortic arch are almost always due to atherosclerosis, rarely syphilis. The diagnosis is usually established by aortography, differentiating the aneurysm from a malignant mediastinal tumor. The degree of involvement of the great vessels arising from the aortic arch also can be determined.

Detailed consideration of the technical management of these aneurysms is beyond the scope of this textbook, but limited pertinent references are listed in the bibliography at the end of the chapter. Because of the complexity of the operative procedure and the high mortality, excision should be attempted only for expanding aneurysms with an obviously impending fatal outcome, usually from tracheal obstruction, unless operation is performed. Surgical excision is a complex undertaking, requiring perfusion of the distal aorta, the great arch vessels, and often the coronary arteries. Hemorrhage and neurologic complications from perfusion of the innominate and carotid arteries have been responsible for an operative mortality often exceeding 60 to 70 percent (Fig. 20-6). Retrograde perfusion of the right brachial artery has been the most satisfactory method of perfusing the right vertebral and right carotid arteries arising from the innominate artery, while perfusion of the left carotid artery has been through direct cannulation. Pressure in the carotid artery should be monitored during perfusion to avoid the extremes of inadequate or excessive perfusion. Surgical techniques have gradually improved and undoubtedly will continue to do so. One remarkable example was published in 1972 by Lefrak et al., who described excision of a massive aneurysm of the aortic arch in a seventy-six-year-old patient which had virtually occluded the trachea. One year later the patient remained well and free of symptoms.

Traumatic Thoracic Aneurysms

ETIOLOGY AND PATHOLOGY. Traumatic aneurysms almost invariably arise from transection of the thoracic aorta associated with closed chest trauma. The section on traumatic rupture of the aorta in this chapter should be read in conjunction with this one, as traumatic rupture and traumatic thoracic aneurysms have a common etiology but a different clinical course. In those few patients fortunate enough not to succumb from exsanguinating hemorrhage an aneurysm will subsequently develop. If a patient survives longer than 6 to 8 weeks following injury, the risk of acute rupture is small. In a review of the English and French literature between 1950 and 1965, Bennett and Cherry found rupture occurring nine times in a total of 105

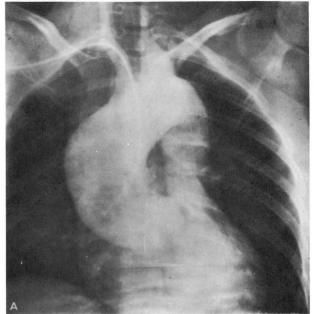

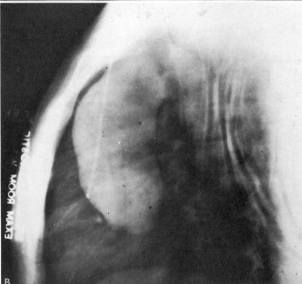

Fig. 20-3. *A.* Posteroanterior view of a thoracic aortogram demonstrating a large aneurysm in the ascending aorta, stopping near the innominate artery. Resection of the aneurysm was successfully performed. The patient was well 5 years following operation. *B.* Lateral view of a thoracic aortogram in the same patient.

aneurysms. The usual course is one of progressive enlargement with compression of adjacent structures.

The aneurysm virtually always arises just distal to the left subclavian artery, opposite the point of insertion of the ligamentum arteriosum. Although a huge aneurysm filling most of the hemithorax may be found, at operation the point of origin is almost invariably found in this area. This localization is a significant one in planning operative therapy, for little disease of the adjacent segments of aorta exists. Reconstruction can usually be done with a short prosthetic graft; occasionally direct anastomosis is possible.

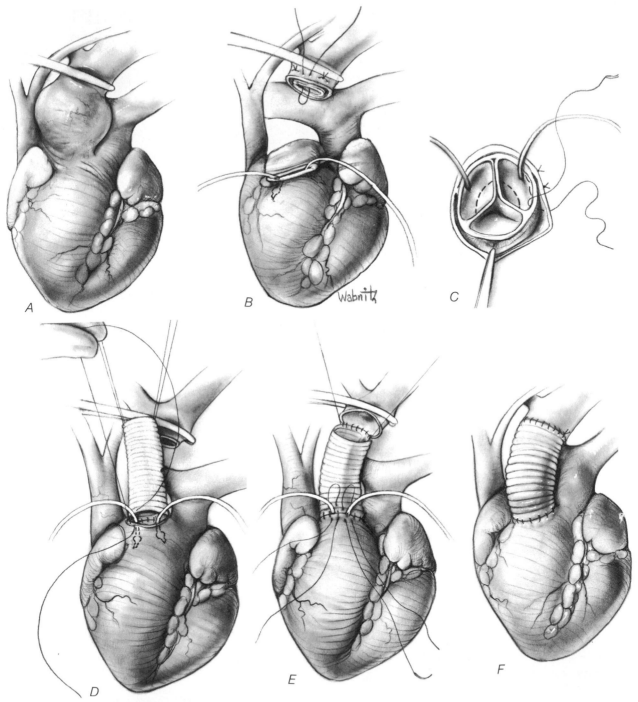

Fig. 20-4. Procedure for excision of dissecting aneurysm of the ascending aorta. *A.* A dissecting aneurysm of the ascending aorta in a patient with the Marfan syndrome. The lesion had produced acute aortic insufficiency. *B.* Initially at operation the aneurysm was excised, and the coronary arteries were perfused to support coronary circulation. Distad the dissected wall of the aorta was approximated with interrupted sutures. *C.* The mechanism of production of aortic insufficiency by an aortic dissection. The area of dissection proceeds proximally to detach the aortic cusps from the aortic wall, permitting them to prolapse into the lumen and cause aortic insufficiency. Prolapse of the right and left coronary cusps is minimized by the location of the coronary artery; hence, dissection of the noncoronary cusp is the most extensive. Reapproximation of the aortic wall may correct the insufficiency. *D.* Aortic reconstruction is performed with a woven Dacron graft, performing the anastomosis with continuous silk sutures. The disease in the aortic wall results in unusual friability, which may make adequate hemostasis difficult. *E.* The proximal anastomosis is completed, leaving the coronary cannulae in position. The distal anastomosis is then similarly performed, after which the coronary catheters are withdrawn and aortic circulation reestablished.

CLINICAL MANIFESTATIONS. Unlike most aneurysms from other causes, traumatic thoracic aneurysms enlarge slowly and in some patients have apparently remained stationary for 10 to 20 years, the diagnosis being made in retrospect after finding an asymptomatic aneurysm with a history of closed-chest trauma 10 to 20 years before. A detailed study of the natural "life history" of such aneurysms was reported by Bennett and Cherry in 1967. As the aneurysm enlarges, compression of the left main bron-

Fig. 20-5. Operative procedure for aortic arch replacement. (*Griepp et al., Thorac Cardiovasc Surg, 70:1051, 1975.*)

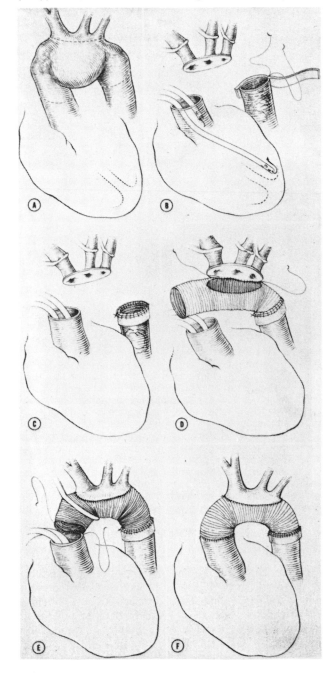

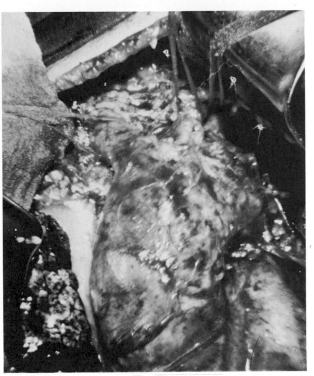

Fig. 20-6. Operative photograph of a patient with aneurysm of the aortic arch. The procedure is a complicated one requiring multiple bypass grafts, temporarily diverting blood through bypass channels to the carotid arteries and distal aorta while the aneurysm is excised and the aortic arch reconstructed.

chus with pain, dyspnea, cough, and atelectasis are the predominant complications. Hoarseness from compression and distortion of the left recurrent laryngeal nerve may appear. These symptoms usually well precede enlargement of the aneurysm to such a degree that rupture occurs. This course of events is emphasized because of the small risk of rupture, which is in direct contrast to factors governing the surgical policy with the majority of aneurysms from atherosclerosis or syphilis, where the threat of rupture constitutes a major reason for recommending elective excision as soon as possible.

Frequently there are no abnormalities on physical examination unless compression of the main bronchus has produced atelectasis of the left lung. A murmur is usually not heard, and there is no abnormality of peripheral pulses.

DIAGNOSTIC FINDINGS. The chest roentgenogram usually discloses an ovoid density near the left subclavian artery. If an aneurysm has been present for several years, calcification is often visible in the wall. The diagnosis can be established by aortography, which is required to delineate the extent of the aneurysm and to differentiate it from other mediastinal tumors (Fig. 20-7).

TREATMENT. The problem of management of acute rupture of the thoracic aorta, with the risk of exsanguinating hemorrhage, is presented in the section on Wounds of the Great Vessels. Elective excision is recommended for the majority of patients, although probably 20 to 30 per-

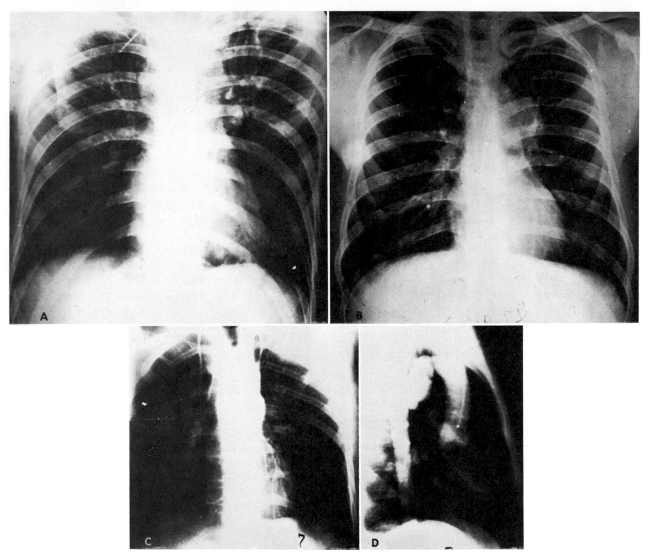

Fig. 20-7. A. Chest roentgenogram following an automobile accident, demonstrating widening of the mediastinum with subcutaneous emphysema. Traumatic rupture of the aorta was not recognized at this time. B. Chest roentgenogram 5 months after the injury demonstrated a left upper mediastinal mass. C. Postero-anterior view of an aortogram demonstrating a localized thoracic aneurysm. This lesion was excised successfully. D. Lateral view of an aortogram in the same patient. E. Chest roentgenogram in a different patient 2 years after an automobile accident demonstrated an asymptomatic mass in the upper mediastinum. F. Aortography demonstrated a saccular thoracic aneurysm, which was subsequently resected successfully. G. Aortogram in the same patient as in F. This film demonstrated the size and extent of the aneurysm as additional contrast material flowed freely within the lesion.

cent of aneurysms remain stationary and asymptomatic for many years. Apparently most aneurysms, despite long latent periods of stability, eventually progressively enlarge. When serious associated disease, such as coronary atherosclerosis, is present, observation with serial chest roentgenograms may be safely employed.

Technique of Operation. A left posterolateral thoracotomy through the fourth or fifth intercostal space is used. Initially the aorta is mobilized and encircled proximal and distal to the aneurysm. Proximal involvement of the left subclavian artery often requires encirclement of the aorta between the left carotid and the left subclavian arteries. This is facilitated by opening the pericardium and dissecting the intrapericardial portion of the aortic arch. The vagus nerve with the recurrent laryngeal nerve should also be mobilized and protected, for the recurrent laryngeal is often adherent to the wall of the aneurysm.

Once the aorta has been encircled proximally and distad and the recurrent laryngeal nerve mobilized as much as possible, further dissection is unnecessary. Some form of

aortic bypass should then be established to maintain flow to the distal aorta during aortic occlusion and prevent ischemic injury of the spinal cord and kidneys. Without an aortic bypass, paraplegia has been reported to develop within as short a time as 20 to 25 minutes of aortic occlusion.

The first effective technique of aortic bypass was the left

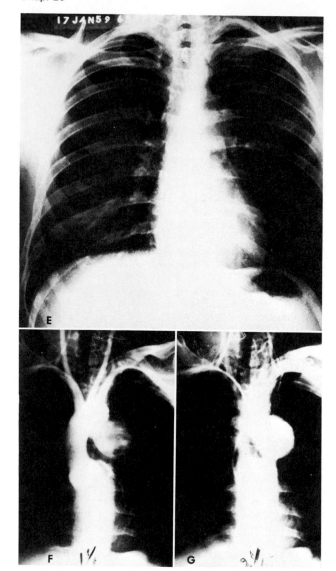

Fig. 20-7 *E-G.* (See legend on facing page.)

shunts was greatly aided by the work by Gott, who developed a method of temporarily binding heparin to the surface of polyvinyl tubes. Different techniques for temporary shunts without any heparin have been reported, but there seems to be little reason not to use the temporary heparin tubes.

In 1972 Krauss and associates described experiences with the Gott shunt in 8 patients. Several reports from that time have described good results with the shunt. A recent report by Donahoo et al. described a ten-year experience.

As described in the following section, Crawford and associates have utilized the interesting approach of not employing any type of shunt at all, simply minimizing the period of ischemia of the aorta. They have properly emphasized that many factors besides the use of a shunt influence paraplegia, such as vessels arising from the aneurysm which may supply the spinal cord and blood pressure before and after excision of the aneurysm, which in turn would influence the rate of flow of blood through the impaired collateral circulation. Although this technique is not one the author would prefer, the Crawford observations are quite significant.

After the type of shunt has been selected and the aorta appropriately localized and occluded proximal and distal to the aneurysm, it is incised, after which the point of origin can be identified as a transverse laceration or transection near the point of insertion of the ligamentum arteriosum. The aorta proximal and distal is usually normal; therefore it is unnecessary to excise any significant length of aorta. The inner lining of the aneurysmal sac may be removed, but it is unnecessary and unwise to attempt complete excision, partly because of vascular adhesions surrounding the wall of the aneurysm. In most patients a 5- to 8-cm segment of woven Dacron graft is sufficient to restore arterial continuity.

Convalescence following operation is usually uneventful, and long-term results are excellent. The risk of operation is probably less than 5 percent. One of the largest groups of patients has been reported by Cooley et al., operating on over 86 such lesions without any operative mortality. The low mortality is due to both the young age and the localized nature of the aneurysm.

Aneurysms of the Descending Thoracic Aorta

ETIOLOGY AND INCIDENCE. Aneurysms in the descending thoracic aorta may result from atherosclerosis, syphilis, trauma, or a dissection of the aortic wall. Most are due to atherosclerosis and are exceeded only by abdominal aneurysms in frequency of occurrence. They are most frequently found in men in the fifth to the seventh decades. Formerly, saccular aneurysms from syphilis were common, but these are now rare. Dissecting aneurysms and traumatic aneurysms are considered in the accompanying sections.

The majority of atherosclerotic aneurysms are located in the proximal part of the descending thoracic aorta, beginning distal to the left subclavian artery. They extend for varying distances and in some instances can involve the entire descending thoracic aorta. They are generally

atrial-femoral bypass, withdrawing blood through a cannula inserted into the left atrium, which in turn is pumped to the distal arterial tree, usually the left iliac, occasionally the distal aorta. Flow rates of 2 to 2.5 liters/minute are required to maintain the base-line pressure in the proximal aorta as well as to maintain distal aortic pressure between 60 and 75 mm Hg. This technique has been widely used but has the disadvantage of increased bleeding associated with systemic heparinization.

If access to the left atrium is awkward, a femoral artery–femoral vein cannulation can be carried out and a pump oxygenator used in the circuit to perfuse the lower half of the body while the aorta is clamped, letting the heart and lungs perfuse the upper half normally.

To avoid the need for heparin, there has been increasing use of different types of temporary shunt inserted between the proximal and distal aorta. This technique has become the one of choice at New York University. The safety of

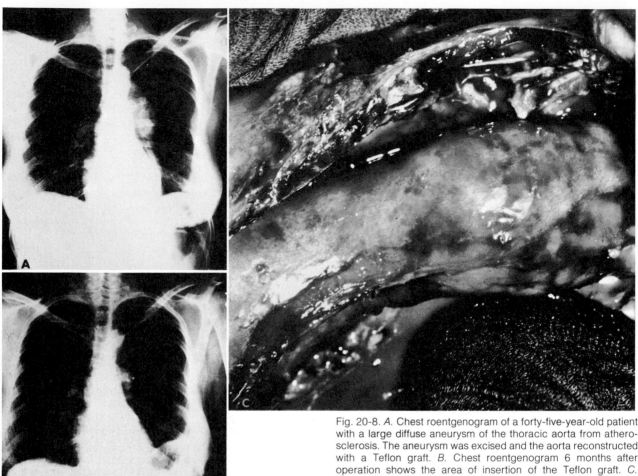

Fig. 20-8. *A.* Chest roentgenogram of a forty-five-year-old patient with a large diffuse aneurysm of the thoracic aorta from atherosclerosis. The aneurysm was excised and the aorta reconstructed with a Teflon graft. *B.* Chest roentgenogram 6 months after operation shows the area of insertion of the Teflon graft. *C.* Operative photograph of atherosclerotic aneurysm demonstrated in the chest roentgenogram seen in *A.*

fusiform (Fig. 20-8), in contrast to syphilitic saccular aneurysms. Their rate of growth is significantly slower than that of abdominal aneurysms, with a less malignant tendency toward rapid enlargement and rupture, but eventual rupture is the outcome in most cases unless other complications of atherosclerosis appear. Syphilitic saccular aneurysms, by contrast, usually rapidly enlarge and rupture, a high percentage rupturing within 2 years after the diagnosis is made. Erosion of bone, commonly seen with saccular syphilitic aneurysms, is unusual with fusiform atherosclerotic aneurysms.

CLINICAL MANIFESTATIONS. In many patients a thoracic aneurysm is found as an asymptomatic mass on a chest roentgenogram made for other reasons. Probably the most common symptoms from enlargement result from compression or erosion of the lung, or compression and obstruction of the left main bronchus with resulting dyspnea and atelectasis. Erosion into the bronchus will produce hemoptysis. Involvement of the left recurrent laryngeal nerve where it encircles the ligamentum arteriosum may lead to paralysis of the vocal cord with hoarseness. In contrast to abdominal aneurysms, where acute rupture may be the first indication of a previously unsuspected aneurysm, such a sequence of events is unusual with a thoracic aneurysm.

Physical examination often yields entirely normal findings. Infrequently, a bruit may be heard over the left chest, loudest in the left paravertebral area. Peripheral pulses are frequently normal, unless involvement of the left subclavian artery produces hypotension in the left arm.

DIAGNOSTIC FINDINGS. The diagnosis can usually be suspected from the appearance of the mass in the region of the aorta on the chest roentgenogram. The differential diagnosis includes other conditions producing an opacity on the chest roentgenogram, such as bronchogenic carcinoma, metastatic carcinoma, or rarely esophageal tumors. Laminar calcification may be visible in the wall of the aorta. Aortography is used both to confirm the diagnosis and to delineate the precise extent of the aneurysm. An electrocardiogram and a blood urea nitrogen determination should be routinely obtained, because atherosclerotic disease in other organs, especially the heart and kidney, is frequent.

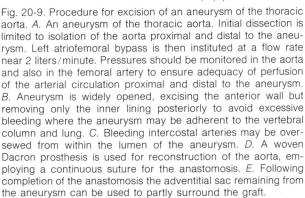

Fig. 20-9. Procedure for excision of an aneurysm of the thoracic aorta. *A.* An aneurysm of the thoracic aorta. Initial dissection is limited to isolation of the aorta proximal and distal to the aneurysm. Left atriofemoral bypass is then instituted at a flow rate near 2 liters/minute. Pressures should be monitored in the aorta and also in the femoral artery to ensure adequacy of perfusion of the arterial circulation proximal and distal to the aneurysm. *B.* Aneurysm is widely opened, excising the anterior wall but removing only the inner lining posteriorly to avoid excessive bleeding where the aneurysm may be adherent to the vertebral column and lung. *C.* Bleeding intercostal arteries may be oversewed from within the lumen of the aneurysm. *D.* A woven Dacron prosthesis is used for reconstruction of the aorta, employing a continuous suture for the anastomosis. *E.* Following completion of the anastomosis the adventitial sac remaining from the aneurysm can be used to partly surround the graft.

TREATMENT. In most patients once the diagnosis of a discrete aneurysm has been made, excision should be recommended. With small aneurysms, associated with significant coronary or cerebrovascular disease, observation with frequent chest roentgenograms to evaluate the rate of enlargement may be safely employed. Serial observations also may be preferable in some patients with a diffuse fusiform dilatation of the entire thoracic aorta.

The technique of operation is detailed in Fig. 20-9. As mentioned in the section on Traumatic Thoracic Aneurysms, the major hazards are operative hemorrhage and ischemic injury to the spinal cord and kidneys while the aorta is clamped and the aneurysm excised. The different methods for perfusing the distal aorta to protect the spinal cord and kidneys are discussed in that section. Either the conventional left atriofemoral bypass, which has the advantage of simplicity but the disadvantage of systemic heparinization, should be used, or some type of temporary shunt without heparin should be employed. Our preference for the last 3 or 4 years has been the Gott shunt, inserted proximally into the ascending aorta and distally into the femoral vessels. In the unusual case where this does not function satisfactorily, one of the forms of bypass with heparin can be employed. Whatever method of perfusion is employed, it is important to monitor pressure in the distal aorta, keeping mean pressure above 60 mm Hg. Pressure in the proximal aorta is similarly monitored to avoid excessive hypertension which may precipitate left ventricular failure, especially in the presence of preexisting coronary disease.

As with aneurysms elsewhere, an important principal in minimizing operative hemorrhage is to avoid an attempt to completely excise the aneurysm, especially when the wall is adherent to the lung or vertebral column. Initial dissection should be limited to encircling the aorta proximally and distad. Once aortic bypass has been instituted, the aorta can be occluded with clamps and the aneurysm opened widely. The inner wall then can be removed, suturing the ostia of any patent intercostal vessels but leaving the outer adventitial layers to avoid bleeding. Following excision of the aneurysm, aortic continuity is reestablished with a vascular prosthesis (Fig. 20-10). Our preference is for woven Dacron prostheses, carefully preclotted, inserted with continuous synthetic sutures. The remaining adventitial wall of the aneurysm then can be wrapped around the prosthesis to further minimize bleeding.

The most serious complication is paraplegia. Fortunately this is rare with adequate aortic bypass. In some instances, however, some degree of spinal cord injury has occurred despite seemingly adequate bypass, probably as a consequence of ligation of intercostal arteries during excision of the aneurysm. As the blood supply to the spinal cord is highly variable, it is impossible to know which, if any, intercostal arteries are vital to spinal cord circulation. Fortunately, with many thoracic aneurysms intercostal arteries arising from the aneurysm have become occluded beforehand by thrombus. Although some patients have tolerated excision of the entire thoracic aorta uneventfully, it is probably wise to limit the degree of excision of adjacent thoracic aorta, even though moderate disease and dilatation are present, especially if large patent intercostal arteries are seen arising from this segment.

Following recovery from operation, the prognosis is favorable and related chiefly to the extent of atherosclerotic disease in other organs. Complications from the prosthetic graft or the adjacent diseased aorta are unusual. With experienced surgical groups, the operative mortality is in the range of 10 to 15 percent. This varies both with

Fig. 20-10. A. Operative photograph of saccular syphilitic aneurysm of distal thoracic aorta. B. Teflon graft used to restore continuity following excision of a syphilitic aneurysm of the lower thoracic aorta. This graft was used in the patient seen in A.

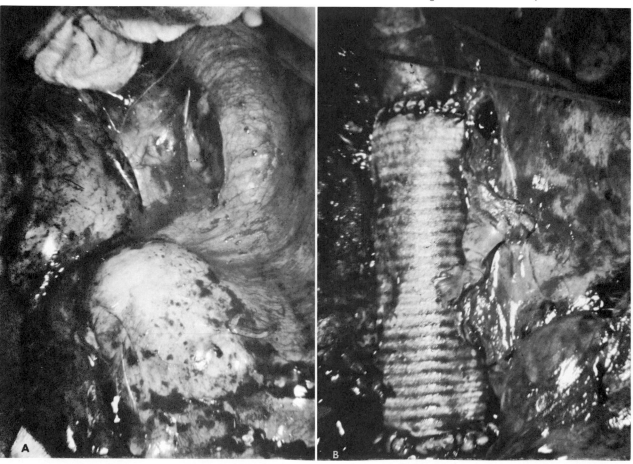

the size of the aneurysm and with the age of the patient; for larger aneurysms there is a greater operative risk from hemorrhage. Actually there is only a limited amount of data in the surgical literature concerning excision. It is probable that infrequently performed operations for thoracic aneurysm have a much higher mortality rate. In a report of 237 aneurysms treated at The Johns Hopkins Hospital between 1952 and 1959 by Vasko and associates, there were only eight patients with thoracic aneurysms due to syphilis or atherosclerosis. All survived operation, but three died within 2 years from further vascular complications. In 1966 Bloodwell and associates described experiences with nearly 400 thoracic aneurysms, but detailed analysis of these cases was not presented. The low mortality reported by Krauss et al. in 1972 in the series of eight patients with seven survivors in whom the temporary heparinized shunt was used indicates the progressive improvement in surgical mortality with improved techniques.

Thoracoabdominal Aneurysms

These aneurysms fortunately are rare, because their excision is a complicated surgical procedure, involving restoration of blood flow to the celiac, superior mesenteric, and renal arteries. Such procedures have usually been performed with multiple bypass techniques to minimize duration of ischemia to different organs, but operative mortality has remained high. More recently some procedures have been performed with a simple left atriofemoral bypass, opening the aneurysm widely and attempting to reestablish flow to different organs with a relatively short period of ischemia.

INCIDENCE AND ETIOLOGY. The rarity of such aneurysms is indicated in the report by DeBakey and associates of experiences with treating over 2,000 aneurysms of the abdominal aorta below the renal arteries, during which less than 50 of these aneurysms above the renal arteries were treated. They are usually due to atherosclerosis, rarely to cystic medial necrosis as in the Marfan syndrome. In the group of 42 patients reported by DeBakey et al., 62 percent resulted from atherosclerosis, and 26 percent were due to syphilis.

CLINICAL MANIFESTATIONS. The rate of enlargement is slow, and excision should be attempted only for expanding aneurysms causing symptoms from compression and displacement of adjacent structures. Often the aneurysm cannot be palpated, because it is concealed in the upper abdomen by the stomach and pancreas. The diagnosis may be suspected from the chest roentgenogram disclosing enlargement of the thoracic aorta near the diaphragm, but aortography is required to confirm the diagnosis.

TREATMENT. Most of the earlier operations have been performed with a multiple bypass technique, inserting an initial bypass graft from the thoracic aorta above the aneurysm to the abdominal aorta below the origin of the renal arteries. From this initial graft, branch grafts are then serially inserted to the celiac artery, superior mesenteric artery, and both renal arteries. Once the grafts have been inserted, avoiding prolonged ischemia of any individual organ, the aneurysm can be opened widely and the inner lining removed. Anastomosis to the right renal artery may be more conveniently performed at this time.

These procedures have been performed through a variety of thoracic and abdominal incisions. A thoracoabdominal incision from a left lateral position has been employed, or a separate midline abdominal incision combined with a left thoracotomy incision.

In recent years Cooley and others have reported the use of left atriofemoral bypass for excision of the aneurysm, establishing bypass and then opening the aneurysm widely, followed by direct anastomoses to the involved visceral arteries with a long straight graft. This technique must be accomplished in a short period of time, however, to avoid significant ischemic injury.

Patients surviving this complex operative procedure have had a fairly good prognosis. In the group of 42 surgically treated patients reported by DeBakey in 1965, 11 died within 1 month of operation, a mortality of 26 percent. There were four deaths subsequently, but the remaining 27 patients were alive without significant disability at the time of the report. The longest individual follow-up was about 10 years (Fig. 20-11).

Fig. 20-11. Angiogram of Dacron graft 1 year after excision of thoracoabdominal aneurysm. The graft was inserted between the thoracic aorta, as an end-to-side anastomosis, and the abdominal aorta, not shown in this illustration. Side branches to the superior mesenteric artery, celiac artery, and right and left renal arteries are individually visible.

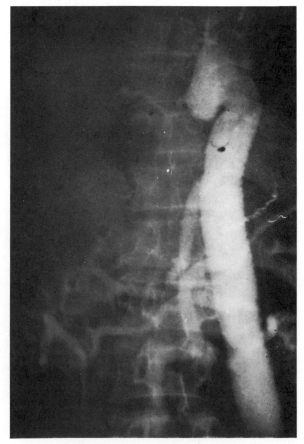

A most significant report came from Crawford and associates in 1973, reporting experiences with 84 patients, 38 in whom some type of bypass was used and 45 more recent cases in which shunting was avoided. The significance of this paper is that with a simplified technique mortality was 8.8 percent versus 21 percent when a shunt was employed. It may be hoped that others can duplicate this impressive record. Basically, their technique avoided heparin or shunting but opened the aneurysm widely and used the "button" technique to anastomose the ostia of the distal vessel to appropriate windows in the side of the aneurysm, minimizing the ischemia time.

DISSECTING ANEURYSMS

ETIOLOGY AND INCIDENCE. Dissecting aneurysms are related to degenerative disease of the media of the aorta, the cause of which is unknown. The disease is about three times as common in males as in females and is most frequently seen in patients in the fifth and sixth decades. However, it can occur in almost any age group, one of the youngest patients being only 14 months of age. The most frequently associated factor is hypertension, present in 75 to 85 percent of patients, although the reported incidence has varied widely.

Conditions associated with abnormalities of connective tissue have a greater frequency with dissecting aneurysm. The most common of these is the Marfan syndrome. Before surgical therapy was available, most patients with the Marfan syndrome succumbed either from a dissecting aneurysm or from aortic insufficiency as a result of dilatation of the aortic annulus. Other conditions occasionally associated with dissecting aneurysm include coarctation of

the aorta, pregnancy, and kyphoscoliosis. Atherosclerosis is not a definite causative factor. The segment of aorta most frequently involved is different in the two diseases, since dissecting aneurysm usually involves the proximal thoracic aorta while atherosclerosis is most severe near the bifurcation of the abdominal aorta. There is also no known relationship to trauma or syphilis.

Experimentally, dissecting aneurysm can be produced in young rats with a diet containing 50 percent sweet peas, which causes a distinct abnormality of connective tissue, known as *lathyrism*. The abnormal chemical agent that weakens the cross-linking of collagen is a β-amino nitrite.

PATHOLOGY. The term "dissecting aneurysm" is actually a misnomer, for the pathologic lesion is more accurately described as a "dissecting hematoma," consisting of a hemorrhagic separation of the layers of the aortic wall (Fig. 20-12). The basic lesion is degeneration of the aortic media, often associated with rupture of the vasa vasorum. Most patients also have a tear in the intima of the aorta, establishing a communication between the lumen of the aorta and the hematoma in the aortic wall. Whether the tear in the intima is a primary or secondary event is uncertain. If it is the primary event, superimposed upon underlying disease of the aortic media, the progressive dissection of the aortic wall which follows may result from establishing a communication between the lumen of the aorta and the aortic wall. The alternative hypothesis is that

Fig. 20-12. *A.* Photograph of dissecting aneurysm of the thoracic aorta operated upon a few days after onset of the dissection. The lung is being separated from the aneurysm. Hematoma in the wall of the dissected aorta is visible. *B.* With a left atriofemoral bypass functioning and the aorta occluded, the aneurysm has been incised. The lacerated edges of the aortic wall from the dissection can be seen. Clot is visible in the wall of the aorta superior to the tip of the metal aspirator.

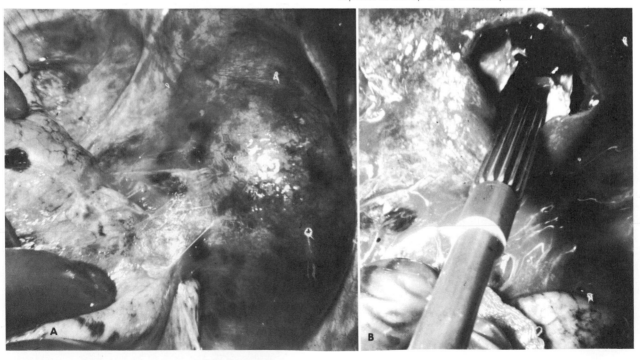

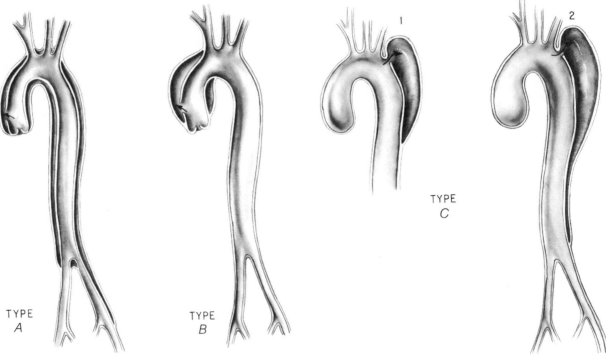

Fig. 20-13. Different types of aortic dissection. *A.* Dissecting aneurysm which begins in the ascending aorta near the aortic valve and extends throughout the aorta down to the external iliac arteries. Unfortunately, this is a common type of dissecting aneurysm. *B.* Dissecting aneurysm limited to the ascending aorta. This is commonly seen in the Marfan syndrome. *C*1. Dissecting aneurysm beginning distal to the left subclavian artery. The localized nature of this aneurysm makes it readily accessible to surgical excision. 2. Dissecting aneurysm arising distal to the left subclavian artery but extending into the abdominal aorta. Only partial excision of the area of dissection is possible.

rupture of the vasa vasorum is the primary event, creating an intramural hemorrhage, which secondarily ruptures through the intima to establish communication with the aortic lumen. Rarely no intimal laceration can be found at autopsy, which indicates that rupture of the vasa vasorum was the primary event. The frequency with which tears of the intima are localized either to the ascending aorta or near the ligamentum arteriosum, however, suggests that laceration of the intima is probably the initial event in the majority of patients.

Two clinical observations indicate that in the majority of patients the tear of the intima is the significant event. First, at operation often not all of the diseased aorta is excised but simply the area in which the intima is torn in the major area of disruption of the aorta. With dissection starting near the left subclavian, the origin is excised and perhaps one-half of the distal thoracic aorta with the remaining dissected aorta is left, approximating the intima to obliterate the false lumen. In these patients the dissection process often extends below the diaphragm. The fact that "recurrent" dissecting aneurysms have not been reported, although corrective operations have now been performed for several years, reinforces the fact that if the tear in the

intima is excised and the hypertension controlled, recurrence is rare. This is particularly noteworthy with Marfan's syndrome, where the primary connective tissue defect cannot be corrected. In such patients, recurrence following successful excision of a dissecting aneurysm is thus far virtually unknown.

In 60 to 70 percent of patients the dissection originates in the ascending aorta, while in about 25 percent it originates beyond the left subclavian artery near the ligamentum arteriosum (Fig. 20-13). Infrequently it may originate in the aortic arch or at more distal locations in the aorta.

Once a dissection has begun, it may extend progressively to involve all of the thoracic and abdominal aorta as well as many of the arterial tributaries. This occurs in a high percentage of patients. As dissection progresses, branch vessels are sheared off, either becoming obliterated or establishing a communication with the false lumen created by the dissection. Proximally, the coronary arteries may be involved, and frequently one or more aortic valve cusps are detached and prolapse into the lumen, creating aortic insufficiency. More distad the vessels involved may include any tributary of the aorta. Involvement of the carotid arteries may produce neurologic injury. Obstruction of the subclavian arteries produces differences in blood pressure between the two arms. Dissection of intercostal arteries may cause spinal cord injury with paraplegia. Dissection of renal arteries may produce fatal renal insufficiency; in the extremities acute obstruction of the iliac or femoral arteries can result in either claudication or gangrene.

The dissection may terminate fatally at any time by rupture of the false lumen. The usual mode of death is rupture into the pericardial cavity from proximal dissection or rupture into the left pleural cavity. In the extensive review of 425 cases by Hirst et al., 21 percent of the patients died within 24 hours and 74 percent within 2 weeks. Ninety-one percent had succumbed within 6 months. In a group of 50 patients reported from the Massachusetts General Hospital by Austen et al., 45 percent died in the first week, 75 percent in the first month, and 86 percent within the first year. In evaluating mortality statistics, it is important to differentiate dissections arising in the ascending aorta from dissections arising distal to the left subclavian artery. The former have a much higher mortality rate. In a group of 62 patients reported by Lindsay and Hurst, almost all 40 patients with dissection involving the ascending aorta succumbed within 3 weeks, while in the group of 19 patients in whom the disease began distal to the aortic arch the survival was greater than 50 percent.

In patients who survive with a dissecting aneurysm an endothelial lining of the false lumen, termed a *healed dissecting aneurysm,* may develop and establish a so-called "double-barreled" aorta. A wide variety of bizarre circulatory patterns may be found in such patients. For example, one renal artery may arise from the "false" lumen and the other from the true lumen (Fig. 20-14), or alternatively both renal arteries can arise from the false lumen. In other patients, one iliac artery may originate from the false lumen, and the other from the true lumen.

In the few patients surviving an aortic dissection, rupture of the false lumen back into the true aortic lumen has often been found at the termination of the dissection. This spontaneous "reentry" into the aortic lumen suggested that establishing a communication between the false lumen and the true lumen might terminate the dissecting process. These observations led to the development of the aortic fenestration operation, originally attempted by Gurin and by Shaw, and later extensively used by DeBakey and associates. At the time of introduction of this operation, little else could be offered such patients. Significant benefit

from fenestration operations has been meager, however, and the operation has now been almost completely abandoned as more effective methods of therapy have been developed. The failure of development of a reentry area to protect against external rupture was noted by McCloy and associates. In a group of 22 patients who died from external rupture of a dissecting aneurysm, 11 had developed a point of reentry of the dissection into the aortic lumen, but this had not prevented fatal rupture.

CLINICAL MANIFESTATIONS. The abrupt onset of excruciating pain, almost immediately reaching its peak intensity, is very characteristic of a dissecting aneurysm. A myocardial infarction, by contrast, may gradually develop pain of increasing severity over several minutes. Usually anterior chest pain develops with dissection of the ascending aorta, while back pain is more common with dissection beginning distal to the aortic arch. Pain may be in both the front and back of the chest with dissection of either type, but usually predominant back pain suggests dissection beyond the left subclavian artery. Another significant characteristic of the pain is its tendency to migrate into different areas as dissection extends distad. As might be predicted from the wide variation in the extent of the dissection process, many pain syndromes may occur. Pain

Fig. 20-14. *A.* Aortogram showing an unusual pattern of aortic dissection in which dissection extended from the thoracic aorta into the abdominal aorta, creating two lumens, with the right renal artery arising from one and the left renal artery from the other. Focal stenosis of the right common iliac artery is seen at the lower part of the field producing intermittent claudication, which was the presenting complaint of the patient. *B.* Aortogram performed by a different root opacifies the left kidney and the left common iliac artery. The condition of the dissected aorta is illustrated in the accompanying drawing. Circulation was reestablished by excising the septum between the two channels at the aortic bifurcation. (*Adapted from W. Gryboski and F. C. Spencer, Intermittent Claudication Caused by a Dissecting Aneurysm of the Aorta, South Med J, 58:593, 1965.*)

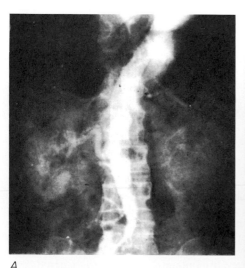

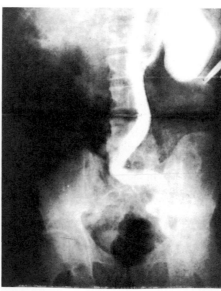

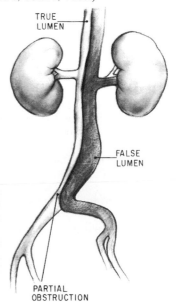

A

B

may radiate to the neck, the arm, the epigastrium, or the leg. Seldom is pain completely absent, probably in no more than 10 percent of patients.

Syncope occurs in 10 to 20 percent of patients, and some neurologic symptoms are present in 20 to 40 percent. These may result from ischemia of the brain, spinal cord, or a peripheral nerve, depending upon whether a carotid artery, an intercostal artery, or a peripheral artery has been compromised.

Hypertension, often of severe degree, is present in 75 to 85 percent of patients. Often the hypertension with severe vasoconstriction contrasts with the clinical picture of an acutely ill patient, pale, sweating, and in acute distress. An aortic diastolic murmur appears in 20 to 30 percent of patients and is of great diagnostic significance, usually originating from detachment of an aortic valve cusp. Less frequently a pericardial friction rub may be audible due to leakage of blood into the pericardial cavity. Inequality of the carotid or subclavian pulses may be found, caused by unequal compression of these vessels. A variety of neurologic abnormalities may be detected, the most common being either a monoplegia or paraplegia.

DIAGNOSTIC FINDINGS. On the chest roentgenogram a widened mediastinum or a left pleural effusion from extravasation of blood is frequently seen. In some patients, however, the roentgenogram may be completely normal. The electrocardiogram is of particular value in distinguishing dissecting aneurysm from myocardial infarction, but there are no characteristic features of aortic dissection. The most common abnormality is left ventricular hypertrophy from the antecedent hypertension.

Aortography to demonstrate the double lumen created by the dissection is the most definitive diagnostic procedure. In some patients a diagnosis cannot be established by any other technique, especially if there are no abnormal physical findings and the only abnormality is a history of severe back pain.

The importance of aortography in any patient with unexplained sustained severe pain cannot be overemphasized. The history of pain may be the *only* abnormality found on subsequent examination. Occasionally a patient is seen a few days or weeks after an acute dissection with no symptoms and no abnormality on physical examination, electrocardiogram, or chest x-ray. Only aortography provides the diagnosis. Similarly, severe pain without abnormal findings in patients in whom aortography was not done has been followed by exsanguination within a few hours or days.

TREATMENT. The most effective treatment for acute dissecting aneurysm has not yet been determined. The ideal form of therapy, drug or surgical, is still uncertain, but with improvement in surgical techniques, the trend is toward the emergency use of drug therapy until the patient is stabilized, followed by prompt operation. How promptly operation should be performed varies among different centers, with Najafi et al. operating on some such patients with the same urgency as for a ruptured abdominal aneurysm, while others may wait for 2 to 7 days.

There is no question that emergency institution of antihypertensive therapy is the top priority in treatment, for this may arrest the dissection process and lessen the risk of fatal hemorrhage. Unfortunately, fatal hemorrhage has occurred in some patients who were asymptomatic and seemingly stable with drug therapy. Hence the prevailing trend is for operation at an appropriate time, probably the sooner the better, once the patient's condition has stabilized, perhaps earlier if drug therapy is not satisfactory and signs of rupture persist such as continued pain, hemothorax, or other signs of leakage of blood into the body cavities. As mentioned earlier, the appearance of a diastolic murmur, indicating detachment of an aortic cusp, is a particularly ominous finding. In 1976 Kirklin reported experiences from the University of Alabama, a total of 108 cases, and concluded that operation was the therapy of choice. The urgency of treatment is well emphasized by the grim mortality statistics, with 40 to 50 percent of patients dying within 2 weeks and the majority of those surviving the first 2 weeks succumbing within 1 year. Only about 10 percent of untreated patients survive beyond this time.

It is important in evaluating different forms of therapy to separate patients with dissections of the ascending aorta from patients in whom the dissection is distal to the aortic arch. The prognosis is much worse with dissections in the ascending aorta, with an acute mortality exceeding 90 percent in some series.

A significant addition to the therapy of dissecting aneurysms was made by Wheat and associates in 1965 when they reported the successful treatment of six patients with antihypertensive drugs. These studies were partly stimulated by observations from the poultry industry that certain flocks of turkeys had a high fatality rate from spontaneous dissecting aneurysm which could be reduced dramatically by adding to the food a small amount of reserpine (0.1 part to 1 million). Wheat et al. noted that their patients often lived a few hours to a few days following onset of the aortic dissection, only to succumb from continued dissection with eventual rupture. Because of the high frequency of hypertension in this group of patients, antihypertensive drugs were utilized to ameliorate the dissecting process. The therapeutic program included the immediate lowering of blood pressure by an intravenous infusion of Arfonad (trimethaphan), combined with the simultaneous administration of reserpine, chlorothiazide (Diuril), and guanethidine (Ismelin). Other investigators employing this form of therapy have substituted methyldopa (Aldomet) for guanethidine. Harris et al. stated that 19 of 21 patients had survived treatment with induced hypotension, 18 of whom were living and well with no progression of the disease. Austen and associates, in contrast, had a 60 percent mortality in patients with acute dissection.

At this time the ultimate role of drug therapy remains uncertain. Although Wheat and associates have obtained an impressively low mortality in their series of patients, others have been unable to duplicate these findings. With improved surgical techniques there has been an increasing tendency to perform early operation, within either a few hours or a few days after onset of symptoms. Data supporting an early operative approach were published in 1970 by Daily et al. and in 1972 by Liotta et al., by Shumacker, and by Najafi and associates.

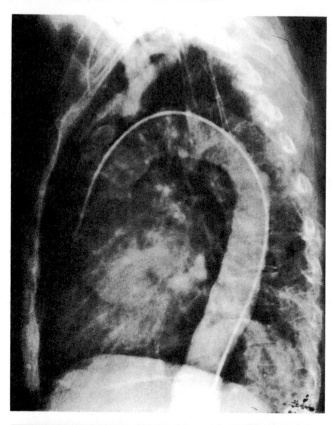

Fig. 20-15. *Opposite.* Thoracic aortogram, performed with a catheter introduced retrograde through the femoral artery, showing a dissecting aneurysm arising distal to the left subclavian artery. The outer channel is faintly visualized as a double density beyond the left subclavian artery. *Lower left.* Operative photograph of dissecting aneurysm arising distal to the left subclavian artery. A clamp is visible on the aorta proximal to the left subclavian artery, which has been encircled with an umbilical tape. The vagus nerve is visible proximally. Laminated clot was found in the lumen of the aneurysm. *Lower right.* Dacron graft inserted to restore aortic continuity following excision of the aneurysm.

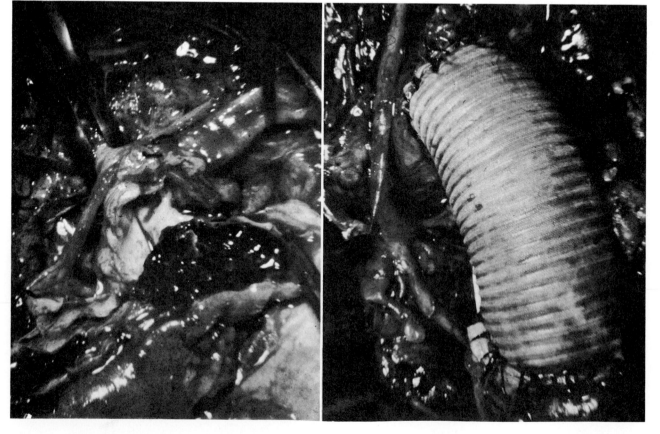

Although the final role of antihypertensive therapy is uncertain, its value is obvious as emergency therapy in the presence of severe hypertension to slow or reduce the dissecting process. Once the patient's condition is stabilized, emergency aortography can be performed to identify the area of dissection. From the location of the dissection, a decision can be made whether to perform emergency operation or not. Operation is simpler if dissection is located distal to the left subclavian artery. At New York University most patients in this category have been operated upon promptly, excising the area of dissection and restoring arterial continuity with a woven Dacron prosthesis (Figs. 20-15 and 20-16). If the dissection extends throughout the thoracic aorta, only the major area of involvement is removed, and the layers of the dissected aorta are sewed together distad before insertion of the prosthetic graft.

When operation is performed upon patients with dissection of the ascending aorta, the preferred treatment is excision of the ascending aorta and reconstruction with a Dacron prosthetic graft. Concomitant aortic insufficiency may be treated by reattachment of the prolapsed aortic valve cusps, occasionally by prosthetic valve replacement (Fig. 20-4). If the dissection has extended into the transverse arch and involves the origin of the great vessels, excision is probably best limited to the ascending aorta, sewing the layers of the dissected aorta together before the prosthetic graft is inserted. The long-term prognosis for these dissected aortas is yet unknown, but data thus far available indicate that prognosis is reasonably good if hypertension is controlled. More than 10 years have now elapsed since some surviving patients underwent excision of dissecting aneurysms.

Several years ago DeBakey and associates reported an extensive series of 142 patients with a mortality of 20 percent. Austen and associates had a similar mortality of 22 percent in 23 patients, while Harris et al. reported a mortality near 50 percent in 22 patients. In 1975, Reul et al. described experiences with 91 patients over a period of 10 years. Those operated on for acute dissection had an operative mortality of 25 percent; with chronic dissection the mortality was 17 percent. Only 1 of 31 patients with simple aneurysms above the diaphragm, operated on electively, died. According to recent reports, with improved techniques mortality rates have been significantly improved.

WOUNDS OF THE GREAT VESSELS

Penetrating Injuries

Penetrating injuries of the aorta or venae cavae are a frequent cause of death with penetrating chest injuries. Fatal hemorrhage occurs so quickly that only a few patients survive long enough for treatment. Patients alive with such injuries when first seen are usually in profound shock with signs of massive intrathoracic bleeding. Immediate thoracotomy offers the only chance for survival. In some instances this must be employed in the emergency department, often with conditions less than ideal. Once hemorrhage has been stopped, the patient is often transferred to the operating room for more definitive surgical exploration and subsequent closure of the incision. Depending upon the location of the injury, a variety of thoracic incisions have been used, including thoracotomy, median sternotomy, resection of the clavicle to expose the subclavian artery, or a cervicothoracic approach. In all likelihood a median sternotomy should be employed far more frequently than in the past, as was emphasized by Brawley et al. in 1970. Injuries involving the origin of the innominate or left common carotid artery, with cerebral ischemia, may be most safely managed with a temporary shunt. Experiences with shunts for injuries of this type were described recently by Ecker et al.

A number of recent case reports have described successful repair of unusual injuries of the aortic arch or its branches from either penetrating or nonpenetrating trauma. These successful experiences result from the avail-

Fig. 20-16. *Left.* Operative photograph of dissecting aneurysm of upper thoracic aorta, starting a few days before operation. The hematoma in the aortic wall is visible. *Center.* With a functioning left atrial bypass, the aorta has been occluded and the aneurysm incised. A tape encircles the left subclavian artery. The vagus nerve with the recurrent nerve encircling the aorta is visible. The aneurysm began in the classic location, just beyond the left subclavian artery. A large thrombus is present in the aortic wall. *Right.* Aortic reconstruction was accomplished with a short woven Dacron graft. The proximal anastomosis is immediately beyond the left subclavian artery.

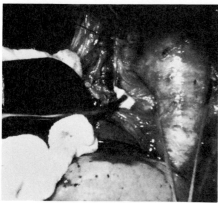
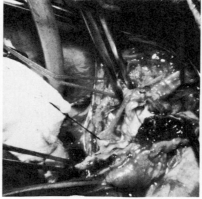
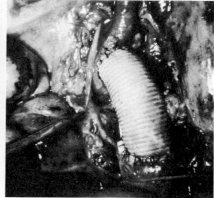

ability of excellent angiography and the increasing trend to prompt thoracotomy with a sternotomy which provides excellent exposure of the vessels of the aortic arch. Undoubtedly in the next few years such injuries will be treated even more successfully than they have been in the past.

An unusual type of penetrating injury is one involving the intrapericardial portion of the ascending aorta; devel-

Fig. 20-17. *A.* Transected aorta found at autopsy when the patient was exsanguinated 24 hours following injury. The patient had only minor chest pain before the terminal event. The sharp, transverse laceration of the aorta is the usual finding, resulting from the deceleration forces at the time of injury. *B.* Partial transection of the aorta found at autopsy when the patient was suddenly exsanguinated 3 weeks following an automobile accident. An aortic lesion had not been previously suspected.

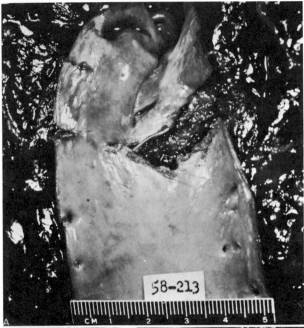

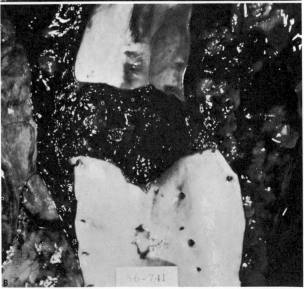

opment of cardiac tamponade may temporarily control bleeding and allow more time for operation. In 1961 Dively et al. reported successful treatment of three patients with this type of unusual injury and described published experiences with others. Rarely a small penetrating injury may produce a fistula between the aorta and right ventricle, between the aorta and vena cava, or between the aorta and pulmonary artery.

Nonpenetrating Injuries

Traumatic injury of the aorta following blunt trauma is important to recognize, because effective surgical therapy is possible in many patients. Unfortunately the diagnosis is often not considered because of the unusual nature of the lesion. It is a frequent finding at autopsy following a fatal injury, but careful analysis of 171 cases by Parmley et al. emphasized that surgical therapy was often possible because 20 percent of the patients lived longer than 30 minutes after injury and several survived for several days before fatal hemorrhage occurred. Only in the past decade has increasing familiarity with the lesion occasionally resulted in early diagnosis and successful therapy.

ETIOLOGY AND PATHOLOGY. A rupture of the aorta is usually produced from a deceleration-type injury, typically in an automobile accident. In 70 to 75 percent of patients the aortic laceration occurs just distal to the left subclavian artery. Apparently the descending thoracic aorta and the aortic arch decelerate at different rates because of differences in anatomic structure, and a transverse tear of the aorta is produced near the site of insertion of the ligamentum arteriosum. The tear may involve part or all of the layers of the aortic wall, varying from laceration of the intima to transection of the aorta with retraction of the two ends. Part or all of the circumference of the aortic wall may be involved (Fig. 20-17). Fatal hemorrhage is prevented in some patients by the adventitia, which has been reported to constitute 60 percent of the tensile strength of the aortic wall.

The next most frequent site of injury is in the ascending aorta near its origin from the left ventricle. Other sites are very unusual and may be produced by various forms of injury, such as direct trauma or vertical deceleration injuries as in a fall from a building. A dissecting aneurysm following trauma is extremely rare.

In patients who do not exsanguinate soon after injury, a hematoma forms in the mediastinum and produces a characteristic roentgenographic appearance due to enlargement of the mediastinum. Disturbances in blood flow through the aorta usually do not occur. Only a few instances of paraplegia appearing after aortic injury from acute interruption of blood flow have been described. Following the acute injury, a latent period is often present before the mediastinal hematoma surrounding the aortic laceration suddenly ruptures into the pleural cavity and causes fatal hemorrhage. The fatal rupture almost always occurs within 4 weeks after injury. Spencer et al. described a few examples of rupture 30 to 90 days after injury.

In patients who survive longer than 2 months after injury a false aneurysm of the aorta gradually develops and may pursue an unusually benign course. Unlike the more common atherosclerotic or syphilitic aneurysms, traumatic aneurysms may remain as asymptomatic mediastinal masses for many years, or even decades, until enlargement occurs. Calcification develops in most such lesions after varying periods of time and may provide the first clue to the diagnosis when first recognized on a chest roentgenogram made for other reasons. Only a moderate amount of data is available about the long-term course of traumatic aneurysms, probably because many have been misdiagnosed as calcified atherosclerotic or syphilitic aneurysms. In 1961, in a detailed review of reported experiences with traumatic aneurysms Spencer et al. found only about 60 reported cases. Apparently most such lesions tend to enlarge after months or years, producing compression of the left main bronchus and the recurrent laryngeal nerve. With such enlargement, symptoms from obstruction of the left bronchus appear and require therapy. Usually enlargement of traumatic aneurysms proceeds slowly for a long period of time before rupture occurs, providing ample time for diagnosis and therapy.

Associated injuries are common. Most patients have fractures of the ribs, and fractures of the extremities occur in about 50 percent of patients, reflecting the severity of trauma producing the aortic injury.

CLINICAL MANIFESTATIONS. Following injury to the thorax, there are usually no symptoms or signs to indicate that an aortic injury has occurred. Dyspnea and chest pain are usually present, but these commonly result from the almost universally present rib fractures and do not aid in recognizing rupture of the aorta. A hemothorax, with varying degrees of shock, is also frequent, but again such findings frequently arise from rib fractures and pulmonary lacerations which do not involve the aorta. A murmur has been present in only a few patients. Rarely, signs of acute obstruction of the aorta, apparently from prolapse of a segment of intima with obstruction of the lumen, have occurred, with weak or absent femoral pulses and even acute paraplegia.

Patients with a traumatic aortic aneurysm who are first seen months or years following injury are often asymptomatic and are evaluated because of the accidental discovery of a mediastinal mass on a chest roentgenogram. Symptoms, if present, are usually due to compression of the left main bronchus from an expanding aneurysm, causing cough, wheeze, dyspnea, and pneumonia. Compression and paralysis of the left recurrent laryngeal nerve may produce hoarseness. (See the section on Traumatic Thoracic Aneurysms.)

DIAGNOSTIC FINDINGS. The chest roentgenogram provides the best clue to the diagnosis. In acutely injured patients with rupture of the aorta, widening of the mediastinum (Fig. 20-18) is almost invariably present. It is important to realize, however, that this may result from a hematoma arising from some cause other than rupture of the aorta. When widening of the mediastinum is recognized on the chest roentgenogram, *an aortogram should be performed immediately,* for only with an aortogram can the diagnosis be firmly established (Fig. 20-19). In 1976 Marsh and Sturn described six radiologic abnormalities which

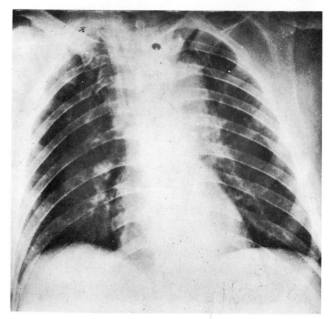

Fig. 20-18. Chest roentgenogram of a patient with traumatic rupture of the thoracic aorta, illustrating the characteristic widening of the mediastinum. When this is observed following a chest injury, emergency aortography should be performed to establish the diagnosis of rupture of the thoracic aorta.

Fig. 20-19. Aortogram demonstrating traumatic rupture of the thoracic aorta distal to the left subclavian artery. The point of rupture can be seen as an irregular border of the thoracic aorta, in association with localized bulging. This angiogram represents the first instance in which emergency aortography was employed to establish firmly the diagnosis of traumatic rupture of the aorta.

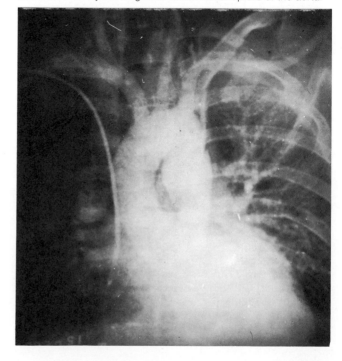

were indications for the prompt performance of thoracic aortography following chest trauma. These observations were obtained from a study of 100 patients without trauma and 47 consecutive patients who underwent aortography following blunt trauma. Postponing aortography may be fatal, for the mediastinal hematoma surrounding the lacerated aorta often ruptures without any warning symptoms. In asymptomatic patients who are seen because of an undiagnosed mediastinal mass, aortography also provides the most definitive means of establishing the diagnosis.

TREATMENT. Thoracotomy should be performed as soon as possible after the diagnosis has been established. A 1961 review of all reported experiences found only one patient who had survived repair of an aortic laceration. In the subsequent 16 years, fortunately, many patients have been sucessfully treated, a result of increasing familiarity with the clinical picture combined with the availability of emergency aortography and thoracotomy.

As with thoracic aneurysms, the surgical approach is through a left posterolateral thoracotomy in the fourth intercostal space. The preference in our unit is some form of aortic bypass, usually the Gott intraaortic shunt, to minimize the risk of paraplegia during occlusion of the aorta (Fig. 20-9). An alternate approach was recently reported by Applebaum et al., describing experiences with 25 patients. In 18 treated by some method of perfusing the distal aorta, two developed paraplegia, while seven treated with simple aortic cross-clamping recovered satisfactorily. Their conclusion was that simple aortic cross-clamping might be preferable to attempts to insert a shunt. The author would disagree with this conclusion, but our data clearly indicate that a shunt per se may not prevent paraplegia. The operation was initially performed with the conventional left atriofemoral bypass, but more recently systemic heparinization has been avoided by the use of aortic shunts. A report by Kirsh et al. in 1976 described experiences with 43 patients treated over a period of 10 years. Overall survival was 70 percent with five patients dying without undergoing operation. Twenty-eight patients underwent operation within 12 hours, with the remaining nine patients undergoing operation from 24 hours to more than 5 days after hospital admission. Most repairs were completed using an external shunt. Successful repair was accomplished in 30 of the 37 patients operated on.

OBSTRUCTION OF THE SUPERIOR VENA CAVA

Obstruction of the superior vena cava produces an unusual but distinctive clinical syndrome which can be easily recognized once the diagnosis is considered. Diagnostic errors are surprisingly common, however, partly because of the infrequent occurrence and partly because of a lack of familiarity with the distinctive clinical features.

ETIOLOGY. In 70 to 80 percent of patients superior vena cava obstruction is due to a malignant neoplasm. This was true in 48 of 64 patients described by Effler and Groves and in 90 percent of 60 cases reported by Hanlon and Danis. Usually the neoplasm is a bronchogenic carcinoma

of the right upper lobe which is invading the mediastinum. Less frequently seen are primary mediastinal tumors, such as thymoma or lymphoma. Metastatic neoplasms from a distant source are unusual.

In the past, saccular aneurysms were found in about 30 percent of patients with vena cava obstruction, but with the marked decrease in frequency of syphilitic aneurysms, these are now infrequently seen. If superior vena cava obstruction is not due to a malignant tumor, a chronic fibrosing mediastinitis, usually of unknown origin, is the most common cause. Probably many of the cases undiagnosed in the past were due to histoplasmosis. Obstruction from a benign tumor, such as a substernal thyroid, is unusual.

PATHOPHYSIOLOGY. With obstruction of the superior vena cava there is an increase in venous pressure in its tributaries in the arms and head to levels ranging between 200 and 500 cm of water. The degree of increase in venous pressure varies with the rate of development and the site of the obstruction. Obstruction proximal to the site of entry of the azygos vein is more disabling than more distal sites of obstruction in which a patent azygos vein can function as a collateral pathway. Acute obstruction of the vena cava, as during a thoracic operation, can produce fatal cerebral edema within a few minutes. At the opposite extreme are instances where superior vena cava obstruction develops slowly, permitting time for the development of collateral circulation, as a result of which symptoms are mild.

CLINICAL MANIFESTATIONS. With mild obstruction, frequent symptoms are headache, swelling of the eyelids, puffiness of the face, or enlargement of the neck. In males there may be a noticeable increase in collar size. The severity of symptoms is closely related to posture, for the patient quickly notes that his symptoms increase if he bends over or lies down. If obstruction of the vena cava develops rapidly, as with hemorrhage into a rapidly growing neoplasm, more serious symptoms of cerebral congestion are present, including drowsiness and blurring of vision. Edema of the vocal cords may produce hoarseness or dyspnea. As the majority of cases are due to a rapidly growing bronchogenic carcinoma, pulmonary symptoms such as cough and hemoptysis are also frequently present. In most patients death results in a few months.

In the minority of patients in whom obstruction is due to a benign process, collateral circulation may enlarge sufficiently to where little disability is present. Prominent features include dilated veins with edema and cyanosis, the degree varying with the degree of stasis. Venous hypertension is manifested by prominence and distension of the veins. Effler and Groves have reported 16 patients with obstruction from a benign process, all of whom eventually developed sufficient collateral circulation to have minimal symptoms; there were no fatalities as a direct result of the chronic venous obstruction. We have observed one patient over a period of 20 years in whom the superior vena cava was obstructed following an intracardiac operation for correction of anomalous pulmonary veins entering the superior vena cava. Initially there was serious venous hypertension to levels of 350 cm of water, producing a bilateral chylothorax ultimately controlled by ligation of the thoracic duct. Within a few months, however, all symptoms subsided, and the patient, now a young married woman with children, has no limitation of physical activities.

DIAGNOSTIC STUDIES. Although the clinical picture is characteristic when fully developed, early manifestations of the disease, such as swelling of the eyes or headache, may be confused with angioneurotic edema, congestive heart failure, or constrictive pericarditis. The diagnosis can be confirmed by measuring the venous pressure, which is usually in the range of 200 to 500 cm of water. The location and extent of the obstruction can be best outlined by venography. In some patients the underlying disease process is uncertain, although usually signs of a bronchogenic carcinoma are visible on a chest roentgenogram. Bronchoscopy and biopsy may be helpful in confirming the diagnosis. Aortography can be used if necessary to exclude the presence of an aneurysm.

TREATMENT. With a malignant process, involvement of the superior vena cava almost precludes surgical resection, although isolated exceptions have been reported. Thoracotomy is a serious undertaking, encountering serious bleeding from the venous hypertension. If a diagnosis can be established without thoracotomy—e.g., by bronchoscopy, mediastinoscopy, or biopsy of a peripheral node—it may be preferable to proceed directly to radiation rather than perform a thoracotomy.

Significant palliation can be obtained by intensive radiation therapy, often in combination with diuretics and chemotherapy. Improvement in symptoms soon occurs, probably from diminution in edema associated with a growing neoplasm. Death from the neoplasm, however, usually occurs within a few months.

With benign obstructions, the report of Effler and Groves clearly indicates that there is no urgency in performing an operation if symptoms are mild. In all likelihood symptoms will improve or subside completely as collateral circulation develops. A number of ingenious attempts have been made to reconstruct an obstructed superior vena cava. Prosthetic grafts have been almost uniformly unsuccessful, with the possible exception of a crimped Teflon graft, which experimentally has given the best results. The most favorable graft is a composite one of autogenous veins, prepared by combining both superficial femoral veins into a graft of larger diameter. Good results lasting for several years have been reported by Hanlon and Danis in three patients in whom such grafts were used.

A good collective review was published by Gomes and Hufnagel in 1975, describing experiences with two patients and reviewing previous reports by others. Methods of constructing a large composite vein graft from the saphenous vein were described by Doty and Baker in 1976. The experimental studies with Gore-Tex, a type of polyethylene, may eventually find applicability in treatment of this unusual condition.

Rarely a localized granuloma may compress and thrombose the vena cava; patency can be restored by opening the vein and removing the clot. Three such cases have been reported by Pate and Hammon and one such patient by Hanlon and Danis. Other ingenious attempts to bypass the obstructed vena cava, applicable in certain specific instances, have been reported. Cooley and Hallman rotated the azygos vein to provide a bypass route for draining blood directly into the atrium, while Schramel and Olinde reversed the saphenous vein in a subcutaneous tunnel to drain blood from the superior vena cava system to the common femoral vein.

References

Aneurysms of the Ascending Aorta

Bahnson, H. T., and Spencer, F. C.: Excision of Aneurysm of the Ascending Aorta with Prosthetic Replacement during Cardiopulmonary Bypass, *Ann Surg,* **151:**879, 1960.

Bloodwell, R. D., Hallman, G. L., and Cooley, D. A.: Aneurysm of the Ascending Aorta with Aortic Valvular Insufficiency, *Arch Surg,* **92:**588, 1966.

Connors, J. P., Ferguson, T. B., Weldon, C. S., and Roper, C. L.: The Use of the TDMAC Heparin Shunt in Replacement of Descending Thoracic Aorta, *Ann Surg,* **181:**735, 1975.

Griepp, R. B., Stinson, E. B., Hollingsworth, J. F., and Buehler, D.: Prosthetic Replacement of the Aortic Arch, *J Thorac Cardiovasc Surg,* **70:**1051, 1975.

Kidd, J. N., Reul, G. J., Cooley, D. A., Sandeford, F. M., Kyger, E. R., III, and Wukasch, D. C.: Surgical Treatment of Aneurysms of the Ascending Aorta, *Circulation,* **54**(Suppl. III):118, 1976.

Kouchoukos, N. T., Karp, R. B., and Lell, W. A.: Replacement of the Ascending Aorta and Aortic Valve with a Composite Graft: Results in 25 Patients, *Ann Thorac Surg,* **24:**140, 1977.

Liddicott, J. E., Bekassy, S. M., Rubio, P. A., Noon, G. P., and DeBakey, M. E.: Ascending Aortic Aneurysms: Review of 100 Consecutive Cases, *Circulation,* **51-52**(Suppl. 1):202, 1975.

Liotta, D., Hallman, G. L., Milam, J. D., and Cooley, D. A.: Surgical Treatment of Acute Dissecting Aneurysm of the Ascending Aorta, *Ann Thorac Surg,* **12:**582, 1971.

Shumacker, H. B., Jr.: Operative Treatment of Aneurysms of the Thoracic Aorta Due to Cystic Medial Necrosis, *J Thorac Cardiovasc Surg,* **63:**1, 1972.

Spencer, F. C., and Blake, H. A.: A Report of the Successful Surgical Treatment of Aortic Regurgitation from a Dissecting Aortic Aneurysm in a Patient with the Marfan Syndrome, *J Thorac Cardiovasc Surg,* **44:**238, 1962.

Weldon, C. S., Ferguson, T. B., Ludbrook, P. A., and Mcknight, R. C.: A New Operation for Far-Advanced Cystic Medial Necrosis of the Aortic Root, *Ann Thorac Surg,* **23:**499, 1977.

Zubiate, P., and Kay, J. H.: Surgical Treatment of Aneurysm of the Ascending Aorta with Aortic Insufficiency and Marked Displacement of the Coronary Ostia, *J Thorac Cardiovasc Surg,* **71:**415, 1976.

Aneurysms of the Transverse Aortic Arch

Allard, J. R., Williams, R. L., and Dobell, A. R. C.: Interrupted Aortic Arch: Factors Influencing Prognosis, *Ann Thorac Surg,* **21:**243, 1976.

Bloodwell, R. D., Hallman, G. L., and Cooley, D. A.: Total Replacement of the Aortic Arch and the "Subclavian Steal" Phenomenon, *Ann Thorac Surg,* **5:**236, 1968.

DeBakey, M. E., Beall, A. C., Jr., Cooley, D. A., Crawford, E. S., Morris, G. C., Jr., and Garrett, H. E.: Resection and Graft

Replacement of Aneurysms Involving the Transverse Arch of the Aorta, *Surg Clin North Am,* **46:**1057, 1966.

Griepp, R. B., Stinson, E. B., Hollingsworth, J. F., and Buehler, D.: Prosthetic Replacement of the Aortic Arch, *J Thorac Cardiovasc Surg,* **70:**1051, 1975.

Lefrak, E. A., Stevens, P. M., and Howell, J. F.: Respiratory Insufficiency Due to Tracheal Compression by an Aneurysm of the Ascending, Transverse, and Descending Thoracic Aorta: Successful Surgical Management, *J Thorac Cardiovasc Surg,* **63:**956, 1972.

Traumatic Thoracic Aneurysms

Bennett, D. E., and Cherry, J. K.: The Natural History of Traumatic Aneurysms of the Aorta, *Surgery,* **61:**516, 1967.

Connors, J. P., Ferguson, T. B., Weldon, C. S., and Roper, C. L.: The Use of the TDMAC Heparin Shunt in Replacement of Descending Thoracic Aorta, *Ann Surg,* **181:**735, 1975.

Cooley, D. A.: Discussion of R. J. Stoney, B. B. Roe, and J. V. Redington, Rupture of Thoracic Aorta Due to Closed-Chest Trauma, *Arch Surg,* **89:**840, 1964.

Donahoo, J. S., Brawley, R. K., and Gott, V. L.: The Heparin-Coated Vascular Shunt for Thoracic Aortic and Great Vessel Procedures: A Ten Year Experience, *Ann Thorac Surg,* **23:**507, 1977.

Kirsh, M. M., Behrendt, D. M., Orringer, M. B., Gago, O., Gray, L. A., Jr., Milts, L. J., Walter, J. F., and Sloan, H.: The Treatment of Acute Traumatic Rupture of the Aorta: A 10 Year Experience, *Ann Surg,* **184:**308, 1976.

Marsh, D. G., and Sturm, J. T.: Traumatic Aortic Rupture: Roentgenographic Indications for Angiography, *Ann Thorac Surg,* **21:**337, 1976.

Spencer, F. C., Guerin, P. F., Blake, H. A., and Bahnson, H. T.: A Report of Fifteen Patients with Traumatic Rupture of the Thoracic Aorta, *J Thorac Cardiovasc Surg,* **41:**1, 1961.

Aneurysms of the Descending Thoracic Aorta

Bahnson, H. T.: Definitive Treatment of Saccular Aneurysms of the Aorta with Excision of the Sac and Aortic Suture, *Surg Gynecol Obstet,* **96:**382, 1953.

Bloodwell, R. D., Hallman, G. L., Beall, A. C., Jr., Cooley, D. A., and DeBakey, M. E.: Aneurysms of the Descending Thoracic Aorta: Surgical Considerations, *Surg Clin North Am,* **46:**901, 1966.

Connolly, J. E., Kountz, S. L., and Boyd, R. J.: Left Heart Bypass: Experimental and Clinical Observations on its Regulation with Particular Reference to Maintenance of Maximal Renal Blood Flow, *J Thorac Cardiovasc Surg,* **44:**577, 1962.

Crawford, E. S., and Rubio, P. A.: Reappraisal of Adjuncts To Avoid Ischemia in the Treatment of Aneurysms of Descending Thoracic Aorta, *J Thorac Cardiovasc Surg,* **66:**693, 1973.

DeBakey, M. E., Cooley, D. A., Crawford, E. S., and Morris, G. C., Jr.: Aneurysms of the Thoracic Aorta. Analysis of 179 Patients Treated by Resection, *J Thorac Surg,* **36:**393, 1958.

Donahoo, J. S., Brawley, R. K., and Gott, V. L.: The Heparin-Coated Vascular Shunt for Thoracic Aortic and Great Vessel Procedures: A Ten Year Experience, *Ann Thorac Surg,* **23:**507, 1977.

Gerbode, F., Braimbridge, M., Osborn, J. J., Hood, J., and French, S.: Traumatic Thoracic Aneurysms: Treatment by Resection

and Grafting with the Use of Extracorporeal Bypass, *Surgery,* **42:**975, 1957.

Kahn, D. R., Vathayanon, S., and Sloan, H.: Resection of Descending Thoracic Aneurysms without Left Heart Bypass, *Arch Surg,* **97:**336, 1968.

Krauss, A. H., Ferguson, T. V., and Weldon, C. S.: Thoracic Aneurysmectomy Using the Tedmac Heparin Shunt, *Ann Thorac Surg,* **14:**123, 1972.

Reul, G. J., Jr., Cooley, D. A., Hallman, G. L., Reddy, S. B., Kyger, E. R., III, and Wukasch, D. C.: Dissecting Aneurysm of Descending Aorta: Improved Surgical Results in 91 Patients, *Arch Surg,* **110:**632, 1975.

Vasko, J. S., Spencer, F. C., and Bahnson, H. T.: Aneurysm of the Aorta Treated by Excision: Review of 237 Cases Followed Up to Seven Years, *Am J Surg,* **105:**793, 1963.

Wechsler, A. S., and Wolfe, W. G.: Heparinless Shunting during Cross-clamping of the Thoracic Aorta, *Ann Thorac Surg,* **23:**497, 1977.

Thoracoabdominal Aneurysms

Crawford, E. S., and Rubio, P. A.: Reappraisal of Adjuncts to Avoid Ischemia in the Treatment of Aneurysms of Descending Thoracic Aorta, *J Thorac Cardiovasc Surg,* **66:**693, 1973.

DeBakey, M. E., Crawford, E. S., Garrett, H. E., Beall, A. C., Jr., and Howell, J. F.: Surgical Considerations in the Treatment of Aneurysms of the Thoraco-abdominal Aorta, *Ann Surg,* **162:**650, 1965.

Garrett, H. E., Crawford, E. S., Beall, A. C., Jr., Howell, J. F., and DeBakey, M. E.: Surgical Treatment of Aneurysm of the Thoracoabdominal Aorta, *Surg Clin North Am,* **46:**913, 1966.

Dissecting Aneurysms

Appelbaum, A., Karp, R. B., and Kirklin, J. W.: Ascending versus Descending Aortic Dissection, *Ann Surg,* **183:**296, 1976.

Austen, W. G., Buckley, M. J., McFarland, J., DeSanctis, R. W., and Sanders, C. A.: Therapy of Dissecting Aneurysms, *Arch Surg,* **95:**835, 1967.

Daily, P. O., Trueblood, H. W., Stinson, E. B., Wuerflein, R. D., and Shumway, N. E.: Management of Acute Aortic Dissections, *Ann Thorac Surg,* **10:**337, 1970.

DeBakey, M. E., Henly, W. S., Cooley, D. A., Morris, G. C., Crawford, E. S., and Beall, A. C.: Surgical Management of Dissecting Aneurysms of the Aorta, *J Thorac Cardiovasc Surg,* **49:**130, 1965.

Gryboski, W., and Spencer, F. C.: Intermittent Claudication Caused by a Dissecting Aneurysm of the Aorta, *South Med J,* **58:**593, 1965.

Harris, P. D., Malm, J. R., Bigger, J. T., and Bowman, F. O.: Follow-up Studies of Acute Dissecting Aortic Aneurysms Managed with Antihypertensive Agents, *Circulation,* **35** (*Suppl* 1): I-183, 1967.

Hirst, A. E., Johns, V. J., and Kime, S. W.: Dissecting Aneurysm of the Aorta: A Review of 505 Cases, *Medicine (Baltimore),* **37:**217, 1958.

Lindsay, J., and Hurst, J. W.: Clinical Features and Prognosis in Dissecting Aneurysm of the Aorta, *Circulation,* **35:**880, 1967.

Liotta, D., Hallman, G. L., Milam, J. D., and Cooley, D. A.: Surgical Treatment of Acute Dissecting Aneurysm of the Ascending Aorta, *Ann Thorac Surg,* **12:**582, 1971.

McCloy, R. M., Spittell, J. A., and McGoon, D. C.: The Prognosis of Aortic Dissection (Dissecting Aortic Hematoma or Aneurysm), *Circulation,* **31**:665, 1965.

Najafi, H., Dye, W. S., Javid, H., Hunter, J. A., Goldin, M. D., and Julian, O. C.: Acute Aortic Regurgitation Secondary to Aortic Dissection: Surgical Management without Valve Replacement, *Ann Thorac Surg,* **14**:474, 1972.

Schumacker, H. B., Jr.: Operative Treatment of Aneurysms of the Thoracic Aorta Due to Cystic Medial Necrosis, *J Thorac Cardiovasc Surg,* **63**:1, 1972.

Spencer, F. C., and Blake, H. A.: A Report of the Successful Surgical Treatment of Aortic Regurgitation from a Dissecting Aortic Aneurysm in a Patient with the Marfan Syndrome, *J Thorac Cardiovasc Surg,* **44**:238, 1962.

Wheat, M. W., Jr., and Palmer, R. F.: Dissecting Aneurysms of the Aorta, *Curr Probl Surg,* July 1971.

———, ———, Bartley, T. D., and Seelman, R. C.: Treatment of Dissecting Aneurysms of the Aorta without Surgery, *J Thorac Cardiovasc Surg,* **50**:364, 1965.

Wounds of the Great Vessels

Applebaum, A., Karp, R. B., and Kirklin, J. W.: Surgical Treatment for Closed Thoracic Aortic Injuries, *J Thorac Cardiovasc Surg,* **71** (3): 458, 1976.

Bennett, D. E., and Cherry, D. K.: The Natural History of Traumatic Aneurysms of the Aorta, *Surgery,* **61**:516, 1967.

Blake, H. A., Inmon, T. W., and Spencer, F. C.: Emergency Use of Antegrade Aortography in Diagnosis of Acute Aortic Rupture, *Ann Surg,* **152**:954, 1960.

Brawley, R. K., Murray, G. F., Crisler, C., and Cameron, J. L.: Management of Wounds of the Innominate, Subclavian, and Axillary Blood Vessels, *Surg Gynecol Obstet,* **131**:1130, 1970.

Castagna, J., and Nelson, R. J.: Blunt Injuries to Branches of Aortic Arch, *J Thorac Cardiovasc Surg,* **69**:521, 1975.

Clarke, C. P., Brandt, P. W. T., Cole, D. S., and Barratt-Boyes, B. G.: Traumatic Rupture of the Thoracic Aorta: Diagnosis and Treatment, *Br J Surg,* **54**:353, 1967.

DeMuth, W. E., Jr., Roe, H., and Hobbie, W.: Immediate Repair of Traumatic Rupture of Thoracic Aorta, *Arch Surg,* **91**:602, 1965.

Dively, W. L., Daniel, R. A., and Scott, H. W.: Surgical Management of Penetrating Injuries of the Ascending Aorta and Aortic Arch, *J Thorac Cardiovasc Surg,* **41**:23, 1961.

Ecker, R. R., Dickinson, W. E., Sugg, W. L., and Rea, W. J.: Management of Injuries of the Innominate and Proximal Left Common Carotid Artery, *J Thorac Cardiovasc Surg,* **64**:618, 1972.

Gerbode, F., Braimbridge, M., Osborn, J. J., Hood, M., and French, S.: Traumatic Thoracic Aneurysm: Treatment by Resection and Grafting with the Use of Extracorporeal Bypass, *Surgery,* **42**:975, 1957.

Jahnke, E. J., Jr., Fisher, G. W., and Jones, R. C.: Acute Traumatic Rupture of the Thoracic Aorta: Report of Six Consecutive Cases of Successful Early Repair, *J Thorac Cardiovasc Surg,* **48**:63, 1964.

Kahn, A. M., Joseph, W. L., and Hughes, R. K.: Traumatic Aneurysms of the Thoracic Aorta: Excision and Repair without Graft, *Ann Thorac Surg,* **4**:175, 1967.

Kirsh, M. M., Behrendt, D. M., Orringer, M. B., Gago, O., Gray, L. A., Jr., Mills, L. J., Walter, J. F., and Sloan, H.: The Treatment of Acute Traumatic Rupture of the Aorta: A 10 Year Experience, *Ann Surg,* **184**:308, 1976.

Marsh, D. G., and Sturm, J. T.: Traumatic Aortic Rupture: Roentgenographic Indications for Angiography, *Ann Thorac Surg,* **21** (4): 337, 1976.

Parmley, L. F., Mattingly, T. W., and Manion, W. C.: Penetrating Wounds to the Heart and Aorta, *Circulation,* **17**:953, 1958.

———, ———, ———, and Jahnke, E. J., Jr.: Non-penetrating Traumatic Injury of the Aorta, *Circulation,* **17**:1086, 1958.

Spencer, F. C., Guerin, P. F., Blake, H. A., and Bahnson, H. T.: A Report of 15 Patients with Traumatic Rupture of the Thoracic Aorta, *J Thorac Cardiovasc Surg,* **41**:1, 1961.

Steenburg, R. W., and Ravitch, M. M.: Cervico-thoracic Approach for Subclavian Vessel Injury from Compound Fracture of the Clavicle: Considerations of Subclavian Axillary Exposures, *Ann Surg,* **157**:839, 1963.

Symbas, P. N., Tyras, D. H., Ware, R. E., and Hatcher, C. R., Jr.: Rupture of the Aorta: A Diagnostic Triad, *Ann Thorac Surg,* **15**:405, 1973.

Obstruction of the Superior Vena Cava

Cooley, D. A., and Hallman, G. L.: Superior Vena Caval Syndrome Treated by Azygos Vein–Inferior Vena Cava Anastomosis: Report of Successful Case, *J Thorac Cardiovasc Surg,* **47**:325, 1964.

Doty, D. B., and Baker, W. H.: Bypass of Superior Cava with Spiral Vein Graft, *Ann Thorac Surg,* **22**:490, 1976.

Effler, D. B., and Groves, L. K.: Superior Vena Caval Obstruction, *J Thorac Cardiovasc Surg,* **43**:574, 1962.

Gomes, M. N., and Hufnagel, C. A.: Superior Vena Cava Obstruction: Review of Literature and Report of Two Cases Due to Benign Intrathoracic Tumors, *Ann Thorac Surg,* **20**:344, 1975.

Hanlon, C. R., and Danis, R. K.: Superior Vena Caval Obstruction: Indications for Diagnostic Thoracotomy, *Ann Surg,* **161**:771, 1965.

Heydorn, W. H., Zajtchuk, R., Miller, F., and Schuchmann, G. F.: Gore-Tex Grafts for Replacement of the Superior Vena Cava, *Ann Thorac Surg,* **23**:539, 1977.

Pate, J. W., and Hammon, J.: Superior Vena Cava Syndrome Due to Histoplasmosis in Children, *Ann Surg,* **161**:778, 1965.

Schramel, R., and Olinde, H. D. H.: A New Method of Bypassing the Obstructed Vena Cava, *J Thorac Cardiovasc Surg,* **41**:375, 1961.

Chapter 21

Peripheral Arterial Disease

by **Anthony M. Imparato and Frank C. Spencer**

INTRODUCTION

Progress in vascular surgery has been so rapid since 1950 that it is difficult for a student of medicine at this time to realize that most of the vascular operations commonly performed today scarcely had been considered 30 years ago. For perspective, an historical review is worthwhile.

Prior to 1900, progress was greatly hampered by the lack of anesthesia and asepsis. Nevertheless in 1888 Matas reported his successful operation upon a patient with a traumatic aneurysm of the brachial artery upon whom he performed the first endoaneurysmorrhaphy. Nine years later (1897) Murphy performed the first end-to-end arterial anastomosis in man following excision of an arteriovenous fistula in the thigh. He performed a total of 34 experiments in dogs, sheep, and calves to evaluate methods of vascular suture prior to performing this first procedure in man. By 1906, Carrel and Guthrie developed many of the techniques of vascular surgery which are still in use today. Soon thereafter autogenous vein grafts were successfully used following excision of aneurysms. In 1915 Bernheim used a vein graft in man for the first time in the United States in treating a patient with a syphilitic popliteal aneurysm.

After World War I a curious lag occurred in vascular surgery until the 1940s, when the epochal work of Blalock, Gross, and Crafoord with tetralogy of Fallot, patent ductus arteriosus, and coarctation of the aorta launched the modern era of vascular surgery. The development of atraumatic vascular clamps by Potts, in conjunction with fine arterial sutures with swaged needles, greatly facilitated the techniques of vascular operations. The introduction of aortic homografts for repair of coarctation of the aorta by Gross stimulated intensive investigation of vascular prostheses. The successful excision of an abdominal aneurysm with replacement by an aortic homograft was reported by Dubost et al. in 1952, and in the same year Voorhees et al. reported the first use of a cloth material, Vinyon-N, as a vascular prosthesis. Within the next 5 years this stimulated the development of the presently used vascular prostheses of Dacron and Teflon, with many contributions made by DeBakey, Cooley, Bahnson, Wesolowski, and others. The increasing use of arteriography, along with the development of safer radiopaque media, greatly enhanced further development of reconstructive surgery. Between 1955 and 1960 operations for carotid artery stenosis and renal artery stenosis were first done. With these many advances in both diagnostic and therapeutic surgical techniques the scope of vascular surgery has increased to the stage where it has become an increasingly large segment of surgical practice.

Since peripheral arterial diseases lend themselves to broad classification as occlusive, aneurysmal, and vasospastic the topics in this chapter are grouped in a sequence representing these three broad categories.

OCCLUSIVE DISEASE OF THE LOWER EXTREMITIES

Clinical Manifestations

HISTORY. The ischemic basis for symptoms can be strongly suspected from the history, which varies markedly depending upon whether ischemia develops acutely, as in embolic occlusion of arteries, or slowly, which is more characteristic of thrombotic occlusions. The key symptom which requires elaboration is *pain.* The characteristics of pain are related to the abruptness of the onset of arterial occlusion and the severity of the ischemia. When arterial interruption occurs abruptly, pain is usually sudden in onset and severe, and involves the entire portion of the extremity supplied by that artery. Characteristically, acute popliteal occlusion results in excruciating pain of the entire extremity below the knee, while common femoral occlusion produces a painful foot, calf, and thigh. Aortoiliac occlusions may result in pain in the lower half of the body. The pain, often associated with numbness, persists until one of three events occurs: (1) the ischemia is relieved by reopening the artery surgically, (2) the opening of the collateral channels over periods of days or weeks, (3) persistence of ischemia, resulting in nerves which are destroyed and consequent anesthesia of the affected limb. When arterial occlusion develops over longer periods of time ischemia may be subtle and may not become manifest until there are demands for blood beyond basal requirements, such as with exercise. Pain is experienced during exertion and gradually disappears within minutes upon cessation of activity. This represents the characteristic symptom of *intermittent claudication,* the most common complaint produced by limb ischemia. The areas which are felt to be painful are usually those requiring the largest amount of blood during exertion, viz., muscle groups.

With acute arterial occlusions, the level of arterial obstruction can often be diagnosed from the history, since exertional muscle pain occurs approximately one joint distal to the site of occlusion. Characteristically, superficial femoral occlusion causes pain in the calf, while external iliac occlusion results in thigh pain, and aortic occlusion is manifest by buttock pain. A characteristic finding in the diabetic who may have only tibial arterial occlusion is that of tightening of the ankle and foot on exertion.

Chronic arterial occlusion may progress, and intermittent pain involving muscle groups may be supplanted by continuous *pain at rest* referred to the sites most distal to the arterial occlusion, viz., toes, feet, fingers, hands. The large muscle groups which are the first to express the ischemic state are almost never the site of rest pain in chronic arterial occlusions. Even rest pain is distinguishable by history from other types of foot or hand pain. Rest pain is worsened by elevation of the extremity, even to the supine position, and is relieved by placing the extremity in the dependent position. Patients with pain related to diabetic neuropathy report no such positional dependence.

Other aspects of history which are critically important include smoking, diabetes, cardiac disorders, trauma, familial disease, and occupational history, as well as drug therapy.

PHYSICAL EXAMINATION. Physical examination is of paramount importance in assessing the presence and severity of vascular disease. In this regard physical examination is relatively of greater importance than with abdominal or thoracic problems, where laboratory investigations play a more dominant role. Particular attention to the color, temperature, and pulse pattern of the extremities involved is required and usually permits estimation of the level of arterial occlusion, the severity of ischemia, and the abruptness of the onset. Acute arterial occlusion characteristically produces marked color and temperature differences; chronic occlusion may produce no visible changes but only a difference in palpable pulses early in the course of disease. When acute occlusion progresses to gangrene it is manifest frequently as "wet" gangrene, with blebs, bullae, and violaceous discoloration. When chronic occlusion progresses gradually to severe ischemia, characteristic changes associated with atrophy appear and progress to localized tissue necrosis, manifested by ulceration. The final stage is usually the mummification characteristic of dry gangrene, which starts peripherally in the toes and extends proximally to involve the entire foot and leg. Palpation of the peripheral pulses is the most important feature of the examination. In the lower extremity, the femoral, popliteal, posterior tibial, and dorsalis pedis pulses should be noted. It is important to remember that the common femoral artery extends only about 5 cm below the inguinal ligament before bifurcating into the profunda femoris and superficial femoral arteries. In the upper extremity the brachial, radial, and ulnar pulses should be noted. In many patients it is possible to feel the digital pulses at the bases of the phalanges. The integrity of the palmar arterial arches can be tested by the performance of the Allen test. This is done by having the patient make a tight fist, then occluding the radial and ulnar arteries at the wrist and having the patient slowly open the hand. With the hand in a relaxed position, the integrity of the radial artery in the hand is determined by releasing radial compression and noting the return of color. The maneuver is repeated releasing the ulnar artery while the radial remains compressed. The ability to determine definitely the presence or absence of a peripheral pulse is one of the most essential features of an adequate evaluation of the peripheral circulation.

With chronic ischemia, characteristic nutritional changes

develop in the feet. These include the loss of hair from the toes, the development of brittle, opaque nails, the appearance of atrophy and rubor in the skin, and atrophy of muscles of the feet with increasing prominence of the interosseous spaces. Hence, a simple glance at a foot can determine the presence or absence of serious vascular disease. The importance of this evaluation is emphasized by the fact that gangrene seldom appears in an extremity with chronic vascular disease until these stigmata of chronic ischemia have appeared.

Characteristic color changes also appear with advanced arterial insufficiency, consisting of a purplish rubor in dependency, changing to pallor when the extremity is elevated. The colors are quite different from the chronic congested extremity with venous insufficiency.

The location of ulcerations offers a major clue to cause, for ulceration from venous insufficiency is virtually unknown below the level of the malleolus. By contrast, most ulcers from arterial insufficiency begin over the toes, corresponding to the most distal parts of the arterial tree. Rarely ischemic ulcers develop on the leg or about the ankle without involvement of the toes, perhaps as a result of local tissue infarction, especially after localized trauma, or from arterioarterial embolization.

Palpation of the extremity for temperature and moisture may provide useful information, especially with vasospastic conditions with increased sympathetic tone, where the cool, sweaty extremity affords an important clue to the diagnosis.

Auscultation is of value for certain disorders, particularly arteriovenous fistulas, where detection of the classic continuous murmur quickly establishes the diagnosis. With localized stenotic lesions in peripheral arteries, usually from atherosclerotic plaques, a systolic bruit may be heard, promptly confirming the presence of arterial stenosis.

Estimation of venous filling time is of some value in the diagnosis of arterial insufficiency, but the test is of no value where incompetent valves are present in the venous system. In the absence of varicosities, the test is performed by elevation of the extremities until collapse of the veins has occurred. The extremities are then quickly lowered, and the time required for the veins to fill, usually on the dorsum of the foot or hand, is noted. Normally venous filling will occur within 10 to 15 seconds. Prolonged filling frequently denotes arterial insufficiency. Venous filling times of longer than 1 minute denote a very high degree of arterial compromise.

An oscillometer may be of some value in extremities with edema where peripheral pulses may be difficult to palpate. This instrument consists of a blood pressure cuff attached to a manometer and provides a method for evaluating pulsatile oscillations when the cuff is inflated to just above diastolic pressure. It is of value for specific problems such as determining that a palpable pulse is distal to a markedly stenotic or occluded artery. Other special instruments which can be used in the office or at the bedside to quantify the degree of ischemia and determine prognosis have limited usefulness. Doppler instruments, as well as other types of pulse recorders, may give information regarding the patency of particular distal arteries such as the

dorsalis pedis or the posterior tibial. Pressures in these arteries may be determined by the use of a standard blood pressure cuff applied to the calf or ankle, inflated to above arterial systolic pressure, and released as one listens with the Doppler instrument over the vessel. As with the oscillometer, these determinations are most useful for defining arterial occlusions or stenoses proximal to palpable distal pulses.

The general physical examination is important to determine whether there are any underlying or associated disorders and whether there are additional areas of arterial involvement detectable by finding absent pulses elsewhere or bruits over arteries such as the carotids. It is vital to know about the presence of aneurysms in the abdomen, groins, or thorax. Examination of the heart is essential to determine whether there are valvular lesions, rhythm disorders, or congenital lesions which might serve as the nidus for thromboemboli.

LABORATORY EXAMINATION. The most important laboratory examination by far is selective arteriography to outline the location and extent of arterial obstruction. Selection of the appropriate method of examination varies with the disease present, for virtually every artery in the body can now be successfully outlined by appropriate catheter angiography. Percutaneous introduction of the arterial catheter is the most frequently employed technique. Arteriography may not be essential to confirm the diagnosis but is important to evaluate the possibilities of successful therapy. Illustrative angiograms are shown in specific disease sections in this chapter.

Other techniques for evaluating peripheral circulation are of little clinical value and are utilized mostly for investigative studies. These include precise measurements of skin temperature, sweating, plethysmography, radioactive isotope clearing rates, and various Doppler studies.

Manifestations of Acute Arterial Occlusion

Recognition of acute arterial occlusion is vital, since it may progress to ischemic necrosis within hours. A thrombus propagates distally as well as proximally to the point where it lodges, occluding collateral channels, thereby worsening the ischemia. Thrombosis may occlude the venous system as well, making restoration of flow impossible.

Acute occlusion usually appears without specific warning symptoms. Prompt diagnosis can be made only if the clinical picture is quickly recognized. This is essential for successful therapy, because within 4 to 8 hours after acute occlusion ischemic necrosis in the involved muscles may become irreversible. An additional feature in the pathogenesis of acute arterial occlusion that emphasizes the time factor is the tendency for thrombi to develop in the arteries distal to the point of occlusion where the flow of blood is either decreased or stagnant. This development, superimposed upon the acute obstruction, makes surgical therapy to restore circulation much more difficult. With persisting ischemia, thrombosis finally develops in the venous system as well, making surgical therapy impossible.

The usual causes of acute arterial occlusion are embolism, trauma, or thrombosis. Thrombosis of a previously undiagnosed aneurysm, such as a popliteal aneurysm, is a less frequent cause. Each of these is discussed in subsequent sections. Embolism is noteworthy in that it often appears without any previous signs of underlying disease as an acute catastrophe involving an extremity. In many it is the first symptom of serious underlying heart disease: mitral stenosis, atrial fibrillation, or myocardial infarction. Arterial trauma, when occurring as an isolated injury, may be easily recognized. When complicated with associated fractures or head injuries, the diagnosis may be difficult.

FIVE P's. For emphasis the five prominent features of acute arterial occlusion may be summarized as five p's: *p*ain, *p*aralysis, *p*aresthesia, *p*allor, and absence of *p*ulses.

Pain is present in 75 to 80 percent of patients with acute arterial occlusion, representing the onset of ischemia in the involved tissues. It is absent in some patients, apparently from the prompt onset of complete anesthesia and paralysis. In others, when collateral circulation minimizes the degree of ischemia produced, pain may also be minimal.

Paralysis and paresthesias (or anesthesia) are the most important symptoms in evaluating the severity of arterial occlusion. The importance of these features is based on the fact that the peripheral nerve endings are the most sensitive tissues to anoxia in an extremity. A familiar illustration of the sensitivity of sensory nerve endings to anoxia is the common experience of one's foot "going to sleep" while one sits with the extremity flexed in an unusual position. The sensitivity of striated muscles to anoxia is almost as great as that of nerve endings. Hence, an extremity with paralysis and paresthesia will almost surely develop gangrene, while, conversely, if motor and sensory function are intact even though signs of ischemia are present, gangrene probably will not occur. The neurologic findings then are an important clue both to the urgency of prompt therapy and in the evaluation of the effectiveness of therapy in restoring circulation. Recognition that a paralysed anesthetic extremity will develop gangrene in most patients within 6 to 8 hours after onset emphasizes the urgency of immediate treatment.

Pallor is a less important sign, representing varying degrees of decreased circulation. Associated with visible pallor may be the sensation of coldness.

Absence of pulses confirms the diagnosis and localizes the point of occlusion. With uncertainty, as in an edematous extremity, an oscillometer may be of some value in confirming the absence of pulses. When palpation is indeterminate, the presence of neurologic symptoms indicates the urgency of deciding whether arterial occlusion is present. A frequent example is seen in a patient with a swollen extremity with a fracture of the femur in whom swelling of the extremity may make palpation of the pulses difficult. To determine whether or not an associated injury of the femoral artery is present may require arteriography. If neurologic symptoms are present, angiography should be performed on an emergency basis.

Manifestations of Chronic Arterial Occlusion

The picture of chronic progressive arterial ischemia is typically seen with atherosclerosis involving the abdominal aorta and its branches to the lower extremities, including the iliac, femoral, and popliteal arteries. The course of the disease may be a gradual, progressive one, or it may be interrupted with acute episodes of segmental arterial thrombosis or minor traumatic injuries to the toes resulting in gangrene. The disease almost always is due to atherosclerosis with its protean variations. Diabetic patients in general tend to have more distal arterial involvement of the popliteal and tibial arteries. Their clinical syndromes are further modified by the not infrequent presence of diabetic neuropathy and by characteristic susceptibility to necrotizing infections. This is more fully discussed in a subsequent section, The Diabetic Foot. In the upper extremities Buerger's disease, Raynaud's disease, and cervical rib are unusual causes of chronic ischemia.

The hallmark of chronic arterial insufficiency is claudication, the pathophysiology of which was discussed earlier. This is a highly specific symptom, virtually diagnostic of chronic arterial insufficiency. Hence, a carefully taken history to establish the presence of claudication is essential to establishing the diagnosis. For a long period of time the only measure of progression of arterial insufficiency is the appearance of claudication with progressively smaller amounts of exercise, usually measured in terms of walking two blocks, one block, or even shorter distances.

An important subsequent feature of progressive arterial insufficiency is the appearance of trophic changes in the feet, including loss of hair from the toes, the appearance of brittle, opaque nails, and atrophy of the skin with the development of rubor in dependency. These objective changes are associated with few symptoms except for an increasing susceptibility to cold. However, their presence in association with claudication indicates a much more advanced state of arterial insufficiency.

The importance of recognizing these changes in management of chronic ischemic disease is the fact that gangrene will readily occur in a foot or hand with advanced trophic changes following trivial trauma, such as trimming of a callus or corn, a blister from improper shoes, or minor exposures to extremes of heat or cold. Thirty to forty percent of patients with gangrene of the extremities ultimately requiring amputation may date the onset of gangrene in a toe to such trivial trauma. Apparently local trauma results in increased metabolic demands and perhaps in regional thrombosis of collateral circulation. The latter may be progressive despite all therapy unless immediate surgical revascularization can be carried out.

The end stages of chronic arterial insufficiency are represented by ischemic rest pain, usually in association with ulceration. Rest pain is due to ischemic neuritis and may be associated with tissue necrosis, often with superficial ulceration. It is seen in its most severe forms in patients with Buerger's disease, probably with superimposed ischemic neuritis. The recognition of ischemic rest pain and its ominous prognosis is of great significance, because unless ulceration or gangrene are already present, they will develop shortly if arterial circulation cannot be improved. Hence, surgical therapy if feasible should be done as soon as possible. Prolonged nonsurgical measures, consisting principally of rest to avoid trauma, vasodilators, and avoidance of tobacco, may be successful in a limited number of patients over a period of many weeks, probably because of the development of additional collateral circulation. In many patients, however, rest pain inevitably progresses to gangrene and amputation unless the occluded vascular bed can be reconstructed.

Fortunately, in the upper extremity, in contrast to the lower extremity, atherosclerosis which progresses to rest pain and gangrene is unusual. Claudication of the arm with exercise may be moderately disabling, but more serious symptoms are uncommon. Rest pain and tissue necrosis when present usually denote digital vessel occlusion either due to embolization from proximal atherosclerotic plaques or end-stage Raynaud's phenomenon.

Atherosclerotic Disease of the Lower Extremities

Atherosclerotic disease of the arteries to the lower extremities may be divided into three large groups, dependent upon the level of involvement. These are aortoiliac, femoropopliteal, and tibioperoneal. There are distinctive clinical features about each of the categories; more than one area is involved in at least one-third of patients seen. Aortoiliac disease in the fifth and sixth decades is characterized by relatively mild atherosclerosis with aortic occlusion from superimposed thrombosis, but in the seventh and eighth decades atherosclerosis is severe and thrombosis is relatively mild. Isolated femoropopliteal disease is especially frequent in cigarette smokers, while tibioperoneal disease occurs predominantly in diabetics. No matter where the obstruction is located, the physiologic deficit is decreased blood flow to the lower extremities, with symptoms ranging from intermittent claudication to gangrene. Tissue necrosis is more prone to occur with distal arterial disease and occlusive disease which progresses rapidly without time for collateral circulation to develop.

The choice of surgical therapy for the three different types depends upon several variables. These include the natural history of the arterial disease and the severity of the ischemic symptoms; the age and responsibilities of the patient; and the reliability of arterial reconstructive procedures, which varies greatly from one area to another.

AORTOILIAC DISEASE

HISTORICAL DATA. The ischemic syndrome produced by atherosclerotic disease of the bifurcation of the abdominal aorta has been recognized with increasing frequency over the past 30 years. Leriche is credited with emphasizing in the early 1940s the clinical characteristics of occlusion of the abdominal aorta, i.e., claudication, impotence, and absence of gangrene. The development of angiography, pioneered by dos Santos, greatly facilitated diagnosis.

ETIOLOGY AND PATHOLOGY. Some degree of atherosclerosis is almost universally seen at autopsy in the abdominal aortas of patients over sixty years of age, but symptoms from decrease in blood flow do not occur unless the diameter of the aorta has been greatly narrowed by as much as 90 percent. The process may simply be athero-

sclerosis with intimal thickening and fibrosis, or it may be complicated by ulceration of atherosclerotic plaques with superimposed thrombosis or embolization of portions of atherosclerotic plaques. As in other arteries, the disease often begins at bifurcations where flow patterns conducive to intimal thickening occur. Hence, involvement is often greatest at the aortic, the iliac, and the common femoral bifurcations. It may extend proximally in the abdominal aorta up to the level of the renal arteries, but fortunately occlusion proximal to the renal arteries is rare.

Patients are frequently seen in the fifth and sixth decades with thrombosis of the abdominal aorta but only mild atherosclerosis of the common iliac arteries. The thrombus often propagates up to the level of the renal arteries, rarely occluding one renal artery, and extending up to near the superior mesenteric artery. These patients contrast to a curious degree with patients in the seventh and eighth decades who may have unusually severe atherosclerosis but without thrombosis and total occlusion despite advanced stenosis. This variation with age suggests that some unrecognized factor in the younger group may precipitate the thrombotic process.

Fortunately clinically significant atherosclerosis of the abdominal aorta is virtually always segmental. Proximally it stops at the level of the renal arteries; distad the profunda femoris artery is almost always patent, though not infrequently involved with correctible stenotic lesions even in the presence of a totally occluded superficial femoral artery. Hence, reconstruction can be done in over 95 percent of patients, directing flow distad into the patent profunda femoris artery, which, however, may require either bypass or endarterectomy to serve as a suitable outflow tract. If the superficial femoral artery is also occluded, additional reconstruction is usually not required unless tissue necrosis is present. Otherwise simple aortoiliac or aorto-profunda femoris will suffice.

A separate therapeutic consideration is the 10 percent of persons with aortoiliac occlusive disease who have small aneurysms as well. This group must be treated by aortic graft replacement of the aneurysmal segment, for aneurysmal dilatation may develop following endarterectomy.

Concomitant coronary or cerebral atherosclerosis occurs frequently, probably in 30 to 50 percent of patients with symptomatic aortoiliac disease. Coronary disease is by far the principal cause of death in the 5-year period following surgical aortoiliac reconstruction. This has led to an increased interest in overcoming the effects of aortoiliac occlusions without invading the abdominal cavity, through the performance of so-called extraanatomical bypass grafts, popularized by Blaisdell et al. In these procedures one or both axillary arteries serve as the takeoff vessels for grafts leading to the groin. To overcome unilateral iliac arterial occlusions, cross-femoral grafts also have been used successfully.

In addition, patients with detectable involvement of cerebral or coronary arteries are evaluated for possible angiographic studies of those arteries and for possible cerebrovascular or coronary arterial reconstructive procedures.

PATHOPHYSIOLOGY. Aortoiliac disease decreases blood

flow to the pelvic viscera and lower extremities. Collateral circulation develops to an extensive degree when the aorta becomes completely occluded. The principal collaterals are through the lumbar arteries, anastomosing distad with the branches of the gluteal arteries and the profunda femoris arteries. Fortunately this collateral circulation is sufficient to prevent ischemia at rest, so symptoms appear only with exercise. In men impotence is frequent because of decreased blood flow through the hypogastric arteries. Claudication is present in the lower extremities, but as blood flow is adequate at rest, the extremity remains well nourished. Only with additional occlusions in the superficial femoral, profunda femoris, or popliteal and tibial arteries do nutritional changes with ulceration and gangrene appear. Rarely a few patients develop occlusion of the aorta at a rapid rate, before collateral circulation develops; these may show severe ischemic changes in the legs, even though no additional disease is present distad. Necrotic toe and foot lesions secondary to embolization of minute particles (atheroemboli) from the aorta or iliac arteries are being recognized with increasing frequency. These may occur in the presence of nonoccluding or even nonstenosing atherosclerotic plaques which give rise to emboli which occlude pedal or digital arteries, resulting in so-called "blue or purple toe" syndromes.

CLINICAL MANIFESTATIONS. The classic symptoms are intermittent claudication and impotence of varying severity in males. Claudication may be symmetric or asymmetric, depending upon the pattern of involvement of the iliac arteries. Characteristically with walking, discomfort is felt in the calf, thigh, and buttock muscles. The symptoms vary in severity from difficulty after walking three to four blocks to inability to walk even indoors. Rest pain, ulceration, or gangrene almost always indicate additional distal disease. This is particularly true in diabetics, where disease of the tibial arteries is common.

Symptoms may remain stable for years and progress only with progression of distal atherosclerosis. In some patients the symptoms improve with exercise as collateral vessels enlarge. Conversely, symptoms may worsen, sometimes dramatically, with hypotension secondary to myocardial infarction or cardiac arrhythmias. Impotence is a complex syndrome which may arise from multiple causes. Its presence or absence cannot be relied upon to diagnose aortoiliac disease. Although it may improve after successful arterial reconstruction, the likelihood in any particular patient is unpredictable.

Physical Examination. The principal finding is diminution or absence of the femoral pulses, combined with absence of popliteal and pedal pulses. Pulsations in the abdominal aorta may be palpable if occlusion is limited to near the aortic bifurcation, but these are absent if the abdominal aorta is occluded up to the renal arteries. A systolic bruit is often audible over the aorta or iliac arteries, confirming the presence of atherosclerosis. However, it does not correlate with the degree of stenosis. Nutrition in the extremities is usually normal. With signs of chronic ischemia, such as absence of hair, brittle nails, or rubor, additional atherosclerotic disease in the femoral or popliteal arteries is probably present.

Occasionally patients are seen with aortoiliac disease with acute episodes of severe ischemia of the toes or feet, often with cyanosis and rest pain. The diagnosis may be especially puzzling if the aortoiliac obstruction is not severe. Occasionally pedal pulses are palpable. The syndrome probably arises from arterioarterial embolization of fragments of atherosclerotic plaques or thrombi dislodged from the surface of such plaques. The diagnosis may be suspected if a localized bruit in the abdomen or groin is found.

As multiple areas of atherosclerosis are frequent, particular care should be taken to search for bruits over the carotid or subclavian arteries, as well as to note the adequacy of pulses in the upper extremities.

LABORATORY STUDIES. With the exception of patients experiencing arterioarterial embolization, the diagnosis usually can be established by the history and physical examination. Roentgenograms often show calcification in the wall of the aorta, but as the calcification is in the media, it does not correlate with the degree of flow obstruction. An unsuspected abdominal aortic aneurysm, however, may be outlined by the calcification within its wall. Aortography is performed if surgical reconstruction is being considered. It delineates the proximal extent of the occlusion and may outline the patent arteries beyond the obstruction, especially the profunda femoris vessels.

TREATMENT. Nonsurgical. The need for surgical reconstruction depends upon the severity of the symptoms and the age of the patient. Intermittent claudication in most instances denotes mild ischemia even in the presence of extensive arterial occlusions and, of itself, is a relative indication for surgical intervention. In 80 percent of patients affected, the course is relatively benign, the claudication either improving or disappearing over a period of months or remaining stable. Two-thirds of all patients affected can be managed successfully without operative intervention; 14 percent require an operation for "social" reasons. For example, mild claudication in a forty-five-year-old patient whose occupation necessitates frequent walking is a strong indication for operation. By contrast, a retired patient of seventy with angina pectoris and claudication does not require operation. The presence of trophic changes in the feet, rubor, absence of hair, and brittle nails is a useful guide to the risk of gangrene, for gangrene is rare except with acute arterial occlusion as long as trophic changes are absent. Only 2.5 percent of claudicators develop gangrene. These usually are the patients with the most severe claudication and the most marked involvement of the tibial arteries, in whom surgical reconstructions either cannot be done or, if done at higher levels, do not result in control of the necrotizing ischemia. Thus, prophylactic intervention in claudicators probably does not avert the appearance of gangrene at a later date (see Table 21-1).

If operation is not recommended, daily exercise to the point of claudication should be encouraged, for this may enhance collateral circulation, as manifested by gradual increase in walking tolerance. If walking is not feasible, a similar exercise can be performed indoors by having the patient raise himself on his toes and then rock back on his heels, repeating the sequence rapidly until calf cramps

Table 21-1. FATE OF 104 CLAUDICATORS*

>600 claudicators ⟶ >500 claudicators; no angiograms

104 claudicators
+
angiograms

6 mo to 8 yr
(average, 2.5 yr)

Stable 82 (79%)   Worsened 22 (21%)

No surgery   Elective   Gangrene   No surgery   Arterial
66 (63%)   surgery   recon-
             16 (15%)   struction

Improved   6 (5.8%)   10 (9.1%)   6 (5.8%)

*These patients had arteriograms and were followed for 6 months to 8 years (average, 2.5 years) in an attempt at nonsurgical management.
SOURCE: From A. M. Imparato, G. E. Kim, and J. G. Crowley, Intermittent Claudication: Its Natural Course, *Surgery,* **78**:795, 1975, Table II, p. 796.

occur. Following a rest period the exercise is repeated, as often as twenty or more times daily.

Abstinence from tobacco in any form is mandatory. There is reasonable statistical evidence that claudication improves when smoking is stopped and that the risk of gangrene is greater in patients who smoke. The precise mechanism is unknown, but tobacco is a potent vasoconstrictor. Robichek et al. have reported that continued smoking after arterial reconstructions results in premature failures. Drug therapy with vasodilators may be tried, but unfortunately few patients have had any improvement in the claudication. Alcohol, orally administered, is employed for its peripheral vasodilator effect.

With severe ischemia, one of the most crucial points in management is educating the patient to protect the feet from any form of trauma. This includes extremes of heat or cold, improperly fitting shoes, or vigorous trimming of calluses, corns, or toenails. A familiar tragedy is that a trauma that would be minor in a foot with normal circulation will produce gangrene of a toe in a severely ischemic foot which not only fails to heal but may gradually progress upward to result in a low thigh amputation. Infection associated with unguis incarnatus or dermatophytosis similarly may cause decompensation of the circulation with gangrene, probably from an increase in local tissue metabolism.

Therapy directed toward lowering blood lipid concentrations by diet, drugs, or even surgical procedures remains of uncertain benefit. Anticoagulant therapy with heparin or warfarin sodium has not been helpful. The recent exciting discovery that acetylsalicylic acid in small doses strikingly alters platelet aggregation and may thereby prevent intravascular thrombosis is now undergoing clinical evaluation and holds considerable therapeutic promise.

Lumbar Sympathectomy. In patients with trophic changes

in the feet not amenable to direct arterial reconstruction, lumbar sympathectomy may be of benefit both in improving symptoms and in protecting from gangrene. Unfortunately, the benefits of sympathectomy are variable and unpredictable although on occasion dramatic. In several reports objective signs of improvement were demonstrated in only 20 to 30 percent of patients, usually consisting of increased circulation in the skin which provides some protection from ulceration. Increased blood flow to the leg muscles, associated with improvement in claudication, is unfortunately rare.

Due to the great variability of the morphologic features of the lumbar sympathetic chain, lumbar sympathectomies should involve near-total denervation, removing the sympathetic chain from the level of the crus of the diaphragm superiorly down to the level of the common iliac inferiorly. Bilateral excisions of the uppermost lumbar ganglia may cause impairment of sexual function, usually disturbances in ejaculation, and must be considered in deciding the extent of bilateral sympathectomy in young men.

Aortic Reconstruction. The most frequently performed surgical procedures are thromboendarterectomy and a bypass graft, usually with Dacron or Teflon. As mentioned earlier, the almost uniform patency of the profunda femoris vessels makes reconstruction feasible in the vast majority of patients. The risk of operation is between 5 and 10 percent, determined principally by the degree of associated coronary or cerebral atherosclerosis. The superiority of one operative procedure over the other has not been demonstrated conclusively, although the late complications associated with each procedure differ considerably. Long-term patency rates after either procedure range from 65 to 90 percent. Though tedious, endarterectomies have been successfully performed from the level of the renal arteries proximally to the mid-profunda femoris vessels distad. Concomitant aneurysmal disease of the aorta is a definite contraindication to endarterectomy. In some instances the procedures are combined, performing an aortofemoral bypass in combination with localized endarterectomy of the common femoral and profunda femoris arteries.

The most frequent late complications after bypass procedures are false aneurysms developing at the suture lines, which have continued to occur since the introduction of synthetic suture material, and graft infection, which may occur years after implant. The most frequent complication after endarterectomy is a recurrent stenosis from progressive fibrosis and narrowing of the arterial lumen.

Extraanatomical Bypass Grafts. A number of factors have led to a growing interest in the use of extraanatomical bypass grafts to overcome the effects of aortoiliac occlusions. The magnitude of the direct aortic operation makes it less suitable for aged, debilitated patients, and has led to the development of the axillofemoral and femorofemoral bypass grafts. The high success rate of these grafts and the long-term course of the patients have made extraanatomical grafts attractive for use in this group of patients, in whom early death from coronary or other vascular disease is quite high. In many series these operations are being performed preferentially in patients with advanced arterial disease and severe ischemia.

Preoperative Considerations. An aortogram is usually performed to determine the extent of disease in the external iliac and femoral arteries. As it is not needed to confirm the diagnosis, which is readily made on physical examination, the aortogram is of little value unless the distal circulation is visualized. In some instances the authors perform operative angiograms of the common femoral artery to delineate the extent of disease in the proximal profunda femoris artery, for endarterectomies may be successfully

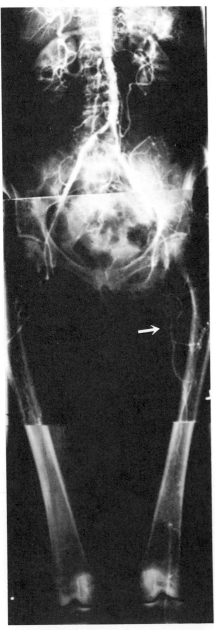

Fig. 21-1. Angiogram illustrating that the profunda femoris artery is usually patent in the presence of aortoiliac occlusive disease. Advanced lesions may be present, however, requiring surgical correction to render the profunda femoris suitable for an outflow tract. Arrow points to patent mid-profunda femoris artery.

performed down to the midportion of this artery (Fig. 21-1).

Operative Technique. A midline abdominal incision, usually extending from the xiphoid process to the pubis symphysis, is preferred. The intestines are retracted onto the right abdominal wall and placed in a plastic bag, after which the retroperitoneal tissues are incised to expose the aorta proximally up to the level of the left renal vein. Once the proximal and distal extent of arterial disease has been defined, a choice is made between a bypass graft or an endarterectomy.

As mentioned earlier, the presence of small aneurysms in the aorta or common iliac artery are absolute contraindications to endarterectomy. A small external iliac artery or severe atherosclerosis in the external iliac artery has influenced many surgeons to perform a bypass procedure to the common femoral artery because of the technical difficulties with endarterectomy of a small diseased external iliac artery. The availability of arterial strippers, as well as the eversion endarterectomy popularized by Conley, however, has extended the scope of endarterectomy and made the operation more satisfactory in these circumstances.

Thromboendarterectomy. A typical pattern of atherosclerotic involvement is extension of disease proximally to within 2 to 3 cm of the renal arteries and distad into the common iliac arteries, stopping in about 50 percent of patients just beyond the bifurcation of the common iliac arteries. Initially the aorta proximally and the external and hypogastric arteries distad are encircled with plastic tapes. The lumbar and inferior mesenteric arteries are similarly exposed. Fifty milligrams of heparin is then given by intravenous injection before occlusive clamps are applied to avoid thrombus formation during the periods of stasis. External iliac clamps are applied before clamping the abdominal aorta to protect from distal embolization. Incisions are made over the distal common iliac arteries, and cleavage planes between the plaques and media are developed. A longitudinal incision is made into the aorta above the level of the inferior mesenteric artery and an appropriate cleavage plane near the junction of the arterial intima and media identified. Using various techniques, including arterial strippers, the core of atherosclerotic material is freed proximally. Usually by blunt dissection the aortic and iliac cores can be mobilized and removed in one piece. A critical aspect of the operative procedure distad is careful inspection of the intima of the proximal external iliac artery to eliminate ledges of thickened intima by suturing. The caliber of the external iliac arteries may be measured with catheters. A diameter smaller than a #16 F catheter often indicates the necessity of extending the endarterectomy to the common femoral arteries. In the hypogastric arteries, endarterectomy is limited to removal of the occluding material near the ostia, for distal dissection of this artery is usually technically unsatisfactory.

The aortotomy incision is closed with a simple continuous suture of 4-0 or 5-0 Tevdek. The iliac arteriotomies may be closed similarly or with a patch graft of either autologous saphenous vein or a prosthetic patch of knitted Dacron. The choice depends upon both the diameter of the artery and the rigidity of the wall. After the incisions are sutured, the occluding clamps are sequentially removed to permit flushing initially into the hypogastric arteries and subsequently into the external iliacs. Strong pulses should be palpable immediately. Weak or absent pulsations indicate obstruction from either retained plaques or stenotic suture lines, in which case the arteriotomy should be promptly reopened and the obstruction corrected. Occasionally in such circumstances operative angiography is needed.

Once blood flow is restored, heparin may be neutralized with protamine, giving 1 to 1.5 mg for each mg heparin used. Often, unless bleeding appears to be excessive, heparin is not neutralized by protamine administration. The posterior peritoneum is sutured over the reconstructed aorta (Fig. 21-2). A concomitant bilateral lumbar sympathectomy is a simple adjunct to the reconstructive procedure but not clearly beneficial. Many uncontrolled data, including higher patency rates, are available regarding the beneficial effects of sympathectomy performed with arterial reconstruction. In our own series, sympathectomy has been performed on rare occasions in association with arterial reconstruction, with no apparent detrimental effect on patency. When it is performed, the sympathetic chain can be identified by palpation as cordlike nodular structures parallel to the aorta on the left and just under the lateral border of the vena cava on the right.

Bypass Grafting. When a bypass procedure is chosen, a knitted rather than a woven Dacron prosthesis is preferred, because of firmer adherence of the neointima which forms subsequently to the wall of the graft. In some tightly woven prostheses, the neointima remains loose, gelatinous, and relatively nonadherent.

After initial determination of where the occlusive disease stops distad, the femoral arteries are exposed if disease extends to the inguinal ligament. The aorta is then isolated proximally and incised longitudinally for 4 to 5 cm. The anastomosis is simpler if a short segment of aorta is identified and clamped, rather than employing a tangential clamp on the anterior wall, which is particularly awkward if the aorta is small and stiff.

The anastomosis is constructed end to side with a continuous suture of 3-0 or 4-0 Tevdek. The graft then can be clamped adjacent to the anastomosis and flow restored to the iliac vessels. Soft tissue tunnels are then developed by blunt dissection anterior and parallel to the iliac vessels, after which the limbs of the prosthesis are brought through the tunnels, lying parallel to the iliac arteries. If the distal anastomosis is performed to the common femoral artery, the graft is brought beneath the inguinal ligament, and the common femoral is incised near the origin of the profunda femoris artery to be certain that there is no obstruction of flow into either the deep or the superficial femoral artery. A continuous suture of 4-0 or 5-0 Tevdek is used. The graft is placed under slight tension at the time of performing the anastomosis to avoid buckling of the graft when it is distended with arterial pressure after the clamps are removed (Figs. 21-3 and 21-4).

A major technical hazard in bypass grafting is the formation of thrombi in the proximal or distal arterial tree with subsequent embolization into the extremity when blood flow is restored. This can be avoided by carefully flushing the graft and routinely inserting a balloon catheter down the distal arterial tree before the distal anastomosis is completed. As the knitted prostheses are porous, they should be preclotted with blood before insertion.

Antibiotics in large amounts are routinely begun at the start of the operation to have circulating blood levels at bactericidal concentrations during the operation. Antibiotics are repeated at appropriate intervals during long procedures.

In performing the axillofemoral bypass graft procedures, the outflow tract is the femoral artery, usually in the groin. This vessel must be made ready to accept a 10- to 12-mm Dacron graft, as for direct aortofemoral grafting. After suitable outflow tracts have been prepared, either unilaterally or bilaterally as the degree of ischemia of the extremities dictates, the axillary artery is exposed in the infraclavicular region. Care must be taken to select axillary arteries which are fully patent. Comparisons of bilateral upper extremity blood pressures are mandatory, since the relatively high incidence of subclavian arterial lesions, usually on the left side, may lead to graft failure. If a blood pressure differential exists or if supraclavicular bruits are heard, arch aortography is indicated. We now favor the right axillary artery, since the innominate, right subclavian complex seems to be involved less often by advanced atherosclerosis. An incision is made over the coracoid process parallel to the clavicle, exposing the pectoralis major muscle, which is divided in the direction of its fibers, exposing the tendon of the pectoralis minor muscle. This is severed from its attachment to the coracoid process, exposing the axillary artery surrounded by the brachial plexus. The artery is dissected free of these nerves, sometimes producing transient and seemingly inevitable brachial plexus neuropathies. The subscapular artery serves as a useful landmark, which is usually though not invariably preserved. A curved tunneler is used to create a subcutaneous tunnel between the infraclavicular incision and the groin incision. When indicated, a suprapubic tunnel is made to connect groin incisions, thereby permitting an additional femorofemoral bypass graft. This latter addition to unilateral axillofemoral grafts is said by some to have a higher late patency rate than the unilateral axillofemoral alone or than bilateral separate axillofemoral grafts.

It is advisable to check the condition of the entire system with operative angiograms, since there are many pitfalls to the procedure. These include not only the usual problems with operations upon atherosclerotic arteries but also accumulations of clot within the prosthesis caused by leakage of tissue thromboplastins from the subcutaneous tunnel into the prosthesis.

Postoperative Care. Peripheral pulses should be closely monitored, for sudden disappearance of a previously palpable pulse usually indicates thrombosis of the graft or an embolus, either of which should be treated by prompt reoperation. Ileus, the most frequent postoperative complication of the intraabdominal procedures, is simply managed by nasogastric suction until adequate peristalsis returns. Antibiotics are given for about 3 to 5 days.

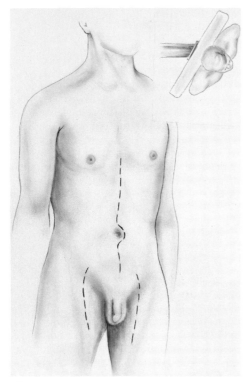

A

Fig. 21-2. Endarterectomy for atherosclerotic obstruction of the aortoiliac segments. *A.* A midline incision from xiphoid process to pubis symphysis is employed. Rotation of the operating table 30 to 40° to the right side facilitates retraction of the intestines. The thighs should be included in the operative field to permit exposure of the bifurcation of the common femoral arteries. *B.* The intestines are either encased in a plastic bag or covered with moist pads. The retroperitoneal tissues are incised exposing the aorta up to the left renal vein. *C.* The arteriotomy incisions are shown placed according to the distribution of the disease. *D.* Endarterectomy strippers may be used to separate the atherosclerotic cores in the iliac arteries. *E.* Following endarterectomy the distal intima is carefully attached to the arterial wall with vertically oriented interrupted sutures to prevent its dissection when circulation is reestablished. *F.* The multiple arteriotomies are either closed by direct suture or with roof patches of autologous vein or Dacron if the vessels are narrow.

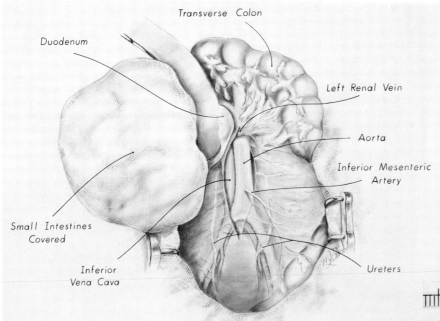

Transverse Colon

Duodenum

Left Renal Vein

Aorta

Inferior Mesenteric Artery

Small Intestines Covered

Inferior Vena Cava

Ureters

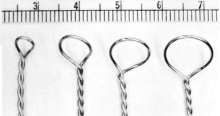

B

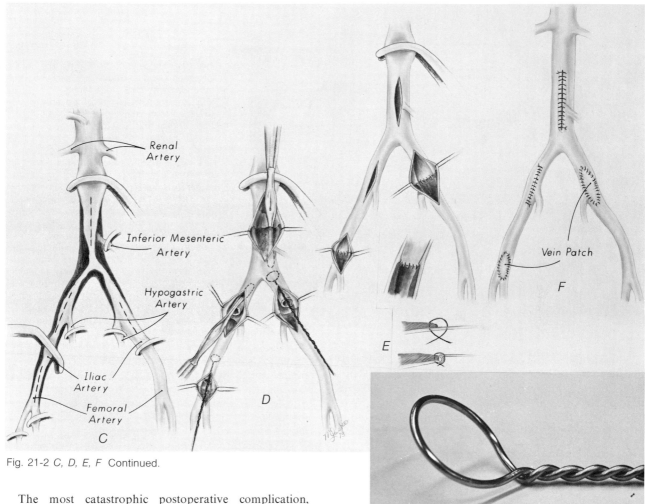

Fig. 21-2 *C, D, E, F* Continued.

The most catastrophic postoperative complication, fortunately extremely rare, is infection developing around the prosthetic graft. In such circumstances the graft usually must be removed to prevent fatal hemorrhage. This can result in unilateral or bilateral amputation of the extremities unless another graft can be inserted. Probably the best form of management is the temporary insertion of axillary-femoral bypass grafts through long subcutaneous tunnels, followed by removal of the infected retroperitoneal prosthesis. Although a single axillary artery has been employed successfully to maintain circulation to the lower half of the body through axillofemoral, femorofemoral grafts, the end-type aortic closures following removal of aortic grafts have frequently ruptured as late as 1 year postoperatively.

Results and Prognosis. Immediate results of aortoiliac reconstructions are excellent. A nearly 100 percent patency rate can be achieved by meticulous technique and proper selection of operative procedures. The immediate functional results are predictable from the angiographic patterns of arterial involvement and the functional status of patients (Fig. 21-5). Claudication is almost always relieved. If tissue loss with gangrene is present, however, additional reconstructive procedures in the distal arterial tree are needed in about 50 percent of the patients.

Numerous data have been published about the long-term results following endarterectomy or bypass grafting. In general, good to excellent results have been sustained in the majority of patients for at least 5 years after operation. If reconstruction is limited to the aorta and common iliac arteries, the 5-year results are similar for endarterectomy and bypass grafts. In a study of 420 patients, Wylie reported that 108 patients with aortoiliac endarterectomy had a 10-year patency of 90 percent. Kouchoukos et al. reported a series of 206 patients treated either by endarterectomy or bypass grafting, after which the 5-year patency rates were virtually identical, 62 and 63 percent. Szilagyi et al. reported similar results 5 years after operation with patency rates of 89 and 85 percent, respectively, when comparing bypass grafting and endarterectomy. Gomes et al. described good results in 84 percent of 401 patients 5 years after operation, and Garrett et al. reported that in over 3,000 operations performed for aortoiliac disease using bypass grafts in the majority of patients good results approached 90 percent 5 years after operation. The results of axillofemoral grafts are not as well documented because of their more recent introduction and failure to receive

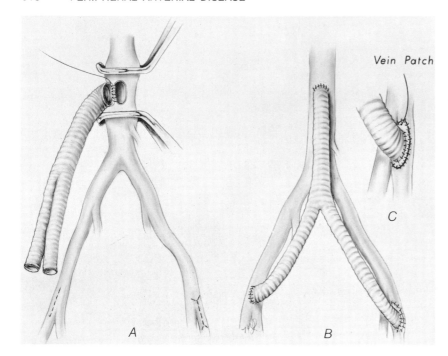

Fig. 21-3. Bypass graft of abdominal aorta. Dissection and exposure are similar to that for endarterectomy procedures. *A.* The proximal anastomosis is performed end to side to the aorta proximal to the point of obstruction. End-to-end aortic anastomosis is preferred by many to lessen the risk of distal embolization. Knitted Dacron is preferred. *B.* The distal anastomoses are performed as end-to-side anastomoses either to the iliac artery proximal to the inguinal ligament or to the common femoral artery at the point of origin of the profunda femoris artery depending upon the degree of atherosclerotic involvement of the external iliac artery. Anastomoses distal to the inguinal ligament are avoided whenever possible to avoid trauma to the prosthesis passing under the inguinal ligament and to lessen the risk of infection posed by having a plastic prosthesis in the groin. *C.* A vein roof patch may be employed to facilitate suture of the prosthesis to small arteries.

immediate universal acceptance. There are now series from Blaisdell, Mannick, and Parsonett which suggest that the immediate and long-term patency rates are comparable to those for aortofemoral grafts, while operative mortality is lower. They are subject to the same complications as other prostheses anastomosed in the groin, viz., false aneurysms and infection.

Hence, it is clear from the data available that the procedure chosen for an individual patient must vary with the disease present and the experience of the surgeon. Whichever technique is used, immediate patency rates should approach 100 percent. False aneurysms following the use of bypass grafts have greatly decreased in frequency with the use of synthetic sutures and the avoidance of excessive tension on the suture lines, although they still occur too frequently. False aneurysms generally do not occur following endarterectomy, and infection with endarterectomy in which autologous tissue only is used is rare.

The principal cause of late deaths after operation is coronary arterial disease, approximately 12 percent within 2 years at New York University. It is hoped that recent advances with coronary bypass operations will improve this poor prognosis.

FEMOROPOPLITEAL OCCLUSIVE DISEASE

PATHOLOGY. The most common site for atherosclerotic occlusion in the lower extremities is the distal superficial femoral artery within the adductor canal. The reason for this characteristic localization is unknown but may be related to the anatomic relationship between the distal femoral artery and the adductor magnus tendon as the artery traverses the adductor foramen to enter the popliteal fossa. The usual sequence of atherosclerotic occlusion is to extend gradually proximally in the superficial femoral artery until the artery is occluded at its origin from the

common femoral. Fortunately, involvement of the profunda femoris artery is infrequent, a complete contrast to the frequency of involvement of the superficial femoral. For this reason atherosclerotic occlusion of the superficial femoral artery alone usually produces claudication but no more serious circulatory impairment.

The importance of the profunda femoris artery in arterial reconstructions of the aortoiliac system has been realized for many years, and correction of ostial stenoses, incident to femoral popliteal reconstructions, has been routinely performed by some. Recently Martin emphasized its importance as a valuable contributor of blood to the extremity in the presence of superficial femoral arterial occlusions, suggesting that the profunda femoris ostium be enlarged even in the absence of high-grade stenosis. Few direct measurements of flow have been made before and after this reconstruction.

When more extensive occlusive disease develops, usually from occlusion of the popliteal artery or its branches, the anterior and posterior tibial arteries, more serious circulatory insufficiency appears. With occlusion of this extent, ulceration and gangrene are common. Such diffuse patterns of atherosclerosis are particularly common in diabetic patients.

CLINICAL MANIFESTATIONS. Segmental occlusion of the superficial femoral artery produces claudication in the leg with moderate exercise, but no symptoms at rest. Physical examination finds a normal femoral pulse but absent popliteal and pedal pulses. Rarely pedal pulses are present at rest but disappear with exercise. The nutrition of the foot is normal. If additional occlusive disease is present beyond the femoral artery, claudication is more severe, perhaps associated with rest pain and trophic changes in the foot, and ulceration and gangrene ultimately ensue. Fortunately, the rate of progression of atherosclerotic occlusion is slow in many patients, and the risk of gangrene developing within 5 years in an extremity with claudication as the only symptom is only about 5 percent.

LABORATORY STUDIES. Arteriography is required to determine the segmental nature of the occlusive disease and the consequent possibilities of arterial reconstruction. Adequate visualization of the popliteal artery and its branches is essential (Fig. 21-6). Fortunately, with current techniques, revascularization procedures extended to the popliteal artery are quite satisfactory if the anterior or posterior tibial branches are patent. The peroneal artery, which does not directly contribute to the formation of the pedal arch, is less satisfactory. If all three branches are occluded, under special circumstances reconstructive procedures may be extended down to the pedal arches of the foot. This is discussed under Tibioperoneal Occlusive Disease.

TREATMENT. If claudication is the only symptom, operation is an elective decision, determined from the age and occupation of the patient. As the risk of gangrene with claudication alone is small, this alone does not constitute an indication for operation. Only when trophic changes appear in the feet is operation indicated because of the risk of gangrene. Care to avoid trauma to the foot, described in the section on aortoiliac occlusive disease, is similarly applicable, avoiding even minor trauma or exposure to extremes of heat or cold. Recommendations regarding tobacco, alcohol, exercise, and vasodilator drugs similar to those made for aortic occlusive disease are applicable. In patients able to walk at least one city block, or 300 feet, a vigorous exercise program of walking at least 1 mile daily has resulted in marked improvement in claudication in at least 50 percent of patients within 6 to 12 months.

Sympathectomy. Unfortunately, when claudication is the only symptom, sympathectomy is of little value. It may enhance the development of collateral circulation and thereby lessen the hazard of more serious insufficiency, but this is primarily theoretic. When trophic changes are pres-

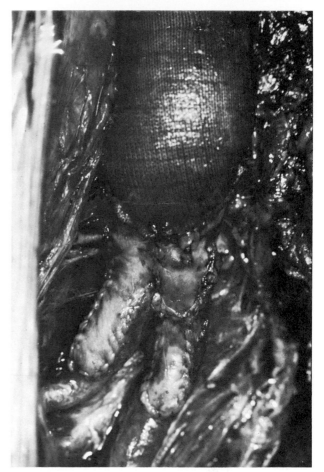

Fig. 21-4. Interposition of vein roof patches over the profunda femoris and superficial femoral arteries facilitates suture of plastic prostheses to the common femoral artery in aortofemoral bypass procedures.

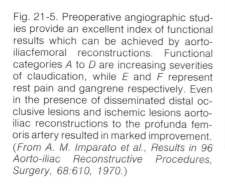

Fig. 21-5. Preoperative angiographic studies provide an excellent index of functional results which can be achieved by aorto-iliacfemoral reconstructions. Functional categories A to D are increasing severities of claudication, while E and F represent rest pain and gangrene respectively. Even in the presence of disseminated distal occlusive lesions and ischemic lesions aorto-iliac reconstructions to the profunda femoris artery resulted in marked improvement. (*From A. M. Imparato et al., Results in 96 Aorto-iliac Reconstructive Procedures, Surgery, 68:610, 1970.*)

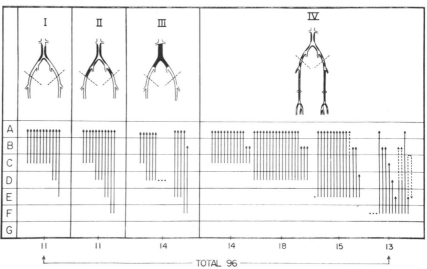

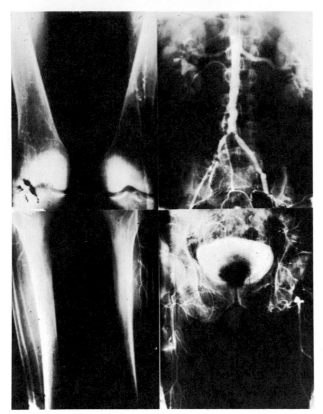

Fig. 21-6. Representative angiographic study required to evaluate patients for arterial reconstruction for claudication. Only in this manner can the inflow and outflow tracts be critically evaluated and arterial reconstructions planned.

ent, however, and direct arterial reconstruction is not possible because of diffuse occlusive disease, a sympathectomy should be performed. The vasodilating effect of sympathectomy on the vessels of the skin provides some protection from ulceration of the ischemic foot. Statistically the results are disappointing, however, for objective improvement can be demonstrated in little more than 20 percent of patients receiving operation.

Direct Arterial Reconstruction. *Bypass Grafting; Endarterectomy.* The basic principle of arterial reconstruction is that there must be both adequate inflow and adequate outflow of blood from the area of reconstruction. Early operative failures are almost always due either to obvious technical faults or to inadequate inflow or outflow. Most groups have become dissatisfied with bypass prosthetic grafts. Although Crawford and associates reported in 1966 that crimped Dacron prostheses, 8 mm or more in diameter, employed in over 2,500 cases gave adequate long-term function, up to 10 years, in about 75 percent of patients, most others have had less satisfactory results. Szilagyi et al. reported a patency rate of only 40 percent in 193 cases 4 years after operation, and Linton achieved only a 6 percent patency 5 years after operation. These poor results contrast markedly to the excellent results following aorto-iliac reconstruction.

The bypass operation with the autologous saphenous

vein is used most commonly though not by all groups. Wylie described similar 5-year results following either endarterectomy or vein bypass. At New York University, three different techniques—venous bypass, long endarterectomy procedures with a venous roof patch, and endarterectomy performed through multiple arteriotomies with multiple vein roof patches—had almost identical results 5 to 7 years later. Analysis of the cause of late failures after reconstruction found that about one-third were due to progressive distal atherosclerosis and one-third to intimal proliferation in the areas of arterial reconstruction. Tissue specimens were not obtained to determine the cause of failure in the other one-third of the cases.

With prosthetic grafts, failure is due to stiffening of the prosthesis from the ingrowth of fibrous tissue, especially when the graft crosses a joint, as well as extensive scarring about the graft which results in poor adherence of the neointima. Venous bypass is favored if a saphenous or cephalic vein can be dilated to an internal diameter greater than 4 mm. If a suitable vein is not available, endarterectomy with wire strippers and multiple vein roof patches has given comparable results, even in diabetic patients. If, for some reason, this is not possible, usually due to a previous operative procedure, then a long endarterectomy with a long vein roof patch, originally described by Edwards et al., is favored. The least satisfactory choices are either a prosthetic graft, usually Dacron, or a homologous vein (Fig. 21-7).

Other techniques have been proposed but lack substantial experience. This includes carbon dioxide ("gas") endarterectomy, developed by Sawyer et al., bovine heterografts, or autologous tissue tubes prepared with a silicone mandril.

Bypass Grafting. The technique of bypass grafting is illustrated in Fig. 21-8. It is particularly attractive because of its simplicity and ease of performance. The precision required for obtaining nearly 100 percent immediate patency can best be evaluated by operative angiography. Relatively small imperfections in the anastomotic suture lines or within the body of the graft can lead to deposition of platelet-fibrin aggregates with occlusion within a few hours.

The saphenous vein is carefully removed from the inguinal ligament to the knee, reversed to permit blood to flow in the direction of the venous valves, and then attached with end-to-side anastomoses to the femoral and popliteal arteries proximal and distal to the obstruction. As mentioned earlier, the vein should be at least 4 to 5 mm in diameter. In 15 to 25 percent of patients a satisfactory vein is not available, because of either previous surgical removal or anatomic variations. A suitable cephalic vein is an acceptable substitute, though a lot of data are not yet available. Otherwise one of the techniques previously described is used.

Endarterectomy. Since its introduction over 20 years ago, between 1951 and 1953, endarterectomy has been modified several times. A completely open technique, incising the artery throughout its length, removing the atherosclerotic core, and suturing the long arteriotomy, had a very high failure rate. Similarly, closed techniques with mechanical

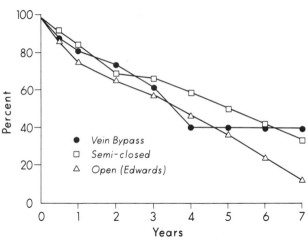

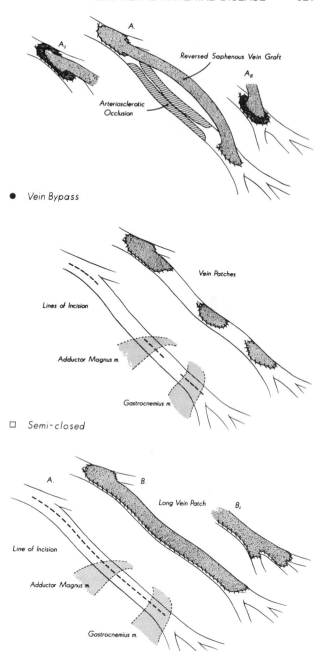

Fig. 21-7. Cumulative patencies of femoropopliteal arterial reconstructions performed by one of three techniques employing only autologous tissue are nearly statistically identical. The three groups are otherwise comparable for indications for operation and grading of severity of involvement of the outflow tracts. Inserts show the three basic techniques employed in reconstructions. (*From A. M. Imparato et al., Comparisons of Three Technics for Femoral-Popliteal Arterial Reconstructions, Ann Surg, 177(3):375, 1973.*)

strippers often failed, usually from leaving loose fragments of intima or atherosclerotic plaque in the lumen. Closure of the long arteriotomy with a vein roof patch, developed by Edwards et al., gave significantly better results. A subsequent modification was the use of multiple vein roof patches to close multiple arteriotomies used for semiclosed endarterectomy. This technique is illustrated in Fig. 21-9. Operative angiography is essential to be certain that atherosclerotic debris has been entirely removed from the lumen.

A technique utilized in some patients is the so-called "in situ" vein graft, in which the saphenous vein is not removed from its bed but is mobilized proximally and distad to be anastomosed end to side to the femoral artery proximally and the popliteal artery or its branches distad. Before the anastomoses are performed, however, the valves in the vein are disrupted by passage of a mechanical instrument along the course of the vein. One limitation of the technique is the production of small arteriovenous fistulas from tributaries of the saphenous vein. Another objection is incomplete disruption of the venous valves with the production of turbulent flow. Some such grafts have been successfully inserted from the common femoral artery proximally to the posterior tibial artery near the ankle, but in general long-term results with the technique have been found unsatisfactory by most groups.

TIBIOPERONEAL ARTERIAL DISEASE

PATHOLOGY. Occlusive disease of the tibial arteries occurs most commonly in patients with diabetes mellitus. It is also seen in patients with Buerger's disease. Some instances of arterioarterial embolism are almost surely incorrectly diagnosed initially and considered as primary occlusive disease of the tibial arteries.

In the diabetic patient there are different patterns of

disease which can be recognized, though the reason for development of such patterns is unclear. All tibial arteries may be involved, as well as occlusion of the pedal arches formed by branches of the anterior and posterior tibial vessels. In such instances surgical reconstruction is impossible. In other patients one or more of the tibial arteries may be entirely patent, or there may be proximal occlusion with patent vessels starting at the level of the malleoli. With this pattern of involvement, arterial reconstruction is possible if grafts are extended to the ankles. Unfortunately, in some diabetic patients there is additional disease in the aortoiliac or femoral areas.

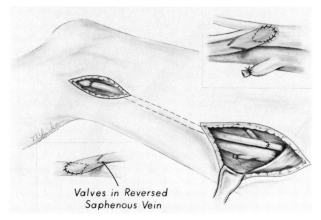

Valves in Reversed
Saphenous Vein

Fig. 21-8. Bypass graft procedure for occlusion of the superficial femoral artery. *A.* Incisions employed for exposure of the major vessels. A proximal incision is made over the saphenous vein from just below the inguinal ligament to the apex of Scarpa's triangle, avoiding undermining of adjacent skin flaps which might result in ischemic necrosis. The distal incision is made on the medial aspect of the popliteal fossa to expose the popliteal artery. The adductor magnus tendon, the site often of most severe superficial femoral arterial involvement, is shown. It is frequently cut to facilitate passing the vein graft from adductor canal to popliteal fossa. *B.* Completed bypass graft of the reversed saphenous vein. The anastomoses are performed end to side to the common femoral and popliteal arteries. The vein is brought either subcutaneously or through the subsartorial canal. Inserts show details of the bevel created in the vein bypass and reversal of the valves. An alternative technique is to leave the saphenous vein in its usual location, without reversal, destroying the valves, accomplishing an in situ nonreversed bypass graft.

CLINICAL MANIFESTATIONS. Occasionally occlusive disease of the tibial arteries merely produces claudication of the foot. Usually, however, there are signs of advanced ischemia. With diabetes there is the additional problem of diabetic neuropathy, difficult to differentiate from ischemic rest pain. Characteristically, ischemic pain is relieved by placing the foot in a dependent position, while that of diabetic neuropathy is not. A frequent problem in the diabetic patient is ulceration on the plantar surface of the foot, secondary to pressure associated with diabetic neuropathy. A more serious problem is a spreading necrotizing infection, with absent pedal pulses. Because of associated ischemia the infection is often refractory to both antibiotic therapy and surgical debridement unless revascularization can be done. This type of progressive, refractory infection may lead to amputation before tissue ischemia per se has caused widespread necrosis. Infection undoubtedly increases the metabolic requirements of the tissue and thereby accentuates the degree of ischemia. A third type of terminal event in the ischemic diabetic foot is soft tissue atrophy to a severe degree, terminating with progressive ischemic dry gangrene of the toes and foot.

LABORATORY STUDIES. Precise angiography is essential to determine the adequacy of the proximal circulation in the aorta and iliac arteries, as well as in the distal arterial tree, especially the small arteries of the ankle and foot. Significant advances in the technique of angiography have

permitted excellent delineation of small arterial branches in these areas. Such studies may be done by direct needle puncture of the femoral artery, followed by injection of a large bolus (50 ml) of contrast medium with serial films made over a long period of time (Fig. 21-10). An alternative technique is to produce ischemic vasodilation by temporary arterial occlusion with an inflated blood pressure cuff for 5 minutes or longer, injecting the dye immediately after deflation of the cuff. This almost invariably produces excellent opacification of distal vessels.

TREATMENT. Unless the extremity is in jeopardy, arterial reconstructions into the tibial arteries are avoided because of the unpredictable outcome in any particular patient. When a reconstruction fails, amputation is usually necessary because the trauma of surgical dissection usually impairs collateral circulation to a significant degree. If operation is not considered indicated, treatment is primarily directed at careful avoidance of foot trauma, as emphasized in the preceding sections.

Surgical reconstruction may be undertaken if only a single tibial artery remains patent or if the pedal arch is found patent on angiogram, usually seen at the ankle as a communication between the anterior and posterior tibial arteries across the dorsum of the foot.

When a necrotizing infection is present, characteristically extending as a necrotic phlegmon rather than an abscess and requiring debridement as opposed to drainage, therapy is almost hopeless without arterial reconstruction. A combined approach of revascularization into the distal tibial and malleolar vessels, followed soon thereafter by debridement of all infected tissue, has been successful. As a practical guideline, if more than one-half of the sole of the foot has been destroyed, the limb will never be suitable for weight bearing, despite effective arterial reconstruction; so amputation is the primary choice. In all such difficult problems intensive antibiotic therapy for the specific organism involved is essential.

Direct Arterial Reconstruction. Bypass venous grafts, usually the greater saphenous vein, have been effective in some patients when connected distad to the anterior or posterior tibial arteries at the level of the malleolus. Tyson and Reichle recently described a substantial experience with the technique performed over the last 4 years. In our experience endarterectomy procedures are not feasible in the small vessels beyond midcalf, although they are quite satisfactory up to that level. However, they have succeeded in the proximal portion in the anterior tibial down to where it passes through the tibiofibular interosseous membrane and down the posterior tibial and peroneal arteries for about 2 in. beyond their origins, removing the overlying soleus muscle to expose the vessels in this area.

These procedures are performed by widely exposing the bifurcation of the popliteal artery through a long medial incision over the calf and lower thigh, a surgical approach described by Imparato and Kim. The endarterectomy is performed with a longitudinal arteriotomy, followed by endarterectomy and closure of the vessels with venous roof patches up to the level of the distal popliteal artery. If arterial reconstruction proximal to this level is required,

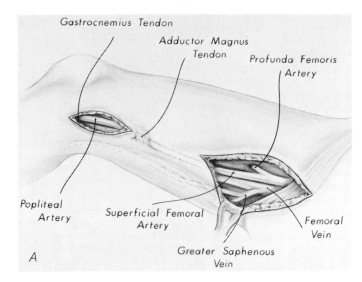

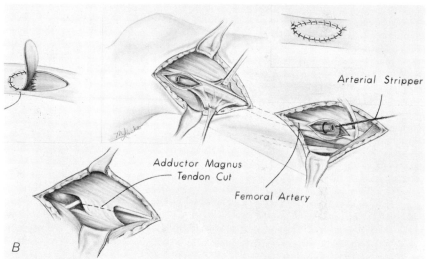

Fig. 21-9. *A.* Femoral popliteal endarterectomy performed by exposing the femoral artery proximally and the popliteal artery distad. *B.* An endarterectomy stripper is used to detach atherosclerotic material via a plane in the media or between media and adventitia. Cutting the adductor magnus tendon facilitates passage of the arterial stripper. The distal intima in the popliteal artery is carefully sutured to prevent detachment and dissection of this free edge when circulation is restored. Arteriotomies are closed with autologous vein roof patches. Angiographic studies are performed to ensure that all debris has been removed, since even minute fragments left behind may result in immediate rethrombosis. Alternative techniques are exposing the entire femoral artery, opening it longitudinally in its entirety and suturing a long roof patch for closure, or utilizing CO_2 intramural injection to accomplish endarterectomy.

a bypass procedure or an endarterectomy can be combined with a distal endarterectomy. Similarly if reconstruction is required distad down to the ankle, the reversed autologous vein bypass technique is employed. Although the arteries at the malleolus are small, with an internal diameter of 1 to 2 mm, the anastomoses can be performed with fine suture material (7-0) and optical magnification. Operative angiography is quite useful when such small anastomoses are performed (Fig. 21-11).

Prognosis. As mentioned earlier, arterial reconstructions in this area are performed only when ulceration and gangrene threaten amputation. Arterial reconstruction is initially successful in about 75 percent of patients, both with reconstruction at the proximal tibioperoneal level and with reconstruction extending down to the malleolus. Immediate failures are almost always due to inadequate outflow tracts. Failures occur invariably if the dorsal arch at the ankle is not complete. When the reconstruction is initially successful, limb salvage is excellent, for the necrotic tissue

can be debrided and the wound subsequently closed by skin grafting. If the arterial reconstruction fails before complete healing is obtained, however, amputation is usually required.

If healing is complete and the arterial reconstruction subsequently becomes occluded, a significant percentage of patients remain with a viable functional extremity. Some reconstructions into the proximal tibial arteries so far have remained patent for as long as 5 to 7 years. Fewer data are available for bypass grafts extending down to the ankle, but the failure rate within 2 years after operation seems to exceed 50 percent.

Lumbar Sympathectomy. Lumbar sympathectomy is often tried in desperation as an alternative to amputation when arterial reconstruction cannot be performed. It also may be combined with reconstruction, although its value in this case cannot be determined. As an isolated procedure, improvement can be significant in more than 50 percent of patients in this group. Occasionally a brilliant result occurs,

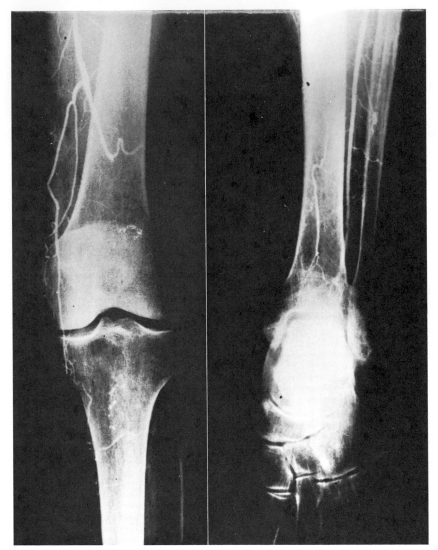

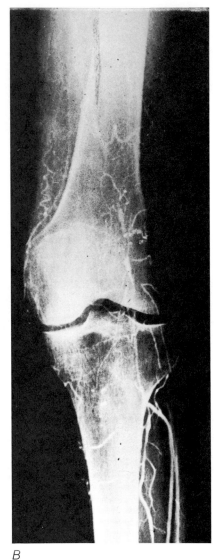

A

B

Fig. 21-10. Preoperative angiographic studies in the presence of tibial disease. *A.* Angiographic studies routinely performed showing poor visualization of tibial arteries. *B.* Angiograms in the same patient obtained 6 weeks later, when an ischemic lesion developed in the foot, showing patency of the anterior tibial artery. This degree of opacification was obtained using the ischemic hyperemia technique described in the text.

consisting of relief of rest pain and marked increase in temperature of the foot. Unfortunately it has not been possible to predict which patients with impending limb loss would respond favorably. Therefore, in our series all patients, whether diabetic or not, whose conditions were considered inoperable from the point of view of arterial reconstruction on the basis of angiographic studies had lumbar sympathectomies. Some 60 percent responded favorably for longer than 6 months, while 40 percent came to early amputation within 2 months.

Infected Prosthesis. The large number of patients now alive with artificial, plastic blood vessel replacements has introduced a numerically significant new pathologic entity, viz., the infected plastic prosthesis. Plastic blood vessel substitutes, especially if placed in the groins, are subject to infection, which usually cannot be eradicated unless the plastic material is removed from the infected area. Axillofemoral bypass grafts have been employed to permit removal of infected intraabdominal grafts. Infections in the

groin, in the presence of noninfected intraabdominal arteries, have been treated by performing iliac to superficial femoral or popliteal bypass grafts, avoiding the infected groins by leading the grafts through the obturator foramen to the posteromedial aspect of the thigh or to the medial aspect of the popliteal fossa, thus permitting the radical debridement of infected tissue and grafts from the groins. These have been highly successful when properly planned in association with prolonged antibiotic therapy. These procedures are indicated at a stage when infection may appear relatively innocuous. Injection of a radiopaque contrast medium into the sinuses has been helpful in delineating the true nature and extent of the problem. Aggressive and extensive surgical procedures are required to prevent exsanguinating hemorrhage from breakdown of suture lines secondary to the local infection. Although obturator bypass grafts have been successful in dealing with infections in the groins, removal of aortic prosthesis with end closure of the infrarenal aorta has resulted frequently in subsequent rupture of the aorta.

Amputation. Some important guidelines should be emphasized when amputation threatens because of progressive ulceration of the foot: First, an arterial reconstructive procedure may be successful if only one major arterial tributary is patent, a branch of the popliteal artery, the anterior tibial, the posterior tibial, or even the peroneal artery. Second, a foot will remain useful for weight bearing as long as the posterior half, including the heel, is intact. If more than 50 percent of the sole has been lost, however, the foot is probably useless for weight bearing even if arterial reconstruction is successful. With these two guidelines, angiograms should be seriously considered for virtually all patients in whom amputation is being considered. Data published by Dale in 1967 are quite significant in this regard. Of 100 patients threatened by amputation, either because of rest pain (38 percent) or ulceration with gangrene (62 percent), arterial reconstructive procedures were performed in 73 and lumbar sympathectomy in 13. The leg was salvaged in 64, and a minor amputation was possible in 10 others.

Both morbidity and mortality are surprisingly high in patients requiring amputation for peripheral vascular disease. Mortality is related to the advanced age in many and to a rate of severe coronary occlusive disease exceeding 50 percent. Morbidity is primarily related to failure of wound healing from improper selection of the site of amputation. In general, as long as gangrene is limited to a toe, the amputation should be delayed and the ischemic toe permitted to mummify and undergo virtual autoamputation. Delay permits growth of collateral circulation in the more proximal tissues so that wound healing may occur if the toe is allowed to gradually separate over a period of weeks; a definitive amputation often results in failure and extension of the wound onto the foot. A transmetatarsal amputation may be effective in some diabetic patients when infection superimposed upon a gangrenous toe requires operation. This is successful if pedal pulses are palpable but ineffective if gangrene has extended into the forefoot. Foot amputations proximal to the transmetatarsal level are generally unsatisfactory for weight bearing except for the Syme amputation, which is almost never successful in the presence of peripheral vascular disease.

A fortunate and surprising development in the past few years has been the demonstration by several groups that below-knee amputations can be successfully performed in a high percentage of patients, even in the absence of a popliteal pulse. Preservation of the knee joint greatly facilitates the wearing of a prosthesis. Guidelines are still being sought to determine the likelihood of wound healing if a below-knee amputation is performed in the absence of a popliteal pulse. The degree of skin bleeding is one of the most useful guidelines, though not infallible, that has yet appeared. An attempted below-knee amputation is a

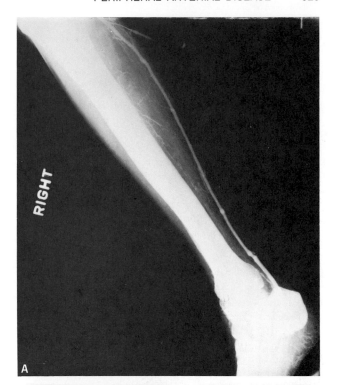

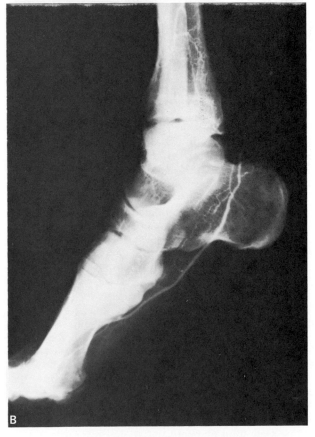

reversed autologous femoral-dorsal pedal bypass graft. *A.* Posterior tibial artery forming pedal arch. *B.* Bypass graft in place.

significant benefit to the patient if successful but is detrimental if the wound fails to heal and a subsequent above-knee amputation must be performed.

THE DIABETIC FOOT

The foot of the diabetic patient has distinct problems, characteristic of the diabetic state, which can quickly progress to conditions that threaten limb and life. Three distinct characteristics can be delineated:

First, the diabetic has an extraordinary susceptibility to infection. This can develop after minor trauma to the toe, the sole of the foot, or the heel. After a seemingly trivial injury, within hours or days a virulent necrotizing infection can appear which rapidly spreads along musculofascial planes. It characteristically begins in an interdigital space, spreads along the plantar fascia, and may continue along tendon sheaths into the muscles of the leg. Frequently the infecting organism is gas-producing and may be of the clostridial group. A life-threatening infection quickly evolves. This same susceptibility to infection manifests itself in the development of carbuncles in the neck and in different types of necrotizing infections of the abdominal wall after elective abdominal operations. These infections often occur with patent major arteries and seemingly are not closely related to local ischemia.

A second peculiarity of the diabetic is diabetic neuropathy. Characteristically this appears as hypalgesia or true anesthesia of some portion of the sole of the foot, subsequently complicated by trophic ulcers. These also are unrelated to ischemia and often develop with strongly palpable pedal pulses. The trophic ulcer, anesthetic and painless initially, then becomes a portal of entry for necrotizing infection.

The third peculiarity of the diabetic foot is the type of arterial occlusive disease which typically involves the popliteal artery and its branches down to the pedal arches. The process may be diffuse, or one or more arteries may be spared. Arteries proximal to the popliteal may be normal or may show a typical "nondiabetic" pattern of atherosclerosis.

CLINICAL MANAGEMENT. Infection. In some unfortunate instances a rampant uncontrolled infection with clostridia may necessitate immediate open amputation through the midcalf or midthigh to prevent death from septic shock. If patients are seen earlier, immediate widespread incision and drainage with debridement of infected tissue may prevent amputation. At an earlier stage, when infection is the dominant process without extensive tissue necrosis, localized debridement combined with intensive antibiotic therapy may be successful. A basic guideline is that all necrotic tissue must be extensively debrided, for simple drainage is hopelessly inadequate in the presence of extensive tissue necrosis, as is radical debridement alone because of the underlying tissue ischemia. In such instances the combination of radical debridement with arterial reconstruction down to the ankle may permit salvage of the extremity. These considerations were discussed in the preceding section on tibioperoneal arterial reconstruction.

Gangrene. If gangrene of a toe is present and not complicated by infection, a much more leisurely approach is indicated, quite in contrast to the urgency of therapy if spreading infection is present. As discussed earlier, localized dry gangrene of a toe is best treated by postponing operation, often permitting autoamputation over a period of weeks, during which time the development of collateral circulation may permit wound healing to occur. In all likelihood such instances of gangrene of a digit represent occlusion of a critical digital vessel. This may be followed by the development of enough collateral circulation to salvage the foot, but such circulation requires time to develop.

Trophic Ulcers. A trophic ulcer can be readily recognized by several characteristics. It is usually a sharply demarcated, punched out area on the sole of the foot overlying a pressure point, usually the metatarsal heads. A location over the first or third metatarsal head is particularly common. Often the ulcers are completely anesthetic and hence relatively free of pain until secondary infection develops. Similarly, the pedal pulses may be entirely normal.

Treatment in the majority of patients consists of local cleansing, protection from trauma, and most important of all, avoidance of weight bearing. Reconstruction of shoes to distribute weight differently is often effective. Special types of shoes, such as those lined with lamb's wool, are useful. Effective therapy requires long-term careful periodic observation to readjust the weight-bearing characteristics of the foot so that pressure on the area of ulceration is avoided. Any superimposed infection requires antibiotics and local debridement. As most patients fortunately do not have any vascular occlusion, arterial reconstruction is not needed.

SUMMARY OF THERAPEUTIC CONCEPTS FOR ARTERIAL OCCLUSIVE DISEASE OF THE LOWER EXTREMITIES

Intermittent claudication with normal nutrition in the extremity is a comparatively benign disease in many patients. The risk of gangrene within 5 years is no more than 5 percent. If a patient stops smoking and exercises regularly, claudication may improve to a significant degree within months or years. This, combined with the fact that arterial reconstructions are not curative, indicates that a conservative approach can be applied to many patients with claudication, depending upon the patient's age and occupation.

A quite different approach is indicated when the nutrition of the foot is impaired from chronic ischemia, for the likelihood of ulceration and gangrene within 1 to 2 years is great. In these patients, the possibilities of arterial reconstruction should be carefully investigated by detailed angiography, examining the arterial tree from the abdominal aorta to the pedal arches at the ankle. This has been especially productive when ulceration and gangrene already have appeared and amputation appears imminent.

ARTERIAL EMBOLISM

It has been long recognized that the majority of arterial emboli originate in the heart. The embolus originated from the heart in 86 percent of 426 emboli reported by Darling and associates and in 91 percent of 214 emboli reported by Cranley et al. In the past few years there has been increasing recognition of emboli which originate in atherosclerotic arteries, either fragments of a plaque or thrombi adherent to the surface of an ulcerated plaque which subsequently dislodge. For simplicity in presentation, emboli arising from the heart, constituting the majority of emboli seen, are referred to as *cardioarterial embolization.* As a separate entity, the frequency of which is yet unknown, emboli arising from an atherosclerotic artery and lodging in the distal branches are referred to as *arterioarterial emboli.*

Cardioarterial Embolization

HISTORICAL CONSIDERATIONS. Emboli have been long recognized as a cause of acute arterial occlusion resulting in gangrene. Several unsuccessful embolectomies were attempted near the end of the nineteenth century, but the first successful embolectomy is credited to Lahey in 1911. For many years embolectomies performed within 4 to 6 hours after lodging of the embolus were successful, while those performed later had a progressively higher failure rate. Less than 15 years ago a serious proposal was made that emboli which had lodged more than 12 hours earlier should not be operated upon. It is now well established that such a viewpoint is erroneous. The difficulties with late operation have been found due to inadequate removal of distal thrombi. With the combination of operative angiography and the balloon catheter developed by Fogarty et al. in 1963, viability can be preserved in well over 90 percent of patients operated upon if operation is performed before the muscles become necrotic, regardless of whether the embolus lodged 3 hours or 3 days beforehand.

INCIDENCE AND ETIOLOGY. In about 90 percent of patients with emboli, the embolus originates in the heart from one of three causes: mitral stenosis, atrial fibrillation, or myocardial infarction. In some patients it is the first sign of previously unrecognized heart disease. Hence, an embolus, though a serious or catastrophic event, is best regarded as a symptom of serious heart disease which must be treated separately.

With mitral stenosis emboli originate from thrombi which have formed in the left atrium because of restriction of blood flow through the stenotic mitral valve. Most such patients also have atrial fibrillation with impaired contractility of the atrium. Atrial fibrillation from atherosclerosis without mitral stenosis can occur and becomes increasingly frequent in older patients. Emboli have been recognized to occur following the spontaneous or induced conversion of fibrillation to sinus rhythm, probably because the contractions of the atrial appendage expel thrombi which have accumulated during the impaired contractility from fibrillation. Emboli following a myocardial infarction originate from mural thrombi forming over the endocardial surfaces of the infarcts. Their frequency is greatest in the first 2 to 3 weeks following infarction, and in some patients they are the first sign that an infarction has occurred.

Unusual causes of peripheral emboli include a paradoxic embolus in which a thrombus arising in the venous circulation passes through a congenital atrial or ventricular septal defect and lodges in a peripheral artery. Other unusual causes include bacterial endocarditis, mural thrombi in subclavian or popliteal aneurysms, and atrial myxoma. In 4 to 5 percent of patients, despite the most diligent search, the source is never found.

PATHOLOGY. Most emboli ejected from the heart, 70 percent of the 426 emboli reported by Darling, lodge in the arteries of the lower extremities. Unfortunately 20 to 25 percent lodge in the cerebral circulation, usually intracranially, and are surgically inaccessible. Five to ten percent lodge in visceral arteries, the superior mesenteric or renal, and an unknown number lodge in silent areas of the circulation, such as the spleen, for which clinical signs are obscure.

Emboli usually lodge at bifurcations of major arteries where the diameter abruptly narrows. Common sites are the bifurcation of the abdominal aorta, the common iliac artery, the common femoral artery, and the popliteal arteries (Fig. 21-12). In the upper extremities similar patterns are found, including the distal subclavian artery and the bifurcation of the common brachial. The severity of the ischemia produced is due both to the abrupt occlusion and the fact that the site of occlusion involves two major arteries whereas an occlusion either immediately proximal or distal to a site of bifurcation would permit collateral circulation through the bifurcation.

PATHOPHYSIOLOGY. The physiologic consequences of an arterial embolus are the immediate onset of severe ischemia of the tissues normally supplied by the occluded artery. Depending upon the artery involved, if untreated, an embolus results in gangrene in about 50 percent of patients. The prominent early symptoms of pain, paralysis, and paresthesia all result from the great sensitivity of peripheral nerves to oxygen deprivation. Striated muscle is secondary only to peripheral nerves in susceptibility to anoxia. Necrosis may appear within 4 to 6 hours after onset of ischemia but varies with a number of factors. These include the size of the artery occluded, the collateral circulation around the site of occlusion, blood pressure, and temperature. If collateral circulation is well developed, necrosis may not appear for 8 to 12 hours; occasionally moderate ischemia is present but necrosis does not develop. The fact that muscle necrosis often begins within 4 to 6 hours is the reason that surgical embolectomy is uniformly successful within 4 to 6 hours but considerably less effective after longer periods of time.

Sluggish flow of blood in arteries distal to the embolus results in secondary thrombosis within the distal arterial tree. This may be a thrombus in continuity with the original embolus, or separate thrombi may develop in areas of severe stasis, varying with the degree of blood flow through collateral circulation. Secondary thrombi further occlude major collateral channels and intensify the ischemia. Effective therapy becomes more difficult because not only the primary embolus but also the secondary thrombus must be removed. Eventually the progressive circulatory stasis is further complicated by extensive venous thrombosis.

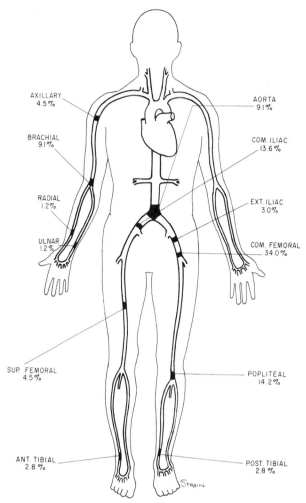

Fig. 21-12. Frequency of involvement of different arteries by arterial emboli. In the majority of patients arteries in the lower extremity are involved. (*Redrawn from H. Haimovici, Peripheral Arterial Embolism, Angiology, 1:20, 1950.*)

CLINICAL MANIFESTATIONS. The five p's discussed earlier under manifestations of acute arterial occlusion, pain, paralysis, paresthesia, absent pulses, and pallor, describe the principal clinical features of arterial embolism. The onset is abrupt in most cases, gradual in a few. In 75 to 80 percent of patients there is severe and unremitting pain, usually referred to the most peripheral portions of the limb. The color may be extreme pallor or mottling from alternate areas of pallor and cyanosis. Sensory disturbances vary from anesthesia to paresthesia. Paralysis may be the most prominent feature; complete paralysis and anesthesia mask the true nature of the disorder, diverting the physician into investigations for neurologic disease while muscle necrosis is occurring.

The neurologic symptoms are the crucial prognostic signs for muscle necrosis usually appearing within 6 to 8 hours after onset unless therapy is effective. Conversely, if motor and sensory function is intact, the extremity will survive even though chronic ischemia may persist.

Physical Examination. The extremity is often pale and

cold with collapsed peripheral veins. With less severe degrees of ischemia there may be cyanosis instead of pallor. A temperature level may be detected which coincides with the level at which the color changes. The arterial pulse is absent at the site of occlusion, frequently with accentuation of the pulse immediately proximal to this point. Sensory impairment varies from hypesthesia to anesthesia, and motor disturbances from weakness to paralysis.

The level of occlusion can often be estimated from the color, temperature level, and pulse findings. Ordinarily acute ischemia develops one joint below the site of occlusion. An iliac embolus produces ischemia at the level of the hip joint, while a common femoral embolus produces ischemia distal to the knee. These, of course, vary with the effectiveness of collateral circulation. Muscle turgor in the ischemic limb is most important. Shortly after the onset of ischemia, the muscles are soft. With continuing ischemia, edema appears, progresses to necrosis, and finally to rigor mortis. Early ischemic edema creates a "doughy" sensation on palpation, termed by some "football calf." The importance of this physical finding is the fact that as long as the muscles are soft to palpation, the extremity can be salvaged with effective embolectomy and thrombectomy, regardless of how long the embolus has been present. Conversely, the presence of stiff muscles warns that necrosis has occurred. This is most clearly apparent in the leg where the muscle tone of the gastrocnemius and soleus group can be easily evaluated. Some limbs with early muscle necrosis can be salvaged by embolectomy and thrombectomy, combined with extensive fasciotomy and later debridement of localized muscle necrosis, but failure is frequent.

An additional important aspect of physical examination is the cardiac examination for underlying heart disease. The cardiac rhythm, murmurs, or friction rubs may provide clues to atrial fibrillation, mitral stenosis, or acute myocardial infarction. Examination of other peripheral arteries for pulses and bruits provides additional clues to underlying cardiac or arterial disease.

LABORATORY STUDIES. A critical decision to be made when the patient is first encountered is whether an angiogram should be performed or not. The diagnosis of acute arterial occlusion can be readily made from the history and physical findings. An electrocardiogram and a chest roentgenogram should both be done to evaluate the presence of heart disease. If performance of angiography delays surgical therapy beyond the 4- to 6-hour "golden period" of therapy, it should be omitted. Intraoperative angiography is one alternative. Angiography is particularly useful where the site of the embolus is uncertain or in distinguishing between arterial embolism and arterial thrombosis superimposed upon an atherosclerotic plaque.

DIAGNOSIS. The condition most easily confused with an arterial embolus is acute thrombosis of an artery previously diseased with atherosclerosis. The importance of differentiating the two conditions is to determine the method of surgical therapy, for a more extensive operative procedure is required with thrombosis. Certain clinical findings suggest thrombosis rather than embolism. Atherosclerosis is usually seen in an older age group, and often symptoms of chronic ischemia, such as claudication, have been present for some time. The involved extremity may show signs of chronic ischemia such as loss of hair from the toes and atrophy of the skin and nails. The absence of heart disease which could cause an arterial embolus further supports the diagnosis of thrombosis. At times differential diagnosis is difficult or even impossible, because an embolus may occur in an older patient with atrial fibrillation who also has claudication from femoral atherosclerosis. Then, an arteriogram is of great value. With atherosclerosis and secondary arterial thrombosis, diffuse changes of atherosclerosis can be seen throughout the peripheral arteries, often with the development of prominent collateral circulation. By contrast, with embolism, the distal arteries are usually normal except at the site of occlusion.

Rarely, acute extensive thrombophlebitis may be confused with an embolus. Thrombophlebitis may be associated with extensive vasospasm, causing pain and peripheral vasoconstriction with diminished pulses. A bluish extremity, termed *phlegmasia cerulea dolens,* is also characteristic of venous thrombosis. With arterial embolism edema appears only after extensive gangrene has developed.

Even more rarely, acute dissecting aneurysm of the thoracic aorta with obliteration of peripheral pulses may suggest multiple peripheral emboli. A dissecting aneurysm can be suspected because of pain in the chest or back, often with a left pleural effusion.

TREATMENT. Indications for Operation. Because patients with arterial emboli usually have serious heart disease, the operative procedure must be planned with regard to the influence of anesthesia and operation on the heart disease. This is particularly critical when the embolus has resulted from a myocardial infarction. With modern vascular techniques, however, embolectomy can be performed in most patients with minimal trauma, often with local anesthesia. Hence, a decision not to operate because of heart disease should be made only if death is imminent. The reason for this is that failure to remove a peripheral embolus, which subsequently produces gangrene, of necessity requires a major amputation, a much greater surgical stress than simple embolectomy.

As repeated frequently in this chapter for emphasis, the urgency for performing arterial embolectomy can be simply estimated from the presence of paralysis and anesthesia. When these are present, muscle necrosis often occurs within 4 to 6 hours. If they are absent, a more conservative approach may be undertaken. However, their absence does not guarantee that claudication will not subsequently develop in the extremity with resumption of normal physical activity.

An unusual indication for nonsurgical therapy occurs with a migrating embolus. An embolus may lodge in a proximal artery, such as the common femoral, then fragment spontaneously within a few hours and migrate distad. Rarely such patients may recover completely, but most remain with significant residual occlusion of peripheral arteries. Peripheral pulses should be unequivocally present before simple observation is continued for a long period of time.

Preoperative Therapy. The prompt intravenous administration of heparin to inhibit the development of thrombi distal to the embolus is the most important therapeutic measure in the treatment of an arterial embolus. Heparin, 5,000 to 10,000 units, is given intravenously by continuous drip or repeated at 3- to 6-hour intervals, depending upon the clotting time, if embolectomy is delayed. Lumbar sympathetic blocks are of dubious value and cannot be safely performed in the presence of systemic anticoagulation. Other measures to influence collateral circulation, such as orally administered vasodilator drugs, are of little value. Intraarterial administration of drugs such as reserpine and priscoline sometimes dramatically improves the appearance of acutely ischemic extremities by eliminating functional arterial resistance to flow.

Operative Technique. For operations on the extremities, local anesthesia can be used in seriously ill patients. Frequently the operative incisions are short, for the location of the embolus can be accurately predicted from the clinical picture. The Fogarty balloon catheter has permitted removal of propagated clot both distal and proximal to emboli, making possible performance of the entire operative procedure through limited surgical incisions. Frequently, it is possible to perform the entire embolectomy and thrombectomy through incision in the upper thigh over the common femoral artery. Emboli and thrombi can be removed from the aorta and both iliac arteries by a retrograde approach. With emboli at the common femoral bifurcation, it is possible to remove thrombi from the arterial tree down to the ankle through the same incision. Rarely is it necessary to enter the peritoneal cavity for aortoiliac embolectomy and thrombectomy. This should be avoided when possible, for these patients are usually quite ill from their cardiac disease. Many have had a large myocardial infarction which in turn produced an embolus large enough to occlude the abdominal aorta. On other occasions, because of difficulty in passing Fogarty balloon catheters from the common femoral artery into the anterior tibial artery, a separate incision is made at the level of the knee joint to expose the origin of the anterior tibial from the popliteal artery.

In general, surgical incisions are placed directly over the uppermost level of arterial occlusion unless the aortoiliac system is involved, in which case incisions are placed over both common femoral arteries. Once the artery has been isolated proximal and distal to the embolus, 5,000 units heparin should be given intravenously. A transverse or a longitudinal arteriotomy is then made in the artery immediately proximal to its bifurcation, where the embolus is usually lodged. The embolus characteristically "pops" out as soon as the lumen is entered and can be recognized by its gray appearance and nonadherence to the arterial wall. Hence, removal is a simple procedure, but removal of thrombi which have formed distad or even proximally may be unusually complex. Fogarty balloon catheters have virtually eliminated the need to make multiple incisions along the course of the arterial tree for the laborious retrograde washing out of thrombi. The preferred technique is to pass the catheter into the distal artery as far as possible, inflate the balloon, and withdraw it in its inflated state. Comparison of the length of the catheter inserted with the length of the extremity indicates how far the catheter has been advanced. Passage of catheters into the aorta for the removal of aortoiliac thrombi is similarly performed. Occasionally it is impossible to pass the balloon catheter into various distal tributaries, either the anterior and posterior tibial in the calf or the radial and ulnar in the forearm. In such instances separate distal incisions are made over these vessels, followed by separate introduction of the catheter into each branch. Dale has used polyethylene catheters to aspirate clot. With these techniques, retrograde flushing of the artery through a distal incision is rarely necessary.

As indicated, the most crucial aspect of the operation is determining the completeness of removal of propagated thrombus. Back-bleeding is a notoriously unreliable indicator. Obviously if there is no back-bleeding, thrombus is still present. Back-bleeding can occur, however, through the nearest arterial branch, while the major artery distad is still occluded. Failure to remove all residual thrombus usually results in reocclusion (Fig. 21-13). The operative procedure should be continued until, by an appropriate combination of techniques, all pulses are restored at the ankle or wrist, or an operative arteriogram has demon-strated that the arteries are patent. On occasion, restoration of a pulse can be misleading, and bounding pulses may be felt in an artery partly reopened but with persisting distal obstruction. For this reason operative angiography is often critical to success.

If severe ischemic injury has been present beforehand, wide fasciotomy of the fascial envelop containing the major muscles may help preserve limb viability. This should be particularly considered if embolectomy has been delayed beyond the golden first 4 to 6 hours and definite change in muscle turgor was palpable before operation.

Postoperative Care. The most important aspect of post-operative care is to be certain that peripheral circulation is adequate. A palpable pulse is the best clinical sign. This should be identified immediately after operation and its presence periodically confirmed by palpation. Pulses which

Fig. 21-13. Embolic material and secondary clot. The embolic material which was deposited in the heart chambers during active blood flow is gray to salmon-colored, of firm consistency, and unattached to the arterial wall. It is composed mainly of fibrin and degenerated platelets. The gelatinous clot which appears homogeneous is a secondary stasis clot and was formed when blood flow ceased. It contains all the blood elements, and is dark red in color.

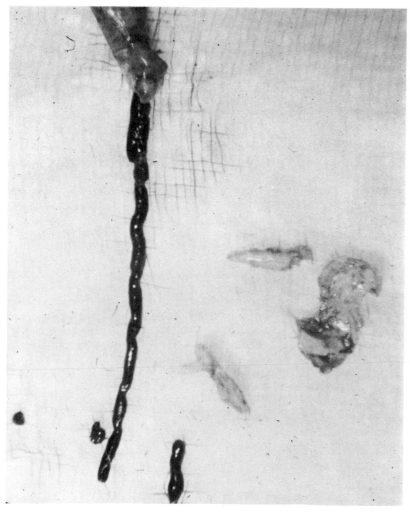

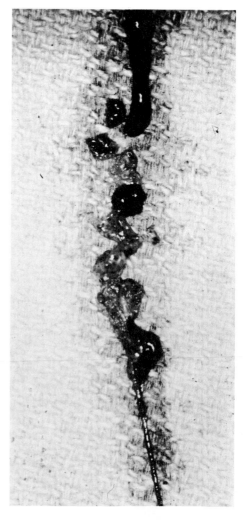

are difficult to feel can be checked with the Doppler instrument, which permits not only auscultation over pedal arteries but also measurement of pressures within those vessels. Disappearance of a previously palpable pulse or a change in Doppler measurements associated with unsatisfactory appearance of the extremity is an indication for either arteriography or immediate reoperation.

The persistence of paralysis and anesthesia following operation is ominous; gangrene is almost a certainty. Conversely, restoration of normal neurologic function indicates adequate circulation for muscle viability. This is particularly reassuring either when pulses cannot be restored or palpation is inconclusive because of edema and swelling.

The mode of heparin administration in the postoperative period is critical, since fresh surgical wounds are subject to hemorrhage, while delay of anticoagulation may predispose to further embolization. Some surgeons give no heparin for 6 hours postoperatively and then administer it by intermittent intravenous injection in doses of 5,000 units every 4 to 6 hours. Oral therapy with Coumadin derivatives is begun after 3 to 4 days and continued as long as the patients are at risk. Salzman et al. have reported that continuously administered intravenous heparin, avoiding peak effects which reach infinity during the intermittent administration, is associated with a lesser incidence of hemorrhage. Thrombolysis may accompany heparin administration, especially when porous knitted vascular prostheses are employed. The importance of prompt and continuous anticoagulant therapy cannot be overemphasized, for the arterial embolus is only a symptom of serious heart disease. Recurrence of embolization, each incident associated with a 25 to 30 percent likelihood of lodging in the brain, is distressingly common unless the heart disease is effectively treated. Patients with intractable atrial fibrillation should be maintained on permanent anticoagulant therapy. Those with mitral stenosis should have a mitral valvulotomy performed soon. Those with myocardial infarction should receive anticoagulants for several weeks, by which time the endocardial surface of the infarct will have healed and the likelihood of embolism is small.

Antibiotic therapy, usually penicillin or methicillin, generally is started at the time of operation and continued for 2 to 4 days.

PROGNOSIS. The most important feature influencing survival of the extremity following embolectomy is the time elapsing between the occurrence of embolization and successful restoration of flow at operation. As mentioned repeatedly, removal within 4 to 6 hours after onset is almost always associated with an excellent prognosis, having the two great advantages of avoiding muscle necrosis and limiting the secondary thrombus formation beyond the site of embolism. In both of the large series reported by Darling et al. and by Cranley et al. excellent results were obtained in 85 to 95 percent of patients. When more than 6 hours elapsed between embolization and embolectomy, unsuccessful results were more common. These particularly occur with inexperienced vascular surgeons and limited facilities. The crucial concept is that as long as the calf muscles are "soft" before operation, indicating that muscle necrosis has not occurred, salvage of the extremity should

approach 95 percent or higher, regardless of the duration of ischemia. However, in delayed cases achieving this goal taxes the resources, skills, and ingenuity of the vascular surgeon to the utmost, for thrombi may have accumulated from the aortic bifurcation to the posterior tibial artery at the ankle and complete removal requires a combination of careful surgical exploration, frequently multiple incisions, and serial operative angiography. If muscle necrosis is present before operation, indicated by a rigid calf muscle, possibilities of limb salvage are small, though these findings are seldom clear enough to warrant primary amputation. Rarely, a functional extremity may be salvaged in which virtually all the calf muscles are lost from necrosis but a viable foot is preserved.

The crucial long-term feature determining prognosis is the ability to prevent further emboli. Without adequate prophylactic anticoagulation recurrence is dismally inevitable, eventually terminating with fatal or crippling cerebral thrombosis. Vigilance to prevent emboli can be relaxed only when a myocardial infarction has healed or mitral stenosis has been treated by valvulotomy.

In any large series of patients with arterial embolism, death occurs in 25 to 30 percent of patients during that hospitalization. This is almost always due to the underlying heart disease causing the embolus, indicating the gravity of the basic illness. In some instances death is due to either inadequate management of the embolic episode, with the complications of sepsis from gangrene, or to recurrent embolism to the brain or viscera, a result of inadequate anticoagulant therapy.

Arterioarterial Embolization

HISTORICAL CONSIDERATIONS. In the past decade there has been increasing awareness of the entity of arterioarterial embolism to produce ischemic syndromes previously unexplained. With cerebrovascular insufficiency, the ophthalmologic visualization of minute particles of atherosclerotic plaque or platelet fibrin emboli in the retina in association with an ulcerated atherosclerotic plaque at the bifurcation of the carotid artery indicated the genesis of minute emboli. In the lower extremities, sudden onset of toe and foot ischemia, the "blue toe" syndrome, with little or no impairment of peripheral pulses led to the finding that minute emboli were the mechanism, having originated in aortic or iliac atherosclerotic plaques. The occasional finding of peripheral emboli beyond aneurysms has been described periodically. Miles et al. have cited observations suggesting that small emboli in the coronary circulation could come from ulcerated plaques, producing diffuse myocardial scarring from myriads of tiny emboli.

PATHOGENESIS. The basic process seems to be ulceration of an atherosclerotic plaque with discharge of minute fragments of atherosclerotic debris into the circulation. The ulcerated surface may become covered by platelets and fibrin which in turn are intermittently dislodged. How often these are subsequently resorbed is unknown. The emboli may arise from an atherosclerotic artery near the end organ where the emboli lodge or may originate some distance away, occasionally seen when emboli in the toes

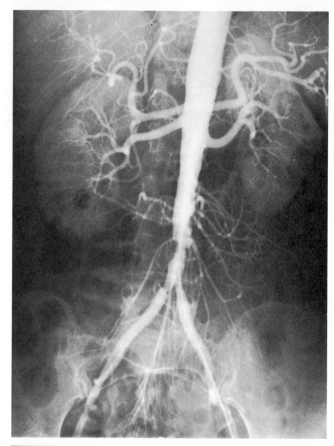

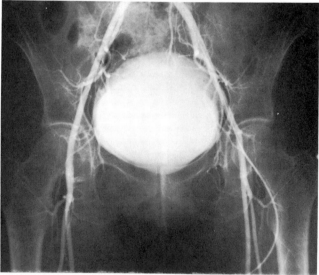

A

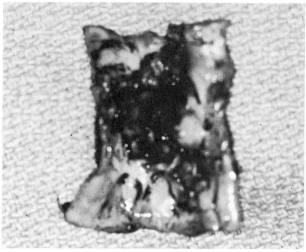

B

Fig. 21-14. Arterioarterial embolization, also known as athero-embolization, in a patient in whom marked ischemia of the toes developed in the presence of palpable pedal pulses. Several attacks occurred with progressive ischemia. *A.* Angiograms showing infrarenal abdominal aortic plaques. Occlusion of small calf arteries without involvement of renal arteries suggested that this infrarenal plaque was the source of emboli. *B.* Aortic plaque removed by endarterectomy. There has been no recurrence of embolization since operation 7 years ago.

apparently originate from plaques in the abdominal or thoracic aorta. Repeated embolic episodes are frequent, at times with almost complete recovery from ischemia between each episode; in other patients progressively greater degrees of ischemia occur, ultimately terminating in necrosis.

CLINICAL FINDINGS. A most striking syndrome occurs with emboli from the distal thoracic aorta, the "blue toe" syndrome. There is severe ischemia of the toes and feet, bilaterally, in association with renal failure. Before the pathogenesis was understood, the diagnosis remained an enigma, for pulses often remained palpable even while distal ischemia progressed to gangrene. There is a wide range in severity, from complete clearing of ischemia to progressive occlusion and gangrene.

Similar episodes occur in the cerebrovascular circulation with any combination of neurologic symptoms from the most transient, fleeting symptoms to complete stroke with cerebral infarction. In the upper extremity the subclavian artery is most frequently involved, with repeated attacks simulating Raynaud's phenomenon.

DIAGNOSIS. The diagnosis can be suspected from the combined findings of severe ischemia of a digit with palpable pulses. Determining the source of the emboli is crucial, for many can be corrected surgically, often by simple endarterectomy. Hence, detailed angiographic studies are necessary. The source of the embolus can be estimated by noting the peripheral circulation in other areas, where previous emboli may have lodged. For example, involvement of branches of the profunda femoris artery indicate emboli arising proximal to this level. Concomitant involvement of renal artery branches suggests that the emboli originated in the thoracic aorta. Similarly in the upper extremity emboli may arise from the subclavian artery or alternatively from lesions located far distad, such as small aneurysms in the palm of the hand. These diagnostic possibilities can be resolved only by precise, extensive angiography.

TREATMENT. When the atherosclerotic plaque can be related to the pattern of distal embolization (Fig. 21-14), arterial reconstruction of the atherosclerotic segment either by endarterectomy or replacement with a prosthetic graft has prevented further embolism. In the carotid system, there is now extensive experience with arterial reconstruction to prevent recurrent ischemic episodes, so-called transient ischemic attacks (TIA). The operation is effective and durable. Similar procedures have been performed in the subclavian artery to prevent TIA in the upper extremity. In the lower extremity experience is still limited, but good results in a series of 10 cases operated upon at New York University have confirmed both the validity of the concept and the surgical approach.

Theoretically emboli from platelet or fibrin aggregates should be inhibited or prevented by anticoagulants, but their effectiveness is yet uncertain. Paradoxically, anticoagulant therapy might prevent healing of an ulcerated plaque and thereby increase the tendency for embolization. This may explain the infrequent clinical puzzle of an embolus developing *after* heparin therapy has been started.

ACUTE ARTERIAL THROMBOSIS

ETIOLOGY AND PATHOLOGY. Acute arterial thrombosis usually occurs in an artery previously narrowed by atherosclerosis. In some patients the process of occlusion is gradual; no acute symptoms appear, but chronic arterial insufficiency slowly becomes more severe. In others, however, sudden thrombosis precipitates acute symptoms, closely mimicking an arterial embolus.

Unusual causes of arterial thrombosis are a cervical rib or repeated occupational trauma, such as operation of a pneumatic tool, the vibrations of which locally injure the arterial wall and produce thrombosis. Very rarely arterial thrombosis develops within a normal artery. This can happen with debilitating infections, especially in infants, usually with diarrhea and dehydration. It may also occur with primary hematologic disorders, such as polycythemia vera.

Iatrogenic thrombosis has become much more common from percutaneous introduction of catheters for cardiac catheterization or selective angiography. Thrombosis develops from detachment of a flap of intima from the arterial wall with subsequent formation of an occluding thrombus. Acute lower extremity arterial thrombosis also has been seen following long periods of immobilization such as in long automobile or plane trips, similar to acute venous thrombosis, which occurs more commonly.

CLINICAL MANIFESTATIONS. When thrombosis occurs suddenly, the findings are similar to those occurring with arterial trauma or embolism: pain, absence of pulses, paresthesias, and paralysis.

The usual question in differential diagnosis is the distinction between an arterial embolus and an arterial thrombosis. Such a distinction cannot always be made with accuracy, but several clues are helpful. A history of claudication in the involved extremity indicates chronic arterial disease. Similarly, examination of the extremity may show the stigmata of chronic arterial insufficiency, including ab-

sence of hair and trophic changes in the skin and nails. Significant findings may also be present in the contralateral, asymptomatic extremity. The absence of heart disease commonly associated with an arterial embolus is indirect evidence that thrombosis is the most likely cause.

Before successful techniques of arterial reconstruction were developed, the distinction between arterial thrombosis and arterial embolism in a patient in whom acute arterial occlusion suddenly developed was an important one. Surgical exploration of patients with arterial thrombosis usually was futile, because the underlying cause of the thrombosis, atherosclerotic stenosis of the artery, could not be treated. Futile surgical exploration often made the condition worse through interruption of collateral circulation. With present surgical techniques, differentiation between the two conditions is much less important, because operation is necessary with either if circulation is impaired to such an extent that gangrene is imminent. The main reason for recognizing which condition is present before operation is to anticipate the degree of vascular reconstruction which will be required. Restoration of blood flow in an extremity with chronic occlusive disease, with an arterial thrombosis superimposed upon an artery previously narrowed by atherosclerosis, is much more difficult than the performance of simple embolectomy upon an artery with no intrinsic vascular disease. Patients with arterial thrombosis should have an arteriogram before operation to assess the extent of occlusive disease and to evaluate the patency of the vascular bed beyond the point of occlusion in order to determine where a bypass graft can be inserted distad.

TREATMENT. Operative correction of the arterial occlusion requires both removal of the thrombus and correction of the atherosclerotic stenosis. The operative techniques are described in detail in the section on chronic arterial disease. Usually either the atherosclerotic narrowing is removed directly with an endarterectomy, or a bypass graft is inserted around the area of obstruction.

BUERGER'S DISEASE

HISTORICAL DATA. The entity referred to as Buerger's disease was first described by Winiwarter in 1879 and elaborated upon by Buerger in 1908 and again in 1924. The descriptive term *thromboangiitis obliterans* (TAO) emphasizes the inflammatory reaction in the arterial wall, with involvement of the neighboring vein and nerve, terminating in thrombosis of the artery. In 1960 doubt was cast upon the specificity of the pathologic findings when Wessler et al. pointed out that arterial occlusion from any cause, be it atherosclerosis or even embolic occlusion, may result in a similar type of angiitis, indistinguishable from what is usually considered to be specific for TAO. The relatively widespread use of arteriography has shown that many cases of so-called Buerger's disease probably represented presenile atherosclerosis occurring in the third, fourth, and fifth decades of life.

INCIDENCE AND ETIOLOGY. In our experience, we have made the diagnosis in fewer than 0.25 percent of all the patients with occlusive arterial disease of the extremities. The disease is found most frequently in men between twenty and forty years of age. In a Mayo Clinic series exceeding 500 patients, the youngest patient seen was seventeen years of age. The disease is uncommon in women, only 5 to 10 percent of patients with Buerger's disease being women. It is also rare in Negroes; of 936 cases found in the Armed Forces and analyzed by DeBakey and Cohen, only 2 percent were in Negroes. Initially it was felt that the disease was much more common in the Jewish race; subsequent statistical studies have shown that this frequency has been greatly exaggerated and the incidence is only slightly greater if at all.

Heavy tobacco smoking, usually 20 or more cigarettes per day, has been almost universally associated with this disease. The Mayo Clinic group found only three non-smokers in a 30-year period. The tobacco habit is so entrenched in these individuals that very few successfully forego smoking although often warned of the dire consequences and in spite of obvious remissions which occur upon cessation. DeBakey and Cohen analyzed 936 patients and found that only 10 percent successfully stopped smoking over a 10-year period.

Although the correlation between Buerger's disease and smoking is strong, the mechanisms involved are not clear. There is either a particular response to tobacco (since there are so many more smokers than patients with Buerger's disease) or, as in the Orient, particular brands of cigarettes are associated with the disease. This has never been noted in the West.

PATHOLOGY. The gross features of Buerger's disease are characteristic of an inflammatory process. The diseased artery is usually surrounded by a dense fibrotic reaction, often incorporating the adjacent vein, less often the neighboring nerve. Although this is usually considered to be characteristic of thromboangiitis obliterans, it also occurs occasionally with atherosclerosis obliterans and very frequently in association with aneurysmal disease.

The distribution of arterial involvement is different from that of atherosclerosis in that smaller, more peripheral arteries, usually in segmental distribution, are involved. In the lower extremities the disease generally occurs beyond the popliteal arteries, starting in tibial vessels extending into the vessels of the foot, similar to the typical arterial involvement in the diabetic. In the upper extremities, where atherosclerotic and diabetic involvement are extremely rare, TAO is manifested by arterial involvement usually distal to the forearm in about 30 percent of these patients. The visceral and cardiac circulations can be involved but this occurs rarely.

Early in the course of Buerger's disease there is involvement of superficial veins, producing the characteristic migratory, recurrent superficial phlebitis, while the larger and deeper veins (such as femoral and iliac) are affected rarely.

Although some doubt has been raised about the specificity of the histologic findings, most observers consider them to be characteristic. Precise retrospective diagnoses have been made on the bases of histologic examination of amputated extremities.

Microscopic examination of small thrombosed arteries shows extensive proliferation of intimal cells and fibroblasts throughout all segments of the arterial wall, with preservation of the basic architecture of the artery. Lipid deposition and calcification, frequently seen in atherosclerosis, are absent. Inflammatory cells, usually lymphocytes, are observed, while giant cells, whose presence was noted originally by Buerger, generally are absent. Necrosis of the arterial wall is very unusual, as is abscess formation. The thrombus in the arterial wall shows an unusual degree of fibroblastic activity with endothelial proliferation, suggesting the presence of a primary antigen in the blood, though none has been found. Spaces within the thrombus, interpreted as partial though functionally ineffectual recanalization, are common but not particularly characteristic of Buerger's disease, since this is seen with all thrombotic occlusions.

Involvement of the neighboring vein and nerve by the inflammatory and fibrotic reactions completes the histologic appearance of the lesions.

Periods of exacerbation of the acute process may be manifested by acute superficial phlebitis, with eventual progression of arterial occlusions and ischemia counterbalanced by remissions, during which collateral circulation becomes effective in the younger patients. The ultimate severity and extent of the extremity ischemia are determined by the frequency and duration of the acute attacks and the length of the quiescent periods. The cycles can usually be broken by cessation of smoking.

DeBakey and Cohen studied this progression in a group of 936 patients followed during a 10-year period after the diagnosis had been made and noted a three times higher mortality rate (10 percent), predominantly from cardiovascular disease, than in a control population. Postmortem examination revealed the familiar pattern of atherosclerotic disease in coronary and cerebral vessels, rather than the characteristic histologic pattern of thromboangiitis obliterans found in upper and lower extremity vessels. The limb amputation rate was 20 to 30 percent in 10 years, with an additional 40 percent showing some progression of ischemia but not requiring amputation. The Mayo Clinic series showed a somewhat better prognosis in that the amputation rate in a 10-year follow-up period was only 20 percent, while the overall survival was similar to that in the control group.

CLINICAL MANIFESTATIONS. There may be a phase of recurrent migratory superficial phlebitis involving superficial veins of the feet, which may occur over a period of years before there is any suspicion of arterial involvement. Invariably the patient is a cigarette smoker, and with continued smoking intermittent claudication appears as the first manifestation of ischemia. Reflecting the peripheral involvement of pedal arteries, pain while walking is usually referred to the arch of the foot, somewhat less often to the calf of the leg, but almost never to the thigh or buttock unless there is associated atherosclerosis obliterans. Upper extremity claudication is rare, probably a reflection of the distribution of arterial involvement, which is usually distal to the wrist. Progression of ischemia is similar to that in all chronic progressive arterial occlusions, in which the initial pain induced by exercise progresses to rest pain, postural color changes, trophic changes, and eventually ulceration and gangrene of one or more digits and finally of an entire foot or hand, necessitating major amputations. Patients with Buerger's disease may eventually require quadruple extremity amputations.

One variant of the typical syndrome is first manifest by painful vesicles of the pulp of fingers with surrounding intensive hyperemia and hypersensitivity, recurring as acute attacks over 2- to 4-year intervals, associated with progressive claudication of the feet and calves. The prognosis appeared to be worsened not only by continued smoking but by smoking certain types of cigarettes.

Pain in Buerger's disease, as in other ischemic conditions of the extremities, is common and may result from phlebitis, ischemia neuritis, or progressive skin and muscle ischemia manifested by the typical ischemic rest pain. This is unremitting and prevents patients from sleeping but is somewhat ameliorated by placing the affected limb in the dependent position. There may be blanching on elevation and rubor on dependence, as well as marked blanching on exposure to cold.

Physical Examination. The most frequent finding is absence of the posterior tibial and dorsalis pedis pulses in the feet. Often the popliteal pulse is palpable, especially in the early stages of the disease. Absence of the posterior tibial pulse is highly suggestive of the diagnosis, especially when bilateral. In the upper extremity, the radial pulse may be congenitally absent in 5 to 10 percent of patients, but absence of both pulses again is very suggestive of the disease. Signs of chronic tissue ischemia include loss of hair from the digits, atrophy of the skin, brittle nails, and rubor on dependency. In more advanced cases there may be ulceration or gangrene in the digits, often beginning near the nail and involving only the distal portion of the digit. With more extensive disease, gangrene extends into the foot. In the upper extremity, fortunately, extension of gangrene beyond the fingers is rare, and amputation of the hand is almost never necessary.

Edema is also frequently seen with advanced ischemia. It may result from keeping the extremity in a dependent position for many hours in an attempt to relieve rest pain. Other mechanisms causing edema include abnormal dilatation of the capillaries, producing rubor, and, rarely, significant venous obstruction. Superficial phlebitis involving segments of superficial veins is frequent, but rarely is phlebitis found in the large veins, such as the femoral or iliac. Accordingly, edema on the basis of phlebitis is unusual.

Another helpful distinction from atherosclerosis is the fact that a bruit is virtually never heard over the involved arteries, whereas such a bruit is frequently audible over the iliac or femoral arteries when atherosclerotic plaques are present.

Laboratory Studies. The most significant laboratory examination is arteriography. Plain roentgenograms of the extremity are helpful only if calcification can be demonstrated in the diseased arteries. This virtually excludes the diagnosis of Buerger's disease. The arteriographic findings, as emphasized by McKusick et al., are frequently characteristic. Typically, the intimal lining of the large arteries is smooth, without the characteristic irregularities seen from cholesterol plaques in atherosclerosis. In the small arteries, there are abrupt areas of occlusion, frequently surrounded by extensive collateral circulation. The collateral circulation, which evolves over many years, is unusually tortuous and has been termed "tree root" or "spiderlike." A "corkscrew" deformity also has been noted in peripheral arteries, probably representing partial recanalization of an artery previously occluded by a thrombus. The combination of extensive occlusive disease in small arteries with large vessels which remain smooth and normal in appearance, especially in association with extensive collateral circulation, is highly characteristic of Buerger's disease and is most useful in differentiating it from atherosclerosis (Fig. 21-15).

DIAGNOSIS. Buerger's disease can be differentiated from atherosclerosis without undue difficulty. Other entities with occlusive disease of small arteries, however, closely resemble Buerger's disease. These include diabetes mellitus or popliteal aneurysms, repeated episodes of arterioarterial embolization from proximal atherosclerotic plaques, and different collagen disorders. Patients with any of these may have palpable popliteal pulses, absent pedal pulses, and severe ischemia in the digits. In most of these, however, the upper extremities are not involved. Positive factors supporting the diagnosis of Buerger's disease are its onset in men between the ages of twenty and forty years, a history of migratory phlebitis, strong dependence upon tobacco, usually cigarettes, and frequent involvement of the upper extremities.

Factors suggesting that the disease is not Buerger's disease include diabetes mellitus, palpable popliteal or abdominal aneurysms, audible bruit over a major artery, high blood cholesterol, calcification of peripheral arteries, and onset after forty years of age.

Usually the diagnosis can be made from the history and physical examination. Angiographic studies are needed for confirmation and to define the possibilities of arterial reconstruction. Final proof of the diagnosis may require gross and microscopic examination of the diseased arteries.

TREATMENT. The most important aspect of treatment is to have the patient forego the use of tobacco in any form. Simply decreasing the frequency of cigarette smoking is ineffective. The great difficulty in getting the patient to stop smoking cannot be overemphasized, for the pernicious addiction to smoking in this disease closely resembles the tenacity of a heroin addict. In most teaching institutions there are one or more pathetic individuals who have undergone amputation of both legs and most of the fingers of each hand but who are trying to get someone to light a cigarette for them! The statistical facts cited by DeBakey and Cohen that a 10-year follow-up demonstrated that only 10 percent of patients had stopped smoking completely further indicates the magnitude of the problem. In the experience of one of the authors with a few patients with histologically proved Buerger's disease, almost none stopped smoking completely for a significant period of time.

A sympathectomy should be performed routinely in the involved extremity to limit the degree of vasospasm which,

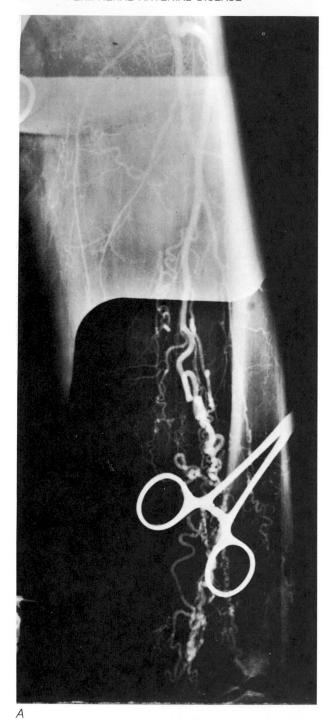

A

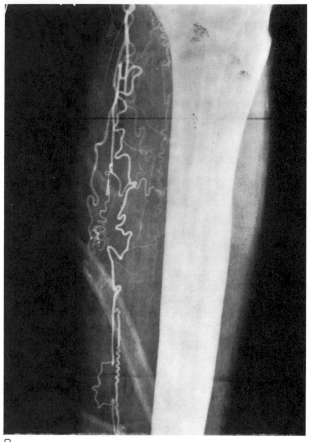

B

Fig. 21-15. *A.* Femoral arteriogram in a patient with Buerger's disease, demonstrating extensive tortuous collateral circulation in the lower thigh which has developed over a period of years as a result of occlusion of the superficial femoral and popliteal arteries. *B.* Angiogram of vessels below the knee, demonstrating the usual tortuosity of small arterial tributaries and illustrating the extensive collateral circulation which may develop with Buerger's disease or any other long-standing arterial occlusion.

when superimposed on ischemia from organic occlusion, may precipitate tissue necrosis. The benefit from sympathectomy is difficult to measure because of the episodic characteristics of Buerger's disease, but at least 50 percent of patients significantly benefit from the procedure. Vasodilating drugs, such as alcohol or Arlidin, may be tried but are of less benefit than sympathectomy.

Exposure to extremes of cold or heat should be avoided. Education regarding foot care similar to that described for

the atherosclerotic patient is very important. Often gangrene is precipitated by minor trauma to the foot, such as unwise trimming of a callus or wearing tight shoes, which a foot with normal circulation can tolerate uneventfully. The patient must recognize that his foot has to be carefully protected from all forms of even minor trauma permanently if ulceration and gangrene are to be avoided.

Arteriography should be performed to confirm the diagnosis and exclude other forms of smaller arterial occlusions which may require surgical therapy. If a popliteal pulse is absent, it may indicate the possibility of performing local direct arterial reconstruction.

Occasionally patients with Buerger's disease develop atherosclerotic obstruction of major arteries which are surgically accessible to reconstruction. Such a combination of arterial disease is suggested if the popliteal pulse is absent. In these patients arterial reconstruction may be successfully done upon the atherosclerotic disease, with marked circulatory improvement. Direct surgical approach to the vessels primarily involved by Buerger's disease, however, is not possible.

A conservative procedure is indicated when amputation is required. Often the patients are among the younger of the twenty-to-forty age group, and the episodic nature of the disease indicates that conservatism may be rewarded by subsidence of the acute episodes with subsequent partial revascularization by the growth of collateral circulation. As long as gangrene is confined to a toe, amputation should be postponed as long as possible unless rest pain or infection cannot be controlled otherwise. Delaying amputation of a gangrenous digit can permit sufficient development of collateral circulation to allow healing following amputation, whereas amputation soon after gangrene has appeared is often followed by failure of wound healing and the necessity for a more extensive amputation.

Once gangrene has involved the foot extensively, there is little point in delaying amputation, because a functional foot can rarely be obtained if the point of amputation is more proximal than the base of the metatarsal bones. Often a below-knee amputation can be performed, rather than an above-knee, because the popliteal artery is frequently patent.

Long-term anticoagulant therapy has not been of measurable benefit. Therapy with adrenal steroids, so effective for many inflammatory conditions, has similarly not been of consistent value and may aggravate the intimal changes in the tibial arteries.

PROGNOSIS. As stated earlier, 10-year follow-up studies have not agreed upon the prognosis. The Mayo Clinic group have found the survival similar to that of the general population, whereas the group studied by DeBakey and Cohen had a 10-year mortality about three times greater than the normal population. The risk of amputation within 10 years after onset of symptoms is probably near 20 percent, although this varies with the continued use of tobacco as well as the degree to which the ischemic foot is carefully protected. In the few patients who stop smoking completely, progression of the disease may be greatly restricted. A marked advance in therapy would be the discovery of a method by which abstinence from tobacco could be achieved uniformly in this unfortunate group of individuals.

ARTERIAL TRAUMA

HISTORICAL DATA. The feasibility of routinely repairing injured arteries in military casualties was first demonstrated in the Korean conflict in 1952. Earlier attempts in World War II were generally unsuccessful, and rather pessimistic conclusions were reached concerning the possibilities. Following the Korean conflict experiences, injured arteries have been repaired almost routinely, for ligation of major arteries has an overall incidence of subsequent gangrene of about 50 percent. The advances in therapy in the Korean conflict were due to several factors. The most significant was the almost routine prevention of infection in traumatic wounds by extensive debridement, followed by antibiotics and secondary wound closure 4 to 10 days later. Familiarity with techniques of vascular surgical treatment, in combination with the availability of vascular instruments, was also important. The prompt evacuation of wounded men by helicopter, often bringing a wounded patient to the hospital within 2 to 4 hours after injury, also was a significant factor.

ETIOLOGY. Most arterial injuries result from penetrating wounds which partly or completely disrupt the wall of the artery. Nonpenetrating injuries, usually associated with a fracture in an adjacent bone, are less frequent but often have a more serious prognosis, partly related to extensive crushing injury to the wall of the artery and partly due to delay in diagnosis.

PATHOLOGY. Most injuries are either lacerations or transections of the arterial wall. Uncommon injuries include arterial spasm, arterial contusion with thrombosis, and arteriovenous fistula. With lacerations or transections, the extent of injury varies with the type of trauma, which is an important consideration in subsequent debridement and surgical therapy. With clean incised wounds, such as those made by a knife or an icepick, injury to the arterial wall is minimal. In contrast, trauma from a high-velocity missile will disrupt the intima and media for a short distance away from the actual laceration in the arterial wall and requires a wider debridement at the time of surgical repair.

Contusion or spasm often occurs in association with fractures and extensive soft tissue injuries from blunt trauma. The presence of multiple injuries obscures recognition of the arterial injury, especially with extensive comminuted fractures. With such problems arteriography has been found of increasing value. Arterial spasm is an infrequent response to injury in which sustained contraction of the smooth muscle in the wall of the artery may obstruct blood flow and precipitate thrombosis. The cause is obscure. The spasm results from direct muscular contraction rather than a neurogenic stimulus. It occurs most frequently in the brachial artery associated with fracture of the humerus.

Arterial contusion from a blunt injury may be characterized by multiple areas of fragmentation of the arterial wall with intramural hemorrhage. The intima may become detached and prolapse into the lumen, creating an intraluminal obstruction which can be detected only by performing an arteriotomy and inspecting the intima. A serious error occurs when a contusion is misdiagnosed as "spasm." The delay in treatment as a consequence of this diagnostic error can result in gangrene. The well-known Volkmann ischemic contracture of the muscles of the forearm is due to an untreated spasm or contusion of the brachial artery in association with a supracondylar fracture of the humerus.

PATHOPHYSIOLOGY. The severity of the ischemic response following an arterial injury varies with the tolerance of different tissues for anoxia. In the extremity the peripheral nerves are the most sensitive to anoxia; hence, paralysis and anesthesia quickly develop when arterial blood flow is seriously decreased. Striated muscle is almost equally sensitive to anoxia and will usually become necrotic if arterial blood flow is decreased to such a degree that anesthesia and paralysis are present. Skin, tendon, and bone all have a greater tolerance for anoxia and may survive an ischemic injury which has produced irreversible extensive muscle necrosis. This is seen in an extremity in which an arterial repair is performed several hours after injury. The skin may appear viable, but the extremity is anesthetic and paralyzed, and after a period of time will be found to have widespread necrosis of the muscles.

The period of tolerance of striated muscle for ischemia is in the range of 6 to 8 hours. Experimental studies by Miller and Welch found arterial repair successful in about 90 percent of experiments when performed within 6 hours after injury, but the success rate decreased to 50 percent when repair was delayed for 12 hours. Therefore, every effort should be made to complete arterial repair within 6 hours after injury if anesthesia or paralysis are present, indicating a severe degree of anoxia. A definite time limit does not exist, however, beyond which arterial repair is futile, for the importance of the time interval varies with the collateral circulation. The collateral circulation, in turn, varies with the artery injured, with the degree of soft tissue injury which has interrupted collateral circulation, with associated shock, and with ambient temperature. In some patients with little disturbance of collateral circulation, arterial repair may be successfully performed 12 to 15 hours after injury, but in general successful repairs are obtained much more frequently when accomplished within 6 hours after injury.

CLINICAL MANIFESTATIONS. Shock, from loss of blood, is present in over 50 percent of patients with an arterial injury, either as a result of hemorrhage from the injured artery or because of associated injuries. The degree of shock varies with the severity of the blood loss or the severity of other injuries. When profound shock is present, the severe peripheral vasoconstriction may conceal the presence of an arterial injury until blood pressure has been restored to near-normal levels.

With blunt trauma, multiple organ injuries are commonly present. These include skull fractures, rib fractures, or blunt abdominal injuries. Careful assessment of each injury, with subsequent assignment of priorities in therapy, is a critical part of initial evaluation of the patient.

In the injured extremity, fractures and nerve injuries are commonly present with either penetrating wounds or following blunt trauma. The presence of a fracture or extensive soft tissue injury greatly influences the prognosis of an arterial injury. For example, in one series of arterial injuries the presence of a fracture of a femur in association with an injury of the femoral artery raised the incidence of gangrene from 11 to 55 percent.

In the extremity, the arterial injury frequently produces four abnormal findings, conveniently remembered as four p's: *p*aralysis, *p*aresthesia or anesthesia, loss of *p*ulses, and *p*allor. Of these four, the neurologic findings, paralysis and paresthesia, are the most important, because, as previously stated, loss of neurologic function indicates a degree of tissue ischemia which will progress to gangrene unless arterial blood flow is improved. Absence of a pulse in the presence of a normal pulse in the contralateral extremity immediately suggests an arterial injury. If serious vasoconstriction is ascribed to hypotension, evaluation of peripheral pulses may be difficult until blood volume is restored. It is important to emphasize, however, that the presence of a peripheral pulse does not exclude an arterial injury. This is frequently seen with a tangential laceration of the wall of an artery which is sealed by a blood clot with preservation of some flow through the arterial lumen.

With penetrating wounds, bright red bleeding, even in small amounts, immediately suggests an arterial injury. In the absence of hemorrhage, a tense hematoma may be palpated around the wound, evolving from extravasation of blood under significant pressure beneath the fascia. Occasionally a systolic bruit may be audible over the wound, or rarely a continuous bruit if an acute arteriovenous fistula has been produced.

It should be emphasized that an arterial injury can be present with virtually no abnormalities in the extremity. Hence, the presence of a penetrating injury near a major artery should alert the physician to the possibility of an arterial injury. In a series of 85 arterial injuries reported by Dillard and associates, the correct diagnosis was delayed in 15 of the patients. Usually the diagnosis is missed if serious hemorrhage is not present or if a peripheral pulse can be felt. In unrecognized cases a secondary hemorrhage from the wound may subsequently develop a false aneurysm, or an arteriovenous fistula may form in the area where the hematoma has formed around the lacerated artery.

With uncertain cases, an arteriogram should be performed. This is of particular value with blunt trauma producing a fracture of the extremity. A critical question in such patients is whether a decreased or absent pulse is due to an arterial injury or to angulation of the artery from the fractured bone.

TREATMENT. Preoperative Considerations. Control of bleeding is the most urgent immediate problem. This can usually be accomplished by tightly packing the wound with gauze and applying a pressure dressing. A large amount of packing may be required, for the efficacy of the packing depends upon compression of the artery between the overlying skin and the underlying bone. Tourniquets are best avoided for most injuries. When used they must be carefully padded to avoid the risk of permanent injury to a peripheral nerve.

Shock, which is present in 50 to 60 percent of patients, should be treated by the rapid infusion of fluids (500 ml every 5 to 10 minutes) until the systolic blood pressure rises to 80 mm Hg, after which additional fluids can be infused more gradually. Usually 1,000 to 2,000 ml of fluid will be required. Blood is preferable, but until the necessary cross matching has been done, Ringer's lactate solution, plasma, or dextran may be used.

Antibiotic therapy should be started promptly and appropriate prophylactic therapy for tetanus begun. Sympathetic blocks and anticoagulant therapy have no significant role in preoperative care.

Operative Technique. An important basic attitude regarding arterial trauma is that almost all injuries can be repaired successfully with available surgical techniques. The prognosis then becomes a question of whether or not the repair was performed before irreversible muscle necrosis developed. The only special instruments required are atraumatic vascular clamps and arterial sutures, usually of synthetic fiber (Dacron, polypropylene) fashioned to be monofilamentous, sizes 4-0 to 5-0, with swaged needles. The surgical incision should be placed to expose the artery proximal and distal to the site of injury in order to avoid hemorrhage when clots are evacuated from the wound. Once proximal and distal control of the artery has been obtained, the hematoma surrounding the injury can be widely opened and the site of injury mobilized. Most injuries are best treated by excision of the injured area followed by end-to-end anastomosis. With injuries from high-velocity missiles, 2 to 4 mm of adjacent arterial wall should be excised. Tangential repairs of lacerations are deceptive in that the suture of the laceration often results in constriction and subsequent thrombosis. Usually excision followed by direct anastomosis is preferable.

With transection of an artery, elastic recoil will separate the two ends of the vessel for 1 cm or more, giving the erroneous impression that a segment of artery has been destroyed. In most instances application of gentle traction on the ends of the artery with vascular clamps will demonstrate that direct anastomosis can be performed. Normally 1 to 2 cm of a peripheral artery can be excised and the vessel ends still approximated after limited mobilization of the two ends. For example, in 180 arterial reconstructions for civilian injuries reported by Patman and associates, grafts were necessary in only 20 patients. Similarly, in a series of 190 arterial reconstructions reported by Morris et al., primary repair was done in 167 patients and vascular grafts in 23. Before the anastomosis is performed, the degree of back-bleeding from the distal artery should be noted and any blood clots removed with a catheter. The anastomosis should be performed with 4-0 or 5-0 arterial sutures, using a continuous suture interrupted in two or three areas to avoid a purse-string effect. Individual sutures should be 1 to 1.5 mm in depth and a similar distance apart. With small arteries, interrupted or horizontal mattress sutures may be employed. Either a continuous over-and-over suture or an everting suture is satisfactory (Fig. 21-16).

A vascular graft is needed only when direct anastomosis cannot be performed because of loss of 2 cm or more of artery; this occurs in about 10 to 15 percent of injuries. An autogenous vein is the preferable graft, reversing the ends of the vein which is employed, usually the saphenous. If for some reason a vein cannot be utilized, a graft of knitted Dacron is preferable. If a prosthetic graft is used, the diameter rarely should be less than 8 mm, for throm-

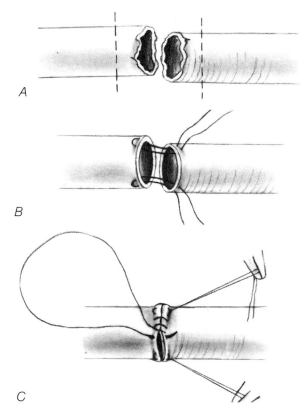

Fig. 21-16. A. Repair of traumatic transection of a peripheral artery. Initially the edges of the injured artery are debrided, removing 1 to 2 mm of normal arterial wall, especially if the injury was from a high-velocity missile which would traumatize adjacent segments of arterial wall. B. Initially the two ends of the artery are aligned with mattress sutures of 4-0 or 5-0 synthetic, monofilament material placed about 180° apart. C. Anastomosis is then performed with a continuous suture of the same material, usually as a simple over-and-over suture. Alternatively, an everting suture can be employed. With small vessels, simple interrupted or horizontal mattress sutures can be used to lessen the risk of constriction of the lumen.

bosis occurs much more frequently with smaller grafts.

With contaminated wounds, the best protection from infection following adequate debridement and arterial reconstruction is approximation of the adjacent soft tissues over the arterial repair and leaving the remaining wound open, to be closed by secondary suture 4 to 7 days later. This technique will almost routinely prevent the development of infection.

Ligation of an injured artery should be performed only for minor arteries, such as a radial or an ulnar artery which is not essential to survival of the limb. Back-bleeding is an inadequate guide to ligation of major arteries, indicating that some collateral circulation is present but not guaranteeing that collateral flow will be large enough to prevent gangrene. In the Korean conflict "good" or "fair" back-bleeding was recorded in 9 of 20 arterial ligations performed in one group of patients, all of which resulted in gangrene.

Arterial spasm, an unusual injury, may be treated by the topical application of 2 to 5% papaverine. Another technique, reported by Mustard and Bull, is the forceful dilatation of the area of spasm by the injection of saline solution into the lumen of the artery. The importance of differentiating spasm from contusion with disruption of the wall of the artery has been mentioned previously. Unless the area of constriction can be satisfactorily corrected, it should be excised and continuity reestablished by direct anastomosis or a vascular graft.

Postoperative Care. Anticoagulant therapy is not recommended after arterial repair, for it provides little protection from thrombosis but does increase the risk of bleeding into the wound. Sympathetic blocks are similarly of little value. The most important consideration following operation is to detect peripheral pulses, which indicate satisfactory restoration of arterial flow. If pulses cannot be detected or if previously palpable pulses disappear, an arteriogram should be performed, or alternatively the site of anastomosis should be reexplored. The important principle to reemphasize is that with modern vascular techniques a traumatic injury of a normal artery can almost always be successfully repaired.

When a femoral artery is repaired hours after injury, ischemic swelling may occur in the leg muscles in the anterior and posterior tibial compartments. The swelling can progress to such an extent that ischemic necrosis results. Prompt fasciotomies over the muscle compartments, decompressing the edematous, turgid muscles, may be of great value.

When an arterial repair is performed several hours after an injury, a peripheral pulse may be restored, but the extremity remains paralyzed and anesthetic. In such patients the skin may be viable, but the status of the underlying muscles is uncertain. Such patients must be carefully observed, because extensive muscle necrosis will result in serious toxic manifestations, with high fever and occasionally renal insufficiency. A decision to amputate such extremities, as opposed to widespread debridement of the necrotic muscles, is a difficult one to make, and each individual case must be evaluated carefully. In some patients the extremity may be salvaged following extensive debridement of necrotic calf muscles, with preservation of a limited but useful foot.

The development of a postoperative infection around the site of arterial repair is a grave complication, because frequently the anastomosis will disrupt with life-threatening hemorrhage. The infection should be treated promptly by widespread drainage, for there is usually inadequate removal of necrotic tissue. If infection involves the arterial reconstruction, ligation of the artery is usually required to prevent fatal hemorrhage or sepsis. Occasionally bypass grafts may be inserted through channels circumventing the area of infection, an anastomosis being performed between the artery proximal and distal to the point of injury. As mentioned earlier, the Korean conflict experiences well emphasized that despite massive contamination, the policy of widespread debridement, followed by secondary wound closure, almost always prevented postoperative wound infections.

PROGNOSIS. With present vascular techniques, arterial reconstruction almost always can be performed successfully if undertaken within 6 hours after injury. In 209 patients with arterial injuries reported by Patman and associates, the amputation rate was 3.8 percent. In another series of 67 arterial reconstructions reported by Dillard et al., only two amputations were necessary. If a vein graft is needed for arterial reconstruction, the long-term patency is probably in the range of 80 to 85 percent, varying with the experience of the surgeon and the circumstances of the injury. If subsequent occlusion of a vein graft does occur, viability of the extremity is rarely jeopardized, although claudication may develop. In such patients a subsequent vascular reconstruction may be performed electively.

Popliteal Artery Entrapment Syndrome

Popliteal artery entrapment syndrome consists of intermittent claudication caused by an abnormal relation of that artery to the muscles, usually the medial head of the gastrocnemius, resulting in ischemia of the leg at an unusually early age.

HISTORICAL DATA. In 1879, a medical student named Stuart recognized an anatomical abnormality associated with a thrombosed aneurysm of the popliteal artery which led to amputation of the extremity. A number of reports, beginning with Hamming in 1959, documented approximately 60 cases. Inshua in 1970 was able to classify the anatomic abnormalities of the structures in the popliteal fossa which led to the development of the syndrome.

ETIOLOGY AND PATHOLOGY. Normally the popliteal artery enters the popliteal fossa through the arch of the adductor magnus muscle and passes along a longitudinal place accompanied by the popliteal vein and tibial vein. The artery exits dorsal to the popliteus muscle, having passed approximately midway between the lateral and medial heads of the gastrocnemius muscle, and divides into its branches at the terminal portion of the popliteal fossa. As a consequence of developmental abnormalities, the popliteal artery may be severely compressed by portions of the medial head of the gastrocnemius muscle, at times continuously and at other times only during tensing of that muscle. As repeated trauma to the vessel ensues, typical arteriosclerotic changes appear, with irreversible stenosis and thrombosis. On occasion, poststenotic dilatation and aneurysm formation may be seen.

CLINICAL MANIFESTATIONS. Almost all patients experience either gradual or sudden onset of progressive intermittent claudication of the leg and sometimes of the foot; the remaining few present with acute ischemia of the leg. Ischemic gangrene has been encountered very rarely. The symptoms are usually unilateral but may be bilateral.

On physical examination there are the usual findings of popliteal arterial stenosis or occlusion with diminished or absent popliteal, dorsalis pedis, and posterior tibial pulses. On occasion all pulses appear to be normal but can be made to disappear on dorsiflexion of the foot, and a pulsatile mass may be noted in the fossa.

DIAGNOSIS. It is essential to establish the diagnosis early, since correction of the abnormality may present irreversible changes which may require more complex arterial reconstructions. Any individual in the preatherosclerotic age group who presents with typical ischemic intermittent claudication or who is found to have a pulsatile popliteal mass should be suspected of having a popliteal artery entrapment syndrome. The physical findings may be minimal or nil; therefore angiographic studies are essential to making the diagnosis. Angiography may demonstrate stenosis, occlusion, or poststenotic dilatation of that artery. Occasionally there may be no visible abnormalities on the angiographic study until the foot is passively dorsiflexed, after which stenosis of the popliteal artery may be seen.

The differential diagnosis requires exclusion of all other causes of popliteal artery occlusion, including thromboangiitis obliterans, embolic occlusion, cystic degeneration of the popliteal artery, atherosclerosis obliterans, as well as other trauma to the vessel.

TREATMENT. Surgical correction is required. The type of surgical procedure which should be performed depends entirely upon the condition of the popliteal artery. When the popliteal artery has had no permanent structural changes, various types of myotomy procedures which can be determined only at the operating table may prove to be curative. In instances in which structural changes have already occurred, in addition to the correction of the anatomic abnormalities, replacement of the artery with vein or thromboendarterectomy angioplasty may be required to restore flow. The results in these young people, who ordinarily have normal arteries above and below the site of compression, are excellent. In most instances the reported case histories indicate that unilateral correction is sufficient, but it is essential that both limbs be studied, since bilateral corrections may be necessary.

PROGNOSIS. The prognosis for immediate restoration of flow to the extremity is excellent in these young people. The long-term prognosis will depend upon the material employed to reconstruct occluded arteries. It would appear desirable to avoid the use of plastic prostheses and employ autologous tissue for the arterial reconstruction.

Anterior Compartment Syndrome

The anterior tibial compartment syndrome is a progressive neuromuscular disability related to pressure from tissue fluid within the closed anterior tibial compartment.

ETIOLOGY. Any condition which increases the presence of fluid or compromises the outflow of fluid from this closed space may result in augmented pressure and clinical consequences. The swelling continues until the intracompartmental pressure exceeds arterial pressure. The critical structures coursing through the closed compartment and subjected to the effects of the intracompartmental pressure include the tibial artery, the anterior tibial nerve, and the anterior tibial, extensor digitorum longus, peroneus tertius, and extensor hallucis longus muscles. The unyielding walls of the compartment are composed of the tibia, the interosseous membrane, and the anterior crural fascia.

In some cases, there is a readily demonstrable arterial lesion; the syndrome has been associated with arterial trauma, arterial embolism, and acute arterial thrombosis; and it has been a complication of femoropopliteal bypass procedures and also of cardiopulmonary bypass. In a second group of patients, the syndrome is caused by severe exertion, and there is no proved anatomic lesion.

CLINICAL MANIFESTATIONS. In young patients with idiopathic anterior tibial syndrome, a history of marked exertion should be investigated. Characteristically, in most cases, the pain is the first and dominant symptom. Initially, it begins as a dull ache which soon becomes severe and is primarily located over the anterior compartment, where palpation may elicit tenderness. Motion of the leg or foot increases the severity of pain. Subsequently, erythema of the skin over the anterior compartment becomes apparent, and there is measurable increase in the size of the calf. As the syndrome progresses, these signs become more apparent. The dorsalis pedis pulse may be normal, diminished, or absent. Actually, its absence is a late sign and occasionally follows the loss of motor power of the muscles of the anterior compartment. The anterior tibial muscle and the extensor hallucis longus usually become paralyzed first, whereas the extensor digitorum longus loses its function later and is usually the first to return after release of pressure. Loss of the extensor digitorum brevis is an ominous sign. Loss of sensation is confined to the area served by the deep peroneal nerve.

The syndrome must be differentiated from a common condition known as "shin splints." The pain in the latter condition is usually over bone and can be relieved by rest, elevation, and application of cold. There is no associated marked swelling and muscle paresis with shin splints. Other conditions to be differentiated include cellulitis, thrombophlebitis, and stress fractures of the tibia.

TREATMENT. This is directed at decompressing the anterior tibial compartment and should be performed early to avoid anoxic necrosis of the muscle mass. Treatment can be effected with fasciotomy. The skin is incised lateral to the tibial crest over the midportion of the anterior tibial muscle, and the incision is carried through subcutaneous tissue and the fascia. Muscle bellies are then allowed to bulge. The skin may be closed over the bulging muscle or can be left open for secondary closure. A variation of the procedure employs two small incisions, one in the craniad and the other in the caudad portion of the anterior compartment. The fascia is then incised blindly between these two small incisions.

PROGNOSIS. If decompression is performed before muscle necrosis is present, return of function is complete. Thus, in many instances, fasciotomy is indicated prior to total disappearance of the pedal pulse. If fasciotomy is delayed until muscle necrosis occurs or neurologic findings are advanced, total recovery of function is not to be anticipated, and rehabilitation is required.

Traumatic Arteriovenous Fistulas

HISTORICAL DATA. The true nature of an arteriovenous fistula was first recognized by William Hunter in 1764. Previously the lesion had not been distinguished from a traumatic aneurysm. In a careful description of two patients in whom fistulas developed following phlebotomy, he described the typical clinical findings of a thrill, continuous murmur, dilated artery proximal to the fistula, and dilated pulsating veins. He first recognized that the lesion was basically a communication between an artery and a vein. Attempted therapy by proximal ligation of the involved artery, which was frequently effective for traumatic aneurysms, was often disastrous for arteriovenous fistulas, because gangrene resulted. The gangrene developed because blood flowing through collateral circulation around the ligated artery would flow through the fistula instead of into the distal extremity.

Matas in 1888 established effective therapy with his

Fig. 21-17. *A.* Immediately following the development of an arteriovenous fistula there is shunting of blood from the artery through the fistula into the vein, from which it returns to the heart. This results in a decrease in peripheral vascular resistance, a fall in diastolic blood pressure, and an increase in heart rate. The venous pressure rises in the involved vein. Peripheral blood flow is decreased in the involved artery. *B.* After several weeks, collateral circulation enlarges around the fistula because of the decreased vascular resistance at the site of the fistula. As the collateral circulation develops, the involved artery and vein also dilate, increasing the amount of blood flowing through the fistula. *C.* After several years, extensive dilatation may develop about a fistula with marked enlargement of collateral circulation. In addition there is enlargement of the artery immediately distal to the fistula, through which blood flows in a retrograde fashion through the fistula toward the heart. The vein may enlarge to marked proportions, creating varicosities in the extremity. Ultimately such progressive dilatation after a period of years may result in congestive heart failure from the increased cardiac output.

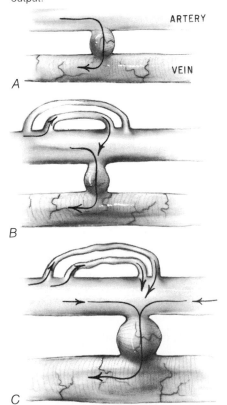

technique of endoaneurysmorraphy. Directly incising the fistulous sac, followed by suture of the communication between the artery and the vein, was more effective than indirect therapy of proximal and distal ligation of the involved artery and vein. The abnormal physiology of an arteriovenous fistula was carefully analyzed in a scholarly monograph published by Holman in 1937.

Although the collateral circulation which develops with an arteriovenous fistula made it possible to treat such fistulas by excision without gangrene resulting, intermittent claudication was frequently permanent. Consequently, after World War II, reconstruction of the injured artery became the preferable form of treatment.

ETIOLOGY AND PATHOLOGY. An arteriovenous fistula usually results from a penetrating injury which simultaneously injures an artery and an adjacent vein, permitting blood to flow directly from the injured artery into the vein. A fistula may be established immediately, in which case there is little external loss of blood, or the fistula may become apparent days or weeks following injury as clot surrounding the lacerated artery and vein is liquefied.

Unusual forms of arteriovenous fistulas have been reported following different surgical operations. Injury of the iliac artery and vein is a well-recognized, fortunately rare complication of removal of an intervertebral disc. Arteriovenous fistulas have been reported following thyroidectomy, nephrectomy, or even thoracentesis, in all instances representing a concomitant injury of an artery and a vein, sometimes due to simultaneous ligation of artery and vein by the same ligature.

PATHOPHYSIOLOGY. A series of anatomic and physiologic changes begin to evolve when an arteriovenous fistula is produced (Fig. 21-17). The immediate effects are a decrease in blood flow to tissues distal to the lesion and an increase in venous pressure. The peripheral vascular resistance is lowered as a result of blood flowing directly through the newly created arteriovenous shunt. This results in a decrease in systolic and diastolic blood pressure, an increase in heart rate, and an increase in cardiac output.

In the ensuing days, several compensatory events occur as a result of the decrease in peripheral vascular resistance: The blood volume is increased, systolic blood pressure increases with a corresponding increase in pulse pressure, and a decrease in pulse rate occurs. Locally there is the progressive development of extensive collateral circulation around the fistula, because the decreased vascular resistance at the site of the fistula is a very potent stimulus to development of collateral circulation. Within a few weeks the blood flow to the distal extremity may approach normal limits. There is a progressive dilatation of the "fistulous circuit," including the heart, the arteries leading to the fistula, the fistula itself, and the venous channels leading from the fistula to the heart.

In subsequent months or years, additional changes evolve. The artery both proximal and distal to the fistula may dilate in response to blood flowing through the fistula. The involved veins progressively dilate with marked tortuosity; external rupture with hemorrhage, however, is very rare. Chronic venous congestion may develop in the extremity, causing skin ulcerations resembling those from varicose veins. In growing children, there may be hypertrophy of the involved limb from increased growth of the bones and soft tissues. With large fistulas, involving vessels as large as the iliac artery and vein, continued dilatation of the heart eventually terminates in heart failure. This, however, is an unusual complication with the majority of arteriovenous fistulas, because the volume of blood shunted is not enough to produce heart failure. Only with large arteries and veins do cardiac symptoms appear.

Two rare complications with arteriovenous fistulas are bacterial endarteritis in the fistula and spontaneous closure. Bacterial endarteritis has been reported in only a few patients and is similar to bacterial endocarditis. Usually with intensive chemotherapy the infection can be controlled or eliminated, after which surgical excision of the fistula should be promptly carried out. A fistula may close spontaneously, occasionally after it has been present for several months. Shumacker reported eight such experiences in 245 patients.

CLINICAL MANIFESTATIONS. A penetrating injury producing an arteriovenous fistula often causes surprisingly few symptoms. External loss of blood can be small, and few disturbances of peripheral circulation develop. Subsequently the patient may be entirely asymptomatic. He is usually aware of a soft mass in the area of the fistula, which transmits a buzzing sensation when the fingers are placed over it. Rarely the patient is totally unaware of the presence of a fistula. In the experience of one of the authors, a fifty-five-year-old patient was admitted for congestive heart failure, presumably due to atherosclerotic heart disease, and was found on physical examination to have a popliteal arteriovenous fistula resulting from trauma many years before. Surgical correction of the fistula promptly eliminated the signs of congestive failure.

In some patients the venous hypertension produces varices with peripheral pigmentation and ulceration from venous insufficiency. Surgical mishaps have resulted from unwise attempts to remove such varices without recognizing their origin.

On physical examination, a soft, diffuse mass is usually palpable and often visible. Dilated veins may surround the area. On palpation a thrill is usually felt, maximal in systole. Auscultation reveals a continuous murmur, loudest in systole, which has been described as a "machinery" murmur, emphasizing the rhythmic rise and fall in intensity and pitch during systole and diastole. It is similar to the murmur of a patent ductus arteriosus. Detection of this classic finding establishes the diagnosis and differentiates the lesion from an arterial aneurysm.

Another significant finding is the demonstration of slowing of the pulse when the fistula is obliterated by digital compression, as evidenced by disappearance of the murmur. This phenomenon, generally known as Branham's sign, was first described by Nicoladoni in 1875. The slowing of the pulse results from the increase in peripheral vascular resistance when the fistula is digitally occluded causing the blood pressure to rise with reflex slowing of the heart rate. The bradycardia results from a neurogenic reflex mediated through pressure-sensitive receptors in the great vessels and carotid sinuses; it can be blocked by atropine.

Usually there are no signs of arterial insufficiency in the extremity. With large fistulas, the pulse pressure is increased, both from an elevation of systolic pressure and a decrease in diastolic pressure. If cardiac enlargement has occurred, a systolic murmur may be audible at the apex of the heart. Usually cardiac failure is found only with fistulas between large vessels, such as the aorta and the vena cava, or when the fistula has been present for many years, allowing time for progressive enlargement of the fistulous opening. In World War II cardiac failure was rarely seen in a collected series of 593 patients treated surgically.

The physical findings are usually sufficient to establish the diagnosis, but if uncertainty exists, an arteriogram readily demonstrates the rapid opacification of adjacent veins and the greatly increased collateral circulation. As the veins fill rapidly, the exact site of the fistula may be obscured unless serial angiograms are obtained. A common problem in differential diagnosis in the cervical area is with a venous "hum," an auscultatory curiosity resulting from flow of blood in the jugular veins. The murmur of a venous hum promptly disappears when intrathoracic pressure is raised by forced expiration against a closed glottis, which will differentiate it from the murmur of an arteriovenous fistula.

TREATMENT. Formerly treatment was delayed for 2 to 4 months to permit the development of collateral circulation in order for the extremity to survive following ligation of the involved artery. Although gangrene virtually never occurred following ligation, claudication frequently resulted, often in as many as 50 percent of patients, despite the abundant collateral circulation. Presently, the majority of patients are treated by division of the fistula and reconstruction of the involved artery, and preferably the injured vein. Excision is performed only for fistulas involving small vessels not essential to normal circulation of the extremity, such as the radial or ulnar arteries. Most fistulas are treated at the time of the arterial injury if the proper diagnosis is made. Otherwise operation is performed within 2 or 3 weeks, after the immediate effects of the injury on the soft tissues have subsided.

Operative Technique. The incision should be placed so as to permit exposure of the artery and vein proximal and distal to the fistula before the fistula is dissected. Once these vessels are isolated and temporarily occluded, the fistulous sac can be incised and the opening directly isolated. Although a large aneurysmal sac may be present, the basic lesion is usually an incomplete laceration of the arterial wall, involving only a short length of artery. A long segment of artery may be incorporated in the wall of the aneurysmal sac, however, which must be freed and mobilized to perform arterial repair. Once the involved vessels have been mobilized, most of the remaining sac may be left, for complete excision is difficult and of little benefit.

In many patients the artery can be repaired by direct anastomosis. In a group of 29 aneurysms and arteriovenous fistulas resulting from civilian injuries reported by Craw-

ford et al., all were treated by end-to-end arterial anastomosis. In 134 fistulas treated by Hughes and Jahnke, an
anastomosis was performed in 61, a vessel graft in 23, a
lateral repair in 4, and simple division of the fistula in
10.

Repair of the involved vein is indicated if the vein is
a large one, such as an iliac or common femoral vein.
Permanent edema has been frequent following ligation of
such large veins. Repair can often be done by lateral
suture.

PROGNOSIS. Convalescence following operation is
usually uneventful, and long-term results are excellent if
arterial continuity is preserved. Hughes and Jahnke published a 5-year follow-up of 148 such lesions treated during
the Korean conflict with satisfactory results in the majority
of patients.

CONGENITAL ARTERIOVENOUS FISTULAS

Congenital arteriovenous fistulas are very uncommon
lesions. In 1963 Tice et al. estimated that only about 200
cases had been reported in the American surgical literature. In 1956 Coursley and associates reported experiences
with 69 patients, and Robertson in a Hunterian Lecture
referred to 40 patients.

ETIOLOGY AND PATHOLOGY. As the name indicates, the
basic lesion is a congenital abnormality of multiple communications between arteries and veins. A single communication is unfortunately very rare, for the multiplicity of
lesions precludes surgical cure in most patients. The extent
of the lesion varies from an angiomatous mass localized
in a foot or a finger to diffuse involvement of an entire
arm or leg. In addition to the presence of multiple lesions,
the almost uniform recurrence suggests that a basic defect
exists in the peripheral vascular tree as a result of which
additional arteriovenous fistulas develop throughout the
life of the patient.

The extremities are a common site for such fistulas.
When present in childhood, there is increased growth of
the affected extremity. Hemihypertrophy of moderate degree was found in over one-half of patients reported by
Coursley and associates and also by Robertson. Fortunately, cardiac difficulties from the arteriovenous shunting
are uncommon; an increase in heart size has been recorded
in only about 15 percent of the patients. The dilated veins
associated with the lesions tend to enlarge gradually, causing difficulty from periodic external rupture and bleeding.
With involvement of the digits, ischemic pain may occur
with gangrene of the tips of the fingers because of shunting
of blood proximally through the fistulas.

CLINICAL MANIFESTATIONS. The finding of multiple
dilated veins or small angiomas may suggest simple varicosities, but the location of the dilated veins in unusual
areas should raise suspicion of congenital arteriovenous
fistulas. Detection of a continuous bruit over the lesion
establishes the diagnosis, but with some diffuse multiple
fistulas involving an entire extremity a bruit may not be
audible. In contrast to traumatic single arteriovenous fistulas, it is impossible to obliterate the bruit completely by

digital compression. Often a bruit is audible in several
widely separated areas, indicating the presence of multiple
fistulas.

Occasionally a patient first becomes aware of his condition following an injury, and an error can easily be made
by concluding that a traumatic fistula with a single communication is present. Careful inquiry concerning earlier
dilatation of the regional veins may give a clue to the
correct diagnosis and prevent a long, futile surgical exploration for a single fistula. The finding of multiple bruits
which cannot be eliminated by digital compression also
suggests a congenital origin. Arteriography is needed to
confirm the diagnosis, demonstrating many tortuous arteries with rapid opacification of numerous dilated veins (Fig.
21-18).

TREATMENT. The keynote to therapy is conservatism.
Operation should be undertaken only when the lesion is
of sufficient size to threaten with ulceration or bleeding,
because surgical excision must be considered as palliative
in the majority of patients. Only when the lesion is localized sufficiently to permit complete excision of adjacent
soft tissue is a curative procedure possible. With most
lesions, thorough understanding should be reached with
the patient beforehand regarding the palliative nature of
the surgical procedure.

On the other hand, amputation merely to remove the
lesion is unwarranted, for excellent palliation can be obtained for many years by serial surgical procedures to
excise all accessible varicosities. Cross et al. has reported
eight patients successfully managed with such measures.

At operation, in contrast to traumatic arteriovenous
fistulas, a widespread en bloc excision of the soft tissue
should be planned, because excision of an isolated fistula
is seldom possible. Amputation of one or more digits may
be required. Precise arterial control is often impossible;
so, a pneumatic tourniquet should be applied proximal to
the lesion if possible. In some patients serious bleeding
has been encountered which could be controlled only by
resection of adjacent bone.

Some of the most difficult lesions to treat are those
involving the head and neck. Ravitch and Gaertner described a remarkable patient treated for an extensive recurrence 48 years after the patient was originally operated
upon by Halsted. Rosenfeld has described experiences with
seven patients which well emphasize the value of conservative therapy. By prolonged, painstaking dissection, the
facial nerve was preserved in most of these patients, but
resection of the mandible was frequently required (Fig.
21-19).

A lesion operated upon by one of the authors, after
several previous surgical procedures had been ineffective,
required amputation of an ear to prevent hemorrhage.
When the cartilage of the ear was divided adjacent to the
skull, numerous large arteries closely adherent to the cartilage were transected. Within a year additional bruits were
audible over the head and neck, but fortunately no symptoms were present.

Another area in which lesions generally are not resectable is in the pelvis and flank. One of the authors operated
upon one such patient at the Walter Reed Army Hospital

in 1958. Previous operation several years before with division of the iliac artery had resulted in only temporary improvement. During a surgical procedure which lasted several hours, numerous large vessels, including the internal iliac artery and vein, were excised and ligated, but it was obvious that a definitive procedure could not be accomplished. Within a week following operation a loud continuous murmur was again audible. Six years later the murmur persisted, but fortunately there was little disability. Such a course emphasizes the value of conservatism with these lesions.

Fig. 21-18. Series of angiograms demonstrating congenital arteriovenous fistulas. *A*. This series of three views shows a popliteal arteriogram in the same patient. The first view is a posteroanterior view which demonstrates the great degree of enlargement of the calf. The next two views are early and late exposures in the arterial phase in a lateral projection. The extensive staining in the late arterial phase is highly suggestive of congenital arteriovenous fistulas. *B*. Arteriogram in the thigh area of a second patient. Note the diffuse staining produced by injection into the profunda femoris vessel. *C*. These two views demonstrate early and late arteriograms in the shoulder area. In this patient the fistulas originate from the circumflex humeral vessels.

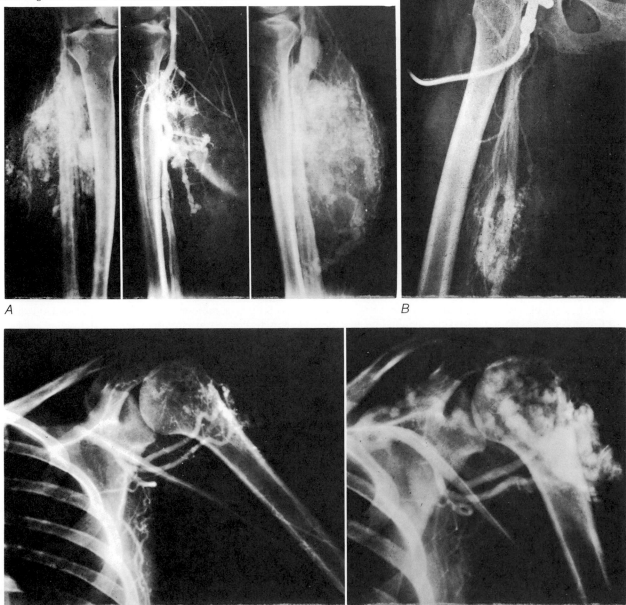

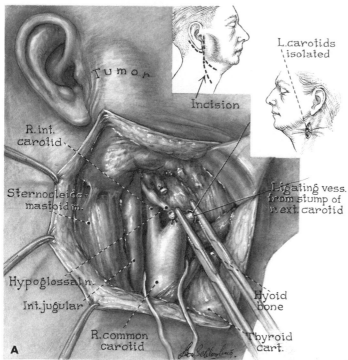

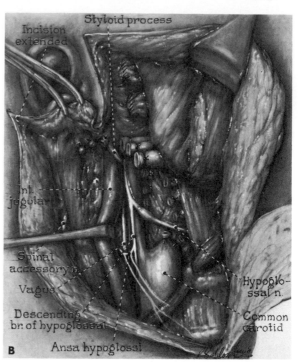

Fig. 21-19. *A.* The usually extensive nature of these lesions is illustrated by the following case history. Large recurrent congenital arteriovenous fistula operated upon by Ravitch 48 years after the lesion had been removed by Halsted. Extensive collateral vessels were found in the neck around tributaries of the external carotid artery. *B.* Operative field following completion of the dissection, indicating the numerous unnamed collateral vessels which had developed over many years, causing recurrence of the lesion. (*Reprinted from M. M. Ravitch and R. A. Gaertner, Congenital Arteriovenous Fistula in the Neck: 48 Year Follow-up on a Patient Operated upon by Dr. Halsted in 1911, Bull Johns Hopkins Hosp, 107:31, 1960.*)

Increasingly favorable experiences with intraarterial embolization have been reported. Combinations of Gelfoam, pellets, and autologous muscle have been injected by the Seldinger technique. Inoperable lesions may be treated by embolization alone, while extensive lesions may be managed by embolization followed by excision.

THORACIC OUTLET SYNDROMES

A variety of physical abnormalities have been recognized which constrict or compress the brachial plexus, the subclavian artery, or the subclavian vein near the first rib and clavicle. Several descriptive terms have been employed, indicating the causative mechanism thought to be present. These include cervical rib, scalenus anticus syndrome, costoclavicular syndrome, and hyperabduction syndrome. The disability is dependent upon which of the major neural or vascular structures is compressed. Regardless of the specific mechanism involved, all such abnormalities may be conveniently grouped together as neurovascular compression syndromes occurring near the thoracic outlet.

HISTORICAL DATA. Cervical ribs have been reported as anatomic curiosities for hundreds of years. They occur in about 0.5 percent of the normal population. Murphy in 1905 described a successful operation upon a patient whose subclavian artery was compressed by a cervical rib. By 1916 Halsted was able to find reports of more than 500 cases of symptoms from a cervical rib. Attention was focused on the scalenus anticus muscle in 1927 when Adson and Coffey observed constriction of the subclavian artery by a scalenus anticus muscle and subsequently pro-

posed that compression by an abnormal scalenus anticus muscle created a syndrome identical to that caused by cervical rib. They also emphasized the role of the scalenus anticus muscle in producing symptoms from a cervical rib, the two structures jointly compressing the brachial plexus between them.

Subsequently the frequency of compression between the clavicle and first rib was recognized and the mechanisms well defined in 1943 by the report of Falconer and Weddel, who named this type of compression the *costoclavicular syndrome.* A short time later, in 1945, Wright observed patients in whom vascular symptoms resulted from hyperabduction and introduced the term *hyperabduction syndrome.*

Some degree of compression of the subclavian artery may be demonstrated in a high percentage of normal individuals in whom no symptoms whatever are present, but it formerly was thought that compression syndromes producing significant disability were rare. Recently, however, since the publication of Roos of a simplified approach to relieve compression syndromes at the thoracic outlet and since the introduction of peripheral nerve conduction velocity determinations, the conditions have been recognized with increasing frequency. It has even been suggested that for certain patients who have thoracic outlet syndromes a diagnosis of angina pectoris is erroneously made. Further experience will be needed to determine the exact frequency of these disorders, for the nerve conduction velocity studies have only recently been developed. The aforementioned transaxillary approach to resection of the first rib, first emphasized by Clagett in 1962, may help define the frequency of the condition more exactly, as removal of the first rib effectively decompresses the thoracic outlet.

REGIONAL ANATOMY. The subclavian artery leaves the thorax by passing over the first rib between the scalenus anticus muscle anteriorly and the brachial plexus and scalenus medius posteriorly. It then passes under the clavicle and subclavius muscle to enter the axilla beneath the pectoralis minor muscle. The subclavian vein has an almost identical course except that it passes anterior to the scalenus anticus muscle. The route of the brachial plexus nearly parallels that of the subclavian artery in the neck, lying posterolaterally between it and the scalenus medius muscle.

A potential area of compression exists in the interscalene triangle between the scalenus anticus anteriorly, the scalenus medius posteriorly, and the first rib inferiorly. Only slightly distal to this area, in the narrow space between the clavicle and the first rib, is another potential site of compression. Finally, in the axilla, where the pectoralis minor tendon attaches to the coracoid process, an area of potential obstruction of the axillary artery exists where it travels around the coracoid process. Lord and Rosati have emphasized that during hyperabduction the axillary vessels and brachial plexus are bent at an angle of approximately 90° in this area.

When a cervical rib persists, there may be in addition either a bony or a ligamentous structure, originating on the lowermost cervical vertebra, coursing between the anterior and medial scalene muscles, passing under the brachial plexus and subclavian artery, and attaching to the first rib.

ETIOLOGY. Although cervical ribs are found in about 0.5 percent of the normal population, only about 10 percent of these produce symptoms. Asymptomatic anomalies of the first rib are also frequently seen. Thus, additional factors other than the presence of a cervical rib or anomalous first rib must contribute to the compression syndrome. Symptoms are very rare in children and most frequently are seen in thin women in the third and fourth decades. An unusually well-developed musculature seems also to predispose to compression. A congenital variation in the anatomy of the head and neck has been suggested by Adson as a predisposing factor, a familiar type of patient being a thin woman with a long, narrow neck. The onset of symptoms in the second and third decade could be due to gradual descent of the shoulder girdle, perhaps from atrophy of the regional musculature.

Local anatomic variations are probably of particular significance. The width of the first rib in individuals in whom we have resected this structure has appeared to be unusually great. The width of the scalene anticus muscle at its insertion into the first rib varies greatly. A wide scalenus anticus muscle, which narrows the space in the interscalene triangle, has often been found at operation in symptomatic patients. Cervical ribs vary from short and rudimentary to completely formed and articulating anteriorly with the first rib. Some incomplete ribs are connected by fascial bands to the first rib which compress the brachial plexus.

Fractures of the clavicle or first rib may subsequently produce a large bony callus, especially if there is poor alignment of the ends of the fractured bone. One patient treated by one of the authors for severe ischemia of the hand was found to have peripheral emboli from a small subclavian aneurysm, produced by fracture of the first rib in an automobile accident.

PATHOLOGY. Disability from compression may be produced in several ways and depends upon which portions of the neurovascular bundle are involved. Compression of the brachial plexus usually causes pain, paresthesias, and a feeling of numbness. Often these symptoms are greatest in the C_8-T_1 distribution, because the ulnar nerve is derived from this most caudad portion of the plexus which rides over the first rib. Muscular weakness, paralysis, or atrophy of muscles are less frequent and appear only in far advanced cases. Vascular symptoms may be intermittent from compression or temporary occlusion of the subclavian artery, producing claudication with exercise, pallor, or a sensation of coldness, numbness, or paresthesia. In chronic cases, a different and more serious mechanism evolves, for intermittent compression and trauma of the subclavian arteries produce atheromatous changes in the artery and, rarely, a poststenotic aneurysm. From either arterial abnormality, emboli may be dislodged into the peripheral circulation and produce ischemia in the hand, even with focal areas of gangrene requiring amputation of digits. Thrombosis of the subclavian artery may eventually result. On occasion Raynaud's phenomenon may occur. Schein and associates found a total of 29 cases of subclavian arterial involvement previously reported. Eleven of these lost part or all of one digit from gangrene, while two required more extensive amputation. Restoration of continuity of the subclavian artery following thrombosis was reported for the first time in a case cited by Schein and associates.

A third group of vascular symptoms are intermittent episodes of vasoconstriction, similar to those seen in Raynaud's disease. The unilateral appearance of the Raynaud's phenomenon, however, almost always suggests a focal disturbance in the blood supply to the involved extremity. Such vasomotor phenomena are uncommon. A possible explanation for this infrequent occurrence has been proposed by Telford and Mottershead, who, on anatomic dissection, found that in 10 to 15 percent of patients the sympathetic innervation of the extremity traveled in a separate cord not incorporated in the main trunks of the brachial plexus. This isolated filament of fibers presumably would be more prone to direct compression and irritation. Finally, intermittent compression of the subclavian vein may cause signs of venous hypertension in the upper extremity with edema and the development of varicosities.

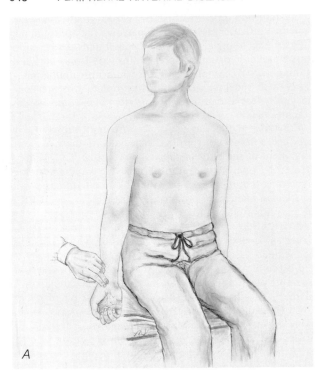

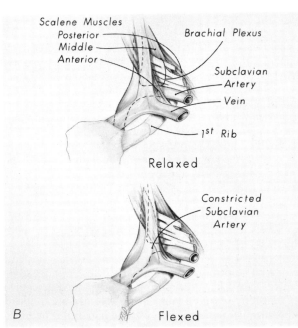

Fig. 21-20. Technique of performance of the Adson test for obstruction of the subclavian artery by the scalenus anticus muscle. *A.* The patient should be seated with his elbows at his sides and his neck extended. During deep inspiration his chin is turned to the affected side, while the intensity of the radial pulse is palpated. All these positions increase the tension on the scalenus anticus muscle. *B.* Course of the brachial plexus and subclavian artery between the scalenus anticus and medius muscles. A localized dilatation of the subclavian artery distal to the scalenus anticus is illustrated. Immediately distal to the scalenus anticus and medius muscles is another potential area of constriction, between the clavicle and the first rib. When the scalenus

The so-called "effort thrombosis," a condition of acute thrombosis of the subclavian vein, may be a result of a neurovascular compression syndrome, but the pathologic mechanisms have not been clearly identified.

CLINICAL MANIFESTATIONS. The symptomatology of the thoracic outlet syndrome depends on whether nerves, blood vessels, or both are compressed. Usually compression of one of these dominates the clinical picture. As reported in a paper by Urschel et al., symptoms of nerve compression manifested by pain and paresthesia were present in all but 6 of 138 patients, the pain usually being of insidious onset, commonly involving the neck, shoulder, arm, and hand with occasional radiation to the anterior chest or parascapular area. Paresthesias in specific nerve distribution occurred in 102 of their patients, the ulnar nerve being involved in 90 percent.

Symptoms of arterial compression were observed less frequently, in about one-quarter of their patients. Thirteen had symptoms of venous compression, including edema, venous distension, and discoloration; only three had the classic effort thrombosis, or Paget-Schroetter syndrome. Raynaud's phenomenon was present in 17 patients, all of whom were women.

Chronic ischemic pain has been observed in three of our patients following embolic occlusion of the radial or ulnar arteries with localized gangrene of one finger in one patient.

Physical Examination. Objective physical signs are more common in patients with vascular compression than in those with neural disorders. In only about 20 percent of patients with nerve compression are objective signs of decreased sensation found; some of these show additional muscle weakness or even atrophy. In the presence of neurologic symptoms at least one of the vascular compression signs can be expected, consisting essentially of loss of radial pulse with either Adson's maneuver, hyperabduction, or hyperextension. In the Adson maneuver, the patient sits with his hands on his knees, inspires deeply, extends his head backward, and turns his chin toward the affected side. Deep inspiration, extension of the neck, and turning of the head all tense the scalene anticus muscle and may decrease or obliterate the radial pulse (Fig. 21-20). Simultaneous auscultation of the supraclavicular space for bruit should be performed. In certain patients, a bruit will appear as the head is turned, reach a peak intensity, and cease as compression is increased to the point of obliterating the radial pulse. In other patients turning the head to the opposite side may demonstrate compression more effectively. The possibility of compression of the neurovascular bundle between the first rib and the clavicle also may be tested by displacing the shoulders backward and downward. The test is considered positive

anticus muscle is relaxed, there is minimal compression of the subclavian artery. With tension on the scalenus anticus muscle, compression of the subclavian artery results in decrease in the radial pulse, in some patients resulting in disappearance of the pulse. A bruit may become audible in the supraclavicular area as the scalenus anticus muscle is progressively stretched to compress the subclavian artery.

if the radial pulse is obliterated. The hyperabduction maneuver is performed by fully abducting the arm above the head and noting the effect upon the radial pulse.

The signs of arterial compression may be evident by direct physical examination. There may be differences in the qualities of the pulses between the two arms when the subclavian, brachial, radial, and ulnar arteries are compared. A localized supraclavicular bruit may be present. On occasion a particularly wide pulse, denoting a subclavian or axillary aneurysm, is palpable. With mild forms of ischemia there may be only pallor on elevation while in the more severe forms, especially with embolization, there may be atrophy of the skin, brittle nails, or even focal ulceration. In approximately 5 percent of patients frank Raynaud's phenomenon can be induced by application of cold to the extremity. In the approximately 10 percent of patients who have signs of venous obstruction, edema and venous distension are apparent.

In evaluating the maneuvers to detect neurovascular compression, it is important to remember that they are positive in a high percentage of normal individuals. This is particularly true of the costoclavicular compression or the hyperabduction test. A positive result, therefore, does not in itself establish a thoracic outlet syndrome; absence of any positive findings, however, suggests some other diagnosis.

LABORATORY STUDIES. Chest and cervical spine roentgenograms may demonstrate bony abnormalities in as many as one-third of the patients, either as cervical ribs, bifid first ribs, fusion of the first and second ribs, or clavicular deformities either congenital or traumatic.

For diagnosing arterial abnormalities, arteriography may be especially useful in demonstrating intimal irregularities, stenoses, or aneurysms of the subclavian artery. The arteriographic studies are of no value where there is no evidence of arterial compression or occlusion. Venographic studies are useful in patients with signs of venous compression, especially in establishing a differential diagnosis between thoracic outlet compression and other entities which mimic the condition.

The determination of nerve conduction velocities through the thoracic outlet as well as electromyographic determinations have been used to attempt to establish objective criteria for diagnosing neural compression. By applying electrical stimulation to various of the distal components of the brachial plexus and measuring conduction velocities to pinpoint areas of abnormal conduction, it is possible to evaluate sites of involvement of various neural structures. This technique used in conjunction with the specific determination of the ulnar nerve conduction velocity has been employed by Urschel to make diagnoses of thoracic outlet syndromes as well as to establish the differential diagnosis. Where atypical thoracic outlet neural compression syndromes are present, other nerves such as the median and the musculocutaneous can be similarly studied. Differential diagnoses between compression at the thoracic outlet, at the carpal tunnel at the wrist, and at the pronator level are possible. When this is combined with carefully performed electromyographic studies, very specific diagnoses are possible. With increasing experience,

correlating the results of electrical studies with postoperative results may permit more precise selection of patients for different types of therapy available.

DIAGNOSIS. Formerly, thoracic outlet syndromes have been erroneously diagnosed on purely clinical criteria, frequently in the presence of neural compression occurring at sites other than the thoracic outlet. Cervical disc disease, arthritis of the cervical spine, and nerve and spinal cord tumors, especially of the extramedullary type, can produce similar symptoms. The most easily diagnosed of the neurologic syndromes is that involving the lowermost portion of the brachial plexus. In this, there are subjective symptoms along the course of the ulnar nerve; relief obtained frequently on moderate abduction at the shoulder joint and a positive vascular compression test confirm the diagnosis. Electrical studies of ulnar nerve conduction velocity, with or without electromyographic studies, can firmly establish the diagnosis. With atypical neural compression syndromes the diagnosis is more difficult in the absence of positive physical signs except for signs of vascular compression during one of the compression maneuvers. An extensive investigation may be required, looking for bony abnormalities in the region of the thoracic outlet and performing nerve conduction and electromyographic studies to establish the probable site of the neural disorder. In many, the diagnosis will be a combination of exclusion of other diagnostic entities associated with positive findings on the specific electrical studies.

Diagnosis of the occlusive vascular disorders is less difficult. Physical findings suggesting arterial or venous compression are usually present. Appropriate angiographic studies may be required to delineate the nature, the specific mechanism, and the indicated therapy.

Diagnosis of the vasospastic disorders (Raynaud's) is clear-cut, but other conditions associated with it must also be considered.

TREATMENT. The treatment can be divided into that for the arterial, venous, and neurologic compressions. Treatment of the arterial compression depends upon the specific entity produced: embolization, stenosis and thrombosis, aneurysm formation, or intermittent vasospasm (Raynaud's). Occlusion of the subclavian artery, if not associated with severe ischemia, may require no therapy except an exercise program to promote development of collateral circulation. With atherosclerotic plaques or aneurysms of the subclavian artery, frequently associated with embolic episodes, therapy should correct the underlying compression mechanism. This usually involves resection of the first rib, preferably by the transaxillary approach, as well as removing the source of emboli. The presence of a thrombus in an aneurysm or ulceration in an atherosclerotic plaque requires resection of the involved artery and replacement, preferably with autologous tissue; composite grafts of saphenous veins have been useful. On occasion direct exposure of the arteries in the arm or forearm is necessary to remove emboli.

The venous occlusions are more difficult to treat, for the compressing mechanism may not be apparent from either physical examination or laboratory studies. It appears clear from results of transaxillary resection of the first rib that the most proximal part of the vein can be decompressed by this procedure, but the roles of the clavicle, the pectoralis minor, and clavipectoral fascia in producing compression cannot be evaluated by this approach. Those patients with effort thrombosis seen within the first day or two of its occurrence should be considered for combined surgical procedures of venous thrombectomy and relief of the compressing mechanism. Anticoagulation therapy then should be used, perhaps for as long as 1 year.

The management of the neural compression syndromes generally involves a conservative, nonsurgical approach. An exercise program designed to strengthen the muscles of the shoulder girdle and lessen the tendency of the shoulder to droop has been of value in some patients with mild to moderate symptoms. A series of such exercises are carefully described by Allen et al. As an example of this approach, fewer than half of a group of 300 patients with thoracic outlet syndromes required surgical intervention. The selection of patients for operation should depend upon the severity of the symptoms, failure to respond to a nonsurgical program, and the specificity of the diagnosis.

Operative Technique. It is important to include the entire extremity in the sterile operative field, permitting manipulation of the extremity in order to define the most likely area of compression. Whether or not a cervical rib is present, the transaxillary approach is favored for its simplicity, the clarity with which the compression mechanisms can be diagnosed, the excellent cosmetic result, and the ease with which cervical ribs together with the first rib can be excised. If vasomotor symptoms are prominent, sympathectomy can be performed through the same transaxillary approach, exposing the third and second thoracic ganglia as well as the lower third of the stellate ganglion; this includes the first thoracic ganglion but avoids the production of Horner's syndrome. If removal of the second and third intercostal nerves with their ganglia is thought necessary, since the demonstration by Skoog that 10 to 15 percent of the sympathetic ganglia to the upper extremity is contained in these nerves, it can be similarly carried out.

The transaxillary approach is performed by making an incision in the lowermost portion of the axilla from the pectoralis major anteriorly to the latissimus dorsi posteriorly (Fig. 21-21). The incision is deepened to the muscles of the chest wall, the serratus anterior and the intercostal muscles coming into view. The dissection is continued upward, avoiding the intercostobrachial nerve, with the arm hyperabducted to raise the neurovascular bundle off the first rib. By gentle dissection, it is possible to outline the scalene muscles and identify the attachment of the cervical rib to the first rib if one is present. The scalene muscles are transected and permitted to retract, and the muscles along the inferior border of the first rib are similarly incised. The first rib and cervical rib usually can be removed in their entirety, including periosteum, from the costochondral junction anteriorly to the posterior angle of the rib. The parietal pleura lies deep to the dissection; care must be taken to avoid puncturing it. If the pleura is punctured, the wound is closed around a catheter in the axilla while the anesthetist expands the lung. This usually suffices to correct the pneumothorax. On occasion it has

been necessary to aspirate air from the pleural cavity in the early postoperative period.

If a sympathectomy is indicated, the parietal pleura is stripped from the chest wall attachments and the sympathetic chain exposed, dissected free, and excised.

The postoperative course is usually benign, with the patient ready for discharge by the third postoperative day.

Other approaches have been described for excising the first rib. The posterior approach has been advocated by many but is an operation of greater magnitude. The anterior transthoracic approach has been proposed by others for more extensive exposure. However, most agree that the supraclavicular approach is probably archaic, since it does not permit thorough exploration of the area and easy excision of the first rib, which has become of paramount importance in treatment.

PROGNOSIS. The prognosis is dependent upon the specific syndrome present. The arterial compression syndromes can be quite satisfactorily relieved and arterial reconstructions performed with a high degree of precision, although a large series of patients treated with arterial compression has not been reported. In our experience it has been possible to stop embolic episodes and restore circulation to the upper extremity by standard arterial reconstructive procedures. However, patients with Raynaud's phenomena and cervical rib in whom associated sympathectomies have been performed have had variable results. Although immediate effects of sympathectomy have been excellent, relapses have occurred quite abruptly as early as 6 months following operation.

The venous compression disorders also have given variable results. It is not clear at present whether thrombectomy, with or without relief of the venous compression mechanism, is any better than prolonged anticoagulant therapy. Those patients with chronic venous occlusions of the subclavian and axillary veins who have been followed for years have shown remarkable recovery, with subsidence of edema coincident with the appearance of a prominent venous pattern on the chest wall and little or no resulting disability.

The surgical approach has often changed through the years. Other procedures include scalenotomy performed through the supraclavicular approach, then resection of the clavicle proposed by Lord and Rosati, and now resection of the first rib. Adson, predominantly performing scalenotomy through the supraclavicular approach, reported in 1947 that over a period of 22 years 142 patients had been operated upon with excellent results in about 50 percent and improvement in another 20 to 30 percent. In another series from the Mayo Clinic, Love reported that of 700 patients seen over a 5-year period with a wide variety of thoracic outlet syndromes, only about 3 percent underwent operation. Roos has reported from a wide experience with transaxillary resection of the first rib that 80 to 90 percent of those with predominantly neurologic symptoms obtained complete relief, while approximately 50 percent of those with predominantly vascular symptoms became free of symptoms.

The recent development of electrical conduction studies provides an objective method not only for making the

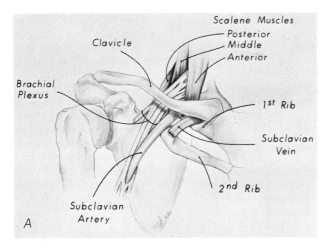

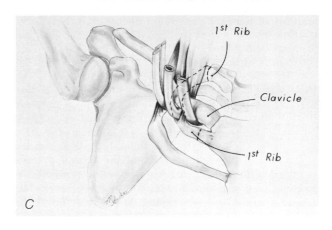

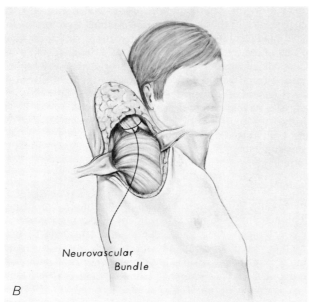

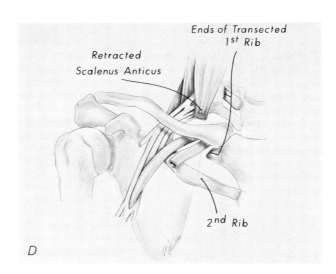

Fig. 21-21. Technique of transaxillary resection of the first rib. *A.* The critical relations of the first rib, clavicle, scalene muscles and neurovascular structures are shown. The lowermost portion of the brachial plexus which gives rise to the ulnar nerve is in contact with the first rib and explains the most characteristic neurologic symptoms usually involving the ulnar aspect of the forearm and fourth and fifth fingers. *B.* Operative incision below the axillary hairline with hyperabduction of the arm which raises the neurovascular bundle out of the operative field. *C.* Effect of hyperabduction in exposing the first rib and scalene muscles, retracting the neurovascular bundle. *D.* Effect of first rib resection, which requires cutting all three scalene muscles, in relieving the compression of artery, vein, and brachial plexus.

diagnosis but for evaluating the results of therapy. The wide variation in frequency of diagnosis and results with operation from different groups is perhaps due to variation in diagnostic criteria. Urschel emphasized the usefulness of electrical conduction studies; in a series of 300 patients seen between 1946 and 1970, only 138 were operated upon. Seventeen of these had bilateral operations. Employing the electrical conduction studies, 96 percent of patients im-

proved after resection of the first rib. There were only five cases of failure, in two of which a cervical disc subsequently was removed. The most favorable group were those with pain and paresthesia in the distribution of the ulnar nerve, diminution of the pulse by one of the various compression tests, and slowing of ulnar nerve conduction velocity below 60 m/second. Failures following operation were more common in those with atypical pain distributions, often with associated cervical syndromes secondary to whiplash or trauma. Usually, pulse changes with the compression tests were minimal or absent, and there was less slowing of ulnar nerve conduction velocity.

EXTRACRANIAL OCCLUSIVE CEREBROVASCULAR DISEASE

HISTORICAL CONSIDERATIONS. One of the most astonishing historical medical facts of the twentieth century relates to the belated recognition 25 years ago that the majority of ischemic strokes are due to occlusive athero-sclerotic disease of the extracranial arteries in the neck, not to intravascular arterial occlusions. The earliest recorded recognition of this possible relationship was made by Savory in 1856. This concept was rediscovered in 1914 by Hunt, who described the postmortem findings of infarction of a cerebral hemisphere in a patient with patent territorial (middle cerebral) arteries but a thrombosed extracranial internal carotid artery. This fact was considered to be a curiosity for almost four more decades, because of both the unavailability of techniques for studying afflicted patients in vivo and the practice of performing incomplete postmortem examinations in order to preserve the cervical carotid arteries for the injection of embalming fluid. The intracranial arteries were examined, as were the origins of the great vessels from the aortic arch, but the critical carotid bifurcation in the neck was left untouched.

The development of safe techniques for cerebral angiography, combined with careful clinical pathologic studies of the type of vascular disease in large numbers of patients with strokes, led to recognition of the frequency with which stroke syndromes were due to extracranial vascular disease. Classic studies were reported by Fischer between 1951 and 1954 and by Hutchinson and Yates in 1956.

The report of Eastcott, Pickering, and Rob documenting the successful operation for carotid bifurcation disease stimulated wide interest in the surgical management of this condition, although three groups, including Carre et al, Stuly et al, and DeBakey, claimed priority in having performed earlier operations. The first significant series in the United States was reported by Lyons and Galbraith in 1957. It was soon established that the operation of endarterectomy for carotid bifurcation atherosclerotic lesions could be performed in large numbers of afflicted individuals with a high degree of safety, in spite of the unmatched sensitivity of the brain to ischemia, and that long-term patency could be expected. The effects of the surgical approach on the natural history of stroke syndromes, which were many and varied, however, had not been evaluated. Therefore, a "Joint Study of Extracranial Arterial Occlusion as a Cause of Stroke" was begun in 1961. Many universities throughout the country participated in a patient-informed prospective randomized study of the effects of surgical reconstructive procedures upon the natural history of the disease. In the ensuing 10 years, on the basis of the carefully collected protocols of 11,000 patients and frequent workshop meetings among the members, understanding of the natural history of the disease, the indications, contraindications, and hazards of diagnostic and surgical procedures were developed. The randomized nature of the study was fully justified by the rapidity with which understanding developed, permitting the elimination, as surgical candidates, of those patients in whom the surgical procedure was detrimental, and vastly improving the management of those in whom the surgical procedure was beneficial.

ETIOLOGY AND PATHOLOGY. Although the term *stroke* encompasses a variety of clinical situations in which major neurologic deficits occur because of involvement of the brain, the term *ischemic stroke* refers to cerebral infarction occurring as a result of impairment of regional blood flow. Atherosclerosis is the basis for this in the vast majority of patients. Smaller percentages are (1) secondary to cerebral embolization of thrombi which originate in the heart, (2) due to fibromuscular hyperplasia, (3) associated with obliterative arteritis of the great vessels as they originate from the aortic arch (see Aortic Arch Occlusive Disease, in Chap. 20), (4) due to blunt or penetrating trauma, (5) secondary to forceful hyperextension of the neck resulting in dissection and tearing of the carotid intima, and (6) due to dissecting thoracic aortic aneurysms which involve the carotid arteries.

A clinical pathologic correlation between the appearance of surgically removed plaques and the specific syndromes presented by patients operated on at New York University confirmed the early findings of Millard Fisher, showing that patients with generalized symptoms of cerebral ischemia had major stenotic fibrotic lesions which had smooth surfaces, while those with focal symptoms were found to have plaques with either frank ulcerations or cul de sacs which could have been the source of emboli. Intramural hemorrhage was the most common single, pathologic finding and could be responsible for fragmentation of plaques, development of sudden stenosis, breakdown of the plaque, and subsequent thrombosis. If patients with stroke syndromes are studied with four-vessel angiography, opacifying both carotid and both vertebral arteries from their origins to their point of entry into the skull, significant extracranial occlusive disease will be found in about 75 percent of the group (Fig. 21-22). The segmental localization is impressive. In the carotid artery, almost all plaques are found at the carotid bifurcation, starting in the distal centimeter of the common carotid and involving the proximal external carotid and the proximal 1 to 2 cm of the internal carotid. Fortunately for surgical reconstruction, and also a striking example of segmental localization of atherosclerosis, the internal carotid beyond the first 1 to 2 cm is usually uninvolved to beyond its point of entry into the skull, the area of the so-called carotid siphon. Because of the freedom of involvement of this portion, arterial reconstruction almost always can be done if the internal carotid is not thrombosed. Disease in the middle cerebral artery is rare. In the basilar-vertebral system, plaques are usually at the origin of the vertebrals from the subclavian, but disease of the vertebral beyond its origin is unusual. In the basilar artery localized atherosclerosis is more common. Within the thorax, the great vessels are infrequently diseased. The lesions are multiple in more than 50 percent of patients.

Soon after the recognition of the frequency of extracranial vascular disease, it became apparent that simple reduction in cerebral blood flow was not an adequate explanation for many of the neurologic syndromes encountered. As a result of several years of investigation by the National Cooperative Stroke Study, it now seems clear that arterioarterial embolization of fragments of plaque or platelet-fibrin aggregates is probably the most frequent mechanism of neurologic injury (Fig. 21-23). These plaques form on the irregular surface of atherosclerotic plaques, usually at the carotid bifurcation, and subse-

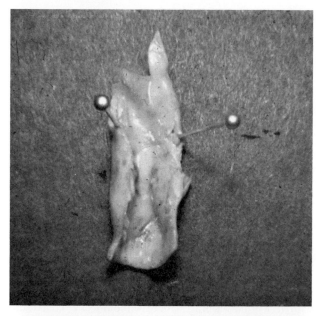

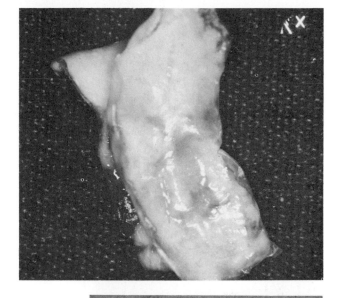

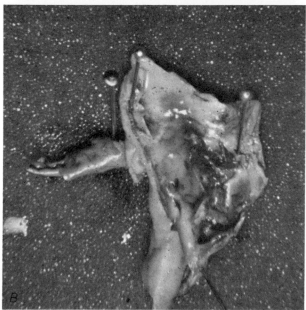

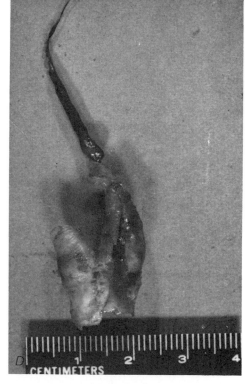

Fig. 21-22. Carotid plaque dynamics in the pathogenesis of stroke syndromes are suggested by the variations in the appearances of lesions surgically removed. *A.* Smooth fibrous plaque producing marked stenosis and decreased blood flow. *B.* Ulcerated plaque giving rise to embolization. *C.* Hemorrhage into the wall of a plaque which can result in sudden stenosis or ulceration and subsequent ulceration and embolization. *D.* Total occlusion of an internal carotid artery secondary to thrombosis.

quently embolize. Ophthalmologic visualization of these plaques suddenly appearing in the retina during transient ischemic attacks was one of the first clues to the mechanism of the syndrome. The second method for production of symptoms is the obvious one of simple decrease in flow from marked stenosis or occlusion. Because of abundant collateral circulation in the brain, major arteries may be-

come narrowed or occluded without any symptoms whatever unless multiple areas are diseased. As with stenotic lesions in the vascular system elsewhere there is little decrease in blood flow until the cross-sectional area of the vessel is narrowed by more than 75 percent. If collateral circulation is adequate, even complete occlusion may be harmless. Routine postmortem studies by Martin and associates of a large group of patients dying from different causes at the Mayo Clinic found that in as many as 40 percent of the patients at least one of the four major extracranial arteries significantly was narrowed or oc-

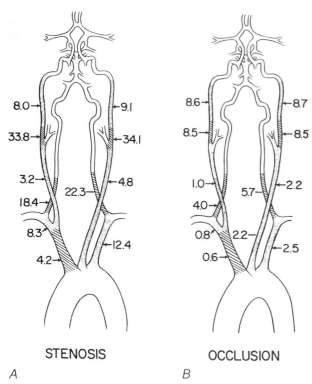

STENOSIS   OCCLUSION

A   B

Fig. 21-23. Frequency distribution of lesions according to anatomic locations and stenosis versus occlusion. The predominance of stenotic lesions over occlusions favors embolization as a
common mechanism for the production of cerebral ischemia. The
predominance of extracranial lesions renders surgical intervention feasible.

cluded, even though there were no neurologic symptoms
before death.

The atherosclerotic plaques removed from the vessels
of symptomatic patients have varied greatly in composition
and appearance. Some were principally fibrotic, with
smooth internal surfaces; others showed advanced degenerative changes, with intramural hemorrhage and little
stenosis, but with ulceration of the intimal surface. Plaques
with a smooth intimal surface are probably harmless until
the cross-sectional area of the artery is reduced to a
marked degree. An ulcerated plaque, however, even
though the lumen is compromised little, may cause serious
or even catastrophic injury from repeated embolization.

CLINICAL MANIFESTATIONS. A great variety of clinical
syndromes result from the different patterns of occlusive
disease in the carotid, vertebral, and subclavian arteries.
These will be only briefly summarized here, for they are
described in considerable detail in standard texts of neu-
rology. The classic stroke from unilateral carotid disease
is ipsilateral blindness and contralateral hemiplegia. The
presence of aphasia depends upon the dominant cerebral
hemisphere. The other extreme is the most fleeting focal
neurologic defect such as a transient monoplegia, transient
hemiplegia, or transient ipsilateral blindness. These episodes, clearing within minutes to hours after an abrupt
onset, are termed *transient ischemic attacks.* Between such

episodes the patient may be completely well, but unfortunately such attacks often precede a catastrophic
stroke. One retrospective study of patients with severe
strokes found that almost 75 percent had such premonitory symptoms in the weeks or months before the stroke
appeared.

Between the transient ischemic attack on the one hand
and the massive stroke on the other, a wide variety of
motor and sensory syndromes are seen. Their unilateral
localization is strongly suggestive of carotid artery disease.
They may be precipitated by hypotension, hypoxia, or
changes in position or posture, or they may be unrelated
to any known cause.

With disease of the vertebral-basilar system, a number
of brainstem symptoms occur. In contrast to carotid disease, the symptoms are often bilateral, involving either
both arms or both legs, but may alternate in severity from
one side of the body to the other. Tinnitus, dizziness,
vertigo, diplopia, and dysarthria are also common. One
type of characteristic syndrome is the so-called "drop attack," in which the patient may literally fall to the ground
with little or no warning, with or without loss of consciousness, and recover equally rapidly with only residual dizziness or mild ataxia.

Disease of the subclavian artery proximal to the origin
of one of the vertebral arteries, more commonly the left,
produces the so-called "subclavian steal" syndrome. The
proximal obstruction in the subclavian artery decreases the
pressure in that artery at the point of origin of the vertebral
artery; this results in an actual reversal of flow in the
vertebral artery, with blood draining out of the basilar
artery into the arm. Although this phenomenon is seen
frequently on angiographic studies, production of symptoms from ischemia of the brainstem by exercising the arm
is uncommon.

Physical Examination. Examination is directed primarily
at determining the presence of any neurologic deficit as
well as the pattern of arterial involvement. Palpation of
the carotid pulses is useful only for the rare instance of
intrathoracic occlusion of the common carotid artery. Palpation for the internal carotid pulse in the pharynx posterior to the tonsillar pillars is no longer advised. Separate
palpation of the external and internal carotid arteries is
impossible because of their location next to one another.
Hence, the carotid pulses are normal on palpation in almost all patients with occlusive disease at the carotid bifurcation. However, auscultation over the carotid bifurcation for a bruit is essential. With high-grade stenoses at the
bifurcation, a bruit is audible just anterior to the sternocleidomastoid muscle near the level of the angle of the
mandible in at least 50 percent of patients with stenosis.
Auscultation in the supraclavicular fossae may find bruits
from subclavian-vertebral disease. When bruits are detected, they must be differentiated from cardiac valvular
lesions, such as aortic stenosis, which produce murmurs
transmitted along the great vessels. If occlusive disease of a
subclavian artery is present, the blood pressure will be
significantly different in the two arms.

Ophthalmodynomometry is a useful screening procedure when there is high-grade stenosis or total occlusion

of one of the internal carotid arteries. The technique is simple comparison of the pressure in the retinal arteries of the two eyes; though not quantitative, it is a useful screening technique.

DIAGNOSIS. The differential diagnosis of cerebrovascular insufficiency syndromes is extremely complex and involves exclusion of a variety of intracranial lesions in addition to generalized conditions which can effect cerebral hypoxia. The latter include myocardial infarction, cardiac arrhythmias, Stokes-Adams syndrome, Ménière's syndrome, and a number of metabolic disorders such as diabetic ketosis and hypoglycemia.

The diagnosis of ischemic stroke syndromes ultimately depends upon angiographic delineation of the intra- and extracranial cerebral arteries. The risks related to angiography generally are assumed by the patients most seriously afflicted with arterial disease, particularly those who have already developed serious neurologic deficits. The overall risk of stroke or death incident to cerebral angiography is about 0.5 to 1 percent. Less serious complications, such as hematomas and temporary or permanent loss of arterial pulses distal to puncture sites, occur with greater frequency.

The presence of amaurosis fugax, transient paralysis or weakness of the extremity, weakness of facial muscles, and transient disorders of speech all require more extensive investigation, which should include skull x-rays, lumbar puncture, computed axial tomography of the head, and electroencephalograms. Electrocardiography with prolonged cardiac monitoring may be appropriate to rule out transient cardiac arrhythmias. The ultimate study in these patients is cerebral angiography.

The major questions related to cerebral angiography concern patients with massive and persistent neurologic deficits and those with asymptomatic bruits. Both cerebral angiographic studies and carotid-vertebral reconstructive procedures assume grave risks in patients who have had full-blown ischemic stroke within the week.

On the other side of the spectrum, the finding of neck bruits in asymptomatic patients during routine examination increasingly poses a problem. Doppler examination of the supraorbital arteries or ultrasound scanning of the cervical carotid arteries may permit detection of hemodynamically significant carotid lesions. However, it is clear that many carotid lesions which produce stroke manifest no local hemodynamic disturbances and act rather as a source of emboli. Thus, there are difficult decisions regarding performance of cerebral angiography in these patients.

The study by Thompson, in which patients with asymptomatic bruits were shown to have "significant" lesions by angiography and appeared to be protected from future stroke by operative intervention, suggests a more aggressive attitude. However, Gaspar and Movius, among others, report that patients who had neck bruits and underwent major abdominal procedures did not develop an increased incidence of postoperative strokes.

The attitude of the authors of this chapter toward asymptomatic bruits, in the face of conflicting data, is to study angiographically those patients with "loud, high-pitched" carotid bruits who are physiologically fit and therefore thought to have long life expectancies. Operations are offered to patients who have 70 percent stenosis or lesions with irregular contour. Any patient with an asymptomatic carotid bruit discovered prior to a major intraabdominal or intrathoracic procedure is studied in a similar manner.

TREATMENT. General Considerations. Data accumulated from several years of study by the National Cooperative Stroke Study clearly show that effective surgical treatment must be performed before major neurologic deficits are produced from cerebral infarction. Hence, surgical therapy must be basically prophylactic. Operations are generally performed on patients who have had transient ischemic attacks. Operation upon patients with acute strokes is associated with a high mortality, considerably higher than that for patients treated medically. If operation for acute stroke is for an ulcerated plaque which does not narrow the artery, there is little benefit at all to the patient except prevention of subsequent episodes. If a totally obstructed internal carotid artery is reopened, the patient's condition may be exacerbated from edema or hemorrhage developing in the infarct as a result of restoring perfusion pressure. The question of operating on patients with asymptomatic bruits has not been resolved.

Recently, as the prevalence of arterioarterial embolization in the production of stroke syndromes has become clear, there has been renewed interest in altering the coagulability of the blood. The striking finding of the influence of acetylsalicylic acid on platelet aggregation may be of considerable therapeutic significance. Clinical trials are now in progress to determine the possible value of aspirin in preventing stroke syndromes.

Treatment of Atherosclerotic Disease of the Internal Carotid Artery. Atherosclerosis of the origin of the internal carotid artery is the most common form of extracranial vascular disease. As stated earlier, the disease fortunately is limited only to the first 1 to 2 cm of the origin of the internal carotid and hence is ideal for surgical correction (Fig. 21-24).

When complete occlusion develops in the carotid artery, however, an organized thrombus develops above the atherosclerotic plaque which extends superiorly into the intracranial internal carotid, making successful operation impossible. In approximately 10 percent of patients with complete occlusion, however, the thrombus has not propagaged more than 2 to 3 cm, and surgical removal is still possible.

As stated earlier, the ideal patient for operation is one with transient ischemic attacks without any permanent neurologic abnormality. In such patients operation can be performed under regional cervical block with little risk. Mortality and major neurologic complications are in the range of 1 to 4 percent. Details of the operation are shown in Fig. 21-25.

The hazards of operation are greater and the likelihood of benefit much less when a stroke has occurred. If the internal carotid has become totally occluded, producing a major neurologic deficit, operation performed within 6 hours after onset of symptoms may produce dramatic recovery. The operative mortality, however, especially with altered states of consciousness, is considerably higher than with elective operations. If operation is delayed much beyond 6 hours after the onset of symptoms, reopening a totally obstructed carotid artery may be followed first by transient improvement, then worsening of symptoms and even death from hemorrhage into the area of infarction precipitated by the restoration of arterial perfusion pressure. It has been suggested by Warren and Triedman that this catastrophe might be prevented by careful avoidance of blood pressure elevation during operation and for some weeks afterward.

If the acute stroke has resulted from embolization of atheromatous debris or platelet aggregates, with occlusion of small intracerebral vessels, emergency operation upon the nonstenosing ulcerated plaque at the carotid bifurcation is neither helpful nor harmful. At a later time such patients perhaps should be considered for operation to prevent future embolization if the permanent neurologic deficit is not severe.

In patients with chronic strokes in whom acute injury weeks or months earlier produced a permanent neurologic deficit indicative of total hemispheric infarction, operation is of little value. A challenging group consists of asymptomatic patients with loud bruits. Thompson et al. have reported a lowered stroke incidence in such patients if angiographic studies revealed significant carotid lesions.

Following endarterectomy of the stenotic carotid artery, the likelihood of long-term patency of the reconstructed artery is excellent. In a group of 100 patients reported by

Blaisdell et al., 21 were evaluated by angiography more than 5 years later. There was only one late occlusion, an asymptomatic one found at autopsy. In 1968 Edwards and associates studied 75 patients operated upon 5 to 9 years earlier. Only five of the 75 had subsequently had a stroke. Three of the group had developed recurrent stenosis at the site of endarterectomy, but all experienced successful reoperation.

The effect of prophylactic carotid endarterectomy in altering the incidence of mortality in future stroke has been analyzed in detail by the National Cooperative Stroke Study. Although the results of the study were not completely definitive, certain facts emerged. The natural history of the disease definitely can be changed if the operative mortality and stroke rate can be kept at low levels (1 to 5 percent). Those patients with the most severe and extensive involvement, viz., those with bilateral carotid

Fig. 21-24. Angiographic studies of the cerebral circulation for stroke syndromes should outline the major extracranial as well as the intracranial arteries. This facilitates planning operative procedures and aids in making differential diagnoses of the various causes of stroke syndromes. Cervical carotid and vertebral arteries are outlined by retrograde right brachial arterial injection. *A.* Arrow points to significant lesion in the internal and external carotids. *B.* Arrow points to typical stenotic lesion at the origin of the vertebral with an associated kink.

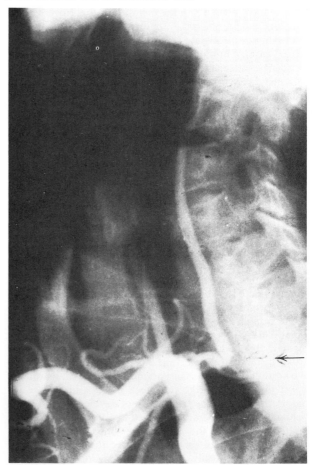

A   *B*

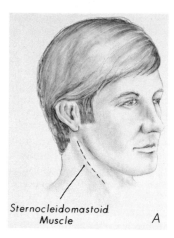

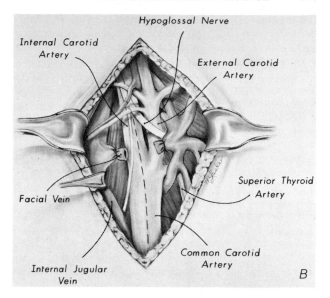

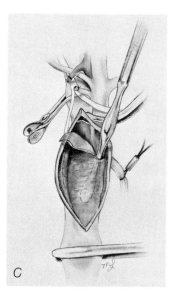

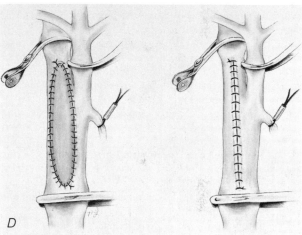

Fig. 21-25. Technique of carotid endarterectomy. *A.* A skin incision is made anterior to the sternocleidomastoid muscle. *B.* The carotid artery branches are widely mobilized. The internal carotid artery is clamped before widely mobilizing the frequently thrombus-containing bulb, thereby protecting the brain from embolization, which may occur during the dissection. The vagus and hypoglossal nerves are carefully protected. Mobilization of the hypoglossal is facilitated by dividing the sternocleidomastoid artery and vein. A longitudinal arteriotomy is made extending above and below the plaque at the carotid bifurcation. *C.* After division of the intima above the plaque, the plaque can be easily dissected from the underlying media or from the adventitia. The distal intima is carefully inspected and sutured if necessary. *D.* The arteriotomy is either closed primarily with 5-0 Tevdek, or a vein roof patch fashioned from autologous saphenous vein is used to avoid producing stenosis. The technique for restoring flow after completion of the closure is crucial to avoid embolization to the brain. The internal carotid clamp is temporarily removed and reapplied. The common and external carotid clamps are removed, and after 1 or 2 minutes of flushing of the carotid bulb the internal carotid clamp is removed.

lesions or with stenosis opposite complete occlusion, who survive operations enjoy the greatest protection from future stroke and from death from stroke. Strokes in the neurologic area corresponding to the surgically repaired artery are virtually eliminated.

In a series of 800 carotid and vertebral operations performed at our institution during a 15-year period, 70 had unilateral and 20 had bilateral carotid operations, 3 percent in conjunction with vertebral arterial reconstructions.

The combined death and stroke rate was 4 percent, being highest for patients with acute strokes (40 percent), 11 percent for strokes in evolution, and 0 for 106 patients who were neurologically intact and asymptomatic at the time of operation. Although patients with multiple extracranial arterial lesions have the highest operative risks, they enjoy the greatest long-term benefits from carotid surgery. Late mortality is primarily due to coronary artery disease.

Treatment of Subclavian-Vertebral Disease. Stenosis involving only the vertebral artery is infrequent. It is physiologically significant only when bilateral or if one vertebral is congenitally hypoplastic or absent. The disease is frequently limited to the site of origin of the vertebral from the subclavian. The atherosclerotic plaques in this area usually have a smooth intimal surface, contrasting to the frequency of ulcerated plaques in the carotid artery. In addition, there are frequently tortuous kinks in the first few centimeters of the vertebral artery, which can be shown to result in total occlusion when the head is turned to one side. Symptoms are probably due to decreased flow through the basivertebral system, although embolization cannot be entirely excluded. Concomitant disease in the basilar artery is frequent.

Atherosclerotic stenosis or occlusion of the subclavian artery proximal to the site of origin of the vertebral artery produces the clinical picture termed the subclavian steal syndrome. This abnormality was well defined by Reivich et al. in 1961, following an angiographic description in 1960 by Contorni of retrograde flow in the involved vertebral artery. The reduction in pressure in the subclavian artery beyond the stenosis results in retrograde flow from the brainstem down the vertebral artery to the arm; hence the term "subclavian steal." The clinical picture is that of ischemic neurologic symptoms in association with mild ischemia in the involved arm. Diagnosis can be easily made by finding a decreased pulse and blood pressure in the symptomatic arm, often in association with a localized bruit in the supraclavicular space. Serial angiograms after injection of contrast media into the opposite brachial artery or the ascending aorta will demonstrate reversal of flow in the involved vertebral artery by initially opacifying the opposite vertebral artery in a normal fashion, followed by retrograde opacification of the involved vertebral. Although this phenomenon is not infrequent on angiographic examination, clinical symptoms are not common, perhaps because collateral circulation in the brain can readily compensate for the amount of blood diverted away from the brain by the retrograde vertebral flow.

Operations upon the vertebral artery usually can be performed without thoracotomy. Surgical exposure of the subclavian-vertebral junction is obtained through a transverse supraclavicular incision which divides the clavicular head of the sternocleidomastoid muscle and the underlying scalenus anticus muscle. If the stenosing plaque has a smooth intimal surface, endarterectomy may not be necessary. The artery can be simply widened with a patch angioplasty with autologous saphenous vein. If the vertebral artery is significantly tortuous and redundant, predisposing to kinking, plication can be performed. In approximately 50 arterial reconstructions of the vertebral artery performed at New York University, there has been no neurologic deficit and no evidence of cerebral ischemia during the period of reconstruction.

Operations for the subclavian steal syndrome are seldom necessary. When done, a transthoracic approach to the subclavian artery can be avoided by employing a bypass graft from the ipsilateral common carotid artery to the distal subclavian artery. This is physiologically possible because the common carotid is large enough to deliver sufficient blood to supply both the brain and the upper extremity. On occasion, when the common carotid or in-nominate arteries are markedly stenotic and not suitable, axilloaxillary bypass grafting has been useful.

Treatment of Aortic Arch Occlusive Disease. In 1962 a report by Crawford et al. stated that during a period of 100 years since the first clinical description of the aortic arch syndrome by Savory in 1854, only about 90 patients were reported. In the report by Crawford et al., operative experiences with 67 patients in the 4-year period between 1957 and 1961 well indicated the increased recognition of the disease through the widespread use of angiography. Atherosclerosis was the most frequent cause. Formerly syphilitic arteritis was common, but this is now unusual. In the Orient a peculiar arteritis of unknown cause occurs, especially in young women. One eponym referring to this disease, Takayasu's disease, originated from an early description of the clinical syndrome by a Japanese ophthalmologist. An arteritis of this type is rarely seen in the United States.

For several years the occlusive lesions were approached directly with a transthoracic exposure. As the atherosclerotic process was often multiple and diffuse, endarterectomy was seldom possible. Bypass grafts were employed from the ascending aorta proximally to the carotid or subclavian arteries distad. This operative approach is extensive, requiring a thoracotomy incision and separate cervical or supraclavicular incisions.

In more recent years short bypass procedures in the neck establishing grafts from the normal artery to the obstructed artery have become increasingly popular. In a report of 125 patients, Dietrich and his associates expressed a preference for cervical carotid-subclavian bypass rather than the thoracic approach. A left carotid subclavian bypass was employed in 91 patients and a right carotid subclavian bypass in 20. The operative mortality was 5 percent, with good results in the majority of patients. This operative technique avoids an intrathoracic procedure but has the theoretic disadvantage of siphoning blood from a normal artery to a diseased artery. Apparently this theoretic objection is of limited clinical significance, for significant neurologic syndromes have not been produced from the shunting procedure.

ABDOMINAL ANEURYSMS

HISTORICAL DATA. The modern era of treatment of abdominal aneurysms began with the first successful excision of an abdominal aneurysm and replacement with an aortic homograft by Dubost in 1951. Previous therapeutic efforts, such as wiring to promote clotting, wrapping or coating with plastics, and other techniques to induce thrombosis, are now of historic interest only. Following the report of Dubost et al., advances in operative therapy came rapidly, especially those achieved by Cooley, DeBakey and his associates, and Bahnson. Late complications of aortic homografts soon appeared, following which replacement of the aorta with a prosthetic graft was developed. Although nylon was used briefly, Dacron or Teflon has been the preferred reconstruction material since 1957 (Fig. 21–26).

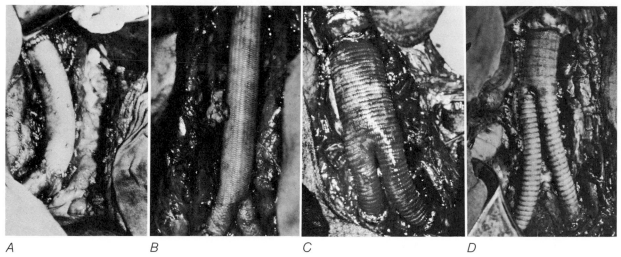

A   *B*   *C*   *D*

Fig. 21-26. Replacement of abdominal aorta. *A.* Aortic homograft inserted following excision of aneurysm of abdominal aorta by Bahnson in 1953. Homografts were among the earliest materials used for arterial grafts but were subsequently discontinued because of late degeneration of the homograft. *B.* Nylon graft used following excision of an abdominal aneurysm in 1954. Nylon was subsequently discontinued because experience found a marked loss in tensile strength 1 year after implantation. (*Courtesy of Dr. Henry T. Bahnson, Department of Surgery, University of Pittsburgh.*) *C.* Operative photograph of knitted Dacron graft inserted following excision of abdominal aneurysm. Dacron has been satisfactorily used since 1967 with excellent long-term results. *D.* Operative photograph of Teflon graft inserted following excision of abdominal aneurysm. Teflon, like Dacron, has given excellent long-term results with large vessels, but with small vessels, such as the femoral artery, results have been less satisfactory.

INCIDENCE. Abdominal aneurysms are the most common of the arteriosclerotic aneurysms. With the increasing age of the population, abdominal aneurysms are increasing in frequency, for most patients are in the sixth or seventh decade. Men are affected more frequently than women, in a ratio approximating 10:1.

ETIOLOGY AND PATHOLOGY. The vast majority of abdominal aneurysms are arteriosclerotic in origin. This is probably related to the frequency of involvement of the abdominal aorta by atherosclerosis, and perhaps to mechanical factors creating turbulent flow at the bifurcation of the abdominal aorta. The authors have never seen an abdominal aneurysm arising below the renal arteries from any cause except arteriosclerosis, although they have been reported from syphilis, trauma, the Marfan syndrome, or bacterial endocarditis.

The aneurysms characteristically originate just below the renal arteries and extend beyond the aortic bifurcation into the common iliacs. Fortunately, they seldom involve the external iliac arteries. Small aneurysms may be limited just to the abdominal aorta. The anatomic location of abdominal aneurysms, therefore, makes them accessible to surgical therapy, for a graft can be inserted proximally from the abdominal aorta below the renal arteries to the common iliac arteries distad. The size of abdominal aneurysms varies greatly, small ones 2 to 3 cm in diameter being

detected accidentally by aortography while others may enlarge to a diameter of 10 to 15 cm before being discovered accidentally by palpation. The usual course of untreated aneurysms was well documented in the classic report by Estes in 1950. Without treatment there is a 20 percent chance of rupture within 1 year after diagnosis and a 50 percent chance within 4 or 5 years. Complications seldom arise from expanding aneurysms until rupture occurs. Erosion of bone, so common in syphilitic aneurysms, virtually never occurs with abdominal aneurysms. There is usually no impairment of peripheral circulation, although larger aneurysms commonly are composed principally of laminated clot with a small central lumen. Emboli from the shaggy laminated clot lining abdominal aneurysms occur but rarely.

Although aneurysms frequently originate within 1 to 2 cm of the origin of the renal arteries, actual involvement of the origin of the renal arteries in the aneurysm, necessitating reconstruction of the renal arteries during surgical excision, is rare. In a series of over 170 abdominal aneurysms at the Johns Hopkins Hospital, only 3 aneurysms involving the renal arteries were found.

An abdominal aneurysm is often associated with generalized atherosclerosis. In a series of 1,400 patients operated upon by DeBakey and associates, some signs of coronary artery disease were present in 30 percent of the patients, and 40 percent of the patients had some increase in systolic blood pressure. Associated occlusive disease of the carotid arteries was found in 7 percent, of the renal arteries in 2 percent, and of the iliac arteries in 16 percent of the patients. Concomitant clinically significant aneurysms were found in the thoracic aorta in 4 percent, in the femoral artery in 3 percent, and in the popliteal artery in 2 percent of the group.

CLINICAL MANIFESTATIONS. Symptoms. Most patients are unaware of their abdominal aneurysms until a mass is accidentally discovered by the patient or his physician. The importance of careful deep palpation of the abdomen on routine physical examination, outlining the abdominal aorta when possible, is obvious. Occasionally, low back pain caused by an abdominal aneurysm may be diagnosed erroneously as due to an orthopedic condition. The pain apparently arises from tension on retroperitoneal tissues from the aneurysm; erosion of bone almost never happens. Virtually any intraabdominal condition may be simulated by an abdominal aortic aneurysm, such as renal colic, acute appendicitis, diverticulitis, peptic ulcer, pancreatitis, or cholecystitis. Rarely, there is gastrointestinal bleeding. With beginning leakage of the aneurysm or frank rupture momentarily contained retroperitoneally, acute abdominal conditions such as perforated ulcer, hemorrhagic pancreatitis, or generalized peritonitis may be simulated.

Sometimes, sudden vascular collapse with shock is the first indication. Most patients, however, have some premonitory symptoms. The absence of signs preceding fatal rupture is a strong reason for removing most abdominal aneurysms as soon as the diagnosis is made, even though the condition is asymptomatic. Symptoms from an aneurysm are an urgent indication for operation and are sometimes called a *syndrome of impending rupture.*

Physical Examination. On physical examination an abdominal aneurysm larger than 5 cm in diameter can be diagnosed with reasonable certainty. Once the patient has relaxed the muscles of the abdominal wall, careful deep palpation can usually outline the abdominal aorta near the bifurcation, generally slightly inferior to the umbilicus. The aorta may be traced proximally into the upper abdomen, where it is concealed beneath the pancreas and transverse colon. A normal aorta is seldom over an inch in diameter. Careful palpation can usually distinguish the lateral walls of the aorta and hence provide an estimate of the width. Finding a pulsating mass greater than an inch in diameter usually establishes the diagnosis of aneurysm.

Confusion may arise in thin females with diastasis of the rectus muscles in whom the aortic pulsations are abnormally prominent. This is particularly true if an increased pulse pressure is present. Such patients may come to the physician because of concern over the prominent pulsations, and vague tenderness may be elicited in palpating the aorta. Formerly the unwary surgeon was led to perform a laparotomy on such patients because of the prominent pulse. Almost always careful palpation will demonstrate that the aorta is of normal diameter. When palpation is uncertain, an echogram or an aortogram may be required to exclude the presence of a small aneurysm. In the majority of patients palpation either establishes or excludes the diagnosis; confirmation by laboratory studies is often superfluous.

During the physical examination, peripheral pulses should be carefully examined, for associated occlusive vascular disease may be present. The presence of a bruit over the bifurcation of the carotid arteries is particularly

Fig. 21-27. X-ray films of the abdomen with the gastrointestinal tract opacified often reveal the calcific rim of abdominal aortic aneurysms quite clearly. The lateral film is most helpful since the thin shadow of the calcification is separated from the shadows of the spinal column. *A.* Anteroposterior view. *B.* Lateral view.

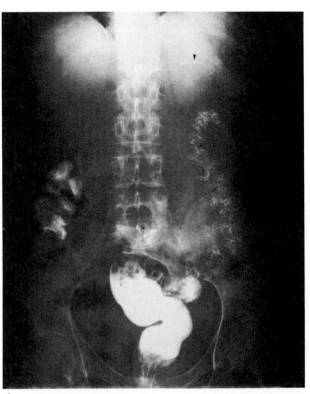

A

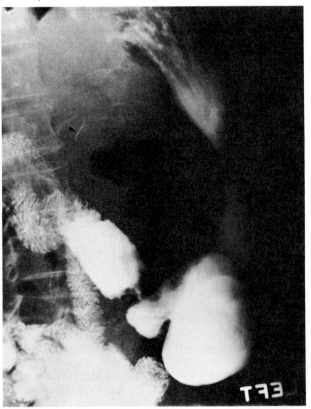

B

significant, because an asymptomatic stenosis of a carotid artery can significantly increase the risk of hypotension occurring during operation.

Laboratory Studies. A roentgenogram of the abdomen, including anteroposterior and lateral views, will establish the diagnosis in many patients by demonstrating calcification in the wall of the aneurysm. The lateral view is particularly helpful, since it permits visualization of the usually thin calcific rim of the aneurysm wall, which may be obscured by the shadows of the vertebral bodies in the frontal projections (Fig. 21-27). An accurate estimate of the size of the aneurysm is obtainable by measuring the distance from the anterior border of the vertebral bodies to the calcium in the anterior wall of the aneurysm and making the appropriate correction for the usual 20 percent magnification produced by the diverging x-rays. The uppermost extent of the aneurysm can be determined from this view. If combined with left lateral views of the chest it permits recognition of upper abdominal and thoracoabdominal aneurysms. A rapid-sequence excretory urogram may also be useful in detecting renal involvement. The use of ultrasound and CAT scan (computed axial tomography) also helps to delineate aneurysms, assisting in differentiation from other abdominal masses.

Aortography is now used infrequently by most vascular surgeons because of the small but definite risk it entails and because the diagnosis can usually be established by these other means. In addition, a laminated thrombus within the aneurysm may mask the true size of the lesion. Formerly, it was thought that in order to establish the relationship of the renal arteries to the aneurysm aortography was essential, but accumulated experiences have found renal artery involvement in only about 1 percent of patients. Nevertheless, some highly experienced vascular groups insist upon performing angiographic studies on all abdominal aortic aneurysm patients to delineate associated vascular lesions. It has not been shown that this has resulted in either increased survival or decreased morbidity.

Our own preference is to perform aortography only for specific indications, avoiding it in the majority of patients. These indications include uncertainty of diagnosis in the presence of small aneurysms (Fig. 21-28), the suspicion of an extensive lesion involving the upper abdominal and thoracic aorta as well, and the presence of lower extremity arterial occlusions manifested by absent pulses. Markedly depressed renal function, or controlled hypertension, though somewhat increasing the risk of aortography, are additional indications for this diagnostic procedure.

TREATMENT. Indications for Operation. Aneurysms smaller than 5 cm in diameter can be relatively safely observed unless they expand or become symptomatic. An asymptomatic aneurysm, measuring at least 5 to 6 cm in diameter, constitutes an indication for operation unless there are other conditions which either markedly increase the operative risk or promise to markedly shorten life expectancy. Asymptomatic aneurysms smaller than 5 to 6 cm are usually considered to carry a very small risk of rupture, while those 5 to 6 cm and larger carry at least a 20 percent yearly risk of rupture. There is very little correla-

tion between the size of the asymptomatic aneurysms beyond 5 to 6 cm, the absence of symptoms, and the tendency to rupture. Operative mortality with a ruptured aneurysm is nearly ten times greater than that for elective excision.

On the other hand, when the aneurysm becomes painful, operation ceases to be elective, for pain often denotes either rupture or impending rupture. The pain may be located in the back, the flank, or the abdominal region and may vary in both intensity and character, simulating many other intraabdominal and musculoskeletal conditions. Abdominal tenderness should increase the suspicion of impending or frank rupture. In such situations the indications for operation are extended to include conditions which might otherwise preclude an elective operation.

Preoperative evaluation should include, in addition to the studies already mentioned, an electrocardiogram, renal clearance studies, coagulation studies including platelet counts and, if indicated, platelet function studies. If carotid bruits are heard, cerebral angiograms may be indicated, and severe carotid stenotic lesions may have to be corrected first. If severe angina pectoris is present, coronary angiograms may be indicated, and coronary arterial surgery may be necessary as the initial procedure.

Technique of Operation for Abdominal Aneurysms. The operative procedure for excision of abdominal aneurysms is illustrated in Fig. 21-29. Separate from the obvious risk of hemorrhage, avoidable with careful technique, there are several common hazards. These include infection, renal failure, declamping shock, peripheral embolization, and ischemic necrosis of the colon. Infection of a plastic prosthesis is an ever-present and serious complication. It may be prevented by meticulous aseptic technique and by the administration of large doses of antibiotics, preoperatively, during the operation, and for about 5 days postoperatively. Renal insufficiency has virtually been eliminated (except in the presence of ruptured aneurysm) by careful attention to renal function during the entire operative procedure, especially during the phase of aortic clamping. Normal quarter-hourly urine output is achieved by carefully maintaining normal cardiodynamics and state of hydration, replacing lost blood promptly, and administering electrolyte solutions to compensate for the known fluid shifts which occur intraoperatively. Diuretics are not administered routinely but only to evaluate the function of the kidneys if anuria is encountered, or to expand circulating volume rapidly. An intrapulmonary catheter of the Swan-Ganz type is an invaluable aid to determine normal cardiodynamics and states of hydration.

Declamping hypotension varies with several factors, such as duration of aortic occlusion, adequacy of blood volume, and degree of collateral circulation to the lower extremities. While the aorta is occluded, the lower extremities are relatively ischemic as a result of which there is pooling of blood in dilated vessels and accumulation of ischemic products of metabolism. If the aorta is unclamped suddenly when ischemia has been severe, profound hypotension, cardiac arrhythmias, and even cardiac arrest can occur. Such problems can be almost completely avoided by different techniques. Hypotension is uncommon if the

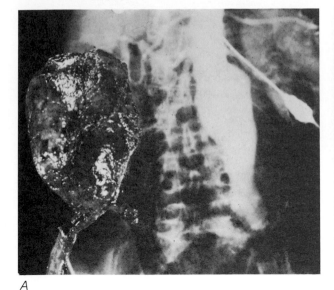

A

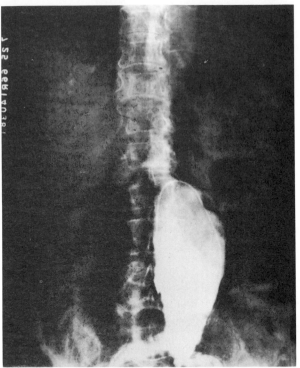

B

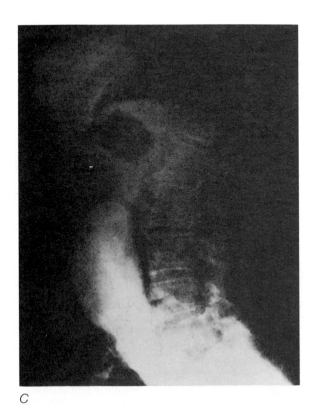

C

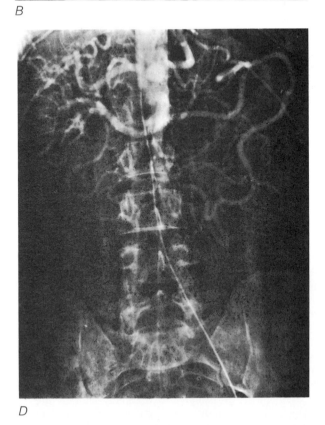

D

aorta is occluded for less than 1 hour. With longer periods gradual restoration of the circulation is useful. An effective approach has been as follows: Once the proximal aortic anastomosis and one iliac anastomosis have been completed, flow is restored to that hypogastric artery, permitting gradual reopening of the circulation. When adjustment has occurred, the ipsilateral iliac artery is similarly unclamped while anastomoses are performed on the contralateral side, and the same sequence is repeated. In a series of 202 aortic operations reported by Imparato et al., declamping shock did not occur with this technique, vasopressors were not needed, and sodium bicarbonate was not required.

Distal embolization of atherosclerotic or thrombotic debris can be particularly hazardous, varying with the friability of the contents of the aneurysm. The following guidelines have been useful: The external and internal iliac arteries are mobilized and occluded before the aorta is clamped proximally. At this time 10 to 20 mg heparin is injected into the distal iliac vessels, or 50 mg heparin is given intravenously. Subsequently, as the individual iliac anastomoses are completed, retrograde flushing of the iliac arteries is allowed to occur. If this cannot be accomplished, a rubber catheter is passed into the external iliac arteries in order gently to pry apart the walls which may have been deformed by application of arterial clamps. Fogarty catheters are not routinely passed into the distal arteries because if aneurysmal disease is present in the femoral and popliteal arteries or if there is atherosclerosis, a thrombus or plaque may be dislodged. The selective iliac "flush" technique described above has been very effective. Finally, at the conclusion of the operation, the peripheral pulses are examined to be certain that they are the same as before operation.

Ischemic injury of the colon can be avoided by dissecting within the wall of the aneurysm rather than outside it and ligating the inferior mesenteric artery at its origin, carefully avoiding injury to any collateral vessels in the mesentery of the left colon. The technique of removing only the inner portion of the aneurysm, leaving the adventitial sheath, facilitates dissection, avoids injury to adjacent structures such as the vena cava, and provides a soft tissue covering of the prosthesis to prevent erosion of the duodenum or other structures subsequently. As the inferior mesenteric artery has been ligated, at least one hypogastric artery must be preserved to maintain collateral circulation to the colon through the middle hemorrhoidal arteries. If one or both

hypogastric arteries have been ligated, either transplanting to the aortic prosthesis a button of aneurysm wall containing the inferior mesenteric artery or bypassing from the prosthesis to the inferior mesenteric artery should be performed. With these guidelines, significant ischemic injury of the colon is very rare, occurring probably only when atherosclerosis has compromised the collateral circulation. If ischemic injury is suspected, however, then a "second-look" laparotomy procedure is indicated to detect irreversible colon ischemia before bowel perforation and peritonitis occur.

An alternative technique to abdominal aortic aneurysm operation has been a retroperitoneal approach which avoids manipulation of the abdominal viscera. Postoperative recovery is said to be smoother by avoiding the problems of prolonged intestinal atony.

Postoperative Complications. The operative mortality for excision of an abdominal aneurysm is now 5 to 10 percent, varying with the age of the patient and the degree of associated atherosclerosis. Paralytic ileus for 2 to 4 days following operation is the most frequent complication. It is best treated by gastric decompression through a nasogastric tube until bowel function returns. Antibiotic therapy, usually with large amounts of penicillin or methicillin, is begun during operation and continued for 4 to 6 days. In uncomplicated aneurysms, convalescence is usually uneventful once postoperative ileus has subsided.

Following operation particular attention should be given to pedal pulses which were palpable before operation. Absence of a pedal pulse is usually an indication for prompt reoperation, for this is commonly due to embolization of atherosclerotic or thrombotic material during removal of the aneurysm. Renal insufficiency is now infrequent following uncomplicated operations. An unusual but often lethal cause of renal insufficiency is embolic occlusion and infarction of the kidneys from atherosclerotic material dislodged during manipulation of the proximal aorta during operation.

PROGNOSIS. The reported 5-year survival following resection of an abdominal aneurysm has varied from 30 to 60 percent. Fatalities are usually due to cardiac or cerebral complications of atherosclerosis. Complications from the prosthetic graft are unusual. The most frequent of these is development of a false aneurysm, often at the proximal suture line, with subsequent rupture or erosion into the duodenum. This can be minimized by limiting dissection of the proximal aorta at the time that the aneurysm is resected, covering the graft with the adventitia of the aneurysm, and subsequently carefully separating the prosthetic graft from the intestine.

Ruptured Abdominal Aneurysm

CLINICAL MANIFESTATIONS. A ruptured abdominal aneurysm constitutes a grave surgical emergency, for irreversible renal injury develops with great rapidity. The onset is characterized by acute vascular collapse, usually with abdominal or flank pain. With severe collapse, the diagnosis initially may be uncertain, because a stuporous or comatose patient cannot describe pain. Until a pul-

Fig. 21-28. *A*. Aortogram showing abdominal aneurysm in the distal aorta. Superimposed on the film is a photograph of a lesion excised at operation, indicating the large laminated clot filling the aneurysm. (*Courtesy of Dr. Henry T. Bahnson, Department of Surgery, University of Pittsburgh.*) *B*. Anteroposterior lumbar aortogram performed by percutaneous introduction of an arterial catheter, illustrating a large abdominal aneurysm arising in the lower abdominal aorta. Linear calcification of the lower thoracic and upper abdominal aorta is also visible. *C*. Lateral view in same patient. *D*. Abdominal aortogram in a patient with atherosclerotic occlusion of the abdominal aorta which has extended up to the level of the renal arteries. The superior mesenteric artery is visible as well as the right renal artery. Extensive collateral circulation has developed, particularly in the left flank.

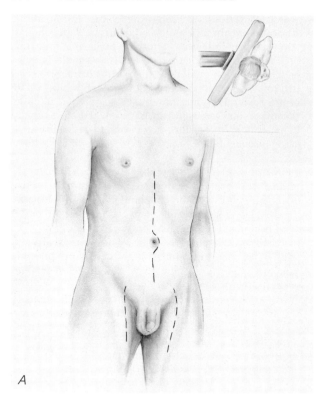

A

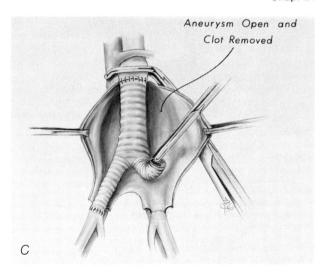

Aneurysm Open and
Clot Removed

C

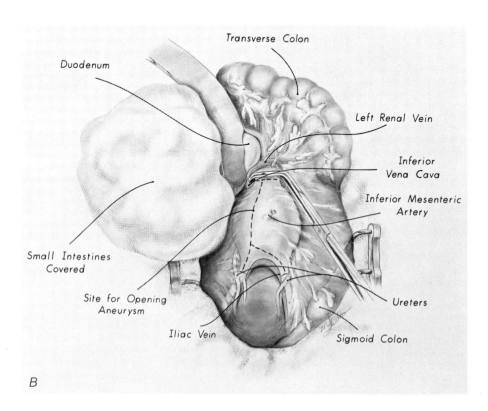

Transverse Colon

Duodenum

Left Renal Vein

Inferior
Vena Cava

Inferior Mesenteric
Artery

Small Intestines
Covered

Site for Opening
Aneurysm

Ureters

Iliac Vein

Sigmoid Colon

B

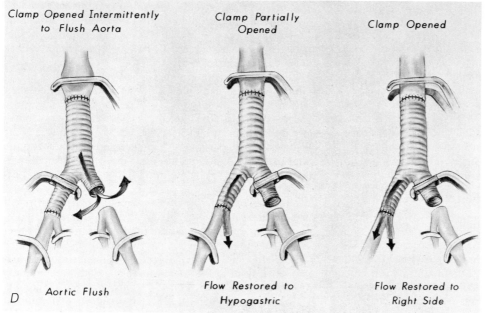

Clamp Opened Intermittently
to Flush Aorta

Clamp Partially
Opened

Clamp Opened

D   Aortic Flush

Flow Restored to
Hypogastric

Flow Restored to
Right Side

Fig. 21-29. Procedure for substituting aortoiliac bifurcation prosthesis for abdominal aortic aneurysm. *A.* A midline incision extending from xiphoid process to pubis symphysis is usually employed. Insert shows rotation of the table to the patient's right
side, which facilitates retraction of the small bowel. *B.* Surgical
exposure of vital structures and lines of incision of the aneurysm
are shown. *C.* Endarterectomy of the aneurysm wall is performed;
the lumbar arteries transfixed with sutures and the prosthesis in
place are shown. *D.* Technique for preventing embolization of
atherosclerotic debris to the lower extremities and gradually
restoring lower extremity circulation to avoid declamping shock.
(1) Aorta is flushed through one open limb of the prosthesis. (2)
Flow gradually restored to one hypogastric artery and, when the
blood pressure has been stabilized, to the ipsilateral external iliac
artery. (3) The sequence is repeated on the opposite side. *E.*
The remains of the aneurysm wall and the base of the left colon
mesentery are carefully sutured over the prosthesis and suture
lines to prevent adherence of the bowel and to bolster the suture
lines to prevent aorticointestinal fistulas. (*From A. M. Imparato et
al., Avoidance of Shock and Peripheral Embolism during Surgery
of the Abdominal Aorta, Surgery, 73(1):68, 1973.*)

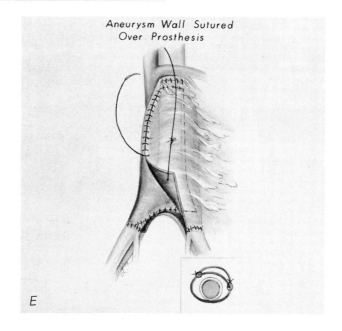

Aneurysm Wall Sutured
Over Prosthesis

E

sating mass is palpated, a frequent erroneous diagnosis is
renal colic from a ureteral stone or massive myocardial or
pulmonary infarction. The diagnosis usually can be established by careful, deep palpation of the abdomen, which
should outline a pulsating, ill-defined mass in the epigastrium or flank.

TREATMENT. Operation should be performed as quickly
as possible, infusing 500 to 1000 ml of fluid every few
minutes until serious hypotension has been corrected. A
midline incision is preferred. Proximal control of the aorta
generally can be obtained by isolating the aorta above the
stomach just below the diaphragm. This should be done
initially, because once the posterior peritoneum is incised
and the hematoma surrounding the ruptured aneurysm is
evacuated, massive hemorrhage can occur with exsanguination. The aorta can be safely clamped below the diaphragm for 20 to 30 minutes without serious ischemic
injury to the intestines or liver. Once it has been clamped,

the ruptured aneurysm can be widely incised, intraabdominal clots evacuated, and the proximal aorta below the renal
arteries isolated, after which a clamp can be applied to
the infrarenal aorta and the previously applied clamp
below the diaphragm released. Reconstruction is then similar to that with elective excision of an abdominal aneurysm, although excision of the wall of the aneurysm should
be limited because of the serious condition of the patient.
On occasion, the infradiaphragmatic portion of the aorta
cannot be clamped, because of either the massive amount
of retroperitoneal hematoma or free rupture into the peritoneal cavity. In this case, left thoracotomy is required to
achieve control. Consequently, in preparing the patient for

emergency operation for abdominal aneurysm, the chest as well as the abdomen must be made surgically accessible. Unfortunately, despite successful removal of the aneurysm, death results from renal insufficiency in 30 to 50 percent of patients.

The value of prompt excision of ruptured abdominal aneurysms is reflected by high survival rates if operation is performed within 1 to 2 hours of rupture. If operation is performed 8 to 10 hours after rupture, there is a very high fatality rate from renal insufficiency. The unheralded rupture of asymptomatic aneurysms, with resulting high fatality rates, is the most urgent reason for recommending routine excision of abdominal aneurysms as soon as the diagnosis is made.

PERIPHERAL ANEURYSMS

Aneurysms outside the major body cavities, the skull, thorax, and abdomen, are rare. If traumatic and congenital malformations, considered in different chapters, are excluded, almost all such aneurysms result from arteriosclerosis, for syphilitic aneurysms now are seldom seen. Similarly, mycotic aneurysms associated with bacterial

Fig. 21-30. Femoral angiogram indicating the presence of a popliteal aneurysm. Characteristic tortuosity of the involved artery is present. Such tortuosity often makes it possible to establish continuity by direct anastomosis following excision of the aneurysm.

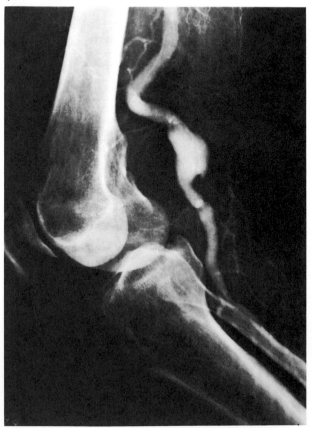

endocarditis are infrequent with present methods of antibiotic therapy. The majority of peripheral arteriosclerotic aneurysms are in the popliteal artery. Infrequent sites include the femoral, carotid, or subclavian arteries. Each of these is considered separately.

The aneurysms in different locations are similar in that they usually occur in men in the fifth to seventh decades, often with hypertension and signs of atherosclerosis in other organs. Multiple aneurysms are frequent. In contrast to abdominal or thoracic aneurysms, where rupture is the greatest threat, peripheral aneurysms infrequently rupture but cause disability due to distal embolization or thrombosis with subsequent ischemia and gangrene of the extremity.

Because of their superficial location, peripheral aneurysms are readily amenable to successful therapy if operated upon electively before embolization and acute ischemia develop in the extremity. Tortuosity of the involved artery often makes it possible to mobilize the artery proximal and distal to the aneurysm and reestablish continuity following excision by end-to-end anastomosis. Continuity also can be established with a short graft, preferably of the saphenous vein. If this is not possible, a knitted Dacron prosthesis is preferred. In 1966 Howell and associates stated that over 400 such aneurysms had been treated at Baylor University during the previous 14 years with serious complications in only 3 percent of the patients. In patients with a distal pulse before operation, distal circulation was restored in all but one.

Popliteal Aneurysms

Almost all popliteal aneurysms originate from arteriosclerosis, usually in men in the sixth or seventh decade. As with other peripheral arteriosclerotic aneurysms, complications of arteriosclerosis in other organs are frequent. Bilateral popliteal aneurysms occur in at least 25 percent of patients. Aneurysms at other sites such as the abdominal aorta also are common. Hypertension is present in 40 to 50 percent of patients.

The aneurysms are often small, 3 by 4 cm, and asymptomatic. Nonetheless they pursue a malignant course of peripheral embolization with subsequent gangrene of the extremity. The marked tendency to progress rapidly to embolization and gangrene may be related to intermittent compression of the aneurysm by flexion of the knee. In one group of 29 aneurysms reported by Hara and Thompson, 18 progressed to acute ischemic occlusion despite their small size and lack of symptoms preceding acute vascular occlusion. In an extensive study of 100 popliteal aneurysms, Gifford et al. found that only about 20 percent remained free of symptoms within 5 years following diagnosis. In some patients, the tendency for silent aneurysms to embolize is demonstrated by the unheralded development of acute ischemic symptoms from occlusion of the popliteal artery; on subsequent physical examination the aneurysm is discovered.

CLINICAL MANIFESTATIONS. The clinical findings in most patients are characteristic enough to permit an accurate diagnosis. Some patients are unaware of the aneurysm, while others note a vigorous pulse behind the knee joint in a small mass which is otherwise asymptomatic. Rarely, the aneurysm may enlarge sufficiently to cause local pain and tenderness. Actual rupture is unusual.

A pulsating mass is usually found. If the aneurysm is thrombosed, pulsation may be absent, and a mass may or may not be felt. Differential diagnosis must include other cystic tumors about the knee joint, such as Baker's cyst, as well as other causes of tibial arterial occlusion, such as emboli, Buerger's disease, and diabetes mellitus. The presence or absence of pedal pulses should be carefully noted.

Calcification in the wall of the aneurysm is often visible on a roentgenogram. The diagnosis can be confirmed by arteriography, although much of the cavity of the aneurysm may be filled with thrombus (Fig. 21-30).

When a patient is seen with symptoms of acute ischemia in an extremity, such as pain, paralysis, or discoloration, the presence of pedal pulses is of particular importance, because the ischemic symptoms usually result from embolization of thrombotic material from the aneurysm distad into the posterior and anterior tibial arteries.

TREATMENT. Because of the hazard of thrombosis, embolization, and gangrene, operation should be performed as soon as possible after the diagnosis is made even though the aneurysm is small, asymptomatic, and seemingly stable. A retrospective study of gangrene and amputation from popliteal aneurysms which have embolized found no warning signs that such a catastrophe was imminent.

Operative Technique. With the patient in a prone position, an incision across the popliteal crease readily exposes the artery proximal and distal to the aneurysm. An alternative exposure, particularly useful when the femoral artery needs to be exposed for some distance from the popliteal, has been described by Imparato and Kim. An incision is made on the medial aspect of the lower thigh and extended across the knee joint into the upper calf, transecting the muscles inserting into the upper medial tibial plateau as well as the head of the gastrocnemius tendon. Transection of these muscles provides unusually wide exposure and has not resulted in any late impairment of function of the extremity.

Once the artery has been isolated distal to the aneurysm, vascular clamps are applied and the aneurysm widely opened. Any laminated thrombus is removed, as well as the inner lining of the wall of the aneurysm, preserving the adventitial sheath. The origins of the geniculate branches of the popliteal artery are sutured from within the lumen. This technique preserves branches of the popliteal vein which are usually stretched over the wall of the aneurysm, and also the collateral circulation is less disturbed. A small amount of heparin should be given either systemically or into the distal artery at the time that the clamps are applied.

If the aneurysm is small and the popliteal artery tortuous, an end-to-end anastomosis is sometimes possible. Most patients, however, require a short graft, preferably a reversed autologous saphenous vein (Fig. 21-31). Short grafts of knitted Dacron also have been satisfactory. As the anastomoses are completed, the distal popliteal artery

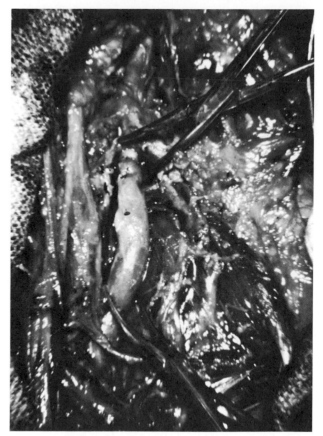

Fig. 21-31. Operative photograph of saphenous vein graft used to restore continuity of the popliteal artery following excision of a popliteal aneurysm. Long-term results of saphenous vein grafts following excision of such aneurysms have been excellent. At present, since most aneurysms of the popliteal artery are small, excision is no longer required and bypass with exclusion is practiced most often.

is cleared with a Fogarty balloon catheter to remove any laminated thrombus.

In a series of 48 popliteal aneurysms reported by Crichlow and Roberts, a vein graft was used in 21 and a Teflon graft in 14. The 21 saphenous vein grafts remained free of complications. Similar experiences were described by Hunter et al. for 27 patients with a total of 31 aneurysms.

Acute Ischemia. When operation is required because thrombosis has produced severe ischemia with impending gangrene, a different approach is needed. Simple excision of the aneurysm, of course, is futile with the obstructed distal circulation. The major consideration is removal of these distal thrombi followed by restoration of arterial continuity across the occluded aneurysm as in elective procedures. Operative incision and exposure should be planned to permit precise cannulation of the anterior and posterior tibial arteries with balloon-tipped catheters to remove propagated thrombus. Retrograde flushing with saline solution from the posterior and anterior tibial arteries is far less satisfactory than the Fogarty catheter technique. Operative angiography should be available to be certain that all thrombi have been removed. In some patients the distal thrombi have become adherent to the arterial wall and require repeated efforts for removal. If thrombi are not completely removed, as confirmed by angiography, rethrombosis terminating in gangrene and amputation is almost a certainty (Fig. 21-32).

Femoral Aneurysms

INCIDENCE AND PATHOLOGY. Femoral aneurysms are virtually all due to arteriosclerosis, with frequent signs of

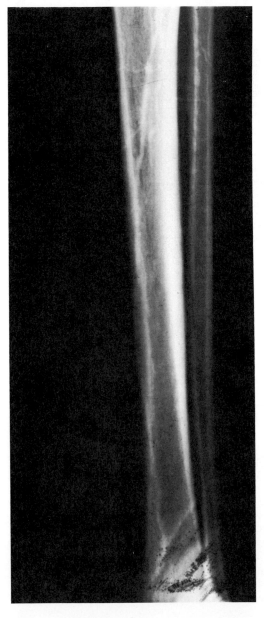

Fig. 21-32. Angiographic study of tibial arteries after surgical repair of popliteal aneurysm showing persistent thrombi in the tibial arteries subsequently removed with Fogarty catheters. Such thrombi almost inevitably lead to occlusion of the tibial arterial outflow tract and may involve the arterial reconstruction itself.

atherosclerosis in other organs. In one series of 89 patients with 115 aneurysms, 86 of the 89 were men with an average age of sixty-four years. In this large series, 36 percent of the aneurysms were bilateral. At least one other aneurysm was present besides a single femoral aneurysm in 69 percent of the patients. Twenty-eight percent of the group had abdominal aneurysms, and 54 percent had hypertension.

In the femoral artery, the aneurysm was limited to the common femoral in 27 percent and to the superficial femoral in 26 percent, and involved both areas in the remainder. In only 1 percent of the entire group was the aneurysm limited to the profunda femoris artery.

As with popliteal aneurysms, the usual course is that of thrombosis, embolization, and ischemia. Rupture is rare. Of the two events producing ischemia, thrombosis is more common than embolization, in contrast to the usual course of popliteal aneurysms. This occurred in 26 percent of the 89 patients reported by Papas and associates, while rupture occurred only five times. Similar experiences were reported in a smaller series of 12 patients by Tolstedt et al. Eight of the twelve thrombosed, resulting in amputation in each patient.

CLINICAL MANIFESTATIONS. Symptoms usually consist of an awareness of a pulsating mass in the upper thigh until thrombosis or embolization produces ischemic symptoms in the extremity. The diagnosis can often be easily made on physical examination, outlining the pulsating mass in the femoral artery. A roentgenogram may show calcification in the wall of the aneurysm. Arteriography is useful to delineate the relationship of the aneurysm to the profunda femoris artery, as well as to define the patency of the distal circulation.

TREATMENT. Surgical correction should be performed promptly, unless coexisting cerebral or coronary artery disease makes the risk of operation prohibitive. If operation is postponed because of concomitant disease, such decisions should be made with the full realization that a subsequent amputation because of gangrene may entail an even greater operative risk to the patient.

At operation the arteries can be mobilized proximal and distal to the point of aneurysm and the aneurysm excised. Vascular continuity may be restored with either a saphenous vein graft or an 8- or 10-mm knitted Dacron prosthesis. Patency of the profunda femoris artery should be maintained by using a Y-bifurcation graft if necessary. Complications following operation are unusual unless peripheral arterial occlusion has already produced severe ischemic signs. In most patients following operation the prognosis is determined by the coexisting atherosclerotic disease, rather than the femoral aneurysm.

Carotid Artery Aneurysms

INCIDENCE AND PATHOLOGY. The infrequent occurrence of carotid aneurysms has been documented by several reports. Reid found only 12 cases in a 30-year survey at the Johns Hopkins Hospital ending in 1922. At the University of Pennsylvania in a 20-year period ending in 1947, five cases were encountered. Raphael and associates reported six patients seen at the Mayo Clinic in a 25-year period, and Beall et al. in 1962 stated that seven carotid aneurysms had been seen at Baylor University over a period of time during which 2,300 operations for aneurysms had been performed.

Most carotid aneurysms result from arteriosclerosis. As in other arteries, syphilis once was the most common cause but is now rare. Unusual causes include trauma, bacterial infection, or cystic medial necrosis. The most frequent location is in the common carotid artery near its bifurcation into the internal and external carotid arteries. Less frequently aneurysms are localized to the internal carotid. The main hazard from an aneurysm is embolization of thrombotic material into the cerebral circulation with production of cerebral infarcts. Infrequently such aneurysms may enlarge and rupture, but treatment is usually undertaken before this has occurred.

CLINICAL MANIFESTATIONS. Patients are usually seen because of a mass in the neck. Pulsations are often prominent and provide an easy clue to the diagnosis. A more difficult problem arises if pulsations are absent, because of laminated thrombus occupying most of the cavity of the aneurysm. Arteriography is the most definitive laboratory technique, establishing the diagnosis and also defining the relationship of the common and internal carotid arteries to the aneurysm (Fig. 21-33). The differential diagnosis should include prominent pulsations from buckling of the carotid artery, a condition seen in hypertensive women, and other solid tumors of the neck, such as a lymph node or a carotid body tumor.

TREATMENT. Because of the constant risk from cerebral infarction, the aneurysm should be excised as soon as possible. The major consideration in planning operation is protection of the brain from ischemic injury while the carotid artery is occluded during excision. In a review of reported experiences by Raphael and associates, 12 patients were described in whom the aneurysm was excised without any protection of the brain from ischemia. Six of the twelve had a transient neurologic injury, while four developed a permanent neurologic deficit.

The safest surgical technique is excision of the aneurysm under local or regional block anesthesia, keeping the patient awake to assess constantly the tolerance of the brain for temporary occlusion of the carotid artery. If ischemic symptoms develop, an internal shunt may be utilized to maintain cerebral blood flow. Even with a large aneurysm, regional block anesthesia is adequate.

The limited surgical experiences with carotid aneurysms was indicated by the report by Kianouri in 1967, who found a total of 28 patients in whom the aneurysm had been excised and arterial continuity reestablished. The first such report of successful excision of a carotid aneurysm, followed by end-to-end anastomosis, was published by Shea in 1955. Experiences at present indicate that in over one-half of the patients there is sufficient tortuosity and elongation of the carotid artery proximal and distal to the site of involvement of the aneurysm to permit mobilization of the ends of the carotid artery and direct anastomosis (Fig. 21-34). Following excision of the aneurysm with reconstruction of the carotid artery, convalescence has usually been uncomplicated, and long-term results are excellent.

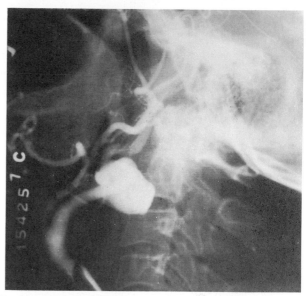

Fig. 21-33. Carotid arteriogram illustrating saccular aneurysm of the internal carotid artery. The internal carotid proximal and distal to the aneurysm is opacified.

Subclavian Aneurysms

The majority of subclavian aneurysms develop as secondary complications of a cervical rib and are discussed in the section on Thoracic Outlet Syndromes. The extremely rare subclavian aneurysm which results from atherosclerosis is similar to other peripheral atherosclerotic aneurysms, occurring in older men, often with atherosclerotic aneurysms elsewhere. The diagnosis is usually readily made from physical examination. The most important differential diagnosis is from the frequently seen tortuosity of the innominate and subclavian arteries which occurs in hypertensive patients. Careful examination of the bulge will differentiate a true aneurysm from a tortuous vessel. If aneurysm cannot be excluded, an arteriogram should be done. Excision with reconstruction of the involved artery can be easily performed.

Visceral Aneurysms

SPLENIC ARTERY ANEURYSMS

Significant aneurysms of the splenic artery are uncommon. Because of their rarity and unusual manifestations, several detailed reviews have been published. In 1953 Owens and Coffey reported six patients and found a total of 198 cases in previous reports. Of historical interest is the fact that President Garfield in 1881 died from a traumatic aneurysm of the splenic artery 2 months after being shot by an assassin.

INCIDENCE AND PATHOLOGY. A report of unusual interest is that of Bedford and Lodge in 1960 who published findings from 250 consecutive postmortem examinations in older patients. Routine dissection of the splenic artery

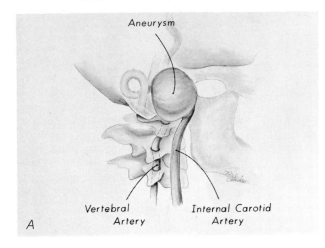

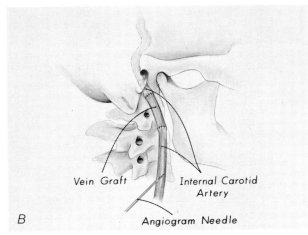

Fig. 21-34. Carotid aneurysmectomy is possible even when the internal carotid artery is involved in its upper extracranial portion, since the artery can be exposed through lateral neck incisions to the base of the skull. *A.* Internal carotid aneurysm. *B.* Replacement with vein graft. *(From G. M. Sanoudos et al., Internal Carotid Aneurysm, Am Surg, 39:118, 1973.)*

found 26 aneurysms, an incidence of nearly 10 percent. All had been asymptomatic. Their size was small, ranging from a few millimeters to as large as 2.5 cm; most were near 1 cm in diameter. In the 204 cases reviewed by Owens and Coffey, the average diameter was 3 cm. This great discrepancy between the high autopsy incidence and the rarity of clinically symptomatic aneurysms indicates that small aneurysms are probably of no clinical significance and are usually overlooked.

These aneurysms, like other atherosclerotic aneurysms, occur in older patients with an average age near fifty. Atherosclerosis is present in the splenic artery in over 95 percent of patients. Surprisingly, though, the aneurysms are more frequent in women, in contrast to the overwhelming predominance of the usual atherosclerotic aneurysm in men. In the Owens and Coffey series, 127 patients were women and 63 were men. Bedford and Lodge noted that the aneurysms tended to develop at bifurcations of the splenic artery and suggested that degeneration of the

media as well as atherosclerosis might be a predisposing factor.

The aneurysms are usually single and in the main trunk of the splenic artery. Rupture is more likely to occur during pregnancy. The actual risk of rupture is uncertain, for many are recognized only after rupture. Rupture is obviously a grave event, for of 131 symptomatic patients reported by Owens and Coffey 94 died from rupture and only 7 from other causes. In 37 female patients, rupture occurred during late pregnancy.

CLINICAL MANIFESTATIONS. Pain in the epigastrium or left flank is the most frequent symptom, occurring in 93 of 131 symptomatic patients in the Owens series. Other symptoms are nonspecific gastrointestinal symptoms, usually interpreted as due to peptic ulcer. These include nausea, vomiting, dyspepsia, and constipation or diarrhea. Gastrointestinal hemorrhage has occurred in about one-third of patients. For unknown reasons gastrointestinal symptoms may exist for months or years before the diagnosis is made. Perhaps this is fortuitous.

In one patient treated by one of the authors several years ago, acute gastrointestinal bleeding led to the erroneous performance of a subtotal gastrectomy a few days earlier, though an ill-defined mass suggesting an aneurysm was noted. When bleeding returned several days later, reoperation was performed. Recovery eventually ensued after a long and difficult convalescence.

Often rupture is the first sign of the aneurysm, in 46 percent of the patients in one series. A "double" rupture is a significant clinical sequence, recognized in about one-half of patients. The first rupture is hemorrhage into the lesser omental sac; this ceases temporarily but is followed in 1 to 2 days by secondary hemorrhage and exsanguination.

With the small size of the splenic aneurysms, physical abnormalities are usually not found. For unknown reasons, moderate splenomegaly has been reported in 40 to 50 percent of patients. However, a mass has been palpated in only 20 percent, and pulsations or a bruit in 10 percent. Roentgenographic identification of a mass with calcium in the walls suggestive of an aneurysm has been reported in 15 percent of the group.

TREATMENT. Obviously symptomatic aneurysms should be excised as soon as the diagnosis is made, usually with concomitant splenectomy. The widespread use of aortography for investigating many abdominal conditions has disclosed aneurysms smaller than 1 cm which are asymptomatic. Their treatment is uncertain because of the rarity of rupture. On the other hand, it is disquieting to note that rupture without preceding symptoms is the first event in one-half of the patients with splenic aneurysms. From data available, surgical treatment does not seem indicated for asymptomatic aneurysms smaller than 1 cm, but those greater than 3 cm should be excised. Further data are needed to be certain of these guidelines.

RENAL ARTERY ANEURYSMS

INCIDENCE AND PATHOLOGY. Aneurysms of the renal artery are similar to aneurysms of the splenic artery in that recognition has greatly increased with the use of vascular angiography. A collective review in 1957 by Garritano found only 180 patients. Nine years later, Cerny et al. found a total of 345 reported cases and described 25 patients from the University of Michigan alone. In discussing this report, Smith described 17 aneurysms at the Henry Ford Hospital, and Morris described operative experience with 58 patients at Baylor Medical Center. The widespread use of renal angiography to investigate patients with hypertension has been chiefly responsible for the increasing recognition of renal aneurysms. Apparently, about 1 percent of hypertensive patients will be found on angiography to have a small aneurysm of one renal artery.

These aneurysms are equally common in males and females, usually in the fifth and sixth decades, but they have been found in all age groups, even in patients as young as nine months. Anatomically they may be saccular or fusiform. Unusual varieties include a false aneurysm from trauma, a dissecting aneurysm, or an arteriovenous fistula. The saccular aneurysm is apparently congenital, arising from a defect in elastic tissue of the wall of the artery, often near a bifurcation. It varies from 1 to 3 cm in size and often develops extensive eccentric calcification, a so-called "signet ring" on the roentgenogram. It is infrequently associated with hypertension and rarely ruptures. The fusiform aneurysm develops distal to an area of constriction of the renal artery and is basically a poststenotic aneurysm similar to that seen in other parts of the arterial circulation. Because of the proximal stenosis, it is frequently seen with hypertension.

The aneurysms occur with equal frequency in either renal artery, usually in the main renal artery or one of its branches. An intrarenal location is uncommon. In one report, 92 aneurysms were in the main renal artery, 44 were in an extrarenal branch, and 15 were intrarenal.

Rupture has been reported in at least 24 patients with

Fig. 21-35. Renal artery aneurysms are frequently saccular, as shown in the angiographic study, and may be associated with arterial hypertension.

a fatal outcome in 20. Eight of these episodes occurred during pregnancy. Rupture has been recognized only three times in a calcified aneurysm.

CLINICAL MANIFESTATIONS. Abdominal or flank pain has occurred in about 50 percent of the patients but is probably unrelated to the aneurysm. Investigation of the symptom subsequently led to finding the aneurysm. Hematuria, gross or microscopic, has also been reported in 30 to 40 percent of patients. As expected, hypertension has been frequently seen with poststenotic aneurysms and has been improved or cured in over one-half of these after operation. By contrast, hypertension in one series was present in only 7 of 12 with a saccular aneurysm and improved after operation in only 1 of the 7. A mechanism by which a saccular aneurysm can produce hypertension is not clear except for the rather nebulous possibility of compression or distortion of the renal artery. The association may simply be fortuitous.

There are usually no abnormalities on physical examination. Occasionally a localized bruit is audible. Roentgenographic examination may show signet ring calcification which must be differentiated from calcification of mesenteric lymph nodes or calcification of other visceral arteries. The intravenous pyelogram is abnormal in about one-half of the patients because of ischemia, infarction, or localized pressure defects. Aortography is essential to establish the diagnosis and define the precise location (Fig. 21-35). As mentioned earlier, most aneurysms have been found during aortography performed for other purposes.

TREATMENT. Prompt operation is indicated whenever an aneurysm is found during investigation of a patient for hypertension. With poststenotic aneurysms the aneurysm can be excised and the renal artery reconstructed, with an excellent likelihood of improving the hypertension. With a saccular aneurysm and hypertension, operation is probably indicated to reconstruct the renal artery, although the prognosis for improving the hypertension is less favorable. Of the 25 patients reported by Cerny et al., 20 were oper-

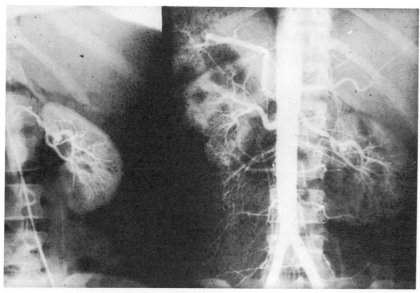

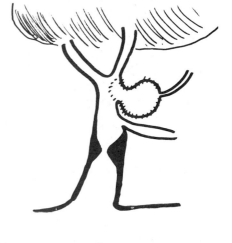

ated upon. Unfortunately 9 required a nephrectomy, but there was no operative mortality. In the 17 patients reported by Smith, 5 had successful operations, while 12 with small aneurysms of questionable significance had been followed for an average of 3 years without complications. Morris stated that reconstructive operations had been performed on 58 patients with renal artery aneurysms, representing about 5 percent of all reconstructive operations upon the renal artery for patients with hypertension. In this group of 58 patients, 8 had previously lost the contralateral kidney, perhaps from complications of an aneurysm in that kidney. The "bench" technique, in which the kidney is removed from its bed by transecting the main arteries and veins and leaving the ureter intact, performing microsurgical arterial repair on branch arteries, and then reattaching the main vessels to the iliac vessels, has permitted removal of branch artery aneurysms without sacrifice of kidneys. In a patient with a small calcified aneurysm without symptoms or hypertension, there probably is little indication for operation, for the risk of rupture is almost negligible. With larger aneurysms, certainly with symptoms present, operation should be performed.

Traumatic Aneurysms

Several milestones in vascular surgery evolved from treatment of traumatic aneurysms produced in military combat. In the second century Antyllus treated an arterial aneurysm by ligature immediately above and below the lesion, followed by incision of the aneurysm, evacuation of the clot, and exteriorization of the cavity. John Hunter, in 1786, electively ligated a femoral artery proximal to a popliteal aneurysm to minimize blood loss during subsequent attempts at extirpation. The anatomic term *Hunter's canal,* referring to the distal third of the superficial femoral artery in the thigh, originated from this surgical episode. In 1888 Rudolf Matas described his operation of endoaneurysmorrhaphy, in which the aneurysm was widely opened and the communications into the artery were sutured. This imaginative approach promptly became the standard treatment and was modified little during the next 55 years; even during World War II it was the operation performed for most traumatic aneurysms. Subsequently, as techniques of vascular reconstruction developed, the policy of restoring arterial continuity became preferred.

ETIOLOGY AND PATHOLOGY. A traumatic aneurysm is produced from a tangential laceration of the wall of an artery. Usually continuity of flow through the lacerated artery is maintained. By contrast, injuries that transect an artery often require immediate treatment because of hemorrhage or ischemia in the affected limb and consequently seldom evolve into an aneurysm.

Following the laceration, blood extravasates into adjacent soft tissues to form a hematoma that compresses and seals the point of injury. If the artery is confined within a small space surrounded by fascia, the hematoma may be small enough to escape recognition. Both the patient and the physician are unaware that an arterial injury has occurred. After days or weeks, the blood clot gradually liquefies; then the firm, immobile mass surrounding the

artery begins to pulsate. A descriptive term for these lesions was "pulsating hematoma." With the appearance of pulsation, the aneurysm begins to enlarge. This is ominous, for enlargement is progressive and relentless, destroying nerves, even eroding bone, and eventually terminating in rupture and death.

Traumatic aneurysms are often termed *false* aneurysms, as distinguished from *true* aneurysms, for the wall is composed of fibrous tissue rather than components of normal arterial wall, as with arteriosclerotic or syphilitic aneurysms.

As the hematoma enlarges in a recent wound, the tissues are firm, tender, perhaps warm. These findings of redness, tenderness, and heat are, of course, the usual characteristics of an abscess. Occasional vivid reports appear in the surgical literature in which an unsuspecting physician widely incised such a red, tender mass to drain an abscess, with resultant violent hemorrhage.

A similar therapeutic catastrophe occasionally occurs when a traumatic aneurysm stabilizes for years and is subsequently confused with a neoplasm. If the previous history of trauma is not available, the differential diagnosis is difficult, for the aneurysm is partly filled with clot and closely resembles a solid tumor. Attempted biopsy of such lesions, with frightening consequences, has been reported.

Usually there is no disability from a traumatic aneurysm except for the local mass until it enlarges to compress adjacent nerves, causing pain, paresthesias, and eventually paralysis. The peripheral arterial circulation is usually normal. Peripheral embolization of thrombi from the aneurysm is unusual except for the rare aneurysm of the subclavian artery following trauma. Here, intermittent compression by the clavicle may dislodge emboli. One of the authors treated such a patient in whom ischemic symptoms in the arm dominated the clinical picture. Arteriography disclosed a small traumatic aneurysm of the subclavian artery which had developed following an automobile accident some months before.

CLINICAL MANIFESTATIONS. A localized mass is often the only finding. As it enlarges, there is pain or paralysis from compression of nerves. On physical examination the borders of the mass are ill defined because the hematoma surrounding the aneurysm is beneath the deep fascia. Pulsations may or may not be present, depending upon the amount of thrombus in the lumen. A systolic bruit is frequently audible. Peripheral pulsations are normal.

If the mass pulsates, the diagnosis is reasonably certain from the physical findings. Otherwise arteriography is required to differentiate it from a neoplasm or a cyst. On arteriography the full size is not disclosed, as much of the cavity is filled with thrombus.

TREATMENT. Operation should be performed as soon as the diagnosis has been established because of the inevitable outcome of enlargement and rupture. If neurologic symptoms are present, operation should be done urgently, within hours, to prevent irreversible pressure injury of crucial nerves. At operation the incision should be placed to permit exposure of the uninvolved artery proximal and distal to the aneurysm. With these vessels temporarily occluded, the aneurysm can be widely incised, clots evacuated, and the point of origin from the artery identified. Dissection around the aneurysm before it is opened should be avoided; it is unnecessary, complicated, and often dangerous.

With unusually large aneurysms, it is important to remember that there is only one small opening in the wall of the aneurysm, the tangential laceration of the arterial wall from which the aneurysm began. Hence, if the aneurysm is inadvertently entered, this small opening can be digitally occluded to control bleeding while further exposure is obtained. This approach was once employed in desperation during emergency treatment of a badly neglected traumatic aneurysm of the proximal subclavian artery which had involved the brachial plexus and compressed the trachea to a near fatal degree.

Once the aneurysm has been opened and the inner contents removed, the site of communication with the parent artery can be mobilized and the injured area excised. Complete excision of the wall of the aneurysm is unnecessary and should be avoided because of the surrounding dense fibrotic reaction. Once the involved artery has been mobilized, arterial continuity can usually be restored by end-to-end anastomosis or by insertion of a short graft, preferably autologous vein. Ligation should be performed only for small arteries, such as the radial, not essential to normal circulation.

PROGNOSIS. Convalescence after operation is usually uneventful and long-term results excellent. Crawford et al. described experiences with a group of 29 patients with aneurysms or arteriovenous fistulas, all of whom were treated by excision and end-to-end anastomosis with a uniformly good result. Hughes and Jahnke similarly reported continuing good results 5 years after surgical treatment of 67 traumatic aneurysms during the Korean conflict.

VASOSPASTIC DISORDERS

Raynaud's Disease

A syndrome of intermittent vasospasm in the upper extremities without permanent vascular obstruction was described by Maurice Raynaud in 1862. The initial description included several disorders which subsequent observation found were not primary Raynaud's disease, but attention was focused on the disorder by this report. The syndrome described by Raynaud, now termed *Raynaud's phenomenon,* consists of recurrent episodes of vasoconstriction in the upper extremities, initiated by exposure to cold or emotional stress. Three sequential phases classically occur: pallor, cyanosis, and rubor. It is now recognized that Raynaud's phenomenon may exist as a primary disorder, termed *Raynaud's disease,* or may be a secondary manifestation of a more serious vascular disease, often not evident for 1 or 2 years after the initial appearance of the recurrent color changes. The more common disorders associated with Raynaud's phenomenon include Buerger's disease (thromboangiitis obliterans), scleroderma, cervical rib or other thoracic outlet syndrome, and atherosclerosis.

It occasionally results from recurrent minor trauma, such as the use of mechanical vibrating tools. Rarely, other collagen diseases, such as periarteritis nodosa or disseminated lupus erythematosus are found. Hence, in the evaluation of a patient the critical decision is to determine whether the disease is primary Raynaud's disease or a secondary manifestation of a more serious disorder. Some suspect that it is always secondary to some other underlying disorder.

ETIOLOGY. The cause of primary Raynaud's disease is unknown. It is much more frequent in women, with a ratio of about 5:1, and appears in over 90 percent of patients before forty years of age. In men, it is usually much less severe in intensity. DeTakats and Fowler observed abnormal electroencephalograms in some patients, suggesting a primary disease in the midbrain, but the existence of a primary neurologic disease has not been established.

PATHOLOGY. The clinical picture of Raynaud's phenomenon is related to the anatomy and physiology of the arteriolar circulation in the dermis. The arterioles penetrate the dermis at right angles with an irregular reticulate pattern and arborize into a capillary network. Some fluctuation in vasomotor tone, as with pallor or blushing, is a normal physiologic variation. In Raynaud's disease, vasospasm occurs with such severity that dermal circulation momentarily ceases, with the production of severe pallor. If the vasospasm is less severe, with slowing but not cessation of the dermal circulation, cyanosis appears, a result of sluggish flow of blood with an increase in the percentage of reduced hemoglobin in the capillaries. When the vasospasm subsides, a reactive hyperemia with vasodilatation develops, probably from the accumulation of tissue metabolites during the anoxic period, producing an unusual redness or rubor.

The basis for the increased tendency of the dermal arterioles to vasoconstriction is unknown. It may be a sensitivity in the arterioles themselves, or possibly may result from hyperactivity of the sympathetic nervous system. Initially the arterioles are normal on histologic examination. With chronic disease, there is progressive hypertrophy of the arteriolar walls and ultimate occlusion. Detailed histologic observation of early phases of Raynaud's disease are not available, because tissue biopsies are seldom performed at this time.

In the majority of patients the episodes of vasoconstriction are precipitated by exposure to cold. In about 25 percent of patients intense emotion, as well as cold, may be the initiating factor. Only rarely is emotion alone the significant stimulus without an abnormal sensitivity to cold.

In most patients the upper extremities are symmetrically involved. Unilateral involvement by Raynaud's phenomenon almost always denotes a proximal mechanical cause, either occlusion of one of the major proximal arteries, recurrent embolization, or neurovascular compression. In 10 to 15 percent of patients the legs are involved as well as the arms. This was found in 51 of 474 patients seen over a period of years at the Mayo Clinic.

With repeated episodes of vasoconstriction and ischemia, trophic changes gradually appear. These include atrophy of the skin with loss of elasticity and hair. The term *sclero-dactylia* has been applied to this appearance, since it resembles the changes found in scleroderma in other organs. However, long-term studies by Gifford et al. have demonstrated conclusively that the presence of sclerodactylia in the fingers does not indicate that generalized scleroderma will appear in the future. Focal areas of ulceration develop and leave characteristic scars with healing. Recurrent superficial infections, such as paronychia, may occur. In the more extreme forms of ischemia, gangrene may require amputation of one or more digits, but fortunately gangrene almost never progresses to involve the hands.

CLINICAL MANIFESTATIONS. The patient is usually a young woman who has noted that episodes of cold precipitate vasoconstriction with a repetitive sequence of pallor, cyanosis, and rubor. Several variations in the color phenomena may occur with less severe disease. For example, there may be only cyanosis followed by rubor or only episodes of mild cyanosis.

In addition to the color changes, the patient may have paresthesias and localized pain in the digits. If infection or ulceration is present, pain is more severe. Except for the discomfort in the hands, the patients usually have no other symptoms.

Physical Examination. In the early phases of the disease, the extremities may be entirely normal with peripheral pulses of equal volume. The best index to the severity of the disease is the extent of trophic changes in the fingers, such as atrophy of the skin and nails with loss of hair over the terminal phalanges. In more advanced disease, signs of chronic ischemia are obvious, with punctate scars from healed ulcerations, chronic rubor, and absence of a radial or ulnar pulse.

Arteriography is of value in establishing the diagnosis by revealing the absence of occlusive arterial disease. The most critical examination is demonstration of the vasoconstrictor response to cold. Induction of the characteristic pallor-cyanosis-rubor sequence in both hands following exposure to cold establishes the diagnosis, although it does not differentiate between primary and secondary Raynaud's phenomenon. An electroencephalogram should be obtained to pursue the observation made by DeTakats that abnormal electroencephalographic tracings are present in some patients.

Once the presence of Raynaud's phenomenon has been confirmed, the principal question is whether the vasomotor changes are primary or secondary to some other vascular disease. The possibility of early scleroderma can be evaluated by study of the motility of the esophagus and small bowel. Other blood tests to screen for collagen disorders, such as lupus, should be done. The presence of cervical ribs can be easily determined by roentgenograms of the cervical spine and thorax. Other compression syndromes of the subclavian artery can be detected by performing the maneuvers described under Thoracic Outlet Syndromes. Complete angiographic studies to opacify the arterial circulation from the aortic arch to the small arteries of the hand should be done to exclude the possibility of proximal atherosclerotic plaques producing distal emboli. Occasionally skin and lymph node biopsies are useful.

An important principle in diagnosis is continued observation of the patient over a period of several years. Even after a thorough examination has failed to detect any underlying vascular disease, such a disease may appear in the next 2 to 3 years. In the Mayo Clinic series the diagnosis of Raynaud's disease is simply considered a tentative one for as long as 2 years.

TREATMENT. In the majority of patients the disability is mild. Avoiding cold or other stimuli which precipitate vasoconstriction is adequate. Moving to a warm climate may be considered, but this does not eliminate the attacks. Tobacco certainly should be avoided because of its potent vasoconstrictor action, but this alone does not abolish the syndrome. Various vasodilator drugs have been repeatedly tried, but none have been of consistent benefit. The most recent medications are orally administered methyldopa, employed for patients with ulceration of the fingers and severe pain, and intraarterially administered reserpine. Significant long-term data are not yet available, but one of the authors has used this therapy in some patients, with occasional dramatic and prolonged relief. Therapy for several weeks is required in increasing doses to be effective.

The most effective therapy is cervicodorsal sympathectomy. This is accomplished by removing the first, second, and third thoracic ganglia, preserving the cervical portion of the stellate ganglion to avoid a Horner's syndrome.

The immediate results after sympathectomy in patients with severe vasospasm is quite encouraging, but relapses are common. For this reason, sympathectomy is usually employed only when symptoms are severe and other therapy ineffective. In Gifford's series of 474 patients, only 77 were operated upon; about one-half of these had excellent to good results. DeTakats and Fowler tabulated reports from different groups, including 40 cases of their own, and found an average of 55 percent good results in 424 sympathectomies performed. More radical sympathectomies have not given any better results. Proximally all of the stellate ganglion has been removed, producing Horner's syndrome; distad the fourth thoracic ganglion has been included. Another technical modification has been to include the second and third intercostal nerves with the third ganglion because of the demonstration by Skoog that 10 to 15 percent of sympathetic ganglia to the upper extremity are contained in these two intercostal ganglia. Also there has been considerable discussion about differences in preganglionic and postganglionic sympathectomy. None of these variations have been found significant, however, and the conservative sympathectomy involving the first, second, and third thoracic ganglia is usually performed. Severe trophic changes before operation are unfortunately often associated with a poor result. Patients with scleroderma also obtain little benefit.

Operative Technique. At least four different surgical techniques have been employed at different times for sympathectomy. Originally most were done through a posterior approach, with the patient in a prone position and an incision similar to that for a thoracoplasty. The sympathetic chain was exposed by resecting a short segment of the second or third rib, followed by an extrapleural dissection to isolate the sympathetic chain. In large muscular individuals this approach is quite difficult and provides only limited exposure. It has been virtually abandoned.

A second technique, a supraclavicular approach, provides excellent exposure in patients of small stature with long thin necks. However, in those with short, thick necks, significant trauma to the brachial plexus, resulting in a painful neuritis, may complicate the postoperative course. An excellent description of the technique was published by Nanson.

Ideal exposure can be obtained by an anterior transthoracic incision, opening the hemithorax in the third or fourth intercostal space. This, of necessity, involves a major thoracotomy, though a simple one. It has been favored by Palumbo, who also emphasized that removal of the lower one-third of the stellate ganglion would adequately sympathectomize the extremity without producing a Horner's syndrome.

In recent years the transaxillary approach has become preferred. This is done through a short incision in the axilla, followed by resection of a short segment of the second or third rib and exposure of the sympathetic chain. Good technical descriptions have been published by Roos and by Kirtley et al. The thoracotomy is of much less magnitude than that through the anterior approach, and the incision is in an inconspicuous location.

PROGNOSIS. The prognosis in most patients with primary Raynaud's disease is good with the exception of the discomfort associated with the abnormal sensitivity to cold. Even in the more advanced forms, tissue loss seldom exceeds the loss of one or more digits. More serious systemic vascular disease does not develop, and although symptoms may continue for many years, there is no known impairment of longevity or health.

Uncommon Vasomotor Diseases

Rare, unusual vasomotor diseases include livedo reticularis and acrocyanosis, which primarily result from vasoconstriction, and erythromelalgia, apparently a result of vasodilatation. The disability with these disorders is usually episodic and mild. Their clinical significance is primarily in differentiating them from more serious underlying disease, such as Buerger's disease, scleroderma, or disseminated lupus erythematosus. Only salient clinical features of these bizarre diseases will be presented here.

LIVEDO RETICULARIS

This unusual vasomotor condition is characterized by a persistent mottled reddish blue discoloration of the skin of the extremities. It is more prominent in the legs and feet than in the hands or arms and only infrequently involves the trunk. Although the severity varies with temperature, becoming worse on exposure to cold, it never entirely disappears spontaneously.

ETIOLOGY AND PATHOLOGY. The cause is unknown, although miscellaneous associated vascular diseases such as hypertension or emotional disorders have been found in different patients.

The pathophysiologic feature apparently is a stenosis of the arterioles which pierce the cutis at right angles and arborize into the peripheral capillaries of the skin. The obstruction of the arterioles, either spastic or organic, therefore affects the peripheral capillary arborizations and accounts for the peculiar reticular nature of the discoloration.

The pathologic change in the arterioles varies from no visible abnormality to proliferation of the intima, in some patients progressing to complete occlusion. With severe organic obstruction, focal ulceration of the skin, usually over the lower legs, may occur.

CLINICAL MANIFESTATIONS. Patients with livedo reticularis complain of the persistent reddish blue mottling over the legs and feet, varying somewhat with temperature. Often the cosmetic appearance is the only concern of the patient. In some there are localized symptoms of coldness, numbness, dull aching, and paresthesias. With severe forms and localized tissue ischemia, there may be pain from local ulceration. These symptoms are more prone to appear during the winter in association with cold temperatures.

The diagnosis is usually made from physical examination, with observation of the persistent blotchy discoloration, and a history of prolonged persistence in association with some variation with environmental temperature. Peripheral pulsations are normal, and trophic changes are not present in the digits. Only with more extreme forms are ischemic ulcers present over the lower legs. These usually heal after a short period of time.

TREATMENT. In most patients no treatment is necessary except reassurance regarding the benign nature of the condition. Only one patient is described in the Mayo Clinic series in whom gangrene developed in the legs. Avoiding extremes of cold is beneficial in some patients. Vasodilating agents may be tried, but none has been found of consistent benefit. Sympathectomy should be employed if the disability is severe enough to produce local ulceration. After sympathectomy the discoloration may decrease in extent and remain pink rather than blue. In most patients the disorder is a permanent one, remaining as a moderate cosmetic disturbance, but fortunately with no other disability.

ACROCYANOSIS

Acrocyanosis is a disorder characterized by persistent but painless cold and cyanosis of the hands and feet. The cause and the pathologic and pathophysiologic features are virtually unknown, for the disease consists primarily of persistent color changes. Usually it is confused with Raynaud's syndrome because of the prominent localized cyanosis. Detailed investigation of the pathophysiologic features by Lewis and Landis concluded that the fundamental disorder was a localized abnormality in vasomotor tone in the circulation of the hands and feet. Apparently the basic physiologic condition is a slow rate of blood flow through the skin, the result of chronic arteriolar constriction, which results in a high percentage of reduced hemoglobin in the blood in the capillaries and production of the cyanotic color. Endocrine dysfunction has been found in some patients, but no consistent pattern has been established.

Usually the disorder is found in a young woman who has noted persistent coldness and blueness of the fingers and hands for many years, often with symptoms of less severity in the toes and feet. The abnormalities are more prominent in cold weather, but the extremities are never completely normal. With heat the color may change from deep purple to red, but there are no episodes of blanching, such as occurs with Raynaud's disorder. The peripheral pulses are normal, and there are no trophic changes indicative of chronic tissue ischemia, such as atrophy of the skin, sclerosis, or ulceration.

The principal differential diagnosis is from Raynaud's disease because of the prominent color changes in both disorders. The absence of pallor, as well as the absence of signs of chronic ischemia, are the most useful features. Similarly, the constant presence of the color changes in acrocyanosis, as opposed to the intermittent episodic occurrence in Raynaud's disease, is characteristic.

Usually reassurance is the only treatment needed, with the avoidance of cold temperatures when possible. Sympathectomy can be employed with reasonably good results if the disability is more serious. Prognosis is excellent, with tissue loss virtually never occurring. Usually the color changes remain for many years or permanently.

ERYTHROMELALGIA

This rare disorder is characterized by red, warm, painful extremities. The clinical characteristics were described by S. Weir Mitchell in 1872 and the disorder named by him in 1878. The cause of the primary disease is unknown. Similar phenomena, so-called "secondary erythromelalgia," can occur as a result of hypertension or polycythemia vera.

The basic abnormality is an unusual sensitivity to warmth, for skin temperatures of 32 to 36°C, which produce no effects in normal individuals, will regularly induce the painful burning sensation. The exact temperature at which the distress can be produced varies with different patients but may be a precise one for any individual patient. It was termed by Lewis a "critical point." The increase in temperature is usually a result of vasodilatation with increase in blood flow. The exact basis for the spontaneous vasodilatation with the rise in temperature and the burning sensation is not known.

The disease is equally prevalent in men and women, usually of middle age. The distress may be greater in the summer months, but only a general relationship to extremes of heat or cold may be present. The patient soon learns that exposing the extremities to cold, such as by immersing them in ice water, may abort an attack.

Physical examination usually reveals no abnormalities of the peripheral arteries. The diagnosis is usually established by demonstration of a close relationship between the symptoms and skin temperature. This may be induced by direct application of heat, noting the skin temperature at which distress appears. Erythromelalgia should be differentiated from the painful red but cold extremities which occur with Buerger's disease and also with peripheral neuritis.

Aside from the troublesome symptoms, the disorder is a benign one. Avoiding extremes of heat is one of the most useful therapeutic measures. Acetylsalicylic acid, 0.65 Gm, has been found beneficial in many patients, although the mode of action is uncertain. A trial of therapy with vasoconstrictor drugs, such as ephedrine, should be employed, but consistent value from one drug has not been found. The disorder is usually a permanent one, but no permanent disability results.

FROSTBITE

Several forms of cold injury have been described, usually varying with the environmental conditions under which exposure occurs. These different syndromes include acute pernio (chilblains), chronic pernio, trench foot, immersion foot, and frostbite. Acute and chronic pernio are focal injuries of the skin and subcutaneous tissue resulting from exposure to cold of moderate intensity, representing an increased susceptibility to cold injury in a particular individual. The disorder is seldom a surgical problem, because the lesions are focal, superficial ones which heal readily. Trench foot and immersion foot are primarily military injuries produced by prolonged exposure to cold in damp surroundings, often with temperatures well above freezing, but in circumstances where there is an element of prolonged immobility. Immersion foot is probably simply the seagoing counterpart of trench foot. Such injuries are rarely seen in civilian practice. For practical purposes frostbite is the type of injury usually encountered and will be discussed in detail. The tissue response in the other disorders mentioned, however, is a similar type of response to cold, modified somewhat with the environmental conditions.

ETIOLOGY. Frostbite results when tissues are exposed to cold for varying periods of time. The severity varies both with the temperature and the duration of exposure. Experimentally, it has been demonstrated that freezing begins in mammalian tissues when the temperature in the deeper parts reaches 10°C and that −5°C is the lowest temperature to which cells may be slowly frozen and still survive. Frostbite injury usually results from exposure over a period of several hours. In the Korean conflict, 90 percent of the cases occurred at temperatures near −7°C after exposure for 7 to 18 hours. A different form of frostbite is produced by acute exposures to below zero temperatures, commonly occurring in airplanes at high altitudes and hence termed "high altitude" frostbite. In such injuries the exposed part is acutely frozen with deposition of ice crystals in the tissues. This unusual form of injury is different from the usual case of frostbite, where a "slow freeze" results.

Several factors influence the injurious effect of cold. Two of the most significant ones are humidity and the presence of wind, both of which accelerate the withdrawal of heat from body tissues. Immobility or occlusive vascular disease also are significant factors, both influencing the rate of peripheral blood flow. Acclimatization has been demonstrated in some persons repeatedly exposed to cold, such as those who live in northern latitudes, and probably is a localized vasomotor adaptation. By contrast, extremities previously injured by cold may remain permanently susceptible to future cold injury, perhaps from an intensified vasoconstrictor response.

PATHOLOGY. The degrees of severity of a frostbite injury have been conventionally grouped into four clinical types: a first-degree injury consists of edema and redness of the affected part without necrosis; formation of blisters represents a second-degree injury; necrosis of the skin constitutes a third-degree injury; in a fourth-degree injury gangrene of the extremity develops, requiring amputation.

As frostbite occurs, the injured tissue becomes numb and moderately stiff without extensive discomfort. Often the patient is unaware that frostbite is occurring. With subsequent rewarming the tissues become reddened, hot, and edematous. At this time blisters erupt and gangrene gradually appears in the more seriously injured tissues. Edema increases to a maximum within 24 to 48 hours and then gradually is resorbed as gangrenous tissue begins to demarcate. The extent of gangrene is difficult to estimate initially and requires observations for as long as 30 days or more. Fortunately the degree of gangrene is often much less than that initially feared, because the skin may be gangrenous but the underlying tissue viable. For this reason amputation is delayed until the extent of gangrene is definitely known.

Following recovery of the extremity, there is frequently a permanent increase in vasoconstrictor tone resulting in hyperhidrosis, and an abnormal sensitivity to cold. Pain and paresthesias are also common, perhaps as residuals from ischemic neuritis.

It is uncertain whether the fundamental injury from cold results from direct freezing with disruption of cell membranes or whether the injury is primarily an ischemic necrosis from widespread thrombosis of arterioles and capillaries. Certainly vascular occlusion is a prominent feature, whether it is a primary or a secondary event. With exposure to cold, there is severe vasoconstriction, decreasing the rate of blood flow in the chilled extremity, with resulting stasis, sludging of blood, and eventual widespread thrombosis. In clinical experiments, immersion of the arm for 2 hours in water at 13°C decreases blood flow to about 3 percent of normal, while immersion of a finger in water at 7°C stops blood flow altogether. In addition to sludging and capillary thrombosis, there is an increase in capillary permeability, resulting in the formation of edema when blood flow is increased after rewarming.

On histologic examination of the injured tissues, edema, infiltration of inflammatory cells, and deposition of fibrin are prominent findings. Widespread thrombosis of small vessels is frequently seen. In addition focal areas of necrosis may be evident in skin, muscle, and other tissues.

CLINICAL MANIFESTATIONS. Frequently, the patient is unaware that frostbite is occurring. The usual injury occurs with exposure to near freezing temperatures for several hours, often combined with wind, high humidity, damp or wet shoes, or immobility from tightly constricting shoes or confinement in a cramped position. All these factors influence the rate of heat transfer between the extremity and the environment. Initially there may be mild discomfort, but as the extremity becomes numb and somewhat stiff, frequently discomfort is minimal.

When rewarmed, the extremity quickly becomes red, edematous, hot, and painful. This is due to vasodilatation and widespread extravasation of fluid through the walls of capillaries whose permeability has been increased from injury. Edema reaches its peak intensity within 48 hours and then gradually subsides over several days. As described under Pathology, gangrene gradually becomes evident and slowly demarcates over a period of many days. An ominous sign, indicating that gangrene will develop, is the persistence of coldness and numbness in an area while surrounding tissues become edematous, hot, and painful. The persistent coldness and numbness indicate cessation of all circulation with the certain outcome of ischemic necrosis.

Following recovery from frostbite, a high percentage of extremities remain with an increased vasoconstrictor tone, manifested by increased susceptibility to cold, hyperhidrosis, paresthesias, and localized pain.

TREATMENT. Frostbite seldom occurs during exposure to cold if proper precautions are taken. This includes the wearing of dry, insulated, loosely fitting clothing and carefully avoiding long periods of immobility of the exposed extremities. Most cases of clinical frostbite occur in circumstances where exposure to cold inadvertently occurs for long periods of time because of coma from injury, alcohol, or other factors.

Rapid warming of the injured tissue is the most important aspect of treatment. Several studies have clearly demonstrated the advantages of the rapid-rewarming method over any other. The frozen tissue should be placed in warm water, with a temperature in the range of 40 to 44°C. Complete rewarming usually requires about 20 minutes. Higher temperatures are more injurious than beneficial. A frostbitten part should never be exposed to hot water, an open fire, or excessive dry heat, as in an oven, for the loss of sensitivity in the frozen area makes it especially vulnerable to injury. Warming in water is much more rapid than application of warm blankets, which require three or four times as long as the immersion method.

Following rewarming, the injured extremity should be elevated to minimize formation of edema and carefully protected in a sterile environment. Usually it is left exposed but surrounded by a protective cradle. Blisters are opened only when necessary to remove necrotic skin. Antibiotic therapy and tetanus antiserum are routinely given to lessen the risk of infection. Demarcation of gangrenous areas should be carefully observed, often for several weeks, before amputation is performed. Often a gangrenous area which initially appears to involve the foot will gradually regress with the separation of superficial areas of gangrenous skin, ultimately with the loss of one or more digits but preservation of the foot.

Dramatic reversal of the vasospasm has been achieved by the use of intraarterial reserpine, the effects being monitored angiographically. Angiography of the frostbite patient can define the extent of organic vascular stenosis and the degree of functional vasospasm, thus aiding the choice of therapy. The use of other fast-acting vasodilators such as papaverine might also be appropriate.

The role of sympathectomy has been studied by Shumacker and Kilman and by Golding et al. Both experimental and clinical experiences indicate a beneficial effect from sympathectomy, especially when employed in the first few days after frostbite has occurred. Shumacker and Kilman reported 66 sympathectomies in 38 patients, 24 of which were performed soon after injury. Their experience indicated that sympathectomy should be performed for injuries severe enough to produce necrosis of tissue, both to minimize the extent of necrosis and to prevent the usual late vasomotor sequelae. Golding et al. found in experimental and clinical studies (68 patients) that the proper time for sympathectomy was between 36 and 72 hours after injury. Earlier sympathectomies accelerated the rate of edema formation, while sympathectomies performed following the peak intensity of edema seemed to hasten absorption of edema and minimize eventual tissue necrosis. Sympathectomy is also beneficial in alleviating the late sequelae from cold injury, i.e., paresthesias, coldness, and hyperhidrosis.

If vascular injury is the primary event, therapeutic measures to decrease vasoconstriction or blood clotting, such as sympathectomy or the administration of heparin, should be of routine benefit. The theoretic benefit from sympathectomy is the release of vasospasm, which may precipitate thrombosis in injured capillaries and arterioles. Heparin and dextran have also been given in attempts to lessen the degree of small vessel thrombosis which is such a prominent feature on histologic examination of the injured tissues. Although theoretically plausible, consistent benefit has not been demonstrated from the routine use of either heparin or dextran.

PROGNOSIS. Following recovery from injury, all studies have found a significant percentage of residual disability in the extremity. Simeone evaluated 1,061 limbs 4 months after frostbite while the patients were still in the hospital and found painful feet and hyperhidrosis the most common complaints. Ervasti described similar sequelae in 812 cases of frostbite 5 to 18 years after injury. Orr and Fainer reported that gangrene occurred in only 6 percent of 1,880 cases from the Korean conflict, but some disability remained in 10 to 20 percent of patients.

References

Occlusive Disease: General

Barker, W. F.: Peripheral Vascular Disease in Diabetes: Diagnosis and Management, *Med Clin North Am,* **55**(4):1045, 1971.

Baumann, F. G., Imparato, A. M., and Kim, G. E.: The Evolution of Early Fibromuscular Lesions Hemodynamically Induced in the Dog Renal Artery: 1. Light and Transmission Electron Microscopy, *Circ Res,* **39**:809, 1976.

Beebe, H. G., Clark, W. F., and DeWeese, J. A.: Atherosclerotic Change Occurring in an Autogenous Venous Arterial Graft, *Arch Surg,* **101**:85, 1970.

Berardi, R. S., and Siroospour, D.: Lumbar Sympathectomy in the Treatment of Peripheral Vascular Occlusive Disease: Ten Year Study, *Am J Surg,* **130**:309, 1975.

Boyd, A. M.: The Natural Course of Arteriosclerosis of the Lower Extremities, *Angiology,* **11**:10, 1960.

Brewster, D. C., Retana, A., Waltman, A. C., and Darling, C.: Angiography in the Management of Aneurysms of the Abdominal Aorta: Its Value and Safety, *N Engl J Med,* **292**(16):822, 1975.

Cohen, S. I., Goldman, L. D., Salzman, E. W., and Glotzer, D. J.: The Deleterious Effect of Immediate Postoperative Prosthesis in Below-Knee Amputation for Ischemic Disease, *Surgery,* **76**(6):992, 1974.

Dale, W. A.: The Beginnings of Vascular Surgery, *Surgery,* **76**(6):849, 1974.

Friedman, S. A., Freiberg, P., and Colton, J.: Vasomotor Tone in Diabetic Neuropathy, *Ann Intern Med,* **77**:353, 1972.

Goldenfarb, P. B., Cathey, M. H., and Cooper, G. R.: The Determination of ADP Induced Platelet Aggregation in Normal Men, *Atherosclerosis,* **12**:335, 1970.

Greenhalgh, R. M., Rosengarten, D. S., and Mervart, I.: Serum Lipids and Lipo Proteins in Peripheral Vascular Disease, *Lancet,* **2**:947, 1971.

Hamaker, W. R., Doyle, W. F., O'Connel, T. J., Jr., and Gomez, A. C.: Subintimal Obliterative Proliferation in Saphenous Vein Grafts. A Cause of Early Failure of Aorta to Coronary Artery By-pass Grafts, *Ann Thorac Surg,* **13**:488, 1972.

Hardy, J. D., Conn, J. H., and Fain, W. R.: Nonatherosclerotic Occlusive Lesions of Small Arteries, *Surgery,* **57**(1):1, 1965.

Hill, G. L.: A Rational Basis for Management of Patients with the Buerger Syndrome, *Br J Surg,* **61**:476, 1974.

Honour, A. J., Pickering, G. W., and Sheppard, B. L.: Ultrastructure and Behavior of Platelet Thrombi in Injured Arteries, *Br J Exp Pathol,* **52**:482, 1971.

Imparato, A. M., Baumann, F. G., Pearson, J., Kim, G. E., Davidson, T., and Ibrahim, I.: Electron Microscopic Studies of Experimentally Produced Fibromuscular Arterial Lesions, *Surg Gynecol Obstet,* **68**:683, 1976.

——, Bracco, A., Hammond, R., Kaufman, B., Kim, G. E., Migrassi, P., Pearson, W., Baumann, G., and Nathan, I.: The Effect of Intimal and Neo-Intimal Fibromuscular Fibroplasia on Arterial Reconstructions, *J Cardiovasc Surg.,* (Torino), Special Issue, **488**, 1975.

——, Kim, G. E., Davidson, T., and Crowley, J. G.: Intermittent Claudication: Its Natural Course, *Surgery,* **78**(6):795, 1975.

Jamieson, C. W., and Hill, D.: Amputation for Vascular Disease, *Br J Surg,* **63**:683, 1976.

Karayannacos, P. E., Yahson, D., and Vasko, J. S.: Narrow Lumbar Spinal Canal with Vascular Syndromes, *Arch Surg,* **111**:803, 1976.

Kelly, J. P., and James, J. M.: Criteria for Determining the Proper Level of Amputation in Occlusive Vascular Disease: A Review of 323 Amputations, *J Bone Joint Surg [AM],* **39A**:883, 1957.

Kim, G. E., Ibrahim, I. M., and Imparato, A. M.: Lumbar Sympathectomy in End Stage Arterial Occlusive Disease, *Ann Surg,* **183**(2):157, 1976.

————, Imparato, A. M., Chu, D. S., and David, S. W.: Lower Limb Amputation for Occlusive Vascular Disease, *Am Surg,* **42:**598, 1976.

Lassen, N. A., and Holstein, P.: Use of Radioisotopes in Assessment of Distal Blood Flow and Distal Blood Pressure in Arterial Insufficiency, *Surg Clin North Am,* **54**(1):39, 1974.

Otteman, M. E., and Stahlgren, L. H.: Evaluation of Factors Which Influence Mortality and Morbidity following Major Lower Extremity Amputations for Arteriosclerosis, *Surg Gynecol Obstet,* **120:**1217, 1965.

Raskin, N. H., Levinson, S. A., Hoffman, P. M., Pickett, J. B., and Fields, H. L.: Postsympathectomy Neuralgia: Amelioration with Diphenylhydantoin and Carbamazepine, *Am J Surg,* **128:**75, 1974.

Rich, N. M., Hobson, R. W., and Fedde, W.: Vascular Trauma Secondary to Diagnostic and Therapeutic Procedures, *Am J Surg,* **128:**715, 1974.

Robinson, K.: Long-Posterior-Flap Myoplastic Below-Knee Amputation in Ischemic Disease, *Lancet,* **1:**183, 1972.

Salzman, E. W.: The Limitations of Heparin Therapy after Arterial Reconstructions, *Surgery,* **57:**131, 1965.

Schatz, I. J.: Classification of Primary Hyperlipidemia, *JAMA,* **210:**701, 1969.

Schnetzer, G. W.: Platelets and Thrombogenesis: Current Concepts, *Am Heart J,* **83:**552, 1972.

Scott, H. W., Jr.: Metabolic Surgery for Hyperlipidemia and Atherosclerosis, *Am J Surg,* **123:**3, 1972.

Sethi, G. K., Scott, S. M., Takaro, T.: Multiple-Plane Angiography for More Precise Evaluation of Aortoiliac Disease, *Surgery,* **78**(2):154, 1975.

Stanley, J. C., Gewertz, B. L., Bove, E. L., Scottiurai, V., and Fry, W. J.: Arterial Fibrodysplasia: Histopathologic Character and Current Etiologic Concepts, *Arch Surg,* **110:**561, 1975.

Strandness, D. E.: Evaluation of the Patient for Vascular Surgery, *Surg Clin North Am,* **54**(1):13, 1974.

Tomatis, L. A., Fierens, E. E., and Verbrugge, G. P.: Evaluation of Surgical Risk in Peripheral Vascular Disease by Coronary Arteriography: A Series of 100 Cases, *Surgery,* **71**(3):429, 1972.

Vlodaver, Z., and Edwards, J. E.: Pathologic Changes in Aortic Coronary Arterial Saphenous Vein Grafts, *Circulation,* **44:**719, 1971.

Wray, C. H., Still, J. M., and Moretz, W. N.: Present Management of Amputations for Peripheral Vascular Disease, *Am Surg,* **38:**87, 1972.

Wright, C. J., and Cousins, M. J.: Blood Flow Distribution in the Human Leg following Epidural Sympathetic Blockade, *Arch Surg,* **105:**334, 1972.

Yao, J. S. T., and Bergan, J. J.: Application of Ultrasound to Arterial and Venous Diagnosis, *Surg Clin North Am,* **54**(1):25, 1974.

Aortoiliac Occlusive Disease

Cohn, L. W., Moore, W. S., and Hall, A. D.: Extra-abdominal Management of Late Aortofemoral Graft Thrombosis, *Surgery,* **67**(5):755, 1970.

Garrett, H. E., Crawford, E. S., Howell, J. F., and DeBakey, M. E.: Surgical Considerations in the Treatment of Aorto-iliac Occlusive Disease, *Surg Clin North Am,* **46:**949, 1966.

Guida, P. M., and Moore, S. W.: Obturator Bypass Techniques, *Surg Gynecol Obstet,* **128:**1307, 1969.

Imparato, A. M., Sanoudos, G., Epstein, H. Y., Abrams, R. M., and Beranbaum, E. R.: Results in 96 Aortoiliac Reconstructive Procedures: Pre Operative Angiographic and Functional Classifications Used as Prognostic Guides, *Surgery,* **68:**610, 1970.

Inihara, T.: Endarterectomy for Occlusive Disease of the Aorto-iliac and Common Femoral Arteries: Evaluation of Results of the Eversion Technique Endarterectomy, *Am J Surg,* **124:**235, 1972.

Kwaan, J. H. M., Molen, R. V., Stemmer, E. A., and Connolly, J. E.: Peripheral Embolism Resulting from Unsuspected Atheromatous Aortic Plaques, *Surgery,* **78**(5):583, 1975.

LoGerfo, F. W., Johnson, W. C., Corson, J. D., Vollman, R. W., Wasel, R. D., Davis, R. C., Nabseth, D. C., and Mannick, J. A.: Comparison of the Late Patency Rates of Axillobilateral Femoral and Axillounilateral Femoral Grafts, *Surgery,* **81:**33, 1977.

Lorentsen, E., Hael, B. L., and Hal, R.: Evaluation of the Functional Importance of Atherosclerotic Obliterations in the Aorto-iliac Artery by Pressure-Flow Measurements, *Acta Med Scand,* **191:**399, 1972.

Mannick, J. A., Williams, L. E., and Nabseth, D. C.: The Late Results of Axillofemoral Grafts, *Surgery,* **68**(6):1038, 1970.

May, A. G., Van de Berg, L., DeWeese, J. A., and Rob, C. G.: Critical Arterial Stenosis, *Surgery,* **54:**250, 1963.

Szilagyi, D. E., Smith, R. F., Elliott, J. P., and Varndecic, M. P.: Infection in Arterial Reconstruction with Synthetic Grafts, *Ann Surg,* **176**(3):321, 1972.

————, Smith, R. F., Elmquist, J. G., Gonzalez, A., and Elliott, J. P.: Angioplasty in the Treatment of Peripheral Occlusive Arteriopathy: A Summary of 12 Years' Experience, *Arch Surg,* **90:**617, 1965.

Femoropopliteal Occlusive Disease

Allan, J. S., and Taylor, G. W.: The Relationship between Blood Flow and Failure of Femoropopliteal Reconstructive Arterial Surgery, *Br J Surg,* **59:**549, 1972.

Brief, D. K., Brener, B. J., Alpert, J., and Parsonnet, V.: Crossover Femoropopliteal Grafts Followed up Five Years or More. An Analysis, *Arch Surg,* **110:**1294, 1975.

Crawford, E. S., Garrett, H. E., DeBakey, M. E., and Howell, J. F.: Occlusive Disease of the Femoral Artery and Its Branches, *Surg Clin North Am,* **46:**991, 1966.

Cutler, B. S., Thompson, J. E., Kleinsasser, L. J., and Hempel, G. K.: Autologous Saphenous Vein Femoropopliteal Bypass: Analysis of 298 Cases, *Surgery,* **79**(3):324, 1976.

Dale, W. A.: Autogenous Vein Grafts for Femoropopliteal Arterial Repair, *Surg Gynecol Obstet,* **123:**1282, 1966.

————: Salvage of Arteriosclerotic Legs by Vascular Repair, *Ann Surg,* **165:**844, 1967.

DeWeese, J. A., and Rob, C. G.: Autogenous Venous Bypass Grafts Five Years Later, *Ann Surg,* **174**(3):346, 1971.

Imparato, A. M., Bracco, A., and Kim, G. E.: Comparisons of Three Technics for Femoral-Popliteal Arterial Reconstructions, *Ann Surg,* **177**(3):375, 1973.

Koontz, T. J., and Stausel, H. C., Jr.: Factors Influencing Patency of the Autogenous Vein Femoropopliteal By-pass Graft: An Analysis of 74 Cases, *Surgery,* **71:**753, 1972.

Linton, R. R., LeRoy, S., and Wirthlin, M. D.: Femoropopliteal Composite Dacron and Autogenous Vein Bypass Grafts: A Preliminary Report, *Arch Surg,* **107**:748, 1973.

Martin, P., and Jamieson, C.: The Rationale for and Measurement after Profundaplasty, *Surg Clin North Am,* **54**(1):95, 1974.

Plecha, F. R., and Pories, W. J.: Intraoperative Angiography in the Immediate Assessment of Arterial Reconstruction, *Arch Surg,* **105**:902, 1972.

Poliwoda, H.: Treatment of Acute and Chronic Arterial Occlusions with Streptokinase, *Aust Ann Med,* **19**(Suppl 1):25, 1970.

Rosenberg, N., Thompson, J. E., Keshishian, J. M., and Vander-Werf, B. A.: The Modified Bovine Arterial Graft, *Arch Surg,* **111**:222, 1976.

Sawyer, P. N., Kaplitt, M. J., Sobel, S., Golding, M. R., and Dennis, C.: Analysis of Peripheral Gas Endarterectomy in 127 Patients, *Arch Surg,* **97**:859, 1968.

Skinner, J. S., and Strandness, D. E., Jr.: Exercise and Intermittent Claudication: Effects of Physical Training, *Circulation,* **36**:23, 1967.

Szilagyi, D. E., Smith, R. F., Elliott, J. P., and Allen, H. M.: Long-Term Behavior of a Dacron Arterial Substitute: Clinical, Roentgenologic and Histologic Correlations, *Ann Surg,* **162**:453, 1965.

Vollmar, J., Frede, M., and Laubach, K.: Principles of Reconstructive Procedures for Chronic Femoro-popliteal Occlusions: A Report of 546 Operations, *Ann Surg,* **168**:215, 1968.

Tibioperoneal Occlusive Disease

Imparato, A. M., Kim, G. E., and Chu, D. S.: Surgical Exposure for Reconstruction of the Proximal Part of the Tibial Artery, *Surg Gynecol Obstet,* **136**:453, 1973.

———, ———, Madayag, M., and Haveson, S.: Angiographic Criteria for Successful Tibial Arterial Reconstructions, *Surgery,* **74**(6):830, 1973.

———, ———, ———, and ———: The Results of Tibial Artery Reconstruction Procedures, *Surg Gynecol Obstet,* **138**:33, 1974.

Kahn, S. P., Lindenauer, M., Dent, T. L., Kraft, R. O., and Fry, W. J.: Femorotibial Vein Bypass, *Arch Surg,* **107**:309, 1973.

Reichle, F. A., and Tyson, R. R.: Comparison of Long-Term Results of 364 Femoropopliteal or Femorotibial Bypasses for Revascularization of Severely Ischemic Lower Extremities, *Ann Surg,* **182**(4):449, 1975.

Arterial Embolism

Billig, D. M., Hallman, G. L., and Cooley, D. A.: Arterial Embolism, *Arch Surg,* **95**:1, 1967.

Cranley, J. J., Krause, R. J., Strasser, E. S., Hafner, C. D., and Fogarty, T. J.: Peripheral Arterial Embolism: Changing Concepts, *Surgery,* **55**:57, 1964.

Crawford, E. S., and DeBakey, M. E.: The Retrograde Flush Procedure in Embolectomy and Thrombectomy, *Surgery,* **40**:737, 1956.

Darling, R. C., Austen, W. G., and Linton, R. R.: Arterial Embolism, *Surg Gynecol Obstet,* **124**:106, 1967.

Fisher, E. R., Hellstrom, H. R., and Myers, J. D.: Disseminated Atheromatous Emboli, *Am J Med,* **29**:176, 1960.

Flory, C. M.: Arterial Occlusions Produced by Emboli from Eroded Aortic Atheromatous Plaques, *Am J Pathol,* **21**:549, 1945.

Fogarty, T. J., Cranley, J. J., Krause, R. J., Strasser, E. S., and

Hafner, C. D.: A Method for Extraction of Arterial Emboli and Thrombi, *Surg Gynecol Obstet,* **116**:241, 1963.

Haimovici, H.: Peripheral Arterial Embolism, *Angiology,* **1**:20, 1950.

Kassirer, J. P.: Atheroembolic Renal Disease, *N Engl J Med,* **280**:817, 1969.

Miles, R. M., Dale, D., and Booth, J. L.: The Dynamics of Peripheral Arterial Embolism, *Ann Surg,* **167**:801, 1968.

Spencer, F. C., and Eiseman, B.: Delayed Arterial Embolectomy: A New Concept, *Surgery,* **55**:64, 1964.

Buerger's Disease

Kjeldsen, K., and Mozes, M.: Buerger's Disease in Israel: Investigations on Carboxyhemoglobin and Serum Cholesterol Levels after Smoking, *Acta Chir Scand,* **135**:495, 1969.

McKusick, V. A., Harris, W. S., and Ottesen, O. E.: The Buerger Syndrome in the United States: Arteriographic Observations, with Special Reference to Involvement of the Upper Extremities and the Differentiation from Atherosclerosis and Embolism, *Bull Johns Hopkins Hosp,* **110**:145, 1962.

———, ———, ———, Goodman, R. M., Shelley, W. M., and Bloodwell, R. D.: Buerger's Disease: A Distinct Clinical and Pathologic Entity, *JAMA,* **181**:5, 1962.

McPherson, J. R., Guergels, J. L., and Gifford, R. W., Jr.: Thromboangiitis Obliterans and Arteriosclerosis Obliterans: Clinical and Prognostic Differences, *Ann Intern Med,* **59**:288, 1963.

Silbert, S.: The Etiology of Thromboangiitis Obliterans, *JAMA,* **129**:5, 1945.

Wessler, S.: Buerger's Disease Revisited, *Surg Clin North Am,* **49**:703, 1969.

———, Si-Chun, M., Gurewich, V., and Freiman, D. G.: Critical Evaluation of Thromboangiitis Obliterans: Case against Buerger's Disease, *N Engl J Med,* **262**:1149, 1960.

Arterial Trauma

Hughes, C. W., and Cohen, A.: The Repair of Injured Blood Vessels, *Surg Clin North Am,* **38**:1529, 1958.

Miller, H. H., and Welch, C. S.: Quantitative Studies on Time Factor in Arterial Injuries, *Ann Surg,* **130**:428, 1949.

Morris, G. C., Jr., Beall, A. C., Jr., Roof, W. R., and DeBakey, M. E.: Surgical Experience with 220 Acute Arterial Injuries in Civilian Practice, *Am J Surg,* **99**:775, 1960.

Mustard, W. T., and Bull, C. A.: A Reliable Method for Relief of Traumatic Vascular Spasm, *Ann Surg,* **155**:339, 1962.

Patman, R. D., Poulos, E., and Shires, G. T.: The Management of Civilian Arterial Injuries, *Surg Gynecol Obstet,* **118**:725, 1964.

Spencer, F. C.: Vascular Injury and Arteriovenous Fistula, in "Lewis-Walters Practice of Surgery," vol. XI, chap. 8, W. F. Prior Co., Inc., Hagerstown, Md., 1965.

——— and Grewe, R. V.: The Management of Arterial Injuries in Battle Casualties, *Ann Surg,* **141**:304, 1955.

Popliteal Artery Entrapment Syndrome

Albertazzi, V. J., Elliott, T. E., and Kennedy, J. A.: Popliteal Artery Entrapment, *Angiology,* **20**:119, 1969.

Brightmore, T. G. J., and Smellie, W. A. B.: Popliteal Artery Entrapment, *Br J Surg,* **58**:481, 1971.

Hamming, J. J.: Intermittent Claudication at an Early Age, due to an Anomalous Course of the Popliteal Artery, *Angiology,* **10**:369, 1959.

Harris, J. D., and Jepson, R. P.: Entrapment of the Popliteal Artery, *Surgery,* **69:**246, 1971.

Inshua, J. A., Young, J. R., and Humphries, A. W.: Popliteal Artery Entrapment Syndrome, *Arch Surg,* **101:**771, 1970.

Stuart, A. T. P.: Note on Variation in the Course of the Popliteal Artery, *J Anat Physiol,* **XIII:**162, 1879.

Anterior Compartment Syndrome

Carter, A. B., Richards, R. L., and Zachary, R. B.: The Anterior Tibial Syndrome, *Lancet,* **2:**928, 1949.

Getzen, L. C., and Carr, J. E., III: Etiology of Anterior Tibial Compartment Syndrome, *Surg Gynecol Obstet,* **125:**347, 1967.

Mavor, G. E.: The Anterior Tibial Syndrome, *J Bone Joint Surg [Br],* **38B:**513, 1956.

Moretz, W. H.: The Anterior Compartment (Anterior Tibial) Ischemia Syndrome, *Am Surg,* **19:**728, 1953.

Traumatic Arteriovenous Fistulas

Creech, O., Jr., Gantt, J., and Wren, H.: Traumatic Arteriovenous Fistula at Unusual Sites, *Ann Surg,* **161:**908, 1965.

Hughes, C. W., and Jahnke, E. J., Jr.: The Surgery of Traumatic Arteriovenous Fistulas and Aneurysms: A Five-Year Follow Up Study of 215 Lesions, *Ann Surg,* **148:**790, 1958.

Shumacker, H. B., Jr.: Arterial Aneurysms and Arteriovenous Fistulas: Report on Spontaneous Cures, in D. C. Elkin, and M. E. DeBakey (eds.), "Vascular Surgery," Office of the Surgeon General, U.S. Public Health Service, 1955.

Spencer, F. C.: Vascular Injury and Arteriovenous Fistula, in "Lewis-Walters Practice of Surgery," vol. XI, chap. 8, W. F. Prior Co., Inc., Hagerstown, Md., 1965.

Congenital Arteriovenous Fistulas

Cross, F. S., Glover, D. M., Simeone, F. A., and Oldenburg, F. A.: Congenital Arteriovenous Aneurysms, *Ann Surg,* **148:**649, 1958.

Fry, W. J.: Surgical Considerations in Congenital Arteriovenous Fistula, *Surg Clin North Am,* **54**(1):165, 1974.

Olcott, C., Newton, T. H., Stoney, R. J., and Ehrenfeld, W. K.: Intra-arterial Embolization in the Management of Arteriovenous Malformations, *Surgery,* **79**(1):3, 1976.

Robertson, D. J.: Congenital Arteriovenous Fistulae of the Extremities: Hunterian Lecture, *Ann R Coll Surg Engl,* **18:**73, 1956.

Rosenfeld, L.: Experiences with Vascular Abnormalities about the Parotid Gland and Upper Neck, *Arch Surg,* **79:**553, 1959.

Spencer, F. C.: Vascular Injury and Arteriovenous Fistula, in "Lewis-Walters Practice of Surgery," vol. XI, chap. 8, W. F. Prior Co., Inc., Hagerstown, Md., 1965.

Szilagyi, E. D., Smith, R. F., Elliott, J. P., and Hageman, J. H.; Congenital Arteriovenous Anomalies of the Limbs, *Arch Surg,* **111:**423, 1976.

Tice, D. A., Clauss, R. H., Kierle, A. M., and Reed, G. E.: Congenital Arteriovenous Fistulae of the Extremities: Observations Concerning Treatment, *Arch Surg,* **86:**460, 1963.

Thoracic Outlet Syndromes

Adams, J. T., and DeWeese, J. A.: Effort Thrombosis of the Axillary and Subclavian Veins, *J Trauma,* **11:**923, 1971.

Adson, A. W.: Surgical Treatment for Symptoms Produced by Cervical Ribs and the Scalenus Anticus Muscle, *Surg Gynecol Obstet,* **85:**687, 1947.

Beyer, J. A., and Wright, I. S.: The Hyperabduction Syndrome: With Special Reference to Its Relationship to Raynaud's Syndrome, *Circulation,* **4:**161, 1951.

Dale, W. A.: Thoracic Outlet Syndrome, *J Tenn Med Assoc,* **64:**941, 1971.

Falconer, M. A., and Weddell, G.: Costoclavicular Compression of the Subclavian Artery and Vein: Relation to the Scalenus Anticus Syndrome, *Lancet,* **2:**539, 1943.

Jochamisen, P. R., and Hartfall, W. G.: Per Axillary Upper Extremity Sympathectomy: Technique Reviewed and Clinical Experience, *Surgery,* **71**(5):686, 1972.

Kirtley, J. A., Riddell, D. H., Stoney, W. S., and Wright, J. K.: Cervico-sympathectomy in Neurovascular Abnormalities of the Upper Extremities: Experiences in 76 Patients with 104 Sympathectomies, *Ann Surg,* **165:**869, 1967.

Lord, J. W., Jr., and Rosati, L. M.: Neurovascular Compression Syndromes of the Upper Extremity, *Ciba Found Clin Symp.* **10:**35, 1958.

Nanson, E. M.: The Anterior Approach to Upper Dorsal Sympathectomy, *Surg Gynecol Obstet,* **104:**118, 1957.

Patman, R. D., Thompson, J. E., and Persson, A.: Management of Post-traumatic Pain Syndromes: Report of 113 Cases, *Ann Surg,* **177**(6):780, 1973.

Roos, D. B.: Transaxillary Approach for First Rib Resection to Relieve Thoracic Outlet Syndrome, *Ann Surg,* **163:**354, 1966.

———— and Owens, J. C.: Thoracic Outlet Syndrome, *Arch Surg,* **93:**71, 1966.

Ross, J. P.: The Vascular Complications of Cervical Rib, *Ann Surg,* **150:**340, 1959.

Schein, C. J., Haimovici, H., and Young, H.: Arterial Thrombosis Associated with Cervical Ribs: Surgical Considerations: Report of a Case and Review of the Literature, *Surgery,* **40:**428, 1956.

Telford, E. D., and Mottershead, S.: Pressure at the Cervicobrachial Junction: An Operative and Anatomical Study, *J Bone Joint Surg [Br],* **30B:**249, 1948.

Urschel, H. D., Paulson, D. L., and McNamara, J. J.: Thoracic Outlet Syndrome, *Ann Thorac Surg,* **6:**1, 1968.

Extracranial Occlusive Cerebrovascular Disease

Bahnson, H. T., Spencer, F. C., and Quattlebaum, J. K., Jr.: Surgical Treatment of Occlusive Disease of the Carotid Artery, *Ann Surg,* **149:**711, 1959.

Baker, Dennis J., Gluecklich, B., Watson, W., Marcus, E., and Vijaylakshmi, K.: An Evaluation of Electroencephalographic Monitoring for Carotid Study, *Surgery,* **78**(6):787, 1975.

Barner, H. B., Kaiser, G. C., and Willman, V. L.: Hemodynamics of Carotid-Subclavian Bypass, *Arch Surg,* **103:**248, 1971.

Barnes, R. W., Bone, G. E., Reinertson, J., Slaymaker, E. E., Hokanson, E., and Strandness, E.: Noninvasive Ultrasonic Carotid Angiography: Prospective Validation by Contrast Arteriography, *Surgery,* **80**(3):328, 1976.

Bernhard, V. M., Johnson, W. D., and Peterson, J. J.: Carotid Artery Stenosis, *Arch Surg,* **105:**837, 1972.

Blaisdell, F. W., Lim, R., and Hall, A. D.: Technical Result of Carotid Endarterectomy: Arteriographic Assessment, *Am J Surg,* **114:**239, 1967.

Bone, G. E., and Barnes, R. W.: Limitations of the Doppler

Cerebrovascular Examination in Hemispheric Cerebral Ischemia, *Surgery,* **79**(5):577, 1976.

Capistrant, T. D.: Thermographic Facial Patterns in Carotid Occlusive Disease, *Radiology,* **100**:85, 1971.

Cervantes, F. D., and Schneiderman, L. J.: Anticoagulants in
Cerebrovascular Disease. A Critical Review of Studies, *Arch
Intern Med,* **135**:875, 1975.

Cohen, A., Manion, W. C., Spencer, F. C., Czarnecki, S. W., and
DeBakey, M. E.: Occlusive Lesions of the Great Vessels of the
Aortic Arch, *Arch Surg,* **84**:628, 1962.

Crawford, E. S., DeBakey, M. E., Garrett, H. E., and Howell, J.:
Surgical Treatment of Occlusive Cerebrovascular Disease,
Surg Clin North Am, **46**:873, 1966.

———, ———, Morris, G. C., Jr., and Cooley, D. A.: Thrombo-
obliterative Disease of the Great Vessels Arising from the
Aortic Arch, *J Thorac Cardiovasc Surg,* **43**:38, 1962.

Dent, T. L., Thompson, N. W., and Fry, W. J.: Carotid Body
Tumors, *Surgery,* **80**(3):365, 1976.

Fields, W. M.: Selection of Stroke Patients for Arterial Reconstructions, *Am J Surg,* **125**:527, 1973.

Ford, J. J., Baker, W. H., and Ehrenhaft, J. L.: Carotid Endarterectomy for Nonhemispheric Transient Ischemic Attacks, *Arch
Surg,* **110**:1314, 1975.

Gresham, G. E., Fitzpatrick, T. E., Wolf, P. A., McNamara P. M.,
and Dawber, T. R.: Residual Disability of Survivors of
Stroke—the Framingham Study, *N Engl J Med,* **293**(19):954,
1975.

Hachinski, V. C., Lassen, N. A., and Marshall, J.: Multi-Infarct
Dementia, a Cause of Mental Deterioration in the Elderly,
Lancet, **2**:207, 1974.

Hays, R. J., Levinson, S. A., and Wylie, E. J.: Intraoperative
Measurement of Carotid Back Pressure as a Guide to Operative Management for Carotid Endarterectomy, *Surgery,*
72(6):953, 1972.

Higgs, W. A., and Bullington, S. J.: Correlation between Opthal-
modynamometry and Arteriography in Diagnosing Carotid
Arterial Occlusive Disease, *Eye Ear Nose Throat Mon,* **49**:369,
1970.

Humphries, A. W., Young, J. R., Beven, E. D., LeFevre, F. A., and
deWolfe, V. G.: Relief of vertebrobasilar symptoms by carotid
endarterectomy, *Surgery,* **57**(1):48, 1965.

Imparato, A. M.: Bracco, A., Kim, G. E., and Bergmann, L.: The
Hypoglossal Nerve in Carotid Arterial Reconstructions,
Stroke, **3**:576, 1972.

——— , Kricheff, I., Capetillo, A., and Post, K.: Circulatory Dynamics of the Cerebrovascular System in Surgery for Stroke,
Circulation, **42**(*Suppl* 3):94, 1970.

——— and Lin, J. P. T.: Vertebral Arterial Reconstruction, Internal Plication and Patch Vein Angioplasty, *Ann Surg,* **166**:213,
1967.

Jacobson, J. H., Mozersky, D. J., Mitty, H. A., and Brothers, M. J.:
Axillary-Axillary Bypass for the Subclavian Steal Syndrome,
Arch Surg, **106**:24, 1973.

Joint Study of Extracranial Arterial Occlusion as a Cause of
Stroke:
  I. Fields, W. S., North, R. R., Hass, W. K., Galbraith, J. G.,
  Wylie, E. J., Ratinov, G., Burns, M. H., MacDonald, M. C.,
  and Meyer, J. S.: Organization of Study and Survey of Patient
  Population, *JAMA,* **203**:955, 1968.
  II. Hass, W. K., Fields, W. S., North, R. R., Kricheff, I. I.,

Chase, N. E., and Bauer, R. B.: Arteriography, Techniques,
  Sites and Complications, *JAMA,* **203**:961, 1968.
  III. Bauer, R. B., Meyer, J. S., Fields, W. S., Remington, R.,
  MacDonald, M. C., and Callen, P.: Progress Report of Con-
  trolled Long Term Survival in Patients With and Without
  Operation, *JAMA,* **208**:509, 1969.
  IV. Blaisdell, W. F., Clauss, R. H., Galbraith, J. G., Imparato,
  A. M., and Wylie, E. J.: A Review of Surgical Considerations,
  JAMA, **209**:1889, 1969.
  V. Fields, W. S., Maslenikov, V., Meyer, J. S., Hass, W. K.,
  Remington, R. D., and MacDonald, M.: Progress Report of
  Prognosis Following Surgery or Non Surgical Treatment for
  Transient Cerebral Ischemic Attacks and Cervical Carotid
  Lesions, *JAMA,* **211**:1993, 1970.

Killen, D. A., Foster, J. H., Gobbel, W. G., Jr., Stephenson, S. E.,
Jr., Collins, H. A., Billings, F. T., and Scott, H. W., Jr.: The
Subclavian Steal Syndrome, *J Thorac Cardiovasc Surg,*
51:539, 1966.

Kollarits, C. R., Lubow, M., and Hissong, S. L.: Retinal Strokes: I.
Incidence of Carotid Atheromata, *JAMA,* **222**(10):1275, 1972.

Lazar, M. L., and Clark, K.: Microsurgical Cerebral Revascularization: Concepts and Practice, *Surg Neurol,* **1**(6):355, 1973.

Lyons, C., and Galbraith, G.: Surgical Treatment of Atherosclerotic Occlusion of the Internal Carotid Artery, *Ann Surg,*
146:487, 1957.

Millikan, C. H.: The Pathogenesis of Transient Focal Cerebral
Ischemia, *Circulation,* **32**:438, 1965.

Najafi, H., Javid, H., Dye, W. S., Hunter, J. A., Wideman, F. E.,
and Julian, O. C.: Emergency Carotid Thromboendarterectomy: Surgical Indication and Results, *Arch Surg,* **103**:610,
1971.

Ranson, J. H. C., Imparato, A. M., Clauss, R. H., Reed, G., and
Hass, W. K.: Factors in Mortality and Morbidity Associated
with Surgical Treatment of Cerebrovascular Insufficiency,
Circulation, **39**(*Suppl* 1):269, 1969.

Reivich, M., Holling, E., Roberts, B., and Toole, J. F.: Reversal of
Blood Flow through the Vertebral Artery and Its Effect on
Cerebral Circulation, *N Engl J Med,* **265**:878, 1961.

Rhodes, L. E., Stanley, J. C., Hoffman, G. L., Cronenwett, J. L.,
and Fry, W. J.: Aneurysms of Extracranial Carotid Arteries,
Arch Surg, **111**:339, 1976.

Rosenberg, J. C., and Spencer, F. C.: Subclavian Steal Syndrome:
Surgical Treatment of Three Patients, *Am Surg,* **31**:307,
1965.

Rosenthal, J. J., Gaspar, M. R., and Movius, H. R.: Intraoperative
Arteriography in Carotid Thromboendarterectomy, *Arch
Surg,* **106**:806, 1973.

Ross, R. S., and McKusick, V. A.: Aortic Arch Syndrome, *Arch
Intern Med,* **92**:701, 1953.

Sand, B. J., Barker, W. F., Freeman, W. L., and Hummell, S.:
Ophthalmic Arterial Blood Pressures Measured by Ocular
Plethysmodynamography, *Arch Surg,* **110**:813, 1975.

Santschi, D. R., Frahm, C. J., Pascale, L. R., and Dumanian,
A. V.: The Subclavian Steal Syndrome: Clinical and Angio-
graphic Considerations in 74 Cases in Adults, *J Thorac
Cardiovasc Surg,* **51**:103, 1966.

Spencer, F. C., and Eiseman, B.: Technique of Carotid Endarterectomy, *Surg Gynecol Obstet,* **115**:114, 1962.

Thompson, J. E., Austin, D. J., and Patman, R. D.: Carotid Endarterectomy for Cerebrovascular Insufficiency: Long-Term

Results in 592 Patients Followed up to Thirteen Years, *Ann Surg,* **172**(4):663, 1970.

———, Kartchner, M. M., Austin, D. J., Wheeler, C. G., and Patman, R. D.: Carotid Endarterectomy for Cerebrovascular Insufficiency (Stroke): Follow Up of 359 Cases, *Ann Surg,* **163**:751, 1966.

——— and Patman, R. D.: Endarterectomy for Asymptomatic Carotid Bruits, *Heart Bull,* **19**:116, 1970.

———, Patman, R. D., and Persson, A. V.: Management of Asymptomatic Carotid Bruits, *Am Surg,* **42**(2):77, 1976.

Thompson, N. W., Olsen, W., Schmidt, C. M., and Kraft, R. O.: Occlusive Disease of the Subclavian Artery and the Subclavian Steal Syndrome, *Univ Mich Med Cent J,* **33**:8, 1967.

Warren, R., and Triedman, L. J.; Pulseless Disease and Carotid-Artery Thrombosis: Surgical Considerations, *N Engl J Med,* **257**:685, 1957.

Wylie, E. J., Hein, M. F., and Adams, J. E.: Intracranial Hemorrhage following Surgical Revascularization for Treatment of Acute Strokes, *J Neurosurg,* **21**:212, 1964.

Abdominal Aneurysms

Bahnson, H. T.: Surgical Treatment of Abdominal Arteriosclerotic Aneurysms, *Surg Clin North Am,* **36**:983, 1956.

DeBakey, M. R., Crawford, E. S., Cooley, D. A., Morris, G. C., Royster, T. S., and Abbott, W. P.: Aneurysm of Abdominal Aorta: Analysis of Results of Graft Replacement Therapy One to Eleven Years after Operation, *Ann Surg,* **160**(4):622, 1964.

Dent, T. L., Lindenauer, M., Ernst, C. B., and Fry, W. J.: Multiple Arteriosclerotic Arterial Aneurysms, *Arch Surg,* **105**:338, 1972.

Estes, J. E., Jr.: Abdominal Aortic Aneurysm: A Study of One Hundred and Two Cases, *Circulation,* **2**:258, 1950.

Hardy, J. D., and Timmis, H. H.: Abdominal Aortic Aneurysms: Special Problems, *Ann Surg,* **173**(6):945, 1971.

Imparato, A. M., Berman, I. R., Bracco, A., Kim, G. E., and Beaudet, R.: Avoidance of Shock and Peripheral Embolism during Surgery of the Abdominal Aorta, *Surgery,* **73**(1):68, 1973.

Jarrett, F., Darling, C. R., Mundth, E. D., and Austen, G.: Experience with Infected Aneurysms of the Abdominal Aorta, *Arch Surg,* **110**:1381, 1975.

Lawrence, R. J., Ferguson, M. D., Bergan, J. J., Conn, J., Jr., and Yao, J. S. T.: Spinal Ischemia following Abdominal Aortic Surgery, *Ann Surg,* **181**(3):267, 1975.

Mehrez, I. O., Nabseth, D. C., Hogan, E. L., and Deterling, R. A., Jr.: Paraplegia following Resection of Abdominal Aortic Aneurysm, *Ann Surg,* **156**:890, 1962.

Porter, J. M., McGregor, F., Acinapura, A. J., and Silver, D.: Renal Function following Abdominal Aortic Aneurysmectomy, *Surg Gynecol Obstet,* **123**(4):819, 1966.

Sethi, G. K., Hughes, R. K., and Takaro, T.: Dissecting Aortic Aneurysms, *Ann Thorac Surg,* **18**(2):301, 1974.

Shumacker, H. B., Barnes, D. L., and King, H.: Ruptured Abdominal Aortic Aneurysms, *Ann Surg,* **177**(6):772, 1973.

Smith, R. F., and Szilagyi, D. E.: Ischemia of the Colon as a Complication in Surgery of the Abdominal Aorta, *Arch Surg,* **80**:806, 1960.

Stanley, J. C., and Fry, W. J.: Pathogenesis and Clinical Significance of Splenic Artery Aneurysms, *Surgery,* **76**(6):898, 1974.

Szilagyi, D. E., Elliot, J. P., and Smith, R. F.: Clinical Fate of the Patient with Asymptomatic Abdominal Aortic Aneurysm and Unfit for Surgical Therapy, *Arch Surg,* **104**:600, 1972.

Szilagyi, D. E., Smith, R. F., De Russo, F. J., Elliott, J. P., and Sherrin, F. W.: Contribution of Abdominal Aortic Aneurysmectomy to Prolongation of Life, *Ann Surg,* **164**(4):678, 1966.

Thompson, J. E., Hollier, L. H., Patman, R. D., and Persson, A. V.: Surgical Management of Abdominal Aortic Aneurysms: Factors Influencing Mortality and Morbidity—a 20 Year Experience, *Ann Surg,* **181**(5):654, 1975.

Vasko, J. S., Spencer, F. C., and Bahnson, H. T.: Aneurysm of the Aorta Treated by Excision: Review of 237 Cases Followed Up to Seven Years, *Am J Surg,* **105**:793, 1963.

Peripheral Aneurysms: General

Howell, J. F., Crawford, E. S., Morris, G. C., Jr., Garrett, H. E., and DeBakey, M. E.: Surgical Treatment of Peripheral Arteriosclerotic Aneurysm, *Surg Clin North Am,* **46**:979, 1966.

Popliteal Aneurysms

Alpert, J.: Aneurysms of the Popliteal Artery, *J Med Soc NJ,* **67**:791, 1970.

Edmunds, L. H., Darling, R. C., and Linton, R. R.: Surgical Management of Popliteal Aneurysm, *Circulation,* **32**:517, 1965.

Gifford, R. W., Jr., Hines, E. A., Jr., and Janes, J. M.: Analysis and Follow-up Study of 100 Popliteal Aneurysms, *Surgery,* **33**:284, 1953.

Hunter, J. A., Julian, O. C., Javid, H., and Dye, W. S.: Arteriosclerotic Aneurysms of the Popliteal Artery, *J Cardiovasc Surg,* **2**:404, 1961.

Femoral Aneurysms

Crawford, E. S., Edwards, W. H., DeBakey, M. E., Cooley, D. A., and Morris, G. C., Jr.: Peripheral Arteriosclerotic Aneurysm, *J Am Geriatr Soc,* **9**:1, 1961.

Papas, G., Janes, J. M., Bernatz, P. E., and Schirger, A.: Femoral Aneurysms: Review of Surgical Management, *JAMA,* **190**:489, 1964.

Stoney, R. J., Albo, R. J., and Wylie, E. J.: False Aneurysms Occurring after Arterial Grafting Operations, *Am J Surg,* **110**:153, 1965.

Tolstedt, G. E., Radke, H. N., and Bell, J. W.: Late Sequela of Arteriosclerotic Femoral Aneurysms, *Angiology,* **12**:601, 1961.

Carotid Artery Aneurysms

Beall, A. C., Jr., Crawford, E. S., Cooley, D. A., and DeBakey, M. E.: Extracranial Aneurysms of the Carotid Artery: Report of Seven Cases, *Postgrad Med,* **32**:93, 1962.

Kianouri, M.: Extracranial Carotid Aneurysms, *Ann Surg,* **165**:152, 1967.

Sanoudos, G. M., Ramp, J., and Imparato, A. M.: Internal Carotid Aneurysm, *Am Surg,* **39**:118, 1973.

Spencer, F. C.: Aneurysm of the Common Carotid Artery Treated by Excision and Primary Anastomosis, *Ann Surg,* **145**:254, 1957.

Subclavian Aneurysms

Howell, J. F., Crawford, E. S., Morris, G. C., Jr., Garrett, H. E., and DeBakey, M. E.: Surgical Treatment of Peripheral Arteriosclerotic Aneurysm, *Surg Clin North Am,* **46**:979, 1966.

Splenic Artery Aneurysms

Bedford, P. D., and Lodge, B.: Aneurysm of the Splenic Artery, *Gut,* **1:**312, 1960.

Owens, J. C., and Coffey, R. J.: Aneurysm of the Splenic Artery, Including a Report of 6 Additional Cases, *Int Abstr Surg,* **97:**313, 1953.

Renal Artery Aneurysms

Cerny, J. C., Chang, C., and Fry, W. J.: Renal Artery Aneurysms, *Arch Surg,* **96:**653, 1968.

Garritano, A. P.: Aneurysm of the Renal Artery, *Am J Surg,* **94:**638, 1957.

Poutasse, E. F.: Renal Artery Aneurysm: Report of 12 Cases, Two Treated by Excision of the Aneurysm and Repair of Renal Artery, *J Urol,* **77:**697, 1957.

Traumatic Aneurysms

Crawford, E. S., DeBakey, M. E., and Cooley, D. A.: Surgical Considerations of Peripheral Arterial Aneurysms, *Arch Surg,* **78:**226, 1959.

Dickinson, E. H., Hood, R. H., and Spencer, F. C.: Traumatic Aneurysm of the Innominate Artery, *U.S. Armed Forces Med J,* **3:**1871, 1952.

Hughes, C. W., and Jahnke, E. J., Jr.: The Surgery of Traumatic Arteriovenous Fistulas and Aneurysms: A Five Year Follow-up Study of Lesions, *Ann Surg,* **148:**790, 1958.

Raynaud's Disease

Burton, E. E., Jr., et al.: Raynaud's Phenomenon: Treatment with Intraarterial Reserpine, *Cutis (N.Y.),* **9:**464, 1972.

DeTakats, G., and Fowler, E. F.: The Neurogenic Factor in Raynaud's Phenomenon, *Surgery,* **51:**9, 1962.

Farmer, R. G., Gifford, R. W., Jr., and Hines, E. A., Jr.: Raynaud's Disease with Sclerodactylia: A Follow-up Study of Seventy-one Patients, *Circulation,* **23:**13, 1961.

Gifford, R. W., Jr., Hines, E. A., Jr., and Craig, W. McK.: Sympathectomy for Raynaud's Phenomenon: Follow-up Study of 70 Women with Raynaud's Disease and 54 Women with Secondary Raynaud's Phenomenon, *Circulation,* **17:**5, 1958.

Kirtley, J. A., Riddell, D. H., Stoney, W. S., and Wright, J. K.: Cervicothoracic Sympathectomy in Neurovascular Abnormalities of the Upper Extremities: Experiences in 76 Patients with 104 Sympathectomies, *Ann Surg,* **165:**869, 1967.

Palumbo, L. T.: Anterior Transthoracic Approach for Upper Thoracic Sympathectomy, *Arch Surg,* **72:**659, 1956.

Varadi, D. P., and Lawrence, A. M.: Suppression of Raynaud's Phenomenon by Methyldopa, *Arch Intern Med,* **124:**13, 1969.

Willerson, J. T., and Decker, J. L.: Raynaud's Disease and Phenomenon, a Medical Approach, Am Heart J, **82:**572, 1971.

Uncommon Vasomotor Diseases

Estes, J. E.: Vasoconstrictive and Vasodilative Syndromes of the Extremities, *Mod Concepts Cardiovasc Dis,* **25:**355, 1956.

Lewis, T., and Landis, E. M.: Observations upon the Vascular Mechanism in Acrocyanosis, *Heart,* **15:**229, 1930.

Frostbite

Ervasti, E.: Frostbites of the Extremities and Their Sequelae: A Clinical Study, *Acta Chir Scand Suppl,* **299,** 1962.

Couch, N. P., Sullivan, J., and Crane, C.: Predictive Accuracy of Renal Vein Renin Activity in Surgery of Renovascular Hypertension, *Surgery,* **79:**70, 1976.

Golding, M. R., Martinez, A., deJong, P., Mendosa, M., Fries, C. C., Sawyer, P. N., Hennigar, G. R., and Wesolowski, S. A.: The Role of Sympathectomy in Frostbite, with a Review of 68 Cases, *Surgery,* **57:**774, 1965.

Mundth, E. D., Long, D. M., and Brown, R. B.: Treatment of Experimental Frostbite with Low Molecular Weight Dextran, *J Trauma,* **4:**246, 1964.

Penn, I., and Schwartz, S. I.: Evaluation of Low Molecular Weight Dextran in the Treatment of Frostbite, *J Trauma,* **4:**784, 1964.

Shumacker, H. B., Jr., and Kilman, J. W.: Sympathectomy in the Treatment of Frostbite, *Arch Surg,* **89:**575, 1964.

Simeone, F. A.: A Preliminary Follow-up Report on Cases of Cold Injury from World War II, in M. I. Ferrer, Cold Injury, *Trans 4th Conf Josiah Macy Jr. Found NY,* 1956, pp. 197-223.

Snider, R. L., and Porter, J. M.: Treatment of Experimental Frostbite with Intra-arterial Sympathetic Blocking Drugs, *Surgery,* **77(4):**557, 1975.

Chapter 22

Venous and Lymphatic Disease

by James A. DeWeese

VENOUS THROMBOSIS AND PULMONARY EMBOLISM

Venous thrombosis is a common direct and indirect cause of morbidity and mortality. During its acute phase, pain and swelling may be incapacitating. The threat of embolization of the thrombus to the pulmonary artery constantly exists. Postthrombotic scarring of the veins may lead to venous insufficiency with chronic discomfort and ulceration. The relatively frequent occurrence of venous thrombosis following operations or trauma arouses the surgeon's interest in the problem. In addition, operative intervention may be indicated to prevent or treat the complications of the thrombosis.

Etiology

Virchow, in the mid 1800s, first recognized three general causes of vascular thrombosis: stasis; injury to the vessel wall; and increased coagulability of the blood. Much more detailed information is now available regarding each of these general causes. Identification of the specific cause for a venous thrombosis seen in a given patient, however, may be very difficult. For example, a patient may present with a deep venous thrombosis following a long car ride, with-

out any history of trauma and without measurable abnormalities of coagulation factors. It is currently popular to incriminate stasis of blood as the etiologic agent. However, thousands of people may be in similar positions for equally long periods without developing thrombi. In other words, at the present time the reasons for thrombotic tendencies in certain patients are not known. The situations (as recorded by DeBakey and by Coon and Coller) in which thrombosis is more likely to occur, however, can be identified: following major injuries, following operations, during pregnancy, after previous thrombosis, with cancer, following long periods of sitting or bed rest, with infection, with varicose veins, and in obese females.

The incidences of at least minor thrombosis in these high-risk states have recently been emphasized in the studies of Kakkar. Using a radioiodinated fibrinogen test, venous thrombi were identified in the legs of 27.8 percent of elective surgery patients, in 54 percent of patients with hip fractures, in 3 percent of postpartum women, and in 19 percent of patients with myocardial infarction.

Pathophysiology

Venous thrombosis may be associated with an acute inflammatory response causing pain, local swelling, redness, tenderness, and tachycardia; the syndrome may then be labeled *thrombophlebitis*. Although acute inflammatory changes are present in the vein wall, bacteria are rarely present. The thrombus, on the other hand, may produce no local signs or symptoms and may be loosely attached to a vein wall which microscopically contains only a few chronic inflammatory cells; the condition may then be labeled *phlebothrombosis*. The differentiation of the two types of venous thrombosis, however, is only of academic interest. From a practical viewpoint it is the thrombus which is responsible for the early and late pathologic and physiologic changes, and it is the thrombus which may become a pulmonary embolus.

The thrombus initially causes obstruction of the vein; if the vein is a major one or if many veins are involved, there may be an increase in distal venous pressure. If the pressure in the venous capillaries becomes sufficiently high, water and solutes are not resorbed, and edema occurs. If the pressure becomes higher than local arterial pressures, blood flow ceases and venous gangrene occurs.

Some veins may remain obstructed following thrombosis; others may recanalize. In either case the venous valves are destroyed, leading to chronic venous valvular insufficiency. Thrombi which break loose in the moving venous bloodstream may be swept through the right heart and lodge in the pulmonary arteries as pulmonary emboli.

Although it is not important to differentiate thrombophlebitis and phlebothrombosis, it is important to differentiate superficial and deep venous thrombosis. Thrombi in the superficial veins rarely, if ever, embolize to the lung and can be treated symptomatically unless they propagate into a deep vein. Thrombi in the deep veins frequently embolize, cause permanent damage to the vein, and should be diagnosed early and treated aggressively.

Types of Venous Thrombosis

SUPERFICIAL VENOUS THROMBOSIS

SYMPTOMS. Patients usually complain of aching and swelling localized to a "knot" or "bump" on the leg or arm.

PHYSICAL FINDINGS. The diagnosis can usually be made by palpation of a firm mass or cord along the known course of a superficial vein. In the leg it is helpful to examine the patient in a standing position, since a distended or varicose vein may be palpated above and below the thrombus. In addition, redness, tenderness and *local* induration frequently are present (Fig. 22-1).

DIFFERENTIAL DIAGNOSIS. Insect bites may mimic superficial phlebitis but usually can be differentiated by the history of exposure, the presence of itching, and their lack of relation to the usual anatomic course of the significant superficial veins. Cellulitis or abscesses may at times be difficult to differentiate from thrombophlebitis, but in general, the more marked erythema, tenderness, and finally fluctuance define the diagnosis. The presence of a

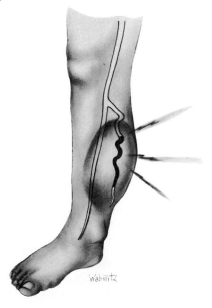

Fig. 22-1. Superficial venous thrombosis. There is usually redness, tenderness, and swelling surrounding a palpable thrombosed superficial vein.

red lymphatic streak or tender lymphadenopathy may also make the diagnosis of infection more obvious. It may be difficult to differentiate a subcutaneous hematoma from a bland thrombus unless a clear-cut history of trauma is present or the site of injury is away from the course of a major vein.

TREATMENT. Nonoperative management is the method of choice in patients with localized disease, since embolization almost never occurs and late morbidity is insignificant. However, superficial venous thrombosis may be present in patients with deep venous thrombosis. The presence of significant distal swelling or of tenderness over the deep veins should make one suspect deep venous thrombosis. A phlebogram may be helpful in ruling out deep-vein involvement.

Nonoperative Management. In general the acute discomfort of the process is over within a few days and symptomatic therapy is adequate. Bed rest is rarely indicated. Hot baths or compresses may be helpful in relieving discomfort. Propagation of the thrombus can usually be prevented by preventing venous stasis. The patient is advised to be either walking with elastic support or lying down with the legs elevated above the level of the heart. Sitting and standing are discouraged. Anticoagulants are not needed. The various enzymatic "clot dissolvers" have little if any effect on the outcome. Expensive and potentially dangerous "anti-inflammatory" drugs do not appear any more effective than aspirin. Antibiotics are not indicated, despite the presence of redness and tenderness, unless a septic cause is obvious.

Operative Treatment. *Ligation.* Thrombi in the greater saphenous system above the level of the knee may propagate into the common femoral vein, and any evidence of the ascension of such thrombi should be treated by ligation of the vein at the saphenofemoral junction, using local anesthesia. Similarly, the lesser saphenous vein may be ligated in the popliteal fossa.

Excision or Stripping. Veins which are the site of recurrent phlebitis and are stubbornly symptomatic can be ligated at their junctions with the deep system and then excised or in some instances "stripped," as suggested by Herrmann.

DEEP VENOUS THROMBOSIS

The deep veins are hidden within their muscular compartments, and the diagnosis of thrombosis, particularly of the bland type, may be difficult. DeBakey, as well as Barner and DeWeese, have reported that venous thrombosis is recognized prior to death in less than 55 percent of patients with fatal pulmonary emboli. This poor record exists despite the fact that the sources of approximately 85 percent of pulmonary emboli are the veins of the lower extremity, according to the experiences of Byrne and O'Neil, Ravdin and Kirby, and Short.

CLINICAL MANIFESTATIONS. Symptoms. There may be an aching pain, which is aggravated by muscular activity, at the site of a deep venous thrombus. In the presence of a massive thrombosis, there may be an extremely severe aching or cramping pain in the calf and thigh. At other times, however, only a feeling of "heaviness," accentuated by standing, will be noticed. Depending on the site of thrombosis, noticeable swelling may be absent, minimal, or marked. Few, if any, symptoms may be noticed by a patient confined to bed.

Physical Findings. The three signs most frequently described as being useful in the diagnosis of deep venous thrombosis include swelling, tenderness, and Homans' sign. Swelling must be searched for with the aid of a measuring tape; the eye cannot be trusted to tell small or even moderate differences in the size of two extremities. When properly looked for, this sign appears to be the most reliable in making a positive diagnosis of deep venous thrombosis. Tenderness over the thrombosed vein is also usually present if carefully looked for by palpation of the calf, popliteal space, adductor canal, and groin.

Homans was one of the first physicians to emphasize the importance of venous thrombosis in the legs as a source of pulmonary emboli. He popularized a simple test for detecting early thrombosis which is now known as Homans' sign. It is performed by dorsiflexing the foot and is considered positive if the patient complains of calf pain. It is thought that passive elongation of the gastrocnemius and soleus muscles causes irritative pain in the calf when the veins of the calf contain thrombi. Although this test is the easiest to perform, it is unfortunately the least reliable, according to the author's personal experience and to McLachlin et al.

The presence of superficial venous dilatation due to deep vein obstruction is considered by some to be a useful observation, but deep venous obstruction can be more objectively determined by measurement of the venous pressure.

Relation to Site of Involvement. The most frequent site of thrombosis is probably in the veins of the calf, particularly in the venous sinuses of the soleus muscle. Untreated, the thrombi may propagate to involve the femoral vein or even the iliac vein. Actually, however, thrombi that involve the iliac and femoral veins most frequently begin in the valve pockets of those veins and propagate distally, according to Gibbs and to McLachlin and Paterson. The signs and symptoms differ according to the veins involved, and it is worthwhile to consider each of the more common sites individually.

Calf Vein Thrombosis (Fig. 22-2*A*). Although the calf is the most frequent site of thrombosis, diagnosis in this location is probably the one most frequently missed. Calf pain and calf tenderness are usually present, but swelling is present in only 70 percent of cases. If present, the swelling is almost always minimal, the circumference of the involved calf and ankle being less than 1.5 cm greater than the normal limb. Homans' sign may or may not be present. The venous pressure is usually normal, which explains why there is little if any edema.

Femoral Vein Thrombosis (Fig. 22-2*B*). Although combined thrombosis of the calf veins and femoral veins is frequently seen, in some instances the thrombus is localized to the femoral vein. There is usually tenderness in the calf, popliteal region, or adductor canal. Swelling is usually present at the ankle and calf level, as might be predicted from the fact that the venous pressure is usually

two to five times normal. Homans' sign may or may not be present.

Iliofemoral Venous Thrombosis (Fig. 22-2*C*). Thrombosis which involves the iliac and femoral veins may also involve the calf veins, but it is frequently sharply localized to the iliofemoral or even iliac level. The left leg is involved two or three times more frequently than the right leg, apparently due to the longer course of the vein, its constriction by the right iliac artery, and the occasional presence of congenital webs at its junction with the vena cava. Iliofemoral venous thrombosis is the most dramatic of the thromboses, since pain, tenderness, and marked swelling of the entire leg are usually present. The venous pressure is considerably elevated, which explains the marked edema and also the bluish discoloration frequently observed during the early course of the process. When pain and cyanosis are present, the process may be termed *phlegmasia cerulea dolens*. This syndrome may progress to venous gangrene secondary to massive thrombosis of all the venous drainage of the part involved. Arterial spasm may also be present in some instances.

Pelvic Vein Thrombosis. Thrombosis of the pelvic veins, including the branches of the internal iliac veins, may be seen in women with pelvic inflammatory disease or in men with involvement of the prostatic plexus. The diagnosis is best made by pelvic or rectal examination plus a high degree of suspicion. Leg signs are not present unless the external and common iliac veins are also involved.

Primary Deep Venous Thrombosis of the Upper Extremity. Although this process of deep thrombosis may be seen in patients with congestive heart failure or with terminal carcinomas, it is more dramatic when it appears in otherwise normal individuals. It has been termed "Paget-Schroetter syndrome," "axillary vein thrombosis," or "effort thrombosis," since it most frequently occurs after some unusual muscular activity of the arm. In otherwise healthy patients, the thrombosis apparently originates in the subclavian vein at the point where the vein can be compressed between the first rib and clavicle. The diagnosis is usually made from swelling of the arm and the presence of tenderness over the axillary vein. Phlebography can confirm the diagnosis and determine the site of the obstruction.

SPECIAL TESTS. Special tests which are helpful in the diagnosis of deep venous thrombosis include (1) phlebography, (2) venous pressure measurements, and (3) noninvasive techniques.

Phlebography. Phlebography provides a means of visualizing the deep veins of the extremities (Fig. 22-3*A,B,C*). It is particularly useful in the patient with equivocal signs or symptoms, since it can provide ancillary evidence for or against the diagnosis of venous thrombosis. It is also helpful in determining the source of pulmonary emboli in patients without significant signs of venous thrombosis. It is helpful in determining the extent of thrombosis in patients who will undergo operative treatment, and it offers an objective means of evaluating any form of therapy.

Since the technique of phlebography was first described by Dos Santos and popularized by Bauer, there have been continued improvements in methods. The following tech-

CALF

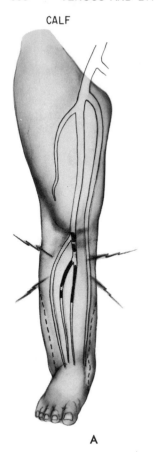

A

FEMORAL

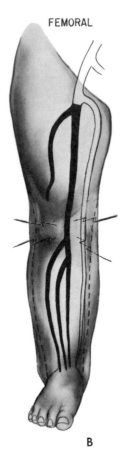

B

ILIO-FEMORAL

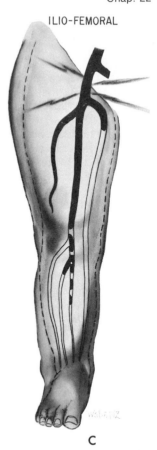

C

nique has been used in over 400 patients with suspected deep venous thrombosis and has been found safe, reliable, and relatively simple to perform.

1. A #21 scalp-vein needle is inserted into a superficial vein on the dorsum of the foot and a slow infusion of saline solution begun to maintain patency of the needle. With experience, a cut-down to expose a vein is rarely necessary.
2. The patient is placed in a semierect position 15 to 45° from the horizontal on a tilt table.
3. A snug rubber tourniquet is placed around the ankle.
4. Over a 1- to 2-minute period, 50 to 100 ml of an angiographic contrast material is injected.
5. Two sets of 14- by 34-in. radiographs are exposed about 30 seconds apart. If the patient was ambulatory prior to the test, he is asked to stand on his toes five times between exposures.

Thrombi are identified as globular or serpentine defects in well-opacified veins. Lack of filling of a vein is considered evidence of venous thrombosis, but only if clots are also seen in the vein, or if the lack of filling of a major vein is associated with visualization of numerous collateral veins at the same level.

Venous Pressure Measurements. Venous pressure is easily measured by inserting a needle into a superficial vein of the foot or ankle and connecting it to a saline solution manometer. The pressure should be compared with those in the other leg and the arm; the test will be positive in the presence of significant venous obstruction only early in the course of the disease before sufficient collaterals have developed.

Fig. 22-2. *A.* Calf vein thrombosis. Thrombosis is localized to veins of calf and popliteal vein. There is minimal, if any, swelling at level of ankle. Calf pain and tenderness are usually present. Homans' sign may or may not be present. *B.* Femoral vein thrombosis. There is thrombosis of femoral vein and usually associated thrombosis of calf vein. Swelling is usually present and extends to just above level of knee. Popliteal tenderness and calf tenderness may be present. Homans' sign may or may not be present. *C.* Iliofemoral venous thrombosis. There is thrombosis of iliac and proximal femoral vein, and frequently calf veins also are involved. Edema is present from foot to level of inguinal ligament. There is usually tenderness in groin and sometimes popliteal and calf tenderness. Homans' sign may or may not be present.

Noninvasive Technique. During the past few years, progress has been made in developing noninvasive methods for diagnosing venous thrombosis, i.e., those which require neither incision nor the introduction of needles into the involved extremity. These methods include isotope studies, the Doppler ultrasound technique, and an electrical impedance test, and presently are most valuable in screening patients. The ^{125}I-labeled fibrinogen test is particularly helpful in identifying small areas of thrombosis in the calf, while the Doppler technique is best for identifying significant venous occlusion in the femoral region. However, phlebography may still be necessary in cases where equivocal results are obtained by noninvasive methods, and it is still recognized as the most definitive test for the diagnosis of deep venous thrombosis.

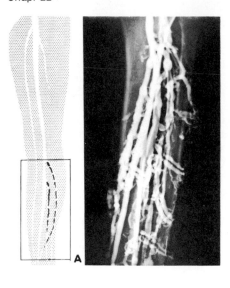

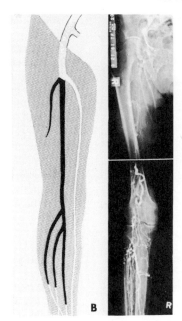

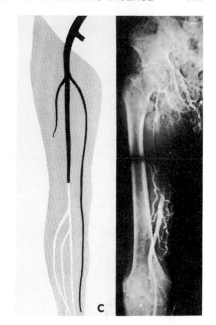

Fig. 22-3. *A.* Phlebogram demonstrating calf thrombi. Note areas of relative radiolucency in opaque-filled veins. *B.* Phlebogram demonstrating femoral and calf thrombosis. *C.* Phlebogram demonstrating iliofemoral thrombosis without involvement of calf vein. Note extensive formation of collaterals in upper thigh. (*From J. A. DeWeese and S. M. Rogoff, Surgery, 53:99, 1963.*)

Isotope Studies. Gomez et al. and Schwartz described methods for the scanning detection of venous thrombi in which radioactive elements are attached to thrombi by either tagged fibrinolytic enzymes or fibrinogen antibodies (Fig. 22-4). Kakkar and Browse more recently reported extensive clinical experience with the use of ^{125}I-labeled fibrinogen to detect venous thrombi.

Human fibrinogen is fractionated from the plasma of a restricted pool of accredited donors to minimize the risk of transmitting viral hepatitis. The fibrinogen is labeled with ^{125}I under sterile conditions and stored at $-20°C$. The patient is given 100 mg of sodium iodide 24 hours before the test to prevent excessive accumulation of the radioactive iodine in the thyroid gland. The test is performed by injecting 100 μCi of the labeled fibrinogen into a femoral vein, and the radioactivity over the legs is measured 2 hours later. Portable bedside equipment is available for this measurement.

The test cannot differentiate thrombi from an inflammatory fibrinous exudate and, therefore, is of no value for patients with superficial thrombophlebitis, recent operative incisions, traumatic wounds, hematomas, cellulitis, active arthritis, or primary lymphedema. In addition, thrombi cannot be accurately diagnosed in the upper thigh and pelvis because of high background counts.

The test is positive only during the active formation or propagation of a thrombus. It is most valuable in detecting the onset of thrombosis in patients at risk, such as during the postoperative period when the test is performed daily with corroborated accuracy in the range of 90 percent. Test accuracy falls to the 80 percent range when it is used for

patients with suspected established deep venous thrombosis.

Doppler Ultrasound Technique. The Doppler ultrasound blood velocity detector emits a sound beam which alters frequency when moving blood cells are encountered. When reflected and detected, the altered frequencies are amplified to drive a loudspeaker or for display on a recorder. Manual compression of the leg augments flow through the veins, producing characteristic "A" sounds for Doppler detection which are hampered or obliterated when venous thrombosis significantly occludes the deep veins.

Sigel et al. have had extensive experience with this technique. The ultrasound method recognized 78.1 percent of new thrombotic venous occlusion corroborated by phlebography. However, the technique cannot differentiate new occlusion from old, and small areas of thrombosis which do not significantly occlude major venous channels cannot be diagnosed.

Impedance Tests. Significant venous obstruction and replacement of blood by thrombi decreases the venous volume changes occurring with respiration. Liquid blood conducts electric currents, and instruments capable of measuring small changes in the electrical resistance of the leg can indirectly assess changes in venous volume. Wheeler et al. have devised an electrical impedance test which uses these principles to detect venous thrombosis indirectly. Cranley et al. use a modified plethysmographic technique for measurement of these venous volume changes.

Unfortunately, several factors other than patency of the major veins may influence venous volume changes. These include venous tone, extravascular compression which may vary with leg position, and adequacy of the collateral circulation, plus the ventilatory excursion. Dmochowski et al. were able to demonstrate only 53.5 percent test accu-

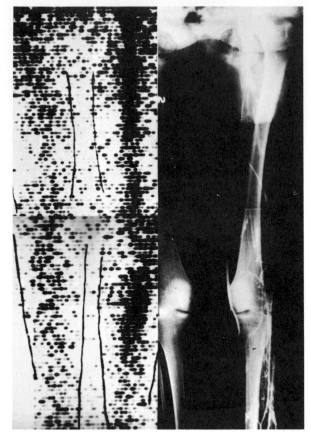

Fig. 22-4. Isotope scan following injection of ^{131}I-labeled anti-fibrinogen. Right leg normal; left leg shows femoral and popliteal thrombus confirmed by phlebography. (*From I. L. Spar, M. I. Varon, R. L. Goodland, and S. I. Schwartz, Arch Surg, 92:752, 1966.*)

racy, and for the present the test must be considered experimental.

DIFFERENTIAL DIAGNOSIS. Superficial venous thrombosis may be associated with deep venous thrombosis. This should be suspected if there is edema other than at the site of thrombosis; if there is calf, popliteal, or groin tenderness; and if Homans' sign is positive. A superficial thrombosis extending to the popliteal space or groin should also arouse suspicion.

A tear of the gastrocnemius, soleus, or plantaris muscles may mimic a calf vein thrombosis and cause edema, calf tenderness, and a positive Homans' sign. A history of a sharp stinging pain in the calf associated with walking or running and the appearance of ecchymosis over the calf and below the malleoli will usually make the diagnosis of muscle tear obvious. An effusion of the knee joint may produce distal edema and popliteal tenderness but can be differentiated from venous thrombosis by detection of a ballotable patella. A cellulitis in a lymphedematous limb may cause edema of the entire limb and tenderness, but the presence of erythema, high fever, and leukocytosis usually differentiates this condition from an iliofemoral or subclavian vein thrombosis. Phlebography is helpful in

differentiating deep venous thrombosis from all these conditions.

PREVENTION. Attempts to prevent venous thrombosis have been aimed at avoidance of venous intimal injury, minimization of venous stasis, and use of anticoagulants. Venous intimal injury can occur with rough handling of vessels during operations. This should be avoided. Hypertonic or irritating intravenous solutions should not be introduced into the veins of the lower extremity and are best given by an indwelling catheter in the high-flow superior vena cava.

Elevation of legs above heart level during operations and in the postoperative period can decrease venous stasis. Although the value of elastic stockings has been questioned, recent studies, including phlebographic studies of Lewis et al., confirm that properly fitting compression stockings can increase flow and clear stagnant blood from behind venous valves. In addition, Flanc and Tsapogas, in separate studies, have demonstrated significant decreases in thrombosis as diagnosed by phlebography or ^{125}I-labeled fibrinogen scanning techniques when elevation, elastic stockings, and bed exercises were used following major operations. Cotton and Roberts have demonstrated that either pedaling of the foot or the intermittent compression of the leg during an operation decreases the incidence of isotopically detectable deep venous thrombosis postoperatively.

Dextran, Coumadin, and heparin have been used in operative patients in hopes of preventing venous thrombosis. The occasional occurrence of pulmonary edema following a dextran fluid load and increased incidence of bleeding and hematomas following the use of dextran or anticoagulants has hampered their routine use. The use of small doses of heparin—5,000 units of concentrated aqueous heparin (25,000 units/ml) subcutaneously 2 hours prior to operation and every 8 hours thereafter for 7 days—was evaluated by Kakkar et al. in a prospective randomized trial. The miniheparin regimen significantly decreased the incidence of deep venous thrombosis as diagnosed by the ^{125}I-labeled fibrinogen test. Many surgeons are now using prophylactic heparin, 5,000 units twice or three times a day, and others are awaiting reports of larger clinical trials before committing their patients to the regimen.

TREATMENT. This generally relies on a medical regimen but occasionally requires an aggressive surgical approach.

Nonoperative Treatment. The primary aims of nonoperative therapy are to prevent thrombi which have already formed from embolizing and to prevent new thrombi from forming.

Bed Rest and Elevation. It is generally agreed that bed rest is indicated for approximately 7 days after onset or progression of symptoms to allow thrombi which are present to become firmly adherent to the vein wall. Bed rest prevents the fluctuations of pressure in the deep venous system that occur with walking. Unfortunately, it does not prevent the more marked fluctuations that may occur with straining during defecation, which all too commonly precipitates a fatal pulmonary embolus. Elevation of the legs above the level of the heart to a height equal to the venous pressure in a superficial vein of the foot, if possible, decreases the pressure in the veins and relieves the edema and pain. In addition, the increased rate of flow in the nondistended veins prevents venous stasis and formation of new thrombi. Elastic support is not required with adequate elevation. When ambulation begins, it is limited to walking with elastic support. The elastic support compresses the superficial veins, and, with walking, the rate of flow in the veins is increased and the venous pressure is kept at a minimum, which impedes the development of edema. Standing and sitting are initially forbidden, since the additional hydrostatic pressure in the veins would increase edema and discomfort. Limitation of the amount of standing and sitting may be necessary for periods of 3 to 6 months in patients with extensive iliofemoral venous thrombosis. In this way edema can be reduced until recanalization of the major veins and/or dilation of collaterals has occurred.

Anticoagulation. The propagation of established thrombi may be prevented with anticoagulants such as heparin or one of the coumarin derivatives.

Heparin. Heparin is believed to prevent thrombus formation by inhibiting the formation of thromboplastin and acting as an antithrombin to inactivate thrombin. Its effect can be determined by measuring the whole blood clotting time and partial thromboplastin time (PTT). Propagation of thrombi can be prevented if the clotting time or the PTT is at least twice normal. Such times can be achieved by the administration of aqueous heparin intravenously, either continuously or every 4 hours in 5,000- to 10,000-unit amounts. Similar results can be obtained by administering 15,000 to 20,000 units of concentrated aqueous heparin (20,000 units/ml) into the deep fat of the abdominal wall every 12 hours. Continuous intravenous administration is the preferred method if a reliable infuser is available. Heparin therapy is advised for varying lengths of time, but it seems reasonable to use it for a period of 7 days, until the thrombi have become firmly adherent to the vein; the amounts given are then tapered off over a 3- to 5-day period. If the drug is discontinued abruptly, new thrombosis is frequently observed within the next few days. This is described as "heparin rebound" by some but may merely be a return of a pretreatment thrombotic tendency. It is advisable to continue anticoagulant therapy with the coumarin derivatives after discontinuing heparin. Possible complications of heparin therapy are bleeding and arterial emboli. Bleeding is most apt to occur in fresh surgical wounds. If necessary the heparin effect can be reversed by injecting protamine sulfate intravenously in 50- to 100-mg amounts. Platelet emboli have been observed by Roberts et al. in patients receiving heparin, but at this time the mechanism is unknown.

Controlled and comparative studies indicate that heparin therapy is superior to no anticoagulation but that pulmonary emboli may still occur. The incidence of pulmonary emboli in patients with venous thrombosis during treatment with heparin is variously reported as 0.9 to 7.7 percent.

Coumarin Derivatives. The coumarin derivatives may interfere with four factors in the clotting mechanism, but the effect of clinical importance is its reduction of the plasma concentration of prothrombin. Its effect can therefore be determined by measuring the prothrombin time, which must be less than 10 percent of normal to inhibit the propagation of thrombi as effectively as heparin does. This, unfortunately, is the level at which bleeding complications are most likely to occur. However, somewhat higher prothrombin times are apparently able to prevent formation of new thrombi. Coumarin derivatives can be administered orally and at the present time are the drugs of choice for prophylactic therapy or long-term therapy following initial heparin therapy. It appears logical to continue anticoagulation with the coumarin derivatives for approximately 4 weeks after an acute venous thrombosis or pulmonary embolism, since recurrence is most likely within that period. Patients with iliofemoral venous thrombosis may be maintained on therapy for 6 months after the onset, since recurrence is most likely during this period when venous stasis is still being decreased by the enlargement of collaterals.

Other Medications. The administration of fibrinolytic drugs or dextran for the treatment of venous thrombosis shows some promise. At present, however, it would seem best to consider their use experimental until further clinical studies are available.

Operative Treatment. Thrombi can be successfully removed from major veins such as the subclavian, iliac, or femoral. Iliofemoral venous thrombectomy is performed through an incision in the groin, using a local anesthetic (Fig. 22-5), via a femoral venotomy. The iliac system is cleared with forceps and suction applied to polyethylene tubing or long fine catheters with an inflatable balloon on

Fig. 22-5. Venous thrombectomy. (*Courtesy of C. Rob and R. Smith.*)

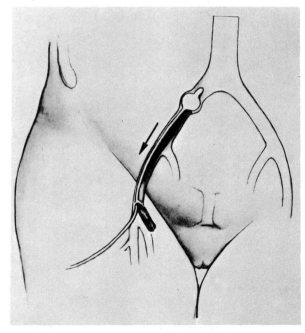

the end. Thrombi can be removed from the femoral vein by the same method plus tight wrapping of the leg with an elastic bandage. The venotomy is then closed with fine arterial suture. In general, venous interruptions are not necessary. Heparin is administered after the operation. The best results are obtained in patients operated on within 1 week of onset and in those in whom the thrombus is segmental in nature as determined by an ascending phlebogram. Care must be taken not to push thrombi into the moving flow of blood in the common iliac vein or inferior vena cava, but pulmonary embolization has rarely if ever occurred during the operation. Despite the use of heparin, thrombosis occasionally recurs, probably secondarily to the mechanical or inflammatory processes which initiated the thrombosis originally. In general, thrombectomy has successfully decreased the early and late morbidity of massive venous thrombosis, and phlebograms have demonstrated restoration of patent veins with normal valves in at least one-third of patients. Mavor et al. demonstrated 85 percent of 42 iliac veins to be patent 14 days after successful venous thrombectomy.

Subclavian Venous Thrombosis. Primary subclavian venous thrombosis is probably secondary to localized thrombosis of the vein at the site where the vein passes between the clavicle and first rib. This theory is supported by the facts that patients may be seen with intermittent venous obstruction at this site and that this obstruction may be relieved by removal of the first rib or clavicle. This theory

Fig. 22-6. Chest x-ray demonstrating peripheral wedge-shaped area of infarction.

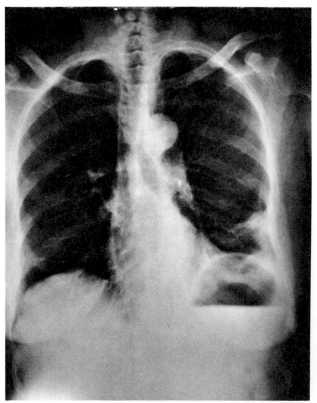

is further supported by observations at the time of subclavian venous thrombectomy that the older thrombi and venous scarring are also found at the point where the vein passes between the clavicle and first rib. Thrombectomy with removal of the clavicle or first rib may provide definitive therapy. Patients who have had a subclavian venous thrombosis develop large collaterals between the axillary vein and the internal jugular venous system, which also passes between the clavicle and first rib. These collaterals may be obstructed by hyperextension of the arm or hyperabduction of the shoulder, and this condition may also be relieved by removal of the clavicle or first rib.

Pulmonary Emboli

INCIDENCE. Complete autopsy studies by Hunter et al. indicate that deep venous thrombi may be found in approximately 50 percent of patients who die in a hospital. Approximately 1 in 5 of these patients demonstrated nonfatal emboli, while 1 in 10 had fatal emboli.

PATHOPHYSIOLOGY. Thrombi, which break loose from their point of origin, pass through the right atrium and ventricle and lodge in the pulmonary arteries. Large thrombi which lodge in major pulmonary arteries may cause immediate death secondary to vasovagal shock, right ventricular failure, and inadequate transfer of oxygen and carbon dioxide in the pulmonary circulation. It is debatable whether small emboli lodging in a lobar or segmental artery can cause death, and if so, by what mechanisms. It is postulated, and supported by some laboratory data, that intense bronchoconstriction and vasoconstriction might explain such an occurrence. Such single small emboli may also result in infarctions. Infection and even abscesses and empyema may ensue. Multiple small emboli may eventually produce enough arterial obstruction to cause pulmonary hypertension and right ventricular failure.

Various autopsy series indicate that the lower extremity (including the iliac veins) is the source of pulmonary emboli in approximately 85 percent of patients. Approximately 10 percent of emboli arise from the right atrium. The remaining 5 percent come from the pelvic veins, vena cava, or upper extremities.

SYMPTOMS. Classically, patients with pulmonary emboli complain of dyspnea, pain, and hemoptysis. The dyspnea is usually the first and may be the only symptom. There may be crushing substernal pain in the presence of a massive embolus lodged in the main pulmonary artery. The pain may be sharp, localized, and stabbing, occurring with breathing, in the presence of a peripheral infarct. This is referred to as *pleuritic* pain. Epigastric pain is occasionally described. Hemoptysis, with coughing up of small flecks or even massive amounts of blood, may occur in the presence of infarction of segments of the lung.

PHYSICAL FINDINGS. Tachycardia is frequently observed, and tachypnea is common. Shock is an ominous sign of a massive embolus. Cyanosis may be present if there is a massive embolus. Splinting of the chest and pleural friction rubs are observed in the presence of peripheral infarcts. Râles may be heard in the region of infiltrates or may be bilateral and bubbling with secondary pulmonary edema. Small pleural effusions are frequently present and sometimes large enough to be recognized on examination.

Less than 50 percent of all pulmonary embolisms found at autopsy had been suspected before death. A retrospective study by Coon and Coller of patients later shown at autopsy to have pulmonary emboli indicates the following frequency of certain signs and symptoms: dyspnea, 58 percent; chest pain, 22 percent; hemoptysis, 11 percent; shock, 28 percent; friction rub, 16 percent. Epigastric pain, cough, fever, and cyanosis are less frequently seen. The classic triad of dyspnea, pain, and hemoptysis was observed in only 3 percent of the patients, and 27 percent appeared to have had no signs or symptoms.

SPECIAL TESTS. Chest X-rays. Since pulmonary emboli do not always cause infarction, the wedge-shaped infiltrate may not be seen (Fig. 22-6). Other signs such as areas of decreased vascularity, dilated pulmonary arteries, or pleural fluid may be found. Stein et al. state that the diagnosis can be suspected from x-rays in approximately 50 percent of patients with pulmonary emboli.

Electrocardiogram. The classic finding of right heart strain is usually not present. However, Henderson reports some significant abnormality concomitant with the acute event in over 60 percent of patients.

Chemical Tests. The triad of elevated serum lactic dehydrogenase (LDH) and serum bilirubin in the presence of normal serum glutamic oxalacetic transaminase (SGOT) level is no longer considered reliable in the diagnosis of pulmonary embolism. Szucs et al. found the triad to be positive in only 18 percent of pulmonary emboli proved by pulmonary arteriogram.

Pulmonary Angiograms. Pulmonary angiography provides the most effective means of diagnosing pulmonary emboli. It is indicated in patients with unexplained pulmonary infiltrates and in those with recurrent symptoms suggestive of pulmonary emboli. It is most helpful in diagnosing the presence and extent of a massive pulmonary embolus. The procedure may be performed by rapidly injecting a radiopaque material into the right atrium or main pulmonary artery through a catheter threaded into position through a peripheral vein. It can also be performed by the simultaneous rapid injection of a bolus of radiopaque material through needles placed in superficial veins in both arms. Visualization of the significant pulmonary arteries can be obtained by either technique, and occlusion of the arteries can be identified by the lack of filling (Fig. 22-7).

Gas Analysis. Pulmonary arterial obstruction with decreased perfusion of the lung results in a decrease in the alveolar carbon dioxide tension (P_{CO_2}). Therefore, the gradient between the brachial arterial P_{CO_2} and the end-tidal ("alveolar") P_{CO_2}, which is usually minimal, is increased in the presence of significant pulmonary emboli.

Radioisotope Scanning. The rapid intravenous injection of radioactive substances such as [131]I- tagged macroaggregated albumin accompanied by scintillation scanning of the chest may be used to diagnose areas of decreased vascularity in the lung field. Obstruction of the pulmonary

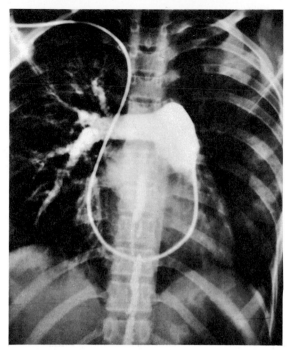

Fig. 22-7. Pulmonary angiogram demonstrating absence of filling of left pulmonary arterial branches, indicative of large embolus obstructing left main pulmonary artery.

arteries by emboli usually results in the appearance of crescent-shaped defects along the lateral borders of the lung (Fig. 22-8). A normal ventilation scan can provide confirmatory evidence that the perfusion scan is demonstrating pulmonary emboli.

DIFFERENTIAL DIAGNOSIS. Inflammatory infiltrates of the lung may mimic recurrent pulmonary emboli, particularly on the chest roentgenogram. Significant fever, leukocytosis, and positive sputum cultures usually differentiate the inflammatory from the embolic lesions. Pulmonary edema may result from pulmonary emboli as well as heart disease. The differentiation is easy only in the absence of heart disease or murmurs. It is frequently difficult to differentiate a massive pulmonary embolism from acute myocardial infarction, and in this situation it may be necessary to perform pulmonary angiography to make an accurate diagnosis.

TREATMENT. Venous Interruption. It is generally agreed that interruption of the veins of the lower extremity is indicated if a pulmonary embolus occurs in a patient receiving adequate anticoagulant therapy or in one for whom anticoagulant therapy is contraindicated. In some centers, venous interruptions are even performed prophylactically or instead of administering anticoagulants. The interruption, which can be performed at the femoral vein level if the thrombi are localized in the distal veins, would be the procedure of choice in the desperately ill patient. Phlebography is routinely used in the author's clinic to assist in localizing the thrombi. The interruption should always be performed at the vena cava level in the presence of pelvic vein or iliac vein thrombosis.

Ligation or Division. Ligation or division of the femoral

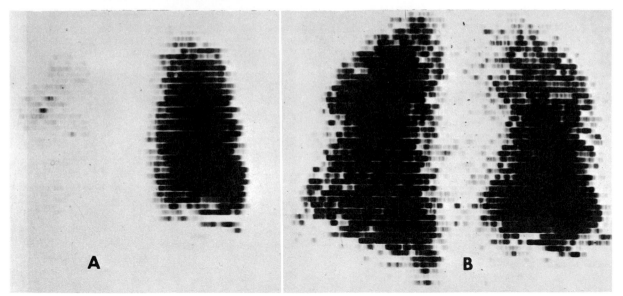

Fig. 22-8. Radioisotope scans following intravenous injection of macroaggregated albumin tagged with [131]I. *A.* Massive pulmonary embolus to right lung. *B.* Small bilateral emboli evidenced by crescent-shaped defects.

vein is variously performed below the entrance of the deep femoral vein or below the entrance of the greater saphenous vein. The postligation sequelae are less severe if only the superficial femoral vein is ligated. However, the deep femoral vein is also frequently the site of thrombosis, and in such instances ligation of the superficial femoral vein would offer no protection. Donaldson et al. report that approximately 4 percent of patients treated by femoral vein interruption alone develop pulmonary emboli. This is an incidence approximately equal to that following anticoagulation therapy alone.

Ligation or division of the vena cava should be performed just distal to the right renal vein to prevent forming a pocket in which thrombi might develop. The operation requires a general or spinal anesthetic, as opposed to femoral vein ligation, which can be performed under local anesthesia. The incidence of pulmonary embolism following this procedure is generally lower than the reported incidence following femoral vein ligation. Its routine use in desperately ill patients, however, can result in an increased mortality rate which may equal that from pulmonary embolism following femoral vein ligation.

The ligation of a vein in which there is distal venous thrombosis usually results in propagation of the thrombus to the site of the ligature. Recurrent phlebitis, pain, edema, and ulceration may ensue. Adams and DeWeese report a 30 to 35 percent incidence of these distressing postligation sequelae.

Partial Vein Interruption. In the hope of preventing postligation sequelae, partial interruptions of the femoral vein or inferior vena cava have been performed to allow normal venous flow and yet trap potential pulmonary emboli (Figs. 22-9, 22-10). The methods described include creation of a grid filter of silk sutures [DeWeese], compartmentalization of the vein with sutures [Spencer et al.], constriction of the vein with a plastic clip [Moretz], and compartmentalization of the vein with a plastic clip having serrated edges [Miles et al.]. Although thrombosis may occur at the site of the partial interruption or the vein may be occluded by a trapped embolus, the results of such an occurrence would be no worse than if the vein were ligated. Mobin-Uddin et al. devised a filter which can be introduced under local anesthesia through a small incision into the jugular vein. Under fluoroscopic control, the collapsed filter is passed to the lower vena cava on the tip of a catheter. As the catheter is withdrawn, the filter is dislodged, opens like an umbrella, and is impinged against the wall of the vena cava distal to the renal vein. However, the umbrella can be misplaced or subsequently dislodged, and at present it appears to be ideally suited for the desperately ill patient who requires interruption at the vena cava level. Greenfield has described the use of an intraluminal steel wire filter that can be introduced through the femoral vein and positioned in the inferior vena cava.

Fig. 22-9. Partial interruption of inferior vena cava: grid and compartmentalization.

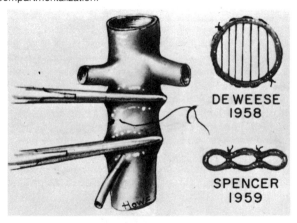

DE WEESE
1958

SPENCER
1959

Table 22-1. VENA CAVA INTERRUPTIONS:
COMPARISON OF LIGATIONS AND
PARTIAL INTERRUPTIONS*

	Ligation	Partial interruptions
Operations	1,159	569
Operative mortality	14.0%	10.3%
Fatal emboli.	1.3%	0.7%
Fatal shock	2.9%	0
Nonfatal emboli	4.1%	6.7%
Patent vena cava.	0†	72.0%†
Disabling symptoms	23.0%‡	7.0%‡

*A summary of 30 reports.
†In patients who had postoperative vena cavagrams.
‡When late follow-up information was available.

Comparison of the reported results of all types of vena cava interruption indicates a slightly higher incidence of nonfatal pulmonary emboli following partial interruption than following ligation (6.7 versus 4.1 percent) (Table 22-1). The incidence of fatal emboli following both procedures is about 1 percent. However, fatal shock secondary to ligation of the vena cava with sudden decrease in venous return or massive distal venous thrombosis occurred in 2.9 percent of cases, compared to no observed occurrence following partial interruption.

When postoperative vena cavagrams are performed following partial interruptions, at least 70 percent are patent, and the incidence of significant late postphlebitic sequelae is only 7 percent following partial interruption compared to 23 percent following ligation. In addition, the large collaterals observed by Parrish et al. following vena cava ligation are capable of transmitting fatal pulmonary emboli from the lower extremities within a few weeks after operation.

Partial interruption of the femoral veins was also found by Adams et al. to be at least as effective as ligation in preventing pulmonary embolism and associated with less late extremity morbidity.

Urokinase Therapy. Urokinase activates the available plasminogen which causes lysis of thrombi. Treatment of pulmonary embolism with materials of high specific activity which are much less toxic and pyrogenic than previously available plasminogen activators was evaluated in a cooperative study. Twelve-hour urokinase infusion followed by at least 5 days of heparin was more effective than heparin alone in lysing thrombi, as seen by significantly greater improvement in pulmonary arteriograms, lung scans, and right heart pressure measurements. Unfortunately, bleeding complications were sufficiently frequent and severe that Sautter et al. felt urokinase therapy to be contraindicated within 10 days of childbirth or any operation within the major body cavity. Severe systemic hypertension, a recent cerebrovascular accident, active gastrointestinal bleeding, renal or hepatic insufficiency, active rheumatic disease, bacterial endocarditis, a history of nephritis, or pregnancy at any stage were also considered contraindications. No significant differences in the rate of pulmonary embolism recurrence or in the 2-week mortality rate were observed. The report concluded that further evaluation of urokinase in the treatment of pulmonary thromboembolism is indicated before specific therapeutic recommendations can be made.

Pulmonary Embolectomy. Approximately 95 percent of patients with a pulmonary embolism massive enough to cause hypotension die. Although most of them die within a few minutes, at least 25 percent live longer than 1 hour. In 1908 Trendelenburg first advocated the emergency removal of large emboli from the pulmonary artery. From 1908 to 1962 only 17 survivors of such a procedure were reported. Since the development of cardiopulmonary bypass, however, pulmonary embolectomies are performed much more frequently. With this technique the main pulmonary arteries can be opened leisurely and emboli removed. Peripheral emboli can also be evacuated by massaging the lung and by the use of catheters to which suction is applied. It may be possible to use a portable temporary

Fig. 22-10. Partial interruption of inferior vena cava using serrated clip. *A.* Transperitoneal approach is preferred to permit high interruption of vena cava and concomitant ligation of the left spermatic or ovarian veins. *B.* Kocher maneuver. *C.* Vena cava cleared immediately below renal veins. *D.* Clip applied. *E.* Clip closed. *F.* Final position of clip in the immediate infrarenal region to prevent cul-de-sac. (*From J. T. Adams and J. A. DeWeese, Surg Gynecol Obstet, 123:1087, 1966.*)

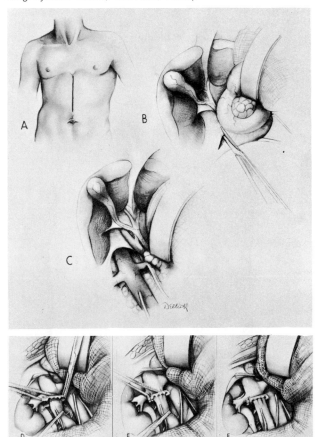

cardiopulmonary bypass to sustain desperately ill patients until they can be transported to the operating room. The studies of Sautter et al. suggest that urokinase therapy is preferable to pulmonary embolectomy for patients recovering from shock. Patients with cardiac arrest or unresponsive shock are still candidates for emergency cardiopulmonary bypass and pulmonary embolectomy.

VENOUS INSUFFICIENCY AND VENOUS ULCERS

There are three conditions of the veins of the lower extremities associated with venous ulcers. These are varicose veins, incompetent perforators, and deep venous abnormalities. Venous ulcers usually appear in the presence of one, two or all three of these conditions, and they are therefore best discussed together. The abnormality common to all is reflux of blood from the deficiency or absence of competent valves.

Hippocrates (460–377 B.C.) is credited with first noting the association between varicose veins and ulcers of the leg and recommending the use of compression bandages in their treatment. However, many centuries elapsed before the role of deep venous abnormalities in the etiology of venous ulcers was appreciated. Gay and Homans demonstrated the relation between postthrombotic changes including the destruction of venous valves, and venous ulcers. More recently Linton and also Dodd and Cockett have emphasized the role of the incompetent perforator in causing ankle ulceration.

Anatomy and Physiology

The veins of the lower extremity consist of superficial veins, deep veins, and perforating veins which join the superficial and deep systems. The superficial veins consist of the greater saphenous and lesser saphenous veins. The greater saphenous vein begins on the dorsum of the foot, passes *anterior* to the medial malleolus, ascends the medial calf and thigh lying close to the deep fascia, and enters the common femoral vein in the groin through the fossa ovalis. Several smaller veins join the greater saphenous vein along its course. The important branches, clinically, include the anterior and posterior branches of the lower leg, which enter the major vein in the upper medial calf region, and the lateral and medial branches of the upper leg, which join the saphenous in the upper thigh (Fig. 22-11*A*). The lesser saphenous vein begins posterior to the lateral malleolus, ascends the posterior calf, where it pierces the deep fascia, usually near the popliteal fossa, and enters the popliteal vein (Fig. 22-11*B*).

The deep veins, in general, follow the course of the major arteries and carry the same names. In the lower leg, however, the veins are routinely paired. The paired anterior tibial, posterior tibial, and peroneal veins join to form the popliteal vein in the region of the knee. The popliteal vein passes beneath the adductor tendon, where it becomes the superficial femoral vein and is joined by the deep femoral vein in the upper thigh to become the common femoral vein. The common femoral veins become the external iliac veins as they pass beneath the inguinal ligament and are joined in the pelvis by the internal iliac

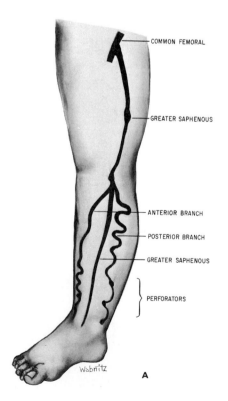

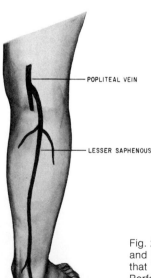

Fig. 22-11. *A*. Usual course of greater saphenous vein and its major branches in lower leg, emphasizing fact that branch varicosities are the ones usually seen. Perforating veins, posterior and superior to medial malleoli, are indicated. *B*. Usual course of lesser saphenous vein in lower leg.

veins to become the common iliac veins; these veins join to become the inferior vena cava.

There are numerous veins perforating the deep fascia connecting the superficial and deep veins. The most constant and clinically important of these perforators are those posterior and superior to the medial malleoli. These perforators, which usually are three in number, connect the posterior branch of the greater saphenous vein to the paired posterior tibial veins. One perforator usually lies posterior to the medial malleolus, the second is 5 to 10 cm superior to the first, and the third is 5 to 10 cm higher (Fig. 22-11*A*). A similar perforator connects the lesser saphenous and peroneal veins posterior and superior to the lateral malleolus.

Normal veins contain bicuspid valves, which, although sometimes found in other areas, are almost always just distal to major branches. In the upper leg only a few valves are found, whereas in the lower leg they are numerous in both the superficial and deep systems. The valves are oriented to permit flow of blood superiorly in the superficial and deep veins. More important is the fact that the valves in the perforators normally allow flow only from the superficial to the deep veins (Fig. 22-12).

There is normally a progressive decrease in mean pressure in the bloodstream beginning in the left ventricle and ending in the right atrium. It is this force from behind, or vis a tergo, that guarantees the continued flow of blood in the venous system. The actual pressure in any one vessel, however, is also dependent on the effect of gravity. In the standing resting position, therefore, the actual pressure in any vein includes a hydrostatic pressure approximately equivalent to the distance between the vein and the heart. The actual pressures in the arteries are also increased by hydrostatic pressure, and venous flow continues.

In addition to vis a tergo, venous return is aided by muscular action and possibly by respiration. Contraction of the calf muscles, for example, squeezes blood from the intramuscular veins into the deep veins. In addition, the veins which pass through the relatively rigid fascial compartment about the muscle are also compressed by the muscle. The combined result is an increase in pressure and flow in the popliteal vein and increased venous return with muscular contraction. During relaxation of the muscles the popliteal venous pressure falls below the resting pressure, and increased emptying of the superficial veins into the deep veins occurs, so that with repeated muscular activity the quantity of blood in the superficial veins decreases and superficial venous pressure decreases to below normal resting pressures. It must be emphasized that these normal variations in venous pressure and flow are dependent upon normal valves. Valves in the calf veins prevent reflux of blood distad when the venous pressure is increased by muscle contraction. Valves in the perforators prevent reflux of blood from the deep into the superficial veins during muscular contraction. The negative intrathoracic pressure which is accentuated by inspiration is believed by some to increase venous return. This positive effect is probably offset by the increased abdominal pressure secondary to descent of the diaphragm, which slows venous return.

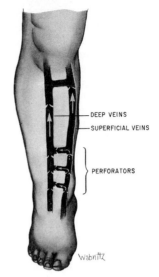

Fig. 22-12. Orientation of valves and flow of blood in superficial, deep, and perforating veins of lower leg.

Etiology of Venous Insufficiency

The causes of venous insufficiency are varicose veins, incompetent perforators, and deep vein abnormalities.

VARICOSE VEINS. The term *varicose veins* is usually applied to dilated, tortuous, elongated branches of the greater and lesser saphenous veins. These branches are quite superficial and are, therefore, most easily seen. The same changes occur to a much lesser extent in the greater and lesser saphenous veins themselves. The important abnormality in both the branches and the major superficial veins is the incompetency of their valves.

It is not known whether the valvular incompetency is the cause of the dilatation of the veins in varicosities or whether the dilatation of the valvular ring occurs first and causes secondary valvular incompetence. There are probably several causes of varicose veins. The rare presence of varicose veins in very small children without other visible arterial and venous malformations indicates that they may be congenital. The occurrence of severe varicosities in several members of a family suggests that heredity may be important in some cases. The frequent appearance of varicosities during pregnancy is well known, but it is not known whether hormonal influence, increased pelvic venous blood flow, or the mechanical effect of the enlarged uterus is the primary cause of these varicosities. The appearance of varicose veins in patients with congenital or acquired arteriovenous shunts implicates these as causative factors. The appearance of branch varicosities following superficial venous thrombosis indicates that trapping and fragmentation of the valves by the thrombus as it retracts to the wall and becomes organized is of importance in some instances. The predilection of varicose veins for the lower extremities in human beings, as opposed to quadrupeds, and for people in professions requiring long periods of standing indicates that the hydrostatic pressure in the veins of the lower extremities in the standing resting position aggravates and may actually cause varicosities.

INCOMPETENT PERFORATORS. There are numerous perforators between the superficial and deep veins. The largest and most constant are those posterior and superior to the medial and lateral malleoli. Normally these perforators cannot be demonstrated clinically. When their valves are incompetent, however, they become dilated and may form rather large localized dilatations at their junctions with the superficial vein. Defects in the deep fascia of the leg at the site where the dilated perforators pierce the fascia may be palpated. The frequent occurrence of incompetent perforators following deep venous thrombosis suggests that the valvular damage in these instances is secondary to recanalization of the perforators. Incompetent perforators, however, may be found in patients without known previous venous thrombosis but with varicose veins. It is likely, therefore, that the factors which cause venous dilatation and valvular incompetency in the valves of other veins may also cause incompetency of the valves of the perforating veins.

DEEP VEIN ABNORMALITIES. The most common abnormalities of the deep veins result from thrombosis of the veins. Following thrombosis, the major deep veins may become patent by gross recanalization, or they may remain functionally occluded, with only microscopic recanalization. With gross recanalization, the veins have the phlebographic appearance of irregular walled valveless tubes. If the veins remain occluded, numerous dilated collaterals *without apparent valves* are visualized. Examination of the occluded major veins demonstrates only microscopic recanalization. The deficiency or absence of valves and the dilatation of the deep veins is observed also in many patients with complicated varicose vein problems. This suggests that the congenital or familial causes of varicosities may also cause deep vein abnormalities.

Symptoms of Venous Insufficiency

The symptoms most frequently attributed to venous insufficiency of the lower extremities include aching, swelling, and night cramps.

An "aching" discomfort in the lower legs is frequently described by patients with severe venous insufficiency. With lesser degrees of insufficiency, "tenderness" of the legs or a "heaviness" may be described. The discomfort may occur soon after arising in the morning but usually begins after a period of relatively inactive standing or sitting. In many women the symptoms are worse just before and during the first part of the menstrual period. The symptoms are relieved by elevation of the legs.

Edema of the lower leg may also occur in venous insufficiency. Although it may occur with varicose veins alone, it is almost always seen in patients with deep venous abnormalities and incompetent perforators. It usually appears during the course of the day and is aggravated by prolonged standing or sitting. It usually disappears or is markedly decreased during a night's sleep.

The explanation for the heaviness, tiredness, and aching is the increase in the weight of the lower extremities secondary to an increase in volume of blood and edema fluid. In a normal individual the erect position is associated with an increased volume of blood in the legs. This volume is increased in venous insufficiency, where dilated veins increase the potential storage space and incompetent valves hinder venous return. Normally the erect position is also associated with an increased amount of interstitial fluid, transferred across the capillary membrane. This fluid is normally resorbed by the capillaries or lymphatics. Resorption by the veins is primarily due to the osmotic force exerted by the intravascular protein, but an increase in venous pressure can overcome the osmotic force and prevent resorption. The venous pressure at the ankle in the normal erect individual is sufficient to prevent resorption, and an increase in interstitial fluid is observed. In normal individuals, however, the venous pressure is markedly decreased by the frequent muscular contractions occurring with daily living. The same exercise in patients with venous insufficiency causes lesser decreases in the pressure and hence more significant increases in interstitial fluid (or edema). Lymphatic abnormalities can also decrease the resorption of the interstitial fluid. Such abnormalities may be observed in patients following venous thrombosis.

Night cramps are due to sustained contractions of muscles and most frequently occur in the muscles of the calf and feet. They usually appear after a few hours of sleep. They are relieved by massage or by standing and walking. Night cramps may be associated with a number of other abnormalities besides venous insufficiency. Night cramps secondary to venous insufficiency, however, can be relieved by proper management. The underlying cause of the increased muscular irritability or increased muscular stimulation is unknown.

Physical Findings

The changes which may be observed in patients with venous insufficiency include edema, brawny induration, brownish discoloration, dermatitis, and ulceration.

Edema may not be observed in patients with varicose veins, but it is almost always present to some degree in patients with deep vein pathologic conditions and incompetent perforators. It may be soft and pitting initially and may completely disappear overnight. In the presence of long-standing venous insufficiency, however, the edema becomes more firm and may decrease slowly and minimally with elevation. It then acquires a "woody" feeling, termed *brawny induration,* due to increased connective tissue in the subcutaneous tissue. This scarring may be secondary to excess protein in the interstitial tissue (see section below on lymphedema) or to repeated trauma, infection, and phlebitis.

Brown pigmentation of the lower leg is frequently observed in long-standing venous insufficiency, particularly about healed ulcers. It is known to be secondary to hemosiderin in the subcutaneous tissue, presumably derived from the breakdown of extravasated blood.

Various types of dermatitis may be seen in patients with venous insufficiency. Dryness and scaling with some pruritis may be seen over prominent varices, particularly at the ankle level. Although the cause is unknown, this condition is apparently related to the underlying venous abnormalities, since it will disappear with treatment of the venous insufficiency alone. Skin infections secondary to dermatophytosis (athlete's foot) may be seen. The most frequent dermatitis, however, is secondary to local medications. The allergic dermatitis may be particularly difficult to control.

Venous ulcers are almost always found in the lower third of the lower leg and are particularly common posterior and superior to the medial and lateral malleoli (Fig. 22-13). Characteristically they are shallow ulcerations with surrounding rims of bluish discoloration and erythema. They may penetrate to the level of the deep fascia or tendons, but not through them. They can, however, erode veins or even arteries. They may on occasion encircle the leg.

The ulcers may appear spontaneously or follow trivial trauma. The underlying problem, however, is venous insufficiency, a point frequently forgotten by the patient and ignored by the physician treating him. Their occurrence in the ankle region incriminates the high venous pressure of the superficial veins in that region as a prime cause. Further support for this hypothesis is the fact that ulcerations are more common in patients with deep vein abnormalities and incompetent perforators than in patients with varicose veins alone. The high venous pressure results in localized varicosities and edema, with consequent increased deposition of fibrous tissue. A localized area of redness, tenderness, and brawny induration frequently precedes an ulcer. Dodd and Cockett present interesting pathologic material to support the thesis that this preulcer state is due to thrombosis of small end veins in the subcutaneous tissue resulting in fat necrosis. A contusion, laceration, or necrosis of the skin over this area results in a deep ulceration because of the underlying fat necrosis.

Although the above chain of events may occur rapidly after the onset of venous insufficiency, it more commonly occurs several years later. Bauer followed a group of patients with known deep venous thrombosis for several years: ulcers appeared in 20 percent of the patients within 5 years, in 52 percent within 10 years, and in 79 percent at a later date.

Tests for Venous Insufficiency

There are a number of tests for diagnosing of venous insufficiency which are also helpful in understanding the pathophysiology of the condition and differentiating the various causes.

PERCUSSION TEST. This test was originally described as a means of determining the incompetency of valves in superficial veins. The saphenous vein is tapped near the saphenofemoral junction and the opposite hand placed over the knee to feel the impulse transmitted through an unbroken column of blood if the valves are incompetent. The percussion of veins may actually be more helpful in other ways. The greater saphenous vein in the thigh usually lies quite close to the deep fascia and is neither visible nor palpable, particularly in obese individuals. Percussion of a varix in the region of the knee, with the opposite hand

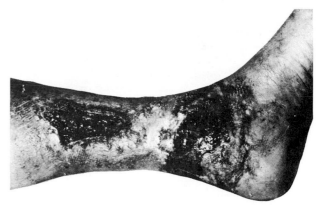

Fig. 22-13. Venous ulcers of lower leg.

following the expected course of the greater saphenous vein, can confirm the association of the varix with the greater saphenous vein. In addition, once the varicose saphenous vein is found by percussion, its size can be estimated. In a similar fashion the size, position, and importance of the lesser saphenous vein in the popliteal space can be determined by tapping varicosities on the posterior calf.

COMPRESSION TESTS. These tests are usually associated with the name of Trendelenburg. The patient lies down and elevates the involved leg until the superficial veins are collapsed. The saphenous vein is then compressed high in the thigh with the fingers of the hand or with a *tight* tourniquet (part 1). With the hand or tourniquet in place, the patient stands up. The sites of previously noted varicosities are carefully observed for 20 to 30 seconds (part 2). The tourniquet is then removed and the veins again carefully observed. There are four possible results of the test:

1. Negative-negative (Fig. 22-14A). In the presence of normal veins there is gradual ascending filling of the superficial veins when the patient stands up; part 1 is negative. With release of compression the gradual filling continues; part 2 is negative.
2. Negative-positive (Fig. 22-14B). In the presence of incompetent valves in the greater saphenous vein without incompetent valves in the perforators, part 1 is negative. With release of compression, however, there is rapid reflux of blood from the femoral vein into and down the greater saphenous vein, with rapid distension of the varicosities; part 2 is positive.
3. Positive-negative (Fig. 22-14C). In the presence of incompetent valves in the perforators, there is reflux of blood from the deep to the superficial system when the patient stands up. The varices in the region of the perforator becomes rapidly filled, and part 1 is positive. If the saphenofemoral valve is competent, there is no further rapid distension of the veins when the compression is released, and part 2 is negative.
4. Positive-positive (Fig. 22-14D). In the presence of incompetent valves in the perforators and also in the greater saphenous vein, filling of the varices occurs on standing, and further rapid filling occurs after the compression is released. Both part 1 and part 2 are positive.

Thus the test can detect the presence of an incompetent saphenous vein and determine the site of incompetent perforators.

VENOUS PRESSURE. The normal standing resting pressure in the saphenous vein at the level of the ankle is

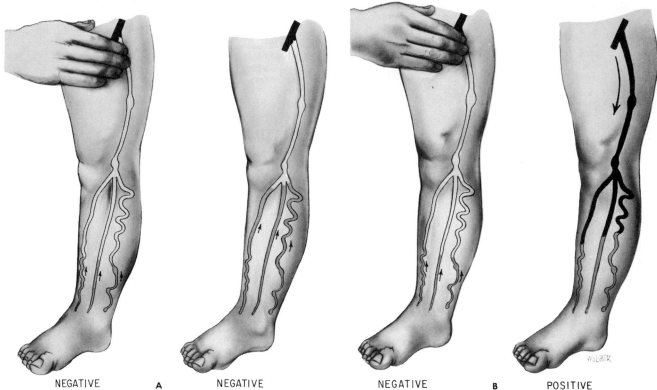

NEGATIVE   A   NEGATIVE   NEGATIVE   B   POSITIVE

Fig. 22-14. Four possible results of Trendelenburg compression test. Patient has been lying down with leg elevated; he then stands up with compression over saphenofemoral junction. *A.* Negative-negative response, in which there is gradual filling of veins from below over a 30-second period and there is continued slow filling after release of hand. *B.* Negative-positive response. On standing, there is gradual filling of distal veins; on release of compression there is rapid retrograde filling of saphenous vein. *C.* Positive-negative response. With hand in place, filling of superficial varicosities through incompetent perforators occurs; with release of compression there is further slow filling of the veins. *D.* Positive-positive response. On standing with hand in place, there is filling of varices through incompetent perforators. On release of compression there is additional rapid filling of saphenous vein.

slightly higher than the hydrostatic pressure of a column of blood reaching from the tip of the catheter to the level of the right midatrium. There are no significant differences in the standing resting pressures for normal extremities and for extremities with varicose veins, incompetent perforators, or abnormal deep vein valves. With walking or rhythmic contraction of the calf muscles, different venous pressure responses are noted (Fig. 22-15). Normally there is a marked decrease in the saphenous vein pressure with exercise, indicating that the muscular action has increased the flow of blood in the deep veins and allowed increased drainage of blood from the superficial to the deep veins during muscular relaxation. When exercise stops, there is a gradual return of venous pressure to normal levels, indicating that the valves in the deep and the superficial systems are competent, preventing rapid reflux of blood. Extremities with varicose veins demonstrate lesser decreases in venous pressure with exercise and more rapid return to normal levels when walking ceases; that is, some of the effect of the rapid emptying of the superficial veins with exercise is counteracted by reflux of blood from the femoral vein into the saphenous vein with its incompetent valves. When exercise stops, there is rapid reflux of blood down the saphenous vein. In the presence of uncomplicated varicose veins, pressure on the saphenofemoral junction or operative removal of the varicosity can result in a normal venous pressure response. Extremities with postthrombotic veins demonstrate little if any decrease in pressure with exercise. After cessation of exercise the venous pressure rapidly returns to normal. The normal decrease in pressure with exercise is prevented by the reflux of blood

back down the abnormal valveless deep veins during muscular relaxation and the propulsion of blood through incompetent perforators during muscular contraction. Ligation of the femoral vein in these patients does not significantly improve the venous pressure response. In the presence of significant obstruction of the deep veins, such as may be seen following a major venous thrombosis or during some pregnancies, the venous pressure actually increases with exercise. Following exercise, the pressure slowly decreases to normal.

FUNCTIONAL PHLEBOGRAPHY. Phlebograms performed with the patient in the semierect position before and immediately after a standard active exercise may demonstrate important pathologic and physiologic abnormalities:

1. The patient lies on a table tilted 60° from the horizontal.
2. A #21 needle is inserted into any superficial vein on the dorsum of the foot and a tourniquet applied snugly to the ankle.

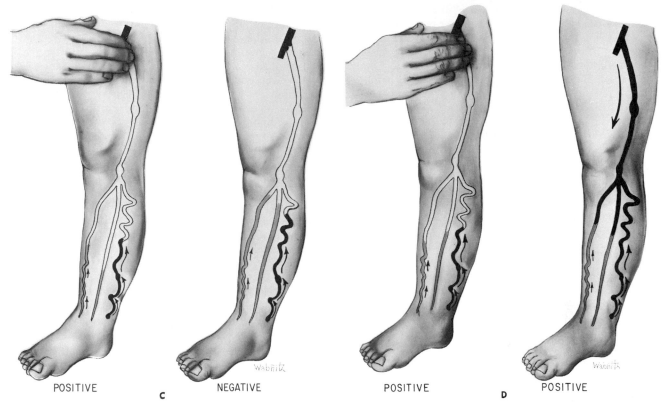

POSITIVE   NEGATIVE
C

POSITIVE   POSITIVE
D

Fig. 22-14 (continued)

3. Over a 1-minute period, 50 ml of any suitable angiographic contrast material is injected.
4. Radiographs of the entire lower extremity are taken before and after the patient stands on his toes ten times.

Normally, slender veins with prominent valves are visualized, and after exercise little radiopaque material is seen except in the cusps of the valves. In the presence of varicose veins alone, the appearance of the deep veins before and after exercise is usually the same as with normal veins. If the superficial veins are visualized, tortuosity and dilatation of the veins may be seen. Following deep venous thrombosis, the veins may be completely recanalized but valveless. They may also remain obstructed, in which case numerous dilated valveless collaterals are visualized. Following exercise there is poor emptying of the radiopaque material from the deep veins, and increased filling of collateral veins, perforating veins, and superficial veins may be seen. Similar changes and responses to exercise may be seen in patients with dilated valveless deep veins presumably of congenital or familial origin. The poor emptying of the radiopaque dye from the veins and dye reflux through perforators into the superficial veins is another demonstration of the abnormal valvular function seen in patients with venous insufficiency.

Differential Diagnosis

Lymphedema may be confused with the edema of venous insufficiency in the early postthrombotic phase

Fig. 22-15. Responses in venous pressure of superficial veins at ankle with exercise. In standing position, venous pressure is slightly higher than hydrostatic pressure in column extending from ankle to heart. This pressure is approximately the same for normal persons and for those with venous insufficiency or chronically obstructed veins in which collaterals have formed. With walking, however, normal persons demonstrate rapid decrease in venous pressure and slow return to normal when exercise stops; patients with varicose veins show lesser decrease in pressure with walking but more prompt return to normal following cessation of exercise; patients with postthrombotic veins demonstrate little if any decrease in venous pressure with walking and rapid return to normal; patients with obstructed veins show increase in pressure with walking and slow return to normal.

AMBULATORY VENOUS PRESSURE CHANGES

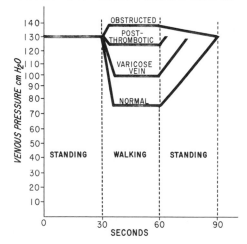

before brawny induration, brownish discoloration, and ulceration occur. Lymphedema, however, generally is of a rubbery consistency and is nonpitting. The edema of congestive heart failure and renal failure is usually bilateral and should also be differentiated by the history and physical examination. Phlebography is particularly helpful in ruling out deep venous thrombosis as a cause of edema.

Venous ulcers almost always occur behind the medial and lateral malleoli. Their positions and associated brawny induration and brownish discoloration generally differentiate them from arterial ulcers, which may occur anywhere on the lower leg, usually have a surrounding blue and then erythematous ring, and are much more painful than venous ulcers. It should also be noted that venous ulcers do not penetrate fascia as arterial ulcers commonly do. A malignant tumor should be suspected in ulcerations of long duration, particularly if they do not respond to proper management.

Treatment

The management of these patients is demanding but rewarding. A single operative procedure is rarely curative except in the mildest cases. Careful education of the patient in the nonoperative management is of utmost importance. In addition, the patients must be seen periodically in order to be sure that they are continuing proper elastic support and periodic elevation.

NONOPERATIVE MANAGEMENT. The nonoperative management of patients with venous insufficiency is based on decreasing the amount of blood sequestration in the veins of the lower extremities and decreasing the venous pressure in the superficial veins.

Elevation of the legs overcomes the hydrostatic pressure in the veins and thereby decreases the pressure and the amount of blood in the dilated valveless veins. It should be emphasized that this is accomplished ideally only when the legs are elevated above the level of the heart, which is facilitated by having the patient sleep with the foot of the bed or the foot of the mattress elevated. During the day, the patient should lie on a couch with the feet elevated on pillows. A sitting posture in a chair with the legs outstretched does not provide adequate elevation.

Active exercise, except in the presence of obstruction, also decreases the volume and pressure in the veins of the lower extremities. Walking is excellent exercise. Standing, without muscular contraction, and sitting increase the volume and pressure of the peripheral venous blood.

Compression of the superficial veins also decreases the volume of the venous pool and if strong enough overcomes the venous pressure transmitted through the superficial veins via incompetent perforators. Means of providing compression vary in strength and, in order of increasing effectiveness, include nylon support hose, ordinary cotton elastic stockings, snugly applied Ace bandages, heavy-duty cotton elastic stockings (Truform), specially constructed pressure-gradient stockings (Jobst), Gelucast, Unna's paste, or Elastoplast boots, and canvas boots containing an inflatable rubber bladder (Aeropulse). The goals of any compression therapy are the relief of symptoms and the pre-

vention of measurable evening swelling of the legs. The importance of proper elastic support in accomplishing this goal cannot be overemphasized. Nylon support hose and ordinary cotton elastic stockings are effective only in the management of patients with very mild venous insufficiency. Ace bandages are only as good as the care with which they are applied. The management of patients with moderate to severe insufficiency and particularly those with ulceration demands the use of one of the stronger means of support.

The severity of the venous insufficiency governs the type of therapy prescribed. A patient with mild symptomatic varicosities might find relief of symptoms and edema with ordinary cotton elastic stockings and elevation of the legs whenever there is a choice between lying down and sitting down. A patient with severe venous insufficiency would need more aggressive treatment similar to the "new way of life" described by Luke. The patient may require overnight elevation of the legs, planned periodic elevation of the legs during the day, and strong elastic support. The nonoperative management of patients with venous ulcers is primarily an aggressive management of the venous insufficiency as outlined above. The use of local medications should be avoided unless a definite secondary infection is present. Increasing the local pressure over the ulcer by means of a sponge rubber pad beneath a strong elastic support can usually heal ulcers of silver-dollar size and sometimes larger.

OPERATIVE MANAGEMENT. Surgical treatment may in some instances be curative, but in most instances is merely helpful as an adjunct to the conservative management of venous insufficiency.

Ligation and Stripping of Greater or Lesser Saphenous Veins. The ligation and stripping of the saphenous veins should not be performed unless incompetency of the vein is demonstrated by the Trendelenburg test. The indications for the procedure are (1) moderate to severe symptomatic varicosities, (2) severe varicosities, even though the patient does not admit to symptoms, (3) severe venous insufficiency with recurrent ulcerations, in association with aggressive nonoperative management. Patients with mild varicosities and significant symptoms usually do not benefit from the procedure, and it is usually found that the symptoms are due to some unrelated cause or to deep venous abnormalities. Significant edema rarely accompanies greater saphenous varicosities alone and is not appreciably helped by vein stripping. Treatment of other underlying conditions or the aggressive nonoperative management of deep venous abnormalities is necessary.

The operative procedure (Fig. 22-16) consists of ligation of the greater saphenous vein at its junction with the femoral vein and ligation of its four major branches at the margin of the transverse groin incision. The entire vein is then stripped from its bed by making a separate incision at the ankle, passing a wire within the lumen in a craniad direction the length of the vein, transecting the vein in the ankle, and avulsing the entire vein by pulling on the wire from the groin incision. The branches of the veins break off near their junctions with the saphenous vein, but bleeding is minimal, particularly if the feet are markedly ele-

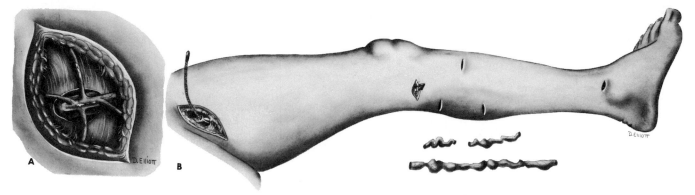

Fig. 22-16. Ligation and stripping of saphenous vein. *A*, Groin incision, showing junction of greater saphenous and femoral veins. Note four major branches of saphenous vein which required ligation and division. *B*, counterincision at knee or ankle to permit stripping of saphenous vein. Additional incisions to permit removal of branch varicose veins.

vated during the operation. As noted before, however, the visible varicosities are usually found in the branches of the vein, and attention must also be directed toward them. Some surgeons prefer to remove the veins through separate incisions at the time of the original operation, others prefer to inject the remaining branches with sclerosing solutions at a later date. These solutions produce a localized phlebitis and thrombosis of the veins. The veins will remain obstructed unless complete recanalization of the lumen occurs.

Fegan has advocated the injection of veins, followed by 6 weeks of continuous elastic compression, for the treatment of varicosities. Doran and White, in a randomized study, concluded that patients who were treated by Fegan's method required significantly less additional treatment at 1 year than those who underwent operation. Long-term results were not available, however, and it is still generally agreed that an operation followed by injection, if necessary, is the treatment of choice.

Following operation, snug elastic stockings are applied, and the foot of the bed is elevated above the level of the heart. During the first week after operation patients are allowed up to walk or allowed to lie in bed with the feet elevated. Sitting is prohibited except for bathroom privileges. During the second week patients find it necessary to elevate the legs during a portion of the day to avoid discomfort. During the third or fourth week after operation they gradually increase their activities to their preoperative level.

Ligation of Incompetent Perforators. Incompetent perforators rarely occur without other types of venous insufficiency. Their ligation, however, may be a valuable adjunct to the nonoperative management of patients with venous insufficiency. It is particularly effective if performed before the patient develops an ulcer. This preulcer state may be recognized by the presence of telangiectasia, brownish pigmentation, or mild brawny induration behind the medial or lateral malleoli. The operation is also indicated

after the nonoperative healing of recurrent ulcers. It should not be performed in the presence of an active infected ulcer.

Various techniques for ligation of the perforators in the lower leg have been described by Linton, Felder and associates, and Dodd and Cockett. Dodd and Cockett point out that the perforators most frequently associated with ulcers are those posterior and superior to the medial and lateral malleoli. Longitudinal incisions are made posterior and superior to the malleoli; then the perforators are interrupted above or below the fascia near their communication with the deep veins (Fig. 22-17). Extensive undermining of the tissue should be avoided, since there is a risk of sloughing of the overlying skin. Ligation of perforators is only an adjunctive measure, and aggressive nonoperative treatment of the underlying deep venous abnormalities is still indicated.

Ligation of the Superficial Femoral or Popliteal Veins. Some surgeons advocate the ligation of the superficial femoral or popliteal veins in the presence of deep venous abnormalities. The procedure was originally advocated to prevent reflux of blood down valveless normal deep veins. However, postoperative phlebograms in patients who have had this type of operation indicate that the obstructed deep veins are only replaced by dilated valveless collaterals. In addition, venous pressure measurements indicate that after such ligations increased venous hypertension occurs.

LYMPHATICS AND LYMPHEDEMA

Anatomy and Physiology of Lymphatic Return

The lymphatic system provides a means of returning certain extravascular materials in the interstitial space to the bloodstream. Normally there is a constant leakage of fluid and protein through the arterial capillary membrane into the interstitial space. The water and solutes can be resorbed by the vascular capillaries; the protein cannot. Proteins, however, can readily enter the lymphatic capillaries. Other materials, including red blood cells, bacteria, and small particulate matter, can also pass through the lymphatic capillary membrane.

The lymphatic capillaries form a superficial plexus within the dermis which covers the whole body surface.

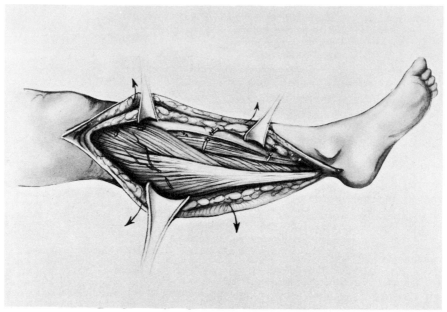

Fig. 22-17. Perforating veins interrupted subfascially. Skin flaps are carefully developed, and the great and small saphenous veins and the subcutaneous tissue, with many communicating veins, are excised. (*After D. Silver, J. J. Gleysteen, G. R. Rhodes, N. G. Georgiade, and W. G. Anlyan, Surgical Treatment of the Refractory Postphlebitic Ulcer, Arch Surg, 103:554, 1971. Copyright 1971, American Medical Association.*)

Another similar plexus lies in the deep dermis or subdermal region. These join other deeper lymphatics to form larger vessels which, in general, follow the course of the major blood vessels to the neck, where they empty into the bloodstream at the junction of the internal jugular and the subclavian vein. The continuity of the larger lymphatics is interrupted by lymph nodes, which acts as filters and also contribute lymphocytes to the lymph. The lymph vessels contain valves which direct the flow of lymph toward the neck. The movement of the lymph is aided by extrinsic factors such as muscle contraction, arterial pulsations, respiratory movement, and massage.

Information regarding the normal or altered anatomy and physiology of the lymphatics can be obtained from special examinations, including (1) dye injections of the superficial dermal lymphatics, (2) lymphangiography, and (3) analysis of the protein content of edema fluid.

DYE INJECTIONS. Hudack and McMaster introduced patent blue dye, and Butcher and Hoover used 4% direct sky blue dye for the intradermal injection of the human superficial dermal lymphatics; 0.2 ml is inserted via a 30-gauge needle, and in normal skin a network of very fine intradermal lymphatic capillaries is demonstrated within 30 to 60 seconds after injection (Fig. 22-18).

LYMPHANGIOGRAPHY. Kinmonth demonstrated the feasibility of obtaining radiographs of the lymphatics. Patent blue dye or direct sky blue dye is injected into the subcutaneous tissue of the foot. The dye rapidly enters the lymphatics. Massage of the foot and muscular contractions increase the lymph flow. An incision is then made on the dorsum of the foot and a cannula inserted into a blue-dye-filled lymphatic; 10 ml of radiopaque dye is injected, and x-rays of the entire extremity are made.

Normally the slender lymphatics, unlike veins, appear of uniform caliber throughout their course. Unlike veins, they bifurcate as they proceed proximally. As with veins,

slight dilatations at the level of the valves are visualized (Fig. 22-18).

ANALYSIS OF THE PROTEIN CONTENT OF EDEMA FLUID. Edema fluid can be collected by the insertion of a special Southey tube into the subcutaneous tissue. The protein content of peripheral edema fluid secondary to venous, heart, or renal disease is less than 1.5 Gm/100 ml. Since the lymphatics are responsible for removal of protein from the interstitial space, abnormally high levels of protein would reflect abnormal lymphatic function.

Lymphedema

Congenital or acquired abnormalities of the lymphatics may hinder the lymphatic capillaries from absorbing materials such as proteins or prevent the main channels from carrying sufficient quantities of tissue fluid from a limb. The result is an accumulation of plasma protein in the tissue spaces. This protein concentration is of high osmotic pressure, causing absorption of fluid into the extravascular space. Edema, or in other words lymphedema, is the result.

ETIOLOGY. The various types of lymphedema have been outlined by Taylor as follows:

1. Primary lymphedema
   a. Congenital
   b. Lymphedema precox
2. Secondary lymphedema
   a. Neoplastic invasion
   b. Surgical excision

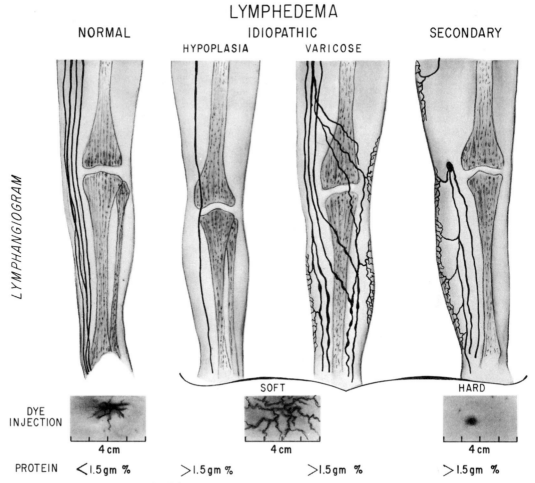

Fig. 22-18. Diagnostic procedures for lymphedema: dye injections, lymphangiograms, and protein analysis.

    c. Radiotherapy
    d. Inflammation or parasitic invasion
    e. Motor paralysis

Primary Lymphedema. Primary lymphedema of the lower extremities is caused by abnormal development of the lymph vessels. The edema may be present at birth and is then called *congenital lymphedema.* More frequently the edema appears during the teens and is then termed *lymphedema precox.* It may appear insidiously or may follow minor trauma or infection. Primary lymphedema is about three times more common in females than in males. It involves both legs in about 50 percent of patients.

Secondary Lymphedema. Secondary lymphedema is usually due to obstruction or destruction of normal lymphatic channels. It may, therefore, follow obstruction of the lymphatics by tumor, repeated infection, or parasitic infestation. It may also follow the excision of lymph nodes, as during a radical mastectomy or radical groin dissection. Radiation therapy, particularly for malignant disease, may similarly destroy the lymphatics.

PATHOPHYSIOLOGY. Primary Lymphedema. Kinmonth et al. performed lymphangiograms on 87 patients with pri-

mary lymphedema. Aplasia, or the absence of any significant lymphatic trunks in the subcutaneous tissue, was observed in 14 percent of the extremities. Dye injected beneath the skin, however, would travel great distances through dilated dermal vessels. Hypoplasia, a deficiency in size or number of lymphatic vessels, was seen in 55 percent of the extremities. Dye injected subcutaneously in the interdigital webs would frequently appear in the dermal plexus of the dorsum of the foot. Varicose lymphatics which were broader and more tortuous than normal were observed in 24 percent of the patients. Dye injected subcutaneously would frequently appear in dermal lymphatics some distance from the site of the injection. This "dermal backflow" in the lymphatics is assumed to be secondary to incompetency of valves in the lymphatics. It can be demonstrated also by the intradermal injection of dye, when "skip areas" in the filling of the dermal lymphatics is observed. The protein content of the edema fluid of patients with primary lymphedema, studied by Crockett and by Taylor et al., was found to be greater than 2 Gm/100 ml in 41 of 48 patients. It would appear, therefore, that the underlying cause of the edema is the inability of the lymphatic system to remove protein from the interstitial fluid at a normal rate. In primary lymphedema this lymphatic insufficiency may be due to aplasia, hypoplasia, or varicosities of the lymphatic vessels (Fig. 22-18).

Secondary Lymphedema. Lymphangiograms of patients with acquired lymphedema demonstrate the point of obstruction of the lymphatics. The remaining vessels appear normal, but there is considerable dermal backflow of the radiopaque material. Intradermal dye injections demonstrate dilatations and prominence of the dermal lymphatics. The inability of the lymphatics to effectively remove protein from the interstitial fluid can be demonstrated by measurements of the protein content of the edema fluid (Fig. 22-18).

CLINICAL MANIFESTATIONS. Symptoms. The usual symptoms of primary and secondary lymphedema are the same. Edema increases during the course of the day and decreases overnight, but the limb always remains larger. There is gradual increase in the degree of swelling over a period of years. The edema may cause some fatigue and be cosmetically objectionable but in most instances causes no real concern. In others the disability is significant, particularly in those with elephantiasis secondary to filariasis.

Physical Findings. Lymphedema is characteristically a firm, rubbery, nonpitting edema. Early in the course of the disease the edema is somewhat softer, and much of it will disappear overnight with elevation of the legs. With the passage of time the edema may become woody in character. This is a result of an increase of fibrous tissue within the subcutaneous tissue, which is believed to be secondary to the increase in protein-rich edema fluid. Repeated infections will hasten growth of fibrous tissue. Some patients develop small blisters containing edema fluid of high protein content. These blisters may occur on the lower abdomen and upper thigh and contain a milky white fluid with the characteristics of chyle; they are believed to be secondary to reflux from the retroperitoneal lymphatics. Hyperkeratosis of the skin is common in long-standing lymphedema.

COMPLICATIONS. Recurrent Cellulitis and Lymphangitis. The major complication of lymphedema is recurrent attacks of cellulitis and lymphangitis. These attacks may occur without warning or may follow minor injuries or infections in the extremity. They are characterized by an elevated temperature, constitutional symptoms of malaise, nausea and vomiting, and local symptoms of redness, pain, and increased swelling of the involved limb. Betahemolytic streptococci are the offending organisms and, if carefully looked for, may be found at the site of minor injuries, in the nose and throat, in blood cultures, or in edema fluid. The protein-rich edema fluid is apparently an excellent culture medium, since the lymphedematous limb is very susceptible to repeated infections. Once the infection starts it spreads rapidly.

Lymphangiosarcoma. A rare but serious complication of lymphedema is the appearance of lymphangiosarcoma. This malignant tumor is most frequently described in patients with lymphedema following a radical mastectomy for breast cancer but is also seen in long-standing lymphedema due to other causes. It is usually first recognized as a bruiselike blue or reddish purple nodule in the skin of the lymphedematous extremity. As the primary lesion enlarges, satellite tumors appear about it. Metastases appear early in the course of the disease, particularly to the lung.

Protein-losing Enteropathy. Very rarely patients with primary lymphedema of their legs may also develop a protein-losing enteropathy. Using mesenteric lymphangiography, Kinmonth and Cox have been able to demonstrate localized lymphatic obstructions of bowel wall treatable by resection of a segment of bowel.

DIFFERENTIAL DIAGNOSIS. The firm, rubbery, nonpitting character of unilateral lymphedema usually differentiates it from the soft, pitting, bilateral edema secondary to heart failure, renal failure, hypothyroidism, or aldosteronism. Some deep cavernous hemangiomas may be confused with lymphedema, but the presence of overlying birthmarks, the sponginess of the hemangiomas, and their decrease in size on elevation usually indicate the correct diagnosis. The edema of an acute postoperative or infectious lymphedema may be confused with deep venous thrombosis, and a phlebogram may be most helpful in establishing the correct diagnosis. The edema of chronic venous insufficiency can usually be differentiated from lymphedema because of its brawniness, overlying brownish discoloration, and telangiectasia. However, lymphedema is commonly a complication of acute thrombophlebitis, and venous insufficiency and lymphedema may coexist. Streptococcal infection should be carefully searched for in the patient with a postphlebitic extremity who is repeatedly admitted to the hospital with high fever and redness, tenderness, and marked swelling of the leg. In the author's experience these cases are usually labeled "recurrent phlebitis" but in actuality are recurrent cellulitis and lymphangitis secondary to lymphedema.

Whenever there is a question of deep venous disease versus lymphedema, a phlebogram may be helpful in establishing the diagnosis of deep venous disease, and the author has found dye injections of the superficial dermal lymphatics helpful in confirming the diagnosis of lymphedema. Lymphangiograms and, in confusing cases, analysis of the protein content of the edema fluid may be necessary to establish the diagnosis.

TREATMENT. Nonoperative Management. The conservative management of lymphedema is directed toward control of the edema and prevention of recurrent infection. Elevation of the involved extremity above the level of the heart will increase lymph drainage by reducing the hydrostatic pressure within the lymph vessels. Patients are therefore instructed to elevate the foot of the bed; they are also instructed to lie down and elevate the extremity whenever they have the opportunity. Massage is also known to increase lymph flow. Special apparatuses are available to accomplish this: one is a cloth sleeve containing a plastic bladder that can be alternately inflated and deflated to produce a rhythmic pneumatic compression of the entire extremity; another is a series of bladders that can be sequentially inflated and deflated to give a massaging effect beginning at the hand or foot and extending to the shoulder or thigh. When the maximal decrease in edema is achieved by these methods, very tight elastic stockings or canvas boots containing an inflatable rubber bladder can be applied. These supports can prevent reaccumulation of edema fluid. In addition they provide a semirigid encasement of the extremity so that muscular action, which causes alterations in the volume of the leg, can produce a massaging effect on the lymphatics. Diuretics may be helpful in reducing the size of the limb temporarily. However, none of the procedures mentioned can completely return the limb to its normal size, particularly in long-standing cases; they can only delay or prevent progression of the process.

The control of the recurrent bouts of infection associated with lymphedema is important. Ideally it should be possible to prevent these by control of edema, local hygiene, avoidance of trauma, and prevention of athlete's foot. These procedures alone are usually not sufficient, however, and the use of prophylactic antibiotics may be indicated. Since the offending organism is almost always the streptococcus, oral penicillin is the drug of choice.

Surgical Treatment. Surgical treatment is indicated for a very small percentage of patients with lymphedema. The indications include excessive edema, when the weight and size of the limb interfere with normal activities, and recurrent bouts of cellulitis. Surgery for cosmetic reasons alone is rarely indicated, since after an effective operation a disproportion in the size of the two limbs will still usually remain, and in addition the scars resulting from the operation may still call attention to the limb.

Numerous surgical approaches to the problem are described, including (1) insertion of silk threads, Teflon wicks, or polyethylene tubing into the subcutaneous tissue in the hope of draining the edema fluid into normal tissue; (2) removal of long strips of fascia in the hope that new anastomoses will form between the superficial and deep lymphatics, as advocated by Thompson; (3) construction of pedicle grafts from the involved limb to the trunk in the hope of bypassing obstructed lymphatics; (4) excision of long strips of subcutaneous tissue and deep fascia to reduce the size of the limb; (5) complete excision of all the skin, subcutaneous tissue, and deep fascia from the limb, followed by application of split-thickness skin grafts to the exposed muscle and periosteum, as originally described by Charles.

The Charles procedure is, in the author's opinion, the most effective of the surgical procedures. The size and weight of the limb are effectively reduced, and there is lower incidence of recurrent cellulitis and lymphangitis after removal of the edematous subcutaneous tissue. It should be reemphasized, however, that this, like other treatments for lymphedema, cannot return the limb to a normal appearance.

References

Venous Thrombosis and Pulmonary Embolism

Adams, J. T., and DeWeese, J. A.: Experimental and Clinical Evaluation of Partial Vein Interruption in the Prevention of Pulmonary Emboli, *Surgery,* **57:**82, 1965.
——— and ———: Comparative Evaluation of Ligation and Partial Interruption of the Femoral Vein in the Treatment of Thromboembolic Disease, *Ann Surg,* **172:**795, 1970.
——— and ———: "Effort" Thrombosis of the Axillary and Subclavian Veins, *J Trauma,* **11:**923, 1971.
———, Feingold, B. E., and DeWeese, J. A.: Comparative Evaluation of Ligation and Partial Interruption of the Inferior Vena Cava, *Arch Surg,* **103:**272, 1971.
Allen, E. V., Hines, E. A., Jr., Kvale, W. F., and Barker, N. W.: The Use of Dicumarol as an Anticoagulant: Experience in 2,307 Cases, *Ann Intern Med,* **27:**371, 1947.
Artz, C. P., and Amspacher, W. H.: Evaluation of Various Methods of Administration of Heparin, *Surg Forum,* **3:**530, 1952.
Barner, H. B., and DeWeese, J. A.: An Evaluation of the Sphygmomanometer Cuff Pain Test in Venous Thrombosis, *Surgery,* **48:**915, 1960.
Barritt, D. W., and Jordan, S. C.: Anticoagulant Drugs in the Treatment of Pulmonary Embolism: A Controlled Trial, *Lancet,* **1:**1309, 1960.
Bauer, G. A.: Roentgenological and Clinical Study of the Sequels of Thrombosis, *Acta Chir Scand [Suppl],* **86:**74, 1942.
Bauer, G.: Clinical Experiences of a Surgeon in the Use of Heparin, *Am J Cardiol,* **14:**29, 1964.
Berger, R. L.: Pulmonary Embolectomy with Preoperative Circulatory Support, *Ann Thorac Surg,* **16:**217, 1973.
Brockman, S. K., and Vasko, J. S.: Phlegmasia Cerulea Dolens, *Surg Gynecol Obstet,* **121:**1347, 1965.
Browse, N. L.: The ¹²⁵I Fibrinogen Uptake Test, *Arch Surg,* **104:**160, 1972.
Byrne, J. J., and O'Neil, E. E.: Fatal Pulmonary Emboli: A Study of 130 Autopsy-proven Fatal Emboli, *Am J Surg,* **83:**47, 1952.
Carey, L. C., and Williams, R. D.: Comparative Effects of Dicumarol, Tromexan, and Heparin on Thrombus Propagation, *Ann Surg,* **152:**919, 1960.
Cegelski, F. C., DeWeese, J. A., and Lund, C. J.: Deep Iliofemoral Venous Thrombosis during Pregnancy, *Am J Obstet Gynecol,* **89:**510, 1964.
Cooley, D. A., and Beall, A. C., Jr.: A Technic of Pulmonary Embolectomy Using Temporary Cardio-pulmonary Bypass, *J Cardiovasc Surg (Torino),* **2:**469, 1961.
Coon, W. W.: The Spectrum of Pulmonary Embolism: Twenty Years Later, *Arch Surg,* **111:**398, 1976.
——— and Coller, F. A.: Clinicopathologic Correlation in Thromboembolism, *Surg Gynecol Obstet,* **109:**259, 1959.
——— and ———: Some Epidemiologic Considerations of Thromboembolism, *Surg Gynecol Obstet,* **109:**487, 1959.
———, Mackenzie, J. W., and Hodgson, P. E.: A Critical Evaluation of Anticoagulant Therapy in Peripheral Venous Thrombosis and Pulmonary Embolism, *Surg Gynecol Obstet,* **106:**129, 1958.
Cosgriff, S. W.: Thromboembolism, *Am J Med,* **3:**758, 1947.
Cotton, L. T., and Roberts, V. C.: The Prevention of Deep Vein Thrombosis, with Particular Reference to Mechanical Methods of Prevention, *Surgery,* **81:**228, 1977.
Crane, C.: Deep Venous Thrombosis and Pulmonary Embolism, *N Engl J Med,* **257:**147, 1957.
———: Femoral vs. Caval Interruption for Venous Thromboembolism, *N Engl J Med,* **270:**819, 1964.
Cranley, J. J., Gay, A. Y., Grass, A. M., and Simeone, F. A.: Plethysmographic Technique for the Diagnosis of Deep Venous Thrombosis of the Lower Extremities, *Surg Gynec Obstet,* **136:**385, 1973.

Dale, W. A.: Inferior Vena Caval Ligation for Venous Thrombo-embolism, *Rev Surg,* **19:**1, 1962.

Deaton, H. L., Anlyan, W. G., Silver, D., and Webster, J.: Thrombosis: Prevention and Treatment, *Surgery,* **49:**130, 1961.

DeBakey, M. E.: A Critical Evaluation of the Problem of Thromboembolism, *Surg Gynecol Obstet,* **98:**1, 1954.

DeWeese, J. A.: Current Status of Plastic Procedures on the Venous System, *NJ Acad Med Bull,* **7:**1, 1961.

———: The Role of Pulmonary Embolectomy in Venous Thromboembolism, *J Cardiovasc Surg (Torino),* **17:**348, 1976.

———: Thrombectomy for Acute Iliofemoral Venous Thrombosis, *J Cardiovasc Surg (Torino),* **5:**703, 1964.

———, Adams, J. T., and Gaiser, D. L.: Subclavian Venous Thrombectomy, *Circulation,* **41, 42** (*Suppl* II):158, 1970.

———, Kraft, R. O., Nichols, W. K., Six, H. H., and Thompson, N. W.: Fifteen-Year Clinical Experience with the Vena Cava Filter, *Ann Surg,* **178:**247, 1973.

——— and Rogoff, S. M.: Phlebographic Patterns of Acute Deep Venous Thrombosis of the Leg, *Surgery,* **53:**99, 1963.

———, ———, Phillips, C. E., Jr., and Pories, W. J.: Deep Venous Thrombosis, *Postgrad Med,* **29:**614, 1961.

DeWeese, M. S., and Hunter, D. C.: A Vena Cava Filter for the Prevention of Pulmonary Embolism, *Arch Surg,* **86:**852, 1963.

Dmochowski, J. R., Adams, D. F., and Couch, N. P.: Impedance Measurement in the Diagnosis of Deep Venous Thrombosis, *Arch Surg,* **104:**170, 1972.

Donaldson, G. A., Linton, R. R., and Rodkey, G. V.: A Twenty-Year Survey of Thromboembolism at the Massachusetts General Hospital, 1939–1959, *N Engl J Med,* **265:**208, 1961.

Edwards, W. H., Sawyers, J. L., and Foster, J. H.: Iliofemoral Venous Thrombosis: Reappraisal of Thrombectomy, *Ann Surg,* **171:**961, 1970.

Engelberg, H., and Berk, M. Z.: Prolonged Anticoagulant Therapy with Subcutaneously Administered Concentrated Aqueous Heparin, *Surgery,* **36:**762, 1954.

Flanc, C., Kakkar, V. V., and Clarke, M. B.: Postoperative Deep-Vein Thrombosis: Effect of Intensive Prophylaxis, *Lancet,* **1:**477, 1969.

Fogarty, T. J., and Krippaehne, W. W.: Catheter Technique for Venous Thrombectomy, *Surg Gynecol Obstet,* **121:**362, 1965.

Fontaine, R., and Tuchmann, L.: The Role of Thrombectomy in Deep Venous Thromboses, *J Cardiovasc Surg (Torino),* **5:**298, 1964.

Gibbs, N. M.: Venous Thrombosis of the Lower Limbs with Particular Reference to Bed-Rest, *Br J Surg,* **45:**15, 1957.

Gomez, R. L., Wheeler, H. B., Belko, J. S., and Warren, R.: Observations on the Uptake of a Radioactive Fibrinolytic Enzyme by Intravascular Clots, *Ann Surg,* **158:**905, 1963.

Greenfield, L. J., Peyton, M. D., Brown, P. P., and Elkins, R. C.: Transvenous Management of Pulmonary Embolic Disease, *Ann Surg,* **180:**461, 1974.

Hafner, C. D., Cranley, J. J., Krause, R. J., and Strasser, E. S.: A Method of Managing Superficial Thrombophlebitis, *Surgery,* **55:**201, 1964.

Haller, J. A., and Abrams, B. L.: Use of Thrombectomy in the Treatment of Acute Iliofemoral Venous Thrombosis in Forty-five Patients, *Ann Surg,* **158:**561, 1963.

Henderson, R. R.: Pulmonary Embolism and Infarction, *Med Clin North Am,* **48:**1425, 1964.

Herrmann, L. G.: Superficial Venous Thrombosis (Saphenous Thrombophlebitis): Should Treatment be Empirical or Definitive? *J Cardiovasc Surg (Torino),* **5:**239, 1964.

Hughes, E. S. R.: Venous Obstruction in the Upper Extremity (Paget-Schroetter's Syndrome): A Review of 320 Cases, *Int Abstr Surg,* **88:**89, 1949.

Hume, M.: The Relation of "Hypercoagulability" to Thrombosis, *Monogr Surg Sci,* **2:**133, 1965.

Hunter, W. C., Sneeden, V. D., Robertson, T. D., and Snyder, G. A. C.: Thrombosis of the Deep Veins of the Leg, *Arch Intern Med,* **68:**1, 1941.

Jorpes, J. E.: Heparin: Its Chemistry, Pharmacology and Clinical Use, *Am J Med,* **33:**692, 1962.

Kakkar, V.: The Diagnosis of Deep Vein Thrombosis Using the ^{125}I Fibrinogen Test, *Arch Surg,* **104:**152, 1972.

———: Prevention of Fatal Postoperative Pulmonary Embolism by Low Doses of Heparin, *Lancet,* **2:**45, 1975.

Lawen, A.: Weitere Erfahrungen über operative Thrombenentfernung bei Venenthrombose, *Arch Klin Chir,* **193:**723, 1938.

Lewis, C. E., Jr., Antoine, J., Mueller, C., Talbot, W. A., Swaroop, R., and Edwards, W. S.: Elastic Compression in the Prevention of Venous Stasis, *Am J Surg,* **132:**739, 1976.

Mahorner, H., Castleberry, J. W., and Coleman, W. O.: Attempts to Restore Function in Major Veins Which Are the Site of Massive Thrombosis, *Ann Surg,* **146:**510, 1957.

Mavor, G. E.: Deep Vein Thrombosis, *Postgrad Med J,* **47:**311, 1971.

McLachlin, J., and Paterson, J. C.: Some Basic Observations on Venous Thrombosis and Pulmonary Embolism, *Surg Gynecol Obstet,* **93:**1, 1951.

———, Richards, T., and Paterson, J. C.: An Evaluation of Clinical Signs in the Diagnosis of Venous Thrombosis, *Arch Surg,* **85:**738, 1962.

Miles, R. M., Chappell, F., and Renner, O.: A Partially Occluding Vena Caval Clip for Prevention of Pulmonary Embolism, *Am Surg,* **30:**40, 1964.

Mobin-Uddin, K., McLean, R., Bolooki, H., and Jude, J. R.: Caval Interruption for Prevention of Pulmonary Embolism: Long Term Results of a New Method, *Arch Surg,* **99:**711, 1969.

———, Trinkle, J. K., and Bryant, L. R.: Present Status of the Inferior Vena Cava Umbrella Filter, *Surgery,* **70:**914, 1971.

Moretz, W. H., Rhode, C. M., and Shepherd, M. H.: Prevention of Pulmonary Emboli by Partial Occlusion of the Inferior Vena Cava, *Am Surg,* **25:**617, 1959.

Moser, K. M., Guisan, M., Cuomo, A., and Ashburn, W. L.: Differentiation of Pulmonary Vascular from Parenchymal Diseases by Ventilation/Perfusion Scintiphotography. *Ann Int Med,* **75:**597, 1971.

———, Houk, V. N., Jones, R. C., and Hufnagel, C. C.: Chronic, Massive Thrombotic Obstruction of the Pulmonary Arteries: Analysis of Four Operated Cases, *Circulation,* **32:**377, 1965.

Murray, G.: Anticoagulants, in Venous Thrombosis and the Prevention of Pulmonary Embolism, *Surg Gynecol Obstet,* **84:**665, 1947.

Nabseth, D. C., and Moran, J. M.: Reassessment of the Role of Inferior-Vena-Cava Ligation in Venous Thromboembolism, *N Engl J Med,* **273:**1250, 1965.

Parrish, E. H., Adams, J. T., Pories, W. J., Burget, D. E., and DeWeese, J. A.: Pulmonary Emboli Following Vena Caval Ligation, *Arch Surg,* **97:**899, 1968.

Ravdin, I. S., and Kirby, C. K.: Experiences with Ligation and Heparin in Thromboembolic Disease, *Surgery,* **29:**334, 1951.

Robb, G. P., and Steinberg, I.: Visualization of the Chambers of the Heart, the Pulmonary Circulation, and the Great Blood Vessels in Man, *Am J Roentgenol Radium Ther Nucl Med,* **41:**1, 1939.

Roberts, B., Rosato, F. E., and Rosato, E. F.: Heparin—A Cause of Arterial Emboli? *Surgery,* **55:**803, 1964.

Robin, E. D., Julian, D. G., Travis, D. M., and Crump, C. H.: A Physiologic Approach to the Diagnosis of Acute Pulmonary Embolism, *N Engl J Med,* **260:**586, 1959.

Sautter, R. D., Myers, W. O., Ray, J. F., III, and Wentzel, F. J.: Pulmonary Embolectomy: Review and Current Status, *Prog Cardiovasc Dis,* **17:**371, 1975.

———, ———, and Wenzel, F. J.: Implications of the Urokinase Study Concerning the Surgical Treatment of Pulmonary Embolism, *J Thorac Cardiovasc Surg,* **63:**54, 1972.

Sawyer, R. B., Moncrief, J. A., and Canizaro, P. C.: Dextran Therapy in Thrombophlebitis, *JAMA,* **191:**740, 1965.

Schwartz, S. I.: Diagnosis of Thromboembolic Disease, *J Cardiovasc Surg (Torino),* suppl. issue, VII Congress of International Cardiovascular Society, Philadelphia, Sept. 5–18, 1965.

Sharp, E. H.: Pulmonary Embolectomy: Successful Removal of Massive Pulmonary Embolus with Support of Cardiopulmonary Bypass: Case Report, *Ann Surg,* **156:**1, 1962.

Short, D. S.: A Survey of Pulmonary Embolism in a General Hospital, *Br Med J,* **1:**790, 1952.

Sigel, B., Felix, W. R., Jr., Popky, G. L., and Ipsen, J.: Diagnosis of Lower Limb Venous Thrombosis by Doppler Ultrasound Technique, *Arch Surg,* **104:**174, 1972.

Spencer, F. C., Quattlebaum, J. K., Quattlebaum, J. K., Jr., Sharp, E. H., and Jude, J. R.: Plication of the Inferior Vena Cava for Pulmonary Embolism: A Report of 20 Cases, *Ann Surg,* **155:**827, 1962.

Stein, G. N., Chen, J. T., Goldstein, F., Israel, H. L., and Finkelstein, A.: The Importance of Chest Roentgenography in the Diagnosis of Pulmonary Embolism, *Am J Roentgenol Radium Ther Nucl Med,* **81:**255, 1959.

Szucs, M. M., Jr., Brooks, H. L., Grossman, W., Banas, J. S., Jr., Meister, S. G., Dexter, L., and Dalen, J. E.: Diagnostic Sensitivity of Laboratory Findings in Acute Pulmonary Embolism, *Ann Int Med,* **74:**161, 1971.

Templeton, J. Y.: Endvenectomy for the Relief of Obstruction of the Superior Vena Cava, *Am J Surg,* **104:**70, 1962.

Trenwith, B. J., and Dooss, T. W.: Soleus Rupture: Differential Diagnosis of Calf Thrombosis, *NZ Med J,* **82:**18, 1975.

Tsapogas, M. J., Goussous, H., Peabody, R. A., Karmody, A. M., and Eckert, C.: Postoperative Venous Thrombosis and the Effectiveness of Prophylactic Measures, *Arch Surg,* **105:**561, 1971.

Urokinase-Streptokinase Embolism Trail, Phase 2 Results, *JAMA,* **229:**1606, 1974.

Wagner, H. N., Sabiston, D. C., Jr., McAfee, J. G., Tow, D., and Stern, H. S.: Diagnosis of Massive Pulmonary Embolism in Man by Radioisotope Scanning, *N Engl J Med,* **271:**377, 1964.

Wessler, S., and Morris, L. E.: Studies in Intravascular Coagulation: IV. The Effect of Heparin and Dicumarol on Serum-induced Venous Thrombosis, *Circulation,* **12:**553, 1955.

Wheeler, H. B., Pearson, D., O'Connel, D., and Mullick, S. C.: Impedance Phlebography: Technique, Interpretation, and Results, *Arch Surg,* **104:**164, 1972.

Williams, J. R., Wilcox, W. C., Andrews, G. J., and Burns, R. R.: Angiography in Pulmonary Embolism, *JAMA,* **184:**473, 1963.

Williams, R. D., and Zollinger, R. W.: Surgical Treatment of Superficial Thrombophlebitis, *Surg Gynecol Obstet,* **118:**745, 1964.

Zilliacus, H.: On the Specific Treatment of Thrombosis and Pulmonary Embolism with Anticoagulants, with Particular Reference to the Post-thrombotic Sequelae, *Acta Med Scand [Suppl],* **171:**13, 1946.

Venous Insufficiency and Ulcers

Bauer, G.: A Roentgenological and Clinical Study of the Sequels of Thrombosis, *Acta Chir Scand,* **86**(Suppl 74):1, 1942.

DeCamp, P. T., Schramel, R. J., Ray, C. J., Feibleman, N. D., Ward, J. A., and Ochsner, A.: Ambulatory Venous Pressure Determinations in Postphlebitic and Related Syndromes, *Surgery,* **29:**44, 1951.

DeWeese, J. A.: Functional Popliteal Phlebography in the Patient with a Complicated Varicose Vein Problem, *Surgery,* **44:**390, 1958.

———, and Rogoff, S. M.: Clinical Uses of Functional Ascending Phlebography of the Lower Extremity, *Angiology,* **9:**268, 1958.

——— and ———: Functional Ascending Phlebography of the Lower Extremity by Serial Long Film Technique: Evaluation of Anatomic and Functional Detail in 62 Extremities, *Am J Roentgenol Radium Ther Nucl Med,* :841, 1959.

Dodd, H., and Cockett, F. B.: "The Pathology and Surgery to the Veins of the Lower Limb," E. & S. Livingstone Ltd., Edinburgh and London, 1956.

Doran, F. S. A., and White, M.: Clinical Trial Designed to Discover if Primary Treatment of Varicose Veins Should be by Fegan's Method or by Operation, *Br J Surg,* **62:**72, 1975.

Edwards, E. A., and Edwards, J. E.: The Effect of Thrombophlebitis on the Venous Valve, *Surg Gynecol Obstet,* **65:**310, 1937.

Felder, D. A., Murphy, T. O., and Ring, D. M.: A Posterior Subfascial Approach to the Communicating Veins of the Leg, *Surg Gynecol Obstet,* **100:**730, 1955.

Fell, S. C., McIntosh, H. D., Hornsby, A. T., Horton, C. E., Warren, J. V., and Pickrell, K.: The Syndrome of the Chronic Leg Ulcer: The Phlebodynamics of the Lower Extremity; Physiology of the Venous Valves, *Surgery,* **38:**771, 1955.

Gay, J.: On Varicose Diseases of the Lower Extremities, in "The Lettsomian Lectures of 1867," J. & A. Churchill Ltd., London.

Homans, J.: The Etiology and Treatment of Varicose Ulcer of the Leg, *Surg Gynecol Obstet,* **24:**300, 1917.

Linton, R. R.: The Post-thrombotic Ulceration of the Lower Extremity: Its Etiology and Surgical Treatment, *Ann Surg,* **138:**415, 1953.

Luke, J. C.: The Deep Vein Valves, *Surgery,* **29:**381, 1951.

Myers, T. T.: Results and Technique of Stripping Operation for Varicose Veins, *JAMA,* **163:**87, 1957.

Pollack, A. A., Taylor, B. E., Myers, T. T., and Wood, E. H.: The Effect of Exercise and Body Position on the Venous Pressure at the Ankle in Patients Having Venous Valvular Defects, *J Clin Invest,* **28:**559, 1949.

Schneewind, J. H.: The Walking Venous Pressure Test and Its Use in Peripheral Vascular Disease, *Ann Surg,* **140:**137, 1954.

Scott, W. J. M., and Radakovich, M.: Venous and Lymphatic Stasis in the Lower Extremities: I. A. Test for Incompetence in the Perforating Veins; II. A Simple Method of Adequate Control, *Surgery,* **26:**970, 1949.

Staffon, R. A., and Buxton, R. W.: Deep Vein Ligation in the Postphlebitic Extremity, *Surgery,* **41:**471, 1957.

Veal, J. R., and Hussey, H. H.: The Venous Circulation in the Lower Extremities during Pregnancy, *Surg Gynecol Obstet,* **72:**841, 1941.

Warren, R., White, E. A., and Belcher, C. D.: Venous Pressures in the Saphenous System in Normal Varicose and Postphlebitic Extremities: Alterations following Femoral Vein Ligation, *Surgery,* **26:**435, 1949.

Lymphatics and Lymphedema

Brush, B. E., Wylie, J. H., Jr., and Beninson, J.: Some Devices for the Management of Lymphedema of the Extremities, *Surg Clin North Am,* **392:**1493, 1959.

Butcher, H. R. Jr., and Hoover, A. L.: Abnormalities of Human Superficial Cutaneous Lymphatics Associated with Stasis Ulcers, Lymphedema, Scars, and Cutaneous Autografts, *Ann Surg,* **142:**633, 1955.

Charles, R. H.: In A. Latham and T. C. English (eds.), "A System of Treatment," vol. 3, p. 516, J. & A. Churchill, Ltd., London, 1912.

Crockett, D. J.: The Protein Levels of Oedema Fluids, *Lancet,* **2:**1179, 1956.

Gibson, T., and Tough, J. S.: The Surgical Correction of Chronic Lymphoedema of the Legs, *Brit J Plast Surg,* **7:**195, 1954.

Hudack, S. S., and McMaster, P. D.: The Lymphatic Participation in Human Cutaneous Phenomena: A Study of the Minute Lymphatics of the Living Skin, *J Exp Med,* **572:**751, 1933.

Jantet, G. H., Taylor, G. W., and Kinmonth, J. B.: Operations for Primary Lymphedema of the Lower Limbs: Results after 1–9 Years, *J Cardiovasc Surg (Torino),* **2:**27, 1961.

Khodadadeh, M., and Johnson, R.: Lymphangiosarcoma Arising from Postmastectomy Lymphedema, *JAMA,* **186:**1097, 1963.

Kinmonth, J. B.: Lymphangiography in Man: A Method of Outlining Lymphatic Trunks at Operation, *Clin Sci,* **11:**13, 1952.

——— and Cox, S. J.: Protein-Losing Enteropathy in Primary Lymphoedema: Mesenteric Lymphography and Gut Resection, *Br J Surg,* **61:**589, 1974.

———, Taylor, G. W., Tracy, G. D., and Marsh, J. D.: Primary Lymphoedema: Clinical and Lymphangiographic Studies of a Series of 107 Patients in Which the Lower Limbs Were Affected, *Br J Surg,* **45:**1, 1957.

Scott, W. J. M., and Radkovich, M.: Venous and Lymphatic Stasis in the Lower Extremities: I. A Test for Incompetence in the Perforating Veins; II. A Simple Method of Adequate Control, *Surgery,* **26:**970, 1949.

Taylor, G. W.: Lymphoedema, *Postgrad Med J,* **35:**2, 1959.

———, Kinmonth, J. B., and Dangerfield, W. G.: Protein Content of Oedema Fluid in Lymphoedema, *Br Med J,* **1:**1159, 1958.

Wakim, K. G., Martin, G. M., and Krusen, F. H.: Influence of Centripetal Rhythmic Compression on Localized Edema of an Extremity, *Arch Phys Med Rehabil,* **36:**98, 1955.

Yoffey, J. M., and Courtice, F. C.: "Lymphatics, Lymph and Lymphoid Tissue," Harvard University Press, Cambridge, Mass., 1956.

Name Index

Subject Index

Infection(s):
  gynecologic, 1733–1734
  hand, 2088–2091
  hyperbaric therapy for, 189
  intracranial, 1793–1800
  mycotic, 210–212
  nosocomial, 186
  opportunistic, 192
  prostatic, 1682–1684
  pseudomycotic, 209–210
  pulmonary, 694–705
    in etiology of adult respiratory distress syn-
      drome, 153
  and rejection of transplanted kidney, 455
  renal, staphylococcal, 1681–1682
  as sign of tumor necrosis, 345
  spinal cord, pain in, 1813
  staphylococcal, 201–203
  stimuli from, 3
  streptococcal, 199–201
  surgical, 186, 187, 189–190
    antibiotics for, 193
    therapy for, 188–189
  following transplantation, prevention of, 412
  urinary tract, differentiation of, from acute ap-
    pendicitis, 1261
  vascular prosthetic, management of, 924–925
  venereal, 1734
  viral, effect of immunosuppressive therapy on,
    411–412
  wound, 496–498
    clostridial, 203–204
Infectious arthritis, rehabilitation for, 2113
Infertility:
  evaluation of, 1730–1731
  in uterine fibroids, 1736
Infiltrating duct carcinoma of breast with productive fibrosis, 576
Infiltrating papillary carcinoma of breast, 576
Infiltration anesthesia, 491
Infiltrative growth of tumor, signs of, 345
Inflammation:
  of appendix, 1257–1264
    (See also Appendicitis)
  of bile duct, 1338–1340
    (See also Cholangitis)
  of biliary tract, 1338–1341
  of colon, 1192–1205
    (See also Colitis)
  of gallbladder, 1334–1338
    (See also Cholecystitis)
  of mediastinum, 734–735
  membrane, in peritonitis, 1398–1399
  of mesenteric lymph nodes, 1445–1446
  of muscles, 1831
  of neck, 622
  of pancreas, 1358–1363
    (See also Pancreatitis)
  of pericardium, 868–870
    (See also Pericarditis)
  of prostate, urinary retention in, 1670
  of thyroid, 1559–1562
  of urethra, acute, 1682
Inflammatory diseases of small intestine, 1169–
  1175
Inflammatory hyperplasia of oral cavity, 603
Infrared radiation in heat therapy, 2109
Infundibulum of gallbladder, 1318
Infusions:
  arterial, administration of chemotherapy by,
    355–356
  intraarterial, in therapy of hypovolemic shock,
    167
Inguinal hernias, 1460–1462
Inguinal orchiectomy, 1710
Inguinal region:
  anatomy of, 1460
  hernias of, 1460–1462
    in infants, surgery for, 1656–1657

Inhalation anesthesia, 487–492
Inheritance of hemostatic defects, 110
Injections, dye, in evaluation of lymphatic return,
  1004
Injury (see Trauma; Wounds)
Innominate osteotomy for congenital hip disloca-
  tion, 1864–1865
Innovar for intravenous anesthesia, 485
Insects, bites and stings of, 239–242
Insensible water loss, 549
Inspection of breast, 567
Inspissated bile syndrome, jaundice in, 1322
Instrumentation in diagnosis of urologic disor-
  ders, 1674–1675
Insufficient antigenicity in evasion of immune
  surveillance, 336
Insulin:
  in metabolism of starvation, 22
  for postoperative control of diabetes, 508–509
  secretion of, decreased, in trauma, 16, 18
Intensity duration curve in diagnosis of muscle
  denervation, 1829
Intensive care delirium, 515
Intercellular matrix, 1875
Interloop abscess, 1419–1420
Intermittent positive-pressure breathing (IPPB):
  for postoperative respiratory failure, 500–501
  to prevent postoperative pulmonary complica-
    tions, 45
Internal jugular vein, catheterization of, for car-
  diovascular monitoring, 534
Interparietal hernia, definition of, 1459
Interphalangeal joint flexors, distal, function of,
  in evaluation of hand injury, 2041, 2042
Intersexual abnormalities, surgery for, 1657–
  1658
Intersphincteric space, 1233–1234
Interstitial emphysema, 654
Interstitial fluid:
  composition of, 66–67
  volume of, 66
Interstitial pulmonary edema in adult respiratory
  distress syndrome, 152
Intertrochanteric fractures, 1956–1957
Intervertebral disc:
  anatomy of, 1802
  degenerative disease of, 1802–1805
  protrusion of, 1820–1823
  mechanisms of, 1820
Intestinal antisepsis, 192
Intestinal bypass, 1186–1187
Intestinal obstruction in newborn, surgery for,
  1642–1645
Intestinal phase:
  in inhibition of gastric secretion, 1133
  in stimulation of gastric secretion, 1132
Intestine(s):
  activity of, changes in, in gastrointestinal dis-
    ease, 1048–1051
  angina of, 1440–1441
  large, 1191–1255
    (See also Anus; Cecum; Colon; Rectum)
  motility in, in mechanical small bowel obstruc-
    tion, 1053
  obstruction of, 1051–1062
    clinical manifestations of, 1055–1057
    closed-loop, 1054–1055
    complicating appendectomy, 1265
    complicating gastrointestinal surgery, 517
    etiology of, 1052
    incidence of, 1052
    management of, 1057–1061
    in newborn, surgery for, 1642–1645
    pathophysiology of, 1052–1055
    strangulated, 1054
  radiation damage to, 1201–1202
  response of, in peritonitis, 1399
  small, 1169–1190
    blind loop syndrome of, 1183–1184

  diverticular disease of, 1181–1182
  fistulas of, 1182–1183
    complicating gastrointestinal surgery, 519
  foreign bodies in, ingested, 1182
  inflammatory diseases of, 1169–1175
  injuries to, 256–257
  mechanical obstruction of, 1052–1054
  Meckel's diverticulum of, 1181
  neoplasms of, 1175–1181
    benign, 1176–1177
    malignant, 1177–1181
  obstruction of, complicating partial gastrec-
    tomy, 1144
  Peutz-Jeghers syndrome of, 1176–1177
  pneumatosis cystoides intestinalis of, 1183
  regional enteritis of, 1169–1175
  short bowel syndrome of, 1184–1186
  tuberculous enteritis of, 1175
  typhoid enteritis of, 1175
  ulcer of, 1182
  (See also Duodenum; Ileum; Jejunum)
  transit of food through, 1048–1049
  transplantation of, 427–428
Intoxication:
  alcohol, complicating anesthesia following
    trauma, 227
  drug, complicating anesthesia following
    trauma, 227
Intrabdominal abscesses, 1414–1417
Intraaortic balloon pumping for assisted circulation, 875
Intraarterial infusions in therapy of hypovolemic
  shock, 167
Intracellular fluid, 66
Intracellular transmembrane potential, effect of
  shock on, 140
Intracerebral hematoma, posttraumatic, 1770–
  1771
Intracranial hemorrhage, posttraumatic, 1768
Intracranial infections, 1793–1800
Intracranial pressure and cerebral edema, 1768
Intracranial space, anatomy of, 1800
Intractability as indication for surgery for
  duodenal ulcer, 1140
Intractable abdominal pain in gastrointestinal
  disease, 1041–1042
Intradermal nevus, 556
Intradural-extramedullary tumors of spinal cord,
  1780–1781
Intrahepatic obstructive jaundice, 1072
Intramedullary tumors of spinal cord, 1781
Intramembranous ossification, 1877–1878
Intramural hematoma of duodenum following
  trauma, 255–256
Intraperitoneal antibiotic therapy, 192–193,
  232
Intraperitoneal bile, effects of, 1328
Intrathoracic goiter, surgery for, 1570–1571
Intrauterine device, pelvic inflammatory disease
  due to, 1734
Intravenous anesthesia, 482–487
Intravenous cholecystography in diagnosis of
  biliary tract disease, 1326
Intravenous hyperalimentation, 30–34, 92–96
  (See also Parenteral alimentation)
Intravenous resuscitation in immediate burn
  therapy, 286–288
Intrinsic factor, organic constituents of, 1131
Intubation:
  endotracheal, for airway obstruction following
    trauma, 226
  in intestinal obstruction, 1058
  nasogastric, in diagnosis and management of
    abdominal injury, 223
  in preparation for surgery for peritonitis, 1408
Intussusception:
  differentiation of, from acute appendicitis,
    1262
  in infants, surgery for, 1645–1646

Pseudohermaphrodites, male, familial, disorders of sexual development in, 1508
Pseudohermaphroditism:
in congenital adrenogenital syndrome, 1505
female, 1729–1730
male, 1729
Pseudohyperparathyroidism, 1587
Pseudohypertrophic muscular dystrophy, 1830
Pseudohypoparathyroidism, 1620
Pseudomembranous enterocolitis, 202, 1202–1203
Pseudomonas aeruginosa, 207
Pseudomycotic infections, 209–210
Pseudomyxoma peritonei, 1746
Pseudopseudohypoparathyroidism, 1620
Psoas sign in appendicitis, 1259
Psychiatric complications, postoperative, 511–515
Psychiatric problems, management of, in rehabilitation, 2110–2111
Psychogenic constipation, 1049
Psychologic management of cancer patient, 376
Psychologic problems following head trauma, 1771
Psychoses:
postoperative, 511–515
postperfusion, 823
PTA, deficiency of, 101, 114
PTC, deficiency of, 101–102
Puberty, 1722
Pulmonary [*see* Lung(s)]
Pulmonary artery, stenosis of, 751
Pulmonary artery sling, 806
Pulmonary capillary wedge pressure monitoring in management of gram-negative septic shock, 177
Pulmonary care, ancillary, in ventilatory support for adult respiratory distress syndrome, 158
Pulmonary edema:
complicating transfusions, 130
interstitial, in adult respiratory distress syndrome, 152
in mitral stenosis, 828
postoperative, 503–504
in septic peritonitis, 1405
Pulmonary embolectomy, 995–996
Pulmonary embolism:
complicating total hip replacement, 2003
complicating transplantation, 413
differential diagnosis of, 993
incidence of, 992
pathophysiology of, 992
physical findings in, 992–993
special tests for, 993
symptoms of, 992
treatment of, 993–996
venous thrombosis and, 985–996
Pulmonary hypertension:
in left-to-right shunts, 741–742
in ventricular septal defect, 775–776
Pulmonary insufficiency, posttraumatic, 46–47, 661–662
Pulmonary osteoarthropathy, hypertrophic, 2009–2010
Pulmonary procedures, rehabilitation for, 2121
Pulmonary responses to shock, 150–158
(*See also* Adult respiratory distress syndrome)
Pulmonary shunting in adult respiratory distress syndrome, 151–152
Pulmonary support in therapy of hypovolemic shock, 166
Pulmonary therapy for gram-negative septic shock, 178–179
Pulmonary veins, anomalous drainage of, 769–771
Pulmonic stenosis, 747–751
clinical manifestations of, 749
diagnosis of, 749–750
historical data on, 747

incidence and etiology of, 747
laboratory findings in, 749
pathologic anatomy of, 747–748
pathophysiology of, 748–749
treatment of, 750–751
Pulse rate, change in, in shock, 137
Pulses:
absence of, in occlusive disease of lower extremities, 910
loss of, in arterial trauma, 938
peripheral, in diagnosis of acquired heart disease, 814
Pumping, intraaortic balloon, for assisted circulation, 875
Pumps for extracorporeal circulation, 817
Puncture wounds, local care of, 229
Purine analogues in prevention of rejection, 402–403
Puromycin in prevention of rejection, 405
Purpura:
Henoch-Schönlein, differentiation of, from acute appendicitis, 1262
thrombocytopenic: idiopathic: splenectomy for, 1389–1390
treatment of, 118
thrombotic, splenectomy for, 1390
transfusion, 109
Pus, staining of, in diagnosis of suppurative peritonitis, 1409
Pyelography:
antegrade, 1677
in diagnosis: of blunt abdominal trauma, 247
of retroperitoneal tumors, 1453
of urinary calculi, 1685
excretory, in diagnosis of renal tumors, 1694
Pyelonephritis:
kidney transplant for, 440
staphylococcal, 1681
Pyeloureterography, retrograde, 1677
Pyemia, 189
Pylethrombophlebitis in appendiceal rupture, 1260
Pyloric gland area of gastric mucosa, 1129
Pyloric mucosa, 1130
Pyloric obstruction:
complicating surgery for duodenal ulcer, 1147
as indication for surgery for duodenal ulcer, 1141
Pyloric stenosis in children, surgery on, 1641
Pyloric ulcer, duodenal, surgery for, elective, 1142–1146
Pyloromyotomy, Fredet-Pamstedt, for pyloric stenosis in infants, 1641
Pyloroplasty:
for AGM lesions, 1156
for duodenal ulcers, 1145
Pyogenic arthritis, 1984–1986
Pyogenic liver abscesses, 1276–1278
Pyogenic osteomyelitis of vertebral column, 1825–1826
Pyogenic pericarditis, acute, 868–869
Pyrexia, malignant, due to succinylcholine, 486
Pyrimidine analogues in prevention of rejection, 403
Pyruvate, metabolism of, in shock, 44

Quadriplegia, rehabilitation for, 2119–2120
Quick test for prothrombin time, 105
as screening device, 107
Quinidine for postoperative atrial fibrillation, 505

Rabies, 232–236
diagnosis of, 233
epidemiology of, 233
exposure of persons previously immunized for, 233
incidence of, 232–234

management of biting animals in, 233
manifestations of, 235
preexposure prophylaxis for, 233, 235
treatment of, 236
Rabies immune globulin, 235
Rad, definition of, 356
Radial nerve:
injuries of, rehabilitation for, 2118
palsy of, management of, 2047
Radiation:
in immunosuppression, 408–409
infrared, in hear therapy, 2109
ionizing, as carcinogen, 329, 330
ultraviolet, as carcinogen, 329, 330
Radiation enterocolitis, 1201–1202
Radiation sterilization, 213
Radiation therapy:
for bronchogenic carcinoma, 714
for carcinoma, 356–360
for cervical cancer, 1739–1741
combined with surgery, 359–360
complications of, 358
for endometrial carcinoma, 1743
for esophageal carcinoma, 1108
for hemangiopericytoma, 555
indications for, 358–360
for lip cancer, 601–602
for malignant obstruction of superior vena cava, 903
following mastectomy for breast cancer, 581–582
prognosis for, 585–586
mechanism of action of, 356–357
for osteosarcoma, 1912
for ovarian carcinoma, 1747
for Paget's disease, 1902
palliative, 359
of pituitary for Cushing's syndrome, 1502
postoperative, 360
preoperative, 359–360
rehabilitation for, 2123
for retroperitoneal tumors, 1454
for sarcomas, 367–368
for skin cancer, 554
for Wilms' tumor, 1690
Radical local resection for carcinoma, 352–353
Radical mastectomy:
prognosis for, 583–587
rehabilitation for, 2121–2122
vs. total mastectomy, controversy over, 580–581
Radical neck dissection, 625–626
Radical resection with en bloc excision for lymphatics for carcinoma, 353–354
Radicular cyst of mandible, 618
Radicular pain in musculoskeletal disorders, 1810
Radioactive brain scan in diagnosis of neurologic disorders, 1761
Radioactive iodine for thyrotoxicosis, 1556
Radiocurability of tumors vs. radiosensitivity of tumors, 357–358
Radiodensity of bone, changes in, in bone disorders, 1878
Radiography (*see* Roentgenography)
Radioimmunoassay of serum gastrin levels in diagnosis of Zollinger-Ellison syndrome, 1136
Radioisotope scanning in diagnosis of pulmonary emboli, 993, 994
Radioisotope studies in evaluation of thyroid function, 1550–1551
Radiosensitivity of tumors vs. radiocurability of tumors, 357–358
Radioulnar synostosis, congenital, 1871
Radium implants for cervical cancer, 1740–1741
Radius:
absence of, 1872
distal, fractures of, 1949–1950
fractures of, 1943
head of, subluxation of, in children, 1947